CORE CURRICULUM *for* CRITICAL CARE NURSING

SIXTH EDITION

American Association of Critical–Care Nurses

CORE CURRICULUM *for* CRITICAL CARE NURSING

Edited by

JOANN GRIF ALSPACH, RN, MSN, EDD, FAAN
Consultant, Staff Development and
Competency-Based Performance Appraisal Systems
Editor, *Critical Care Nurse*
Annapolis, Maryland

**AMERICAN
ASSOCIATION
*of*CRITICAL-CARE
NURSES**

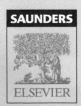

SAUNDERS

ELSEVIER

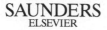

SAUNDERS
ELSEVIER

11830 Westline Industrial Drive
St. Louis, Missouri 63146

CORE CURRICULUM FOR CRITICAL CARE NURSING,
SIXTH EDITION

ISBN-13: 978-0-7216-0450-3
ISBN-10: 0-7216-0450-1

Notice

Knowledge and best practice in this field are constantly changing. As new research and experience broaden our knowledge, changes in practice, treatment and drug therapy may become necessary or appropriate. Readers are advised to check the most current information provided (i) on procedures featured or (ii) by the manufacturer of each product to be administered, to verify the recommended dose or formula, the method and duration of administration, and contraindications. It is the responsibility of the practitioner, relying on their own experience and knowledge of the patient, to make diagnoses, to determine dosages and the best treatment for each individual patient, and to take all appropriate safety precautions. To the fullest extent of the law, neither the Publisher nor the Editor assume any liability for any injury and/or damage to persons or property arising out or related to any use of the material contained in this book.

The Publisher

ISBN-13: 978-0-7216-0450-3
ISBN-10: 0-7216-0450-1

Executive Publisher: Barbara Nelson Cullen
Associate Developmental Editor: Mayoor Jaiswal
Publishing Services Manager: Deborah L. Vogel
Senior Project Manager: Deon Lee
Design Direction: Jyotika Shroff

Printed in United States of America

Last digit is the print number: 9   8   7   6   5   4   3   2   1

Contributors

Jan Marie Belden, MSN, APRN, BC, FNP
Nurse Practitioner, Pain Management
Advanced Practice Nursing Department
Loma Linda University Medical Center
Loma Linda, California
The Neurologic System (Pain section only)
Psychosocial Aspects of Critical Care
(Pain section only)

Nancy Blake, RN, MN(Nursing Administration), CCRN, CNAA
Director, Critical Care Services
Children's Hospital Los Angeles
Los Angeles, California
Critical Care Patients with Special Needs:
Pediatric Patients

Pamela J. Bolton, RN, MS, ACNP, CCNS, CCRN, PCCN
College of Nursing and Health
University of Cincinnati
Cincinnati, Ohio;
Acute Care Nurse Practitioner
St. Elizabeth Hospital
Crestview Hill, Kentucky;
The Jewish Hospital
Cincinnati, Ohio;
St. Luke West Hospital
Florence, Kentucky;
Clinical Nurse
The University Hospital
Cincinnati, Ohio
Multisystem

Dennis J. Cheek, RN, PhD, FAHA
Abell-Hanger Professor of Gerontological
   Nursing
Harris School of Nursing
Texas Christian University
Fort Worth, Texas
Hematologic and Immunologic Systems

Kathleen Ellstrom, RN, PhD, APRN, BC
Pulmonary Clinical Nurse Specialist
VA Loma Linda Healthcare System
Loma Linda, California;
Part-Time Lecturer
California State University
Fullerton, California
The Pulmonary System

Susan Gallagher, RN, MSN, CNS, PhD
Clinical Affairs Coordinator
SIZEWise Rentals
Ellis, Kansas
Critical Care Patients with Special Needs:
Bariatric Patients

Mary A. Hall, RN, MSN
Adjunct Faculty
University of North Carolina–School
   of Nursing
Chapel Hill, North Carolina;
Legal Nurse Consultant/Staff
Faison & Gillespie Law Firm
Durham, North Carolina;
Chatham Hospital
Siler City, North Carolina
Hematologic and Immunologic
Systems

Elizabeth A. Henneman, RN, PhD, CCNS
Assistant Professor, School
   of Nursing
University of Massachusetts
Amherst, Massachusetts;
Staff RN, Intensive Care Unit
Baystate Medical Center
Springfield, Massachusetts
Psychosocial Aspects of Critical
Care

Renee Holleran, RN, PhD, CEN, CCRN, CFRN, FAEN
Nurse Manager
Adult Transport Services, IHC Life Flight
LDS Hospital
Salt Lake City, Utah
Critical Care Patients with Special Needs: Patient Transport

M. Lindsay Lessig, BSN, MSEd, MBA(Health Care Administration)
Staff Nurse, Clinical Care Float Pool
Swedish Medical Center/Providence Campus
Seattle, Washington
The Cardiovascular System

Kim Litwack, PhD, RN, CFNP, FAAN
Associate Professor of Nursing
University of Wisconsin–Milwaukee
Milwaukee, Wisconsin;
Family Nurse Practitioner
Advanced Pain Management
Middleton, Wisconsin
The Endocrine System

Karen A. McQuillan, RN, MS, CCRN, CNRN
Clinical Nurse Specialist
R Adams Cowley Shock Trauma Center
University of Maryland Medical Center
Baltimore, Maryland
The Neurologic System

Nancy C. Molter, RN, MN, PhD
Adjunct Faculty—Acute Care Nursing
University of Texas Health Science Center
San Antonio
San Antonio, Texas;
Clinical Research Coordinator Program
Manager
US Army Institute of Surgical Research
Fort Sam Houston, Texas
Professional Caring and Ethical Practice

Amy A. Nichols, RN, CNS, EdD
Associate Professor, School of Nursing
San Francisco State University
San Francisco, California;
Interim Director, Center of Nursing Excellence
Lucile Packard Children's Hospital at
Stanford
Palo Alto, California
Critical Care Patients with Special Needs: High-Risk Obstetric Patients

Jan Odom-Forren, MS, RN, CPAN, FAAN
Perianesthesia Nursing Consultant
and Educator
Louisville, Kentucky
Critical Care Patients with Special Needs: Sedation in Critically Ill Patients

Ginette A. Pepper, PhD, RN, FAAN
Professor and Colby Endowed Chair
in Gerontological Nursing
University of Utah College of Nursing
Salt Lake City, Utah
Critical Care Patients with Special Needs: Geriatric Patients

Patricia Radovich, RN, MSN, CNS, FCCM
Assistant Clinical Professor
Loma Linda University;
Clinical Nurse Specialist
Loma Linda University Medical
Center
Loma Linda, California
The Gastrointestinal System

Marilyn Sawyer Sommers, RN, PhD, FAAN
Professor of Nursing
University of Cincinnati College
of Nursing
Cincinnati, Ohio
Multisystem

June L. Stark, RN, BSN, MEd
Continuing Education Nurse Educator
Adult Continuing Education Department
University of Southern Maine
Portland, Maine;
Director, Case Management
North Shore Medical Center–Salem
Hospital
Salem, Massachusetts
The Renal System

Reviewers

Bizhan Aarabi, MD, FRCSC, FACS
Associate Professor, Department
    of Neurosurgery
University of Maryland School
    of Medicine;
Director of Neurotrauma
R Adams Cowley Shock Trauma Center
University of Maryland Medical Center
Baltimore, Maryland

James D. Anholm, MD
Chief, Pulmonary Section
Loma Linda Veterans Healthcare System
Loma Linda, California

Mona Bahouth, MSN, CRNP
Nurse Practitioner, Neurology
Director, Clinical Programs and Research
The Maryland Brain Attack Center
Baltimore, Maryland

Deborah L. Barnes, RN, MSN
Clinical Nurse Specialist for Nursing
    Quality Improvement
Palomar Pomerado Health
Escondido, California

Linda J. Bell, RN, MSN
Clinical Practice Specialist
American Association of Critical-Care
    Nurses
Aliso Viejo, California;
Per Diem Staff Nurse
Medical-Surgical ICU
Loma Linda University Medical Center
Loma Linda, California

G. Carpinito, MD
Chief of Urology and Minimally Invasive
    Surgery
Associate Professor, Tufts School of Medicine
New England Medical Center
Boston, Massachusetts

Christopher B. Cooper, MD
Professor of Medicine and Physiology
David Geffen School of Medicine
University of California
Los Angeles, California

Anthony Dash, MD
Associate Professor, Tufts School
    of Medicine
Division of Nephrology
St. Elizabeth's Medical Center
Boston, Massachusetts

Lorrie Frankel, MD
Professor, Stanford School of Medicine
Lucile Packard Children's Hospital
Palo Alto, California

Donald J. Hillebrand, MD
Associate Professor of Medicine
Chief of Hepatology
Medical Director, Liver Transplantation
Loma Linda University Transplantation
    Institute
Loma Linda University Medical Center
Loma Linda, California

James Hurst, MD, FACS
Professor, Department of Surgery
University of Cincinnati
Cincinnati, Ohio

Evelyn Hutt, MD
Associate Professor
Divisions of Health Care Policy
    and Geriatrics
Department of Medicine
University of Colorado at Denver;
Health Sciences Director
Program to Improve Quality of Life
    and Care for Veterans
LTC Denver Veteran Affairs Medical Center
Denver, Colorado

Preface

As a dynamic specialty nursing organization, the American Association of Critical-Care Nurses (AACN) has continually evolved to better meet the needs of its members and the patients they serve. As the healthcare industry, healthcare services, and traditional boundaries of healthcare institutions have been altered so rapidly and pervasively over recent years, AACN has continued its vital growth and development to remain at the forefront of these changes.

The AACN Synergy Model of Patient Care affords an elegant yet clear conceptual framework for certified practice in critical care. The most fundamental premise of the Synergy Model is that patient characteristics drive the competencies that nurses need in order to provide holistic, healing care that achieves optimal patient outcomes.* A knowledge base of critical care nursing underlies clinical practice and reflects a foundational requirement for the development of these nursing competencies.

The purpose of the *Core Curriculum for Critical Care Nursing* in this, its sixth edition, remains as it was in its inception, to articulate the knowledge base that underlies acute, progressive, and critical care nursing practice. Each edition of this work attempts to redefine that knowledge base for nurses who practice in this ever-expanding specialty area.

A number of similarities exist between the fifth and sixth editions of the *Core Curriculum*. The current edition continues to use the CCRN examination blueprint and task statements as a starting point for determining relevant content and its apportionment throughout the book. The presentation format continues to be an embellished outline, and body systems are again used to segregate the major content areas into chapters. Subsections related to physiologic anatomy, pathophysiology, and patient assessment have also been retained.

A number of noteworthy additions and modifications can be found in this edition. The most striking difference is that the *Core Curriculum* now includes 11 rather than 9 chapters. The new Chapter 1, Professional Caring and Ethical Practice, provides an encompassing description of AACN's perspective of critical care nursing as well as a thorough summary of the origin and elements that compose the AACN Synergy Model of Patient Care. Content includes AACN's mission, vision, and values statements; its characterization of what critical care nurses do; and its organizational model for a humane, caring, and healing patient and practice environment. Related materials pertaining to patient safety as well as ethical and legal aspects of critical care nursing practice are also presented.

The second major addition is Chapter 11, a mosaic of six patient populations who merit special nursing care considerations as acute, progressive, or critical care patients. These special patient population categories include bariatric patients, geriatric patients, high-risk obstetric patients, pediatric patients (in an adult ICU or stepdown unit), sedated patients, and patients requiring intrafacility or interfacility transport.

---

*Villaire M: The Synergy Model© of certified practice: creating safe passage for patients, *Crit Care Nurse* 16(4):94-99, 1996.

The fundamentals of capnography and ventilator waveform analysis now augment the Pulmonary System chapter. The Cardiovascular System chapter incorporates extensive updating in covering acute coronary syndromes and their related diagnostic study findings; determining stages, classification, and treatment of heart failure; managing complications of pericarditis, myocarditis, and endocarditis; developing discharge planning for infective endocarditis; managing cardiovascular emergencies according to the latest ACLS standards; and providing pharmacologic management of valvular disorders as well as hypertensive crises. Additions to coverage include laboratory tests for cardiac troponin T and troponin I, myoglobin, and brain natriuretic peptides; bubble echocardiography; myocardial perfusion imaging; and electron beam computed tomography.

The Neurologic System chapter has been revised considerably to include the physiologic aspects of pain as the fifth vital sign as well as to include pain assessment and pharmacologic management of pain. Other neuroassessment monitoring parameters now incorporated include partial pressure of brain tissue oxygen ($Pbto_2$); near-infrared cerebral spectroscopy (NIRS); transcranial Doppler (TCD) studies; continuous cerebral blood flow (CBF) monitoring; diagnostic studies such as computed tomography (CT) angiogram, pre- and post-CT scan patient care, and spinal and digital subtraction angiography; and some additions to physical assessment parameters (e.g., muscle group testing, muscle strength grading, sensory function scoring; expansion of the Hunt-Hess classification for subarachnoid hemorrhage, and the Fisher and Spetzler-Martin AVM grading scales).

Revisions to the Renal System chapter include a description of the aging kidney and updated information related to renal radiologic diagnostic studies, diuretics, intrarenal failure, anticoagulation, vascular access for hemodialysis, continuous renal replacement therapies, maintenance renal transplant immunosuppressive therapy, and treatment of renal trauma. Updates to the Hematologic and Immunologic Systems chapter reflect advancements in understanding of clotting factors and coagulation.

The Gastrointestinal System chapter has been extensively revised by addition of a new patient health problem, carcinoma of the pancreas, and considerable additions in coverage of carcinoma of the gastrointestinal tract and liver, gastroesophageal reflux, selected types of gastrointestinal surgery, hepatitis D, hepatitis E, and autoimmune and drug-related hepatitis. Augmented coverage of the physiologic anatomy of the esophagus, colon, hepatic vascular supply, and pancreatic physiology is provided together with updates to management of acute abdomen and chronic liver failure, as well as pathophysiology and management of acute pancreatitis and acute gastrointestinal bleeding.

Additions to the Multisystem chapter include quantification of organ failure via the multiorgan dysfunction syndrome (MODS) score and sequential organ failure assessment (SOFA) score, burn-specific physical assessment, and induced hypothermia. Areas notably updated are definitions related to sepsis and severe sepsis; epidemiology, pathophysiology, and treatment of sepsis; pharmacologic therapies for infection; pathophysiology of MODS; pathophysiology, assessment, and management of patients with multisystem trauma; and etiology and statistics related to toxic ingestions.

The Psychosocial Aspects of Critical Care chapter has been completely reorganized to align more closely to the format of other chapters, to integrate the AACN Synergy Model of Patient Care, and to incorporate the critical care patient's experience of pain. This last element includes a description of pain as well as its etiology, clinical manifestations, diagnosis, nonpharmacologic management, and desired outcomes.

A few structural changes have been introduced in this edition. The major segment that appeared under the heading of "Commonly Encountered Nursing Diagnoses" has been replaced by the heading "Patient Care" and followed by various common health problems listed in their approximate order of clinical priority. Nursing diagnoses are no longer incorporated because of their declining use in clinical settings. Within the "Patient Assessment" sections, the eight patient characteristics identified in the Synergy Model are now incorporated under the section "Appraisal of Patient Characteristics." In addition to each characteristic, clinical scenarios are provided as examples of levels 1, 3, and 5 along the continuum of that characteristic.

The contributors, reviewers, and I have made every attempt to provide the most current and relevant knowledge base of information related to acute, progressive, and critical care nursing. I welcome your comments related to this edition and your suggestions for the next edition of the *Core Curriculum*.

Grif Alspach, RN, MSN, EdD, FAAN
Editor-in-Chief, *Core Curriculum* Series
GrifCCN@comcast.net

Contents

1. PROFESSIONAL CARING AND ETHICAL PRACTICE, 1

Nancy C. Molter, RN, MN, PhD

4. THE NEUROLOGIC SYSTEM, 381

Karen A. McQuillan, RN, MS, CCRN, CNRN, and Jan Marie Belden, MSN, APRN, BC, FNP (Contributor for content related to pain)

5. THE RENAL SYSTEM, 525

June L. Stark, RN, BSN, MEd

10.   PSYCHOSOCIAL ASPECTS OF CRITICAL CARE, 849

Elizabeth A. Henneman, RN, PhD, CCNS, and Jan Marie Belden, MSN, APRN, BC, FNP (Contributor for content related to pain)

11.   CRITICAL CARE PATIENTS WITH SPECIAL NEEDS, 883

Bariatric Patients: *Susan Gallagher, RN, MSN, CNS, PhD;* Geriatric Patients: *Ginette A. Pepper, PhD, RN, FAAN;* High-Risk Obstetric Patients: *Amy A. Nichols, RN, CNS, EdD;* Patient Transport: *Renee Holleran, RN, PhD, CEN, CCRN, CFRN, FAEN;* Pediatric Patients: *Nancy Blake, RN, MN, CCRN, CNAA;* and Sedation in Critically Ill Patients: *Jan Odom-Forren, MS, RN, CPAN, FAAN*

1 Professional Caring and Ethical Practice

NANCY C. MOLTER, RN, MN, PhD

AMERICAN ASSOCIATION OF CRITICAL-CARE NURSES (AACN) VISION, MISSION, AND VALUES (AACN, 2002)

Vision

A health care system driven by the needs of patients and families in which nurses can make their optimal contribution

Mission

Building on decades of clinical excellence, AACN provides and inspires leadership to establish work and care environments that are respectful, healing, and humane. The key to AACN's success is its members. Therefore, AACN is committed to providing the highest-quality resources to maximize nurses' contribution to caring and improving the health care of critically ill patients and their families.

Values

As AACN works to promote its mission and vision, it is guided by values that are rooted in, and arise from, the association's history, traditions, and culture. Therefore, AACN and its members, volunteers, and staff will

1. **Be accountable** to uphold and consistently act in concert with ethical values and principles
2. **Advocate** for organizational decisions that are driven by the needs of patients and their families
3. **Act with integrity** by communicating openly and honestly, keeping promises, honoring commitments, and promoting loyalty in all relationships
4. **Collaborate** with all essential stakeholders by creating synergistic relationships to promote common interest and shared values
5. **Provide leadership** to transform thinking, structures, and processes to address opportunities and challenges
6. **Demonstrate stewardship** through fair and responsible management of resources
7. **Embrace lifelong learning, inquiry, and critical thinking** to enable each to make optimal contributions
8. **Commit to quality and excellence** at all levels of the organization, meeting and exceeding standards and expectations
9. **Promote innovation** through creativity and calculated risk taking
10. **Generate commitment** to and passion for the organization's causes and work

SYNERGY OF CARING

What Nurses Do (American Nurses Association [ANA], 2003)

1. **Attend** to the full range of human experiences of and responses to health and illness
2. **Integrate** objective data with knowledge of the patient as a person and understanding of the patient's subjective experience
3. **Apply** scientific knowledge to the process of diagnosis and treatment of the responses to health and illness
4. **Establish** a caring relationship that facilitates healing

What Critical Care Nurses Do (Medina, 2000)

1. **Critical care nurses** deal with human responses to life-threatening problems
2. **The Scope of Practice** includes all ages and involves a dynamic interaction between the critically ill patient, the patient's family, the critical care nurse, and the environment
3. **The framework of practice** includes the scientific body of specialized knowledge, an ethical model for decision making, a commitment to interdisciplinary collaboration, and the AACN Synergy Model for Patient Care. Critical care nurses rely on this framework to do the following (Bell, 2002, p. 44):
   a. Support and maintain the physiologic stability of patients
   b. Assimilate and prioritize information sources to take immediate and decisive patient-focused action
   c. Respond with confidence and adapt to rapidly changing patient conditions
   d. Respond to the unique needs of patients and families coping with unanticipated treatment, quality of life, and end-of-life decisions
   e. Manage appropriately the interface between the patient and technology that may be threatening, invasive, and complex so that human needs for a safe, respectful, healing, humane, and caring environment are established and maintained
   f. Monitor and allocate critical care services, recognizing the fiduciary role of nurses working in a resource-intensive environment

The Environment of Critical Care

1. **Complexity requiring vigilance:** Critically ill patients require complex assessment and therapies, high-intensity interventions, and continuous vigilance
2. **Organizational model** for a humane, caring, and healing environment
   a. The critical care nurse works with an interdisciplinary team to create a humane, caring, and healing environment. There are five elements of an organizational model for health and healing (Malloch, 2000; Molter, 2003):
      i. Common values of health as a function of mind-body-spirit interrelationships
      ii. Patient and family–centered philosophy
      iii. Physical environment that supports healing
      iv. Use of complementary and alternative therapies as well as conventional therapies
      v. Organizational culture that promotes personal growth
   b. The critical care nurse is a constant in the environment and works to develop an organizational culture that supports the following (Bell, 2002, p. 45):
      i. Providers that act as advocates on behalf of patients, families, and communities
      ii. The dominance of the patient's and family's values
      iii. Practice based in research and driven by outcomes

        iv. Ethical decision making

        v. Collaboration

        vi. The fostering of leadership at all levels and in all activities

        vii. Lifelong learning as fundamental to professional growth

        viii. Optimization of existing talents and resources

        ix. The rewarding of innovation and creativity

        x. Respect for diversity

3. **Patient safety**

    a. An Institute of Medicine (IOM) study notes the occurrence of a significant number of deaths related to health care service delivery processes (IOM, 1999)

    b. The Joint Commission on Accreditation of Healthcare Organizations (JCAHO) established National Patient Safety Goals in 2005 (JCAHO, 2006). The goals include the following*:

        i. Improve the accuracy of patient identification by using at least two patient identifiers when administering medications or blood products, taking blood samples and other specimens for clinical testing, or providing any other treatments or procedures.

        ii. Improve the effectiveness of communication among caregivers by reading back verbal or telephone orders and critical laboratory results; standardizing abbreviations, acronyms, and symbols not to be used in the organization; improving the timeliness of receiving critical test results and values; and standardizing the "hand off" of communications.

        iii. Improve the safety of using medications by standardizing and limiting the number of drug concentrations available in the organization, identifying and reviewing a list of look-alike/sound-alike drugs, taking action to prevent errors involving the interchange of these drugs, and labeling all medications, medication containers, or other solutions in perioperative and other procedural settings.

        iv. Reduce the risk of health care–associated infections by complying with current Centers for Disease Control and Prevention hand hygiene guidelines and managing as sentinel events all identified cases of unanticipated death or major permanent loss of function associated with a health care–associated infection.

        v. Accurately and completely reconcile medications across the continuum of care by implementing a process to obtain and document a complete list of the patient's current medications upon the patient's admission to the organization, by comparing the medications on the list to those available in the organization and by communicating the list to the next provider of service when a patient is referred or transferred.

        vi. Reduce the risk of patient harm resulting from falls by implementing a fall-reduction program and evaluating its effectiveness.

The "Synergy" of the AACN Synergy Model for Patient Care

1. **Synergistic practice and patient and family safety:** The AACN Synergy Model for Patient Care (Curley, 1998) describes nursing practice in terms of the needs and characteristics of patients. The model's premise is that the needs of the patient and family system drive the competencies required by the nurse. When this occurs, synergy is produced and optimal outcomes can be achieved. Buckminster Fuller stated that "synergy is the only word in our language that means behavior of whole systems unpredicted by the separately observed behaviors of any of the

---

*National Patient Safety Goals change every year. Go to the JCAHO website (http://www.jcaho.org) for the most current goals.

system's separate parts or any subassembly of the system's parts" (cited in Carlson, 1996, p. 92). The synergy created by practice based on the Synergy Model helps the patient-family unit safely navigate the health care system.

2. **The Synergy Model and ethical practice:** The Synergy Model provides a foundation for addressing ethical concerns related to critical care nursing practice (McGaffic, 2001). The model focuses on the characteristics of patients, the competencies needed by the critical care nurse to meet the patient's needs based on these characteristics, and the outcomes that can be achieved through the synergy that develops when nursing competencies are driven by the patient's needs. AACN is committed to helping members deal with ethical issues through education (Glassford, 1999).

AACN SYNERGY MODEL FOR PATIENT CARE

Origin of the Synergy Model

In 1992, AACN developed a vision of a health care system driven by the needs of patients and their families in which critical care nurses can make their optimal contribution. AACN Certification Corporation in tandem was rethinking the contributions of certification to the care of patients. Patient needs and outcomes must be the central focus of certification. A think tank was convened in 1992 to reconceptualize certified practice (Caterinicchio, 1995; Villaire, 1996).

Purpose

Prior to development of the Synergy Model, the certification process conceptualized nursing practice according to the dimensions of the nurse's role, the clinical setting, and the patient's diagnosis. The Synergy Model reconceptualized certified practice to recognize that the needs and characteristics of patients and families influence and drive the competencies of nurses. The synergy that develops when this occurs influences the outcomes of individual patients, the nurse's practice, and the organization. A separate think tank in 1996 identified the potential outcomes (Biel, 1997).

Overview of the Synergy Model (AACN Certification Corporation, 2003, 2004)

1. **Description of the Synergy Model** (Figure 1-1): The synergy that occurs when patient and family characteristics or needs drive the competencies that nurses need to achieve optimal outcomes for the patient, nurse, and organization
2. **Assumptions of the Synergy Model** (AACN Certification Corporation, 1998)
   a. All patients are biologic, psychologic, social, and spiritual entities who have similar needs and experiences at a particular developmental stage across wide ranges or continua from health to illness. The whole patient must be considered. More compromised patients have more complex needs.
   b. The dimensions of a nurse's practice as determined by the needs of a patient and family can also be described along continua
   c. The patient, family, and community all contribute to providing a context for the nurse-patient relationship
   d. Optimal outcomes can be achieved through the synergy effected by alignment of nurse competencies with patient and family needs. A peaceful death can be an acceptable outcome.
3. **Patient characteristics:** Characteristics unique to each patient and family span the continua of health and illness. The first five are intrinsic to the patient and the last three are extrinsic. Each characteristic is described in terms of a range of levels from 1 to 5 in Table 1-1 (AACN Certification Corporation, 1997, 2004).

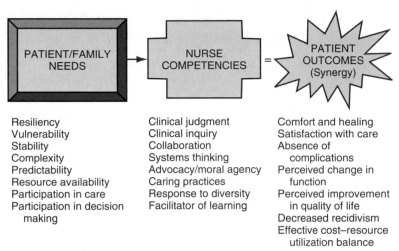

FIGURE 1-1 ■ Patient and family characteristics drive nurse competencies to achieve optimal (synergistic) outcomes.

■ **TABLE 1-1**
■ ■ **The Synergy Model—Patient Characteristics**

Characteristic and Description	Continua of Health and Illness*
INTRINSIC CHARACTERISTICS	
Resiliency The capacity to return to a restorative level of functioning using compensatory and coping mechanisms; the ability to bounce back quickly after an insult	*Level 1: Minimally resilient* • Unable to mount a response • Failure of compensatory/coping mechanisms • Minimal reserves • Brittle *Level 3: Moderately resilient* • Able to mount a moderate response • Able to initiate some degree of compensation • Moderate reserves *Level 5: Highly resilient* • Able to mount and maintain a response • Intact compensatory/coping mechanisms • Strong reserves • Endurance
Vulnerability Susceptibility to actual or potential stressors that may adversely affect patient outcomes	*Level 1: Highly vulnerable* • Susceptible • Unprotected, fragile *Level 3: Moderately vulnerable* • Somewhat susceptible • Somewhat protected *Level 5: Minimally vulnerable* • Safe; out of the woods • Protected, not fragile

Continued

■ **TABLE 1-1**
■ ■ **The Synergy Model—Patient Characteristics—cont'd**

Characteristic and Description	Continua of Health and Illness*
Stability The ability to maintain a steady-state equilibrium	*Level 1: Minimally stable* • Labile; unstable • Unresponsive to therapies • High risk of death *Level 3: Moderately stable* • Able to maintain steady state for limited period of time • Some responsiveness to therapies *Level 5: Highly stable* • Constant • Responsive to therapies • Low risk of death
Complexity The intricate entanglement of two or more systems (e.g., body, family, therapies)	*Level 1: Highly complex* • Intricate • Complex patient/family dynamics • Ambiguous/vague • Atypical presentation *Level 3: Moderately complex* • Moderately involved patient/family dynamics *Level 5: Minimally complex* • Straightforward • Routine patient/family dynamics • Simple/clear-cut • Typical presentation
Predictability A characteristic that allows one to expect a certain course of events or course of illness	*Level 1: Not predictable* • Uncertain • Uncommon patient population or illness • Unusual or unexpected course • Does not follow critical pathway, or no critical pathway developed *Level 3: Moderately predictable* • Wavering • Occasionally noted patient population or illness *Level 5: Highly predictable* • Certain • Common patient population or illness • Usual and expected course • Follows critical pathway
EXTRINSIC CHARACTERISTICS	
Resource availability Extent of resources (e.g., technical, fiscal, personal, psychologic, and social) the patient, family, and community bring to the situation	*Level 1: Few resources* • Necessary knowledge and skills not available • Necessary financial support not available • Minimal personal/psychologic supportive resources • Few social systems resources *Level 3: Moderate resources* • Limited knowledge and skills available • Limited financial support available • Limited personal/psychologic supportive resources • Limited social systems resources

■ TABLE 1-1
■ ■ The Synergy Model—Patient Characteristics—cont'd

Characteristic and Description	Continua of Health and Illness*
	Level 5: Many resources • Extensive knowledge and skills available and accessible • Financial resources readily available • Strong personal/psychologic supportive resources • Strong social systems resources
Participation in care Extent to which patient and/or family engage in aspects of care	*Level 1: No participation* • Patient and/or family unable or unwilling to participate in care *Level 3: Moderate participation* • Patient and/or family need assistance in care *Level 5: Full participation* • Patient and/or family fully able and willing to participate in care
Participation in decision making Extent to which patient and/or family engages in decision making	*Level 1: No participation* • Patient and/or family have no capacity for decision making; require surrogacy *Level 3: Moderate participation* • Patient and/or family have limited capacity; seek input/advice from others in decision-making *Level 5: Full participation* • Patient and/or family have capacity, and make decisions themselves

From AACN Certification Corporation.
*Note that the continua of health and illness levels vary in order of rating based on the characteristic.

3. **Patient characteristics—cont'd**
   a. Resiliency: The capacity to return to a restorative level of functioning using compensatory and coping mechanisms; the ability to bounce back quickly after an insult
   b. Vulnerability: Susceptibility to actual or potential stressors that may adversely affect patient outcomes
   c. Stability: The ability to maintain a steady-state equilibrium
   d. Complexity: The intricate entanglement of two or more systems (e.g., body, family, therapies)
   e. Predictability: A characteristic that allows one to expect a certain course of events or course of illness
   f. Resource availability: Extent of resources (e.g., technical, fiscal, personal, psychologic, and social) the patient, family, and community bring to the situation
   g. Participation in care: Extent to which the patient and/or family engages in aspects of care
   h. Participation in decision making: Extent to which the patient and/or family engages in decision making
4. **Nurse characteristics:** Nursing care is an integration of knowledge, skills, experience, and individual attitudes. The continua of nurse characteristics needed are derived from the patient's needs and range from a competent to expert level as outlined in Table 1-2.
   a. Clinical judgment: Clinical reasoning, which includes clinical decision making, critical thinking, and a global grasp of the situation, coupled with nursing skills acquired through a process of integrating education, experiential knowledge, and evidence-based guidelines

■ **TABLE 1-2**
■ ■ **The Synergy Model—Nurse Characteristics**

Characteristic and Description	Continua of Level of Expertise (Levels 1-5 Range from Competent to Expert)
Clinical judgment Clinical reasoning, which includes clinical decision making, critical thinking, and a global grasp of the situation, coupled with nursing skills acquired through a process of integrating education, experiential knowledge, and evidence-based guidelines.	*Level 1* • Collects and interprets basic-level data • Follows algorithms, protocols, and pathways with all populations and is uncomfortable deviating from them • Matches formal knowledge and clinical events to make basic care decisions • Questions the limits of one's ability to make clinical decisions and defers the decision making to other clinicians • Recognizes expected outcomes • Often focuses on extraneous details *Level 3* • Collects and interprets complex patient data focusing on key elements of case; able to sort out extraneous detail • Follows algorithms, protocols, and pathways and is comfortable deviating from them with common or routine patient population • Recognizes patterns and trends that may predict the direction of illness • Recognizes limits and utilizes appropriate help • Reacts to and limits unexpected outcomes *Level 5* • Synthesizes and interprets multiple, sometimes conflicting, sources of data • Makes judgments based on an immediate grasp of the "big picture," unless working with new patient populations; uses past experiences to anticipate problems (applies principles from old situations to new situations) • Helps patient and family see the "big picture" • Recognizes the limits of clinical judgment and seeks multidisciplinary collaboration and consultation with comfort • Recognizes and responds to the dynamic situation (following patient/family lead) • Anticipates unexpected outcomes • Acts on and directs others to act on identified clinical problems • Assists nursing staff in identifying daily goals for patients
Advocacy/moral agency Working on another's behalf and representing the concerns of the patient/family and nursing staff; serving as a moral agent in identifying and helping to resolve ethical and clinical concerns within and outside the clinical setting.	*Level 1* • Works on behalf of the patient and self • Begins to self-assess personal values • Aware of ethical conflicts/issues that may surface in clinical setting • Makes ethical/moral decisions based on rules/guiding principles and on own personal values • Represents patient if consistent with own framework • Aware of patient rights • Acknowledges death as an outcome *Level 3* • Works on behalf of patient and family • Considers patient values and incorporates in care, even when differing from personal values

■ **TABLE 1-2**
■ ■ **The Synergy Model—Nurse Characteristics—cont'd**

Characteristic and Description	Continua of Level of Expertise (Levels 1-5 Range from Competent to Expert)
	• Supports patients, families, and colleagues in ethical and clinical issues, identifying internal resources • Moral decision making can deviate from rules • Demonstrates give and take with patients/family, allowing them to speak/represent themselves when possible • Aware of and acknowledges patient and family rights • Recognizes that death may be an acceptable outcome • Facilitates patient/family comfort in the death and dying process *Level 5* • Works on behalf of patient, family, and community • Advocates from patient/family perspective, whether similar to or different from personal values • Advocates for resolution of ethical conflict and issues from patient's, family's, or colleague's perspective; utilizes and participates in internal and external resources • Recognizes rights of patient/family to drive moral decision making • Empowers the patient and family to speak for/represent themselves • Achieves mutuality within patient/family/professional relationships
Caring practices Nursing activities that create a compassionate, supportive, and therapeutic environment for patients and staff, with the aim of promoting comfort and healing and preventing unnecessary suffering. These caring behaviors include but are not limited to vigilance, engagement, and responsiveness. Caregivers include family and health care personnel.	*Level 1* • Focuses on basic and routine needs of the patient • Bases care on standards and protocols • Maintains a safe physical environment *Level 3* • Responds to subtle patient and family changes • Engages with the patient to provide individualized care • Employs caring and comfort practices to provide individualized care for patient/family • Optimizes patient/family environment *Level 5* • Has astute awareness and anticipates patient/family changes and needs • Fully engaged with and senses how to stand alongside the patient/family, and community • Patient/family needs determine caring practices • Anticipates hazards, and promotes safety, care, and comfort throughout transitions along the health care continuum • Initiates the establishment of an environment that promotes caring • Provides patient/family the skills to navigate transitions along the health care continuum (i.e., facilitates safe passage)

Continued

■ **TABLE 1-2**
■ ■ **The Synergy Model—Nurse Characteristics—cont'd**

Characteristic and Description	Continua of Level of Expertise (Levels 1-5 Range from Competent to Expert)
Collaboration Working with others (e.g., patients, families, health care providers) in a way that promotes each person's contributions toward achieving optimal and realistic patient/family goals. Collaboration involves intradisciplinary and interdisciplinary work with colleagues and community.	*Level 1* • Willing to be taught, coached, and/or mentored • Participates in team meetings and discussions regarding patient care and/or practice issues • Open to various team members' contributions *Level 3* • Willing to be taught/mentored • Participates in preceptoring and teaching • Initiates and participates in team meetings and discussions regarding patient care and/or practice issues • Recognizes and critiques multidisciplinary participation in care decisions *Level 5* • Seeks opportunities to role model, teach, mentor, and to be mentored • Facilitates active involvement and contributions of others in team meetings and discussions regarding patient care and/or practice issues • Involves/recruits multidisciplinary resources to optimize patient outcomes • Role models, teaches, and/or mentors professional leadership and accountability for nursing's role within the health care team and community
Systems thinking Body of knowledge and tools that allow the nurse to manage whatever environmental and system resources exist for the patient/family and staff, within or across health care and non–health care systems.	*Level 1* • Utilizes previously learned strategies or standardized processes • Identifies problems but unclear of health care systems to resolve problems • Sees patient and family within the isolated environment of the unit • Sees self as key resource for patient/family • Applies personal experiences to identify patient/family needs *Level 3* • Develops processes/strategies based on needs and strengths of patient/family • Able to make connections within pieces or components of the health care system • Sees and begins to use negotiation as a tool for practice-based decisions • Recognizes and reacts to needs of patient/family as they move through health care systems • Recognizes how to obtain and utilize resources within the health care system *Level 5* • Develops, integrates, and applies a variety of strategies that are driven by the needs and strengths of the patient/family • Recognizes global or holistic interrelationships that exist within and across both health care and non–health care systems • Knows when and how to negotiate and navigate through the system on behalf of patients and families

■ **TABLE 1-2**
■ ■ **The Synergy Model—Nurse Characteristics—cont'd**

Characteristic and Description	Continua of Level of Expertise (Levels 1-5 Range from Competent to Expert)
	• Develops core plans based on anticipated needs of patients/families • Utilizes a variety of resources as necessary to optimize patient/family outcomes
Response to diversity The sensitivity to recognize, appreciate, and incorporate differences into the provision of care. Differences may include, but are not limited to, cultural, spiritual, gender, race, ethnicity, lifestyle, socioeconomic, age, and values.	*Level 1* • Assesses diversity and acknowledges differences, but uses standardized plans of care • Provides care based on own belief system • Practices within the culture of the health care environment • Recognizes barriers • Recognizes practices based upon diversity that have potential negative outcomes *Level 3* • Inquires about cultural differences and considers their impact on care • Accommodates personal and professional differences in plans of care • Helps patient/family understand the culture of the health care system • Recognizes barriers and seeks strategies for resolution • Identifies and utilizes resources that promote and support diversity *Level 5* • Anticipates needs of patient/family based on identified diversities and develops plans accordingly • Acknowledges and incorporates differences • Adapts health care culture, to the extent possible, to meet the diverse needs and strengths of the patient/family • Anticipates and intervenes to reduce/eliminate barriers • Incorporates patient/family values with evidence-based practice for optimal outcomes
Clinical inquiry The ongoing process of questioning and evaluating practice and providing informed practice; creating changes through evidence-based practice, research utilization, and experiential knowledge.	*Level 1* • Follows polices, procedures, standards and guidelines without deviation • Uses research-based practices as directed by others • Recognizes the need for further learning to improve patient care • Recognizes obvious changing patient situation (e.g., deterioration, crisis) and seeks assistance to identify patient problems and solutions • Participates in data collection (e.g., research, continuous quality improvement [CQI], quality improvement [QI]) *Level 3* • Utilizes policies, procedures, standards, and guidelines, adapting to patient needs • Applies research findings when not in conflict with current clinical practice • Accepts advice or information to improve patient care • Recognizes subtle changes in patient condition and begins to compare and contrast possible care alternatives • Participates on team (e.g., CQI, survey, research)

Continued

■ **TABLE 1-2**
■ ■ **The Synergy Model—Nurse Characteristics—cont'd**

Characteristic and Description	Continua of Level of Expertise (Levels 1-5 Range from Competent to Expert)
	Level 5 • Improves, modifies, or individualizes policies, procedures, standards, and guidelines for particular patient situations or populations based on experiential or published data • Questions and/or evaluates current practice based on patient/family's responses, review of the literature, research, and education/learning • Seeks to validate whether research answers clinical questions • Embraces lifelong learning and acquires knowledge and skills needed to address questions arising in practice to improve patient care • Evaluates outcomes of studies and implements changes (converging of clinical inquiring and clinical judgment allows for anticipation of patient needs)
Facilitator of learning The ability to facilitate learning for patients and families, nursing staff, other members of the health care team, and community; includes both formal and informal facilitation of learning.	*Level 1* • Follows planned educational programs using standardized educational materials • Sees patient/family education as a separate task from delivery of care • Provides information without seeking to assess learner's readiness or understanding • Has basic knowledge and/or understanding of the patient/family's educational needs • Focuses educational plan on nurse-identified patient/family needs • Sees the patient/family as a passive recipient *Level 3* • Adapts planned educational programs to meet individual patient's needs • Begins to recognize and integrate different ways of implementing education into delivery of care • Assesses patient's/family's readiness to learn, develops education plan based on identified needs, and evaluates learner understanding • Recognizes the benefits of educational plans from different health care providers' perspectives • Sees the patient/family as having input into educational goals • Incorporates patient's/family's perspective into individualized education plan *Level 5* • Creatively modifies or develops patient/family education programs • Integrates patient/family education throughout delivery of care • Evaluates patient/family readiness to learn and provides comprehensive individualized education evaluating behavior changes related to learning, adjusting to meet the educational goal. • Collaborates and incorporates all health care providers' ideas into ongoing educational plans for the patient/family • Sees patient/family as having choices and consequences that are negotiated in relation to education

From AACN Certification Corporation and PES: *Final report of a comprehensive study of critical care nursing practice.* Aliso Viejo, Calif, 2004, The Corporation.

    b. Advocacy/moral agency: Working on another's behalf and representing the concerns of the patient/family, and nursing staff; serving as a moral agent in identifying and helping to resolve ethical and clinical concerns within and outside the clinical setting

    c. Caring practices: Nursing activities that create a compassionate, supportive, and therapeutic environment for patients and staff, with the aim of promoting comfort and healing and preventing unnecessary suffering. These caring behaviors include but are not limited to vigilance, engagement, and responsiveness. Caregivers include family and health care personnel.

    d. Collaboration: Working with others (e.g., patients and families, health care providers) in a way that promotes each person's contributions toward achieving optimal and realistic patient and family goals. Collaboration involves intradisciplinary and interdisciplinary work with colleagues and community.

    e. Systems thinking: The body of knowledge and tools that allow the nurse to manage whatever environmental and system resources exist for the patient, family, and staff within or across health care and non–health care systems

    f. Response to diversity: The sensitivity to recognize, appreciate, and incorporate differences into the provision of care. Differences may include, but are not limited to, cultural, spiritual, gender, race, ethnicity, lifestyle, socioeconomic, age, and values.

    g. Clinical inquiry or innovation and evaluation: The ongoing process of questioning and evaluating practice and providing informed practice; creating changes through evidence-based practice, research utilization, and experiential knowledge

    h. Facilitator of learning: The ability to facilitate learning for patients and families, nursing staff, other members of the health care team, and community; includes both formal and informal facilitation of learning

5. Outcomes of patient-nurse synergy (Figure 1-2) (Curley, 1998)

    a. Patient-derived outcomes

        i. Behavior change: Based on the dispensing and receiving of information. Requires caregiver trust. Patients and families grow in their knowledge about health and take greater responsibility for their own health.

            (a) Functional change and quality of life: Multidisciplinary measures that can be used across all populations of patients but provide specific information to a population of patients when analyzed separately

            (b) Satisfaction ratings: Subjective measures of individual health and quality of health services. Satisfaction measures query about expectations (technical care provided, trusting relationships, and education experiences) and the extent to which they are met. Often linked with functional change and quality-of-life perceptions.

            (c) Comfort ratings and perceptions: Quality-of-care outcomes based on caring practices with the aim of promoting comfort and alleviating suffering

    b. Nurse-derived outcomes

        i. Physiologic changes: Require monitoring and managing instantaneous therapies and noting changes. The nurse expects a specific trajectory of changes when he or she "knows" the patient (Tanner, Benner, and Chesla, 1993).

        ii. The presence or absence of preventable complications: Through vigilance and clinical judgment, the nurse creates a safe and healing environment

        iii. Extent to which care and treatment objectives were attained: Reflects the nurse's role as an integrator of care that requires a high degree of collaboration

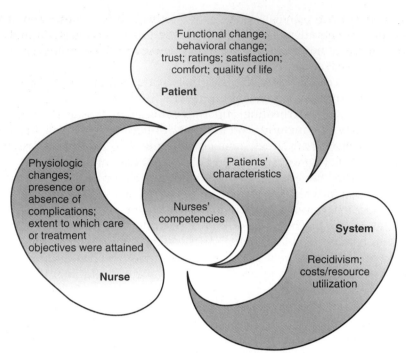

FIGURE 1-2 ■ Three levels of outcomes delineated by the AACN Synergy Model for Patient Care: those derived from the patient, those derived from the nurse, and those derived from the health care system. (From Curley M: Patient-nurse synergy: optimizing patients' outcomes, *Am J Crit Care* 7:69, 1998.)

   c. System-derived outcomes
      i. Recidivism: Decrease in rehospitalization or readmission, which adds to the personal and financial burden of care
      ii. Cost and resource utilization: Organizations usually evaluate financial cost based on an episode of care. Achieving cost-effective care requires knowing the patient and providing continuity of care. Resource utilization can affect patient outcomes when there is not enough care given by competent nurses (Aiken et al, 2001). When nurses cannot provide care at an appropriate level to meet patient needs, they are dissatisfied and turnover is high, which results in increased costs for the organization (Cornerstone Communication Group, 2001).

Validation

1. **National validation study methodology**
   a. Synergy Model originally validated in large-scale national study of practice (Muenzen and Greenberg, 1998)
   b. Survey methodology used to determine predicted relationships among patient-family and nurse characteristics and their interactions in the Synergy Model
   c. Surveys sent to 3924 nurses (adult, pediatric, and neonatal nurses in subacute, acute, and critical care settings); response rate of 24%
2. **Findings**
   a. Respondents accurately perceived acuity of patients' conditions in the profiles developed for the study
   b. Respondents perceived that the critically ill patients described in the patient profiles required care by nurses with higher levels of the nurse characteris-

tics listed in Table 1-2 than did the less acutely ill patients described in the profiles; respondents perceived that "clinical judgment" was most strongly related to patient need and that the nurse requires a higher level of this characteristic to achieve optimal outcomes

  c. The eight patient characteristics and their associated rating scales were useful in differentiating acuity levels

  d. Acuity-of-care levels were not differentiated based on the patient's and family's ability to participate in decision making and care, and the patient's and family's level of technical, fiscal, personal and psychologic, and social resources

  e. Patients whose care requires critical care skills are not found solely in critical care units. They may be located in progressive care units, postanesthesia units, rehabilitation facilities, and the home environment.

  f. The eight patient characteristics fall into two groups: Intrinsic (resiliency, vulnerability, stability, complexity, and predictability) and extrinsic (participation in decision making, participation in care, and resource availability)

  g. The eight nurse characteristics are all intercorrelated and may reflect overall nurse competency

Application of the Synergy Model

There are many applications for the model in clinical operations, clinical practice, education, and research*

1. **Clinical operations**
   a. Leadership: Using the model for organizational infrastructure for achieving excellence in practice, improving financial outcomes, and establishing clinical advancement programs (Cohen et al, 2002; Czerwinski, Blastic, and Rice, 1999; Doble et al, 2000; Kerfoot, 2001)
   b. Development of continuity-of-care models (Ecklund, 2002; Edwards, 1999)
   c. Foundation model for family-centered care practice (Collopy, 1999; Henneman and Cardin, 2002; Stannard, 1999)
   d. Basis for making care assignments and making nursing rounds (Hartigan, 2000; Mullen, 2002)

2. **Clinical practice**
   a. Development of clinical strategies (Markey, 2001)
   b. Direct patient care (Annis, 2002; Hardin and Hussey, 2003)

3. **Education**
   a. Curricula design: Serves as the basis for the graduate nursing program curriculum at Duquesne University[†]
   b. Basis for CCRN (critical care nurse) and CCNS (critical care clinical nurse specialist) certification examinations since 1999 (Moloney-Harmon, 1999)
   c. Potential use as a foundation for education of health care teams (Molter, 1997)

4. **Research**
   a. Validated in the AACN Certification Corporation Study of Practice (1998, 2004)
   b. Underwent theoretical review (Sechrist, Berlin, and Biel, 2000)
   c. Further research needed related to consumer perspective, staffing and productivity implications for nursing, patient outcomes measurement, and development of a quantitative tool based on the model for rapidly assessing patients and determining nursing characteristics needed

---

*Refer to the AACN Certification Corporation website (http://www.certcorp.org) for up-to-date applications.
[†]For more information, go to the nursing school website (http://www.nursing.duq.edu/).

GENERAL LEGAL CONSIDERATIONS RELEVANT TO CRITICAL CARE NURSING PRACTICE

State Nurse Practice Acts

1. **Purpose:** To protect the public
2. **Statutory laws:** Written by the individual states
3. **Usual authorization:** Board of nursing to oversee nursing (by use of regulations or administrative law)
4. **Content:** Define scope of practice for nurses

Scope of Practice

Provides guidance for acceptable nursing roles and practices, which vary from state to state

1. **Nurses are expected to follow the nurse practice act** and not deviate from usual nursing activities
2. **Advanced nursing practice:** Expanded roles for nurses include nurse practitioner, clinical nurse specialist, certified registered nurse anesthetist, and certified nurse-midwife. These roles require education beyond the basic nurse education and usually involve a master's degree. Certain responsibilities associated with these roles are not interchangeable (ANA, 1997)
3. **A scope of practice and standards for the acute care nurse practitioner** was developed by AACN and the ANA
4. **A scope of practice and standards for the acute care clinical nurse specialist** based on the Synergy Model was published by AACN (Bell, 2002)

Standards of Care

1. **A standard of care** is any established measure of extent, quality, quantity, or value; an agreed-upon level of performance or a degree of excellence of care that is established
2. **Standards are established** by usual and customary practice, institutional guidelines, association guidelines, and legal precedent
3. **Standards of care, standards of practice, policies, procedures, and performance criteria** all establish an agreed-upon level of performance or degree of excellence
   a. AACN standards for acute and critical care nursing practice (Medina, 2000)
   d. ANA standards: The ANA has generic standards and also specialty standards (e.g., for medical-surgical nursing)
   c. Standards of clinical practice for acute care certified nurse practitioners
   d. AACN Scope of Practice and Standards of Professional Performance for the Acute and Critical Care Clinical Nurse Specialist (Bell, 2002)
4. **National facility standards:** Include those published by JCAHO and the National Committee for Quality Assurance*
5. **Community and regional standards:** Standards prevalent in certain areas of the country or in specific communities
6. **Hospital and medical center standards:** Standards developed by institutions for their staff and patients
7. **Unit practice standards, policies, and protocols:** Specific standards of care for specific groups or types of patients or specific procedures (e.g., insulin or massive blood transfusion protocols)

---

*The National Committee for Quality Assurance website contains the various standards the committee endorses and/or publishes (http://www.ncqa.org/index.asp).

8. **Precedent court cases:** Standard of a "reasonable, prudent nurse" (i.e., what a reasonable, prudent nurse would have done in the given situation)
9. **Other nursing and interdisciplinary specialty organization standards** (such as those of the American Heart Association, the Society of Critical Care Medicine, the Association of periOperative Registered Nurses)

Certification in a Specialty Area

1. **Certification** is a process by which a nongovernmental agency, using predetermined standards, validates an individual nurse's qualification and knowledge for practice in a defined functional or clinical area of nursing
2. **A common goal** of specialty certification programs is to promote consumer protection and to promote high standards of practice
3. **The certified nurse** may be held to a higher standard of practice in the specialty than the noncertified nurse; certification validates the nurse's knowledge and experience in a specialty area
4. **Critical care certifications** are awarded by AACN Certification Corporation, established in 1975. AACN Certification Corporation is accredited by the National Commission for Certifying Agencies, the accreditation arm of the National Organization for Competency Assurance
   a. CCRN certification: Separate certification processes for critical care nurses practicing with neonatal, pediatric, or adult populations
   b. CCNS: Advanced practice certification of nurses in acute and critical care clinical nurse specialist practice

Professional Liability

1. **Professional negligence:** An unintentional act or omission; the failure to do what the reasonable, prudent nurse would do under similar circumstances, or an act or failure to act that leads to an injury of another. Six specific elements are necessary for professional negligence action and must be established by a person bringing a suit against a nurse (plaintiff) (Giordano, 2003; Guido, 1997):
   a. Duty: To protect the patient from an unreasonable risk of harm
   b. Breach of duty: Failure by a nurse to do what a reasonable, prudent nurse would do under the same or similar circumstances. The breach of duty is a failure to perform within the given standard of care. The standard defines the nurse's duty to the patient.
   c. Proximate cause: Proof that the harm caused was foreseeable and that the person injured was foreseeably a victim. This element can determine the extent of damages for which a nurse may be held liable.
   d. Injury: The harm done
   e. Direct cause of injury: Proof that the nurse's conduct was the cause of or contributed to the injury to the patient
   f. Damages: Proof of actual loss, damage, pain, or suffering caused by the nurse's conduct
2. **Malpractice:** A specific type of negligence that takes account of the status of the caregiver as well as the standard of care (Giordano, 2003; Guido, 1997). Professional negligence is malpractice. It is differentiated from ordinary negligence (e.g., failure to clean up water from the floor).
   a. Professional misconduct, improper discharge of professional duties, or a failure by a professional to meet the standard of care that results in harm to another person
   b. Malpractice is the failure of a professional person to act in accordance with prevailing professional standards or a failure to foresee consequences that a professional person who has the necessary skills and education would foresee

    c. Most common types of malpractice or negligence in critical care settings include medication errors, failure to prevent patient falls, failure to assess changes in clinical status, and failure to notify the primary provider of changes in patient status

3. **Delegation and supervision**
   a. Definitions (National Council of State Boards of Nursing, 1995)
      i. Delegation: Transferring to a competent individual the authority to perform a selected nursing task in a selected situation; the nurse retains accountability for the delegation
      ii. Accountability: Being responsible and answerable for actions or inactions of self or others in the context of delegation
      iii. Authority: Deemed present when a registered nurse (RN) has been given the right to delegate based on the state nurse practice act and also has the official power from an agency to delegate
      iv. Unlicensed assistive personnel (UAP): Any unlicensed personnel, regardless of title, to whom nursing tasks are delegated
      v. Delegator: The person making the delegation
      vi. Delegatee: The person receiving the delegation
      vii. Competent: Demonstrating the knowledge and skill, through education and experience, to perform the delegated task
   b. The five "rights" of delegation
      i. Right task: The RN ensures that the task to be delegated is appropriate to be delegated for that specific patient. Example: Delegating suctioning of a tracheostomy in a stable patient to a licensed practical nurse is appropriate. If the patient is a head injury patient who becomes bradycardic and hypotensive during suctioning, then delegation of this task for this patient may not be appropriate.
      ii. Right circumstances: The RN ensures that the setting is appropriate and that resources are available for successful completion of the delegated task
      iii. Right person: The RN delegates the right task to the right person to be performed on the right person
      iv. Right direction and communication: The delegating nurse provides a clear explanation of the task and expected outcomes; the RN sets limits and expectations for performance of the task
      v. Right supervision: The RN does appropriate monitoring and evaluation, and intervenes as needed; the RN provides feedback to the delegatee and establishes parameters for receiving feedback about the outcome of the task
   c. Model of the delegation decision-making process: The nurse must ensure that delegation of nursing tasks is based on appropriate assessment, planning, implementation, and evaluation. Box 1-1 describes the model for delegation established by the National Council of State Boards of Nursing.
   d. Nurse executives must ensure the following:
      i. Policies and procedures concerning supervision and delegation are in place and are consistent with state nurse practice acts
      ii. Job descriptions for UAPs do not include responsibilities for whose performance a license is required
      iii. Adequate training and consistent orientation for UAPs are provided
      iv. A mechanism for regular evaluation of UAPs is in place
   e. In the complex critical care environment, many of the concepts for delegation to UAPs can also be applied to delegation of care to other professional nurses

■ **BOX 1-1**
■ **NATIONAL COUNCIL OF STATE BOARDS OF NURSING MODEL FOR DELEGATION DECISION-MAKING PROCESS**

I. Delegation criteria
  A. Nursing Practice Act
    1. Permits delegation
    2. Authorizes task(s) to be delegated or authorizes the nurse to decide to delegate
  B. Delegator qualifications
    1. Within scope of authority to delegate
    2. Appropriate education, skills, and experience
    3. Documented or demonstrated evidence of current competency
  C. Delegatee qualifications
    1. Appropriate education, training, skills, and experience
    2. Documented or demonstrated evidence of current competency
Provided that this foundation is in place, the licensed nurse may enter the continuous process of delegation decision making.
II. Assess the situation.
  A. Identify the needs of the patient, consulting the plan of care.
  B. Consider the circumstances and setting.
  C. Assure the availability of adequate resources, including supervision.
    If patient needs, circumstances, and available resources (including supervisor and delegatee) indicate that patient safety will be maintained with delegated care, proceed to step III.
III. Plan for the specific task(s) to be delegated.
  A. Specify the nature of each task and the knowledge and skills required to perform it.
  B. Require documentation or demonstration of current competence by the delegatee for each task.
  C. Determine the implications for the patient, other patients, and significant others.
    If the nature of the task, competence of the delegatee, and patient implications indicate that patient safety will be maintained with delegated care, proceed to step IV.
IV. Assure appropriate accountability.
  A. As delegator, accept accountability for performance of the task(s).
  B. Verify that delegatee accepts the delegation and the accountability for carrying out the task correctly.
    If delegator and delegatee accept the accountability for their respective roles in the delegated patient care, proceed to steps V-VII.
V. Supervise the performance of the task.
  A. Provide directions and clear expectations of how the task(s) is(are) to be performed.
  B. Monitor performance of the task(s) to assure compliance with established standards of practice, policies, and procedures.
  C. Intervene if necessary.
  D. Ensure appropriate documentation of the task(s).
VI. Evaluate the entire delegation process.
  A. Evaluate the patient.
  B. Evaluate the performance of the task(s).
  C. Obtain and provide feedback.
VII. Reassess and adjust the overall plan of care as needed.

and licensed practical or vocational nurses (through assignments made by charge nurses or nurse managers)
  i. The job descriptions and scope of practice for personnel with various levels of expertise and for various roles must be clearly defined

    ii. When assignments are made, the patient's characteristics (as defined by the Synergy Model) and required care procedures guide the decision regarding the competency level of the nurse who should provide the care

    iii. Nurse executives and nurse managers must ensure that nurses have demonstrated and documented levels of expertise necessary to provide the care required by specific patients

    iv. Additional training and experience are required for performance of many of the complex therapies needed by vulnerable critically ill patients

4. Adequate staffing

  a. Staffing is a process and an outcome. The term can refer to the process by which human resources are used within a nursing care unit or to the number of staff members required to provide care. The individuals managing health care services have ethical responsibilities to ensure that policies and processes are in place to ensure the safety of the patients and the staff (Box 1-2) (Curtin, 2002a, 2002b).

  b. The optimal use of RN time and expertise depends on a number of variables: allocating acute and critical care beds based on patient need; ensuring availability of adequate numbers of qualified, competent nursing and support staff; establishing sufficient support systems; following and adhering to legal and regulatory requirements; and evaluating services through outcome and quality measures

  c. Patient and family–focused care requires matching the right caregiver to each patient, identifying systems that provided the right support in delivering care, incorporating legal and regulatory considerations, and measuring the outcomes of care

  d. AACN (2000) recommendations for staffing policy include the following:

    i. Develop a comprehensive strategic plan that links patient and family needs, cost of delivery, competency of providers, and staff mix with patient outcomes. Such a plan is required by the JCAHO standards. The plan must be flexible to adjust staffing to the unpredictability of increasing patient acuity in the critical care setting. It is difficult to state a single national staffing ratio or mix because staffing must be adjusted to meet the needs of a specific group of patients at a given time.

    ii. The foundation for minimum staffing levels is clearly articulated in standards for acute and critical care nursing practice that prescribe a competent level of nursing practice, as well as in standards of professional performance that articulate the roles and behaviors of nursing professionals

▤ **BOX 1-2**
▤ **ETHICAL RESPONSIBILITIES OF HEALTH CARE DELIVERY MANAGERS**

In order of priority, the following are the ethical responsibilities of those managing health service delivery systems:

1. Ensuring the safety of the services delivered
2. Ensuring a safe environment for those receiving and those delivering the health care services
3. Ensuring the responsible use, care, and distribution of the materials needed for safe delivery of services
4. Carefully developing and implementing a budget
5. Developing responsible institutional policies
6. Intelligently interpreting and implementing institutional policies
7. Knowing and adhering to all applicable laws governing practice and personnel management

---

Adapted from Curtin L: The ethics of staffing—part 1. *J Clin Syst Manage* 4(3):6-7, 2002.

Documentation

1. **Mandates of regulatory agencies**
   a. Federal requirements: Related to narcotics, controlled substances, organ transplantation
   b. National voluntary requirements: JCAHO's requirements related to quality improvement activities
   c. State requirements: May exist in specific situations (e.g., in relation to minors)
   d. Community (regional or local) standards: May include enhanced documentation in specific areas of practice (e.g., epidural medication)
   e. Hospital, medical center, or health maintenance organization requirements
2. **Purposes of nursing care documentation in the patient record**
   a. To provide clear and concise communication between providers
   b. To facilitate planning and evaluation of care, and demonstrate use of the nursing process
   c. To show progress of patient treatment, changes in condition, and continuity of care, and to record patient status, appearance, and behavior
   d. To protect the patient; the medical record may be used in litigation
   e. To protect health care professionals and institutions, and reduce risk for possible litigation
3. **Documentation requirements**
   a. General requirements regarding patient records
      i. Should contain accurate, factual observations
      ii. Should include times, dates, and signatures for notations and events entered
      iii. Reflects patient status and unusual events
      iv. Should reflect documentation of the nursing process on a continuing basis throughout the hospitalization
      v. Should note omissions of care and rationale
      vi. Should show that the physician was informed of unusual or adverse situations and record the nature of the physician's response
      vii. Should note deviations from standard hospital practice and the rationale for such deviations
      viii. Should be legible
      ix. Should carefully document method of the patient's admission, condition on admission, discharge planning, and condition on discharge
   b. Specific JCAHO requirements regarding patient records
      i. Patient's name, address, date of birth, and name of any legally authorized representative
      ii. Legal status of patient receiving mental health services
      iii. Emergency care, if any, provided to the patient before arrival
      iv. Findings of the patient assessment, including assessment of pain status, learning needs and barriers to learning, and cultural or religious needs that may affect care
      v. Conclusions or impressions drawn from the medical history and physical examination
      vi. Diagnosis or diagnostic impression
      vii. Reasons for admission or treatment
      viii. Goals of treatment and the treatment plan; evidence of interdisciplinary plan of care
      ix. Evidence of known advance directives or documentation that information about advance directives was offered

    x. Evidence of informed consent, when required by hospital policy
    xi. Diagnostic and therapeutic orders, if any
    xii. Records of all diagnostic and therapeutic procedures and all test results
    xiii. Records of all operative and other invasive procedures performed, with acceptable disease and operative terminology that includes etiology, as appropriate
    xiv. Progress notes made by the medical staff and other authorized persons
    xv. All reassessments and any revisions of the treatment plan
    xvi. Clinical observations and reports of patient's response to care
    xvii. Evidence of patient education
    xviii. Consultation reports
    xix. Records of every medication ordered or prescribed for an inpatient
    xx. Records of every medication dispensed to an ambulatory patient or an inpatient on discharge
    xxi. Records of every dose of medication administered and any adverse drug reaction
    xxii. All relevant diagnoses established during the course of care
    xxiii. Any referrals and communications made to external or internal care providers and to community agencies
    xxiv. Conclusions at termination of hospitalization
    xxv. Discharge instructions to the patient and family
    xxvi. Clinical discharge summaries, or a final progress note or transfer summary. Discharge summary contains reason for hospitalization, significant findings, procedures performed and treatment rendered, patient's condition at discharge, and instructions to the patient and family, if any, including pain management plan.

Good Samaritan Laws

1. **Various states have enacted laws** to allow health care personnel and citizens trained in first aid to deliver needed emergency care without fear of incurring criminal and civil liability (Guido, 1997, pp. 103-104)
2. **Laws vary among states;** thus, nurses should be familiar with the relevant state law. Look for these elements when evaluating the state's law:
   a. Who is covered under the law?
   b. Where does the coverage extend?
   c. What is covered?
3. **Most laws require that care be given in good faith** and that it be gratuitous
4. **There is no legal duty to render care** to strangers in distress

ETHICAL CLINICAL PRACTICE

Foundation of Ethical Nursing Practice

1. **ANA Code of Ethics** (ANA, 2001)
   a. The foundation of ethical practice for nursing is the ANA Code of Ethics (Box 1-3). The ANA code is a statement of the ethical obligations and duties of every nurse, a nonnegotiable ethical standard for the profession, and an expression of the nursing profession's commitment to society.
   b. The preface to the ANA Code of Ethics states: "Ethics is an integral part of the foundation of nursing. Nursing has a distinguished history of concern for the welfare of the sick, injured, and vulnerable and for social justice. This con-

▓ BOX 1-3
▓ PROVISIONS OF THE AMERICAN NURSES ASSOCIATION CODE OF ETHICS

The nurse, in all professional relationships, practices with compassion and respect for the inherent dignity, worth, and uniqueness of every individual, unrestricted by considerations of social or economic status, personal attributes, or the nature of health problems.

The nurse's primary commitment is to the patient, whether an individual, family, group, or community.

The nurse promotes, advocates for, and strives to protect the health, safety, and rights of the patient.

The nurse is responsible and accountable for individual nursing practice and determines the appropriate delegation of tasks consistent with the nurse's obligation to provide optimum care.

The nurse owes the same duties to self as to others, including the responsibility to preserve integrity and safety, to maintain competence, and to continue personal and professional growth.

The nurse participates in establishing, maintaining, and improving health care environments and conditions of employment conducive to the provision of quality health care and consistent with the values of the profession through individual and collective action.

The nurse participates in the advancement of the profession through contributions to practice, education, administration, and knowledge development.

The nurse collaborates with other health professionals and the public in promoting community, national, and international efforts to meet health needs.

The profession of nursing, as represented by associations and their members, is responsible for articulating nursing values, for maintaining the integrity of the profession and its practice, and for shaping social policy.

cern is embodied in the provision of nursing care to individuals and the community. Nursing encompasses the prevention of illness, the alleviation of suffering, and the protection, promotion and restoration of health in the care of individuals, families, groups, and communities. Nurses act to change those aspects of social structures that detract from health and well-being. Individuals who become nurses are expected not only to adhere to the ideals and moral norms of the profession but also to embrace them as a part of what it means to be a nurse. The ethical tradition of nursing is self-reflective, enduring, and distinctive. A code of ethics makes explicit the primary goals, values and obligations of the profession." (ANA, 2001)

2. **AACN Ethic of Care** (AACN, 2002): AACN's mission, vision, and values are framed within an ethic of care and ethical principles. An ethic of care is a moral orientation that acknowledges the interrelatedness and interdependence of individuals, systems, and society. An ethic of care respects individual uniqueness, personal relationships, and the dynamic nature of life. Essential to an ethic of care are compassion, collaboration, accountability, and trust. Within the context of interrelationships of individuals and circumstances, traditional ethical principles provide a basis for deliberation and decision making. These ethical principles include the following:

  a. Respect for persons: A moral obligation to honor the intrinsic worth and uniqueness of each person; to respect self-determination, diversity, and privacy

  b. Beneficence: A moral obligation to promote good and prevent or remove harm; to promote the welfare, health, and safety of society and individuals in accordance with beliefs, values, preferences, and life goals

    c. Justice: A moral obligation to be fair and promote equity, nondiscrimination, and the distribution of benefits and burdens based on needs and resources available; to advocate on another's behalf when necessary

Emergence of Clinical Ethics

1. **Definition of clinical ethics:** "The systematic identification, analysis, and resolution of ethical problems associated with the care of particular patients" (Ahronheim, Moreno, and Zuckerman, 2001, p. 2)
2. **Goals**
   a. Promote patient-centered decision making that honors the rights and interests of the patient
   b. Facilitate the involvement of all clinicians (e.g., physicians, nurses, social workers, and other health care professionals) who require assistance in this complex field
   c. Promote organizational commitment as well as cooperation among all involved parties to implement plans on behalf of the patient
3. **Foundation of clinical ethics** (Jonsen, 1998)
   a. Article by Shana Alexander (1962), "They Decided Who Lives, Who Dies"; described the work of a committee of ordinary citizens in Seattle, Washington, tasked with determining who would receive hemodialysis
   b. Article in the *New England Journal of Medicine* by Duff and Campbell (1973) on ethical problems in the intensive care nursery; described the deliberate decision to withhold treatment from 43 babies with significant problems.
   c. New Jersey Supreme Court decision in 1976 that allowed Karen Ann Quinlan's family to withdraw medical treatment they believed she would not have wanted; laid the foundation for "ethics committees" (Cert denied, 1976)
   d. Movement of bioethics out of the classroom into the clinical arena in the 1980s
   e. Development in 1998 by the American Society for Bioethics and Humanities of core competencies recommended for all ethics consultants (Society for Health and Human Values–Society for Bioethics Consultation Task Force on Standards for Bioethics Consultation, 1998)
   f. Progress in clinical ethics has been significant; however, many issues that have been evident for several years continue to be unresolved (Singer, Pellegrino, and Siegler, 2001)
4. **Religion and clinical ethics** (Ahronheim et al, 2001)
   a. "Clinical ethics" now refers to secular bioethics
   b. Religious leaders continue to play a role in the deliberation of moral and ethical dilemmas; often provide wisdom to secular community
   c. Religious convictions of competent adults should be honored and respected (Brett and Jersild, 2003). This can be difficult for health care providers when it involves decision making by parents for dependent children.
   d. Spiritual values (apart from religious beliefs) may affect health. Health care providers should be sensitive to the spirituality of their patients (Lynn and Harrold, 1999).
5. **Cultural competence and clinical ethics:** Cultural competence is the ability to identify the effects of a patient's culture on the health of the patient (Ahronheim et al, 2001). The health care provider should use a framework of ethical decision making that factors in the patient's culture while avoiding cultural stereotyping.
6. **Organizational ethics and clinical ethics:** Spencer et al (1999) define organizational ethics in terms of articulating, evaluating, and applying consistently the values of an organization as these are defined internally and externally. The mission of the organization should be consistent with the expectations of the employees.

The health care provider's ethical obligations supersede any organization's processes or requirements (Ahronheim et al, 2001).

7. **Ethics across the life span:** Issues include the following (Ahronheim et al, 2001):
   a. Before pregnancy: Carrier screening for genetic disorders; testing for human immunodeficiency virus; in vitro fertilization and related technologies; potential for human cloning; stem cell research; and surrogacy
   b. During pregnancy: Manipulation of embryos; substance abuse during pregnancy; abortion; prenatal genetic diagnosis; implications of multiple births due to reproductive technologies
   c. Infants: Treatment of infants born with severe impairments
   d. Children and adolescents: Role in decision making
   e. Elderly: Issues related to truth telling and confidentiality have shifted for this generation; planning with patient for potential lapses in decision making; emphasis on advance directives for this age group; end-of-life care issues
   f. Caring for the family: Although the rights of the individual patient are still presumed to outweigh those of the family, this is being challenged in many situations and often leads to significant ethical conflicts. Conflicts center on autonomy and confidentiality. A philosophy of family-centered care has the potential to prevent such conflicts or reduce their effects on the care provided patients (Clarke et al, 2003; Curtis et al, 2001; Henneman and Cardin, 2002; Levine and Zuckerman, 1999; Levy and Carlet, 2002).

Standard Ethical Theory (Ahronheim et al, 2001)

1. **Deontology**
   a. Duty-based ethics; health care providers have special duties of care to their patients
   b. Associated with German philosopher Immanuel Kant
2. **Utilitarianism**
   a. Belief that actions are morally evaluated based on the extent to which they facilitate or promote happiness or well-being; health care providers' actions often based on achieving a desired outcome or preoccupation with consequences of an intervention
   b. Associated with English philosophers John Locke and John Stuart Mill

Ethical Principles (Ahronheim et al, 2001; Beauchamp and Childress, 2001; Stanton, 2003)

1. **Patient autonomy and self-determination**
   a. Principle that a competent adult patient has the right to make his or her own health care decisions
   b. Autonomy refers to the potential to be self-determining; clinically supported through the informed consent process, which facilitates decision making that is individualized based on the patient's own values
   c. *Paternalism* is the term used when health care providers make the decisions for the patient based on the rationale that it is in the patient's best interest. This practice denies the patient the autonomy to make his or her own decisions.
2. **Beneficence**
   a. Principle that the competent patient or appropriate surrogate is the best judge of the patient's best interests
   b. Source of common ethical conflicts when there are disagreements between physician and patient or surrogate. Conflict may arise between the physician's

perceived obligation to do good and obligation to respect the patient's expressed wishes.
3. **Nonmaleficence**
   a. Principle to "do no harm"
   b. Often considered same principle as beneficence
4. **Justice**
   a. Principle that everyone fundamentally deserves equal respect
   b. Point of reference for social policy related to access to health care
   c. Distributive justice in health care usually involves how resources are allocated (e.g., scarcity of organs for donation, availability of intensive care unit [ICU] beds or health care staff, futility of care versus patient autonomy, cost-benefit ratio of treatments, and limiting of access to expensive treatments)
      i. Macroallocation decisions (e.g., public health policy)
      ii. Microallocation decisions (e.g., triage during wartime); area of distributive justice involving the clinician role

Common Ethical Distinctions

Should common ethical distinctions be used in clinical ethics assessments? According to Ahronheim et al (2001, pp. 51-56) there are four common distinctions used in clinical ethics discussions. These authors believe it is important to determine if these distinctions are logically valid (i.e., capable of sorting actions into two different groups without ambiguity) and morally relevant (i.e., one of the actions identified is morally justifiable whereas the other is not).
1. **Active versus passive means to an end** (or commission versus omission)
   a. Often associated with euthanasia
   b. Validity questioned because the decision to omit medical interventions to bring about a certain end often involves active behaviors (such as calling a meeting)
   c. Involves serious moral issues similar to those in the distinction between "killing" and "letting die." (For instance, it can be argued that it is justifiable to actively hasten a death if the alternative is to passively stand by while a patient suffers a prolonged death.)
   d. Recommended not to use this distinction in clinical ethics assessments
2. **Ordinary versus extraordinary means**
   a. Attempts to identify interventions based on whether they are standard of practice or not
   b. Practice standards reflect what is being done, not necessarily what should or should not be done based on scientific principles. Should a patient be required to accept any kind of standard means of extending life even if properly grounded in science?
   c. Not recommended as part of a clinical ethics assessment unless a patient adheres to a particular faith that prohibits a specific intervention(s)
3. **Killing versus letting die**
   a. "Killing" infers a deliberate and physically active process such as giving a lethal injection; "letting die" refers to letting the disease process take its course. No one has a moral obligation to rescue a person if the attempt would not prolong life or the attempt would put the rescuer at risk for significant harm.
   b. The distinction appears to be valid and morally relevant but creates significant ethical dilemmas, especially in relation to assisted suicide
4. **Withholding versus withdrawing**
   a. "Withholding" means never starting a given treatment; "withdrawing" means removing or stopping a treatment already started

   b. Logical validity is questionable because there are only a few situations in which the distinction between the two actions is clear. There is no legal basis for the distinction.

   c. No clear distinction in terms of moral relevance. Is it more justifiable not to intubate a patient than to extubate a patient when the end point is similar in both situations?

   d. Despite the lack of logical validity and moral relevance, this distinction is commonly applied in clinical ethics

The Law in Clinical Ethics (Guido, 1997)

1. Informed consent for clinical care: Physicians or independent licensed practitioners have a separate duty to provide needed facts to a patient so that the patient can make an informed health care decision. The right to treat a patient is based on a contractual relationship grounded in mutual consent of the parties.

   a. Types of consent

      i. Expressed consent: Given directly by written or verbal words

      ii. Implied consent: Presumed in emergency situations or implied by the patient's behavior (such as presenting an arm to the practitioner to have blood drawn)

      iii. Partial or complete consent: A patient may give consent for only part of a proposed therapy, for example, consenting to a breast biopsy but not to a mastectomy should it be needed

   b. Elements of informed consent for clinical treatment

      i. Explanation of treatment or procedure

      ii. Name and qualifications of the person to perform the procedure and those of any assistants

      iii. Explanation of significant risks (those that may lead to serious harm, including death)

      iv. Explanation of alternative therapies to the procedure or treatment, including the risk of doing nothing at all

      v. Explanation that the patient can refuse the treatment or procedure without having alternative care or support discontinued

      vi. Explanation that the patient can still refuse the treatment or procedure even after it has started

   c. Standards of informed consent disclosure

      i. Medical community standard (reasonable medical practitioner standard): Disclosure of facts related to the treatment or procedure that a reasonable medical practitioner in a similar community would disclose

      ii. Objective patient standard (prudent patient standard): Disclosure of risks and benefits based on what a prudent person in the given patient's situation would deem material

      iii. Subject patient standard (individual patient standard): Disclosure of facts relevant to a particular patient's situation and what he or she would deem important to know to make an informed decision

      iv. Medical disclosure laws: Requirement by some states that certain risks and consequences be printed on a consent form

      v. Evolving standard proposed by Piper (1994, p. 310): Patient and physician determine together what informed consent means to them; patient must communicate his or her values and expectations of the procedure or treatment to the physician, ask questions and seek clarification of the physician-patient discussion, evaluate symptoms and report impressions of how well the treatment or procedure is working or worked, and make good-faith efforts to participate in the treatment

    d. Exceptions to informed consent

        i. Emergency situations: Consent is implied if there is no time for disclosure and informed consent

        ii. Therapeutic privilege: Primary health care providers are allowed to withhold information that they feel would be detrimental to the patient's health (i.e., likely to hinder or complicate necessary treatment, cause severe psychologic harm, or cause enough anxiety to make a rational decision by the patient impossible)

        iii. Patient waiver: The patient may waive full disclosure while consenting to the procedure, but this cannot be suggested by the health care provider; the waiver must be initiated by the patient

        iv. Prior patient knowledge: If the patient has had the same procedure previously and knows the risks and benefits as explained for the first procedure, then consent can be waived

    e. Accountability for obtaining informed consent

        i. The physician or independent practitioner has full accountability for obtaining informed consent

        ii. A hospital is responsible for informed consent only if those obtaining the consent are employed by the hospital or if the hospital fails to take appropriate actions when informed consent was not obtained and the hospital is aware it was not obtained

        iii. The nurse's role in obtaining informed consent varies with the situation, institution, and state law

            (a) Nurses should explain all nursing care procedures to patients and families. Such procedures rely on orally expressed consent or implied consent. If a patient refuses a procedure or care, this must be honored.

            (b) Physicians can delegate the obtaining of informed consent to nurses. They do so at their own risk, but the nurse must ensure that all aspects of an informed consent are disclosed. Some hospitals do not allow nurses to obtain informed consent to limit the hospital's liability.

            (c) If a nurse has knowledge that an already signed consent form does not meet the criteria for informed consent or the patient revokes the consent, the nurse must notify the supervisor and/or physician

        iv. To obtain blood at the request of law enforcement personnel without consent, five conditions must be present and documented (Guido, 1997, p, 130):

            (a) The suspect is under arrest

            (b) The likelihood exists that the blood drawn will produce evidence for criminal prosecution

            (c) A delay in drawing blood would lead to destruction of evidence

            (d) The test is reasonable and not medically contraindicated

            (e) The test is performed in a reasonable manner

2. Consent forms

    a. Blanket consent: Required prior to admission and covers routine and customary care

    b. Specific consent forms: Often mandated by states; a detailed consent form with the following elements:

        i. Signature of a competent patient or legally authorized representative; "competent" means that the patient has not been declared incompetent by a court of law and the person is able to understand the consequences of his or her actions

            (a) The signature cannot be coerced

            (b) The patient cannot be impaired due to medications previously received

      ii. Name and description of procedure in lay language

     iii. Description of risks and alternatives to treatment (including nontreatment)

     iv. Description of probable consequences of proposed procedure

      v. Signatures of one or two witnesses as mandated by state law; the witness is attesting that the patient actually signed the form

3. Informed consent in human research

  a. Since 1974, the Department of Health and Human Services has required an institutional review board to approve protocols for human research*

  b. Special precautions are in place to protect vulnerable patient populations such as minors, mentally disabled persons, children, and prisoners

  c. Informed consent must include the following basic elements (Guido, 1997, pp. 131, 132):

      i. A description of the purpose of the research, procedures that are experimental and those that are part of regular care, and expected duration of the subject's participation

     ii. The number of subjects to be enrolled in the study

     iii. Description of foreseeable risks or discomforts

     iv. Benefits, if any, to the subject

      v. Disclosure of alternatives courses of treatment available

     vi. Description of how confidentiality of information will be maintained

    vii. Explanation of any compensation that will be provided and explanation of medical care that will be provided if injury occurs

   viii. Contact information for further questions about the research and the subject's rights as a research volunteer

     ix. A clear statement that the subject understands that he or she is a volunteer and has not been coerced into participating; also a statement that the subject may withdraw consent to participate any time during the procedure without loss of benefits or penalties to which the subject is entitled

      x. Language that is easy to understand and includes no exculpatory wording (such as that the researcher has no liability for the patient's outcome)

     xi. Notification of any additional cost that the subject may incur from participating in the research

4. Advance directive: A document in which a person gives directions in advance about medical care or designates who should make medical decisions if he or she should lose decision-making capacity

  a. Living will: Generic term for an advance directive; some states do not recognize these

      i. Not binding for medical practitioners

     ii. Does not protect practitioner from criminal or civil liability

  b. Natural death acts: Enacted by many states to protect practitioners from civil and criminal lawsuits and to ensure that the patient's wishes are followed if the patient is not competent to make his or her own health care decisions.

      i. A legally recognized living will

        (a) Must be developed by a competent adult 18 years of age or older

        (b) Must be witnessed by two persons; some states put restrictions on who can witness

---

*For comprehensive resources related to the protection of human research subjects, see the website for the Office for Human Research Protections, Department of Health and Human Services (http://www.hhs.gov/ohrp/).

      (c) May be revoked by physically destroying, revoking in writing, or verbally rescinding

      (d) Remains valid until revoked

      (e) Becomes effective only when the person becomes qualified (i.e., is terminally ill or has an irreversible condition with loss of decision-making capacity). Usually two physicians must certify that procedures or treatments will not prevent death but merely prolong it

      (f) Does not apply to medications and therapies given to prevent suffering and to provide comfort

  c. Durable power of attorney for health care: Allows competent adults to designate someone to make their health care decisions for them if they become unable to make their own decisions

  d. Medical or physician directive: Allowed in some states; lists a variety of treatments and procedures that the patient may want depending on the patient's condition at the time he or she cannot make his or her own decisions; similar to a living will and with equal legal worth

  e. Uniform Rights of the Terminally Ill Act: Adopted in 1980 and revised in 1989

    i. Similar to natural death acts

    ii. Narrow in scope and limited to treatment that is life prolonging in patients with a terminal or irreversible condition

    iii. Patients who are in a persistent vegetative state are not qualified to use the provisions of this act

  f. Patient Self-Determination Act of 1990

    i. Mandates patient education about advance directives and provides assistance in executing such directives

    ii. States that providers may not discriminate against a patient based on the presence or absence of an advance directive

  g. Do-not-resuscitate (DNR) directives: Institution-based policies that allow patients and physicians to make a decision not to resuscitate in the event of cardiopulmonary arrest

    i. Some states have out-of-hospital DNR laws that allow an individual to request not to be resuscitated by emergency personnel. These orders are still in effect for outpatient treatment, including emergency department care, unless revoked.

    ii. Some hospitals do not recognize DNR orders during surgery. Others believe that the decision to resuscitate or not to resuscitate should be made together by the patient, the physician, and the anesthesiologist. Whatever decision is made should be clearly documented in the medical record prior to surgery.

5. Declaration of death

  a. World Medical Association Declaration on Death*

  b. Uniform Determination of Death Act (UDDA) guidelines developed by the President's Commission for the Study of Ethical Problems in Medicine and in Biomedical and Behavioral Research state that "any individual who has sustained either irreversible cessation of circulatory and respiratory functions, or irreversible cessation of all functions of the entire brain, including the brainstem, is dead."† Most states have adopted these guidelines.

---

*For the text of the declaration, go to http://www.wma.net/e/policy/d2.htm.
†Actual determination approved in 1989; the text can be found at http://www.law.upenn.edu/bll/ulc/fnact99/1980s/urtia89.pdf.

    c. Confusion and controversy still exist over the term *brain death* and the relation of such death to donorship for organ transplantation (Capron, 2001; Truog, 2003)

    d. Procedural guidelines for the declaration of death

        i. Triggering of a neurologic evaluation: As soon as the responsible physician has a reasonable suspicion that an irreversible loss of all brain functions has occurred, he or she should perform the appropriate tests and procedures to determine the patient's neurologic status

        ii. Obligation to declare a patient dead

           (a) Cardiopulmonary criteria for determining death are recognized in all states. When the physician determines that the patient has experienced an irreversible cessation of cardiopulmonary functions, he or she declares the patient dead. Consent of the surrogate, family, or concerned friends is not required.

           (b) Sensitivity to family or surrogate needs is required in declaring brain death. Family members have the option to obtain a second opinion about brain death.

        iii. Cessation of treatment after a declaration of death: Once the declaration of death has been made, all treatment of the patient ordinarily should cease; exceptions to this might be when efforts are made to use the body or body parts for purposes stated in the Uniform Anatomical Gift Act (education, research, advancement of medical or dental science, therapy, transplantation) or when the patient is pregnant and efforts are being made to save the life of the fetus

        iv. In cases involving organ donation, health care professionals who make the declaration of death

           (a) Should not be members of the organ transplantation team

           (b) Should not be a member of the patient's family

           (c) Should not have malpractice charges pending against them that are related to the case

           (d) Should not have any other special interest in declaration of the patient's death (i.e., stand to inherit anything according to patient's will)

6. Organ donation

    a. World Medical Association Statement on Human Organ and Tissue Donation and Transplantation (World Medical Association, 2000)*

    b. Types of organ donors

        i. Tissue donor or living organ donor: Donor may be alive (e.g., bone marrow, kidney donor) or deceased (e.g., eye donor); organ donation by living donors poses special concerns due to the increased risk to donors' lives (Benner, 2002)

        ii. Heart-beating donor: Donor is brain dead but respiratory function is supported mechanically while cardiac function continues spontaneously

        iii. Non–heart-beating donor: Organs are procured immediately after cessation of cardiorespiratory function

    c. A recent study (Exley, White, and Martin, 2002) indicated that the following characteristics significantly influence the likelihood that families will make a decision to donate tissues or organs:

        i. Anglo-American ethnicity

        ii. Any religious affiliation

---

*Adopted in 2000 to address the professional obligations of physicians and hospitals related to organ donation and transplantation. The complete statement can be found at http://www.wma.net/e/policy/wma.htm.

      iii. Someone initiates discussion of donation: This person could be family member, physician, or organ procurement organization coordinator, but it is helpful to include the organ procurement organization coordinator early in the process

      iv. Death caused by gunshot or suicide

      v. Issuing of request before or during declaration of brain death

      vi. Presence of signed donor card

7. Emergency Medical Treatment and Labor Act (EMTALA)

    a. A 1986 law requiring hospitals participating in Medicare to screen patients for emergency medical conditions and stabilize them or provide protected transfers for medical reasons (Center for Medicaid and State Operations, 2004; Frank, 2001)

    b. Failure to adhere to the law results in large fines or loss of Medicare funding

    c. Patients may sue hospitals in federal or state court for damages under EMTALA's private right of action provision

    d. First case was decided by the U.S. Supreme Court in 1998

8. Futile care

    a. Concept is an evolving standard (Ahronheim, 2001, pp. 72-74)

    b. Definitions of futility lack consensus and are value laden, but futile care involves interventions that sustain life for prolonged periods even when there is no hope of improvement or achieving the goals of therapy (American Medical Association Council on Ethical and Judicial Affairs, 1999). Many questions remain unresolved and lead to ethical dilemmas and conflict.

      i. Who establishes the goals of therapy? Is it the physician, the patient, the family, or all of them?

      ii. What does the physician or hospital do if the medical decision is in conflict with that of the patient and family, who may have an unrealistic expectation for improvement (Curtis and Burt, 2003; Lofmark and Nilstun, 2002)?

    c. The American Medical Association Council on Ethical and Judicial Affairs (1999) recommends resolution of futility conflicts using a process-based framework

    d. There is some evidence that bioethics consultation resulting in cessation of therapy shortens the length of therapy significantly (Rivera et al, 2001; Schneiderman, Gilmer, and Teetzel, 2000; Schneiderman et al, 2003)

9. Legal barriers to end-of-life care (Meisel et al, 2000)

    a. The legal context of care affects interventions and outcomes

    b. Legal myths and counteracting reality

      i. *Myth:* Forgoing life-sustaining treatment for a patient without decision-making capacity requires evidence that this is the patient's wish
Reality: Only a few states require "clear and convincing evidence." Most states will allow forgoing life-sustaining treatment based on a surrogate's word that it was the patient's wish. Some states even allow termination of such treatment if no one knows the patient's wishes and it is deemed in the patient's "best interest."

      ii. *Myth:* Withholding or withdrawing artificial nutrition or hydration from terminally ill or permanently unconscious patients is illegal
Reality: Just like any other therapy, fluids and nutrition may be withheld if it is the patient's or surrogate's wish

      iii. *Myth:* Risk management personnel must be consulted before life-sustaining medical treatment can be stopped
Reality: This may be a hospital policy, but there is no legal requirement to notify risk management personnel

      iv. *Myth:* Advance directives must be developed using specific forms, are not transferable to other states, and govern all future decisions. Advance directives given orally are not enforceable.

Reality: Oral statements made by the patients may be legally valid directives. The patient does not have to be competent to revoke an advance directive but does have to be competent to make one. There are no specific forms required by any law to be used to document advance directives. Most states honor directives developed in other states.

v. *Myth:* Physicians will be criminally prosecuted if they prescribe high dosages of medication for palliative care (to relieve pain or discomfort symptoms) that result in death

Reality: In 1997 the U.S. Supreme Court ruled on the constitutionality of laws making physician-assisted suicide a crime. The physician has not committed assisted suicide or homicide if the pain medications were ordered to relieve pain. The doctrine of "double effect" states that if an intervention is used for its intended purpose (such as pain relief) but has an unintended effect that would be illegitimate if it were intended (such as the death of the patient), then the physician is not morally responsible for the unintended effect. In reality the application of this doctrine can be ambiguous, and acting under the double-effect doctrine does not eliminate the risk of prosecution. Although a good defense can be made under the doctrine, such defense takes a toll on the physician. As a result, undertreatment of pain at the end of life often occurs.

vi. *Myth:* There are no legal options for easing suffering in a terminally ill patient whose suffering is overwhelming despite palliative care

Reality: Terminal sedation is an option to treat otherwise intractable symptoms in patients imminently dying. Only Oregon gives physicians the right to prescribe oral medication to competent patients who intend to commit suicide with the medication. The patient must take his or her own medication. The physician can only prescribe the drugs. The 1997 Supreme Court decision on assisted suicide leaves other states free to legalize or prohibit the practice.

Clinical Ethics Assessment

1. **Identification of ethical issues and ethical decision-making models**
   a. Distinction between ethical and nonethical problems and dilemmas: Three characteristics must be present for a problem to be deemed an ethical one (Curtin as cited in Stanton, 2003):
      i. The problem cannot be resolved with just empirical data
      ii. The problem is inherently perplexing
      iii. The result of the decision making will affect several areas of human concern
   b. Elements of ethical decision-making models (Ahronheim et al, 2001; Stanton, 2003): There are many decision-making models. Common elements include the following actions:
      i. Gather all data (including information from all the stakeholders) related to the issue
      ii. Analyze and interpret the data: Is it an ethical issue versus a legal or policy issue? What ethical principles are involved? What ethical conflicts are present? What are the capabilities of the stakeholders involved?
      iii. Identify courses of action and analyze the benefits and burdens of each course; project the consequences of the action
      iv. Choose a plan of action and implement the plan; provide support to the stakeholders as needed
      v. Evaluate the consequences of the actions taken
      vi. Evaluate the ethical decision-making process
2. **Ethical conflicts**
   a. Conflicts between moral principles

    b. Conflicts between interpretations of a patient's best interest

    c. Conflicts between moral principles and institutional policy or the law

3. Institutional ethics committees

    a. Multidisciplinary team resource for patients and families, clinicians, and the institution

        i. Assist with clarifying issues

        ii. Assist with the development of institutional policies and procedures related to clinical ethical issues

    b. Goals include promoting the rights of patients, fostering shared decision making between patients and clinicians, promoting fair policies and procedures that maximize the likelihood of good patient-centered outcomes; and enhancing the ethical practice of health care professionals and health care institutions

    c. Educate staff and the community to achieve goals

    d. Ethics consultation: The most common situations triggering consultations by physicians include the following (DuVal et al, 2001):

        i. End-of-life care

        ii. Patient autonomy

        iii. Conflicts among persons involved

    e. Composition: Should include representatives of all disciplines and of the institution administration, and community-at-large members

4. Ethics consultation: Process elements

    a. Who has access to the process (all clinicians, patients, and/or families) should be delineated

    b. Patients (or surrogates), if appropriate, and attending physicians should be notified (providing reason for the consultation, describing the process, and inviting participation)

    c. Documentation should be in patient record or some other permanent record

    d. Case review or process evaluation should be done to promote accountability

5. Core skills and knowledge required for effective ethics consultations (Society for Health and Human Values, 1998)

    a. Core skills (Table 1-3)

        i. Ethical assessment skills required to identify the nature of the ethical dilemma or conflict

        ii. Process skills required to focus on efforts to resolve the ethical dilemma or conflict

        iii. Interpersonal skills critical to the consultation process

    b. Core knowledge areas

        i. Moral reasoning and ethical theory as it relates to consultation

        ii. Bioethical issues and concepts that typically emerge in ethical consultations

        iii. Health care systems as they relate to ethics consultation

        iv. Clinical knowledge as related to the ethics consultation

        v. Knowledge of the health care institution and institution policies in the context of the ethical consultation

        vi. Beliefs and perspectives of the patient and staff populations served by the ethics consultation

        vii. Relevant code of ethics, standards of professional conduct, and guidelines of accrediting organizations as they relate to ethics consultation

        viii. Health law relevant to ethics consultation

Nurse's Role as Patient Advocate and Moral Agent

1. Organizational ethics and the nurse as patient advocate: AACN takes the position that the role of the critical care nurse includes being a patient advocate

■ **TABLE 1-3**
■ ■ **Core Skills for Ethics Consultation**

Skill Category	Specific Skills
Ethical assessment skills	***Ability to:*** Discern and gather relevant data Assess social and interpersonal dynamics Distinguish ethical dimensions of case from other dimensions (i.e., legal, medical, psychiatric) Identify the assumptions that stakeholders bring to the situation Identify values held by the various stakeholders (requires knowledge to access and analyze the relevant laws, policies, and bioethical knowledge needed) Use relevant moral considerations in case analysis Identify and justify a range of morally acceptable options and their consequences Evaluate evidence for and against the options presented for action Recognize and acknowledge personal limitations and potential areas of conflict between personal views and role as ethics consultant (may involve accepting group decisions that are morally acceptable but in conflict with personal viewpoint)
Process skills	***Ability to:*** Identify key stakeholders and involve them in the process Set ground rules for formal meetings Stay within the limits of the consultant's role Create an atmosphere of trust that respects privacy and confidentiality and promotes honest discussion of issues Build moral consensus by helping individuals analyze the values underlying their assumptions and decisions, negotiating and resolving conflicts, and engaging in creative problem solving Use institutional structure and resources to facilitate the implementation of the selected course of action Document the consultation and elicit feedback about the process for evaluation
Interpersonal skills	***Ability to:*** Listen well and communicate respect, support, and empathy to stakeholders Educate about the ethical dimensions of the case Elicit the moral views of stakeholders Represent the views of all involved parties to the others Enable involved parties to communicate effectively and be heard by others Recognize and attend to communication barriers

Adapted from Society for Health and Human Values–Society for Bioethics Consultation Task Force on Standards for Bioethics Consultation: *Core competencies for health care ethics consultation*, Glenview, Ill, 1998, American Society for Bioethics and Humanities, pp. 12-14.

(AACN, 2003). The health care institution is instrumental in providing an environment in which patient advocacy is expected and supported. Patient advocacy is a fundamental nursing characteristic in the Synergy Model (Hayes, 2000). As a patient advocate, the critical care nurse does the following:

a. Respects and supports the right of the patient or the patient's designated surrogate to autonomous, informed decision making

b. Intervenes when the best interest of the patient is in question

    c. Helps the patient obtain necessary care

    d. Respects the values, beliefs, and rights of the patient

    e. Provides education and support to help the patient or the patient's designated surrogate make decisions

    f. Represents the patient in accordance with the patient's choices

    g. Supports the decisions of the patient or the patient's designated surrogate or transfers care to an equally qualified critical care nurse

    h. Intercedes for a patient who cannot speak for himself or herself in situations that require immediate action

    i. Monitors and safeguards the quality of care the patient receives

    j. Acts as liaison among the patient, the patient's family, and health care professionals

2. **Patient rights**

    a. American Hospital Association (AHA) Patient Bill of Rights (AHA, 1992); first published in 1973, revised in 1992; posted in all hospitals in the United States

    b. Ethics of restraints: The use of restraints in critical care has the potential to violate several ethical principles (Reigle, 1996) and thus should be undertaken with caution

        i. Nonmaleficence, or preventing harm; and beneficence, or doing good. Restraints are often used to prevent harm, but unintended consequences may violate this principle. The patient's autonomy is breached, and restraints often cause significant physical harm. In many cases use of restraint does not prevent the disruption of medical therapy.

        ii. Informed consent should be obtained from the patient and/or family prior to use of restraints. A discussion of alternative treatments should be included. A patient with decision-making capacity should be able to choose to forego restraint. Paternalism is involved in situations in which one overrides another's decision to prevent harm to the person or maximize the benefits of treatment. There may be justifications for such actions in the critical care environment. If the patient lacks decision-making capacity and no surrogate decision maker is available, the nurse is obligated to use restraints to prevent significant or irreversible harm.

        iii. Trust is important to the patient and family members. They trust nurses, and thus ongoing communication about restraint decisions is crucial. Family members become upset when the patient is restrained without their knowledge.

    c. Ethics of pain management (American Pain Society Task Force on Pain, Symptoms and End of Life Care, n.d.; McCaffery and Pasero, 1999)

        i. Patients have the right to have their reports of pain believed

        ii. Patients have the right to have pain addressed appropriately

        iii. Clinicians, patients, and families must be educated about pain treatment

        iv. Pain and pain management must be made visible and emphasized in organizations

        v. Policies on reimbursement for the services of health professionals, medications, and other palliative treatments must be designed so that they do not create barriers to symptom treatment

        vi. Development of policies to ensure adequate treatment of symptoms should take precedence over legalization of physician-assisted suicide and euthanasia

3. **Family-centered care versus patient-centered care**

    a. Family members are not visitors (Molter, 2003)

    b. The family has a vital role in supporting the patient through a critical illness (Simpson, 1991). When family members' needs are not attended to or met, significant conflict occurs (Chesla and Stannard, 1997; Levine and Zuckerman, 1999).

   c. Family-centered care focuses on the whole patient as a member of a family unit. It incorporates the family as a team member in the healing process. Improving family communications at the end of life can be cost effective for the family and institution (Aherns et al, 2003).

   d. The family-centered care philosophy was developed by pediatric practitioners (Edelman, 1995). Box 1-4 summarizes the key tenets of the family-centered care philosophy. It is a collaborative approach to care and not a unilateral approach on the part of the clinicians or the family. It can be practically established in critical care units (Henneman and Cardin, 2002).

4. End-of-life care

   a. AACN organized a consortium to develop an agenda for the nursing profession on end-of-life care (EOLC) (Nursing Leadership Consortium on End-of-Life Care, 1999). Nine priorities were identified:

      i. Education: Integrate EOLC into all curricula and develop interdisciplinary education on palliative care

      ii. Professionalism: Create an environment for collaboration among health care systems, educational institutions, associations, and government agencies to meet the needs of EOLC

      iii. Clinical and patient care: Establish practice guidelines that incorporate supportive strategies to prevent pain and suffering and promote comfort and well-being

      iv. Research: Provide health care staff with research-based information on EOLC

      v. Patient and family advocacy: Educate and empower the consumer of health care services about EOLC

      vi. Decision making: Develop a dynamic process for making decisions about EOLC

■ BOX 1-4
■ EIGHT ELEMENTS OF FAMILY-CENTERED CARE

1. Incorporating into policy and practice the recognition that the family is the constant in a person's life, while the service systems and support personnel within those systems fluctuate.
2. Facilitating family/professional collaboration at all levels of hospital, home, and community care.
3. Exchanging complete and unbiased information between families and professionals in a supportive manner at all times.
4. Incorporating into policy and practice the recognition and honoring of cultural diversity, strengths, and individuality within and across all families.
5. Recognizing and respecting different methods of coping and implementing comprehensive policies and programs that provide developmental, educational, emotional, environmental, and financial supports to meet the diverse needs of families.
6. Encouraging and facilitating family-to-family support and networking.
7. Ensuring that hospital, home, and community service and support systems for individuals and their families needing specialized health and development care are flexible, accessible, and comprehensive in responding to diverse family-identified needs.
8. Appreciating families as families and individuals as individuals, recognizing that they possess a wide range of strengths, concerns, emotions, and aspirations beyond their need for specialized health services and support.

From Edelman L, editor: *Getting on board: training activities to promote the practice of family-centered care,* ed 2, Bethesda, MD, 1995, Association for the Care of Children's Health, pp. 4-5.

     vii. Culture: Create a national environment in which EOLC is freely discussed

  viii. Systems of care: Structure a health care system that allows all dying patients and their families access to pain management and hospice care

    ix. Resource allocation policy: Enact legislation that provides comprehensive financing for palliative care that is not limited to skilled nursing episodes or hospice care

b. Quality indicators for EOLC (Clarke et al, 2003, p. 2258). Consensus was established by the Robert Wood Johnson Foundation Critical Care End-of-Life Peer Workgroup. Seven domains were identified with specific indicators:

  i. Patient and family–centered decision making

    (a) Recognize the patient and family as the unit of care

    (b) Assess the patient's and family's decision-making style and preferences

    (c) Address conflicts in decision making within the family

    (d) Assess, together with appropriate clinical consultants, the patient's capacity to participate in decision making about treatment and document this assessment

    (e) Initiate advance care planning with the patient and family

    (f) Clarify and document the status of the patient's advance directive

    (g) Identify the health care proxy or surrogate decision maker

    (h) Clarify and document resuscitation orders

    (i) Assure the patient and family that decision making by the health care team will incorporate their preferences (Heyland et al, 2003)

    (j) Follow ethical and legal guidelines for patients who lack both capacity and a surrogate decision maker

    (k) Establish and document clear, realistic, and appropriate goals of care in consultation with the patient and family

    (l) Help the patient and family assess the benefits and burdens of alternative treatment choices as the patient's condition changes

    (m) Forgo life-sustaining treatments in a way that ensures that patient and family preferences are elicited and respected

  ii. Communication within the team and with patients and families

    (a) Meet as an interdisciplinary team to discuss the patient's condition, clarify goals of treatment, and identify the patient's and family's needs and preferences (Curtis et al, 2001)

    (b) Address conflicts among the clinical team before meeting with the patient and/or family

    (c) Use expert clinical, ethical, and spiritual consultants when appropriate

    (d) Recognize the adaptations in communication strategy required for the patient and family depending on the chronic versus acute nature of illness, cultural and spiritual differences, and other influences

    (e) Meet with the patient and/or family on a regular basis to review the patient's status and to answer questions

    (f) Communicate all information to the patient and family, including distressing news, in a clear, sensitive, unhurried manner, and in an appropriate setting

    (g) Clarify the patient's and family's understanding of the patient's condition and goals of care at the beginning and end of each meeting

    (h) Designate a primary clinical liaison(s) who will communicate with the family daily

    (i) Identify a family member who will serve as the contact person for the family

    (j) When indicated, prepare the patient and family for the dying process

   iii. Continuity of care
       (a) Maximize continuity of care across clinicians, consultants, and settings
       (b) Orient new clinicians regarding the patient and family status
       (c) Prepare the patient and/or family for a change of clinician(s) and introduce new clinicians
   iv. Emotional and practical support
       (a) Elicit and attend to the needs of the dying person and his or her family
       (b) Distribute written material for families that includes orientation to the ICU environment and open visitation guidelines, logistical information (nearby hotels, banks, restaurants; directions), listings of financial consultation services, and bereavement programs and resources
       (c) Facilitate strengthening of patient-family relationships and communication
       (d) Maximize privacy for the patient and family
       (e) Value and support the patient's and family's cultural traditions
       (f) Arrange for social support for a patient without family or friends
       (g) Support the family through the patient's death and their bereavement
   v. Symptom management
       (a) Emphasize the comprehensive comfort care that will be provided to the patient rather than the removal of life-sustaining treatments
       (b) Institute and use uniform quantitative symptom assessment scales appropriate for communicative and noncommunicative patients on a routine basis
       (c) Standardize and follow best clinical practices for symptom management
       (d) Use nonpharmacologic as well as pharmacologic measures to maximize comfort as appropriate and desired by the patient and family
       (e) Reassess and document symptoms following interventions
       (f) Know and follow best clinical practices for withdrawing life-sustaining treatments to avoid patient and family distress
       (g) Eliminate unnecessary tests and procedures (laboratory work, weighing, routine monitoring of vital signs) and maintain intravenous catheters only for symptom management in situations in which life support is being withdrawn
       (h) Attend to the patient's appearance and hygiene
       (i) Ensure the family's and/or clinician's presence so the patient is not dying alone
   vi. Spiritual support
       (a) Assess and document spiritual needs of the patient and family on an on-going basis
       (b) Encourage access to spiritual resources
       (c) Elicit and facilitate spiritual and cultural practices that the patient and family find comforting
   vii. Emotional and organizational support for ICU clinicians
       (a) Support health care team colleagues caring for dying patients
       (b) Adjust nursing staff and medical rotation schedules to maximize continuity of care providers for dying patients
       (c) Communicate regularly with the interdisciplinary team regarding the goals of care
       (d) Establish a staff support group, based on the input and needs of ICU staff and experienced group facilitators, and integrate meeting times into the routine of the ICU
       (e) Enlist palliative care experts, pastoral care representatives, and other consultants to teach and model aspects of EOLC

      (f) Facilitate the establishment of rituals for the staff to mark the death of patients

5. **Resuscitation and family presence**
   a. DNR order policies first appeared in hospital policies in 1976 (Burns et al, 2003)
   b. Survival statistics for patients requiring cardiopulmonary resuscitation are poor; thus, early discussions with the patient and/or family are essential to avoid futile intervention (Agich and Arroliga 2000; Khalafi, Ravakhah, and West, 2001; van Walraven, Forster, and Stiell, 1999)
   c. Some evidence exists that DNR forms can assist in defining the limits of intervention (DePalo, Iacobucci, and Crausman, 2003)
   d. There are many advantages and disadvantages to the practice of allowing family to be present during resuscitation, as identified in the adult and pediatric literature (MacLean et al, 2003; McGahey, 2002)
      i. Advantages
         (a) Family members can observe the efforts of the health care team: Promotes trust by removing "secrecy"
         (b) Family can provide support to their family member and feel as if they are participating in the healing process
         (c) The practice is consistent with a holistic family-centered approach to care that sees the patient and family as the unit of care
      ii. Disadvantages
         (a) Family members may disrupt resuscitation efforts
         (b) Fear of litigation may inhibit the actions of the health care team
         (c) Long-term effects on family's emotional status are unknown
         (d) Patient's privacy may be violated
         (e) Additional stress is put on the health care staff
   e. The practice of allowing family to witness resuscitation remains controversial; however, recent research indicates that more families are requesting presence and recommends the development of policies or guidelines for this practice (MacLean et al, 2003)
6. **Good palliative care practice** (Kirchhoff, 2002)
   a. Goals to enable the patient to achieve a peaceful end of life (Ruland and Moore, 1998)
      i. The patient will be pain free
      ii. The patient will feel comfortable
      iii. The patient will experience dignity and respect
      iv. The patient will be at peace
      v. The patient will be close to significant others
   b. Precepts of palliative care*
      i. Respect patient goals, preferences, and choices
      ii. Provide comprehensive care
      iii. Utilize the strengths of interdisciplinary resources
      iv. Acknowledge and address caregiver concerns
      v. Build systems and mechanisms of support
   c. Develop the competencies needed to provide care to patients at the end of life[†]

---

*The actual document developed by the Last Acts Task Force on Palliative Care in 1997 can be found at https://www.aacn.org/AACN/practice. nsf/Files/ep/$file/2001Precep.pdf.

[†]Competencies recommended by the American Association of Colleges of Nursing are found at http://www.aacn.nche.edu/Publications/deathfin.htm.

REFERENCES

Environment of Professional Caring and the AACN Synergy Model for Patient Care

Agich GJ, Arroliga AC: Appropriate use of DNR orders: a practical approach, *Cleve Clin J Med* 67:392, 395, 399-400, 2000.

Ahrens T, Yancey V, Kollef M: Improving family communications at the end of life: implications for length of stay in the intensive care unit and resource use, *Am J Crit Care* 12:317-324, 2003.

Aiken LH, Clarke SP, Sloane DM, et al: Nurses' reports on hospital care in five countries, *Health Affairs* 20:43-53, 2001, retrieved May 4, 2005, from http://www.healthaffairs.org.

American Association of Critical-Care Nurses: Maintaining patient-focused care in an environment of nursing staff shortages and financial constraints, statement approved Nov 2000, retrieved May 4, 2005, from http://www.aacn.org/aacn/pubpolcy.ns/vwdoc/pmp?opendocument.

American Association of Critical-Care Nurses: Role of the critical care nurse, updated Feb 24, 2003, retrieved May 4, 2005, from http://www.aacn.org/aacn/pubpolcy.nsf/vwdoc/pmp?opendocument.

American Association of Critical-Care Nurses: Vision, mission, values and ethic of care statement, updated Feb 12, 2005, retrieved Aug 14, 2005, from http://www.aacn.org/aacn/aacnhome.nsf/vwdoc/aacninformation.

AACN Certification Corporation: *Resource booklet: AACN Certification Corporation study of practice survey booklet,* Aliso Viejo, Calif, 1997, American Association of Critical-Care Nurses.

AACN Certification Corporation: Summary of results, AACN Certification Corporation study of practice, Unpublished report, Aliso Viejo, Calif, 1998, American Association of Critical-Care Nurses.

AACN Certification Corporation: The AACN synergy model for patient care, 2003, retrieved May 4, 2005, from http://www.aacn.org/certcorp/certcorp.nsf/vwdoc/SynModel?opendocument.

AACN Certification Corporation and PES: *Final report of a comprehensive study of critical care nursing practice,* Aliso Viejo, Calif, 2004, The Corporation.

American Nurses Association: *Nursing facts. Advanced practice nursing: a new age in health care,* 1997, retrieved Aug 14, 2005, from http://www.nursingworld.org/readroom/fsadvprc.htm.

American Nurses Association: *Nursing's social policy statement,* ed 2, Washington DC, 2003, The Association.

Annis TD: The interdisciplinary team across the continuum of care, *Crit Care Nurse* 22:76-79, 2002.

Bell L, editor: *Scope of practice and standards of professional performance for the acute and critical care clinical nurse specialist,* Aliso Viejo, Calif, 2002, American Association of Critical-Care Nurses.

Biel M: *Reconceptualizing certified practice: envisioning critical care practice of the future,* Aliso Viejo, Calif, 1997, AACN Certification Corporation.

Carlson MB: Engaging synergy: kindred spirits on the edge, *J Humanist Psychol* 36(3):85-102, 1996.

Caterinicchio MJ, for the AACN Certification Corporation: Redefining nursing according to patients' and families' needs: an evolving concept, *AACN Clin Issues* 6:153-156, 1995.

Chesla CA, Stannard D: Breakdown in the nursing care of families in the ICU, *Am J Crit Care* 6:64-71, 1997.

Collopy KS: Advance practice nurses guiding families through systems, *Crit Care Nurse* 19:80-85, 1999.

Cohen SS, Crego N, Cuming RG, et al: The Synergy Model and the role of clinical nurse specialists in a multihospital system, *Am J Crit Care* 11:436-445, 2002.

Cornerstone Communications Group: *Analysis of American Nurses Association staffing survey,* Washington, DC, 2001, American Nurses Association.

Curley MAQ: Patient-nurse synergy: optimizing patients' outcomes, *Am J Crit Care* 7:64-72, 1998.

Curtis JR, Patrick DL, Shannon SE, et al: The family conference as a focus to improve communication about end-of-life care in the ICU: opportunities for improvement, *Crit Care Med* 29(2 suppl): N40-45, 2001.

Czerwinski S, Blastic L, Rice B: The Synergy Model: building a clinical advancement program, *Crit Care Nurse* 19:72-77, 1999.

Doble RK, Curley MAQ, Hession-Leband E, et al: Using the Synergy Model to link nursing care to diagnosis-related groups, *Crit Care Nurse* 20:86-92, 2000.

Ecklund MM, Stamps DC: Promoting synergy in progressive care, *Crit Care Nurse* 22:60-66, 2002.

Edelman L, editor: *Getting on board: training activities to promote the practice of family-centered care,* ed 2, Bethesda, MD, 1995, Association for the Care of Children's Health.

Edwards DF: The Synergy Model: linking patient needs to nurse competencies, *Crit Care Nurse* 19:97-99, 1999.

Exley M, White N, Martin JH: Transplantation: Why families say no to organ donation, *Crit Care Nurse* 6:44-51, 2002.

Glassford BA: Goals aimed at helping to integrate ethics into practice, *AACN News* 16(11), 1999.

Hardin S, Hussey L: AACN Synergy Model for patient care: case study of CHF patient, *Crit Care Nurse* 23:73-76, 2003.

Hartigan RC: Establishing criteria for 1:1 staffing ratios, *Crit Care Nurse* 20:114-116, 2000.

Hayes C: Strengthening nurses' moral agency, *Crit Care Nurse* 20:90-94, 2000.

Henneman EA, Cardin S: Family-centered critical care: a practical approach to making it happen, *Crit Care Nurse* 22:12-16, 18-19, 2002.

Institute of Medicine: *To err is human: building a safer health care system,* Washington DC, September 1, 1999, Institute of Medicine.

Joint Commission on Accreditation of Healthcare Organizations: 2006 National patient safety goals, 2006, retrieved October 3, 2005, from http://www.jcaho.org/ general+public/patient+safety/gp_06_ npsgs.htm.

Kaplow R: Applying the Synergy Model to nursing education, *Crit Care Nurse* 22:77-81, 2002.

Kerfoot K: The Synergy Model in practice: the leader as synergist, *Nurs Econ* 19:29-30, 2001.

Kirchhoff KT: Promoting a peaceful death in the ICU, *Crit Care Nurs Clin North Am* 14:201-206, 2002.

Last Acts Palliative Care Task Force: *Precepts of palliative care,* Washington DC, 1997, Last Acts.

Levy MM, Carlet J: Compassionate end-of-life care in the intensive care unit, *Crit Care Med* 29(2 suppl):N1, 2002.

Malloch K: Healing models for organizations: description, measurement, outcomes, *J Healthc Manag* 45:332-345, 2000.

Markey DW: Applying the Synergy Model: clinical strategies, *Crit Care Nurse* 21:72-76, 2001.

McCaffery M, Pasero C: *Pain: clinical manual,* ed 2, St Louis, 1999, Mosby.

McGahey PR: Family presence during pediatric resuscitation: a focus on staff, *Crit Care Nurse* 22:29-34, 2002.

Medina J, editor: *Standards for acute and critical care nursing practice,* Aliso Viejo, Calif, 2000, American Association of Critical-Care Nurses.

Moloney-Harmon P: The Synergy Model: contemporary practice of the clinical nurse specialist, *Crit Care Nurse* 19:101-104, 1999.

Molter NC: The Synergy Model: creating safe passage in healthcare. In Biel M, editor: *Reconceptualizing certified practice: envisioning critical care practice of the future,* Aliso Viejo, Calif, 1997, American Association of Critical-Care Nurses Certification Corporation.

Molter NC: Creating a healing environment for critical care, *Crit Care Nurs Clin North Am* 15:295-304, 2003.

Muenzen PM, Greenberg S: Final report for phase 1 in the development of a certification examination program for clinical nurse specialists (CNSs). In *Role delineation study for CNSs caring for acute and critically ill patients,* New York, 1998, Professional Examination Service, Department of Research and Development.

Mullen JE: The Synergy Model as a framework for nursing rounds, *Crit Care Nurse* 22:66-68, 2002.

National Council of State Boards of Nursing: Delegation: concepts and decision-making process. 1995, retrieved Oct 30, 2003, from http://www.ncsbn.org/regulation/uap_ delegation_documents_delegation.asp.

Nursing Leadership Consortium on End-of-Life Care: *Designing an agenda for the nursing profession on end-of-life care,* Aliso Viejo, Calif, 1999, American Association of Critical-Care Nurses.

Ruland CM, Moore SM: Theory construction based on standards of care: a proposed theory of the peaceful end of life, *Nurs Outlook* 46:169-175, 1998.

Sechrist KR, Berlin LE, Biel M: Overview of the theoretical review process, *Crit Care Nurse* 20:85-86, 2000.

Simpson T: The family as a source of support for the critically ill adult, *AACN Clin Issues Crit Care Nurs* 2:229-235, 1991.

Stannard D: Being a good dance partner, *Crit Care Nurse* 19:86-87, 1999.

Tanner CA, Benner P, Chesla C, et al: The phenomenology of knowing the patient, *Image* 25:273-280, 1993.

van Walraven C, Forster AJ, Stiell IG: Derivation of a clinical decision rule for the discontinuation of in-hospital cardiac arrest resuscitation, *Arch Intern Med* 159:129-134, 1999.

Villaire M: The Synergy Model of certified practice: creating safe passage for patients, *Crit Care Nurse* 16:95-99, 1996.

Legal Aspects of Care

Benner P: Living organ donors: respecting the risks involved in the "gift of life," *Am J Crit Care* 11:266-268, 2002.

Capron AM: Brain death—well settled yet still unresolved, *N Engl J Med* 344:1244-1246, 2001.

Center for Medicaid and State Operations, Survey and Certification Group: Revised Emergency Medical Treatment and Labor Act (EMTALA) interpretive guidelines, May 13, 2004, retrieved Aug 14, 2005, from http://www.cms.hhs.gov/medicaid/survey-cert/SC0434.pdf.

Frank G: EMTALA: an expert tells us what it's all about, *J Emerg Nurs* 27:65-67, 2001.

Giordano K: Legal counsel: examining nursing malpractice: a defense attorney's perspective, *Crit Care Nurse* 23:104-106, 108, 2003.

Guido GW: *Legal issues in nursing*, ed 2, Stamford, CT, 1997, Appleton & Lange.

Meisel A, Snyder L, Quill T, et al: Seven legal barriers to end-of-life care: myths, realities, and grains of truth, *JAMA* 284:2495-2501, 2000.

Piper A Jr: Truce in the battlefield: a proposal for a different approach to medical informed consent, *J Law Med Ethics* 22(4):301-313, 1994.

Truog RD: Role of brain death and the dead donor rule in the ethics of organ transplantation, *Crit Care Med* 31:2391-2396, 2003.

World Medical Association: World Medical Association declaration on death, Aug 1968, revised Aug 1983, retrieved May 4, 2005, from http://www.wma.net/e/policy/d2.htm.

World Medical Association: World Medical Association statement on human organ and tissue donation and transplantation, Jan 2000, retrieved May 4, 2005, from http://www.wma.net/e/policy/wma.htm.

Ethical Aspects of Care

Ahronheim JC, Moreno JD, Zuckerman C: *Ethics in clinical practice*, ed 2, Gaithersburg, MD, 2001, Aspen.

Alexander S: They decide who lives, who dies, *Life* 11:102, Nov 9, 1962.

American Hospital Association: Patient bill of rights, Chicago, 1992, The Association.

American Medical Association, Council on Ethical and Judicial Affairs: Medical futility in end-of-life care: report of the Council on Ethical and Judicial Affairs: 1999, *JAMA* 281:937-941, 1999.

American Nurses Association: *Code of ethics with interpretive statements*, Washington, DC, 2001, The Association, retrieved May 4, 2005, from http://www.nursingworld.org/ethics/code/protected_nwcoe303.htm.

American Pain Society Task Force on Pain, Symptoms, and End of Life Care: Treatment of pain at the end of life. A position statement from the American Pain Society, no date, retrieved Nov 30, 2003, from http://www.ampainsoc.org/advocacy/treatment.htm.

Beauchamp TL, Childress JF: *Principles of biomedical ethics*, ed 5, New York, 2001, Oxford University Press.

Brett AS, Jersild P: "Inappropriate" treatment near the end of life: conflict between religious convictions and clinical judgment, *Arch Intern Med* 163:1645-1649, 2003.

Burns JP, Edwards J, Johnson J, et al: Do-not-resuscitate order after 25 years, *Crit Care Med* 31:1543-1550, 2003.

Cert denied, 429 US: 1992 In re Quinlan, 355 A 2d 647 (NJ 1976).

Clarke EB, Curtis JR, Luce JM, et al: Quality indicators for end-of-life care in the intensive care unit, *Crit Care Med* 31:2255-2262, 2003.

Curtin L: The ethics of staffing—part 1, *J Clin Syst Manage* 4:6-7, back cover, 2002a.

Curtin L: The ethics of staffing—part 2, *J Clin Syst Manage* 4:13, 18, 2002b.

Curtis JR, Burt RA: Why are critical care clinicians so powerfully distressed by family demands for futile care? *J Crit Care* 18:22-24, 2003.

DePalo V, Iacobucci R, Crausman RS: Do-not-resuscitate and stratification-of-care forms in Rhode Island, *Am J Crit Care* 12:239-241, 2003.

Duff R, Campbell AGM: Ethical dilemmas in the special care nursery, *N Engl J Med* 289:890-894, 1973.

DuVal G, Sartorius L, Clarridge B, et al: What triggers requests for ethics consultations? *West J Med* 175:24, 2001.

Heyland DK, Tranmer J, O'Callaghan CJ, et al: The seriously ill hospitalized patient: preferred role in end-of-life decision-making, *J Crit Care* 18:3-10, 2003.

Jonsen AR: *The birth of bioethics,* New York, 1998, Oxford University Press.

Khalafi K, Ravakhah K, West BC: Avoiding the futility of resuscitation, *Resuscitation* 50:161-166, 2001.

Levine C, Zuckerman C: The trouble with families: toward an ethic of accommodation, *Ann Intern Med* 130:148-152, 1999.

Lofmark R, Nilstun T: Conditions and consequences of medical futility—from a literature review to a clinical model, *J Med Ethics* 28:115-119, 2002.

Lynn J, Harrold J, Center to Improve the Care of the Dying, George Washington University: *Handbook for mortals,* New York, 1999, Oxford University Press.

MacLean SL, Guzzetta CE, White C, et al: Family presence during cardiopulmonary resuscitation and invasive procedures: practices of critical care and emergency nurses, *Am J Crit Care* 12:246-257, 2003.

McGaffic C: Family care giving: the Synergy Model as a foundation of ethical practice, *AACN News* 18(10), 2001, retrieved May 4, 2005, from http://www.aacn.org/ aacn/aacnsite.nsf/htmlmedia/aacn_news. html.

Reigle J: The ethics of physical restraints in critical care, *AACN Clin Issues* 7:585-591, 1996.

Rivera S, Kim D, Morgenstern L, et al: Motivating factors in futile clinical intervention, *Chest* 119:1944-1947, 2001.

Scanlon C: Ethical concerns in end-of-life care: when questions about advance directives and the withdrawal of life-sustaining interventions arise, how should decisions be made? *Am J Nurs* 103:48-55, 2003.

Schneiderman LJ, Gilmer T, Teetzel HD: Impact of ethics consultations in the intensive care setting: a randomized controlled trial, *Crit Care Med* 28:3920-3924, 2000.

Schneiderman LJ, Gilmer T, Teetzel HD, et al: Effects of ethics consultations on nonbeneficial life-sustaining treatments in the intensive care setting: a randomized controlled trial, *JAMA* 290:1166-1172, 2003.

Singer PA, Pellegrino ED, Siegler M: Clinical ethics revisited, *BMC Med Ethics* 2:1, 2001, retrieved May 4, 2005, from http://biomedcentral.com/1472-6939/2/1.

Society for Health and Human Values–Society for Bioethics Consultation Task Force on Standards for Bioethics Consultation: *Core competencies for health care ethics consultation,* Glenview, IL, 1998, American Society for Bioethics and Humanities.

Spencer EM, Mills A, Rorty MV, et al: *Organization ethics for healthcare organizations,* New York, 1999, Oxford University Press.

Stanton K: Nursing management of end-of-life issues: ethical and decision-making principles, *AACN News* 20(4):12-13, 15, 2003.

2 The Pulmonary System

KATHLEEN ELLSTROM, RN, PhD, APRN, BC

SYSTEMWIDE ELEMENTS

Physiologic Anatomy

1. **Respiratory circuit**
   a. The pulmonary system exists for the purpose of gas exchange. Oxygen (O_2) and carbon dioxide (CO_2) are exchanged between the atmosphere and the alveoli, between the alveoli and pulmonary capillary blood, and between the systemic capillary blood and all body cells.
   b. Atmospheric O_2 is consumed by the body through cellular aerobic metabolism, which supplies the energy for life
   c. CO_2, a by-product of aerobic metabolism, is eliminated primarily through lung ventilation
   d. The respiratory circuit includes all structures and processes involved in the transfer of O_2 between room air and the individual cell, and the transfer of CO_2 between the cell and room air
   e. Cellular respiration cannot be directly measured but is estimated by the amount of CO_2 produced ($\dot{V}\mathrm{CO_2}$) and the amount of O_2 consumed ($\dot{V}\mathrm{O_2}$). Ratio of these two values is called the *respiratory quotient*. Respiratory quotient is normally about 0.8 but changes according to the nutritional substrate being burned (i.e., protein, fats, or carbohydrates). Patients fully maintained on intravenous (IV) glucose alone will have a respiratory quotient approaching 1.0 as a result of the metabolic end product, CO_2.
   f. Exchange of O_2 and CO_2 at the alveolar-capillary level (external respiration) is called the *respiratory exchange ratio* (R). This is the ratio of the CO_2 produced to the O_2 taken up per minute. In homeostasis, the respiratory exchange ratio is the same as the respiratory quotient, 0.8.
   g. Proper functioning of the respiratory circuit requires efficient interaction of the respiratory, circulatory, and neuromuscular systems
   h. In addition to its primary function of O_2 and CO_2 exchange, the lung also carries out metabolic and endocrine functions as a source of hormones and a site of hormone metabolism. In addition, the lung is a target of hormonal actions by other endocrine organs.

2. **Steps in the gas exchange process**
   a. *Step 1—Ventilation:* Volume change, or the process of moving air between the atmosphere and the alveoli and distributing air within the lungs to maintain appropriate concentrations of O_2 and CO_2 in the alveoli
      i. Structural components involved in ventilation
         (a) Lung
            (1) Anatomic divisions: Right lung (three lobes—upper, middle, lower); left lung (two lobes—upper, lower). Lobes are divided into bronchopulmonary segments (ten right, nine left). Bronchopulmonary segments are subdivided into secondary lobules.
            (2) Lobule: Smallest gross anatomic units of lung tissue; contain the primary functional units of the lung (terminal bronchioles, alveolar ducts and sacs, pulmonary circulation). Lymphatics surround the lobule, keep the lung free of excess fluid, and remove inhaled particles from distal areas of the lung.
            (3) Bronchial artery circulation: Systemic source of circulation for the tracheobronchial tree and lung tissue down to the level of the terminal bronchiole. Alveoli receive their blood supply from the pulmonary circulation.
         (b) Conducting airways: Entire area from the nose to the terminal bronchioles where gas flows, but is not exchanged, is called *anatomic dead space* (VD_{anat}). Amount is approximately 150 ml but varies with patient size and position. Airways are a series of rapidly branching tubes of ever-diminishing diameter that eventually terminate in the alveoli.
            (1) Nose
               a) Serves as a passageway for air movement into the lungs
               b) Preconditions air by the action of the cilia, mucosal cells, and turbinate bones
                  1) Warms air to within 2° to 3° of body temperature; humidifies it to full saturation before it reaches the lower trachea
                  2) Filters by trapping particles larger than 6 μm in diameter
               c) Has voice resonance, olfaction, sneeze reflex functions
            (2) Pharynx: Posterior to nasal cavities and mouth
               a) Separation of food from air is controlled by local nerve reflexes
               b) Opening of eustachian tube regulates middle ear pressure
               c) Lymphatic tissues control infection
            (3) Larynx: Complex structure consisting of incomplete rings of cartilage and numerous muscles and ligaments
               a) Vocal cords: Speech function
                  1) Narrowest part of the conducting airways in adults
                  2) Contraction of muscles of the larynx causes the vocal cords to change shape
                  3) Vibration of the vocal cords produces sound. Speech is a joint function of the vocal cords, lips, tongue, soft palate, and respiration, with control by temporal and parietal lobes of the cerebral cortex.
                  4) Rima glottis: Opening between the vocal cords
               b) Valve action by the epiglottis helps to prevent aspiration
               c) Cough reflex: Cords close and intrathoracic pressure increases to permit coughing or Valsalva maneuver
               d) Cricoid cartilage
                  1) Only complete rigid ring
                  2) Narrowest part of the child's airway

3) Inner diameter sets the limit for the size of an endotracheal tube passed through the larynx
(4) Trachea: Tubular structure consisting of 16 to 20 incomplete, or C-shaped, cartilaginous rings that stabilize the airway and prevent complete collapse with coughing
   a) Begins the conducting system, or tracheobronchial tree
   b) Warms and humidifies air
   c) Mucosal cells trap foreign material
   d) Cilia propel mucus upward through the airway
   e) Cough reflex present, especially at the point of tracheal bifurcation (carina)
   f) Smooth muscle innervated by the parasympathetic branch of the autonomic nervous system
(5) Major bronchi and bronchioles
(6) Terminal bronchioles
   a) Smooth muscle walls (no cartilage); bronchospasm may narrow the lumen and increase airway resistance
   b) Ciliated mucosal cells become flattened, with progressive loss of cilia toward the alveoli
   c) Sensitive to CO_2 levels: Increased levels induce bronchiolar dilation, decreased levels induce constriction
(c) Gas exchange airways: Semipermeable membrane permits the movement of gases according to pressure gradients. These airways are not major contributors to airflow resistance but do contribute to the distensibility of the lung. The *acinus* (terminal respiratory unit) is composed of the respiratory bronchiole and its subdivisions (Figure 2-1).

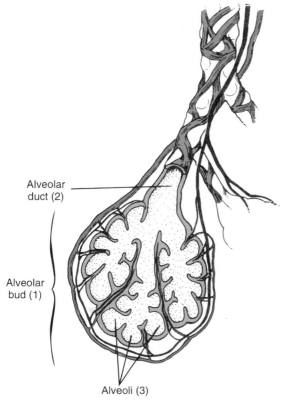

Alveolar duct (2)

Alveolar bud (1)

Alveoli (3)

FIGURE 2-1 ■ Components of the acinus. (From Eubanks DH, Bone RC: *Comprehensive respiratory care: a learning system*, ed 2, St Louis, 1990, Mosby, p 168.)

(1) Respiratory bronchioles and alveolar ducts
   a) Terminal branching of airways
   b) Distribution of inspired air
   c) Smooth muscle layer diminishes

(2) Alveoli and alveolar bud
   a) Most important structures in gas exchange
   b) Alveolar surface area is large and depends on body size. Total surface area is about 70 m^2 in a normal adult. Thickness of the respiratory membrane is about 0.6 μm. This fulfills the need to distribute a large quantity of perfused blood into a very thin film to ensure near equalization of O_2 and CO_2.
   c) Alveolar cells
     1) Type I: Squamous epithelium, adapted for gas exchange, sensitive to injury by inhaled agents, structured to prevent fluid transudation into the alveoli
     2) Type II: Large secretory, highly active metabolically; origin of surfactant synthesis and type I cell genesis
     3) Alveolar macrophages: Phagocytize foreign materials
   d) Pulmonary surfactant
     1) Phospholipid monolayer at the alveolar air-liquid interface; able to vary surface tension with alveolar volume
     2) Enables surface tension to decrease as alveolar volume decreases during expiration, which prevents alveolar collapse
     3) Decreases the work of breathing, permits the alveoli to remain inflated at low distending pressures, reduces net forces causing tissue fluid accumulation
     4) Reduction of surfactant makes lung expansion more difficult; the greater the surface tension, the greater the pressure needed to overcome it
     5) Surfactant also detoxifies inhaled gases and traps inhaled and deposited particles
   e) Alveolar-capillary membrane (alveolar epithelium, interstitial space, capillary endothelium)
     1) Bathed by interstitial fluid; lines the respiratory bronchioles, alveolar ducts, and alveolar sacs; forms the walls of the alveoli
     2) About 1 μm or less thick (less than one red blood cell); permits rapid diffusion of gases; any increase in thickness diminishes gas diffusion
     3) Total surface area of about 70 m^2 in an adult is in contact with about 60 to 140 ml of pulmonary capillary blood at any one time
   f) Gas exchange pathway (Figure 2-2): Alveolar epithelium → alveolar basement membrane → interstitial space → capillary basement membrane → capillary endothelium → plasma → erythrocyte membrane → erythrocyte cytoplasm

ii. Alveolar ventilation ($\dot{V}_A$): That part of total ventilation taking part in gas exchange and, therefore, the only part useful to the body
  (a) Alveolar ventilation is one component of minute ventilation
    (1) Minute ventilation ($\dot{V}_E$): Amount of air exchanged in 1 minute. Equal to exhaled tidal volume (V_T) multiplied by respiratory rate (RR or f). Normal resting minute ventilation in an adult is about 6 L/min:

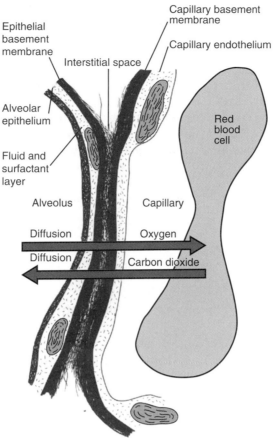

FIGURE 2-2 ■ Ultrastructure of the respiratory membrane. (From Guyton AC, Hall JE: *Textbook of medical physiology*, ed 9, Philadelphia, 1996, Saunders, p 508.)

$$V_T \times RR = \dot{V}_E \ (500 \text{ ml} \times 12 = 6000 \text{ ml})$$

Tidal volume is easily measured at the bedside by hand-held devices or a mechanical ventilator. Exhaled minute ventilation is a routinely measured parameter for patients on ventilators.

(2) Minute ventilation is composed of both alveolar ventilation ($\dot{V}_A$) and physiologic dead space ventilation ($\dot{V}_D$):

$$\dot{V}_E = \dot{V}_D + \dot{V}_A$$

where $\dot{V}$ = volume of gas per unit of time

Physiologic dead space ventilation is that volume of gas in the airways that does not participate in gas exchange. It is composed of both anatomic dead space ventilation ($\dot{V}D_{anat}$) and alveolar dead space ventilation ($\dot{V}D_A$).

(3) Ratio of dead space to tidal volume (V_D/V_T) is measured to determine how much of each breath is wasted (i.e., does not contribute to gas exchange). Normal values for spontaneously breathing patients range from 0.2 to 0.4 (20% to 40%).

(b) Alveolar ventilation cannot be measured directly; it is inversely related to arterial CO_2 pressure (Pa_{CO_2}) in a steady state by the following formula:

$$\dot{V}_A = \frac{\dot{V}_{CO_2} \times 0.863}{Pa_{CO_2}}$$

where 0.863 = correction factor for differences in measurement units and conversion to STPD (standard temperature [0° C] and pressure [760 torr], dry)

(c) Since $\dot{V}_{CO_2}$ remains the same in a steady state, measurement of the patient's Pa_{CO_2} reveals the status of the alveolar ventilation

(d) Pa_{CO_2} is the only adequate indicator of effective matching of alveolar ventilation to metabolic demand. To assess ventilation, Pa_{CO_2} must be measured.

(e) If Pa_{CO_2} is low, alveolar ventilation is high; hyperventilation is present

$$\downarrow Pa_{CO_2} = \uparrow \dot{V}_A$$

(f) If Pa_{CO_2} is within normal limits, alveolar ventilation is adequate

$$Normal\ Pa_{CO_2} = normal\ \dot{V}_A$$

(g) If Pa_{CO_2} is high, alveolar ventilation is low and hypoventilation is present

$$\uparrow Pa_{CO_2} = \downarrow \dot{V}_A$$

iii. Defense mechanisms of the lung
  (a) Although an internal organ, the lung is unique in that it has continuous contact with particulate and gaseous materials inhaled from the external environment. In the healthy lung, defense mechanisms successfully defend against these natural materials by the following means:
    (1) Structural architecture of the upper respiratory tract, which reduces deposited and inhaled materials
    (2) Processing system, including respiratory tract fluid alteration and phagocytic activity
    (3) Transport system, which removes material from the lung
    (4) Humoral and cell-mediated immune responses, which may be the most important bronchopulmonary defense mechanisms
  (b) Loss of normal defense mechanisms may be precipitated by disease, injury, surgery, insertion of an endotracheal tube, or smoking
  (c) Upper respiratory tract warms and humidifies inspired air, absorbs selected inhaled gases, and filters out particulate matter. Soluble gases and particles larger than 10 μm are aerodynamically filtered out. Normally, no bacteria are present below the larynx.
  (d) Inhaled and deposited particles reaching the alveoli are coated by surface fluids (surfactant and other lipoproteins) and are rapidly phagocytized by pulmonary alveolar macrophages
  (e) Macrophages and particles are transported in mucus by bronchial cilia, which beat toward the glottis and move materials in a mucus-fluid layer, eventually to be expectorated or swallowed. This process is referred to as the *mucociliary escalator*. Pulmonary lymphatics also drain and transport some cells and particles from the lung.
  (f) Antigens activate the humoral and cell-mediated immune systems, which add immunoglobulins to the surface fluid of the alveoli and activate alveolar macrophages

      (g) Disruption of or injury to these defense mechanisms predisposes to acute or chronic pulmonary disease

    iv. Lung mechanics

      (a) Muscles of respiration: Act of breathing is accomplished through muscular actions that alter intrapleural and pulmonary pressures and thus change intrapulmonary volumes

        (1) Muscles of inspiration: During inspiration, the chest cavity enlarges. This enlargement is an active process brought about by the contraction of the following:

          a) Diaphragm: Major inspiratory muscle

            1) Normal quiet breathing is accomplished almost entirely by this dome-shaped muscle, which divides the chest from the abdomen

            2) Divided into two "leaves"—the right and left hemidiaphragms

            3) Downward contraction increases the superior-inferior diameter of the chest and elevates the lower ribs

            4) Innervation is from the C3 to C5 level through the phrenic nerve

            5) Normally, accounts for 75% of tidal volume during quiet inspiration

            6) Facilitates vomiting, coughing and sneezing, defecation, and parturition

          b) External intercostal muscles

            1) Increase the anterior-posterior (A-P) diameter of the thorax by elevating the ribs

            2) A-P diameter is about 20% greater during inspiration than during expiration

            3) Innervation is from T1 to T11

          c) Accessory muscles in the neck: Scalene and sternocleidomastoid

            1) Lift upward on the sternum and ribs and increase A-P diameter

            2) Are not used in normal, quiet ventilation

        (2) Muscles of expiration: During expiration, the chest cavity decreases in size. This is a passive act unless forced, and the driving force is derived from lung recoil. Muscles used when increased levels of ventilation are needed are the following:

          a) Abdominals: Force abdominal contents upward to elevate the diaphragm

          b) Internal intercostals: Decrease A-P diameter by contracting and pulling the ribs inward

      (b) Pressures within the chest: Movement of air into the lungs requires a pressure difference between the airway opening and alveoli sufficient to overcome the resistance to airflow of the tracheobronchial tree (Table 2-1)

        (1) Air flows into the lungs when intrapulmonary air pressure falls below atmospheric pressure

        (2) Air flows out of the lungs when intrapulmonary air pressure exceeds atmospheric pressure

        (3) Intrapleural pressure is normally negative with respect to atmospheric pressure as a result of the elastic recoil of the lungs, which tend to pull away from the chest wall. This "negative" pressure prevents the collapse of the lungs.

        (4) Increased effort (forced inspiration or expiration) may produce much greater changes in intrapulmonary and intrapleural pressures during inspiration and expiration

■ **TABLE 2-1**
■ ■ **Example of Changes in Pressures Throughout the Ventilatory Cycle**

Pressure	At Rest (No Airflow) (mm Hg)	Inspiration (mm Hg)	Expiration (mm Hg)
Atmospheric (P_B)	760	760	760
Intrapulmonary or intraalveolar (P_{alv})	760	757	763
Intrapleural (P_{pl}) or intrathoracic	756	750	756

   (c) Structural components of the thorax
      (1) For protection: Sternum, spine, ribs
      (2) Pleura
         a) Visceral layer next to the lungs; parietal layer next to the chest wall
         b) Pleural fluid between layers: Allows smooth movement of the visceral layer over the parietal layer
         c) Adherence: Pleural space is normally a potential space (vacuum); because of a constant negative pressure (less than atmospheric pressure by 4 to 8 mm Hg), any change in the volume of the thoracic cage is reflected by a similar change in the volume of the lungs
         d) Nerve supply: Parietal pleura has fibers for pain transmission, but visceral pleura does not
   (d) Resistances
      (1) *Elastic resistance* (static properties)
         a) Lung, if removed from the chest, collapses to a smaller volume because of lung elastic recoil. This tendency of the lungs to collapse is normally counteracted by the chest wall tendency to expand. Volume of air in the lungs depends on the equal and opposite balance of these forces.
         b) Compliance (C_L) is an expression of the elastic properties of the lung and is the change in volume (ΔV) accomplished by a change in pressure (ΔP):

$$C_L = \frac{\Delta V}{\Delta P}$$

         If compliance is high, the lung is more easily distended; if compliance is low, the lung is stiff and more difficult to distend
      (2) *Flow resistance* (dynamic properties)
         a) Airway resistance must be overcome to generate flow through the airways
         b) Changes in airway caliber affect airway resistance. Examples are changes caused by bronchospasm or secretions.
         c) Flow through the airway depends on pressure differences between the two ends of the tube as well as resistance. Driving pressure for flow in airways is the difference between atmospheric and alveolar pressures.
   (e) Work of breathing
      (1) To minimize the work required to maintain a given level of ventilation, the body automatically changes the respiratory pattern
      (2) Work performed must be sufficient to overcome the elastic resistance and the flow resistance

(3) In diseased states, the workload increases

v. Control of ventilation: Although the process of breathing is a normal rhythmic activity that occurs without conscious effort, it involves an intricate controlling mechanism within the central nervous system (CNS). Basic organization of the respiratory control system is outlined in Figure 2-3.

(a) Respiratory generator: Located in the medulla and composed of two groups of neurons

(1) One group initiates respiration and regulates its rate

(2) One group controls the "switching off" of inspiration and thus the onset of expiration

(b) Input from other regions of the CNS

(1) Pons: Input is necessary for normal, coordinated breathing

(2) Cerebral cortex: Exerts a conscious or voluntary control over ventilation

(c) Chemoreceptors: Contribute to a feedback loop that adjusts respiratory center output if blood gas levels are not maintained within the normal range

(1) Central chemoreceptors: Located near the ventrolateral surface of the medulla (but are separate from the medullary respiratory center)

a) Respond not directly to blood partial pressure of carbon dioxide (P_{CO_2}) but, rather, to the pH of the extracellular fluid (ECF) surrounding the chemoreceptor

b) Feedback loop for CO_2 can be summarized as follows: Increased arterial P_{CO_2} → increased brain ECF P_{CO_2} → decreased brain ECF pH → decreased pH at chemoreceptor → stimulation of central chemoreceptor → stimulation of medullary respiratory center → increased ventilation → decreased arterial P_{CO_2}

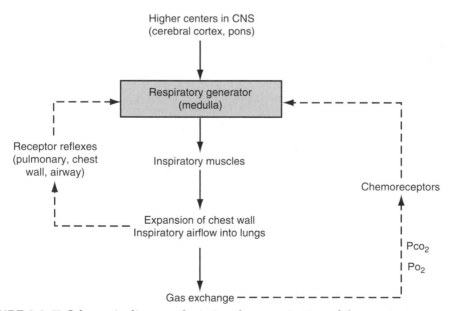

FIGURE 2-3 ■ Schematic diagram depicting the organization of the respiratory control system. The dashed lines show feedback loops affecting the respiratory generator. P_{CO_2}, Partial pressure of carbon dioxide; P_{O_2}, partial pressure of oxygen. (From Weinberger SE: *Principles of pulmonary medicine*, ed 2, Philadelphia, 1992, Saunders, p 206.)

        (2) Peripheral chemoreceptors: Located in the carotid body and aortic body
           a) Sensitive to changes in the partial pressure of oxygen (PO_2),with hypoxemia stimulating chemoreceptor discharge
           b) Minor role in sensing PCO_2

    (d) Other receptors
        (1) Stretch receptors in the bronchial wall respond to changes in lung inflation (Hering-Breuer reflex)
           a) As the lung inflates, receptor discharge increases
           b) Contribute to the start of expiration
        (2) Irritant receptors in the lining of the airways respond to noxious stimuli, such as irritating dust and chemicals
        (3) "J" (juxtacapillary) receptors in the alveolar interstitial space
           a) Cause rapid shallow breathing in response to deformation from increased interstitial volume due to high pulmonary capillary pressures (such as in heart failure or inflammation)
           b) Stimulation can also cause bradycardia, hypotension, and expiratory constriction of the glottis
        (4) Receptors in the chest wall (in the intercostal muscles)
           a) Involved in the fine tuning of ventilation
           b) Adjust the output of the respiratory muscles for the degree of muscular work required

b. *Step 2—Diffusion:* Process by which alveolar air gases are moved across the alveolar-capillary membrane to the pulmonary capillary bed and vice versa. Diffusion occurs down a concentration gradient from a higher to a lower concentration. No active metabolic work is required for the diffusion of gases to occur. Work of breathing is accomplished by the respiratory muscles and the heart, which produce a gradient across the alveolar-capillary membrane.

    i. Ability of the lung to transfer gases is called the *diffusing capacity* of the lung (D_L). Diffusing capacity measures the amount of gas (O_2, CO_2, carbon monoxide) diffusing between the alveoli and pulmonary capillary blood per minute per millimeter Hg mean gas pressure difference.

    ii. CO_2 is 20 times more diffusible across the alveolar-capillary membrane than O_2. If the membrane is damaged, its decreased capacity for transporting O_2 into the blood is usually more of a problem than its decreased capacity for transporting CO_2 out of the body. Thus, the diffusing capacity of the lungs for O_2 is of primary importance.

    iii. Diffusion is determined by several variables:
        (a) Surface area available for gas exchange
        (b) Integrity of the alveolar-capillary membrane
        (c) Amount of hemoglobin (Hb) in the blood
        (d) Diffusion coefficient of gas as well as contact time
        (e) Driving pressure: Difference between alveolar gas tensions and pulmonary capillary gas tensions (Table 2-2). This is the force that causes gases to diffuse across membranes.
           (1) During the breathing of 100% O_2, the alveolar O_2 tension (PAO_2) becomes so large that the difference between PAO_2 and $P\bar{v}O_2$ (mixed venous O_2 tension) significantly increases, proportionately increasing the driving pressure
           (2) Therefore, hypoxemia due solely to diffusion defects is usually improved by breathing 100% O_2

■ **TABLE 2-2**
■ ■ **Driving Pressures**

Alveolar Gas	Alveolar-Capillary Membranes	Pulmonary Capillaries
PA_{O_2} 104 mm Hg	Diffusion →	$P\bar{v}_{O_2}$ 40 mm Hg
Pa_{CO_2} 40 mm Hg	Diffusion →	$P\bar{v}_{CO_2}$ 45 mm Hg

Pa_{CO_2}, Arterial partial pressure of carbon dioxide; *PA_{O_2}*, alveolar partial pressure of oxygen; *$P\bar{v}_{CO_2}$*, mixed venous partial pressure of carbon dioxide; *$P\bar{v}_{O_2}$*, mixed venous partial pressure of oxygen.

    iv. A–a gradient ($PA_{O_2} - Pa_{O_2}$) is the alveolar to arterial O_2 pressure difference (i.e., the difference in the partial pressure of O_2 in the alveolar gas spaces [PA_{O_2}] and the pressure in the systemic arterial blood [Pa_{O_2}]). This gradient is always a positive number.

      (a) Normal gradient in young adults is less than 10 mm Hg (on room air) but increases with age and may be as high as 20 mm Hg in people over age 60 years

      (b) A–a gradient provides an index of how efficient the lung is in equilibrating pulmonary capillary O_2 with alveolar O_2. It indicates whether gas transfer is normal.

      (c) Large A–a gradient generally indicates that the lung is the site of dysfunction (except with cardiac right-to-left shunting)

      (d) Formula for calculation (on room air)

$$\text{A–a gradient} = PA_{O_2} - Pa_{O_2}$$

$$PA_{O_2} = PI_{O_2} - (Pa_{CO_2} \div 0.8)$$

$$PI_{O_2} = (P_B - 47) \times FI_{O_2}$$

where
47 = vapor pressure of water at 37° C (in mm Hg)
PI_{O_2} = pressure of inspired O_2
0.8 = assumed respiratory quotient (ratio of CO_2 produced to O_2 consumed per unit time)
P_B = barometric pressure (sea level normal P_B is 760 mm Hg)
FI_{O_2} = fraction (percent) of inspired O_2
Therefore,

$$FI_{O_2} (P_B - 47) - (Pa_{CO_2} \div 0.8) - Pa_{O_2} = \text{A–a gradient}$$

Example of calculation:

$$0.21 (760 - 47) - (40 \div 0.8) - 90 = 10$$

      (e) Normally, A–a gradient increases with age and increased FI_{O_2}

      (f) Pathologic conditions that increase the A–a gradient (difference) include the following:

        (1) Mismatching of ventilation ($\dot{V}$) to perfusion ($\dot{Q}$) ($\dot{V}/\dot{Q}$ abnormalities)

        (2) Shunting

        (3) Diffusion abnormalities

  c. *Step 3—Transport of gases in the circulation*

    i. Approximately 97% of O_2 is transported in chemical combination with Hb in the erythrocyte and 3% is carried dissolved in the plasma. Pa_{O_2} is a measurement of the O_2 tension in the plasma and is a reflection of the driving pressure that causes O_2 to dissolve in the plasma and combine with Hb. Thus, O_2 content is related to PaO_2.

  ii. Oxyhemoglobin dissociation curve (Figure 2-4)

    (a) Relationship between O_2 saturation (and content) and PaO_2 is expressed in an S-shaped curve that has great physiologic significance. It describes the ability of Hb to bind O_2 at normal PaO_2 levels and release it at lower PO_2 levels.

    (b) Relationship between the content and pressure of O_2 in the blood is not linear

      (1) Upper flat portion of the curve is the arterial association portion. Dissociation relationship in this range protects the body by enabling Hb to retain high saturation with O_2 despite large decreases (down to 60 mm Hg) in PaO_2.

      (2) Lower steep portion of the curve is the venous dissociation portion. Dissociation relationship in this range protects the body by enabling the tissues to withdraw large amounts of O_2 with small decreases in PaO_2.

    (c) Hb O_2 binding is sensitive to O_2 tension. The binding is reversible; the affinity of Hb for O_2 changes as PO_2 changes.

      (1) When PO_2 is increased (as in pulmonary capillaries), O_2 binds readily with Hb

      (2) When PO_2 is decreased (as in tissues), O_2 unloads from Hb

    (d) Increase in the rate of O_2 utilization by tissues causes an automatic increase in the rate of O_2 release from Hb

    (e) Shifts of the oxyhemoglobin curve

      (1) Shifts to the right: More O_2 is unloaded for a given PO_2, which thus increases O_2 delivery to the tissues. These shifts are caused by the following:

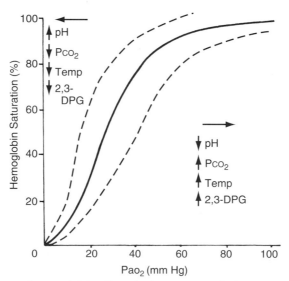

FIGURE 2-4 ■ The oxyhemoglobin dissociation curve, relating percent hemoglobin saturation and arterial partial pressure of oxygen (PaO_2). The normal curve is depicted by the solid line; the curves shifted to the right or left (along with the conditions leading to them), by the dashed lines. *2,3-DPG,* 2,3-Diphosphoglycerate; *PCO_2,* partial pressure of carbon dioxide; *Temp,* temperature. (From Weinberger SE: *Principles of pulmonary medicine,* ed 2, Philadelphia, 1992, Saunders, p 10.)

      a) pH decrease (acidosis), the Bohr effect
      b) P_{CO_2} increase
      c) Increase in body temperature
      d) Increased levels of 2,3-diphosphoglycerate (2,3-DPG)

  (2) Shifts to the left: O_2 is not dissociated from Hb until tissue and capillary O_2 are very low, which thus decreases O_2 delivery to the tissues. These shifts are caused by the following:
      a) pH increase (alkalosis), the Bohr effect
      b) P_{CO_2} decrease
      c) Temperature decrease
      d) Decreased levels of 2,3-DPG
      e) Carbon monoxide poisoning

  (3) 2,3-DPG is an intermediate metabolite of glucose that facilitates the dissociation of O_2 from Hb at the tissues. Decreased levels of 2,3-DPG impair O_2 release to the tissues. This may occur with massive transfusions of 2,3-DPG–depleted blood and anything that decreases phosphate levels.

iii. Ability of Hb to release O_2 to the tissues is commonly assessed by evaluating the P_{50}
  (a) P_{50} = the partial pressure of O_2 at which the Hb is 50% saturated, standardized to a pH of 7.40
  (b) Normal P_{50} is about 26.6 mm Hg; varies with the disease process

iv. Each gram of normal Hb can maximally combine with 1.34 ml of O_2 when fully saturated (values of 1.36 or 1.39 are sometimes used)

v. Amount of O_2 transported per minute in the circulation is a factor of both the arterial O_2 concentration (CaO_2) and cardiac output. This amount reflects how much O_2 is delivered to tissues per minute and is dependent on the interaction of the circulatory system (delivery of arterial blood), erythropoietic system (Hb in red blood cells), and respiratory system (gas exchange) according to the following equations:
  (a) O_2 content (CaO_2) is calculated from O_2 saturation, O_2 capacity, and dissolved O_2
    (1) O_2 capacity is the maximal amount of O_2 the blood can carry. It is expressed in milliliters of O_2 per deciliter (100 ml) of blood (ml/dl) and is calculated by multiplying Hb in grams by 1.34.
    (2) O_2 saturation is the percentage of Hb actually saturated with O_2 (SaO_2 or $S\bar{v}O_2$) and is usually measured directly. It is equal to the O_2 content divided by the O_2 capacity multiplied by 100.
    (3) O_2 content is the actual amount of O_2 the blood is carrying (oxyhemoglobin plus dissolved O_2)

$$O_2 \text{ content} = (O_2 \text{ capacity} \times O_2 \text{ saturation}) + (0.0031 \times PaO_2)$$

  (b) Systemic O_2 transport

$$\text{ml/min} = \text{arterial } O_2 \text{ content (ml/dl)} \times \text{cardiac output (L/min)} \times 10 \text{ (conversion factor)}$$

    (1) Normal cardiac output = approximately 5 to 6 L/min (range, 4 to 8 L/min)
    (2) Normal arterial O_2 content = approximately 20 ml/dl
    (3) Therefore, systemic O_2 transport averages about 1000 to 1200 ml/min

vi. Focusing only on the O_2 tension of the blood is unwise because an underestimation of the severity of hypoxemia may result. O_2 content and transport are more reliable parameters because they take into account the Hb concentration and cardiac output.

vii. Arterial–mixed venous differences in O_2 content ($CaO_2 - C\bar{v}O_2$) is the difference between arterial O_2 content (CaO_2) and mixed venous O_2 content ($C\bar{v}O_2$) and reflects the actual amount of O_2 extracted from the blood during its passage through the tissues

  (a) Of the 1000 to 1200 ml of O_2 delivered per minute to tissues, cells typically use only about 250 to 300 ml ($\dot{V}O_2$ or O_2 consumption). If $\dot{V}O_2$ remains constant, changes in cardiac output can be related to changes in the $CaO_2 - C\bar{v}O_2$ gradient or difference. Mixed venous O_2 values are measured from the distal tip of pulmonary artery catheters.

  (b) Normal $CaO_2 - C\bar{v}O_2$ is 4.5 to 6 ml/dl

$$(Hb \times 1.34)\ (SaO_2 - S\bar{v}O_2) + (PaO_2 - P\bar{v}O_2)\ (0.0031)$$

  (c) Fall in $C\bar{v}O_2$ resulting in a rise in the $CaO_2 - C\bar{v}O_2$ gradient signifies decreased cardiac output and inadequate tissue perfusion if $\dot{V}O_2$ is constant

  (d) These are average values; actual O_2 utilization is different for different tissues. The heart uses almost all the O_2 it receives.

viii. CO_2 transport: CO_2 is carried in the blood in three forms, as follows:

  (a) Physically dissolved ($PaCO_2$), which accounts for 7% to 10% of CO_2 transported in the blood

  (b) Chemically combined with Hb as carbaminohemoglobin. This reaction occurs rapidly, and reduced Hb can bind more CO_2 than oxyhemoglobin. Thus, unloading of O_2 facilitates loading of CO_2 *(Haldane effect)* and accounts for about 30% of CO_2 transport.

  (c) As bicarbonate (HCO_3^-) through a conversion reaction:

$$CO_2 + H_2O \xrightleftharpoons{CA} H_2CO_3 \rightleftharpoons H^+ + (Hb\ buffer) + HCO_3^-$$

  where CA = carbonic anhydrase

  (1) Reaction accounts for 60% to 70% of CO_2 in the body

  (2) Reaction is slow in plasma and fast in red blood cell owing to the CA enzyme

  (3) When the concentration of these ions increases in red blood cells, HCO_3^- diffuses but H^+ remains

  (4) To maintain electrical neutrality, chloride diffuses from the plasma (the "chloride shift")

ix. Pulmonary circulation (pulmonary artery, arterioles, capillary network, venules, and veins)

  (a) Pulmonary vessels are peculiarly suited to maintaining a delicate balance of flow and pressure distribution that optimizes gas exchange. They are richly innervated by the sympathetic branch of the autonomic nervous system.

  (b) In contrast to the systemic circulation, the pulmonary circulation is a low-resistance system. Pulmonary arteries have far thinner walls than systemic arteries do, and vessels distend to allow for increases in volume from systemic circulation. Intrapulmonary blood volume increases or decreases of approximately 50% occur with changes in the relationship between intrathoracic and extrathoracic pressure.

(c) Pulmonary arteries accompany the bronchi within the lung and give rise to a rich capillary network within the alveolar walls. Pulmonary veins are not contiguous with the bronchial tree.

(d) Primary function of the pulmonary circulation is to act as a transport system

(1) Transport of blood through the lung

a) Flow resistance through vessels (R) is defined by *Ohm's law:*

$$R = \frac{\Delta P}{F}$$

where

ΔP = the pressure difference between the two ends of the vessel (upstream and downstream pressures)

F = flow

Driving pressure for flow in the pulmonary circulation is the difference between the inflow pressure in the pulmonary artery and the outflow pressure in the left atrium

b) In the lung, measurement of flow resistance is pulmonary vascular resistance (PVR)

PVR = [mean pulmonary artery pressure
   − mean left atrial (or pulmonary wedge) pressure]
   ÷ cardiac output

c) About 12% of the total blood volume of the body is in the pulmonary circulation at any given time

d) Normal pressures in the pulmonary vasculature

1) Mean pulmonary artery pressure: 10 to 15 mm Hg

2) Mean pulmonary venous pressure: 4 to 12 mm Hg

3) Mean pressure gradient: Approximately 10 mm Hg (considerably less than the systemic gradient)

4) Pressures are higher at the base of the lung than at the apex

5) Perfusion is better in the dependent areas of the lung

e) Unique characteristic of the pulmonary arterial bed is that it constricts in response to hypoxia. Diffuse alveolar hypoxia causes generalized vasoconstriction, which results in pulmonary hypertension. Localized hypoxia causes localized vasoconstriction that does not increase pulmonary hypertension. This localized vasoconstriction directs blood away from poorly ventilated alveoli and thus improves overall gas exchange.

f) Chronic pulmonary hypertension (increased PVR) can result in right ventricular hypertrophy (cor pulmonale)

1) Transvascular transport of fluids and solutes

a) Transvascular fluid filtration in the lung (and all other organs) is described by the Starling equation. This means that fluid and solutes move due to increases or decreases in hydrostatic or osmotic filtration pressures or due to changes in the permeability of vessel walls to fluids or proteins.

b) Thus, excess fluid in the lung (pulmonary edema) can result from either a net increase in hydrostatic pressure forces (favoring filtration) or a decreased resistance to filtration

2) Metabolic transport

    a) All cardiac output passes through the lung before reaching systemic circulation. Therefore, pulmonary circulation can influence the composition of the blood supplying all organs.

    b) Several humoral substances are added, extracted, or metabolized in the lung. Examples are inactivation of vasoactive prostaglandins, conversion of angiotensin I to angiotensin II, and inactivation of bradykinin.

d. *Step 4—Diffusion between the systemic capillary bed and body tissue cells*

    i. Pressure gradients allow for the diffusion of O_2 and CO_2 among systemic capillaries, interstitial fluid, and cells (Figures 2-5 and 2-6)

    ii. Within the mitochondria of each individual cell, O_2 is consumed through aerobic metabolism. This process produces the energy bonds of adenosine triphosphate and the waste products of CO_2 and water.

3. Hypoxemia: Hypoxemia is a state in which the O_2 pressure or saturation of O_2 in arterial blood, or both, is lower than normal. *Hypoxemia* is generally defined as PaO_2 less than 55 mm Hg or SaO_2 below 88% at sea level in an adult breathing room air. Disorders that lead to hypoxemia do so through one or more of the following processes.

    a. Low inspired O_2 tension

        i. Reduced ambient pressure (P_B) or reduced O_2 concentration of inspired air (FIO_2)

        ii. If the lungs are normal, the A–a gradient will be normal

        iii. Rarely a clinically important cause of arterial hypoxemia. Reduced P_B occurs at high altitudes in healthy humans and in enclosed spaces such as mine cave-ins where fresh air is not replenished; FIO_2 remains normal, however.

    b. Alveolar hypoventilation (increased $PaCO_2$)

        i. Decrease in alveolar ventilation from disorders of the respiratory center, peripheral nerves that supply the muscles of respiration, the respiratory muscles of the chest wall, or the lungs; medications that diminish ventilation

        ii. This causes an increase in $PaCO_2$, which results in a fall in PAO_2 according to the alveolar air equation

        iii. If the lungs are normal, the A–a gradient will be normal. Hypoxemia will improve with ventilation.

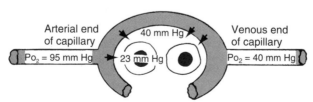

FIGURE 2-5 ▪ Diffusion of oxygen from a tissue capillary to the cells. *PO_2*, Partial pressure of oxygen. (From Guyton AC, Hall JE: *Textbook of medical physiology*, ed 9, Philadelphia, 1996, Saunders, p 514.)

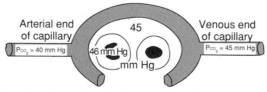

FIGURE 2-6 ▪ Uptake of carbon dioxide by the blood in the capillaries. (Guyton AC, Hall JE: *Textbook of medical physiology*, ed 9, Philadelphia, 1996, Saunders, p 515.)

c. $\dot{V}/\dot{Q}$ mismatch

   i. Most common cause of hypoxemia; A–a gradient increased

   ii. Ideally, ventilation of each alveolus is accompanied by a comparable amount of perfusion, which yields a $\dot{V}/\dot{Q}$ ratio of 1.00. Usually, however, there is relatively more perfusion than ventilation, which yields a normal $\dot{V}/\dot{Q}$ ratio of 0.8. Normal amount of blood perfusing the alveoli ($\dot{Q}$) is 5 L/min, and normal amount of air ventilating the alveoli ($\dot{V}$) is 4 L/min. Figure 2-7 presents in simplified form the possible relationships between ventilation and perfusion in the lung.

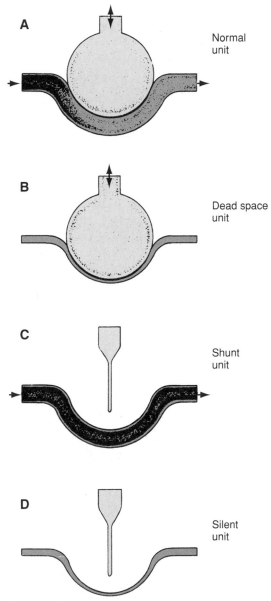

FIGURE 2-7 ■ The theoretical respiratory unit. **A,** Normal ventilation, normal perfusion. **B,** Normal ventilation, no perfusion. **C,** No ventilation, normal perfusion. **D,** No ventilation, no perfusion. (From Shapiro BA, Peruzzi WT, Templin R, et al: *Clinical application of blood gases,* ed 5, St Louis, 1994, Mosby, p 22.)

iii. When $\dot{V}/\dot{Q}$ is decreased (<0.8), a decrease of ventilation in relation to perfusion has occurred. This is similar to a right-to-left shunt because more deoxygenated blood is returning to the left side of the heart. Low $\dot{V}/\dot{Q}$ ratios and hypoxemia occur together, because good areas of the lung cannot be overventilated to compensate for the underventilated areas. (Hb cannot be saturated to more than 100%.) Atelectasis, pneumonia, and pulmonary edema are clinical examples of intrapulmonary shunt.

iv. When $\dot{V}/\dot{Q}$ is increased (>0.8), a decreased perfusion relative to ventilation exists, the equivalent of dead space or wasted ventilation. Examples of cases in which this occurs are pulmonary emboli and cardiogenic shock.

v. Hypoxemia that is thought to be due to $\dot{V}/\dot{Q}$ mismatch can be corrected by giving the patient a simple incremental FIO_2 test. For example, if the PaO_2 increases significantly in response to an FIO_2 change from 0.30 to 0.60, the primary problem is low $\dot{V}/\dot{Q}$. If the PaO_2 does not increase significantly, a right-to-left shunt exists.

d. Shunting

i. Shunting occurs when a portion of venous blood does not participate in gas exchange. An anatomic shunt may occur (a portion of right ventricular blood does not pass through the pulmonary capillaries) or a portion of pulmonary capillary blood may pass by airless alveoli.

ii. Normal physiologic shunting amounts to 2% to 5% of cardiac output (this is bronchial and thebesian vein blood)

iii. Shunting occurs in arteriovenous malformations, adult respiratory distress syndrome (ARDS), atelectasis, pneumonia, pulmonary edema, pulmonary embolus, vascular lung tumors, and intracardiac right-to-left shunts

iv. Breathing at an increased FIO_2 level does not correct shunting because not all blood comes into contact with open alveoli and shunted blood passes directly from pulmonary veins to arterial blood (venous admixture). Lack of improvement of hypoxemia with O_2 therapy is a hallmark of shunting.

v. Usually, shunting does not result in elevated $PaCO_2$, even though shunted blood is rich in CO_2. Brain chemoreceptors sense elevated $PaCO_2$ and respond by increasing ventilation.

vi. Shunting is measured by comparing mixed venous O_2 (from the pulmonary artery catheter) to arterial O_2 ($CaO_2 - C\bar{v}O_2$). Amount of true shunt can be estimated by having the patient breathe 100% O_2 for 15 minutes, which eliminates the effects of abnormal $\dot{V}/\dot{Q}$ and diffusion defects. Normal shunt is 5 vol% (5 ml/dl).

e. Diffusion defects

i. Seen in patients with a thickened alveolar-capillary membrane, as in pulmonary fibrosis, which enlarges the distance between alveolar gas and the pulmonary capillaries

ii. May be overcome by diffusion because the rate of diffusion always depends on the pressure gradient

iii. Is rarely a cause of hypoxemia by itself at rest but may contribute to hypoxemia in patients with $\dot{V}/\dot{Q}$ mismatch and/or shunting caused by a disease state or in certain patients during exercise

4. **Acid-base physiology and blood gases**

a. Terminology

i. *Acid:* Donor of hydrogen ions (H^+); substance with a pH below 7.0

ii. *Acidemia:* Condition in which the blood pH is below 7.35

iii. *Acidosis:* Process (metabolic or respiratory) that causes acidemia

iv. *Base:* Acceptor of H^+ ions; any substance with a pH above 7.0

    v. *Alkalemia:* Condition in which the blood pH is above 7.45

    vi. *Alkalosis:* Process (metabolic or respiratory) that causes alkalemia

    vii. *pH:* Negative logarithm of the H^+ ion concentration

      (a) Increase in $[H^+]$ = lower pH, more acidic

      (b) Decrease in $[H^+]$ = higher pH, more alkaline

b. Buffering: Normal body mechanism that occurs rapidly in response to acid-base disturbances to prevent changes in $[H^+]$

    i. Bicarbonate (HCO_3^-) buffer system

$$[H^+] + HCO_3^- \longleftrightarrow H_2CO_3 \longleftrightarrow CO_2 + H_2O$$

This system is very important because HCO_3^- can be regulated by the kidneys and CO_2 can be regulated by the lungs

    ii. Phosphate system

    iii. Hb and other proteins

c. Henderson-Hasselbalch equation: Defines the relationship between pH, P_{CO_2}, and bicarbonate. Arterial pH is determined by the logarithm of the ratio of bicarbonate concentration to arterial P_{CO_2}. Bicarbonate is regulated primarily by the kidney and P_{CO_2} is regulated by alveolar ventilation:

$$pH = pK + \log \frac{[HCO_3^-]}{Pa_{CO_2}}$$

where pK = a constant (6.1)

    i. As long as the ratio of HCO_3^- to CO_2 is about 20:1, the pH of the blood will be normal. It is this ratio, rather than the absolute values of each, that determines blood pH.

    ii. pH must be maintained within a narrow range of normal because the functioning of most enzymatic systems in the body depends on the H^+ concentration (Figure 2-8)

d. Normal adult blood gas values (at sea level): See Table 2-3. *Note:* Knowledge of blood gas values neither supersedes nor replaces sound clinical judgment.

e. Effect of altitude on blood gas values

    i. Pa_{O_2} and Sa_{O_2} are lower at high altitudes because of a lower ambient O_2 tension

    ii. Normal for 5280 feet (Denver) = Pa_{O_2} of 65 to 75 mm Hg, Sa_{O_2} of 94% to 95%

f. Respiratory parameter (Pa_{CO_2}): If the primary disturbance is in the Pa_{CO_2}, the patient is said to have a respiratory disturbance

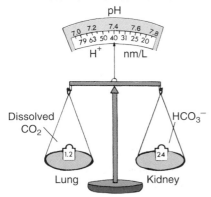

FIGURE 2-8 ■ The balance between bicarbonate (HCO_3^-) (24) and dissolved carbon dioxide (CO_2) (1.2 of arterial partial pressure of CO_2 [Pa_{CO_2}] = 40) is normally 20:1, and this is usually associated with a pH of about 7.40 and an H^+ concentration of about 40 nmol/L. (From Cherniack RM, Cherniack L: *Respiration in health and disease,* ed 3, Philadelphia, 1983, Saunders, p 85.)

■ **TABLE 2-3**
■ ■ **Normal Adult Blood Gas Values (at Sea Level)**

	Arterial	Mixed Venous
pH	7.40 (7.35-7.45)	7.36 (7.31-7.41)
Po_2	80-100 mm Hg	35-40 mm Hg
Sao_2	≥95%	70%-75%
Pco_2	35-45 mm Hg	41-51 mm Hg
HCO_3^-	22-26 mEq/L	22-26 mEq/L
Base excess	−2 to +2	−2 to +2

HCO_3^-, Bicarbonate; Pco_2, partial pressure of carbon dioxide; Po_2, partial pressure of oxygen; Sao_2, arterial oxygen saturation.

    i. $Paco_2$ is a reflection of alveolar ventilation
       (a) If increased, hypoventilation is present
       (b) If decreased, hyperventilation is present
       (c) If normal, adequate ventilation is present
       (d) To assess relationships, measurements of both $Paco_2$ and minute ventilation are needed
    ii. Respiratory acidosis (elevated $Paco_2$), caused by hypoventilation of any etiology (may be acute or chronic). Treatment generally consists of improving alveolar ventilation.
       (a) Obstructive lung disease, sleep apnea, and other lung diseases resulting in inadequate excretion of CO_2
       (b) Oversedation, head trauma, anesthesia, and drug overdose
       (c) Neuromuscular disorders: Guillain-Barré syndrome
       (d) Pneumothorax, flail chest, or other types of chest wall trauma that interfere with breathing mechanics
       (e) Inappropriate mechanical ventilator settings
   iii. Respiratory alkalosis (low $Paco_2$) caused by hyperventilation of any etiology. Treatment consists of correcting the underlying cause.
       (a) Nervousness and anxiety
       (b) Hypoxemia, interstitial lung disease
       (c) Excessive ventilation with mechanical ventilator, as a response to metabolic acidosis (diabetic ketoacidosis) or from respiratory stimulant drugs, such as salicylates, theophylline, catecholamines
       (d) Pregnancy
       (e) Pulmonary embolus, pulmonary edema
       (f) Bacteremia (sepsis), liver disease, or fever
       (g) CNS disturbances, such as brainstem tumors and infections
  g. Nonrespiratory (renal) parameters (HCO_3^-): If the primary disturbance is in the bicarbonate level, the patient has a metabolic disturbance
    i. Concentration influenced by metabolic processes
       (a) When HCO_3^- is elevated, metabolic alkalosis results
          (1) Loss of nonvolatile acid
          (2) Gain of HCO_3^-
       (b) When HCO_3^- is decreased, metabolic acidosis results
          (1) H^+ is added in excess of the capacity of the kidney to excrete it
          (2) HCO_3^- is lost at a rate exceeding the capacity of the kidney to regenerate it

    ii. Causes of metabolic alkalosis (elevated HCO_3^-)

        (a) Chloride depletion (vomiting, prolonged nasogastric suctioning, diuretic therapy)

        (b) Cushing's syndrome, hyperaldosteronism, potassium deficiency, renal artery stenosis, licorice ingestion

        (c) Exogenous administration of alkali (massive blood transfusions containing citrate, bicarbonate administration, ingestion of antacids)

    iii. Causes of metabolic acidosis (decreased HCO_3^-)

        (a) Increase in unmeasurable anions (acids that accumulate in certain diseases and poisonings); high anion gap

            (1) Diabetic ketoacidosis, starvation

            (2) Drugs: Salicylates, ethylene glycol, methanol alcohol, paraldehyde

            (3) Lactic acidosis resulting from tissue hypoperfusion and subsequent anaerobic metabolism (shock, sepsis)

            (4) Renal failure, uremia

            (5) Easy mnemonic is MULEPAK—methanol, uremia, lactic acidosis, ethylene glycol, paraldehyde, aspirin (salicylates), and ketoacidosis

        (b) No increase in unmeasurable anions, normal anion gap

            (1) Diarrhea, ureterosigmoidostomy (long or obstructed ileal conduit)

            (2) Drainage of pancreatic juices

            (3) Rapid IV infusion of non–bicarbonate-containing solutions causing a dilutional acidosis

            (4) Certain drugs, renal tubular acidosis

            (5) Hyperalimentation (causes hyperchloremic acidosis)

  h. Compensation for acid-base abnormalities: Physiologic response to minimize pH changes by maintaining a normal bicarbonate to PCO_2 ratio

    i. pH returned to near normal by changing component that is not primarily affected

    ii. Respiratory disturbances result in kidney compensation, which may take several days to become maximal

        (a) Compensation for respiratory acidosis

            (1) Kidneys excrete more acid

            (2) Kidneys increase HCO_3^- reabsorption

            (3) Compensation is slow (days)

        (b) Compensation for respiratory alkalosis

            (1) Kidneys excrete HCO_3^-

            (2) Compensation is slow (days)

    iii. Metabolic disturbances result in pulmonary compensation, which begins rapidly but takes a variable amount of time to reach maximal levels

        (a) Compensation for metabolic acidosis

            (1) Hyperventilation to decrease $PaCO_2$

            (2) Compensation is rapid (begins in 1 to 2 hours and reaches maximum in 12 to 24 hours)

        (b) Compensation for metabolic alkalosis

            (1) Hypoventilation (limited by the degree of the rise in $PaCO_2$)

            (2) Compensation is rapid (minutes to hours)

    iv. Body does not overcompensate. Therefore, the acidity or alkalinity of the pH identifies the primary abnormality if there is only one. Abnormalities may be multiple; each is not a discrete entity. Mixed acid-base disturbances often occur.

  i. Correction of acid-base abnormalities: Caused by a physiologic or therapeutic response

    i. pH returned to normal by altering the component primarily affected; blood gas values are returned to normal

   ii. Correction for respiratory acidosis: Increased ventilation, treatment of cause

  iii. Correction for respiratory alkalosis: Decreased ventilation, treatment of cause

  iv. Correction for metabolic acidosis

    (a) Treatment of underlying cause

    (b) Administration of bicarbonate intravenously or orally (given only under specific circumstances)

   v. Correction for metabolic alkalosis

    (a) Treatment of underlying cause

    (b) Direct reduction by isotonic hydrochloric acid solution (cautious IV administration required) via a central line at a rate no higher than 0.2 mEq/kg/hr)

    (c) Arginine monohydrochloride or ammonium chloride used rarely; acetazolamide (carbonic anhydrase inhibitor–diuretic) used in certain situations

j. Arterial blood gas (ABG) analysis

   i. Purpose

    (a) Shows end result of what occurs in the lung

    (b) Confirms the presence of respiratory failure and indicates acid-base status

    (c) Absolutely necessary in monitoring patients in acute respiratory failure (ARF) and patients on ventilators

  ii. Main components: PaO_2, $PaCO_2$, pH, base excess, HCO_3^-, SaO_2, O_2 content, Hb. Both FIO_2 and body temperature must be measured for proper interpretation. It is also essential to know whether HCO_3^- and SaO_2 are directly measured or are calculated.

k. Guidelines for interpretation of ABG levels and acid-base balance

   i. Examine pH first (Table 2-4)

    (a) If pH is reduced (<7.35), the patient is acidemic

      (1) If $PaCO_2$ is elevated, the patient has respiratory acidosis

      (2) If HCO_3^- is reduced, the patient has metabolic acidosis

      (3) If $PaCO_2$ is elevated and HCO_3^- is reduced, the patient has combined respiratory and metabolic acidosis

    (b) If pH is elevated (>7.45), the patient is alkalemic

■ **TABLE 2-4**
■ ■ **Analysis of the Acid-Base Balance of an Arterial Blood Gas**

pH	↑	Alkalemia
	↓	Acidemia
$PaCO_2$	↑	Acidemia: pH should be ↓
	↓	Alkalemia: pH should be ↑
HCO_3^-	↑	Alkalemia: pH should be ↑
	↓	Acidemia: pH should be ↓

© K. Ellstrom, 1998. Used by permission.
pH and $PaCO_2$ go in opposite directions; pH and HCO_3^- go in the same direction.
HCO_3^-, Bicarbonate; $PaCO_2$, arterial partial pressure of carbon dioxide.

(1) If Pa_{CO_2} is decreased, the patient has respiratory alkalosis

(2) If HCO_3^- is elevated, the patient has metabolic alkalosis

(3) If Pa_{CO_2} is decreased and HCO_3^- is elevated, the patient has combined metabolic and respiratory alkalosis

  (c) Expected change in pH for changes in Pa_{CO_2}: Commonly used rule is that the pH rises or falls 0.08 (or 0.1) in the appropriate direction for each change of 10 mm in the Pa_{CO_2}

  (d) If the pH is normal (7.35 to 7.45), alkalosis or acidosis may still be present as a mixed disorder (Box 2-1)

  ii. Assess the hypoxemic state and tissue oxygenation state (Box 2-2)

    (a) Arterial oxygenation is considered compromised when Hb saturation is less than 88% (Pa_{O_2} is <60 mm Hg). If the Pa_{O_2} is below 55 mm Hg, hypoxemia is present.

    (b) If the patient is receiving supplemental O_2 therapy, Pa_{O_2} values must be interpreted in relation to the FI_{O_2} delivered. One way involves examination of the two as a ratio (Pa_{O_2}/FI_{O_2}). Normal Pa_{O_2}/FI_{O_2} ratio is 286 to 350, although levels as low as 200 may be clinically acceptable. Another way to assess oxygenation is to use the following formula to calculate the A–a arterial P_{O_2} gradient ($PA_{O_2} - Pa_{O_2}$):

$$PA_{O_2} = [FI_{O_2}(P_B - 47) - Pa_{CO_2}]/R$$

where

47 = vapor pressure of water at 37° C (in mm Hg)

R = respiratory quotient, the ratio of CO_2 production to O_2 consumption ($\dot{V}_{CO_2}/\dot{V}_{O_2}$); assumed to be 0.8

Normal $PA_{O_2} - Pa_{O_2}$ difference is less than 10 to 15 mm Hg. Although it provides an estimate of oxygenation, the gradient does not take into account the normal increasing gradient as a function of increasing FI_{O_2}

■ BOX 2-1
■ ARTERIAL BLOOD GAS ANALYSIS: ACID-BASE EXAMPLE

MEASUREMENTS
pH: 7.38
Pa_{CO_2}: 70 mm Hg
HCO_3^-: 32 mEq/L
Pa_{O_2}: 65 mm Hg
Sa_{O_2}: 92%

ANALYSIS
pH: Normal, but on acidic side
Pa_{CO_2}: Elevated—acidotic
HCO_3^-: Elevated—alkalotic
Primary disorder is respiratory acidosis (pH is on the acidic side and Pa_{CO_2} is elevated).
Secondary disorder is metabolic alkalosis (HCO_3^- is elevated) as compensation.

INTERPRETATION
Compensated respiratory acidosis (e.g., patient with stable chronic obstructive pulmonary disease).

HCO_3^-, Bicarbonate; *Pa_{CO_2}*, arterial partial pressure of carbon dioxide; *Pa_{O_2}*, arterial partial pressure of oxygen; *Sa_{O_2}*, arterial oxygen saturation.

■ **BOX 2-2**
■ **ARTERIAL BLOOD GAS ANALYSIS: OXYGENATION EXAMPLE**

MEASUREMENTS
pH: 7.38
$Paco_2$: 70 mm Hg
HCO_3^-: 32 mEq/L
Pao_2: 65 mm Hg
Sao_2: 92%
Cao_2: 19.0 g/dl
Hb: 18 g/dl
Hct: 54%
On 2 L/min O_2 by nasal cannula, at sea level

ANALYSIS
pH: Normal, not in lactic acidosis from hypoxia
Pao_2: Low but adequate
Sao_2: Low but adequate
Cao_2: Within normal limits
Hb: Elevated
Hct: Elevated

INTERPRETATION
Adequate oxygenation on 2 L/min O_2. Hb/Hct elevated as compensatory mechanism to increase O_2-carrying capacity and compensate for underlying lung disease (chronic obstructive pulmonary disease) producing hypoxemia.

Cao_2, Arterial oxygen concentration; *Hb*, hemoglobin level; *Hct*, hematocrit; HCO_3^-, Bicarbonate; $Paco_2$, arterial partial pressure of carbon dioxide; Pao_2, arterial partial pressure of oxygen; Sao_2, arterial oxygen saturation.

levels. The higher the FIO_2, the larger the increase in the A–a gradient can be without changing the level of intrapulmonary shunt or oxygenation. (*Note:* Primarily used for patients on a ventilator when the FIO_2 is known. FIO_2 is unknown [and its value therefore unreliable] with other O_2 delivery methods, but it can be estimated.)

(c) Excessively high Pao_2 (>100 mm Hg) is generally not necessary and in such cases FIO_2 should be reduced

(d) Assessment of cardiac output and O_2 transport determines tissue oxygenation. $P\bar{v}o_2$ and $S\bar{v}o_2$ may be useful guides in evaluating the adequacy of overall tissue oxygenation.

(e) Effectiveness of O_2 transport may be judged clinically by examining the patient carefully for mental status, skin color, urine output, and heart rate. Tests that measure end-organ function are also important clinical assessment tools.

Patient Assessment

1. **Nursing history:** Nursing history follows the sequence and length of the standard history-taking process and is modified as needed for acutely ill patients
   a. Patient health history: Patient's interpretation of his or her signs and symptoms and the emotional response to them play a significant role in the development or exacerbation of symptoms, especially as related to dyspnea

  i. Common symptoms

    (a) Dyspnea: *Subjective* feeling of shortness of breath or breathlessness; considered the sixth vital sign in pulmonary patients, in whom it may be more significant than pain

      (1) Difficult to quantify objectively

        a) Count the average number of words the patient is able to speak between breaths, or whether the patient can speak in full sentences

        b) Ask the patient to rate breathing comfort on a visual analogue or dyspnea scale from 1 to 10

      (2) Emotional problems may cause an increased awareness of respirations and complaints of inability to get enough air, despite normal blood gas values

      (3) Dyspnea caused by increased work of breathing accompanies both obstructive and restrictive lung diseases as well as the dysfunction of nerves, respiratory muscles, or thoracic cage

      (4) Question the patient regarding exercise tolerance; some dyspnea is normal with exercise but is abnormal if exercise tolerance is decreased

      (5) Assess whether the patient's dyspnea is acute or chronic, and whether it has recently increased or decreased

      (6) Determine all circumstances under which dyspnea occurs (walking, stair climbing, eating) and how long the patient has experienced dyspnea with those activities

      (7) Assess orthopnea or dyspnea when the patient is lying flat; ask how many pillows the patient generally uses for sleep and whether for comfort or shortness of breath

      (8) Assess for paroxysmal nocturnal dyspnea by asking whether dyspnea ever awakens the patient from sleep

      (9) Determine whether dyspnea is accompanied by other symptoms, such as cough, wheezing, or chest pain

     (10) In some patients, it is difficult to differentiate cardiac from pulmonary dyspnea

    (b) Cough: Normal when it occurs as a lung defense mechanism

      (1) Determine whether cough is acute and self-limiting or chronic (lasting more than 6 weeks) and persistent

      (2) Note any change in character and frequency

      (3) Determine what the timing is (both daily and seasonal) and whether the cough is accompanied by sputum production, hemoptysis, wheezing, chest pain, blackouts or falls, or dyspnea

      (4) Most common etiologic mechanisms

        a) Inhaled irritants or airway diseases (asthma, bronchitis)

        b) Aspiration or lung diseases (pneumonia, lung abscess, tumor)

        c) Left ventricular failure (pulmonary edema)

        d) Side effect of medications (some angiotensin-converting enzyme inhibitors)

    (c) Sputum production

      (1) Quantify amount by asking how many teaspoons, cups, or shot glasses of sputum are coughed up daily

      (2) Determine aggravating and alleviating factors

      (3) Assess the character of the sputum (color, odor, consistency)

      (4) Determine whether current sputum characteristics (quantity and quality) are changed from usual

     (d) Hemoptysis: Expectoration of blood from the lungs or airways

        (1) Determine whether the material coughed up is grossly bloody, blood streaked, or blood tinged (pinkish)

        (2) Try to differentiate from hematemesis. Product of *hemoptysis* is often frothy, alkaline, and accompanied by sputum; product of *hematemesis* is nonfrothy, acidic, and dark red or brown, with food particles.

        (3) Determine the approximate amount of blood produced in hemoptysis using a reasonable measurement guideline, such as the number of teaspoons or shot glasses per day. Assess whether all expectorated specimens contain blood or whether this is an isolated event.

        (4) Blood may originate from the nasopharynx, airways, or lung parenchyma; blood from these sites remains red because of the contact with atmospheric O_2

        (5) Etiologic mechanisms of hemoptysis fall into three categories by location: Airways, pulmonary parenchyma, and vasculature

           a) Airways disease: Most common; bronchitis, bronchiectasis, and bronchogenic carcinoma

           b) Parenchymal causes: Often infectious—tuberculosis (TB), lung abscess, pneumonia

           c) Cardiovascular disease: Mitral stenosis, pulmonary embolism, pulmonary edema

           d) Autoimmune disorders: Wegener's granulomatosis, Goodpasture's syndrome

        (6) Suspect neoplasm if hemoptysis occurs in a patient without prior respiratory symptoms

     (e) Chest pain: As a reflection of the respiratory system, does not originate in the lung, because the lung is free of sensory nerve fibers

        (1) Chest wall pain: Arises from the parietal pleura, intercostal muscles, ribs, or overlying skin

           a) Well localized

           b) Often exacerbated by deep inspiration

        (2) Diaphragm pain: Often caused by an inflammatory process; pain often referred to the ipsilateral shoulder

        (3) Mediastinal pain: Caused by a mass or air under the mediastinum (pneumomediastinum); pain is substernal and dull

  ii. Miscellaneous symptoms of respiratory disease: Postnasal drip, sinus pain, epistaxis, hoarseness, general fatigue, weight loss, fever, sleep disturbances, night sweats, anxiety, nervousness, anorexia

iii. Past medical history

     (a) Question the patient regarding the presence of any allergy to either medications (herbal, over the counter) or food. Obtain a description of the type and severity of the reaction.

     (b) Determine past instances of the present illness, with treatment and outcome. Assess for previous episodes of TB, exposure to TB, or positive TB skin test result. Assess for childhood lung diseases or infections such as asthma, pneumonia, and whooping cough. Record the treatment given (if any) and the length of time the patient followed the medication regimen.

     (c) Identify past surgeries or hospitalizations: Dates, diagnosis, and complications; previous use of O_2 or mechanical ventilation

     (d) Question about previous chest radiographs: Dates, reasons, findings

   (e) Determine whether any pulmonary function tests were performed previously and the results if known

 b. Family history (extremely important)

  i. Assess for similar illness or signs and symptoms in the patient's parents, siblings, and grandparents

  ii. Determine the current state of health or cause of death for parents, siblings, and grandparents

  iii. Find out if there is a family history of diseases such as asthma, cystic fibrosis, bronchiectasis, and α_1-antitrypsin deficiency (emphysema)

  iv. Determine whether a family member ever had TB with consequent exposure of the patient

 c. Social history and habits

  i. Personal status: Assess education, socioeconomic class, marital status, general life satisfaction, interests

  ii. Health habits

   (a) Smoking

    (1) Determine whether the patient is a current or past smoker of cigarettes, cigars, or pipe

     a) Calculate pack-year history:

$$\text{No. of packs/day} \times \text{No. of years smoked} = \text{pack-years}$$

     b) Determine whether the patient has tried to quit and, if so, what methods were used and whether the effort was successful. If the patient is a former smoker, determine the time since the last cigarette; otherwise, determine the desire for information on smoking cessation resources and readiness to quit.

    (2) Ascertain whether the patient has smoked marijuana or another inhaled recreational drug (e.g., crack cocaine). If so, attempt to quantify the amount and frequency of drug use.

    (3) Determine whether the patient chews tobacco. If so, quantify the type chewed and the amount per day.

   (b) Drinking habits: Determine the frequency and amount consumed, and the type of alcoholic and caffeine-containing beverages

   (c) Eating habits: Assess the quality of meals (adequacy or excess) and determine whether any respiratory symptoms occur with eating (i.e., meal-induced dyspnea or cough)

   (d) Sexual history: Question about sexual activity and orientation

  iii. Home conditions: Assess economic conditions, housing quality, presence of any pets and their health, presence of allergens

  iv. Occupational history: Assess past and present work conditions

   (a) Determine whether the patient was exposed to heat and cold, industrial toxins, or pollutants during work or military duty

   (b) Assess the duration of exposure and the use of protective devices

 d. Medication history (prescription and over-the-counter medications or home remedies)

  i. Determine current and recent medications, dosage, and the reason for prescribing

  ii. Assess whether the patient is using any inhaled medications

   (a) Identify the device used: Metered-dose inhaler (MDI), nebulizer, or other delivery device (e.g., Spinhaler, HandiHaler)

   (b) Assess the frequency of use—on an as-needed basis or on a regular schedule

(c) If possible, have the patient demonstrate the technique for inhaling medication. Many patients use an incorrect technique when inhaling their medications, which results in reduced deposition of the drug in the lung and reduced efficacy. Patients should exhale completely, inhale the drug slowly and deeply, and then hold the breath for 10 seconds if possible.

(d) Preferred delivery methods: Powder delivery devices (nonaerosol), MDI with spacer, nebulizer, MDI with open mouth, MDI with closed mouth (least amount of medication delivered)

2. **Nursing examination of patient**
   a. Physical examination data
      i. Inspection
         (a) Ensure that the patient is stripped to the waist and, if possible, seated
            (1) Warm room and good lighting should be available
            (2) Nurse must have a thorough knowledge of anatomic landmarks and lines (Figure 2-9)
               a) Manubrium, body, and xiphoid process of the sternum, right and left sternal borders
               b) Angle of Louis, point of maximal impulse, suprasternal notch
               c) Interspaces, ribs, costal margins, costal angle, and spinous processes
               d) Pulmonary lobes and areas of contact with the chest wall (Figure 2-10)
               e) Lines: Midclavicular, midsternal, anterior-axillary, midaxillary, posterior-axillary, vertebral, and midscapular
         (b) Observe general condition and musculoskeletal development
            (1) State of nutrition, debilitation, evidence of chronic disease
            (2) Pectus carinatum: Sternum protrudes instead of being lower than the adjacent hemithoraces

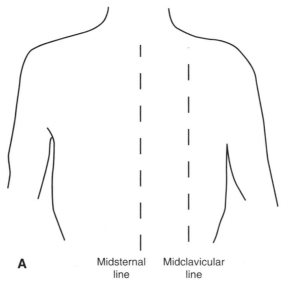

A   Midsternal   Midclavicular
          line   line

FIGURE 2-9 ■ Landmarks of the chest. **A,** Anterior chest wall.

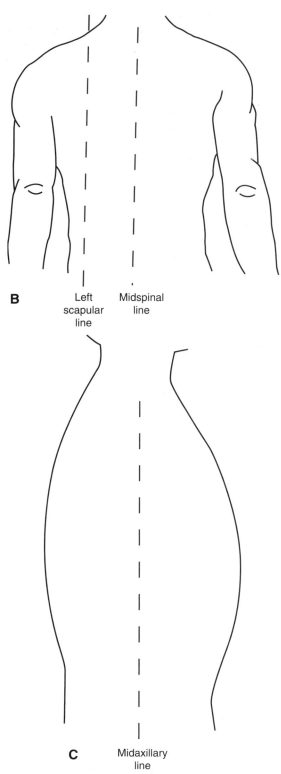

FIGURE 2-9 cont'd ■ **B,** Posterior chest wall. **C,** Lateral chest wall. (Courtesy American Association of Critical-Care Nurses, Aliso Viejo, Calif.)

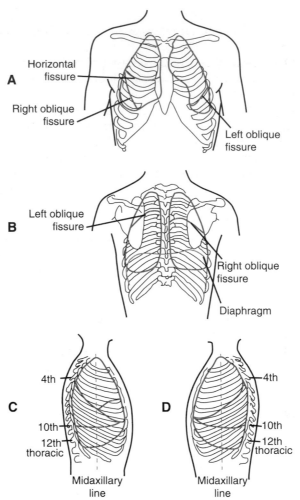

FIGURE 2-10 ■ Topographic position of lung fissures. **A,** Anterior chest. **B,** Posterior chest. **C,** and **D,** Lateral chest. (From Ahrens TS: Pulmonary data acquisition. In Kinney MR, Packa DR, Dunbar SB, editors: *AACN's clinical reference for critical care nursing,* ed 3, St Louis, 1993, Mosby, p 690.)

      (3) Pectus excavatum: Sternum is abnormally depressed between the anterior hemithoraces

      (4) Kyphosis: Exaggerated A-P curvature of the spine

      (5) Scoliosis: Lateral curvature of the spine, causing widened intercostal spaces on the convex side and crowding of the ribs on the concave side; when accompanied by kyphosis, it is called *kyphoscoliosis*. If severe, it can result in restrictive lung disease.

   (c) Observe the A-P diameter of the thorax; normal A-P diameter is approximately one third the transverse diameter. In patients with obstructive lung disease, the A-P diameter may be as great as or greater than the transverse diameter ("barrel chest").

   (d) Observe the general slope of the ribs

      (1) Ribs are normally at a 45-degree angle in relation to the spine

      (2) In patients with emphysema, the ribs may be nearly horizontal

(e) Observe for asymmetry
   (1) One side may be larger because of tension pneumothorax or pleural effusion
   (2) One side may be smaller because of atelectasis or unilateral fibrosis
   (3) If asymmetry is present, the abnormal side will move less than the normal side
(f) Look for retraction or bulging of the interspaces
   (1) Retraction of the interspaces, which can be observed during inspiration, indicates more negative intrapleural pressure due to obstruction of the inflow of air or increased work of breathing
   (2) Bulging of the interspaces may result from a large pleural effusion or pneumothorax, often seen during a forced expiration in patients with asthma or emphysema
(g) Observe the ventilatory pattern
   (1) Assess the level of dyspnea and the work of breathing
      a) Position in which the patient can breathe most comfortably. Patients with chronic obstructive pulmonary disease (COPD) often assume a forward-leaning position, resting the arms on the knees or a bedside table.
      b) Use of accessory muscles of breathing
      c) Use of pursed-lip breathing
      d) Flaring of the ala nasi during inspiration, a common sign of air hunger, especially in ventilated patients
      e) Paradoxical movement of the diaphragm
   (2) Assess for *inspiratory stridor*—low-pitched or crowing inspiratory sounds that occur when the trachea or major bronchi are obstructed for one of the following reasons:
      a) Tumor (intrinsic or extrinsic), foreign body
      b) Severe laryngotracheitis or crushing injury
      c) Goiter, scar, or granulation tissue
   (3) Observe for *expiratory stridor*—low-pitched crowing sound heard on expiration. Causes include foreign body or intrathoracic, tracheal, or main-stem tumor.
   (4) Observe for unusual movements with breathing; on inspiration, the chest and abdomen should expand or rise together. *Paradoxical breathing* occurs with respiratory muscle fatigue: On inspiration, the chest rises and the abdomen is drawn in because the fatigued diaphragm does not descend on inspiration as it should. Instead, the diaphragm is drawn upward by the negative intrathoracic pressure during inspiration.
   (5) Observe and assess the ventilatory pattern
      a) *Eupnea:* Normal, quiet respirations
      b) *Bradypnea:* Abnormally slow rate of ventilation
      c) *Tachypnea:* Rapid rate of ventilation
      d) *Hyperpnea:* Increase in the depth and, perhaps, in the rate of ventilation. Overall result is increased tidal volume and minute ventilation.
      e) *Apnea:* Complete or intermittent cessation of ventilation
      f) *Biot's breathing:* Two to three short breaths alternating with long, irregular periods of apnea
      g) *Cheyne-Stokes respiration:* Periods of increasing ventilation, followed by progressively more shallow ventilations until apnea

occurs; pattern typically repeats itself. Sometimes occurs in normal persons when asleep, and usually indicates CNS disease, heart failure, or sleep apnea.

(6) Splinting of respirations—act of resisting full inspiration in one or both lungs as a result of pain

(7) Flail chest—inward movement of a portion of the chest on inspiration, usually associated with trauma to the chest; from fracture of the rib cage in two or more sections

(h) Other observations

(1) General state of restlessness, pain, altered mental status, fright, or acute distress. Earliest signs of hypoxemia often include a change in mental status and restlessness.

(2) If O_2 is being administered, record the amount (flow in liters per minute), type of device (liquid, compressed gas), method of delivery (nasal cannula, Oxymizer, mask)

(3) Inspect the extremities

a) Clubbing of the fingers is a late sign of a chronic pulmonary or cardiac disease

b) Cigarette stains on the fingers suggest a current smoking habit

c) Lower-extremity edema indicates possible right-sided heart failure from chronic pulmonary disease and hypoxemia-induced pulmonary hypertension

(4) Observe for cyanosis

a) Fundamental mechanism of cyanosis is an increase in the amount of reduced (deoxygenated) Hb in the vessels of the skin caused by one of the following:

1) Decrease in the O_2 saturation of the capillary blood

2) Increase in the amount of venous blood in the skin as a result of the dilation of venules and capillaries

b) Visible cyanosis requires the presence of at least 5 g of reduced Hb per deciliter of blood

1) This is an absolute, not a relative, value. It is not the percentage of deoxygenated Hb that causes cyanosis but the amount of deoxygenated Hb without regard to the amount of oxyhemoglobin. Presence or absence of cyanosis may be an unreliable clinical sign.

2) In anemia, cyanosis may be difficult to detect because the absolute amount of Hb is too low. Conversely, patients with polycythemia may be cyanotic at higher levels of arterial O_2 saturation than those with normal Hb levels.

c) Discoloration suggestive of cyanosis may occur in patients with abnormal blood or skin pigments (methemoglobinemia, sulfhemoglobin, argyria)

d) Factors influencing cyanosis include the rate of blood flow, perfusion, skin thickness and color, the amount of Hb, cardiac output, and the perception of the examiner

e) *Central* versus *peripheral* cyanosis

1) Central cyanosis implies arterial O_2 desaturation or an abnormal Hb derivative. Both mucous membranes and skin are affected.

2) Peripheral cyanosis without central cyanosis may result from the slowing of perfusion to the tissues (cold exposure, shock, decreased cardiac output). O_2 saturation may be normal.

        f) In carbon monoxide poisoning, O_2 saturation may be dangerously low without obvious cyanosis because carboxyhemoglobin causes the skin to turn a cherry red

  (i) Assess for neck vein distention, neck masses, and enlarged nodes

  (j) Look for *superior vena caval syndrome*: Distention of the neck veins and edema of the neck, eyelids, and hands; often seen with lung cancer

  (k) In elderly patients, examination shows flattening of the ribs and diaphragm, decreased chest expansion, use of accessory muscles, marked bony prominences, loss of subcutaneous tissue, pronounced dorsal curve of the thoracic spine, increased A-P diameter relative to lateral diameter, dyspnea on exertion, dry mucous membranes, decreased ability to clear mucus, and hyperresonance from increased distensibility of the lung

ii. Palpation

  (a) Palpate the thoracic muscles and skeleton, feeling for any of the following: Pulsations, palpable fremitus, tenderness, bulges, or depressions in the chest wall

  (b) Expansion of the chest wall

    (1) Examiner's hands should be placed over the lower lateral aspect of the chest, with the thumbs along the costal margin anteriorly or meeting posteriorly in the midline

    (2) Movement of the hands is noted on inspiration and expiration. Asymmetry of movement is always abnormal. Reduced chest wall movement is often seen in patients with barrel chest and emphysema.

  (c) Position and mobility of the trachea

    (1) Deviations of the trachea toward the defect are seen in atelectasis, unilateral pulmonary fibrosis, pneumonectomy, hemidiaphragm paralysis, and the inspiratory phase of flail chest

    (2) Deviation of the trachea to the side opposite the lesion is seen with neck tumors, thyroid enlargement, tension pneumothorax, pleural effusion, mediastinal mass, and the expiratory phase of flail chest

  (d) Point of maximal impulse: Deviates with mediastinal shift

  (e) Palpation of ribs and chest for tenderness, pain, or air in subcutaneous tissue (crepitus)

  (f) Vocal fremitus, palpable vibration of the chest wall, produced by phonation

    (1) Patient should be instructed to say the word *ninety-nine* loud enough so that the fremitus can be felt with uniform intensity. Some soft-spoken women may need to falsely lower their voice so that the fremitus can be felt. Examiner should place the hands on the patient's chest wall.

    (2) Diminished fremitus is seen in any condition that interferes with the transference of vibrations through the chest

      a) Pleural effusion or thickening, pleural tumors

      b) Pneumothorax with lung collapse or emphysema

      c) Obstruction of the bronchus (sputum plugs or tumors)

    (3) Increased fremitus results from any condition that increases the transmission of vibrations through the chest, such as the following:

      a) Pneumonia, consolidation

      b) Atelectasis (with open bronchus)

      c) Pulmonary infarction or pulmonary fibrosis

      d) Secretions with a patent airway

(g) Pleural friction fremitus
   (1) Occurs when inflamed pleural surfaces rub together during ventilation, producing a "grating" sensation that coincides with the respiratory excursion
   (2) May be palpable during both phases of ventilation but sometimes is felt only during inspiration
(h) Rhonchal fremitus
   (1) Produced by the passage of air through thick exudate, secretions, or an area of stenosis in the trachea or major bronchi
   (2) Unlike friction fremitus, rhonchal fremitus can be relieved by coughing, suctioning, or clearing the secretions from the tracheobronchial tree
(i) Subcutaneous emphysema: Indicates a leak of air under the skin due to a communication with the airway, mediastinum, or pneumothorax
   (1) May be palpated over the area
   (2) On auscultation, may be mistaken for crackles (rales)
iii. Percussion: Tapping or thumping of parts of the body to produce sound. Nature of the sound produced depends on the density of the structures immediately under the area percussed.
   (a) Sound vibrations produced by percussion probably do not penetrate more than about 4 to 5 cm below the surface; therefore, solid masses deep in the chest cannot be outlined with percussion. In addition, because a lesion must be several centimeters in diameter to be detectable by percussion, only large abnormalities can be located.
   (b) Procedure: Accomplished by striking the dorsal distal third finger of one hand, which is held against the thorax, with the distal tip of the flexed middle finger of the other hand
      (1) Striking finger must strike only the stationary finger instantaneously and then be immediately withdrawn
      (2) All movement is executed at the wrist
      (3) Examiner must be sensitive to the sounds that are received from the chest wall
      (4) One side of the chest is compared with the other side
      (5) Percussion of the posterior chest: Patient inclines the head forward and rests the forearms on the thighs to move the scapulae laterally
      (6) Percussion begins at the apices and continues downward to the bases, alternating side to side
   (c) Percussion sounds over the lung
      (1) *Resonance:* Sound heard normally over the lungs
      (2) *Hyperresonance:* Sound heard over the lungs in normal children, in the apices of the lungs relative to the base in an upright adult, and throughout the lung fields in adults with emphysema or pneumothorax
         a) Lower in pitch than normal resonance
         b) Relatively intense and easy to hear
         c) Indicates increased air (less dense)
      (3) *Tympany:* Produced by air in an enclosed chamber; does not occur in the normal chest except below the dome of the left hemidiaphragm, where it is produced by air in the underlying stomach or bowel
         a) Relatively musical sound
         b) Usually higher-pitched than normal resonance; the higher the tension within the viscus, the higher the pitch

       (4) *Dullness:* Sound that is heard with lung consolidation, atelectasis, masses, pleural effusion, or hemothorax
          a) Short, not sustained
          b) Soft, not loud; similar to a dull thud
          c) Indicates that more dense material (fluid or solid) is in the underlying thorax
          d) Normally heard over the liver and heart
   (d) Percussion for diaphragmatic excursion: Range of motion of the diaphragm may be estimated with percussion
       (1) Instruct the patient to take a deep breath and hold it
       (2) Determine the lower level of resonance-to-dullness change (the level of the diaphragm) by percussing downward until a definite change is heard in the percussion note. Mark the spot with a felt-tipped marker.
       (3) After instructing the patient to exhale and hold the breath, repeat the procedure
       (4) Distance between the levels at which the tone change occurs is the diaphragmatic excursion
          a) Normal diaphragmatic excursion is about 3 to 4 cm; partial descent or hemidescent of the diaphragm may be due to paralysis of the diaphragm or hemidiaphragm. Suspect nerve injury in postoperative patients with these signs following thoracic surgery.
          b) Diaphragm is normally higher on the right than the left
          c) Diaphragm is elevated in conditions that increase intraabdominal pressure (pregnancy, ascites) and conditions that decrease thoracic volume (atelectasis)
          d) Diaphragm is fixed and lower than normal in emphysema
          e) It is difficult to differentiate between an elevated diaphragm and a thoracic disease that causes dullness to percussion (e.g., pleural effusion). Paralysis of one or both hemidiaphragms may be present.
iv. Auscultation: Listening to sounds produced within the body
   (a) Basic points
       (1) Examiner should always compare one lung to the other by moving the stethoscope back and forth across the chest starting at the top of the thorax and moving downward
       (2) Listening to the anterior chest will cover the upper and middle lobes; listening to the back covers the bases (see Figure 2-10)
       (3) Patient should be asked to breathe through the mouth a little more deeply than usual. This minimizes turbulent flow sounds produced in the nose and throat.
       (4) Diaphragm of the stethoscope is more sensitive to higher-pitched tones and is thus best for hearing most lung sounds
       (5) Stethoscope earpieces should fit snugly to exclude extraneous sounds but should not be so tight that they are uncomfortable
       (6) Stethoscope tubing should be no longer than 20 inches. Optimal length is 12 to 14 inches.
       (7) Place the stethoscope firmly on the chest to exclude extraneous sounds and eliminate sounds that result from light contact with the skin or air. Confusing sounds may be produced by moving the stethoscope on the skin or hair, breathing on the tubing, sliding the fingers on the tubing or chest piece, or listening through clothing.

(b) Normal breath sounds vary according to the site of auscultation
   (1) *Vesicular* (always normal)
      a) Soft sounds heard over the anterior, lateral, and posterior chest
      b) Heard primarily during inspiration
   (2) *Bronchial* (may be normal or abnormal, depending on the location of the sounds)
      a) Heard normally over the trachea
      b) High-pitched, harsh sound with long and loud expirations
      c) When heard over the lung fields, the sound is abnormal and suggests consolidation
   (3) *Bronchovesicular* (normal or abnormal, depending on the location)
      a) Heard over large bronchi (near the sternum, between the scapulae, over the right upper lobe apex)
      b) Abnormal when heard over the lung fields; signifies consolidation
(c) Abnormalities of breath sounds
   (1) Absent or diminished sounds caused by decreased airflow (airway obstruction, COPD, muscle weakness, splinting) or increased insulation blocking the transmission of sounds to the stethoscope (obesity, pleural disease or fluid, pneumothorax)
   (2) Bronchial sounds heard over the lung fields suggest consolidation or increased density of lung tissue (e.g., atelectasis, pulmonary infarction, pneumonia, large tumors with no airway obstruction)
(d) *Adventitious* sounds: Abnormal sounds that are superimposed on underlying breath sounds
   (1) Evaluate whether position and coughing affect the sounds
   (2) Terminology
      a) *Crackles* (rales): Signify the opening of collapsed alveoli and small airways
         1) Described as fine or coarse
         2) Heard as small pops or crackles; the sound of fine crackles can be mimicked by rubbing together a few pieces of hair near one's ear. Sound of coarse crackles can be mimicked by pulling open Velcro material.
         3) Fine crackles occurring late in inspiration imply conditions that cause restrictive ventilatory defect
         4) Fine crackles heard early in inspiration are often atelectatic, due to small airway closure
         5) Coarse early inspiratory crackles are associated with bronchitis or pneumonia
      b) *Wheeze:* Indicates an obstruction to airflow or air passing through narrowed airways
         1) Continuous high-pitched sound with musical quality; also called "sibilant" wheeze
         2) Commonly heard during expiration but may be heard during inspiration
         3) Causes: Asthma, bronchitis, foreign body, tumor, pulmonary edema, pulmonary emboli, poorly mobilized secretions
      c) *Gurgles* (rhonchi): Result from the passage of air through secretions in the large airways
         1) Low-pitched, continuous sounds
         2) May have a snoring quality when very large airways are involved ("sonorous" wheezes)

3) Tend to improve or disappear after coughing
d) *Pleural friction rub:* Indicates inflammation and loss of pleural fluid
1) Grating, harsh sound in inspiration and expiration; disappears with breath holding. Sound can be mimicked by cupping a hand over one's ear and rubbing the fingers of the other hand over the cupped hand.
2) Heard with pleural infections, infarction, pulmonary emboli, fractured ribs. Located in the area of most intense chest wall pain.
e) *Mediastinal crunch:* Indicates air in the pericardium, mediastinum, or both. Heard synchronously with systole; often associated with pericardial friction rubs.
f) *Pericardial friction rub*
1) Occurs at atrial and ventricular systole with or without a diastolic component
2) Sounds persist with breath holding; heard most clearly at the left lower sternal border
(e) Voice sounds: Spoken words are modified by disease in a manner similar to breath sounds, which results in the increased or decreased conduction of sound
(1) Increased conduction occurs when normal lung tissue is replaced with denser, more solid tissue; it is associated with bronchial breathing
a) Bronchophony: Spoken word (e.g., *ninety-nine*) is heard distinctly but normal sound is muffled
b) Egophony: *E* sound changes to *A*; sound has the quality of sheep bleating
c) Whispered pectoriloquy: Whispered sounds are heard with clarity, as if the patient were speaking into the diaphragm of the stethoscope, but normal sound is muffled
(2) Decreased conduction of sound occurs in the presence of obstructed bronchi, pneumothorax, or large collections of fluid or tissue between the lung and the chest wall
a) Decreased ability to hear voice sounds
b) Accompanied by decreased fremitus
b. Monitoring data
i. Pulse oximetry
(a) Noninvasive estimate of arterial O_2 saturation (SpO_2) using an infrared light source placed at the finger or other acceptable extremity, forehead, or earlobe
(b) Uses two principles for measurement
(1) *Spectrophotometry* measures the infrared light absorption of Hb (to distinguish saturated from reduced Hb)
(2) *Photoplethysmography* uses light to measure the arterial pressure waveforms generated by the pulse (pulse rate and strength) in the capillaries of the tissue at the measurement site
(c) Pulse oximeters are generally accurate in the SpO_2 range of 70% to 100% but are inaccurate in states of low blood flow (decreased perfusion due to hypovolemia, hypotension, or vasoconstriction)
(d) SpO_2 reading is adversely affected by the following:
(1) Motion of the extremity (false pulse rate and waveform artifact)

(2) Light dilution (interferes with the probe's ability to detect the correct light wavelength)

(3) Abnormal Hb (device cannot distinguish between oxyhemoglobin and carboxyhemoglobin and thus overestimates saturation); methemoglobin may interfere with light absorption

(4) IV dyes, some fingernail polish colors (e.g., metallic, dark colors such as black), or abnormal skin pigmentation (interfere with light absorption)

(5) Anemia (Hb level below 5 g/dl may result in insufficient signal to process readings)

(e) Useful for identifying the trend of changes in PaO_2 or acute desaturation episodes, especially when weaning from a ventilator

(f) Extreme caution must be exercised not to overrely on a normal SpO_2 level to indicate normal oxygenation in all cases. Numerous clinical situations (e.g., COPD) may cause erroneous readings. If in doubt, get an ABG.

ii. $S\bar{v}O_2$ monitoring

(a) Mixed venous oxygen saturation ($S\bar{v}O_2$) is monitored in the pulmonary artery, at the distal end of a flow-directed thermodilution pulmonary artery catheter

(b) Catheter holds an optical module that contains a light-emitting source, a photodetector, and a microprocessor to analyze reflected light

(c) Reflectance spectrophotometry is used to differentiate oxygenated blood from deoxygenated blood through light wavelengths in the red and infrared spectra

(d) Continuous $S\bar{v}O_2$ monitoring allows for assessment of global oxygenation. It can detect cardiopulmonary instability and changes prior to changes in other hemodynamic parameters (Table 2-5). Some specific indications include the following:

(1) High-risk cardiovascular surgery, end-stage heart failure, acute myocardial infarction

(2) Acute hypoxemic respiratory failure (e.g., ARDS, pulmonary embolus)

(3) Severe burns, multisystem organ failure

(4) Neurosurgery

(5) High-risk obstetrics

(e) $S\bar{v}O_2$ reflects the delicate balance between O_2 delivery and O_2 utilization. Identifying the trend in measurements allows for real-time assessment and intervention. Because of this, the measure can be used for the following:

(1) Evaluate the adequacy of tissue oxygenation

(2) Detect adverse changes in O_2 delivery and O_2 consumption or impaired tissue oxygenation

(3) Evaluate the effectiveness of interventions to improve the balance between O_2 delivery and consumption, including administration of fluids or drugs and the use of mechanical assistance (e.g., intraaortic balloon pump [IABP], positive end-expiratory pressure [PEEP])

(4) Evaluate the effects of routine medical and nursing procedures on tissue oxygenation (Figures 2-11 and 2-12)

(5) Diagnose intracardiac shunting, cardiac tamponade

(6) Assist in the differential diagnosis of pathologic conditions

(f) Normal $S\bar{v}O_2$ value is 70%

■ **TABLE 2-5**
■ ■ **Factors Associated with Fluctuations in Mixed Venous Oxygen Saturation (S$\bar{v}$o$_2$)**

Changes	Causative Factors
CHANGES THAT DECREASE S$\bar{v}$o$_2$	
Decrease in cardiac output	Hypovolemia or cardiac tamponade
	Shock
	Myocardial infarction
	Arrhythmias
	Increases in positive end expiratory pressure (PEEP)
Decrease in oxygen saturation	Pulmonary edema
	Adult respiratory distress syndrome
	Decrease in inspired oxygen
Decrease in hemoglobin level	Anemia
	Hemorrhage
	Dysfunctional hemoglobin
Increase in oxygen consumption	Pain
	Anxiety or fear
	Agitation or restlessness
	Hyperthermia or burns
	Tachycardia
	Shivering
	Activity (positioning, suctioning)
CHANGES THAT INCREASE S$\bar{v}$o$_2$	
Decrease in oxygen consumption	Use of analgesics and anesthetics
	Neuromuscular blockade or use of paralytics
	Use of β-antagonists
	Hypothermia
	Hypothyroidism
	Sepsis (dysoxia, shunting)
	Cyanide poisoning
	Sleep or rest
Increase in oxygen saturation	Increase in fraction of inspired oxygen or hyperoxia
	Intracardiac shunt or arteriovenous fistula
	Severe mitral valve regurgitation
	Distal migration of a pulmonary artery catheter
Increase in cardiac output	Optimal preload
	Use of positive inotropic agents
	Use of mechanical-assist devices

From Jesurum J: S$\bar{v}$o$_2$ monitoring. In Chulay M, Gawlinski A, editors: *Hemodynamic monitoring protocols for practice*, Aliso Viejo, Calif, 1998, American Association of Critical-Care Nurses. Used with permission.

(1) Values lower than 60% may indicate either inadequate delivery of O$_2$ or increased O$_2$ consumption (e.g., decreased Hb level, decreased Sao$_2$, decreased cardiac output, increased tissue metabolic demands)

(2) Values higher than 80% may indicate either increased O$_2$ delivery or decreased O$_2$ demand (e.g., increased cardiac output, decreased metabolic demand, reduced ability of the cells to utilize oxygen)

(g) Accuracy of S$\bar{v}$o$_2$ monitoring may be affected by the following:

(1) Blood pH and hematocrit level

(2) Blood flow characteristics and blood temperature (including the flow of IV fluid past the catheter tip)

(3) Motion artifacts due to catheter "whip" against the vessel wall

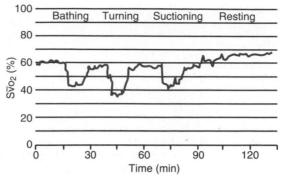

FIGURE 2-11 ■ Effects of routine nursing procedures (bathing, turning, and endotracheal suctioning) on mixed venous oxygen saturation ($S\bar{v}o_2$). (From Jesurum J: $S\bar{v}o_2$ monitoring. In Chulay M, Gawlinski A, editors: *Hemodynamic monitoring protocols for practice*, Aliso Viejo, Calif, 1998, American Association of Critical-Care Nurses. Used with permission.)

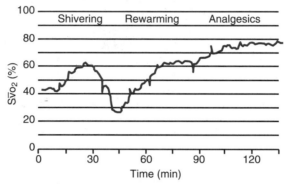

FIGURE 2-12 ■ Effects of shivering, active rewarming, and analgesics on mixed venous oxygen saturations ($S\bar{v}o_2$) after cardiac surgery. (From Jesurum J: $S\bar{v}o_2$ monitoring. In Chulay M, Gawlinski A, editors: *Hemodynamic monitoring protocols for practice*, Aliso Viejo, Calif, 1998, American Association of Critical-Care Nurses. Used with permission.)

   iii. End-tidal CO_2 monitoring (Petco_2)
      (a) Noninvasive sampling and measurement of exhaled CO_2 tension at the patient-ventilator interface
      (b) Devices (capnographs) typically employ infrared analysis of respired gas using different light wavelengths to measure the absorption of CO_2 molecules
         (1) Requires either a simple transducer or a tubing connection to the ventilator circuitry, which is then tied into a standard hemodynamic pressure monitoring module or, by ventilator electronic interface, directly into a physiologic monitoring system
         (2) Displayed airway pressure tracings can be helpful in identification of patient-ventilator dyssynchrony, assessment of the inspiratory work of breathing, and detection of auto-PEEP
      (c) Graphic display of exhaled CO_2 generated during the ventilatory cycle (Figure 2-13)
      (d) Provides both numerical and graphic display of CO_2 waveform on a breath-by-breath basis or at a slower speed for identification of trends (Figure 2-14)
         (1) Normal speed shows the phases of CO_2 elimination
         (2) Slow speed shows trends over minutes to hours

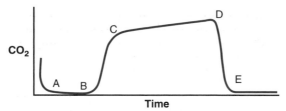

FIGURE 2-13 ■ Typical normal carbon dioxide waveform. *A* to *B*, Exhalation of carbon dioxide–free gas from dead space. *B* to *C*, Combination of dead space and alveolar gases. *C* to *D*, Exhalation of mostly alveolar gas (alveolar plateau). *D*, End-tidal point; that is, exhalation of carbon dioxide at maximum point. *D* to *E*, Beginning of inspiration and rapid fall of carbon dioxide concentration to baseline or zero. (From St. John RE: End-tidal carbon dioxide monitoring, *Crit Care Nurse* 23:83-88, 2003.)

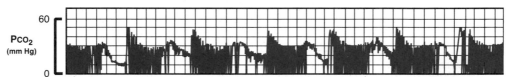

FIGURE 2-14 ■ Slow speed capnogram showing Cheyne-Stokes respirations in a 72-year-old woman who required mechanical ventilation after a cerebral vascular accident. Note the changes in breathing pattern associated with periods of apnea that consistently repeat. P_{CO_2}, Partial pressure of carbon dioxide. (From St. John RE: End-tidal carbon dioxide monitoring, *Crit Care Nurse* 23:83-88, 2003.)

    (e) Pa_{CO_2} to Pet_{CO_2} gradient is 1 to 4 mm Hg (normal $\dot{V}/\dot{Q}$ matching is assumed in the lungs); in critically ill patients, the gradient may exceed 20 mm Hg

    (f) Application is limited for reliably predicting changes in alveolar ventilation except in patients with normal pulmonary perfusion and $\dot{V}/\dot{Q}$ ratios

    (g) Measurement of Pet_{CO_2} depends on adequate blood flow to the lungs to eliminate CO_2

    (h) Gradual narrowing of the gradient over time represents improved ventilation-perfusion matching, decreased CO_2 production, or decreased pulmonary perfusion

    (i) Increased gradient may indicate hypoventilation, increased production of CO_2 (e.g., in fever, seizures), or absorption of CO_2 from an outside source. Rapid rise in the gradient may indicate malignant hyperthermia.

    (j) Sudden drop to a low level indicates incomplete sampling, possibly due to a system leak or partial air obstruction; a zero value indicates a disconnect in the system

    (k) Pulse oximetry assesses oxygenation only; Pet_{CO_2} measurement should be considered for monitoring ventilation in patients undergoing deep sedation and may be useful to detect changes over time in other patients, even those not on ventilators

  iv. Blood gas analysis

    (a) Acid-base balance (pH, Pa_{CO_2}, HCO_3^-): See Tables 2-3 and 2-4

    (b) Oxygenation status (Pa_{O_2}, Sa_{O_2}, Ca_{O_2})

v. Respiratory (ventilator) waveform analysis (Figure 2-15)
  (a) Provides real-time information to assess changes in lung mechanics over time. Less useful in high-frequency or oscillation ventilation modes.
  (b) Visual representation of respiratory waveforms is available with most newer ventilators
    (1) Volume mode—volume is preset, pressure varies with patient compliance and resistance
    (2) Pressure mode—pressure is preset, volume varies
  (c) Pressure-time waveforms
    (1) Used to assess the following:
      a) Ventilator mode
      b) Patient-ventilator synchrony
      c) Inspiratory attempts in heavily sedated or paralyzed patients
      d) End expiration for hemodynamic monitoring
    (2) Positive pressure or upward stroke is the ventilator breath
    (3) Negative deflection is from the patient's spontaneous breathing (or attempts)
    (4) Volume breath waveform starts at zero or the preset PEEP, builds gradually, looks like a shark fin (see Figure 2-15, *A*)
    (5) Pressure waveform shows a constant pressure, a characteristic "square wave" (see Figure 2-15, *B*)
    (6) Modes of ventilation can be identified through the waveform signature (Figure 2-16)
    (7) Patient-ventilator synchrony
      a) Normal ratio of inspiration to expiration is 1:2 or 1:3
      b) Flow rate can be adjusted faster or slower to match the patient's need
      c) Inadequate flow rate is identified by a "scooped-out" appearance on the inspiratory waveform
    (8) Auto-PEEP occurs when expiration is not long enough to empty the lungs. If auto-PEEP is present, the baseline pressure will rise when an end-expiratory hold maneuver is performed.
  (d) Flow-time waveforms (Figure 2-17)
    (1) Used to assess auto-PEEP and patient response to therapy
    (2) Volume breath: Flow of gas is constant throughout the breath; referred to as a *square-flow waveform*

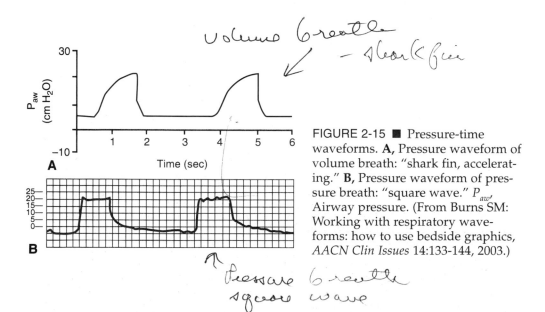

FIGURE 2-15 ■ Pressure-time waveforms. **A,** Pressure waveform of volume breath: "shark fin, accelerating." **B,** Pressure waveform of pressure breath: "square wave." P_{aw}, Airway pressure. (From Burns SM: Working with respiratory waveforms: how to use bedside graphics, *AACN Clin Issues* 14:133-144, 2003.)

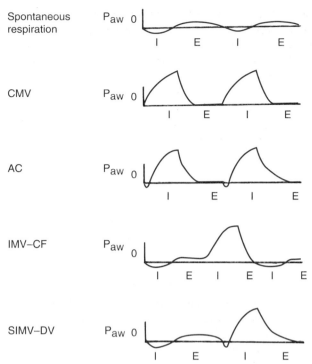

FIGURE 2-16 ■ Airway pressure (P_{aw}) during various modes of ventilation. *AC*, Assist control; *CMV*, controlled mechanical ventilation; *E*, expiration; *I*, inspiration; *IMV-CF*, intermittent mandatory ventilation by a continuous flow circuit; *SIMV-DV*, synchronized intermittent mandatory ventilation by a demand valve circuit. (From Dantzker DR: *Cardiopulmonary critical care*, ed 2, Philadelphia, 1991, Saunders, p 269.)

    (3) Pressure breath: Flow is higher at the beginning and slower at the end; referred to as a *decelerating flow pattern*

    (4) Spontaneous breaths: Decelerating but more rounded; referred to as *sinusoidal*

    (5) Auto-PEEP is identified when the expiratory waveform does not reach baseline

    (6) Bronchospasm reduces expiratory flow. If therapy is effective, expiratory flow will be faster and reach baseline more quickly.

  (e) Pressure-volume and flow-volume loops

    (1) Pressure-volume loops: Pressure and volume are plotted on different axes; result looks like a loop (Figure 2-18)

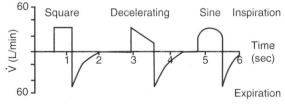

FIGURE 2-17 ■ Square flow waveform associated with a volume breath. Decelerating flow waveform associated with a pressure breath. Sine flow waveform associated with a spontaneous breath. (From Burns SM: Working with respiratory waveforms: how to use bedside graphics, *AACN Clin Issues* 14:133-144, 2003.)

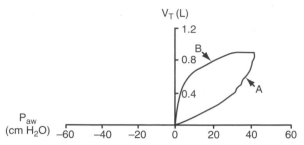

FIGURE 2-18 ■ Pressure-volume loop: Mandatory breath. *A,* Inspiration. *B,* Expiration; P_{aw}, airway pressure. (From Burns SM: Working with respiratory waveforms: how to use bedside graphics, *AACN Clin Issues* 14:133-144, 2003.)

        a) Spontaneous breaths show negative movement (to left of graph) on inspiration, positive movement (to right) on expiration

        b) Ventilator breaths (volume and pressure) have loops that go counterclockwise on the right (positive) side of the graph; the lower portion shows inspiration, the higher portion shows expiration

        c) Monitor resistance and compliance over time

           1) Increased compliance shifts the slope to the right and down

           2) Increased resistance produces a bow-shaped inspiratory curve

     (2) Flow-volume loops plot flow and volume on different axes. Expiratory portion of the loop helps assess the effectiveness of bronchodilator therapy.

   (f) Continuous airway pressure monitoring (CAPM)

     (1) Allows continuous monitoring of waveforms integrated with hemodynamic monitoring

     (2) Useful as a backup to monitor system disconnects

     (3) Zeroing should occur with initial setup and any disconnection

     (4) Damping of the waveform occurs with fluid in the tubing or leaks; check for disconnects and leaks, clear the tubing by flushing with an air-filled syringe

3. **Appraisal of patient characteristics:** Patients with acute, life-threatening pulmonary problems may present in critical care units with an array of clinical findings that represent the highest priority of patient needs. Their clinical course may resolve quickly, slowly, or not at all. Important clinical features that the nurse needs to assess when providing care for these patients include the following:

  a. Resiliency

    i. Level 1—*Minimally resilient:* A malnourished 82-year-old man, disabled by a series of strokes, is admitted with smoke inhalation and partial thickness burns

    ii. Level 3—*Moderately resilient:* A 45-year-old tourist has a near-drowning episode when he falls overboard from a cruise ship after heavy alcohol intake and celebratory dancing

    iii. Level 5—*Highly resilient:* An adolescent female who received plastic surgery as a high school graduation present is now febrile, with rapid, shallow respirations and a rising white blood cell (WBC) count, and continues to refuse to cough, deep breathe, or ambulate postoperatively

b. Vulnerability

 i. Level 1—*Highly vulnerable:* A 62-year-old engineer with lung cancer remains intubated following thoracotomy for evacuation of a large pleural effusion. Radiation therapy has not been successful.

 ii. Level 3—*Moderately vulnerable:* A 32-year-old day care provider, who is 5 ft 2 inches tall and weighs 394 lb, is being admitted for possible aspiration during extubation following appendectomy

 iii. Level 5—*Minimally vulnerable:* An otherwise healthy 47-year-old woman who suffered steering wheel contusion 72 hours earlier when she rear-ended another car has no fractures or cardiac contusion

c. Stability

 i. Level 1—*Minimally stable:* A 28-year-old roofer who suffered severe blunt chest trauma, multiple rib fractures with flail chest, hemothorax, and severe blood loss is admitted with an intermittently audible systolic pressure of 62 mm Hg measured via Doppler ultrasonography

 ii. Level 3—*Moderately stable:* A 67-year-old patient with type 1 diabetes mellitus and hypertension hospitalized with viral pneumonia shows slowly improving ABG levels following extubation

 iii. Level 5—*Highly stable:* A 42-year-old patient whose deep venous thrombosis has now resolved continues to complain of dyspnea

d. Complexity

 i. Level 1—*Highly complex:* An 18-year-old member of a street gang received multiple thoracic and abdominal stab wounds before he was dropped into a dumpster, where he remained overnight

 ii. Level 3—*Moderately complex:* A 60-year-old diabetic woman with severe rheumatoid arthritis complains of moderate chest pain and dyspnea shortly after arriving on a flight from Hong Kong

 iii. Level 5—*Minimally complex:* A patient newly diagnosed with asthma became acutely dyspneic when he toured a recently painted and carpeted apartment and could not get his inhaler to work

e. Resource availability

 i. Level 1—*Few resources:* A 58-year-old Vietnam veteran with chronic bronchiectasis is admitted following two episodes of hemoptysis. He does not qualify for Veterans Administration benefits, is estranged from his only sibling, and subsists on meals at the local shelter.

 ii. Level 3—*Moderate resources:* A 49-year-old cab driver recovering from ARDS after a motor vehicle crash will need continued pulmonary therapy after discharge. His son, a respiratory therapist, will visit his father twice daily to provide that care.

 iii. Level 5—*Many resources:* The wife of a 67-year-old architect who developed ARF when influenza was superimposed on his COPD has contacted a home care coordinator to make any necessary care arrangements

f. Participation in care

 i. Level 1—*No participation:* A 43-year-old woman in a persistent vegetative state requires ventilatory support

 ii. Level 3—*Moderate level of participation:* A nursing home resident recovering from community-acquired pneumonia is eager to ambulate and use the incentive spirometer but requires assistance with the former and repeated instruction in the latter

      iii. Level 5—*Full participation:* A 37-year-old science teacher who suffered toxic inhalation injury when a student inadvertently "blew up the lab" plans to develop lessons that demonstrate what happened to him and how his treatments facilitate his recovery

  g. Participation in decision making

      i. Level 1—*No participation:* A patient is in fulminant ARDS after falling from scaffolding five stories high 16 days earlier

      ii. Level 3—*Moderate level of participation:* A patient who underwent lung transplantation 48 hours earlier is making a concerted yet not fully effective effort postoperatively to perform the self-care she demonstrated preoperatively

      iii. Level 5—*Full participation:* A generation X software sales representative whose pulmonary embolism was recognized and treated in time requests the intranet programs related to the prevention of deep venous thrombosis

  h. Predictability

      i. Level 1—*Not predictable:* A 66-year-old passenger involved in a train derailment shows blunt head trauma, crushing chest injuries, fractured pelvis, and no discernible inspiratory effort

      ii. Level 3—*Moderately predictable:* A high school football player requires open reduction of a compound fracture of the left clavicle as well as rib fractures with pneumothorax

      iii. Level 5—*Highly predictable:* A 74-year-old former smoker develops pneumonia whenever a new strain of influenza appears

4. Diagnostic studies

  a. Laboratory

      i. Sputum examination

         (a) Obtain a specimen through voluntary coughing and expectoration, induction of sputum by inhalation of an aerosol, nasotracheal or endotracheal suctioning, transtracheal aspiration, or bronchoscopy

         (b) Assess characteristics: Compare to the patient's normal state

            (1) Color and consistency: Green—*Pseudomonas* infection; yellow—bacterial infection; rust colored—pneumococcal infection

            (2) Volume: More than 25 ml/day is excessive

            (3) Odor: Should be odorless

               a) Foul smell may indicate an anaerobic putrefactive process

               b) Musty odor may indicate *Pseudomonas* infection

            (4) Microscopic examination

               a) Cytologic study for malignant cells

               b) Smear for examination for bacteria (e.g., Gram stain) or fungi

               c) Sputum cultures to diagnose infection and assess drug resistance

               d) Stains on cultures for mycobacteria (acid-fast bacilli), *Pneumocystis carinii, Legionella pneumophila*

      ii. Pleural fluid examination

         (a) Diagnostic thoracentesis or pleural biopsy is performed to obtain a specimen

         (b) Determination of whether the fluid is a transudate or an exudate is based on the protein and lactate dehydrogenase (LDH) levels in the pleural fluid and blood

         (c) Specimen is examined for cell counts, protein and LDH levels, glucose level, amylase level, and pH; Gram staining for bacteria is performed; cytologic analysis for malignant cells and microorganisms is conducted

         (d) Biopsy of parietal pleura may be performed

        iii. Skin tests

           (a) Type I hypersensitivity (mediated by immunoglobulin E): To pollens, molds, grass

           (b) Type II hypersensitivity (mediated by T lymphocytes): Purified protein derivative testing for TB

           (c) Fungal diseases

           (d) As controls to assess anergy: Mumps, *Candida* infection

        iv. Serologic tests are used to determine the causative pathogen in bacterial, viral, mycotic, and parasitic diseases

    b. Radiologic

        i. Chest radiographic examination precedes all other studies

           (a) Posteroanterior and lateral views most common

           (b) Portable anteroposterior views are obtained in the intensive care unit (ICU) when the patient cannot be moved. These radiographs are generally of lesser quality than an erect posteroanterior film for the following reasons:

               (1) Difficulty in positioning the patient

               (2) Short film distance from the chest; variable distances in serial films

               (3) Less powerful x-ray generator; interference from attached tubes, lines, equipment

           (c) Lateral decubitus views are used if fluid levels need to be identified (as with pleural effusions and abscesses)

           (d) Oblique views may be used to localize lesions and infiltrates

           (e) Lordotic views are used to evaluate the apical portion of the lung and the middle lobe or lingula and can help determine whether a lesion is anterior or posterior

           (f) Expiratory films are used for visualizing pneumothorax or air trapping

        ii. Fluoroscopy

           (a) Shows the movement of pulmonary and cardiac structures and the diaphragm, localizes pulmonary lesions

           (b) Used to monitor during special procedures—catheter or chest tube insertion, bronchoscopy, thoracentesis

           (c) Exposure of the patient to radiation is greater during fluoroscopy than during a standard radiographic examination

        iii. Tomography: Provides views at different planes through the lungs

           (a) Gives better definition of small or questionable lesions; particularly useful for determining whether a lesion has calcification. Plain tomography is rarely used.

           (b) Computed tomography (CT) scan: All chest CTs are spiral CTs now

               (1) To scan axial cross sections of the body

               (2) Particularly useful in detecting subtle differences in tissue density

               (3) High-resolution CT (HRCT) for three-dimensional images of the lung to detect a pattern of emphysema, progression of fibrosis

        iv. Magnetic resonance imaging (MRI)

           (a) Can distinguish tumors from other structures, such as blood vessels, spinal cord, and bronchial walls

           (b) Can differentiate pleural thickening, pleural fluid, and chest wall tumors from each other

        v. Pulmonary angiography: Visualizes the pulmonary arterial tree through the injection of radiopaque dye

           (a) Useful to investigate thromboembolic disease of the lung, congenital circulatory abnormalities, masses

      (b) Some risks; dangerous to perform in pulmonary hypertension; O_2 desaturation has occurred in some patients with the injection of contrast medium. Hemodynamic parameters should be measured before the procedure.

    vi. Ventilation-perfusion lung scanning

      (a) Involves injection or inhalation of radioisotopes; performed to obtain information on pulmonary blood flow and ventilation

      (b) Can detect pulmonary emboli and assess regional lung function preoperatively

    vii. Ultrasonography

      (a) Useful in evaluating pleural disease

      (b) Can detect small amounts of pleural fluid and loculations within the pleural space

      (c) Can distinguish fluid from pleural thickening

      (d) Can localize the diaphragm and detect disease immediately below it, such as a subphrenic abscess

      (e) Not useful for defining structures or lesions within the pulmonary parenchyma (the ultrasonic beam penetrates air poorly)

c. Pulmonary function studies: See Box 2-3 and Figure 2-19

d. Lung biopsy

    i. Needle biopsy is used for the diagnosis of malignancy or infection; pneumothorax may be a complication

    ii. Open lung biopsy requires a thoracotomy or thoracoscopic examination but has better diagnostic yields

e. Bronchoscopy: Insertion of a fiberoptic scope into the airways for direct visualization and possible obtaining of specimens

    i. Indicated for diagnosis of lung malignancy, evaluation of hemoptysis, removal of foreign body or secretions, and sampling of lung tissue via washings, brushings, or biopsy

    ii. After the procedure, the patient must be observed for respiratory depression (due to sedatives), decreased ventilation, and hypoxemia

    iii. Supplemental O_2 is administered during the procedure

    iv. If transbronchial biopsy is performed, hemoptysis or pneumothorax is a possible complication

f. Mediastinoscopy is performed for the diagnostic exploration of the mediastinum and to obtain biopsy specimens

Patient Care

1. Inability to establish or maintain a patent airway

a. Description of problem: Blocked airway due to physiologic or mechanical obstruction and the inability of the patient to clear or maintain the airway. Clinical findings vary with the degree of obstruction and include abnormal breath sounds, altered respiratory rate or depth, cough, cyanosis (late), dyspnea.

b. Goals of care

    i. Airway patency is maintained

    ii. Breath sounds are clear with no adventitious sounds

    iii. Secretions are easily expectorated or suctioned

c. Collaborating professionals on health care team: Nurse, physician, anesthesiologist, respiratory therapist

d. Interventions

    i. Assist the patient to deep breathe

■ **BOX 2-3**
■ **PULMONARY FUNCTION STUDIES**

PURPOSE
- Classify pulmonary function as normal or exhibiting a restrictive or obstructive defect
- Describe disease early and in physiologic terms
- Follow the patient in quantitative terms for future comparisons
- Assist in evaluation of the risk of surgery

LUNG VOLUMES AND CAPACITIES
- Measured with the patient in the upright position; values obtained are compared with predicted values (see Figure 2-19)
- Volumes: There are four discrete and nonoverlapping lung volumes
  1. Tidal volume (V_T): Volume of gas inspired and expired during each respiratory cycle
  2. Inspiratory reserve volume (IRV): Maximal volume of gas that can be inspired after a tidal breath is taken
  3. Expiratory reserve volume (ERV): Maximal volume of gas that can be expired from the end-expiratory position
  4. Residual volume (RV): Volume of gas remaining in the lungs at end of a maximal expiration
- Capacities: There are four capacities, each of which includes two or more of the primary volumes
  1. Total lung capacity (TLC): Volume of gas contained in the lung at the end of a maximal inspiration

$$TLC = V_T + IRV + ERV + RV$$

  2. Vital capacity (VC): Maximal volume of gas that can be expelled from the lungs following a maximal inspiration

$$VC = V_T + IRV + ERV$$

  3. Inspiratory capacity (IC): Maximal volume of gas that can be inspired from the resting expiratory level

$$IC = V_T + IRV$$

  4. Functional residual capacity (FRC): Volume of gas remaining in the lungs at resting end expiration

$$FRC = ERV + RV$$

VENTILATORY MECHANICS
- Provide information about dynamic lung function. Subjects perform forced breathing maneuvers.
- Forced expiratory spirograms
  FVC: Forced vital capacity; reduced in restrictive disease or in obstructive disease if there is air trapping
  FEV_t: Forced expiratory volume in t (seconds); usually measured at 0.5, 1, and 3 seconds. Reduced in obstructive disease. Most useful measurements are FEV_1 and FEV_6.
  $FEV_1/VC\%$: Forced expiratory volume at 1 second as a percentage of vital capacity. Evaluates obstruction to flow. FEV_1/VC: Normally >75% in adults.
  FEF: Forced expiratory flows ($FEF_{25\%-75\%}$, $FEF_{75\%-85\%}$). These tests assess flows over a range of lung volumes.
  Values for timed flow studies are decreased out of proportion to vital capacity in obstructive disease
- Flow-volume loop studies: Volume and flow during inspiration and expiration are graphically plotted. Obstructive disease produces abnormal flow-volume loops; restrictive disease produces normal-appearing but smaller flow-volume loops.

Continued

■ **BOX 2-3**
■ **PULMONARY FUNCTION STUDIES—cont'd**

VENTILATORY MECHANICS—cont'd
- Maximum voluntary ventilation (MVV)
  - Volume of air ventilated with maximal effort over a short period of time
  - May be used to predict the patient's ability to undergo procedures that require ventilatory reserve (i.e., surgery, extubation)

LUNG COMPLIANCE STUDIES
- Assess the distensibility of the lungs; lung compliance (C_L) is the reciprocal of elastance
- Expressed as the increase in volume (V) per increase in transpulmonary pressure (P)

$$C_L = \frac{\Delta V}{\Delta P}$$

- Static compliance (C_{st}) is measured in the absence of airflow
  - In the patient on a ventilator, it is measured by dividing V_T by the plateau pressure (minus positive end-expiratory pressure [PEEP]) and is called the *effective static compliance*
  - Normal values are around 100 ml/cm H_2O
- Dynamic compliance (C_{dyn}) is measured under conditions of flow
  - In patients on a ventilator, it is measured by dividing V_T by the peak inspiratory pressure (minus PEEP) and is called the *effective dynamic compliance*
  - Normal range is between 40 and 50 ml/cm H_2O
- Compliance is decreased in conditions that make the lungs or thorax stiffer or reduce expansibility. Such conditions include atelectasis, pneumonia, pulmonary edema, fibrotic changes, pleural effusion, pneumothorax, kyphoscoliosis, obesity, abdominal distention, flail chest, and splinting due to pain.
- Increases in compliance occur with age or emphysema
- Compliance curves (serial changes in volume plotted against changes in pressure) are useful in monitoring patients on volume ventilators. Determinations of the best pressure-volume combinations for the patient may be made. Comparisons of static and dynamic pressure-volume curves help to determine which component (airway, lung, or chest wall) is contributing to changes in compliance.

GAS TRANSFER AND EXCHANGE STUDIES
- Blood gas and acid-base analysis
  - Fundamental to the diagnosis and management of pulmonary problems
  - See Physiologic Anatomy
- Diffusing capacity (D_L)
  - Measures the amount of functioning alveolar-capillary surface area available for gas exchange
  - Values decrease with ventilation-perfusion mismatching and membrane problems and with decreases in pulmonary capillary blood volume

GUIDELINES FOR INTERPRETATION OF PULMONARY FUNCTION TEST RESULTS
- Values are compared with predicted values for age, height, and gender
- Restrictive pulmonary impairment generally results in decreased volumes and capacities
- Decreased static lung compliance suggests parenchymal disease
- Obstructive defect generally results in decreased values on tests of dynamic ventilatory function. This change may be reversible with the use of bronchodilators.
- Chronic obstructive pulmonary disease with long-term air trapping and destruction of parenchyma results in increased FRC, RV, and TLC
- Patient preparation and cooperation are necessary to obtain reliable and valid data for most pulmonary function tests

      (a) Position to maximize inspiratory muscle length and to maximize ventilation (semi-Fowler's to high Fowler's position, depending on patient comfort)

      (b) Ask the patient to take slow, deep breaths; assess volume (i.e., functional residual capacity [FRC] to total lung capacity [TLC]); ask the patient to hold the breath several seconds

      (c) Provide the patient with cues or devices to motivate independent deep-breathing exercises (e.g., incentive spirometer)

  ii. Position the patient to facilitate coughing

      (a) Help the patient assume a comfortable cough position (high Fowler's), with knees bent and a lightweight pillow over the abdomen to augment the expiratory pressures and minimize discomfort

      (b) Teach the patient alternate cough techniques (controlled cough, the forced expiratory technique known as "huff coughing" or quad-assist cough). For controlled cough, the patient takes a slow maximal inspiration, holds the breath for several seconds, and follows with two or three coughs. Huff cough consists of one or two forced exhalations (huffs) from middle to low lung volumes with the glottis open.

      (c) Guaifenesin (an expectorant) may help to liquefy secretions

  iii. Provide an artificial airway and ventilation if indicated

      (a) Oropharyngeal airway

          (1) Maintains the airway by holding the tongue anteriorly

          (2) Technique: Correct size measures from the corner of the patient's mouth to the angle of the jaw following the natural curve of the airway. Apply a jaw lift to help displace the tongue. Rotate the airway 180 degrees before insertion. As the tip of the airway reaches the hard palate, rotate the airway again by 180 degrees, aligning it as before in the pharynx.

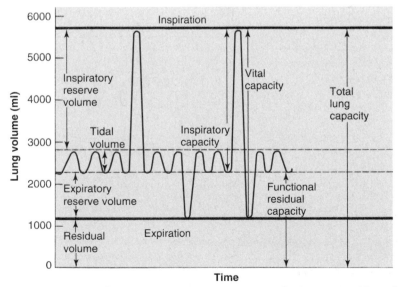

FIGURE 2-19 ■ Diagram showing respiratory excursions during normal breathing and during maximal inspiration and maximal expiration. (From Guyton AC, Hall JC: *Textbook of medical physiology,* ed 9, Philadelphia, 1996, Saunders, p 483.)

      (3) Complications: Vomiting and aspiration with an intact gag reflex; malpositioning due to improper length; worsening of obstruction by pushing the tongue back further into the pharynx due to incorrect placement

   (b) Nasopharyngeal airway

      (1) Purpose: Useful in facial and jaw fractures when an oral airway cannot be used; more readily tolerated than the oropharyngeal airway

      (2) Complications: Nosebleed, nasal mucosa irritation

      (3) Adequate humidification is essential to ensure the patency of a narrow lumen

      (4) Airway should be taped in place to prevent inadvertent displacement. Tube should be removed periodically to prevent skin breakdown.

   (c) Cricothyroidotomy: Restricted to extreme emergencies when other methods fail or are unavailable. Incision must be made through the cricothyroid membrane.

   (d) Laryngeal mask airway (Figure 2-20)

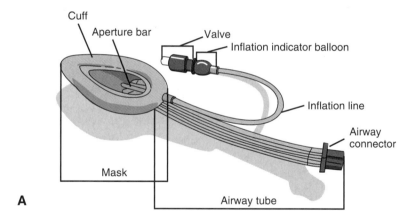

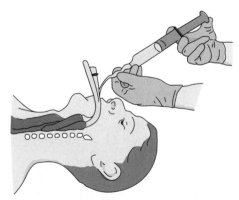

FIGURE 2-20 ■ **A,** Laryngeal Mask Airway (LMA). **B,** Placement of LMA. (Courtesy LMA North America, San Diego, Calif.)

(1) For use by experienced, trained physicians only—usually an anesthesiologist

(2) Can be used with spontaneous respirations or mechanical ventilation

(3) Laryngeal mask airway sits tightly over the larynx

(4) Disadvantages: Suctioning is difficult, may not prevent aspiration, the patient may dislodge it if agitated

(e) Esophageal obturator airway and esophageal gastric obturator airway: Generally not used because of the potential for complications and lack of experience in practice

(f) Endotracheal intubation: See Box 2-4 and Figure 2-21

(g) Tracheostomy

(1) Purpose and indications

a) To facilitate removal of secretions from the tracheobronchial tree

b) To decrease dead space ventilation

c) To bypass an upper airway obstruction or provide an alternate airway

d) To prevent or limit the aspiration of oral or gastric secretions (cuffed tubes)

e) To aid in patient comfort when assisted or controlled ventilation is needed for an extended period of time

(2) Principles of care

a) Stoma is kept clean and dry

b) Frequency of inner cannula tube exchanges with disposable tubes and of routine cleaning of inner cannulas with reusable inner cannulas follows hospital or institutional guidelines

1) Be prepared for complications during any cleaning procedure

2) Keep the following equipment at the bedside:

   a) Self-inflating manual resuscitation bag and mask

   b) Suction equipment (include catheters, O_2 flowmeter, tubing)

   c) Intubation materials

   d) Tracheal tube and stoma cleaning supplies

3) Be prepared to intubate or otherwise support ventilation

4) Have an extra tracheostomy tube of the same size and type at the bedside; keep a tube obturator at the bedside in case the tube must be reinserted emergently

c) *Uncuffed tubes* are commonly used in children and adults with laryngectomies and are sometimes used during decannulation or weaning (progressive downsizing of tube)

d) *Cuffed tubes* are typically used when the patient is receiving artificial ventilation (Figure 2-22). Tube may have an air filled or self-inflating foam cuff, depending on the brand.

e) Suctioning is always a sterile procedure except at home, where a clean technique may be used

(3) Weaning from the tracheostomy tube

a) Criteria (see discussion of extubation criteria in Box 2-4)

b) Patient must demonstrate physiologic and psychologic independence from an artificial airway. Techniques include the use of the following:

1) Cuff deflation periods, with the tube opening capped to allow breathing through the upper airway

2) Tracheostomy button

■ BOX 2-4
■ ENDOTRACHEAL INTUBATION AND EXTUBATION

KEY PRINCIPLES FOR INTUBATION
- Thorough training and retraining in this procedure are absolute necessities for competency
- Preoxygenate with 100% O_2 for at least 2 minutes if possible
- Check for correct placement of the tube after insertion (see Figure 2-21)
  1. Feel air movement through the tube opening
  2. Assess for bilateral chest excursion during inspiration and expiration
  3. Auscultate both sides of the chest peripherally as well as the abdomen
  4. Use an exhaled CO_2 detector-monitor or esophageal balloon to confirm lung versus esophagus placement
  5. Obtain a chest radiograph (gold standard); tip of the tube should be about 2 to 3 cm above the carina
  6. Provide manual ventilation using a self-inflating resuscitation bag connected to a 100% O_2 source set at 10 to 15 L/min

NASOTRACHEAL INTUBATION
- Sometimes used when the oral route is not available
- Risk of paranasal sinusitis as well as bleeding is increased
- Should not be used if the patient has a bleeding abnormality

NURSING CARE CONSIDERATIONS FOR THE INTUBATED PATIENT
- Provide frequent mouth care including dental care (absolutely necessary)
- Check the placement of the tube immediately after insertion and after tube position adjustments
- Carefully secure the tube to prevent movement and to decrease tracheal damage
- Provide adequate humidity regardless of whether nasal or oral intubation is used
- Assess the oral mucosa at least daily and move oral tubes from side to side when necessary. Note and document the centimeter marking on the tube at the teeth or gum line as a reference point.
- Be aware that infection may result from contaminated equipment or nonsterile procedures
- Suction as required according to the patient's need, not at a routine interval. Use a sterile technique.
  1. Use either a single-use or closed-suction catheter system, depending on hospital policy
  2. Provide presuctioning and postsuctioning oxygenation with three to five deep inflations of 100% O_2 for 30 seconds using either the manual two-handed technique or the manual demand breath by ventilator
  3. Keep the duration of suctioning brief (10 to 15 seconds) to minimize the amount of O_2-containing air that is evacuated from the lungs; apply suction only when withdrawing the catheter
  4. Monitor the electrocardiogram for arrhythmias during and after suctioning; observe for changes in O_2 saturation by pulse oximetry if available
  5. Observe and document the amount and type of secretions
- For a prolonged intubation procedure, the person performing the intubation may instill lidocaine into the tube or inject it onto the vocal cords to increase patient tolerance

TRACHEAL TUBE CUFFS
- Cuff design characteristics
  - Low sealing pressure; intracuff pressure should not exceed the capillary filling pressure of the trachea (≤25 cm H_2O or ≤20 mm Hg) to avoid tracheal mucosal injury
  - Cuff pressure is distributed over a large contact area
  - Large volumes of air are accepted with minor increases in balloon tension
  - Provides sufficient pressure to maintain an adequate seal during inspiration and expiration (necessary to allow positive pressure ventilation and the use of positive end-expiratory pressure [PEEP]). Also may help prevent pulmonary aspiration of large food particles but does not protect against aspiration of liquids, such as water and enteral formula feedings.
  - Does not distort tracheal wall
- Low-pressure, high-volume cuffs generally meet the desired characteristics and have replaced low-residual-volume, high-pressure cuffs

Continued

- Special cuffs (e.g., Fome-cuf, Bivona) are available for both endotracheal and tracheal tubes (see Figure 2-22). These devices inflate passively to fill a spongelike cuff which produces little or no pressure against the trachea. May be difficult to maintain a seal with positive pressure ventilation and increased PEEP or peak pressures.
- Principles of cuff inflation and deflation
  - Inflation of low-pressure cuffs:
    Inflate with sufficient air to ensure no leak (minimal occlusive volume technique) or only minimal leak during peak inspiration (minimal leak technique).
    Need for increasing amounts of air to obtain a seal may be due to tracheal dilation or to a leak in the cuff or pilot balloon valve; the condition should be corrected
  - Routine deflation is not necessary. Periodic deflation may be useful so that the patient can breathe around the tube to facilitate speech (often difficult to accomplish when the patient is receiving mechanical ventilation).
  - Regardless of cuff design or pressure characteristics, all cuff pressures should be routinely measured at least every 8 to 12 hours and whenever the cuff is reinflated or the tube position is changed

KEY PRINCIPLES FOR EXTUBATION

- Extubation will depend on whether or not the underlying patient condition that led to the need for intubation has improved or reversed to the extent that the artificial airway is no longer necessary. Generally accepted criteria for extubation include the following:
  - Stable vital signs and hemodynamic parameters without vasopressor support
  - Patient awake and alert
  - Absence of copious secretions
  - Ventilatory parameters or measurements (such as maximum inspiratory pressure and negative inspiratory force, spontaneous tidal volume, minute ventilation, and vital capacity) within acceptable limits
- Postextubation monitoring
  1. Repeat blood gas studies 30 minutes after extubation or sooner as indicated and periodically thereafter
  2. Observe for laryngospasm. Auscultate the trachea with a stethoscope for stridor and breathing difficulties. Treatment may consist of racemic epinephrine inhalation, administration of steroids to reduce laryngeal edema, and possibly reintubation.
  3. Postextubation stridor may occur immediately or take several hours to develop
  4. Monitor the patient's tolerance of extubation by clinical observation, auscultation of breath sounds, measurement of arterial blood gas levels, observation for stridor, and ventilatory measurements

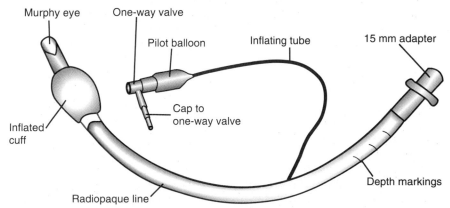

FIGURE 2-21 ■ Components of the endotracheal tube. (From Kirsten LD: *Comprehensive respiratory nursing: a decision making approach,* Philadelphia, 1989, Saunders, p 637.)

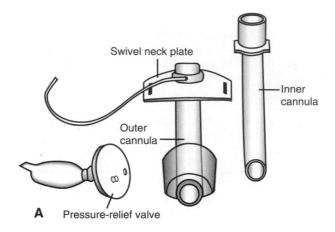

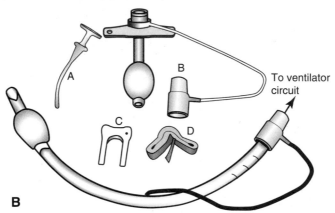

FIGURE 2-22 ■ Tracheostomy tubes. **A,** Shiley tracheostomy tube with disposable inner cannula. **B,** Bivona foam-cuffed tubes. *A,* Obturator; *B,* sideport airway connector; *C,* wedge; *D,* fabric tape. (From Kirsten LD: *Comprehensive respiratory nursing: a decision making approach,* Philadelphia, 1989, Saunders, pp 656, 659.)

        3) Fenestrated tube with the cuff inflated or deflated, with the external tube opening capped or occluded to permit airflow to be directed to the upper airway

        4) Progressive downsizing of the tube from the original size to a smaller one

    c) Patient is monitored carefully to see how weaning is tolerated; blood gas studies and clinical observations are used

    d) Complete sealing of the tracheotomy incision may occur within 72 hours of extubation. Patients cannot produce adequate coughing pressure until this is accomplished.

  iv. Prevent complications of airway intubation: See Box 2-5

e. Evaluation of patient care

  i. Breath sounds are clear bilaterally with no adventitious sounds

  ii. Patient is able to expectorate or suction secretions

  iii. ABG levels and ventilatory parameters are within acceptable limits

  iv. Patient or caregiver is able to care for the artificial airway

■ **BOX 2-5**
■ **PREVENTION OF COMPLICATIONS OF AIRWAY INTUBATION**

PHYSIOLOGIC ALTERATIONS CAUSED BY AIRWAY DIVERSION
- Inspired air is inadequately conditioned and is irritating to delicate pulmonary membranes
- Plastic or metal tubes are foreign bodies; they cause greater mucus production and impair ciliary movement
- Accumulated oral bacteria and secretions provide a good medium for bacterial growth and may precipitate ventilator-associated pneumonia
- Bypassing the larynx produces aphonia
- Eliminating the glottis from the air route prevents the development of increased intrathoracic pressures, which makes effective coughing difficult

COMPLICATIONS DURING PLACEMENT OF THE AIRWAY
ENDOTRACHEAL TUBE
- Mucous membrane disruption and tooth damage or dislodgment
- Right main-stem bronchial intubation; tube must be repositioned immediately
  - Decreased or absent breath sounds on the left side
  - Decreased arterial partial pressure of oxygen (Pao_2) or arterial O_2 saturation by pulse oximetry (Spo_2)
  - Arrhythmias, including pulseless electrical activity
  - Shift of the trachea to the left (late)
- With the nasotracheal route, one may see the following:
  - Nosebleed
  - Submucosal dissection
  - Introduction of a polyp or plug from the nose into the lungs, which results in infection or obstruction
  - Sinusitis

TRACHEOSTOMY AND CRICOTHYROTOMY
(Problems are fewer and less severe with tracheostomy if it is an elective procedure done in the operating room.)
- Mediastinal emphysema
- Hemorrhage
- Pneumothorax
- Cardiac arrest
- Damage to adjacent structures in the neck

COMPLICATIONS OCCURRING WHILE THE TUBE IS IN PLACE
OBSTRUCTION DUE TO
- Plugging with secretions that have become dried and inspissated; this is entirely preventable by systemic hydration and proper use of humidification and suctioning
- Herniation of the cuff over the end of the tube
- Kinking of the tube
- Cuff overinflation

DISPLACEMENT OR DISLODGEMENT
Displacement or dislodgement out of the trachea (endotracheal or tracheostomy tube) and inadvertent movement into a false passage or pretracheal space (tracheostomy tube)
- Especially hazardous during the first 3 to 5 days of tracheostomy. Avoid by using a tube of the proper length and fixing it securely to the patient. Although securing the tube is important, care of the stoma and surrounding skin to prevent skin breakdown or pressure sores from the tube neck plate is also important.
- Dislodgement out of the trachea into tissue causes mediastinal emphysema, subcutaneous emphysema, and pneumothorax. Diagnosis is determined by observation of reduced or absent airflow movement from the tube opening, deterioration in blood gas values and/or

Continued

■ **BOX 2-5**
■ **PREVENTION OF COMPLICATIONS OF AIRWAY INTUBATION—cont'd**

DISPLACEMENT OR DISLODGEMENT—cont'd
vital signs, observations of neck and local tissue swelling with crepitations by palpation, poor chest excursion and respiratory distress, and inability to pass a suction catheter properly through the tube.
■ Low tube placement into one bronchus or at the level of the carina results in obstruction or atelectasis of the nonventilated lung. Check the placement of the endotracheal tube by auscultation, followed by radiographic examination or use of a fiberoptic scope.
  ● Displacement into one bronchus: Signs and symptoms are as follows:
    Decreased or delayed motion on one side of the chest
    Unilateral diminished breath sounds
    Excessive coughing
    Localized expiratory wheeze
■ Placement at the level of the carina: Signs and symptoms are as follows:
  ● Excessive coughing
  ● Localized expiratory wheeze
  ● Difficulty in introducing the suction catheter
  ● Bilateral diminished breath sounds

OTHER COMPLICATIONS
■ Poor oral hygiene; mouth care is absolutely essential
■ Local infection of tracheostomy wound, tracheal tissue, or lungs; tracheostomy should be treated as a surgical wound and specimens for culture should be obtained if active infection is suspected
■ Massive hemorrhage resulting from erosion of the tracheostomy tube into the innominate vessels; may be fatal. Occurs most often with low placement of the tube, excessive "riding" of the tube within the trachea, or pulling torsion on the tube; watch for pulsations moving the tube with the heartbeat.
■ Disconnection between the tracheal tube and ventilator
  ● Most likely to occur when the patient is being turned
  ● All ventilators must have adequate alarms
  ● Frequent checking of all connections should be routine
■ Leaks caused by broken or malfunctioning cuff balloon or pilot valve
  ● Diagnosis is confirmed by the ability of a previously aphonic patient to talk, detection of air movement at the nose and mouth, pressure changes on the ventilator, and decreased exhaled volumes as measured with a hand-held portable respirometer or ventilator spirometer
  ● Tube must be removed and replaced. Always check the cuff for leaks before inserting; note the cuff pressure and amount of air required to fill the cuff and compare with later values.
■ Tracheal ischemia, necrosis, dilation
  ● Because of the oval shape of the trachea and the round shape of the tube, there is a tendency for erosion in the anterior and posterior trachea
  ● Diagnosis is indicated by the necessity to use larger and larger amounts of air to inflate the balloon to maintain the seal
  ● May progress to tracheoesophageal fistula; this is indicated if food is aspirated through the trachea or air is in the stomach or if the results of a methylene blue dye test are positive
  ● Prevention is through the use of low-pressure cuffs and routine monitoring of cuff pressures

EARLY POSTEXTUBATION COMPLICATIONS
ACUTE LARYNGEAL EDEMA
■ Most frequently seen in children
■ In adults, is commonly associated with the use of an oversized tube or with preexisting inflammation of the upper airway

Continued

- Prevention
  - Close observation for several hours after extubation
  - Patient may require supplemental O_2 following prolonged intubation; use of a bland aerosol, such as highly humidified air via a face mask or face tent, is controversial and of no proven benefit
- Treatment
  - Oxygen, steroids
  - Introduction of a smaller endotracheal tube, tracheotomy
  - Racemic epinephrine administered via small volume nebulizer; intent is to reduce subglottic edema by inhalation of a potent vasoconstrictor

HOARSENESS

- Common following either short-term or long-term endotracheal intubation
- Usually disappears during the first week

ASPIRATION

Aspiration of food, saliva, or gastric contents if the swallowing mechanism is impaired

- Presence of the tube over extended periods results in a loss of the usual protective reflexes of the larynx
- Monitor the patient carefully during feedings; watch for excessive coughing; start with clear liquids after tube removal

DIFFICULTY IN REMOVING THE TRACHEOSTOMY TUBE

- More frequently seen in infants but occurs in adults as well
- Related to the narrow lumen of the trachea, which is further reduced by swelling

LATE POSTEXTUBATION COMPLICATIONS

FIBROTIC STENOSIS OF THE TRACHEA

- Caused by prolonged use of any tube with a rigid inflatable cuff
- Follows earlier ulceration and necrosis of the site
- Lesions may become advanced before the appearance of clinical evidence (dyspnea, stridor); a tracheoesophageal fistula may form
- Prevented by the use of low-pressure cuffs and proper monitoring of cuff pressures

STENOSIS OF THE LARYNX

- Caused by the discrepancy between the anatomy of the larynx and the size and shape of the tube
- Treatment
  - Dilation or surgical intervention
  - Permanent tracheostomy

2. **Impaired respiratory mechanics**
   a. Description of problem: Patient is unable to maintain adequate oxygen supply due to structural impediments (e.g., airway constriction, closure, or obstruction by secretions; a flattened diaphragm; respiratory muscle fatigue; loss of structural integrity of the thoracic cage). Clinical findings may include dyspnea, tachypnea, fremitus, abnormal ABG values, cyanosis (late finding), cough, nasal flaring, use of accessory muscles of respiration, assumption of a three-point position or the use of pursed-lip breathing, prolonged expiratory phase, increased A-P chest diameter, and altered chest excursion.
   b. Goals of care
      i. Respiratory rate, tidal volume, and maximal inspiratory pressure are within normal limits for the patient
      ii. Dyspnea at rest is minimal; exertional dyspnea is decreased
      iii. Patient takes bronchodilator medications as prescribed

    iv. Patient is able to pace the activities of daily living (ADLs) in line with ventilatory function

  c. Collaborating professionals on health care team: Physician, pulmonologist, nurse, respiratory therapist, possibly physical or occupational therapist

  d. Interventions

    i. Teach pursed-lip breathing, abdominal stabilization, and directed or controlled coughing techniques to minimize the energy expenditure of respiratory muscles. Pursed-lip breathing forces the patient to breathe slowly and establishes a back pressure in the airway, which helps to stabilize the airway and diminish dyspnea, especially after exertion.

    ii. Evaluate the status of the inspiratory muscles and, if appropriate, initiate inspiratory muscle training

      (a) Inspiratory muscle training may improve the conscious control of the respiratory muscles and decrease the anxiety associated with increased respiratory effort

      (b) Improved respiratory muscle strength may improve exercise tolerance and decrease dyspnea

      (c) Monitor O_2 saturation via pulse oximetry as a measure of tolerance during training

    iii. Teach the patient medication names, doses, method of administration, schedule, and appropriate behavior should an adverse effect occur. Instruct in the consequences of improper use of medications.

      (a) β-agonists and anticholinergics are bronchodilators commonly prescribed to decrease airflow resistance and the work of breathing. Methylxanthines are less commonly prescribed but may also be used for COPD exacerbations.

      (b) Patient should be able to demonstrate the proper technique for MDI self-administration. Spacer may be attached to the MDI to optimize medication delivery. If technique is poor or the patient is unable to use an MDI, assess the need for an alternative delivery device, such as a small-volume nebulizer.

    iv. Teach the patient to modify ADLs within ventilatory limits

      (a) Encourage periodic hyperinflation of the lungs with a series of slow, deep breaths

      (b) Hyperinflation therapy helps to prevent atelectasis and reduced lung compliance by expanding the alveoli, which are partially closed, and by mobilizing airway secretions

    v. Monitor the rate and pattern of respiration, breath sounds, use of accessory muscles of respiration, and sensation of dyspnea. Clinical manifestations of respiratory muscle fatigue include the following:

      (a) Shallow, rapid breathing in early stages

      (b) Use of accessory muscles and a paradoxical breathing pattern

      (c) Active use of expiratory muscles, magnified sense of dyspnea

      (d) Respiratory alternans

  e. Evaluation of patient care

    i. Rate, depth, and pattern of ventilation are in the normal range for the patient

    ii. Patient reports decreased dyspnea at rest and with exertion

    iii. When inspiratory muscle training is appropriate, the patient's use of this training improves maximal inspiratory pressures

    iv. Patient demonstrates safe and correct inhalation of respiratory medications and identifies side effects to be reported

3. Impaired alveolar ventilation
  a. Description of problem: Inability to maintain spontaneous ventilation. Clinical findings include an ineffective breathing pattern, dyspnea, tachypnea or apnea, accessory muscle use, abnormal ABG levels, excess work of breathing.
  b. Goals of care
    i. Respiratory rate and breathing pattern are normal for the patient
    ii. ABG levels are within acceptable limits for the patient
    iii. Dyspnea is decreased with no air trapping at the end of expiration
    iv. No evidence of ventilator-related complications is apparent
  c. Collaborating professionals on health care team: Nurse, physician, anesthesiologist, respiratory therapist, infection control specialist, home care service aide
  d. Interventions
    i. Promote normal rest and sleep patterns. Plan activities to allow rest periods. Rest allows energy reserves to be replenished. Sleep deprivation blunts the patient's respiratory drive.
    ii. Provide an appropriate level of mechanical ventilatory support as warranted (Box 2-6 and Table 2-6)
    iii. Prevent the development of complications associated with the use of positive pressure ventilation (Box 2-7)
    iv. Provide optimal methods for weaning (also called *liberating*) patients from continuous mechanical ventilation
      (a) Indications for weaning or liberation (term usually reserved for the gradual withdrawal of ventilatory support, although it includes the overall process of discontinuing ventilator support)
        (1) Underlying disease process is resolved; original signs of the need for ventilatory support are no longer present
        (2) Patient's strength, vigor, and nutritional status are adequate
        (3) Patient does not require more than 5 cm H_2O of PEEP or an FIO_2 greater than 0.5 to maintain an acceptable PaO_2 (usually at least 55 to 60 mm Hg)
        (4) Patient has stable, acceptable hemodynamic parameters and Hb level
        (5) Patient has stable and acceptable values for ABGs, V_T, vital capacity, respiratory rate, minute ventilation, maximum inspiratory and expiratory pressures, A–a gradient or PaO_2/FIO_2 ratio, and compliance; V_D/V_T ratio is within minimal acceptable range (<0.6)
        (6) Level of consciousness is acceptable
        (7) Patient is psychologically prepared, emotionally ready, and cooperative
        (8) Predictors of successful weaning and criteria for liberation trial
          a) Resting minute volume ($\dot{V}_E$) of less than 10 L and ability to double this value during a maximum voluntary ventilation effort
          b) Maximum inspiratory pressure more negative than −20 cm H_2O
          c) Spontaneous V_T greater than 5 ml/kg
          d) Spontaneous respiratory frequency (f) equal to or less than 30 breaths/min
          e) Vital capacity above 10 ml/kg body weight
          f) PaO_2/FIO_2 ratio higher than 200
          g) f/V_T ratio less than 105 (rapid shallow breathing index)
          h) Acceptable scores on integrative indices such as the Burns Wean Assessment Program (BWAP), CROP index (*c*ompliance, *r*ate, *o*xygenation, *p*ressure)

Text continues on p. 120

■ **BOX 2-6**
■ **LEVELS OF VENTILATORY SUPPORT**

OBJECTIVES OF MECHANICAL VENTILATION
PHYSIOLOGIC OBJECTIVES
- To support or otherwise manipulate pulmonary gas exchange
  - Alveolar ventilation (e.g., arterial partial pressure of carbon dioxide [$Paco_2$] and pH)
  - Arterial oxygenation (e.g., partial pressure of oxygen [Pao_2], arterial oxygen saturation [Sao_2], and oxygen content [Cao_2])
- To increase lung volume
  - End-inspiratory lung inflation
  - Functional residual capacity
- To reduce or otherwise manipulate the work of breathing

CLINICAL OBJECTIVES
- To reverse hypoxemia
- To reverse acute respiratory acidosis
- To relieve respiratory distress
- To prevent or reverse atelectasis
- To reverse ventilatory muscle fatigue
- To permit sedation and/or neuromuscular blockade
- To decrease systemic or myocardial oxygen consumption
- To reduce intracranial pressure
- To stabilize the chest wall

MAJOR TYPES OF MECHANICAL VENTILATORS
(See Table 2-6 for ventilator types and modes.)

NEGATIVE EXTERNAL PRESSURE VENTILATORS
- These ventilators attempt to duplicate spontaneous breathing
- Entire body, up to the neck, is placed within an "iron lung" or tank respirator, while the head and neck protrude to the atmosphere. Beneath the tank, electrically powered bellows create subambient pressure within the tank.
- Intermittently applied negative pressure creates a pressure gradient that promotes air entry into the lungs. Minute ventilation (V_E) can be altered by changing the negative pressure (and thus the tidal volume) or the respiratory rate, but inspiratory flow rate cannot be adjusted.
- Use is restricted to patients who have normal lung parenchyma (e.g., patients with poliomyelitis)
- Modified approach to negative-pressure ventilation: Chest cuirass ventilator, consisting of a rigid shell or poncho wrap placed around the rib cage, with a hose attached to a vacuum pump that regulates the negative pressure setting as well as the ventilation rate
- Regardless of the type of negative pressure ventilator, failure to maintain a proper seal around the chest may result in inadequate alveolar ventilation

POSITIVE PRESSURE VENTILATORS
- Most common type of ventilatory support used in critical care. Apply positive pressure to the airways during the clinician-selected pattern of ventilation.
- Response of the breath delivery system to patient efforts
  - Triggering: Initiation of gas delivery. Significant ventilatory loads can be imposed by insensitive or unresponsive ventilator triggering systems. Oversensitive valves can result in spontaneous ventilator cycling independent of patient effort.
  - Gas delivery: Flow from the ventilator is governed (or limited) by a set flow (flow limited) or set pressure (pressure limited) on most machines
  - Cycling: Gas delivery can be terminated at a preset volume, time, or flow
- Response of patient efforts to ventilator settings
  - Alteration of the activity of mechanoreceptors in the airways, lungs, and chest wall
  - Alteration of arterial blood gas (ABG) values

Continued

- Elicitation of respiratory sensations in conscious or semiconscious patients
- Result is a change in rate (ventilatory demand), depth, and timing of respiratory efforts (synchrony between patient and ventilator) through neural reflexes, chemical (chemoreceptors), and behavioral responses

STANDARD MODES OF MECHANICAL VENTILATION

Modes of mechanical ventilation are classified according to initiation of the inspiratory cycle (see Figure 2-16)

- *Spontaneous respiration:* With most ventilators, the patient can breathe spontaneously through the ventilator circuit when the ventilator rate is set at zero. Positive airway pressure can be applied when the patient is breathing through the circuit.
- *Controlled mandatory ventilation (CMV):* Ventilator delivers a preset number of breaths per minute of a predetermined tidal volume. Patient cannot trigger additional breaths, so this mode may lead to patient apprehension and air hunger and therefore it is not used clinically. However, it may be used to provide complete control of ventilation in certain situations when the patient requires chemical sedation, paralysis, or both in order to gain total control of ventilation.
- *Assist control (A/C):* Every breath is supported by the ventilator. Backup control ventilatory rate is set, but the patient may choose any rate above the set rate. Most ventilators deliver A/C ventilation using volume-cycled or volume-targeted breaths. Pressure-limited or pressure-targeted A/C is available on certain ventilators.
- *Intermittent mandatory ventilation (IMV):* Mode of ventilation and weaning that combines a preset number of ventilator-delivered mandatory breaths of predetermined tidal volume with the capability for intermittent patient-generated spontaneous breaths. In a subtype of this mode, called *synchronized intermittent mandatory ventilation* (SIMV), a demand valve is incorporated into the IMV system that senses the start of a patient breath. The demand valve opens, and the mandatory breath is delivered in synchrony with the patient's effort.
- *Pressure support ventilation (PSV):* Pressure-targeted, flow-cycled mode of ventilation in which each breath must be triggered by the patient. Application of positive pressure to the airway is set by the clinician. This augmentation to inspiratory effort starts at the initiation of inhalation and typically ends when a minimum inspiratory flow rate is reached. There are two applications for this mode:
  1. Used in conjunction with SIMV to improve patient tolerance and decrease the work of spontaneous breaths, especially from demand-flow systems and endotracheal tubes with a narrow inner diameter
  2. Used as a stand-alone ventilatory mode for patients under consideration for weaning or during the stabilization period
- *Continuous positive airway pressure (CPAP):* Designed to elevate end-expiratory pressure to above atmospheric pressure to increase lung volume and oxygenation. All breaths are spontaneous, and therefore an intact respiratory drive is required. Can be used in intubated as well as nonintubated patients via a face or nasal mask. Depending on machine type, CPAP is delivered via a continuous flow or demand valve system.
- *Bilevel positive airway pressure* (BiPAP, Respironics, Inc.): This noninvasive ventilatory assist device employs a spontaneous breathing mode with the baseline pressure elevated above zero. Unlike CPAP, BiPAP allows separate regulation of inspiratory and expiratory pressures. Application of BiPAP is essentially a combination of PSV with CPAP. The differences between inspiratory and expiratory positive airway pressures (IPAP and EPAP, respectively) contribute to the total ventilation. Enhances the capabilities of home CPAP for obstructive sleep apnea to provide nocturnal support in a variety of restrictive and obstructive disorders. Affords a noninvasive means of augmenting alveolar ventilation in hypercapnic respiratory failure.

SERVO-CONTROLLED MODES OF MECHANICAL VENTILATION

Servo-controlled ventilation modes are used both for ventilating and for weaning patients from mechanical ventilators by incorporating a feedback system to control a specific variable within a narrow range

Continued

■ **BOX 2-6**
■ **LEVELS OF VENTILATORY SUPPORT—cont'd**

SERVO-CONTROLLED MODES OF MECHANICAL VENTILATION—cont'd

■ *Mandatory minute ventilation (MMV):* Ensures delivery of a preset minimum minute volume, with the patient allowed to breathe spontaneously. Should the patient's minute volume fall below an established level, mechanical breaths at a predetermined volume are delivered at a rate sufficient to reach the target level.

■ *Servo-controlled PSV:* Ventilatory support strategy in which the underlying mode is PSV and the targeted parameter is either respiratory rate or tidal volume. If the target level is not met, the ventilator modifies either the target pressure level or the cycling. Depending on the ventilator, these modalities can include volume-ensured pressure support (PS), pressure augmentation, volume support, and volume assisted breaths.

ALTERNATE MODES OF MECHANICAL VENTILATION

Some ventilatory support strategies are aimed at limiting or reducing lung inflation volumes and/or pressures to avoid ventilator-associated lung injury

■ *High-frequency ventilation:* Provides a faster respiratory rate (60 to 3000 breaths/min) and lower tidal volume (1 to 3 ml/kg) than other ventilator systems, to reduce barotrauma-volutrauma and cardiac depression. Three types of mechanical system are capable of delivering high-frequency ventilation:

High-frequency positive pressure ventilation (HFPPV): Time-cycled, volume-limited ventilation that delivers a preset tidal volume 60 to 100 times per minute

High-frequency jet ventilation (HFJV): Delivers jets of high-pressure gas through a small catheter in the trachea or an endotracheal tube at frequencies of 60 to 600 breaths/min

High-frequency oscillation (HFO): Moves a volume of gas to and fro in the airway, through laminar flow at rates of 600 to 3000 cycles/min (50 Hz) throughout the lungs

■ *Inverse-ratio ventilation (IRV):* Ventilatory support strategy that employs a prolonged inspiratory to expiratory ratio (I/E) greater than or equal to 1:1. Breath delivery is either pressure controlled (PC-IRV) or volume controlled (VC-IRV).

● Major function of prolonged inspiratory time is to allow for recruitment of alveolar units with long time constants

● Increase in mean airway pressure is key to the beneficial effects related to oxygenation as well as to potential adverse hemodynamic effects (decreased cardiac output)

● Because of the abnormal I/E ratio, patient dyssynchrony with the ventilator is common, and sedation and/or paralysis is usually required

● Development of auto–positive end-expiratory pressure (auto-PEEP) is common and should be routinely monitored; during PC-IRV, tidal volume varies according to respiratory mechanics

■ *Differential lung ventilation (DLV):* Each lung is ventilated independently. A double-lumen endobronchial tube is inserted, usually with the distal tip threaded into the left main-stem bronchus, which permits isolation of each lung for the purposes of mechanical ventilation.

● Typically, there are two separate ventilators; each has ventilator settings based on the degree of injury in each lung. Machine breaths are delivered synchronously or asynchronously, depending on the type of ventilator used.

● Meticulous care of the endobronchial tube is critical. Malposition may result in tracheal injury, and overinflation of the endobronchial tube cuff may result in bronchial rupture. Sedation or muscle paralysis may be required to avoid patient agitation and inadvertent tube movement. The tube is left in place for only a limited period of time.

● Independent lung ventilation outside the operating room setting is sometimes used for unilateral lung disorders unresponsive to conventional ventilation techniques. This modality is extremely labor intensive, and adequate room space is necessary because two ventilators are used.

■ Other modes have been tried experimentally and are listed in Table 2-6

Continued

GUIDELINES FOR VENTILATOR ADJUSTMENT DURING VOLUME-TARGETED (VOLUME-CYCLED) VENTILATION

All ventilator controls and settings are adjusted according to the patient's underlying disease process and the results of ABG analysis.

- *Minute ventilation:* Usually 6 to 10 L/min but may be much higher, depending on patient needs
- *Tidal volume:* Governed by estimated tidal volume; normally varies from 8 to 10 ml/kg ideal body weight to prevent lung overinflation and potential stretch injury to the lung tissue. Preset tidal volume may be reduced to 6 to 8 ml/kg. Intentional use of lower tidal volumes may cause an increase in arterial CO_2 levels and is therefore referred to as *permissive hypercapnia*. Low tidal volume has been shown to lower mortality in some settings. Use of intermittent sighs during mechanical ventilation is no longer routinely recommended.
- *Respiratory rate:* Varies from 8 to 12 breaths/min for most clinically stable patients; rates above 20 breaths/min are sometimes necessary
- *Flow rate:* Adjusted so that inspiratory volume delivery can be completed in a time frame that allows adequate time for exhalation. Inspiratory flow rate range of about 40 to 100 L/min is most commonly employed. Slow flow rates are preferred for optimal air distribution in normal lungs; faster flow rates are beneficial in patients with obstructive lung disease. Altering the flow rate may reduce the work of breathing, improve patient-ventilator synchrony, and increase the comfort of patients who are restless while undergoing mechanical ventilation.
- *I/E ratio:* Normal ratio is 1:2 to 1:3
- *Inspiratory flow* of gas from the ventilator: Depending on the model, can be delivered using one of several flow patterns, such as decelerating, square wave, or sine wave
- *Oxygen concentration:* Initially, the fraction of inspired oxygen (FIo_2) is deliberately set at a high value (often 1.0) to ensure adequate oxygenation. An ABG sample is obtained, and the FIo_2 is adjusted according to the patient's arterial partial pressure of oxygen (Pao_2) and Sao_2. Inspired partial pressure of O_2 is adjusted so that Pao_2 is acceptable for the patient's condition. This is usually a Pao_2 higher than 55 mm Hg or an Sao_2 of 88% or higher. Excessively high levels for prolonged periods can cause oxygen toxicity. The lowest FIo_2 that achieves an acceptable Pao_2 and Sao_2 should be used.
- *PEEP:* Used as appropriate to reduce the FIo_2 to safe levels
- *Humidification:* Continuous humidification is mandatory, with inspired air warmed to near body temperature. Standard humidifiers using a water feed system must be monitored closely for water condensation in the tubing and emptied routinely. Heat and moisture exchanges (HME) are sometimes used.
- *Sensitivity:* Established parameters are followed for sensitivity settings (when the patient can trigger the machine for "assistance"); sensitivity is adjusted so that minimal patient effort is required, usually −0.50 to −1.5 cm H_2O; certain ventilators allow for a flow-triggering mechanism and should be set to their maximum sensitivity (1 to 3 L/min)
- *Pressure limit alarms:* Should be set at approximately 10 to 15 cm H_2O above the patient's normal peak inflation pressure (PIP) or airway pressure. Goal is to keep PIP below 35 to 40 cm H_2O if possible. Peak inspiratory plateau is equal to or less than 35 cm H_2O. Certain ventilators provide a low-airway-pressure alarm feature. Check that all other alarms are operational and on at all times (Joint Commission on Accreditation of Healthcare Organizations patient safety goal).

ASSESSMENT OF THE EFFECTIVENESS OF MECHANICAL VENTILATION

- Some general measures include the following:
  - All patients on life support equipment should be monitored and clinically observed routinely according to institutional policy
  - Physical assessment should be performed each shift
  - Ventilator system and its current settings should be assessed
  - Manual self-inflating resuscitation bag should be open and ready for use
  - Suction equipment should be in working order and ready for use
  - When medications are to be given, orders must be written clearly and precisely (e.g., a bronchodilator can be administered continuously by aerosol or via the ventilator circuit by metered dose inhaler)

Continued

■ **BOX 2-6**
■ **LEVELS OF VENTILATORY SUPPORT—cont'd**

ASSESSMENT OF THE EFFECTIVENESS OF MECHANICAL VENTILATION—cont'd
- Many patients have an arterial line, cardiac monitor, intravenous line, and urinary catheter if they are on continuous ventilatory support
- General monitoring for patients on continuous ventilatory support
  - Hemodynamic monitoring (arterial or pulmonary artery catheter) if indicated
  - Cardiac monitoring, heart sounds, pulses, pulse pressures, electrocardiogram as needed or as part of standard intensive care unit routine
  - Pulmonary function studies: Vital capacity, negative inspiratory pressure, minute ventilation, maximum voluntary ventilation, as required
  - Biochemical, hematologic, and electrolyte studies
  - Cardiac output assessment, blood volume status
  - Measurement of intake and output, body weight
  - Respiratory pattern assessment, breath sounds, symmetry in chest movement, vital signs
  - Inspection of dressings and drainages, tubes, and suction apparatus
  - Assessment of neurologic state, level of consciousness, pain, level of anxiety
  - Evaluation of response to treatments and medications

VENTILATORY MONITORING OF ANY PATIENT ON CONTINUOUS VENTILATION
- Ventilation checks performed routinely
  - When blood gas samples are drawn
  - When changes are made in ventilator settings
  - Hourly or more frequently for any patient in unstable condition
  - Routinely throughout each shift
- Components of the ventilator sheet to be recorded on the nursing flow sheet
  - Blood gas values
    Record source (arterial, mixed venous) with ventilator settings and measurements so that decisions about changes may be made
    It often is valuable to document the patient's position at the time of the blood gas drawing, because position changes (side lying, upright, supine) influence ventilation-perfusion relationships and, hence, blood gas analysis results
  - Ventilator settings to be read from the machine
    Ventilator mode (e.g., SIMV or A/C)
    Tidal volume, machine preset rate, pressure support level (if used), preset minute volume, inspiratory flow rate or time and preset I/E ratio (depending on mode and ventilator)
    Temperature of the humidification device, temperature of the inspired gas
    Oxygen concentration
    Peak inflation airway pressure limit
    PEEP level set
    Alarms on
  - Ventilator measurements to be taken
    PIP, plateau, and/or mean airway pressures if requested, and PEEP level (measurement of auto-PEEP may be required for some patients)
    FIO_2, alveolar to arterial gradient or PaO_2/FIO_2 ratio, shunt fractions (if ordered)
    Minute ventilation (exhaled), respiratory rate (both patient and machine), tidal volume (exhaled)
    Effective compliance, static and dynamic; compliance curves (depending on institutional policy)
    I/E ratio (displayed), dead space/tidal volume ratio (if requested)
  - Respiratory monitoring techniques during mechanical ventilation
    Pulse oximetry: Noninvasive estimate of arterial oxygen saturation (SpO_2). See discussion in Monitoring Data under Patient Assessment.
    End-tidal CO_2 ($PETCO_2$) monitoring: Noninvasive sampling and measurement of exhaled CO_2 tension at the patient-ventilator interface. See discussion in Monitoring Data under Patient Assessment.

TABLE 2-6
Ventilator Modes and Types

Mode	Indications	Advantages	Disadvantages	Patient Monitoring
Negative pressure ventilation • "Iron lung" or cuirass shell • Uses negative pressure to pull out chest	Neuromuscular or acute muscle fatigue or paralysis in patient with normal lung parenchyma Experimentally has been used in adult respiratory distress syndrome (ARDS), chronic obstructive pulmonary disease (COPD)	In specific patients can improve oxygenation Avoids complications related to invasive means of ventilatory support	Inspiratory flow rate cannot be adjusted Unable to provide adequate support to patients with lung disease Available only in controlled mode Noisy, bulky machines Physician and staff unfamiliar with negative pressure Patient physically constrained	Patient comfort Cardiovascular parameters, which may be affected by negative pressure cycling Nursing care of patient in tank is logistically difficult
Controlled mandatory ventilation (CMV) • Preset number of breaths • Preset tidal volume (V_T) • Cannot be triggered	Minimal or no respiratory effort (central nervous system dysfunction) Sedation or neuromuscular blockade Severe flail chest Anesthesia	Can be used to manage or manipulate acid-base balance Rests patient	Patient-ventilator asynchrony is likely May lead to respiratory muscle weakness and atrophy May produce altered hemodynamics Acid-base balance must be monitored closely	Peak inspiratory pressure (PIP) Exhaled V_T Acid-base balance Patient-ventilator synchrony

Continued

TABLE 2-6
Ventilator Modes and Types—cont'd

Mode	Indications	Advantages	Disadvantages	Patient Monitoring
Assist/control (A/C) • Preset number of breaths • Preset V_T • Variable pressure	Weak respiratory muscles Increased metabolic demands Weaning or for rest after weaning trials Respiratory muscle strengthening for each breath if needed	Rests patient Allows patient to trigger breaths Affords security of controlled ventilation with support awake, nonsedated Responsive to patient effort; can augment support on demand	Carries danger of barotrauma May produce altered hemodynamics May be poorly tolerated in patients due to dyssynchrony of patient and machine cycle lengths; increases work of breathing if settings not appropriate May be associated with respiratory alkalosis and worsen air trapping in patients with COPD If pressure-targeted A/C is used, V_T may be variable and potentially decreased	PIP Acid-base balance
Synchronized intermittent mandatory ventilation (SIMV) • Predetermined number of breaths • Preset V_T, pressure • Spontaneous breaths	Minimal spontaneous respirations postoperatively Respiratory muscle conditioning Weaning	Improves patient comfort Hyperventilation less of a problem Leads to less atrophy of respiratory muscles Patient can perform a variable amount of work with security of preset level of mandatory ventilation	Intermittent mandatory ventilation has risks of ventilator dyssynchrony between patient effort and machine-delivered volume SIMV has risks of hyper-ventilation and respiratory alkalosis (similar to A/C), excessive work of breathing due to poorly responsive	Respiratory rate PIP Exhaled V_T of mandatory and spontaneous breaths (V_E) Patient comfort

Mode and characteristics	Indications	Advantages / Disadvantages	Monitoring
Pressure support ventilation (PSV) • Preset inspiratory positive pressure • Variable V_T	Weaning Long-term mechanical ventilation Small-diameter endotracheal tube Respiratory muscle conditioning	Useful for weaning: Can vary from partial ventilatory support to near total support to spontaneous breathing Decreased work of breathing roughly proportional to level of PSV delivered Since patient has significant control over delivery, overt dyssynchrony is less likely than with A/C or SIMV Provides greater patient comfort Can be used to compensate for demand valve and endotracheal tube size demand valve, worsening dynamic hyperinflation in patients with COPD May lead to increased work of breathing with spontaneous breaths V_T is not controlled, so can vary Careful monitoring is needed for patients in unstable condition Excessive air leak during inspiration may cause delay in the flow-cycling mechanism of pressure support Poorly tolerated by some patients with high airway resistance (may improve with adjustment of initial inspiratory flow)	Exhaled V_T Airway cuff leaks Spontaneous respiratory rate Hemodynamic status
Continuous positive airway pressure (CPAP) • Positive pressure throughout respiratory cycle • No other ventilatory assistance	Adequate ventilation but poor oxygenation due to atelectasis or secretions Adequate ventilation but need to maintain airway Weaning	Offers benefits of positive end-expiratory pressure (PEEP) to spontaneously breathing patients by recruiting and stabilizing previously closed alveoli May help reduce work of breathing in patients with dynamic hyperinflation or auto-PEEP Reduces atelectasis; maintains and promotes respiratory muscle strength Ventilator alarms present May increase inspiratory work of breathing if CPAP levels set too high or if PEEP device has high flow resistance Risk of barotrauma: • Decreased cardiac output, venous return • May increase intracranial pressure	Blood pressure Respiratory rate Exhaled V_T Patient comfort

Continued

■ TABLE 2-6
■ ■ Ventilator Modes and Types—cont'd

Mode	Indications	Advantages	Disadvantages	Patient Monitoring
Mandatory minute ventilation (MMV) • Preset MMV • Ventilator adjusts rate and volume to supplement spontaneous breaths	Fluctuations in ventilatory drive (drug overdose, severe neuromuscular disease) Weaning	Varies ventilatory support according to patient need	Alveolar ventilation not monitored Less clinical evaluation (changes made by protocols or algorithms) MMV level not well defined (experimental)	Alveolar ventilation, arterial blood gas (ABG) levels
High-frequency ventilation • Small V_T (1-5 ml/kg) • High respiratory frequencies (60-3000 breaths/min)	Hypoxemia secondary to diffuse lung injury Persistent bronchopleural or tracheal-esophageal fistulas	In specific patients, can improve oxygenation when nothing else works May limit barotrauma and volutrauma Produces more uniform distribution of ventilation Reduces ventilation-perfusion (V/Q) mismatching	Conventional ventilators do not provide this mode Experimental ventilators needed for jet and oscillation ventilation Specific endotracheal tube needed for jet ventilation Experimental, last resort No studies have shown a decrease in mortality or morbidity	Hemodynamics Patient comfort
Pressure control • Preset pressure, rate, and inspiratory time • Variable V_T	Noncompliant lungs with high airway pressures and poor oxygenation Requirement for more flow during assisted breaths Presence of high PIPs in volume ventilation	Patient able to initiate spontaneous breaths Spontaneous breaths delivered at preset pressure Promotes laminar flow Maintains open airways and improves gas distribution	May result in "stacking" of breaths May lead to respiratory alkalosis May produce altered hemodynamics Auto-PEEP may occur	PIP Exhaled V_T Patient comfort Acid-base balance

Mode	Indications	Advantages	Disadvantages	Complications
Pressure-controlled inverse-ratio ventilation (PC-IRV) • Preset respiratory rate • Augmented by preset inspiratory pressure • Reverses I/E ratio • V_T varies with resistance and compliance • Auto-PEEP splints unstable alveoli	Noncompliant lungs with high airway pressures and poor oxygenation with volume-cycled ventilation	Can be used with conventional or inverse inspiration/expiration (I/E) ratio Patient can be awake In specific patients can improve oxygenation when nothing else works Increases functional reserve capacity Reduces intrapulmonary shunt and PIP Improves oxygenation Reduces dead space ventilation	Extremely uncomfortable for patients (patient should be paralyzed) Barotrauma a major risk	PIP Pneumothorax, subcutaneous emphysema Patient comfort
Differential lung ventilation (DLV) • Independent ventilation of each lung	Unilateral lung disease (infection) Bronchopleural fistula Bilateral lung disease (different) Airway hemorrhage Surgery	Corrects $\dot{V}/\dot{Q}$ abnormalities Increases compliance and improves tissue oxygen delivery Decreases shunt and transbronchial contamination	Very labor intensive (two ventilators) Very uncomfortable for patient (large endotracheal tube, asynchronous ventilation for each lung—patient should be paralyzed and sedated)	Hemodynamics Barotrauma Patient comfort
Pressure regulated volume control (PRVC) • Control mode with preset respiratory rate and V_T given as pressure breath	Complete ventilatory control Resting mode during weaning	Ventilator uses lowest pressure to achieve desired V_T Ventilator adjusts pressure based on lung mechanics Provides guaranteed V_T Reduces risk of barotrauma	Only available on computer-controlled ventilators Only available in control mode	Patient comfort Barotrauma PIP

Continued

■ **TABLE 2-6**
■ **Ventilator Modes and Types—cont'd**

Mode	Indications	Advantages	Disadvantages	Patient Monitoring
Airway pressure release ventilation • Pressure release valve in ventilation circuit	Acute lung injury with risk of barotrauma (high PEEP)	Reduces risk of barotrauma (auto-PEEP) Has low peak airway pressure Has low intrathoracic pressure Improves V̇/Q̇ matching	Special circuit required Uses pressure control of ventilation Airway and circuit resistance affects ventilation Decreases transpulmonary pressure Interferes with spontaneous ventilation	Airway pressure Synchrony of patient with ventilator Patient comfort
Proportional assist ventilation • Ventilator generates pressure in proportion to patient effort	Presence of spontaneous respiratory efforts but with development of respiratory distress and/or failure without ventilatory support (neuromuscular weakness)	Patient fits ventilation and breathing pattern to own needs Easy to match patient and ventilator Ventilator sensitive to patient changes	Computerized ventilation required Sensitive to leaks in system Potential for excessive pressure or volume delivery Auto-PEEP may occur	PIP Leaks Barotrauma Patient comfort
Permissive hypercapnia • Hypercapnia but not acidemia	Weaning Chronic ARDS (fibrosis) Acute lung injury Severe airflow obstruction	Avoids barotrauma, volutrauma Decreases work of breathing	Acute hypercapnia affects other organ systems (heart, kidney)	Acid-base status Patient comfort
Extracorporeal membrane oxygenation (ECMO)/ extracorporeal carbon dioxide removal (ECO$_2$R)/ intravascular oxygenation (IVOX) • Uses capillary membrane oxygenation	Rescue oxygenation (last ditch)	In specific patients can improve oxygenation when nothing else works	Basically experimental No studies have shown improved outcomes	Infection control Patient comfort

© K. Ellstrom, 2000. Used by permission.

■ BOX 2-7
■ **COMPLICATIONS ASSOCIATED WITH POSITIVE PRESSURE VENTILATION**

CARDIAC EFFECTS
DECREASED CARDIAC OUTPUT
■ Caused by decreased venous return to the heart and reduced transmural pressures (intracardiac minus intrapleural pressures). In addition, there are increases in pulmonary vascular resistance and juxtacardiac pressure from the surrounding distended lungs.
■ Pulse changes, decreased urine output and blood pressure
■ Treatment
   ● Positioning with the head flat and legs elevated (modified Trendelenburg's position)
   ● Administration of fluids to increase preload
   ● Adjustment of volumes delivered by ventilator
   ● Careful positive end-expiratory pressure (PEEP) titration; avoidance of auto-PEEP

POSSIBLE DYSRHYTHMIAS
■ Causes: Hypoxemia and pH abnormalities
■ Patients in unstable condition on ventilators should have cardiac monitoring

PULMONARY EFFECTS
BAROTRAUMA (PNEUMOTHORAX, PNEUMOMEDIASTINUM, SUBCUTANEOUS EMPHYSEMA)
■ Occurs when a high pressure gradient between the alveolus and adjacent vascular sheet causes the overdistended alveolus to rupture. Gas is forced into the interstitial tissue of the underlying perivascular sheet. The gas may dissect centrally along the pulmonary vessels to the mediastinum and into the fascial planes of the neck and upper torso; high inflation volumes, or volutrauma, has also been described as an important risk factor.
■ Positive pressure ventilation, especially with PEEP, subjects patients to the risk of pneumothorax, particularly if high pressures and volumes are used
■ Barotrauma can occur with main-stem intubation, in patients with adult respiratory distress syndrome or chronic obstructive pulmonary disease (COPD), and in other patients with acute lung injury
■ *Diagnosis*
   ● Increases in airway peak pressure
   ● Decreased breath sounds and chest movement on the affected side
   ● Changes in vital signs, restlessness, possible cyanosis
   ● Chest radiographic changes

ATELECTASIS
■ Collapse of lung parenchyma from the occlusion of air passage, with reabsorption of gas distal to the occlusion
■ Causes
   ● Obstruction
   ● Possible lack of periodic deep inflations in patients ventilated with small tidal volumes
■ Diagnosis
   ● Diminished breath sounds or bronchial breath sounds, rales or crackles
   ● Chest radiographic evidence
   ● Alveolar to arterial (A–a) gradient increases, ratio of arterial partial pressure of oxygen (Pao_2) to fraction of inspired oxygen (Flo_2) decreases, and compliance decreases
■ Prevention
   ● Use of lower tidal volumes
   ● Humidification, vigorous tracheal suctioning based on need
   ● Chest physical therapy, repositioning

TRACHEAL DAMAGE, TRACHEOESOPHAGEAL FISTULA, VESSEL RUPTURE
■ Cause: Excessive tube cuff pressures due to overinflation or reduced tracheal blood flow causing ischemia

Continued

■ **BOX 2-7**
■ **COMPLICATIONS ASSOCIATED WITH POSITIVE PRESSURE VENTILATION—cont'd**

TRACHEAL DAMAGE, TRACHEOESOPHAGEAL FISTULA, VESSEL RUPTURE—cont'd
■ Prevention
  ● Careful monitoring of intracuff pressures or volumes
  ● Avoidance of frequent manipulation and pulling of endotracheal tube

OXYGEN TOXICITY
■ Pathology: Impaired surfactant activity, progressive capillary congestion, fibrosis, edema and thickening of interstitial space
■ Cause: Prolonged administration of high oxygen concentrations (FlO_2 of >0.50)
■ Prevention: Careful monitoring of blood gas levels. Goal is to use the lowest FlO_2 that achieves adequate oxygenation (PaO_2 over 55 mm Hg and arterial oxygen saturation [SaO_2] over 88%).

INABILITY TO LIBERATE (WEAN) FROM VENTILATOR
■ Can occur in any patient, particularly those with COPD, cystic fibrosis, debilitation, malnutrition, and musculoskeletal disorders
■ Mechanical ventilation eases the work of breathing for these patients, which makes the transition to breathing off the ventilator (i.e., weaning) difficult

HYPERCAPNIA–RESPIRATORY ACIDOSIS
■ Inadequate ventilation leads to acute retention of carbon dioxide and decreased pH
■ Patients can tolerate increased arterial partial pressure of carbon dioxide ($PaCO_2$) and decreased pH under certain circumstances
■ Corrected by improving alveolar ventilation and treating the underlying cause

HYPOCAPNIA–RESPIRATORY ALKALOSIS
■ Due to hyperventilation, which causes increased elimination of carbon dioxide and increased pH
■ If carbon dioxide is decreased too rapidly, shock or seizures may result, particularly in children. Maintain ventilation to produce a normal pH, not necessarily a normal partial pressure of carbon dioxide ($PaCO_2$).
■ Treatment
  ● Decrease the respiratory rate
  ● Decrease the tidal volume if inappropriately high
  ● Add mechanical dead space

FLUID IMBALANCE
■ Fluid retention: Due to overhydration by airway humidification and decreased urinary output because of possible antidiuretic hormone effects. Symptoms include the following:
  ● Increased A–a gradient, decreased PaO_2/FlO_2 ratio
  ● Decreased vital capacity and compliance
  ● Weight gain, intake greater than output
  ● Increased dead space/tidal volume ratio
  ● Hemodilution (decreased hematocrit and decreased sodium values)
  ● Increased bronchial secretions
■ Dehydration related to decreased enteral or parenteral intake in relation to urinary and/or gastrointestinal output, and overdiuresis. In addition, insensible losses average 300 to 500 ml/day and increase with fever. See Chapters 5 and 6 for clinical findings.
■ Signs and parameters to be monitored
  ● Daily weight changes (often more accurate than intake and output measurement)
  ● Skin turgor, moistness of the oral mucosa
  ● Hemoglobin and hematocrit values
  ● Character of pulmonary secretions
  ● Airway humidification

Continued

INFECTION AND VENTILATOR-ASSOCIATED PNEUMONIA

- Patients at risk: Debilitated, aged, immobile, early postoperative, or immunocompromised individuals
- Intubation bypasses normal upper airway defenses and makes oral care more difficult
- Ventilatory equipment and therapy, particularly aerosols, may be the carrier
- Suctioning technique may not be sterile
- There may be cross-contamination between patients and staff or autocontamination
- Pulmonary patients may have indwelling catheters of various types
- Nonsterile solutions may be left out in open containers
- Patients may be improperly positioned so that aspiration is possible, or the endotracheal tube cuff may not be inflated to minimal occlusive volume
- Preventive measures
  - Aseptic airway and tracheostomy technique
  - Sterile suction technique using an open-suction or closed-suction catheter system
  - Elevation of the head of the bed to 30 to 45 degrees continuously or as patient condition warrants
  - Rigorous hand washing, which is mandatory and critical, as well as the use of personal protective equipment as necessary
  - Meticulous oral care to assist in prevention, including teeth brushing to remove dental bacteria, which should be performed regularly and frequently
  - Bronchial hygiene, chest physical therapy as indicated
  - Isolation techniques as needed
  - Routine cultures of specimens from patients and machines
  - Avoidance of routine tracheal instillation of normal saline for lavage
  - Antibiotics as indicated
  - Restriction of the number of patient contacts (staff and visitors)
  - Early recognition and response to clinical and laboratory signs of infection
  - Change of ventilator tubing, including humidifier reservoirs, according to institutional policy; verify the length of time that the ventilator circuit is left in place before changing
  - Emptying and changing of reservoir water per institutional policy; empty water in tubing into a waste receptacle every 1 to 2 hours and as needed

GASTROINTESTINAL EFFECTS

COMPLICATIONS

- Stress ulcer and bleeding
- Adynamic ileus
- Gastric dilatation from loss of adequate nerve supply; fluid shifts may lead to shock

PREVENTION AND TREATMENT

- Routine auscultation of bowel sounds
- Antacids, histamine antagonists
- Hemoccult or Gastroccult and pH stomach aspirate testing; stool check for blood

PATIENT "FIGHTING" OF THE VENTILATOR, AGITATION, AND DISTRESS

CAUSES

- Incorrect ventilator setup for the patient's needs (e.g., inspiratory flow rate less than needed)
- Acute change in patient status
- Obstructed airway, pneumothorax
- Ventilator malfunction
- Acute anxiety
- Acute pain

MANAGEMENT

- Perform a rapid bedside check of the patient and ventilator
- Disconnect the patient from the ventilator and provide manual ventilation with 100% oxygen via a self-inflating bag

Continued

■ **BOX 2-7**
■ **COMPLICATIONS ASSOCIATED WITH POSITIVE PRESSURE VENTILATION—cont'd**

MANAGEMENT—cont'd
- Check vital signs, chest expansion, and bedside monitoring equipment
- Suction the airway and check the patency of the endotracheal or tracheostomy tube
- Obtain arterial blood gas values
- Sedate the patient if indicated and order for acute anxiety, and give analgesics if pain is present; observe for hypoventilation and be prepared to adjust the ventilator setting to meet the patient's needs

PRINCIPLES FOR MATCHING VENTILATION TO PATIENT NEEDS
- Do not assume that the patient will adjust to the ventilator; the reverse is desirable
- Vary the cycle frequency, tidal volume, triggering sensitivity, and inspiratory flow rate until the correct combination is achieved
- Provide calm reassurance and moderate sedation as indicated

(b) Principles of liberation
  (1) Explain the procedure. Place the patient in an upright position for better lung expansion. Obtain baseline measurements of vital signs.
  (2) Obtain ventilatory measurements or weaning parameters while the patient is *off* the ventilator. Measure minute ventilation, rate, V_T, maximum inspiratory pressure, V_C, and maximum voluntary ventilation.
  (3) Be prepared to give periodic manual ventilations
  (4) Consider returning the patient to the ventilator with baseline settings if signs of patient intolerance or tiring occur, including the following:
    a) Decreased V_T, increased respiratory rate
    b) Increasing $PaCO_2$ and/or decreasing pH
    c) O_2 desaturation by blood gas analysis or pulse oximetry
    d) Patient apprehension, diaphoresis, fatigue, decreasing level of consciousness
    e) Cardiac dysrhythmias, changes in blood pressure or heart rate, or hemodynamic changes
  (5) Mechanisms contributing to failure to wean include insufficient ventilatory drive, hypoxemia, high ventilatory requirement, respiratory muscle weakness, low compliance, and excessive work of breathing. The longer it takes to resolve the problem that precipitated the need for ventilatory support, the more difficult it may be to wean.
(c) Techniques of discontinuing ventilator support (T tube, intermittent mandatory ventilation, pressure-supported ventilation, continuous positive airway pressure [CPAP]): See Box 2-8
(d) Treatment of the difficult-to-wean patient
  (1) Some patients pose significant problems in terms of costs, health care resources, and ethical dilemmas when ventilator removal is attempted
  (2) Evaluate for and, if appropriate, initiate inspiratory muscle training (the benefit of this step is controversial)
  (3) Monitor O_2 saturation via oximeter during the training session to verify that the patient's blood does not desaturate

■ **BOX 2-8**
■ **TECHNIQUES FOR DISCONTINUING VENTILATOR SUPPORT**

T-TUBE TRIAL

T-tube trial is also known as a Briggs, T-piece, or T-bar adapter trial. Patient is disconnected from the ventilator and attached to a high-humidity oxygen or air source by a T-shaped airway adapter.

- Total unassisted spontaneous breathing occurs, usually for 5 to 120 minutes depending on tolerance, followed by periods of rest
- Optimal duration of the T-tube trial has not been standardized; patients are usually extubated once they can tolerate several hours of unassisted breathing
- Arterial blood gas (ABG) levels are periodically measured to assess alveolar ventilation status
- Careful visual observation is required because the ventilator is on standby status and without integral alarms in case of T-tube system disconnection

INTERMITTENT MANDATORY VENTILATION

In intermittent mandatory ventilation (IMV), the amount of support provided by the ventilator is gradually reduced and the amount of respiratory work done by the patient is progressively increased.

- Transition period may be several hours to several days, depending on the length of time ventilatory support was required as well as institutional policy
- Pace of decreasing the IMV rate is determined by clinical assessment and ABG analysis
- Pressure support ventilation (PSV) is often used with IMV in lower amounts (5 to 10 cm H_2O); the IMV rate is reduced while the PSV level is held constant

PRESSURE SUPPORT VENTILATION

Stand-alone mode of PSV is also used as a means of gradually reducing the level of ventilator support.

- PSV level is initially titrated to a spontaneous tidal volume of 10 to 12 ml/kg and then reduced in increments of 3 to 6 cm H_2O based on clinical assessment and ABG analysis
- PSV is titrated down until a low level of support is reached (5 to 10 cm H_2O)

CONTINUOUS POSITIVE AIRWAY PRESSURE

With continuous positive airway pressure (CPAP) ventilatory support, the patient breathes spontaneously (with no mechanical assistance) against a threshold resistance, with pressure above atmospheric levels maintained at the airway throughout breathing.

- CPAP level is initially set at 3 to 5 cm H_2O
- May be helpful for patients with dynamic hyperinflation and auto–positive end-expiratory pressure
- When weaning trials are completed, the patient is usually extubated from CPAP at 3 to 5 cm H_2O

In theory, CPAP prevents or limits the deterioration in oxygenation that often occurs when patients switch from mechanical ventilation to spontaneous breathing. Some data refute this notion.

(4) Monitor the color, consistency, and volume of sputum. Change in sputum characteristics may indicate infection, which may increase the work of breathing.

(5) Physical therapy and rehabilitation efforts are very important (with both physical and psychologic advantages)

(6) Monitor the rate and depth of respiration, breath sounds, use of accessory muscles of respiration, and dyspnea

(7) Monitor the patient for clinical signs of respiratory muscle fatigue, including shallow, rapid breathing (early); increased $Paco_2$, decreased respiratory rate (late)

(8) Monitor the ratio of inspiratory time (T_i) to total duration of respiration (T_{tot}); an increase in the T_i/T_{tot} ratio indicates decreased respiratory muscle endurance

(9) Observe for abnormal chest wall motion as an indication of respiratory muscle dysfunction

    a) Paradoxical motion of the chest wall is characterized by expansion of the rib cage and inward motion of the abdomen during inspiration

    b) Asynchronous chest wall motion is characterized by disorganized and uncoordinated respiratory motion

(10) Administer appropriate drug therapy for maintenance of ventilation (Box 2-9)

  v. Assist the patient in maintaining adequate nutrition

    (a) Assess nutritional status (see Chapter 8)

    (b) Provide nutritional support

      (1) Oral feedings with calorie supplements; small, frequent feedings are often better tolerated by dyspneic patients

      (2) Enteral feedings via nasogastric, small-bore nasoenteral, or gastric feeding tubes for patients who cannot eat but have a functional gastrointestinal tract or have endotracheal tubes and cannot take oral feedings. See pp. 156-158 and Chapter 8 for precautions to avoid pulmonary aspiration.

      (3) Total parenteral nutrition (TPN): Indicated for patients with a nonfunctional gastrointestinal tract

    (c) Provide general patient care and personal hygienic measures (especially meticulous oral care), which may improve the patient's appetite

e. Evaluation of patient care

  i. Acid-base and oxygenation parameters remain within normal limits

  ii. Patient is comfortable and well rested on the ventilator with no air trapping or auto-PEEP

  iii. No clinical evidence of ventilator-associated infections or complications is present (Table 2-7)

4. Impaired respiratory gas exchange

a. Description of problem: Inability to maintain adequate respiratory gas exchange. Clinical findings include confusion, anxiety, somnolence, restlessness, irritability, inability to mobilize secretions, hypercapnia, hypoxemia, hypoxia, dyspnea, cyanosis, tachycardia, and dysrhythmias.

b. Goals of care

  i. Hypoxemia resolves or improves

  ii. Eucapnia is present or the patient's usual compensated $Paco_2$ and pH levels are observed

  iii. Patient performs ADLs and modifies self-care activity with or without supplemental O_2

  iv. Patient indicates that he or she is able to breathe comfortably

c. Collaborating professionals on health care team: Nurse, physician, respiratory therapist, dietitian, physical therapist, social worker, discharge coordinator

d. Interventions

  i. Assess oxygenation status

    (a) Hypoxia-hypoxemia relationships

▨ **BOX 2-9**
▨ **DRUG THERAPY FOR MAINTENANCE OF VENTILATION**

NARCOTICS
- Morphine sulfate, meperidine, and fentanyl, dosed to effect
- Act as a respiratory depressant; good euphoric agents and excellent analgesics
- Provide sedation and good control of ventilation without adverse side effects in a well-ventilated, well-oxygenated, acid-base–balanced patient; often used in combination with a benzodiazepine for sedative effects
- Sensation of dyspnea is reduced
- Large dosages may cause increased venous capacitance
- Drug tolerance may develop with prolonged use

NARCOTIC ANTAGONISTS
- Used in cases of narcotic overdose to reverse the effects of narcotics
- They are not stimulants but compete with narcotic molecules for cellular receptors in drug-depressed neurons

BENZODIAZEPINES
- Lorazepam and midazolam are the most commonly used agents in the critical care setting
- These drugs cause a central nervous system (CNS) depressant effect, which can lead to alveolar hypoventilation and respiratory acidosis, particularly in geriatric patients and in those with liver disease
- Severe respiratory depression and apnea can result if they are used with other CNS depressant drugs
- As with any sedative agent, the routine use of a validated sedation scale for monitoring and assessing the degree of sedation is important

ANESTHETIC AGENTS
- Propofol is a phenolic compound with general anesthetic properties when administered intravenously (IV). It is used as a sedative agent in the intensive care unit setting. It is unrelated to any of the currently used barbiturate, opioid, and benzodiazepine agents.
- IV bolus dose of 0.25 to 1.00 mg/kg is usually required, followed by a continuous infusion at a rate of 50 to 100 mcg/kg/min. Onset of action is approximately 15 to 60 seconds. Drug has a relatively short half-life.
- Respiratory and hemodynamic monitoring are essential during continuous infusion

PARALYTIC AGENTS
- Provide pharmacologic intervention at the myoneural junction, which results in muscle paralysis
- If the patient is conscious, sedation is mandatory

NONDEPOLARIZING MUSCLE RELAXANTS
- Administered IV
- Compete with acetylcholine at the receptor site
- Vecuronium and atracurium are the most common agents used in the critical care setting
- Loading doses given (different for each drug), followed by maintenance doses, with careful monitoring
  - Use of peripheral nerve stimulator for determining train-of-four at least every 2 hours; the goal is one or two out of four twitches
  - Use of end-tidal carbon dioxide monitoring for visual detection of respiratory efforts; in-line airway pressure graphic monitoring may also be helpful
  - Skeletal muscle weakness and disuse atrophy occur when these agents are administered for prolonged periods; full recovery of muscles may take from weeks to months
  - Neuromuscular blockade and sedation should be stopped at least once daily to assess the patient's underlying level of sedation and also to reevaluate the need for continued paralysis or sedation

Continued

■ **BOX 2-9**
■ **DRUG THERAPY FOR MAINTENANCE OF VENTILATION—cont'd**

DEPOLARIZING MUSCLE RELAXANT (SUCCINYLCHOLINE)
- Attaches to the muscle cell wall and causes depolarization
- Used primarily for inducing short-duration muscle relaxation in anesthesia and endotracheal intubation
- Bolus dose is typically 1.0 to 1.5 mg/kg IV; onset of action is approximately 45 to 60 seconds; duration of action after a single dose is approximately 2 to 10 minutes

BRONCHODILATORS
METHYLXANTHINES
- Theophylline, aminophylline (80% theophylline), used primarily in exacerbation of chronic obstructive pulmonary disease
- Actions: Stimulate the CNS, act on the kidney to produce diuresis, stimulate cardiac muscle, and relax bronchial smooth muscle
- Serum levels: Therapeutic range, 8 to 20 mcg/ml

β-AGONISTS
- Stimulate β-receptors in the bronchial smooth muscle, which results in bronchial smooth muscle relaxation; the most potent bronchodilators currently available
- Epinephrine: Stimulates β_1- and β_2-receptors; given by inhalation or parenterally, with rapid action either way; duration of action is 0.5 to 2 hours
- Isoproterenol: Stimulates both β_1- and β_2-receptors; given IV, sublingually, or inhaled; duration of action is 0.5 to 2 hours; generally used in cases of cardiogenic pulmonary edema
- Metaproterenol: Has equal β_1 and β_2 effects; given in inhaled or oral form; duration of action is 3 to 4 hours
- Isoetharine: Mainly β_2 effects; given by inhalation; duration of action is 3 to 4 hours
- Terbutaline: Mainly β_2 actions; given subcutaneously, orally, or inhaled; duration of action is 2 to 4 hours for subcutaneous route, 3 to 7 hours inhaled, 5 to 8 hours orally; however, side effects are worse with oral doses
- Albuterol: Mostly β_2 selective; given in inhaled and oral forms; duration of action is 4 to 6 hours inhaled and 5 to 8 hours in oral form
- Bitolterol: Mostly β_2 selective; given in inhaled and oral forms; duration of action is 4 to 8 hours
- Pirbuterol: Mostly β_2 selective; given by inhalation; duration of action is 4 to 6 hours
- Salmeterol and formoterol: Mostly β_2 selective; given by inhalation; duration of action is 12 hours; because of the delay in the onset of action, this drug is never to be used in an acute bronchospasm attack

ANTICHOLINERGIC BRONCHODILATORS
- Block cholinergic constricting influences on bronchial muscle
- Work predominantly on the large airways
- Atropine and ipratropium: Given in inhaled form
- Tiotropium (Spiriva): 24-hour duration of action, given by powder inhalation

ANTIALLERGY MEDICATIONS
- Block immunoglobulin E–dependent mast cell release of mediators of bronchoconstriction, such as histamine and leukotrienes
- Cromolyn sodium: Does not actively bronchodilate but prevents bronchoconstriction; inhaled liquid given by metered dose inhaler, inhaled powder given by Spinhaler, or liquid nasal spray
- Nedocromil sodium: Given by inhalation aerosol (similar to cromolyn sodium)
- Montelukast: Given orally in the evening to counteract hormonal variation in bronchoconstriction

Continued

ADRENOCORTICOSTEROIDS

- Augment the effects of β-agonist bronchodilators and are antiinflammatory; often started at high dosage, then tapered off
- Dosage should be kept low to minimize adrenocortical and pituitary suppression and side effects
- Prednisone: Oral dose often given once daily, in the early morning to minimize systemic side effects
- Hydrocortisone: Methylprednisolone given IV
- Inhaled steroids (beclomethasone, flunisolide, fluticasone triamcinolone): Given after inhaled β-agonists
  - Provide beneficial pulmonary steroid effects with minimal systemic absorption
  - When steroids are taken by inhalation, the patient must use a spacer device and rinse the mouth with water after each use to prevent fungal infection (candidiasis) of the oropharynx or larynx

---

(1) *Hypoxia:* Decrease in oxygenation at the tissue level (a clinical diagnosis); must be corrected; in some cases O_2 therapy alone may not correct tissue hypoxia

(2) *Hypoxemia:* Decrease in arterial blood O_2 tension (a laboratory diagnosis). A normal PaO_2 alone does not guarantee adequate tissue oxygenation.

(3) Organs most susceptible to lack of O_2: Brain, adrenal glands, heart, kidneys, liver, and retina of the eye

(4) Factors governing effective oxygenation

   a) Sufficient O_2 supply in inspired air

   b) Sufficient ventilation to enable gas exchange between the atmosphere and the alveoli of the lungs

   c) Ready diffusion of gases across the alveolar-capillary membrane

   d) Adequate circulation of blood from the lungs to tissues; adequate volume of blood and Hb level. Falling cardiac output leads to a compensatory rise in O_2 extraction at the tissue level.

   e) O_2 brought to tissues must be readily released from the Hb molecule and be readily diffused into and taken up by various tissues

---

■ **TABLE 2-7**

■ ■ **Patient Safety and Prevention of Complications of Mechanical Ventilation**

Possible Complication	Preventive Measures
Ventilator-associated pneumonia	Elevation of head of bed 30 degrees
	Meticulous oral care, including teeth brushing
Gastrointestinal effects	Prophylactic agents (e.g., famotidine, sucralfate)
Deep venous thrombosis	Compression stockings
	Heparin or fractionated heparin
Overmedication or undermedication for sedation and pain relief	Continual assessment using a validated sedation scale and administration of medications
	Daily "wake up" from continuous sedation-paralysis
Delirium	Ongoing assessment using a validated assessment scale (e.g., Confusion Assessment Method for the Intensive Care Unit [CAM-ICU])
	Alarms audible at nursing station (Joint Commission on Accreditation of Healthcare Organizations patient safety goal)

   (b) Assessment of hypoxemia-hypoxia

     (1) Clinical signs and symptoms: See Description of Problem; may also include apprehension, headache, angina, impaired judgment, hypotension, abnormal respirations, hypoventilation, yawning

     (2) ABG analysis, including oxyhemoglobin saturation, and content; Hb level; arteriovenous O_2 content differences (if pulmonary artery catheter is in place)

     (3) Noninvasive O_2 monitoring

       a) Transcutaneous O_2 tension ($TcPO_2$, measures the O_2 concentration at the skin with an electrode). Heat is applied to improve blood flow. Skin blood flow, thickness, and temperature, and skin O_2 consumption influence readings. This technique becomes less accurate and reliable as the patient becomes older. Careful calibration and monitoring of electrode temperature are critical, as is periodic site rotation to prevent possible blistering and local tissue injury. $TcPO_2$ normally tends to underestimate PaO_2. In cases of compromised hemodynamic status, PaO_2 may be significantly underestimated.

       b) Pulse oximetry (SpO_2): See Patient Assessment

  ii. Provide O_2 therapy

    (a) Principles of O_2 therapy

     (1) *Remember the airway*; no O_2 treatment is of any use without a patent and adequate airway

     (2) *O_2 is a drug* and should be administered in a prescribed dose (the FIO_2 is the dose)

     (3) Response to O_2 administration should be interpreted in terms of its effect on tissue oxygenation rather than only its effect on ABG values

     (4) Disease pathology is the major determinant of the effectiveness of O_2 therapy

     (5) Delivered concentration of gas from any appliance is subject to the condition of the equipment, the application technique, and the cooperation and ventilatory pattern of the patient

     (6) *Low-flow O_2 systems* do not provide the total inspired gas (the patient breathes some room air) and therefore are adequate only if tidal volume is adequate, respiratory rate is not excessive, and ventilator pattern is stable. Variable O_2 concentrations (21% to 90%) are provided, but FIO_2 varies greatly with changes in tidal volume and ventilatory pattern.

     (7) *High-flow O_2 systems* provide the total inspired gas (the patient breathes only gas supplied by the apparatus) and are adequate only if flow rates exceed the inspiratory flow rate and minute ventilation. Both high and low O_2 concentrations (24% to 100%) may be delivered.

    (b) Rationale for the use of low-flow O_2 systems in patients with COPD and chronic CO_2 retention

     (1) Central chemoreceptors become desensitized to chronically high blood CO_2 levels, so CO_2 no longer serves as a respiratory stimulus; the only remaining stimulus to increase ventilation is hypoxemia. As a result, high concentrations of O_2 *depress* the ventilatory drive, which leads to $\dot{V}/\dot{Q}$ mismatching, the Haldane effect, depressed minute ventilation, and increased $PaCO_2$.

     (2) Nursing implications

       a) Administer only enough O_2 to keep PaO_2 at adequate levels for the patient (50 to 60 mm Hg)

  b) Safety lies in the use of controlled low flow rates, monitoring of ABG levels, and careful observation

(c) Hazards of O_2 therapy

 (1) O_2-induced hypoventilation

  a) Prevent by the use of low flow rates and O_2 concentrations (FIO_2 of 0.24 to 0.30)

  b) Patient is at greatest risk when the $Paco_2$ is chronically elevated above normal

  c) Use O_2 therapy with caution in patients with chronic CO_2 retention (see earlier); priority is to correct hypoxemia; if $Paco_2$ increases and pH decreases, may need to intubate or use BiPAP

 (2) Absorption atelectasis: Due to the elimination of nitrogen (nitrogen washout) and the effect of O_2 on pulmonary surfactant

 (3) Retinopathy of prematurity (retrolental fibroplasia) in neonates

 (4) O_2 toxicity: Rarely seen in adults

  a) Due to lung exposure to a high concentration (exact level is controversial; usually considered to be FIO_2 >0.50 to 0.70) over an extended time (longer than 48 to 72 hours)

  b) May be mild or fatal

  c) Early signs and symptoms

   1) Retrosternal distress, dyspnea, coughing

   2) Restlessness, paresthesias in the extremities

   3) Nausea, vomiting, anorexia

   4) Fatigue, lethargy, malaise

  d) Late signs and symptoms include progressive respiratory difficulty to asphyxia, cyanosis

  e) Pathologic process

   1) Local toxicity to the capillary endothelium leads to interstitial edema, which thickens the alveolar-capillary membrane. Type I alveolar cells are destroyed by an exudative response. In the end stages, hyaline membranes form in the alveolar region, followed by fibrosis and pulmonary hypertension.

   2) Biochemical changes are most likely due to the overproduction of oxygen free radicals, which produce oxidation reactions that inhibit enzyme functions and/or kill cells. High Po_2 values can also release additional free radicals from neutrophils and platelets, which instigate the capillary endothelial damage described.

  f) Both the concentration and duration of O_2 administration are critical (50% O_2 or higher over several days is potentially dangerous). Even low-flow O_2 (1 to 2 L/min) has been shown to produce cellular changes over time.

  g) Clinical changes in O_2 toxicity: Decreased compliance and vital capacity, increased A–a gradient, reduced Pao_2/FIO_2 ratio

 (5) Prevention of complications caused by O_2 therapy

  a) O_2 is a potent drug that should be used only when indicated and according to preestablished goals of therapy

  b) If high concentrations are necessary, the duration of administration should be kept to a minimum and the concentration reduced as soon as possible

  c) Objective: Maintain Pao_2 of at least 55 to 60 mm Hg to produce an acceptable Sao_2 of 88% to 90% without causing lung injury or inducing CO_2 retention

d) Reassessment of ABG levels is mandatory during the initial titration of O_2 therapy and when pulse oximetry values are questionable

e) Depending on the O_2 delivery device used, the exact concentration of FIO_2 should be measured when appropriate with an O_2 analyzer

f) Patients should never be exposed to dangerous levels of hypoxemia for fear of development of O_2 toxicity. Hypoxia is far more common than O_2 toxicity and must be corrected. Pure O_2 (100%) should never be withheld in an emergency.

(d) Methods of O_2 delivery (low-flow and high-flow systems): See Box 2-10

iii. Administer PEEP: Major oxygenation adjunct treatment modality

(a) Pressure above the atmospheric level is maintained at the airway opening at the end of expiration to prevent alveolar collapse

(b) At the end of quiet expiration, lung volume is increased; therefore, FRC is increased. Increase in FRC depends on both the amount of PEEP used and the functional state of the lungs. Alveolar volume is increased; recruitment of alveoli occurs.

(c) Major goal of PEEP is enhanced O_2 transport by improvement in PaO_2 and SaO_2. PEEP reduces the shunt effect of collapsed alveoli and may increase PaO_2 dramatically. Another important goal of PEEP is to avoid increasing FIO_2, which could lead to O_2 toxicity.

(d) Clinical use of PEEP

(1) ARDS and the presence of diffuse pulmonary infiltrates, characterized by closure of the airways or the collapse of alveoli at end expiration, which results in refractory hypoxemia and increased FIO_2 requirements

(2) ARF that has caused a persistent hypoxemia with an FIO_2 of 0.5 or greater

(3) Cardiogenic pulmonary edema

(4) Avoidance of pulmonary O_2 toxicity from high FIO_2 values

(e) Dose: Amount of PEEP is tailored to the patient's need; there is no arbitrary upper limit. Determination of the optimal level requires accurate assessment of cardiopulmonary function, including measurement of peak and plateau airway pressures, blood pressure, and cardiac output when available. PEEP levels above 10 to 12 cm H_2O are generally considered high.

(f) Side effects of PEEP

(1) Exacerbation of the same hemodynamic consequences that occur with positive pressure breathing (see Box 2-7). Patients with poor cardiovascular dynamics are at most risk. Adequate intravascular volume is essential.

(2) Barotrauma or volutrauma: Rupture of lung tissue at high PEEP levels, especially in patients with acute lung injury. Associated with high peak and plateau inflation pressures and high mean airway pressures.

(g) Monitoring guidelines

(1) It is essential to monitor the parameters that indicate the status of cardiac output and tissue perfusion (see Chapter 3)

(2) Patients should undergo routine arterial pressure monitoring and, if indicated, more complex cardiovascular monitoring (pulmonary artery catheter) if available. Urinary output should be closely monitored.

■ **BOX 2-10**
■ **METHODS OF OXYGEN DELIVERY**

MASKS
GENERAL POINTS
■ Useful if O_2 is needed quickly and for short periods
■ Concentrations of 24% to 100% O_2 are delivered, depending on the device

DISADVANTAGES
■ Uncomfortable and hot
■ Irritation of the skin caused by tight fit
■ Difficult to control the fraction of inspired O_2 (FIO_2) precisely, except when the Venturi mask is used
■ Must be removed when the patient eats, so that O_2 delivery is lost

POSSIBLE COMPLICATIONS
■ Patients who are prone to vomit may experience aspiration
■ Obstruction by a flaccid tongue may occur in comatose patients; use an oral airway and secure it
■ May cause CO_2 retention and hypoventilation if the flow is too low and exhalation ports are obstructed

TYPES OF MASK
■ Simple
  ● 35% to 60% O_2 at flows of 6 to 10 L/min
  ● FIO_2 varies considerably with changes in tidal volume, ventilatory pattern, and inspiratory flow rate and with a tight or loose fit of the mask
■ Partial rebreathing
  ● Delivers 35% to 60% O_2 or higher at flows of 6 to 10 L/min
  ● Portion of exhaled breath enters the reservoir bag to be rebreathed with incoming 100% O_2 in the next breath
  ● Flows must be adjusted so that the reservoir bag does not completely collapse during inspiration; otherwise, CO_2 retention may occur
■ Nonrebreathing
  ● Delivers 90% or more O_2 concentration, provided there are no leaks in the system; a one-way valve between the reservoir bag and mask prevents rebreathing from the 100% O_2 gas source
  ● Ideal method of delivering a high O_2 gas concentration for the short term
  ● Reservoir bag must not collapse during inspiration
■ Air entrainment (Venturi mask)
  ● Adjustments allow for the delivery of precise O_2 concentrations of 24% to 50%
  ● Total airflow must be adequate for the ventilatory needs of the patient
  ● Best suited to patients who must have a consistent FIO_2

NASAL CANNULA
■ Low O_2 concentrations are delivered (<40%), but level depends on the patient's tidal volume
■ FIO_2 can be estimated as a 4% increase in FIO_2 for each liter of O_2 flow; generally not run at flow rates beyond 5 or 6 L/min
■ Humidifier not necessary unless flow rates exceed 4 L/min

ADVANTAGES
■ Easy to apply
■ Light
■ Economical
■ Disposable
■ Patient mobility allowed

Continued

■ **BOX 2-10**
■ **METHODS OF OXYGEN DELIVERY—cont'd**

DISADVANTAGES
- Easily dislodged
- High flow rates uncomfortable (dryness and bleeding)
- Possible skin breakdown around the ears caused by tubing, nasal dryness, and breakdown of mucous membranes from the prongs

NASAL CATHETER
- Low O_2 concentrations delivered (<40%)
- Catheter should not be forced through the nose; periodic rotation of a new catheter to the opposite nares should be done at least every 8 hours; rarely used in adults
- Eventual delivery of O_2 to blood is not significantly different regardless of whether a cannula or a catheter is used or whether the patient's mouth is open or closed. Variability in FIo_2 is caused by the O_2 flow rate setting and the patient's rate and depth of respiration.

DISADVANTAGES
- Technique of insertion
- Potential for gastric distention
- Potential for nasopharyngeal injury

TRANSTRACHEAL CATHETER
Small catheter is percutaneously inserted transtracheally through the anterior neck for low-flow O_2 delivery

ADVANTAGES
- Economical (less O_2 is used to maintain a given arterial oxygen saturation than with other methods)
- Very cosmetically appealing to some patients (catheter may be concealed by clothing) with improved compliance with therapy
- Improved sense of taste, smell, and appetite
- Avoidance of nasal and ear irritation

DISADVANTAGES
- Technique of insertion (minor)
- Need for meticulous care (major)
- Risk of infection
- Possibility of subcutaneous emphysema if the catheter dislodges before a transtracheal tract is established
- Need for the patient to be capable of recognizing and troubleshooting common problems

RESERVOIR CANNULA
Combines the concepts of low flow and reservoir delivery systems. Reservoir cannula stores about 20 ml of O_2 during exhalation. Pendant reservoir delivery system is situated over the anterior chest wall.

ADVANTAGES
- Decreased flow needed for a given FIo_2
- Reduced O_2 costs
- Allows longer periods away from a stationary O_2 source

DISADVANTAGES
- Patients may object to the appearance of a reservoir "mustache" cannula
- FIo_2 variability still exists
- Amount of O_2 savings varies greatly, depending on individual patient needs

Continued

AIR ENTRAINMENT NEBULIZER

Air entrainment nebulizer, a pneumatically powered device containing sterile water, is capable of providing high-level humidification in the form of an aerosol and heat control as well as delivering O_2 at a preset Flo_2. Dilution of the 100% O_2 source from the flow meter occurs via a fixed or adjustable air entrainment port located on the nebulizer canister. Flo_2 can be set from 0.21 to 1.0.

ADVANTAGES

- Ideal for providing humidification for a patient with an artificial airway
- Humidified air or O_2 is delivered using a variety of attachments, including the following:
  - Aerosol mask
  - Face tent
  - Tracheostomy collar
  - T-tube or Briggs adapter

DISADVANTAGES

- Air entrainment nebulizers generate consistent Flo_2 delivery to the patient only when their output flow meets or exceeds the patient's inspiratory flow demands
- Because water condensation in large-bore tubing obstructs total flow and decreases air entrainment, Flo_2 increases
- Delivered Flo_2 is more variable at O_2 concentrations above 40%

HYPERBARIC OXYGEN THERAPY

- O_2 is administered at pressures greater than 1 atmosphere
  - Administered in a multiplace (12 or more patients) or monoplace (single patient) chamber
  - Monitoring systems and ventilators can be adapted to allow treatment of critically ill patients
- Indications: Primary treatment for decompression of divers, air or gas embolism, carbon monoxide and/or cyanide poisoning, acute traumatic ischemias (compartment syndrome, crush injury), clostridial gangrene, necrotizing soft tissue infection, ischemic skin grafts or flaps, enhanced healing of problem wounds, refractory osteomyelitis
- Complications: Barotrauma, tympanic membrane rupture, pneumothorax, air embolism, O_2 toxicity, fire risk, reversible visual changes, claustrophobia, sudden decompression, radiation necrosis, central nervous system toxic reaction (rare)

OTHER MEDICAL GAS THERAPIES

- Helium therapy: Used as an adjunct in managing large airway obstruction and status asthmaticus. Because of helium's low density, the driving pressure to move gas in and out of the larger airways is decreased and, therefore, the work of breathing is reduced.
  - Administered in prepared gas cylinders delivering a mixture with a helium/O_2 ratio of either 80%:20% or 70%:30%
  - Because of the high diffusibility of helium, the gas is generally administered via a nonrebreathing mask; it can be used with mechanical ventilation
  - In a nonintubated patient, speech may be distorted during helium administration
- Nitric oxide therapy: Used in the treatment of diseases characterized by pulmonary hypertension and hypoxia. Not approved by the U.S. Food and Drug Administration for these applications except as an investigational drug. In very low concentrations (2 to 20 parts per million) mixed with O_2, nitric oxide selectively dilates pulmonary blood vessels, reduces intrapulmonary shunt, and improves arterial oxygenation.
  - Commonly administered via ventilator with a special analyzer for precise and stable nitric oxide dose titration; can be given to a nonintubated patient through a tight-fitting face mask
  - Toxic effects are possible with inhaled nitric oxide, including production of nitrous dioxide, methemoglobinemia, production of peroxynitrite, platelet inhibition, increased left ventricular filling pressure, rebound hypoxemia, and pulmonary hypertension

(3) If a significant drop in cardiac output occurs, PEEP may need to be reduced, or vasoactive drug support for blood pressure may be indicated. Hypovolemia, if present, must be corrected when this is a contributing factor to decreased cardiac output. Short-term inotropic therapy may sometimes be employed to correct decreased cardiac output in a normovolemic patient with known or suspected ventricular dysfunction.

(4) PEEP is lost if the patient is disconnected from the ventilator for suctioning. For this reason, closed-suction catheter systems are often used for mechanically ventilated patients to maintain PEEP levels during suctioning. If a precipitous drop in SpO_2 occurs during suctioning, preoxygenation before the procedure becomes critical.

 iv. Administer CPAP (see Boxes 2-6 and 2-8)

   (a) Similar to PEEP but used in spontaneously breathing patients via a nasal mask. May also be used in ventilator-dependent patients to improve PaO_2 and saturation levels.

   (b) Used during weaning from mechanical ventilation, for obstructive sleep apnea, and in select pediatric patients

  v. Encourage the patient to take deep breaths (see Inability to Establish or Maintain a Patent Airway)

 vi. Position the patient to facilitate $\dot{V}/\dot{Q}$ matching ("good side down")

vii. Provide rest periods between activities to minimize O_2 demands

viii. Alleviate or minimize anxiety, which may increase O_2 demands

 ix. Monitor the patient's response to any activity. If deterioration occurs, assist the patient with care, including helping with turning and transfer, and passive range-of-motion exercises.

  x. Teach the patient and significant others techniques of self-care that will minimize O_2 consumption

 xi. Maintain body temperature at a normal level; avoid patient shivering

e. Evaluation of patient care

  i. ABG and vital sign values are within normal limits for the patient with or without supplemental O_2 or mechanical ventilation

 ii. Cyanosis and dyspnea are absent

iii. Patient performs techniques that maximize ventilation-perfusion matching

SPECIFIC PATIENT HEALTH PROBLEMS

Acute Respiratory Failure

1. **Pathophysiology**
   a. Respiratory system cannot carry out its two major functions: (1) delivery of an adequate amount of O_2 into the arterial blood and (2) removal of a corresponding amount of CO_2 from mixed venous blood. As an "acute" disorder, the onset must be relatively sudden; however, the onset can occur over *days*, as may be seen in patients with preexisting lung disease, or within *minutes to hours*, as may be seen in patients with no preexisting lung disease.
   b. ARF can be categorized according to the extent to which ABG values are abnormal. Abnormalities can exist in PO_2, PCO_2, or both; the more severe the hypoxemia or hypercapnia, the greater the consensus about categorization. However, the interpretation of ABGs must take into consideration two important aspects of the clinical situation: Blood gas values before the onset of ARF

(which depend on whether preexisting lung disease was present) and the rapidity with which the ABG abnormalities developed.

c. As mentioned, the abnormalities in ABG levels may be in P_{O_2} (hypoxemic respiratory failure), in P_{CO_2} (hypercapnic respiratory failure), or both. Critical value for the diagnosis based on arterial hypoxemia is Pa_{O_2} lower than 55 mm Hg or Sa_{O_2} lower than 88%; lower values can cause a marked decrease in oxyhemoglobin saturation and, therefore, a considerable drop in O_2 content. Corresponding critical value for the diagnosis of acute hypercapnic respiratory failure is Pa_{CO_2} above 50 to 55 mm Hg (with an accompanying acidemia, or pH of <7.30).

d. Four major pathophysiologic mechanisms cause ARF—hypoventilation, ventilation-perfusion mismatching, shunt, and diffusion impairment. Of these, the first three mechanisms are by far the most common; diffusion limitation is a relatively unimportant cause of clinically significant hypoxemia. These physiologic abnormalities result from structural processes that comprise the pathologic background for the abnormalities of gas exchange. Two major processes involved are the following:

  i. Increase in extravascular lung water
    (a) Characterized by severe hypoxemia with normal to low Pa_{CO_2}
    (b) Occurs in patients with cardiogenic or noncardiogenic pulmonary edema and other parenchymal infiltrates
  ii. Impaired ventilation
    (a) Characterized by elevated Pa_{CO_2} and decreased Pa_{O_2}
    (b) Occurs with intrapulmonary disorders (airway disease) or extrapulmonary problems (neuromuscular or chest wall diseases, alterations in respiratory drive). Other causes include low Pi_{O_2} due to high altitude or inhalation of toxic gases and low mixed-venous oxygenation secondary to anemia, hypoxemia, inadequate cardiac output, or increased O_2 consumption.

2. **Etiology and risk factors**
  a. Increase in extravascular lung water (ARDS, pulmonary edema, aspiration, pneumonia, atelectasis)
  b. Impaired ventilation
    i. Intrapulmonary problems (see causes listed under Impaired Respiratory Mechanics and Impaired Alveolar Ventilation)
    ii. Extrapulmonary problems: Pleural effusion, kyphoscoliosis, multiple rib fractures, thoracic surgery, peritonitis; neuromuscular defects such as polio, Guillain-Barré syndrome, multiple sclerosis, myasthenia gravis, brain or spinal injuries; drug effects (narcotics, barbiturates, tranquilizers, anesthetic agents); cerebral infarction
  c. Patient history
    i. Past medical history—chronic airway obstruction, restrictive defects, neuromuscular defects, or respiratory center damage; history of conditions that impair gas exchange and diffusion
    ii. Family history—any significant pulmonary disease in parents, grandparents, or siblings. One form of emphysema caused by a deficiency of the enzyme α_1-antitrypsin is an inherited disorder.
    iii. Social history—current or past smoking; calculate the pack-year history for smokers (number of cigarettes smoked per day times the number of years smoked)
    iv. Medication history—prescribed and over-the-counter medications, their dosages, and last time taken. Assess for evidence of noncompliance in taking prescribed medications (i.e., missed doses or overdoses).

3. Signs and symptoms
  a. Patient's chief complaint
    i. Most often dyspnea or increased work of breathing
    ii. Other symptoms include the following:
      (a) Increased pulmonary secretions
      (b) Manifestations of hypoxemia
      (c) Manifestations of hypercapnia with acidemia: Headache, confusion, inability to concentrate, irritability, somnolence, dizziness
  b. Nursing examination of patient
    i. Inspection
      (a) General observations
        (1) Posture, skin color, cyanosis, tissue perfusion, lung expansion
        (2) Signs of right-sided heart failure, such as pitting edema of the lower extremities, jugular venous distention
        (3) Signs of hypercapnia with acidemia: Muscle twitching, asterixis, miosis, papilledema, engorged fundal veins, diaphoresis
      (b) Thoracic abnormalities such as increased A-P diameter (barrel chest), intercostal retractions, bulging interspaces on expiration (obstruction to air outflow), pectus carinatum or excavatum, spinal deformities
      (c) Pattern of ventilation
        (1) Use of accessory muscles of respiration
        (2) Abnormal rate, depth, or rhythm of breathing
        (3) Inspiration to expiration ratio (normal ratio is 1:2 or 1:3)
        (4) Inspiratory and/or expiratory stridor, indicative of upper airway airflow obstruction
    ii. Palpation
      (a) Skin temperature and texture
      (b) Vocal fremitus
    iii. Percussion
      (a) Dullness over dense lung tissue (consolidation or pulmonary edema)
      (b) Hyperresonance with air trapping (COPD) or pneumothorax
    iv. Auscultation
      (a) Decreased breath sounds with less air movement or less dense lung tissue (COPD)
      (b) Bronchial and bronchovesicular breath sounds over areas of consolidation, atelectasis, pulmonary edema
      (c) Adventitious sounds: Crackles or rales, rhonchi or gurgles, wheezes, pleural friction rub with pleuritis
4. Diagnostic study findings
  a. Laboratory: ABG analysis
    i. Respiratory failure is defined by ABG measurements as hypoxemic (decreased Pao_2) and/or hypercapnic (increased $Paco_2$ and decreased Pao_2)
    ii. Criteria: Pao_2 below 55 mm Hg, $Paco_2$ above 50 mm Hg, or both
      (a) Acute: Acidosis, normal or mildly increasing blood buffer (HCO_3^-) levels
      (b) Chronic: Relatively normal pH, elevated blood buffer levels
    iii. Shunt studies: Demonstrate intrapulmonary shunt greater than 15%
  b. Radiologic: Findings depend on the primary disease
5. Goals of care
  a. Impaired respiratory gas transport: Fio_2 is sufficient for the patient's O_2 supply needs; respiratory rate, tidal volume, ABG levels are within normal limits for the patient
  b. Impaired alveolar ventilation

      i. Respiratory rate and breathing pattern are normal for the patient

      ii. Patient has a minimal sensation of dyspnea with no auto-PEEP

      iii. No ventilator-associated infections or other complications are present

    c. Impaired respiratory gas exchange

      i. Hypoxemia resolves or improves

      ii. Eucapnia or the usual compensated $Paco_2$ and pH levels are observed

      iii. Mental status is normal and the patient is breathing comfortably

      iv. Patient performs techniques that maximize $\dot{V}/\dot{Q}$ matching

6. **Collaborating professionals on health care team:** Nurse, physician, respiratory therapist, infection control specialist, dietitian, clinical pharmacologist

7. **Management of patient care**

    a. Anticipated patient trajectory

      i. Positioning: Keep the head of the bed elevated at least 30 degrees to maximize ventilation and prevent aspiration; turn as warranted to maximize $\dot{V}/\dot{Q}$ matching

      ii. Skin care: Turn the patient frequently to mobilize secretions and maintain skin integrity

      iii. Pain management: Administer pain medication or sedative to relieve the discomfort of tubes and treatment and prevent treatment interference

      iv. Nutrition: Obtain dietary consult and collaboration; provide adequate nutrition to maintain cellular function and healing with the increased work of breathing

      v. Infection control: Follow all measures to avoid ventilator-associated pneumonia, including thorough oral care with brushing at regular intervals; hand washing hygiene; and meticulous care with vascular lines, airways, humidification systems, and the like to prevent hospital-associated infection. Maintain the integrity of invasive line systems and urinary drainage system; use aseptic technique as warranted.

      vi. Transport: Same level of care and all precautions as on the unit need to be maintained if the patient requires transport within or outside the facility

      vii. Discharge planning: Initiate early with the patient and family, especially if the patient will require continued care at home; evaluate the need for support and rehabilitation on discharge; anticipate home care equipment needs; provide a social services consult to arrange for the transition to home care, if warranted

      viii. Pharmacology: Antibiotics, sedatives, and analgesics as warranted. Instruct the patient and family in medications, inhalers, spirometry, and so on, to be used at home.

      ix. Psychosocial issues: Psychosocial impact is affected by the circumstances of the patient's admission (abrupt due to trauma vs. slow deterioration at a skilled care facility), prior hospitalizations in acute care units, the effects on family dynamics and household income, and many other variables. Degree, nature, and extent of support must be tailored to patient and family needs and incorporate as wide an array of health care services as warranted.

      x. Treatments

        (a) Noninvasive

          (1) Bilevel positive airway pressure (BiPAP), CPAP

          (2) O_2 delivery systems

        (b) Invasive

          (1) Intubation and mechanical ventilation

(2) IV medications, vascular monitoring lines, drainage systems

(3) Nutrition via nasogastric feeding tube, percutaneous endoscopic gastrostomy (PEG) tube, or small-bore feeding tube

   xi. Ethical issues: Issues related to the use and withdrawal of artificial means of ventilation represent a common source of ethical decision-making requirements involving the patient (with or without an advance directive in place), family members, members of the health care team, and possibly others such as a hospital ethics committee (see Chapter 1 coverage of these issues)

  b. Potential complications

   i. Hospital-associated infections: Aspiration, urinary tract infection, pneumonia

    (a) Mechanism: Patient vulnerable due to position changes and possible need for enteral feedings, probable use of a urinary catheter, foreign airway object, recumbency, and the need for cleansing and removal of oropharyngeal secretions

    (b) Management: See Positioning, Skin Care, and Infection Control (covered earlier)

   ii. Complications related to the therapies used for ventilatory support (i.e., O_2 toxicity, barotrauma, volutrauma, tracheal damage, gastric ulcers, inability to wean from the ventilator)

    (a) Mechanism: See Box 2-7

    (b) Management: See Box 2-7

   iii. Ethical issues: See coverage in Chapter 1

8. Evaluation of patient care

  a. Arterial and mixed-venous blood gas values are within the desired range for the patient

  b. Ventilatory parameters are within acceptable limits for the patient

  c. Rate, depth, and pattern of ventilation remain within normal limits for the patient with minimal or no use of accessory muscles of respiration

  d. Patient reports decreased dyspnea at rest and with exertion

  e. When inspiratory muscle training is appropriate, the patient's use of the training results in improved maximal inspiratory pressures

  f. Patient demonstrates correct and effective administration of inhaled respiratory medications and identifies side effects that need to be reported to a health care provider

  g. No signs of ventilator-associated infections or other complications are noted

  h. Patient performs ADLs with or without supplemental O_2

Acute Respiratory Distress Syndrome

1. Pathophysiology

  a. ARDS refers to a group of manifestations of an evolving severe diffuse lung injury. Acute form of ARDS nearly always occurs suddenly. Some patients survive and recover completely, although may have some residual impairment, however slight. Others—notably those with sepsis (particularly of abdominal origin)—have a high mortality because their ARDS evolves into a chronic form.

  b. *Acute* phase of ARDS is characterized by damaged integrity of the blood-gas barrier. There is extensive damage to type I alveolar epithelial cells with increased endothelial permeability. Interstitial edema is found along with the leakage of protein-containing fluid into the alveoli. This alveolar fluid contains erythrocytes and leukocytes in addition to amorphous material comprising strands of fibrin. There is also impaired production and function of surfactant. Resultant physiologic abnormalities are as follows:

    i. Shunting of blood through atelectatic or fluid-filled lung units causes a widening of the A–a difference in Po_2; the resultant hypoxemia is resistant to high FIo_2 but is often responsive to PEEP

    ii. Physiologic dead space is increased, frequently exceeding 60% of each breath; consequently, very large minute ventilation may be required to maintain acceptable levels of arterial Pco_2

    iii. Compliance of certain portions of lung parenchyma is reduced. Increased stiffness of the lungs is associated with decreased FRC and a requirement for high peak inspiratory pressures during mechanical ventilation. Other lung areas have relatively normal specific compliance and thus are not so much stiff as they are small.

    iv. Resistance to blood flow through the lungs is increased by narrowing or obstruction of pulmonary vessels. As a result, peak airway pressure (PAP) is often increased while pulmonary capillary occlusive pressure (PCOP) remains normal or low. Chest radiographs reveal diffuse bilateral infiltrates suggesting noncardiogenic pulmonary edema (i.e., filling pressures in the left side of the heart are low or normal).

  c. *Chronic* phase of ARDS is characterized by thickening of the endothelium, epithelium, and interstitial space. Type I cells are destroyed and replaced by type II cells (neutrophils), which proliferate but do not differentiate into type I cells as normal. Interstitial space is greatly expanded by edema fluid, fibers, and a variety of proliferating cells. Fibrosis commences after the first week. Within the alveoli, the protein-rich exudate may organize to produce the characteristic "hyaline membrane," which effectively destroys the structure of the alveoli.

  d. Resultant physiologic abnormalities are the following:

    i. Increased vascular resistance

    ii. Hypoxemia due to $\dot{V}/\dot{Q}$ mismatch or possible diffusion defect

    iii. Decreased tissue compliance

2. Etiology and risk factors

  a. *Direct injury:* Pulmonary contusion, gastric aspiration, near-drowning, inhalation of toxic gases and vapors, some infections, fat embolus, amniotic fluid embolus, radiation, bleomycin

  b. *Indirect injury:* Septicemia, shock or prolonged hypotension, nonthoracic trauma, cardiopulmonary bypass, drug overdose, head injury, pancreatitis, diabetic coma, multiple blood transfusions

3. Signs and symptoms

  a. Patient's chief complaint is severe dyspnea

  b. Increased work of breathing manifested by tachypnea, hyperpnea, nasal flaring, intercostal retractions, use of accessory muscles

  c. Production of frothy, pink sputum, dullness to percussion, bronchovesicular breath sounds over most lung fields, and diffuse crackles and gurgles over all lung fields if substantial pulmonary edema is present

  d. Diminished lung expansion

  e. Diminished level of consciousness if hypoxemia is severe

4. Diagnostic study findings: To exclude other causes of pulmonary edema

  a. Laboratory: ABG analysis

    i. Hypoxemia is the hallmark of ARDS and is due to intrapulmonary shunting. Hypoxemia is refractory to O_2 therapy (i.e., Pao_2 is below 60 mm Hg or Sao_2 is below 90% with FIo_2 above 0.5).

    ii. Respiratory alkalosis occurs in the early phases of ARDS because of hyperventilation

        iii. Hypercapnia not usually seen initially; it is an ominous sign if present

        iv. Shunt studies demonstrate large right-to-left shunt (usually >20% of cardiac output) measured during 100% O_2 breathing

        v. Increased A–a gradient, reduced PaO_2/FIO_2 ratio

    b. Radiologic: Chest radiograph demonstrates diffuse bilateral interstitial and alveolar infiltrates without cardiomegaly or pulmonary vascular redistribution in the acute phase; a fine or coarse reticular pattern evolves in the chronic phase

    c. Pulmonary function

        i. Reduced pulmonary compliance and FRC

        ii. Reduced FRC secondary to microatelectasis and edema

        iii. Increased dead space ventilation (V_D/V_T)

    d. Hemodynamic monitoring: Pulmonary artery occlusive pressure may be normal or low, but PAP is often elevated

5. Goals of care

    a. Hypoxemia resolves or improves with or without O_2 supplementation or mechanical ventilation

    b. Respiratory rate, depth, and breathing pattern are normal for the patient

    c. Arterial pH, PCO_2, and PO_2 normalize to acceptable values

    d. Patient has minimal or no sensation of dyspnea

    e. There is no clinical evidence of any complications related to equipment or therapies

6. Collaborating professionals on health care team

    a. Nurse, advanced practice nurse, home care nurse

    b. Physician, intensivist, pulmonologist as warranted

    c. Respiratory therapist

    d. Dietitian

    e. Clinical pharmacologist

    f. Infection control specialist

    g. Discharge coordinator, home care aide

    h. Social service personnel

    i. Occupational and/or physical therapist, as indicated

7. Management of patient care

    a. Anticipated patient trajectory: See also Acute Respiratory Failure and Patient Care

        i. Treatments (additional)

            (1) ABG monitoring: Notify the physician immediately if PaO_2 drops below 60 mm Hg or if $PaCO_2$ shows an upward trend

            (2) BiPAP, CPAP

            (3) Decreased V_T to protect lung; permissive hypercapnia may be used

    b. Potential complications (see also Acute Respiratory Failure)

        i. Fluid overload

            (a) Mechanism: Same mechanisms responsible for producing pulmonary infiltrates

            (b) Management: Monitor input and output closely; observe for signs of fluid overload; use the lowest intravascular volume compatible with adequate tissue perfusion

8. Evaluation of patient care: Underlying condition(s) that precipitated the development of ARDS is(are) reversed or effectively managed; see also Acute Respiratory Failure

Chronic Obstructive Pulmonary Disease

1. Pathophysiology

  a. COPD is an inclusive and nonspecific term referring to a condition in which patients have chronic cough and expectoration and various degrees of dyspnea either at rest or with exertion, with a significant and progressive reduction in expiratory airflow as measured by the forced expiratory volume in 1 second (FEV_1). This airflow abnormality does not show major reversibility in response to pharmacologic agents. Terms such as *chronic obstructive airway disease, chronic obstructive lung disease, chronic airflow obstruction* or *chronic airway obstruction,* and *chronic airflow limitation* all mean the same thing.

  b. COPD is usually divided into two subtypes: Chronic bronchitis and emphysema. However, other diseases such as cystic fibrosis, bronchiectasis, or bronchiolitis obliterans are associated with chronic airflow limitation. The separate pathophysiology of these subtypes (chronic bronchitis and emphysema) is described here, but most patients exhibit signs and symptoms of both clinical conditions. Asthma has an obstructive component but is no longer classified with COPD.

  i. *Chronic bronchitis:* Clinical diagnosis defined as the presence of chronic cough with sputum production on a daily basis for a minimum of 3 months a year for not less than 2 successive years. Many patients exhibit chronic hypoxemia with resultant episodes of cor pulmonale. They may also have reduced responsiveness of the respiratory center to hypoxemic stimuli, a trait that is probably inherited. Some of the pathophysiologic findings of chronic bronchitis are the following:

   (a) Increase in the size of the tracheobronchial mucus glands (increased Reid index) and goblet cell hyperplasia, which results in increased sputum production

   (b) Epithelial mucus cell metaplasia, which results in a decreased number of cilia. Hypersecretion of mucus and impaired cilia lead to a chronic productive cough.

   (c) Increase in bronchial wall thickness with progressive obstruction to airflow (chronic obstructive bronchitis)

   (d) Exacerbations are usually due to infection, with the following clinical picture:

    (1) Increased amount of sputum and retained secretions

    (2) Increased $\dot{V}/\dot{Q}$ abnormalities, which increase hypoxemia, CO_2 retention, and acidemia

    (3) Hypoxemia and acidemia increase pulmonary vessel constriction, raising PAP and ultimately leading to right-sided heart failure (cor pulmonale)

  ii. *Emphysema:* Anatomic alteration of the lung characterized by an abnormal enlargement of the air spaces distal to the terminal, nonrespiratory bronchioles, accompanied by destructive changes in the alveolar walls. Emphysema patients often exhibit increased dyspnea and breathing effort owing to an inherent increased responsiveness to hypoxemia. Resultant clinical picture is typically that of a well-oxygenated and dyspneic patient. Pulmonary abnormalities seen in emphysema are the following:

   (a) Gas exchange surface of the respiratory bronchioles, alveolar ducts, and alveoli is reduced

   (b) Air trapping is increased because of the loss of elastic recoil in airway support structures (causes increased A-P diameter)

(c) Air sacs are replaced by bullae and capillary area is proportionately diminished

(d) $\dot{V}/\dot{Q}$ inequality occurs and FRC is increased

(e) Increased work of breathing results in greater resting O_2 consumption

2. **Etiology and risk factors** (chronic bronchitis and emphysema)
   a. Cigarette smoking—the most important factor and the major toxic stimulus
   b. Environmental pollution, occupational exposure
   c. Predisposition due to genetic makeup, especially if there is known α_1-antitrypsin deficiency. Should be considered in nonsmokers or young patients (<50 years of age) with emphysema. Current guidelines recommend testing every COPD patient for this genetic finding.

3. **Signs and symptoms:** These diseases may present as pure entities, but it is common for patients to have a combination of the symptoms of the two
   a. Chronic bronchitis
      i. Chief complaint is usually chronic cough and sputum production
      ii. Wheezing, peripheral edema
      iii. Observe for signs of right-sided heart failure: Peripheral edema, distended neck veins, skin color that is dusky or cyanotic. Patients with chronic bronchitis show little sign of respiratory distress or dyspnea at rest.
      iv. Chest expansion may be normal; vocal fremitus may be normal or increased due to copious bronchial secretions
      v. Resonance may be heard on percussion if there are no areas of secretion retention or consolidation
      vi. Dullness to percussion is heard in areas of increased lung density (consolidation)
      vii. Coarse crackles and gurgles, expiratory wheezes are commonly heard
   b. Emphysema
      i. Chief complaint is dyspnea on exertion (early symptom) and eventually dyspnea at rest
      ii. Skin color often pinkish because the patient is well oxygenated
      iii. Weight loss, inability to perform ADLs
      iv. Barrel chest; note posture and work of breathing both at rest and during exercise; use of accessory muscles of respiration is common
      v. Pursed-lip breathing
      vi. Reduced chest excursion due to hyperinflated lungs and flattened diaphragm from chronic air trapping
      vii. Reduced vocal fremitus due to less dense, more hyperinflated lungs
      viii. Hyperresonance throughout all lung fields
      ix. Distant, quiet breath sounds due to reduced air movement and air trapping; wheezes heard on occasion

4. **Diagnostic study findings**
   a. Chronic bronchitis
      i. Laboratory
         (a) ABG analysis: Hypoxemia and often hypercapnia with compensated respiratory acidosis
         (b) Other laboratory findings: Polycythemia on complete blood count (CBC) in some patients
      ii. Pulmonary function: Reduction in FEV_1 and all other measures of expiratory airflow; some reversibility following bronchodilator therapy in selected patients
   b. Emphysema
      i. Laboratory: ABG analysis—may be normal or abnormal, depending on the type and severity of $\dot{V}/\dot{Q}$ abnormalities. Hypoxemia, if present, may be mild with normal Pa_{CO_2}; greatest during sleep.

ii. Radiologic: Chest radiographs often show low, flattened diaphragms. In severe emphysema, lung fields may be hyperlucent and show hyperinflation, with diminished vascular markings and bullae. Disease is most prominent in the upper lung zones except in α_1-antitripsin deficiency, in which a basilar predominance may be seen. Chest radiographs are of value during acute exacerbation to exclude complications such as pneumonia and pneumothorax.

iii. Pulmonary function: Increased FRC, residual volume, and TLC. Reduced FEV_1 with the ratio of FEV_1 to forced vital capacity (FVC) of less than 75% (greater than 80% is normal) and reduction in other expiratory airflow measures, which is typically nonreversible following administration of bronchodilators. Increased lung compliance and decrease in static recoil. Decreased diffusion capacity indicating a reduction in alveolar capillary gas exchange area (not a specific indicator of emphysema, however).

5. **Goals of care**
   a. Both disorders
      i. Major through terminal airways remain patent and free of secretions
      ii. Oxygenation improves
      iii. Alveolar ventilation improves
      iv. Work of breathing is minimized; ABG levels, vital signs, and tidal volume are within normal limits for the patient
   b. Chronic bronchitis
      i. Constricted airways are dilated
      ii. Patient is able to effectively clear secretions
      iii. There are minimal to no signs and symptoms of right-sided heart failure
      iv. Patient reports taking bronchodilator medications as prescribed
   c. Emphysema
      i. Breathing pattern is normal for the patient
      ii. Sensation of dyspnea is decreased
      iii. There is no air trapping at the end of expiration (auto-PEEP)
6. **Collaborating professionals on health care team:** See Acute Respiratory Failure
7. **Management of patient care**
   a. Anticipated patient trajectory
      i. Positioning: Keep the head of the bed elevated 30 to 45 degrees unless medically contraindicated to improve ventilation and prevent aspiration. Allow the patient to assume a position of comfort for breathing to diminish dyspnea. Patients with emphysema may need an overbed table for best positioning.
      ii. Skin care: Many of these patients have little adipose tissue owing to the increased work of breathing associated with these disorders. Others may exhibit peripheral edema related to right-sided heart failure. In either case, skin integrity warrants frequent monitoring and active care so that pressure ulcers or other breaks do not lead to infection.
      iii. Nutrition: Labored ventilation and the increased work of breathing associated with these disorders often precipitate the need for dietary consultation to ensure that sufficient protein and calorie intake are paired with judicious fluid intake
      iv. Infection control: These patients are especially vulnerable to hospital-associated infections; see coverage in Acute Respiratory Failure. Consultation with an infection control specialist on an ongoing basis may be warranted.
      v. Transport: If transport is necessary, ensure that optimal levels of patient care, patient monitoring, O_2 supply, humidification, and positioning are maintained throughout transport

    vi. Discharge planning: See Acute Respiratory Failure. In addition, discuss the need for smoking cessation; instruct in the proper use of an inhaler, effective coughing techniques, follow-up care at home. Secure consultation with social services to address the medical and social services support needed.

    vii. Pharmacology: Bronchodilators, steroids, and antibiotics as needed; sedatives and pain medication sufficient to enable therapies to be performed and to keep the patient comfortable. For patients with documented α_1-antitrypsin deficiency receiving α_1-proteinase inhibitor (Prolastin), provide medication monitoring instruction.

    viii. Psychosocial issues: Determine patient and family needs for support, because COPD can have a major impact on family roles, dynamics, and income. Identify issues important to the patient and family and communicate these to the social services member of the team.

    ix. Treatments (see also Acute Respiratory Failure)

        (a) Carefully administer O_2 using the lowest FIO_2 that produces adequate oxygenation; observe for CO_2 retention

        (b) Observe for signs of fluid overload; monitor intake and output closely

        (c) Monitor ABG levels; notify the physician immediately if PaO_2 drops below the patient's known baseline or target level (usually PaO_2 of 55 to 60 mm Hg or higher) or if $PaCO_2$ rises significantly beyond the established baseline value. In a patient with chronic CO_2 retention, monitoring $PaCO_2$ is less important than observing pH changes. Be prepared for the possibility of endotracheal intubation and the need for mechanical ventilatory support.

        (d) Consider administration of influenza and pneumococcal vaccine

    x. Ethical issues: See Acute Respiratory Failure; determine if an advance directive is in place because intubation may be a terminal event

  b. Potential complications

    i. Hospital-associated infections: See Acute Respiratory Failure

    ii. Inability to wean or liberate from the ventilator: See prior coverage

    iii. Deconditioning secondary to steroid use or lack of muscle work

        (a) Mechanism: Chronic increased work of breathing may not be compensated sufficiently by diet and—together with right-sided heart failure—may make ambulation virtually impossible, so COPD patients have a tenuous ability to maintain muscle strength

        (b) Management: Dietary consult to develop a comprehensive plan to replace the nutritional deficit and enable the patient to regain muscle strength; physical and/or occupational therapy to provide strength training

    iv. Cor pulmonale

        (a) Mechanism: Right-sided heart failure develops secondary to increased resistance to blood flow and increased pressures in the right side of the heart, the pulmonary artery, and the venous circuit owing to COPD

        (b) Management: Symptomatic management of problems such as fluid balance, peripheral edema, cough

8. Evaluation of patient care

  a. Airways are clear with minimal constriction and secretions

  b. Patient experiences minimal dyspnea at rest, lessened dyspnea on exertion

  c. ABG levels and pulmonary parameters are within acceptable ranges for the patient

  d. Tidal volume and respiratory excursion are optimal for the patient

   e. Overt signs and symptoms of right-sided heart failure are minimal or absent
   f. No ventilator-associated infections or other complications are present

Asthma and Status Asthmaticus (Severe Asthmatic Attack)

1. **Pathophysiology**
   a. *Asthma:* Chronic disease of variable severity characterized by airway hyperreactivity that produces airway narrowing of a *reversible* nature
      i. Increased responsiveness of the airways to various stimuli
      ii. Widespread narrowing of the airway with changes in severity; airway closure may occur
      iii. Cellular infiltration and mucosal edema
      iv. Airway hyperreactivity, with smooth muscle contraction and excessive mucus production and diminished secretion clearance
      v. $\dot{V}/\dot{Q}$ abnormalities
      vi. Increased work of breathing and airway resistance
      vii. Hyperinflation of the lung, with an increase in residual volume
      viii. Host defect of altered immunologic state
      ix. Some patients develop airway remodeling, then respond as in COPD
   b. *Status asthmaticus:* Severe asthma attack that is refractory to bronchodilator therapy, including β-adrenergic agents and IV aminophylline
      i. Severely reduced spirometric values for peak expiratory flow rate (PEFR), FVC, and FEV_1
      ii. Hypoxemia is present with a widened A–a O_2 tension gradient or reduced Pao_2/FIo_2 ratio
      iii. Airway narrowing due to the following:
         (a) Bronchial smooth muscle spasm (minor component)
         (b) Inflammation of bronchial walls, which leads to increased mucosal permeability and basement membrane thickening
         (c) Mucus plugging from airways due to increased production and reduced clearance of secretions. Mucus plugging, mucosal edema, and inspissated secretions account for the apparent resistance to bronchodilator therapy in patients in status asthmaticus.

2. **Etiology and risk factors** (for development of an asthma attack)
   a. Respiratory infection
   b. Allergic reaction to inhaled antigen (pollen, grass, perfume, smoke)
   c. Inappropriate bronchodilator management
   d. Idiosyncratic reaction to aspirin or other nonsteroidal antiinflammatory drugs
   e. Emotional stress, exercise
   f. Occupational or environmental exposure (air pollution, ingestion of metabisulfite [food preservative])
   g. Use of nonselective β-blocking agents (propranolol, timolol maleate)
   h. Mechanical stimulation (coughing, laughing, and cold air inhalation)
   i. Sinusitis, reflux esophagitis
   j. Genetic predisposition

3. **Signs and symptoms**
   a. Chief complaints are usually dyspnea, wheezing, cough, and chest tightness; severity ranges from intermittent, mild symptoms to severe respiratory symptoms despite intensive therapy
   b. Physical exhaustion, inability to sleep or rest, anxiety
   c. Difficulty speaking in sentences, minimal chest excursion with inspiration
   d. Production of thick, tenacious sputum
   e. Increased work of breathing evidenced by the following:

  i. Posture—habitus often leaning forward, with head lowered

  ii. Respiratory distress, tachypnea, hyperpnea at rest, expiratory stridor

  iii. Use of pursed-lip breathing with prolonged expiration

  iv. Nasal flaring, bulging of interspaces on expiration, diaphoresis

 f. Pulsus paradoxus may be present; pulse rate higher than 110 beats/min with pulsus paradoxus greater than 12 mm Hg in the presence of tachypnea (respiratory rate of >30/min) indicates a severe episode

 g. Signs of dehydration

 h. Vocal fremitus may be decreased (decreased density with lung hyperinflation); rhonchal fremitus with copious secretions

 i. Hyperresonance throughout the lung fields, low diaphragm, and limited diaphragmatic excursion on percussion

 j. Expiratory wheezes or rhonchi (as air and secretions move through narrowed airways). Severe wheezing may be audible without a stethoscope.

 k. Decreased breath sounds throughout constitute an ominous sign. Asthmatic patient is then not moving enough air and will likely need to be intubated.

4. Diagnostic study findings

 a. Laboratory

  i. Evidence of infection (i.e., positive sputum culture results), elevated WBC count

  ii. ABG analysis

   (a) May initially show low normal or decreased $PaCO_2$, increased pH, and decreased PaO_2 (<60 mm Hg)

   (b) In severe asthmatic attacks, progression to a "normal" or increased $PaCO_2$ level may be a sign of impending respiratory failure

 b. Radiologic: Chest radiograph may be normal or hyperlucent. Used to confirm or rule out a diagnosis of pneumonia, atelectasis, pneumothorax, or other condition that mimics asthma.

 c. Pulmonary function: Reduced FEV_1 and PEFRs. Serial measurements of these parameters indicating the response to bronchodilators are essential to establish the severity of the obstruction and assess the adequacy of the response to therapy. In patients requiring hospitalization, PEFR may be less than 60 L/min initially or may not improve to more than 50% of the predicted value after 1 hour of treatment. FEV_1 may be less than 30% of the predicted value or may not improve to at least 40% of the predicted value after 1 hour of aggressive therapy.

5. Goals of care

 a. Diameter and patency of the airways are improved

 b. Airway secretions and coughing are reduced

 c. Dyspnea and the work of breathing are reduced

 d. Oxygenation and ABG values are optimized

6. Collaborating professionals on health care team: See Acute Respiratory Failure

7. Management of patient care

 a. Anticipated patient trajectory

  i. Positioning: Keep the head of the bed elevated 30 to 45 degrees to maximize ventilation, enhance coughing effectiveness, and prevent aspiration. Assist the patient to his or her own position of comfort.

  ii. Nutrition: See coverage under Chronic Obstructive Pulmonary Disease. Dietary consult may be needed to arrange dietary supplements, treat any malnourishment, and restore positive nitrogen balance and adequate hydration.

      iii. Infection control: See Acute Respiratory Failure and Chronic Obstructive Pulmonary Disease. Patients are particularly susceptible to pulmonary infection because of the copious volume of thick secretions, inspissated secretions that plug the airways, and airway constriction.

      iv. Transport: See Chronic Obstructive Pulmonary Disease

      v. Discharge planning: See Chronic Obstructive Pulmonary Disease. In addition, teach correct inhaler technique, teach peak flow and symptom monitoring, and instruct the patient and family on avoidance of allergens and situations that trigger episodes and on the importance of taking medications properly.

      vi. Pharmacology: Administer bronchodilators and monitor effects (use of salmeterol is contraindicated during an acute asthma attack because of its delayed onset of action; albuterol or some other bronchodilator with a rapid onset of action should be used); administer steroids and antibiotics as needed

      vii. Psychosocial issues: Asthmatic attacks are stressful and frightening to the patient and family; the ICU environment may only add further anxiety. Need to work with the family as a unit because the ramifications of asthma may extend to the physical home environment and interpersonal dynamics, and ability to work and function in customary roles.

      viii. Treatments: See Chronic Obstructive Pulmonary Disease

        (a) Administer BiPAP, CPAP, heliox (helium and oxygen mixture)

        (b) For cases in which intubation and mechanical ventilation become necessary: See Acute Respiratory Failure

        (c) Administer fluids and humidification to keep airway secretions thin and easily expectorated

        (d) Follow designed dietary plan for nutrition

        (e) Perform close objective monitoring of ABG values, acid-base status, and ventilatory parameters (especially FEV_1 or peak flow rates if spirometry is not available)

  b. Potential complications: See Chronic Obstructive Pulmonary Disease. Note that asthma is a reversible condition, so avoidance of allergens and other triggers, sufficient fluid intake, effective coughing, air humidification, and proper use of an MDI should enable the patient to reverse most problems and resume normal activities.

8. Evaluation of patient care

  a. Airways remain patent and significantly less constricted

  b. Airway secretions are diminished in volume and readily expectorated

  c. Patient experiences minimal dyspnea at rest with significantly reduced work of breathing

  d. ABG values and pulmonary parameters are acceptable for the patient

Pulmonary Embolism

1. Pathophysiology

  a. Pulmonary embolism (PE), an obstruction of the pulmonary artery by an embolus, affects lung tissue, the pulmonary circulation, and the function of the right and left sides of the heart. Degree of compromise correlates with the extent of embolic vascular occlusion and the degree of preexisting cardiopulmonary disease.

  b. Most emboli (>90%) arise from deep venous thromboses (DVTs) in the iliofemoral system. Other sites include the right side of the heart and the pelvic area. Nonthrombotic emboli, such as fat, air, and amniotic fluid, also occur but are relatively uncommon.

c. Factors favoring venous thrombosis (Virchow's triad) include the following:
   i. Blood stasis
   ii. Blood coagulation alterations
   iii. Vessel wall abnormalities

d. Distribution of emboli is related to the size of emboli and blood flow. Very large emboli have an impact in a large artery; however, the thrombus may break up and block several smaller vessels. Lower lobes are frequently involved because they have greater blood flow.

e. Pulmonary infarction (death of the embolized tissue) occurs infrequently. More often, there is distal hemorrhage and atelectasis, but alveolar structures remain viable. Infarction is more likely if the embolus completely blocks a large artery or if there is preexisting lung disease. Infarction results in alveolar filling with extravasated red blood cells and inflammatory cells and causes opacity on a radiograph. Occasionally, the infarct becomes infected, which leads to an abscess.

f. Effects of acute pulmonary artery obstruction
   i. Altered gas exchange due to right-to-left shunting and $\dot{V}/\dot{Q}$ inequalities. Possible etiologic mechanisms for these alterations include the following:
      (a) Overperfusion of the uninvolved lung, which lowers $\dot{V}/\dot{Q}$ ratios
      (b) Eventual reperfusion of atelectatic areas distal to the embolic obstruction
      (c) Development of postembolic pulmonary edema
   ii. Degree of hemodynamic compromise correlates with the degree of vascular occlusion in patients with no underlying heart or lung disease
      (a) Initial hemodynamic consequence is acute reduction in the pulmonary vascular cross-sectional area with a subsequent increase in the resistance to blood flow through the lungs
      (b) If cardiac output remains constant or increases, pulmonary arterial pressure must rise
   iii. If cardiac or pulmonary disease exists and has already impaired the pulmonary vascular reserve capacity, a small degree of vascular occlusion will result in greater pulmonary artery hypertension and more serious right ventricular dysfunction

2. **Etiology and risk factors** (for DVT then PE)
   a. Previous pulmonary embolus or venous disease of a lower extremity
   b. Surgery or anesthesia, prolonged immobilization
   c. Diabetes mellitus, polycythemia vera, dysproteinemia
   d. Central line disconnection (air embolus)
   e. Trauma (especially fractures of the spine, pelvis, or legs with fat emboli) or recent pelvic or lower abdominal surgery
   f. Heart failure, acute myocardial infarction
   g. Shock (bacteremic or nonbacteremic), burns
   h. Obesity, malignancy
   i. Estrogen administration, pregnancy, recent childbirth (amnionic fluid embolus)

3. **Signs and symptoms**
   a. Patient's chief complaint varies considerably, depending on the severity and type of embolism. Sudden onset of chest pain (usually pleuritic), cough, and hemoptysis (which suggests pulmonary infarction) are commonly reported.
   b. Massive PE (>50% vascular occlusion): Mental clouding, anxiety, feeling of impending doom and apprehension
   c. Other symptoms may be vague and nonspecific
      i. Dyspnea, tachypnea, increased work of breathing

    ii. Tachycardia, diffuse chest discomfort, reduced blood pressure

    iii. Anxiety, restlessness, apprehension, agitation, syncope

    iv. Asymmetric chest expansion due to pleuritic pain

    v. Petechiae over the thorax and upper extremities (fat emboli)

    vi. Diaphoresis, cold and clammy skin, and cyanosis

    vii. Increased fremitus with a large hemorrhagic pulmonary infarct; pleural friction fremitus may be palpated in patients with pleural inflammation distal to an infarct

    viii. Resonance heard throughout the lung fields except dullness to percussion over the area of infarction

    ix. Pleural friction rub; inspiratory crackles (rales) may be heard; increased intensity of the pulmonic second sound (P_2); fixed splitting of the second heart sound (S_2) is an ominous finding caused by marked right ventricular overload. Murmur is heard over the affected lung field, augmented by inspiration, and is generated by flow through a partially obstructed pulmonary artery. Murmur may be absent initially and then develop as an embolus resolves.

4. Diagnostic study findings

  a. Laboratory: ABG levels may indicate respiratory alkalosis (caused by hyperventilation) and hypoxemia; A–a gradient is increased; in a small percentage (6%) of patients, the A–a gradient may be normal

  b. Radiologic

    i. Chest radiograph: Nonspecific, frequently normal. Pleural effusion occurs in 30% to 50% of cases but is small; atelectasis and elevated hemidiaphragm on the affected side may be seen. Useful to defect other things causing similar symptoms.

    ii. Lower-extremity Doppler ultrasonography: To evaluate for DVT as a possible cause. Negative findings on serial ultrasonographic scans reduce the likelihood of PE to less than 2%.

    iii. Pulmonary angiography: Most definitive test (gold standard) for PE; should be considered when results of noninvasive tests are equivocal or contradictory or as an initial diagnostic test if the patient is hemodynamically unstable

    iv. CT-angio or CT-PA may also be done.

  c. Electrocardiogram (ECG): Usually normal, but in massive PE may reveal "P pulmonale," right-axis deviation, or incomplete or new righty bundle branch block. ECG often demonstrates sinus tachycardia or, less frequently, atrial fibrillation or flutter.

  d. Radionuclide testing: Lung ventilation-perfusion scan not definitive but suggestive of PE; less risky than angiography; performed for all clinically stable patients with suspected PE; about 60% of $\dot{V}/\dot{Q}$ scans will show indeterminate findings

5. Goals of care

  a. Pulmonary artery blood flow is restored

  b. Hemodynamic parameters return to normal

  c. Recurrence or worsening of embolization and thrombosis is prevented

  d. Chest pain is relieved

6. Collaborating professionals on health care team: Nurse, physician, pulmonologist, respiratory therapist, clinical pharmacologist

7. Management of patient care

  a. Anticipated patient trajectory

    i. Positioning: Keep the head of the bed elevated at 30 to 45 degrees to enhance ventilation and prevent aspiration. Avoid using knee elevation on a Gatch bed; instruct the patient to avoid crossing the legs or sitting with the feet dependent for long periods. Vary position and do range-of-motion manipulations to enhance peripheral blood flow.

ii. Skin care: Inspect skin integrity regularly, especially on the lower legs. Promptly report the patient's development of pain, swelling, tenderness, rubor, and localized warmth in a lower extremity (suggestive of phlebitis, possible thrombosis). Have the patient perform active or passive range-of-motion exercises, ambulate when able, wear antiembolism stockings as ordered.

iii. Pain management: Administer analgesics for relief of chest pain (can be severe)

iv. Nutrition: Ensure adequate fluid intake to avoid dehydration and increased blood viscosity

v. Discharge planning: Provide patient education and follow-up related to the prevention of phlebitis and DVT, facilitation of venous return, and safe use of anticoagulants

vi. Pharmacology: Administer anticoagulants as ordered; monitor for signs of bleeding; administer thrombolytic therapy, sedatives, and pain medication as ordered

vii. Treatments
   (a) O_2 administration, as needed
   (b) Early ambulation, turning, promotion of coughing and deep breathing
   (c) Use of elastic stockings, pneumatic compression stockings (if not contraindicated with systemic anticoagulation), leg elevation
   (d) Adequate fluid intake
   (e) Thrombolytic and anticoagulant therapy, heparin or low-molecular-weight heparin
   (f) IV medications
   (g) Placement of filter device in inferior vena cava
   (h) Surgical embolectomy

b. Potential complications
   i. Hospital-acquired infection: Aspiration; see Acute Respiratory Failure
   ii. Bleeding
      (a) Mechanism: Risk of anticoagulation therapy
      (b) Management: Judicious, closely monitored use of anticoagulants

8. **Evaluation of patient care**
   a. Respiratory rate, breathing pattern, and hemodynamic parameters are normal for the patient
   b. Arterial pH, P_{CO_2}, and P_{O_2} indicate desired levels of oxygenation, ventilation, and acid-base balance for the patient
   c. Coagulation profile is within the desired range for the patient
   d. Patient reports a decrease in the sensation of dyspnea
   e. Patient denies chest pain and dyspnea

Chest Trauma

1. **Pathophysiology:** Depends on the type and extent of injury. Trauma to the chest or lungs may interfere with any of the components involved in inspiration, gas exchange, and expiration.
   a. *Blunt injuries:* Chest wall damage must be evaluated in conjunction with the accompanying intrathoracic and intraabdominal visceral injuries. Injuries seen with blunt trauma include the following:

       i. Visceral injuries without chest wall damage
         (a) Pneumothorax, hemothorax
         (b) Lung contusion
         (c) Diaphragmatic injury
         (d) Myocardial contusion, aortic rupture
         (e) Rupture of the trachea or bronchus
      ii. Soft tissue injuries—possibly a sign of severe underlying damage
         (a) Cutaneous abrasion
         (b) Ecchymosis
         (c) Laceration of superficial layers
         (d) Burns
         (e) Hematoma
     iii. Fracture of the sternum: Occurs either as a result of direct impact or as the indirect result of overflexion of the trunk
     iv. Rib fractures as a result of overflexion or straightening. Rib fractures can be unifocal or multifocal. Multiple fractures result in *flail chest* and are often complicated by injuries to the soft tissues and pleura.
      v. Separation or dislocation of ribs or cartilage from a blow to the anterior chest
  b. *Penetrating injuries*
       i. Pleural cavity as well as the chest wall has been entered. Damage to deeper structures is a serious consequence.
      ii. Extent of injury and the organs injured generally can be predicted by the course of the wound and the nature of the penetrating instrument. High-velocity projectiles do more damage than is apparent from the surface.
     iii. Injuries seen with penetrating trauma
         (a) Open sucking chest wounds with air entering the pleural space during inspiration
         (b) Hemothorax, hemopneumothorax, or chylothorax
         (c) Combined thoracoabdominal injuries (esophageal, diaphragmatic, or abdominal viscus injuries)
         (d) Damage to the trachea and large airways
         (e) Wounds of the heart or great vessels

2. Etiology and risk factors
  a. Blunt trauma: Automobile crashes, falls, assaults, explosions
  b. Penetrating trauma: Automobile crashes; falls; assaults; explosions; injury by bullets, knives, shell fragments, free-flying objects; industrial accidents

3. Signs and symptoms
  a. Chief complaint varies with the specific injury. Tachypnea, dyspnea, pain, and respiratory distress may occur with any injury. Other symptoms vary with the type of trauma.
  b. Fractures of the ribs, sternochondral junction, or sternum: Pain accentuated by chest wall movement, deep inspiration, or touch
  c. Flail chest: Dyspnea and localized pain
  d. Trauma to the lung parenchyma, trachea, or bronchi: Hemoptysis, respiratory distress
  e. Contusion of the heart: Angina
  f. Rupture of the aorta and major vessels: Dyspnea and backache, intense pain in the chest or back unaffected by respirations; rapid exsanguination may occur
  g. Open sucking chest wound: If the opening in the chest wall is smaller than the diameter of the trachea, the patient may have minimal subjective symptoms. If the opening is larger, more air enters the pleural space, which collapses the lung, impairs ventilation and gas exchange, and results in dyspnea.

    h. Skin: Ecchymosis, hematomas, abrasions, burns, and lacerations

    i. Increased work of breathing: Use of accessory muscles, intercostal retractions

    j. Shallow respirations (seen with pain from rib fractures); tachypnea often accompanies pain and apprehension

    k. Chest wall asymmetry seen with tension pneumothorax or hemothorax. In flail chest, chest wall movement is paradoxical—sinks on inspiration and flails out on expiration.

    l. Subcutaneous emphysema: May be palpable in pneumothorax or rupture of the trachea or bronchus

    m. Position of the trachea may be displaced—toward the injured side in pneumothorax, toward the contralateral side in hemothorax or tension pneumothorax

    n. Ipsilateral tympany or hyperresonance in pneumothorax and tension pneumothorax

    o. In rupture of the diaphragm, the left hemidiaphragm is usually involved, which results in dullness (from fluid-filled bowel) or tympany (from gas-filled bowel) heard over the left chest

    p. Dullness to percussion with hemothorax, hemopneumothorax, or parenchymal hemorrhage

    q. Reduced breath sounds heard in any condition in which there are shallow respirations; diminished or absent breath sounds heard in pneumothorax, tension pneumothorax, flail chest, hemothorax, or hemopneumothorax; bronchial breath sounds heard with parenchymal hemorrhage

    r. Bowel sounds may be heard in the chest with rupture of the diaphragm

4. Diagnostic study findings

    a. Radiologic

        i. Chest radiography is performed for all injuries if the patient is stable

            (a) Visualizes rib fractures, parenchymal hemorrhage, hemothorax, or hemopneumothorax

            (b) Pneumothorax: Expiratory chest films are often used in the diagnosis

            (c) Tension pneumothorax: Shows a shift in the mediastinum to the unaffected side in addition to pneumothorax

            (d) Rupture of the diaphragm: Shows bowel loops in the thorax

            (e) Rupture of the aorta or major vessels: Revealed by a widening of the mediastinum

        ii. MRI or CT if the patient is stable: Can further identify specific injuries that may need to be surgically corrected

        iii. Aortography: Confirms the diagnosis of rupture of the aorta or other major vessels

    b. ECG: To evaluate heart contusion, in which tachycardia, dysrhythmias, and electrocardiographic changes may be found

    c. Bronchoscopy: May confirm a diagnosis of rupture of the trachea or bronchus

5. Goals of care

    a. Patent airway is maintained

    b. ABG levels and pulmonary parameters are restored to and maintained within acceptable limits for the patient

    c. Chest wall integrity and stability are restored

    d. Integrity of the pleural space is reestablished

    e. Chest pain and dyspnea are minimized

6. Collaborating professionals on health care team: See Acute Respiratory Failure

7. Management of patient care

    a. Anticipated patient trajectory

i. Positioning: Keep the head of the bed elevated 30 to 45 degrees to optimize ventilation and prevent aspiration; provide symptomatic treatment for uncomplicated rib fractures to ensure the ability to cough and deep breathe

ii. Skin care: Clean and remove debris from wounds; reinforce dressings as necessary; provide wound care around chest tubes and at other invasive sites

iii. Pain management: Pain medication and sedatives to relieve the discomfort of tubes and treatment and prevent treatment interference. Administer analgesia judiciously to avoid compromise of ventilation.

iv. Nutrition: Provide adequate nutrition to promote healing; secure pharmacologic and dietary consults for composition and administration of parenteral and/or enteral feeding. Maintain accurate input and output records and monitor fluid balance.

v. Infection control: See Acute Respiratory Failure. Patient with a history of penetrating trauma with "dirty" or contaminated instruments and/or multiple wounds may be especially at risk.

vi. Transport: Initial and any subsequent transport must maintain appropriate levels of care, support of vital functions, body alignment, and readiness for emergencies as provided in units. See Patient Transport in Chapter 11.

vii. Discharge planning: Evaluate the need for rehabilitation on discharge; anticipate home care equipment needs

viii. Pharmacology: Antibiotics as needed, sedatives and pain medication

ix. Psychosocial issues: Unanticipated nature of the trauma may increase the difficulty of the patient and family in adjusting to the patient's current circumstances. Especially early on, family members need considerable support and information to ease their concerns and prepare them for the patient's likely prognosis. Securing assistance from pastoral care staff, social services, or other support staff may ease in provision of support to the family. Once the patient is able to comprehend what has transpired, he or she will need comparable support throughout hospitalization.

x. Treatments

(a) Intubation, mechanical ventilation, suctioning, O_2 therapy, O_2 delivery devices. See Acute Respiratory Failure.

(b) Provide nutrition via TPN or nasogastric, PEG, or small-bore feeding tube

(c) Perform suctioning as needed to stimulate cough and clear the airways of blood and secretions

(d) Intrapleural chest tubes drainage system: Monitor water seal chest drainage in the treatment of pneumothorax or hemothorax; observe for the absence or presence of bubbling in the water seal chamber; if suction is ordered, maintain the appropriate suction setting; monitor and record the volume and nature of drainage; notify the physician if the volume of bloody drainage exceeds the limit set by protocol, unit routine, or written order

(e) Avoid dependent loops in chest drainage tubing to facilitate drainage; properly secure the chest tube insertion site. Observe for signs of leaking pleural fluid or bleeding at the insertion site; routinely check the system for loose connections.

(f) Be prepared for an inadvertent break in a closed chest drainage system set for negative pressure; follow unit procedure in the event of a break in system integrity

(g) Assist with emergency decompression of tension pneumothorax through insertion of a large-bore needle into the second anterior interspace or insertion of a chest tube

    xi. Ethical issues: If relevant to the case, see discussion in Acute Respiratory Failure, Chronic Obstructive Pulmonary Disease; see also Chapter 1

  b. Potential complications

    i. Hospital-associated infection via aspiration, urinary tract infection, wound contamination; see Acute Respiratory Failure, Chronic Obstructive Pulmonary Disease

    ii. Trauma related: See Chapter 9

8. Evaluation of patient care

  a. Respiratory rate, breathing pattern, and ABG values are normal for the patient

  b. Chest wall motion and expansion are normal in both phases of ventilation

  c. All blood, air, chyle, or other foreign matter is evacuated from the pleural space; negative pressure is restored; both lungs are fully expanded

  d. Patient denies chest pain, shortness of breath, and dyspnea

Acute Pneumonia

1. Pathophysiology

  a. Inflammatory process of the alveolar spaces caused by infection

  b. Possible pathogenic mechanisms for the development of pneumonia include the following:

    i. Aspiration

    ii. Inhalation

    iii. Inoculation

    iv. Direct spread from contiguous sites

    v. Hematogenous spread

    vi. Colonization in chronic lung disease (e.g., COPD, cystic fibrosis)

  c. Acquisition of infection depends on the nature of the infecting organism, the immediate environment, and the defense status of the host

  d. Important constituents of the pulmonary defense system

    i. Upper airway defenses: Adversely affected by nasotracheal intubation, endotracheal intubation, suction catheters, nasogastric tubes

      (a) Nasopharyngeal filtration

      (b) Mucosal adherence

      (c) Bacterial interference

      (d) Saliva

      (e) Secretory immunoglobulin A

    ii. Lower airway defenses: May be impaired or inactivated by old age; underlying diseases such as diabetes, chronic bronchitis, malnutrition; and drug or O_2 therapy

      (a) Cough reflex

      (b) Mucociliary clearance

      (c) Humoral factors

      (d) Cellular factors

2. Etiology and risk factors

  a. Normal host infected with usual organisms

    i. *Streptococcus pneumoniae* (pneumococcus): Most common cause, especially in older patients and those with a variety of chronic diseases

    ii. *Mycoplasma pneumoniae* ("walking pneumonia"): Spread by droplet nuclei; may occur in epidemics

iii. *Haemophilus influenzae:* With encapsulated type B organisms, is more likely to cause bacteremia; nontypable *H. influenzae* is seen more in the elderly population

iv. Viruses: Relatively uncommon cause of pneumonia in adults, accounting for 25% to 50% of nonbacterial pneumonias; influenza A virus is the most common cause; others include adenovirus and coxsackievirus; pneumonia caused by cytomegalovirus (CMV), respiratory syncytial virus, and herpes simplex virus are often seen in immunocompromised patients

v. *Chlamydia pneumoniae:* Causes a spectrum of illnesses from mild upper respiratory symptoms to pneumonia

vi. Fungi: Inhalation of *Histoplasma capsulatum* results in acute severe pulmonary histoplasmosis. Similar reactions occur in patients infected with *Blastomyces dermatitidis, Cryptococcus, Coccidioides immitis, Aspergillus fumigatus*, and *Candida albicans*. Geographic location is important in identifying certain organisms.

b. Normal host infected with unusual organisms

i. *Legionella pneumophila* infections may be sporadic or occur in localized outbreaks in institutions

ii. *Bacillus anthracis* infects humans who have been in contact with anthrax-infected animals

iii. *Yersinia pestis* causes plague; transmitted from wild animals and their fleas, or via the respiratory route

iv. *Francisella tularensis* causes pleuropulmonary tularemia, endemic in certain parts of the United States; transmitted by ticks or, possibly, by inhalation from infected animals

v. Group A *Streptococcus* and *Meningococcus* bacteria reside in the upper respiratory tract; pneumonia occurs in individuals housed in groups, such as in military service. *Streptococcus pyogenes* causes pneumonia typically after outbreaks of viral infections.

vi. *Mycobacterium tuberculosis* infection or atypical TB can produce life-threatening pulmonary complications in hosts whose only risk factor is age

c. Abnormal host infected with usual organisms: Compromised states can result from the presence of chronic underlying disease, poor nutrition, trauma, or surgery, or subsequent to immunosuppression

i. Pneumococcal pneumonia is more severe in this population

ii. Gram-negative bacilli, such as *Escherichia coli, Pseudomonas aeruginosa, Serratia, Proteus vulgaris, Acinetobacter* and *Klebsiella pneumoniae,* and *Moraxella catarrhalis,* can be the causative organisms

iii. Anaerobic bacteria, such as *Bacteroides,* cause severe pulmonary infections in the abnormal host

iv. *Staphylococcus aureus* pneumonia is seen in diabetic patients, in patients with a recent history of influenza, and institutionalized or hospitalized patients

v. *K. pneumoniae* causes a virulent, necrotizing pneumonia often seen in alcoholic or debilitated patients; abscess formation is common

d. Abnormal host infected with unusual organisms

i. Enterococcal pneumonia is associated with the use of third-generation cephalosporins

ii. Group B *S. pneumoniae* pneumonia is often seen in older patients with underlying diseases

iii. Hospital-acquired *L. pneumophila* pneumonia occurs in renal transplant patients and those who are debilitated and immunocompromised

       iv. *Legionella micdadei,* the Pittsburgh pneumonia agent, may infect renal transplant patients during corticosteroid therapy

       v. Fungi, including *A. fumigatus* and *Aspergillus flavum,* produce pneumonia mostly in patients who have received high doses of steroids and broad-spectrum antibiotics

      vi. *Nocardia asteroides* pneumonia is seen in renal transplant patients and patients with hematologic malignancies

     vii. *Pneumocystis carinii* infections, infections with typical and atypical mycobacteria, and CMV infections are seen in patients with acquired immunodeficiency syndrome

   e. Multidrug-resistant organisms, vancomycin-resistant enterococci, and penicillin-resistant *S. pneumoniae* are becoming more prevalent in the community, so that patients may enter facilities with the infection rather than acquire it in the hospital

   f. Pneumonias can be categorized by their mode of origin as follows:

       i. Ventilator-associated pneumonia

      ii. Hospital-acquired pneumonia

     iii. Health care–associated pneumonia

     iv. Community-acquired pneumonia

3. Signs and symptoms

   a. Chief complaint varies, depending on the organism. Some common presentations include the following:

       i. Pneumococcal pneumonia: Abrupt shaking chills or rigor, fever, dyspnea, pleuritic pain, and cough productive of rusty sputum

      ii. *Mycoplasma*: Fever, myalgias, headache, minimally productive cough, and nonpleuritic chest pain

     iii. *H. influenzae*: Fever, chills, and cough with purulent sputum

     iv. *Klebsiella*: Sudden onset, blood-tinged sputum, and tachypnea

   b. Clinical features: See Acute Respiratory Failure; also hypoxemia, increased work of breathing, impaired alveolar ventilation, impaired respiratory gas exchange

       i. Asymmetric chest expansion with dullness or flatness to percussion over affected areas

      ii. Breath sounds may be decreased; fine inspiratory crackles or bronchial breath sounds over areas of consolidation (lobar pneumonia)

     iii. Bronchophony; whispered pectoriloquy and egophony may also be heard with consolidation

4. Diagnostic study findings

   a. Laboratory

       i. Sputum examination

          (a) Color and consistency vary with the pathogen

          (b) Initial Gram staining and microscopic examination

            (1) Good sputum specimen contains few (less than five) squamous epithelial cells picked up in transit through the upper respiratory tract. When sputum cannot be expectorated, a specimen may be obtained by other means such as suctioning, transtracheal aspiration, fiberoptic bronchoscopy, needle aspiration of the lung, or open lung biopsy.

            (2) Examination of expectorated sputum specimens has relatively poor sensitivity and specificity

            (3) Staining demonstrates polymorphonuclear leukocytes (PMNs) and bacterial agents; large numbers of PMNs are seen in most bacterial pneumonias; fewer PMNs and more mononuclear inflammatory cells are seen in mycoplasmal and viral pneumonias

(4) Sputum cultures are done with initial Gram staining and microscopic examination; however, some bacteria are relatively difficult to grow, so the initial Gram stain result is just as important in making the etiologic diagnosis

   ii. Blood cultures

     (a) Obtaining a blood sample is very important in patient evaluation because of the high specificity of a positive culture result, especially in hospitalized patients with pneumococcal pneumonia

     (b) Blood and sputum cultures are obtained before antibotic administration

     (c) Patients with documented bacteremic pneumonia have a worse prognosis than those with nonbacteremic pneumonia

   iii. Leukocyte counts

     (a) Often elevated in lobar pneumonia; may be normal with atypical pneumonia

     (b) Normal or reduced in the elderly, in immunocompromised patients, in patients with overwhelming infections, and in those with viral infection

   iv. ABG analysis: May indicate hypoxemia and hypocapnia in lobar pneumonia

  b. Radiologic: Chest radiographic findings vary with involvement

   i. Segmental or lobar consolidation, infiltrates

   ii. Particularly helpful in detecting parapneumonic effusions, abscesses, and cavities

  c. Thoracentesis: May be indicated when significant pleural effusion is present

5. Goals of care

  a. Pulmonary infection is halted and reversed

  b. Oxygenation and ventilation are improved

  c. Removal of airway secretions is facilitated

  d. Vital signs, ABG values, and respiratory dynamics are restored to within normal limits for the patient

  e. Dyspnea at rest and with exertion are minimized

  f. Positive nitrogen balance is established and maintained to promote regaining of strength and healing

6. Collaborating professionals on health care team: See Acute Respiratory Failure, Chronic Obstructive Pulmonary Disease

7. Management of patient care

  a. Anticipated patient trajectory:

   i. Positioning: See Acute Respiratory Failure, Chronic Obstructive Pulmonary Disease; change position to mobilize secretions; avoid the supine position

   ii. Skin care: Turn frequently to drain lungs and maintain skin integrity

   iii. Pain management: Pleuritic chest pain control may be achieved by antiinflammatory agents, analgesics, or intercostal nerve blocks; pain medication and sedatives need to relieve the discomfort of tubes and treatment and prevent interference with turning, coughing, deep breathing, incentive spirometry, ambulation

   iv. Nutrition: Enlist assistance from a dietitian to ensure that nutritional intake is adequate to restore strength, facilitate ventilator weaning, and support healing and recovery; if possible, use the enteral route to reduce infection risk

   v. Infection control: Regular, thorough oral care with brushing (versus swabbing) and cleansing appears to reduce morbidity and mortality from pneumonia. Use strict infection control procedures; avoid unnecessary invasive procedures or limit their duration of use.

   vi. Transport: See Chronic Obstructive Pulmonary Disease

      vii. Pharmacology: Administer antibiotics within 8 hours of admission, pre-ferrably within 4 hours, and monitor response; administer sedatives and pain medication as needed

      viii. Treatments: See Acute Respiratory Failure

  b. Potential complications

      i. Superimposed hospital-associated infection(s): See Acute Respiratory Failure

      ii. Difficulty weaning or liberating from mechanical ventilation: See Impaired Alveolar Ventilation Respiratory Failure, Chronic Obstructive Pulmonary Disease

8. Evaluation of patient care

  a. No clinical, laboratory, or radiologic evidence of pulmonary infection is present

  b. Secretions are minimal and the patient able to expectorate readily

  c. Blood gas values and ventilatory parameters are within acceptable limits

  d. Breath sounds are clear bilaterally and no adventitious sounds are present

Pulmonary Aspiration

1. Pathophysiology (varies with the type of aspiration)

  a. Pulmonary aspiration may result from vomiting or regurgitation. *Vomiting* is an active mechanism that interrupts breathing, causes the diaphragm to descend, contracts the anterior abdominal wall, elevates the diaphragm, closes the pylorus, and opens the esophageal sphincter, which results in ejection of contents from the stomach. *Regurgitation* is completely passive and may occur even in the presence of paralyzed muscles. Powerful laryngeal and cough reflexes normally prevent aspiration of gastric contents into the tracheobronchial tree. Any impairment or depression of these normal reflexes increases the risk of pulmonary aspiration.

  b. Large particles: Can obstruct major airways and cause immediate asphyxiation and death

  c. Clear acidic liquid: pH of aspirated material largely determines the extent of pulmonary injury. If the pH decreases below 2.5 or if the volume of acidic fluid is large, the severity of lung injury increases.

      i. Chemical burns destroy type II alveolar cells that produce surfactant and increase alveolar capillary membrane permeability, with subsequent extravasation of fluid and blood into the interstitium and alveoli

      ii. As fluid and blood accumulate in the alveolar space, the lung volume diminishes; thus, both FRC and compliance decrease. Reflex airway closure may also occur.

      iii. Alveolar ventilation decreases relative to perfusion, which results in intra-pulmonary shunting. Hypoxia can occur minutes after acid aspiration.

      iv. Extensive irritation of the airways by acidic fluid may induce intense bron-chospasm

      v. Widespread peribronchial hemorrhage along with pulmonary edema and necrosis may occur

  d. Clear nonacidic liquid: Nature and extent of pulmonary damage depends on the volume of the aspirate and its composition

      i. Aspiration of less acidic or neutral pH liquids can induce hypoxia with acute respiratory decompensation. Reflex airway closure, pulmonary edema, and changes in the characteristics of surfactant may occur. There is little necrosis.

      ii. Sequelae are more frequently transient and more easily reversible than with aspiration of acidic liquid

e. Foodstuff or small particles: May produce a severe subacute inflammatory pulmonary reaction with extensive hemorrhage

    i. Within 6 hours of aspiration, there may be extensive hemorrhagic pneumonia

    ii. Extravasation of fluid from the intravascular space into the lungs usually occurs but is generally not as intense or rapid as after acid aspiration

    iii. Severe intrapulmonary shunting may result, and arterial Po_2 may be as low as or lower than that seen after the aspiration of acidic liquid

    iv. Arterial Pco_2 is usually much higher after the aspiration of food. This may indicate a higher degree of hypoventilation.

    v. Aspiration of acidic foodstuff may produce even more tissue necrosis as a result of the combined effects of acid and foods

f. Contaminated material: Aspiration of material grossly contaminated with bacteria (i.e., in bowel obstruction) can be fatal

2. **Etiology and risk factors:** Aspiration is usually associated with specific predisposing conditions

a. Altered consciousness: Drug or alcohol use, anesthesia, seizures, CNS disorders, shock, use of sedatives

b. Altered anatomy: Tracheostomy, esophageal or tracheal abnormalities, nasogastric or nasointestinal tube, endotracheal tube, intestinal obstruction

c. Protracted vomiting or coughing

d. Improper positioning of the patient, especially if the patient is receiving enteral hyperalimentation

3. **Signs and symptoms**

a. Patient's chief complaints: Cough, dyspnea, wheezing. With fluid or solid object aspiration, there can be an abrupt onset of acute respiratory distress.

b. Hypoxemia: See Acute Respiratory Failure, Inability to Establish or Maintain a Patent Airway, Impaired Respiratory Mechanics

c. Increased work of breathing (depends on the nature and extent of aspiration): See Chronic Obstructive Pulmonary Disease, Asthma

d. Increased respiratory secretions, hypotension, tachycardia, tachypnea, fever

e. Inspiratory stridor due to foreign body obstruction of a large bronchus; may be accompanied by cyanosis, tachypnea, use of accessory respiratory muscles

f. Wheezing heard with aspiration of both liquids and solid objects. Crackles and possible wheezing heard in the affected lung with aspiration. Absent breath sounds if a major bronchus is occluded.

4. **Diagnostic study findings**

a. Laboratory

    i. Sputum examination: Induced cough or tracheal suction to obtain specimens for stain and culture; cytologic examination is sometimes diagnostic. Fiberoptic bronchoscopy is sometimes used in infectious processes.

    ii. ABG analysis: May demonstrate hypoxemia

b. Radiologic: Dependent lobe infiltrates and atelectasis. Gravity-dependent areas of the lungs most prone to aspiration include the superior segments of the lower lobes and the posterior segments of the upper and lower lobes. If a nasogastric or nasointestinal tube is in place, radiographs should verify their proper location and position, particularly if medications and/or enteral formula feedings are being administered.

c. Pulmonary function: May show decreased compliance or decreased diffusing capacity

d. Open lung biopsy: Reserved for patients who are unable to safely undergo transbronchial biopsy

5. **Goals of care**
   a. Patent airway is established and maintained
   b. Oxygenation and alveolar ventilation return to normal values
   c. Harmful effects of the aspirant on pulmonary function are minimized
   d. Recurrence of aspiration is prevented
6. **Collaborating professionals on health care team:** See Acute Respiratory Failure, Chronic Obstructive Pulmonary Disease
7. **Management of patient care**
   a. Anticipated patient trajectory: See also Acute Pneumonia, Acute Respiratory Failure
      i. Positioning: Elevate head of the bed 30 to 45 degrees to prevent recurrence of aspiration; avoid the supine position or any posture that predisposes to regurgitation or aspiration, especially if enteral feedings are administered
      ii. Nutrition: See Acute Pneumonia. If the patient is being fed nasoenterally, carefully verify the location of the feeding tube and routinely assess for pulmonary aspiration by clinical findings as well as routine testing of tracheal aspirates for the presence or absence of glucose. False-positive readings may be caused by blood or other unknown factors.
      iii. Infection control: Monitor carefully because many aspirants may cause chemical irritation and/or infection
      iv. Transport: Maintain precautions to prevent aspiration throughout transport
      v. Discharge planning: If the patient will return home with a feeding tube in place, provide patient and family education regarding safe administration of tube feedings; supervision by home care services may need to be arranged
      vi. Pharmacology: Antibiotics may be necessary if infection ensues; corticosteroids may be of benefit if given immediately after aspiration of acid
      vii. Treatments: See Pneumonia, Acute Respiratory Failure
   b. Potential complications: See Pneumonia, Acute Respiratory Failure
8. **Evaluation of patient care**
   a. Airway remains patent and free of secretions
   b. ABG values and ventilatory parameters are within acceptable limits
   c. No clinical evidence of complications from aspirated material is present

Near-Drowning

1. **Pathophysiology**
   a. Near-drowning is defined as immersion in a liquid that necessitates the victim's being transported to a hospital emergency department but is not severe enough to result in death within the first 24 hours after submersion
   b. Electrolyte change: There is a tendency toward hemoconcentration in salt water drowning and toward hemodilution in fresh water drowning; however, dangerous changes in plasma electrolyte levels are very unusual
   c. Pulmonary effects: 90% of victims aspirate fluid, and most victims (85%) aspirate less than 25 ml/kg of body weight; however, the water aspirated may contain mud, sand, algae, chemicals, and/or vomitus
      i. In fresh water aspiration, water rapidly enters the circulation; in salt water aspiration, the hypertonic sea water draws fluid from the circulation into the lungs. However, near-drowning victims of salt water and fresh water immersion have the same initial pathophysiologic aberrations: Major insults include hypoxemia and tissue hypoxia, hypoxic brain injury with cerebral edema, hypercapnia, and acidemia. Hypothermia, pneumonia, and (rarely) disseminated intravascular coagulation (DIC), acute renal failure, and hemolysis may also occur.

      ii. Organic and inorganic contents of the aspirated fluid, regardless of the type of water, produce an inflammatory reaction in the alveolar-capillary membrane that leads to an outpouring of plasma-rich exudate into the alveolus, displacement of air, and deposition of proteinaceous material

      iii. There is destruction of surfactant by aspirated water and proteinaceous exudate, which results in large areas of atelectasis

      iv. Regional hypoxia promotes hypoxic vasoconstriction, which raises pulmonary intravascular pressures, promotes further interstitial fluid flux, and frequently gives rise to pulmonary edema

      v. In some patients, hyaline membranes develop on the walls of injured bronchioles, alveolar ducts, and alveoli. This results in reduced compliance and increased ratio of dead space to tidal volume, increased respiratory work, and $\dot{V}/\dot{Q}$ mismatch.

2. Etiology and risk factors

  a. Fresh water or salt water immersion due to young age and inability to swim

  b. Prior alcohol or drug ingestion

  c. Head and neck trauma and loss of consciousness associated with epilepsy, diabetes, syncope, or dysrhythmias

  d. Barotrauma associated with scuba diving; CO_2 narcosis ("the bends")

3. Signs and symptoms

  a. Patient's chief complaint: Respiratory distress, coughing

  b. Unconsciousness, neurologic deficits if cerebral anoxia has occurred

  c. Tachypnea and intercostal retractions in the conscious patient (must generate greater negative inspiratory forces to inflate fluid-filled, less compliant lungs)

  d. Apnea in the unconscious patient; may also see cyanosis, other signs of hypoxemia, anoxia

  e. Hypothermia or fever

  f. Diminished chest expansion owing to low lung compliance; dullness to percussion over most lung zones (possible diffuse pulmonary edema); possible diffuse crackles on inspiration

4. Diagnostic study findings

  a. Laboratory

      i. Minimal electrolyte and Hb changes

      ii. ABG levels: Hypoxemia and metabolic acidosis

      iii. Leukocytosis

      iv. Coagulation studies: Coagulation disorders, including DIC, have been reported in near-drowning victims; screening studies of prothrombin time, activated partial thromboplastin time, and platelet count are often done. If these results are abnormal, fibrinogen levels, fibrin split product levels, and euglobulin clot lysis time should be tested.

  b. Radiologic: Chest radiograph shows aspiration or pulmonary edema

  c. ECG: May show dysrhythmias, nonspecific changes. Few victims die of ventricular fibrillation. Acidemia, CO_2 retention, and hypoxemia result in marked irregular bradycardia, which precedes asystole and cardiac arrest.

5. Goals of care

  a. Effective ventilation and perfusion are restored (Advanced Cardiac Life Support at the scene)

  b. Patient is rewarmed to normothermia if hypothermic

  c. Gastric contents are evacuated

  d. ABG levels, oxygenation, electrolyte levels, and fluid balance values are normalized

  e. Early complications are minimized and late complications are prevented

6. **Collaborating professionals on health care team:** See Acute Pneumonia and Respiratory Failure
7. **Management of patient care**
   a. Anticipated patient trajectory
      i. Positioning: Keep the patient's head and neck in the neutral position and avoid hyperextension of the cervical spine until spinal cord and head trauma injuries have been ruled out
      ii. Skin care: If the patient was submerged in cold water, use core rewarming to gradually return body temperature to the normal range. Monitor and maintain skin integrity via hypothermia-hyperthermia devices.
      iii. Nutrition: Patient may require insulin for hyperglycemia; nasogastric tube may be needed for gastric decompression
      iv. Infection control: Use good hand hygiene to prevent transmission of infection
      v. Transport: See Positioning earlier
      vi. Pharmacology: Patient may require vasopressors for blood pressure support, sodium bicarbonate for metabolic acidosis, β-agonists for bronchospasm, diuretics for fluid balance
      vii. Psychosocial issues: If incident was not accidental, the circumstances of the near-drowning episode may warrant follow-up and counseling. Patient prognosis will affect the need for family support and home care issues.
      viii. Treatments: See Acute Pneumonia, Acute Respiratory Failure
   b. Potential complications
      i. Early: See each respective disorder (Chapters 4, 5, and 8)
         (a) Hyperglycemia
         (b) Hypothermia
         (c) Fluid and electrolyte imbalances
         (d) Seizures
      ii. Late: See each respective condition (Chapters 3 and 9 and relevant sections of the present chapter)
         (a) ARDS
         (b) Aspiration pneumonia
         (c) Pulmonary edema
         (d) Sepsis
8. **Evaluation of patient care**
   a. ABG levels and O_2 saturation are within normal limits for the patient
   b. Normothermia and fluid and electrolyte balance are restored
   c. Neurologic status is normal
   d. No clinical evidence of complications from the incident are present

Pulmonary Problems in Surgical Patients

1. **Pathophysiology**
   a. Surgery represents a stress to the respiratory system. Pulmonary problems are the major cause of morbidity after surgery.
   b. Changes in pulmonary function occur normally during the immediately postoperative period. These changes are most evident following abdominal or thoracic surgery.
      i. Reduction in FVC is consistent with a restrictive defect; it is significant but usually temporary
      ii. Reduction in lung volumes, especially FRC, also occurs, due in part to pain and the supine position

      iii. Reduced lung compliance is present, resulting in reduced tidal volume and increased respiratory frequency

  c. Microatelectasis is the most common cause of hypoxemia; the increased respiratory frequency leads to respiratory alkalosis

  d. Bacterial invasion of the lower airways and reduced clearance postoperatively predispose to respiratory infection

  e. Aspiration of gastric and oropharyngeal contents occurs postoperatively in patients who have a disturbance in consciousness

  f. Arterial hypoxemia due to $\dot{V}/\dot{Q}$ mismatching is common in the postoperative period in normal patients and is exaggerated in patients with COPD

2. Etiology and risk factors

  a. History of COPD or cigarette smoking is the most important risk factor. Preoperative hypercapnia is a serious risk factor.

  b. Obesity results in decreased vital capacity

  c. Very young and elderly persons are at increased risk for these complications

  d. People with underlying chronic diseases are at greater risk

  e. Prolonged anesthesia time increases risk

  f. Thoracic and abdominal surgery are especially hazardous to patients at risk. Maximal inspirations are voluntarily limited because of pain, which thereby increases the risk of atelectasis.

3. Signs and symptoms

  a. Patient's chief complaint varies with the type of surgery but is often incisional pain

  b. Cough with or without sputum production and fear of or reluctance to cough, deep breathe, and move about after surgery

  c. Tachypnea, shallow respirations due to splinting with incisional pain may progress to signs of respiratory distress, increased work of breathing, dyspnea

  d. If atelectasis progresses to pneumonia, clinical signs include those related to fever and infection (e.g., crackles from small airway collapse due to shallow breathing, rhonchi or gurgles from secretions in the larger airways, wheezing indicating airflow obstruction, bronchial breath sounds with consolidation)

4. Diagnostic study findings

  a. Preoperative medical evaluation includes chest radiography, ECG, sputum examination, and pulmonary function tests

      i. FEV_1, FVC, and PEFR values are used to predict the development of postoperative pulmonary complications

      ii. Split pulmonary function studies estimate the amount of pulmonary function remaining postoperatively

      iii. Other diagnostic tests may be ordered preoperatively, depending on preexisting pulmonary or cardiac disease. These include CT scan of the chest and $\dot{V}/\dot{Q}$ scan.

  b. For patients with abnormal pulmonary function study results, ABG analysis is performed preoperatively. Presence of hypoxemia or CO_2 retention at baseline indicates that postoperative ABG levels should be followed closely.

  c. Cardiac stress test, possible cardiac catheterization if the stress test results are positive

5. Goal of care: Prevent or minimize postoperative pulmonary complications

6. Collaborating professionals on health care team: Nurse, physician, anesthesiologist, respiratory therapist

7. Management of patient care

  a. Anticipated patient trajectory: See Pulmonary Aspiration, Acute Pneumonia, Chronic Obstructive Pulmonary Disease

i. Treatments
    (a) Provide preoperative training in effective techniques for turning, deep breathing, coughing, ambulation, activity exercises, and active and passive range of motion exercises; suggest oral hygiene care
    (b) Encourage cessation of smoking at least 48 hours before surgery. If surgery can be postponed or is elective, cessation 4 to 6 weeks prior to surgery may be indicated.
    (c) Familiarize the patient with respiratory therapy equipment and techniques, such as incentive spirometry, chest physiotherapy, and the postoperative exercise program
    (d) Provide early ambulation and leg exercises, chest physiotherapy, and postural drainage
    (e) Guide the patient to perform intensive deep breathing exercises and incentive spirometry, and support chest and abdominal incisions during coughing
  b. Potential complications (see previous coverage of each complication listed)
    i. Acute pneumonia
    ii. Acute respiratory failure
    iii. Difficulty weaning from ventilator
8. **Evaluation of patient care**
  a. Patient evidences no clinical signs of pulmonary complications postoperatively
  b. Patient's pulmonary function is equivalent to or better than preoperative function

Acute Pulmonary Inhalation Injuries

1. **Pathophysiology**
  a. Inhalation injuries include smoke inhalation, thermal burns, and carbon monoxide poisoning
  b. Asphyxiants such as carbon monoxide displace O_2 from ambient air and from Hb O_2 binding sites
    i. Effects range from mild irritation of the eyes, throat, and upper respiratory tract to fatal respiratory failure
    ii. Toxic exposure causes irritation and edema of the mucous membranes, inflammatory capillary damage, bronchospasm, pulmonary edema (may be delayed up to 24 hours after exposure), and hypoxia
    iii. Inhalation injuries above the glottis may lead to upper airway obstruction
  c. Thermal injury to lung tissues produces mucosal sloughing, bronchorrhea, and pulmonary edema
  d. Systemic absorption of carbon monoxide or other chemical asphyxiants or irritants
    i. Carbon monoxide toxicity is related to dose, duration, alveolar ventilation (activity, cardiac output), and preexisting cardiovascular disease
    ii. Carbon monoxide is normally attached to Hb at levels of about 1% but has an affinity for the Hb molecule that is 200 to 250 times that of O_2. Small amounts of inspired carbon monoxide have major effects on the O_2-carrying capacity of blood and cause severe tissue hypoxia. Elimination of carbon monoxide is via the lungs only.
2. **Etiology and risk factors**
  a. Exposure to smoke or toxic gases
  b. Closed-space injury
  c. Prolonged exposure to injurious substances

    d. Unconsciousness

    e. Preexisting respiratory or cardiovascular disease

    f. Solubility of gas

3. Signs and symptoms

    a. Patient's chief complaint varies with the type of inhalation. Headache is often seen with carbon monoxide inhalation; cough, wheezing, and dyspnea are seen with inhalation of smoke and other noxious agents.

    b. Supraglottic injury evidenced by erythematous and edematous mucosa, blisters and ulcerations; worst 24 to 48 hours after inhalation

    c. Facial burns, singed nares, soot on tongue, and pharyngeal and oral blistering (signs of severe exposure)

    d. Edema of the lips and face, cyanosis

    e. Dizziness, headache, weakness, nausea and vomiting, diminished visual acuity, depressed mentation

    f. Tachypnea, use of accessory respiratory muscles

    g. Diffuse adventitious sounds bilaterally: Wheezes, crackles, and rhonchi

    h. Carbon monoxide poisoning: Cognitive, memory, visual, and personality changes; cherry-red color of the skin is a rare and late finding

4. Diagnostic study findings

    a. Laboratory

        i. Serial ABG analysis

            (a) Carbon monoxide poisoning does not cause a decrease in measured PaO_2 but impairs the O_2-carrying capacity of Hb. Directly measured SaO_2 is markedly reduced.

            (b) Hypoxemia is present in thermal injury and toxic exposure with a widened A–a gradient or decreased PaO_2/FIO_2 ratio

            (c) Determine whether saturation is measured or calculated; if calculated, severe hypoxemia may be missed

        ii. Serial carboxyhemoglobin analysis for carbon monoxide poisoning. Healthy nonsmoking individuals have a carboxyhemoglobin level of less than 2%, whereas smokers may have a level of 5% to 10%. Severe carbon monoxide poisoning is present when levels are higher than 20% to 40%. Levels above 60% are associated with coma and death.

    b. Radiologic: Chest studies—diffuse pulmonary edema in thermal injury and toxic inhalation; no change in carbon monoxide inhalation

    c. ECG: Tachycardia, ST-segment changes, conduction blocks, atrial or ventricular arrhythmias

    d. Fiberoptic bronchoscopy: To rule out and assess life-threatening upper airway injury. Presence of soot below the cords indicates more severe injury.

5. Goals of care

    a. Patent airway is established and maintained

    b. Adequate oxygenation and ventilation are restored

    c. Major complications of inhalation injury are avoided or minimized

6. Collaborating professionals on health care team: Physician, nurse, respiratory therapist

7. Management of patient care

    a. Anticipated patient trajectory: See Pulmonary Aspiration, Near-Drowning

        i. Positioning: Keep the head of the bed elevated at least 30 degrees to prevent aspiration

        ii. Skin care: Patient may require specialized care if related injury such as burns or caustic inflammation is present

        iii. Pain management: Pain medication and sedatives as warranted

      iv. Infection control: Infection is the primary complication of inhalation injuries, so due diligence with meticulous attention to its prevention is of paramount importance

      v. Pharmacology: Antibiotics only if a specific organism is identified; bronchodilators may be used; sedatives and pain medication as indicated

      vi. Treatments

         (a) Humidified 100% O_2 administration by tight-fitting mask or endotracheal tube for carbon monoxide poisoning to shorten the half-life of carboxyhemoglobin

         (b) Hyperbaric oxygenation for carbon monoxide poisoning if the patient has neurologic signs or symptoms, ECG changes consistent with ischemia, severe metabolic acidosis, pulmonary edema, or shock. Transfer to a hyperbaric treatment facility should occur only after the patient's condition has been stabilized.

         (c) Spo_2 values may be unreliable (this test measures the amount of saturated Hb but cannot distinguish whether the Hb is saturated with O_2 or carbon monoxide); need to correlate with Sao_2 values

  b. Potential complications

    i. Pulmonary edema: See Adult Respiratory Distress Syndrome

    ii. Infection: See Acute Pneumonia, Pulmonary Aspiration

8. Evaluation of patient care

  a. Airway is patent

  b. ABG levels and pulmonary function test results are within normal limits

  c. Toxic effects of the inhalant have subsided or are resolved

  d. No evidence exists of persisting complications

Neoplastic Lung Disease

1. Pathophysiology: Almost all lung cancers fall within one of four histologic categories: Squamous cell carcinoma, small cell carcinoma, adenocarcinoma, and large cell carcinoma. In addition, two other forms of neoplastic lung disease are discussed: Bronchial carcinoids and malignant mesothelioma.

  a. *Squamous cell carcinoma:* Constitutes approximately one third of all bronchogenic carcinomas. These tumors originate in the epithelial layer of the bronchial wall. Series of progressive histologic abnormalities results from chronic or repetitive cigarette smoke–induced injury.

    i. Initially, there is metaplasia of the normal bronchial columnar epithelial cells, which are replaced by squamous epithelial cells

    ii. Squamous cells become more atypical until a well-localized carcinoma (carcinoma in situ) develops

    iii. These cells tend to be located in relatively large or proximal airways, most commonly at the subsegmental, segmental, or lobar level. With the growth of tumor into the bronchial lumen, the airway may become obstructed and the lung distal to the obstruction frequently becomes atelectatic and may develop a postobstructive pneumonia.

    iv. At times a cavity develops within the tumor mass; cavitation is more common with squamous cell carcinoma than other bronchogenic carcinomas

    v. Metastasis beyond the airway usually involves the following:

       (a) Direct extension to the pulmonary parenchyma or to other neighboring structures

       (b) Invasion of the lymphatics, with spread to local lymph nodes in the hilum or mediastinum

     vi. Squamous cell tumors tend to remain within the thorax and cause problems by intrathoracic complications rather than by distant metastasis. Overall prognosis for 5-year survival is better for squamous cell carcinoma than for any of the other cell types.

b. *Small cell carcinoma:* Comprises about 20% of all lung cancers and consists of several subtypes. These tumors generally originate within the bronchial wall, most commonly at a proximal level.

     i. Oat cell carcinoma, the most common subtype, shows a submucosal growth pattern, but the tumor quickly invades the lymphatics and submucosal blood vessels. Hilar and mediastinal nodes are involved early in the course of the disease and these involved nodes are frequently the most prominent aspect of the radiographic presentation.

     ii. Metastasis to distant sites is a common early complication; common sites are the brain, liver, bone (and bone marrow), and adrenal glands

     iii. Propensity for early metastasis gives small cell carcinoma the worst prognosis among the major categories of bronchogenic carcinoma

c. *Adenocarcinoma:* Accounts for more than one third of all lung tumors, with the majority occurring in the periphery of the lung

     i. Characteristic tendency to form glands and to produce mucus

     ii. Usually presents as a peripheral lung nodule or mass. Occasionally, tumors can arise within a relatively large bronchus and therefore may present with complications of localized bronchial obstruction.

     iii. May spread locally to adjacent regions of the lung, to the pleura, or to the hilar or mediastinal lymph nodes; may metastasize to distant sites—liver, bone, CNS, and adrenal glands. In contrast to small cell carcinoma, it is more likely to be localized at the time of presentation.

     iv. Overall prognosis is intermediate between that of squamous cell and that of small cell carcinoma

d. *Large cell carcinoma:* Accounts for 15% to 20% of all lung cancers. These carcinomas are defined by the characteristics that they lack (i.e., the specific features that would otherwise classify them as one of the other three cell types). It is difficult to pinpoint the cells of origin from which these tumors arise.

     i. Behavior is similar to that of adenocarcinoma

     ii. Found in the periphery of the lungs, although it tends to be somewhat larger than adenocarcinoma

     iii. Tumor spread and prognosis are the same as for adenocarcinoma

e. *Bronchial carcinoid:* Viewed as a low-grade malignancy; constitutes approximately 5% of primary lung tumors

     i. Arises in the relatively central airways of the tracheobronchial tree from the neurosecretory Kulchitsky cells (K cells)

     ii. In some carcinoid tumors, the histology has more atypical features suggestive of frank malignancy; the overall prognosis for these tumors is poorer than for those tumors without such features

     iii. Patients with bronchial carcinoids are younger than patients with other pulmonary malignancies

     iv. Treatment is surgical resection, if possible, with an excellent prognosis; however, in patients with carcinoid tumors of atypical histology, metastatic disease is commonly found and the prognosis is worse

f. *Malignant mesothelioma*

     i. Involves the pleura rather than the airways or pulmonary parenchyma

     ii. Eventually traps the lung and spreads to mediastinal structures

      iii. No clearly effective form of therapy is available, and fewer than 10% of patients survive 3 years

2. Etiology and risk factors

  a. Smoking is the single most important risk factor for the development of carcinoma of the lung. Duration of smoking, the number of cigarettes smoked per day, the depth of inhalation, and the amount of each cigarette smoked all correlate with the risk for lung cancer. Each of the four major categories of carcinoma is associated with cigarette smoking; however, the statistical association between smoking and the individual cell types is greatest for squamous cell and small cell carcinomas, which are seen almost exclusively in smokers. Even though smoking increases the risk for adenocarcinoma and large cell carcinoma, these cell types are also observed in nonsmokers. In addition, smoking does not appear to be a risk factor for bronchial carcinoids or malignant mesothelioma.

  b. Occupational factors

    i. Asbestos, a fibrous silicate used for its fire resistant and thermal insulatory qualities, is the most widely studied of the environmental and occupationally related carcinogens. Carcinoma of the lung is the most likely malignancy to complicate asbestos exposure, although other tumors, especially mesothelioma, are strongly associated with prior asbestos exposure. Risk for development of lung cancer is particularly high in a smoker exposed to asbestos, in which case the two risk factors have a multiplicative effect. There is a long time lag (>20 years) after exposure before the tumor becomes apparent.

    ii. Other occupational exposures implicated in the development of lung cancer also have a long latent period of at least two decades between exposure and presentation of the tumor. Examples include exposure to arsenic, ionizing radiation (uranium, gamma radiation, x-rays), haloethers (chemical industry), polycyclic aromatic hydrocarbons (mineral oils, soots, coal tar, and foundry work), synthetic mineral fibers (rock wool or slag wool), diesel exhaust, and crystalline silica.

  c. Radon decay products: Radon gas is a decay product of naturally occurring uranium in the earth that may cause bronchogenic carcinoma or contribute to cancer risk only when inhaled into the respiratory system, where it interacts with pulmonary epithelial or other cells

  d. Diet

    i. A number of epidemiologic studies have convincingly shown a relation between greater dietary intake of vegetables and modestly lower risk for lung and other cancers

    ii. Low dietary intake of fruits and vegetables without β-carotene is associated with increased lung cancer risk. Low serum β-carotene level is associated with risk of later development of lung cancer.

  e. Nonmodifiable risk factors: Gender, race, inherited predisposition

3. Signs and symptoms

  a. Patient's chief complaints: Cough and hemoptysis are the most common presenting symptoms in patients with lung cancer. Other symptoms vary, depending on the region of tumor involvement.

  b. Dyspnea secondary to an obstructed bronchus or large pleural effusion

  c. Chest pain from pleural involvement

  d. Dysphagia from tumor involvement of the adjacent esophagus

  e. Hoarseness from vocal cord paralysis

  f. Edema of the face and upper extremities from superior vena cava obstruction

g. Nonspecific symptoms: Anorexia, weight loss, wasting, dyspnea, diminished chest expansion, bronchial breath sounds over a large tumor or postobstructive pneumonia, dullness over a large tumor near the chest wall or a pleural mass, signs of pleural effusion

4. **Diagnostic study findings**
   a. Laboratory: Cytologic examination of sputum, washings, or brushings or of material aspirated from the tumor with a small-gauge needle
   b. Radiologic
      i. Chest radiograph: May reveal a nodule or mass in the lung, involvement of the hilar or mediastinal nodes, or pleural involvement
      ii. CT and MRI: Help to define the location, extent, and spread of tumor
   c. Bronchoscopy: Allows direct examination of the airways intrabronchially and sampling for cytologic evaluation. Forceps biopsy specimens used for both histologic and cytologic analysis; bronchial washings used extensively in the diagnosis of bronchogenic carcinoma (usefulness is controversial). Cytologic analysis of bronchial brushings is an effective diagnostic procedure, especially when used in combination with forceps biopsy.
   d. Transbronchial needle aspiration can be useful in the diagnosis of a tumor presenting as a submucosal lesion or as a mass that compresses the bronchial lumen externally. Patients with necrotic lesions or lesions from which significant bleeding is anticipated are candidates for this technique.
   e. Mediastinoscopy: For staging of lung cancer if CT is not diagnostic of lymph node involvement
   f. Staging of lung cancer is based on the following:
      i. Size, location, and local complications, such as direct extensions to adjacent structures or obstruction of the airway lumen
      ii. Mediastinal lymph node involvement
      iii. Distant metastasis

5. **Goals of care**
   a. Patent airway is established and maintained
   b. Ventilation and respiratory gas exchange are maximized to the extent possible
   c. Every effort is made to ensure that the patient is pain free
   d. Hospital-acquired and surgery-related complications are prevented

6. **Collaborating professionals on health care team:** See Acute Respiratory Failure, Pulmonary Problems in Surgical Patients; in addition, oncologist, radiation oncologist, clinical pharmacologist, home care aide, social worker, American Cancer Society personnel

7. **Management of patient care** (see also Acute Respiratory Failure, Pulmonary Problems in Surgical Patients)
   a. Anticipated patient trajectory: Follows the course for specific clinical problems related to the nature, extent, and location of the tumor and the surgery and other treatments employed. See those specific conditions.
      i. Pain management: Some forms of lung cancer can be exquisitely painful, so special attention to this aspect of care is warranted. See content related to pain in Chapters 4 and 10.
      ii. Nutrition: Patients with significant weight loss and wasting require dietary consult for planning nutritional needs. May need to revisit this aspect of care if chemotherapy and/or radiation therapy precipitates the need for nutritional supplementation.
      iii. Infection control: Of major concern, especially when the patient may be imminently in need of undergoing chemotherapy and/or radiation therapy, which will further weaken the immune system

      iv. Discharge planning: Nature and extent of postdischarge needs must be evaluated, including outpatient follow-up care, chemotherapy or radiation therapy, home care supplies, equipment and care needs, and the nature of health care required in relation to the ancillary staff resources. If appropriate, provide referral to hospice care services.

      v. Pharmacology: Chemotherapy may prolong survival; antibiotics are administered as needed and the results monitored; pain medication needs to ensure patient comfort

      vi. Psychosocial issues: Patient and/or family may require considerable support in dealing with this diagnosis, its treatment both in the hospital and in the community and home, its potential outcomes, and its prognosis. Pastoral care may be supportive and comforting if the patient and/or family desires this. Other means of support include working with social services or the American Cancer Society in arranging for another patient with a similar diagnosis who has successfully coped with this situation to visit the patient to provide encouragement and sharing of experiences.

      vii. Treatments: See therapies for specific problems; in addition, initial planning for chemotherapy or radiation therapy may be completed while the patient is in the ICU

      viii. Ethical issues: Determine if an advance directive is in place, if the patient situation warrants it; see Chapter 10

   b. Potential complications (see also Acute Respiratory Failure, Acute Pneumonia)

      i. Hospital-acquired infection: Aspiration, urinary tract infection

      ii. Vary with the nature, extent, location, and staging of the neoplasm as well as the patient's response to treatment

8. Evaluation of patient care

   a. ABG values and ventilatory parameters are within acceptable limits

   b. Rate, depth, and pattern of ventilation remain within normal limits for the patient

   c. No evidence of air hunger or shortness of breath is present

   d. Patient and/or family or caregivers are able to provide the necessary follow-up care, including care of artificial airways

Obstructive Sleep Apnea

1. Pathophysiology

   a. *Apnea* is defined as cessation of airflow for more than 10 seconds. *Sleep apnea* is defined as repeated episodes of upper airway obstruction associated with obstructive apnea and hypopnea during sleep together with daytime sleepiness or altered cardiopulmonary function. Epidemiologic studies estimate that the condition affects 2% to 4% of middle-aged adults.

   b. Upper airway dysfunction and the specific sites of narrowing or closure are influenced by the underlying neuromuscular tone, upper airway muscle synchrony, and the stage of sleep

      i. These events are most prominent during rapid eye movement sleep secondary to hypotonia of the upper airway muscles characteristic of this stage of sleep

      ii. Definitive event in obstructive sleep apnea is the posterior movement of the tongue and palate into apposition with the posterior pharyngeal wall, which results in occlusion of the nasopharynx and oropharynx

      iii. Following the obstruction and resultant apnea, progressive asphyxia develops until there is a brief arousal from sleep, restoration of upper airway patency, and resumption of airflow. Patient quickly returns to sleep, only to experience the sequence of events over and over again.

    iv. Patients with sleep apnea are at increased risk for diurnal hypertension, pulmonary hypertension, nocturnal dysrhythmias, right and left ventricular failure, myocardial infarction, and stroke

    v. Hypoxemia, hypercapnia, polycythemia, and cor pulmonale may complicate the late stages of the disease

2. **Etiology and risk factors**
   a. Obesity—increased upper body obesity, as reflected by neck circumference (neck size 17 inches and larger in males, 16 inches and larger in females)
   b. Nasal obstruction such as severe septal deviation or nasopharyngeal infection or blockage
   c. Adenoidal or tonsillar hypertrophy (seen in children)
   d. Micrognathia, retrognathia, or macroglossia
   e. Vocal cord paralysis
   f. Genetically determined craniofacial features or abnormalities of ventilatory control (CNS) may be the reason that sleep apnea is common in some families

3. **Signs and symptoms**
   a. Patient's chief complaint: Excessive daytime sleepiness
   b. Fatigue as well as related personality changes and cognitive difficulties (patient may come to the hospital following an accident caused by daytime sleepiness)
   c. Chronic loud snoring
   d. Morning headaches
   e. Loss of libido

4. **Diagnostic study findings**
   a. Laboratory: ABG analysis is not diagnostic of sleep apnea but is performed as part of a diagnostic workup to determine baseline ventilation and oxygenation
   b. Polysomnography (sleep study) for sleep staging, airflow and ventilatory effort, arterial O_2 saturation, ECG, body position, and periodic limb movement evaluation
   c. Home evaluation and testing
          i. Pulse oximetry, portable (home) monitoring of cardiopulmonary channels, such as airflow, ventilatory effort, and heart rate
          ii. Sensitivity and specificity of pulse oximetry findings alone for the diagnosis of sleep apnea are controversial
   d. Pulmonary function studies may be done to exclude or confirm concomitant intrinsic lung disease, such as obstructive or restrictive lung disease

5. **Goals of care:** Apneic episodes during sleep are prevented

6. **Collaborating professionals on health care team:** Nurse; ear, nose, and throat physician; sleep study staff; respiratory therapist

7. **Management of patient care:** If the patient is obese, see Bariatric Patients in Chapter 11 for all aspects of care
   a. Anticipated patient trajectory
          i. Positioning: Keep the head of the bed elevated 30 to 45 degrees; avoid the supine position; maintain a neutral position for head and neck alignment; avoid neck flexion
          ii. Nutrition: Obtain a dietary consult to initiate a weight reduction program if obesity is a contributing factor
          iii. Transport: Maintain body alignment, especially of the head and upper torso, to keep the airway patent at all times
          iv. Discharge planning: Educate the patient regarding the proper use and care of oral or dental devices or CPAP equipment. Side effects of the use of oral

or dental devices include excessive salivation and temporomandibular joint discomfort.

    v. Pharmacology: Instruct the patient to avoid alcoholic beverages and sedatives before sleep

    vi. Psychosocial issues: Daytime demeanor and social interactions may improve considerably after the disorder is effectively treated

    vii. Treatments

        (a) O_2 delivery via a CPAP or BiPAP device as ordered

            (1) Instruct on the proper use and maintenance of equipment

            (2) Teach care of the skin surrounding the nose area where the mask is applied

            (3) Assess for intolerance to nasal CPAP machine noise and airway pressure

        (b) Postoperative monitoring and instruction following surgical treatment or correction for sleep apnea if indicated

            (1) Preoperative and postoperative teaching for patients requiring tracheostomy; if the neck is thick, the decannulation process may be difficult

            (2) Repeat the sleep study or nocturnal oximetry following tracheostomy tube placement, because the patient may still hypoventilate secondary to central sleep apnea or intrinsic lung disease

            (3) Provide tracheostomy tube and stoma care instruction to the patient and family

  b. Potential complications: Hospital-acquired infection. See Pulmonary Aspiration, Acute Pneumonia.

8. Evaluation of patient care

  a. Repeat sleep study verifies that no further episodes of obstructive sleep apnea have occurred

  b. Patient reports feeling well rested with no headache on awakening

  c. Patient's presenting symptoms and related signs of fatigue no longer persist

End-Stage Pulmonary Conditions Eligible for Lung Transplantation

1. Pathophysiology: Specific pathophysiologic mechanisms responsible for end-stage pulmonary disease depend on the underlying etiologic factors

  a. Transplantation of one or both lungs as a treatment for end-stage pulmonary failure has become a commonly accepted practice. Since 1983, the number of transplantations performed annually (about 1100) and the number of centers performing lung transplantation have continued to increase and the spectrum of diseases treated with lung transplantation has broadened.

  b. Primary underlying diagnoses for patients with end-stage lung disease

    i. Emphysema: 40% of the total

    ii. Pulmonary fibrosis: 22%

    iii. Cystic fibrosis: 16%

    iv. α_1-anitrypsin deficiency: 6%

    v. Pulmonary hypertension: 4%

    vi. Other disorders (bronchiectasis, eosinophilic granuloma, lymphangioleiomyomatosis, obliterative bronchiolitis, sarcoidosis): 12%

  c. United Network for Organ Sharing (UNOS) reports that nearly 4000 people in the United States await lung transplantation, yet only about 1000 receive a transplant and 500 die waiting. Median wait time in the United States is slightly more than 3 years.

  d. Survival rates following lung transplantation are 80% at 1 year and 60% at 4 years. Survival rates are highest for those with pulmonary fibrosis or pulmonary hypertension and lowest for those with emphysema.

2. **Etiology and risk factors:** Pulmonary transplantation is appropriate for patients with irreversible, progressively disabling, end-stage pulmonary disease whose life expectancy is projected to be less than 18 months despite the use of appropriate medical or alternative surgical therapies. These include patients with the following disorders:

  a. Emphysema and α_1-antitrypsin deficiency (which together account for 46% of all cases)
    i. Patients with COPD and an FEV_1 lower than 20% to 25% of the predicted value, hypercarbia ($Paco_2$ of >50 mm Hg), or mean pulmonary artery pressure without O_2 of more than 30 mm Hg have a 2-year survival rate of less than 70%
    ii. Usually, patients who receive a transplant have an FEV_1 of less than 20% of the predicted value

  b. Cystic fibrosis
    i. Patients with cystic fibrosis who have an FEV_1 of less than 30% of that predicted, a Pao_2 of less than 55 mm Hg, or a $Paco_2$ of more than 50 mm Hg have a 2-year survival rate of approximately 70%
    ii. Women and younger patients with cystic fibrosis have lower survival rates than men or the elderly, and so should be considered for transplantation earlier

  c. Pulmonary hypertension (primary and secondary)—patients with a mean pulmonary artery pressure of more than 45 mm Hg

  d. Idiopathic pulmonary fibrosis or interstitial lung disease
    i. Such patients tend to have the highest mortality while awaiting transplantation
    ii. These patients often have an FEV_1 and FVC of less than 50% of the predicted values

3. **Signs and symptoms** (see also specific underlying disorder)
  a. Patient's chief complaint: Varies, depending on the type of underlying respiratory disorder and the degree of disability. At the initial screening or clinic visit virtually all patients have some degree of dyspnea and shortness of breath, either at rest or on minimal exertion.

  b. Physical findings vary widely, depending on the underlying pulmonary condition and the degree to which pulmonary function is impaired

  c. *Traditional* selection criteria for lung transplant recipients used until recently are the following:
    i. Age of 65 years or younger for a single lung transplant; age of 60 years or younger for a bilateral lung transplant
    ii. No other underlying significant systemic disease such as renal or hepatic insufficiency or neoplastic disease
    iii. Demonstrated past and current compliance with medical regimens
    iv. No evidence of serious psychiatric illness such as functional psychosis or organic brain disease, major depression, or severe characterologic disturbances with a history of self-destructive acts (alcohol, drug abuse)
    v. No immune markers or contraindication to immunosuppression
    vi. Abstinence from tobacco use for longer than 6 months
    vii. No extrapulmonary site of infection
    viii. Ambulatory with rehabilitation potential with O_2 as required
    ix. Significant coronary artery disease
    x. Longer time on the wait list

    d. *"Transplant benefit":* Revised lung allocation system instituted by the Organ Procurement and Transplantation Network and UNOS to provide an evidence-based, individualized, clinical data–driven system for allocating lungs for transplantation

        i. Replaces the system heavily based on the length of time on that waiting list with an approach that balances the waiting list urgency and the likely duration of benefit from transplantation

        ii. Intention is that candidates who are most urgently in need of a transplant *and* who are expected to receive the greatest survival benefit from the transplant will receive priority for available lungs

        iii. Patient's health data are entered online into the UNOS database system, called UNet, to generate a lung allocation score (LAS), which ranges from 0 to 100. If data change, new or revised data can be entered online by health care staff. Time on the waiting list is used only to select among candidates with equal LASs. Candidate with the highest LAS in his or her particular age group gets priority.

        iv. Some of the criteria used in determining the LAS include the following:

            (a) Need for continuous mechanical ventilation

            (b) Presence of type 1 or 2 diabetes mellitus

            (c) Need for O_2 at rest

            (d) Cardiac catheterization data (pulmonary artery systolic pressure, mean PAP, PCOP), FVC

            (e) Pulmonary diagnoses

            (f) Age

            (g) Body mass index

            (h) New York American Heart Association class

        v. Verify the patient's commitment to transplant candidacy

            (a) Discussion among the patient, family, and transplant team about the transplantation process and provision of the opportunity to explore options, ask questions, and voice concerns

            (b) Decision by the patient as to whether or not to proceed with the formal evaluation

            (c) Formal evaluation performed on either an inpatient or outpatient basis, depending on the degree of pulmonary impairment

4. Diagnostic study findings

    a. Laboratory

        i. Infectious disease testing: Purified protein derivative, mumps, *Candida* testing

        ii. Serologic studies: CMV titer, varicella-zoster titer, herpes simplex titer, Epstein-Barr titer

        iii. Human immunodeficiency virus antigen-antibody levels, hepatitis screen, blood type and cross-match

        iv. Serum electrolyte levels, CBC with differential, prothrombin time, partial thromboplastin time, platelet count, creatinine clearance, liver function tests, levels of nutritional markers (albumin, total protein), urinalysis

        v. Thyroid and endocrine function tests

        vi. ABG levels

    b. Radiologic

        i. Chest radiograph, posteroanterior and lateral

        ii. High-resolution or spiral CT of the chest (considered the gold standard)

        iii. Quantitative $\dot{V}/\dot{Q}$ scan

    c. Pulmonary function

      i. Spirometry (includes prebronchodilator and postbronchodilator studies if obstruction is present)

      ii. Lung volumes using nitrogen washout and plethysmography

      iii. Diffusion capacity of carbon monoxide

   d. Cardiovascular studies: ECG, echocardiogram with pulse Doppler imaging, cardiac catheterization studies except in patients who have no history of smoking and are younger than 35 years of age (then only for the right side of the heart)

5. Goals of care

   a. Alveolar ventilation and tissue oxygenation are optimized

   b. Hemodynamic stability, acid-base balance, electrolyte levels, and fluid balance are maintained

   c. Family is prepared for and supported during the preoperative, postoperative, and discharge events related to lung transplantation

   d. Patient is able to manage postdischarge care and follow-up

   e. Potential complications related to lung transplantation, immunosuppressive therapy, and related hospitalization are prevented or minimized

6. Collaborating professionals on health care team: All members of the lung transplantation team—pulmonologist, thoracic surgeon, anesthesiologist, nurse, pharmacologist, dietitian, psychiatric social worker, organ procurement coordinator, physical therapist, respiratory therapist, and infection control specialist

7. Management of patient care

   a. Anticipated patient trajectory: See Acute Respiratory Failure, the discussion of cardiac (thoracic) surgery in Chapter 3, and Pulmonary Problems in Surgical Patients

      i. Positioning: Keep the head of the bed elevated at least 30 to 45 degrees to enhance ventilation, prevent aspiration, and promote drainage from the thoracic pleural space

      ii. Pain management: Pain medication to relieve the discomfort of surgical wounds, tubes, and dressings and to prevent treatment interference

        (a) Provide adequate thoracotomy pain control according to patient needs via IV or epidural pain management, patient-controlled analgesics, or oral analgesics

        (b) Consider pain control needs prior to exercise and chest physiotherapy sessions

        (c) Employ pain control to enhance sleep and rest. Early postoperative phase often results in fragmented sleep, confusion, and irritability, so haloperidol may be administered and then the dosage tapered slowly through the recovery phase.

      iii. Nutrition: Comprehensive nutritional plan via dietary consult

        (a) Administer enteral feedings when the gastrointestinal system is functional and the patient is unable to take food by mouth; advance the diet as tolerated

        (b) Administer TPN when the gastrointestinal tract is not available or nonfunctional

        (c) Avoid excessive carbohydrates to limit CO_2 production and respiratory workload

        (d) Avoid excessive fluids, particularly in patients with renal insufficiency

      iv. Infection control

        (a) Of utmost importance, especially when immunosuppressive therapy will be utilized and when the patient is already malnourished

        (b) Maintain sterile technique when caring for arterial or venous access devices or any invasive line

     v. Discharge planning

        (a) Initiate patient and family education early in the preoperative phase. (See details under Psychosocial Issues later.)

        (b) Early postoperative period: Encourage patient participation in inpatient rehabilitation

           (1) Range-of-motion exercises (12 to 24 hours postoperatively)

           (2) Progressive resistance exercises within the first 2 to 3 days after transplantation if cardiovascular stability is established

           (3) Ambulation for short distances; if mechanical ventilation is required, the patient may ambulate short distances using a manual resuscitation bag for assisted ventilations

        (c) After the patient leaves the ICU: Ambulation progresses as rapidly as tolerated

           (1) Special walker to hold O_2 tanks and IV pole or pumps, a urinary drainage bag, chest tubes, portable suction, and pulse oximeter

           (2) Weaning from O_2 therapy or to the level of O_2 flow required to maintain SpO_2 equal to or above 92%

           (3) Return of the patient to the treadmill for endurance training (if able)

        (d) Conduct comprehensive education as part of the discharge planning process. Teach the patient the benefits of participating in an outpatient rehabilitation program following discharge.

           (1) Endurance program progresses to home exercise

           (2) Progression of musculoskeletal program: Improved functional ability to perform ADLs. Instruct on the need for the patient to continue ongoing medical follow-up with a private doctor and the transplant center.

              a) Periodic pulmonary function, O_2 assessment

              b) Signs and symptoms to report

              c) Maintenance of logs of laboratory and spirometry records, medication dosages

              d) Medication regimen: See Pharmacology

    vi. Pharmacology: Antibiotics as needed, sedatives and pain medication

        (a) Reduce pulmonary artery pressures with epoprostenol (Flolan) administered via continuous ambulatory drug delivery (CADD) pump, sildenafil, or nitrates

        (b) Teach self-administration of medication, as with MDIs

        (c) Teach the role of immunosuppression therapy in survival

        (d) Teach medication dose scheduling, monitoring for side effects, and the importance of early reporting of adverse reactions to the physician or nurse

    vii. Psychosocial issues: Provide psychosocial support throughout the hospital stay via active involvement of the patient and family in all aspects of the process

        (a) Prepare the patient and support person or family for the preoperative evaluation and waiting period: Relocation to a transplant center for lung transplantation

           (1) Living arrangements

           (2) Support group

           (3) Consent forms signed with the surgeon

           (4) Medical follow-up and ongoing care while transplantation is awaited

        (b) Conduct preoperative education of the patient and support person or family concerning the rationale for the preoperative tests, responsibilities of the patient while awaiting transplantation, operative procedure, and expected postoperative course, including activity and medication regimen

    (1) Familiarize with the organization or program coordinating organ availability (i.e., placement on a national computerized waiting list; donor availability, selection, and preparation; donor-recipient matching [ABO compatibility, size]; lung allocation process and priorities)

    (2) Use of beepers for coordination of transplantation

       a) Gather information regarding the available donor

       b) Notify the retrieval team and the patient

    (3) Role of the transplant nurse coordinator and when to call

    (4) Operative procedures and pretransplantation and posttransplantation care, including anticipated hospital surgical and anesthetic preparation, surgical technique, time in the operating room, ICU stay

    (5) Pretransplantation rehabilitation program for conditioning

       a) Goals and expected outcomes

       b) Exercise prescription of O_2 therapy

       c) Supervision and monitoring (i.e., SpO_2 measurement)

    (6) Daily self-assessment by the patient to detect early changes in medical and pulmonary condition

       a) Progression of endurance training

       b) Periodic reevaluation of exercise tolerance

  (c) Postoperative planning

    (1) Discuss anticipated feelings and issues related to the patient's return to independence and to the transition to a less active role on the part of the support person(s) or family

    (2) Encourage the patient's self-care activities, such as making appointments and scheduling laboratory work

    (3) Offer early involvement of the hospital or transplant chaplain or pastoral services

viii. Treatments: See Potential Complications

ix. Ethical issues: Discussions at the time of candidacy and selection need to include planning by the patient and family for decisions regarding ethical issues that may arise at any point in the transplantation process. Advance directive, health care power of attorney, and other necessary documents need to be on file and readily available.

b. Potential complications

  i. Intrathoracic hemorrhage

    (a) Mechanism: Major intrathoracic surgery involving major vascular supply to the cardiopulmonary system

    (b) Management

      (1) Monitor for intrathoracic and/or intraabdominal bleeding postoperatively

      (2) Assess pleural and mediastinal chest tubes, verify that the suction level is as ordered, note the color and consistency of drainage, calculate the volume and rate of drainage output

      (3) Assess the abdomen for distention and tenderness, and volume and consistency of nasogastric drainage

      (4) Monitor chest radiographic changes

(5) Monitor and maintain the stability of hemodynamic parameters (e.g., systemic blood pressure, PAP, cardiac output, cardiac index, stroke volume, systemic vascular resistance, pulmonary vascular resistance, Sao_2, $S\bar{v}o_2$)

  a) Obtain hemodynamic profiles as ordered or routinely if the pulmonary artery catheter is in place

  b) Titrate vasoactive drugs as necessary

(6) Transfuse as ordered using Leukopor filters and CMV-negative blood products; autotransfusion setups must be routinely available to allow quick response to blood loss

ii. Fluid overload

(a) Mechanism: May have preexisting pulmonary infiltrates related to underlying pulmonary disorder, right-sided heart failure owing to pulmonary hypertension and vascular resistance

(b) Management

(1) Monitor intake and output and fluid status with particular attention to avoiding volume overload

  a) Measure urine output; maintain at over 30 ml/hr

  b) Monitor serum blood urea nitrogen and serum creatine levels

  c) Monitor urine and serum electrolyte levels

(2) Administer diuretics as indicated

iii. Infection

(a) Mechanism: Numerous sources, including aspiration, incisional contamination, poor wound healing, surgery, transplant

(b) Management

(1) Optimize pulmonary care in the early postoperative phase

  a) Provide frequent and thorough oral care that includes brushing, cleansing, and removal of secretions; verify that the cuff of the endotracheal tube is sealed properly so oral secretions cannot pass

  b) Provide pulmonary hygiene, positioning, chest physical therapy, inhaled bronchodilator treatment as ordered, suctioning based on need

  c) Monitor trends in peak and mean inspiratory pressures, exhaled V_T, breathing effort, synchrony with ventilator

(2) Discontinue (wean or liberate from) mechanical ventilation as soon as possible

  a) Weaning from mechanical ventilation: See Impaired Alveolar Ventilation under Patient Care

  b) After ventilator is removed: Monitor for respiratory muscle fatigue and distress

iv. Rejection of transplanted lung

(a) Mechanism: Transplanted lung(s) represent foreign body that immune system normally rejects

(b) Management

(1) Monitor for rejection of transplanted lung

  a) Administer immunosuppressive agents

  b) Monitor donor and recipient bronchoscopy culture results

  c) Administer antimicrobial therapy

  d) Maintain proper isolation procedures

(2) Assess pulmonary function via arterial to alveolar ratio, A–a gradient, ABG levels, end-tidal CO_2 level, pulse oximetry; hypoxemia may indicate fluid volume overload, lung infection, or lung rejection

8. **Evaluation of patient care**
   a. Pulmonary function studies and ABG levels indicate adequate alveolar ventilation and tissue oxygenation
   b. Hemodynamic parameters, intake and output, and vital signs reflect acid-base, electrolyte, and fluid balance
   c. No clinical evidence of major complications is present following lung transplantation
   d. Patient, family, and/or caregivers demonstrate effective coping with stressors related to the transplantation process and the ability to carry out follow-up home care, outpatient care, and rehabilitation programs

REFERENCES

Physiologic Anatomy

Boron WF, Boulpaep EL: *Medical physiology*, Philadelphia, 2004, Saunders.

Guyton AC, Hall JE: *Textbook of medical physiology*, ed 11, Philadelphia, 2005, Saunders.

Steingrub J, Kacmarek RM, Stoller J, et al, editors: *Cardiopulmonary critical care*, Oxford, 2002, BIOS Scientific Publishers.

West JB: *Respiratory physiology: the essentials*, ed 6, Philadelphia, 2000, Lippincott Williams & Wilkins.

Patient Assessment

Ahrens T, Sona C: Capnography application in acute and critical care, *AACN Clin Issues* 14:123-132, 2003.

American Thoracic Society: Dyspnea: mechanisms, assessment, and management: a consensus statement, *Am J Respir Crit Care Med* 159:321-340, 1999.

Bigatello LM, Davignon KR, Stelfox HT: Respiratory mechanics and ventilator waveforms in the patient with acute lung injury, *Respir Care* 50:235-245, 2005.

Bridges EJ: Monitoring pulmonary artery pressures: just the facts, *Crit Care Nurse* 20:59-78, 2000.

Burns SM: Working with respiratory waveforms: how to use bedside graphics, *AACN Clin Issues* 14:133-144, 2003.

Chulay M, Gawlinsky A: *Hemodynamic monitoring*, Protocols for practice series, Aliso Viejo, Calif, 1998, American Association of Critical-Care Nurses.

Durbin CG: Applied respiratory physiology: use of ventilator waveforms and mechanics in the management of critically ill patients, *Respir Care* 50:287-293, 2005.

Giulliano KK, Higgins TL: New-generation pulse oximetry in the care of critically ill patients, *Am J Crit Care* 14:26-39, 2005.

Grap MJ: *Pulse oximetry*, ed 2. In MacArthur BG, Burns SM, editors: Noninvasive monitoring series, ed 2, Aliso Viejo, Calif, 2005, American Association of Critical-Care Nurses.

Jesurum J: *Svo$_2$ monitoring*, Protocols for practice series, Aliso Viejo, Calif, 1998, American Association of Critical-Care Nurses.

Jesurum J: Svo$_2$ monitoring, *Crit Care Nurse* 24:73-76, 2004.

Nilsestuen JO, Hargett KD: Using ventilator graphics to identify patient-ventilator asynchrony, *Respir Care* 50:202-234, 2005.

Spector N, Connolly M: *Dyspnea*, Protocols for practice series, Aliso Viejo, Calif, 2003, American Association of Critical-Care Nurses.

Squara P: Matching total body oxygen consumption and delivery: a crucial objective? *Intensive Care Med* 30:2170-2179, 2004.

St. John RE: End-tidal carbon dioxide monitoring, *Crit Care Nurse* 23:83-88, 2003.

St. John RE: *End-tidal CO$_2$ monitoring*, ed 2. In MacArthur BG, Burns SM, editors: Noninvasive monitoring series, ed 2, Aliso Viejo, Calif, 2005, American Association of Critical-Care Nurses.

Patient Care

Bridges EJ: Ask the experts: To turn or not to turn? Patients on mechanical ventilation, *Crit Care Nurse* 21(6):66, 2001.

Burns SM: *Weaning from mechanical ventilation*, Protocols for practice series, Aliso Viejo, Calif, 1998, American Association of Critical-Care Nurses.

Chulay M, Burns SM, editors: *Care of the mechanically ventilated patient*, Protocols for practice series, Aliso Viejo, Calif, 1998, American Association of Critical-Care Nurses.

Fenstermacher D, Hong D: Mechanical ventilation: what have we learned? *Crit Care Nurs Q* 27:258-294, 2004.

Frawley PM, Habashi NM: Airway pressure release ventilation: theory and practice, *AACN Clin Issues* 12:234-246, 2001.

Gattinoni L, Tognoni G, Pesenti A, et al: Effect of prone positioning on the survival of patients with acute respiratory failure, *N Engl J Med* 345:568-573, 2001.

Happ MB: Communicating with mechanically ventilated patients: state of the science, *AACN Clin Issues* 12:247-259, 2001.

Henneman E, Dracup K, Ganz T, et al: Using a collaborative weaning plan to decrease duration of mechanical ventilation and length of stay in the intensive care unit for patients receiving long-term ventilation, *Am J Crit Care* 11:132-140, 2002.

Pate MF, ZapataT: Ask the experts: suctioning ET and TT tubes, *Crit Care Nurse* 22(2): 130-131, 2002.

Acute Respiratory Failure

Burns SM: The science of weaning: when and how? *Crit Care Nurs Clin North Am* 16(3): 379-386, ix, 2004.

Corrado A, Gorini M: Negative-pressure ventilation: is there still a role? *Eur Respir J* 20(1):187-197, 2002.

El-Masri MM, Williamson KM, Fox-Wasylyshyn SM: Severe acute respiratory syndrome: another challenge for critical care nurses, *AACN Clin Issues* 15(1):150-159, 2004.

Keenan SP, Sinuff T, Cook DJ, et al: Does noninvasive positive pressure ventilation improve outcome in acute hypoxemic respiratory failure: a systematic review, *Crit Care Med* 32:2516-2523, 2004.

Luer JM: Sedation and neuromuscular blockade in patients with acute respiratory failure, *Crit Care Nurse* 22(5):70-75, 2002.

MacIntyre NR: Evidence-based ventilator weaning and discontinuation, *Respir Care* 49(7):830-836, 2004.

Markou NK, Myrianthefs PM, Baltopoulos GJ: Respiratory failure: an overview, *Crit Care Nurs Q* 27(4):353-379, 2004.

Acute Respiratory Distress Syndrome

Acute Respiratory Network: Ventilation with lower tidal volumes as compared with traditional tidal volumes for acute lung injury and the acute respiratory distress syndrome, *N Engl J Med* 342:1301-1308, 2000.

Adhikari N, Burns KEA, Meade MO: Pharmacologic therapies for adults with acute lung injury and acute respiratory distress syndrome, *Cochrane Database of Systematic Reviews,* Issue 4, Art No CD004477, pub2, DOI: 10.1002/14651858. CD004477, 2004.

Brower RG, Ware LB, Berthiaume Y, et al: Treatment of ARDS, *Chest* 20:1347-1367, 2001.

Cooper SJ: Methods to prevent ventilator-associated lung injury: a summary, *Intensive Crit Care Nurs* 20(6):358-365, 2004.

Davies P: Guarding your patient against ARDS, *Nursing* 32(3):36-41, 2002.

Dirkes SM, Winklerprins A: Help for ARDS patients, *RN* 65(8):52-58, 2002.

Eisner MD, Thompson T, Hudson LD, et al: Efficacy of low tidal volume ventilation in patients with different clinical risk factors for acute lung injury and the acute respiratory distress syndrome, *Am J Respir Crit Care Med* 164:231-236, 2001.

Gattinoni L, Caironi P, Pelosi P, et al: What has computed tomography taught us about the acute respiratory distress syndrome? *Am J Respir Crit Care Med* 164:1701-1711, 2001.

Kane C, Galanes S: Adult respiratory distress syndrome, *Crit Care Nurs Q* 27(4):325-335, 2004.

McCarthy MS: Use of indirect calorimetry to optimize nutrition support and assess physiologic dead space in the mechanically ventilated ICU patient: a case study approach, *AACN Clin Issues* 11(4):619-630, 2000.

McCormick J, Blackwood B: Nursing the ARDS patient in the prone position: the experience of qualified ICU nurses, *Intensive Crit Care Nurs* 17(6):331-340, 2001.

Munro N: Pulmonary challenges in neurotrauma, *Crit Care Nurs Clin North Am* 12(4): 457-464, 2000.

Munro N: Cardiac bypass without the pump, *RN* 66(10):28-32, 2003.

Powers J, Daniels D: Turning points: implementing kinetic therapy in the ICU, *Nurs Manage* 35(5):suppl 1-7, 2004.

Rance M: Kinetic therapy positively influences oxygenation in patients with ALI/ ARDS, *Nurs Crit Care* 10(1):35-41, 2005.

Respiratory distress following transfusion, *Oncol Nurs Forum* 29(1):23-24, 2002.

Rowe C: Development of clinical guidelines for prone positioning in critically ill adults, *Nurs Crit Care* 9(2):50-57, 2004.

Sevransky JE, Levy MM, Marini JJ: Mechanical ventilation in sepsis-induced acute lung injury/acute respiratory distress syndrome: an evidence-based review, *Crit Care Med* 32:S548-S553, 2004.

Slutsky AS: Basic science in ventilator-induced lung injury: implications for the bedside, *Am J Respir Crit Care Med* 163:599-600, 2001.

Verger JT, Bradshaw DJ, Henry E, et al: The pragmatics of feeding the pediatric patient with acute respiratory distress syndrome, *Crit Care Nurs Clin North Am* 16(3):431-443, 2004.

Vollman KM: Prone positioning in the patient who has acute respiratory distress syndrome: the art and science, *Crit Care Nurs Clin North Am* 16(3):319-336, viii, 2004.

Ware LB, Matthay MA: The acute respiratory distress syndrome, *N Engl J Med* 342:1334-1349, 2000.

Wilson JN, Pierce JD, Clancy RL: Reactive oxygen species in acute respiratory distress syndrome, *Heart Lung* 30(5):370-375, 2001.

Chronic Obstructive Pulmonary Disease

Andenaes R, Kalfoss MH, Wahl A: Psychological distress and quality of life in hospitalized patients with chronic obstructive pulmonary disease, *J Adv Nurs* 46(5):523-530, 2004.

Austan F, Polise M: Management of respiratory failure with noninvasive positive pressure ventilation and heliox adjunct, *Heart Lung* 31(3):214-218, 2002.

Bailey PH, Colella T, Mossey S: COPD-intuition or template: nurses' stories of acute exacerbations of chronic obstructive pulmonary disease, *J Clin Nurs* 13(6):756-764, 2004.

Bernier MJ, Leonard B: Pulmonary rehabilitation after acute COPD exacerbation, *Crit Care Nurs Clin North Am* 13(3):375-387, 2001.

Bhowmik A, Seemungal TAR, Sapsford RJ, et al: Relation of sputum inflammatory markers to symptoms and lung function changes in COPD exacerbations, *Thorax* 55:114-120, 2000.

Booker R: Chronic obstructive pulmonary disease: non-pharmacological approaches, *Br J Nurs* 14(1):14-18, 2005 (review).

Boyle AH, Locke DL: Update on chronic obstructive pulmonary disease, *Medsurg Nurs* 13(1):42-48, 2004.

Burns DM: Tobacco-related diseases, *Semin Oncol Nurs* 19(4):244-249, 2003.

Carrieri-Kohlman V, Gormley JM, Eiser S, et al: Dyspnea and the affective response during exercise training in obstructive pulmonary disease, *Nurs Res* 50(3):136-146, 2001.

Celli BR, MacNee W, ATS/ERS Task Force: Standards for the diagnosis and treatment of patients with COPD: a summary of the ATS/ERS position paper, *Eur Respir J* 23:932-946, 2004.

Chojnowski D: "GOLD" standards for acute exacerbation in COPD, *Nurse Pract* 28(5):26-35, 2003.

Collins EG, Langbein WE, Fehr L, et al: Breathing pattern retraining and exercise in persons with chronic obstructive pulmonary disease, *AACN Clin Issues* 12:202-209, 2001.

Estabrooks CA, Midodzi WK, Cummings GG, et al: The impact of hospital nursing characteristics on 30-day mortality, *Nurs Res* 54(2):74-84, 2005.

Fehrenbach C: Initiatives to improve outcomes for chronic obstructive pulmonary disease, *Prof Nurse* 20(6):43-45, 2005.

Frazier SC: Implications of the GOLD Report for chronic obstructive lung disease for the home care clinician, *Home Healthc Nurse* 23(2):109-114, 2005.

Gronkiewicz C, Borkgren-Okonek M: Acute exacerbation of COPD: nursing application of evidence-based guidelines, *Crit Care Nurs Q* 27(4):336-352, 2004.

Heinzer MM, Bish C, Detwiler R: Acute dyspnea as perceived by patients with chronic obstructive pulmonary disease, *Clin Nurs Res* 12(1):85-101, 2003.

Hogg JC, Chu F, Utokaparch S, et al: The nature of small-airway obstruction in chronic obstructive pulmonary disease, *N Engl J Med* 350:2645-2653, 2004.

Johnstone C: Linking diet and respiratory distress, *Nurs N Z* 7(5):22-23, 2001.

Kanervisto M, Paavilainen E, Astedt-Kurki P: Impact of chronic obstructive pulmonary disease on family functioning, *Heart Lung* 32(6):360-367, 2003.

Lomborg K, Bjorn A, Dahl R, et al: Body care experienced by people hospitalized with severe respiratory disease, *J Adv Nurs* 50(3):262-271, 2005.

Lynes D, Kelly C: The psychological needs of patients with chronic respiratory disease, *Nurs Times* 99(33):44-45, 2003.

O'Connell L: Management of patients with chronic obstructive pulmonary disease in ICU and promotion of smoking cessation, *Nurs Crit Care* 5(3):130-136, 2000.

Saetta M, Turato G, Maestrelli P, et al: Cellular and structural bases of chronic obstructive pulmonary disease, *Am J Respir Crit Care Med* 163:1304-1309, 2001.

Seemungal T, Harper-Owen R, Bhowmilk A, et al: Respiratory viruses, symptoms, and inflammatory markers in acute exacerbations and stable chronic obstructive pulmonary disease, *Am J Respir Crit Care Med* 164:1618-1623, 2001.

Sethi S: Infectious etiology of acute exacerbations of chronic bronchitis, *Chest* 117: 3808-3858, 2000.

Simmons P, Simmons M: Informed nursing practice: the administration of oxygen to patients with COPD, *Medsurg Nurs* 13(2):82-85, 2004.

Spector N, Klein D: Chronic critically ill dyspneic patients: mechanisms and clinical measurement, *AACN Clin Issues* 12(2):220-233, 2001.

Truesdell S: Helping patients with COPD manage episodes of acute shortness of breath, *Medsurg Nurs* 9(4):178-182, 2000.

Wisniewski A: Chronic bronchitis and emphysema: clearing the air, *Nursing* 33(5):46-49, 2003.

Asthma and Status Asthmaticus (Severe Asthmatic Attack)

Alvey Smaha D: Asthma emergency care: national guidelines summary, *Heart Lung* 30(6):472-474, 2001.

Barnes PJ, Adcock IM: How do corticosteroids work in asthma? *Ann Intern Med* 139(5 pt 1):359-370, 2003.

Booker R: The effective assessment of acute breathlessness in a patient, *Nurs Times* 100(24):61-63, 65, 67, 2004.

Busse WW, Lemanske RF Jr: Asthma, *N Engl J Med* 344(5):350-362, 2001.

Conner B, Meng A: Pulmonary function testing in asthma: nursing applications, *Nurs Clin North Am* 38(4):571-583, 2003.

Corbridge SJ, Corbridge TC: Severe exacerbations of asthma, *Crit Care Nurs Q* 27:207-228, 2004.

Cote J, Bowie DM, Robichaud P, et al: Evaluation of two different educational interventions for adult patients consulting with an acute asthma exacerbation, *Am J Respir Crit Care Med* 163:1415-1419, 2001.

Donohue JF: The expanding role of long-acting B-agonists, *Chest* 118:283-285, 2000.

Henderson DP: Coping with asthma: the National Institutes of Health Asthma Guidelines, *J Emerg Nurs* 26(1):70-75, 2000.

Kreutzer ML, Louie S: Pharmacologic treatment of the adult hospitalized asthma patient, *Clin Rev Allergy Immunol* 20:357-358, 2001.

Miracle V, Winston M: Take the wind out of asthma, *Nursing* 30(8):34-41, quiz 42-43, 2000.

Miracle V: Asthma attack, *Nursing* 32(11 pt 1): 104, 2002.

Musto PK: General principals of asthma management: education, *Nurs Clin North Am* 38(4):621-633, 2003.

Mutlu GM, Factor P, Schwartz DE, et al: Severe status asthmaticus: management with permissive hypercapnia and inhalation anesthesia, *Crit Care Med* 30:477-480, 2002.

National Asthma Education and Prevention Program Expert Panel Report: guidelines for the diagnosis and management of asthma, Washington, DC, 2002, US Department of Health and Human Services.

Pruitt B, Jacobs M: Caring for a patient with asthma, *Nursing* 35(2):48-51, 2005.

Ramirez EG: Management of asthma emergencies, *Nurs Clin North Am* 38(4):713-724, 2003.

Roberts J: The new asthma guidelines: a patient-centered approach to asthma, *Prof Nurse* 18(7):379-382, 2003.

Sackesen C, Sekerel B: Severe life threatening asthma, *Thorax* 56:897-898, 2001.

Salvi SS, Krishna MT, Sampson AP, et al: The anti-inflammatory effects of leukotriene-modifying drugs and their use in asthma, *Chest* 119:1533-1546, 2001.

Sims JM: Guidelines for treating asthma, *Dimens Crit Care Nurs* 22(6):247-250, 2003.

Suissa S, Ernst P, Benayoun S, et al: Low-dose inhaled corticosteroids and the prevention of death from asthma, *N Engl J Med* 343:332-336, 2000.

Weir P: Quick asthma assessment: a stepwise approach to treatment, *Adv Nurse Pract* 12(1):53-56, 2004.

Pulmonary Embolism

Ahrens T, Sona C: Capnography application in acute and critical care, *AACN Clin Issues* 14(2):123-132, 2003.

Burgess AW: Death by catheterization? Sudden, unexpected deaths of older adults are often not questioned, *Am J Nurs* 105(4):56-59, 2005.

Costello J, Hogg K: CT pulmonary angiogram compared with ventilation-perfusion scan for the diagnosis of pulmonary embolism in patients with cardiorespiratory disease, *Emerg Med J* 20:547-548, 2003.

Fedullo PF, Tapson VF: Clinical practice: the evaluation of suspected pulmonary embolism, *N Engl J Med* 349:1247-1256, 2003.

Frost SD, Brotman DJ, Michota FA: Rational use of D-dimer measurement to exclude acute venous thromboembolic disease, *Mayo Clin Proc* 78:1385-1391, 2003.

King JE: Could my patient have deep vein thrombosis? *Nursing* 33(9):24, 2003.

Konstantinides S, Geibel A, Heusel G, et al: Heparin plus alteplase compared with heparin alone in patients with submassive pulmonary embolus, *N Engl J Med* 347:1143-1150, 2002.

Koschel MJ: Pulmonary embolism: quick diagnosis can save a patient's life [erratum in *Am J Nurs* 104(10):15, 2004], *Am J Nurs* 104(6):46-50, 2004.

Yang JC: Prevention and treatment of deep vein thrombosis and pulmonary embolism in critically ill patients, *Crit Care Nurs Q* 28(1):72-79, 2005.

Chest Trauma

Keough V, Pudelek B: Blunt chest trauma: review of selected pulmonary injuries focusing on pulmonary contusion, *AACN Clin Issues* 12:270-281, 2001.

Kirkwood P: Ask the experts: closed system chest tube suctioning, *Crit Care Nurse* 20(3):98, 2000.

Morris J: Motor vehicle crash victim with chest injury, *J Emerg Nurs* 30(1):91-93, 2004.

Schrader KL: Ask the experts: instilling medications via chest tubes, *Crit Care Nurse* 21(3):77-78, 2001.

Veronesi JF: Trauma nursing: blunt chest injuries, *RN* 67(3):47-54, 2004.

Acute Pneumonia

American Association of Critical-Care Nurses: *Ventilator associated pneumonia (VAP),* Practice alert series, Aliso Viejo, Calif, 2004, Author.

American Thoracic Society: Consensus statement: guidelines for the management of adults with hospital-acquired, ventilator-associated, and healthcare-associated pneumonia, *Am J Respir Crit Care Med* 171:388-416, 2005.

Boldt MD, Kiresuk T: Community-acquired pneumonia in adults, *Nurse Pract* 26(11):14-16, 19-23, 2001.

Goldrick BA: Infection in the older adult: long-term care poses particular risk, *Am J Nurs* 105(6):31, 33-34, 2005.

Lindgren VA, Ames NJ: Caring for patients on mechanical ventilation: what research

indicates is best practice, *Am J Nurs* 105(5):50-60, 2005.

McQuillan DP, Duncan RA, Craven DE: Ventilator-associated pneumonia: emerging principles of management, *Infect Med* 22(3):104-118, 2005.

Pancorbo-Hidalgo PL, Garcia-Fernandez FP, Ramirez-Perez C: Complications associated with enteral nutrition by nasogastric tube in an internal medicine unit, *J Clin Nurs* 10(4):482-490, 2001.

St. John RE: Airway management, *Crit Care Nurse* 4(2):93-96, 2004.

Vecchiarino P, Bohannon RW, Ferullo J, et al: Short-term outcomes and their predictors for patients hospitalized with community-acquired pneumonia, *Heart Lung* 33:301-307, 2004.

Williams TA, Leslie GD: A review of the nursing care of enteral feeding tubes in critically ill adults: part I, *Intensive Crit Care Nurs* 20(6):330-343, 2004.

Yoneyama T, Yoshida M, Ohrui T, et al: Oral care reduces pneumonia in older patients in nursing homes, *J Am Geriatr Soc* 51:1018-1022, 2003.

Pulmonary Aspiration

Bates N: Acute poisoning: bleaches, disinfectants and detergents, *Emerg Nurse* 8(10):14-19, 2001.

Pancorbo-Hidalgo PL, Garcia-Fernandez FP, Ramirez-Perez C: Complications associated with enteral nutrition by nasogastric tube in an internal medicine unit, *J Clin Nurs* 10(4):482-490, 2001.

St. John RE: Ask the experts: detecting pulmonary aspirations in tube-fed patients, *Crit Care Nurse* 20(4):100-101, 2000

St. John RE: Airway management, *Crit Care Nurse* 24(2):93-96, 2004.

Tablan OC, Anderson LJ, Besser R, et al: Guidelines for preventing health-care-associated pneumonia, 2003, *MMWR Recomm Rep* 53:1-36, 2004.

Williams TA, Leslie GD: A review of the nursing care of enteral feeding tubes in critically ill adults: part I, *Intensive Crit Care Nurs* 20(6):330-343, 2004.

Williams TA, Leslie GD: A review of the nursing care of enteral feeding tubes in critically ill adults: part II, *Intensive Crit Care Nurs* 21(1):5-15, 2005.

Near-Drowning

Bergeron KT: Family members' presence during resuscitation efforts of a 7-year-old victim of a freshwater drowning, *J Emerg Nurs* 29(4):307-308, 2003.

Dueker CW: Immersion in fresh water and survival, *Chest* 126(6):2027-2028, 2004.

Salomez F, Vincent JL: Drowning: a review of epidemiology, pathophysiology, treatment and prevention, *Resuscitation* 63(3): 261-268, 2004.

Williamson JP, Illing R, Gertler P, et al: Near-drowning treated with therapeutic hypothermia, *Med J Aust* 181(9):500-501, 2004.

Pulmonary Problems in Surgical Patients

See also references under Acute Pneumonia.

Brooks JA: Postoperative nosocomial pneumonia: nurse-sensitive interventions, *AACN Clin Issues* 12:305-323, 2001.

Wynne R, Botti M: Postoperative pulmonary dysfunction in adults after cardiac surgery with cardiopulmonary bypass: clinical significance and implications for practice, *Am J Crit Care* 13:384-393, 2004.

Acute Pulmonary Inhalation Injuries

Flynn MB: Identifying and treating inhalation injuries in fire victims, *Dimens Crit Care Nurs* 18(4):18-23, 1999.

Kress T, Krueger D: Identifying carbon monoxide poisoning, *Nursing* 34(11):68-69, 2004.

Merrel P, Mayo D: Inhalation injury in the burn patient, *Crit Care Nurs Clin North Am* 16(1):27-38, 2004.

Sheridan R: Specific therapies for inhalation injury, *Crit Care Med* 30(3):718-719, 2002.

Neoplastic Lung Disease

Bakas T, Lewis RR, Parsons JE: Caregiving tasks among family caregivers of patients with lung cancer, *Oncol Nurs Forum* 28(5): 847-854, 2001.

Bialk JL: Ethical guidelines for assisting patients with end-of-life decision making, *Medsurg Nurs* 13(2):87-90, 2004.

Burns DM: Tobacco-related diseases, *Semin Oncol Nurs* 19(4):244-249, 2003.

Kreamer KM: Getting the lowdown on lung cancer, *Nursing* 33(11):36-42, 2003.

Kuo TT, Ma FC: Symptom distresses and coping strategies in patients with non-small cell lung cancer, *Cancer Nurs* 25(4): 309-317, 2002.

Rawl SM, Given BA, Given CW, et al: Intervention to improve psychological functioning for newly diagnosed patients with cancer, *Oncol Nurs Forum* 29(6):967-975, 2002.

Walker S: Updates in small cell lung cancer treatment, *Clin J Oncol Nurs* 7(5):563-568, 2003.

Winton T, Livingston R, Johnson D, et al: Vinorelbine plus cisplatin vs. observation in resected non–small-cell lung cancer, *N Engl J Med* 352:2589-2597, 2005.

Obstructive Sleep Apnea

Chasens ER, Umlauf MG: Nocturia: a problem that disrupts sleep and predicts obstructive sleep apnea, *Geriatr Nurs* 24(2):76-81, 105, 2003.

Ecklund MM, Kurlak SA: Caring for the bariatric patient with obstructive sleep apnea, *Crit Care Nurs Clin North Am* 16(3): 311-317, 2004.

Merritt SL, Berger BE: Obstructive sleep apnea-hypopnea syndrome, *Am J Nurs* 104(7):49-52, 2004.

End-Stage Pulmonary Conditions Eligible for Lung Transplantation

American Lung Association: Lung transplants: treatment options and support, retrieved July 7, 2005, from http://www.lungUSA.org/site/pp.asp?c=dvLUK9O0 E&b=2301.

Berkowitz DS, Coyne NG: Understanding primary pulmonary hypertension, *Crit Care Nurs Q* 26(1):28-34, 2003.

Cooper JD, Lefrak SS: Surgery for emphysema, *N Engl J Med* 346:860-862, 2002.

Dells PL: Advances in prostacyclin therapy for pulmonary arterial hypertension, *Crit Care Nurse* 24:42-54, 2004.

DeMeester J, Smits JM, Persijn GG, et al: Listing for lung transplantation: life expectancy and transplant effect, stratified by type of end-stage lung disease, the Eurotransplant experience, *J Heart Lung Transplant* 20(5):518-524, 2001.

Duquette SL, LaLonde LC, Traiger GL: Living-donor lobar lung transplantation: a case study, *Crit Care Nurse* 20(1):69-80, 2000.

Elpern EH, Cheatham J: Inpatient care of the adult with an exacerbation of cystic fibrosis, *AACN Clin Issues* 12(2):293-304, 2001.

Mullan B, Snyder M, Lindgren B, et al: Home monitoring for lung transplant candidates, *Prog Transplant* 13(3):176-182, 2003.

Petty M: Lung and heart-lung transplantation: implications for nursing care when hospitalized outside the transplant center, *Medsurg Nurs* 12(4):250-259, 2003.

United Network for Organ Sharing: Information for transplant professionals about the lung allocation score system, retrieved July 7, 2005, from http://www.unos.org.

US Organ Procurement and Transplantation Network (OPTN), Scientific Registry of Transplant Recipients (SRTR): OPTN/SRTR annual report, retrieved July 7, 2005, from http://www.optn.org/AR2004.htm.

Wilmoth D, Walters PE, Tomlin R, et al: Caring for adults with cystic fibrosis, *Crit Care Nurse* 21(3):34-44, 2001.

Yusen RD, Lefrak SS, Gierada DS: A prospective evaluation of lung volume reduction surgery in 200 consecutive patients, *Chest* 123:1026-1037, 2003.

3 The Cardiovascular System

M. LINDSAY LESSIG, BSN, MSEd, MBA

SYSTEMWIDE ELEMENTS

Physiologic Anatomy

1. **Heart** (Figures 3-1 and 3-2)
   a. The heart lies in the mediastinum, on and to the left of the midline
   b. Its long axis is oriented from the right shoulder blade to the left upper quadrant of the abdomen
   c. The base (top wide area) of the heart (atria and great vessels) is located diagonally at the second intercostal space, right and left sternal borders
   d. The apex, or tip, of the heart (junction of the ventricles and ventricular septum) is usually located at the fifth intercostal space, on the left midclavicular line
2. **Cardiac wall structure**
   a. Pericardium: Fibrous sac surrounding the heart and containing small amounts (15 to 50 ml) of pericardial fluid. This lubricated space protects the heart from friction, allowing it to easily change volume and size during contractions. The pericardium also keeps heart muscle anchored within the mediastinum.
   b. Epicardium: Outer surface of the heart (includes epicardial coronary arteries, autonomic nerves, adipose tissue, lymphatics)
   c. Myocardium: Muscular, contractile portion of the heart. Muscle fibers wrap around the heart in multiple, interlacing layers.
   d. Endocardium: Inner surface of the heart
   e. Papillary muscles: Myocardial structures extending into the ventricular chambers and attaching to the chordae tendineae
   f. Chordae tendineae: Strong tendinous attachments from the papillary muscles to the tricuspid and mitral valves; prevent prolapse of the valves into the atria during systole
3. **Chambers of the heart**
   a. Atria: Thin-walled, low-pressure chambers
      i. Right and left atria act as reservoirs of blood for their respective ventricles
      ii. Right atrium (RA), located above and to the right of the right ventricle, receives systemic venous blood via the superior vena cava and inferior vena cava, and venous blood from the heart via the coronary sinus
      iii. Left atrium (LA), superior and posterior to the other chambers, receives oxygenated blood returning to the heart from the lungs via the pulmonary veins

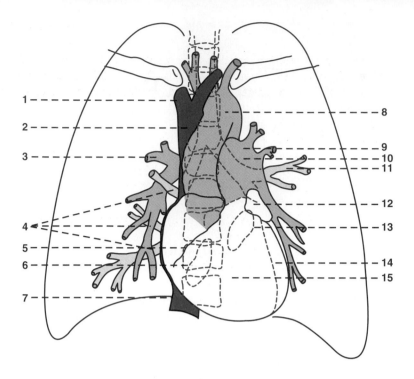

1. Right innominate vein
2. Superior vena cava
3. Right main branch of the pulmonary artery
4. Upper and lower lobe veins
5. Right atrium
6. Tricuspid valve
7. Inferior vena cava
8. Arch of the aorta
9. Left main branch of the pulmonary artery
10. Main pulmonary artery
11. Left upper lobe vein
12. Appendage of the left atrium
13. Mitral valve
14. Left ventricle
15. Right ventricle

FIGURE 3-1 ■ Cardiac silhouette, posteroanterior view. (From Gedgaudas E, Moller JH, Castaneda-Zuniga MD, et al: *Cardiovascular radiology,* Philadelphia, 1985, Saunders, p 38.)

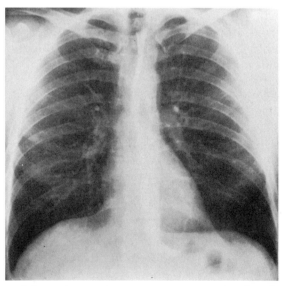

FIGURE 3-2 ■ Normal thoracicoroentgenogram, posteroanterior view. (From Gedgaudas E, Moller JH, Castaneda-Zuniga MD, et al: *Cardiovascular radiology,* Philadelphia, 1985, Saunders, p 38.)

       iv. When the mitral and tricuspid valves open, there is rapid filling of blood passively from atria into ventricles (about 80% to 85% of total filling)

       v. At the end of diastole, atrial contraction ("atrial kick") forcefully adds 15% to 20% more to the ventricular volume

  b. Ventricles: Major "pumps" of the heart

       i. Right ventricle (RV) is anterior under the sternum

          (a) Thin-walled, low-pressure system

          (b) Contracts and propels deoxygenated blood into the pulmonary circulation via the pulmonary artery (the only artery in the body that carries deoxygenated blood)

       ii. Left ventricle (LV) is the main "pump": Conical (ellipsoid) structure behind and to the left of the RV

          (a) Thick-walled, high-pressure system

          (b) Squeezes and ejects blood into the systemic circulation via the aorta during ventricular systole

       iii. Interventricular septum is functionally more a part of the LV than of the RV. It forms the anterior wall of the LV. Its curved shape protrudes into the RV cavity.

4. Cardiac valves

  a. Atrioventricular (AV) valves

       i. Location and structure: Situated between the atria and the ventricles (tricuspid valve on the right, mitral valve on the left)

          (a) Tricuspid valve is composed of three leaflets: The large anterior leaflet, and the two smaller posterior and septal leaflets

          (b) Mitral valve is composed of two leaflets: The long, narrow posterior (mural) leaflet (like a toilet seat) and an oval anterior (aortic) leaflet (like a toilet lid)

       ii. Function: These are one-way "check" valves that permit unidirectional blood flow from the atria to the ventricles during ventricular diastole and prevent retrograde flow during ventricular systole

          (a) With ventricular diastole, the ventricles relax and the valve leaflets open

          (b) With ventricular systole, the valve leaflets close completely

          (c) First heart sound (S_1) is produced as the mitral (M_1) and tricuspid (T_1) valves close. M_1 is the initial and major component of S_1.

  b. Semilunar valves

       i. Location and structure

          (a) Pulmonary valve is situated between the RV and the pulmonary artery. It consists of three semilunar cusps that attach to the wall of the pulmonary trunk.

          (b) Aortic valve is situated between the LV and aorta. It consists of three slightly thicker valve cusps, the bases of which attach to a valve annulus (fibrous ring).

       ii. Function: Permit unidirectional blood flow from the outflow tract during ventricular systole and prevent retrograde blood flow during ventricular diastole

          (a) With ventricular systole, the valves open when the respective ventricle contracts and pressure is greater in the ventricle than in the artery

          (b) After ventricular systole, pressure in the artery exceeds pressure in the ventricles. This and retrograde blood flow cause the valve to close.

          (c) Second heart sound (S_2) is produced when the aortic (A_2) and pulmonic (P_2) valves close. A_2 is normally the initial and major component of S_2.

5. **Coronary vasculature** (Figure 3-3)
   a. Arteries
      i. Two main arteries branch off at the base of the aorta, supplying blood to the heart
      ii. Right coronary artery (RCA)
         (a) Originates behind the right coronary cusp of the aortic valve
         (b) Supplies
            (1) RA and RV
            (2) Sinoatrial (SA) node and AV node
            (3) Inferior-posterior wall of the LV (in 90% of hearts)
            (4) Inferior-posterior third of the interventricular septum
         (c) Main branches
            (1) SA node in 55% of hearts
            (2) RV branch
            (3) AV node in 90% of hearts
            (4) Posterior descending artery (supplying the inferior-posterior wall of the LV in 85% of hearts)
      iii. Left coronary artery (LCA)
         (a) Left main coronary artery (LMCA): Branches into the left anterior descending and circumflex arteries
         (b) Left anterior descending (LAD) artery
            (1) Supplies the anterior two thirds of the interventricular septum and the anterior wall of the LV
            (2) Branches include diagonals (two to six other diagonals may be present), septal perforators (three to five other perforators may be present)
         (c) Left circumflex (LCX) artery also branches from the LMCA
            (1) LCX artery supplies
               a) SA node in 45% of hearts
               b) AV node in 10% of hearts

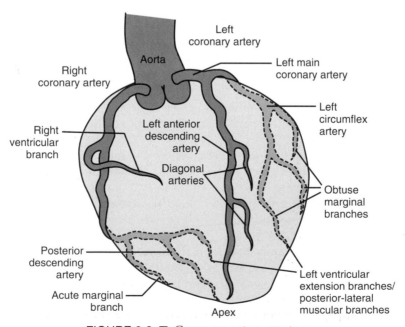

FIGURE 3-3 ■ Coronary artery anatomy.

c) Inferior-posterior LV in 10% of hearts

d) Lateral posterior surface of the LV via the obtuse marginal branches (OMBs)

e) Posterior descending artery arises from the LCX artery in 15% of hearts (see description under RCA)

(2) Branches of the LCX include the OMBs (may be one to three), which supply the lateral wall of the LV and occasionally the posterior lateral muscular branch

iv. Coronary collaterals: Potential vascular connections between the RCA and LCA exist

(a) They may open, if stenosis of one of the coronary arteries occurs, to supply blood from the other artery

(b) They cannot augment flow to meet acute requirements for increased flow

b. Cardiac veins

i. Return deoxygenated blood to the RA, mostly through the coronary sinus

ii. Follow paths similar to those of the arteries; have no valves

c. Coronary blood flow

i. Coronary vascular reserve: Coronary circulation has the ability to increase flow to meet added needs up to approximately six times normal

ii. Coronary blood flow is about 70 to 90 ml/min

iii. The heart uses most of the oxygen available in the coronary circulation; little oxygen reserve exists

iv. Most of coronary blood flow is in diastole, because in systole, coronary artery blood flow usually decreases due to ventricular compression and contraction

v. Coronary blood flow is reduced by

(a) Hypotension

(b) Tachycardia: Decreased LV diastolic filling times

(c) Mechanical obstruction (coronary stenosis or spasm)

6. **Neurologic control of the heart**

a. Autonomic nervous system: Influences contractility, depolarization-repolarization, and rate of conductivity

i. Sympathetic stimulation: Norepinephrine release is the main impetus of stimulation to the heart; its two effects include the following:

(a) α-adrenergic: Causing peripheral arteriolar vasoconstriction

(b) β-adrenergic

(1) Increases SA node discharge, increasing heart rate (positive chronotropy)

(2) Increases the force of myocardial contraction (positive inotropy)

(3) Accelerates AV conduction time

ii. Parasympathetic stimulation: Occurs via the tenth cranial (vagus) nerve. Acetylcholine release is the main parasympathetic impetus to cardiac effects.

(a) Decreases the rate of SA node discharge, slowing heart rate (negative chronotropy)

(b) Slows conduction through AV tissue

iii. Ventricles have mainly sympathetic innervation and only sparse vagal innervation

iv. Parasympathetic influences normally predominate in the conducting system (SA node, AV node)

b. **Chemoreceptors:** Afferent receptors located in the carotid and aortic bodies. Sensitive to changes in partial pressure of oxygen, partial pressure of carbon dioxide, and pH, causing changes in heart rate and respiratory rate via stimulation of vasomotor center in the medulla.

   c. **Baroreceptors:** Stretch receptors in the heart and blood vessels that respond to pressure and volume changes
7. **Cardiac muscle microanatomy and contractile properties:** See Box 3-1 for key elements
8. **Anatomy of the cardiac conduction system** (Figure 3-4)
   a. SA node
      i. Normal pacemaker of the heart, possessing the fastest inherent rate of automaticity (approximately 70 beats/min)
      ii. Located in the right superior wall of the RA at the junction of the superior vena cava and the RA
   b. Internodal atrial conduction
      i. Impulse is conducted from the SA node through the RA and LA musculature to the AV node
      ii. Although the atria do not have specialized high-speed conduction tracts comparable to the ventricular bundles and fascicles, there are preferred conduction pathways (e.g., Bachmann's bundle, which conducts impulses from the SA node to the LA)
   c. AV node
      i. Delays the impulse from the atria before it goes to the ventricles. This allows time for both ventricles to fill before ventricular systole.
      ii. Inherent rate of automaticity is approximately 40 beats/min
      iii. Located in the right interatrial septum, above the tricuspid valve's septal leaflet
   d. Bundle of His: Arises from the AV node and conducts the impulse to the bundle branch system. The bundle of His is close to the annulus of the tricuspid valve.

■ **BOX 3-1**
■ **KEY ELEMENTS OF CARDIAC MUSCLE MICROANATOMY**

CARDIAC MUSCLE FIBERS
Two main contractile properties: Ability to shorten and to develop force
Syncytium: Fibers arranged in latticelike "network": When one fiber is stimulated, all fibers become stimulated
Sarcomere: Contractile unit composed of
   ● Contractile proteins: Myosin and actin (their interactions help to produce contraction, fiber shortening)
   ● Regulatory proteins: Troponin and tropomyosin (they inhibit myosin-actin interactions)
Intercalated discs:
   ● Interlock cardiac muscle fibers together at ends
   ● Provide quick transmission of electrical impulse
Myocardial working cells: Enable chemical energy to be transformed into mechanical actions (contraction and relaxation)

EXCITATION-CONTRACTION PROCESS
1. During excitation (depolarization), calcium enters working cell interior across sarcolemma
2. Calcium binds with troponin, and myosin-actin inhibition is lost
3. Actin and myosin may now interact, using adenosine triphosphate for energy
4. Sarcomeres shorten, which results in muscle fiber shortening and subsequent cardiac muscle contraction
5. Calcium is then pumped out of cell, allowing fiber to relax again until process repeats

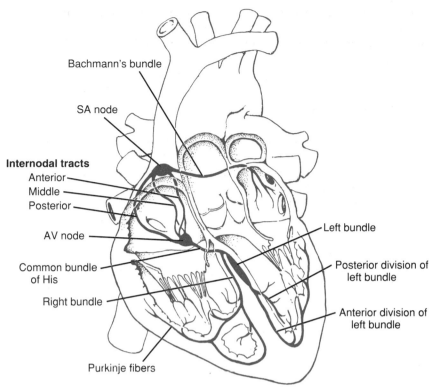

FIGURE 3-4 ■ Anatomy of the cardiac conduction system. *AV*, Atrioventricular; *SA*, sinoatrial.

  e. Bundle branch system: Pathways that arise from the bundle of His and branch at the top of the interventricular septum
    i. Right bundle branch is the smaller, direct continuation of the bundle of His. It transmits the impulse down the right side of the interventricular septum to the RV myocardium.
    ii. Left bundle branch is the larger branch from the bundle of His. It transmits the impulse to the septum and the LV. The left bundle branch divides into three parts:
      (a) Left anterior fascicle: Transmits the impulse to the anterior and superior endocardial surfaces of the LV
      (b) Left posterior fascicle: Transmits the impulse over the posterior-inferior endocardial surface of the LV
      (c) Septal bundle
  f. Purkinje system
    i. Arises from the distal portion of the bundle branches, forming networks on the ventricle's endocardial surface
    ii. Transmits the impulse into the subendocardial and myocardial layers of both ventricles
    iii. Provides for depolarization of the myocardium (from endocardium to epicardium)
    iv. Ventricles have their own inherent rate of automaticity of approximately 20 to 30 beats/min
9. Electrophysiology
  a. Electrophysiologic properties of cardiac muscle cells

    i. Excitability: Ability to depolarize and form an action potential when sufficiently stimulated

    ii. Automaticity: Ability to generate an impulse without an outside stimulus

    iii. Conductivity: Ability to conduct an electrical impulse to neighboring cells, spreading the impulse throughout the heart to achieve total depolarization

    iv. Refractoriness: Temporary inability of the depolarized cell to become excited and generate another action potential

b. Resting membrane potential (RMP): Electrical charge of cardiac muscle cell at rest. Cell ions consist primarily of sodium, potassium, and calcium.

    i. Sodium ion concentration is greater *outside* the cell

    ii. Potassium ion concentration is greater *inside* the cell

    iii. Calcium ion concentration is greater *outside* the cell

c. Depolarization: Change in the electrical charge of a stimulated cell from negative to positive by the flow of ions across the cell membrane. Sodium moves into the cell, potassium moves out.

d. Repolarization: Recovery or recharging of a cell's normal polarity. Sodium moves back out of the cell, potassium moves into the cell. The cell recovers its negative charge.

e. Threshold potential: The electric voltage level at which cardiac cells become activated and produce an action potential, which leads to muscular contraction

f. Stimulation of myocardial cells

    i. Stimulus may be chemical, electrical, or mechanical

    ii. When the cell is stimulated, the electrical charge inside the cell becomes less negative, and depolarization occurs

    iii. When the threshold potential is reached, changes occur in the membrane

    iv. SA and AV nodes achieve threshold potential first

    v. Cell membrane permeability is altered, and specialized channels in the membrane open, which allows the entry of sodium and calcium ions into the cell

g. Action potential: As cardiac cells reverse polarity, the electrical impulse generated during that event creates an energy stimulus that travels across the cell

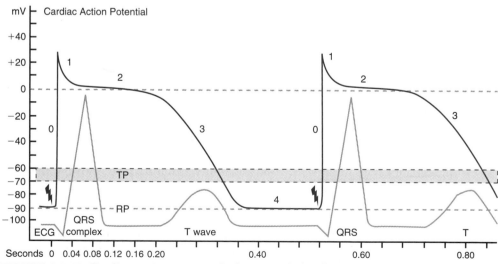

FIGURE 3-5 ■ Cardiac action potential of myocardial cells. *ECG*, Electrocardiogram; *RP*, resting membrane potential; *TP*, threshold membrane potential. (From Huszar RJ: *Basic dysrhythmias: interpretation and management,* ed 3, Philadelphia, 2001, Mosby, p 13.)

membrane—a high-speed, short-lived, self-reproducing current (heart only). This is represented on an action potential curve (Figure 3-5).

     i. *Phase 0*—Depolarization: A quick upstroke (several milliseconds) representing the initial phase of excitation

     ii. *Phase 1*—Initial phase of repolarization

     iii. *Phase 2*—Plateau phase of repolarization: Slow inward current of calcium (and, to a lesser extent, sodium); potassium diffuses out of the cells

     iv. *Phase 3*—Last phase of repolarization: Outward current of potassium increases, and the slow, inward current of sodium and calcium decreases. Cells rapidly repolarize, returning to normal RMP.

     v. *Phase 4*—Membrane at RMP

  h. Cardiac pacemaker cells (SA and AV nodes) action potential

     i. Pacer cells, having increased automaticity, spontaneously depolarize in phase 4 without a stimulus. Other cells of the heart, having repolarized, require another stimulus to become depolarized.

       (a) Rate of automaticity may be altered by increasing or decreasing the slope of phase 4

       (b) Increasing the slope speeds heart rate; decreasing the slope slows heart rate

     ii. Spontaneous depolarization of pacer cells is caused by a steady influx of sodium and efflux of potassium

     iii. SA node has the fastest rate of depolarization

  i. Refractoriness of heart muscle

     i. *Absolute refractory period* (effective refractory period): Another stimulus to the cell will not produce another action potential (phases 0, 1, and 2 and part of phase 3 of the action potential curve)

     ii. *Relative refractory period*: Only a very strong stimulus can initiate an action potential and cause depolarization (latter part of phase 3)

     iii. *Supernormal period*: Weak stimulus (one that would not normally elicit an action potential) can evoke an action potential and cause depolarization (at the end of phase 3)

10. **Events in the cardiac cycle** (Figure 3-6)

  a. Ventricular systole: Contraction and emptying of the ventricles

     i. QRS complex: Represents ventricular depolarization (an electrical event)

     ii. First phase of ventricular contraction (systole) is called isovolumetric contraction. Pressure increases, but no blood is ejected until LV pressure exceeds aortic pressure (and opens the aortic valve).

     iii. As pressure rises in the ventricles, the AV valves close, producing the first heart sound (S_1, composed of mitral [M_1] and tricuspid [T_1] components)

     iv. The "c" wave of the atrial pressure curve is produced when the AV valves are pushed backward toward the atria as ventricular pressure builds

     v. When LV pressure exceeds the pressure in the aorta, the aortic valve opens (comparable events in the RV occur with the pulmonic valve)

     vi. Blood is rapidly ejected into the aorta (systolic ejection)

     vii. LV pressures decrease, falling below the pressure in the aorta, ventricular ejection stops, and the aortic valve closes. (Comparable events occur in the pulmonary artery, closing the pulmonic valve.)

     viii. Closing of the aortic and pulmonic valves produces the second heart sound (S_2, composed of aortic [A_2] and pulmonic [P_2] components)

     ix. Aortic valve closure is represented by the dicrotic notch in the aortic pressure waveform

     x. Repolarization of the ventricles occurs at this time and produces the T wave on the electrocardiogram (ECG)

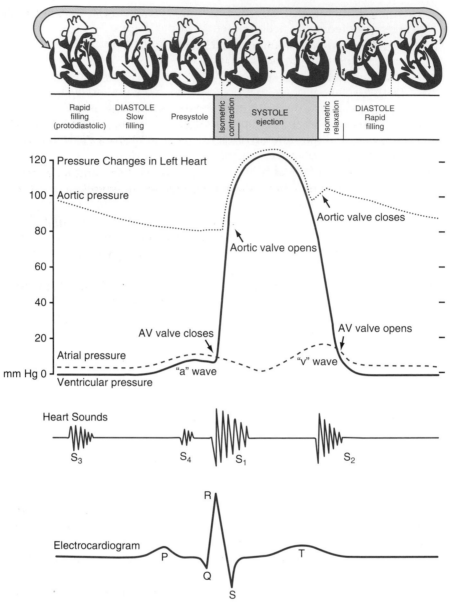

FIGURE 3-6 ■ Events in the cardiac cycle. *AV,* Atrioventricular. (Adapted from Jarvis C: *Physical examination and health assessment,* ed 2, Philadelphia, 1996, Saunders, p 518.)

> **xi.** After the aortic valve closes, pressure in the LV falls rapidly (isovolumetric relaxation phase); no blood enters the ventricle
> **xii.** LA "v" wave is produced by rapid filling of the atria during ventricular systole, against closed AV valves. This marks the end of systole.
>
> **b.** Ventricular diastole: Filling phase of the ventricles
> > **i.** When pressure is lower in the ventricles than in the atria, the AV valves reopen, which initiates the early rapid filling phase of the ventricles during diastole. This marks the start of diastole.
> > **ii.** Pressure in the atria is higher than diastolic pressure in the ventricles, so blood flows from the atria into the ventricles
> > **iii.** "a" wave: Atrial pressure rises with atrial contraction

      iv. P wave (ECG): In late diastole, represents atrial depolarization (an electrical event)

11. **Variables affecting LV function and cardiac output (CO)**
    a. CO: Amount of blood ejected by the LV in 1 minute
      i. CO is the product of stroke volume (SV) and heart rate (HR):
      CO = SV × HR
      ii. SV is the amount of blood ejected by the LV with each contraction, or the difference between left ventricular end-diastolic volume (LVEDV) and left ventricular end-systolic volume (LVESV): SV = LVEDV − LVESV; (60 to 130 ml)
      iii. Normal resting CO = 4 to 8 L/min
      iv. CO is determined by preload, afterload, contractility, and heart rate
    b. Preload: The degree to which muscle fibers are lengthened (stretched) prior to contraction
      i. In the intact heart, preload is secondary to the volume (size) of the chamber. This is determined by the amount of blood filling the chamber.
      ii. Increases in preload increase the CO as described by the *Frank-Starling law* of the heart
      iii. Muscle fibers can reach a point of stretch beyond which contraction is no longer enhanced, and further increases in preload do not yield any further increase in CO
      iv. Increased preload occurs with
        (a) Increased circulating volume
        (b) Venous constriction (decreases venous pooling and increases venous return to heart)
        (c) Drugs: Vasoconstrictors
      v. Decreased preload occurs with
        (a) Hypovolemia
        (b) Mitral stenosis
        (c) Drugs: Vasodilators (e.g., nitrates), diuretics
        (d) Cardiac tamponade
        (e) Constrictive pericarditis
    c. Afterload: Initial resistance that must be overcome by the ventricles to develop force and contract, opening the semilunar valves and propelling blood into the systemic and pulmonary circulatory systems (systolic contraction)
      i. Factors affecting afterload include arterial resistance (wall stress and thickness), aortic impedance, and blood viscosity
      ii. Systemic vascular resistance (SVR) is used as a rough estimate of afterload
      iii. To calculate SVR: Mean arterial pressure (MAP) minus central venous pressure (CVP); this number is divided by CO; the resulting value then is multiplied by 80 and converts into dynes/sec/cm^{-5} (1 dyne is the force that gives a mass of 1 g an acceleration of 1 cm/sec^2):

$$SVR = \frac{MAP - CVP}{CO} \times 80$$

      iv. Normal SVR = 900 to 1400 dynes/sec/cm^{-5}
      v. Excessive afterload: Increases LV stroke work, decreases SV, increases myocardial oxygen demands, and may result in LV failure
      vi. Increased afterload is seen in
        (a) Aortic stenosis
        (b) Peripheral arteriolar vasoconstriction
        (c) Hypertension
        (d) Polycythemia
        (e) Use of arterial vasoconstrictor drugs
      vii. Decreased afterload is seen in

        (a) Hypovolemia
        (b) Sepsis
        (c) Use of arterial vasodilators
    d. Contractility (inotropic state): Heart's contractile strength
        i. There is no way to measure contractility directly. Contractile state can be assessed indirectly through its effects on CO or with noninvasive imaging.
        ii. Factors increasing the contractile state of the myocardium include
            (a) Use of positive inotropic drugs (e.g., digitalis, milrinone, epinephrine, dobutamine)
            (b) Increased heart rate (Bowditch's phenomenon)
            (c) Sympathetic stimulation (via β_1 receptors)
        iii. Factors decreasing the contractile state of the myocardium include
            (a) Negative inotropic drugs (e.g., type 1A antiarrhythmics, β-blockers, calcium channel blockers, barbiturates)
            (b) Hypoxia
            (c) Hypercapnia
            (d) Myocardial ischemia or infarction
            (e) Metabolic acidosis
    e. Heart rate
        i. Influenced by many factors, including
            (a) Blood volume status
            (b) Sympathetic and parasympathetic tone
            (c) Drugs
            (d) Temperature
            (e) Respiration
            (f) Arrhythmias
            (g) Peripheral vascular tone
            (h) Emotions
            (i) Metabolic status (increases with hyperthyroidism)
        ii. Determinant of myocardial oxygen supply and demand
            (a) Increased heart rates increase myocardial oxygen consumption
            (b) Fast heart rates (above 150 beats/min) decrease diastolic coronary blood flow (shorter diastole)
    f. Cardiac index (CI)
        i. CI is CO corrected for differences in body size (CO of 4 L/min may be adequate for a 100-lb woman but inadequate for a 200-lb man)
        ii. Based on body surface area (BSA) as estimated from a height and weight nomogram: CI = CO/BSA
        iii. Normal CI is 2.5 to 4.0 L/min/m^2
    g. Ejection fraction (EF)
        i. Percentage of blood in the ventricle ejected with every beat
            (a) Normal LV EF = 50% to 75%
            (b) Not clinically significant until less than 50%
        ii. Good reflection of LV performance
    h. Ventricular function curve: Shows how to relate the contributions of preload, afterload, and contractility (but *not* heart rate) to ventricular function (Figure 3-7)
12. **Systemic vasculature**
    a. Major functions: Provides tissues with blood, nutrients, and hormones and removes metabolic wastes
    b. Resistance to flow: Depends on diameter of vessels (especially arterioles), viscosity of blood, and elastic recoil in vessel walls

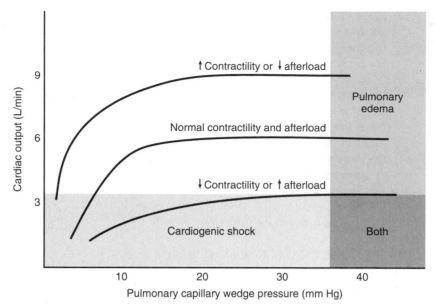

FIGURE 3-7 ■ Ventricular function curve. The ventricular function curve is not a Starling curve. It relates all the contributors to cardiac output, except heart rate, to ventricular function. It is an excellent framework for assessment and decision making.

    c. Circulating blood volume: There is approximately 5 L of total circulating blood volume in the adult body

    d. Major components of the vascular system

      i. Arteries

        (a) Strong, compliant, elastic-walled vessels that branch off the aorta, carry blood away from the heart, and distribute it to capillary beds throughout the body

        (b) A high-pressure circuit

        (c) Able to stretch during systole and recoil during diastole because of elastic fibers in the arterial wall

      ii. Arterioles

        (a) Control systemic vascular resistance and thus arterial pressure

        (b) Have strong smooth muscle walls innervated by the autonomic nervous system

        (c) Autonomic nervous system

          (1) Adrenergic (stimulatory) system: Releases two neurotransmitters (epinephrine, norepinephrine). Epinephrine stimulates β-receptors (increases heart rate, increases contractility, dilates arterioles). Norepinephrine stimulates α-receptors (vasoconstriction).

          (2) Cholinergic (inhibitory) system: Releases acetylcholine (decreases heart rate; releases nitric oxide, causing vasodilatation).

        (d) Lead directly into capillaries, supply tissue beds

      iii. Capillary system

        (a) Tissue bed exchange of oxygen and carbon dioxide and solutes between blood and tissues; site of fluid volume transfer between plasma and interstitium

        (b) Gas exchange caused by diffusion. Diffusion of a substance is from an area of high concentration to an area of low concentration until equilibrium is established.

(c) Fluid homeostasis
(1) Increased capillary hydrostatic pressure moves fluid from the vessel into the interstitium
(2) Greater capillary osmotic pressure moves fluid from the interstitium into the vessels
(3) Plasma protein concentration in the capillaries provides the osmotic gradient
(4) Retains fluid in the intravascular space
(5) Prevents edema formation in the interstitium
(6) Albumin accounts for 75% of total plasma osmotic pressure; fibrinogen accounts for a small amount
(7) Serum albumin level is a good indicator of a patient's colloid osmotic pressure
(d) Capillaries lack smooth muscle
iv. Venous system
(a) Stores about 65% of total blood volume
(b) Receives blood from capillaries
(c) Conducts blood back to the heart within a low-pressure system
(d) No muscle layer: Veins are compressed by the contraction of surrounding skeletal muscle
(e) Valves in the veins prevent reverse blood flow
(f) Venous pressure in the lower extremities is normally 20 mm Hg or less

13. **Control of peripheral blood flow**
   a. Autoregulation: Ability of the tissues to control their own blood flow (vasodilatation, vasoconstriction)
      i. Coronary blood flow remains fairly constant over a wide range of blood pressures
      ii. As coronary perfusion pressure drops below 50 mm Hg, autoregulatory ability becomes impaired
   b. Autonomic regulation of vessels
      i. Vasoconstriction occurs when norepinephrine is released by stimulation of the sympathetic nervous system (adrenergic effect)
      ii. Vasodilatation occurs when acetylcholine is released by stimulation of the parasympathetic nervous system (cholinergic effect) or by inhibition of vasoconstriction
   c. Stretch receptors: Baroreceptors (pressoreceptors) keep MAP constant
      i. Receptor sites in the arteries (aortic arch, carotid sinus, pulmonary arteries, and atria)
      ii. Action with increased blood pressure
         (a) Respond to stretching of arterial walls
         (b) Impulse transmitted from the aortic arch via the vagus nerve to the medulla
         (c) Parasympathetic nervous system stimulated, sympathetic nervous system inhibited
         (d) Result: Decreased heart rate and contractility, dilation of peripheral vessels, decreased SVR, decreased blood pressure
      iii. Action with decreased blood pressure
         (a) Sympathetic nervous system stimulated, parasympathetic nervous system inhibited
         (b) Result: Increased heart rate and contractility, arterial and venous constriction (which preserves blood flow to the brain and heart), and increased blood pressure

14. **Arterial pressure**
   a. Neurohumoral regulation
      i. Renin-angiotensin-aldosterone system also helps control arterial pressure (see Chapter 5)
      ii. Renin is a protease secreted by the kidneys; converts angiotensinogen to angiotensin I
      iii. Renin release from the kidneys is affected as follows:
         (a) Decreased blood pressure (i.e., hemorrhage, dehydration, diuretics, sodium depletion) → increases in renin secretion
         (b) Rise in sympathetic output (β stimulation) → increases in renin secretion
         (c) Fall in sodium concentration → increases in renin secretion (decreased volume)
         (d) Increased blood pressure → decreases in renin secretion
      iv. Angiotensin I is converted to angiotensin II. (These effects are blocked by angiotensin-converting enzyme [ACE] inhibitors.)
      v. Angiotensin II, the most potent vasoconstrictor known, is produced when increased renin secretion stimulates its formation
         (a) Effects of angiotensin II include the following:
            (1) Arteriolar constriction, which increases systolic and diastolic pressures
            (2) Stimulation of the adrenal cortex to secrete aldosterone, which causes sodium and water retention
            (3) Increase in extracellular fluid volume, which shuts off the stimulus that initiated renin secretion so that blood pressure is maintained at the normal level
         (b) Effects of angiotensin II are blocked at its receptors by angiotensin II receptor blockers (ARBs)
   b. Pulse pressure: Difference between systolic and diastolic pressures
      i. Function of SV and arterial capacitance
      ii. Normal pulse pressure: 30 to 40 mm Hg
      iii. Changes in SV (with exercise, shock, heart failure) are reflected in similar changes in pulse pressure
   c. MAP: Average arterial pressure during the cardiac cycle; dependent on mean arterial blood volume and elasticity of the arterial wall
      i. $MAP = \dfrac{(\text{diastolic pressure} \times 2) + \text{systolic pressure}}{3}$
      ii. Example: Blood pressure of 120/60 mm Hg

$$MAP = [(60 \times 2) + 120]/3$$

$$MAP = (120 + 120)/3$$

$$MAP = 240/3 = 80$$

Patient Assessment

1. **Nursing history**
   a. Main complaint: Patient's explanation for seeking medical assistance
   b. History of present illness: Ascertain the following:
      i. Description of complaint
      ii. Onset: Date, time of day, duration, course, precipitating factors
      iii. Signs and symptoms: Exacerbations, remissions
         (a) Discomfort: Character, location, radiation, quality, duration, factors that aggravate or produce, factors that alleviate
         (b) Fatigue: With or without activity

   (c) Edema: Location, degree, duration

   (d) Syncope and presyncope: Onset (presyncopal warning or sudden event), time and circumstances of occurrence (postural, nonpostural, activity), provocative events (cough, micturition, head movement)

   (e) Dyspnea: Orthopnea, paroxysmal nocturnal dyspnea, dyspnea on exertion (determine how much exercise it takes to elicit in number of blocks, flights of stairs, etc.)

   (f) Palpitations: Nature, length, associated symptoms

   (g) Cough, hemoptysis

   (h) Claudication: Hip or calf? How many blocks can you walk?

   (i) Recent weight gain or loss

 c. Medical history: Identify all previous illnesses, injuries, and surgical procedures

  i. Patient's assessment of general health for last several years

  ii. Risk factors: Hypertension, hypercholesteremia, smoking, family history of cardiac disease, diabetes

  iii. Last medical examination, hospitalizations, prior relevant cardiac tests (e.g., echocardiography, catheterization)

  iv. Heart history: Coronary artery disease (CAD), angina, myocardial infarctions (MIs), hypertension, valvular disease, arrhythmias, trauma, peripheral vascular disease, congenital heart defects, heart murmurs, rheumatic fever, cerebrovascular accident (CVA), transient ischemic attacks

 d. Family history: Identify

  i. State of health or cause of death and age at death of immediate family members

  ii. Hereditary, familial diseases pertaining to cardiovascular system

   (a) Diabetes mellitus

   (b) Hypertension

   (c) Cardiovascular disease

   (d) Sudden death or syncope

   (e) Lipid disorders

   (f) Stroke

   (g) Collagen vascular disease

 e. Social history: Identify

  i. Present and past work experiences

  ii. Level of activity, exercise

  iii. Smoking and drinking habits (present, past)

  iv. Daily living patterns

  v. Nutrition: Foods eaten, meals per day, who prepares meals

  vi. Support system: Relationship with significant others

  vii. Cultural issues and language barriers

 f. Medication history: Identify all prescribed or over-the-counter medications. Determine why and how often the patient is taking drug(s), dosages, any side effects, compliance issues.

 g. Allergies: Medications, foods (i.e., shellfish), environmental substances, iodine (potential reaction to contrast medium used during cardiac catheterization procedures)

2. Nursing examination of patient

 a. Physical examination data

  i. General overall appearance: Skin and mucous membranes

   (a) Color

   (b) Temperature

   (c) Moisture

    (d) Turgor

    (e) Edema: Found in dependent areas; pitting versus nonpitting (extremities and sacrum)

    (f) Nail bed: Color, refill

    (g) Angiomas

    (h) Petechiae

    (i) Cyanosis (circumoral, peripheral)

    (j) Clubbing of fingers or toes

ii. Vital signs

    (a) Pulses: Palpate bilaterally

        (1) Check rate, rhythm, character, and volume

        (2) Describe pulses, using scale of 0 to 3

            a) 0 = absent pulses

            b) 1+ = palpable but thready, easily obliterated

            c) 2+ = normal, not easily obliterated

            d) 3+ = bounding, easily palpable, cannot obliterate

        (3) Common sites for palpation of arteries

            a) Radial

            b) Brachial

            c) Femoral

            d) Carotid

            e) Popliteal

            f) Dorsalis pedis

            g) Posterior tibialis

        (4) Describe pulse characteristics

            a) Normal pulse character: Smooth, rounded

            b) Pulse deficit: Inability to palpate all contractions of the heart

                1) Premature or rapid contractions may not generate a peripheral pulse

                2) Determine by comparing radial pulse with auscultated apical pulse; record difference in rates

            c) Pulsus parvus et tardus: Small (parvus) pulse with delayed (tardus) slow upstroke and prolonged downstroke. Noted in

                1) Aortic stenosis: Parvus and tardus

                2) Mitral stenosis: Only parvus

                3) Constrictive pericarditis: Only parvus

                4) Cardiac tamponade: Only parvus

             d) Pulsus alternans: Pulse waves alternate, every other beat is weaker; caused by impaired myocardium; noted in severe LV failure

            e) Water hammer (Corrigan's pulse)

                1) Abrupt, rapid upstroke followed by rapid downstroke

                2) Palpated in patients with aortic insufficiency, patent ductus arteriosus (PDA)

    (b) Blood pressure

        (1) Sphygmomanometer: Key points

            a) Width of cuff important

                1) Ideal width is 40% of the circumference of the arm

                2) For obese patients, use a thigh cuff, 18 cm wide

            b) Positioning of cuff: No less than 2.5 cm from the antecubital fossa

            c) Falsely low measurement: Cuff too large for arm, arm above heart level, inability to accurately hear first Korotkoff sound

d) Falsely high measurement: Cuff too small for arm, loose cuff not centered over brachial artery, arm below heart level
(2) Take blood pressure in both arms. More than a 10- to 15-mm Hg difference in systolic pressures indicates diminished arterial flow on the side with the lower reading (obstruction, dissection)
(3) Orthostatic blood pressure drop: Assess at-risk patients
    a) Check blood pressure supine, sitting, standing
    b) Fall of more than 20 mm Hg of systolic pressure signifies orthostatic hypotension
    c) Caused by vasodilating drugs, volume depletion
(4) Pulsus paradoxus: Exaggeration of the normal physiologic response to inspiration (blood pressure lower on inspiration than on expiration)
    a) Examine with the patient breathing normally
    b) Inflate sphygmomanometer until no Korotkoff sounds are heard; slowly deflate cuff until Korotkoff sounds first heard on expiration; note pressure reading
    c) Continue to deflate cuff until sounds heard during both expiration and inspiration; note reading
    d) Subtract second reading from first to determine pulsus paradoxus
    e) Normally, on inspiration, the difference between inspiration and expiration is less than 11 mm Hg. With pulsus paradoxus, fall in blood pressure on inspiration is 11 mm Hg or greater.
    f) Seen in
        1) Cardiac tamponade
        2) Constrictive pericarditis
        3) Emphysema, asthma
        4) Hemorrhagic shock

iii. Neck examination
    (a) Neck veins give important clues regarding fluid status
        (1) Jugular veins reflect RA and RV filling pressures
        (2) Internal jugular veins are harder to visualize than external jugular veins, but they more accurately reflect pressure and volume changes in the RA (central venous pressure)
        (3) Check for distention and pulsation
            a) Elevate the head of the bed until jugular waves can be seen
            b) Shine a bright light tangentially to illuminate vessels, if not obvious
        (4) Determine jugular venous pressure
            a) The sternal angle (angle of Louis) is roughly 5 cm above the atrium (when the patient is upright or lying down)
            b) Measure the distance in centimeters from the sternal notch to the top of the distended neck vein
            c) The value obtained plus the 5 cm provides a rough estimate of central venous pressure
    (b) Check for hepatojugular reflux
        (1) Place the patient at a 45-degree angle
        (2) Compress the upper right abdomen for 30 to 45 seconds (causes additional venous return from liver to heart)
        (3) If hepatojugular reflux is present, the jugular pulses become more pronounced, and the level of filling of neck veins will rise (signifies inability of the right side of the heart to deal with the added volume)

iv. Chest examination
   (a) Shape and contour of the chest
   (b) Symmetry
   (c) Breathing pattern
v. Cardiac examination
   (a) Palpate three areas: Base, apex, and left sternal border; check for
      (1) Pulsations (e.g., the point of maximal intensity [PMI]; the patient *must be supine*)
      (2) Thrills (palpable vibrations, analogous to the sensation felt on the throat of a purring cat) signify turbulence or murmur loud enough to feel (aortic stenosis, mitral stenosis, PDA, ventricular septal defect [VSD])
      (3) Left peristernal lift: Suggests RV dilatation
      (4) Apical impulse (PMI in the *normal* heart): Not always easy to palpate
         a) Normally located at the fifth left intercostal space, midclavicular line, and is approximately 2 cm in size
         b) PMI that can be palpated over two or more intercostal areas signifies diffuse PMI resulting from
            1) LV dilatation (LV volume overload)
            2) Aortic insufficiency, mitral regurgitation, dilated cardiomyopathy
         c) A forceful, *sustained* apical impulse indicates LV hypertrophy
         d) Nonsustained but forceful apical impulses are created by high-output states (fever, anemia, anxiety, hyperthyroidism)
   (b) Auscultation of the heart
      (1) Use of the stethoscope
         a) Bell: Use to hear low-pitched sounds such as ventricular filling sounds (S_3 and S_4) and filling rumble of mitral and tricuspid stenosis
         b) When using the bell of the stethoscope, press only hard enough to create a seal; otherwise, underlying skin functions as a diaphragm and low-pitched sounds will not be heard
         c) Diaphragm: Use to hear high-pitched sounds such as heart sounds S_1 and S_2, ejection clicks, opening snaps, and most murmurs
         d) Usual listening positions: Supine, left lateral decubitus position, sitting up, and leaning forward
         e) Main auscultation areas on the chest (Figure 3-8)
            1) Aortic area (second intercostal space, right sternal border)
            2) Pulmonic area (second intercostal space, left sternal border)
            3) Tricuspid area (fifth intercostal space, left sternal border)
            4) Mitral or apical area at the PMI (usually the fifth intercostal space, left midclavicular line)
      (2) Origin of heart sounds: Opening and closing of valves (see Figure 3-6) and rapid acceleration or deceleration of blood produce either low- or high-pitched sounds
      (3) Normal heart sounds
         a) First heart sound (S_1): Produced by mitral and tricuspid valve closure
            1) Marks the onset of ventricular systole
            2) LV depolarizes and contracts before the RV
            3) Best heard at the apex

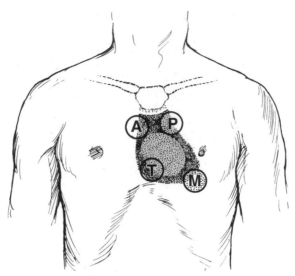

FIGURE 3-8 ▪ Cardiac examination. Auscultation areas: Aortic *(A)*, pulmonic *(P)*, tricuspid *(T)*, and mitral *(M)*.

    4) Component parts of S_1 may be split (mitral component [M_1] before tricuspid component [T_1])

    5) Coincides with carotid artery pulse wave

  b) Second heart sound (S_2): Produced by aortic and pulmonic valve closure

    1) Listen with diaphragm at the pulmonic area

    2) Both component parts of S_2 may be heard: Aortic component [A_2] before pulmonary component [P_2]. Normal P_2 is heard only at pulmonic area.

  c) Fourth heart sound (S_4)

    1) Normal in many adults

    2) Audible only in sinus rhythms (requires atrial contraction)

  d) Physiologic (normal) split of S_2 (A_2P_2)

    1) P_2 is delayed on inspiration when the RV is slower to contract than the LV

    2) Delay due to increased volume loading of the RV in inspiration caused by increased venous return to the heart

    3) RV ejection of blood is prolonged and delays pulmonic valve closure, prolonging the time from aortic closure (A_2) to pulmonic closure (P_2). A resulting split occurs between A_2 and P_2 during quiet inspiration.

    4) A_2 precedes P_2 and is generally louder

    5) Split of S_2 is heard only over the pulmonic area

    6) Best heard in quiet respiration when the patient is sitting or standing

(4) Abnormal heart sounds: See Table 3-1

(5) Extracardiac sounds

  a) Ejection clicks: Sharp, high-pitched sounds just after S_1; caused by tensioning of the great vessels as they distend in early systole

  b) Pericardial friction rubs

    1) Are like leather rubbing or new snow crunching

TABLE 3-1

Abnormal Heart Sounds

Abnormal Heart Sound	Cause/Circumstance	Seen In	Characteristics
Fixed splitting of S_2 Persistent (wide) splitting of S_2	Occurs with any increase in right ventricular (RV) volume or pressure, prolonged RV ejection and delayed pulmonary valve closure, or delay in RV systole (right bundle branch block)	Atrial septal defect Right bundle branch block Pulmonary hypertension of any cause Pulmonary stenosis Ventricular septal defect	Does not change with expiration (no respiratory variation) Second heart sound is split on expiration and more widely split on inspiration
Paradoxical splitting (reversed splitting) of S_2 (e.g., P_2 earlier than A_2)	Occurs when left ventricular (LV) ejection time is prolonged, resulting in delayed aortic closure; therefore, pulmonic valve closes first	Left bundle branch block Severe aortic stenosis Patent ductus arteriosus	Split widens on expiration and narrows on inspiration (P_2 precedes A_2)
Third heart sound (S_3): Ventricular gallop	Occurs during rapid phase of ventricular filling in early diastole; caused by resistance to ventricular filling, resulting from increased volume load or decreased ventricular compliance	Can normally be heard in children and young adults, and in women during the last trimester of pregnancy (physiologic S_3) Abnormal when heard in older age groups or in association with disease states (left-sided heart failure, ischemia, right-sided heart failure, fluid overload) Heard transiently in patients with ischemia	Sound is low pitched (heard best with bell) When originating in LV, heard best at the apex with patient in left lateral decubitus position When originating in RV, heard best along fourth intercostal space, left sternal border, in inspiration Sounds like cadence of "see" in "Tennessee"
Atrial gallop (presystolic or S_4)	Occurs during atrial contraction, just before S_1 during late phase of ventricular filling Occurs when there is volume overload of either ventricle or decreased ventricular compliance	Often a normal finding in adults Heard also in patients with myocardial ischemia or infarction, systemic and pulmonic hypertension, ventricular failure	Left-sided S_4 is usually heard best at the apex (does not change with respirations) Right-sided S_4 (less common) is usually louder on inspiration, over left lower sternal border Sounds like cadence of "a" in "appendix" or "Ken in Kentucky"
Summation gallop	Simultaneous occurrence of atrial (S_4) and ventricular (S_3) gallop	Heard with tachycardias (which cause shortening of diastole) and heart failure	

2) Should be heard with the diaphragm in full expiration (are loudest when the patient is leaning forward)

3) Often have three components (ventricular systole, ventricular filling, and atrial systole)

    c) Opening snaps: Sounds produced by a stenotic mitral valve snapping into the open position

    d) Prosthetic valves: Crisp, sometimes metallic clicking, with both opening and closure heard

  (6) Murmurs

    a) Sounds produced by turbulent blood flow (Box 3-2)

    b) Abnormal murmurs (hemodynamically significant): See Table 3-2

vi. Abdominal examination: Note the following

  (a) Aortic pulsations (expansile in abdominal aortic aneurysm)

  (b) Hepatomegaly

  (c) Ascites

vii. Extremities examination: Note the following

  (a) Edema: Indicates right-sided heart failure, venous stasis, venous insufficiency

  (b) Color, temperature changes: Indicate arterial insufficiency (especially if asymmetrically cool)

  (c) Skin condition: Petechiae, jaundice

  (d) Hair loss: Indicates arterial disease

  (e) Ulcerations: Indicates stasis, ischemia

  (f) Peripheral pulses: Check for bruits

  (g) Motor and sensory function: Numbness, foot drop (in advanced peripheral ischemia)

  (h) Clubbing of nail beds: Cyanotic congenital heart defects

  (i) Varicosities

  (j) Gangrene

b. Monitoring data (Figure 3-9)

  i. See Table 3-3 for types of bedside monitoring and Table 3-4 for hemodynamic pressures

  ii. Complications of bedside hemodynamic monitoring

    (a) Arrhythmias

    (b) Hemorrhage

    (c) Infection

    (d) Thrombi, emboli (air, blood)

    (e) Pneumothorax

    (f) Cardiac perforation

    (g) Pulmonary infarction (balloon left inflated)

    (h) Vascular occlusion or spasm

  iii. To prevent complications associated with these monitoring catheters, ensure the following:

    (a) Balloon is deflated after wedge pressure is obtained, to prevent pulmonary infarction

    (b) Catheter has not wedged when it is deflated or has not slipped back into the RV (risk of ventricular tachycardia [VT])

    (c) Only 0.8 to 1.5 ml of air is used to inflate the balloon (with 3-ml syringe): Risks of balloon overinflation include possible rupture, emboli, infarctions

    (d) Catheter is inserted under sterile technique (use catheter guard to cover catheter)

■ **BOX 3-2**
■ **EVALUATING MURMURS: SOUNDS PRODUCED BY TURBULENT BLOOD FLOW**

DETERMINE WHETHER MURMUR IS SYSTOLIC OR DIASTOLIC
1. Concentrate first on systole (S_1 to S_2); listen at all areas, starting with the base and moving down to the apex
2. Listen to all areas in diastole (S_2 to S_1)
3. Listen to all areas with the bell and diaphragm

DETERMINE CHARACTERISTICS OF THE SOUND TO INCLUDE
- Site of maximal intensity
- Radiation of sound (murmurs radiate in the direction of blood flow)
- Timing, duration, and location
- Effect of respirations on murmur, whether increased or decreased with either inspiration or expiration
- Effect of patient position on the murmur's intensity

DESCRIBE PATTERNS, INTENSITY, AND QUALITY OF MURMURS
- Patterns
  Crescendo: Builds up in intensity
  Decrescendo: Decreases in intensity
  Crescendo-decrescendo: Peaks and then decreases in intensity
- Intensity: Based on a grade of I to VI; recorded with grade over VI to show scale used
  I/VI: Barely audible; the clinician can hear only after listening awhile
  II/VI: Easily audible
  III/VI: Loud; not associated with a thrill
  IV/VI: Loud and may be associated with a thrill
  V/VI: Very loud; can be heard with the stethoscope partly off the chest (tilted); associated with a thrill
  VI/VI: Very loud; can be heard with the stethoscope off the chest; associated with a thrill
- Quality: May be described as blowing, musical, rough, harsh, honking, vibratory, cooing
- Pitch: High pitched, low pitched

CHARACTERISTICS OF SPECIFIC HEART SOUNDS
- Ejection murmurs: Usually rough, extending into or through systole (e.g., aortic stenosis or sclerosis)
- Regurgitant murmurs: Are usually a more pure, uniform sound (e.g., mitral regurgitation)
- Pansystolic (holosystolic) murmurs: Heard from S_1 through S_2

COMMENTS ON FUNCTIONAL, INNOCENT MURMURS
- Hemodynamically insignificant, physiologic; usually ejection murmurs associated with either increased flow or volume
- Not associated with cardiovascular disease
- Common in children and pregnant women
- Heard in hyperthyroidism, anemia
- Diastolic murmurs are never functional or innocent

    (e) Introducer sheath is sutured to the skin to prevent catheter migration, which can cause ventricular ectopy; possible perforation of RA, RV, or pulmonary artery; or pulmonary infarction

    (f) Pressurized, heparinized drip is used to maintain patency and to prevent both clot formation at the end of the catheter and possible embolization

■ TABLE 3-2
■ Abnormal Heart Murmurs: Main Characteristics

Abnormal Murmur	Location Where Heard Best	Characteristics	Comments
SYSTOLIC MURMURS			
Mitral insufficiency or regurgitation	Loudest at apex Radiates to left axilla	Blowing quality, high-pitched	Pansystolic—extends through A_2 May be rough and heard at base (mitral valve prolapse)
Tricuspid insufficiency or regurgitation	Loudest at lower left sternal border Radiates to right sternal border, liver	Blowing quality, low-pitched Variable in intensity (may increase with inspiration)	Pansystolic
Aortic stenosis	Maximal intensity at base of heart, usually at second intercostal space, right sternal border Radiates to neck and apex	Harsh in quality, medium or high-pitched May be crescendo-decrescendo murmur Intensity varies; no relation to severity of murmur	Systolic ejection murmur Extends to S_2 Thrill may be found at second intercostal space, right sternal border
Hypertrophic obstructive cardiomyopathy	Maximal intensity at second to fourth intercostal spaces, right sternal border May radiate to apex	Crescendo-decrescendo Decreases during expiration and squatting Increases with Valsalva maneuver	Ejection murmur Thrill may be found at lower left sternal border
Pulmonic stenosis	Maximal loudness at second intercostal space, left sternal border Louder when patient is supine and during inspiration	Harsh Usually grade III to IV intensity Persistent split of S_2, including expiration; the more severe the stenosis, the more pronounced the split	Pulmonary systolic ejection sound (click) Thrill may be felt at second intercostal space, left sternal border Right ventricular (RV) S_4 possible
Interventricular septal defect	Maximal loudness along lower sternal border Radiates widely	Harsh	Pansystolic or early systolic Thrill often present over left sternal border

Patent ductus arteriosus	Maximal intensity at second intercostal space, left sternal border	Machinery-like murmur	Continuous systolic and diastolic murmur Occasional thrill at second intercostal space, left sternal border
DIASTOLIC MURMURS Mitral stenosis	Maximal intensity at point of maximal intensity (PMI) May be heard only when patient lying on left side at the PMI with bell of stethoscope	Very low pitched Fading rumble Presystolic, crescendo if patient in normal sinus rhythm Intensity not affected by inspiration	Early diastolic and presystolic rumble (if in sinus rhythm) May be associated with an opening snap and accentuated S_1
Tricuspid stenosis	Maximal intensity at fourth intercostal space, left sternal border	Rumbling Low pitched Intensity should increase on inspiration, unless RV has failed	Early diastolic May have an opening snap
Aortic insufficiency or regurgitation	Maximal intensity at third to fourth intercostal space, left sternal border, and at apex Radiates to apex Heard best when patient is sitting up and leaning forward, during exhalation	Blowing quality High pitched Decrescendo Intensity varies with severity	Pandiastolic (unless acute, when it is short, early diastolic murmur)
Pulmonary insufficiency or regurgitation	Maximal loudness along second left intercostal space, left sternal border Radiates along left sternal border	Blowing quality High pitched Decrescendo	Sometimes increases with inspiration

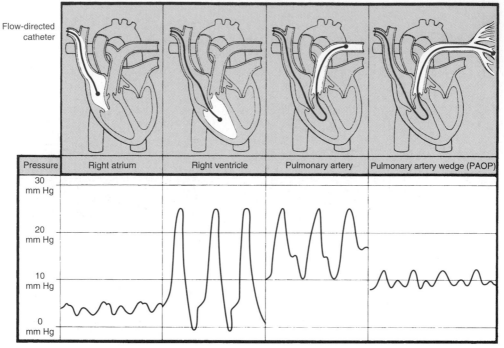

FIGURE 3-9 ■ Bedside hemodynamic monitoring via flow-directed, balloon-tipped catheter capable of thermodilution cardiac output determination. *PAOP,* Pulmonary artery occlusion pressure. (From Urden LD, Stacy KM, Lough ME: *Thelan's critical care nursing: diagnosis and management,* Philadelphia, 2002, Mosby, p 378.)

     (g) Electrical equipment is well grounded and operating correctly (to prevent electrically induced ventricular fibrillation [VF])

3. Appraisal of patient characteristics

   a. Resiliency

      i. Level 1—*Minimally resilient*: Mr A., an 82-year-old male with severe aortic stenosis in rapid atrial fibrillation and recovering from a CVA

     ii. Level 3—*Moderately resilient*: Mrs. B., a 71-year-old obese female with history of insulin-dependent diabetes and hypertension. She is admitted with a blood pressure of 195/110 mm Hg, sinus tachycardia, atypical chest pain, and abdominal discomfort.

    iii. Level 5—*Highly resilient*: Mr. C., a 45-year-old male with a history of hypertension, admitted complaining of left-sided chest and shoulder pain. Cardiac catheterization results are normal.

   b. Vulnerability

      i. Level 1—*Highly vulnerable:* Mr A., whose family reports that he lost his wife (of 60 years) 4 days earlier when she suddenly collapsed at home. Results of his transesophageal echocardiography show several large clots in the LA.

     ii. Level 3—*Moderately vulnerable:* Mr. D., a 53-year-old male with a history of sudden cardiac death (requiring implantation of a cardiac defibrillator), ulcerative colitis, pericardial effusion, and steroid-induced diabetes. He is anemic, with tarry stools. His wife is also very anxious and requires a great deal of attention.

■ TABLE 3-3
■ ■ Common Types of Bedside Monitoring

Type of Monitoring	Uses	Measurements	Comments
Direct arterial BP monitoring: Catheter inserted into artery and attached to pressure transducer that converts and amplifies arterial pressure to electrical waveform for continuous readings	Monitor BP trends (e.g., during cardiac surgery, in critically ill patients, with IABP, potent vasopressors or vasodilators) For ventilated patients, frequent ABG testing, monitoring for acid-base imbalances Radial artery most commonly used	Reference (air fluid interface) stopcock closest to pressure transducer at heart level (phlebostatic axis; see Bedside Hemodynamic Monitoring later in table); radial line should be at same level	**Allen's test:** Check adequacy of ulnar circulation before radial catheter insertion 1. Have patient clench fist tightly 2. Occlude both radial and ulnar arteries 3. Have patient open hand; observe for pallor 4. Release pressure over ulnar artery; color should return within 2-3 sec if artery patent 5. If no capillary filling in 3 sec, test result is negative
CVP monitoring: Use of a single or multilumen catheter positioned in superior vena cava (inferior vena cava for femoral lines) attached to pressure transducer	Continuous monitoring of blood volume, RV function, CVP Fluid, blood, and medication administration Vein sites: Internal or external jugular, femoral, subclavian	Normal CVP varies from patient to patient Monitor trends in CVP Normal CVP: 2-6 mm Hg	Decreased CVP: Hypovolemia, venodilation, negative-pressure ventilators, RV assist devices, central venous obstruction (masses), decreased venous return Increased CVP: Increased blood volume, right-sided heart failure, cardiac tamponade, positive pressure breathing, straining
Bedside hemodynamic monitoring via flow-directed, balloon-tipped catheter capable of thermodilution cardiac output determination (PA catheter); see Figure 3-9 Various catheters are available with capabilities of continuous CO monitoring, transvenous pacing, and mixed venous oxygen saturation measurements, and with additional fluid and medication administration ports	Assess and manage hemodynamics via continuous monitoring: Fluid balance, intracardiac pressures, CO, CI, SVR, Sv_{O_2} Evaluate trends; report significant changes Monitoring RA and PCWP is preferable to assess RV and LV function **PA mean:** Used primarily for hemodynamic calculations of pulmonary vascular resistance	**RA pressure** is measured through proximal port of catheter; reflects RVEDP **RV pressures** are seen when floating catheter into position during insertion; RV waveform is distinct with sharp upstroke after the QRS and downstroke, no dicrotic notch PAP and PCWP measured through distal port (see Figure 3-9 and Table 3-4 **PA systolic pressure** represents pressure produced by RV	**Phlebostatic axis:** Obtain pressure reading with patient in comfortable position (0-60 degrees), as long as transducer is at same phlebostatic level as marked axis (intersection of following two lines): 1. Draw a line from fourth intercostal space at sternum toward edge of chest and down to side 2. Draw second line on side of chest, halfway between anterior and posterior portions of chest (midaxillary), running head to foot 3. Mark intersection of lines on side of chest; place transducer at level horizontal to that mark

Continued

■ **TABLE 3-3**
■ ■ **Common Types of Bedside Monitoring—cont'd**

Type of Monitoring	Uses	Measurements	Comments
		PA diastolic pressure generally reflects LVEDP and is used as measure of LV function and diastolic filling pressures; usually 2-4 mm Hg higher than mean PCWP or mean **LA pressure** PCWP is a reflection of LA pressure and is used to assess LVEDP filling pressure = "a" wave; balloon of catheter is inflated, wedges in small branch of PA (see Figure 3-9); PCWP should be 2-4 mm Hg less than PA diastolic pressure	Catheter must not be left in RV (ventricular tachycardia occurs) PA diastolic pressure: Correlates well with mean PCWP in the normal heart, during myocardial infarction, and in LV failure; often used instead of PCWP if obtaining accurate wedge is impossible **CO** can also be measured manually via proximal port by means of thermodilution (an average of three rapid injections of 10 ml D5W or NS is used to calculate CO, CI, SVR by computer).

ABG, Arterial blood gas; *BP,* blood pressure; *CI,* cardiac index; *CO,* cardiac output; *CVP,* central venous pressure; *D5W,* dextrose 5% in water; *IABP,* intraaortic balloon pump; *LA,* left atrial; *LV,* left ventricular; *LVEDP,* left ventricular end-diastolic pressure; *NS,* normal saline; *PA,* pulmonary artery; *PAP,* pulmonary artery pressure; *PCWP,* pulmonary capillary wedge pressure; *RA,* right atrial; *RV,* right ventricular; *RVEDP,* right ventricular end-diastolic pressure; Svo_2, venous oxygen saturation; *SVR,* systemic vascular resistance.

▓ **TABLE 3-4**
▓ ▓ **Hemodynamic Pressures: Normal Values and Possible Causes of Abnormal Values**

Measurements	Normal Values	Possible Causes for Increase	Possible Causes for Decrease
Right atrial pressure (RAP)/central venous pressure (CVP)	2-6 mm Hg	Pulmonary hypertension Pulmonary embolism Constrictive pericarditis Cardiac tamponade Right heart failure Pulmonic stenosis Chronic obstructive pulmonary disease (COPD) Obstructive sleep apnea (OSA) Right ventricular (RV) infarction	Hypovolemia (e.g., diuretics, blood loss, burns, vomiting) Vasodilatation (e.g., nitrates, morphine, hypersensitivity reactions)
RV pressures	**Systolic:** 15-30 mm Hg **Diastolic:** 2-6 mm Hg	Pulmonary hypertension (e.g., left-sided heart failure, left ventricular [LV] ischemia, infarct, mitral regurgitation or stenosis, cardiomyopathy) Pulmonary disease (e.g., pulmonary embolism, hypoxemia, COPD) OSA Eisenmenger's syndrome: Pulmonary hypertension associated with right-to-left shunt, cyanosis	Same as above
Pulmonary artery (PA) pressures	**Systolic:** 20-30 mm Hg **Diastolic:** 5-10 mm Hg **Mean:** 10-20 mm Hg	Atrial or ventricular septal defects (increased pulmonary blood flow due to left-to-right shunt) Pulmonary hypertension Hypertension Pulmonary emboli COPD LV failure Mitral stenosis or regurgitation Volume overload Ischemia	

Continued

■ TABLE 3-4
■ Hemodynamic Pressures: Normal Values and Possible Causes of Abnormal Values—cont'd

Measurements	Normal Values	Possible Causes for Increase	Possible Causes for Decrease
Pulmonary capillary wedge pressure (PCWP)	4-12 mm Hg	Fluid overload LV failure Ischemia Mitral stenosis or regurgitation Constrictive pericarditis	Hypovolemia Venodilating drugs
Systemic vascular resistance (SVR)	800-1400 dynes/sec/cm^{-5}	Hypovolemia Hypothermia Vasoconstriction	Vasodilating drugs Shock: Septic, neurogenic, or anaphylactic
Pulmonary vascular resistance (PVR)	50-250 dynes/sec/cm^{-5}	Pulmonary embolism, large Pulmonary hypertension Hypoxemia	Pulmonary vasodilating drugs
Cardiac output (CO)	4-8 L/min	Sepsis Intra- and extracardiac shunts	Decreased preload Increased afterload Decreased contractility Arrhythmias
Cardiac index (CI) $S\bar{v}O_2$	2.5-4.0 L/min/m^2 60%-80%	Sepsis Sepsis Left-to-right intracardiac shunt Thyrotoxicosis Anesthesia	Same as for CO Hypoxemia Anemia, bleeding Fever Heart failure Arrhythmias Respiratory failure Right-to-left heart shunts

      iii. Level 5—*Minimally vulnerable:* Mrs. E., 48 years old, admitted with acute pericarditis, responding well to an oral nonsteroidal antiinflammatory drug [NSAID]; her pain is resolving, and her condition is stable

  c. Stability

      i. Level 1—*Minimally stable:* Mr. F., a 47-year-old male with history of scleroderma, Raynaud's disease, and severe pulmonary hypertension. He is presently on intravenous (IV) dobutamine. He has 2+ edema bilaterally in his lower extremities. His lungs have crackles in the bases. He is being evaluated for epoprostenol (Flolan) home therapy to assist in improving his quality of life. He is not eligible for heart transplantation.

      ii. Level 3—*Moderately stable:* Mrs. G., a 78-year-old female with a history of ischemic cardiomyopathy, severe mitral regurgitation, hyperlipidemia, and three-vessel disease. Complained of chest pain at home, relieved with nitroglycerin.

      iii. Level 5—*Highly stable:* Mr. H., a 65-year-old male with a history of third-degree AV block, who received a permanent pacemaker 2 days earlier. His incision site is healing well, and he has minimal discomfort. The pacemaker is functioning appropriately.

  d. Complexity

      i. Level 1—*Highly complex:* Miss P., a 27-year-old female with a history of open heart transplantation 7 years ago and MI 3 years ago. Has had numerous coronary interventions, including recent placements of stents to her LCA. She has a history of a permanent pacemaker, asthma, hypertension, heart failure, and chronic renal insufficiency. She is admitted with a large pericardial effusion.

      ii. Level 3—*Moderately complex:* Mr. S., 63 years old, with a history of open heart transplantation 10 years ago, hospitalized 1 month ago for endocarditis. Admitted from skilled care with an infected right Hickman catheter, an elevated temperature, and a heart rate of 105 beats/min with frequent premature ventricular contractions, and is on several IV inotropic agents; urinary output is marginal.

      iii. Level 5—*Minimally complex:* Mrs. V., who had acute-onset atrial tachycardia and was given IV medications, after which her heart rhythm converted into sinus rhythm. She is up in her room ready for instructions before going home.

  e. Resource availability

      i. Level 1—*Few resources:* Mrs. B., who lives alone and whose family is gone. It is physically hard for her to leave her apartment. She has a small income and cannot afford the combination of drugs prescribed for her hypertension, diabetes, and hyperlipidemia.

      ii. Level 3—*Moderate resources:* Mr. L., 60 years old, with a history of coronary artery bypass graft 3 years ago, who experienced chest discomfort while at his cardiac rehabilitation group. His wife and family are supportive and involved in his care.

      iii. Level 5—*Many resources:* Mrs. R., a 65-year-old woman with MI with ST-segment elevation, who had a percutaneous coronary intervention (PCI) and was given thrombolytics 90 minutes after the onset of symptoms. She is married to a staff physician and her daughter is a nurse.

  f. Participation in care

      i. Level 1—*No participation:* Mrs. Q., a 68-year-old obese female who experienced cardiac arrest on a medical floor and has a history of end-stage renal disease, diabetes, and hypertension. She is unconscious and has a full code status.

    ii. Level 3—*Moderate level of participation:* Miss P., who, although she is a patient with a highly complex condition, is very interested in her diagnosis, medication, and therapy. She attempts to watch her intake and diet. Her parents are also involved in all care aspects. They do, however, verbalize some inaccurate medical information leading to erroneous conclusions.

    iii. Level 5—*Full participation:* Mrs. M., a 40-year-old female with pulmonary hypertension who is awaiting heart transplantation. She is independent in her care activities. She and her husband take full advantage of educational resources and talk with transplant patients.

  g. Participation in decision making

    i. Level 1—*No participation:* Mr. T., 18 years old, homeless, victim of a stab wound to the chest, intubated, unconscious, brought to the operating room for emergency thoracotomy

    ii. Level 3—*Moderate level of participation:* Mr. O., a 60-year-old male admitted with chest pain due to a reoccluded coronary lesion, who decided he did not need to continue his clopidogrel after discharge from the hospital

    iii. Level 5—*Full participation:* Mr. F. (in a highly unstable condition), who with his family is actively involved in end-of-life decision making. In conferences with the physicians and nurses, he and his family have requested that he not be intubated or resuscitated if the situation presents. They want Mr. F. to have only comfort measures.

  h. Predictability

    i. Level 1—*Not predictable:* Mrs. G., who received an automatic implantable cardiac defibrillator during her hospitalization. The day after her discharge home, her defibrillator discharged eight times throughout the evening and night. She is readmitted to reevaluate medical therapy.

    ii. Level 3—*Moderately predictable:* Mr. H., 49 years old, who was admitted for another MI (had his first MI when he was 37 years old) and received brachytherapy and a stent to the CX artery. Eptifibatide (Integrelin) is infusing. Vital sign are stable.

    iii. Level 5—*Highly predictable:* Mr. X., who has a small VSD that does not require surgery. Staff stressed the importance of good dental care and prophylactic antibiotics because of the high risk of infectious endocarditis.

4. **Diagnostic studies**

  a. **Laboratory**

    i. Cardiac troponin T and troponin I: Group of compounds that bind to tropomyosin and help with excitation-contraction in muscle

      (a) Most sensitive cardiac markers; very specific, mark injury to myocytes (not just cell death)

      (b) Levels rise 4 to 6 hours after the onset of ischemic symptoms; peak at 18 to 24 hours after MI; fall slowly, over up to 2 weeks (Figure 3-10)

      (c) Cleared by kidneys, so levels are elevated in chronic renal failure

      (d) Rare for the value to be more than 0.1 ng/ml in a normal individual

      (e) Facilitate quicker decision making in identification, risk stratification, and treatment of patients

      (f) Predictor of high risk for subsequent cardiac events in acute coronary syndromes, postoperative vascular surgery; prognostic indicator for pulmonary embolus

    ii. Creatine kinase (CK): CK-MB isoenzyme

      (a) Enzyme associated with adenosine triphosphate conversion in contractile muscle tissue; found in the heart, brain, and skeletal tissues

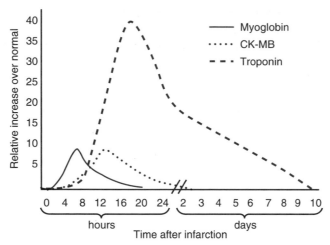

FIGURE 3-10 ■ Time course of the appearance of serum levels of creatine kinase MB isoenzyme *(CK-MB)*, myoglobin, and troponin in a patient with an ST-segment elevation myocardial infarction. (From Henry JB: *Clinical diagnosis and management by laboratory methods*, Philadelphia, 2001, Saunders, p 297.)

  (b) MB isoenzyme levels very sensitive for cardiac tissue; not as sensitive in early MI less than 6 hours after onset
  (c) Level rises 4 to 8 hours after onset, peaks 12 to 24 hours after MI, returns to normal in approximately 24 to 48 hours
  (d) CK-MB concentration of more than 5% of total CK indicates myocardial necrosis
  iii. Myoglobin: Heme-containing protein
  (a) Very sensitive marker but not cardiac specific; can be elevated with cardiopulmonary resuscitation (CPR), falls, and injections
  (b) Level peaks 8 hours after infarct, then rapidly returns to normal in 18 to 24 hours
  (c) Useful in the emergency department for early MI detection, ruling out of MI, reperfusion monitoring
  iv. Brain natriuretic peptide (BNP)
  (a) Released with myocardial stretch
  (b) Level correlates with LV dysfunction
  (c) Used to evaluate heart failure (both LV and RV) and pulmonary emboli and to differentiate cardiac from pulmonary causes of pulmonary distress and dyspnea
  (d) Higher levels indicate poor prognosis
  (e) Falsely low results can occur in obese patients due to clearance in adipose tissue (adipose tissue removes BNP from the circulation)
  (f) Falsely high results can occur in the elderly, hypertensive individuals, females, and patients being given nesiritide
  v. C-reactive protein
  (a) Biomarker of inflammation
  (b) Independent predictor of future cardiovascular risk
  (c) Elevations may also indicate an acute infection, inflammatory disease processes, possible uremia
  vi. Clotting profile
  (a) Partial thromboplastin time (PTT): Used for monitoring heparin levels

    (b) International normalized ratio (INR): Used for measuring the effectiveness of anticoagulant therapy
        (1) For atrial fibrillation, therapeutic range for INR is 2.0 to 3.0
        (2) For prosthetic valves, therapeutic range for INR is 2.5 to 3.5
    (c) Activated clotting time (ACT): Bedside test done to measure the time required for blood coagulation
    (d) Platelet count
  vii. Complete blood cell count (CBC), hemoglobin (Hb) level, hematocrit (HCT)
 viii. Electrolyte levels, blood urea nitrogen (BUN) level, creatinine level, glucose level
   ix. Fasting serum lipid profile: Normal levels
    (a) Total cholesterol level: Goal is less than 200 mg/dl
    (b) High-density lipoprotein (HDL): Goal is HDL level above 40 mg/dl
    (c) Low-density lipoprotein (LDL): Level of less than 100 mg/dl is optimal if CAD is present (otherwise, 130 mg/dl is the goal)
    (d) Triglycerides: Desired level is less than 150 mg/dl; 150 to 199 mg/dl is borderline; 200 to 499 mg/dl is high; more than 500 mg/dl is very high
    (e) Lipoprotein(a): Marker for CAD, not usually followed; levels of more than 30 mg/dl associated with CAD
   x. Homocysteine level: To identify folic acid–responsive hyperlipidemia. Normal level is 5 to 15 μmol/L. Elevated levels considered an independent risk factor for CAD.
  b. Imaging
    i. Chest radiograph is used to visualize
     (a) Cardiac size, position, chamber size
     (b) Abnormalities of the heart, great vessels, lungs, pleura, and ribs
     (c) Pulmonary vasculature
     (d) Position of catheters, lines, and pacemaker leads
    ii. Magnetic resonance imaging (MRI): Safe diagnostic technique involving no ionizing radiation. Used with contrast to produce a magnetic resonance angiogram (MRA).
     (a) Provides a three-dimensional view of cardiovascular structure
     (b) Creates a computer-assisted image, measures tissue proton density
     (c) MRI is used to determine or identify
       (1) Anatomy of the heart
       (2) Congenital heart defects
       (3) Masses in the myocardium or pericardium
       (4) Ventricular aneurysm
       (5) Aortic dissection
       (6) Arterial disease (MRA)
     (d) Safe alternative to radiography for children and pregnant women
     (e) As a magnetic device, MRI machine interferes with pacemaker function
     (f) Not used for patients with prosthetic metallic devices (valves, prosthetic joints). Can displace or damage such devices due to powerful magnet
   iii. Ultrafast (electron beam) computed tomography (EBCT): Form of computed tomography (CT) in which a rapid electron beam is used for high-speed imaging
     (a) Provides two-dimensional image of cardiovascular structures
     (b) Visualizes coronary calcium, silent atherosclerosis

        (1) Amount of calcium can be predictive of multivessel CAD
        (2) Not sufficiently specific
     (c) Cost and specificity limit use at present

  iv. Myocardial imaging: Radioisotope is injected into a peripheral vein and its cardiac uptake can be imaged. Methods include

     (a) Multiple-gated acquisition (MUGA) scan
        (1) Used to measure the EF of the LV
        (2) Very accurate unless the patient has an irregular rhythm, because multiple images cannot be "gated" (superimposed) on ECG

     (b) Myocardial scintigraphy (perfusion imaging)
        (1) Involves the use of thallium-201 or technetium Tc 99m sestamibi to identify ischemia, infarct, and myocardial viability
        (2) Normal myocardium takes up the isotope from the blood
        (3) Decreased myocardial perfusion results in decreased uptake; ischemic sites show normal uptake at rest and decreased uptake on exercise. Infarcted sites show no uptake at all.
        (4) Pharmacologic agents (dipyridamole, adenosine) are used to simulate the effects of exercise (potentially to induce ischemia) in patients who are unable to exercise
        (5) Perfusion imaging is more sensitive and specific (80% to 85%) than exercise ECG–stress testing (70%)

     (c) Infarct-avid imaging (myocardial infarct indicators)
        (1) Technetium Tc 99m pyrophosphate is injected into a peripheral vein
        (2) Infarcted areas of the heart show increased levels of radioactivity as "hot spots." These appear within 4 hours of infarction, may not peak until 12 to 24 hours later, and remain positive for 2 to 7 days.
        (3) Limited usefulness in acute MI; useful when ECG changes are not definitive or when enzyme levels have already returned to normal

     (d) Clinical uses of nuclear medicine: Evaluation of
        (1) Ischemic heart disease (including risk stratification)
        (2) LV function

  v. Cardiac catheterization and angiography: High-quality coronary images produced by x-ray digital imaging. Radiopaque contrast medium is injected into the coronary arteries for visualization; recordings are made on digital media. Still photographs may be produced for patient records.

     (a) Patients selected include
        (1) Asymptomatic patients with
          a) Evidence of significant ischemia or severe LV dysfunction on noninvasive testing
          b) Survival after a sudden cardiac death event
          c) Valvular heart disease
        (2) Symptomatic patients with
          a) Angina—unstable or stable
          b) Atypical chest pain
          c) Recent MI
          d) Valvular disease
          e) Congenital heart defects
          f) Aortic disease
          g) LV failure

     (b) Technique
        (1) Right-sided heart catheterization performed via the right or left femoral or brachial vein with the catheter advanced into the RA and

then past the tricuspid valve through the RV into the pulmonary artery to record pressures, perform angiography, determine CO and resistances, and define anatomy

(2) Left-sided heart catheterization performed in a retrograde manner via the femoral or brachial artery (or transseptal approach through the RA and intraatrial septum); catheter is advanced into the LV to determine pressure

(c) Left ventriculography

   (1) Technique: Radiopaque contrast medium is injected into the LV cavity

   (2) Purposes

     a) Evaluate ventricular wall motion and chamber size

       1) Identify akinetic areas and wall motion abnormalities

       2) Detect hypokinetic areas: Weaker than normal contractions in systole

       3) Detect dyskinetic areas: Areas bulge outward during systole instead of contracting

     b) Assess function, determining

       1) End-diastolic volume

       2) End-systolic volume

       3) Stroke volume

       4) EF

     c) Detect ventricular aneurysms

     d) Evaluate mitral, aortic valves

     e) Demonstrate ventricular-level left-to-right intracardiac shunts (VSD)

(d) Aortography

   (1) Technique: Contrast injected into aortic root or descending aorta

   (2) Purpose: To assess

     a) Aortic valve insufficiency

     b) Aneurysms or dissections of ascending aorta

     c) Coarctation of the aorta

     d) Diseases of the aorta

     e) Presence of saphenous vein grafts

     f) Presence of PDA

(e) Coronary arteriography

   (1) Radiopaque contrast material injected into the ostia of the LCA and RCA, allowing multiple views and recordings of coronary arterial circulation

   (2) Purpose

     a) To assess the extent of significant CAD by identifying the presence and severity of lesions

     b) To guide therapeutic options in ischemic heart disease

     c) To assess possible coronary arterial spasm

     d) To administer intracoronary thrombolytics and drugs

     e) To perform transcatheter interventional procedures: PCI, coronary stent placement, rotational atherectomy, and percutaneous transluminal coronary angioplasty (PTCA)

(f) Complications of diagnostic cardiac catheterization

   (1) Death: Approximately 0.11% incidence (most frequently seen in left main disease)

   (2) MI: Approximately 0.05% incidence

      (3) Neurologic events (stroke): Approximately 0.07% incidence

      (4) Acute renal failure or oliguria caused by contrast medium and inadequate hydration

      (5) Transient cardiac arrhythmias, bradycardia, conduction disturbances

      (6) Hemorrhage or hematoma at insertion site

      (7) Allergic reactions to contrast medium

      (8) Arterial perforation, thrombosis, embolus, and dissection

      (9) Hypovolemia (due to diuresis from contrast medium and nothing-by-mouth [NPO] status)

c. Other

    i. ECG: Records the electrical activity of the heart

      (a) Identifies

        (1) Arrhythmias and conduction defects

        (2) Ischemia or infarction

        (3) Electrolyte abnormalities

        (4) Drug effects

        (5) Hypertrophy of the ventricles and enlargement of the atria

        (6) Anatomic orientation of the heart

      (b) ECG paper (Figure 3-11)

        (1) Measures time along the horizontal axis

          a) Records P wave, QRS complex, and T wave (in time), as well as PR and QT intervals

          b) Each small (1-mm) box = 0.04 second

          c) Each large (5-mm) box = 0.20 second

          d) Normal speed of paper: 25 mm/sec

        (2) Measures voltage in the vertical direction

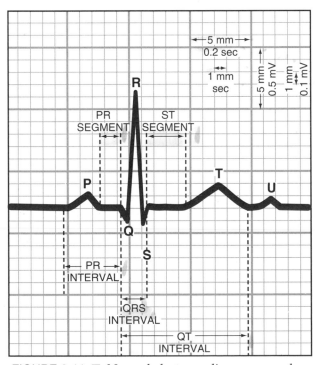

FIGURE 3-11 ■ Normal electrocardiogram complex.

      a) Measures and records amplitude and voltage of P wave, QRS complex, and T wave

      b) Each small box (1 mm) = 0.1 mV

      c) Each large box (5 mm) = 0.5 mV

      d) Usual calibration standard is 10 mm = 1 mV

      e) Useful in detection of atrial and ventricular hypertrophy

(c) Deflections: Waves of the ECG recording are either above or below the isoelectric line

    (1) Positive deflections occur when the heart's depolarization wave *moves toward* the positive electrode of the recording lead

    (2) Negative deflections occur when the heart's depolarization wave *moves away from* the positive electrode of the recording lead

    (3) Biphasic deflections occur when the heart's depolarization wave is moving both toward and away from the positive electrode. If the wave of depolarization is perpendicular to the positive electrode, waves may be small or absent.

(d) ECG waves: Representation, measurement, abnormalities—see Table 3-5, Figure 3-11

(e) 12-Lead ECG (Box 3-3 and Figure 3-12)

    (1) Standard limb leads: Two electrodes of opposing polarity (positive and negative) are used to record electrical activity. These bipolar electrodes are placed on the patient's arms and/or legs.

    (2) Augmented limb leads: Electrical activity is recorded between one positive electrode (unipolar) and the electrical sum of other two standard limb electrodes. The wave's amplitude is augmented (enhanced voltage) for ease of visualization.

    (3) Precordial (chest) V leads: Record electrical activity between one positive electrode (unipolar) and the electrical sum of the three standard limb electrodes.

      a) R waves get progressively larger (normal R-wave progression) moving from V_1 toward V_5 (V_5 is higher than V_6)

      b) V_4R (analogous to V_4, only on right side): Used for RV infarcts.

(f) Miscellaneous monitoring leads

    (1) Modified chest lead (MCL_1)

      a) Electrode placement: Similar to lead V_1

      b) Typical pattern of PQRST is negative

      c) Helps differentiate ventricular arrhythmias from supraventricular arrhythmias with right bundle branch block (RBBB) aberrancy

        1) LV origin of VT is likely with Rsr' pattern: *left peak* is taller than right peak of the "rabbit ears"

        2) Aberrant conduction of SVT is likely if the first beat of a run of ectopic beats has an rsR' pattern: *right peak* of "rabbit ears" is taller

      d) Differentiation between RV and LV ectopy is possible

        1) RV ectopy: Negative QRS complex

        2) LV ectopy: Positive QRS deflection; may also be a biphasic

      e) RBBB and left bundle branch block (LBBB) may be differentiated

        1) RBBB: Classical rSR' pattern or predominately positive in V_1

        2) LBBB: Predominately negative in V_1

    (2) Lewis lead: Used for finding P wave; arm leads are positioned along the sternal border until P waves become evident

TABLE 3-5

Electrocardiogram (ECG) Waves and Intervals: Description, Characteristics, and Abnormalities

ECG	Description	Characteristics	Causes for Abnormalities
P wave	Represents atrial depolarization Right atrium (RA) begins depolarization earlier than the left atrium (LA)	Normal duration: <0.10 sec Normal amplitude: ≤2.5 mm P waves >2.5 mm in amplitude in any lead are abnormal "2.5 × 2.5 rule" (handy rule of thumb): P wave should not be wider than 2.5 mm (LA enlargement) or taller than 2.5 mm (RA enlargement)	Atrial hypertrophy: Increased P amplitude or width RA hypertrophy: • Tall, peaked P waves in lead II, III, and aVF • May show tall or biphasic P waves in V_1 (>2.5 mm in amplitude) LA hypertrophy: • Wide, notched P waves in limb leads and V_4 to V_6 and/or P waves with broad negative deflection in lead V_1 (>1 mm); • P >2.5 mm in width
PR interval	Represents time required for conduction through atrioventricular (AV) node PR segment represents normal delay of impulse in AV node	Normal interval: 0.12-0.20 sec Measure from beginning of P wave to beginning of QRS complex	Prolonged delay (PR interval >0.20 sec) indicates diseased AV node, ischemia, drug effects, or increased vagal tone
QRS complex	Represents ventricular depolarization Atrial repolarization occurs during this time period but is obscured by QRS	Normal duration: 0.06-0.10 sec; borderline at 0.11 sec Measured from onset of Q wave (or R wave if no Q wave is present) to end of QRS	Abnormal if ≥0.12 sec; indicative of intraventricular conduction delay; seen in patients with bundle branch blocks (≥0.12), Wolff-Parkinson-White (WFW) syndrome, and hyperkalemia (sine wave)
Q wave	Present if the first deflection of the QRS is negative	Small physiologic Q waves are usually seen in leads I, aVL, V_5, and V_6; as well as in inferior leads II, III, and aVF	Q waves are pathologic when >0.04 sec wide (>0.03 sec in inferior leads II, III, and aVF) and >25% of R wave amplitude Q waves in leads III, aVR, and V_1 are normal Pathologic Q waves result from myocardial infarction
R wave	First positive deflection occurring in the QRS complex		Prominent R waves may be seen with ventricular hypertrophy and in young adults, persons with thin chests, and patients with WPW syndrome
S wave	Negative deflection that follows an R wave		

Continued

■ TABLE 3-5
■ ■ Electrocardiogram (ECG) Waves and Intervals: Description, Characteristics, and Abnormalities—cont'd

ECG	Description	Characteristics	Causes for Abnormalities
ST segment	Represents initial ventricular repolarization	Measure immediately after QRS complex to beginning of T wave; normally isoelectric	Elevated ST segment is caused by pericarditis, injury, acute infarctions, LV aneurysms, and normal variation (early repolarization) Depressed ST segment may indicate subendocardial injury or ischemia, electrolyte disturbances, drug effect, or early repolarization, or it may be nonspecific
T wave	Represents ventricular repolarization		Inverted T waves may be associated with infarctions, ischemia, injury, or hypertrophy Tall, peaked T waves may be caused by hyperkalemia or acute injury or may be a normal variant
QT interval	Represents complete duration of ventricular depolarization and repolarization QT interval varies with heart rate, gender, and age	Corrected QT interval (QTc) takes heart rate into account and provides a normal range corrected for heart rate In general, QTc of ≥0.44 sec in males and ≥0.45 sec in females is considered abnormal Measure from the beginning of the Q wave to the end of the T wave	Causes of prolonged QTc: Ischemia, electrolyte imbalances (hypocalcemia), hypertrophy, antiarrhythmic drugs (procainamide, amiodarone), and congenital prolongation Prolonged QTc is associated with an increased incidence of polymorphic ventricular tachycardia (torsade de pointes) and, potentially, sudden death Causes of shortened QTc: Acute ischemia, hypercalcemia, and drugs (digitalis)

■ **BOX 3-3**
■ **TWELVE-LEAD ELECTROCARDIOGRAPH AND MCL₁ ELECTRODE PLACEMENT**

Lead I: Right arm (negative electrode), left arm (positive electrode)
Lead II: Right arm (negative electrode), left leg (positive electrode)
Lead III: Left arm (negative electrode), left leg (positive electrode)
aVR: Right arm; normally a negative deflection
aVL: Left arm; usually a positive deflection
aVF: Left leg; usually a positive deflection
V_1: Fourth intercostal space, right sternal border
V_2: Fourth intercostal space, left sternal border
V_3: Halfway between V_2 and V_4
V_4: Fifth intercostal space, left midclavicular line
V_5: Level with V_4, left anterior axillary line
V_6: Level with V_4, left midaxillary line
V_4R: Fifth intercostal space, right midclavicular line
MCL_1 (monitoring lead): Fourth intercostal space, right sternal border (positive electrode);
  below left clavicle, midclavicular line (negative electrode); below right clavicle (ground)

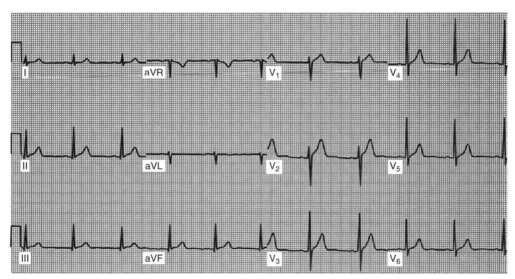

FIGURE 3-12 ■ Twelve-lead electrocardiogram (sinus rhythm).

    (3) Transvenous leads or esophageal pill leads (a small gelatin capsule enclosing an electrode and attached to thin wire) are helpful in looking for P waves or differentiating supraventricular from ventricular rhythms
  (g) See Box 3-4 for ECG and rhythm assessment checklist
  (h) See Table 3-6 for descriptions of cardiac arrhythmias and conduction defects
 ii. Echocardiography: One of the most important noninvasive tools
  (a) High-frequency ultrasonic vibrations are emitted via a transducer on the patient's chest or in the esophagus. The returning echo of sound waves is received. An image is created and recorded for interpretation.
  (b) Provides information on

■ **BOX 3-4**
■ **CARDIAC RHYTHM ASSESSMENT CHECKLIST**

Analyze electrocardiogram rhythms systematically, including
- **Rates:** Atrial and ventricular
- **Rhythm:** Regular, irregular, pattern if irregular
- **P wave:** Identification
  - Relation to QRS (before, after)
  - Configuration or morphology
- **PR interval:** Measurement
- **QRS complex:** Measurement, configuration
- **ST segment:** Isoelectric, depressed, elevated
- **T wave:** Size, shape, direction
- **Arrhythmia origin:** Identify if possible
- **Possible implications:** For patient and nursing care

(1) Chamber size and function, including
    a) LV systolic function: EF
    b) LV wall motion (shows areas of hypokinesis, akinesis, dyskinesis), wall thickness, cavity size
    c) LV diastolic function
    d) Chamber size
(2) Valvular morphology and function
    a) Regurgitation
    b) Prosthetic valve function
    c) Stenotic valves
(3) Intracardiac masses, including tumors, thrombi, and vegetations
(4) Congenital defects and shunts
(5) Pericardial disease
    a) Pericardial effusion
    b) Cardiac tamponade
(c) M mode: Used to measure intracardiac dimensions; measures chamber size and wall thickness
(d) Two-dimensional echocardiography provides real-time imagery of the heart and its structures using a two-dimensional ultrasonic beam
(e) Doppler echocardiography is used to demonstrate the velocity and direction of blood flow through the heart and great vessels
(f) Color flow imaging: Doppler signals are processed to depict real-time velocities superimposed on a two-dimensional echocardiogram. Red represents flow toward the transducer; blue represents flow away from the transducer. Lighter shades mean higher velocity. Used to evaluate shunts, regurgitation, stenosis.
(g) Contrast echocardiography
    (1) Bubble echo (agitated saline): Used to detect congenital or acquired shunts, patent foramen ovale
    (2) Enhancing agents (e.g., Optison): Used to enhance the LV endocardial border and help identify myocardial infarct or ischemia
(h) Stress echocardiography: Images obtained before, during, and after exercise or pharmacologic stress (states of increased myocardial oxygen demand)

Text continues on p. 241

▉ TABLE 3-6
▉ ▉ Cardiac Arrhythmias and Conduction Defects

Rhythm	Mechanism	Characteristics	Comments
SINUS RHYTHMS Sinus rhythm	Originates in sinoatrial (SA) node	Rate: 50-100 beats/min Rhythm: Regular P wave: • Normal and upright in leads II, III, aVF • Precede each QRS • Identical size and shape in any given lead PR interval: 0.12-0.20 sec 	Optimal cardiac rhythm **Sinus arrhythmia:** If rhythm varies (PP or RR interval varies >0.16 sec; usually related to respirations (RR intervals decrease with inspiration) Causes: Vagal responses (children, young adults), SA node disease (in elderly)
Sinus bradycardia		Rate: <50 beats/min PQRST: Complexes and intervals are normal	Causes: May be normal during sleep and in athletes and young hearts; seen in hypothermia, increased intracranial pressure, decreased sympathetic tone, increased parasympathetic tone, Valsalva maneuver, carotid massage, vomiting, drugs, hypothyroidism
Sinus tachycardia		Rate: 100-200 beats/min Rhythm: Regular PQRST: Complexes and intervals normal 	Causes: Secondary to anxiety, exercise, pain, hyperthyroidism, shock, anemia, fever, hypoxia, hypercapnia, heat exposure, drugs, heart failure (early sign)

Continued

■ **TABLE 3-6**
■ **Cardiac Arrhythmias and Conduction Defects—cont'd**

Rhythm	Mechanism	Characteristics	Comments
SINUS RHYTHMS—cont'd			
Sinus arrest or sinus pause	SA node fails, no impulse initiated, atrial standstill	PQRST complex: Not seen Sinus pause: If <3.0 sec Sinus arrest: If >3.0 sec Pause is usually greater than two regular RR intervals	Causes of sinus blocks and pauses: Increased vagal stimulation (i.e., by suctioning), myocardial infarction (MI), myocarditis, drug effects (e.g., from digitalis)
ATRIAL RHYTHMS			
Premature atrial contraction (PAC)	Early atrial impulse, interrupting the inherent regular rhythm	Normal QRS complex if ventricular repolarization was complete Abnormal QRS complex if conducted aberrantly (ventricle partially repolarized)	Causes: Stimulants (caffeine, tobacco, alcohol), hypoxia, drugs, digitalis toxicity, atrial enlargement

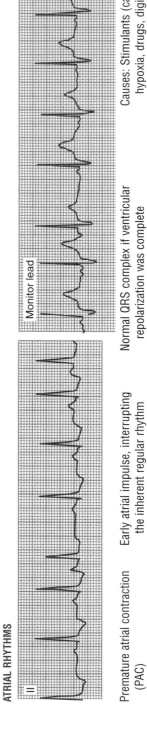

No QRS complex if beat arrived too early during the ventricle's absolute refractory period (i.e., blocked PAC)
Usually no compensatory pause, but may have a partial pause

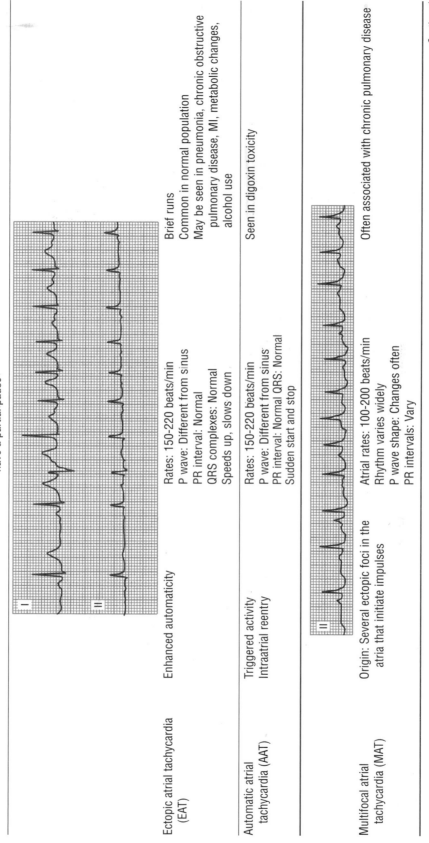

Ectopic atrial tachycardia (EAT)	Enhanced automaticity	Rates: 150-220 beats/min P wave: Different from sinus PR interval: Normal QRS complexes: Normal Speeds up, slows down	Brief runs Common in normal population May be seen in pneumonia, chronic obstructive pulmonary disease, MI, metabolic changes, alcohol use
Automatic atrial tachycardia (AAT)	Triggered activity Intraatrial reentry	Rates: 150-220 beats/min P wave: Different from sinus PR interval: Normal QRS: Normal Sudden start and stop	Seen in digoxin toxicity
Multifocal atrial tachycardia (MAT)	Origin: Several ectopic foci in the atria that initiate impulses	Atrial rates: 100-200 beats/min Rhythm varies widely P wave shape: Changes often PR intervals: Vary	Often associated with chronic pulmonary disease

Continued

■ **TABLE 3-6**
■ ■ **Cardiac Arrhythmias and Conduction Defects—cont'd**

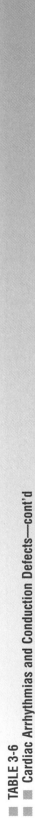

Rhythm	Mechanism	Characteristics	Comments
ATRIAL RHYTHMS—cont'd			
Atrial flutter	Origin: Reentry	Atrial rates: 200-350 beats/min Ventricular rates, along with rhythm, may be constant at 2:1, 3:1, 4:1 or may vary; if there is a variable atrioventricular (AV) conduction block Flutter waves may appear as wide, sawtooth waves representing rapid atrial depolarization, persist through QRS complexes, and are best seen in leads II, III, and aVF	According to the "rule of 150," a supraventricular tachycardia (SVT) at a rate of 150 beats/min is usually atrial flutter with a 2:1 block 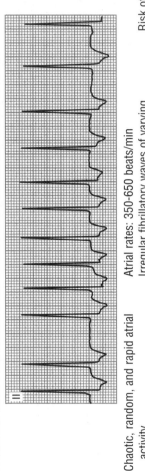
Atrial fibrillation	Chaotic, random, and rapid atrial activity Atrial impulses are randomly conducted through the AV junction	Atrial rates: 350-650 beats/min Irregular fibrillatory waves of varying amplitude; best seen in V_1 P wave: Not seen Ventricular rhythm is irregular QRS complex: Often looks normal, but	Risk of atrial thrombi with atrial fibrillation If ventricular rhythm becomes regular ("regularization of atrial fibrillation"), digitalis toxicity should be suspected

aberrantly conducted beats are often seen when a long RR interval is followed by a short RR interval, before ventricle is fully repolarized (Ashman's phenomenon)

JUNCTIONAL RHYTHMS

AV junctional beats

Originate in AV junction, spreading both antegrade and retrograde

AV junction includes cells in low atrium just above AV node, in AV node itself, and in bundle of His

With origin high in AV junction

If conduction to atria and ventricles is simultaneous, P wave is buried in QRS complex (not visible) and QRS usually normal

Atria depolarize first (retrograde—producing inverted P wave), then ventricles depolarize; inverted P wave precedes QRS

With origin low in AV junction

Ventricles depolarize first, producing QRS; inverted P wave follows QRS

Premature junctional beats (PJBs) and premature junctional contractions (PJCs)

Early beat, disrupts rhythm and sinus pacing cadence

Same characteristics as AV junctional beats, except occur prematurely

PR interval is shortened (<0.12 sec)

Junctional escape rhythm

Origin: SA node automaticity is suppressed and next fastest pacemaker (AV node) takes over

Rate: 40-60 beats/min
RR interval: Extremely regular
P-wave morphology: See PJB
QRS complex: Normal

Common causes: MI, ischemia, electrolyte imbalances, atrial myopathy, parasympathetic stimulation, effects of digitalis, other drugs

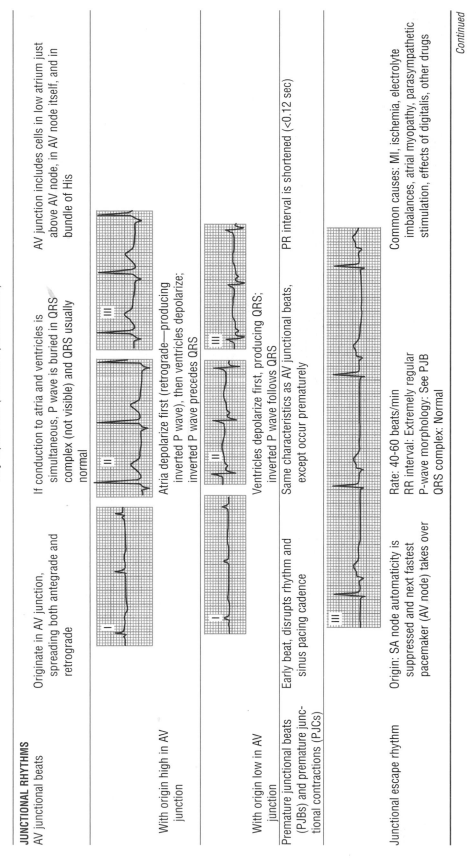

Continued

■ **TABLE 3-6**
■ **Cardiac Arrhythmias and Conduction Defects—cont'd**

Rhythm	Mechanism	Characteristics	Comments
JUNCTIONAL RHYTHMS—cont'd			
AV junctional tachycardia	An usurping rhythm	Rates: 60-120 beats/min Rhythm: Extremely regular P-wave morphology: See PJB QRS complex: Usually normal, narrow	Often caused by digitalis toxicity
AV nodal reentrant tachycardia (AVNRT), previously called paroxysmal supraventricular tachycardia (PSVT) or paroxysmal atrial tachycardia (PAT)	Reentry Where two or more electrical pathways exist, circuit can be formed with rapid circular conduction until broken	Impulse often begins abruptly with a PAC Atrial and ventricular rates: 170-250 beats/min Rhythm: Regular P wave: Retrograde and buried in QRS complex, not visible (80%); seen just after QRS (10%); occur just before QRS (10%)	May have always been present
Atrioventricular reciprocating tachycardia (AVRT)	Macroreentry rhythm using the AV node and an accessory pathway (AC) to complete a reentrant circuit		AVRT may or may not be associated with Wolff-Parkinson-White on baseline ECG (short P-R interval with a delta wave due to ventricular preexcitation
Orthodromic AVRT	Orthodromic circuit goes down the AV node and up the AC	Rates: 170-250 beats/min Rhythm: Regular P wave: Short R-P interval (<½ R-R interval) QRS: Narrow	Rx orthodromic AVRT with IV adenosine, DC shock

Continued

| Antidromic AVRT | Antidromic circuit goes down the AC and up the AV node | Rates: 170-250 beats/min
Rhythm: Regular
P wave: Short R-P interval (<½ R-R interval)
QRS: Wide | Rx antidromic AVRT with IV procainamide, DC shock |

VENTRICULAR RHYTHMS

| Premature ventricular contractions (PVCs) | Usurping, early beat originating in ventricles
Conduction is slowed through muscle
Retrograde conduction to atria may occur
Interpolated PVCs occur early enough to allow ventricles to repolarize prior to the next beat and do not disrupt rhythm; no compensatory pause is seen | 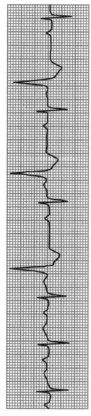 Wide, bizarre QRS complexes (>0.12 sec)
Can have varying morphology
Compensatory pause usually occurs
SA node rate is not altered, so next occurring sinus beat is able to conduct through to ventricles and produces normal QRS complex on time
In MCL₁ lead, QRS complex of a PVC originating in left ventricle is mostly positive deflection; PVC originating from right ventricle is mostly negative | A "full compensatory" pause: RR intervals surrounding the PVC are equal to two sinus-cycle intervals. To measure:
1. Mark off two normal RR intervals (three R waves) with calipers or paper
2. Place first mark on the QRS complex immediately preceding the PVC
3. Third mark should fall on QRS complex of the normal beat immediately following the PVC if fully compensated |
| Ventricular escape rhythm | Impulses from higher centers (SA or AV node) either are not generated or are blocked; ventricles initiate "escape" rhythm based on inherent automaticity of the ventricular tissue | 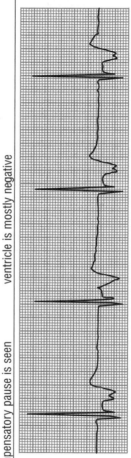 Rate: 20-40 beats/min (usually 20-30 beats/min), rarely <20 beats/min
Rhythm: Usually very regular
QRS complex: Wide, bizarre
No P wave association with QRS complex | |

■ **TABLE 3-6**
■ ■ **Cardiac Arrhythmias and Conduction Defects—cont'd**

VENTRICULAR RHYTHMS—cont'd

Rhythm	Mechanism	Characteristics	Comments
		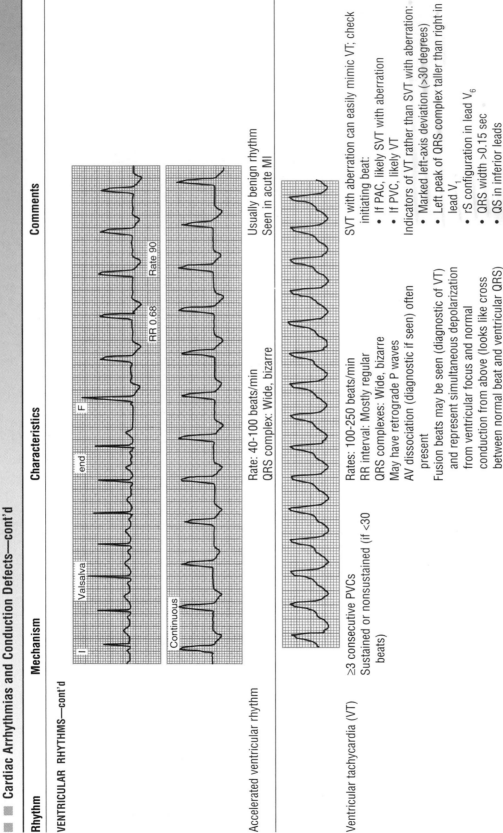	
Accelerated ventricular rhythm		Rate: 40-100 beats/min QRS complex: Wide, bizarre	Usually benign rhythm Seen in acute MI
Ventricular tachycardia (VT)	≥3 consecutive PVCs Sustained or nonsustained (if <30 beats)	Rates: 100-250 beats/min RR interval: Mostly regular QRS complexes: Wide, bizarre May have retrograde P waves AV dissociation (diagnostic if seen) often present Fusion beats may be seen (diagnostic of VT) and represent simultaneous depolarization from ventricular focus and normal conduction from above (looks like cross between normal beat and ventricular QRS)	SVT with aberration can easily mimic VT; check initiating beat: • If PAC, likely SVT with aberration • If PVC, likely VT Indicators of VT rather than SVT with aberration: • Marked left-axis deviation (>30 degrees) • Left peak of QRS complex taller than right in lead V_1 • rS configuration in lead V_6 • QRS width >0.15 sec • QS in inferior leads

Labels in figure: I Valsalva end F RR 0.68 Rate 90 Continuous

Torsade de pointes (twisting of points)	Form of VT (actually halfway between VT and ventricular fibrillation)	Rate: 150–250 beats/min Irregular and wide QRS complexes undulate and twist on isoelectric axis Associated with a prolonged QT interval (QTc >0.46 sec)	Usually terminates spontaneously after 5–30 sec but may continue and degenerate into ventricular fibrillation Seen with electrolyte imbalances (hypomagnesemia, hypokalemia), or in association with antiarrhythmic drug therapy and tricyclic antidepressant use
Ventricular fibrillation (VF)	Uncoordinated chaotic activity of ventricles	Erratic waveforms with no discernible PQRST complexes Coarse VF: Obvious coarse baseline Fine VF: Small or barely discernible waveforms, may be mistaken for asystole	
Ventricular asystole (standstill)	No ventricular activity	QRS complex: Not seen P wave: Seen if sinus rhythm is maintained	
AV CONDUCTION DEFECTS			
First-degree AV block	Impulse is delayed at AV junction	PR interval: >0.20 sec Every sinus beat is conducted to the ventricles, producing normal QRS complex for every P wave	

Continued

TABLE 3-6

■ Cardiac Arrhythmias and Conduction Defects—cont'd

Rhythm	Mechanism	Characteristics	Comments
AV CONDUCTION DEFECTS—cont'd			
Second-degree AV block	Impulses are not all conducted through AV node		
Mobitz type I or Wenckebach	Progressive delay in conduction through AV node until a QRS complex is dropped	PR interval: Gradually increases until impulse fails to conduct through AV junctional tissue; produces dropped QRS at varying or constant intervals PR interval: Shortest after each dropped beat PP interval: Constant if in sinus rhythm (untrue, if sinus arrhythmia) RR interval: Progressively shortens P waves and QRS: Normal	Related to infarction, drug effect, or vagal effect

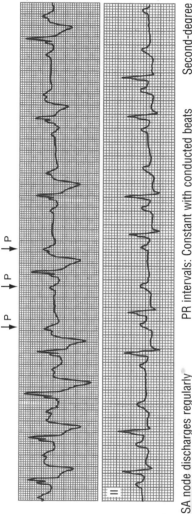

P   P   P

Mobitz type II

SA node discharges regularly
Produces constant PP interval
One or more atrial impulses fails to conduct to ventricles (no QRS complex seen)

PR intervals: Constant with conducted beats (unlike those in type I)
RR interval: Fixed
Ratio of P waves to QRS may vary: 2:1, 3:1, 4:1

Second-degree AV block with 2:1 conduction may be either Mobitz I or II.
• Narrow QRS suggests Wenckebach (type I)
• Wider QRS (i.e., bundle branch block, LV conduction delay) suggests Mobitz type II
Mobitz II is less common, but more serious

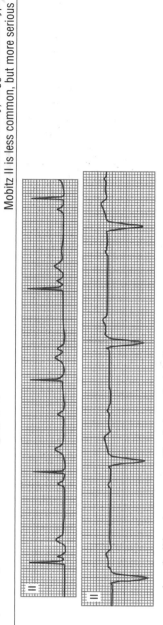

Third-degree (complete) AV block

Occurs anywhere in AV node or bundle of His: No conduction of sinus impulses
Two pacemakers become apparent
Upper: SA node fires normally
Lower: Ventricles respond to an escape pacemaker

Two independent rhythms
P waves, QRS complexes not associated
PP interval: Regular
Rate: 60-100 beats/min, if sinus rhythm
RR interval: Usually very regular, ventricular rate depends on site and inherent rate of escape pacemaker

Continued

■ **TABLE 3-6**
■ **Cardiac Arrhythmias and Conduction Defects—cont'd**

Rhythm	Mechanism	Characteristics	Comments

ECG CHANGES WITH ELECTROLYTE IMBALANCES
POTASSIUM IMBALANCES

×½   ×½

Hypokalemia

Prominent U wave
T-wave amplitude decreased
ST segment depressed
P wave may be prominent
PR interval may be prolonged
Prolonged QTc interval (actually QT-U)

When U-wave height is same as T-wave height, potassium level is usually ≤3.0 mEq/L

Hyperkalemia

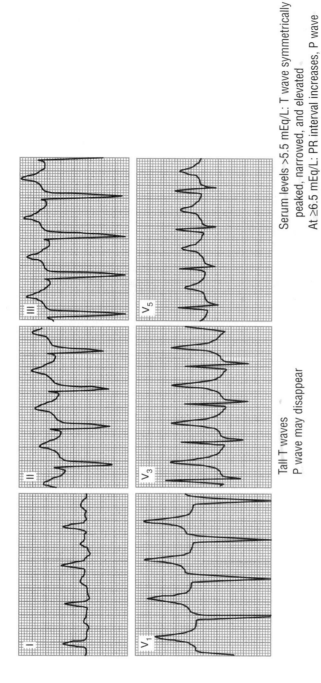

Tall T waves
P wave may disappear

Serum levels >5.5 mEq/L: T wave symmetrically peaked, narrowed, and elevated
At ≥6.5 mEq/L: PR interval increases, P wave gets smaller or disappears

At ≥7.5 mEq/L: QRS pattern widens to sine wave

Continued

■ **TABLE 3-6**
■ ■ **Cardiac Arrhythmias and Conduction Defects—cont'd**

Rhythm	Mechanism	Characteristics	Comments
CALCIUM IMBALANCES			
Hypocalcemia		Prolonged QTc interval and prolonged isoelectric ST segment	
Hypercalcemia		Shortened QTc interval ST segment is shortened or absent T waves are generally unchanged	

Figures from Chou T, Knilans TK: *Electrocardiography in clinical practice*, ed 4, Philadelphia, 1996, Saunders.

(1) Methods used include treadmill (most common) and pharmacologic stressing (dobutamine, dipyridamole, adenosine)

(2) Ischemia results in a region of hypokinesis (decreased wall motion)

(3) Evaluates extent and location of CAD and ischemic mitral regurgitation

(i) Transesophageal echocardiography (TEE): Transducer is placed in the esophagus

   (1) Capable of exquisite definition of cardiac structure and function because of the proximity of the transducer to the heart

   (2) Used in the operating room when the adequacy of valvular repair is to be evaluated and when more detail is needed (in cases of prosthetic valves or suspected patent foramen ovale, LA thrombus, or aortic dissection; in patients with poor acoustic penetration of the ultrasonic signal from the chest, such as patients with chronic obstructive pulmonary disease or a heavy build)

iii. Intravascular ultrasonography (IVUS): A small ultrasonic transducer attached to a catheter tip is threaded into the coronary artery over a guidewire. It provides high-resolution images of the inside of the artery. Invaluable in the catheterization laboratory for interventional procedures. Assesses the following:

(a) Size of the lumen, degree of stenosis

(b) Structure of the arterial wall

(c) Proper coronary stent placement

iv. Exercise electrocardiography (exercise stress testing)

(a) ECG is taken during exercise

(b) Indications for exercise testing

   (1) To identify suspected CAD

   (2) To rule out ischemia

   (3) To perform a functional assessment in patients known to have CAD (such as patients who have had an MI or angioplasty, or are undergoing coronary bypass surgery) to assess risk, severity, and prognosis

   (4) To evaluate the effectiveness of revascularization or medical therapy for CAD

   (5) To evaluate arrhythmias, especially exercise-induced VT

   (6) To evaluate patients with rate-responsive pacemakers

   (7) To screen persons entering physical fitness programs or high-risk professions (e.g., airline pilots) for CAD

(c) Contraindications to exercise testing

   (1) Acute MI

   (2) Unstable (preinfarction) angina (on effort)

   (3) Uncompensated heart failure (HF)

   (4) Severe aortic stenosis

   (5) Uncontrolled, severe hypertension

   (6) Severe illness such as fulminant infection, asthma, renal failure

   (7) Acute pericarditis or myocarditis

(d) Limitations

   (1) Patient must be able to exercise to at least 85% of the maximum predicted heart rate to have a successful test

   (2) Resting ECG must have normal ST segments at baseline

   (3) Test is insensitive to single-vessel disease (will miss 40% of such cases, giving a false-negative result)

(4) False-positive results are frequent in patients at low risk for CAD, patients taking digoxin, and patients with LV hypertrophy

v. Long-term ambulatory monitoring
   (a) Types
      (1) Holter monitor: ECG continuously recorded over a 24- to 48-hour period. Tape scanned and analyzed.
      (2) Cardiac event monitors (e.g., King of Hearts monitor): Looping event recorder kept with the patient for up to 30 days. Patient records ECG tracings when symptoms occur, then transmits over telephone. ECG then forwarded and evaluated by the physician.
      (3) Implanted loop recorders: Cardiac monitors implanted in the patient to identify suspected rhythms that have not otherwise been seen
   (b) Used in documenting the following:
      (1) Arrhythmias not demonstrated by resting or exercise ECG, especially with symptoms of palpitations, syncope
      (2) Efficacy of surgical and medical therapy for arrhythmias
      (3) Pacemaker function
      (4) Silent ischemia (if proper recording equipment is used)
   (c) Records at least two leads: I and V_5 simultaneously
   (d) Diary is kept by the patient to note symptoms (chest pain, palpitations, syncope) and activities during recording to correlate with rhythm

vi. Electrophysiologic studies (EPS): Series of programmed electrical stimuli are applied within the heart to the endothelium through electrodes in the cardiac chambers, under fluoroscopic guidance. Used to induce cardiac arrhythmias.
   (a) Purpose: To reproduce arrhythmias in a controlled environment to assess the best mode of therapy for their control (e.g., medications, pacemaker, ablation)
   (b) Patients selected include
      (1) Patients with ventricular or supraventricular tachyarrhythmias
      (2) Patients at high risk for sudden cardiac death
      (3) Patients with unexplained recurrent syncopal episodes with suspected cardiac cause
      (4) Patients who have survived a cardiac arrest without identified cause
      (5) Candidates for an implantable defibrillator
      (6) Candidates for ablation therapy

Patient Care

1. **Decreased cardiac output (CO)**
   a. Description of problem: Decreased CO can be due to either mechanical or electrical cardiac dysfunction. Findings can include the following:
      i. Changes in the patient's hemodynamics: Blood pressure, heart rate, CO
      ii. ECG changes or arrhythmias
      iii. Chest pain
      iv. Weakness, fatigue, dizziness
      v. Shortness of breath, dyspnea, crackles
      vi. Cold and clammy skin, cyanosis, pallor
      vii. Decreased peripheral pulses
      viii. Decreased or absent urinary output (oliguria, anuria)
      ix. Diminished mentation or loss of consciousness
      x. Jugular vein distention

   b. Goals of care

      i. Work of the heart is decreased by decreasing myocardial oxygen demands

     ii. Myocardial oxygen supply is increased (minimizing ischemia, size of infarct)

    iii. Hemodynamics are normal: CO is adequate

    iv. Heart rate is controlled and arrhythmias are eliminated

     v. Patient is free of chest pain

    vi. Patient has normal urinary output

   c. Collaborating professionals on health care team: Nurse, physician, pharmacist, and physical therapist

   d. Interventions

      i. Monitor heart rate, rhythm, and patient responses (e.g., blood pressure, mental status, diaphoresis, pain, shortness of breath)

     ii. Assess blood pressure at regular intervals and with changes in the patient's condition. Discuss with the physician what drug is to be administered for significant changes in blood pressure.

    iii. Watch the patient's oxygenation by frequently checking pulse oximetry readings and assessing breath sounds, respirations, and circulation. Administer oxygen as needed.

    iv. Assess changes in the patient's neurologic status. Observe for central nervous system disturbances (confusion, restlessness, agitation, dizziness).

     v. Administer fluids as ordered to maintain left ventricular end-diastolic pressure (LVEDP)

    vi. Monitor for heart failure

   vii. Monitor intake and output (urine output should average at least 30 ml/hr), daily weights

   viii. Check presence and quality of peripheral pulses

    ix. Check for other signs of perfusion deficits: Cool skin, sluggish capillary refilling

     x. Monitor hemodynamic pressures, CO readings if the patient has a right-sided heart catheter

       (a) Notify the physician of significant hemodynamic changes

       (b) Collaborate with the physician regarding medication needs, management of hemodynamic status

       (c) Be aware of the rationale for current therapy, parameters, and goals of care

    xi. Have the patient notify the nurse immediately at the onset of chest discomfort and other associated symptoms of distress. Place the patient in a semi-Fowler position or position of comfort. Stress the importance of early recognition and treatment of problems.

   xii. Watch for and identify any ECG changes

       (a) Document the rhythm strip (at least once a shift)

       (b) Obtain a 12-lead ECG if a new arrhythmia is noted

       (c) Determine the patient's response to arrhythmia, verbally and through vital signs

       (d) Administer appropriate emergency drugs if the patient's cardiac rhythm becomes significantly bradycardic or tachycardic, per unit protocols

       (e) Have emergency equipment readily available and fully stocked

       (f) Be knowledgeable about and prepared to use emergency equipment (defibrillator, transcutaneous pacer, transvenous pacer)

       (g) Administer CPR and call code if the patient is pulseless, in VF, or in asystole

    e. Evaluation of patient care

        i. Blood pressure, heart rate, and hemodynamics are within normal limits or those set for the patient

        ii. Sinus rhythm is normal on ECG

        iii. Patient is alert and oriented

        iv. Patient is comfortable and pain free

        v. Skin is warm and dry

        vi. Urinary output is adequate

2. Acute chest pain

    a. Description of problem: Acute pain due to ischemia. Findings can include the following:

        i. Patient communication of discomfort: Description of quality (on a scale of 1 to 10, with 10 being the worst), intensity, location, radiation, timing, and aggravating and alleviating factors (movement, deep inspiration, positioning)

        ii. Anxiety

        iii. Diaphoresis

        iv. Changes in blood pressure, heart rate, respiratory rate

        v. Nausea, vomiting

        vi. ECG changes (ST segment, T waves) or arrhythmias

    b. Goals of care

        i. Pain or discomfort is relieved completely

        ii. Vital signs are stable and within normal limits

    c. Collaborating professionals on health care team: Nurse, physician, physician assistant, advanced registered nurse practitioner, pharmacist, occupational and physical therapists, dietitian, social worker, home health aide

    d. Interventions

        i. Have the patient notify the nurse immediately at the onset of chest discomfort and other associated symptoms of distress. Stress the importance of early recognition and treatment of chest discomfort.

        ii. Administer oxygen per unit protocol

        iii. Check vital signs, monitor ECG

        iv. Do a 12-lead ECG immediately

        v. Ensure that the patient has a patent IV line

        vi. Administer and titrate medications to alleviate angina

        vii. Notify the physician

        viii. Collaborate with the physician on medication needs (types, dosages, frequency, route) and titrations and adjustments of medications, depending on the patient response

        ix. Monitor the patient's pain

            (a) Assess quality, duration, intensity, frequency of the pain

            (b) Assess the effectiveness of medications

            (c) Look for trends and drug interactions, and identify other possible comfort measures

        x. Provide other comfort interventions as appropriate (e.g., back rub, repositioning, special mattresses)

        xi. Alert the physician if pain continues so that further actions can be determined. Cardiac pain means the myocardium is in jeopardy, and immediate interventions are needed.

    e. Evaluation of patient care

        i. Patient is pain free and comfortable (with or without analgesia)

        ii. Vital signs are stable

       iii. Patient reports pain or discomfort, when it occurs, immediately and clearly to the nurse

3. Activity intolerance

  a. Description of problem: Due to cardiac dysfunction, the patient may exhibit the following clinical findings, reflecting a decreased tolerance for the activities of daily living

      i. Fatigue, weakness

      ii. Dyspnea with progressively less exertion

      iii. Leg cramps

      iv. Discomfort in chest, neck, jaw, shoulder, arm

      v. Increased heart rate and/or blood pressure

      vi. Arrhythmias

      vii. ST-segment and T-wave changes signifying ischemia

  b. Goals of care

      i. Cause is identified and treated

      ii. Patient engages in progressive ambulation

      iii. No complications of bed rest are present (skin intact, breath sounds clear, no signs of deep venous thromboembolism)

      iv. Patient is educated regarding the need for routine exercise and weight control (as needed)

  c. Collaborating professionals on health care team: Physical and occupational therapists; cardiac rehabilitation nurse for activity plans in hospital and after discharge; social worker to assist with home equipment acquisition, home visits, nursing home placement (temporary or permanent); dietitian

  d. Interventions

      i. Assess and document the patient's response to progressive ambulation, including monitoring of heart rate and rhythm, respiration, and blood pressure

      ii. Assist the patient with initial increases in ambulation

      iii. Administer pain medication, as needed, before planned ambulation (if the patient is pain free, progression in ambulation will be more successful)

      iv. Plan rest periods between various treatments, visits, and ambulation

      v. Teach the patient how to progress safely: Instruct in correct positioning and efficient use of body for each step

        (a) Active range-of-motion exercises

        (b) Dangling

        (c) Transfers from bed to chair or bedside commode

        (d) Ambulation in room and hallway

      vi. Ensure that the patient is instructed with regard to the availability and use of special equipment to assist in ambulation (walkers, canes, wheelchairs), if needed

      vii. If the patient becomes unstable (ischemic pain, vital signs beyond set limits, arrhythmias), help the patient back to bed and immediately evaluate the need for oxygen, medications (e.g., nitrates, antiarrhythmics), ECG, notification of the physician, emergency equipment

      viii. Arrange consultations with other health professionals, as appropriate

      ix. Encourage the patient and family to openly ventilate feelings and ask questions regarding the ability to ambulate and lifestyle resumption and changes

  e. Evaluation of patient care

      i. Patient has verbalized and demonstrated an understanding of activity capacity and limitations

    ii. Exercise program is incorporated into the patient's lifestyle. Weight control goals are met, if appropriate.

    iii. Activity plan includes a support system and community services, as needed, to achieve the desired lifestyle

4. Inadequate knowledge of cardiac diagnosis, medications, or treatment

  a. Description of problem

    i. Patient and/or family verbalizations indicate a lack of knowledge or inappropriate or incorrect information

    ii. Patient may have been noncompliant with the recommended regimen, which resulted in incorrect or inappropriate care at home

    iii. Patient is easily agitated, hostile, worried, suspicious (because of misinformation, misunderstanding, or misinterpretation)

    iv. Patient and/or family is unable to plan realistic goals or home care

  b. Goals of care

    i. Patient (and family) verbalizes an understanding of the diagnosis, medications, treatment, and follow-up care

    ii. Patient demonstrates proper home care techniques

  c. Collaborating professionals on health care team: See Acute Chest Pain

  d. Interventions

    i. Identify learning needs

    ii. Assess readiness to learn (the patient is alert, pain free, not sleep deprived; information is not given immediately after sedatives are administered)

    iii. Determine the best methods for the patient to learn (group, one to one, videos)

    iv. Reinforce learning with the use of printed materials related to the disease, discharge instructions, procedures, and medications

    v. Instruction sheets should be available in languages other than English

    vi. Arrange for an interpreter if the patient does not understand English (staff, family member, interpretation services)

    vii. Document teaching and the patient's response

    viii. Arrange appropriate consults: Cardiac rehabilitation; dietary, occupational, and physical therapy; home health; social work

    ix. Schedule practice and return demonstrations of psychomotor skills

  e. Evaluation of patient care

    i. Patient or significant other verbalizes an understanding of the medical condition, medications, necessary home care, follow-up, and diet and any other lifestyle changes

    ii. Patient or significant other knows where to seek assistance for information and help

    iii. Patient or significant other demonstrates proper techniques for various applicable home self-care procedures (low-molecular-weight heparin injections, pulse monitoring, wound care, IV therapy)

SPECIFIC PATIENT HEALTH PROBLEMS

Coronary Artery Disease

Coronary artery disease is a progressive disorder in which the coronary arteries become occluded as a result of atherosclerosis

1. Pathophysiology

  a. Injury (due to LDL cholesterol, toxins, infections, or mechanical causes) occurs to the endothelial cells in the intima of the coronary arteries, altering cell structure

b. Platelets adhere and aggregate at the site of injury, and macrophages migrate to the area as a result of injury. Smooth muscle cells and macrophage foam cells enter the intimal layer. These accumulations promote the development over time of a fatty fibrous plaque, or "fatty streak." Migration of LDL into the subintimal space results in "lipid core."

c. This plaque is a pearly white accumulation in the intimal lining, consisting mostly of smooth muscle cells but also collagen-producing fibroblasts and macrophages. These deposits protrude into the lumen, obstructing blood flow.

d. Progressive narrowing of the vessel occurs

e. This process tends to occur at vessel bifurcations and at the proximal end of the artery

f. The fatty fibrous plaque can rupture and form either a mural thrombus or an occlusive thrombus

    i. A mural thrombus can partially or totally obstruct the artery. The disrupted plaque and mural thrombus can develop into a more fibrotic, stenotic lesion, which changes the plaque's geometry.

    ii. An acute, labile, occlusive thrombus can totally obstruct the artery and create clinical complications (MI, unstable angina, sudden cardiac death)

    iii. The ruptured plaque, caused by endothelial injury and exposure to blood flow, activates platelet and fibrin formation, enhancing thrombus formation

g. Coronary blood flow may be further diminished by vasoconstriction (resulting from the release of vasoactive agents [thromboxane A_2, angiotensin II], impaired vasodilatation, and platelet activation)

h. Atherosclerotic process causes

    i. Decreases in blood flow and oxygen supply to the myocardium

    ii. An imbalance between myocardial oxygen supply and demand, which results in myocardial ischemia

2. Etiology and risk factors

a. Heredity: Familial component for premature heart disease; MI or sudden cardiac death in father, mother, or siblings

b. Age: CAD is more prevalent among middle-aged and older persons (males older than 45 years of age; females older than 55 years of age)

c. Gender: CAD is more prevalent among men

    i. Before age 55, prevalence is three to four times higher among men than among women (before menopause)

    ii. After age 55, prevalence rates slowly equalize for both sexes; at age 75, rates are close to equal

d. Smoking

    i. Enhances atherogenic progression; decreases HDL cholesterol level; influences thrombus formation, plaque instability, arrhythmias

    ii. Dose and duration dependent: Risk of death from CAD is two to six times higher among smokers than among nonsmokers

e. Hyperlipidemia: High levels of triglycerides, LDL, and very-low-density lipoproteins are associated with an increased risk of CAD

    i. Triglycerides: Higher than 200 mg/dl

    ii. LDL: Higher than 130 mg/dl

    iii. HDL: Lower than 40 mg/dl (HDL level higher than 60 mg/dl is a negative risk factor)

f. Hypertension

    i. Contributes to direct vascular injury, along with the effects of increased wall stress and oxygen demands

  ii. Approximately 30% of American adults have hypertension (the rate is up to three times higher in African Americans than in the general population). Women have a higher incidence of hypertensive heart disease.

  iii. Defined as systolic blood pressure higher than 140 and/or diastolic pressure higher than 90 mm Hg (Chobanian, Bakris, Black, et al, 2003)

 g. LV hypertrophy: Heart's response to chronic pressure overloads; associated with increased risk for cardiovascular events

 h. Thrombogenic risk factors: Deficiencies in serum coagulation inhibitors (antithrombin III, protein C, and protein S), elevated plasma fibrinogen level, enhanced platelet aggregation

 i. Diabetes mellitus: Patients with diabetes mellitus are twice as likely to develop CAD as persons without diabetes

 j. Obesity: Positively associated with an increased rate of CAD; also contributes to the development of hypertension and diabetes

  i. Fat distribution plays a role (abdominal or central obesity carries a higher risk)

  ii. Metabolic syndrome: Recognized syndrome (also referred to as insulin resistance syndrome) associated with higher risk and identified by the presence of three or more of the following:

   (a) Abdominal obesity: Waist circumference greater than 40 inches in men and greater than 35 inches in women

   (b) Triglyceride level higher than 150 mg/dl

   (c) HDL level lower than 40 mg/dl in men and 50 mg/dl in women

   (d) Blood pressure higher than 130/85 mm Hg

   (e) Glucose level (fasting) higher than 110 mg/dl

 k. Sedentary lifestyle; studies show a positive relationship between inactivity and CAD, mainly resulting from its aggravation of other risk factors

3. Signs and symptoms

 a. History

  i. Assessment of the aforementioned risk factors

  ii. Possible sequelae of CAD include the following:

   (a) Angina pectoris

   (b) MI

   (c) Ventricular aneurysm or rupture

   (d) Heart failure, cardiogenic shock

   (e) Arrhythmias, sudden cardiac death

   (f) Cardiomyopathy

   (g) Mitral insufficiency

 b. Physical examination (see Patient Assessment section): CAD may be asymptomatic and may be diagnosed due to abnormal findings on tests (stress testing, echocardiography)

4. Diagnostic study findings

 a. Laboratory

  i. Fasting lipid profile: Total cholesterol, HDL, LDL, triglyceride levels

  ii. Fasting serum glucose levels

 b. Exercise ECG stress testing: Used to rule out ischemia, to evaluate chest pain symptoms, to stratify the risk of known CAD, to detect arrhythmias, and to assess the efficacy of treatment

 c. Myocardial perfusion imaging (with exercise or pharmacologic stress): Used to detect inadequate myocardial perfusion (ischemia) or the absence of perfusion (infarction) by assessing the degree of uptake in the myocardium of a radioactive tracer

    d. Echocardiography

      i. Exercise stress echocardiography: Ultrasound images taken during or after treadmill or bicycle exercise

      ii. Pharmacologic stress echocardiography: Dobutamine or adenosine is used to increase myocardial oxygen requirements (similar to exercise demands)

    e. EBCT: Done with an ultrafast CT scanner. Measures coronary calcium on artery walls and calculates score, which, if elevated, is associated with increased possibility of CAD

    f. Cardiac catheterization and coronary angiography: Used to define cardiac function and coronary anatomy to guide therapy

    g. IVUS: Catheter-tipped two-dimensional ultrasonic probe is used to define intracoronary anatomy

    h. Intracardiac echocardiography (ICE): Experimental; used to define intracoronary anatomy

5. Goals of care

    a. Modifiable risk factors are under control and/or improved

    b. Risk factor modification is incorporated into the patient's lifestyle

    c. Goals of the treatment program are met

6. Collaborating professionals on health care team: Physician, nurse, dietitian, pharmacist, community service worker (i.e., smoking cessation programs)

7. Management of patient care

    a. Anticipated patient trajectory: Primary prevention is the key to decreasing the morbidity and mortality of CAD

      i. Nutrition

        (a) Nutritional status, dietary habits should be assessed.

        (b) Education should be provided on the rationale for compliance with a cholesterol-controlled diet if lipid levels are above the goals.

        (c) Information should be provided to the patient and family on low-fat, low-cholesterol foods. Referrals should be given to hospital and community resources for follow-up and reinforcement.

        (d) Diet should include the use of monounsaturated and polyunsaturated fats (olive, sunflower, and corn oils; soft oleomargarine) and avoidance of *trans*-fatty acids, which should be less than 7% of total calories. Other dietary additions can include fish and ω-3 fatty acids, fiber, and flaxseed.

        (e) Goals for weight should be discussed. Weight and height should be measured. Body mass index (BMI) should be determined.

$$BMI = \frac{weight\ in\ pounds}{(height\ in\ inches)^2} \times 703$$

          (1) Desirable waist circumference: Less than 41 inches in males and less than 36 inches in females

          (2) BMI: Desired = 18 to 24.9 (25 to 30 indicates overweight; more than 30 indicates obesity)

      ii. Pharmacology

        (a) Antiplatelet agents (such as aspirin [acetylsalicylic acid], 81 mg/day) should be included in the patient's health regimen, if not contraindicated

        (b) Lipid-lowering agents will often be necessary; the patient should be aware of their uses and side effects, and follow-up requirements

        (c) Antihypertensive agents may be necessary (diuretics, ACE inhibitors, β-blockers)

      iii. Psychosocial issues

        (a) An adequate support system to assist in changing to heart-healthy behaviors and lifestyle is important

  (b) Complementary and alternative medical methods to assist with stress reduction include massage therapy, yoga, regular exercise, postural therapy, and acupuncture
  iv. Treatments
  (a) Provide the patient with information regarding the risk factors for CAD
  (b) Encourage the patient and significant others to quit smoking; provide information and help regarding risks, methods for stopping, and nicotine replacement
  (c) Provide information on lipid-lowering diets that have 30% or less fat, with less than 7% saturated fat
  (d) Goals for lipid management
   (1) LDL level of less than 130 mg/dl (less than 100 mg/dl if CAD is present)
   (2) HDL level of more than 40 mg/dl
   (3) Triglyceride level of less than 200 mg/dl
  (e) If the patient is hypertensive
   (1) Blood pressure goal: 140/90 mm Hg or lower
   (2) Modifications include weight control, routine exercise, moderate alcohol consumption, and sodium restriction
  (f) Weight control should be discussed with the patient and a plan for weight loss developed (especially for patients who are more than 120% of their ideal weight for height). Hypertensive patients and/or patients with elevated glucose or triglyceride levels should receive information on achieving ideal body weight.
  (g) Encourage exercise and physical activity (after risks are assessed, often after exercise testing in patients over 40 years of age)
   (1) Goal of 30 minutes, three to four times weekly (minimum); preferably 30 to 60 minutes of moderate exercise, including walking, cycling, jogging, swimming
   (2) Other opportunities for increased physical activity should be explored
  (h) Increased emphasis is being placed on education regarding women and cardiovascular disease and on more aggressive medical management for women along with the inclusion of more female patients in clinical trials
  b. Potential complications: See the following sections for each of the possible sequelae of CAD
8. **Evaluation of patient care**
  a. Patient verbalizes an understanding of how to manage or modify the risk factors contributing to CAD progression
  b. Patient and family have educational resources (i.e., smoking cessation program, medication information sheets, follow-up plan) to assist in implementing new health practices

Chronic Stable Angina Pectoris

1. **Pathophysiology**
  a. Myocardial oxygen demand outstrips oxygen supply
  b. Progressive coronary atherosclerosis increasingly limits coronary blood flow and myocardial perfusion
2. **Etiology and risk factors**
  a. Precipitating factors

   i. Increased myocardial oxygen demand due to
   - (a) Increased heart rate resulting from exertion, tachyarrhythmia, anemia, fever, anxiety, pain, thyrotoxicosis, drugs, digestion, hyperadrenergic states
   - (b) Increased contractility resulting from exercise, tachycardia, anxiety, drugs, hyperadrenergic states
   - (c) Increased afterload resulting from hypertension, aortic stenosis, drugs (pressors)
   - (d) Increased preload resulting from volume overload, drugs

   ii. Decreased oxygen supply due to
   - (a) CAD (fixed narrowing of coronary arteries)
   - (b) Coronary artery spasm (cocaine abuse, cold air, drugs [ergots])
   - (c) Circulatory diversion (digestion, coronary artery steal)
   - (d) Anemia
   - (e) Hypoxemia
   - (f) Hypovolemia
   - (g) Shock
   - (h) Heart failure

   b. Risk factors: The common risk factors of CAD

3. Signs and symptoms
   a. Subjective findings: Anginal discomfort is any exertional, rest-relieved symptom and may be described as burning, squeezing, aching, heaviness, pressure sensation, smothering, indigestion-like, or a "band across the chest." It may occur anywhere between the ears and the umbilicus.

   i. Etiologic or precipitating factors: Elicit pertinent information from the patient

   ii. Characterize the patient's symptoms
   - (a) Duration of discomfort: Chest pain from acute coronary syndromes generally lasts more than 20 minutes
   - (b) Location and radiation of discomfort: Can include the chest, neck, jaws, arms, back, epigastrium
   - (c) Patient is asked to quantify the discomfort by using a scale from 1 (the least) to 10 (the worst pain ever experienced by the patient)
   - (d) Associated symptoms may include nausea, diaphoresis, palpitations, shortness of breath, syncope, and presyncope
   - (e) Effect of exertion and rest: The timing of the discomfort is crucial. Was it with activity, in bed at rest, postprandial? With what kind of activity? How often does it recur? What starts it? What relieves it?
   - (f) Effect of nitrates (if the patient has CAD, nitrates should decrease or abolish the discomfort in 1 to 2 minutes, not 15 to 20 minutes)

   b. Objective findings
   i. Determine the type or form of discomfort
   - (a) Unstable angina: New-onset angina or angina that has changed in frequency, severity, or duration or occurs with less exertion or at rest. Duration of pain is usually more than 20 minutes (see Acute Coronary Syndromes).
   - (b) Chronic, stable angina: Angina that has not increased in frequency or severity over time. Caused primarily by obstructive, fixed atheromatous coronary lesions.
   - (c) Prinzmetal's (variant) angina: Resting angina caused by coronary artery spasm, associated with transient ST-segment elevation

   ii. Determine class of angina: Canadian classification

        (a) Canadian class I: Angina produced by strenuous exertion

        (b) Canadian class II: Angina produced by walking more than two level blocks

        (c) Canadian class III: Angina produced by walking less than two level blocks

        (d) Canadian class IV: Angina at rest

     iii. Other important aspects of the history include the following:

        (a) Presence of risk factors for CAD

        (b) Cardiac review of systems

        (c) Medication history (including use of illicit drugs)

        (d) History of tests, interventions; coronary artery bypass graft (CABG), PTCA

        (e) Allergies to shellfish, iodine (contrast dye)

        (f) If the patient underwent intervention (PCI, CABG), try to elicit the patient's anginal history prior to the intervention

4. Diagnostic study findings

  a. Laboratory: Levels of troponins or CK-MB isoenzymes are not elevated with stable angina

  b. ECG: May be normal or show nonspecific ST or T-wave changes or evidence of prior infarction

  c. Echocardiography: May or may not show transient abnormal wall motion, valve dysfunction, hypertrophy

  d. Treadmill stress testing: Results may or may not be positive for CAD. Very sensitive for left main artery or three-vessel disease but can miss up to 40% of single-vessel disease. Used in low-risk patients who are pain free for 12 to 24 hours and without symptoms of heart failure.

  e. Dobutamine or exercise stress echocardiography: Can demonstrate ischemia (stress-induced wall motion abnormalities), ventricular dysfunction, and ischemic mitral regurgitation

  f. Myocardial scintigraphy (thallium, Tc 99m sestamibi) with exercise or pharmacologic stress (adenosine, dipyridamole): May demonstrate ischemia, infarction, and LV dysfunction

  g. Coronary catheterization: Used to assess the extent and severity of CAD as well as to assess valvular and ventricular function. It facilitates risk assessment and guides therapy (medical or interventional).

5. Goals of care

  a. Ischemia, MI, and death are prevented by

     i. Decreasing myocardial oxygen demand (β-blockers, calcium channel blockers, nitrates)

     ii. Improving myocardial oxygen supply (nitrates)

  b. Disease process is modified

     i. Antiplatelet and antithrombin therapy

     ii. Lifestyle modifications (i.e., smoking cessation, diet, blood pressure control, diabetes control)

6. Collaborating professionals on health care team: Physician (cardiologist, cardiac surgeon), nurse, physical and occupational therapists, social worker, cardiac rehabilitation team, dietitian, pharmacist

7. Management of patient care

  a. Anticipated patient trajectory: Prognosis varies widely depending on LV function, the severity of CAD and associated risk factors. Prompt diagnosis and treatment enables elimination of symptoms and improved longevity.

     i. Discharge planning

(a) Risk factor modification teaching
   (1) Smoking cessation to reduce reoccurrence of cardiac events
   (2) Weight control
   (3) Exercise: Daily routine important
   (4) Blood pressure: Less than 130/85 mm Hg
   (5) Diabetes: Tight glucose control
   (6) Lipid control: If LDL level is higher than 100 mg/dl; discuss lipid target levels, diet, medications
(b) For PCI: Teach discharge activities, symptoms to report (e.g., masses, bleeding, increased localized pain and bruising at the site of insertion, tingling or numbness, extremity weakness, shortness of breath, chest discomfort), medications, diet, risk factors, and actions to take:
   (1) Call physician and apply pressure for bleeding or swelling at catheter site
   (2) Limit activities for 2 days. Do not lift more than 10 lb.
   (3) Do not drive for 1 day
   (4) Recognize the importance of following the medication plan (e.g., antiplatelet therapy)
   (5) Follow discharge follow-up schedule
(c) Give the patient a stent information packet and an identification stent card and ensure that questions regarding care are answered
(d) Provide clear instructions regarding all medications (types, rationales, dosages, side effects) to the patient and significant others

  ii. Pharmacology
(a) Nitroglycerin (NTG): To relieve angina
(b) Aspirin: 81 mg daily (clopidogrel given if unable to take aspirin)
(c) β-blockers: Given unless contraindications exist
(d) Calcium antagonists and/or long-acting nitrates: If β-blockers are unsuccessful or contraindicated
(e) ACE inhibitors: For patients with diabetes, LV systolic dysfunction
(f) Lipid-lowering agents: Statins

  iii. Psychosocial issues: Aggressive risk factor modification and lifestyle changes are necessary. Barriers and challenges to these goals need to be identified. Reduction of emotional stressors may improve long-term prognosis.

  iv. Treatments
(a) PCIs: Used to increase the luminal diameter of coronary arteries that have been stenosed by CAD and to increase coronary blood flow using PTCA, coronary stent placement, and atherectomy (Figures 3-13 and 3-14)
   (1) PTCA
      a) Balloon catheter is placed across stenosis and inflated
      b) Enlarges lumen diameter by mechanically compressing and splitting plaque
   (2) Coronary stent placement
      a) Devices are placed intraluminally to achieve maximal lumen size and maintain the patency of the vessel's lumen. Majority of PCI procedures now include some form of stenting with PTCA.
         1) Stents are made from various metals
         2) Drug-eluding stents: Made of synthetic materials with the ability to deliver drugs to almost eliminate the restenosis of stents

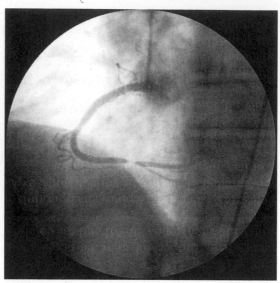

FIGURE 3-13 ■ Stenosis of the right coronary artery before percutaneous coronary intervention. (Courtesy Dr. Steve Ramee, Ochsner Clinic Foundation.)

    b) Indications
        1) Primary stenting to restore the normal luminal diameter
        2) Restenosis: After PCI
        3) Intimal tears: After PCI
(3) Coronary atherectomy: Removal of atheromatous material from the artery (debulking). Procedure is now used less due to improved stenting procedures.
    a) Directional coronary atherectomy: Plaque is cut by a catheter with a rotating cutter and trapped in its chamber for removal

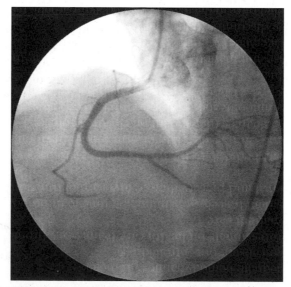

FIGURE 3-14 ■ Right coronary artery revascularization after percutaneous coronary intervention with a coronary stent procedure. (Courtesy Dr. Steve Ramee, Ochsner Clinic Foundation.)

  b) Transluminal extraction atherectomy: Slower rotating cutter is used with vacuum suction to withdraw atheromatous debris
  c) Rotational atherectomy: High-speed, rotating burr grinds atheromatous material into microdebris in the blood stream
(4) Brachytherapy: Intracoronary radiation procedure to treat and prevent in-stent restenosis
(5) Key points for nursing care after PCI procedure: See Box 3-5
(b) CABG: Surgical revascularization of the myocardium with bypass grafting
  (1) Saphenous vein graft: Reversed saphenous vein from leg used to create a conduit. One end of the graft is sewn onto the aorta and the other end is sewn onto the affected coronary artery distal to the obstruction
  (2) Internal mammary artery bypass
    a) Proximal artery remains attached to the subclavian artery from which it arises and the distal end is dissected from the anterior chest wall and sewn onto the coronary artery distal to the obstruction
    b) Long-term patency rate is better (more than 90% at 10 years) than with saphenous vein graft (40%)
    c) Avoids need for leg incisions if only one or two vessels require bypass
  (3) Complications during surgery
    a) MI: 2% to 7%
    b) Intraoperative stroke: 1% to 2%
    c) Death: 1% to 2%
  (4) Immediately postoperative complications
    a) Low CO, hypotension: Due to inadequate volume replacement, fluid shifts (third spacing), hemorrhage. Can decrease systemic perfusion, affecting the kidneys, brain, and heart.
    b) Hemorrhage
    c) Hypertension (increased afterload decreases CO)
    d) Cardiac tamponade: Suspect if decreased CO and hypotension are present with increased CVP (unless hypovolemic), narrowed pulse pressure, distended jugular veins, pulsus paradoxus, distant heart sounds
    e) Arrhythmias: Caused by electrolyte imbalances, hypoxemia, drug toxicity, hypothermia, anesthesia, pulmonary artery catheters. Atrial fibrillation is common (approximately 25% of patients).
    f) Respiratory failure: Associated with hypoxemia, alveolar hypoventilation
    g) Prerenal azotemia: Caused by decreased CO, hypovolemia
    h) Electrolyte imbalances: Hypokalemia, hypocalcemia, hypomagnesemia (common)
    i) Graft closure: Can be prevented by antiplatelet aggregation therapy with risk factor modification
  (5) Early extubation (usually within 6 hours) should be anticipated once the patient meets weaning criteria
  (6) Agents commonly used after CABG
    a) Volume support (albumin, hetastarch, and/or whole and packed red blood cells): To increase the preload, elevate CVP,

■ **BOX 3-5**

■ **KEY POINTS IN NURSING CARE AFTER PERCUTANEOUS CORONARY INTERVENTION PROCEDURES**

GENERAL NURSING CARE
1. Observe for complications.
2. Maintain the patient on bed rest for 2 to 6 hours with progressive elevation of head of bed (initially, less than 30 degrees). Time of restrictions depends on method of postprocedure closure: Manual pressure, mechanical closure (e.g., FemoStop), collagen closure plugs (e.g., Angio-Seal), percutaneous suture devices (e.g., Perclose).
3. Affected limb should be kept straight, immobile; soft leg restraint may be used.
4. Patient may be positioned in reverse Trendelenburg's position to facilitate eating and comfort, and repositioned on side by log rolling, if procedure site is not bleeding.
5. Take electrocardiogram on return from procedure and if chest discomfort is present.
6. Ensure that blood work is done for serial measurement of cardiac markers.
7. Monitor vital signs closely.
8. Monitor pulses, warmth, sensation of affected limb; assess for bleeding and hematoma at femoral site.
9. If there is bleeding or hematoma, hold direct pressure until bleeding has stopped.
10. Mark hematoma and closely watch for signs of increased size. Inflatable femoral compression systems may be applied to maintain hemostasis.
11. Finger foods are easier for patient while head-of-bed elevation is restricted.
12. Assess need for medication for back and groin discomfort.
13. Maintain intravenous (IV) fluids as ordered and encourage drinking of fluids (to facilitate excretion of catheterization dye by kidneys).
14. Ensure adequate output. Foley catheter may be necessary for patients who cannot void (within 2 to 4 hours), for patients who are unable to void in bed at required position, or for patients who are at high risk for bleeding.
15. Patient may be on heparin drip after percutaneous coronary intervention: Monitor partial thromboplastin time for adequate anticoagulation (ordered parameters). Perform other monitoring to detect bleeding problems (check urine, vomit, stools; watch for nosebleeds; monitor neurologic status). Heparin should be stopped 1 to 4 hours before sheath removal.
16. Check activated coagulation time if sheath is to come out (if <150 seconds, sheath may be removed if patient is stable and without ischemic pain).
17. Various closure devices are used, each with its own postcatheter protocol.

POSTPROCEDURE NURSING CARE DURING SHEATH REMOVAL
1. Thoroughly explain removal process to patient.
2. Medicate patient before removal to diminish discomfort. Medications include morphine or other fast-acting analgesics along with local anesthesia to site.
3. Have normal saline bolus and atropine (0.5 mg IV) readily available at bedside for vasovagal reactions (hypotension, bradycardia, diaphoresis, nausea).
4. Gather all other equipment for removal: Suture removal kit; syringes; gloves, goggles, and gown; dressings; Doppler device, compression devices, if used.
5. Aspirating 5 to 10 ml of blood from each sheath (both venous and arterial lines) ensures that there are no clots on the tip of the sheath to embolize on withdrawal and that any heparin is removed from the patient's system.
6. Locate arterial pulse. Apply manual, direct pressure just above puncture site (and over arterial pulse) for a minimum of 20 minutes after sheath removal until hemostasis is complete. Pulling the arterial sheath first and then the venous sheath after hemostasis avoids potential risk of arteriovenous fistula.
7. If using a compression device, follow protocols for safe use during and after sheath removal.

Continued

POSTPROCEDURE NURSING CARE AFTER SHEATH REMOVAL

1. After sheath removal check vital signs every 15 minutes four times, every 30 minutes four times, and then every hour.
2. Continue to monitor and document pulses and assess for bleeding or hematoma; promptly treat with direct pressure until hemostasis is complete. Notify physician if bleeding recurs.
3. Maintain bed rest for 2 to 6 hours after sheath removal per protocol for closure method and procedure site (i.e., radial, femoral). Elevate head of bed progressively (initially less than 30 degrees), with affected limb immobilized.
4. Continue to medicate for discomfort from bed rest.
5. Auscultate for systolic bruit at site of sheath insertion at least every 8 hours: Positive bruit along with localized pain and pulsatile mass suggests possible pseudoaneurysm; notify physician immediately. Surgery or ultrasonographically guided compression is necessary for closure. Patients at high risk for pseudoaneurysm include the following:
   - Obese patients (difficult to apply direct pressure)
   - Patients in whom sheath size larger than No. 8 French was used (larger injury to artery)
   - Patients receiving postprocedure anticoagulants (hemostasis problem)
   - Elderly patients (artery wall changes with age)
   - Females (fat distribution, smaller arteries, potential for multiple punctures during catheterization procedure)

---

                 increase systolic blood pressure if it falls below predetermined parameters, and increase the HCT

    b) Drugs for acute management: See Heart Failure

    c) Antiarrhythmic agents often administered prophylactically to decrease the incidence of atrial fibrillation

  (c) Intraaortic balloon pump (IABP) may be used in conjunction with other therapies for recurrent ischemia, hemodynamic or electrical instability, cardiogenic shock (pump failure); see Heart Failure

  (d) Ventricular assist device (VAD): See Heart Failure

b. Potential complications of PCIs

  i. Recurrent pain: Restenosis

    (a) Mechanism of restenosis: Results from intimal hyperplasia during healing. Factors associated with increased risk of restenosis include multivessel CAD, proximal LAD stenosis, diabetes, final lumen diameter of less than 100%.

    (b) Management: Follow interventions for acute chest pain (see earlier Acute Chest Pain under Patient Care). PCI or CABG may be indicated.

  ii. Iodine contrast reaction

    (a) Mechanism: Allergic reaction (itching, rash, laryngospasm, swelling, or anaphylaxis)

    (b) Management: Treat with diphenhydramine (Benadryl) 25 to 50 mg orally, epinephrine 0.5 to 1 ml (1:1000 IV), IV steroids

  iii. Acute coronary occlusion

    (a) Mechanism: Results from dissection

    (b) Management: Emergency CABG in fewer than 0.5% of cases

  iv. MI: See ST-Segment Elevation Myocardial Infarction

8. Evaluation of patient care

  a. Patient is free from cardiac pain

  b. Patient has no complications associated with the various angina therapies received

c. Patient and significant others have received education and written handouts and demonstrate understanding regarding the disease process, the rationale for therapy (medications, procedures), symptoms to report, applicable risk factors to modify and a plan for accomplishment, and follow-up care

Acute Coronary Syndromes: Unstable Angina Pectoris and Non–ST-Segment Elevation Myocardial Infarction

Unstable angina and non–ST-segment elevation myocardial infarction (NSTEMI) have similar pathophysiology, presentations, and therapy. Unstable angina is not, however, associated with elevations in the levels of cardiac biomarkers (troponins).

1. **Pathophysiology:** Whereas chronic stable angina (ischemia) results when myocardial oxygen demand outstrips supply, acute coronary syndromes result from abrupt, nonexertional plaque rupture, thrombosis, vasoconstriction, or arterial occlusion, often with subsequent reperfusion
   a. Coronary occlusion
       i. Plaque rupture
      ii. Platelet-mediated thrombosis
     iii. Vasoconstriction
      iv. Arterial occlusion (subtotal or total)
   b. Coronary spasm (Prinzmetal's angina) can temporarily occlude coronary artery flow
   c. Restenosis after PCI can create an obstruction to blood flow without spasm or thrombus
   d. Severity and number of obstructions, availability of collateral circulation, and amount of thrombus all factor into the clinical presentation
2. **Etiology and risk factors**
   a. Precipitating factor: Atherosclerotic plaque
   b. Risk factors: The common risk factors of CAD
   c. Identifiers of patients at high risk
       i. Prolonged pain (particularly at rest)
      ii. Arrhythmias: Bradycardias, tachycardias
     iii. Hypotension
      iv. Transient ST changes during pain
       v. New mitral regurgitation murmur, S_3, crackles
      vi. New BBB
3. **Signs and symptoms**
   a. Subjective and objective findings: Same as for chronic stable angina, except for the following:
       i. Symptoms occur at rest
      ii. Symptoms usually last longer than 20 minutes
   b. Physical findings
       i. Fear
      ii. Minimal movement
     iii. Possible clutching of chest
      iv. Tachycardia (increased sympathetic tone)
       v. Transient mitral regurgitation—new murmur
      vi. Transient rales—new symptom
     vii. Transient S_3, S_4
    viii. Hypotension
4. **Diagnostic study findings**
   a. Laboratory

        i. Levels of troponins or CK-MB isoenzymes are not elevated in unstable angina. Levels of troponins (cardiac troponin T and troponin I) are more than 0.1 ng/ml in NSTEMI.

           (a) Elevations noticeable 4 to 12 hours after onset of symptoms

           (b) Follow-up sampling needed at 8 to 12 hours

           (c) Elevations in troponin levels are strong prognostic indicators of mortality risk

       ii. CBC: Check for cause of anemia (decreased oxygen supply)

      iii. Creatinine, BUN levels: Assess renal function (for dye administration, heparinization)

      iv. C-reactive protein (inflammatory marker) and BNP (indicates ventricular dilatation, pressure overload) are markers used to evaluate risk for future events

   b. ECG: May or may not show evidence of myocardial injury or ischemia (see ST-Segment Elevation Myocardial Infarction)

       i. Transient ST changes with pain: Occurrence of ST changes with symptoms and at rest are highly suggestive of ischemia and probably severe CAD

      ii. ST depression

     iii. Inverted T-wave changes

     iv. New BBB

      v. Sustained VT

   c. Echocardiography: May or may not show transient abnormal wall motion, valve dysfunction, hypertrophy. Identifies LV dysfunction.

   d. Dobutamine stress echocardiography: Demonstrates ischemia, stress-induced wall motion abnormalities, ventricular dysfunction, ischemic mitral regurgitation

   e. Myocardial scintigraphy (thallium, Tc 99m sestamibi) with pharmacologic stress (adenosine, dipyridamole) may demonstrate ischemia, infarction, and LV dysfunction

   f. Coronary catheterization

5. Goals of care

   a. Ischemia, MI, and death are prevented by

       i. Decreasing myocardial oxygen demand

      ii. Improving myocardial oxygen supply

   b. Disease process is modified

       i. Antiplatelet and antithrombin therapy

      ii. Lifestyle modifications (smoking cessation; diet; weight, blood pressure, and glucose control)

6. Collaborating professionals on health care team: See Chronic Stable Angina

7. Management of patient care

   a. Anticipated patient trajectory: Therapy with effective antiplatelet agents and prompt angiography have resulted in significant gains in infarct prevention and myocardial preservation

       i. Positioning: See Chronic Stable Angina

      ii. Nutrition: Low-fat, low-sodium diet

     iii. Discharge planning: See Chronic Stable Angina

     iv. Pharmacology: Pain and ischemia management

        (a) NTG: Rapid-acting nitrate

           (1) Actions

             a) Dilates veins and arteries

             b) Decreases venous return by systemic pooling of blood: Decreases preload

          c) Reduces myocardial oxygen demand and consumption

          d) Relieves coronary artery spasm

       (2) Dosages

          a) Sublingually 0.4 mg every 5 minutes; up to three doses

          b) IV drip started at 5 to 10 mcg/min. Titrate until pain is relieved or adverse side effects occur (hypotension).

       (3) IV solution readily absorbed into plastic bags and tubing, so glass bottles used

       (4) Do not stop IV NTG abruptly. Wean gradually; observe for returning symptoms. Once dosage is 10 mcg/min, stop NTG after 15 minutes.

       (5) Side effects include hypotension, headache, sweating, nausea, tachycardia, bradycardia

       (6) If IV NTG results in decreased blood pressure, give fluid bolus and place patient in Trendelenburg's position

       (7) Patients often develop tolerance of NTG's hemodynamic effects after 12 to 24 hours of administration. Infusion rate may need to be adjusted with continued use. If an NTG patch is used, it may be discontinued for 8 to 12 hours each day (usually at nighttime).

       (8) NTG should not be taken within 24 hours of taking sildenafil (Viagra) because severe hypotension may result from the drugs' combined vasodilatory effects

   (b) Morphine sulfate: Analgesic, anxiolytic

       (1) Used when NTG is ineffective for pain relief or symptoms of pulmonary edema are present

       (2) Doses of 1 to 5 mg IV

   (c) β-blockers (e.g., atenolol, metoprolol)

       (1) Action

          a) Decrease angina

          b) Decrease heart rate and contractility

          c) Decrease myocardial oxygen demand

          d) Increase diastolic filling time

          e) Increase exercise tolerance

       (2) IV administration initially is used for continued chest pain

       (3) Contraindications: Bronchial asthma, heart failure (unless caused by ischemia), AV blocks, hypotension

       (4) Side effects: Hypoglycemia, arrhythmias (including conduction blocks), central nervous system effects (decreased energy, decreased libido, nightmares, confusion), gastrointestinal effects (diarrhea, nausea, constipation)

       (5) Sudden withdrawal of the drug can have rebound effects (including angina, hypertension, MI). Gradual withdrawal or adjustment should be made, unless an emergency (e.g., bradycardia) mandates immediate discontinuation.

   (d) Calcium channel antagonists: Nondihydropyridines (e.g., verapamil or diltiazem)

       (1) Actions

          a) Negative inotropic; negative chronotropic effects on SA and AV conductive tissue

          b) Increase angina threshold, reduce ischemia, increase exercise tolerance, decrease afterload

          c) Vasodilators help to improve myocardial blood supply

(2) Use cautiously in combination with β-blockers due to possible adverse effect on heart rate and LV function suppression

(3) Contraindications: Aortic valve disease, severe anemia, AV blocks, Wolff-Parkinson-White (WPW) syndrome (verapamil)

(e) ACE inhibitors: Used if hypertension continues in a patient receiving NTG, β-blockers, especially when caused by LV dysfunction or heart failure symptoms

v. Pharmacology: Antiplatelet and antithrombotic combination therapy (Table 3-7)

(a) Aspirin: Blocks only one pathway to platelet aggregation

(b) Glycoprotein IIb/IIIa (GPIIb/IIIa) receptor blockers

(1) Block the final common pathway of platelet aggregation

(2) Therefore, may be ideal in treating acute coronary syndromes

vi. Psychosocial issues: See Chronic Stable Angina

vii. Treatments (See also Chronic Stable Angina)

(a) PCI: Early invasive strategy is recommended for patients with the following:

(1) Angina or ischemia recurring at rest or with minimal activity with aggressive medical therapy

(2) Angina or ischemia recurring with symptoms of heart failure (S$_3$, pulmonary edema, increased crackles, new or worse mitral regurgitation)

(3) EF of less than 40%

(4) Hemodynamic instability, hypotension with angina at rest

(5) PCI within 6 months previously

(6) Prior CABG

(7) Sustained VT

(b) CABG: See Chronic Stable Angina

(c) IABP: See Heart Failure

(d) VAD: See Heart Failure

b. Potential complications: See Chronic Stable Angina

8. Evaluation of patient care: See Chronic Stable Angina

ST-Segment Elevation Myocardial Infarction

ST-elevation myocardial infarction (STEMI) is characterized by the necrosis of myocardial tissue due to the interruption of coronary perfusion to the myocardium

1. Pathophysiology (see also Coronary Artery Disease)

a. Blood flow may be obstructed acutely by a thrombus in the coronary artery

b. Site and amount of necrosis depend on the location of the arterial occlusion, on collateral circulation, and on the previous occurrence of any infarctions or disease

c. Extent of necrosis

i. Transmural: Full thickness (endocardium to epicardium) STEMI

ii. Nontransmural: Non–Q wave (subendocardial)

d. See also Acute Coronary Syndromes

2. Etiology and risk factors

a. Atherosclerotic CAD (see also Coronary Artery Disease): Slow, progressive coronary artery narrowing with an acute ruptured plaque that develops into an occlusive thrombotic lesion. Most prevalent cause of MI.

b. Coronary artery spasm

c. Severe anemia (decreased oxygen supply)

d. Severe aortic stenosis

■ **TABLE 3-7**
■ ■ **Pharmacologic Antiplatelet and Antithrombotic Combination Therapy**

Drug	Actions	Administration	Comments
Aspirin	Platelet inhibition and antiinflammatory properties	Initial dosing of 325 mg, non–enteric coated, taken as soon as possible after symptom onset Daily doses of 75-160 mg	Adverse side effects of bleeding, gastrointestinal (GI) distress are minimized with lower dosages
Adenosine diphosphate (ADP) antagonist (e.g., clopidogrel, ticlopidine)	Interferes early in process of platelet thrombus development, inhibits and diminishes platelet aggregation	Clopidogrel • Acts rapidly (therapeutic levels within 2 hr) when loading dose of 300-600 mg given • Daily dose of 75 mg is given for up to 1 yr after percutaneous coronary intervention (PCI) Ticlopidine • Requires several days of therapy before reaching maximum effectiveness • Loading dose is 500 mg • Daily dose of 250 mg bid	If patient needs coronary artery bypass graft, clopidogrel ideally should be withheld for 5-7 days before surgery to minimize bleeding complications Used also if patient is intolerant to aspirin (allergy, GI disturbances, bleeding disorders) Routine blood monitoring (platelet and white blood cell counts) required when taking drug to identify neutropenia (occurs in 2% of patients) thrombotic thrombocytopenic purpura (occurs in 0.03%, more fatal)
Heparin: Unfractionated heparin (UFH)	Anticoagulant agents	For UFH a weight-based dose is given, 60-70 units/kg intravenous (IV) bolus (maximum 5000 units) • Initially 12-15 units/kg/hr (maximum 1000 units/hr) to reach activated partial thromboplastin time (aPTT) goal of 1.5-2 times control	Close blood monitoring required routinely (every 6 hr until therapeutic level reached and with dosage changes) to ensure tight PTT goal maintenance control Given in conjunction with aspirin (unless contraindicated) Monitor for heparin-induced thrombocytopenia

Low-molecular-weight heparin (LMWH)		LMWH (e.g., enoxaparin) is administered 1 mg/kg subcutaneously every 12 hr	Advantages: Avoidance of need for close blood monitoring, less likely to induce thrombocytopenia Disadvantages: More frequent minor bleeding events are seen with its use
Glycoprotein IIb/IIIa blockers and receptor inhibitors: (e.g., eptifibatide, tirofiban, abciximab)	Prevent binding of von Willebrand factor and fibrinogen, combating platelet aggregation Significantly reduce death or myocardial infarction in short term Used with aspirin and heparin for patients who undergo early PCI, or are at high risk for intervention	Administered IV only for set time periods and at set dosages (before, during, and after PCI) Present dosing regimens: Eptifibatide: 180 mcg/kg bolus, then 2 mcg/kg/min for 72-96 hr Tirofiban: 0.4 mcg/kg/min for 30 min, then 0.1 mcg/kg/min for 48-96 hr Abciximab: 0.25 mcg/kg bolus, then 0.125 mcg/kg/min (max 10 mcg/min) for 12-24 hr	Oral glycoprotein IIb-IIIa receptor inhibitors have not proven effective or safe to date
Thrombolytics	Not appropriate and harmful in this setting		May increase risk of myocardial infarction

e. Other causes include hyperthyroidism, emboli (endocarditis, atrial fibrillation), trauma, dissection, drugs (cocaine)

f. Other precipitating factors include acute hypotension, ventricular tachyarrhythmias

g. Risk factors: See Coronary Artery Disease

3. **Signs and symptoms**

a. Patient history alone continues to be sufficient to rule in MI, even in the absence of ECG changes; 10% of patients with acute MI have normal ECG initially

b. Discomfort in the chest that has lasted longer than 20 to 30 minutes and is unrelieved by rest or nitrates. May radiate to neck, jaw, arms, and back. These areas may be the only locations of discomfort. Similar to angina in the character of the discomfort, but usually more intense and longer in duration (see Chronic Stable Angina for a description).

c. Other findings vary with the size and extent of the infarction, the patient's status, and the history of previous MI

   i. Pallid, diaphoretic, cool, clammy skin

   ii. Weakness, light-headedness

   iii. Vagal effects (bradycardia, nausea, and vomiting)

   iv. Dyspnea (most common presentation in the elderly)

   v. Arrhythmias

   vi. Low, normal, or high blood pressure

   vii. Irregular, slow, fast, and/or thready pulse

   viii. Apprehension, physically "stillness"

   ix. S_3: Diastolic (ventricular) gallop (in acute LV failure)

   x. Ankle edema

   xi. Crackles in acute LV failure

   xii. Murmurs

   xiii. Pericardial friction rub

4. **Diagnostic study findings**

a. Laboratory

   i. Troponins

     (a) Troponin I level: Diagnostic of MI (false elevations in renal insufficiency)

     (b) Troponin T level: Can be elevated in skeletal muscle injury

     (c) Remain elevated for days

   ii. CK-MB isoenzyme levels elevated within 6 hours. May be dissipated if 24 hours since the onset of symptoms. CK-MB levels have dramatic elevation with reperfusion therapy and decrease quickly.

   iii. Leukocytosis (large MI) due to stress and tissue necrosis; peaks 2 to 4 days after the infarction

b. ECG: Most important diagnostic tool; changes on ECG correlate with the location of the necrosis (as opposed to ST changes) (Table 3-8)

   i. ECG signs of MI: Necrosis (cell death)

     (a) Acute ST elevation

     (b) Abnormal Q wave

       (1) More than 0.04 seconds in duration (0.03 seconds for inferior MI)

       (2) Appears within hours of transmural MI

   ii. Other causes of Q waves

     (a) Normal Q waves; small Q wave in leads I, aVL, V_5, V_6, aVR

     (b) Normal Q wave in lead III: Less than 0.03 seconds, decreased with inspiration

     (c) LBBB

     (d) Myocarditis, cardiomyopathy

■ **TABLE 3-8**
■ ■ **Acute Myocardial Infarction: Infarct Area, Electrocardiographic (ECG) Evidence, Associated Coronary Arteries, and Potential Complications**

Area of Infarct	ECG Evidence		Associated Coronary Artery	Potential Complications
	Leads Reflecting Infarct Area Directly	Leads Reflecting Reciprocal Changes		
Left Ventricle				
Lateral wall, high	I, aVL	II, III, aVF	Left circumflex	Pump failure, conduction disturbances
Inferior wall	II, III, aVF	I, aVL, V_5, V_6	Right coronary, possibly left circumflex	Sinoatrial and atrioventricular nodal conduction disturbances; valve dysfunction
Septal wall	V_1-V_2	II, III, aVF	Left anterior descending	Pump failure, conduction disturbance
Anterior wall	V_2-V_4	II, III, aVF	Left anterior descending	Pump failure, conduction disturbance
Lateral wall, low (apical area)	V_5-V_6	II, III, aVF	Left anterior descending	Pump failure, conduction disturbance
Posterior	V_7-V_9*	V_1-V_3	Posterior descending, right coronary, or left circumflex	Atrioventricular nodal conduction disturbance
Right Ventricle†	V_4R	—	Right coronary	Atrioventricular nodal disturbance, valve dysfunction, hypotension

From Bucher L, Melander S: *Critical care nursing*, Philadelphia, 1999, Saunders, p 230.
*Leads are placed on the left posterior chest wall at the fifth intercostal space, beginning at the left posterior axillary line.
†Right ventricular infarction is present in approximately one third of patients with inferior myocardial infarctions, and assessment of this lead should be performed routinely in all patients diagnosed with an acute inferior myocardial infarction.

    iii. Determination of the age of the infarction (Table 3-9)
    iv. Serial ECGs are essential, along with those done during ischemic pain
  c. Echocardiography: Assesses LV function, wall motion abnormalities, and complications such as VSD, thrombi, aneurysms, mitral regurgitation, pericardial effusions
  d. Coronary catheterization
5. Goals of care
  a. Patient has no pain
  b. Patient has limited myocardial injury due to reperfusion (through thrombolysis or PCI)

■ **TABLE 3-9**
■ **Changes in the Facing Electrocardiographic (ECG) Leads During the Four Phases of a Transmural, Q-Wave Myocardial Infarction**

Phase of Infarction	Q Waves	R Waves	ST Segments	T Waves	ECG
Phase 1 (0-2 hr): Onset of extensive ischemia occurs immediately, subendocardial injury occurs within 20-40 min, and subendocardial necrosis occurs in about 30 min; necrosis extends to about half of the myocardial wall by 2 hr	Unchanged	Unchanged or abnormally tall	Onset of elevation	Amplitude increases; peaking may occur	
Phase 2 (2-24 hr): Transmural infarction is considered complete by 6 hr as necrosis involves about 90% of the myocardial wall; the rest of the necrosis occurs by the end of phase 2	Width and depth begin to increase	Amplitude begins to decrease	Maximum elevation	Amplitude and peaking lessen; T waves still positive	
Phase 3 (24-72 hr): Little or no ischemia or injury remains as healing begins	Reach maximum size	Absent	Return to baseline	Become maximally inverted	
Phase 4 (2-8 wk): Necrotic tissue is replaced by fibrous tissue	Q waves persist	May return partially	Usually normal	Slight inversion	

From Huszar RJ: *Basic dysrhythmias: interpretation and management*, ed 3, St Louis, 2002, Mosby, p 330.

    c. Patient has adequate hemodynamic parameters

    d. Arrhythmias are absent or controlled

6. Collaborating professionals on health care team: See Chronic Stable Angina

7. Management of patient care

    a. Anticipated patient trajectory: Minimizing time to thrombolytic or PCI therapy increases survival and preservation of myocardial function

        i. Positioning

            (a) Maintain bed rest for the first 12 hours, with use of a bedside commode

            (b) Postprocedure issues: Leg or arm immobilization, head of bed lower than 15 degrees (dependent on closure protocols)

            (c) Early immobilization is important: Use of a chair or bedside commode in the first 24 hours (improves well-being, lowers risk of pulmonary embolus)

            (d) Increase ambulation in room as tolerated during the first 48 hours

        ii. Pain management

            (a) Relieve discomfort with analgesics

                (1) Relief of pain decreases elevated sympathetic response and myocardial workload (lowering heart rate and blood pressure) and counters the arrhythmic effect of circulating catecholamines

                (2) Morphine: 2 to 4 mg IV every 5 minutes to relieve pain

                    a) Decrease dosages in the elderly and in patients with respiratory disease

                    b) Respiratory depression with morphine sulfate usually peaks 7 minutes after IV injection and is dose related (not usually a problem in patients with MI)

                    c) Orthostatic hypotension can result from volume depletion: Provide volume support and keep the patient in Trendelenburg's position

                    d) Naloxone, 0.4 mg IV (repeated up to 3 times at 3-minute intervals), may be given to counteract narcotic-induced depressed respirations and hypotension

                (3) Remind the patient to notify the nurse immediately if discomfort recurs

            (b) Antiemetics (e.g., droperidol) may be necessary because of the high degree of acute vagal tone with MI and the emetic side effects of opiate analgesia

            (c) Anxiolytics (e.g., benzodiazepines, haloperidol) may be used if the patient is agitated, delirious, or very anxious, experiences sleep deprivation, or has intensive care unit psychosis

        iii. Nutrition

            (a) Keep the patient on NPO status until the discomfort or pain is gone, then give clear liquids and progress the diet

            (b) Feed a low-fat, low-sodium diet

            (c) Earlier "coronary precautions" have now been abandoned (e.g., restriction of hot and cold fluids, avoidance of caffeine; regular caffeine drinkers develop tolerance and can experience withdrawal symptoms of increased heart rate or headaches; several cups of coffee have no ill effects)

        iv. Discharge planning

            (a) Teaching issues include the rationales for and descriptions of therapy, methods for treating discomfort or pain at home

            (b) Stress smoking cessation after MI. Patient may need nicotine replacement if he or she is a heavy smoker or has withdrawal symptoms.

v. Pharmacology
  (a) Oxygen: 2 to 4 L/min to keep oxygen saturation above 90%. Hypoxemia is due to ventilation-perfusion mismatch and LV failure.
  (b) NTG: Sublingual, IV infusions (see Acute Coronary Syndromes)
  (c) β-blockers: Reduce myocardial ischemia and increase hospital survival rates. Usually IV β-blockers (e.g., metoprolol, 10 mg IV; atenolol, 5 mg IV) given initially to ensure rapid lowering of heart rate, blood pressure.
  (d) ACE inhibitors: For patients with anterior MI, pulmonary congestion, LV EF of less than 40% (unless systolic blood pressure is less than 100 mm Hg). Contraindicated in renal failure.
  (e) ARBs: For patients intolerant of ACE inhibitors
  (f) Antiplatelet-antithrombotic therapy
    (1) Aspirin is given immediately. Usually 325 mg, chewed. Daily dose of 81 mg.
    (2) Clopidogrel used if the patient cannot take aspirin and after PCI
    (3) Heparin (low molecular weight): See Table 3-7
    (4) GPIIb/IIIa receptor blockers if direct PCI planned
  (g) Thrombolytics: See Table 3-10
  (h) Stool softeners
  (i) Statins: Lipid-lowering therapy. Goal is LDL level of less than 100 mg/dl (the lower, the better).

vi. Psychosocial issues
  (a) Denial is an emotion many patients exhibit, both prior to admission and during hospitalization
  (b) Flexible visiting hours can assist in relieving anxiety and other stress that can create a situation promoting pain occurrence (depending on the patient's status, need for rest, procedures, and family dynamics)

vii. Treatments
  (a) Place the patient on a monitor. Watch closely for arrhythmias, because VF is common in the early hours of MI.
  (b) Ensure that the patient has at least two good IV sites for administration of drugs, volume support, reperfusion therapy
  (c) RV MI: Preload is vital for maintaining forward output in RV MI. Ensure that the patient has sufficient volume before giving NTG due to the high risk of hypotension. Goal: CVP of 15 to 20 mm Hg.
  (d) Primary PCI: PCI with stenting to open the occluded artery and limit myocardial necrosis. Indicated if
    (1) Available
    (2) Door to stent is less than 1 hour
    (3) Emergency medical service (EMS) to stent is less than 90 minutes
    (4) Pain is present less than 3 hours
  (e) Thrombolysis (see Table 3-10 and Box 3-6): IV thrombolytic as soon as possible (in the emergency department, EMS, critical care unit)
    (1) If PCI not available
    (2) If door to PCI is more than 1 hour
    (3) If EMS to PCI is more than 90 minutes
    (4) There is no difference between tissue plasminogen activator (t-PA) and streptokinase if used early (within the first hour)
  (f) IABP may be necessary for severe hypotension or cardiogenic shock, especially in patients with low CO and ongoing ischemia (see Heart Failure). IABP is used during MI for the following:

■ **TABLE 3-10**
■ ■ **Thrombolytic Agents**

Agent	Dosing	Comments
Alteplase (t-PA): Recombinant form of human tissue plasminogen activator	Half-life: <5 min Dosage: • 15-mg bolus • Follow with 0.75-mg/kg infusion over 30 min (not >50 mg) • Then 0.5 mg/kg over 60 min (not >35 mg) • Maximum dose = 100 mg	Concurrent heparin required to avoid reocclusion (goal is partial thromboplastin time of 50-75 sec) Aspirin also given Disadvantages: • Complex dosing schedule • Expensive • Contraindicated with gentamicin allergy (drug used in preparation of t-PA)
Reteplase (r-PA): Recombinant plasminogen activator	Half-life: 14-18 min Dosage: Two 10 million unit boluses, 30 min apart	Advantage: Two intravenous (IV) doses Disadvantage: Expensive
Tenecteplase (TNK-tPA): Genetically mutant tissue plasminogen activator	Half-life: 20-24 min Dosage: • 30-50 mg IV push (0.5-0.55 mg/kg) • Maximum dose: 50 mg (for patient >90 kg)	Advantages • Higher clot specificity • Single dose Disadvantage: Expensive
Streptokinase (SK): First-generation thrombolytic	Half-life: 30 min Dosage: 1.5 million units IV over 1 hr	Advantage: Inexpensive Disadvantages: • Lacks specificity • Allergic reactions in 5.8% • Occasional hypotension • Contraindicated if previous SK therapy or if recent streptococcal infection (increases risk of allergy)
Combination therapy	Decreased dose of plasminogen activator plus full dose of glycoprotein IIb/IIIa inhibitor (abciximab, eptifibatide, tirofiban)	Being trialed with good results

      (1) Acute mitral regurgitation
      (2) Refractory ventricular arrhythmias
      (3) Post-MI angina
      (4) As a bridge to revascularization
  b. Potential complications
    i. Postinfarction pain (persistent, recurrent)
      (a) Mechanism: Common causes are ischemia, reinfarction, pericarditis (Dressler's syndrome). Pericarditis does not occur in the first 24 hours.
      (b) Management
        (1) When pain is present, obtain an ECG and compare with previous ECGs
        (2) Pain recurring after MI suggests ongoing ischemia and should be treated promptly
    ii. Cardiogenic shock
      (a) Mechanism: Seen in the first 48 hours, especially with large anterior MI, due to ischemia or with severe mitral regurgitation

■ **BOX 3-6**

■ **CONTRAINDICATIONS AND CAUTIONS FOR THE USE OF FIBRINOLYSIS IN ST-SEGMENT ELEVATION MYOCARDIAL INFARCTION***

ABSOLUTE CONTRADICTIONS
- Any prior intracranial hemorrhage
- Known structural cerebral vascular lesion (e.g., arteriovenous malformation)
- Known malignant intracranial neoplasm (primary or metastatic)
- Ischemic stroke within 3 months *except* acute ischemic stroke within 3 hours
- Suspected aortic dissection
- Active bleeding or bleeding diathesis (excluding menses)
- Significant closed head or facial trauma within 3 months

RELATIVE CONTRAINDICATIONS
- History of chronic, severe, poorly controlled hypertension
- Severe uncontrolled hypertension on presentation (systolic blood pressure higher than 180 mm Hg or diastolic blood pressure higher than 110 mm Hg)†
- History of prior ischemic stroke longer than 3 months ago, dementia, or known intracranial pathology not covered in contraindications
- Traumatic or prolonged (longer than 10 minutes) cardiopulmonary resuscitation or major surgery (less than 3 weeks ago)
- Recent (within 2 to 4 weeks) internal bleeding
- Noncompressible vascular punctures
- For streptokinase or anistreplase: Prior exposure (more than 5 days ago) or prior allergic reaction to these agents
- Pregnancy
- Active peptic ulcer
- Current use of anticoagulants: The higher the international normalized ratio, the higher the risk of bleeding

From Antman DM, Anbe DT, Armstrong PW, et al: ACC/AHA guidelines for the management of patients with ST-elevation myocardial infarction: executive summary: a report of the ACC/AHA Task Force on Practice Guidelines (Committee to Revise the 1999 Guidelines on the Management of Patients with Acute Myocardial Infarction), *J Am Coll Cardiol* 44(3):671-719, 2004.
*Viewed as advisory for clinical decision making and may not be all-inclusive or definitive.
†Could be an absolute contraindication in low-risk patients with ST-segment elevation myocardial infarction (see Section 6.3.1.6.3.2 of the full-text guidelines).

(b) Management: See Heart Failure and Shock
iii. Arrhythmias: Atrial fibrillation, VT, VF, bradyarrhythmias
    (a) Mechanism: See Cardiac Rhythm Disorders
    (b) Management
       (1) Monitor the patient's ECG and watch for hypotension and brady-cardia
       (2) Watch for reperfusion arrhythmias. In the initial period after coronary blood flow is restored, ventricular arrhythmias frequently occur.
       (3) AV sequential pacing may be required for increasing CO (blocks are common)
       (4) Instruct the patient to avoid Valsalva maneuvers: Cause dramatic changes in heart rate and blood pressure (ventricular filling) and can cause arrhythmias (especially in patients younger than 45 years of age)
iv. Other complications

    (a) Reocclusion: Symptoms include ST-segment changes, chest discomfort, arrhythmias, hypotension

    (b) LV thrombus: More likely with a CK rise of more than 3200 IU/L. Treatment includes anticoagulation for 3 to 6 months.

    (c) VSDs: Surgical repair is needed immediately if the patient is hemodynamically unstable or if CO is low (IABP, inotropic drugs, vasodilators, surgical or catheter-based closure)

    (d) LV aneurysm: Surgical repair is often combined with CABG, valve repair

    (e) Severe acute mitral regurgitation: IABP, inotropic drugs, catheterization, surgery

    (f) Rupture of LV free wall or papillary muscle rupture (Table 3-11): Volume support, IABP, vasoactive medications, surgery. Majority of patients with free wall rupture do not survive.

8. Evaluation of patient care

  a. Patient has no pain

  b. Coronary artery flow is restored within 30 to 90 minutes

  c. Patient has adequate hemodynamic parameters (CO) without mechanical support

  d. Arrhythmias are controlled or absent

  e. Peripheral pulses are present and circulation is good

  f. Patient verbalizes knowledge of home care and follow-up requirements

Heart Failure

Heart failure is a clinical presentation of impaired cardiac function in which one or both ventricles are unable to maintain an output adequate to meet the metabolic demands of the body. Heart failure can occur on either the right or the left side of the heart and is due to systolic dysfunction (poor contraction), diastolic dysfunction (impaired filling), increased afterload (increased resistance), or alterations in heart rate (too fast, too slow).

1. Pathophysiology

  a. Left-sided heart failure, systolic dysfunction

    i. Impaired forward output caused by decreased LV contractility (e.g., CAD, cardiomyopathies) in which the EF is reduced to below normal

    ii. To compensate, the LV dilates and the heart rate increases in an attempt to maintain a normal output. This increase in the SV and heart rate may return the CO toward normal despite a poor EF

    iii. LV filling pressures rise because of increased preload or decreased LV compliance (producing LV diastolic dysfunction)

    iv. LA and pulmonary venous pressures rise, producing pulmonary congestion and edema

      (a) When pulmonary capillary oncotic pressure (30 mm Hg) is exceeded, fluid leaks into the pulmonary interstitial space, creating pulmonary edema

      (b) Decreased oxygenation of the blood occurs as oxygen exchange is impeded by the presence of fluid

    v. Right-sided heart pressure increases as a result of increased pressure in the pulmonary system

    vi. Right-sided heart failure may then occur because of the pulmonary hypertension, resulting in peripheral and organ edema

  b. Left-sided heart failure, diastolic dysfunction

    i. A noncompliant, stiff LV (due to hypertrophy, ischemia, infiltration, scarring) has less ability to relax, which interferes with adequate filling and results in rising diastolic (filling) pressures

TABLE 3-11
■ Characteristics of Ventricular Septal Rupture, Rupture of the Ventricular Free Wall, and Papillary Muscle Rupture

Characteristic	Ventricular Septal Rupture	Rupture of Ventricular Free Wall	Papillary Muscle Rupture
Incidence	1%–3% without reperfusion therapy, 0.2%–0.34% with fibrinolytic therapy, 3.9% among patients with cardiogenic shock	0.8%–6.2%; fibrinolytic therapy does not reduce risk; primary percutaneous transluminal coronary angioplasty seems to reduce risk	About 1% (posteromedial more frequent than anterolateral papillary muscle)
Time course	Bimodal peak; within 24 hr and 3-5 days; range, 1-14 days	Bimodal peak; within 24 hr and 3-5 days; range, 1-14 days	Bimodal peak; within 24 hr and 3-5 days; range, 1-14 days
Clinical manifestations	Chest pain, shortness of breath, hypotension	Anginal, pleuritic, or pericardial chest pain; syncope; hypotension; arrhythmia; nausea; restlessness; hypotension; sudden death	Abrupt onset of shortness of breath and pulmonary edema, hypotension
Physical findings	Harsh holosystolic murmur, thrill (positive), S_3, accentuated second heart sound, pulmonary edema, right ventricular (RV) and left ventricular (LV) failure, cardiogenic shock	Jugulovenous distention (29% of patients), pulsus paradoxus (47%), electromechanical dissociation, cardiogenic shock	Soft murmur in some cases, no thrill, variable signs of RV overload, severe pulmonary edema, cardiogenic shock
Echocardiographic findings	Ventricular septal rupture, left-to-right shunt on color flow Doppler echocardiography through the ventricular septum, pattern of RV overload	Greater than 5-mm pericardial effusion not visualized in all cases; layered, high-acoustic echoes within the pericardium (blood clot); direct visualization of tear; signs of tamponade	Hypercontractile LV, torn papillary muscle or chordae tendineae, flail leaflet, severe mitral regurgitation on color flow Doppler echocardiography
Right-heart catheterization findings	Increase in oxygen saturation from right atrium (RA) to RV, large V waves	Ventriculography insensitive, classic signs of tamponade not always present (equalization of diastolic pressures among the cardiac chambers)	No increase in oxygen saturation from the RA to RV, large P waves, * very high pulmonary capillary wedge pressures

From Antman DM, Anbe DT, Armstrong PW, et al: ACC/AHA guidelines for the management of patients with ST-elevation myocardial infarction: executive summary: a report of the ACC/AHA Task Force on Practice Guidelines (Committee to Revise the 1999 Guidelines on the Management of Patients with Acute Myocardial Infarction), *J Am Coll Cardiol* 44(3):671–719, 2004. Modified with permission from Birnbaum Y, Fischbein MC, Blanche C, Siegel RJ: Ventricular septal rupture after acute myocardial infarction, *N Engl J Med* 347:1426–1432, 2002. Copyright 2002 Massachusetts Medical Society.

*Large V waves are from the pulmonary capillary wedge pressure.

      ii. As a consequence, LA, pulmonary venous, and pulmonary capillary pressures increase

      iii. Pulmonary artery and right-sided heart pressures rise if the condition is untreated

      iv. Systolic function is often normal and accounts for the fact that up to 30% to 50% of patients with "heart failure" have normal LV systolic function

  c. Right-sided heart failure, systolic dysfunction

      i. The right side of the heart is unable to pump blood forward adequately, which results in a drop in CO

      ii. Causes include pulmonary hypertension (most common) as well as RV MI

      iii. RV dilatation and elevation of filling pressure develop, which results in peripheral edema

  d. Right-sided heart failure, diastolic dysfunction: Can occur with RV hypertrophy and cardiomyopathies; analogous to left-sided heart diastolic dysfunction, except the consequence is peripheral edema rather than pulmonary edema, associated with elevated right-sided heart filling pressures (increased jugular venous pressures).

  e. Four stages of heart failure progression:

      i. Stage A: High risk of heart failure, no cardiac structural disorders

      ii. Stage B: Structural defect or disorder of the heart, no symptoms of heart failure

      iii. Stage C: Structural defect or disorder of the heart, present or past symptoms of heart failure

      iv. Stage D: End-stage cardiac disease; the patient needs continuous therapy (inotropic drugs, mechanical supports, transplantation, hospice care)

2. Etiology and risk factors: See Table 3-12 for factors related to left- and right-sided heart failure

3. Signs and symptoms: Patients generally have asymptomatic heart failure for an uncertain time before the recognition of symptoms. Decrease in activity tolerance and/or fluid retention are generally the first complaints identified.

  a. History: See Table 3-13 for clinical findings in left- and right-sided heart failure

  b. Physical examination of patient

      i. See Table 3-13

      ii. Functional therapeutic classification of patients with heart failure

         (a) I: Symptoms occur with strong exertion

         (b) II: Symptoms occur with normal exertion

         (c) III: Symptoms occur with minimal exertion

         (d) IV: Symptoms occur at rest

4. Diagnostic study findings

  a. Laboratory

      i. BNP level: Elevations reflect myocyte stretch and increased ventricular pressures; prognostic indicator

      ii. C-reactive protein level: May be elevated

      iii. HCT, Hb level: Assess for anemia

      iv. Electrolyte levels: Imbalances due to diuresis

      v. Thyroid stimulating hormone level: Hypothyroidism, hyperthyroidism causes

      vi. Renal function tests: BUN, creatinine levels

      vii. Liver function tests (right-sided failure)

     viii. Cardiac troponin, enzyme levels (if potential acute MI)

      ix. Human immunodeficiency virus (HIV) testing: If the patient is at high risk for this cause

■ **TABLE 3-12**
■ ■ **Etiologic or Precipitating Factors in Heart Failure**

Left-Sided Heart Failure		Right-Sided Heart Failure	Both Sides
Systolic	**Diastolic**		
Ischemic heart disease (50% of all cases)	Coronary artery disease	Left-sided heart failure	Patient noncompliant regarding
Myocardial infarction	Myocardial ischemia	Atherosclerotic heart disease	• Medications
Myocardial stunning, hibernation	Left ventricular hypertrophy	Acute right ventricular myocardial	• Dietary restrictions
Coronary artery disease	Cardiomyopathy: hypertrophic,	infarction	• Alcohol use
Idiopathic dilated cardiomyopathy	restrictive, dilated	Pulmonary embolism	Medications
Myocardial contusion	Increased circulating volume	Fluid overload, excess sodium intake	• Negative inotropic agents
Aortic insufficiency	Cardiac tamponade	Myocardial contusion	• Causing sodium retention
Arrhythmias: Ventricular tachycardia, atrial	Constrictive pericarditis	Cardiomyopathy	
fibrillation	Left ventricular hypertrophy	Valvular heart disease	
Postpump syndrome	Mitral stenosis or insufficiency	Atrial or ventricular septal defect	
Myocarditis	Aortic stenosis or insufficiency	Pulmonary outflow stenosis	
Infectious: Viral, bacterial, fungal	Age (decreased compliance of heart	Chronic obstructive pulmonary disease	
Acute rheumatic fever	muscle)	Pulmonary hypertension (corpulmonale)	
Drug abuse: Heroin, alcohol, cocaine	Diabetes mellitus	Sleep apnea	
Nutrition deficits: Protein, thiamine	Intracardiac shunts		
Electrolyte disorders: Decrease in calcium,			
sodium, potassium, phosphate			
Diabetes, thyroid disease			
Drugs suppressing contractility (negative inotropic)			

███ **TABLE 3-13**
██ ██ **Clinical Findings in Heart Failure**

Left-Sided Heart Failure		Right-Sided Heart Failure
Systolic	**Diastolic**	
Anxiety	Exercise intolerance	Increased fatigue
Sudden light-headedness	Orthopnea	Hepatomegaly
Fatigue, weakness, lethargy	Dyspnea, dyspnea on	Splenomegaly
Orthopnea	exertion, paroxysmal	Dependent pitting edema
Dyspnea, dyspnea on exertion,	nocturnal dyspnea	Ascites
paroxysmal nocturnal dyspnea	Cough with frothy white or	Cachexia
Tachypnea (on exertion)	pink sputum	Abdominal pain (from congested
Cheyne-Stokes respirations	(in pulmonary edema)	liver)
(if severe)		
Diaphoresis	Tachypnea (on exertion)	Anorexia, nausea, emesis
Palpitations	Basilar crackles, rhonchi,	Weight gain
Sacral edema, pitting of	wheezes	Low blood pressure
extremities	Pulmonary edema	Oliguria, nocturia (increased renal
Basilar rales, rhonchi, crackles,	Symptoms of right-sided	perfusion, blood volume when
wheezes	heart failure	lying in bed)
Cool, moist, cyanotic skin	Hypoxia, respiratory acidosis	Venous distention
Hypoxia, respiratory acidosis	Elevated pulmonary artery	Hepatojugular reflux
Elevated pulmonary artery	diastolic pressure,	Fatigue, weakness
diastolic pressure, pulmonary	pulmonary capillary	Kussmaul's sign (if constriction)
capillary wedge pressure	wedge pressure	Murmur of tricuspid insufficiency
Nocturia	S_3, S_4 heart sounds	S_3, S_4 heart sounds (right-sided)
Mental confusion	Holosystolic murmur	Elevated central venous pressure
Decreased pulse pressure	(if tricuspid, mitral	and right atrial and right
Pulsus alternans	regurgitation)	ventricular pressures
Lateral displacement of point of		
maximal impulse		
S_3, S_4 heart sounds		
Murmur of mitral insufficiency		

    b. Radiologic: Results often normal
        i. Pulmonary vasculature: Edema, congestion
        ii. Cardiac silhouette: May show cardiac chamber enlargement
        iii. Pleural effusion (left-sided failure)
        iv. Valve calcifications
    c. ECG
        i. Nonspecific changes
        ii. Arrhythmias, ischemic disease, conduction abnormalities, drug and electrolyte effects
    d. Echocardiogram: To assess
        i. Chamber size, wall thickness
        ii. Systolic and diastolic function
        iii. Thrombus formation
        iv. Valvular function
        v. Pericardial disease
    e. Radionuclide imaging
        i. Assessment of chamber function and volume
        ii. Myocardial perfusion imaging for ischemia, infarction

      f. Ultrafast CT and MRI: To assess structural abnormalities, tumors, vascular anomalies, pericardial disease

      g. Cardiac catheterization with arteriography: To assess

         i. Coronary anatomy (two thirds of patients have CAD as a contributing cause)

         ii. Pressures in right and left chambers

            (a) High filling pressures represent diastolic dysfunction

            (b) Diuretic and IV NTG use can create a false-negative result by artificially normalizing the filling pressures

         iii. Ventricular contractility

         iv. Valvular function, cardiac defects

5. Goals of care

    a. Symptoms are relieved

    b. Hemodynamics are stabilized rapidly (using diuretics, vasodilators, inotropic agents)

    c. Excess fluid is removed and edema is corrected

    d. Complications from arrhythmias are prevented

6. Collaborating professionals on health care team: See Chronic Stable Angina; also electrophysiologist, psychologist, home health aide, financial aid counselor

7. Management of patient care

    a. Anticipated patient trajectory: A common clinical cardiology problem with a poor prognosis. Quality of life and longevity can be improved dramatically with available medications and therapy.

       i. Positioning

          (a) Placement in reverse Trendelenburg's position and/or use of extra pillows may increase ease of breathing

          (b) Prevent complications of deep venous thrombosis by range-of-motion exercises, use of thromboembolic disease hose, pneumatic antiembolic stockings

      ii. Skin care: If the patient is on prolonged bed rest, institute measures to prevent the hazards of immobility

      iii. Pain management: Administer medications to alleviate discomfort, as ordered

      iv. Nutrition

         (a) Monitor intake and output closely

         (b) Closely observe restrictions on fluid (1000 to 1500 ml/day) and sodium

         (c) Weigh patient daily

      v. Discharge planning: Before discharge, the patient and/or significant others should be able to do the following:

         (a) Explain heart failure and its prognosis

         (b) List symptoms that indicate a worsening of the condition, whether from heart failure or from drug side effects. Patient should know when to call for medical advice to prevent rehospitalizations and complications.

         (c) Describe each current medication: Name, purpose, dosage, frequency, side effects, and benefits of compliance

         (d) Identify the lifestyle changes necessary to prevent recurrence

            (1) Diet and weight control

               a) Sodium restriction (diet, drugs)

               b) Fluid restrictions, as ordered

               c) Foods rich in potassium (important for patients taking loop diuretics)

               d) Daily weight monitoring

(2) Cessation of high-risk activities: Smoking, alcohol, and/or drug use

(3) Routine exercise: Increases exercise tolerance, decreases symptoms

(e) Identify the rationale for the control of blood pressure, lipid levels, diabetes

(f) Demonstrate how to take the pulse; recognize the need to have blood pressure taken routinely

(g) Verbalize the importance of follow-up care

vi. Pharmacology

(a) See Table 3-14 for drugs commonly used in the treatment of heart failure

(b) Avoid drugs that decrease myocardial contractility (except β-blockers)

(1) Antiarrhythmic drugs (except amiodarone)

(2) Calcium channel blocking agents (except for amlodipine, felodipine)

(3) NSAIDs: Cause sodium retention, renal insufficiency

(4) Chemotherapeutic drugs (e.g., daunorubicin, doxorubicin)

vii. Psychosocial issues

(a) Patient will likely need help at home (help arrange home services)

(b) Noncompliance with the prescribed diet, weight, fluid intake, and medications can be devastating with this disorder. Patient and significant others need education, support, and close follow-up

(c) Coping with a long-standing, progressive disease becomes a strain on both patient and caregivers. Assess for signs of depression.

(d) High costs of medications, hospitalizations, interventions create additional strains

viii. Treatments

(a) Biventricular pacing: Cardiac resynchronization therapy (CRT) has been shown to increase LV systolic function by synchronizing ventricular contraction so that the LV walls contract at the same time, which results in increased CO and improved remodeling. Pacemaker education (procedure, rationales, incision care, follow-up) is needed.

(b) IABP placement: May be necessary to stabilize the patient as a bridge to other interventions. Patient and significant others should be prepared for this procedure.

(1) Purposes of IABP

a) Decrease afterload

b) Decrease myocardial oxygen demands

c) Increase coronary perfusion

d) Increase CO and tissue perfusion

e) Prevent cardiogenic shock, limit size of infarctions

f) Limit myocardial ischemia

(2) Uses of IABP

a) Support in acute MI with cardiogenic shock

b) Circulatory support after CABG

c) Support in high-risk cardiac catheterizations

d) In severe ischemia, as a bridge to revascularization

(3) Placed percutaneously via the femoral artery into the descending thoracic aorta

(4) Inflation and deflation of the balloon are synchronized with the patient's ECG or arterial pressure waveform (Figures 3-15 and 3-16)

a) During ventricular diastole, the balloon is inflated. Augments diastolic pressures and increases coronary blood flow. Myocardial oxygen supply and contractility improve.

■ TABLE 3-14
■ Drugs Commonly Used to Treat Heart Failure in the Critical Care Setting

Agent	Action/Indications	Administration	Comments
Nesiritide (BNP)	Causes vasodilatation, ↑ renal blood flow, ↑ urinary output, and improved hemodynamics	Dosage: 2 mcg/kg IV bolus, then infusion starting at 0.01 mcg/kg/min (titrated up to 0.03 mcg/kg/min for maximum of 48 hr)	Drug is expensive at present, used if patient does not respond to first-line drugs ↑ BNP levels (false-positive BNP test result)
INOTROPIC AGENTS			
Phosphodiesterase inhibitors (milrinone)	↑ Myocardial contractility without increasing HR Relaxes vascular (arterial and venous) smooth muscle, producing peripheral vasodilatation (↓ afterload and preload)	Half-life: 20-45 min Dosage: 50 mcg/kg undiluted is administered over 10 min (loading dose), followed by a 0.375-0.75-mcg/kg/min infusion	Untoward effects include tachycardia, arrhythmias, hypotension (to correct hypovolemia)
Dobutamine (Dobutrex)	↑ Myocardial contractility ↑ Stroke volume and CO ↓ SVR No beneficial renal effects	Dosage: Infused at an IV rate of 2.5-15 mcg/kg/min Contraindications: Hypertrophic cardiomyopathy, severe AS	Monitor for tachyarrhythmias, (ventricular ectopy) Can ↓ BP in low dosages (usually associated with volume depletion, excessive diuresis, IV nitroglycerin); check for volume depletion before administering drug
VASOPRESSORS			
Dopamine (Intropin)	Used to support BP	Dosages of 2-10 mcg/kg/min (β-adrenergic effects) ↑ BP, cerebral and renal perfusion Dosages of >10 mcg/kg/min (α-adrenergic effects) cause peripheral vasoconstriction, ↑ SVR, ↑ afterload and BP (possible ↓ CO)	May cause tachycardia Check skin color, temperature, capillary refill; α-adrenergic stimulation causes peripheral venoconstriction. Infuse in central or large vein. Extravasation causes tissue necrosis and sloughing. If this occurs: Stop infusion and immediately inject phentolamine (Regitine), 5-10 mg diluted in 10-15 ml of saline solution, around site to lessen deleterious effects of infiltrated dopamine.

Drug	Effects	Dosage	Monitoring
Phenylephrine (Neo-Synephrine)	Effectively increases BP by arteriolar constriction ↓ HR, ↑ SV	Dosage: 0.1-0.5 mg IV slowly (diluted 1 mg in 10 ml normal saline) Infusion: 0.2-5.0 mcg/kg/min (use lowest therapeutic dose) Onset: Immediate Duration: 15-20 min	Monitor hemodynamic parameters closely, especially when using vasoactive drugs (monitor arterial and hemodynamic pressures often with noninvasive BP monitoring, arterial lines, and pulmonary artery catheter)
Other vasoactive drugs, including vasopressin (antidiuretic hormone), norepinephrine (Levophed)			
AFTERLOAD REDUCTION			
Sodium nitroprusside (Nipride)	↓ Afterload via arterial dilation, also causing ↓ preload and BP and ↑ CO ↓ SVR and PCWP Contraindications: Severe AS, coarctation of aorta	Action: Immediate and very brief; effect ends 1-2 min after infusion stopped Initial dosage: Start at 0.1 mcg/kg/min; rate of infusion is titrated by BP, hemodynamics	Extravasation should be treated with phentolamine (see earlier under dopamine) to avoid necrosis at IV site Watch for cyanide toxicity with methemoglobinemia
ACE inhibitor (e.g., captopril, enalapril)	Used for afterload and preload reduction ↑ Heart function and exercise capacity ↓ Mortality risk Contraindicated in shock, hyperkalemia (K$^+$ >5.5 mEq/L)	Angiotensin II receptor blockers may be used in patients who are unable to tolerate ACE inhibitors, usually due to cough	Monitor for • Symptomatic hypotension • ↑ K$^+$ (increases retention) • ↑ Creatinine (decreased renal function)
PRELOAD REDUCTION			
IV nitroglycerin	Improves left ventricular function by lowering preload via vasodilatation, to relieve discomfort		

Continued

■ **TABLE 3-14**
■ **Drugs Commonly Used to Treat Heart Failure in the Critical Care Setting—cont'd**

Agent	Action/Indications	Administration	Comments
PRELOAD REDUCTION—cont'd			
Diuretics (i.e., torsemide, furosemide, bumetanide)	↓ Intravascular and extravascular fluid volume, and subsequently ↓ preload		Evaluate for patient response: ↑ Urinary output, ↓ edema, improved lung sounds and breathing; ↓ central venous pressure and PCWP Monitor for complications: • Electrolyte imbalances (↓ Na⁺, ↓ K⁺, ↓ Mg⁺⁺) • Impaired renal function (↑ creatinine) • Hypovolemia • Other symptoms: Fatigue, nausea, vomiting, headache, dry mouth, muscle cramps, wooziness
β-blockers	Beneficial in decreasing symptoms of heart failure, increasing patient well-being	Watch for fluid retention, fatigue, hypotension, increased symptoms	Carvedilol combines β-blockade with vasodilatation properties
Digoxin (Lanoxin)	Beneficial in decreasing symptoms, improving exercise tolerance, especially in combination therapy Also used for rate control of atrial fibrillation, atrial flutter		
Spironolactone (Aldactone)	Antagonist to aldosterone ↓ Mortality, hospitalization	Dosages: 12.5-25 mg/day	Watch K⁺ retention Not used in renal insufficiency
Anticoagulation (warfarin)	Used for atrial fibrillation, thromboembolism risk		
Morphine	↓ Preload ↓ Venous return to heart (↑ capacitance) ↓ Pain, anxiety ↓ Myocardial oxygen consumption	3-5 mg IV	

ACE, Angiotensin-converting enzyme; *AS,* aortic stenosis; *BNP,* brain natriuretic peptide; *BP,* blood pressure; *CO,* cardiac output; *HR,* heart rate; *IV,* intravenous; *PCWP,* pulmonary capillary wedge pressure; *SV,* stroke volume; *SVR,* systemic vascular resistance.

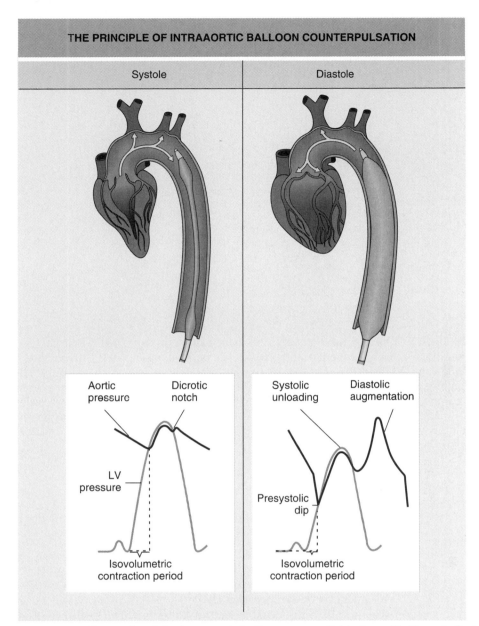

THE PRINCIPLE OF INTRAAORTIC BALLOON COUNTERPULSATION

Systole	Diastole

FIGURE 3-15 ■ Principle of the intraaortic balloon pump. Initiation of balloon inflation is timed to the arterial dicrotic notch, which produces an augmentation in proximal aortic diastolic pressure. Deflation of the balloon is timed to begin just before the onset of the next ventricular systole, which produces the systolic unloading effect (presystolic dip). *LV,* Left ventricular. (From Crawford MH, DiMarco JP, Paulus WJ, editors: *Cardiology,* ed 2, Philadelphia, 2004, Mosby, p 382.)

      b) Just before ventricular systole, the balloon is deflated. Reduces afterload. Myocardial oxygen demand is decreased.

  (5) Contraindications

      a) Aortic insufficiency

      b) Severe aortic disease

      c) Severe peripheral vascular disease in affected limb

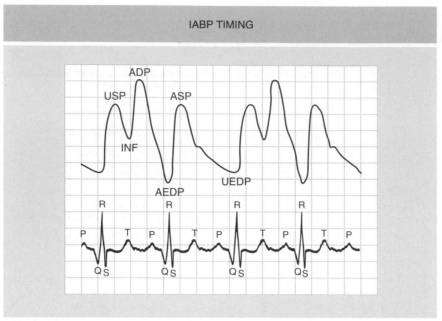

IABP TIMING

FIGURE 3-16 ■ Optimal timing of an intraaortic balloon pump *(IABP)*. Arterial pressure tracing from a patient with an IABP. The balloon was set at 2:1 to evaluate timing. Inflation *(INF)* was timed to the dicrotic notch to follow aortic valve closure. There is augmentation of diastolic pressure *(ADP)* and lowering of the end-diastolic pressure with augmented beats *(AEDP)* compared to the unaugmented end-diastolic pressure *(UEDP)*. The augmented systolic pressure *(ASP)* is often lower than the unaugmented systolic pressure *(USP)* as well. (From Crawford MH, DiMarco JP, Paulus WJ, editors: *Cardiology,* ed 2, Philadelphia, 2004, Mosby, p 867.)

       (6) Complications
          a) Ischemia of limb distal to insertion site: Caused by mechanical occlusion of the artery or thromboembolism
          b) Dissection of the aorta
          c) Thrombocytopenia
          d) Septicemia
          e) Infection at the insertion site
       (7) Key points in the nursing care of patients with IABPs are given in Box 3-7 (see also Figure 3-16)
    (c) VAD, implanted device (in either or both ventricles) that bypasses the affected ventricle, takes over its pumping action, and allows the heart to rest and recover, thus preventing end-organ failure
       (1) Left ventricular assist device (LVAD): Blood is diverted from the LA, bypasses the LV, is sent to the pump, and returns to the patient via cannulation of the ascending aorta (Figure 3-17)
       (2) Indications
          a) Cardiogenic shock
          b) Inability to be weaned from cardiopulmonary bypass during cardiac surgery
          c) Bridge to transplantation: In patients waiting for transplantation
          d) Destination therapy: In patients not eligible for transplantation

■ BOX 3-7
■ **KEY POINTS IN THE NURSING CARE OF PATIENTS WITH AN INTRAAORTIC BALLOON PUMP (IABP)**

1. Monitor all vital signs, especially heart rate. IABP timing is based on heart rate: When rate changes dramatically, duration of balloon inflation must be adjusted.
2. Monitor arterial pressures closely and watch volume status: Improvement should occur with use.
3. Monitor closely for arrhythmias (especially irregular), which can hamper IABP efficacy.
4. Look for signs of improved, effective cardiac output and improved mental status (if patient is not sedated), urinary output, skin color and warmth, capillary refill.
5. Assess peripheral pulses; document presence and changes from baseline. Watch for changes in color, sensation, and temperature.
6. Keep a close watch on insertion site for signs of bleeding, hematomas.
7. Do not elevate head of bed beyond 15 degrees; patient must keep affected limb straight.
8. Assess pulses in upper extremities, especially left arm. Catheter can migrate up and occlude subclavian artery.
9. Heparin anticoagulation is mandatory. Watch for side effects from anticoagulation: Abnormal laboratory coagulation results, positive results on guaiac stool test, or nasogastric secretions and petechiae.
10. Be knowledgeable about IABP controls, safeguards, and protocols for use.
11. Be alert to signs of infection locally or systemically. Prevent infections by following unit protocols for dressing changes and other precautions.
12. Prevent complications from immobility (e.g., skin breakdown, respiratory compromise).

     e) Bridge to recovery: Used with medical management to enable recovery of LV function (reverse remodeling) to the point that the patient can do without the device and avoid transplantation

  (3) Contraindications

     a) Prolonged cardiac arrest with severe neurologic damage

     b) No prospect of being weaned from the VAD: Irreversible, extensive organ damage (renal, hepatic, respiratory)

  (4) Complications of VAD use

     a) Thromboembolism

     b) Bleeding

     c) Infections

  (5) Nursing care for patients with VADs

     a) Be knowledgeable about VAD operation and protocols of use; cardiac perfusionists are great resources and are involved in care

     b) Frequently assess vital signs, hemodynamics, CO, intake and output, circulation

     c) Monitor for arrhythmias and treat promptly

     d) Patient discharged with an LVAD will need a thorough knowledge of the device and its management in the home setting

 (d) Mechanical ventilation: Used in patients with hypoventilation and severe hypoxia

 (e) Surgery

  (1) Revascularization for ischemic heart failure

  (2) Valvular repair or replacement

  (3) Transplantation

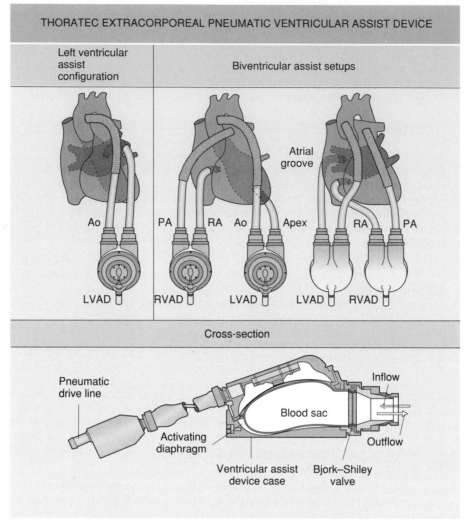

FIGURE 3-17 ■ Thoratec extracorporeal pneumatic ventricular device. The device is shown in left ventricular assist configuration, in two biventricular assist setups, and in cross section. *Ao,* Aorta; *LVAD,* left ventricular assist device; *PA,* pulmonary artery; *RA,* right atrium; *RVAD,* right ventricular assist device. (From Crawford MH, DiMarco JP, Paulus WJ, editors: *Cardiology,* ed 2, Philadelphia, 2004, Mosby, p 925.)

   b. Potential complication: Death
8. Evaluation of patient care
   a. Patient is hemodynamically stable: CO and tissue perfusion are adequate
   b. Decrease in edema and return to normal weight are achieved
   c. Lungs are clear, according to auscultation and radiography
   d. Intake and output are balanced
   e. Arrhythmias are controlled or absent

Pericardial Disease

1. Pathophysiology
   a. Pericarditis
      i. Inflammation of the pericardium with a wide variety of causes
      ii. May be acute or chronic
      iii. Acute pericarditis most commonly of viral or idiopathic origin

(a) Produces acute illness characterized by fever, chest pain (characteristically relieved by sitting up or leaning forward), pericardial friction rub, global ST elevation, little to no pericardial effusion

(b) Is usually self-limited and responds to NSAIDs

(c) May be recurrent with relapses

b. Pericardial effusion

    i. Abnormal amount of pericardial fluid can result when pericardial fluid is produced too rapidly to be reabsorbed

    ii. If pericardial fluid accumulates slowly, the pericardium stretches with little increase in intrapericardial pressure. Cardiac filling and function are not disturbed. If effusion accumulates rapidly, intrapericardial pressure rises and tamponade may result.

    iii. Huge effusions (several liters) may develop slowly without tamponade (especially in uremic pericarditis)

    iv. Same causes as for pericarditis

c. Cardiac tamponade

    i. Common causes are few: Aortic dissection, MI with myocardial rupture, trauma (catheter or pacemaker perforation, contusion during CPR), laceration during pericardiocentesis (postoperative bleeding)

    ii. Results when pericardial fluid accumulates too rapidly to allow the pericardium to stretch. Can occur with small amounts of fluid or blood (approximately 150 ml) in the pericardial space

    iii. Intrapericardial pressure rises dramatically

    iv. Increased intrapericardial pressure exceeds the filling pressures of the right side (pretamponade) and then of both sides, impairing ventricular filling and output

    v. CVP and jugular venous pressures rise (may not be seen in marked hypovolemia)

    vi. Pulsus paradoxus develops

    vii. CO falls dramatically

    viii. Compensatory tachycardia develops

    ix. Hypotension and death result in minutes

d. Constrictive pericarditis

    i. Results from chronic scarring and thickening of the pericardium after pericarditis of any cause

    ii. Most common causes are posttraumatic, postpericardiotomy, and postradiation factors; neoplasm; and tuberculosis

    iii. Epicardium becomes thickened with tough and rigid fibrous tissue that calcifies

    iv. This interferes with filling (especially of the right side of the heart) in mid to late diastole, which results in decreased CO and increased jugular venous filling pressures

    v. Syndrome of right-sided heart failure with decreased output develops

    vi. Pulmonary edema is not seen

    vii. Death is the usual outcome, unless life-saving but high-risk (5% to 15% mortality) pericardiectomy is performed

2. Etiology and risk factors for pericarditis

  a. Idiopathic, acute, or nonspecific (most common)

  b. Infection

    i. Viral: Echovirus and coxsackievirus B (the two most common causes of acute pericarditis); adenovirus, enterovirus, and influenza, mumps, measles, smallpox, and chickenpox viruses

      ii. Bacterial: Pneumococci, staphylococci, *Mycobacterium tuberculosis*, streptococci, *Pseudomonas* species

     iii. Fungal: *Histoplasma, Aspergillus, Candida*

     iv. Rickettsial, spirochetal (Lyme disease, due to *Borrelia burgdorferi*)

      v. HIV infection and acquired immunodeficiency syndrome: Becoming a prevalent cause worldwide

  c. Neoplasms (especially metastatic tumors from the lung and breast; melanomas; lymphomas)

  d. Connective tissue diseases: Systemic lupus erythematosus, rheumatoid arthritis, polyarteritis nodosa, and scleroderma

  e. Radiation therapy to the thorax: Treatments for Hodgkin's disease, breast or lung cancer

  f. Acute MI: Early inflammatory process (24 to 72 hours after) or delayed immunologic response (Dressler's syndrome). Dressler's syndrome (occurring weeks or months after MI) has decreased in incidence due to advanced MI therapy (use of thrombolytics).

  g. Postcardiotomy or postthoracotomy syndrome (occurs 2 to 10 days after surgery). Pericardial effusions are common. In heart transplant patients, effusions are associated with a higher incidence of acute rejection.

  h. Chest trauma, penetrating (stabbing, rib fractures) or nonpenetrating, including surgical procedures such as pacemaker insertion

  i. Dissecting aortic aneurysm

  j. Systemic disease: Uremia, myxedema, sarcoidosis, severe hypothyroidism (pericardial effusions)

  k. Immunologic or hypersensitivity reactions: Drug reactions (e.g., to hydralazine, procainamide, penicillin, phenytoin, isoniazid)

3. Signs and symptoms

  a. Subjective and objective findings

      i. Sharp or stabbing precordial pain, increased with inspiration, lying down, swallowing or belching, or turning of thorax; may be relieved by sitting up and/or leaning forward. Pain may also be dull (hard to distinguish from MI pain).

     ii. Associated trapezius ridge pain (specific for pericarditis)

    iii. Nonspecific influenza-like complaints such as low-grade fever, joint discomfort, fatigue, weight loss, night sweats

    iv. Weakness, exercise intolerance

     v. History of any of the etiologic findings

    vi. Recent history of taking immunosuppressive drugs (e.g., corticosteroids)

    vii. Weight loss

  b. Pulsus paradoxus: In cardiac tamponade, pulsus paradoxus is the result of the influence of respiration on the beat-to-beat filling of the LV by flow from the pulmonary veins

      i. During inspiration, there is less pulmonary venous return to the left side of the heart; this is exaggerated by impaired filling caused by high intrapericardiac pressure

     ii. Result is decreased left-sided heart output and decreased blood pressure during inspiration

    iii. Pulsus paradoxus is an inspiratory decrease in blood pressure of 11 mm Hg or greater

    iv. May not be seen in states in which LV filling is not solely dependent on pulmonary venous return (aortic insufficiency, VSD)

  c. Pericardial friction rub

       i. Has two or three components with scratchy or squeaky sounds. May be very transient. Absence of a rub does not rule out pericarditis.

      ii. Heard best with the stethoscope diaphragm pressed firmly

    iii. Loudest over the left mid-lower sternal border when the patient is sitting up and leaning forward

    iv. Having the patient hold the breath will help differentiate from pleural friction rub

  d. Other physical findings: Depending on the severity, any or all of the following symptoms may be observed:

       i. Dyspnea with or without pain, orthopnea

      ii. Cough, hemoptysis

    iii. Tachycardia

    iv. Fever

     v. Anxiety, confusion, restlessness

    vi. Pallor

   vii. Anorexia

  viii. Jugular venous distention

    ix. Kussmaul's sign (rise in CVP on inspiration): Seen in patients with constrictive pericarditis

     x. Flushing, sweating

    xi. Peripheral edema, abdominal swelling or discomfort (constrictive pericarditis) with prominent Y descent

   xii. Increased cardiac dullness in large effusions

  xiii. Hepatojugular reflux

  xiv. Heart sounds are often normal except muffled and distant sounding with effusion

   xv. Pericardial "knock" in constriction

4. Diagnostic study findings

  a. Laboratory

       i. Troponin: Elevated levels mark myocardial injury

      ii. Moderate leukocytosis, increased sedimentation rate in acute or chronic pericarditis

    iii. C-reactive protein: Elevated levels

    iv. Blood cultures: To identify causative organisms and their sensitivity to antibiotics

     v. Antinuclear antibody test: Results positive in connective tissue diseases

    vi. BUN level: Renal status evaluation

   vii. Purified protein derivative testing: Tuberculosis

  viii. Pericardiocentesis, especially pericardial biopsy and drainage, may be helpful diagnostically

  b. ECG

       i. In acute pericarditis

        (a) Diffuse ST-segment elevation in most leads

        (b) PR segment may be depressed

        (c) ST segment reverts to normal and T wave inverts after several days

      ii. Arrhythmias: Bradycardias, tachycardia (sinus or atrial arrhythmias, atrial fibrillation)

  c. Radiologic: Normal or shows cardiac enlargement resulting from pericardial effusion

  d. Echocardiography: To identify and quantify pericardial effusions, wall motion abnormalities, RA and RV diastolic collapse (pretamponade)

       i. Results usually normal in acute pericarditis unless effusions present

      ii. In tamponade: Identifies pericardial effusions, LA compression, and respiratory variation in LV inflow of more than 25% (tamponade)

      iii. Restriction in ventricular filling (constriction)

   e. MRI, CT: To detect thickening of the pericardium, calcifications

   f. Right-sided heart catheterization: Used to

      i. Evaluate and monitor hemodynamics

      ii. Evaluate the severity of constriction

      iii. Assess the need for pericardiotomy

      iv. Assist in the differential diagnosis of constriction and restrictive cardiomyopathy

      v. Identify increased RV and LV filling pressures with equalization (constriction)

5. Goals of care

   a. Treatment is directed toward the underlying disease

   b. Patient is comfortable, pain free, and without symptoms

   c. Hemodynamics, vital signs, and ECG are within normal limits

   d. Patient is free from complications (heart failure, tamponade)

   e. Laboratory values and clinical findings return to normal

6. Collaborating professionals on health care team: See Chronic Stable Angina; also infectious disease specialist

7. Management of patient care

   a. Anticipated patient trajectory: Cardiac tamponade is a life-threatening condition, and the patient will die if emergent pericardiocentesis is not performed. Constrictive pericarditis is lethal and requires pericardiectomy. Pericarditis is generally self-limited.

      i. Positioning: Position the patient for comfort; sitting up and leaning forward will help to increase comfort

      ii. Pain management

         (a) Frequently ask the patient about pain and discomfort; if present, assess characteristics

         (b) Give medications to relieve pain caused by the inflammatory process, (acetaminophen, aspirin, antiinflammatory agents). Pain is often gone or diminished significantly in 24 to 48 hours but may last weeks. Corticosteroids are given for recurring, severe pain.

         (c) Reassure the patient regarding the nonischemic cause of the pain

      iii. Pharmacology

         (a) Antimicrobial agents: If culture or serologic evidence of a susceptible etiologic agent is present

         (b) NSAIDs: For pericarditis, pleural effusions

         (c) Corticosteroids: If unresponsive to NSAIDs after 48 hours. Used cautiously for short term and tapered quickly. They can contribute to recurrences due to viral proliferation.

         (d) Colchicine: May help prevent recurrences

         (e) Anticoagulants: Withheld with pericardial effusions to lower risk of tamponade. Heparin can be used, if necessary, due to its shorter half-life and reversibility.

         (f) Volume support (IV fluids) and/or inotropic agents (e.g., dobutamine): Used as a temporizing agent to improve CO during tamponade

      iv. Treatments

         (a) Nursing care for cardiac tamponade

            (1) If tamponade occurs, place the patient in Trendelenburg's position, notify the physician

(2) Administer oxygen as ordered

(3) Prepare the patient for pericardiocentesis

(4) Emergency pericardiocentesis is life saving. Removal of 50 to 100 ml of fluid can bring major hemodynamic improvement.

(5) If a pericardial catheter is present, aspirate pericardial fluid, per orders

(6) Give fluids to increase preload

(7) Discontinue agents that decrease preload (diuretics, nitrates, morphine)

(b) Pericardiocentesis: For persistent effusions, tamponade, purulent pericarditis

(1) Echocardiographic guidance of the procedure improves safety

(2) Sclerosing agents may be infiltrated intrapericardially for chronic effusions

(c) Pericardiotomy procedures for effusions and diagnostic biopsy, subxiphoid pericardiotomy, pericardial window surgery

(d) Pericardiectomy: Treatment for constrictive pericarditis. Higher-risk surgery (10% to 25% mortality) in severe or chronic disease.

   b. Potential complications

   i. Cardiac tamponade: Complication of pericarditis (see Treatments earlier)

   ii. Recurrent pericarditis

   (a) Mechanism

   (1) Probable autoimmune response, may reoccur numerous times, over years

   (2) Can be related to tapering or stopping of antiinflammatory agents

   (b) Management

   (1) Corticosteroids often needed to stop painful symptoms. Steroid dependency and adverse side effects are major concerns. Nonsteroidal agents (e.g., colchicine, azathioprine) can be used to help avoid reoccurrence.

   (2) Pericardiectomy is considered when medical therapy is unsuccessful

8. Evaluation of patient care

   a. Patient states that pain is reduced or alleviated

   b. Laboratory values show that antimicrobial therapy is effective (e.g., leukocyte count and CBC returning to normal or within normal limits; blood culture results are negative)

Myocarditis

Myocarditis is an inflammation of the myocardium caused by various microorganisms, drugs, or chemicals. Can be acute or chronic (subacute) and focal or diffuse. It may mimic MI. There may be complete recovery or it can lead to severe cardiovascular compromise and death from dilated cardiomyopathy.

1. Pathophysiology

   a. Myocardial damage occurs due to infection or injury

   b. Interstitial infiltrates develop. Immune responses to inflammation ensue, and myocardial fibers become injured, hypertrophy, and begin to die

   c. Necrosis of the myofibers may be global or spotty

   d. Vascular responses to inflammation include vasculitis and spasm, which contribute to myocardial fibrosis and necrosis

   e. Pericardial involvement often occurs at the same time

   f. Contractility and CO decrease

   g. LV function may be sufficiently impaired to cause heart failure

    h. Myocardial injury can continue after active infection as a result of persistent immune and autoimmune responses

2. Etiology and risk factors

    a. Causes can include viral, bacterial, rickettsial, parasitic, or mycotic organisms. There are also noninfectious causes, which include autoimmune disorders, drugs, and cardiac toxins.

    b. In Europe and North America, viral infection (in particular, infection with coxsackievirus B) is the most common cause of myocarditis.

    c. Viral

        i. Most common types include coxsackievirus A and B, adenovirus, and echovirus

        ii. Others include influenza virus, cytomegalovirus, HIV, hepatitis B virus, and mumps and rubella viruses

    d. Bacterial

        i. Infection with *Salmonella typhi, Coxiella burnetii*

        ii. Diphtheria: Most common cause of death

        iii. Tuberculosis

        iv. Streptococci, meningococci, clostridia, staphylococci

    e. Rickettsial

    f. Fungal: Aspergillosis

    g. Protozoal: Chagas' disease (*Trypanosoma cruzi*), seen in patients traveling to or living in Central and South America; malaria

    h. Autoimmune disorders: Systemic lupus erythematosus, Wegener's granulomatosis

    i. Cardiac toxins (e.g., cocaine, catecholamines)

    j. Drugs: Doxorubicin (Adriamycin), amitriptyline (Elavil)

3. Signs and symptoms: Viral myocarditis is a diagnosis of exclusion. The responsible virus is very difficult to identify.

    a. Clinical manifestations of viral myocarditis

        i. Patient may have complaints of a "common cold," fever, chills, sore throat, abdominal pain, nausea, vomiting, diarrhea, arthralgia, and myalgia up to 6 weeks before overt symptoms of heart failure appear

        ii. Chest pain (two thirds of patients) with no evidence of pericarditis or ischemia. Pain may be pleuritic, precordial, or associated with sweating, nausea, or vomiting. Chest pain can imitate ischemic pain.

        iii. Dyspnea: Dyspnea at rest, exertional dyspnea, paroxysmal nocturnal dyspnea, orthopnea

        iv. Palpitations

        v. Fatigue, weakness

    b. Physical findings

        i. Tachycardia

        ii. Symptoms of heart failure (rapid, fulminant)

        iii. Increased jugular venous pressure

        iv. Enlarged lymph nodes: Seen with sarcoidosis

        v. Pruritic rash (maculopapular): Drug reaction

        vi. Pulsus alternans (extreme heart failure)

        vii. Narrow pulse pressure

        viii. Hypotension

        ix. S_1 diminished (decreased contractility)

        x. S_3 gallop: Common

        xi. Murmurs: Mitral or tricuspid regurgitation (if ventricular dilatation is present)

        xii. Pericardial friction rub: Uncommon

4. **Diagnostic study findings**
   a. Laboratory
      i. Cultures (blood, throat, urine, stool specimens): To rule out bacterial and fungal causes
      ii. Cardiac enzyme levels
      iii. CBC: Slight to moderate leukocytosis
      iv. Erythrocyte sedimentation rate: Elevated
      v. Titers for *Rickettsia*, virus, fungus
      vi. Skin test for tuberculosis
   b. Radiologic: Findings may be normal or
      i. Pulmonary congestion
      ii. Cardiomegaly
   c. ECG
      i. Sinus tachycardia
      ii. ST segment can be elevated, T waves inverted; nonspecific ST, T-wave changes
      iii. QTc interval is prolonged
      iv. ST returns to baseline in several days
      v. T-wave changes may last weeks or months (with severe myocarditis)
      vi. Arrhythmias are seen in one third of patients
         (a) VT, supraventricular tachycardia (SVT), premature ventricular contractions
         (b) Atrial fibrillation
         (c) AV blocks
   d. Echocardiography: Used to rule out other causes of heart failure and evaluate LV function
      i. Diffuse hypocontractility
      ii. Pericardial effusions
      iii. Valvular dysfunction
      iv. Chamber enlargement
      v. Ventricular thrombi
   e. Endocardial biopsy: Although myocarditis is a nonspecific histologic diagnosis, routine biopsy has no proven utility, due to the high level of insensitivity and numerous false-negative results (up to 55% when only five specimens are obtained)
   f. Right-sided heart catheterization: To evaluate CO, CI, SVR, pulmonary vascular resistance (PVR) for LV function
   g. Coronary angiography: To exclude other causes of heart failure; CAD, valvular disease, congenital disorders
   h. EPS: If history of sudden death, VF, and/or VT
5. **Goals of care**
   a. CO, hemodynamics, and vital signs are within normal limits
   b. Patient has no arrhythmias
   c. Patient has no signs or symptoms of heart failure
   d. Plan is developed for progressive activities and exercise
   e. Patient shows a progressive (slow) increase in activity tolerance
6. **Collaborating professionals on health care team:** See Chronic Stable Angina; also infectious disease specialist
7. **Management of patient care**
   a. Anticipated patient trajectory: Usually a mild disease; bed rest is important, along with management of symptoms. Patient is often in a stepdown unit, unless symptoms of heart failure, heart block, or other complications arise.

i. Positioning
   (a) Maintain bed rest at first (the patient needs activities restricted); exception would be use of a bedside commode, if tolerated
   (b) Allow patient to slowly ambulate with assistance
   (c) Monitor heart, respiratory rates, blood pressure, and oxygen saturation with activity

ii. Pain management: Relieve chest pain promptly

iii. Nutrition: Low-sodium diet, fluid restriction, if signs of heart failure are present

iv. Discharge planning
   (a) Instruct the patient about the need for a progressive increase in ambulation over the next 2 months
   (b) Teach the patient which symptoms to look for and report regarding activity tolerance. Patient should be able to monitor his or her pulse.
   (c) Facilitate and assist with the development of an activity and exercise program for the patient, both in the hospital and at home

v. Pharmacology
   (a) Oxygen: Ensure adequate oxygenation; check pulse oximetry results, maintain oxygen saturations at over 92%. Hypoxia is common with myocarditis.
   (b) Afterload reduction agents (ACE inhibitors, ARBs, diuretics): For cardiac failure
   (c) IV pressors and inotropic agents: If hemodynamic support is needed
   (d) Antiarrhythmics: As needed; monitor closely for arrhythmias—high risk for sudden death
   (e) Antiviral therapy (pleconaril): Used for enteroviruses
   (f) β-blockers: To decrease heart rate, arrhythmias
   (g) Immunosuppressive therapy: Has not proved beneficial for preservation of LV function or survival (except in a small number of patients)
   (h) NSAIDs: Ineffective; may facilitate disease process, increase mortality

vi. Treatments: Focused on managing symptoms
   (a) Treat causative agent if known
   (b) Temporary transvenous pacemaker for AV blocks
   (c) Temporary LVADs may be required: IABP, LVAD to assist in CO and as a bridge to transplantation
   (d) Heart transplantation

b. Potential complications
   i. Arrhythmias
      (a) Mechanism: Myocardial injury, infection
      (b) Management
         (1) SVTs: Cardioversion
         (2) Heart blocks: Temporary transvenous pacemaker (transient condition usually not requiring permanent pacemaker)
   ii. Dilated cardiomyopathy, heart failure
      (a) Mechanism: Can develop slowly over time
      (b) Management: Patient with myocarditis routinely followed to evaluate LV function

8. Evaluation of patient care
   a. Plan of care is consistent with the patient's responses to activity and appropriate limits are set
   b. Support services and significant others are actively involved in the patient's rehabilitation

Infective Endocarditis

Infective endocarditis (IE) is an acute or chronic infection of the heart's endocardial surface, including valves, chordae tendineae, septum, and mural endothelium. Median age of affected patients has increased to 50 years, due to the decrease in rheumatic heart disease, increase in longevity, and emergence of nosocomial causes. Disease frequency is 2.5 times greater in men than in women.

1. **Pathophysiology**
   a. Infecting organisms may be present in the blood stream (may be a very transient invasion)
   b. Valves and endothelial surface of the heart can be predisposed to injury. Infecting organisms have an affinity for traumatized areas and preexisting defects such as with valvular disease, prosthetic valves, septal defects, or local trauma (from indwelling catheters)
   c. When traumatic injury from abnormal hemodynamic or endothelial stress has occurred, deposits of platelets and fibrin form microscopic thrombotic lesions
   d. Affected areas are then amenable to colonization by microorganisms. Bacteria and organisms from other infections in the body (skin, genitourinary tract, lungs, mouth) attach to the valves and to these thrombotic lesions.
   e. As the microorganisms colonize, they cause the deposition of platelets, leukocytes, erythrocytes, and fibrin, forming vegetations. Eventually, valvular tissue is destroyed by the infection, and the valve leaflets may become incompetent, ulcerate, rupture, abscess (ring or annular), or perforate.
   f. Valves on the left side of the heart are more often affected (85% of cases). Mitral valve is most commonly affected. Right-sided IE is predominantly caused by IV drug use and generally involves the tricuspid and pulmonic valves.
   g. The bacteria and other microorganisms from the vegetations are circulated systemically, which causes bacteremia
   h. Antibody formation increases the levels of immune complexes in the blood, which causes hypersensitivity reactions (allergic vasculitis) in peripheral parts of the body involving the arterioles, vessel walls, and cutaneous tissue
   i. Embolization of infective material may occur throughout body (left-sided vegetation causes systemic emboli; tricuspid valve vegetation causes pulmonary emboli)
2. **Etiology and risk factors**
   a. A wide variety of microorganisms cause endocarditis. Common organisms include the following:
      i. *Streptococcus* types (50% to 60%)
         (a) *Streptococcus viridans*: Had been the most prevalent causative organism in subacute cases (now involved in only approximately one third of cases)
         (b) Group B, D, or G streptococci
         (c) *Enterococci*: Often a nosocomial cause; resistant to medical therapy
      ii. *Staphylococcus* types (15% to 40%)
         (a) *Staphylococcus aureus*: Most prevalent causative organism in acute and nosocomial cases (i.e., methicillin-resistant strains)
         (b) Coagulase-negative species: Often the cause of prosthetic valve endocarditis
      iii. Gram-negative rods (HACEK organisms [*Haemophilus* species, *Actinobacillus actinomycetemcomitans*, *Cardiobacterium hominis*, *Eikenella corrodens*, *Kingella kingae*])
      iv. Enterobacteriaceae: *Pseudomonas aeruginosa*

       v. Fungi: *Candida albicans, Aspergillus fumigatus*

      vi. Viruses: Coxsackievirus, adenovirus

  b. Surgery or procedures predisposing to IE bacteremia risk

      i. Dental procedures (extractions, surgery, cleaning) that cause mucosal or gingival bleeding: Cause 20% of cases of bacteremia

      ii. Tonsillectomy, adenoidectomy

      iii. Bowel surgeries, esophageal procedures

      iv. Genitourinary surgery, biopsies

  c. Other therapies and procedures predisposing patients to IE bacteremia risk

      i. Invasive tests and monitoring (pulmonary artery catheters)

      ii. Prolonged IV therapy (hyperalimentation)

      iii. Immunosuppressive therapy

      iv. Hemodialysis

  d. Medical conditions that predispose to IE

      i. Prosthetic valve

      ii. Rheumatic valvular disease: Previously most common predisposing condition (accounts for 7% to 18% of cases)

      iii. Previous IE episode

      iv. Congenital heart defect (e.g., PDA, coarctation of the aorta, VSD): About 14% of cases

      v. Degenerative valve disease: About 9% of cases

      vi. Mitral valve prolapse

      vii. Hypertrophic, obstructive cardiomyopathy

      viii. Abscesses on skin

      ix. Inflammatory gastrointestinal disease, gastrointestinal tumors

  e. Other factors: Intravenous drug abuse, unidentified causes of IE bacteremia (30% to 40% of IE cases)

3. Signs and symptoms

  a. Subjective findings: Patient may complain of nonspecific, vague symptoms

      i. Fever (prolonged, unknown source, sudden onset)

      ii. Chills, night sweats

      iii. Fatigue, malaise

      iv. Neurologic dysfunctions: Headache, vision loss, stroke, confusion

      v. Nausea, vomiting, anorexia, weight loss

      vi. Arthralgias, myalgias

      vii. Back pain (cause unknown)

      viii. Dyspnea

  b. Physical findings: Depend on the presence of a systemic versus a local infection, the presence of systemic emboli, immune responses, and the duration of infection

      i. Fever: Higher than 100.4° F (38° C)

      ii. Signs and symptoms of heart failure

      iii. Petechiae (caused by emboli or allergic vasculitis): Seen in 20% to 40% of patients on the conjunctivae, neck, chest, abdomen, and mucosa of the mouth (usually a sign of a long-standing infection)

      iv. Osler's nodes (resulting from immunologically mediated vasculitis): Small, very tender, reddened, raised nodules on fingers and toe pads

      v. Roth's spots (resulting from emboli or allergic vasculitis): Round or oval white spots on the retina

      vi. Purpuric pustular skin lesions (caused by emboli)

      vii. Janeway lesions (caused by septic emboli or allergic vasculitis): Large, nontender nodules on the palms of the hands, toes, and soles of the feet

viii. Splinter hemorrhages of the nails (resulting from emboli or allergic vasculitis)

ix. Conduction disturbances seen on ECG

x. Central nervous system disturbances (e.g., hemiplegia, confusion, headache, seizures, transient ischemic attacks, aphasia, ataxia, changes in the level of consciousness, psychiatric symptoms) if embolization to the brain has occurred

xi. Hematuria, oliguria, flank pain, hypertension, if the kidney is infarcted or abscessed from emboli. Glomerulonephritis frequently caused by allergic or immunologic reactions; kidney involvement is common.

xii. Tachypnea, dyspnea, hemoptysis, sudden pain in the chest or shoulder, cyanosis, and restlessness if the lung is infarcted

xiii. Abdominal pain (caused by mesenteric emboli)

xiv. Decreased or no pulses in cold limbs (emboli)

xv. Splenomegaly or pain caused by splenic infarction

xvi. If heart failure present, possible hepatojugular reflux, jugular venous distension, or peripheral edema

xvii. New murmurs of valvular insufficiency. Murmurs may also develop later, with therapy, and may change character.

xviii. Decreased or absent breath sounds or adventitious breath sounds if the lungs are infarcted

4. **Diagnostic study findings**

   a. Laboratory data

      i. Positive blood culture results (minimum of two separate sample sets initially, drawn 12 hours apart). Negative blood culture results do not necessarily rule out IE.

      ii. Other associated findings

         (a) Elevated sedimentation rate and C-reactive protein level (immune response)

         (b) Anemia (common in subacute endocarditis)

         (c) Leukocytosis, thrombocytopenia (associated with splenomegaly)

         (d) Proteinuria, microscopic hematuria, pyuria

         (e) Rheumatoid factor levels may be elevated, as may circulating immune complex levels

         (f) Hyperglobulinemia (common)

         (g) Abnormal laboratory values associated with affected organs (kidneys, lungs, heart)

   b. ECG

      i. Signs of ischemia or infarction if coronary artery emboli have occurred

      ii. New AV blocks, BBB

   c. Chest radiograph: Occasional pleural effusion; multiple, patchy pulmonary infiltrates

   d. Transthoracic echocardiography: Presence of vegetations on any of the valves; assesses degree of valvular dysfunction and complications (e.g., ruptured chordae tendineae, perforated valve cusps)

   e. MRI or CT of head: With neurologic symptoms, to evaluate for infarction, abscess, or bleeding

   f. TEE: Better sensitivity for vegetations, recommended for prosthetic valves

      i. Excellent views of prosthetic valves, mitral valve, aortic valve, ring abscesses

   ii. Evaluation of ventricular function

   iii. Assessment of the severity of mitral regurgitation

   iv. Negative TEE results does not exclude IE

   g. Catheterization: Preoperative evaluation, if valve replacement planned. Assesses the following:

   i. Valve dysfunction

   ii. Aneurysms, intracardiac shunts

   iii. Underlying CAD

5. Goals of care

   a. Patient is afebrile

   b. Patient has negative blood culture results

   c. Patient is well hydrated, as evidenced by normal skin turgor, balanced intake and output, and moist mucosa

6. Collaborating professionals on health care team: See Chronic Stable Angina; also infectious disease specialist, home health nurse (IV therapy)

7. Management of patient care

   a. Anticipated patient trajectory: Prompt diagnosis is difficult but important for successful treatment. Prognosis is good with effective antibiotic therapy; however, mortality remains approximately 20%. Elderly patients with symptoms of heart failure, renal insufficiency, or systemic embolization have a worse prognosis.

   i. Skin care: Monitor for problems in skin integrity resulting from fever and sweating. Ensure that the patient is turning or turned often while on bed rest.

   ii. Nutrition

   (a) Assess the patient for signs of dehydration

   (b) Monitor caloric and fluid intake and output. Weigh patient daily.

   iii. Infection control

   (a) Monitor vital signs, especially temperature. Persistent or recurring fevers can indicate failure of or hypersensitivity to antimicrobial therapy, nosocomial infections, emboli, abscesses, thrombophlebitis, or drug reaction.

   (b) Assist in reduction of fever (e.g., administer antimicrobials, antipyretics, and cooling measures, as ordered; encourage fluid intake, if no evidence of heart failure)

   (c) Draw several blood culture samples initially and if temperature spikes (proper technique for drawing blood samples for culture is vital because of the difficulty in choosing antibiotics to adequately treat microorganisms)

   (d) Ensure that proper preventative measures are taken against nosocomial causes: Provide meticulous monitoring and care of indwelling catheters (change dressings and tubing; limit the duration of site use)

   iv. Discharge planning

   (a) Preventative teaching includes the following:

   (1) Discussion of the use of prophylactic antibiotics (for predisposing procedures, e.g., dental, bowel, bladder surgery). Provision of written material on high-risk procedures and recommended IE prophylaxis.

   (2) Stress good oral hygiene to decrease the frequency of bacteremia

   a) Stress the importance of close monitoring (physician appointments, laboratory work) during therapy and for several months afterward. Patient needs to be aware of the symptoms (i.e., fever, rash) to report promptly. Relapses generally occur within 2 months after therapy has been completed.

    b) If the patient is to go home with continued outpatient IV antimicrobial therapy, then a demonstrated knowledge of drugs, indwelling catheter care, and home health services is necessary

  v. Pharmacology

    (a) Antimicrobial-antibiotic therapy

      (1) Initiate as soon as possible after initial blood culture results (to halt continued valvular damage and abscess formation). Patient will likely receive prolonged intravenous antibiotic therapy.

      (2) Check antimicrobial peak and trough serum levels to monitor therapeutic effects and prevent toxicity

      (3) Assess for musculoskeletal involvement (arthralgias, back pain, and myalgia are common symptoms). Antibiotic therapy usually helps decrease symptoms.

      (4) Fever usually stops after 3 days of therapy. If fever persists longer than 14 days, secondary infection or antibiotic resistance should be suspected.

      (5) If the patient is responding and stable, home outpatient IV therapy may be considered to finish the course of drug therapy

    (b) Anticoagulants: Do not prevent IE emboli and may increase bleeding risks

  vi. Treatments

    (a) Prolonged IV administration of appropriate antimicrobials

    (b) Valve replacement surgery indicated (30% to 50% of cases) if the patient has significant damage to the valves (prosthetic valves), ring or annular abscesses, heart failure, or refractory bacteremia

      (1) With aortic valve IE, valve replacement is imperative

      (2) In mitral or tricuspid valve IE, repair of valve is possible

b. Potential complications

  i. Heart failure

    (a) Mechanism: Main cause of death from IE. Occurs when aortic and/or mitral valve becomes incompetent or regurgitant, or chordae tendineae rupture. May be progressive or acute (more often caused with aortic regurgitation).

    (b) Management

      (1) Assess the patient for signs and symptoms of heart failure

      (2) Monitor for new murmurs during hospitalization. Murmurs may change or appear during the course of the illness.

      (3) Valve replacement surgery: Immediate surgery is generally required

  ii. Embolization

    (a) Mechanism: Occurs from vegetations on the valves. May be the presenting symptom; can happen at any time and numerous events may occur. Seen in 20% to 50% of cases of IE. Often affects the central nervous system and the lower extremities, kidney, spleen, and bone.

    (b) Management

      (1) Assess the patient for signs and symptoms of systemic embolization

      (2) Monitor level of consciousness: Check for signs of cerebral emboli (e.g., headache, numbness, weakness, tingling, paralysis, ataxia, sudden blindness, or sudden hemiplegia)

      (3) Check for petechiae on neck, upper trunk, eyes, and lower extremities

(4) Observe the extremities for painful nodes, swelling, erythema, decreased or absent pulses, coolness, decreased capillary refill

(5) Assess the patient for signs and symptoms of MI; monitor the ECG

(6) Arrange for guaiac test of stools, tests for blood in urine and nasogastric aspirations

(7) If pulmonary, myocardial, or cerebral embolism occurs, administer oxygen therapy, position the patient for comfort and ease of breathing, and give pain medications as ordered

(8) Ultrasonography, CT, and/or MRI used in diagnosis

(9) This type of embolization is not treated with anticoagulants unless the patient has a previous indication for their use (such as a prosthetic valve). Anticoagulants have not proved to be beneficial in therapy and may result in the complication of intracranial hemorrhage.

(10) Treatment is aimed at the infection and antimicrobials are given

(11) Surgery for valve replacement is considered if embolization occurs more than once, if infection is uncontrolled, or if there is persistent heart failure

iii. Abscess
  (a) Mechanism: Occurs from contaminants, bacteremia
    (1) Cardiac valve ring abscess: Occurs with prosthetic valve endocarditis. Infection at the suture site of the valve can cause valve incompetency and dehiscence.
    (2) Extracardiac abscess: Often involves the spleen
  (b) Management: Splenectomy is the main therapy if the spleen is involved

iv. Neurologic complications
  (a) Mechanism: Due to emboli and subsequent cerebral infarction, hemorrhage, cerebral abscesses, mycotic aneurysms (late complication). Neurologic complications are seen in 30% to 40% of IE patients and are associated with a high (40%) mortality rate.
  (b) Management: Watch for the development of headaches, seizures. See Chapter 4.

v. Renal insufficiency
  (a) Mechanism: Caused by immune-response glomerulonephritis, renal embolic infarcts. Azotemia develops.
  (b) Management: Usually improves with antimicrobial therapy

vi. Conduction defects
  (a) Mechanism: Due to infectious process at the aortic valve; affects the AV node or bundle of His and includes all AV blocks, BBB
  (b) Management: Surgical intervention generally required

8. Evaluation of patient care
  a. Patient's temperature returns to normal
  b. Blood culture results are negative; there are no signs of active infection
  c. Skin has normal turgor and mucous membranes are moist; intake equals output
  d. Cardiac function is normal
  e. Patient has no evidence of systemic embolization, heart failure, or other complications

Cardiomyopathy

Cardiomyopathy is a chronic or acute disorder of the heart muscle. The three classifications include dilated, hypertrophic, and restrictive cardiomyopathy.

1. **Pathophysiology**
   a. Dilated cardiomyopathy (DCM; most common type in the United States): Disorder is 2.5 times more common in males
      i. Myocardial fibers degenerate and fibrotic changes occur
      ii. Severe dilatation of the heart occurs; includes atrial and ventricular dilatation, which creates global enlargement
      iii. Systolic and diastolic dysfunction occur and contractility decreases, which results in decreased SV, decreased EF, low CO, and compensatory increase in heart rate
      iv. Mitral annular dilatation is secondary to LV dilatation and results in mitral insufficiency
      v. Heart failure develops, is often refractory to treatment, and is accompanied by malignant ventricular arrhythmias (often the cause of death)
   b. Hypertrophic cardiomyopathy (HCM)
      i. Increased mass and thickening of the heart muscle, which results in diastolic dysfunction
      ii. Myocytes become abnormal: Lose their geometric parallel arrangement and become fibrotic
      iii. Ventricles become rigid and stiff, restricting filling. Filling volumes decrease, and thus SV decreases
      iv. LV chamber becomes very small (hypertrophy occurs inwardly at the expense of the LV chamber)
      v. LA becomes dilated
      vi. Contractility may be normal or increased
      vii. Obstructive form of HCM can occur: Often associated with an LV outflow tract dynamic obstruction that may be caused by concentric hypertrophy or localized hypertrophy. This obstructive form is referred to as *hypertrophic obstructive cardiomyopathy* (HOCM)
      viii. These processes may continue for years with no obvious problems and delayed onset of symptoms, or they may end with sudden cardiac death as a first sign of the disease process, due to malignant ventricular arrhythmias (VF, VT)
      ix. Men and women equally affected
   c. Restrictive cardiomyopathy (least common)
      i. Restricted filling of ventricles
      ii. Usually caused by an infiltrative process, most often amyloidosis in adults
      iii. Heart loses its compliance, grows stiff, and cannot distend well in diastole or contract well in systole
      iv. LVEDP increases; contractility decreases, which results in low CO, heart failure, and death
2. **Etiology and risk factors**
   a. DCM
      i. Idiopathic
      ii. Familial: 25% to 30% of cases
      iii. Infection (autoimmune reaction): Bacterial, parasitic, fungal, protozoal
      iv. Metabolic disorders: Chronic hypophosphatemia, thiamine deficiency, protein deficiency
      v. Toxins: Alcohol, lead, arsenic, uremic substances
      vi. Connective tissue disorders: Lupus erythematosus, rheumatoid disease, polyarteritis, scleroderma
      vii. Viral myocarditis
      viii. Drugs: Amitriptyline, doxorubicin, cocaine

        ix. Ischemia

        x. Pregnancy (third trimester) or the postpartum period (common in multiparous women who are older than 30 years or have a history of toxemia)

        xi. Neuromuscular disorders: Muscular dystrophy, myotonic dystrophy

        xii. Infiltrative disorders: Sarcoidosis, amyloidosis

        xiii. Beriberi

    b. Hypertrophic cardiomyopathy

        i. Strong familial component (60% to 70% of cases)

        ii. Idiopathic

        iii. Neuromuscular disorders: Friedreich's ataxia

        iv. Metabolic: Hypoparathyroidism

        v. Hypertension

    c. Restrictive cardiomyopathy

        i. Idiopathic

        ii. Infiltrative: Amyloidosis, sarcoidosis, hemochromatosis, neoplasms

        iii. Endomyocardial fibroelastosis in children

        iv. Glycogen and mucopolysaccharide deposition

        v. Radiation

3. Signs and symptoms: See Table 3-15 for physical findings associated with DCM, HCM, and restrictive cardiomyopathy. HCM may present at any age, may remain asymptomatic.

    a. Ascertain the patient's chief complaint and the history of the present illness

    b. Patient may complain of angina, syncope, palpitations, exertional dyspnea, orthopnea, fatigue

    c. Determine whether there is a familial component (family history of cardiomyopathy or sudden death in young adults)

    d. Rule out other disease processes, such as hypertension, ischemic heart disease, amyloidosis, and toxemia

    e. Identify potential etiologic factors such as recent infections, history of alcohol use, current use of medications, use of cocaine, pregnancy, and any endocrine disorders

4. Diagnostic study findings

    a. Laboratory

        i. Arterial blood gas (ABG) levels: Check for hypoxemia

        ii. Electrolyte levels: Decreased potassium, decreased magnesium

        iii. Cardiac enzyme levels: Infarct

        iv. Renal function: BUN, creatinine levels

    b. Radiologic

        i. Heart normal or enlarged

        ii. Pulmonary congestion

    c. ECG

        i. Arrhythmias or conduction defects (e.g., sinus tachycardia, atrial fibrillation, ventricular ectopy, BBBs)

        ii. Atrial fibrillation: High incidence (70% to 80%)

        iii. Evidence of both LA and LV enlargement: Increased QRS voltage

        iv. Abnormal Q waves

        v. VT

        vi. Prolonged QTc interval

    d. Transthoracic echocardiography

        i. LV systolic function: EF of 15% to 30% in DCM

        ii. Valvular dysfunction

        iii. LV hypertrophy (in HCM)

■ TABLE 3-15
■ Physical Findings Associated with Dilated, Hypertrophic, and Restrictive Cardiomyopathy

Cardiomyopathy	Patient Complaint	Inspection	Palpation	Percussion	Auscultation
Dilated	Dyspnea on exertion, orthopnea, fatigue, palpitations	Clinical manifestations of HF, dysrhythmias on monitor, conduction defects	Narrow pulse pressure, pulsus alternans, cool skin, JVD, PMI laterally displaced, left ventricular heave, peripheral edema, hepatomegaly	Cardiac enlargement, dullness in bases of lungs	Irregular heart beat, third and fourth heart sounds, mitral and tricuspid insufficiency, pulmonary rales
Hypertrophic	Dyspnea on exertion, orthopnea, PND, angina, syncope, palpitations	Dyspnea, orthopnea	Forceful and laterally displaced apical impulse, systolic thrill (in HOCM)		Fourth heart sound, a third heart sound may be heard, split-second heart sound, systolic ejection murmur
Restrictive	Fatigue, weakness, dyspnea on exertion, anorexia, poor exercise tolerance	Dysrhythmias, distended neck veins, Kussmaul's sign	Edema, ascites, HJR, right upper quadrant pain	Cardiac enlargement, pulmonary congestion	Third and fourth heart sounds, mitral and tricuspid insufficiency

HF, Heart failure; *HJR*, hepatojugular reflux; *HOCM*, hypertrophic obstructive cardiomyopathy; *JVD*, jugular venous distention; *PMI*, point of maximal impulse; *PND*, paroxysmal nocturnal dyspnea.

      iv. Marked asymmetric septal hypertrophy (in HCM, HOCM) and LV outflow tract pressure gradient (in HOCM)

      v. LA enlargement

  e. Radionuclide tests: May reveal increased ventricular volumes, decreased EF in DCM, increased uptake in patients with amyloidosis, defects in cardiac wall in patients with neoplasms or sarcoidosis

  f. TEE: To evaluate anatomy and rule out thrombosis

  g. Right-sided heart catheterization:

      i. Pulmonary capillary wedge pressure (PCWP) and pulmonary artery pressure (PAP) elevated, CO decreased

      ii. RV end-diastolic pressure and CVP rise in right-sided heart failure or with DCM

  h. Left-sided heart catheterization, angiogram, arteriogram

      i. Rule out CAD

      ii. Mitral regurgitation

      iii. LV outflow tract gradient in HOCM

  i. EPS and Holter study: To identify VF and VT and to guide therapy

  j. Endomyocardial biopsy: Used to identify the cause of restrictive cardiomyopathy

5. Goals of care

  a. Symptoms of heart failure are relieved

  b. Cause (especially if toxin) is determined and removed or treated

  c. Sinus rhythm is maintained, if possible. Atrial fibrillation or other arrhythmias are treated promptly

  d. High risk of sudden death is reduced

6. Collaborating professionals on health care team: See Chronic Stable Angina

7. Management of patient care

  a. Anticipated patient trajectory: In most patients, cardiomyopathy may be stabilized or actually improved with medical management. A few patients will succumb to progressive heart failure unless transplantation is possible.

      i. Positioning: Use preventive measures, especially for patients at high risk

        (a) Assist with passive and active exercises while the patient is confined to bed

        (b) Apply antiembolism stockings

        (c) Encourage ambulation as tolerated

        (d) Position the patient so that angulation at the groin and knees is avoided. Elevate the patient's legs when the patient is out of bed. Patient should be instructed not to cross the legs or ankles. Avoid using the knee joint on a Gatch bed.

        (e) Instruct the patient to avoid activities that may cause straining or increase the obstruction, such as strenuous exercise, Valsalva maneuvers, and sitting or standing suddenly

      ii. Pain management: Administer supportive measures as the situation dictates (e.g., oxygen therapy, pain medications, sedatives, emotional support)

      iii. Nutrition: Sodium-restricted diet, weight control

      iv. Infection control: IE prophylactic therapy

      v. Discharge planning: Patient education regarding the following:

        (a) Activities that aggravate symptoms

        (b) Benefits of weight reduction, sodium restriction, smoking and/or alcohol use cessation, exercise

        (c) Blood pressure control

    (d) Follow-up evaluations

    (e) Screening of family members (physical examination, laboratory tests, ECG, echocardiography) starting at age 12 years

  vi. Pharmacology

    (a) ACE inhibitors: Used to decrease afterload and remodeling, improve LV EF

    (b) β-blockers (e.g., metoprolol, atenolol)

        (1) Function by slowing or reversing the progression of LV dysfunction (due to hyperadrenergic tone)

        (2) Increase LV EF

        (3) Decrease heart rate, increase ventricular filling time

        (4) Decrease hospitalization for heart failure

    (c) Antiarrhythmic agents (atrial fibrillation, VT)

    (d) Anticoagulants: For atrial fibrillation (monitor INR, PTT; observe for bleeding)

    (e) Antibiotics: Because the patient is at risk for IE, instruct the patient to notify the dentist before any dental or surgical procedures (for prophylactic antibiotics)

    (f) Treatment specific to DCM

        (1) Inotropic agents to improve myocardial contractility and decrease heart failure

        (2) Diuretics to relieve pulmonary congestion; monitor volume status

        (3) Afterload- and preload-reducing agents such as ACE inhibitors and ARBs to decrease myocardial workload, improve CO, and decrease pulmonary venous pressure

        (4) Spironolactone: Helpful in decreasing mortality in heart failure

    (g) Treatment specific to HOCM

        (1) Goal is to administer medications to reduce outflow tract obstruction to relieve syncope, angina, dyspnea, and arrhythmias, and prevent sudden cardiac death. β-blockers (i.e., propranolol), calcium channel blockers (verapamil), or a type IA antiarrhythmic (i.e., disopyramide) are used.

        (2) Avoid agents that decrease preload (nitrates, diuretics, or morphine). Hypovolemia can be very detrimental because the LV is very preload dependent for adequate CO.

        (3) Avoid administering isoproterenol, dopamine, or digitalis preparations because they increase contractility and hence worsen the obstruction

    (h) Treatment specific to restrictive cardiomyopathy: Avoid digoxin in patients with cardiac amyloidosis, because it concentrates in the amyloid fibrils and can result in digitalis toxicity

  vii. Psychosocial issues

    (a) Help the patient identify stressors and teach methods of stress reduction

    (b) Counseling may be needed for the patient and family members if alcohol or cocaine use is present and is suspected as a cause

 viii. Treatments

    (a) Closely monitor vital signs, ECG, intake and output, hemodynamics, laboratory values

    (b) For HOCM patients

        (1) Surgical septal myectomy: Septal muscle creating obstruction is surgically excised. Hypertrophied muscle does not regenerate. Many patients can return to their normal lifestyles.

        (2) Septal ablation (alternative to surgery): Alcohol is injected, via a percutaneous transluminal catheter, into the small coronary artery supplying the obstructive area; muscle is destroyed and shrinks, which lessens the obstruction. Potential complications include heart blocks, arrhythmias, VSD, and MI.

    (c) Biventricular synchronized pacemaker used to help improve CO in DCM and HOCM

        (1) Patients with an LV EF of less than 35%, QRS of more than 0.12 mm. Used in older patients.

        (2) Can decrease obstruction. Increases activity tolerance and quality of life, used as a bridge.

        (3) Prepare the patient for this procedure. Be knowledgeable about the pacemaker procedure, equipment, protocols.

    (d) Automatic implantable cardiac defibrillator (AICD): The following patients are candidates:

        (1) Patients who have experienced sudden cardiac death

        (2) All patients with impaired systolic function: Show improved survival with AICD (Multicenter Automatic Defibrillator Implantation Trial [MADIT II])

    (e) Patients with end-stage disease may be candidates for cardiac transplantation (see End-Stage Heart Disease)

  b. Potential complications

    i. Heart failure, LV failure (see Heart Failure)

    ii. Dysrhythmias, particularly atrial and ventricular, on ECG: Atrial fibrillation, ventricular arrhythmias (See Cardiac Rhythm Disorders). Arrhythmias attributed to HCM are a common cause of sudden cardiac death in young adults.

      (a) With atrial fibrillation: Rate and rhythm control by cardioversion, drugs (e.g., amiodarone)

      (b) Patients at high risk for sudden cardiac death evaluated for AICD

      (c) Bradycardias, AV conduction defects may require permanent pacemakers

    iii. IE: See Infective Endocarditis section

    iv. Embolism

      (a) Mechanism: Stasis of blood can cause deep venous thrombosis, pulmonary embolism

        (1) Patients at risk are the elderly and immobile patients on bed rest; patients who are in heart failure or atrial fibrillation, or who have a dilated myocardium

        (2) Yearly risk of systemic embolization and stroke with HOCM and atrial fibrillation is 20%

      (b) Management: Long-term anticoagulation, use of supportive stockings, performance of range-of-motion exercises

8. Evaluation of patient care

  a. Patient is hemodynamically stable; vital signs are within set parameters for the patient

  b. Patient is alert and oriented

  c. Sinus rhythm is maintained, atrial fibrillation is rate controlled

  d. Lungs are clear on auscultation

  e. Patient has no embolic episodes or pulmonary congestion. Sequelae of cardiomyopathy are minimized or absent

  f. Patient can identify and recognize the need for management measures such as prevention of endocarditis, anticoagulation therapy and monitoring of parameters, and follow-up

End-Stage Heart Disease

In end-stage heart disease, the disease has advanced to a point at which all possible medical or surgical interventions have been exhausted. Life expectancy is less than 24 months. Patient is free of other life-threatening disease; dysfunction of other organ systems is reversible.

1. **Pathophysiology**
    a. Severe LV dysfunction with CO; EF is less than 25%
    b. See Pathophysiology subsection under Heart Failure
2. **Etiology and risk factors**
    a. Ischemic heart disease and CAD
    b. DCM: Idiopathic or secondary to pregnancy or viral infections
    c. Valvular disease
    d. Drug-related myocardial injury
    e. Congenital heart disease
    f. Infection (Chagas' disease)
3. **Signs and symptoms:** The number of candidates for transplantation far exceeds the number of donor hearts. Careful assessment and selection are necessary to determine who can potentially return to a functional life after transplantation, as well as to ensure that all conventional remedies have been exhausted.
    a. Subjective findings: Complaints of dyspnea, angina, low exercise tolerance (bed-to-chair existence, bedridden)
    b. Physical findings
        i. Severe heart failure necessitating frequent "tune-ups" and hospitalizations
        ii. Cardiac cachexia: Anorexia, weight loss
        iii. Life-threatening arrhythmias
4. **Diagnostic study findings**
    a. See Heart Failure. Follow-up studies to evaluate disease progression and treatment effectiveness and to prevent complications.
    b. Right-sided heart catheterization: Used to guide therapy
        i. Assess PVR
            (a) Irreversible pulmonary hypertension is a cause of perioperative mortality
            (b) Donor heart cannot generate pressure high enough to maintain a sufficient pulmonary flow
            (c) Patients with irreversible pulmonary hypertension may be candidates for heart-lung transplantation
            (d) Pharmacologic agents (e.g., sildenafil) may be used to evaluate the potential for reversibility of increased PVR
        ii. Assess PAP, PCWP, CO
    c. Cardiac arteriography: Pretransplantation to ascertain the degree of CAD and the potential for revascularization
    d. Cardiac biopsy: To rule out amyloidosis and identify patients with sarcoidosis or myocarditis for possible immunosuppressive therapy
    e. EPS: To assess the effectiveness of antiarrhythmic therapy
5. **Goals of care**
    a. Balanced fluid status, intake, and output are maintained
    b. Patient and family participate in identifying lifestyle changes and support required in coping with transplantation
    c. Patient tolerates the new heart (successful transplantation)
6. **Collaborating professionals on health care team:** See Chronic Stable Angina; also electrophysiologist, transplant coordinator, psychologist, home health aide, financial services counselor

7. Management of patient care

   a. Anticipated patient trajectory: Heart transplantation is the standard of care and is performed on patients of all ages from newborn to 65 years. Mortality rate is as low as 4% from heart transplantation; average survival time is longer than 5 years.

   i. Positioning: Head of bed elevated for patient comfort and breathing ease

   ii. Nutrition

   (a) Assess nutritional status: To optimize the potential for posttransplantation success and facilitate the healing process

   (b) Restrict diet to less than 2 gm sodium, 1000 to 1500 ml fluid

   iii. Infection control

   (a) Observe for and prevent infections (from IV drips, central lines, immunosuppressive therapies). Screen visitors for communicable illnesses due to the patient's suppressed immune system. (Have visitors use masks, wash hands, limit contact.)

   (b) Administer antimicrobial prophylaxis used to prevent nosocomial infections

   iv. Discharge planning

   (a) Discuss with the patient and family the following aspects of the transplantation process:

      (1) Body image changes with the new heart

      (2) Importance of family support

      (3) Unknown waiting period

      (4) Cost: Huge financial burden; insurance coverage

      (5) Frequency of checkups, tests; stress need for regular examinations

      (6) Possibility of failure to be accepted as a transplantation candidate

      (7) Possibility of rejection reaction after transplantation

      (8) Dependency issues

      (9) Arrange for the patient and family to talk with transplantation survivors

   (b) Home oxygen: May be required for dyspnea, pulmonary congestion

   (c) Home health care: Includes IV therapy

   (d) Information on the use of indwelling catheters: For home-based IV therapy to reduce infection risks

   (e) Hospitalizations: Patient and significant others need to be instructed with regard to the following:

      (1) Possible need for frequent hospital visits for "tune-ups," medication changes, close observation

      (2) Need for hemodynamic monitoring

      (3) Need for high-dose medications

      (4) Use of mechanical assists: IABP, VAD, ventilators

   v. Pharmacology: See also Heart Failure

   (a) Preload reduction: Diuretics, nitrates

   (b) IV inotropic drugs (e.g., milrinone, dobutamine to increase CO, improve renal perfusion)

   (c) Afterload reduction

   (d) Antiarrhythmic therapy

   (e) Anticoagulation: For risk of thromboembolism

   (f) Immunosuppressive protocols (e.g., cyclosporine, tacrolimus, steroids)

   (g) Statin therapy: Lowering lipid levels shows positive effects on cardiac allograft rejection; immunosuppressive drugs can cause hyperlipidemia

(h) Antibiotic prophylaxis
vi. Psychosocial issues
  (a) Prepare the patient for the rigors of waiting for transplantation and the care before and after
  (b) Assess emotional status: Psychiatric history, motivational issues. Transplantation is a major stressful undertaking.
  (c) Assess the support system: Strong family, friends, and medical support are needed
  (d) Assess financial issues: Insurance coverage for costly procedure, drugs, follow-up care
  (e) Determine alcohol and drug use history
  (f) Assess the ability to comply with a complex lifelong medical regimen: Frequent follow-up examinations (include endomyocardial biopsies, strict medication protocols, rejection issues). Transplantation requires active patient participation.
  (g) Determine dependency issues. Formulate a plan with the patient and significant others
    (1) Allow the patient to do what he or she can
    (2) Family is included in care in the hospital
    (3) Home services are arranged
    (4) Need for immediate readiness is emphasized. When a donor heart becomes available, ischemic time (time from cross-clamp [donor] to cross-clamp [recipient]) must be less than 5 hours (or the heart is not usable); therefore, the patient must not travel.
vii. Treatments
  (a) Patient refractory to IV inotropic therapy should be transported to a facility with a cardiac transplantation program
  (b) AICD may need to be placed to prevent sudden death
  (c) Extracorporeal devices (e.g., LVAD): Used as a bridge to transplantation or therapy for patients (see Heart Failure)
  (d) Evaluate the potential for posttransplantation success
    (1) In patients with insulin-dependent diabetes, steroid therapy after transplantation can increase blood glucose levels
    (2) In patients with renal disease, cyclosporine therapy is nephrotoxic
  (e) Teaching points for immediately postoperative cardiac transplantation care are similar to those for CABG care
b. Potential complications
  i. Related to ventricular dysfunction: Arrhythmias, heart failure, cardiomyopathy
  ii. Postoperative CABG complications and additional transplantation complications, which include the following:
    (a) Allograft rejection
    (b) RV failure from high pulmonary vascular resistance
    (c) Bradycardia: Pacemaker may be needed; isoproterenol may be used. Atropine will not help denervated transplanted heart.
    (d) Immunosuppressive therapy complications
      (1) Increased susceptibility to infection
      (2) Adverse effects can include nephrotoxicity, hypertension, hyperlipidemia, seizures
8. **Evaluation of patient care**
  a. Balanced fluid status (intake and output) is maintained
  b. Patient and family actively participate in the plan of care

    c. Transplantation process is successful. Patient is tolerating the new heart without signs of infection or rejection.

    d. Patient demonstrates an understanding of the information and skills required for complex home management

Cardiac Trauma

Trauma to the heart can occur from penetrating injuries (e.g., knife, gunshot wounds) or nonpenetrating injuries (deceleration, myocardial contusions from falls and motor vehicle crashes). Injury may be to the pericardium, a single chamber, two or more chambers, the great vessels, and/or the coronary arteries.

1. Pathophysiology

    a. Penetrating cardiac trauma: 50% prehospital mortality

        i. Open wound hemorrhages into the pericardial space. Hypovolemic shock may be present as a result of the hemorrhaging. Most stab wounds (80% to 90%) result in tamponade.

        ii. Gunshot wounds cause cellular damage to adjacent areas of the myocardium

            (a) Myocardial damage is usually extensive, with profuse bleeding

            (b) Most commonly affects the RV; often more than one chamber involved

    b. Nonpenetrating or blunt trauma

        i. Deceleration injury is caused by

            (a) Sternal compression

            (b) Impingement of the heart between the sternum and spinal column

            (c) Rupture or dissection of the aorta at the ligamentum arteriosum, where it is anchored

        ii. Blunt aortic trauma creates a shearing force within the vessel

            (a) Causes laceration

            (b) Intimal tear may cause dissections

            (c) Hemorrhage, cardiac tamponade, and subsequent shock are the most pressing events

            (d) With cardiac tamponade: Decreased ventricular (diastolic) filling volume leads to hypovolemia, hypotension, and death

        iii. Myocardial contusion: Direct damage to the myocardium causes temporary or permanent myocardial dysfunction

            (a) RV is the chamber most commonly injured, because of its anatomic position (behind the sternum). Second in frequency is the LV.

            (b) If significant pulmonary contusion and adult respiratory distress syndrome have occurred, pulmonary hypertension results, causing the right chambers to fail

        iv. Electrical injuries: Tissue damage due to the conversion of electrical energy into thermal energy

            (a) Autonomic nervous system emits a large amount of catecholamines

            (b) Myocytes may be stunned, injured, or damaged, which decreases contractility and CO

2. Etiology and risk factors

    a. Penetrating trauma

        i. Gunshot wounds, knives, ice picks, low-velocity shrapnel, flying objects

        ii. Fractures of ribs and sternum (rare cause)

    b. Nonpenetrating or blunt trauma

        i. Motor vehicle crashes

        ii. Falls

      iii. Physical crushing assaults, direct blows to the chest by the fist or objects such as a steering wheel or baseball

      iv. Kicks from large animals

      v. Blasts, electrical injuries, lightning strikes

   c. Iatrogenic trauma: CPR, endomyocardial biopsy, pericardiocentesis

3. Signs and symptoms

   a. Patient history: Generally provides limited information

      i. Patient is often unconscious

      ii. Have a high index of suspicion when obtaining the patient history. Serious cardiac sequelae may have a delayed onset (hours to days) after trauma.

      iii. Penetrating wounds easier to assess than blunt injuries

      iv. Survival rate is better with stab wounds to the LV (they often seal off, if small), depending on the clinical condition on arrival to the emergency department, the method of injury, and associated injuries. Wounds to the RA and RV cause rapid hemopericardium and tamponade due to their thinner walls.

   b. Physical examination

      i. Symptoms of hemorrhage, shock

      ii. Blunt trauma (aorta): May produce few symptoms

      iii. Most common valve ruptured is the aortic. Observe for signs and symptoms of acute aortic insufficiency—cardiogenic shock, chest pain, dyspnea.

      iv. Urinary output absent or decreased (aortic rupture)

      v. Myocardial contusion: May produce subtle signs of chest pain, similar to those of MI

      vi. Inspect trauma patients for associated injuries: Head, neck, chest, abdomen

      vii. Jugular venous pressure: Increased with tamponade

     viii. Pulses may be decreased in the legs

      ix. Discrepancy between pulses in the upper extremities; no femoral pulses (suspect blunt trauma in high-speed automobile crashes, truncal deceleration—sternal, first rib injuries)

      x. Isolated upper body hypertension (blunt trauma to the aorta)

      xi. New holosystolic murmurs heard with a ruptured ventricular septum, diastolic murmur with aortic insufficiency

      xii. Pericardial rub: Heard in contusions

4. Diagnostic study findings

   a. ECG: If ECG and troponin levels are abnormal, need to monitor the patient closely for at least 24 hours

      i. Sinus tachycardia, atrial flutter or fibrillation, premature ventricular contractions, VT, VF, pulseless electrical activity (PEA)

      ii. Prolonged QTc interval

      iii. Low voltage, electrical alternans (in pericardial effusions)

      iv. RBBB (ruptured ventricular septum)

      v. Right precordial ECG lead V_4R: To check for signs of RV injury

      vi. Infarct patterns with coronary artery lacerations

      vii. ST elevations (pericarditis, coronary lacerations)

   b. Radiologic

      i. Possible enlargement of the cardiac silhouette

      ii. Hemothorax

      iii. Rib fractures, pneumothorax, tension pneumothorax

      iv. Pulmonary edema

v. Aortic trauma: Mediastinal widening; loss of the aortic knob, left pleural effusion

  c. Echocardiography: Helps detect lesions in valves and septum, pericardial effusions, tamponade; evaluates LV function

  d. CT and MRI: For aortic trauma

  e. TEE: Potential for additionally diagnosing aortic dissections

  f. Pericardiocentesis: For treatment of tamponade

5. Goals of care

  a. Oxygenation is adequate

  b. Hemodynamics are stable

  c. Blood pressure is normal

  d. Sinus rhythm is maintained and the patient is free of ectopy and arrhythmias

6. Collaborating professionals on health care team: See Chronic Stable Angina; also emergency medical service personnel, intensive care personnel, rehabilitation services personnel

7. Management of patient care

  a. Anticipated patient trajectory: Rapid transport to a trauma center, if nearby, affords the patient the best chance of survival

  i. Psychosocial issues: Many patients do not survive. Families need help identifying community resources (counseling, spiritual support, social services) for grieving and loss.

  ii. Treatments

  (a) Perform rapid assessment of airway, breathing, circulation, need for cervical immobilization

  (b) Perform CPR as needed

  (c) Ensure adequate oxygenation: Use pulse oximetry, check ABG results, evaluate the need for intubation or mechanical ventilation (there is a high risk of hypoxemia)

  (d) Listen to breath sounds: Check for tension pneumothorax

  (e) Monitor continuously for adequate pulse, blood pressure, hemodynamics

  (f) Closely observe for arrhythmias, PEA

  (g) Ensure that at least two large-bore IV lines are inserted for access. Central line and arterial line are often indicated.

  (h) Prepare the patient for emergency procedures

  (1) Pericardiocentesis: For tamponade

  (2) Chest tube insertion: For tension pneumothorax, hemopneumothorax

  (3) Emergency thoracotomy: At bedside or in the emergency department, if the patient is in extremis (bridge to the operating room)

  (4) Emergency surgery in the operating room for repair of ventricles, valves

  (5) Fasciotomies, débridement in cases of electrical burns

  (i) Treat contusion similarly to MI with rest, close monitoring, oxygenation, maintenance of fluid balance, treatment of arrhythmias

  b. Potential complications

  i. Hypovolemia

  (a) Mechanism: Due to hemorrhage, hypovolemic shock, burns; decreased contractility, which severely lowers CO

  (b) Management

  (1) Monitor vital signs continuously, particularly blood pressure, temperature, heart rate

        (2) Watch for changes in mental status

        (3) Closely watch hemodynamics: CVP, PCWP, MAP

        (4) Elevate the lower extremities to increase preload, if necessary

        (5) Weigh daily; maintain strict intake and output measurements, including all losses plus output of drainage tubes (nasogastric tube, chest tubes)

        (6) Maintain two large-bore (16-gauge) IV lines for administration of volume expanders, drugs

        (7) Administer volume expanders as ordered, including blood, fresh frozen plasma, fluids, crystalloids, colloids (dextran, albumin)

        (8) Observe the condition of the skin: Color, turgor, temperature, refill

        (9) Monitor laboratory values for abnormalities

    ii. Sudden death and arrhythmias (e.g., VF, VT, asystole, PEA): See Cardiac Rhythm Disorders

        (a) Prompt recognition and treatment of arrhythmia. Defibrillate for VF, VT

        (b) Identify reversible causes of PEA (i.e., hypovolemia, hypoxemia, hyperacidosis, tamponade, tension pneumothorax)

    iii. Infection

        (a) Mechanism: Foreign body, trauma, surgery

        (b) Management

            (1) Monitor for elevated temperature, localized pain, swelling, redness at trauma site

            (2) Check temperature often; report if it exceeds parameters (e.g., 101° F [38.3° C] or higher)

            (3) Check laboratory results (i.e., leukocyte count elevated). Monitor culture reports.

            (4) Frequently monitor invasive line and wound sites

            (5) Keep wounds clean; change dressings per unit standards

            (6) Administer antibiotics as ordered to maintain therapeutic blood levels

            (7) Maintain blood and body fluid precautions, good hand-washing technique

            (8) Maintain aseptic technique for bedside procedures

            (9) Monitor age of invasive lines, IV lines, Foley catheter

    iv. Other potential complications include the following:

        (a) Traumatic pericarditis, tamponade due to blunt or penetrating trauma

        (b) Embolization is a potential problem when bullets or fragments remain in chambers

        (c) Coronary artery lacerations cause tamponade, MI, shock, severe hemorrhage, and death

        (d) Late complications with contusions and lacerations: Myocardial fibrosis can cause akinesia, hypokinesia, LV aneurysms, heart failure

        (e) Electrical injuries can cause cardiac arrest, MI, hypertension (due to increased peripheral vasospasm)

8. Evaluation of patient care

  a. CO is within set parameters for the patient

  b. No arrhythmias are present, or arrhythmias are controlled by medications and pacemakers

  c. Fluid volume (intake and output, preload) and electrolyte levels are within normal limits

  d. No signs or symptoms of infection are present

     i. Wound and incision sites are free of signs of infection

     ii. Temperature and vital signs are within normal limits

     iii. Laboratory results (CBC, culture results) are normal

Cardiac Rhythm Disorders

Life-threatening cardiac rhythms are divided into arrhythmias that are either too slow, too fast, or unable to generate an adequate pulse

Symptomatic Bradycardia

Bradycardias, conduction defects, and slow escape rhythms

1. **Pathophysiology**
   a. Dysfunction of the SA node: Result of ischemia, infarction, disease, degeneration, defects, or drug effects (SA exit blocks, severe sinus bradycardia, sinus pause, sinus arrest, sick sinus syndrome)
   b. Dysfunction of the AV node: Result of ischemia, infarction, disease, defects, degeneration, or drug effects; leads to AV conduction defects—second-degree, types I and II, third-degree (complete) heart block
      i. AV nodal tissue slows or fails to propagate electrical impulses to the ventricles
      ii. Slower pacemaker cells in lower sites (junctional, bundle of His, ventricular) escape and take over as the cardiac pacemaker in third-degree blocks
      iii. In acute anterior MI, complete heart block develops in 6% to 10% of patients
      iv. In inferior MI, ischemia or infarction of the AV node may create a temporary conduction defect, which usually resolves in less than a week
   c. Hypersensitivity of the carotid sinus: Exaggerated response to vagal stimulation causes slowing of the heart rate and conductivity and lowering of the blood pressure
2. **Etiology and risk factors**
   a. Parasympathetic or vagal stimulation: Valsalva maneuver, nausea, vomiting, suctioning, pain
   b. Aging: Structural degeneration of the conductive system
   c. MI, ischemic heart disease
   d. Drugs: Calcium channel blockers (verapamil, diltiazem); cardiac glycosides (digoxin); β-blockers (propranolol)
   e. Infectious process: Endocarditis, myocarditis, typhoid fever, rheumatic fever, Chagas' disease
   f. Metabolic disorders: Myxedema, hypothermia, hypercalcemia
   g. Aortic stenosis
   h. Tumors
   i. Trauma (post–cardiac surgery)
   j. Connective tissue disease (sarcoidosis, amyloidosis, systemic lupus erythematous, thyroid disease)
   k. Dive reflex (immersion in cold water)
3. **Signs and symptoms**
   a. Syncope or presyncope
   b. Wooziness, light-headedness
   c. Fatigue, weakness
   d. Shortness of breath
   e. Angina
   f. Pauses in pulse longer than 3 seconds
   g. Heart rates lower than 40 beats/min

      h. Hypotension

      i. Signs of heart failure, cardiogenic shock

      j. Dyspnea

      k. Exercise intolerance

      l. Decreased CO, CI

4. Diagnostic study findings

  a. ECG: See Table 3-6 for arrhythmia features

      i. Correlation of symptoms with documented ECG is main diagnostic tool

      ii. Pauses more than 3 seconds in duration

      iii. Third-degree heart block with inferior MI: Usually narrow QRS complex accompanies bradycardia (higher escape pacemaker)

      iv. Third-degree heart block with anterior MI: Wide QRS complex may be observed (lower escape pacemaker)

  b. Holter monitoring: To identify arrhythmias not documented elsewhere and correlate with symptoms

  c. EPS: To test SA and AV node function, confirm need for permanent pacemaker

5. Goals of care

  a. Hemodynamics are improved via improved heart rate

  b. Symptoms from bradycardia are decreased or absent

6. Collaborating professionals on health care team: See Chronic Stable Angina; also electrophysiologist

7. Management of patient care

  a. Anticipated patient trajectory: Marked bradycardia results in diminished CO, poor tissue perfusion, hypotension, and potentially loss of consciousness and death

      i. Infection control: Proper wound care and site observation (for drainage, redness, tenderness) is necessary to decrease the potential for infection from pacemakers. Monitor temperature, laboratory results (white blood cell count).

      ii. Discharge planning: Patient education regarding the following:

        (a) Rationales, procedure, and wound care for pacer placement

        (b) Daily pulse checks at home (permanent pacemaker)

        (c) Symptoms to report: Wooziness, fainting, prolonged weakness, fatigue, palpitations, chest pain, difficulty breathing, fever, redness, drainage or swelling at surgical site, prolonged hiccups, electrical shocks

        (d) Follow-up care: To assess pacemaker function, adjust pacemaker parameters

        (e) Hazards or interference to avoid: Digital pagers, cellular phones, microwaves less than 1 ft away

        (f) Identification bracelet (medical alert)

        (g) Home (telephonic) pacemaker monitoring

      iii. Pharmacology

        (a) If the patient is symptomatic, administer atropine, 0.5 to 1.0 mg IV

          (1) Given every 3 to 5 minutes IV; total IV dosage of up to 0.04 mg/kg

          (2) Effective for marked sinus bradycardia, second-degree and some third-degree blocks

          (3) Dose of less than 0.5 mg IV can cause paradoxical bradycardia

        (b) Other potential medications include dopamine, epinephrine, isoproterenol

        (c) Isoproterenol is used for heart transplant patients; due to vagal denervation, these patients will not respond to atropine

 iv. Treatments
  (a) If the patient is in stable condition or asymptomatic: Monitor closely, notify the physician, determine possible causes, have medications and transcutaneous pacemaker equipment readily available (especially if the patient is in third-degree block or second-degree AV block type II)
  (b) Ensure adequate oxygenation: Oxygen saturations of 92% or higher
  (c) Check the patency of IV lines
  (d) Pacemakers: If the patient is unable to maintain adequate CO, use of a temporary or permanent pacemaker is indicated
   (1) Purpose: To provide an extrinsic electrical impulse so that depolarization and subsequent contraction occur
   (2) Modes of pacing (see also Figure 3-18)
    a) Fixed rate (asynchronous): Impulses are delivered at a predetermined rate, irrespective of any intrinsic electrical activity
    b) Demand (synchronous): Impulses are delivered at a predetermined rate only if the patient's own heart rate is less than the pacemaker's set rate

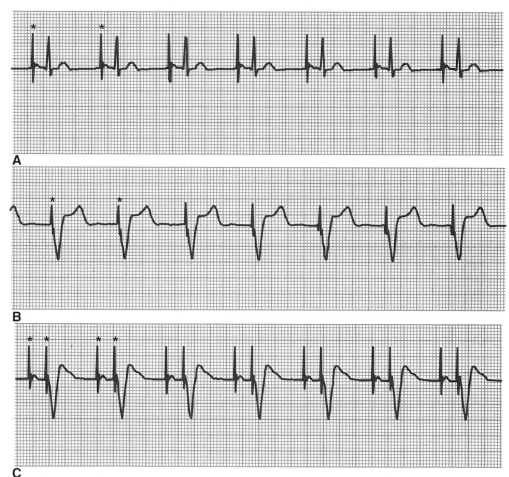

FIGURE 3-18 ■ Pacing examples. **A,** Atrial pacing. **B,** Ventricular pacing. **C,** Dual-chamber pacing. The asterisk indicates the pacemaker impulse. (From Urden LD, Stacy KM, Lough ME: *Thelan's critical care nursing: diagnosis and management,* Philadelphia, 2002, Mosby, p 378.)

c) Dual chamber: Pacemakers that can sense electrical activity in and pace either or both chambers to provide the normal sequence of atrial and ventricular contraction (AV sequential pacing) are the most common

d) Rate responsive: Pacemakers increase the heart rate to meet the demands of increased activity

(3) Components of all pacemakers

a) Battery

1) In temporary pacers, battery longevity depends on use and capabilities. Batteries should be checked routinely and changed per unit standards.

2) Permanent pacemaker batteries last 7 to 10 years (varies with the degree of the patient's pacemaker dependency)

b) Lead system: Transmission of electrical impulse as follows:

1) Unipolar electrode systems: One pole is the pacing lead tip and the other pole is the pacemaker generator; produce large pacing spikes, easily seen on monitors and ECGs

2) Bipolar electrode systems (most common): Both negative and positive electrode poles are at the distal end of the pacing lead; produce small pacing spikes, often not seen on monitors and ECGs

c) Pulse generator; pacemaker's control box

(4) Capture threshold level: Minimum pacemaker output setting required to pace the heart 100%

a) Factors increasing the threshold: Hyperkalemia, hypoxia, drugs (β-blockers, type I antiarrhythmics)

b) Factors decreasing the threshold: Increased catecholamine levels, digitalis toxicity, corticosteroids

(e) Transcutaneous pacemaker: Emergency therapy used until a transvenous pacer can be inserted. Many have monitoring, defibrillation, and pacing capabilities.

(1) One large anterior pacing electrode is ideally placed over the heart, and the other is placed directly posterior on the back. Other models have sternal-apex electrodes.

(2) Pacemaker electrodes are attached to an output cable attached to a pacing unit. Pacing unit is generally part of a portable defibrillator unit.

(3) Pacing rate and output are then set. Rate initially is set at 80 beats/min. Output is gradually increased until a pacer spike with a depolarization (pacer-generated QRS) is seen.

(f) Transvenous pacemaker: Pacing catheter is placed via the percutaneous route to the RA, RV, or both for pacing. The proximal end of the catheter is attached to a pacing generator.

(1) Initial rate usually set at 60 to 80 beats/min

(2) Output is set to an intermediate level (approximately 5 mA) and decreased until capture is lost (usually at less than 2 mA)

(3) Pacing output is then set to two to three times the level required for capture

(g) Epicardial transthoracic pacing: Electrode wires are attached to the epicardium (RA, RV, or both). Used during cardiac surgery in anticipation of conduction defects or arrhythmias. Proximal ends exit through the chest wall for attachment to the pulse generator.

         (1) Electrode wires need to be insulated when not in use

         (2) May have one or two RA and one or two RV wires and a ground wire

      (h) Permanent pacemaker: Leads placed in contact with the endocardium. Generator is implanted in a subcutaneous, subclavicular, or abdominal pocket. Capabilities can include sequential pacing of the RA, RV, or both; programmability and rate responsiveness to allow for heart rate increases during exercise.

       (i) Key points for nursing care of patients with pacemakers: See Box 3-8

b. Potential complications

    i. Monitor for complications of pacemaker insertion

      (a) Pneumothorax

      (b) Myocardial perforation: Can lead to hypotension, tamponade

      (c) Hematoma

      (d) Arrhythmias (premature ventricular contractions)

      (e) Infections (systemic or local)

      (f) Hiccups, muscle twitches (from stimulation of the diaphragm, abdomen)

    ii. Monitor for pacemaker malfunctions (Box 3-9 and Figures 3-19 and 3-20)

■ **BOX 3-8**
■ **KEY POINTS IN THE NURSING CARE OF PATIENTS WITH PACEMAKERS**

TRANSCUTANEOUS PACEMAKERS
■ Patient will need sedation and analgesia because of increased output requirements (50 to 200 mV) for transcutaneous route
■ Cardiopulmonary resuscitation may be performed safely over pacing electrodes, if needed
■ Frequent inspection of skin is needed to prevent potential burns, if pacing is prolonged

TRANSVENOUS PACEMAKERS
1. Ensure that chest radiograph is obtained to rule out pneumothorax if pacemaker is placed via subclavian or internal jugular approach
2. Monitor closely for appropriate sensing and pacing
3. Take appropriate action in case of sudden loss of capture
  ● Can signify that pacing electrode has migrated out of position or perforated right ventricle
  ● Increase output to attempt recapture and notify physician
  ● Do not attempt to reposition pacing electrode
  ● Be prepared to use atropine, isoproterenol, or transcutaneous pacing
4. Ensure electrical safety when using temporary pacemaker
  ● Ensure that all equipment is grounded and in good working order
  ● Wear gloves when handling electrodes
  ● Place pulse generator in plastic bag or glove to protect from bodily fluids, other liquids
  ● Position pulse generator in safe location (i.e., intravenous drip pole, holder strap when ambulating) to avoid dropping it or patient's rolling over on it in bed

EPICARDIAL TRANSTHORACIC PACEMAKER
■ Electrode wires need to be insulated when not in use

PERMANENT PACEMAKER
1. Keep defibrillator paddles 1 to 2 inches away from permanent pacemaker site on chest
2. Ensure pacer is interrogated after defibrillation or code is over
3. Have magnet (doughnut) available: Used over pacer to program to asynchronous mode if pacemaker-mediated tachycardia is suspected or if electrocautery is to be used

■ **BOX 3-9**
■ **COMPLICATIONS ASSOCIATED WITH PACEMAKER FUNCTIONING**

FAILURE TO PACE
No pacer spike seen at appropriate times
Caused by
- Battery failure
- Lead dislodgement
- Wire fracture
- Disconnection of wire or cable
- Generator failure
- Oversensing: No impulse generated because some other activity (often muscular) has been sensed and misinterpreted as a QRS complex

FAILURE TO CAPTURE
Pacer-generated QRS not seen
Caused by
- Lead dislodgement or malposition
- Battery failure
- Pacing at voltage below capture threshold
- Faulty connections
- Lead fracture
- Ventricular perforation

FAILURE TO SENSE
Pacemaker may compete with patient's own intrinsic rhythm
Caused by
- Sensitivity setting that is too high
- Battery failure
- Malposition of catheter lead
- Lead fracture
- Pulse generator failure
- Lead insulation break

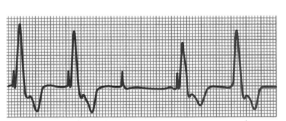

FIGURE 3-19 ■ Failure of the pulse generator to capture. (From Phillips RE, Feeney MR: *The cardiac rhythms*, ed 2, Philadelphia, 1980, Saunders, p 347.)

8. **Evaluation of patient care**
   a. Heart rate is sufficient to maintain stable vital signs and CO
   b. Arrhythmias are controlled or absent
   c. Pacemaker functions properly with no signs of failure to pace, capture, or sense
   d. Patient or significant other verbalizes an understanding of the rationale, procedure, and follow-up for pacemaker use

Symptomatic Tachycardia

Rhythms in this section include SVTs or VTs that cause symptoms necessitating immediate conversion or control

1. **Pathophysiology**
    a. With increased heart rate at rest, diastolic filling period shortens and CO falls because of decreased ventricular filling
    b. Eventually, blood pressure drops
    c. Pulmonary venous pressures increase, causing shortness of breath and dyspnea as the result of pulmonary congestion
    d. Heart rate at which CO declines is variable and depends on the patient's substrate cardiac function
    e. Myocardial oxygen demands increase and myocardial oxygen supply decreases due to diminished coronary perfusion at rapid heart rates; subendocardial ischemia can result
    f. Loss of atrial systole (kick) decreases the ventricular diastolic filling volume; SV and CO fall 10% to 15% in rhythms without a normal atrial-ventricular sequence of contraction
    g. Decreased output can result in end-organ dysfunction (e.g., syncope, presyncope, oliguria, ischemia)
2. **Etiology and risk factors**
    a. SVTs
        i. Acute MI
        ii. Ischemia
        iii. Reentry (most common cause of paroxysmal SVT)
        iv. Valvular heart disease
        v. Use of stimulants: Alcohol, coffee, tobacco
        vi. Congenital heart disease
        vii. Pulmonary disease
        viii. Drug toxicity: Digitalis, antidepressants
        ix. WPW syndrome (accessory pathway)
        x. Cardiomyopathies
    b. VT: Sustained (>30 seconds)
        i. Acute MI
        ii. Ischemia
        iii. Cardiomyopathies
        iv. Tetralogy of Fallot
        v. Drugs: Digitalis, antiarrhythmic agents
        vi. Electrolyte imbalances: Low potassium, magnesium
        vii. Hypoxia
        viii. LV aneurysms
        ix. Congenital long QT syndromes
        x. Valvular heart disease
3. **Signs and symptoms**
    a. Dyspnea
    b. Palpitations
    c. Shortness of breath
    d. Angina
    e. Wooziness, syncope
    f. Weakness, exercise intolerance
    g. Anxiety
    h. Mentation changes
    i. Heart rate exceeding 100 beats/min
    j. Jugular venous distention

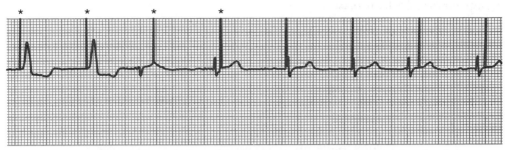

FIGURE 3-20 ■ Pacemaker malfunction: Undersensing. Notice that after the first two paced beats, a series of intrinsic beats occurs; the pacemaker unit fails to sense these intrinsic QRS complexes. These spikes do not capture the ventricle because they occur during the refractory period of the cardiac cycle. The asterisk indicates the pacemaker impulse. (From Urden LD, Stacy KM, Lough ME: *Thelan's critical care nursing: diagnosis and management*, Philadelphia, 2002, Mosby, p 447.)

    k. Polyuria, oliguria

    l. Hypotension

    m. Unconsciousness

    n. Rapid, thready pulse or pulse deficit

4. Diagnostic study findings

    a. Laboratory: To ascertain

        i. Imbalances of electrolytes, include magnesium

        ii. ABG levels: Hypoxia, acidosis

        iii. CBC: To rule out hemorrhage, infection

    b. ECG

        i. See ECG features for VT (see Table 3-6)

        ii. See ECG features for SVTs (see Table 3-6)

    c. Intracardiac electrode

    d. EPS, after the patient's condition is stabilized

5. Goals of care

    a. Rapid rhythm is terminated or rate is controlled to maintain adequate CO and tissue perfusion

    b. Patient has relief of symptoms related to the rapid rhythm

6. Collaborating professionals on health care team: See Chronic Stable Angina; also electrophysiologist, anticoagulation clinic or nurse

7. Management of patient care

    a. Anticipated patient trajectory: Marked tachycardia results in diminished CO, poor tissue perfusion, hypotension, and potentially loss of consciousness and death

        i. Pharmacology

            (a) Stable narrow QRS supraventricular rhythms

                (1) Adenosine may be administered, 6 mg IV, injected over 3 seconds or less, followed by a dose of 12 mg 1 to 2 minutes later

                    a) Adenosine often terminates AV nodal reentry and sinus nodal reentrant tachycardia

                    b) Not used for atrial fibrillation or flutter

                (2) Atrial fibrillation: Most frequently seen supraventricular tachyarrhythmia

                    a) Main goals are to lower ventricular response rate, decrease symptoms, and convert to sinus rhythm if and when possible

b) If the duration of atrial fibrillation is longer than 48 hours (or if unknown), anticoagulation is necessary to decrease the risk of atrial thrombi and CVA. INR of 2 to 3 (for at least 1 month) is necessary prior to elective direct current (DC) cardioversion. IV heparin is initiated and continued until the treatment plan is determined.

c) If the duration is less than 48 hours, diltiazem, digoxin, or β-blockers are used for rate control

d) If the duration is less than 48 hours, amiodarone may be used to convert the rhythm prior to elective cardioversion

e) If the duration is longer than 48 hours, antiarrhythmic drugs (amiodarone, procainamide) are not used, because they could convert the rhythm and place the patient at risk for a thrombotic event prior to adequate anticoagulation

f) Rate control of chronic atrial fibrillation has better long-term outcomes than attempts to maintain sinus rhythm with antiarrhythmics

(3) Atrial flutter: Rate control with β-blockers. Calcium channel blockers and digoxin are given prior to DC cardioversion or radiofrequency ablation.

(4) Automatic atrial tachycardia (produced by enhanced automaticity in atrial tissue): β-blockers, propafenone (amiodarone, if poor LV function)

(5) Multifocal atrial tachycardia (MAT): Metoprolol, verapamil, magnesium

a) Correct the underlying cause

b) MAT is unresponsive to cardioversion

c) Theophylline levels should be checked (toxicity can cause MAT): MAT is often seen in respiratory failure

(6) AV nodal reentrant tachycardia (AVNRT), atrioventricular reciprocating tachycardia (AVRT), orthodromic (WPW syndrome): Adenosine

(b) Stable wide QRS arrhythmias

(1) VT

a) Amiodarone, 150 mg IV over 10 minutes, followed by 1 mg/min infusion for 6 hours, then maintenance infusion of 0.5 mg/min for 18 hours

1) Drug of choice with known LV dysfunction in both supraventricular and ventricular arrhythmias

2) Adverse effects: Hypotension, QT interval prolongation

b) Lidocaine, 0.5 to 0.75 mg/kg IV push, is given every 5 to 10 minutes to a total of 3 mg/kg if desired; maintenance infusion is 1 to 4 mg/min IV

c) Procainamide, if LV function is known to be good (EF of more than 40%)

1) 20 to 30 mg/min IV, injected slowly

2) Maximum dose: 17 mg/kg

3) End points for therapy: Arrhythmia termination; hypotension; widening of QRS by more than 50%

4) If procainamide is successful at terminating VT, infusion is started at 1 to 4 mg/min

      d) Treatment includes correcting the underlying cause. Choice of antiarrhythmic agent, when the patient is in stable condition, is guided by EPS or some other documented test of efficacy (e.g., serial Holter monitoring)

      e) Adenosine is no longer recommended to be used with wide QRS tachycardias as a diagnostic tool

  (2) Torsade de pointes (a polymorphic form of VT)

      a) Often seen as a proarrhythmic arrhythmia as a result of antiarrhythmic drug therapy

      b) Responds to measures that shorten the QT interval (isoproterenol, phenytoin, magnesium, overdrive pacing)

      c) If the patient is unstable, cardioversion is performed immediately per the advanced cardiac life support (ACLS) standards for VT

  (3) AVRT—antidromic (WPW): Wide complex; procainamide used

ii. Treatments

  (a) Evaluate stability by rapid assessment of vital signs, level of consciousness, related symptoms

  (b) Ensure adequate airway, breathing, circulation

  (c) Administer oxygen as needed to provide for oxygen saturations exceeding 92%

  (d) DC cardioversion: If the patient is symptomatic and unstable (heart rate above 150 beats/min), prepare for immediate cardioversion

    (1) Cardioversion is delivery (to the patient) of a selected amount of electrical energy synchronized with the R wave of the patient's intrinsic rhythm

    (2) Amount of energy required to convert tachyarrhythmias varies from 50 J (for reentrant tachycardias) to 360 J (for atrial fibrillation, VF)

    (3) Explain the entire procedure to the patient and significant others, including the risks

    (4) Obtain a consent form, if conditions are not deteriorating too rapidly

    (5) Sedative and anesthetic drugs are given to the patient before the procedure, if the patient is conscious (an anesthesiologist is often used for elective procedures)

    (6) Attach the defibrillator monitor leads to the patient; these leads can be piggybacked to many bedside monitors for quick ECG access

    (7) Make sure the monitor is synchronized to the patient's rhythm: the "Sync" button should be on, and spikes indicating the recognition of R waves should be seen on the monitor. If spikes are not seen, check the gain on the machine, try another lead, and/or adjust the electrodes

    (8) Code cart and suction equipment should be at bedside. Knowledge of the safe use of the defibrillator is vital.

    (9) Place the defibrillator on the left side of the bed if possible, to prevent the operator from leaning over the bed while cardioverting the patient

  (10) If the patient goes into VF, deliver immediate defibrillation; turn off the "Sync" button, if necessary (most machines default to defibrillation mode after a cardioversion attempt). Remember to turn the "Sync" button back on each time, if repeated cardioversion is necessary.

(e) Vagal maneuvers (gagging, cold water immersion) often terminate AVNRT. These are more successful when performed as soon after onset as possible. Patient should be instructed as to a safe procedure for home use.

(f) Radiofrequency ablation: Patient may need to be prepared for radiofrequency catheter ablation of accessory pathways

    (1) In the procedure, done in the EPS laboratory, a catheter is used to deliver low-voltage, high-frequency, alternating current that selectively damages myocardial tissue

    (2) Ablation stops the conduction of electrical impulses and disrupts the reentry circuit

    (3) Uses

        a) Accessory pathways: WPW syndrome

        b) Symptomatic SVT: AVNRT, AVRT with an accessory pathway, rapid AV conduction of atrial fibrillation, sinus node reentrant tachycardias

        c) Junctional tachycardia: Caused by enhanced automaticity; seen in infants and children after surgery for congenital heart defects and in digitalis toxicity

        d) Atrial flutter (treatment of choice)

        e) VT with bundle branch reentry, refractory VT

    (4) Complications of radiofrequency ablation

        a) Bleeding at the catheter site

        b) Deep venous thrombosis

        c) Cardiac tamponade

        d) Myocardial perforation

        e) Infection

        f) Ischemia

        g) Stroke

        h) Complete AV block

        i) Pulmonary embolism

        j) Pneumothorax

    (5) Patient education issues

        a) Procedure description, rationale

        b) Procedure length (2 to 4 hours average, up to 10 hours)

        c) Possible need for a permanent pacemaker

        d) Recurrence rate for tachyarrhythmias: 8% to 12%

        e) Monitor the patient and site (see Box 3-5)

(g) Atrial or transesophageal pacing (antitachycardia) may also be considered for termination of persistent stable tachycardias (atrial fibrillation, AVNRT, atrial tachycardia, AVRT in selected patients)

(h) Surgical endocardial or epicardial techniques for ablation of pathways are used in cases in which radiofrequency catheter ablation is not possible and the patient's symptoms are hindering quality of life. The surgical maze procedure is very successful in abolishing atrial fibrillation.

(i) AICD

    (1) Device is implanted into the patient with sensing leads and defibrillator patches attached to the endocardium and to a pulse generator. This is done by transvenous approach or a thoracotomy.

    (2) Capabilities include the following:

        a) Bradycardia pacing

        b) Overdrive pacing

          c) Cardioversion: At 25 J

          d) Defibrillation

          e) ECG measurement with storage and event logs

          f) Dual chamber pacemaking

        (3) Indications: Recurrent VT, VF; sudden cardiac death; or decreased LV EF of less than 30% (MADIT II trials; Moss et al, 1999)

        (4) Important issues to understand and teach to the patient and significant others:

          a) If the AICD discharges, it is not dangerous to the staff or family

          b) Incidence of spontaneous (appropriate or inappropriate) discharge is 75% the first year

          c) Concurrent use of antiarrhythmic agents is still necessary to decrease the frequency of events

          d) Interrogator units can analyze the history of shocks, battery life, and heart rhythm at the time of shock

8. Evaluation of patient care

  a. Signs of adequate CO are present

  b. Tachycardia is controlled and terminated

Absent or Ineffective Pulse

All cases of absent or ineffective pulse are life threatening and necessitate immediate intervention, usually CPR

1. Pathophysiology

  a. No CO and, subsequently, no tissue perfusion

  b. Respirations cease. Patient is clinically dead.

  c. Rapid cell death. Brain cells start to die after 4 to 6 minutes of circulatory collapse. After 10 minutes, some degree of brain death is inevitable.

  d. VF: Inability to generate an organized impulse for muscular contraction

  e. Asystole: No electrical activity initiated

  f. PEA: Electrical activity and conduction occur, with the absence of a palpable pulse and blood pressure. Rhythms seen are any rhythm except VF or VT.

    i. Caused by lack of ventricular filling volume (hypovolemia, fluid losses, saddle emboli, tamponade)

    ii. Caused by the myocardium's inability to contract effectively: Lack of oxygen, acidotic states, electrolyte disturbances (elevated or decreased potassium levels), physical impairment to contraction (tension pneumothorax, tamponade, pericardial effusion), muscular dysfunction from necrosis (MI), thrombosis, hypothermia, drug overdose

2. Etiology and risk factors

  a. Causes of VF or pulseless VT

    i. MI

    ii. Ischemia

    iii. Myocardial disease: Cardiomyopathies, myocarditis

    iv. Anoxia: Smoke inhalation, drowning, respiratory failure, airway obstruction

  b. Causes of asystole

    i. Hypokalemia

    ii. Hyperkalemia

    iii. Hypothermia

    iv. Acidosis

  c. Causes of PEA

    i. Hypovolemia: Most common cause

    ii. Hypoxia

   iii. Tension pneumothorax

   iv. Acidosis

   v. Acute MI

   vi. Pulmonary embolism

   vii. Hyperkalemia

   viii. Tamponade

   ix. Drug overdose: Calcium channel blockers, digitalis, tricyclic antidepressants, β-blockers

   x. Hypothermia

3. Signs and symptoms

 a. History

  i. History taking is often deferred or performed in conjunction with emergency, life-preserving measures

  ii. Determine whether the patient has a history of any of the aforementioned causes

 b. Physical examination

  i. No pulse

  ii. Unconsciousness or rapidly deteriorating level of consciousness

  iii. No respiration

4. Diagnostic study findings

 a. ABG levels: Measured after immediate actions taken, to check oxygenation, acidosis

 b. Electrolyte levels

 c. ECG or monitor

  i. In PEA, there is organized electrical activity but no significant CO

  ii. VF (coarse versus fine)

  iii. Pulseless VT (very rapid)

 d. No invasive studies are performed until the patient's condition is stabilized

5. Goals of care

 a. Life is preserved

 b. CO and tissue perfusion are restored rapidly without brain death

6. Collaborating professionals on health care team: Physician, nurse, pharmacist, respiratory therapist, chaplain

7. Management of patient care

 a. Anticipated patient trajectory: Patient "clinically dead." Preservation of life and avoidance of brain death require prompt action.

  i. Positioning: Lay patient flat, with a board under the back for support during CPR

  ii. Pharmacology

   (a) Emergency medications for VF and pulseless VT: See the current ACLS standards of the American Heart Association for detailed descriptions, algorithms

    (1) 100% oxygen

    (2) Epinephrine, 1 mg IV push, every 3 to 5 minutes during arrest; start after initial defibrillation

    (3) Vasopressin, 40 units IV, one time, as an alternative drug; half-life is 10 to 20 minutes

    (4) After epinephrine or vasopressin administration, and repeated defibrillation attempts, antiarrhythmic drugs are considered

     a) Amiodarone: Dose is 300 mg IV, diluted in 20 to 30 ml dextrose 5% in water, infused rapidly; dose of 150 mg IV given for recurrent VF

        b) Other antiarrhythmics used include lidocaine, 1 to 1.5 mg/kg IV (up to 3 mg/kg total); procainamide; and magnesium, 1 to 2 g IV (if polymorphic arrhythmia, hypomagnesemia)

   (b) Medications for asystole and PEA

     (1) Emergency medications given in boluses

     (2) Epinephrine, 1 mg IV push, every 3 to 5 minutes during arrest

     (3) Atropine, 1 mg IV, every 3 to 5 minutes (up to a total of 0.04 mg/kg maximum vagolytic dose)

     (4) Vasopressin is not recommended for PEA or asystole

     (5) Sodium bicarbonate, 1 mEq/kg, is used if the patient had prearrest hyperkalemia or drug overdose (i.e., tricyclic antidepressants)

     (6) Defibrillation is reattempted after each drug intervention

     (7) If hypokalemia: Potassium and magnesium are given

     (8) If hyperkalemia: Sodium bicarbonate, glucose and insulin, Kayexalate, digitalis, albuterol may be given

     (9) Thrombolytic agents may be given for massive pulmonary embolism

   (c) IV infusions are not hung during immediate arrest; they can be hung only after the patient's heart rate and rhythm have been restored

iii. Psychosocial issues: Family needs support during this time. Chaplain, social worker, nursing supervisor, and charge nurse can assist with comforting and communicating with significant others.

iv. Treatments

   (a) Immediately call cardiac arrest code team

   (b) Assess *a*irway, *b*reathing, and *c*irculation (ABC); perform CPR

   (c) Ensure that crash cart and emergency equipment are at bedside

   (d) Defibrillate as soon as equipment is available, without delay *if the patient is in VF, pulseless VT, or asystole* (could be fine VF)

     (1) Use 200, 300, and 360 J per ACLS standards

     (2) Be familiar with the safe use of the defibrillator. Always treat it as if it is a weapon and visually ensure that everyone at the bedside is clear from the bed before defibrillating (each time).

     (3) If the monitor shows a flat line, check the power (cables connected?), check the gain (too low?), check the other leads (activity may be seen in a different axis)

   (e) Ensure that CPR is resumed promptly after defibrillation or any assessments

   (f) Automatic external defibrillator may be the only defibrillator available in some areas of the hospital

     (1) Fully or semiautomatic models

     (2) Cables attach to two adhesive conductive pads

     (3) Machine records rhythm, analyzes data, states command to "Clear," and delivers electrical shocks

     (4) CPR must be stopped for the machine to analyze the rhythm (takes 15 to 20 seconds), then it will deliver shocks

     (5) Most problems result from operator difficulties (learn to use the equipment properly)

   (g) Transcutaneous pacemakers for asystole: If considered, should be used early in arrest (less than 5 min after onset) for the best chance of success. May be temporizing, to help the heart pace while the causes are identified and treated.

   (h) Induced hypothermia may be used to improve neurologic outcome after sudden cardiac death survival

      (i) AICD often used if the patient survives arrest

      (j) Promptly assess and treat for the common causes of PEA

          (1) Administer immediate volume replacement. Can lift legs for immediate autoinfusion

          (2) Listen for breath sounds; check for pneumothorax

          (3) Ensure proper oxygenation

          (4) Hyperventilate the patient: Respiratory acidosis usually occurs in arrest as a result of inadequate ventilation

          (5) Check ABG results for acidosis

          (6) Assist the physician with pericardiocentesis for tamponade, needle decompression of pneumothorax

          (7) Draw blood for measurement of electrolyte levels, drug screens

    v. Ethical issues

      (a) Health care professionals should be aware of the patient's wishes regarding CPR before emergencies occur. Advance directives should be identified at admission and "Do not attempt resuscitation" orders initiated and communicated to all appropriate staff. Patient and family need to understand that outpatient directives must be reinstituted as a medical order when the patient is hospitalized in order to be valid.

      (b) Duration of resuscitative efforts depends on many factors (i.e., age, medical condition)

8. Evaluation of patient care

    a. Signs of life are present: Adequate airway, breathing, circulation, and CO, and good mentation

    b. Arrhythmia is controlled and terminated

    c. Cause of arrest is identified and treated

    d. Patient's advance directive is respected by initiating a "Do not attempt resuscitation" order as appropriate.

Mitral Regurgitation

In mitral regurgitation, blood is partially regurgitated back into the LA during ventricular systole because of an incompetent mitral valve. This may happen acutely or develop as a chronic condition.

1. Pathophysiology

    a. With the failure of the mitral valve to close completely during ventricular contraction, some fraction of the LV output is ejected backwards into the LA

    b. Pressures in the LA and pulmonary veins rise (dramatically if the onset is acute), and pulmonary congestion and/or edema results in dyspnea

    c. Reduced forward output results in chronic fatigue (or hypotension if acute)

    d. The pathophysiology and clinical course vary dramatically, depending on whether the onset is acute or chronic

    e. Acute onset

      i. LA diastolic pressures, along with pulmonary pressures, dramatically increase

      ii. LA has no time to compensate and initially remains small and noncompliant (which creates high pressures)

      iii. Forward output falls dramatically, and cardiogenic shock develops

      iv. Pulmonary congestion may develop as a result of high pressures within the pulmonary vascular bed, and pulmonary edema rapidly ensues

    f. Chronic process

      i. LA has time (often years) to enlarge and develop compliance to keep pressures at near-normal levels

      ii. Pulmonary artery pressures remain relatively normal

     iii. Eventually the degree of mitral regurgitation may exceed the capacity of the LA to compensate, and pulmonary congestion and dyspnea may develop

     iv. LV compensates for chronic volume overload by dilating in an attempt to maintain normal forward output, while emptying a large volume of its output backward into the LA

      v. LV can dilate to the extent that it is unable to recover, even after surgical correction of mitral regurgitation

     vi. Pulmonary venous pressures rise, with resulting increases in PCWP and secondary pulmonary hypertension

    vii. Atrial fibrillation often is seen and occurs secondary to LA enlargement

   viii. RV also will progressively hypertrophy, and right-sided heart failure may follow

2. **Etiology and risk factors**
   a. Acute causes
      i. Acute rupture of the chordae tendineae as a result of endocarditis or chronic strain on the mitral valve apparatus by mitral valve prolapse, rheumatic heart disease
      ii. Papillary muscle dysfunction or rupture secondary to acute MI
      iii. Trauma
   b. Chronic causes
      i. Rheumatic heart disease
      ii. Congenital malformations of the mitral valve, chordae tendineae, or mitral annuli
      iii. Mitral valve prolapse
      iv. LV dilatation from other causes
      v. Connective tissue disease (e.g., Marfan's syndrome)
      vi. IE
      vii. Calcified mitral annulus

3. **Signs and symptoms**
   a. Subjective findings: Patient complains of
      i. Shortness of breath
      ii. Orthopnea
      iii. Paroxysmal nocturnal dyspnea
      iv. Weakness or becoming easily fatigued
      v. Palpitations
      vi. Symptoms of RV failure
   b. Objective findings: History of past rheumatic fever, streptococcal infection, endocarditis, ischemia, trauma, mitral valve prolapse
   c. Physical findings
      i. If the patient is in heart failure, the following may be seen:
         (a) Tachypnea
         (b) Anxiety
         (c) Diaphoresis
         (d) Cyanosis
         (e) Confusion
         (f) Edema
         (g) Jugular venous distention (right-sided heart failure)
         (h) Signs of pulmonary edema (frothy, pink sputum)
      ii. Other findings include the following:
         (a) Apical impulse (PMI) is laterally displaced, diffuse, and hyperdynamic (in chronic mitral regurgitation)

      (b) Apical systolic thrill may be felt

      (c) Pulse may be irregular if in atrial fibrillation

      (d) Hepatomegaly (late sign)

    iii. Auscultation

      (a) High-pitched, blowing holosystolic murmur

        (1) Heard best at apex with radiation to axilla

        (2) Begins at S_1 and extends through S_2 (aortic closure)

      (b) Rales if pulmonary congestion or edema present

      (c) S_2 may be widely split or accentuated (P_2) as a result of early closure of the aortic valve, because LV ejection time is shortened; pulmonic closure delayed because of right-sided heart pressure overload

      (d) Possible RV lift secondary to RV pressure overload

4. Diagnostic study findings

  a. Radiologic

    i. LA and LV enlargement in chronic mitral regurgitation

    ii. LA does not enlarge with acute onset

    iii. Calcification of mitral valve

    iv. Pulmonary edema

  b. ECG: Atrial fibrillation

  c. Echocardiography: Helps determine the cause, LV function and dimensions, indications for surgery

    i. Degree of insufficiency

    ii. LA and LV enlargement in chronic mitral insufficiency

    iii. Mitral valve prolapse, mitral annular calcification, flail leaflet, vegetations, rheumatic heart disease

    iv. Abnormal regional wall motion if papillary muscle dysfunction is the cause

  d. TEE: Used in guiding mitral valve reconstructive surgery; superior to transthoracic echocardiography in visualizing the mitral valve leaflets

  e. Cardiac catheterization

    i. Documents the severity of mitral regurgitation

    ii. Screens for CAD

    iii. Documents PCWP and right-sided heart pressures

5. Goals of care

  a. Patient is hemodynamically stable and in sinus rhythm

  b. Symptoms of reduced CO are identified and treated promptly

  c. Patient receives appropriate teaching regarding surgical interventions, medications, and discharge care

6. Collaborating professionals on health care team: See Chronic Stable Angina

7. Management of patient care

  a. Anticipated patient trajectory: Severe mitral regurgitation must be corrected, or progressive left-sided heart failure and early death occur

    i. Discharge planning

      (a) Instructions include the usual postoperative instructions for any heart surgery

      (b) If the valve is replaced, the importance of endocarditis prophylaxis and chronic anticoagulation is stressed (if the patient does not comply with the follow-up medication regimen, stroke and possibly death are highly likely)

    ii. Pharmacology

      (a) Treat atrial fibrillation: Slow the ventricular response, increase exercise capacity with digitalis, β-blockers, calcium antagonists

(b) Antibiotics: For prophylaxis of recurrent rheumatic heart disease, prophylaxis for IE during dental procedures

(c) Acute mitral regurgitation may respond to administration of vasodilators to decrease afterload (e.g., nitroprusside) or as a prelude to valve surgery

(d) Diuretics, nitrates: To lower pulmonary congestion; use carefully, may lower CO

(e) Anticoagulants: Prevent embolization if atrial fibrillation is present. Goal is an INR of 2 to 3.

iii. Treatments

(a) IABP may be a life-saving procedure in severe cases

(b) If the valve is to be surgically reconstructed (surgical mitral valvuloplasty) or replaced, the patient and family must be counseled with regard to the surgery

(1) Explain the disease process, preoperative routines, surgical procedure (including the replacement valve to be used), and expectations during the immediately postoperative period

(2) Mitral valve reconstruction shown to yield improved rest and exercise EFs postoperatively (benefits are partly the result of preserved chordae tendineae, papillary muscles, valve shape) and decreased mortality

(3) Chronic anticoagulant use is not necessary with reconstruction if the patient is in sinus rhythm

(4) Postoperative general care for valve repair is similar to postoperative care for most cardiac surgical operations

b. Potential complications

i. Systemic emboli with atrial fibrillation requiring anticoagulation

ii. IE: IE prophylaxis needed (see Infective Endocarditis)

8. **Evaluation of patient care**

a. Hemodynamic stability is evidenced by normal vital signs and lack of, or control of, arrhythmias

b. Postoperatively, no complications are noted

c. On discharge, the patient and significant others relate an understanding of all postoperative care measures (e.g., wound care, sternal precautions), the need for antibiotic prophylaxis when the patient undergoes future surgical or dental procedures, and, if necessary, chronic anticoagulant therapy

Mitral Stenosis

Mitral stenosis is a progressive narrowing of the mitral orifice that impedes the flow of blood from the LA to the LV during ventricular diastole

1. **Pathophysiology**

a. Progressive fibrosis, scarring, and thickening of the valve leaflets, usually from rheumatic valvular disease

b. Extensive fusion of the leaflets and chordae tendineae develops

c. Area of a normal adult's mitral valve orifice is 4 to 6 cm^2. In mild mitral stenosis, it is 2 cm^2 (symptoms may be experienced only with exercise, atrial fibrillation). In severe mitral stenosis, it is 1 cm^2, with symptoms apparent even at rest.

d. Elevation of LA pressures results from the obstruction to the flow from the LA to the LV. As the valve continues to narrow, the LA slowly dilates and hypertrophies.

e. Intractable atrial fibrillation usually results

    f. As atrial pressures elevate, pulmonary capillary hydrostatic pressure rises above the plasma oncotic pressure, and fluid escapes into the pulmonary interstitium and alveoli

    g. As the valve orifice narrows to smaller than 1 cm^2, pulmonary hypertension occurs and RV pressures increase, with eventual hypertrophy and dilatation. RV failure frequently follows.

    h. Stenotic obstruction impedes forward blood flow and alone is often enough to decrease SV and CO. Loss of atrial kick resulting from atrial fibrillation or tachycardia compound the problem, decreasing LV filling time and further decreasing CO.

    i. Atrial thrombi form in the LA appendage, and systemic or cerebral emboli may ensue

2. Etiology and risk factors: Incidence has decreased in the United States

    a. Rheumatic heart disease (most common cause)

    b. Congenital mitral valve disease (uncommon)

    c. Tumors of the LA (atrial myxoma)

    d. Risk factor: Pregnant women with mitral stenosis often develop cardiac decompensation in the third trimester

3. Signs and symptoms

    a. History

        i. Gradual decline in physical activity over the years

        ii. Palpitations (frequent complaint): Possibly from frequent premature atrial contractions, paroxysmal atrial fibrillation

        iii. Shortness of breath, dyspnea on exertion

        iv. Paroxysmal nocturnal dyspnea

        v. Cough (bronchial irritability), hoarseness

        vi. Orthopnea

        vii. Fatigue

        viii. Hemoptysis (ruptured bronchial vessels)

        ix. Symptoms of right-sided heart failure (occur later)

        x. Dysphagia (enlarged atrium displaces the esophagus)

        xi. History of systemic emboli, rheumatic heart disease

    b. Objective findings: Signs and symptoms of right-sided heart failure occur as late signs (See Heart Failure)

    c. Physical examination: Findings depend on the degree of heart failure present

        i. Inspection

            (a) Any of the signs of heart failure

            (b) Jugular venous distention

        ii. Palpation

            (a) May feel the RV lift if pulmonary hypertension is present; an LV "tap" may be present

            (b) Diastolic thrill may be present at the apex (with the patient in the left lateral recumbent position)

        iii. Auscultation

            (a) Pronounced S$_1$

            (b) Low-pitched apical diastolic murmur (best heard at the apex, radiates to the left sternal border)

            (c) Associated murmur of tricuspid insufficiency may be present if RV failure exists. Listen at the left lower parasternal area.

            (d) Pulmonary component, S$_2$, later and louder if pulmonary hypertension exists

            (e) Mitral opening snap present just after pulmonic component of S$_2$

4. **Diagnostic study findings**
   a. Radiologic: Chest radiograph reveals the following:
      i. LA and RV hypertrophy
      ii. Interstitial edema, pulmonary vascular redistribution to the upper lobes of the lungs (caused by high PCWP)
   b. ECG
      i. If in sinus rhythm, broad P waves: Notched in lead I, biphasic in V_1
      ii. Atrial fibrillation
      iii. RV hypertrophy pattern (with pulmonary hypertension)
   c. Transthoracic echocardiography with Doppler
      i. Reveals thickened, tethered, and doming (stuck together) anterior and posterior mitral valve leaflets
      ii. Calculates mitral valve area
      iii. Shows enlarged LA
      iv. Shows enlarged RV
      v. Assess the degree of pulmonary hypertension and mitral regurgitation, and the function of the other valves
   d. TEE: For identification of an LA appendage thrombus (seen in 20% of cases of atrial fibrillation)
   e. Cardiac catheterization: Used if the echocardiographic results are confusing or questionable given the patient presentation
      i. To assess pulmonary hypertension and CO; to measure PCWP–LV diastolic pressure gradient and calculate mitral valve area
      ii. Coronary arteriography: Used to assess the function of the other valves and rule out CAD
5. **Goals of care**
   a. Hemodynamics improve
   b. Complications (including atrial fibrillation, recurrent infections, atrial thrombus) are treated and/or prevented
6. **Collaborating professionals on health care team:** See Chronic Stable Angina
7. **Management of patient care**
   a. Anticipated patient trajectory: Patient with mitral stenosis will gradually develop limiting symptoms and heart failure, with the likelihood of stroke and early death
      i. Nutrition: Restricted sodium intake
      ii. Infection control: IE prophylactic therapy
      iii. Discharge planning: Patient education regarding the following:
         (a) Activity limitations
         (b) Medications
         (c) Anticoagulation and follow-up requirements
      iv. Pharmacology
         (a) Diuretics, nitrates: To lower pulmonary congestion; use carefully, may lower CO
         (b) Digitalis, β-blockers, calcium antagonists: To treat atrial fibrillation, slow ventricular response, and increase exercise capacity
         (c) β-blocking agents may increase exercise tolerance by slowing the heart rate and lengthening the diastolic filling period. Use carefully in patients with impaired LV function.
         (d) Anticoagulants: Prevent embolization. Goal is an INR of 2 to 3.
         (e) Antibiotics: Prophylaxis for recurrent rheumatic heart disease; prophylaxis for IE during dental procedures
      v. Treatments

(a) Medical management is palliative; mechanical correction is eventually required to improve CO and decrease atrial and pulmonary pressures

(b) Current treatment options include surgical mitral valve replacement, open surgical commissurotomy, percutaneous balloon mitral valvuloplasty

(c) Cardioversion, if atrial fibrillation is present

b. Potential complications

i. Systemic or pulmonary emboli from atrial thrombus

(a) Mechanism: High risk for thrombus formation during atrial fibrillation or heart failure

(1) Central nervous system embolism: Symptoms of stroke (e.g., paralysis, weakness, dysphasia, confusion)

(2) Pulmonary embolism: Symptoms of tachycardia, tachypnea, hypoxia, dyspnea, cough, hemoptysis, elevated PAP, hypotension, chest pain, abnormal ABG values, cyanosis, positive lung scan results

(3) Renal embolism: Hematuria, oliguria, back pain, rising BUN level

(4) Splenic embolism: Left upper quadrant pain with radiation to the left shoulder

(5) Mesenteric embolism: Pain in the lower abdomen, bloody diarrhea, elevated leukocyte count, and elevated erythrocyte sedimentation rate

(b) Management: Dependent on type, anticoagulation

ii. Other complications include heart failure, infection

8. Evaluation of patient care

a. Systemic or pulmonary emboli are absent or resolved

b. Patient is hemodynamically stable

Aortic Regurgitation

In aortic regurgitation (AR), an incompetent aortic valve causes the backward flow of blood from the aorta to the LV during ventricular diastole

1. Pathophysiology

a. Aortic valve can become incompetent as a result of destruction of the cusps (endocarditis), degeneration of the cusps, unhinging of the valvular apparatus (dissection), rheumatic disease, connective tissue disease, congenital heart disease, trauma, or degenerative change

b. Acute onset

i. Increased regurgitation into the LV produces volume overload, *markedly* increasing the LVEDP

ii. CO falls and hypotension develops

iii. There is a drop in the aortic diastolic pressure that diminishes the coronary blood flow

iv. The compensatory increase in heart rate adds to the already elevated myocardial oxygen demand

v. Patient comes for treatment with pulmonary edema, cardiogenic shock. Ischemia and sudden cardiac death may occur.

c. Chronic process

i. LV compensates by dilating to increase its SV to maintain an adequate forward output. This gradually increases myocardial oxygen demands.

ii. LVEDP increases. The LV myocardial fibers stretch and hypertrophy. Preload and EF, at this point, remain relatively normal.

    iii. As the disease progresses, the LV fails and decompensates; SV and EF decrease. LV systolic and diastolic pressures increase.

    iv. Wide pulse pressure develops as a result of low aortic diastolic pressures

    v. Decreased blood flow to the coronary arteries during diastole results in myocardial ischemia

2. **Etiology and risk factors**

   a. Acute causes

     i. IE (most common cause of acute AR): Can also be a chronic cause

     ii. Aortic dissection

     iii. Blunt trauma, causing valve rupture (e.g., motor vehicle collision)

     iv. Prosthetic valve dysfunction

   b. Chronic causes

     i. Idiopathic calcification of the valve

     ii. Congenital malformations (bicuspid aortic valve)

     iii. Hypertension

     iv. Rheumatic disease

     v. Aortic aneurysms (e.g., Marfan's syndrome)

     vi. Diseases of the aortic valve and root

     vii. Systemic lupus erythematosus

     viii. Drugs: Appetite suppressants

     ix. Syphilis (rare)

3. **Signs and symptoms:** Can be well tolerated. Symptoms often do not become evident to the patient until the disease is fairly well advanced.

   a. Subjective findings

     i. Dyspnea (most common symptom): Caused by an increased LVEDP

     ii. Angina pectoris

     iii. Paroxysmal nocturnal dyspnea

     iv. Orthopnea

     v. Presyncope and syncope

   b. Physical examination: Many of physical findings are absent in acute AR. Widening pulse pressure of chronic disease creates these findings. Acute disease has a narrow pulse pressure.

     i. Inspection

       (a) Signs and symptoms of left-sided heart failure

       (b) Distinct carotid artery pulsations

       (c) De Musset's sign (nodding of the head with each beat of the heart)

       (d) Flushed appearance

     ii. Palpation

       (a) Diffuse apical impulse, displaced laterally and downward (in chronic forms); the apical impulse does not change with acute onset

       (b) Water-hammer pulse: Bounding, abrupt rise and fall in the carotid arteries and other peripheral pulses

       (c) Positive Quincke's sign: When the fingertip is pressed, capillary pulsation of the nail beds is visible

     iii. Auscultation

       (a) High-pitched, blowing, decrescendo diastolic murmur

         (1) Loudest at lower left sternal border, third-fourth intercostal space

         (2) Starts immediately after S_2

         (3) Short (early diastole) with acute aortic insufficiency

         (4) Long (through diastole) if chronic

         (5) If hard to hear, have the patient sit up and lean forward. Press firmly with the bell.

(b) S_3 common

(c) S_4 heard in more severe disease (abnormal LV compliance)

(d) Rales at the bases, if the onset is acute

4. **Diagnostic study findings**
   a. Radiologic: Chest radiograph reveals the following:
      i. LV enlargement (normal with acute aortic insufficiency)
      ii. Wide mediastinum (if due to aortic dissection)
      iii. Possible aortic valve calcification
      iv. Possible interstitial pulmonary edema
   b. ECG: Often normal in mild to moderate AR
      i. LV hypertrophy: Increased amplitude of QRS
      ii. As disease progresses, ST segment and T waves invert
      iii. Sinus tachycardia (acutely)
   c. Echocardiography: Very important tool, particularly in the diagnosis of acute cases
      i. Identifies cause and severity of AR
      ii. Shows LV cavity dilatation with chronic cases
      iii. Reveals vegetations
   d. MRI or CT scan: To exclude aortic dissection
   e. Radionuclide imaging: Used to evaluate the severity of AR and LV function
   f. TEE: To assess the ascending and descending thoracic aorta for aneurysms, dissection, and the cause and severity of aortic insufficiency
   g. Cardiac catheterization
      i. Evaluates hemodynamics
         (a) CO assessment
         (b) Increased PCWP
         (c) Increased right-sided heart pressures (late)
      ii. Quantifies the degree of insufficiency
      iii. Assesses LV function and EF, reveals other abnormalities
      iv. Reveals coronary anatomy
      v. Evaluates for aortic dissection

5. **Goals of care**
   a. Stable hemodynamics are maintained
   b. Afterload is reduced
   c. Pulmonary congestion, if evident, is decreased

6. **Collaborating professionals on health care team:** See Chronic Stable Angina; also electrophysiologist, infectious disease specialist

7. **Management of patient care**
   a. Anticipated patient trajectory: When severe, AR will ultimately result in irreversible heart failure and early death if not recognized and corrected with aortic valve replacement prior to LV dysfunction
      i. Positioning: Head of bed elevated, if signs of heart failure are present
      ii. Infection control: Prophylaxis for IE risk
      iii. Discharge planning
         (a) Teach the patient about the need for adherence to the medication regimen and follow-up evaluations
         (b) Prophylactic antibiotics will be used to prevent IE. Patient should understand what types of procedures require antibiotic prophylaxis.
      iv. Pharmacology
         (a) Inotropic agents (dopamine, dobutamine) to increase CO in acute AR (before surgery)
         (b) ACE inhibitors: To decrease LV remodeling and hypertrophy, reduce afterload (if necessary)

       (c) Diuretics, nitrates: With symptoms of heart failure, to decrease pulmonary congestion

       (d) Antibiotics: IE prophylaxis

       (e) β-blockers: Avoided in acute AR; used very cautiously because the patient often needs sinus tachycardia to support output

    v. Treatments

       (a) Cardiac surgery

          (1) If the patient is symptomatic or asymptomatic with LV dysfunction or significant dilatation, valve replacement is the main treatment for the incompetent valve

          (2) AR caused by IE: Does not require a delay in surgery, if the patient is symptomatic

       (b) Bedside hemodynamic monitoring: To assess and monitor CO and responses to medication

       (c) EPS study: If VT is present, AICD implantation because of the high risk of sudden cardiac death

       (d) Atrial pacing: May be needed to increase the heart rate, decrease regurgitation

       (e) IABP contraindicated

  b. Potential complications

    i. IE: Most significant complication to prevent

    ii. Arrhythmias: Ventricular, heart blocks, electromechanical dissociation

    iii. Heart failure, cardiogenic shock, death

8. Evaluation of patient care

  a. Patient is free of signs and symptoms and has improved hemodynamics

  b. Symptoms are improved or relieved if the patient underwent surgical replacement of the aortic valve

  c. Patient demonstrates a knowledge of IE prophylaxis, exercise guidelines, requirements for follow-up care, medications

  d. Patient verbalizes an understanding of anticoagulation therapy (if needed) and has received written guidelines regarding dietary interactions with medication, laboratory testing and anticoagulation follow-ups, and activity

Aortic Stenosis

Aortic stenosis is shown in Figure 3-21. Ejection from the LV during systole is impaired because of an obstructive narrowing. Stenosis may be supravalvular, subvalvular, or valvular. Obstructions above the valve are rare and are usually congenital. Obstructions below the valve are associated with hypertrophic cardiomyopathy. Obstructions at the valve itself are the most common cause.

1. Pathophysiology

  a. Valve becomes thickened and calcified, with a progressive fusing of the cusps. LV afterload gradually increases. Aortic insufficiency often develops.

  b. Systolic pressure gradient develops between the LV and the aorta

  c. To maintain SV and adequate CO, the LV hypertrophies in a concentric manner

  d. LV becomes stiff and noncompliant; the LVEDP increases

  e. LA pressures increase, which increases the pulmonary vascular pressures. Pulmonary congestion develops and eventually increases the pressures in the right chambers.

  f. Because the left side of the heart has to pump against increased afterload, myocardial oxygen demand is greatly increased.

  g. LV hypertrophy and increased LVEDP cause a decrease in subendocardial coronary perfusion, and ischemia can result in angina and arrhythmias

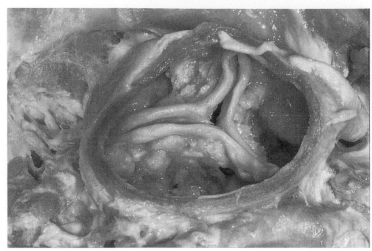

FIGURE 3-21 ■ Gross pathology of degenerative aortic stenosis. (From Crawford MH, DiMarco JP, Paulus WJ, editors: *Cardiology*, ed 2, Philadelphia, 2004, Mosby, p 1122.)

h. Because forward CO cannot be augmented to meet requirements, exertional syncope may result

2. **Etiology and risk factors**
   a. Most common cause: Calcific or degenerative process (progressive disease in patients older than 65 years)
   b. Congenital heart defects: Bicuspid valve (symptoms usually seen in patients in their fifties and sixties); associated with other defects, especially coarctation of the aorta. Most common cause in younger adults.
   c. Rheumatic valvular heart disease (the commissure fuses, leaflets thicken and fibrose; symptoms often seen in patients in their thirties and forties), associated with mitral valve disease
   d. Prevalence of aortic stenosis increases with age

3. **Signs and symptoms**
   a. Dyspnea on exertion (pulmonary congestion)
   b. Syncope on exertion (transient arrhythmias, decreased cardiac and cerebral perfusion) or presyncope
   c. Angina (caused by LV hypertrophy, increased myocardial demands, lowered coronary blood flow)
   d. Symptoms of LV failure
   e. Palpitations
   f. Fatigue or weakness
   g. History of a gradual decrease in physical activity to avoid dyspnea
   h. Inspection
      i. Anxiety
      ii. Labored respiration, tachypnea
      iii. Jugular veins: Presence of an "a" wave (if right-sided heart failure is present and the patient is in sinus rhythm)
   i. Palpation
      i. Forceful, sustained apical impulse
      ii. Systolic thrill felt rarely in the second or third right intercostal space
      iii. Pulsus parvus and tardus (small carotid upstroke and delayed peak) is variably present

   j. Auscultation

      i. Harsh, loud systolic ejection murmur, crescendo-decrescendo, loudest at the second right intercostal space, radiating up to the base of the neck and at apex

      ii. Paradoxical split S_2

      iii. S_3 (in severe LV dysfunction)

      iv. S_4 (with LV hypertrophy)

      v. Rales (LV failure)

4. Diagnostic study findings

   a. Radiologic: Studies may be normal in significant stenosis

      i. Cardiac enlargement in late stages

      ii. Pulmonary vascular congestion

      iii. Calcified aortic valve

      iv. Dilated ascending aorta

   b. ECG: Normal in 20% to 30% of patients

      i. LV hypertrophy and strain pattern (increased QRS voltage, ST changes)

      ii. Conduction defects: LBBB, occasional heart block

      iii. Left axis deviation

      iv. Atrial fibrillation in late stages

   c. Echocardiography: For diagnosis, follow-up

      i. Presence and severity of aortic stenosis

      ii. LV hypertrophy (concentric), impaired LV diastolic function

      iii. LA enlargement

      iv. Other valvular disease

   d. Exercise treadmill study: Unsafe unless aortic stenosis is mild

   e. Cardiac catheterization: Used to assess the following:

      i. CAD: 50% of patients have coexisting CAD

      ii. Hemodynamics

         (a) Increased LV systolic pressure and LVEDP

         (b) Pressure gradient between the LV and the aorta is usually more than 50 mm Hg

         (c) Calculation of the aortic valve area

5. Goals of care

   a. Patient is free of the signs and symptoms of complications (i.e., heart failure, arrhythmias, emboli)

   b. Patient demonstrates a knowledge of the disease progress, medications, and therapies to allow active participation in decision making regarding surgical interventions

6. Collaborating professionals on health care team: See Chronic Stable Angina; also infectious disease specialist, electrophysiologist, stroke team

7. Management of patient care

   a. Anticipated patient trajectory: Aortic stenosis threatens the patient with limiting angina, heart failure, and death, and can be surgically corrected at any age

      i. Nutrition: Diet should be low in sodium

      ii. Infection control: IE prophylaxis

      iii. Discharge planning

         (a) Teach the patient about the symptoms to report promptly and disease progression: The patient is at increased risk for sudden cardiac death.

         (b) Activity restrictions: Moderate aortic stenosis—avoid competition sports. Severe aortic stenosis—low-level activity only.

      iv. Pharmacology: Medical management is palliative. Treatment is based on symptom presentation.

(a) Antibiotics: To prevent IE

(b) Antihypertensives: To control hypertension

(c) Antiarrhythmics: To prevent and control rhythm disturbances (e.g., digoxin, amiodarone for atrial fibrillation)

(d) If signs of heart failure, pulmonary congestion are present: Digitalis, diuretics, ACE inhibitors. Watch preload. These drugs can lower CO, because the LV is very dependent on preload.

(e) Vasodilators: Should be avoided; can cause profound hypotension

(f) Statins: Therapy slows rate of progression of aortic stenosis

v. Psychosocial issues: Patient's goals and wishes are important because of the high risk of mortality. Activity limitations have a major impact on home life, finances, and morale.

vi. Treatments

(a) Surgery is the only effective therapy for critical aortic stenosis

(1) Valve replacement with stented bioprosthetic mechanical valves or pulmonic autograft (Ross procedure)

(2) Lifelong anticoagulant therapy is necessary when prosthetic mechanical valves are used

(b) Aortic percutaneous balloon valvuloplasty and débridement are not an alternative to surgery

(1) Used as a bridge to surgery in patients with pulmonary edema or cardiogenic shock, to improve hemodynamics

(2) Used for patients who are not surgical candidates to improve symptoms

(3) Does not improve survival

(4) Benefits last only a few months

b. Potential complications

i. Sudden cardiac death

(a) Mechanism: High incidence after the patient becomes symptomatic, often resulting from ventricular arrhythmias

(b) Management: AICD may be required

ii. Other complications (see also applicable sections)

(a) LV failure (diastolic dysfunction)

(b) Conduction defects: Heart blocks (especially in degenerative disease)

(c) IE (more common in younger patients)

(d) Emboli: Stroke, vision problems

8. Evaluation of patient care

a. Patient is free of signs and symptoms of heart failure

b. Symptoms are improved or relieved if the patient underwent surgical repair or replacement of the aortic valve

c. Patient verbalizes an understanding of anticoagulation therapy (if needed) and the importance of IE prophylaxis

d. Written guidelines are given regarding dietary interactions with medication, laboratory testing and anticoagulation clinic follow-ups, and exercise

e. Patient can summarize the symptoms to report promptly and disease progression

Atrial Septal Defect

Atrial septal defect (ASD) is a defect in the interatrial septum that allows free communication between the right and left sides of the heart at the atrial level. Found in 7% to 10% of patients with congenital heart defects. Can result in shortened life span and morbidity as a result of dyspnea and right-sided heart failure. Paradoxical emboli (right-to-left circulation) can result after the right side of the heart fails.

1. **Pathophysiology**
    a. Common types of ASD include the following:
        i. Secundum defect (fossa ovalis): Located in the middle of the septum in the area of the foramen ovale. This is the most common type (70%).
        ii. Primum defect (often associated with endocardial cushion defects): Located at the lower end of the septum, superior to the interventricular septum (20%)
        iii. Sinus venosus defect: Located high in the septum at the junction of the RA and superior vena cava. Frequently associated with partial anomalous pulmonary venous return of the right upper lobe vein to the superior vena cava. Least common type (5% to 10%).
        iv. Patent foramen ovale: Open congenital "hole" defect found in up to 27% of adults. Large patent foramina ovales and/or defects with right-to-left shunting are associated with cryptogenic strokes (focal neurologic deficits due to focal ischemia).
    b. As a result of the defects, flow is from the normally higher-pressure LA to the RA, which creates a left-to-right shunt
    c. Right-side heart and pulmonary artery flow increase because these structures handle both the normal systemic venous return from the body and the left-to-right shunt flow through the ASD
    d. This results in volume overload of the right chambers
    e. RA, RV, and pulmonary artery dilate
    f. Systolic murmur of an ASD results from increased flow across the normal pulmonic valve (flow murmur). Diastolic rumble can occur from increased flow across the tricuspid valve.
    g. Spontaneous closure rarely occurs after 2 years of age
    h. Pulmonary hypertension and pulmonary vascular disease may develop over time (seen in 15% to 20% of adults with this defect). In extreme cases, the shunt may reverse, becoming right to left and irreversible (Eisenmenger's syndrome)
    i. RV dilatation, hypertrophy, and failure can result
    j. Atrial fibrillation is often seen
    k. Mitral valve anomalies (with cleft leaflets) often occur in endocardial cushion defects (associated with ostium primum defects), resulting in mitral insufficiency

2. **Etiology and risk factors**
    a. Occurs twice as often among females
    b. Exact cause unknown; may be due to
        i. Genetic factors
        ii. Maternal and fetal infection during the first trimester of pregnancy (e.g., rubella)
        iii. Effects of drugs or medications
        iv. Dietary deficiencies during fetal development

3. **Signs and symptoms:** Symptoms often develop in the fourth to sixth decades of life. Presentations vary, depending on the direction of the shunt. When the shunt reverses to right to left, signs and symptoms of severe heart failure with cyanosis will be present.
    a. Patient may complain of
        i. Mild fatigue
        ii. Exertional dyspnea
        iii. Palpitations
    b. Appearance is generally normal
    c. Symptoms of heart failure may be seen in older patients

    d. Cyanosis, clubbing of the fingers and toes (with right-to-left shunts)

    e. Palpation: Systolic, hyperdynamic lift along the left sternal border, caused by enlarged RV

    f. Auscultation

        i. Systolic ejection murmur: Heard best in the second left intercostal space; caused by increased flow across the pulmonic valve

        ii. Fixed, widely split S_2

        iii. Early, low-pitched diastolic murmur may be heard best at the lower left sternal border or xiphoid area; caused by increased blood flow across the tricuspid valve if shunt flow is large

4. Diagnostic study findings

    a. Radiologic: Chest radiograph may be normal or may reveal the following:

        i. Mild to moderate enlargement of the RA, RV, pulmonary artery

        ii. Increased pulmonary vascular markings

    b. ECG

        i. Atrial fibrillation and/or atrial flutter

        ii. PR prolongation

        iii. Incomplete RBBB

        iv. Left axis deviation in ostium primum defects

    c. Echocardiography

        i. RV enlargement

        ii. Actual defect is occasionally seen with two-dimensional echocardiography, color-flow Doppler studies

        iii. IV injection of contrast medium demonstrates the shunt by the early appearance of contrast medium in the left heart chambers

    d. TEE: Used to evaluate the mitral valve

    e. Cardiac catheterization: Used predominantly to evaluate CAD, hemodynamics, associated heart disease. Can be used for quantifying shunt.

        i. Characteristic finding is an increase (step-up) in oxygen concentration in the RA

        ii. Increased pulmonary artery pressures may be documented

5. Goals of care

    a. Prompt aggressive treatment of heart failure symptoms is provided

    b. Elective repair of the defect is accomplished as soon as possible

6. Collaborating professionals on health care team: See Chronic Unstable Angina; also pediatrician

7. Management of patient care

    a. Anticipated patient trajectory: ASD can rob people of two decades of life and should be corrected as soon as recognized

        i. Pharmacology

            (a) Antibiotics to prevent endocarditis

            (b) Medical management of heart failure

        ii. Treatments

            (a) Surgical repair is the standard treatment for a significant ASD

                (1) Prepare the patient and family (parents, if the patient is a child) for the possibility of surgical repair, including providing an explanation of the disease process, preoperative routines, the surgical procedure, expectations for the postoperative period

                (2) Using a median sternotomy or right thoracotomy, the surgeon closes the defect with a pericardial or Dacron patch or suture

                (3) Early defect repair is recommended to prevent pulmonary hypertension, heart failure, and early death

(4) Repair may be deferred in children but should be performed before they enter school (2 to 5 years of age)

(5) In older children and young adults, the repair should be performed before pulmonary hypertension develops; pathophysiologic changes may be irreversible if the defect is not repaired

(6) Postoperative care for ASD repairs is similar to postoperative care for most cardiac operations; stress the importance of preventing potential complications (atrial fibrillation, embolization)

(b) Transcatheter closure of an ASD and patent foramen ovale is now being used in suitable patients

(c) Heart-lung transplantation: Becomes the only available option if the disease has progressed to include irreversible pulmonary hypertension and pulmonary vascular disease

b. Potential complications

   i. Transient heart block

      (a) Mechanism: Most common complication after closure of a septum primum defect because of edema or injury to the AV node

      (b) Management: Temporary pacing may be required. Occasionally, heart block is permanent

   ii. Other complications include

      (a) Arrhythmias: Watch for atrial fibrillation, flutter, AV blocks (more frequent in older patients). SVTs may continue after surgery.

      (b) Heart failure (left side and right side), pulmonary hypertension

      (c) Pulmonary embolism or thrombosis, stroke

      (d) Brain abscess

8. Evaluation of patient care

  a. Patient is free from associated complications from the interventions

  b. If complications occur, they are promptly identified and treated

Ventricular Septal Defect

VSD is an abnormal opening between the ventricles occurring in the membranous or muscular portion of the ventricular septum. Constitutes 25% of all defects and is frequently associated with other defects.

1. Pathophysiology

  a. Common types of this defect include the following:

   i. Perimembranous defects

      (a) Occur in approximately 80% of patients with VSD

      (b) Located at the base of the septum under the aortic valve

      (c) Aortic insufficiency can result if the valve cusp is poorly supported

   ii. Muscular defects

      (a) Occur in 5% to 20%

      (b) Occasionally multiple defects

  b. Small defects

   i. 75% close spontaneously before the affected individuals are 20 years of age (50% by age 4 years)

   ii. Generally create no hemodynamic disturbance or pulmonary hypertension in adults; low risk of IE

   iii. Small left-to-right shunt with high pressure gradient between the LV and RV causes a high-velocity jet and a loud (usually grade IV/VI) murmur

  c. Large defects

   i. Left-to-right shunting through the defect as a result of the higher LV pressures

    ii. Increased RV pressures and PAP occur

    iii. Increased pulmonary blood flow results in increased pulmonary venous return to the LA. LA pressures, along with the LVEDP, increase. The left heart chambers are volume overloaded, which leads to dilatation, failure, and pulmonary edema.

    iv. Over time, the pulmonary hypertension can become irreversible, often exceeding systemic pressures. The shunt then reverses, becoming right to left, with resulting cyanosis (Eisenmenger's syndrome).

2. Etiology and risk factors

  a. Precise cause of the congenital defect is unknown

  b. Associated with coarctation of the aorta, PDA

  c. Factors contributing to congenital defects

    i. Genetic abnormalities

    ii. Chromosomal abnormalities (e.g., Down syndrome)

    iii. Maternal and fetal infections during the first trimester of pregnancy (e.g., rubella)

    iv. Effects of drugs and medications (e.g., cocaine use) during fetal development

    v. Dietary deficiencies during fetal development

    vi. Effects of maternal smoking and/or alcohol intake during pregnancy

    vii. High altitudes

  d. Acute MI: VSD is a serious but infrequent complication of MI and rapidly leads to heart failure, shock, and death

3. Signs and symptoms: Effects of large defects often become evident at 3 to 12 weeks of age. Symptoms depend on defect size and the patient's age.

  a. Subjective findings

    i. Small defects: Patients are usually asymptomatic

    ii. Large defects

      (a) Fatigue, exercise intolerance

      (b) Exertional dyspnea

      (c) Angina-like symptoms (caused by pulmonary hypertension)

      (d) Eisenmenger's syndrome

  b. Objective findings

    i. Frequently normal growth and development

    ii. Possible difficulty in feeding

    iii. May have a history of slow weight gain, small size

    iv. History of endocarditis

    v. History of frequent respiratory infections, often with bronchopneumonia

    vi. History of heart murmurs from birth

    vii. Family history of heart defects

    viii. Maternal exposure to infectious process or poor nutrition, drugs, and medications in the first trimester

  c. Physical examination of the patient: Signs vary, depending on shunt direction and size. Right-to-left shunts produce signs and symptoms of severe heart failure and cyanosis.

    i. Inspection

      (a) Restlessness, irritability

      (b) Frail appearance, thinness, paleness, waxen complexion

      (c) Tachypnea, air hunger, grunting respirations

      (d) Excessive sweating

      (e) Hemoptysis

      (f) Symptoms of heart failure, cyanosis

(g) Prominent sternum: From large RV while growing

  ii. Palpation

    (a) Systolic thrill over lower LSB, fourth intercostal space

    (b) PMI may be displaced laterally in larger defects

    (c) Lift may be felt over the left sternal border

    (d) Peripheral pulses: Rapid, thready

  iii. Auscultation

    (a) Harsh, loud, high-pitched holosystolic murmur (even with a small VSD)

      (1) Loudest at the left sternum, third to fifth intercostal space

      (2) The louder the murmur, the smaller the defect

      (3) Nonradiating murmur

    (b) Loud S_2, split but not fixed (may be single in Eisenmenger's syndrome)

    (c) Mitral diastolic rumble at the apex (from increased flow through the mitral valve) indicates a large defect

    (d) Aortic insufficiency murmurs (associated with membranous defects) may be heard

    (e) Patient with Eisenmenger's syndrome may not have a murmur (with equalization of right- and left-sided heart pressures)

    (f) Rales with failure

4. Diagnostic study findings

  a. Radiologic (findings may be normal for small VSDs)

    i. LA and LV enlargement

    ii. RA and RV enlargement in the presence of pulmonary artery hypertension

    iii. Increased pulmonary vascular markings

    iv. Pulmonary artery dilatation

  b. ECG

    i. Small defects produce a normal ECG

    ii. Large defects

      (a) LA enlargement and LV hypertrophy

      (b) RV hypertrophy

  c. Echocardiography

    i. Distinguishes shunt flow, increased pulmonary flow, aortic insufficiency; checks prosthetic patches (postoperatively), aneurysms (after closure complication)

    ii. Reveals chamber enlargement

    iii. Demonstrates shunting by the use of echocardiographic contrast material and color-flow Doppler studies

  d. TEE: Identifies residual shunt flow (intraoperatively)

  e. Cardiac catheterization: Can confirm and quantify shunt; assesses hemodynamics; documents the degree of pulmonary hypertension and associated disease (pulmonary stenosis, AR, CAD)

5. Goals of care

  a. Patient's response to the VSD is evaluated to identify the need for interventions

  b. If symptoms or complications occur, they are promptly identified and treated

  c. Patient is taught about infection risks, follow-up care

6. Collaborating professionals on health care team: See Chronic Stable Angina; also pediatrician, dentist

7. Management of patient care

  a. Anticipated patient trajectory: Most VSDs close within the first 2 years of life, but the remainder put patients at risk of endocarditis, limitations due to dyspnea, heart failure, and early death if not corrected

    i. Nutrition: Diet high in calories to assist with infant growth; nasogastric tube may be required

    ii. Infection control: IE prophylaxis

    iii. Discharge planning

      (a) Teach the patient the importance of good dental hygiene

      (b) Instruct regarding the need for antibiotic prophylaxis to prevent IE (if a small, residual VSD)

    iv. Pharmacology

      (a) Antibiotics: For IE prophylaxis

      (b) Diuretics (i.e., furosemide, chlorothiazide): To treat pulmonary edema, lower intravascular volumes. Electrolytes and renal function need monitoring.

      (c) Afterload reduction

    v. Treatments: Depend on defect size

      (a) Asymptomatic patients who have no pathologic changes do not require surgery. Small defects may close spontaneously over time.

      (b) Plasma exchange transfusions (if HCT higher than 65%) for severe polycythemia

      (c) Catheter closure of VSDs now being done with occlusive devices especially for muscular VSDs

      (d) Patients require surgery when

        (1) Patient is symptomatic with heart failure

        (2) Patient is asymptomatic with a ratio of pulmonary to systemic blood flow in the shunt of 1.5:1 or higher

        (3) Patient shows failure to thrive (at 6 months, the prospect of spontaneous closure has diminished considerably)

        (4) Patient experiences repeated, severe respiratory infections or recurrent endocarditis

b. Potential complications (see specific sections in chapter)

    i. Heart failure (causes 11% of deaths from VSD)

    ii. IE: 4% to 10% risk

    iii. Arrhythmias, sudden cardiac death: Frequently seen with Eisenmenger's syndrome

8. Evaluation of patient care

  a. Patient is free of associated complications from the interventions

  b. Complications are promptly identified and treated

  c. Patient complies with the need for IE prophylaxis and good oral hygiene

Patent Ductus Arteriosus

PDA is a persistent patency of the fetal circulation between the aorta and the pulmonary artery that failed to close after birth, seen in 2% of adults

1. Pathophysiology

  a. During fetal circulation: Blood from the pulmonary artery flows through the ductus into the descending aorta to bypass collapsed lungs. Ductus functionally closes within 24 to 48 hours after birth but may remain open up to 8 weeks.

  b. Ductus closure: Contraction of smooth muscles in the ductus wall results from increased arterial oxygen tension. If the smooth muscles do not contract, the ductus remains open (i.e., hypoxia at birth). Prostaglandin inhibitors can stimulate closure.

  c. If the ductus has not closed spontaneously by 3 months of age, it probably will not

    d. Because the aorta has higher pressures, blood flows back through the patent ductus into the lower-pressure pulmonary artery in a *left-to-right* shunt, and oxygenated blood is recirculated to the lungs

    e. Resistance in the ductus to the shunting of blood is caused not only by the diameter of the defect but also by its length

    f. Small PDAs may have no hemodynamic effects and calcify with aging

    g. With larger PDAs, LV workload increases (handles both normal CO and shunt flow), but right-sided heart flow is not increased

        i. Increased blood return to the LA and LV overloads the left side of the heart. LV compensates by enlarging, and symptoms of left-sided heart failure develop.

        ii. Pulmonary hypertension may develop over time

    h. Large shunts can result in equal pressure in the systemic and pulmonary systems (Eisenmenger's syndrome with irreversible pulmonary hypertension)

    i. Increased pulmonary pressures then lead to increased work for the RV (which enlarges and fails)

    j. If obstructive pulmonary vascular lesions develop, pulmonary artery pressure will rise above aortic pressure and the shunt will reverse, becoming right to left. Cyanosis and right-sided heart failure result. Deoxygenated blood is distributed to the left arm and the lower body below the ductus (causing cyanosis and clubbing of the toes), whereas the upper body receives oxygenated blood with no abnormalities

    k. All patients with PDAs are at risk for heart failure and IE. Vegetations may embolize to the lungs, which leads to infarctions and death.

2. Etiology and risk factors

    a. Failure of the ductus to close at birth

    b. Associated anomalies: Atrial and ventricular septal defects

    c. Individuals at risk:

        i. Infants with congenital rubella (acquired in first trimester)

        ii. Infants with birth hypoxia or respiratory distress, lung disease

        iii. Premature infants (weighing less than 1000 g)

        iv. Infants born at high altitudes (chronic hypoxia)

        v. Females (twice as common as among males)

3. Signs and symptoms: Shunt size and PVR determine the hemodynamic effects. Asymptomatic in 50% of cases. Moderate-sized PDA may not become symptomatic until LV failure and pulmonary hypertension develop

    a. Child

        i. Easy fatigability, irritability, poor feeding that results in poor weight gain

        ii. History of maternal rubella during first trimester

        iii. History of hypoxia at birth

        iv. Failure to thrive; growth and developmental problems

        v. High number of respiratory tract infections

    b. Physical findings can include

        i. Dyspnea on exertion, tachypnea, hemoptysis

        ii. Angina-like pain, tachycardia, syncope, signs and symptoms of heart failure

        iii. Deafness, cataracts

        iv. Hoarseness (compression of the laryngeal nerve)

        v. Clubbing, mild cyanosis possible in the left fingers (because of the entry of unsaturated blood into the left subclavian artery); cyanosis in the lower parts of the body and clubbing of the toes (if right- to left-shunting); leg fatigue

    vi. Palpation
        (a) Hyperdynamic precordium: Distinct LV impulse (overload)
        (b) Bounding, brisk peripheral pulses (especially with large defects)
        (c) Prominent apical impulse
        (d) Possible systolic thrill in the second left intercostal space
    vii. Auscultation
        (a) Loud, rough, continuous machinery-like murmur is indicative of a PDA; peaks at S_2, heard in more than 50% of patients
            (1) Is loudest high, at left upper sternal border (pulmonic area), left infraclavicular area
            (2) Caused by pressure gradient between the aorta and the pulmonary artery
            (3) Possible mitral flow rumble at the apex
        (b) Wide pulse pressure

4. Diagnostic study findings
    a. Radiologic: Chest radiograph
      i. LA and LV enlargement (in large left-to-right shunts)
      ii. Increased pulmonary vascular markings, pulmonary edema in failure
      iii. Enlarged aorta; prominent ascending aorta and aortic knob
      iv. Central pulmonary artery enlarged
    b. ECG (normal in small- and medium-sized PDAs)
      i. LV hypertrophy with left axis deviation
      ii. LA enlargement
    c. Transthoracic echocardiography: Detects the PDA, reveals enlarged chambers, shows flow from the aorta to the pulmonary system in diastole. Color-flow Doppler study helps visualize small shunts and associated congenital defects
    d. TEE: To delineate the PDA
    e. Cardiac catheterization: Not usually necessary
      i. Establishes the aortopulmonary communication and shunt size and direction
      ii. Assesses pulmonary pressures and resistance
      iii. Increased pressures will be evident in the pulmonary artery with right-to-left shunts

5. Goals of care
    a. Duct is closed by transcatheter or surgical techniques
    b. Prompt, aggressive treatment is provided for symptoms of heart failure
    c. IE is prevented

6. Collaborating professionals on health care team: See Chronic Stable Angina; also pediatrician, obstetrician-gynecologist

7. Management of patient care
    a. Anticipated patient trajectory: Patients with PDA are at risk of endocarditis, heart failure, and possibly shortened life span unless the congenital defect is closed
      i. Infection control: Antibiotic prophylaxis for IE or endarteritis until surgical repair, generally not needed after closure
      ii. Nutrition: Control of fluid and sodium intake, if heart failure symptoms are present
      iii. Discharge planning: IE prophylaxis, follow-up care and evaluation
      iv. Pharmacology
        (a) Patients usually are asymptomatic and do not require medication (except IE prophylaxis) until PDA closure
        (b) Treatment of heart failure

v. Treatments
- (a) Pharmacologic closure of PDA with prostaglandin inhibitors such as indomethacin (effective only in infancy). Complications of the use of indomethacin are increased bleeding risks due to platelet dysfunction, necrotizing enterocolitis.
- (b) Transcatheter closure with a detachable coil closure device deployed in the duct to occlude the shunt is being used for older children and adults
- (c) Surgical ligation of the PDA is the alternative and long-standing treatment. It is primarily performed on large ducts and in young infants.
    - (1) Surgery is performed through a small left thoracotomy incision
    - (2) In adults, calcification and rigidity of the ductus make closure much more difficult. A patch may be needed.
    - (3) Video-assisted thoracoscopic surgery and robotic techniques are also used
    - (4) Postoperative nursing care involves the same basic care as for thoracotomy
- (d) Heart-lung transplantation may be indicated in cases of fixed pulmonary hypertension and right-to-left shunting

b. Potential complications (see also applicable sections)
- **i.** IE
- **ii.** LV heart failure
- **iii.** Pulmonary hypertension and Eisenmenger's syndrome
- **iv.** Postoperative complications: Uncommon, include recurrent nerve injury, infections, bleeding, possible hemothorax, pneumothorax, or chylothorax
- **v.** Complications of the surgical procedures: Failure to close, emboli, vascular complications

8. Evaluation of patient care
- **a.** Patient is free of associated complications from the interventions and heart failure
- **b.** Complications are promptly identified and treated

Coarctation of the Aorta

Coarctation of the aorta is a congenital deformity of the aorta that creates a narrowing of the lumen and, subsequently, decreased flow. Usually located just beyond the left subclavian artery or just distal to the ligamentum arteriosum. Can be associated with other congenital defects of the heart (e.g., bicuspid aortic valve, VSD).

1. Pathophysiology
- **a.** In the fetus, the smooth muscle of the ductus arteriosus extends into the aorta. After birth, tissue contracts to close the duct, the aorta is pulled inward, and abnormal infolding or narrowing occurs.
- **b.** Thickening of the aortic medial tissue can form a ridge projecting into the lumen of the aorta, obstructing aortic flow
- **c.** Fetal development of the aortic arch may also be abnormal, in conjunction with the formation of other cardiac defects (VSD, mitral valve defects, bicuspid aortic valve)
- **d.** Pressure gradient develops: Pressures proximal to the coarctation are increased and pressures distal are decreased
- **e.** LV pressures increase, as do pressures in all aortic arch vessels
- **f.** Progressively, the LV dilates, hypertrophies, and can fail because of increased afterload

    g. Cerebral and upper extremity systemic hypertension results from the mechanical obstruction and stimulation of the renin-angiotensin system due to decreased renal blood flow

    h. Collateral circulation develops and supports the lower body and extremities, compensating for the decreased blood flow through the aorta. Collaterals involved include the internal mammary, internal thoracic, scapular, epigastric, intercostal, lumbar, and thyrocervical arteries

    i. If the coarctation is left untreated, death is caused by the consequences of the prolonged hypertension (e.g., strokes, CAD, heart failure, aortic rupture, or dissection). Other complications include IE, cerebral hemorrhage.

2. Etiology and risk factors

    a. Incidence higher in males

    b. Associated with the following disorders: VSD, Turner's syndrome, cerebral aneurysms (circle of Willis)

    c. Average life expectancy of an untreated patient with significant coarctation is less than 30 years

3. Signs and symptoms: Usually diagnosed in childhood. Newborns may have heart failure and require intervention. After infancy, many patients are asymptomatic until after 20 to 30 years of age. Coarctation is often discovered on routine examinations as a result of hypertension or murmur (i.e., during school physicals for sports).

    a. Subjective findings: Patient may complain of headaches, visual disturbances, epistaxis, leg cramps or fatigue (with exercise), dizziness, dysphagia

    b. Objective findings: Unremarkable in an asymptomatic patient

        i. Cyanosis in preductal coarctation, more noticeable in the fingers than in the toes

        ii. Possible irritability, poor feeding, tachypnea in a critically ill infant

        iii. Oliguria

        iv. Metabolic acidosis

        v. Hypotension

    c. Physical examination

        i. Inspection

            (a) Forceful thrust may be seen at the apex as a result of LV hypertrophy

            (b) Infants may have lower extremity cyanosis

            (c) Rarely, the upper body may be more developed (athletic) than the lower body, which may be underdeveloped (thin legs, narrow hips)

        ii. Palpation

            (a) Check radial and femoral pulses simultaneously for pulse lag (forceful upper extremity pulses, typically weak and delayed or absent lower extremity pulses). Femoral pulses are absent in about 40% of affected patients (the result of narrow pulse pressure, not of absent flow).

            (b) Blood pressure in the lower extremities is less than that in the upper extremities (often by more 20 mm Hg). Systolic hypertension seen in the upper extremities.

            (c) Blood pressure may vary in the arms, especially if the coarctation is proximal to the left subclavian artery

            (d) Suprasternal notch thrill

            (e) Apical thrust

        iii. Auscultation

            (a) Systolic ejection murmur, heard best at the right upper sternal border

            (b) Loud S_2 (aortic component)

            (c) S_4 present with left hypertrophy

4. **Diagnostic study findings**
   a. Radiologic: Chest radiograph may be the first means of discovery
      i. Enlarged LV
      ii. Notching of ribs (inferior margins of the third through eighth ribs), caused by the collateral circulation of the intercostal arteries
      iii. "3" sign: Dilated ascending aorta followed by the constricted area, followed by the poststenotic dilatation
   b. ECG: LV hypertrophy pattern
   c. Echocardiography: LV hypertrophy—screen for other associated aortic stenoses, VSDs
   d. MRI, CT: Confirms the diagnosis safely in pregnant patients (MRI), provides good images of the thoracic aorta and the site of coarctation
   e. Cardiac catheterization: Used to exclude CAD in adults preoperatively. Aortogram shows the location, degree, and character of the aortic lumen narrowing.
5. **Goals of care**
   a. Prompt, aggressive treatment is provided for symptoms of heart failure
   b. Hypertension is controlled
6. **Collaborating professionals on health care team:** See Chronic Stable Angina; also pediatrician, obstetrician-gynecologist
7. **Management of patient care**
   a. Anticipated patient trajectory: Patients with unrecognized coarctation of the aorta will be exposed to severe hypertension and acceleration of atherosclerosis, which can result in heart failure, stroke, MI, and early death if the defect is not repaired
      i. Infection control: IE antibiotic prophylaxis
      ii. Discharge planning
         (a) Lifelong monitoring for recoarctation, stenosis, hypertension, valvular disease
         (b) Genetic counseling for female patients considering pregnancy
         (c) Pregnancy should be avoided until the repair is accomplished. Close supervision for hypertension issues is necessary.
      iii. Pharmacology: Antihypertensives for blood pressure control with close follow-up monitoring
      iv. Psychosocial issues: Issues regarding contraceptive use and pregnancy are sensitive matters and can cause anxiety and stress in younger patients
      v. Treatments
         (a) Coarctation is relieved by surgery
            (1) If the patient is asymptomatic, surgery is usually delayed until age 1 to 5 years but should be performed as soon as possible to avoid hypertension
            (2) The older the patient, the higher the risk of death from surgery
            (3) Surgical correction decreases the hypertension and reverses LV failure
         (b) When surgery is undertaken, a left thoracotomy incision is performed
            (1) Postoperative nursing involves the basic care for a thoracotomy patient
            (2) Record blood pressure in both arms
            (3) Assess brachial and femoral pulses simultaneously
         (c) Percutaneous transluminal angioplasty, with or without balloon-expandable endovascular stents, is employed more often, especially with recoarctation
   b. Potential complications

      i. IE

      ii. Common causes of death from coarctation in older patients are spontaneous aortic rupture, heart failure, IE, and cerebral hemorrhage

      iii. Postoperative complications are recoarctation, paradoxical or persistent systemic hypertension, aortic dissection or rupture, heart failure, and stroke; 20% of patients have transient postoperative abdominal pain and/or distention (probably due to restoration of normal pulsatile blood flow and pressure)

      iv. Paradoxical systolic hypertension may occur for the first 24 to 36 hours after surgery; caused by increased levels of circulating catecholamines; treated with sodium nitroprusside, β-blockers, ARBs

      v. Complications after percutaneous transluminal angioplasty for restenosis include aneurysms, rupture, recoarctation, stroke

      vi. Pregnancy: Increased risk of aortic dissection

8. Evaluation of patient care

    a. Blood pressure is controlled per predetermined parameters

    b. Patient is free of associated complications from surgery. Any complications are promptly identified and treated.

    c. Patient and significant others discuss the need for follow-up

Hypertensive Crisis

Hypertensive crisis is a life-threatening elevation in blood pressure necessitating emergency treatment (within 1 hour) to prevent severe end-organ damage and death

1. Pathophysiology

    a. Hypertensive pathophysiology and its effects on the heart, brain, and kidneys: See Table 3-16

■ **TABLE 3-16**
■ ■ **Sequelae of Hypertension: Its Effects on End Organs That May Lead to Hypertensive Crisis**

HYPERTENSION
Enhanced sympathetic stimulation
Effects of renin-angiotensin system (increased fluid retention, increased systemic vasoconstriction)
Necrosis of arterioles
Decreased blood flow to end organs

Heart	Brain	Kidney
Tachycardia	Loss of autoregulatory mechanisms	↓ Renal perfusion
↑ Cardiac output	Arterial spasm and ischemia → TIAs	↓ Ability to concentrate urine
↓ Perfusion → angina → MI	Weakened vessels → aneurysms → hemorrhage → CVA	↑ BUN, creatinine levels
CAD		↑ Proteinuria
LV hypertrophy		Kidney failure
LV failure		Uremia
Angina		

→, Leading to; *BUN*, blood urea nitrogen; *CAD*, coronary artery disease; *CVA*, cerebrovascular accident; *LV*, left ventricular; *MI*, myocardial infarction; *TIA*, transient ischemic attack.

    b. Hypertensive encephalopathy: Sudden, excessive elevation of the blood pressure (higher than 250/150 mm Hg) → dysfunction of cerebral autoregulation → vasospasm → ischemia → increased capillary pressure and permeability → cerebral edema, hemorrhage

2. Etiology and risk factors

    a. Untreated or uncontrolled hypertension

    b. Poor compliance with antihypertensive medication regimen

    c. Renal dysfunction (acute glomerulonephritis, acute or chronic renal failure, renal tumors, renovascular hypertension caused by acute renal artery occlusion)

    d. Preeclampsia of pregnancy

    e. Adrenergic crisis: Seen with a sharp rise in catecholamine levels caused by drug reactions (monoamine oxidase [MAO] inhibitor interactions, β-adrenergic agonist ingestion, abrupt withdrawal from antihypertensive therapy), pheochromocytoma

    f. Postoperative complications: CABG surgery, renal transplantation, peripheral vascular surgery

    g. Pituitary tumors

    h. Adrenocortical hyperfunction

    i. Severe burns

    j. Risk factors: Diabetes, obesity, smoking, hyperlipidemia, oral contraceptives, history of hypertension with pregnancy, alcohol abuse

3. Signs and symptoms: Patient may be unable to respond to questions; significant other may need to answer history inquiries (e.g., complaints of severe headache, epistaxis) (Figure 3-22)

    a. History

        i. Chronic hypertension

        ii. Positive family history of hypertension

        iii. Medication history positive for MAO inhibitors, oral contraceptives, appetite suppressants, pressor agents, street drugs

        iv. History of any etiologic factor mentioned

        v. History of CAD, renal dysfunction

    b. Clinical picture in hypertensive encephalopathy

        i. Blood pressure exceeding 250/150 mm Hg

        ii. Retinopathy

        iii. Papilledema of the optic disc

        iv. Severe headache

        v. Vomiting

        vi. Altered level of consciousness (obtunded, comatose)

        vii. Transitory focal neurologic signs (e.g., nystagmus)

        viii. Seizures

        ix. Signs and symptoms of heart failure

        x. Increased MAP

4. Diagnostic study findings

    a. Laboratory

        i. BUN and creatinine values elevated in patients with renal disease

        ii. Electrolyte levels: Hypocalcemia, hyponatremia, hypokalemia

        iii. Enzyme levels for MI

    b. Radiologic: Chest radiograph may show LV enlargement

    c. ECG: LV hypertrophy may be seen

    d. Echocardiogram: Impairment of diastolic function, LV hypertrophy, wall motion abnormalities

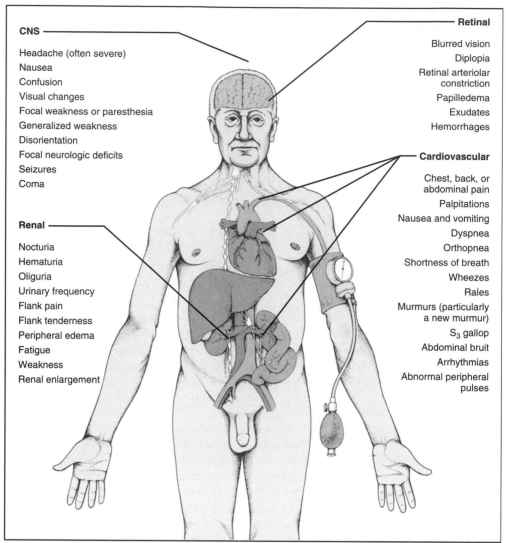

CNS

Headache (often severe)
Nausea
Confusion
Visual changes
Focal weakness or paresthesia
Generalized weakness
Disorientation
Focal neurologic deficits
Seizures
Coma

Renal

Nocturia
Hematuria
Oliguria
Urinary frequency
Flank pain
Flank tenderness
Peripheral edema
Fatigue
Weakness
Renal enlargement

Retinal

Blurred vision
Diplopia
Retinal arteriolar
constriction
Papilledema
Exudates
Hemorrhages

Cardiovascular

Chest, back, or
abdominal pain
Palpitations
Nausea and vomiting
Dyspnea
Orthopnea
Shortness of breath
Wheezes
Rales
Murmurs (particularly
a new murmur)
S₃ gallop
Abdominal bruit
Arrhythmias
Abnormal peripheral
pulses

FIGURE 3-22 ■ Symptoms and signs associated with target-organ damage in hypertensive crisis. *CNS*, Central nervous system. (From Antman EM, editor: *Cardiovascular therapeutics: a companion to Braunwald's heart disease*, Philadelphia, 2002, Saunders, p 821.)

    e. MRI or CT: To exclude stroke or hemorrhage when neurologic symptoms present. Shows diffuse brain edema with hypertensive crisis.
    f. Renal ultrasonography: To identify renal artery stenosis
5. Goals of care
    a. Rapid, life-preserving treatment of elevated blood pressure is provided
    b. MAP is lowered no more than 25% in the first 2 hours, or to 160/100 mm Hg
    c. Blood pressure is lowered in small decrements to avoid causing hypotension, oliguria, and/or mental changes from renal, coronary, or cerebral ischemia
    d. Cause of the hypertension is identified and treated
6. Collaborating professionals on health care team: See Chronic Stable Angina
7. Management of patient care
    a. Anticipated patient trajectory: Immediate blood pressure reduction is essential for the prevention or minimization of end-organ damage

  i. Nutrition
- (a) Obtain accurate intake and output measurements, along with daily weights
- (b) NPO initially, later a sodium-restricted diet
- (c) Dietary consult: For education on weight control, sodium restriction

  ii. Discharge planning: Patient education regarding the following:
- (a) Importance of blood pressure control: High risk for renal, cerebral, coronary problems with uncontrolled hypertension. Compliance with medication regimen essential.
- (b) Need for follow-up to assess the effectiveness of medications and to check for potential side effects from therapy
- (c) Lifestyle modification: Limitation of sodium intake, smoking cessation, moderation in alcohol use, walking program, weight control

  iii. Pharmacology
- (a) Nitroprusside: "Gold standard" for acute malignant hypertensive therapy. Drug of choice for hypertensive encephalopathy, cerebral infarction or bleeding, dissecting aortic aneurysm. Contraindicated in pregnancy (can cause fetal renal impairment).
  - (1) 0.25 to 0.5 mcg/kg/min IV. Titrate every 5 minutes (maximum dose 8 to 10 mcg/kg/min). Titrate to lowest dose for therapeutic effects.
  - (2) Drug acts in seconds, is quickly reversed by stopping infusion (drug action lasts 1 to 5 minutes)
  - (3) Protect bag and lines from light
  - (4) Watch for cyanide toxicity (blurred vision, confusion, tinnitus, seizures) especially after 48 hours of therapy or with renal insufficiency. Thiocyanate blood level should be measured at 48 hours. Level should not exceed 1.7 mmol/L.
  - (5) Closely monitor the patient's response to therapy by frequent assessments of blood pressure, hemodynamics. Titrate IV medications to the patient's responses per established parameters.
- (b) Fenoldopam (selective dopamine receptor agonist): Very potent vasodilator; as effective as nitroprusside in lowering blood pressure
  - (1) Dose: 0.1 mcg/kg/min; titrated every 15 minutes to response
  - (2) Half-life is 10 minutes
  - (3) Side effects include hypokalemia, headache, flushing, dizziness, reflex tachycardia
  - (4) Increases intraocular pressure (contraindicated with glaucoma)
- (c) Sympathetic blocking agents
  - (1) Labetalol (drug of choice for intracranial hemorrhage)
  - (2) Dosage: 20-mg IV bolus, then 20 to 80 mg every 10 minutes or IV infusion
  - (3) An α- and β-adrenergic blocking agent, used especially for adrenergic crisis. Does not increase heart rate (good in CAD).
- (d) ACE inhibitors
  - (1) Drug of choice for LV failure and pulmonary edema
  - (2) Enalapril: 1.25 to 5 mg IV every 6 hours
  - (3) Onset of action: 10 to 15 minutes
- (e) β-blockers: Block the effects of increased adrenergic tone, reduce mortality and morbidity
  - (1) Metoprolol: 5 mg IV every 5 minutes up to 15 mg total
  - (2) Esmolol: 500 mg/kg/min for 4 minutes, then 50 to 300 mg/kg/min IV

(f) IV NTG for hypotension due to cardiac causes (acute MI, failure)

(g) Loop diuretics (torsemide, furosemide, ethacrynic acid) for LV failure, pulmonary edema. Watch for volume depletion.

   iv. Psychosocial issues

(a) Reassure the patient and family

(b) Create a calm, quiet atmosphere, conducive to ample rest for the patient

(c) If the patient has been noncompliant with the medication regimen and has not addressed known risk factors, explore the reasons for noncompliance

    (1) Make sure the patient knows the rationales for medications and the consequences of inaction

    (2) Blood pressure medications are expensive. Help the patient find resources—financial services, drug programs for the indigent, use of pill splitters (buying larger doses and splitting the pills may be more economical), purchase of generics

   v. Treatments

(a) Ensure that the patient has adequate IV access; prepare for central line insertion, if needed

(b) Patient should undergo continuous arterial monitoring while drugs are being titrated and the condition is unstable

(c) Adjust antihypertensive intravenous medications promptly by titration, depending on the patient's response. Watch for side effects of medications.

(d) Accurately monitor fluid and electrolyte status. Observe for abnormalities in laboratory test results (i.e., electrolyte levels)

(e) If symptoms of tissue ischemia develop, reduce the speed with which blood pressure is lowered. *Note*: Most problems that occur in hypertensive crisis occur when treatment is too aggressive for the patient to tolerate.

  b. Potential complications (see also Figure 3-22)

   i. Cerebral dysfunction: Hypertensive encephalopathy, intracerebral or subarachnoid hemorrhage, head injuries, intracranial masses, embolic brain infarction

(a) Mechanism: Increased intracranial pressure (from cerebral edema)

(b) Management: Watch for changes in mentation or vision, headaches, nausea, vomiting. Intracranial pressure monitoring may be needed.

   ii. Cardiac or vascular dysfunction

(a) Mechanism: Caused by LV failure, dissecting aortic aneurysm, acute MI, unstable angina, coarctation of the aorta, arrhythmias

(b) Management: Monitor the ECG, observe for T-wave inversions that occur with rapid blood pressure reductions; ischemia is rare. Sudden chest pain may indicate aortic dissection.

   iii. Renal failure

(a) Mechanism: Can be a cause or a result of severely elevated blood pressure

(b) Management: Close monitoring, blood pressure control; dialysis may be required

8. Evaluation of patient care

  a. Blood pressure is within set parameters

  b. No side effects of medications are evident

  c. Electrolyte levels are normal

  d. No signs of cerebral dysfunction or increased intracranial pressure are noted

    e. ECG is in sinus rhythm

    f. CO is adequate as evidenced by hemodynamic assessments, urinary output, adequate circulation

Aortic and Peripheral Arterial Disease

Diseases of the aorta, cerebral arteries, and peripheral arteries have consequences that include aneurysm formation, dissection, or ischemia in their respective perfusion beds (Figures 3-23 and 3-24)

1. Pathophysiology

    a. Aortic aneurysm

        i. Focal or diffuse weakness of the aortic wall

        ii. Atherosclerosis is the most common cause

        iii. Dilatation, increased pressures, and thinning of the wall all increase wall stress, further weakening and dilating the vessel and producing an aneurysm

ANEURYSMS

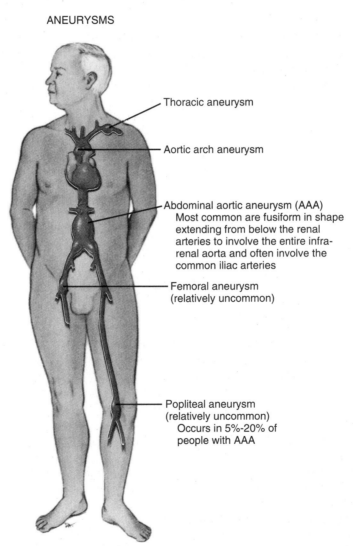

Thoracic aneurysm

Aortic arch aneurysm

Abdominal aortic aneurysm (AAA)
Most common are fusiform in shape extending from below the renal arteries to involve the entire infrarenal aorta and often involve the common iliac arteries

Femoral aneurysm
(relatively uncommon)

Popliteal aneurysm
(relatively uncommon)
Occurs in 5%-20% of people with AAA

FIGURE 3-23 ■ Peripheral artery disease: Aneurysms. (From Jarvis C: *Physical examination and health assessment*, ed 2, Philadelphia, 1996, Saunders, p 597.)

OCCLUSIONS

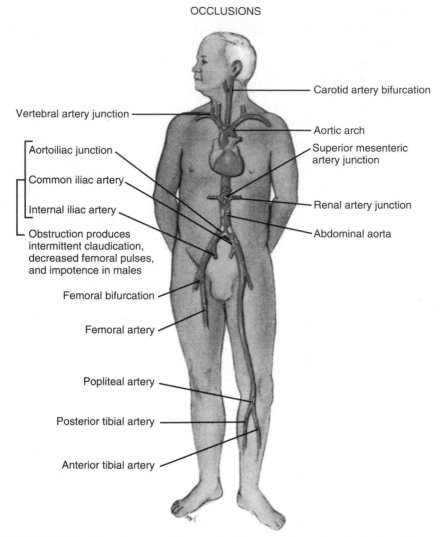

Carotid artery bifurcation

Vertebral artery junction —

Aortic arch

Aortoiliac junction

Superior mesenteric artery junction

Common iliac artery

Internal iliac artery

Renal artery junction

Obstruction produces intermittent claudication, decreased femoral pulses, and impotence in males

Abdominal aorta

Femoral bifurcation

Femoral artery

Popliteal artery

Posterior tibial artery

Anterior tibial artery

FIGURE 3-24 ■ Peripheral artery disease: Occlusions. (From Jarvis C: *Physical examination and health assessment*, ed 2, Philadelphia, 1996, Saunders, p 597.)

 iv. Rupture and death are likely when the diameter exceeds 6 cm for the thoracic aorta or 5 cm for the abdominal aorta
 v. Common sites for aneurysms
  (a) Abdominal aortic aneurysm: Location between the renal and iliac arteries is the most common site
  (b) Thoracic aortic aneurysm
   (1) Ascending, transverse, or descending aorta
   (2) Most common in men aged 60 to 70 years or older
  (c) Aneurysms of the iliac, femoral, and popliteal arteries
 b. Aortic dissection
  i. Intima of the ascending and/or descending aorta weakened by atherosclerosis or congenital disease of the media
  ii. Hypertension causes or contributes to the injury in 80% of cases
  iii. Tear develops through the intima and is propagated up and down the aorta by a dissecting column of blood

       iv. False channel is created

       v. Some organs may be perfused by the true lumen and some by the false lumen

      vi. Occasionally, a dissection of the ascending aorta extends to the aortic valve, and aortic insufficiency and even bleeding into the pericardium can result

      vii. End-organ ischemia and injury can occur

   c. Peripheral artery disease

      i. Atherosclerotic disease develops from the same risk factors and process as those for CAD

      ii. Stenosis and hypoperfusion result, culminating in ischemia, occlusion, and infarction (unless supported by collateral circulation)

      iii. Occluded lesions generally occur at bifurcations

      iv. Occlusions can also result from thrombus or embolus

      v. Common sites for peripheral artery disease include the carotid, renal, popliteal, aortoiliac, and femoral arteries (but any artery including the mesenteric can be involved)

2. Etiology and risk factors

   a. Atherosclerosis

   b. Congenital abnormalities (cystic medial necrosis, Marfan's syndrome)

   c. Trauma: Blunt trauma can create tears in the intima of the thoracic aorta (causing dissecting aneurysm)

   d. Severe hypertension

   e. Arteritis

   f. Raynaud's disease

   g. Risk factors are the same as for CAD (smoking, hypertension, diabetes, hyperlipidemia, family history)

3. Signs and symptoms: Manifestations usually occur at age 60 years or older

   a. Signs and symptoms vary with the location of the aneurysm or occlusion

      i. Aneurysm (most common): Often asymptomatic, found on routine examination

        (a) Abdominal aortic aneurysm

          (1) Pulsation in the abdominal area

          (2) Dull abdominal or low back pain or ache (impending rupture)

          (3) Nausea and vomiting (pressure against the duodenum)

          (4) Severe, sharp, sudden abdominal pain: Continuous, radiates to back, hips, scrotum, pelvis (rupture)

          (5) Abdominal tenderness, if an inflammatory process

          (6) Syncope, hypovolemic shock

        (b) Thoracic aortic aneurysm

          (1) Sudden, tearing chest pain radiating to the shoulders, neck, and back

          (2) Cough, hoarseness, weak voice from pressure against the recurrent laryngeal nerve

          (3) Dysphagia due to pressure on the esophagus

      ii. Aortic dissections

        (a) Marked by acute severe and instantaneous chest pain (in 90% of cases), radiating to the back, neck, jaw, or abdomen, associated with an absence of the affected pulses and evidence of end-organ injury

        (b) "Ripping," "tearing" sensations described

        (c) Pain may be differentiated from that of acute MI by its instantaneous, severe onset and the absence of pulses

        (d) Neurologic symptoms present in 15% of cases

    iii. Peripheral arterial disease

      (a) Intermittent claudication

        (1) Cramping, aching pain with exertion

        (2) Pain in the calf (most often) but may also be in the buttocks

        (3) Reproduced after walking a predictable distance

        (4) Relieved with rest, standing still

      (b) Nonhealing ulcers

      (c) Impotence

      (d) Severe pain in the extremities, pallor, absence of pulses, paresthesias, paralysis (seen in acute thrombosis of an abdominal aortic aneurysm)

      (e) Carotid arteries: Transient ischemic attacks, monocular visual disturbances, sensory or motor deficits, expressive or receptive aphasia, stroke

      (f) 50% of patients with occlusive arterial disease involving the lower extremities are asymptomatic

b. History

    i. History of atherosclerosis (CAD, CVA) and hypertension

    ii. Risk factors for atherosclerosis

    iii. Trauma: Blunt, deceleration type

    iv. History of impotence (seen in severe aortoiliac disease)

c. Physical examination: Manifestations depend on the organ perfused (i.e., cerebral vascular disease, renal vascular disease, ischemic or infarcted bowel, ischemic extremities)

    i. Aneurysms: Often asymptomatic except for rupture, when the patient is in obvious severe pain

      (a) Hypertensive or hypotensive

      (b) Obvious discomfort with rupture or expansion

      (c) Stridor, hoarseness, dysphagia (pressure on the esophagus, trachea, pharyngeal nerve)

      (d) Bruits: Abdominal aorta; femoral, renal, popliteal artery

      (e) Murmur of aortic insufficiency, if the aneurysm involves the aortic ring

    ii. Aortic dissection

      (a) Hypertension or hypotension

      (b) Dyspnea

      (c) Stridor, hoarseness, dysphagia (pressure on the esophagus, trachea, pharyngeal nerve

      (d) Palpation: Wide pulse pressure, absence of various peripheral pulses and pressures (50% of cases)

      (e) Auscultation: Murmur of aortic insufficiency (heard in 50% of cases)

    iii. Peripheral arterial disease

      (a) Pain on elevation of the extremities

      (b) Pale, mottled extremities on elevation: Rubor on dependence of the extremities

      (c) Ulcers, gangrene in the extremities

      (d) Skin changes due to impaired circulation (hair loss, thin and shiny skin)

      (e) Retinal arterial emboli (carotid disease)

      (f) Weak or absent peripheral pulses

      (g) Cool skin

      (h) Sluggish capillary refill

      (i) Pulsatile mass in the popliteal fossa (popliteal aneurysm)

      (j) Auscultation: bruits

4. **Diagnostic study findings**
   a. Laboratory
      i. CBC: Decreased HCT (anemia)
      ii. Elevated BUN and creatinine levels, proteinuria, hematuria (compromised kidneys)
   b. Radiologic
      i. Chest radiograph: Increased aortic diameter, right deviation of the trachea, pleural effusions
      ii. Abdominal films (anteroposterior, lateral views): For abdominal aneurysm
      iii. Provides anatomical information
   c. Doppler duplex ultrasonography: To assess peripheral, cerebrovascular blood flow and velocity
   d. Ankle-brachial index (ABI): Ankle systolic pressure is divided by the systolic pressure at the brachial artery to derive an index. Used to evaluate for the presence and severity of disease.
      i. Normal ABI = 0.9 to 1.3 (pressure normally higher in the ankle)
      ii. ABI less than 0.9 = positive for peripheral artery disease
      iii. ABI less than 0.4 = indicates severe ischemia
   e. CT: Assesses lumen diameter, wall thickness, aneurysm size, mural thrombi, and origin and extent of dissection, including the blood supply to end organs. Three-dimensional CT with angiography gives vivid three-dimensional views of the vascular system.
   f. MRA: Defines the arterial anatomy, shows the presence and severity of the occlusion
   g. TEE: Assesses for the presence of dissection in the aortic root, proximal ascending aorta, or descending thoracic aorta; aortic insufficiency; pericardial effusion. Used intraoperatively to determine the effectiveness of surgery.
   h. Peripheral angiography: Defines the anatomy and severity of lesions and their suitability for intervention
   i. Aortography: Origin and extent of dissection seen
5. **Goals of care**
   a. Patient has no pain at rest or with activity
   b. Perfusion to affected extremities is adequate
   c. No interventional complications are experienced
   d. Blood pressure is controlled at the systolic goal set for the patient
   e. Patient understands medications, follow-up requirements, any limitations on activities, proper diet, when to call for medical help, what symptoms to report
6. **Collaborating professionals on health care team:** See Chronic Stable Angina; also vascular specialist, primary care physician, stroke team
7. **Management of patient care**
   a. Anticipated patient trajectory: Aortic aneurysms and dissections are the most frequently missed preventable causes of sudden cardiac death
      i. Pain management: Relieve pain by administering ordered analgesics
      ii. Skin care: Meticulous attention to the skin because of poor circulation and tissue perfusion. Assess for pressure points, reddened or inflamed areas.
         (a) Frequent repositioning. Turn at least every 2 hours
         (b) Heel protection: Off bed on pillows or foam pads, or in protective boots; elevated
         (c) Ointments, skin barriers as needed
      iii. Nutrition: Dietary consult—assess nutritional status

    iv. Discharge planning: Teach the patient and significant others about the disease process (aneurysm, peripheral arterial occlusive disease), including the following:

      (a) Risk factor modification (e.g., smoking cessation, blood pressure control, diabetes control)

      (b) Discussion of a walking program, identification of resources to help with follow-up

      (c) Good foot care: Daily washing, nail trimming, use of well-fitting shoes, prompt professional attention to corns, calluses, ulcers

      (d) Weight reduction, if overweight

    v. Pharmacology

      (a) β-blockers (e.g., propranolol, labetalol) to lower blood pressure

      (b) Simultaneous use of nitroprusside to further lower blood pressure and to decrease contractility and sheer force

      (c) Antiplatelet agents: Aspirin daily (to lower the risk of CVA, MI). May also prevent reocclusions.

      (d) Cilostazol: For claudication pain, helps activity tolerance (contraindicated in HF)

      (e) Lipid-lowering agents (statins)

   vi. Treatments

      (a) Dissections: Distal dissections (distal to the left subclavian artery) are usually managed medically. Ascending dissections are treated with medications, but require surgery.

      (b) Acute aortic dissections: Surgical emergency

        (1) Goals: Stabilize emergently, prevent complications from rupture. Control systemic blood pressure (100 to 120 mm Hg systolic is the goal)

        (2) Prepare the patient for surgery: Resection, replacement, and/or reconstruction of involved arteries

          a) Continuous blood pressure monitoring

          b) Intubation may be necessary, if the patient's condition is unstable

          c) Assess peripheral pulses and blood pressure, comparing both sides. Pressure differences exceeding 20 mm Hg in the upper extremities indicate possible dissection or occluded subclavian, innominate, brachial, or axillary arteries. Pulses may be impossible to assess by palpating and difficult or impossible to assess with Doppler ultrasonographic studies.

          d) Observe for symptoms of shock

        (3) Proximal dissections carry a high (80%) mortality rate, but survival rate with surgery is also high

        (4) Postoperative nursing care for dissection

          a) Monitor hemodynamics

          b) Watch urinary output, mentation

      (c) Surgery for descending dissections performed only if the patient's condition continues to be unstable after medical therapy, with aortic rupture or Marfan's syndrome

      (d) Endovascular stent grafts are being deployed successfully to cover the descending dissections as a less invasive alternative

      (e) Endovascular revascularization interventions are widely used before surgery in peripheral arterial disease

        (1) Percutaneous transluminal angioplasty is used to open occluded arteries, particularly in proximal lesions (iliac, renal)

        (2) Excimer laser technology has also been used to debulk atherosclerotic material

        (3) Stents are used to reduce restenosis in both native arteries and grafts

        (4) Patients with acute arterial occlusions may be eligible for low-dose catheter-directed thrombolytic therapy (e.g., t-PA)

        (5) Mechanical thrombolysis or catheter-directed thrombectomy may also be performed for rapid thrombus removal

        (6) Watch for signs of bleeding, especially if the patient has received thrombolytic therapy

  b. Potential complications

     i. Aortic aneurysm: Dissection, embolization of thrombus, end-organ compromise

     ii. Large abdominal aneurysms: Disseminated intravascular coagulation is an associated problem

     iii. Ascending aortic dissections: MI, hemorrhagic cerebral infarct, tamponade, AR, death

     iv. Postoperative complications with ascending dissections: Death, CVA, end-organ compromise

     v. Postoperative complications with descending dissections: Ischemia of the spinal cord, paralysis, end-organ compromise

     vi. Postprocedure complications with endovascular intervention: Small bowel infarcts, gangrene

8. Evaluation of patient care

  a. Palpable pulses are felt in the affected extremities

  b. Limbs are warm with good color and brisk capillary refill

  c. No signs of bleeding are noted

  d. Patient is relaxed and free of pain

  e. Patient and family verbalize an understanding of the treatment plan for home care, medication administration, and risk factor modification, and the importance of a walking program

Shock

In shock, tissue perfusion to vital body organs is inadequate (see Chapter 9)

1. Pathophysiology (Table 3-17)

  a. Diminished tissue perfusion deprives cells of oxygen, nutrients, and energy. Cellular dysfunction and potential cell necrosis ensue, because of the lack of oxygenation and resulting acidosis.

  b. Cellular dysfunction is reversible at first but leads to organ damage if untreated

  c. Compensatory mechanisms: To support blood pressure, vasoconstriction is the homeostatic response of the body to hypotension and shock. This response is appropriate for, and probably evolved from, the need to respond to hemorrhagic shock. It is completely inappropriate and detrimental in the management of cardiogenic shock.

  d. Major organs begin to malfunction as they are deprived of oxygen, as a result of hypoxemia and metabolic acidosis (respiratory failure, renal failure, decreased cerebral perfusion, and disseminated intravascular coagulation may be seen)

2. Etiology and risk factors

  a. Cardiogenic shock: Impaired tissue perfusion as a result of severe cardiac dysfunction

TABLE 3-17
Pathophysiology and Clinical Presentations of Shock

Type of Shock	Forward Cardiac	CVP	PCWP	SVR	Clinical Examination	Comments
CARDIOGENIC SHOCK						
PUMP FAILURE						
LV MI	↓↓↓	↑↑	↑↑↑	↑↑	+S₃, +S₄	Extensive infarct (>40% LV)
RV MI	↓↓	↑↑↑	↔ or ↓	↑	Right sided +S₃, +S₄	Concomitant inferior wall MI common, consider if elevated right-sided filling pressures with normal or low PCWP or hypotension with clear lung fields
Non-CAD cardiomyopathy	↓↓↓	↑↑	↑↑↑	↑↑	+S₃, +S₄	Includes myocarditis, idiopathic, inflammatory causes
Allograft failure	↓↓↓	↑↑	↑↑↑	↑↑	+S₃, +S₄	Includes cellular and humoral rejection
Infiltrative disease (late)	↓↓↓	↑↑	↑↑↑	↑ or ↔	+S₄ (early)	Characteristic echocardiographic appearance. Site involved: RA-RV > LA-LV
Trauma	↓↓	↑ or ↔	↑↑	↑ or ↔	Variable	May see combined shock (i.e., hypovolemic vs. obstructive with pump failure)
MECHANICAL CAUSES						
Acute aortic regurgitation Native or prosthetic	↓↓	↔	↑↑ or ↑↑↑	↑↑	EDM	Endocarditis most common cause. IABP contraindicated
Acute mitral regurgitation Native or prosthetic	↓↓	↑ or ↔	↑↑↑	↑↑	ESM	Prominent PCWP V wave. IABP very effective
Aortic stenosis	↔	↑ or ↔	↑↑	↑↑		Symptoms may become manifest with increased metabolic demand (e.g., pregnancy, exercise, thyrotoxicosis, sepsis)
Mitral stenosis	↔	↑ or ↔	↑↑↑	↑↑		
VSD (acute post-MI)	↓ or ↓↓	↑ or ↑↑	↑ or ↑↑	↑↑	HSM, thrill	May be 3-5 days s/p MI, uncommon event but high mortality

Type					Heart sounds	Comments
Free wall rupture (post-MI)	↓ or ↓↓	↑ or ↑↑	↑ or ↑↑	↑↑	Silent	Catastrophic presentation 1-3 days s/p MI, earlier presentation with lytics
OBSTRUCTIVE SHOCK						
Pericardial tamponade	↓↓ (LV)	↑↑↑	↑↑↑	↑↑	Silent	Pressure equalization: RA mean, RV EDP, PA diastolic, PCWP within 5 mm Hg
Pulmonary embolism	↓↓ (RV)	↑↑↑	↔	↑ or ↑↑	RV S_3 or S_4, RV lift	RV dysfunction, moderate increase in PA pressure (40-50 mm Hg)
HYPOVOLEMIC SHOCK						
Blood or volume loss	↓	↓↓↓	↓↓↓	↑ or ↔	Silent	Look for source of blood or volume loss
DISTRIBUTIVE SHOCK						
Septic shock	↑ or ↑↑	Initial ↓↓	↓↓	↓↓↓	Hyperdynamic precordium	Provide early antibiotics, supportive care, identify occult source (e.g., abscess)
Anaphylactic shock Treatment is epinephrine	↔ or ↑		↓↓	↓↓↓	None	Document antigen exposure
COMBINED SHOCK (PRECISE HEMODYNAMICS OFTEN DIFFICULT TO PREDICT)						
Septic + cardiogenic	↓↓	↓ or ↔	↑↑	↓ or ↓↓	Variable — Infection (e.g., pneumonia) after MI	**Common settings:** Sepsis-induced LV dysfunction
Cardiogenic + hypovolemic	↓↓↓	↓ or ↔	↑ or ↑↑	↑↑↑	Variable	Free wall rupture after MI, GI bleeding with thrombolytics after MI
Hypovolemic + obstructive	↓↓	↓ or ↔	↑↑	↑↑↑	Quiet precordium	Ruptured aortic dissection with tamponade

From Crawford MH, DiMarco JP, Paulus WJ, editors: *Cardiology*, ed 2, St Louis 2004, Mosby, p 856.
↔, Unchanged; *CAD*, coronary artery disease; *CVP*, central venous pressure; *EDM*, early diastolic murmur; *EDP*, end-diastolic pressure; *ESM*, early systolic murmur; *GI*, gastrointestinal; *HSM*, holosystolic murmur; *IABP*, intraaortic balloon pump; *LA*, left atrium; *LV*, left ventricle; *MI*, myocardial infarction; *PA*, pulmonary artery; *PCWP*, pulmonary capillary wedge pressure; *RA*, right atrium; *RV*, right ventricle; *s/p*, status post; *SVR*, systemic vascular resistance; *VSD*, ventricular septal defect.

      i. MI, especially if large and/or anterior
      ii. Myocardial ischemia (left main artery disease, multivessel CAD)
      iii. Papillary muscle rupture, acute valvular dysfunction (acute mitral regurgitation, aortic insufficiency)
      iv. Heart failure, cardiac tamponade
      v. Arrhythmias
      vi. Cardiomyopathy
      vii. Other severe forms of myocardial injury (trauma)
      viii. Risk factors: peripheral vascular disease, decreased LV EF, diabetes

  b. Hypovolemic shock: Impaired tissue perfusion resulting from severely diminished circulating blood volume
      i. Hemorrhage: Loss of blood, plasma, and body fluids due to surgery, trauma, gastrointestinal bleeding
      ii. Hypovolemia from fluid shifts (e.g., burns)
      iii. Severe dehydration (vomiting, diarrhea, diabetic ketoacidosis, diabetes insipidus, heat stroke)
      iv. Internal, extravascular fluid loss: Resulting from third-spacing in interstitial space, ascites, ruptured spleen, pancreatitis, hemothorax
      v. Adrenal insufficiency

  c. Obstructive shock: Impaired tissue perfusion resulting from some obstruction to blood flow
      i. Pulmonary embolism (see Chapter 2)
      ii. Aortic dissection

  d. Anaphylactic shock: Impaired tissue perfusion resulting from antigen-antibody reaction that releases histamine into the blood stream. Capillary permeability increases, and arteriolar dilatation occurs. SVR falls. Blood return to the heart is decreased dramatically. Hypotension results.
      i. Contrast media
      ii. Drug reactions
      iii. Blood transfusion reactions
      iv. Food allergies
      v. Insect bites or stings
      vi. Snake bites

  e. Septic shock (systemic inflammatory response syndrome): Impaired tissue perfusion caused by widespread infection and invasion of microorganisms in the body, causing vasodilatation, decreased SVR, and hypotension (see Chapter 9)

  f. Neurogenic shock: Impaired tissue perfusion caused by damage to or dysfunction of the sympathetic nervous system. This type of shock is rare and may be associated with trauma, anesthesia, or spinal shock.

3. Signs and symptoms: History and assessments must be done rapidly so that immediate life-preserving therapy can be initiated; information is often obtained from significant others or previous records (e.g., bleeding, trauma, symptoms, fever, drugs, exposure)
  a. Clinical picture of cardiogenic shock
      i. Inspection
        (a) Hypotension: Systolic blood pressure lower than 90 mm Hg by cuff, lower than 80 mm Hg by arterial line
        (b) Patient confused, restless, or obtunded
        (c) Shallow, rapid respirations
        (d) Distended neck veins (RV MI, tamponade, pulmonary embolism)

    (e) Large differences in extremity pressures
    (f) Oliguria
  ii. Palpation
    (a) Cold, clammy extremities (vasoconstricted)
    (b) Peripheral pulses: Thready, rapid, or absent
    (c) Low temperature
  iii. Auscultation
    (a) Crackles (pulmonary edema)
    (b) S_3: Gallop
    (c) Systolic murmur (heard with acute mitral regurgitation, VSD, aortic stenosis)
    (d) Diastolic murmur of aortic insufficiency may be heard (short in acute aortic insufficiency)
    (e) Heart sounds distant in tamponade
  iv. Hemodynamics
    (a) Elevated CVP with neck vein distention (in RV MI, tamponade, massive pulmonary embolism)
    (b) Decreased CO, CI (<2 L/min)
    (c) Elevated PCWP
    (d) Elevated SVR
 b. Clinical picture of hypovolemic shock
  i. Inspection
    (a) Anxiety, irritability
    (b) Decreased level of consciousness
    (c) Poor capillary refill
    (d) Pale, gray skin
    (e) Increased heart rate
    (f) Hypotension
    (g) Collapsed neck veins
    (h) Tachypnea
    (i) Urinary output decreased or absent
  ii. Hemodynamics
    (a) Decreased CVP, filling pressures, PAP, PCWP, CO, CI
    (b) Increased PVR, SVR
 c. Clinical picture of anaphylactic shock
  i. Inspection
    (a) Altered mental status, headache
    (b) Stridor, tachypnea, wheezing
    (c) Increased heart rate, decreased blood pressure
    (d) Hives; itching; flushed, warm skin
    (e) Abdominal cramping, nausea, vomiting, diarrhea
    (f) Chills
  ii. Hemodynamics
    (a) Decreased CVP
    (b) Decreased PCWP
    (c) Decreased SVR
    (d) Variable CO
 d. Clinical picture of septic shock
  i. Inspection
    (a) Confusion, decreased level of consciousness
    (b) Fever, chills

       (c) Tachycardia

       (d) Tachypnea

       (e) Warm skin

       (f) Cyanosis

       (g) Oliguria

    ii. Hemodynamics

       (a) Decreased CVP

       (b) Decreased PCWP

       (c) Decreased SVR

       (d) Increased CO

e. Clinical picture of neurogenic shock

    i. Inspection

       (a) Mentation changes (restlessness, confusion)

       (b) Warm, dry skin

       (c) Bradycardia

       (d) No sweating (temperature-regulating center altered): Risk for overheating, chilling

       (e) Paralysis

       (f) Apnea, tachypnea, diaphragmatic breathing

       (g) Profound hypotension

       (h) Nausea, vomiting

       (i) Decreased urinary output

    ii. Hemodynamics

       (a) Decreased CVP

       (b) Decreased PCWP

       (c) Decreased SVR

       (d) Decreased CO, CI

       (e) Decreased oxygen saturations by pulse oximetry

4. Diagnostic study findings

    a. Laboratory

       i. ABG levels

         (a) Cardiogenic shock: Metabolic acidosis on ABG testing (hypocapnia, hypoxemia)

         (b) Hypovolemic shock: Respiratory alkalosis, metabolic acidosis

       ii. HCT: Decreased with hemorrhage

       iii. Leukocytosis (bacteremia in septic shock)

       iv. Thrombocytopenia (disseminated intravascular coagulation, septic shock)

       v. Abnormal electrolyte levels: Check potassium, sodium, chloride, magnesium

       vi. Troponin levels elevated in acute MI

    b. Radiologic findings: Chest radiograph for

       i. Cardiomegaly

       ii. Pulmonary congestion

       iii. Dilated aortic arch (see Aortic Dissection and Peripheral Arterial Disease)

       iv. Pleural effusion

       v. Cervical and thoracic spinal evaluation (for neurogenic shock)

    c. ECG

       i. Ischemia, infarction

         (a) RV infarction: ST elevation in RV leads (lead V_4R)

         (b) Anterior MI commonly associated with cardiogenic shock

         (c) Prior MI

       ii. Arrhythmias, conduction defects

iii. New right axis deviation: With tachycardia, pulmonary embolism
  d. Echocardiography
      i. LV and RV dysfunction (abnormal wall motion, chamber sizes)
     ii. Tamponade, pericardial effusions
    iii. Valvular disease
     iv. Hypovolemia (small, hyperdynamic chamber)
      v. VSD
  e. Bedside right-sided heart catheterization: To assess hemodynamics (i.e., CO, CI, SVR, PCWP), monitor volume status; evaluate the effectiveness of vasoactive agents and other therapies
  f. TEE: To look for aortic dissection, valvular disease, VSD
  g. Cardiac catheterization: Assesses
      i. CAD severity
     ii. LV function
    iii. Valvular function
     iv. Hemodynamics
      v. Shunts
     vi. Aortography: Dissection, aortic regurgitation
5. **Goals of care**
  a. Systolic blood pressure is increased to adequately perfuse tissues and vital organs. Blood pressure and pulse are within normal limits for the patient.
  b. Sufficient oxygenation is provided
  c. Pulmonary congestion is decreased
  d. Fluid and electrolyte balances are maintained
  e. Intake and output are balanced
6. **Collaborating professionals on health care team:** See Chronic Stable Angina; also critical care specialist, infectious disease specialist
7. **Management of patient care**
  a. Anticipated patient trajectory: Initial management of all forms of shock start with the ABC of *a*irway, *b*reathing and *c*irculation. Rapid identification and treatment of the cause(s) will help to avoid end-organ damage and death.
      i. Positioning: Place the patient in reverse Trendelenburg's position for severe drop in blood pressure while other measures are being initiated. Legs can be quickly elevated while the patient is lying flat to shift blood volume from the lower periphery to the central organs instantly.
     ii. Nutrition: Patient will need to receive parenteral or enteral nourishment if on NPO status for a prolonged period
    iii. Infection control: If septic shock, the causative microorganism must be identified and properly treated
     iv. Pharmacology
        (a) Cardiogenic shock
            (1) Inotropic agents: Dobutamine, dopamine, norepinephrine, milrinone, nesiritide
            (2) Vasopressors
            (3) Anticoagulants and antiplatelet agents: Heparin, aspirin, GPIIb/IIIa inhibitors
            (4) Avoid negative inotropic agents
            (5) Diuretics, if pulmonary edema present
        (b) Hypovolemic shock
            (1) Administer emergency infusions of volume replacement fluids, blood products

        (2) Observe for and identify symptoms associated with volume over-load, especially if the patient has received large amounts of replacement fluids

    (c) Anaphylactic shock: IV epinephrine, steroids

    (d) Septic shock: Appropriate antibiotics, volume replacement fluids, vasopressors

    (e) Neurogenic shock: Volume replacement fluids, vasopressors, steroids, atropine (for bradycardia)

  v. Treatments

    (a) Treat hypoxemia and acidosis

        (1) Give the patient oxygen to maintain the oxygen saturation at 92% or higher

        (2) Monitor ABG levels, report abnormalities, correct acidotic states: Ensure adequate ventilation

        (3) Hyperventilation with mechanical ventilator may be used to raise pH

        (4) Aggressive respiratory care when the patient is intubated to avoid the complication of pneumonia (especially with neurogenic shock)

        (5) Arterial line may be required

    (b) Treat hypovolemia (inadequate LV filling volumes)

        (1) Ensure that the patient has good IV access: Two patent, large-bore IV lines available and/or a central line

        (2) Give 250 ml normal saline as a trial. May need to repeat the amounts decided upon with the physician. Closely monitor the patient's response to avoid being too aggressive with fluid replacement. Hemodynamic monitoring is helpful to identify fluid status, patient response. If PCWP is less than 15 mm Hg, volume is needed, especially with RV MI (CVP higher than 20 mm Hg preferred).

        (3) Record vital signs at least every hour, more often as warranted

        (4) Monitor heart rate, blood pressure, MAP, CVP, PCWP to evaluate the patient's response to therapy

        (5) Maintain a strict hourly record of all intake and output

        (6) Analyze laboratory results: BUN level, HCT, electrolyte levels; notify the physician of abnormal findings

        (7) Watch for changes in level of consciousness

        (8) Observe skin condition: Color, turgor, temperature

    (c) Early reperfusion in acute MI is vital: Patient will need to be prepared for emergent angiography and coronary revascularization efforts such as primary PCI, thrombolysis, CABG

    (d) IABP can rapidly correct low CO, decreasing afterload and myocardial oxygen demands while assisting in increasing myocardial oxygen supply

    (e) LV or biventricular assist devices can be used as a bridge to potential transplantation

  b. Potential complication: Death. Prevention, rapid identification, and appropriate treatment of shock states are vital. Vigilance is the best management for the prevention of death.

8. Evaluation of patient care

  a. Tissue perfusion and oxygenation are adequate

  b. Vital signs and hemodynamic parameters within normal limits

  c. Fluid volume and electrolyte balance are maintained

  d. Coronary blood flow is restored with revascularization, as needed

REFERENCES

Physiologic Anatomy

Alpert JS, editor: *Cardiology for the primary care physician*, Philadelphia, 2001, Current Medicine.

Antman EM, editor: *Cardiovascular therapeutics: a companion to Braunwald's heart disease*, Philadelphia, 2002, Saunders.

Braunwald E, editor: *Essential atlas of heart diseases*, New York, 2001, McGraw-Hill.

Braunwald E, Zipes DP, Libby P, editors: *Heart disease: a textbook of cardiovascular medicine*, ed 6, Philadelphia, 2001, Saunders.

Chatterjee K, Karliner J, Rapaport E, et al, editors: *Cardiology: an illustrated text/reference*, Philadelphia, 1991, Lippincott.

Crawford MH, DiMarco JP, Paulus WJ, editors: *Cardiology*, ed 2, Philadelphia, 2004, Mosby.

Darovic GO: *Hemodynamic monitoring: invasive and noninvasive clinical application*, ed 3, Philadelphia, 2002, Saunders.

Fuster V, Alexander RW, O'Rourke RA, editors: *Hurst's the heart*, ed 10, New York, 2001, McGraw-Hill.

Goldman L, Ausiello D: *Cecil textbook of medicine*, ed 22, Philadelphia, 2004, Saunders.

Murphy JG, editor: *Mayo Clinic cardiology review*, ed 2, Philadelphia, 2000, Lippincott Williams & Wilkins.

Patient Assessment

Bates B, Bickley LS, Hoeklman RA: *A guide to physical examination and history-taking*, ed 6, Philadelphia, 1995, Lippincott.

Braunwald E, editor: *Essential atlas of heart diseases*, New York, 2001, McGraw-Hill.

Braunwald E, Zipes DP, Libby P, editors: *Heart disease: a textbook of cardiovascular medicine*, ed 6, Philadelphia, 2001, Saunders.

Crawford MH, DiMarco JP, Paulus WJ, editors: *Cardiology*, ed 2, Philadelphia, 2004, Mosby.

Darovic GO: *Hemodynamic monitoring: invasive and noninvasive clinical application*, ed 3, Philadelphia, 2002, Saunders.

Fuster V, Alexander RW, O'Rourke RA, editors: *Hurst's the heart*, ed 10, New York, 2001, McGraw-Hill.

Shub C: Physical examination. In Murphy JG, editor: *Mayo Clinic cardiology review*, ed 2, Philadelphia, 2000, Lippincott Williams & Wilkins, pp 261-284.

Diagnostic Studies

Alpert JS, editor: *Cardiology for the primary care physician*, Philadelphia, 2001, Current Medicine.

Antman EM, editor: *Cardiovascular therapeutics: a companion to Braunwald's heart disease*, Philadelphia, 2002, Saunders.

Braunwald E, Zipes DP, Libby P, editors: *Heart disease: a textbook of cardiovascular medicine*, ed 6, Philadelphia, 2001, Saunders.

Bridges EJ: Monitoring pulmonary artery pressures: just the facts, *Crit Care Nurse* 20(6):59-75, 2000.

Can atherosclerosis imaging techniques improve the detection of patients at risk for ischemic heart disease? Proceedings of the 34th Bethesda Conference, Bethesda, Maryland, USA, October 7, 2002, *J Am Coll Cardiol* 41(11):1855-1917, 2003.

Chatterjee K, Davis KB, Fifer MA, et al: ACC expert consensus document: present use of bedside right heart catheterization in patients with cardiac disease, *J Am Coll Cardiol* 32(3):840-864, 1998.

Chou T, Knilans TK: *Electrocardiography in clinical practice*, ed 4, Philadelphia, 1996, Saunders.

Crawford MH, DiMarco JP, Paulus WJ, editors: *Cardiology*, ed 2, Philadelphia, 2004, Mosby.

Darovic GO: *Hemodynamic monitoring: invasive and noninvasive clinical application*, ed 3, Philadelphia, 2002, Saunders.

Fuster V, Alexander RW, O'Rourke RA, editors: *Hurst's the heart*, ed 10, New York, 2001, McGraw-Hill.

Goldman L, Ausiello D: *Cecil textbook of medicine*, ed 22, Philadelphia, 2004, Saunders.

Henry JB: Clinical diagnosis and management by laboratory methods, Philadelphia, 2001, Saunders.

Huszar RJ: *Basic dysrhythmias: interpretation and management*, ed 3, Philadelphia, 2002, Mosby.

Klocke FJ, Baird MG, Bateman TM: ACC/AHA/ASNC guidelines for the clinical use of cardiac radionuclide imaging—executive summary: a report of the American College of Cardiology/American Heart Association Task Force on Practice Guidelines (ACC/AHA/ASNC Committee to Revise the 1995 Guidelines for the Clinical Use of Cardiac Radionuclide Imaging), *J Am Coll Cardiol* 42(7):1318-1333, 2003. Full text available at http://www.acc.org/clinical/topic/topic.htm#cardiacimaging.

Landesberg G, Shatz V, Akopnik I, et al: Association of cardiac troponin, CK-MB, and postoperative myocardial ischemia with long-term survival after major vascular surgery, *J Am Coll Cardiol* 42(9):1547-1554, 2003.

Murphy JG, editor: *Mayo Clinic cardiology review,* ed 2, Philadelphia, 2000, Lippincott Williams & Wilkins.

Wallach J: *Interpretation of diagnostic tests,* Philadelphia, 2000, Lippincott Williams & Wilkins.

Coronary Artery Disease

Braunwald E, editor: *Essential atlas of heart diseases,* New York, 2001, McGraw-Hill.

Braunwald E, Zipes DP, Libby P, editors: *Heart disease: a textbook of cardiovascular medicine,* ed 6, Philadelphia, 2001, Saunders.

Can atherosclerosis imaging techniques improve the detection of patients at risk for ischemic heart disease? Proceedings of the 34th Bethesda Conference, Bethesda, Maryland, USA, October 7, 2002, *J Am Coll Cardiol* 41(11):1855-1917, 2002.

Cannon CP, O'Gara PT, editor: *Critical pathways in cardiology,* Philadelphia, 2002, Lippincott Williams & Wilkins.

Canto JG, Iskandrian AE: Major risk factors for cardiovascular disease: debunking the "only 50%" myth, *JAMA* 290:947-949, 2003.

Cardenas GA, Lavie CJ, Milani RV: Importance and management of low levels of high-density lipoprotein cholesterol in older adults. Part I: role and mechanism, *Geriatr Aging* 7(3):40-45, 2004.

Cardenas GA, Lavie CJ, Milani RV: Importance and management of low levels of high-density lipoprotein cholesterol in older adults. Part II: screening and treatment, *Geriatr Aging* 7(4):41-48, 2004.

Chobanian AV, Bakris GL, Black HR, et al: The seventh report of the Joint National Committee on Prevention, Detection, Evaluation, and Treatment of High Blood Pressure: the JNC 7 report, *JAMA* 289:2560-2572, 2003.

Coffey M, Crowder GK, Cheek DJ: Reducing coronary artery disease by decreasing homocysteine levels, *Crit Care Nurse* 23(1):25-29, 2003.

Cooper R, Cutler J, Desvigne-Nickens P, et al: Trends and disparities in coronary heart disease, stroke, and other cardiovascular diseases in the United States: findings of the National Conference on Cardiovascular Disease Prevention, *Circulation* 102:3137-3147, 2000.

Crawford MH, DiMarco JP, Paulus WJ, editors: *Cardiology,* ed 2, Philadelphia, 2004, Mosby.

Fuster V, Alexander RW, O'Rourke RA, editors: *Hurst's the heart,* ed 10, New York, 2001, McGraw-Hill.

Greenland P, Knoll MD, Stamler J, et al: Major risk factors as antecedents of fatal and nonfatal coronary heart disease events, *JAMA* 290:891-897, 2003.

Grundy SM, Cleeman JI, Merz CN, et al: Implications of recent clinical trials for the National Cholesterol Education Program Adult Treatment Panel III guidelines, *Circulation* 110:227-239, 2004.

Haskell WL: Cardiovascular disease prevention and lifestyle interventions: effectiveness and efficacy, *J Cardiovasc Nurs* 18(4):245-255, 2003.

Knot UN, Khot MB, Bajzer CT, et al: Prevalence of conventional risk factors with coronary heart disease, *JAMA* 290:898-904, 2003.

Mosca L, Appel LJ, Benjamin EJ, et al: Evidence-based guidelines for cardiovascular disease prevention in women, *J Am Coll Cardiol* 43(5):898-921, 2004.

Ridker PM, Skerrett PJ, Gaziano JM: Primary prevention of ischemic heart disease. In Antman EM, editor: *Cardiovascular therapeutics: a companion to Braunwald's heart disease,* Philadelphia, 2002, Saunders, pp 53-96.

Sharis PJ, Cannon CP: *Evidence-based cardiology,* ed 2, Philadelphia, 2003, Lippincott Williams & Wilkins.

Smith SC, Blair SN, Bonow RO, et al: AHA/ACC scientific statement: AHA/ACC guidelines for preventing heart attack and death in patients with arteriosclerotic cardiovascular disease: 2001 update: a statement for healthcare professionals from the American Heart Association and the American College of Cardiology, *Circulation* 104:1577-1579, 2001.

Stuart-Shor EM, Buselli EF, Carroll DL: Are psychosocial factors associated with pathogenesis and consequences of cardiovascular disease in the elderly? *J Cardiovas Nurs* 18(3):169-183, 2003.

Third report of the National Cholesterol Education Program (NCEP) Expert Panel on Detection, Evaluation, and Treatment of High Cholesterol in Adults (Adult Treatment Panel III), *Circulation* 106:3143-3421, 2002.

Websites

American Diabetes Association: http://www.diabetes.org.

National Heart, Lung and Blood Institute: http://www.nhlbi.nih.gov/. Practice guidelines, excellent patient resources on weight management, blood pressure guidelines, stroke prevention, cholesterol guidelines, Framingham coronary heart disease risk scoring system.

Office of the Surgeon General, US Department of Human Services: http://www.surgeongeneral.gov/tobacco. Smoking information.

Acute Coronary Syndromes: Unstable Angina Pectoris and Non–ST-Segment Elevation Myocardial Infarction

Bertrand ME, Simoons ML, Fox KA, et al: Management of acute coronary syndromes: acute coronary syndromes without persistent ST segment elevation; recommendations of the Task Force of the European Society of Cardiology, *Eur Heart J* 21:1406-1432, 2000.

Blake GJ, Ridker PM: C-reactive protein and other inflammatory risk markers in acute coronary syndromes, *J Am Coll Cardiol* 41(4 suppl S):37S-42S, 2003.

Braunwald E, Antman E, Bedasley J, et al: ACC/AHA 2002 guideline update for the management of patients with unstable angina and non-ST segment elevation myocardial infarction—summary article: a report of the American College of Cardiology/American Heart Association Task Force on Practice Guidelines (Committee on the Management of Patients with Unstable Angina), *J Am Coll Cardiol* 40:1366-1374, 2002. Full text available at http://www.acc.org/clinical/guidelines/unstable/update_index.htm.

Cannon CP: Small molecule glycoprotein IIb/IIIa receptor inhibitors as upstream therapy in acute coronary syndromes, *J Am Coll Cardiol* 41(4 suppl S):-43S-48S, 2003.

Cohen M: The role of low-molecular-weight heparin in the management of acute coronary syndromes, *J Am Coll Cardiol* 41(4 suppl S):55S-61S, 2003.

Conti R, Fuster V, Badimon JJ: Pathogenetic concepts of acute coronary syndromes, *J Am Coll Cardiol* 41(4 suppl S):7S-14S, 2003.

Crawford PA, editor: *The Washington manual cardiology subspeciality consult*, Philadelphia, 2004, Lippincott Williams & Wilkins.

Darovic GO: *Hemodynamic monitoring: invasive and noninvasive clinical application*, ed 3, Philadelphia, 2002, Saunders.

Gibbons RJ, Abrams J, Chatterjee K, et al: ACC/AHA 2002 guideline update for the management of patients with chronic stable angina (summary article): a report of the American College of Cardiology/American Heart Association Task Force on Practice Guidelines (Committee on the Management of Patients with Chronic Stable Angina), *J Am Coll Cardiol* 41(1): 159-168, 2002. Full text available at http://www.acc.org/clinical/guidelines/unstable/update_index.htm.

Jaffe AS, Davidenko J, Clements I: Diagnosis of acute coronary syndromes including myocardial infarction. In Crawford MH, DiMarco JP, Paulus WJ, editors: *Cardiology,* ed 2, Philadelphia, Mosby, 2004, pp 311-348.

Lynn-McHale DJ, Carlson KK, editors: *AACN procedure manual for critical care*, ed 4, Philadelphia, 2001, Saunders.

McKay RG: "Ischemia-guided" versus "early invasive" strategies in the management of acute coronary syndrome/non-ST-segment elevation myocardial infarction, *J Am Coll Cardiol* 41(4 suppl S):96S-102S, 2003.

Mehta LSR, Yusuf S: Short- and long-term oral antiplatelet therapy in acute coronary syndromes, *J Am Coll Cardiol* 41(4 suppl S): 79S-88S, 2003.

Moliterno DJ, Chan AW: Glycoprotein IIb/IIIa inhibition in early intent-to-stent treatment of acute coronary syndromes: EPISTENT, ADMIRAL, CADILLAC, and TARGET, *J Am Coll Cardiol* 41(4 suppl S): 49S-54S, 2003.

Monroe S, Pepine CJ: Management of unstable angina. In Antman EM, editor: *Cardiovascular therapeutics: a companion to Braunwald's heart disease*, Philadelphia, 2002, Saunders, pp 205-232.

Monroe VS, Kerensky RA, et al: Pharmacologic plaque passivation for the reduction of recurrent cardiac events in acute coronary syndromes, *J Am Coll Cardiol* 41(4 suppl S):23S-30S, 2003.

Newby LK, Goldmann BU, et al: Troponin: an important prognostic marker and risk-stratification tool in non-ST-segment elevation acute coronary syndromes, *J Am Coll Cardiol* 41(4 suppl S):31S-36S, 2003.

Opie LH: *Drugs for the heart*, ed 4, Philadelphia, 2001, Saunders.

Sabatine MS, Antman EM: The thrombolysis in myocardial infarction risk score in unstable angina/non–ST-segment eleva-tion myocardial infarction, *J Am Coll Cardiol* 41(4 suppl S):89S-95S, 2003.

Sharis PJ, Cannon CP: *Evidence-based cardiol-ogy,* ed 2, Philadelphia, 2003, Lippincott Williams & Wilkins.

Skah PK: Mechanisms of plaque vulnerability and rupture, *J Am Coll Cardiol* 41(4 suppl S): 15S-22S, 2003.

Skah PK, Chyu K: Unstable angina. In Crawford MH, editor: *Current diagnosis and treatment in cardiology,* New York, 2002, McGraw-Hill, pp 44-56.

Topol EJ: A guide to therapeutic decision-making in patients with non–ST-segment elevation acute coronary syndromes, *J Am Coll Cardiol* 41(4 suppl S):123S-129S, 2003.

Topol EJ, editor: *Textbook of interventional car-diology,* ed 4, Philadelphia, 2004, Saunders.

Waters DD: Diagnosis and management of patients with unstable angina. In Fuster V, Alexander RW, O'Rourke RA, editors: *Hurst's the heart,* ed 10, New York, 2001, McGraw-Hill, pp 1237-1274.

ST-Segment Elevation Myocardial Infarction

Alexander RW, Pratt CM, Ryan TJ, et al: Diagnosis and management of patients with acute myocardial infarction. In Fuster V, Alexander RW, O'Rourke RA, editors: *Hurst's the heart,* ed 10, New York, 2001, McGraw-Hill, pp 1275-1359.

Alpert JS: Defining myocardial infarction: "Will the real myocardial infarction please stand up?" *Am Heart J* 146(3):377-379, 2003.

Antman EM, editor: *Cardiovascular therapeu-tics: a companion to Braunwald's heart dis-ease,* Philadelphia, 2002, Saunders.

Antman EM, Anbe DT, Armstrong PW, et al: ACC/AHA guidelines for the management of patients with ST-segment elevation myocardial infarction: a report of the American College of Cardiology/American Heart Association Task Force on Practice Guidelines (Committee to Revise the 1999 Guidelines for the Management of Patients with Acute Myocardial Infarction), *J Am Coll Cardiol* 44(3):E1-E211, 2004. Full text and pocket guide available at http://www.acc. org/clinical/guidelines/stemi/index.htm.

Antman EM, Braunwald E: Acute myocar-dial infarction. In Braunwald E, Zipes DP, Libby P, editors: *Heart disease: a textbook of cardiovascular medicine,* ed 6, Philadelphia, 2001, Saunders, pp 1114-1231.

Archbold RA, Schilling RJ: Atrial pacing for the prevention of atrial fibrillation after coronary bypass graft surgery: a review of the literature, *Heart* 90:129-133, 2004.

Crawford MH, DiMarco JP, Paulus WJ, edi-tors: *Cardiology,* ed 2, Philadelphia, 2004, Mosby.

Crawford PA, editor: *The Washington manual cardiology subspeciality consult,* Philadelphia, 2004, Lippincott Williams & Wilkins.

Darovic GO: *Hemodynamic monitoring: inva-sive and noninvasive clinical application,* ed 3, Philadelphia, 2002, Saunders.

Fuster V, Alexander RW, O'Rourke RA, edi-tors: *Hurst's the heart,* ed 10, New York, 2001, McGraw-Hill.

Hochman JS, Califf RM: Acute myocardial infarction. In Antman EM, editor: *Cardio-vascular therapeutics: a companion to Braunwald's heart disease,* Philadelphia, 2002, Saunders, pp 233-291.

Jaffe AS, Miller WL: Acute myocardial infarc-tion. In Crawford MH, editor: *Current diag-nosis and treatment in cardiology,* New York, 2002, McGraw-Hill, pp 57-84.

Joint Commission on Accreditation of Healthcare Organizations: Overview of the acute myocardial infarction (AMI) core measure set, March, 22, 2002, retrieved June 10, 2005, from http://www.jcaho.org/ pms/core+measures/ami-overview.htm.

Kontos MC, Fritz LM, Anderson FP, et al: Impact of the troponin standard on the prevalence of acute myocardial infarction, *Am Heart J* 146(3):446-452, 2002.

Meier MA, Al-Badr WH, Cooper JV, et al: The new definition of myocardial infarc-tion: diagnostic and prognostic implica-tions in patients with acute coronary syndromes, *Arch Intern Med* 162:1585-1589. 2002.

Myocardial infarction redefined—a consen-sus document of the Joint European Society of Cardiology/American College of Cardiology Committee for the Redef-inition of Myocardial Infarction, *J Am Coll Cardiol* 36(3):959-969, 2000.

Nguyen TN, Hu D, Saito S, et al, editors: *Management of complex cardiovascular prob-lems,* New York, 2002, Futura.

Ryan TJ, Antman EM, Brooks NH, et al: 1999 update: ACC/AHA guidelines for the man-agement of patients with acute myocardial infarction: executive summary and recom-mendations: a report of the American College of Cardiology/American Heart

Association Task Force on Practice Guidelines (Committee on Management of Acute Myocardial Infarction), *Circulation* 100:1016-1030, 1999.

Schwertz DW, Vaitkus P: Drug-eluding stents to prevent re-blockage of coronary arteries, *J Cardiovasc Nurs* 18(1):11-16, 2003.

Sharis PJ, Cannon CP: *Evidence-based cardiology,* ed 2, Philadelphia, 2003, Lippincott Williams & Wilkins.

Spertus JA, Radford MJ, Every NR, et al: Challenges and opportunities in quantifying the quality of care for acute myocardial infarction: summary from the Acute Myocardial Infarction Working Group of the American Heart Association/American College of Cardiology First Scientific Forum on Quality of Care and Outcomes Research in Cardiovascular Disease and Stroke, *J Am Coll Cardiol* 41(9):1653-1663, 2003.

Topol EJ: *Textbook of interventional cardiology,* ed 4, Philadelphia, 2004, Saunders.

White HD: Things ain't what they used to be: impact of a new definition of myocardial infarction, *Am Heart J* 144(6):933-937, 2002.

Websites

American College of Cardiology: http:// www.acc.org. Cardiology practice guideline updates.

American Heart Association: http://www. americanheart.org.

Cardiology home page of Veterans Health Administration: http://www1.va.gov/ cardiology/. Ischemic heart disease, quality enhancement, research initiative.

Ischemic Heart Disease Quality Enhancement Research Initiative: http://www.hsrd. seattle.med.va.gov/ihdqueri/abstracts.htm.

Joint Commission on Accreditation of Healthcare Organizations: *Acute myocardial infarction,* version 1.02, http://www. jcaho.org/pms/core+measures/aligned_ manual.htm.

Heart Failure

Albert NM: Cardiac resynchronization therapy through biventricular pacing in patients with heart failure and ventricular dyssynchrony, *Crit Care Nurse* 23(3 suppl): 2-16, 2003.

Braunwald E, Zipes DP, Libby P, editors: *Heart disease: a textbook of cardiovascular medicine,* ed 6, Philadelphia, 2001, Saunders, pp 503-658.

Cianci P, Lonergan-Thomas H, Slaughter M, et al: Current and potential applications of left ventricular assist devices, *J Cardiovasc Nurs* 18(1):17-22, 2003.

Darovic GO: *Hemodynamic monitoring: invasive and noninvasive clinical application,* ed 3, Philadelphia, 2002, Saunders.

Eckardt L, Milberg P, Bocker D, et al: Arrhythmias in heart failure. In Crawford MH, DiMarco JP, Paulus WJ, editors: *Cardiology,* ed 2, Philadelphia, 2004, Mosby, pp 905-915.

Frishman WH, Sonnenblick EH, Sica DA, editors: *Cardiovascular pharmacotherapeutics,* ed 2, New York, 2004, McGraw-Hill.

Fuster V, Alexander RW, O'Rourke RA, editors: *Hurst's the heart,* ed 10, New York, 2001, McGraw-Hill, pp 655-724.

Givertz MM, Stevenson LW, Colucci WS: Hospital management of heart failure. In Antman EM, editor: *Cardiovascular therapeutics: a companion to Braunwald's heart disease,* Philadelphia, 2002, Saunders, pp 357-373.

Goldman L, Ausiello D: *Cecil textbook of medicine,* ed 22, Philadelphia, 2004, Saunders.

Hunt SA, Abraham WT, Chin MH, et al: ACC/AHA 2005 guideline update for the diagnosis and management of chronic heart failure in the adult: a report of the American College of Cardiology/American Heart Association Task Force on Practice Guidelines, *Circulation* 112:e154-e235, 2005, www.acc.org/clinical/topic/topic.htm#H.

Joint Commission on Accreditation of Healthcare Organizations: Overview of the heart failure (HF) core measure set, March 22, 2002, retrieved June 10, 2005, from http://www.jcaho.org/pms/core+measures/hf_overview.htm.

Kirklin J, Young J, McGiffin D: *Heart transplantation,* New York, 2002, Churchill Livingstone.

MacKlin M: Managing heart failure: a case study approach, *Crit Care Nurse* 21(2):40-46, 50-51, 2001.

Mehra MR, Uber PA, Potluri S, et al: Is heart failure with reserved systolic function an overlooked enigma? *Curr Cardiol Rep* 4(3):187-193, 2002.

Patel AR, Konstam MA: Assessment of the patient with heart failure. In Crawford MH, DiMarco JP, Paulus WJ, editors: *Cardiology,* ed 2, Philadelphia, 2004, Mosby, pp 845-854.

Prahash A, Lynch T: B-type natriuretic peptide: a diagnostic, prognostic, and therapeutic tool in heart failure, *Am J Crit Care* 13(1):46-55, 2004.

Redfield MM, Rodeheffer RJ: Medical therapy of systolic ventricular dysfunction and heart failure. In Murphy JG, editor: *Mayo Clinic cardiology review,* ed 2, Philadelphia, 2000, Lippincott Williams & Wilkins, pp 75-92.

Rodeheffer RJ, Redfield MM: Congestive heart failure: diagnosis, evaluation, and surgical therapy. In Murphy JG, editor: *Mayo Clinic cardiology review,* ed 2, Philadelphia, 2000, Lippincott Williams & Wilkins, pp 55-74.

Schwarz KA, Elman CS: Identification of factors predictive of hospital readmissions for patients with heart failure, *Heart Lung* 32(2):88-99, 2003.

Websites

Datascope Corp: http://www.datascope.com. Intraaortic balloon counterpulsation.

Heart Failure Society of America: http://www.hfsa.org/. Practice guidelines, patient education.

Pericardial Disease

Bonnefoy E, Godon P, Kirkorian G, et al: Serum cardiac troponin I and S-T segment elevation in patients with acute pericarditis, *Eur Heart J* 21:832-836, 2000.

Cheitlein MD, Armstrong WF, Aurigemma GP, et al: ACC/AHA/ASE 2003 guideline update for the clinical application of echocardiography: summary article: a report of the American College of Cardiology/American Heart Association Task Force on Practice Guidelines (ACC/AHA/ASE Committee to Update the 1997 Guidelines for the Clinical Application of Echocardiography), *Circulation* 108:1146-1162, 2003.

Hoit BD: Diseases of the pericardium. In Fuster V, Alexander RW, O'Rourke RA, editors: *Hurst's the heart,* ed 10, New York, 2001, McGraw-Hill, pp 2061-2085.

Kabbani SS, LeWinter MM: Pericardial disease. In Murphy JG, editor: *Mayo Clinic cardiology review,* ed 2, Philadelphia, 2000, Lippincott Williams and Wilkins, pp 993-1007.

Oh JK: Pericardial diseases. In Murphy JG, editor: *Mayo Clinic cardiology review,* ed 2, Philadelphia, 2000, Lippincott Williams & Wilkins, pp 509-532.

Spodick DH: Pericardial diseases. In Braunwald E, Zipes DP, Libby P, editors: *Heart disease: a textbook of cardiovascular medicine,* ed 6, Philadelphia, 2001, Saunders, pp 1823-1876.

Myocarditis

Felker GM, Boehmer JP, Hruban RH, et al: Echocardiographic findings in fulminant and acute myocarditis, *J Am Coll Cardiol* 36(1):227-232, 2000.

Goldman ME: Infectious myocarditis. In Alpert JS, editor: *Cardiology for the primary care physician,* Philadelphia, 2001, Current Medicine, pp 250-269.

Kirklin J, Young J, McGiffin D: *Heart transplantation,* New York, 2002, Churchill Livingstone, pp 221-222.

Sarda L, Colin P, Boccara F, et al: Myocarditis in patients with clinical presentation of myocardial infarction and normal coronary angiograms, *J Am Coll Cardiol* 37(3): 786-792, 2001.

Schultheiss H-P, Kuhl U: Myocarditis and inflammatory cardiomyopathy. In Crawford MH, DiMarco JP, Paulus WJ, editors: *Cardiology,* ed 2, Philadelphia, 2004, Mosby, pp 937-949.

Infective Endocarditis

Acar J, Michel P-L: Infective endocarditis. In Murphy JG, editor: *Mayo Clinic cardiology review,* ed 2, Philadelphia, 2000, Lippincott Williams & Wilkins, pp 1161-1177.

Cheitlein MD, Armstrong WF, Aurigemma GP, et al: ACC/AHA/ASE 2003 guideline update for the clinical application of echocardiography: summary article: a report of the American College of Cardiology/American Heart Association Task Force on Practice Guidelines (ACC/AHA/ASE Committee to Update the 1997 Guidelines for the Clinical Application of Echocardiography), *Circulation* 108:1146-1162, 2003.

Ewy GA: Infectious endocarditis. In Alpert JS, editor: *Cardiology for the primary physician,* ed 3, Philadelphia, 2001, Current Medicine, pp 271-278.

Karchmer AW: Infective endocarditis. In Braunwald E, Zipes DP, Libby P, editors: *Heart disease: a textbook of cardiovascular medicine,* ed 6, Philadelphia, 2001, Saunders, pp 1723-1750.

Mylonakis E, Callderwood SB: Infective endocarditis in adults, *N Engl J Med* 345:1318-1330, 2001.

Patel R, Steckelberg JM: Infections of the heart. In Murphy JG, editor: *Mayo Clinic cardiology review*, ed 2, Philadelphia, 2000, Lippincott Williams & Wilkins, pp 407-444.

Sande MA, Kartalija M, Anderson, J: Infective endocarditis. In Fuster V, Alexander RW, O'Rourke RA, editors: *Hurst's the heart*, ed 10, New York, 2001, McGraw-Hill, pp 2087-2125.

Cardiomyopathy

Akkad MZ, O'Connell JB: Dilated and toxic cardiomyopathy. In Crawford MH, DiMarco JP, Paulus WJ, editors: *Cardiology*, ed 2, Philadelphia, 2004, Mosby, pp 951-973.

Bristow MR, Mestroni L, Bohlmeyer TJ, et al: Dilated cardiomyopathies. In Fuster V, Alexander RW, O'Rourke RA, editors: *Hurst's the heart*, ed 10, New York, 2001, McGraw-Hill, pp 1947-1966.

Elliott PM, Reith S, McKenna WJ: Hypertrophic cardiomyopathy. In Crawford MH, DiMarco JP, Paulus WJ, editors: *Cardiology*, ed 2, Philadelphia, 2004, Mosby, pp 961-973.

Hoekstra JW, editor: *Handbook of cardiovascular emergencies*, ed 2, Philadelphia, 2001, Lippincott Williams & Wilkins.

Kirklin J, Young J, McGiffin D: *Heart transplantation*, New York, 2002, Churchill Livingstone.

Maron BJ: Hypertrophic cardiomyopathy. In Fuster V, Alexander RW, O'Rourke RA, editors: *Hurst's the heart*, ed 10, New York, McGraw-Hill, 2001, pp 1967-1987.

Maron BJ: Hypertrophic cardiomyopathy, *Circulation* 106:2419-2421, 2002.

Maron BJ, McKenna WJ, et al: ACC/ESC clinical expert consensus document on cardiomyopathy: a report of the American College of Cardiology Task Force on Clinical Expert Consensus Documents and the European Society of Cardiology Committee for Practice Guidelines (Committee to Develop an Expert Consensus Document on Hypertrophic Cardiomyopathy), *J Am Coll Cardiol* 42(9):1687-1713, 2003.

Nishimura RA, Ommen SR, Tajik AJ: Hypertrophic cardiomyopathy: a patient perspective, *Circulation* 108:e133-e135, 2003.

Pereira NL, Dec GW: Restrictive and infiltrative cardiomyopathy. In Crawford MH, DiMarco JP, Paulus WJ, editors: *Cardiology*, ed 2, Philadelphia, 2004, Mosby, pp 983-992.

Sweeney MO, Elloenbogen KA: Implantable devices for the electrical management of heart disease: overview of indications for therapy and selected advances. In Antman EM, editor: *Cardiovascular therapeutics: a companion to Braunwald's heart disease*, Philadelphia, 2002, Saunders, pp 516-528.

End-Stage Heart Disease

Albert NM: Cardiac resynchronization therapy through biventricular pacing in patients with heart failure and ventricular dyssynchrony, *Crit Care Nurse* 23(3 suppl): 2-16, 2003.

Bolno PB, Kresh JY: Physiologic and hemodynamic basis of ventricular assist devices, *Cardiol Clin* 21(1):15-27, 2003.

Holmes EC: Outpatient management of long-term assist devices, *Cardiol Clin* 21: 91-99, 2003.

Hunt SA, Abraham WT, Chin MH, et al: ACC/AHA 2005 guideline update for the diagnosis and management of chronic heart failure in the adult: a report of the American College of Cardiology/American Heart Association Task Force on Practice Guidelines, *Circulation* 112:e154-e235, 2005, www.acc.org/clinical/topic/topic.htm#H.

Hunt SA, Schroeder JS, Berry GJ: Cardiac transplantation, mechanical ventricular support, and endomyocardial biopsy. In Fuster V, Alexander RW, O'Rourke RA, editors: *Hurst's the heart*, ed 10, New York, 2001, McGraw-Hill, pp 725-744.

Jessup M, Brozena SC: Epilogue: support devices for end stage heart failure, *Cardiol Clin* 21:135-139, 2003.

Kirklin J, Young J, McGiffin D: *Heart transplantation*, New York, 2002, Churchill Livingstone.

Mehra MR, Uber PA: The dilemma of late-stage heart failure, *Cardiol Clin* 19(4):627-635, 2001.

Mehra MR, Uber PA: Emergence of Laplace therapeutics: declaring an end to "end-stage" heart failure, *Congest Heart Fail* 8:228-231, 2002.

Mehra MR, Uber PA, et al: Comparative beneficial effects of simvastatin and pravastatin on cardiac allograft rejection and survival, *J Am Coll Cardiol* 40(9):1609-1614, 2002.

Miniati DN, Robbins RC, Reitz B: Heart and heart-lung transplantation. In Braunwald E, Zipes DP, Libby P, editors: *Heart disease: a textbook of cardiovascular medicine*, ed 6, Philadelphia, 2001, Saunders, pp 615-634.

Park MH, Scott RL, Uber PA, et al: Treatment of pulmonary hypertension, *Catheter Cardiovasc Interv* 57:395-403, 2002.

Patel H, Pagani FD: Extracorporeal mechanical circulatory assist, *Cardiol Clin* 21(1): 29-41, 2003.

Remme WJ, Swedberg K: Comprehensive guidelines for the diagnosis and treatment of chronic heart failure, Task force for the diagnosis and treatment of chronic heart failure of the European Society of Cardiology, *Eur J Heart Fail* 4:11-22, 2002.

Young JB: Surgery, assist devices and cardiac transplantation for heart failure. In Crawford MH, DiMarco JP, Paulus WJ, editors: *Cardiology*, ed 2, Philadelphia, 2004, Mosby, pp 917-930.

Cardiac Trauma

Cummins RO, editor: *ACLS for experienced providers*, Dallas, Tex, 2003, American Heart Association.

Mattox KL, Estera AL, Wall MJ: Traumatic heart disease. In Braunwald E, Zipes DP, Libby P, editors: *Heart disease: a textbook of cardiovascular medicine*, ed 6, Philadelphia, 2001, Saunders, pp 1877-1907.

Murphy JG, Nobrega TP: Cardiac trauma. In Murphy JG, editor: *Mayo Clinic cardiology review*, ed 2, Philadelphia, 2000, Lippincott Williams & Wilkins, pp 1129-1138.

Myers ML, Cheung A, Sibbald WJ: Trauma. In Crawford MH, DiMarco JP, Paulus WJ, editors: *Cardiology*, ed 2, Philadelphia, 2004, Mosby, pp 1577-1582.

Poh KK, Tan HC, Chia BL, et al: A case of broken heart from blunt trauma, *Singapore Med J* 43(8): 423-425, 2002.

Symbas PN: Traumatic heart disease. In Fuster V, Alexander RW, O'Rourke RA, editors: *Hurst's the heart*, ed 10, New York, 2001, McGraw-Hill, pp 2219-2226.

Website

www.surgical-tutor.org.uk/core/trauma/chest_trauma.htm

Cardiac Rhythm Disorders

Symptomatic Bradycardia

Crawford MH, DiMarco JP, Paulus WJ, editors: *Cardiology*, ed 2, Philadelphia, 2004, Mosby.

Cummins RO: *ACLS—the reference book. ACLS: principles and practice*, Dallas, Tex, 2003, American Heart Association.

Gregoratos G, Epstein AE, Hayes DL, et al: ACC/AHA/NASPE 2002 guidelines update for implantation of cardiac pacemakers and antiarrhythmia devices: summary article: a report of the American College of Cardiology/American Heart Association Task Force on Practice guidelines (ACC/AHA/NASPE Committee to Update the 1998 Pacemaker Guidelines), *Circulation* 106:2145-2161, 2002.

Hayes DL, Zipes DP: Cardiac pacemakers and cardioverter-defibrillators. In Braunwald E, Zipes DP, Libby P, editors: *Heart disease: a textbook of cardiovascular medicine*, ed 6, Philadelphia, 2001, Saunders, pp 775-814.

Huszar RJ: *Basic dysrhythmias: interpretation and management*, ed 3, Philadelphia, 2001, Mosby.

Lynn-McHale DJ, Carlson KK, editors: *AACN procedure manual for critical care*, ed 4, Philadelphia, 2001, Saunders.

Moss AJ, Cannom DS, Daubert JP, et al: Multicenter Automatic Defibrillator Implantation Trial II (MADIT II): design and clinical protocol, *Ann Noninvasive Electrocardiol* 4:83-91, 1999.

Murphy JG, editor: *Mayo Clinic cardiology review*, ed 2, Philadelphia, 2000, Lippincott Williams & Wilkins.

Symptomatic Tachycardia

Blomstrom-Lundqvist C, Aliot EA, Calkins H: ACC/AHA/ESC guidelines for the management of patients with supraventricular arrhythmias: executive summary: a report of the American College of Cardiology/American Heart Association Task Force on Practice Guidelines and the European Society of Cardiology Committee for Practice Guidelines (Writing Committee to Develop Guidelines for the Management of Patients with Supraventricular Arrhythmias), *J Am Coll Cardiol* 42(8):1493-1531, 2002.

Braunwald E, Zipes DP, Libby P, editors: *Heart disease: a textbook of cardiovascular medicine*, ed 6, Philadelphia, Saunders, 2001.

Crawford MH, DiMarco JP, Paulus WJ, editors: *Cardiology*, ed 2, Philadelphia, 2004, Mosby.

Cummins RO: *ACLS—the reference book. ACLS: principles and practice*, Dallas, Tex, 2003, American Heart Association.

Deaton C, Dunbar SB, Moloney M, et al: Patient experiences with atrial fibrillation and treatment with implantable atrial defibrillation therapy, *Heart Lung* 32(5):291-299, 2003.

Fuster V, Rydén LE, Asinger RW, et al: ACC/AHA/ESC guidelines for the management of patients with atrial fibrillation: executive summary: a report of the American College of Cardiology/American Heart Association Task Force on Practice Guidelines and the European Society of Cardiology Committee for Practice Guidelines and Policy Conferences (Committee to Develop Guidelines for the Management of Patients with Atrial Fibrillation), *J Am Coll Cardiol* 38(4): 1231-1266, 2001. Full text available at http://www.acc.org/clinical/guidelines/atrial_fib/af_index.htm.

Gregoratos G, Epstein AE, Hayes DL, et al: ACC/AHA/NASPE 2002 guidelines update for implantation of cardiac pacemakers and antiarrhythmia devices: summary article: a report of the American College of Cardiology/American Heart Association Task Force on Practice Guidelines (ACC/AHA/NASPE Committee to Update the 1998 Pacemaker Guidelines), *Circulation* 106:2145-2161, 2002. Full text available at http://www.acc.org/clinical/guidelines/pacemaker/incorporated/index.htm.

Hayes DL, Zipes DP: Cardiac pacemakers and cardioverter-defibrillators. In Braunwald E, Zipes DP, Libby P, editors: *Heart disease: a textbook of cardiovascular medicine*, ed 6, Philadelphia, 2001, Saunders, pp 775-814.

Lynn-McHale DJ, Carlson KK, editors: *AACN procedure manual for critical care*, ed 4, Philadelphia, 2001, Saunders.

Murphy JG, editor: *Mayo Clinic cardiology review*, ed 2, Philadelphia, 2000, Lippincott Williams & Wilkins.

Singer DE, Go AS: Antithrombotic therapy in atrial fibrillation, *Clin Geriatr Med* 17(1): 131-147, 2001.

Absent or Ineffective Pulse

Crawford MH, DiMarco JP, Paulus WJ, editors: *Cardiology*, ed 2, Philadelphia, 2004, Mosby.

Cummins RO: *ACLS—the reference book. ACLS: principles and practice*, Dallas, Tex, 2003, American Heart Association.

Gregoratos G, Epstein AE, Hayes DL, et al: ACC/AHA/NASPE 2002 guidelines update for implantation of cardiac pace-makers and antiarrhythmia devices: summary article: a report of the American College of Cardiology/American Heart Association Task Force on Practice Guidelines (ACC/AHA/NASPE Committee to Update the 1998 Pacemaker Guidelines), *Circulation* 106:2145-2161, 2002.

Murphy JG, editor: *Mayo Clinic cardiology review*, ed 2, Philadelphia, 2000, Lippincott Williams & Wilkins.

Myerburg RJ, Castellanos A: Cardiac arrest and sudden cardiac death. In Braunwald E, Zipes DP, Libby P, editors: *Heart disease: a textbook of cardiovascular medicine*, ed 6, Philadelphia, 2001, Saunders, pp 890-931.

Mitral Regurgitation

Bonow RO, Carabello B, de Leon AC, et al: ACC/AHA guidelines for the management of patients with valvular heart disease: report of the American College of Cardiology/American Heart Association Task Force on Practice Guidelines (Committee on Management of Patients with Valvular Heart Disease), *J Am Coll Cardiol* 32:1486-1588, 1998.

Braunwald E: Valvular heart disease. In Braunwald E, Zipes DP, Libby P, editors: *Heart disease: a textbook of cardiovascular medicine*, ed 6, Philadelphia, 2001, Saunders, pp 1643-1722.

Carabello BA: The timing of valve surgery. In Antman EM, editor: *Cardiovascular therapeutics: a companion to Braunwald's heart disease*, Philadelphia, 2002, Saunders, pp 975-993.

Carabello BA: Mitral regurgitation. In Crawford MH, DiMarco JP, Paulus WJ, editors: *Cardiology*, ed 2, Philadelphia, 2004, Mosby, pp 1083-1094.

Enriquez-Sarano M, Schaff HV, Frye RL: Mitral regurgitation: what causes the leakage is fundamental to the outcome of valve repair, *Circulation* 108:253-256, 2003.

Karon BL, Enriquez-Sarano M: Valvular regurgitation. In Murphy JG, editor: *Mayo Clinic cardiology review*, ed 2, Philadelphia, 2000, Lippincott Williams & Wilkins, pp 303-335.

Rahimtoola SH, Enriquez-Sarano M, Schaff HV, et al: Mitral valve disease. In Fuster V, Alexander RW, O'Rourke RA, editors: *Hurst's the heart*, ed 10, New York, 2001, McGraw-Hill, pp 1697-1727.

Mitral Stenosis

Bonow RO, Carabello B, de Leon AC, et al: ACC/AHA guidelines for the management of patients with valvular heart disease: a report of the American College of Cardiology/American Heart Association Task Force on Practice Guidelines (Committee on Management of Patients with Valvular Heart Disease), *J Am Coll Cardiol* 32(5):1486-1588, 1998.

Braunwald E: Valvular heart disease. In Braunwald E, Zipes DP, Libby P, editors: *Heart disease: a textbook of cardiovascular medicine,* ed 6, Philadelphia, 2001, Saunders, pp 1643-1722.

Carabello BA: The timing of valve surgery. In Antman EM, editor: *Cardiovascular therapeutics: a companion to Braunwald's heart disease,* Philadelphia, 2002, Saunders, pp 975-993.

Cardoso LF, Grinberg M, Rati MA, et al: Comparison between percutaneous balloon valvuloplasty and open commissurotomy for mitral stenosis: a prospective and randomized study, *Cardiology* 98(4):186-190, 2002.

Carroll JD, Sutherland JP: Mitral stenosis. In Crawford MH, DiMarco JP, Paulus WJ, editors: *Cardiology,* ed 2, Philadelphia, 2004, Mosby, pp 1071-1081.

Nishimura RA: Valvular stenosis. In Murphy JG, editor: *Mayo Clinic cardiology review,* ed 2, Philadelphia, 2000, Lippincott Williams & Wilkins, pp 285-301.

Rahimtoola SH, Durairaj A, Mehra A, Nuno I: Current evaluation and management of patients with mitral stenosis, *Circulation* 106(10):1183-1188, 2002.

Rahimtoola SH, Enriquez-Sarano M, Schaff HV, et al: Mitral valve disease. In Fuster V, Alexander RW, O'Rourke RA, editors: *Hurst's the heart,* ed 10, New York, 2001, McGraw-Hill, pp 1697-1727.

Aortic Regurgitation

Aurigemma GP, Meyer TE: Acute aortic regurgitation. In Crawford MH, DiMarco JP, Paulus WJ, editors: *Cardiology,* ed 2, Philadelphia, 2004, Mosby, pp 1131-1135.

Bonow RO, Carabello B, de Leon AC, et al: ACC/AHA guidelines for the management of patients with valvular heart disease: a report of the American College of Cardiology/American Heart Association Task Force on Practice Guidelines (Committee on Management of Patients with Valvular Heart Disease), *J Am Coll Cardiol* 32:1486-1588, 1998.

Braunwald E: Valvular heart disease. In Braunwald E, Zipes DP, Libby P, editors: *Heart disease: a textbook of cardiovascular medicine,* ed 6, Philadelphia, 2001, Saunders, pp 1643-1722.

Carabello BA: The timing of valve surgery. In Antman EM, editor: *Cardiovascular therapeutics: a companion to Braunwald's heart disease,* Philadelphia, 2002, Saunders, pp 975-993.

Karon BL, Enriquez-Sarano M: Valvular regurgitation. In Murphy JG, editor: *Mayo Clinic cardiology review,* ed 2, Philadelphia, 2000, Lippincott Williams & Wilkins, pp 303-335.

Rahimtoola SH: Aortic valve disease. In Fuster V, Alexander RW, O'Rourke RA, editors: *Hurst's the heart,* ed 10, New York, 2001, McGraw-Hill, pp 1667-1695.

Aortic Stenosis

Bonow RO, Carabello B, de Leon AC, et al: ACC/AHA guidelines for the management of patients with valvular heart disease: a report of the American College of Cardiology/American Heart Association Task Force on Practice Guidelines (Committee on Management of Patients with Valvular Heart Disease), *J Am Coll Cardiol* 32:1486-1588, 1998.

Braunwald E: Valvular heart disease. In Braunwald E, Zipes DP, Libby P, editors: *Heart disease: a textbook of cardiovascular medicine,* ed 6, Philadelphia, 2001, Saunders, pp 1643-1722.

Carabello BA: The timing of valve surgery. In Antman EM, editor: *Cardiovascular therapeutics: a companion to Braunwald's heart disease,* Philadelphia, 2002, Saunders, pp 975-993.

Nishimura RA: Valvular stenosis. In Murphy JG, editor: *Mayo Clinic cardiology review,* ed 2, Philadelphia, 2000, Lippincott Williams & Wilkins, pp 285-301.

Rahimtoola SH: Aortic valve disease. In Fuster V, Alexander RW, O'Rourke RA, editors: *Hurst's the heart,* ed 10, New York, 2001, McGraw-Hill, pp 1667-1695.

Shavelle DM, Otto CM: Aortic stenosis. In Crawford MH, DiMarco JP, Paulus WJ, editors: *Cardiology,* ed 2, Philadelphia, 2004, Mosby, pp 1121-1129.

Atrial Septal Defect

Freed MD: The pathology, pathophysiology, recognition, and treatment of congenital heart disease. In Fuster V, Alexander RW, O'Rourke RA, editors: *Hurst's the heart,* ed 10, New York, 2001, McGraw-Hill, pp 1837-1938.

Gersony WM, Rosenbaum MS: *Congenital heart disease in the adult*, New York, 2002, McGraw-Hill.

Ishii M: Atrial septal defect. In Crawford MH, DiMarco JP, Paulus WJ, editors: *Cardiology*, ed 2, Philadelphia, 2004, Mosby, pp 1261-1270.

Mullen MP, Landzberg MJ: Care for adults with congenital heart disease. In Antman EM, editor: *Cardiovascular therapeutics: a companion to Braunwald's heart disease*, Philadelphia, 2002, Saunders, pp 1048-1074.

Warnes CA: Adult congenital heart disease. In Murphy JG, editor: *Mayo Clinic cardiology review*, ed 2, Philadelphia, 2000, Lippincott Williams & Wilkins, pp 1049-1066.

Website

www.med.umn.edu/radiology/cvrad/chd/asd.html

Ventricular Septal Defect

Freed MD: The pathology, pathophysiology, recognition, and treatment of congenital heart disease. In Fuster V, Alexander RW, O'Rourke RA, editors: *Hurst's the heart*, ed 10, New York, 2001, McGraw-Hill, pp 1837-1938.

Gersony WM, Rosenbaum MS: *Congenital heart disease in the adult*, New York, 2002, McGraw-Hill.

Krabill KA: Ventricular septal defect. In Crawford MH, DiMarco JP, Paulus WJ, editors: *Cardiology*, ed 2, Philadelphia, 2004, Mosby, pp 1279-1287.

Mullen MP, Landzberg MJ: Care for adults with congenital heart disease. In Antman EM, editor: *Cardiovascular therapeutics: a companion to Braunwald's heart disease*, Philadelphia, 2002, Saunders, pp 1048-1074.

Warnes CA: Adult congenital heart disease. In Murphy JG, editor: *Mayo Clinic cardiology review*, ed 2, Philadelphia, 2000, Lippincott Williams & Wilkins, pp 1049-1066.

Website

www.med.umn.edu/radiology/cvrad/chd/vsd.html

Patent Ductus Arteriosus

Freed MD: The pathology, pathophysiology, recognition, and treatment of congenital heart disease. In Fuster V, Alexander RW, O'Rourke RA, editors: *Hurst's the heart*, ed 10, New York, 2001, McGraw-Hill, pp 1837-1938.

Gersony WM, Rosenbaum MS: *Congenital heart disease in the adult*, New York, 2002, McGraw-Hill.

Mullen MP, Landzberg MJ: Care for adults with congenital heart disease. In Antman EM, editor: *Cardiovascular therapeutics: a companion to Braunwald's heart disease*, Philadelphia, 2002, Saunders, pp 1048-1074.

Redel DA: Patent ductus arteriosus. In Crawford MH, DiMarco JP, Paulus WJ, editors: *Cardiology*, ed 2, Philadelphia, 2004, Mosby, pp 1383-1390.

Warnes CA: Adult congenital heart disease. In Murphy JG, editor: *Mayo Clinic cardiology review*, ed 2, Philadelphia, 2000, Lippincott Williams & Wilkins, pp 1049-1066.

Website

www.med.umn.edu/radiology/cvrad/chd/pda.html

Coarctation of the Aorta

Freed MD: The pathology, pathophysiology, recognition, and treatment of congenital heart disease. In Fuster V, Alexander RW, O'Rourke RA, editors: *Hurst's the heart*, ed 10, New York, 2001, McGraw-Hill, pp 1837-1938.

Gersony WM, Rosenbaum MS: *Congenital heart disease in the adult*, New York, 2002, McGraw-Hill.

Mullen MP, Landzberg MJ: Care for adults with congenital heart disease. In Antman EM, editor: *Cardiovascular therapeutics: a companion to Braunwald's heart disease*, Philadelphia, 2002, Saunders, pp 1048-1074.

Ohkubo M, Ino T: Coarctation of the aorta. In Crawford MH, DiMarco JP, Paulus WJ, editors: *Cardiology*, ed 2, Philadelphia, 2004, Mosby, pp 1391-1396.

Warnes CA: Adult congenital heart disease. In Murphy JG, editor: *Mayo Clinic cardiology review*, ed 2, Philadelphia, 2000, Lippincott Williams & Wilkins, pp 1049-1066.

Hypertensive Crisis

Alper AB, Calhoun DA: Hypertensive emergencies. In Antman EM, editor: *Cardiovascular therapeutics: a companion to Braunwald's heart disease*, Philadelphia, 2002, Saunders, pp 817-831.

Beevers DG, Lip GY: Hypertensive crises. In Crawford MH, DiMarco JP, Paulus WJ, editors: *Cardiology*, ed 2, Philadelphia, 2004, Mosby, pp 545-552.

Black HR, Bakris GL, Elliott WJ: Hypertension: epidemiology, pathophysiology, diagnosis, and treatment. In Fuster V, Alexander RW, O'Rourke RA, editors: *Hurst's the heart*, ed 10, New York, 2001, McGraw-Hill, pp 1553-1604.

Chobanian AV, Bakris GL, Black HR, et al: Seventh report of the Joint National Committee on Prevention, Detection, Evaluation, and Treatment of High Blood Pressure, *Hypertension* 42:1206-1252, 2003.

Goldman L, Ausiello D: *Cecil textbook of medicine*, ed 22, Philadelphia, 2004, Saunders.

Hogan MJ: Hypertension. In Murphy JG, editor: *Mayo Clinic cardiology review*, ed 2, Philadelphia, 2000, Lippincott Williams & Wilkins, pp 1067-1082.

Vaughan CJ, Delanty N: Hypertensive emergencies, *Lancet* 356:411-417, 2000.

Weber MA: *Hypertension medicine*, Totowa, NJ, 2001, Humana Press, pp 429-435.

Websites

American Heart Association Council for High Blood Pressure Research: http://www.americanheart.org/presenter.jhtml?identifier=1115.

American Society of Hypertension: http://www.ash-us.org/.

Aortic and Peripheral Arterial Disease

Braunwald E, Zipes DP, Libby P, editors: *Heart disease: a textbook of cardiovascular medicine*, ed 6, Philadelphia, 2001, Saunders.

Crawford PA, editor: *The Washington manual cardiology subspeciality consult*, Philadelphia, 2004, Lippincott Williams & Wilkins.

Erbel R, Alfonso F, Boileau C, et al: Diagnosis and management of aortic dissection, *Eur Heart J* 22:1642-1681, 2001.

Fagrell B: Arterial disease of the limbs. In Crawford MH, DiMarco JP, Paulus WJ, editors: *Cardiology*, ed 2, Philadelphia, 2004, Mosby, pp 109-122.

Fahey VA: *Vascular nursing*, ed 3, Philadelphia, 1999, Saunders.

Garmany R: Diseases of the aorta. In Crawford PA, editor: *The Washington manual cardiology subspecialty consult*, Philadelphia, 2004, Lippincott Williams & Wilkins, pp 235-242.

Goldman L, Ausiello D: *Cecil textbook of medicine*, ed 22, Philadelphia, 2004, Saunders.

Halperin JL, Fuster V: Meeting the challenge of peripheral arterial disease, *Arch Intern Med* 28:877-878, 2003.

Hirsch AT, Criqui MH, Treat-Jacobson D, et al: Peripheral arterial disease detection, awareness, and treatment in primary care, *JAMA* 281(11):1317-1324, 2001.

McPhail IR, Spittel PC, Weston SA, et al: Intermittent claudication: an objective office-based assessment, *J Am Coll Cardiol* 37:1381-1385, 2001.

Mehta R, O'Gara P, Bossone E, et al: Acute type A aortic dissection in the elderly: clinical characteristics, management, and outcomes in the current era, *J Am Coll Cardiol* 40:685-692, 2002.

Wernly JA: Thoracic aorta disease. In Crawford MH, DiMarco JP, Paulus WJ, editors: *Cardiology*, ed 2, Philadelphia, 2004, Mosby, pp 141-152.

Shock

Alexander RW, Pratt CM, Ryan TJ, et al: Diagnosis and management of patients with acute myocardial infarction. In Fuster V, Alexander RW, O'Rourke RA, editors: *Hurst's the heart*, ed 10, New York, 2001, McGraw-Hill, pp 1275-1359.

Braunwald E, Zipes DP, Libby P, editors: *Heart disease: a textbook of cardiovascular medicine*, ed 6, Philadelphia, 2001, Saunders.

Crawford MH, DiMarco JP, Paulus WJ, editors: *Cardiology*, ed 2, Philadelphia, 2004, Mosby.

Darovic GO: *Hemodynamic monitoring: invasive and noninvasive clinical application*, ed 3, Philadelphia, 2002, Saunders.

Goldman L, Ausiello D: *Cecil textbook of medicine*, ed 22, Philadelphia, 2004, Saunders.

Hochman JS, Califf RM: Acute myocardial infarction. In Antman EM, editor: *Cardiovascular therapeutics: a companion to Braunwald's heart disease*, Philadelphia, 2002, Saunders, pp 233-291.

Hoekstra JW, editor: *Handbook of cardiovascular emergencies*, ed 2, Philadelphia, 2001, Lippincott Williams & Wilkins.

Murphy JG, editor: *Mayo Clinic cardiology review*, ed 2, Philadelphia, 2000, Lippincott Williams & Wilkins.

The Neurologic System

KAREN A. MCQUILLAN, RN, MS, CCRN, CNRN
JAN MARIE BELDEN, MSN, APRN, BC, FNP (Contributor for content related to pain)

SYSTEMWIDE ELEMENTS

Physiologic Anatomy

1. **Brain**
   a. Coverings
      i. Scalp
         (a) Dermal layer: Skin
         (b) Subcutaneous fascia: Fibrous fatty layer between the skin and galea that contains blood vessels
         (c) Galea aponeurotica: Freely movable, tendinous tissue; covers the vertex of the skull; absorbs the force of external trauma
         (d) Subaponeurotic or subgaleal space: Contains the diploic and emissary veins
         (e) Periosteum: Thin layer of tissue that covers the skull
      ii. Cranium
         (a) Part of the skull that houses and protects the brain (Figure 4-1)
         (b) Bones: Frontal, sphenoid, ethmoid, occipital, two temporal and two parietal bones
         (c) Basilar skull: Base of the skull has three depressions—the anterior, middle, and posterior fossae (Figure 4-2)
      iii. Meninges (Figure 4-3)
         (a) Dura mater
            (1) Outermost covering of the brain; consists of two layers of tough fibrous tissue
            (2) Outer layer forms the periosteum of the bone
            (3) Inner layer folds to form the falx cerebri, tentorium cerebelli, falx cerebelli, and diaphragma sella
            (4) Meningeal arteries and venous sinuses lie in clefts formed by the inner and outer layers of the dura mater
            (5) Subdural space: Lies between the inner dura mater and the arachnoid mater
         (b) Arachnoid mater
            (1) Fine, fibrous, elastic layer between the dura mater and pia mater
            (2) Subarachnoid space
               a) Lies between the arachnoid mater and pia mater; expanded areas of this space form cisterns at the base of the brain

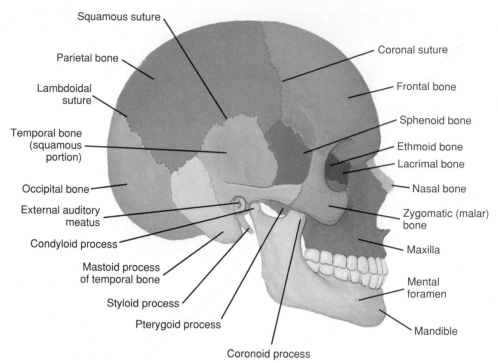

FIGURE 4-1 ■ The skull as seen from the side. (From Slazinski T, Littlejohns LR: Anatomy of the nervous system. In Bader MK, Littlejohns LR, editors: *AANN core curriculum for neuroscience nursing*, ed 4, St Louis, 2004, Saunders, p 31; modified from Thibodeau GA, Patton K: *Anatomy and physiology*, ed 5, St Louis, 2003, Mosby.)

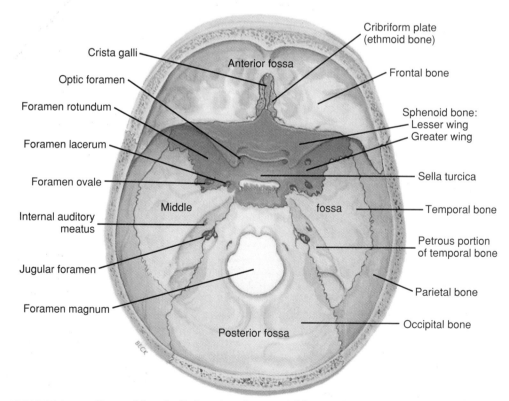

FIGURE 4-2 ■ Base of the skull showing the cranial fossae. (From Slazinski T, Littlejohns LR: Anatomy of the nervous system. In Bader MK, Littlejohns LR, editors: *AANN core curriculum for neuroscience nursing*, ed 4, St Louis, 2004, Saunders, p 32; modified from Thibodeau GA, Patton K: *Anatomy and physiology*, ed 5, St Louis, 2003, Mosby.)

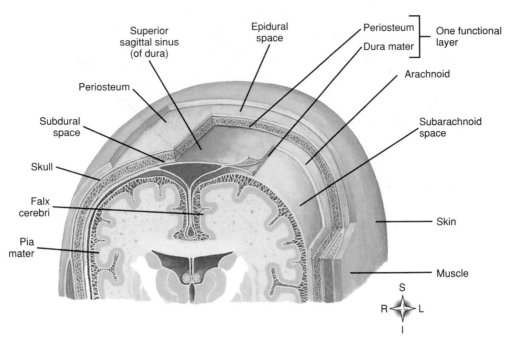

FIGURE 4-3 ■ Coverings of the brain. *I*, Inferior; *L*, left; *R*, right; *S*, superior. (From Thibodeau GA, Patton K: *Anatomy and physiology*, ed 5, St Louis, 2003, Mosby, p 376.)

      b) Contains blood vessels, including the circle of Willis
      c) Contains cerebrospinal fluid (CSF), which completely surrounds the brain and spinal cord; acts as a shock absorber
      d) Contains the arachnoid villi: Projections of the arachnoid mater that absorb CSF into the venous system
  (c) Pia mater
    (1) Delicate vascular layer that covers the brain surface, following the sulci and gyri
    (2) Surrounds surface blood vessels and emerging nerves
    (3) Blood vessels of the pia mater form the choroid plexus
b. Divisions of the brain
  i. Cerebrum
    (a) Telencephalon: Two cerebral hemispheres separated by a longitudinal fissure; joined by the corpus callosum
      (1) Functional localization in the cerebral cortex, including *cerebral dominance* (Table 4-1)
      (2) Corpus callosum: Commissural fibers that transfer learned discriminations, sensory experiences, and memory from one cerebral hemisphere to corresponding parts of the other
      (3) Basal ganglia (basal nuclei) (Figure 4-4)
        a) Masses of gray matter; includes the caudate, putamen, globus pallidus, claustrum, amygdaloid, and, functionally, the subthalamic and substantia nigra nuclei
        b) Functions: Exert regulating and controlling influences on the coordination of voluntary motion, motor integration, movement initiation, muscle tone, and postural reflexes. A major center of the extrapyramidal motor system.

■ **TABLE 4-1**
■ ■ **Functional Localization in the Cerebral Cortex**

Lobe	Functions
Frontal	Higher mental functions
	Concentration
	Abstract thinking
	Foresight and judgment
	Behavior and tactfulness
	Inhibition
	Memory
	Personality
	Affect
	Conjugate eye movements
	Voluntary motor function
	Motor control of speech (dominant hemisphere*)
Temporal	Hearing
	Comprehension of spoken language (dominant hemisphere*)
	Visual, olfactory, and auditory perception
	Memory
	Learning and intellect
	Emotion
Parietal	Sensory perception of touch, pain, temperature, position, pressure, and vibration
	Body awareness
	Sensory interpretation
Occipital	Visual perception and interpretation
	Control of some visual and ocular movement reflexes

*Cerebral dominance: In right-handed and most left-handed people, the left cerebral hemisphere is dominant for language, mathematical, and analytic functions. The opposite nondominant hemisphere is thought to be concerned with nonverbal, geometric, spatial, visual, and musical functions.

    (b) Diencephalon (Figure 4-5)
        (1) Thalamus: Two egg-shaped masses of gray matter that abut the lateral walls of the third ventricle; subdivided into several nuclei
           a) Certain nuclei receive, integrate, and process sensory input for relay to the cerebral cortex
           b) Other nuclei participate in affective aspects of brain function; are functionally related to the association areas of the cortex; or have a role in conscious pain, temperature, and touch awareness, motor function, and the ascending reticular activating system
        (2) Hypothalamus: Below the thalamus; regulates
           a) Body temperature
           b) Food and water intake
           c) Behavior: Part of the limbic system; concerned with aggressive and sexual behavior; elicits physical expressions associated with emotions; may be involved with sleep-wake cycles and circadian rhythm control
           d) Autonomic responses: Control center for the autonomic nervous system (ANS); controls numerous visceral and somatic activities (e.g., heart rate, pupil constriction and dilation)

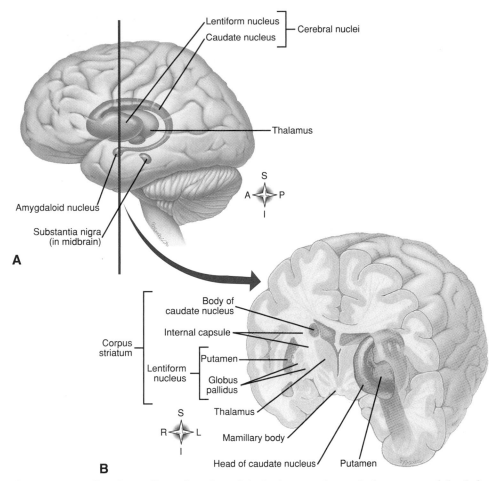

FIGURE 4-4 ■ Basal ganglia or basal nuclei. **A,** As seen through the cortex of the left cerebral hemisphere. **B,** As seen in a frontal (coronal) section of the brain. *A,* Anterior; *I,* inferior; *L,* left; *P,* posterior; *R,* right; *S,* superior. (From Thibodeau GA, Patton K: *Anatomy and physiology,* ed 5, St Louis, 2003, Mosby, p 392.)

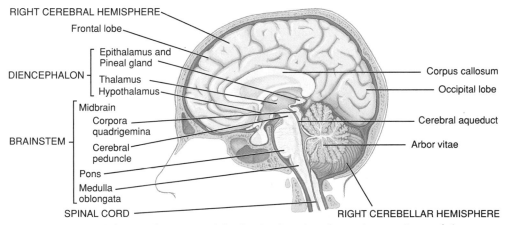

FIGURE 4-5 ■ Midsagittal section of the brain showing the major portions of the diencephalon, brainstem, and cerebellum. (From Applegate EJ: *The anatomy and physiology learning systems textbook,* ed 2, Philadelphia, 2000, Saunders, p 167.)

e) Hormonal secretion of the pituitary gland (see Chapter 6)
  1) Posterior pituitary gland (neurohypophysis): Stores and releases antidiuretic hormone (ADH) and oxytocin, produced by the hypothalamus. ADH causes vasoconstriction and increases renal water reabsorption. Oxytocin stimulates uterine contraction and milk ejection.
  2) Anterior pituitary gland (adenohypophysis): Secretes prolactin and growth-stimulating, thyroid-stimulating, adrenal-stimulating, follicle-stimulating, and luteinizing hormones; hormonal secretion is under the control of pituitary releasing and inhibiting factors produced in the hypothalamus and transported to the anterior pituitary via a pituitary portal system (see Chapter 6)
(3) Subthalamus: Functionally related to the basal ganglia
(4) Epithalamus: Dorsal part of the diencephalon
  a) Contains the pineal gland
  b) Thought to regulate circadian rhythms and the food-getting reflex; probable role in growth and development
(c) Limbic system (Figure 4-6)
  (1) Composed of the limbic lobe (cingulate and parahippocampal gyri) plus structures to which it is anatomically and functionally connected such as the amygdala, hippocampus, fornix, hypothalamus, olfactory tract, and thalamus
  (2) Responsible for emotional behavioral responses and accompanying visceral, endocrine, and somatic responses; has a role in basic instinctual drives (e.g., mating, hunger, motivation) and in some aspects of memory and learning
ii. Brainstem (Figure 4-7; also see Figure 4-5)
  (a) Midbrain (mesencephalon): Located between the diencephalon and pons

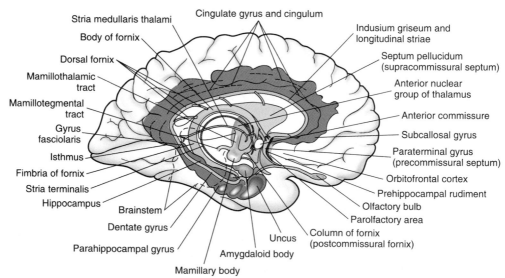

FIGURE 4-6 ■ Anatomy of the limbic system illustrated by the shaded areas of the figure. (From Slazinski T, Littlejohns LR: Anatomy of the nervous system. In Bader MK, Littlejohns LR, editors: *AANN core curriculum for neuroscience nursing*, ed 4, St Louis, 2004, Saunders, p 41.)

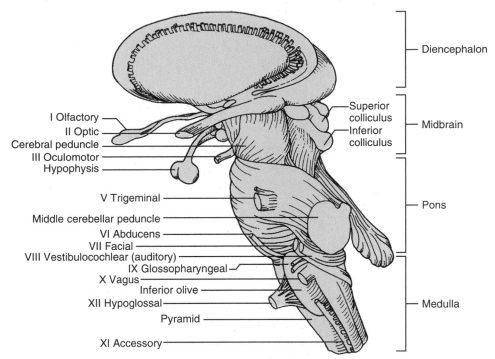

I Olfactory
II Optic
Cerebral peduncle
III Oculomotor
Hypophysis

Superior colliculus
Inferior colliculus

Diencephalon

Midbrain

V Trigeminal
Middle cerebellar peduncle
VI Abducens
VII Facial
VIII Vestibulocochlear (auditory)
IX Glossopharyngeal
X Vagus
Inferior olive
XII Hypoglossal
Pyramid

XI Accessory

Pons

Medulla

FIGURE 4-7 ■ Lateral view of the brainstem showing the main subdivisions, surface landmarks, and cranial nerves. (From Barker E: *Neuroscience nursing: a spectrum of care*, ed 2, St Louis, 2002, Mosby, p 23.)

    (1) Contains nuclei of cranial nerve (CN) III (oculomotor) and CN IV (trochlear) and some CN V (trigeminal) nuclei
    (2) Contains motor and sensory pathways
    (3) Holds respiratory control centers
    (4) Tectal region (inferior and superior colliculi): Concerned with the auditory and visual systems
    (5) Connects to the cerebellum via the superior cerebellar peduncles
  (b) Pons (metencephalon): Between the midbrain and medulla
    (1) Contains nuclei of CN V, VI (abducens), and VII (facial), and some CN VIII (acoustic) nuclei
    (2) Middle cerebellar peduncles on its basal surface provide extensive connections between the cerebral cortex and cerebellum, ensuring maximal motor efficiency
    (3) Contains motor and sensory pathways
    (4) Holds respiratory control centers that help coordinate breathing patterns
  (c) Medulla (myelencephalon): Between the pons and spinal cord
    (1) Contains nuclei of CN IX (glossopharyngeal), X (vagus), XI (spinal accessory), and XII (hypoglossal) and some nuclei from CN V, VII, and VIII.
    (2) Motor and sensory tracts of spinal cord continue into the medulla
    (3) Attaches to the cerebellum via inferior the cerebellar peduncles
    (4) Holds respiratory, cardiac, and vasomotor control centers
  (d) Reticular formation (RF) (Figure 4-8): Diffuse cellular network in the brainstem, with axons projecting to the thalamus and into the cortex;

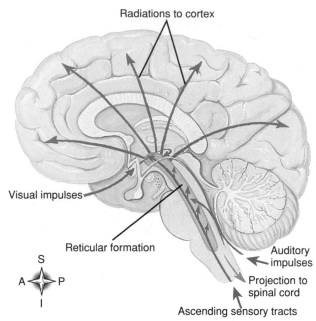

FIGURE 4-8 ▪ Reticular activating system. Consists of centers in the brainstem reticular formation plus fibers that conduct to the centers from below and fibers that conduct from the centers to widespread areas of the cerebral cortex. Functioning of the reticular activating system is essential for consciousness. *A*, Anterior; *I*, inferior; *P*, posterior; *S*, superior. (From Thibodeau GA, Patton K: *Anatomy and physiology*, ed 5, St Louis, 2003, Mosby, p 395.)

receives input from the cerebrum, spinal cord, other brainstem nuclei, and the cerebellum; has a role in the control of autonomic and endocrine functions, skeletal muscle activity, and visceral and somatic sensation. The reticular activating system is part of the RF.

(1) *Ascending* reticular activating system is essential for arousal from sleep, alert wakefulness, focusing of attention, and perceptual association

(2) *Descending* reticular activating system may inhibit or facilitate motor neurons controlling the skeletal musculature

iii. Cerebellum: Lies in the posterior fossa behind the brainstem; separated from the cerebrum by the tentorium cerebelli

(a) Influences muscle tone in relation to equilibrium, locomotion, posture, and nonstereotyped movements

(b) Important in the synchronization of muscle action to enable coordinated movement

(c) Input is from the spinal cord, brainstem, vestibular system, and cerebral centers; output to the brainstem and thalamus influences spinal and cerebral activities

c. Cerebral circulation (Figure 4-9)

i. Arterial system: Supplied by the internal carotid and vertebral arteries

(a) Circle of Willis: Anastomosis of arteries at the base of the brain formed by a short segment of the internal carotid and anterior and posterior cerebral arteries, which are connected by an anterior communicating

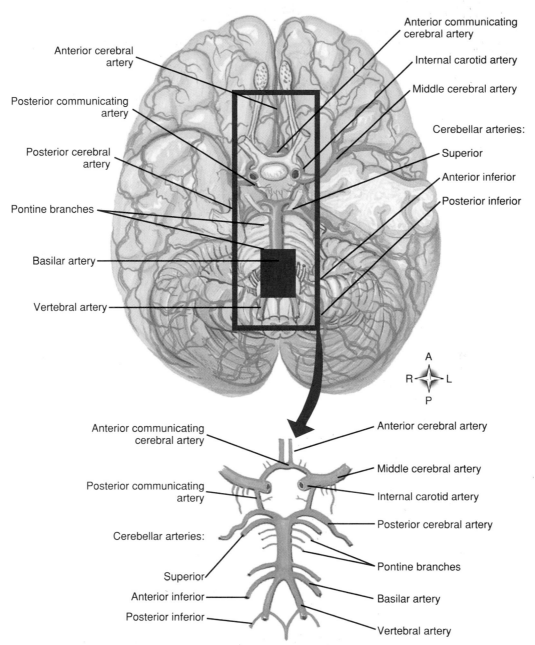

FIGURE 4-9 ■ Arteries at the base of the brain. The arteries that compose the circle of Willis are the two anterior cerebral arteries joined to each other by the anterior communicating cerebral artery and to the posterior cerebral arteries by the posterior communicating arteries. *A*, Anterior; *L*, left, *R*, right, *P*, posterior. (From Thibodeau GA, Patton K: *Anatomy and physiology*, ed 5, St Louis, 2003, Mosby, p 573.)

artery and two posterior communicating arteries. This anastomosis may permit collateral circulation if a carotid or vertebral artery becomes occluded.

(b) Internal carotid system: Internal carotid arteries arise from the common carotid arteries. Table 4-2 shows the branches of this system and the areas they supply.

■ **TABLE 4-2**
■ ■ **Major Cerebral Arteries and Areas They Supply**

Artery	Area of the Brain Supplied
INTERNAL CAROTID ARTERY BRANCHES	
Anterior cerebral artery (ACA)	Medial aspect of the frontal and parietal lobes; part of the cingulate gyrus and corpus callosum; via the recurrent artery of Heubner supplies part of the basal ganglia and a portion of the internal capsule
Anterior communicating artery (Acom)	Connects the right and left anterior cerebral arteries
Middle cerebral artery (MCA) (largest branch of the internal carotid artery)	Most of the lateral surfaces of the frontal, temporal, and parietal lobes; via the lenticulostriate artery, supplies the majority of the basal ganglia and internal capsule
Posterior communicating artery (Pcom)	Connects the posterior cerebral artery with the internal carotid artery; connects the carotid with the vertebrobasilar circulation
VERTEBRAL ARTERY BRANCHES	
Anterior spinal artery	Anterior one half to three quarters of the spinal cord
Posterior inferior cerebellar artery (PICA)	Undersurface of the cerebellum; choroid plexus of the fourth ventricle; medulla
BASILAR ARTERY BRANCHES	
Posterior cerebral artery (PCA)	Occipital lobes and the inferior and medial portion of the temporal lobes; thalamus and part of the hypothalamus; choroid plexuses of the lateral and third ventricles; midbrain
Superior cerebellar artery (SCA)	Upper surface of the cerebellum; midbrain
Anterior inferior cerebellar artery (AICA)	Inferior surface of the cerebellum; portion of the pons

(c) Vertebral system: Vertebral arteries arise from the subclavian arteries and join at the lower pontine border to form the basilar artery. Branches of this system and the areas they supply are summarized in Table 4-2.

(d) Branches of the internal carotid, external carotid, and vertebral arteries (e.g., anterior, middle, posterior meningeal arteries) provide blood supply to the meninges

ii. Cerebral blood flow (CBF)

(a) Normal CBF averages 50 ml/100 g of brain tissue per minute

(b) Cerebral perfusion pressure (CPP) and intrinsic regulatory mechanisms affect CBF

(1) CPP: Pressure gradient that drives blood into the brain; calculated as the difference between the mean arterial pressure (MAP) and the intracranial pressure (ICP): CPP = MAP − ICP

(2) Regulatory mechanisms influence the diameter of the cerebrovasculature

a) Pressure or myogenic autoregulation: Alteration in the diameter of the brain's resistance vessels (arterioles) that maintains a constant CBF over a range of pressures between 50 and 150 mm Hg. Chronic hypertension can increase the upper and lower pressure ranges for the range of autoregulation.

  b) Elevated arterial partial pressure of carbon dioxide ($Paco_2$) and hypoxemia (arterial partial pressure of oxygen [Pao_2] of <50 mm Hg) cause vasodilatation and increased CBF; decreased $Paco_2$ causes vasoconstriction and reduced CBF

  c) Metabolic autoregulation: CBF varies with metabolic activity. Factors that increase the metabolic rate (e.g., seizures, fever) increase CBF; reduced metabolic requirements (e.g., hypothermia) decrease CBF.

 (3) Inadequate CBF results in brain tissue ischemia (CBF <18 to 20 ml/100 g/min) and death (CBF <8 to 10 ml/100 g/min)

 (4) CBF higher than metabolic demand is called *hyperemia*

iii. Venous system: Brain surface drains into the superficial veins; the central interior cerebrum drains into the internal veins beneath the corpus callosum (Figure 4-10). Veins have no valves.

 (a) Veins empty into venous sinuses between dural layers (Table 4-3)

 (b) Internal jugular veins collect blood from the large dural venous sinuses and return blood to the heart

iv. Blood-brain barrier: Specialized permeability of the brain capillaries that limits transfer of certain substances from blood into brain tissue. Barrier formed by tight junctions between brain capillary endothelial cells, reduced transport mechanisms of these cells, and footlike projections from the astrocytes that encase the capillaries.

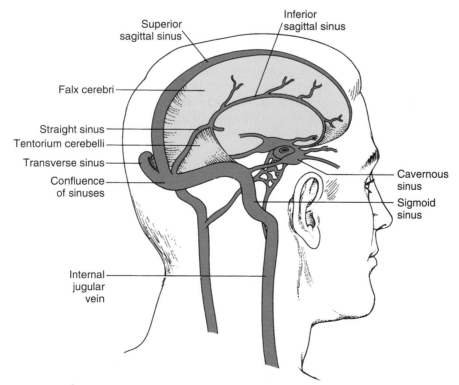

FIGURE 4-10 ■ Diagram showing the pattern of distribution of the major dural venous sinuses and their connection to the internal jugular veins. (From Barker E: *Neuroscience nursing: a spectrum of care*, ed 2, St Louis, 2002, Mosby, p 36.)

■ **TABLE 4-3**
■ ■ **Major Venous Drainage Structures, Their Locations, and Areas Drained**

Venous Structure	Location and Area Drained
Superior sagittal sinus	Courses along the midline at the superior border of the falx cerebri; superior cerebral veins empty into it
Straight sinus	Lies in the midline attachment of the falx cerebri and the tentorium; drains the system of internal cerebral veins (including the inferior sagittal sinus and great cerebral vein of Galen)
Transverse sinuses	Lie in the bony groove along the fixed edge of the tentorium cerebelli; drain the straight sinus and the superior sagittal sinus
Sigmoid sinuses	Lie on the mastoid process of the temporal bone and jugular process of the occipital bone; receive blood from the transverse sinuses and empty into the internal jugular veins
Inferior sagittal sinus	Lies along the free inferior border of the falx cerebri just above the corpus callosum; receives blood from the medial aspects of the hemispheres
Emissary veins	Connect the dural sinuses with veins outside the cranial cavity

    (a) Water, carbon dioxide, oxygen, glucose, and lipid-soluble substances cross the cerebral capillaries with ease. Uptake of other substances, such as dyes and ions (e.g., Na^+, K^+), is much slower.

    (b) Regulates the entry or removal of various substances to maintain a homeostatic environment for the central nervous system (CNS)

    (c) Clinically significant in treating and diagnosing CNS disease. Blood-brain barrier disruption and increased permeability occurs with brain injury, tumors, infections, and stroke.

  d. Ventricular system and CSF (Figure 4-11)

    i. Ventricles: Four cavities containing CSF

      (a) Lateral ventricles: Largest ventricles, one in each cerebral hemisphere. The anterior (frontal) horns lie in the frontal lobes; the bodies extend back through the parietal lobes to the posterior (occipital) horns, which project into the occipital lobes; the inferior (temporal) horns lie in the temporal lobes.

      (b) Third ventricle: Midline between the two lateral ventricles, surrounded by the diencephalon

      (c) Fourth ventricle: In the posterior fossa bordered by the pons, medulla, and superior cerebellar peduncles; continuous with the cerebral aqueduct (aqueduct of Sylvius) superiorly and the central spinal canal inferiorly

    ii. CSF functions

      (a) Cushions the brain and spinal cord from injury

      (b) Provides support and buoyancy for the brain, decreasing its effective weight on the skull

      (c) Its displacement out of the cranial cavity (and, to an extent, its increased reabsorption) compensates for increases in intracranial volume and pressure

      (d) Regulates the nervous system chemical environment to preserve homeostasis

      (e) Enables water-soluble metabolites to diffuse from the brain

      (f) Serves as a channel for neurochemical communication within brain

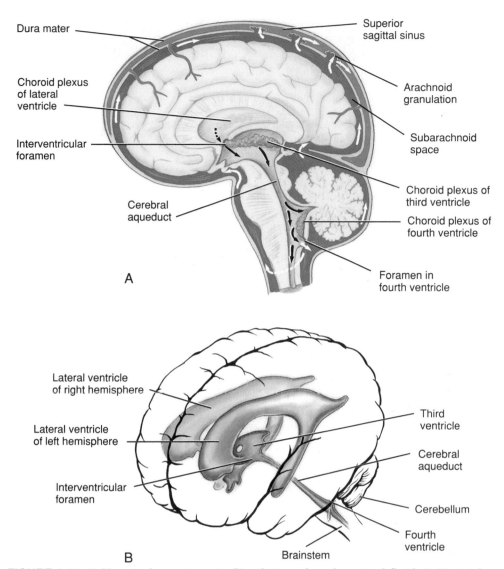

FIGURE 4-11 ■ Ventricular system. **A,** Circulation of cerebrospinal fluid. **B,** Ventricles of the brain. (From Applegate EJ: *The anatomy and physiology learning systems textbook*, ed 2, Philadelphia, 2000, Saunders, p 169.)

    iii. CSF properties: See Table 4-4
    iv. CSF formation
        (a) Rate of synthesis estimated as 500 ml/day or 22 to 25 ml/hr
        (b) Choroid plexus: Tuft of capillaries covered by epithelial cells found in all ventricles; principal source of CSF; lateral ventricles produce most
        (c) Small amounts of CSF are produced by the blood vessels of the brain and meningeal linings
    v. Circulation and absorption of CSF (see Figure 4-11)
        (a) CSF circulates from the lateral ventricles through the interventricular foramina (foramina of Monro) to the third ventricle and to the fourth ventricle via the aqueduct of Sylvius; CSF then circulates to the subarachnoid space via the foramina of Luschka and Magendie

■ **TABLE 4-4**
■ ■ **Normal Properties of Cerebrospinal Fluid (CSF)**

Characteristic	Normal Finding
Appearance	Clear, colorless
Specific gravity	1.007
Glucose level	50-75 mg/dl or approximately 60% of serum glucose level
Protein level	Lumbar: 15-45 mg/dl (*Note:* Increases when blood is present in CSF)
Cells	White blood cells: 0-5/mm³ Red blood cells: 0/mm³
Lactate level	10-20 mg/dl
pH	7.35
Pressure	70-180 mm water, measured at the lumbar level, with the patient in the lateral decubitus position
Volume	Ventricular system and subarachnoid space contain approximately 125 to 150 ml of CSF

        (b) Most CSF is absorbed via the arachnoid villi into the dural sinuses
        (c) When CSF pressure exceeds venous pressure, CSF is absorbed through the unidirectional valves of the arachnoid villi
    vi. Blood-CSF barrier: Choroid plexus epithelium imposes a barrier analogous to the blood-brain barrier; permits selective transport of substances from the blood into the CSF
  e. Brain metabolism
    i. Brain has high metabolic energy requirements; energy primarily used for neuronal conductive and metabolic activities
    ii. At rest, the brain consumes 25% of body glucose and 20% of body oxygen; cerebral oxygen consumption averages 49 ml/min
    iii. Brain utilizes glucose as its principal energy source
    iv. Minimal storage of oxygen and glucose in the brain necessitates a constant supply for normal neuronal function
    v. Anaerobic glucose metabolism (glycolysis) yields insufficient adenosine triphosphate (ATP) to meet cerebral energy demands. Rate of glycolysis increases markedly during hypoxia in an attempt to maintain functional neuronal activity.
    vi. Within seconds to minutes of anoxia, the energy-dependent sodium-potassium pump fails; cytotoxic cerebral edema results
    vii. Hypoglycemia causes neuronal dysfunction and may lead to convulsions, coma, and death
  f. Cells of the nervous system
    i. Neuron: Basic functional unit of the nervous system; transmits nerve impulses
        (a) Components of each cell (Figure 4-12)
            (1) Cell body: Carries out the metabolic functions of the cell; contains a nucleus, cytoplasm, and organelles surrounded by a lipoprotein cell membrane
            (2) Dendrites: Short branching extensions of the cell body; conduct impulses toward the cell body
            (3) Axon hillock: Thickened area of the cell body from which the axon originates

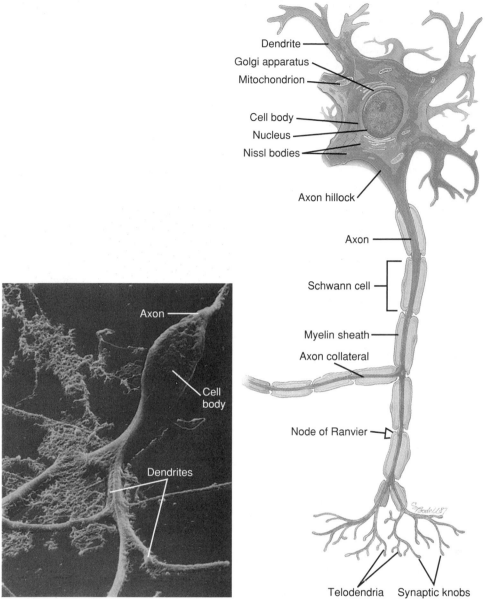

Dendrite

Golgi apparatus

Mitochondrion

Cell body

Nucleus

Nissl bodies

Axon hillock

Axon

Schwann cell

Myelin sheath

Axon collateral

Node of Ranvier

Axon

Cell body

Dendrites

Telodendria   Synaptic knobs

FIGURE 4-12 ■ Structure of a typical neuron. (From Thibodeau GA, Patton K: *Anatomy and physiology*, ed 5, St Louis, 2003, Mosby, p 348.)

(4) Axon: Long extension of the cell body; conducts impulses away from the cell body; usually myelinated. Outside the brain, axons are also covered with neurilemma. Branch into several processes at the terminal end.

(5) Myelin sheath: White protein-lipid complex that surrounds some axons; laid down by oligodendrocytes in the CNS and by Schwann cells in the PNS

(6) Nodes of Ranvier: Periodic interruptions in the myelin covering along the axon. Impulses are conducted from node to node (saltatory conduction), which makes conduction more rapid and efficient.

(7) Synaptic knobs: At the terminal ends of the axon; contain vesicles that store neurotransmitter substances

(b) Functions

(1) Receive input from other neurons, primarily via the dendrites and cell body

(2) Conduct action potentials or impulses along the axon

(3) Transfer information by synaptic transmission to other neurons, muscle cells, or gland cells

ii. Neuroglial cells: Support, nourish, and protect the neurons; about 5 to 10 times as numerous as neurons. Four types:

(a) Microglia: Phagocytize tissue debris when nervous tissue is damaged

(b) Oligodendroglia: Responsible for myelin formation on axons in the CNS

(c) Astrocytes: Contribute to the structure of the blood-brain barrier. Provide nutrients for neurons. Constitute the structural and supporting framework for nerve cells and capillaries. Remove excess potassium and neurotransmitters. Contribute to scar formation in response to neuronal cell injury or death.

(d) Ependyma: Line the ventricles of the brain and the central canal of the spinal cord. Regulate the flow of substances from these cavities into the brain. Aid in CSF production.

g. Synaptic transmission of impulses: Unidirectional conduction of an impulse from a presynaptic neuron across a junction or synapse to a postsynaptic neuron

i. *Resting membrane potential* (RMP): Voltage difference across the cell membrane when the neuron is resting. Determined by the difference in ion concentrations on either side of the membrane. At rest, cells are positively charged outside and negatively charged inside.

ii. *Depolarization:* Stimulus causes sodium channels to open, which results in an intracellular influx of sodium ions (Na^+)

(a) These ionic fluxes decrease RMP

(b) This depolarization is called the *excitatory postsynaptic potential* (EPSP)

iii. *Action potential:* If a transient voltage change that occurs with depolarization is of sufficient magnitude (threshold level), an action potential is produced and transmitted (conducted as an impulse) along the nerve fibers in an active, self-propagating process

iv. *Summation:* Simultaneous excitation of numerous excitatory presynaptic terminals (or rapidly successive discharges from the same presynaptic terminal) can add together to cause a progressive increase in the postsynaptic potential that may eventually reach threshold to generate an action potential

v. Neurotransmitters (Table 4-5): Chemicals secreted by presynaptic knobs or vesicles (usually located at the axon terminal) that excite, inhibit, or modify the response of a postsynaptic neuron. When an action potential reaches the synaptic knob, calcium channels are opened, allowing Ca^{++} influx into the knob, which triggers neurotransmitter release.

(a) Transmitter diffuses across the synapse and binds with postsynaptic membrane receptors, which causes certain ion channels to open

(b) Excitatory neurotransmitters: Open sodium and potassium channels, which results in postsynaptic membrane depolarization

Neurotransmitter	Location	Action*
Acetylcholine (ACh)	Distributed throughout the body, including concentrations in the following locations: • Many areas of the brain (e.g., motor cortex, some basal ganglia cells, hypothalamus) • Motor neurons innervating muscles or glands • Cholinergic fibers of the autonomic nervous system (ANS)	Usually excitation Inhibitory effect on some of the parasympathetic nervous system (PNS) (e.g., vagus nerve on the heart) Primary neurotransmitter of the PNS
AMINES		
Norepinephrine (NE)	Distributed throughout the central nervous system (CNS) In the brain, produced by neurons with cell bodies in the pons (in the locus ceruleus nuclei) and medulla, which send axons to all areas of the CNS, including the brainstem, spinal cord, cerebellum, cortex, hypothalamus, and thalamus Found in the adrenergic fibers of the ANS	Excitation and inhibition Primary neurotransmitter of the sympathetic nervous system (SNS); regulates SNS effectors Implicated in numerous functions, including motor control, emotional responses, mood, feeding behavior, temperature regulation, and sleep
Dopamine (DA)	Produced by neurons of the substantia nigra and distributed throughout the CNS, particularly the basal ganglia Found in the ANS	Mostly inhibition Regulates motor control Also involved in other functions, including emotions, mood, behavior control, and mental functions
Serotonin (5-HT)	Produced in the raphe nuclei of the brainstem that project to several regions in the CNS, including the hypothalamus, brainstem, spinal cord, cortex, basal ganglia, and cerebellum	Mostly inhibition Implicated in a number of functions, including sensory processing, control of body heat, behavior, hunger, emotions, and sleep
AMINO ACIDS		
γ-aminobutyric acid (GABA)	Distributed over much of the CNS including neuron terminals in the spinal cord, cerebellum, basal ganglia, and some areas of the cortex	Inhibition
Glutamate	Found in many areas of the CNS High concentrations in the cortex, particularly the hippocampus and basal ganglia Released in large amounts when brain cells are injured by trauma or hypoxia-ischemia; hypoxic-ischemic changes are attributed in part to glutamate, which affects the hippocampus in particular	Excitation Excessive glutamate receptor stimulation opens ionic channels, causing neuronal disintegration from calcium influx through N-methyl-D-aspartate (NMDA) receptors and cellular swelling from influx of sodium and water

*Action is determined by the postsynaptic receptor rather than the neurotransmitter.

vi. Refractory period

(a) *Absolute refractory period:* Membrane is unresponsive to any stimulus, so that the neuron is incapable of producing an action potential. Occurs for a fraction of a second after the membrane surpasses the threshold potential. Limits the frequency of the impulses that a cell can generate.

(b) *Relative refractory period:* Neuron can be excited again but only by a very strong stimulus (i.e., summation above threshold); occurs during membrane repolarization

vii. Repolarization

(a) At the peak of an action potential, the cell membrane again becomes impermeable to Na^+; potassium channels open and allow rapid efflux of K^+ from the cell, which thereby reestablishes the RMP

(b) RMP returns with the aid of the sodium–potassium–adenosine triphosphatase (ATPase) pump, which pumps Na^+ out of the cell and K^+ into the cell

viii. Inhibition

(a) *Inhibitory postsynaptic potential (IPSP)*

(1) Inhibitory neurotransmitters open potassium and/or chloride channels; this causes increased negativity of the membrane potential, which results in hyperpolarization of the cell membrane

(2) Decreases excitability and inhibits impulse transmission

(b) Presynaptic inhibition: Reduced amount of neurotransmitter is released; this reduces the magnitude of the EPSP to subthreshold levels

2. Spine and spinal cord

a. Vertebral column (Figure 4-13)

i. Composed of 33 vertebrae

(a) Cervical: Seven vertebrae

(1) Support the head and neck; smallest vertebrae

(2) Atlas (first cervical vertebra): Supports the head; articulates with the occipital bone superiorly and the axis inferiorly

(3) Axis (second cervical vertebra)

a) Odontoid process (dens): Projection of the axis that protrudes upward through the anterior arch of atlas

b) Allows for rotation of the head

(b) Thoracic: Twelve vertebrae; articulate with the ribs; support the chest muscles

(c) Lumbar: Five vertebrae; support the lower back muscles; the largest and strongest vertebrae

(d) Sacral: Five fused vertebrae; form a large triangular bone, the sacrum

(e) Coccygeal: Four fused rudimentary vertebrae

ii. Anatomic features of a typical vertebra

(a) Body: Flat round, solid portion; lies anteriorly

(b) Arch: Posterior part of the vertebra. Consists of:

(1) Pedicles: Two short bony projections that extend posterior from the body

(2) Lamina: Join each pedicle and fuse posteriorly at the midline to complete the arch; processes project from the laminae

(3) Spinous process: Midline projection protruding posteriorly from the laminae

(4) Transverse processes: Projections from the laminae on each side of the vertebrae

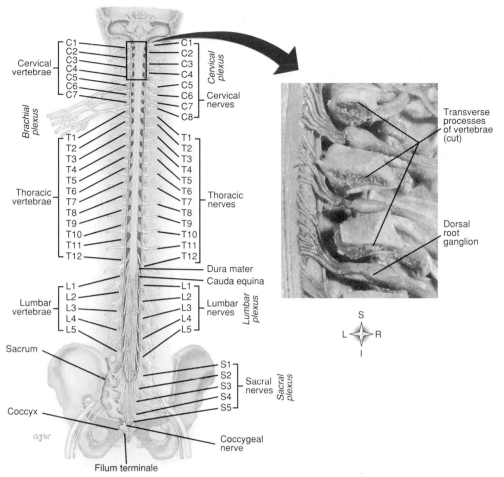

FIGURE 4-13 ■ Spinal nerves. Each of the 31 pairs of spinal nerves exits the spinal cavity from the intervertebral foramina. The names of the vertebrae are given on the left and the names of the corresponding spinal nerves on the right. Note that after leaving the spinal cavity, many of the spinal nerves interconnect to form plexuses. *I*, Inferior; *L*, left; *R*, right; *S*, superior. (From Thibodeau GA, Patton K: *Anatomy and physiology*, ed 5, St Louis, 2003, Mosby, p 414.)

       (5) Articular processes (facets): Projections from the laminae that protrude upward or downward (superior or inferior articulating processes); inferior processes articulate with the superior processes of the vertebra directly below

   (c) Intervertebral foramina: Openings between the vertebrae through which spinal nerves pass

   (d) Spinal foramina: Opening between the arch and the body through which the spinal cord passes

  iii. Intervertebral discs

   (a) Fibrocartilage layer between the bodies of adjoining vertebrae

   (b) Act as shock absorbers

   (c) Composed of the annulus fibrosus (tough outer layer) and nucleus pulposus (gelatinous inner layer)

 iv. Spinal ligaments: Hold the vertebrae and discs in alignment; prevent excessive spinal flexion or extension

   b. Spinal cord
   i. Location: Extends from the superior border of the atlas to the first or second lumbar vertebra
      (a) Continuous with the medulla oblongata
      (b) Conus medullaris: Caudal end of the spinal cord
      (c) Central canal: In the center of the spinal cord; contains CSF and is continuous with the fourth ventricle
      (d) Filum terminale: Nonneural filament that extends downward from the conus medullaris and attaches to the coccyx; helps maintain the position of spinal cord during trunk movement
   ii. Meninges: Continuous with the layers covering the brain
   iii. Gray matter (Figure 4-14)
      (a) An H-shaped, internal mass of gray substance surrounded by white matter; consists of cell bodies and their dendrites and axons
      (b) Anterior gray column (anterior horn): Contains cell bodies of efferent motor fibers
      (c) Lateral column: Contains preganglionic fibers of the ANS
      (d) Posterior gray column (posterior horn): Contains cell bodies of afferent sensory fibers
   iv. White matter (see Figure 4-14)
      (a) Composed of three longitudinal columns (funiculi): Anterior, lateral, and posterior
      (b) Contains mostly myelinated axons
      (c) Funiculi contain tracts (fasciculi): Composed of axons with similar origin, course, and termination that perform specific functions; clinically significant tracts are summarized in Table 4-6; classified as follows (Figure 4-15):
         (1) Ascending or sensory tracts: Pathways to the brain for impulses that enter the cord via the dorsal roots of the spinal nerves

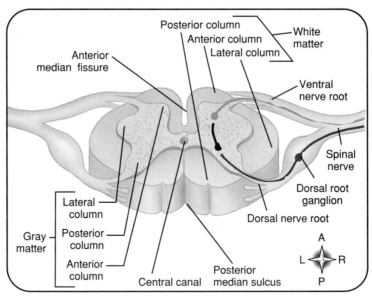

FIGURE 4-14 ■ Transverse section of the spinal cord. *A,* Anterior; *L,* left, *R,* right, *P,* posterior. (From Ozuna JM: Nursing assessment neurologic system. In Lewis SM, Heitkemper MM, Dirksen SR: *Medical surgical nursing assessment and management of clinical problems,* ed 5, St Louis, 2000, Mosby, p 1584.)

TABLE 4-6
Major Spinal Cord Tracts

Name	Origin	Termination	Cross	Function
ASCENDING TRACTS				
Posterior dorsal columns: Fasciculus gracilis and fasciculus cuneatus	Fasciculus gracilis: Spinal cord at the lumbar and sacral levels Fasciculus cuneatus: Spinal cord at the cervical and thoracic levels	Medulla → thalamus → sensory strip of the cerebral cortex	Ascend in the posterior funiculus and cross over in the lower medulla	Conveys position and vibratory sense, joint and two-point discrimination, tactile localization, pressure and discriminating touch Fasciculus gracilis: Carries impulses from the lower body Fasciculus cuneatus: Carries impulses from the upper body
Lateral spinothalamic tract	Posterior horn	Thalamus → cerebral cortex	Crosses over in the spinal cord to the contralateral anterolateral funiculus before ascending	Conveys pain and temperature sensation
Anterior spinothalamic tract	Posterior horn	Thalamus → cerebral cortex	Crosses over in the spinal cord to the contralateral anterolateral funiculus before ascending	Conveys light touch and pressure sensation
Posterior spinocerebellar tract	Posterior horn	Cerebellum	Ascends uncrossed in the lateral funiculus	Conveys proprioceptive data that influence muscle tone and synergy necessary for coordinated muscle movements
Anterior spinocerebellar tract	Posterior horn	Cerebellum	Mostly crosses in the spinal cord before ascending in the lateral funiculus	Conveys proprioceptive data that influence muscle tone and synergy necessary for coordinated muscle movements
Spinotectal tract	Posterior horn	Tectum (roof) of the midbrain	Ascends crossed in the lateral funiculus	Conveys general sensory information that influences pupil reaction and head and eye movement in response to stimuli

Continued

■ TABLE 4-6
■ Major Spinal Cord Tracts—cont'd

Name	Origin	Termination	Cross	Function
DESCENDING TRACTS				
Rubrospinal tract	Red nucleus of the midbrain	Anterior horn	Crosses in the midbrain and descends in the lateral funiculus	Conveys impulses to control muscle tone and synergy and to maintain posture
Lateral corticospinal tract	Cerebral cortical motor areas	Anterior horn	Up to 90% crosses in the medulla and descends in the lateral funiculus	Carries impulses for voluntary movement
Anterior corticospinal tract	Cerebral cortical motor areas	Anterior horn	Descends in the anterior funiculus and crosses in the cord at the level at which it terminates	Carries impulses for voluntary movement
Tectospinal tract	Superior colliculus of the midbrain	Anterior horn in the cervical spinal cord	Crosses in the midbrain and descends in the anterior funiculus	Mediates optic and auditory reflexes (e.g., reflexive head turning in response to visual or auditory stimuli)

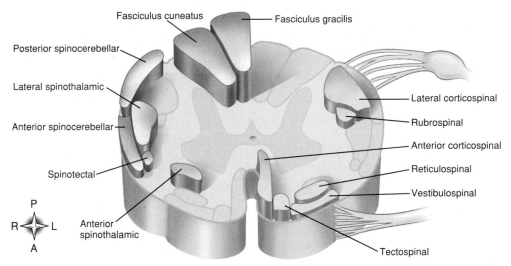

FIGURE 4-15 ■ Major ascending (sensory) and descending (motor) tracts of the spinal cord. *A*, Anterior; *L*, left; *R*, right; *P*, posterior. (From Thibodeau GA, Patton K: *Anatomy and physiology*, ed 5, St Louis, 2003, Mosby, p 382.)

   (2) Descending or motor tracts: Transmit impulses from the brain to the motor neurons of the spinal cord that exit via the ventral root of the spinal nerves
   (d) Most tracts are named to indicate the column in which the tract travels, the location of its cells of origin, and the location of axon termination
   v. Upper and lower motor neurons
   (a) Lower motor neurons (LMNs): Spinal and cranial motor neurons that directly innervate muscles. LMN lesions cause flaccid paralysis, muscular atrophy, absent reflexes.
   (b) Upper motor neurons (UMNs): Located completely in the CNS; regulate LMN activity. UMN lesions are associated with spastic paralysis, clonus, increased tone, hyperactive reflexes, Babinski's sign.
 c. Reflexes
   i. Reflex arc: Requires a receptor, sensory neuron, motor neuron, and effector (e.g., muscle or gland) (Figure 4-16)
   ii. Monosynaptic reflex arc: Direct synapse between the afferent and efferent neurons
   (a) Stimulation of afferent nerve fibers sends impulses to the spinal cord through the dorsal roots of spinal nerves
   (b) Impulse synapses with anterior motor neurons, sending out an efferent discharge confined to the axons supplying the muscle from which the afferent impulse originated
   iii. Polysynaptic reflex arc
   (a) More than one synapse required to complete the reflex arc
   (b) Most reflexes are polysynaptic; may involve interneurons (neurons in the CNS that transmit impulses from a sensory neuron to or toward a motor neuron) and multiple spinal segments and/or areas of brain
   iv. Reciprocal innervation: Impulses that excite motor neurons supplying a particular muscle also inhibit motor neurons of antagonistic muscles

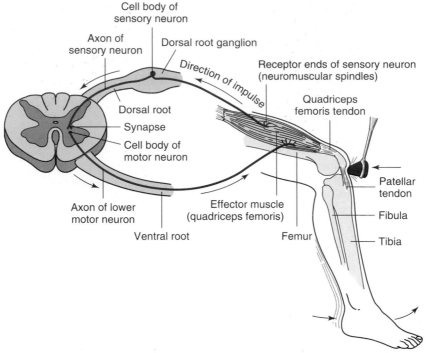

FIGURE 4-16 ■ The two-neuron patellar reflex or "knee jerk." (From Phipps WJ, Marek JF, Monahan FD, et al: *Medical-surgical nursing health and illness perspectives*, ed 7, St Louis, 2003, Mosby, p 1311.)

3. **Peripheral nervous system (PNS)**
   a. Spinal nerves
      i. Thirty-one symmetrically arranged pairs of nerves, each possessing a sensory (dorsal) root and a motor (ventral) root: 8 cervical pairs, 12 thoracic pairs, 5 lumbar pairs, 5 sacral pairs, 1 coccygeal pair (see Figure 4-13)
      ii. Fibers of the spinal nerves
          (a) Motor fibers: Originate in the anterior gray column of the spinal cord, form the ventral root of the spinal nerve, and pass to skeletal muscles
          (b) Sensory fibers: Originate in the spinal ganglia of the dorsal roots; peripheral branches distribute to visceral and somatic structures as mediators of sensory impulses to the CNS
          (c) Autonomic fibers
              (1) Sympathetic
                  a) Originate from cells between the posterior and anterior gray columns from the first thoracic to second lumbar cord segment
                  a) Innervate the viscera, blood vessels, glands, and smooth muscle
              (2) Parasympathetic
                  a) Arise from sacral cord segments S2 to S4
                  b) Pass to the pelvic and abdominal viscera
          (d) Cauda equina: Spinal nerves that arise from the lumbosacral portion of the spinal cord contained within the lumbar cistern
      iii. Dermatomes (Figure 4-17): Skin areas supplied by the dorsal root (sensory fibers) of a given spinal nerve; adjacent dermatomes overlap
      iv. Plexuses: Network of spinal nerve roots (Table 4-7)

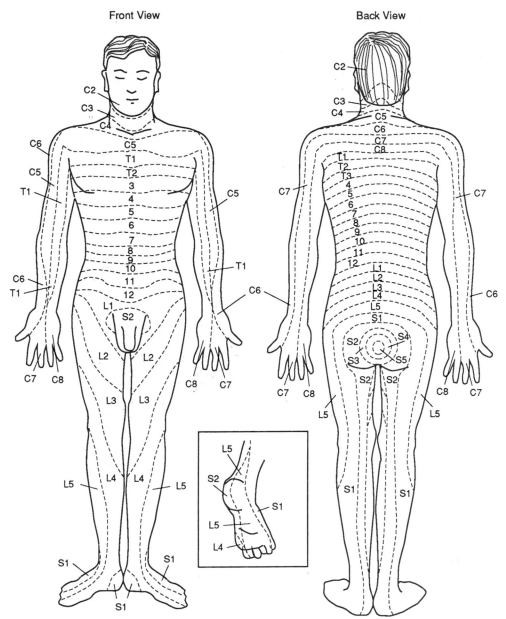

FIGURE 4-17 ■ Dermatomes. (From Russo-McCourt TA: Spinal cord injuries. In McQuillan KA, Von Rueden KT, Hartsock RL, et al, editors: *Trauma nursing from resuscitation through rehabilitation*, ed 3, St Louis, 2002, Saunders, p 522.)

b. Neuromuscular transmission (Figure 4-18)
  i. Physiologic anatomy at the neuromuscular junction
    (a) Motor end plate: Distal end of motor axon loses its myelin sheath and flattens out at the end lying close to the muscle fiber membrane (sarcolemma)
    (b) Synaptic cleft: Space between the motor endplate and the muscle fiber membrane
    (c) Synaptic gutter: Invagination of the muscle fiber membrane where numerous folds increase the surface area available for neurotransmitter to act

■ **TABLE 4-7**
■ ■ **Plexuses and Their Locations and Areas of Innervation**

Name	Spinal Nerve Anterior Branches That Comprise Plexus	Location of Plexus	Important Nerves That Emerge	Areas of Innervation
Cervical	C1-C4	Deep within the neck	Portion of the phrenic nerve	Muscles and skin of a portion of the head, neck, and upper shoulders; diaphragm
Brachial	C5-C8 and T1	Deep within the shoulder	Phrenic, circumflex, musculocutaneous, ulnar, median, and radial nerves	Shoulder, arm, and hand; diaphragm
Lumbar	L1-L4	Lumbar region of the back	Femoral cutaneous, femoral and genitofemoral branches	Anterior abdominal wall and genitalia; thigh and leg
Sacral	L4 and L5 and S1-S4	Inner surface of the posterior pelvic wall	Tibial, common peroneal, sciatic, and pudendal nerves	Skin of the leg; muscles of the posterior thigh, leg, and foot

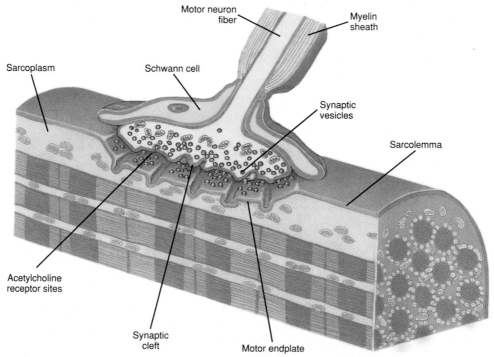

FIGURE 4-18 ■ Neuromuscular junction. This figure shows how the distal end of a motor neuron fiber forms a synapse, or "chemical junction," with an adjacent muscle fiber. Neurotransmitters (specifically, acetylcholine) are released from the neuron's synaptic vesicles and diffuse across the synaptic cleft. There they stimulate receptors in the motor endplate region of the sarcolemma. (From Thibodeau GA, Patton K: *Anatomy and physiology*, ed 5, St Louis, 2003, Mosby, p 316.)

(d) Vesicles: Nerve terminal structures that store and release the neuro-transmitter acetylcholine (ACh)

　　ii. When an action potential reaches the neuromuscular junction, vesicles release ACh into the synaptic cleft. Amount released depends on the magnitude of the action potential and the presence of calcium. ACh attaches to receptor sites on the postjunctional muscle membrane and increases its permeability to Na^+, K^+, and other ions.

　　iii. End-plate potential: Motor nerve action potential that is local (e.g., non-propagated) and graded, rather than all or nothing

　　iv. Muscle contraction: Action potentials subsequently form on either side of the endplate and conduct in both directions along the muscle fiber, initiating a series of events that result in muscle contraction

　　v. Acetylcholinesterase: Catalyzes the hydrolysis of ACh to choline and acetic acid and thus limits the duration of ACh action on the endplate, which ensures production of only one action potential

c. Cranial nerves: 12 pairs of nerves considered part of the PNS (Figure 4-19 and Table 4-8)

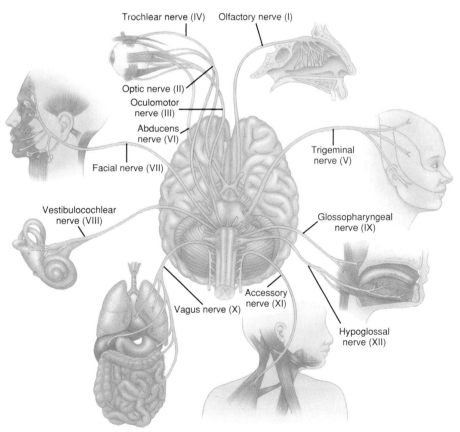

FIGURE 4-19 ■ Cranial nerves. Ventral surface of the brain showing the attachment of the cranial nerves. (From Thibodeau GA, Patton K: *Anatomy and physiology*, ed 5, St Louis, 2003, Mosby, p 421.)

■ **TABLE 4-8**
■ ■ **Cranial Nerves: Origin, Course, and Function**

Cranial Nerve	Origin and Course	Function
Olfactory (I)	Receptor cells located in the nasal mucosa. Axons from these cells form the olfactory nerve, which passes to the olfactory bulb and then forms the olfactory tract.	Smell
Optic (II)	Fibers originate from the ganglion cells of the retina. At the optic chiasm, optic nerve fibers from the nasal half of the retina cross; those from the temporal half do not. Fibers continue as optic tracts to the lateral geniculate bodies of the thalamus and then as geniculocalcarine tracts to the occipital cortex.	Vision
Oculomotor (III)	Nuclei are located in the midbrain. Preganglionic parasympathetic fibers originate in the Edinger-Westphal nucleus and accompany other oculomotor fibers into the orbit, where they terminate in the ciliary ganglion. Postganglionic fibers pass to the constrictor papillae and ciliary muscles of the eye.	Pupil constriction Levator palpebrae innervation raises the upper eyelid Innervates extraocular muscles to move the eye as follows: • Inferior rectus: moves eye downward and outward • Medial rectus: Moves eye medially • Superior rectus: Moves eye upward and outward • Inferior oblique: Moves eye upward and inward
Trochlear (IV)	Originates in the midbrain.	Supplies the superior oblique muscle, which moves the eye downward and inward
Trigeminal (V)	Sensory fibers arise from cells in the semilunar (trigeminal) ganglion. Axons from the ganglion attach to the lateral aspect of the pons. Motor fibers leave the pons ventromedial to the sensory roots. Components of this nerve are also located in the midbrain and medulla.	Three sensory divisions 1. Ophthalmic branch provides sensation to the forehead, upper eyelid, cornea, conjunctiva, nose, and part of the nasal mucosa 2. Maxillary branch provides sensation to the lower eyelid, upper jaw, teeth, gums and lip, upper cheek, hard and soft palates, some of the nasal mucosa, and the lower side of the nose 3. Mandibular branch provides sensation to the lower jaw, teeth, gums and lip, buccal mucosa, tongue, part of the external ear, and auditory meatus All three divisions contribute sensory fibers to the meninges Motor fibers innervate the muscles of mastication

Continued

Abducens (VI)	Arises from nuclei in the pons. Emerges anteriorly at the border of the pons and medulla. Enters the orbit through the superior orbital fissure with cranial nerves III, IV and the ophthalmic branch of V.	Supplies the lateral rectus muscle, which abducts the eye horizontally
Facial (VII)	Fibers originate in the pons and emerge at the junction of the pons and medulla. The smaller nerve root containing the sensory and parasympathetic fibers is called the *nervus intermedius*. Sensory fibers originate in the geniculate ganglion located within the facial canal of the temporal bone, and parasympathetic fibers originate in the superior salivary nucleus located within the medulla.	Motor portions of the nerve innervate all muscles of facial expression Sensory portion conveys taste from the anterior two thirds of the tongue and skin sensation from the external auditory meatus and the auricle Parasympathetic fibers innervate the salivary and lacrimal glands
Acoustic (VIII) (also known as vestibulo-cochlear)	Nerve enters the brainstem at the pontomedullary junction. Two divisions: • Cochlear nerve: Cell bodies of these bipolar neurons are located in the spiral ganglion of the cochlea. Peripheral fibers of these neurons innervate hair cells located in the organ of Corti of the cochlea, which transduce sounds into neural signals. Central fibers of the neurons project to the ventral and dorsal cochlear nuclei in the medulla. Fibers from these nuclei synapse in the medial geniculate nuclei of the thalamus and then on the auditory cortex of the temporal lobe. • Vestibular nerve: Cell bodies of these bipolar neurons are located in the vestibular ganglion. Peripheral fibers of the vestibular ganglion receive input from receptors in the semicircular canals, the utricle, and the saccule of the inner ear. Central fibers project from the vestibular ganglion to the vestibular nuclei located in the pons and medulla. These nuclei send out projections to the spinal cord, cerebellum, reticular formation and nuclei of cranial nerves III, IV, and VI.	Cochlear nerve: Hearing Vestibular nerve: Aids in maintaining equilibrium or balance and coordinating head and eye movements
Glossopharyngeal (IX)	Sensory fibers arise from cells at the back of the tongue, the pharynx, and the palate and enter the medulla. Motor fibers originate from the	Sensory fibers provide sensation to the pharynx, soft palate, and posterior third of the tongue. They also supply special receptors

Continued

■ **TABLE 4-8**
■ ■ **Cranial Nerves: Origin, Course, and Function—cont'd**

Cranial Nerve	Origin and Course	Function
	ambiguus nucleus in the medulla to innervate the stylopharyngeus muscle of the pharynx. Preganglionic fibers terminate in the otic ganglion, which is the parasympathetic ganglion that innervates the parotid gland.	in the carotid body and carotid sinus, which are concerned with reflex control of respiration, blood pressure, and heart rate. Motor fibers participate with the vagus nerve in swallowing
Vagus (X)	Sensory fibers originate in the cells of ganglia just below the jugular foramen and enter the medulla. Motor fibers leave the medulla and join the sensory part of the nerve. Preganglionic parasympathetic fibers are distributed to the abdominal and thoracic viscera.	Sensory fibers convey sensation from the palate and pharynx (along with IX) and from the larynx, external auditory meatus, and thoracic and abdominal viscera Motor fibers innervate muscles of the palate, pharynx (along with IX), and larynx Provides parasympathetic functions to the abdominal and thoracic organs
Spinal accessory (XI)	Motor fibers arise from the medulla and upper cervical spinal cord.	Supplies the trapezius muscle to enable shoulder elevation, and the sternocleidomastoid muscle, which allows the head to tilt, turn, and be thrust forward
Hypoglossal (XII)	Motor fibers originate in the hypoglossal nucleus of the medulla.	Innervates muscles of the tongue

    d. ANS (Figure 4-20)
      i. Structure
        (a) Composed of two neuron chains
        (b) Preganglionic cell bodies are located within the lateral gray column of the spinal cord or brainstem nuclei
        (c) Most preganglionic axons are myelinated and synapse on the cell bodies of postganglionic neurons outside the CNS
        (d) Axons of postganglionic neurons terminate on visceral effectors (i.e., smooth and cardiac muscle, glandular epithelium)
      ii. Divisions
        (a) Sympathetic (thoracolumbar)
          (1) Preganglionic axons emerge from cell bodies within the lateral horn of the spinal cord gray matter at the thoracic and upper two lumbar levels. Axons leave the spinal cord via the ventral roots and pass to
            a) Paravertebral sympathetic ganglion chain via white rami communicantes, ending on cell bodies of postganglionic neurons
            b) Collateral ganglia, ending on postganglionic neurons closer to the viscera

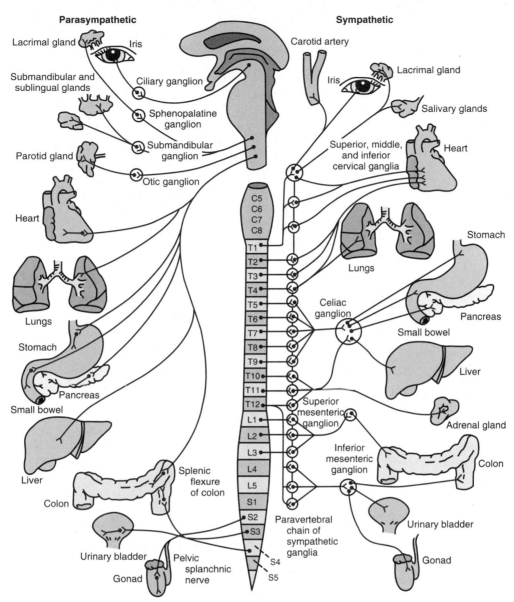

FIGURE 4-20 ■ Diagram of the autonomic nervous system. The parasympathetic nervous system division *(left)* arises from cranial nerves III, VII, IX, and X and from spinal cord segments S2 to S4. The sympathetic division *(right)* arises from spinal cord segments T1 to T12. (From DeMyer W: *Neuroanatomy,* ed 2, Baltimore, 1998, Williams & Wilkins, p 99.)

   c) Adrenal medulla, ending on modified postganglionic neurons that are secretory endocrine cells
  (2) Postganglionic axons pass to
   a) Viscera via the sympathetic nerves
   b) Gray rami communicantes, which return to the spinal nerve and are distributed to autonomic effectors in areas supplied by these nerves
  (3) Functions (Table 4-9)

■ **TABLE 4-9**
■ ■ **Autonomic Nervous System Effects on Various Effector Sites**

Effector Organ		Sympathetic Influence	Parasympathetic Influence
Eyes	Pupils	Dilation (mydriasis)	Constriction (miosis)
Glands	Lacrimal	Decreased	Increased
	Nasal	Decreased	Increased
	Salivary	Decreased	Increased
	Sweat	Increased	None
Heart		Increased rate	Decreased rate
		Increased conduction velocity	
		Increased contractility	Decreased contractility
Blood vessels	Coronary	Vasodilation	Minimal dilation
	Skeletal	Vasodilation	None
	Abdominal viscera	Vasoconstriction	None
	Cutaneous	Vasoconstriction	None
Blood pressure		Increased	Decreased
Lungs		Bronchodilation	Bronchoconstriction
Gastrointestinal	Motility	Decreased peristalsis	Increased peristalsis
system	Sphincter	Increased tone	Relaxation
	Secretions	Inhibition	Stimulation
Bladder		Decreased detrusor tone	Increased detrusor tone
Sex organs		Ejaculation	Erection
Skin	Pilomotor muscles	Excited (contraction)	None

From Russo-McCourt T: Spinal cord injuries. In McQuillan KA, Von Rueden KT, Hartsock RL, et al, editors: *Trauma nursing: from resuscitation through rehabilitation*, ed 3, Philadelphia, 2002, Saunders, p 512.

a) Come into widespread activity under emergency conditions ("fight or flight")
b) Generally antagonistic to parasympathetic activity
c) Synapse with many postganglionic fibers

(b) Parasympathetic (craniosacral) (see Table 4-9)
  (1) Preganglionic cell bodies are located in brainstem nuclei and the lateral gray columns of the middle three sacral spinal cord segments (S2 to S4)
  (2) Preganglionic fibers end on short postganglionic neurons located on or near visceral structures
  (3) Supplies visceral structures in the head via the oculomotor (III), facial (VII), and glossopharyngeal (IX) cranial nerves and those in the thorax and upper abdomen via the vagus (X) nerve
  (4) Sacral outflow supplies the pelvic viscera via the pelvic branches of S2 to S4
  (5) Produces localized reactions rather than the mass action of sympathetic stimulation

iii. Chemical mediation: ANS is divided into *cholinergic* and *adrenergic* divisions based on the neurotransmitter released
  (a) Cholinergic neurons release ACh and include
    (1) All preganglionic neurons
    (2) Parasympathetic postganglionic neurons
    (3) Sympathetic postganglionic neurons to the sweat glands and skeletal muscle blood vessels (vasodilation)

(b) Adrenergic neurons release norepinephrine and include
  (1) Sympathetic postganglionic endings, except as noted earlier
  (2) Constrictor fibers of the skeletal muscle blood vessels

4. **Physiology of pain**
  a. *Core Curriculum* focuses primarily on acute (nociceptive or physiologic) pain. Chronic pain is discussed briefly because unrelieved acute pain can result in the development of chronic (pathologic) pain.
  b. Acute pain results when mechanisms such as surgery, trauma, or disease cause inflammation and cellular damage
    i. Warns of potential for, or extent of, tissue damage; initiates protective behaviors to minimize damage and promote tissue repair
    ii. Usual characteristics include the following:
      (a) Activates sympathetic nervous system (autonomic, involuntary) responses, such as increased heart rate, blood pressure (BP), respiratory rate
      (b) Proportional to intensity and extent of stimuli; however, wide variations exist among patients
      (c) Has a beginning and end, with resolution or healing of the underlying pathologic condition. Research indicates that
        (1) Long-term alterations in neural tissue are initiated within the first few hours after injury (Blakely and Page, 2001)
        (2) Inadequately managed acute pain can persist after injured tissue is repaired (McCaffery and Pasero, 1999)
    iii. Classifications of acute pain
      (a) *Somatic*: Arising from tissues (e.g., skin, muscle, bone). Descriptors include *sharp, dull, aching, cramping*. Is localized or diffuse; may radiate.
      (b) *Visceral*: Arising from organs (e.g., liver, pancreas, bowel). Descriptors include *sharp, stabbing, deep ache*. Is well or poorly localized; may be referred.
    iv. Key physiologic concepts
      (a) *Nociception:* Neurochemical process of transmitting the pain response to a peripheral noxious (thermal, mechanical, or chemical) stimulus to an intact spinal cord and brain
        (1) Pain perception requires cortical integration of many factors (e.g., physiologic factors, psychosocial factors, past experiences); often results in emotional responses (e.g., anger, anxiety)
        (2) Nociception does not always result in pain (e.g., pain perception can be blunted by endogenous endorphin release); pain can occur without nociception (e.g., phantom limb pain)
      (b) *Nociceptors*: Peripheral neurons (primary afferent peripheral fibers) that sense unpleasant or potentially damaging noxious stimuli. Examples are
        (1) *A delta*: Large, thinly myelinated fibers that rapidly conduct impulses generated in response to mechanical or thermal stimuli; usually results in sharp, well-localized pain
        (2) *C*: Smaller, unmyelinated fibers that slowly conduct impulses generated in response to all noxious stimuli; usually poorly localized, dull, aching pain; 75% of nociceptors are C fibers (Munden, Eggenberger, Goldberg, et al, 2003)
      (c) *Peripheral sensitization*: Lowering of nociceptor activation threshold following exposure to chemical mediators or repeated noxious stimuli
      (d) Four basic stages of nociception are described in Table 4-10 and illustrated in Figure 4-21

Stage	Steps	Mechanisms of Action for Interventions
Transduction	1. Cells damaged by noxious stimuli release nociceptor activating substances (e.g., prostaglandins, serotonin, substance P, histamine), which cause inflammation, peripheral sensitization, and primary hyperalgesia (increased sensitivity around the area of tissue damage). 2. An action potential leads to generation of an electrical impulse in response to the stimulus.	1. Nonsteroidal antiinflammatory drugs target the inflammatory response. 2. Anticonvulsants and local anesthetics can block various ion exchanges involved in the generation of an action potential.
Transmission	1. Sensitized fibers release neurotransmitters (e.g., glutamate, substance P), which facilitate impulse travel to dorsal horn neurons in the spinal cord. Glutamate binds N-methyl-D-aspartate (NMDA) receptors and facilitates transmission. 2. Impulses travel on to the brainstem, thalamus (relay station between the brain and spinal cord), and cortex via different ascending tracts.	1. Opioids reduce release of substance P. 2. NMDA receptor antagonists (e.g., ketamine, dextromethorphan, possibly methadone) inhibit glutamate binding.
Perception	Once impulses reach the brain, pain processing is thought to include the following: • Reticular activating system: Autonomic response and alerting of the individual to respond to pain • Somatosensory cortex: Localization, characterization, and preservation of information about pain • Limbic system: Site of emotional-behavioral response to pain	1. Opioids binding to their receptors in the brain can alter the perception of pain. 2. Strategies like distraction or relaxation may modify pain perception by limiting the number of signals the brain has to process.
Modulation	1. Neurons descending from the brainstem synapse on dorsal horn neurons and release inhibitory neurotransmitters: Inhibitory amino acids (e.g., γ-amino-butyric acid [GABA], glycine) and neuropeptides (e.g., endogenous opioids), serotonin, and norepinephrine. • These substances bind with receptors to raise the threshold for nociceptor activation and prevent the release of other neurotransmitters (e.g., substance P). • Neurotransmitters are then recycled and stored for future use. 2. Emotions (e.g., fear, anxiety, anticipation, stress) can increase pain.	1. Baclofen binds to GABA receptors and mimics its inhibitory effects. 2. Opioids activate descending inhibitory pathways. 3. Tricyclic antidepressants prevent the reuptake and storage of serotonin and norepinephrine, which makes them more available.

Compiled from Ballantyne J, Fishman SM, Abdi S, editors: *The Massachusetts General Hospital handbook of pain management,* Philadelphia, 2002, Lippincott Williams & Wilkins; Blakely WP, Page GG: Pathophysiology of pain in critically ill patients, *Crit Care Nurs Clin North Am* 12(2):167-179, 2001; McCaffery M, Pasero C: *Pain: clinical manual,* ed 2, St Louis, 1999, Mosby; Melzack R, Wall PD, editors: *Handbook of pain management,* Edinburgh, 2003, Churchill Livingstone; and National Pharmaceutical Council: Pain: current understanding of assessment, management, and treatment, Reston, Va, 2001, Author.

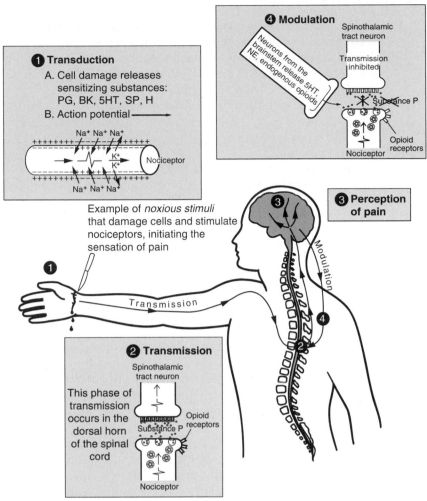

FIGURE 4-21 ■ Four basic processes involved in nociception. *BK*, Bradykinin; *5HT*, 5-hydroxytryptamine (serotonin); *H*, histamine; *NE*, norepinephrine; *PG*, prostaglandin; *SP*, substance P. (From McCaffery M, Pasero C: *Pain: clinical manual*, St Louis, 1999, Mosby, p 21.)

   c. Chronic pain: Pain state persisting beyond the period of healing
      i. Serves no useful purpose (St. Marie, 2002)
     ii. Usual characteristics (McCaffery and Pasero, 1999)
        (a) Neither tissue pathology nor sympathetic nervous system activation is identifiable
        (b) Represents a disproportionate response to the stimulus and/or physical findings
        (c) Possibly indicates interpersonal or psychologic problems
    iii. Often involves *neuropathic pain*: Abnormal processing of sensory input in PNS or CNS due to injury or impairment
        (a) Described as either continuous or intermittent sensations (e.g., burning, shooting, shocklike, tingling, jabbing)
        (b) Examples include pain caused by nerve root compression, diabetic neuropathy, Guillain-Barré syndrome; phantom limb pain, complex regional pain syndrome

    iv. Key physiologic concepts
       (a) *Neuroplasticity:* Ability of neurons to change their subsequent response to stimuli following long-term or sustained exposure to noxious stimuli
       (b) *Central sensitization:* State of heightened excitability resulting in an exaggerated response to stimuli and an expanded distribution of pain
          (1) *Hyperalgesia:* Lowered threshold for noxious stimuli
          (2) *Allodynia:* Perception of normally benign stimuli as painful

Patient Assessment

1. **Nursing history**
   a. Current health issues
      i. Current symptoms, including chronologic sequence of onset, duration, location, and frequency
      ii. Factors that relieve or exacerbate symptoms
      iii. Difficulties performing activities of daily living (ADLs)
   b. Patient health history: Significant medical and surgical history, including traumatic injury and childhood diseases
   c. Medication history: Use of over-the-counter and prescription drugs, nutritional and herbal supplements, including amount, frequency, duration, last dose, effectiveness, adverse response. Especially note use of analgesics, anticonvulsants, tranquilizers, sedatives, anticoagulants, platelet aggregation inhibitors, stimulants, antihypertensives, cardiac medications.
   d. Allergies
   e. Family history: Note history of disease that may impact current illness (e.g., cardiac disease, stroke [especially early onset], aneurysms, arteriovenous malformations, seizures, migraines, dementia, autoimmune disorders)
   f. Social history and habits
      i. Significant others affected by the patient's illness
      ii. Support systems available to assist the patient and family
      iii. Alcohol and tobacco use: Past and present, amount, duration
      iv. Illicit drug use or abuse: Particularly cocaine, amphetamines
      v. Type of work; impact of symptoms on work
      vi. Hobbies, recreational activities
      vii. Current dwelling, including layout and number of stairs
2. **Nursing examination of patient**
   a. Physical examination data
      i. First ABC: Evaluate *a*irway patency, sufficiency of *b*reathing and *c*irculation
      ii. Inspection then palpation of the head, face, and spine: Shape, symmetry, bony contour, coloration and skin integrity; irregularities may indicate injury, ventricular shunt, previous surgery, or congenital abnormality. Note nares or ear drainage.
      iii. Auscultation: Heart for murmurs and clicks; carotid arteries and over eyes for bruits
      iv. Assessment of neurologic function
         (a) Level of consciousness (LOC) (Box 4-1)
         (b) Glasgow Coma Scale (GCS) (Table 4-11): Used to assess LOC; total score also used to classify severity of brain injury. Limitations include inability to assess eye opening in patients with periorbital swelling or verbal response in intubated patients. Hypoxia, hypotension, hypothermia, drug intoxication, postictal state, and administration of sedatives, analgesics, or paralytic agents can interfere with GCS

■ **BOX 4-1**
■ **ASSESSMENT OF LEVEL OF CONSCIOUSNESS**

Consciousness is an awareness of self and the environment. A disturbance in consciousness is a sensitive indicator of neurologic dysfunction. Unconsciousness (coma) can result from extensive bilateral cerebral lesions, injury to the diencephalon or pontomesencephalic (pons-midbrain) reticular formation, or metabolic abnormalities. Unilateral lesions of the cerebrum (without prior contralateral injury) and lesions of the medulla or spinal cord do not cause coma.

Arousal: Evaluate what stimulus is necessary to elicit a response. Determine if the patient responds spontaneously; if not, apply the following stimuli in progressive order until a response is obtained: Address the patient by name, shake the patient, apply a peripheral pain stimulus (i.e., nail bed pressure), apply a deep central pain stimulus (i.e., sternal rub, supraorbital pressure).

Awareness or the content of consciousness reflects higher cortical functions; can be assessed via the following:

- General behavior and appearance; appropriateness to the situation
- Attention span, long- and short-term memory, insight, orientation, and calculation
- Intellectual capacity appropriate for educational level, judgment
- Emotional state, affect
- Thought content: Illusions, hallucinations, delusions
- Execution of intentional motor activity: *Apraxia* is the inability to perform these movements
- Recognition and interpretation of sensations
- Language: Fluency, clarity, content, comprehension of written and spoken word, ability to name objects and repeat phrases, patient's awareness of a language disorder

   Aphasia: Difficulty in the expression of language (expressive aphasia) or understanding of language (receptive aphasia) indicates dominant hemisphere dysfunction

   Motor speech apraxia: Inability to perform the mouth movements to produce the sounds for the intended words; a motor speech programming disorder indicates a lesion in Broca's speech area

   Dysarthria: Difficulty with articulation due to impaired movement of the speech musculature may result from dysfunction of cranial nerves V, VII, IX, X, or XII or cerebellar dysfunction that interferes with the coordination of the muscles innervated by these nerves; represents speech impairment without a language deficit

responses. Presence of any confounding variable should be noted when reporting score. Neurologic deterioration that affects only one side of the body is not reflected in GCS score.

(c) Motor function

   (1) Assess size and contour of muscles: Note atrophy, hypertrophy, asymmetry, and joint malalignments

   (2) Observe for involuntary movements, such as fasciculations, tics, tremors, abnormal positioning

   (3) Determine motor response to stimuli

      a) Ability to follow simple commands such as "Hold up two fingers." Do not ask the patient to squeeze your hand because this may be a reflex response to palmar stimulation.

      b) Localization: Able to locate a noxious stimulus (e.g., deep pain stimulus) and attempt to remove it; indicates cortical dysfunction

      c) Withdraws: Pulls limb(s) away from painful stimuli with normal flexor movement; indicates extensive cortical damage

■ **TABLE 4-11**
■ ■ **Glasgow Coma Scale**

Response	Score
EYE OPENING	
Assesses arousal state	
"Spontaneously": Patient opens eyes without stimulation	4
"To voice": Patient opens eyes when spoken to	3
"To pain": Patient opens eyes when a noxious stimulus is applied	2
"None": Patient does not open eyes to any stimulus	1
BEST VERBAL RESPONSE	
Assesses the content of consciousness in terms of the ability to produce speech and quality of speech. It is controversial whether points should be added to the score when patients nod or gesture indicating they would speak appropriately if able.	
"Oriented": Patient can state his or her name, where he or she is, and the date	5
"Confused": Patient speaks words but cannot state either who he or she is, where he or she is, or the date	4
"Inappropriate words": Patient speaks words with no specific intent at communicating	3
"Incomprehensible sounds": Patient grunts, groans, or makes other sounds	2
"None": Patient makes no attempt to vocalize. (*Note:* A "T" may be written after the score to indicate the presence of a tracheal tube.)	1
BEST MOTOR RESPONSE	
Assesses both arousal and the content of consciousness. Ensure consistent stimuli and limb position with each assessment to avoid influencing the patient's response.	
"Obeys": Follows commands	6
"Localizes": Attempts to remove noxious stimulus	5
"Withdraws": Pulls away from noxious stimulus	4
"Abnormal flexion": Decorticate posturing*	3
"Abnormal extension": Decerebrate posturing†	2
"No response": No motor movement of any kind to any stimulus	1

SCORING
The patient's responses are graded and the best scores achieved for the eye opening, verbal, and motor categories are summed.
Total score ranges from 3 to 15, with 15 being normal.

*Rigid flexion, internal rotation, and adduction of the upper extremity; extension, internal rotation, and plantar flexion of the lower extremity.
†Rigid extension, adduction, and internal rotation of the upper extremity; extension, internal rotation, and plantar flexion of the lower extremity.

    d) Abnormal flexion (decorticate posturing; see Table 4-11): Associated with lesions to the corticospinal tract just above the brainstem near or in the cerebral hemispheres, in the area of the diencephalon

    e) Extensor (decerebrate) posturing (see Table 4-11): Indicates damage to the midbrain or upper pons

    f) No response: Associated with lower brainstem or high spinal cord dysfunction

  (4) Strength testing (if the patient is able to follow commands)

    a) Evaluate the integrity and function of UMNs and LMNs that innervate a specific muscle or muscle group (Table 4-12)

■ **TABLE 4-12**
■ ■ **Muscle Groups, Associated Level of Spinal Cord Innervation, and Method of Testing**

Muscle(s) Tested	Primary Level(s) of Spinal Nerve Innervation	Method of Testing
Deltoids	C5	Raising of arms
Biceps	C5	Flexion of elbow
Wrist extensors	C6	Extension of wrist
Triceps	C7	Extension of elbow
Hand intrinsics	C8-T1	Hand squeezing, finger flexion, finger abduction
Iliopsoas	L1, L2	Hip flexion
Hip adductors	L2-L4	Adduction of hips (squeezing legs together)
Hip abductors	L4, L5, S1	Abduction of hips (separating hips)
Quadriceps	L3, L4	Knee extension
Hamstrings	L5, S1, S2	Knee flexion
Tibialis anterior	L4, L5	Dorsiflexion of foot
Extensor hallucis longus	L5	Extension of great toe
Gastrocnemius	S1	Plantar flexion of foot

Adapted from McIlvoy L, Meyer K, McQuillan KA: Traumatic spine injuries. In Bader MK, Littlejohns LR, editors: *AANN core curriculum for neuroscience nursing,* ed 4, St Louis, 2004, Saunders, p 345.

b) Grade strength on a 0 to 5 scale (Table 4-13)
c) Note whether weakness follows a distributional pattern (proximal-distal, right-left, or upper-lower extremity)
(5) Strength testing for a patient unable to follow commands:
a) Observe which extremities move spontaneously or to noxious stimuli
b) *Hemiparesis* or *hemiplegia* may be detected by lifting both arms off the bed and releasing them simultaneously. The limb on the hemiparetic side will fall more quickly and more limply than that on the normal side.
(6) Muscle tone: State of muscle tension assessed by palpating muscles at rest and during passive range-of-motion (ROM) movement; possible abnormalities include:
a) *Rigidity:* Increased muscular resistance throughout passive ROM movement; seen with a basal ganglia lesion

■ **TABLE 4-13**
■ ■ **Muscle Strength Grading Scale**

Score	Muscle Function
0	Absent, no muscle contraction
1	Contraction of muscle felt or seen
2	Movement through full range of motion with gravity removed
3	Movement through full range of motion against gravity
4	Movement against resistance but can be overcome
5	Full strength against resistance

b) *Spasticity:* Increased muscular resistance to joint movement, often followed by release of resistance; increased tone indicates corticospinal tract lesion

c) *Hypotonia* (flaccidity): Decreased muscle tone associated with LMN lesions, cerebellar dysfunction, or spinal shock related to acute spinal cord injury

(7) Deep tendon or muscle stretch reflexes: Elicited by percussing the tendon with a reflex hammer, which causes stretching of the muscle spindles and subsequent contraction of muscle fibers when the monosynaptic reflex arc is intact. Compare responses side to side.

a) Hyperreflexia usually indicates UMN lesion

b) May be diminished initially after an acute intracranial injury due to cerebral shock or at and below the level of spinal cord injury due to spinal shock

c) Areflexia most often due to LMN lesions

d) Deep tendon reflexes commonly tested: See Table 4-14

e) Grade deep tendon reflexes on a 0 to 4 scale: See Table 4-15

(8) Superficial reflexes: Tested by stroking the skin with a moderately sharp object (Table 4-16). These reflexes are lost or abnormal with UMN or LMN lesions.

(9) Pathologic reflexes: See Box 4-2

(10) Abnormal movements: See Box 4-2

(11) Balance and coordination: See Box 4-2

(d) Sensory function

(1) In an unresponsive or uncooperative patient, a cursory sensory examination is performed by noting the patient's response to painful stimuli applied while performing various interventions (e.g., venipuncture)

■ **TABLE 4-14**
■ ■ **Deep Tendon or Muscle Stretch Reflexes and Level of Spinal Cord Innervation**

Reflex	Level of Spinal Cord Innervation
Biceps	C5, C6
Brachioradialis	C5, C6
Triceps	C7, C8
Quadriceps (patellar)	L2-L4
Achilles (ankle jerk)	S1, S2

■ **TABLE 4-15**
■ ■ **Grading Scale for Strength of Deep Tendon Reflexes**

Score	Reflex Response
4+	Hyperreactive, clonus
3+	Very brisk
2+	Normal, average
1+	Diminished
0	No response, flaccid

From McIlvoy L, Meyer K, McQuillan KA: Traumatic spine injuries. In Bader MK, Littlejohns LR, editors: *AANN core curriculum for neuroscience nursing,* ed 4, St Louis, 2004, Saunders, p 346.

■ TABLE 4-16
■ ■ Superficial Reflexes, Level of Spinal Nerve Innervation, and Method for Assessment

Reflex	Spinal Nerve Innervation	Stimulus	Response
Upper abdominal	T8-T10	Stroke upper abdomen	Abdominal wall contraction that causes umbilicus to move toward the stimulus
Lower abdominal	T10-T12	Stroke lower abdomen	Abdominal wall contraction that causes umbilicus to move toward the stimulus
Cremasteric	L1, L2	Stroke medial thigh	Testicular elevation
Bulbocavernous	S3, S4	Apply pressure to glans penis	Contraction of the anus
Perianal	S3-S5	Stroke perianal area	Contraction of the external anal sphincter

Adapted from McIlvoy L, Meyer K, McQuillan KA: Traumatic spine injuries. In Bader MK, Littlejohns LR, editors: *AANN core curriculum for neuroscience nursing,* ed 4, St Louis, 2004, Saunders, p 347.

■ BOX 4-2
■ ASSESSMENT OF PATHOLOGIC REFLEXES, ABNORMAL MOVEMENTS, BALANCE, AND COORDINATION

Pathologic reflexes
■ Primitive reflexes present in infants but normally absent in adults may reappear in association with frontal lobe impairment. Examples include the following:
  ● Grasp reflex: In response to palmar stimulation
  ● Sucking reflex: In response to lip stimulation
  ● Rooting reflex: Mouth opens, head deviates toward a stimulus applied to the lower lip or cheek
■ Babinski's sign
  ● Stroking the lateral aspect of the sole of the foot from the heel upward and across the ball causes abnormal dorsiflexion of the great toe and extensor fanning of the other toes
  ● In an adult, indicates a lesion of the corticospinal tract anywhere from the motor cortex to the anterior horn of the spinal cord
Abnormal movements: Note the distribution, rate, duration, and relationship to activity of any involuntary movements, such as the following:
■ Seizures (refer to Seizures under Specific Patient Health Problems)
■ Tremors: Rhythmic trembling movement of muscles
■ Clonus: Abrupt onset of brief jerking movements of a muscle or muscle group (e.g., oscillation of the foot between flexion and extension with sudden passive extension of the foot)
Balance and coordination: Primarily evaluate cerebellar function; tested in patients able to perform voluntary movements
■ Romberg's test: Patient stands erect with the feet together, first with the eyes open and then with the eyes closed. Positive test result indicating posterior column or cerebellar dysfunction occurs when the patient loses balance and sways or falls when the eyes are closed.
■ Observe the patient while sitting; swaying indicates cerebellar dysfunction
■ Evaluate for *dystaxia* or *ataxia* (muscle incoordination with volitional movements) and *dysmetria* (inability to halt a movement at a desired point), which indicate cerebellar dysfunction
  ● Have the patient first touch the examiner's finger, positioned at the length of patient's arm from the face, and then touch his or her nose
  ● Have the patient slap the thigh first with the palm and then with the back of the hand in quick, alternating movements
  ● Have the patient run the heel from the opposite knee down the shin

Continued

■ **BOX 4-2**
■ **ASSESSMENT OF PATHOLOGIC REFLEXES, ABNORMAL MOVEMENTS, AND BALANCE AND COORDINATION—cont'd**

- Rebound test: Have the patient extend the arms forward while the examiner taps the patient's wrist; in cerebellar disease, the arm moves markedly out of place and overshooting occurs as the patient attempts to move the arm back into position
- Gait
  - Observe the gait and have the patient perform tandem (heel-to-toe) walking
  - A wide-based, staggering gait and the inability to perform tandem walking indicate cerebellar dysfunction
  - Gait disturbances with different clinical characteristics can be correlated with other specific neurologic or muscular dysfunction (e.g., spastic hemiparesis following an upper motor neuron lesion causes the patient to walk with the arm flexed close to the body and the spastic leg to move outward and forward in a semicircle, often with the toe dragged)

    (2) In an awake, cooperative patient able to understand and follow commands, a complete sensory assessment can be performed. Test with the patient's eyes closed and compare one side of the body with the other
    (3) Sensory function is scored using a 0 to 2 scale: See Table 4-17
    (4) When possible, delineate sensory impairments based on dermatome distribution (see Figure 4-17)
    (5) Spinothalamic tracts: See Box 4-3
    (6) Posterior columns: See Box 4-3
    (7) Cortical discriminatory sensation: See Box 4-3
  (e) Cranial nerves: See Table 4-18 and Figure 4-22
  (f) Eye and pupil signs: In addition to cranial nerve assessment, other findings may include the following:
    (1) Pupil abnormalities (Table 4-19)
    (2) Gaze deviation or gaze preference: Horizontal or vertical gaze deviations indicate a cortical or brainstem lesion
      a) Eyes deviate toward the side of a destructive hemispheric lesion affecting the frontal gaze centers
      b) Gaze deviates away from irritative foci (seizures) affecting the frontal gaze centers
      c) Inability to gaze upward is associated with dorsal midbrain lesions
      d) Eyes deviate away from the side of a unilateral pons lesion

■ **TABLE 4-17**
■ ■ **Sensory Function Scoring**

Score	Sensory Function
0	Absent
1	Impaired or hyperesthetic
2	Normal or intact

Adapted from McIlvoy L, Meyer K, McQuillan KA: Traumatic spine injuries. In Bader MK, Littlejohns LR, editors: *AANN core curriculum for neuroscience nursing*, ed 4, St Louis, 2004, Saunders, p 344.

■ **BOX 4-3**
■ **ASSESSMENT OF SPINOTHALAMIC TRACTS, POSTERIOR COLUMNS, AND CORTICAL DISCRIMINATORY SENSATION**

Lesions or dysfunction of the peripheral nerves, ascending nerve tracts, or sensory perceptive areas of the cerebral cortex (i.e., parietal lobe) may impair sensory function

SPINOTHALAMIC TRACTS (ANTERIOR AND LATERAL)
■ Test either pain or temperature sensation, because both functions are carried in the same lateral spinothalamic tracts
■ Pain: Have the patient distinguish sharp from dull stimuli randomly applied; gently touch the skin using a clean pin for sharp sensation and using a blunt edge (head of a pin) for dull sensation
■ Temperature: Ask the patient to distinguish between hot and cold stimuli when randomly touched with test tubes filled with hot or cold water
■ Light touch: Lightly touch the patient with a wisp of cotton

POSTERIOR COLUMNS (FASCICULUS GRACILIS AND FASCICULUS CUNEATUS)
■ Test either proprioception or vibration sense, because both are carried in the same tracts
■ Vibration: Apply a vibrating tuning fork to bony prominences; ask the patient to report when vibration is felt; apply first to the distal aspect of each extremity and move proximally
■ Proprioception (position sense): Ask the patient to close the eyes and report whether a finger or toe is being moved up or down; assess in all four extremities

CORTICAL DISCRIMINATORY SENSATION
In addition to the sensory pathways, assesses the association portions of the cortex (i.e., the parietal lobe). Deficits are called *agnosias* (not knowing). Examples include the following:
● *Stereognosis:* Ask the patient, without the aid of vision, to identify familiar objects placed in his or her hand. The inability to identify objects is *astereognosia.*
● *Graphesthesia:* Ask the patient to identify numbers or letters traced on the palm. Inability to discern what is written is *agraphesthesia.*
● *Simultaneous double stimulation:* With the patient's eyes closed, touch the patient's limb and then touch both sides of the body in corresponding locations. Determine if the patient can detect the number and location of stimuli. Inability to identify that he or she is being touched on both sides of body simultaneously is *tactile inattention.* Inability to locate a single touch sensation is *atopognosia.*

     (3) Nystagmus (rhythmic, oscillatory eye movements)
        a) Detected by having the patient follow your finger through the fields of gaze
        b) Due to lesions of the cerebellum, vestibular system, or brainstem pathways, or toxic-metabolic disorders; clinical features vary with the part of the pathway affected
   (g) Vital signs
     (1) Temperature
        a) Hyperthermia increases cerebral oxygen consumption by 10% for every 1.8° F (1° C) elevation. Higher metabolic demand increases the risk for CNS ischemia. *Neurogenic fever* can be caused by damage to the hypothalamus, where the thermoregulation center is located.
        b) Hypothermia, if extreme, can lead to cardiac dysrhythmias, coagulopathies, other complications. Seen with hypothalamic

■ **TABLE 4-18**
■ ■ **Cranial Nerve Assessment and Anticipated Deficits**

Cranial Nerve (CN)	Assessment in Conscious Patient	Assessment in Unconscious or Uncooperative Patient	Anticipated Deficit
Olfactory (I)	Test each nostril separately. Ask the patient to identify familiar nonirritating odors, such as coffee or perfume.	Unable to assess.	Loss of sense of smell (*anosmia*)
Optic (II)	1. Inspect the optic disc (fundus), macula, and blood vessels with an ophthalmoscope. 2. Test visual acuity with a Snellen chart or printed material; test each eye individually. 3. Determine visual field using the confrontation test. Have the patient cover one eye and fixate on you with the other. Position yourself about 24 inches directly in front of the patient and close your eye that is opposite the patient's covered eye. With your finger halfway between yourself and the patient, bring your finger from the periphery into the patient's field of vision, evaluating the upward, downward, nasal, and temporal fields. Compare your visual field with the patient's. Repeat the test with the other eye.	Evaluate the pupillary light reflex (provides the sensory limb for this reflex) as part of the assessment with CN III described below.	1. Papilledema (optic disc swollen and distorted with a reddish hue), which is indicative of increased intracranial pressure 2. Decrease or loss of central vision; blindness 3. Visual field defect (see Figure 4-22)
Oculomotor (III)	1. Evaluate the width and symmetry of the palebral fissures and eyelid position. 2. Assess pupil shape, size, and equality. Describe size in millimeters. 3. Test the direct light reflex (constriction of the pupil when stimulated by light). This tests the afferent limb of CN II and the efferent limb of CN III. Describe the reflex as brisk, sluggish, or nonreactive.	1. Assess pupil shape, size, equality, and reactivity to light as was done for a conscious patient. 2. Evaluate extraocular movement as described later.	1. Eyelid droops (*ptosis*) 2. Irregularly shaped pupils can be caused by direct trauma, cataracts, or other ocular dysfunction; an irregularly shaped or oval pupil may accompany tentorial herniation that compresses CN III 3. Disruption or compression of parasympathetic fibers from CN III and/or the nucleus (e.g., from a mass lesion or

			tentorial herniation) cause the ipsilateral pupil to dilate, which results in unequal pupils (*anisocoria*)
	4. Test the consensual light reflex (constriction of the opposite pupil when light stimulates one eye). Differentiates CN II and CN III lesions. Reflex is "present" or "absent."		4. The direct light reflex is lost with oculomotor (parasympathetic) or optic nerve injury but retained with sympathetic disruption
	5. Test the accommodation reflex: Have the patient look at an object (e.g., finger, pen) positioned 2-3 ft in front of the patient; as the object is moved toward the patient, the patient's eyes converge toward the midline, pupils constrict, and the lenses thicken.		5. A blind eye (CN II lesion) does not have a direct light reflex; it has a consensual light reflex if CN III and midbrain connections are intact; cortical blindness does not affect either direct or consensual reflexes
	6. Assess extraocular movement as part of the assessment for CN IV and VI described later.		6. The accommodation reflex is lost
Oculomotor (III), trochlear (IV), and abducens (VI)	1. Check the range of extraocular movements (EOMs) by having the patient's eyes follow your finger through all fields of gaze. Observe for nystagmus at rest and during ocular movements. 2. Ask the patient whether double vision is experienced in any visual field.	In patients who open their eyes, determine whether they can move both their eyes medially (CN III), laterally outward (CN VI), or up and down (more difficult to elicit) in response to a verbal or noxious stimulus. Evaluate whether the eyes move together (conjugate movement).	1. Impairment of EOM • Inability to move eye(s) downward and outward, medially, upward and inward, or upward and outward indicates CN III involvement • Impaired downward and inward movement indicates CN IV involvement • Inability to move the eye(s) horizontally outward indicates CN VI involvement 2. Diplopia
Trigeminal (V)	Sensory examination 1. Test the forehead, cheeks, and jaw on each side of the face. To evaluate light touch sensation, use a wisp of cotton; to evaluate temperature sensation, use test tubes of warm and cold water. 2. Corneal reflex: Touch the cornea of each eye with a wisp of cotton. Observe for reflex blinking. This tests the afferent limb of CN V and the efferent limb of CN VII.	Test the corneal reflex.	1. Absent, unequal, or uncomfortable sensation when the face is stimulated 2. Absence or weakness of blink response to corneal stimuli 3. Weakness of masseter and/or temporal muscles

Continued

■ **TABLE 4-18**
■ ■ **Cranial Nerve Assessment and Anticipated Deficits—cont'd**

Cranial Nerve (CN)	Assessment in Conscious Patient	Assessment in Unconscious or Uncooperative Patient	Anticipated Deficit
	Motor examination 1. Ask the patient to clench his or her teeth and palpate the masseter and temporal muscles. Assess the symmetry and strength of muscle contraction. Assess the strength of the masseter muscles by pushing down on the mandible (chin) against the patient's resistance. 2. Assess the patient's ability to chew.		
Facial (VII)	1. Ask the patient to raise his or her eyebrows, frown, smile, and open the eyes against resistance. Note the strength and symmetry of facial movement. 2. Test taste on the anterior two thirds of the tongue by applying salt and then sugar to both sides of the tongue. Ask the patient to identify the taste prior to closing the mouth. 3. Assess the corneal reflex.	Test the corneal reflex.	1. Weakness on one or both sides of the upper and/or lower face; if only the lower portion of the face is weak the cause is an upper motor neuron lesion (e.g., stroke) on the contralateral side of the facial weakness; weakness of the entire side of the face is due to an ipsilateral lower motor neuron lesion of the facial nerve 2. Loss of taste sensation 3. Absence or weakness of the corneal reflex
Acoustic (vestibulocochlear) (VIII)	Cochlear (hearing) 1. Hearing acuity: Cover one ear, and test the other with a watch or a whisper. 2. Weber's test: Place the stem of a vibrating tuning fork on the midline vertex of the skull. Ask the patient if the sound is heard equally in both ears or more on one side. Normally, there is no lateralization of sound. 3. Rinne's test: Place the stem of a vibrating tuning fork on the mastoid bone. When sound is no longer heard, invert the tuning fork and place	The vestibular portion of CN VIII and its connections via the medial longitudinal fasciculus with CN III, IV, and VI provide information regarding the integrity of the brainstem; can be tested by the oculocephalic or oculovestibular reflex: 1. Oculocephalic reflex (doll's eye test): In a comatose patient who has had a cervical spine injury ruled out, turn the patient's head	1. Impaired hearing 2. Negative result on Weber's test: When sound is referred to the better-hearing ear, decreased hearing is due to impaired function of the cochlear nerve 3. Negative result on Rinne's test: Because air conduction is normally greater than bone conduction, middle ear disease is suspected in a patient who can hear the tuning fork as well or better when it is placed on the mastoid bone than near the ear

it in front of the ear. Ask the patient to tell you when sound is no longer heard.

Vestibular (balance)

1. Assess the patient for complaints of vertigo, nausea, anxiety, nystagmus, postural deviation, and vomiting. All may indicate vestibular nerve dysfunction.
2. Observe gait.
3. Evaluate balance.
4. Perform the caloric irrigation test (to test the oculovestibular reflex): Position the patient with the head of the bed elevated 30 degrees. After checking to ensure an unoccluded ear canal and intact tympanic membrane, irrigate the canal with cold water. In the awake patient, when the pathway from the vestibular portion of CN VIII through the brainstem to CN III and CN VI is intact, the response will consist of slow conjugate eye deviation toward the irrigated ear and then rapid eye movement away from the irrigated ear. The cerebral cortex controls the fast phase. Awake patients may also experience vertigo, nausea, and vomiting.

quickly from side to side while holding open the patient's eyes and noting the direction of eye movement. With intact connections between CN VIII and CN III and VI, the eyes move bilaterally in the opposite direction of the head movement. This is described as "doll's eyes present."

2. Oculovestibular reflex (caloric irrigation test): Tested the same as described for a conscious patient. Conjugate eye deviation toward the irrigated ear indicates that the pathway from the vestibular portion of CN VIII to CN III and VI is intact. (When the cerebral cortex is depressed, the fast eye deviation is lost.)

4. Presence of complaints seen with vestibular dysfunction
5. Imbalance
6. Abnormal oculocephalic reflex: There is no eye movement or the eyes move asymmetrically in response to head rotation
7. Abnormal oculovestibular reflex (showing the brainstem pathways to be impaired): The eyes stay in midposition when the ear is irrigated

---

Glossopharyngeal (IX) and vagus (X)

1. Ask the patient to open his or her mouth and say, "Ahh." Observe for symmetric elevation of the palatal arch and midline uvula.
2. Test for the gag reflex: Stroke the palatal arch with a tongue blade. The palate should elevate, and the patient should have a gag response. This tests the afferent limb of CN IX and the efferent limb of CN X.
3. Appraise articulation and voice quality.
4. Assess the ability to swallow.
5. Evaluate the ability to taste salt and sugar placed on the posterior third of the tongue.

1. Test by evaluating the gag and cough reflexes, usually accomplished by observing the patient's response to suctioning or movement of the endotracheal tube or to direct stimulation of the palatal arch.
2. Evaluate the patient's ability to handle oral secretions by swallowing.

1. Deviation of the uvula to the unaffected side
2. Palate does not rise on the affected side
3. Absent gag reflex
4. Difficulty with vocalization (dysphonia):
   • No voice
   • Hoarseness related to vocal cord paralysis; laryngoscopic examination may be indicated
   • Whisper, nasal-sounding voice indicates soft palate paralysis
5. Difficulty swallowing (dysphagia)
6. Loss of taste sensation on the posterior third of the tongue

Continued

TABLE 4-18

Cranial Nerve Assessment and Anticipated Deficits—cont'd

Cranial Nerve (CN)	Assessment in Conscious Patient	Assessment in Unconscious or Uncooperative Patient	Anticipated Deficit
Spinal accessory (XI)	1. Assess the sternocleidomastoid (SCM) and trapezius muscles for size, symmetry, and spasticity. 2. Ask the patient to turn his or her head to one side. Place one hand on the patient's cheek and the other on the patient's shoulder for stability. Instruct the patient to resist your attempt to forcibly turn the head back to midline. Repeat on other side. 3. Ask the patient to push the head forward against your hand. Assess the strength of both SCM muscles. 4. Ask the patient to shrug his or her shoulders upward against the resistance of your downward pressure on the shoulders. Note the strength of the trapezius muscles.	Not typically assessed in the unconscious patient.	1. Atrophy or spasticity of the SCM or trapezius muscles 2. Weakness or inability to turn or lift the head or shrug the shoulder
Hypoglossal (XII)	1. Inspect the tongue for atrophy or fasciculation with the patient at rest. 2. Have the patient protrude the tongue and assess for alignment and symmetry. 3. Ask the patient to move the tongue to the right and left and then press the tongue against the inside of the cheek while you assess its strength. 4. Note articulation.	Not typically assessed in the unconscious patient.	1. Tongue deviation to the paralyzed side 2. Tongue movement weakness or paralysis 3. Dysarthria

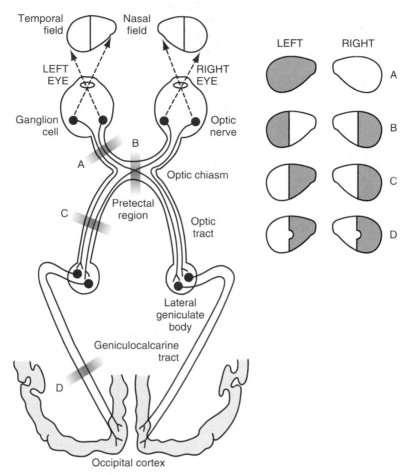

FIGURE 4-22 ■ Visual pathways. Transection of the pathways at the locations indicated by the letters causes the visual field defects shown in the diagrams on the right. Occipital lesions may spare fibers from the macula (as in *D*) because of the separation in the brain of these fibers from the others subserving vision. (From Ganong WF: *Review of medical physiology*, ed 21, New York, 2003, Lange Medical Books/McGraw-Hill, p 153.)

       lesions, spinal cord injury with autonomic dysfunction, and metabolic or toxic encephalopathy.

(2) Respirations: Respiratory dysrhythmias often correlate with lesions at specific locations in the brain, although effects may vary and may be influenced by other factors (Table 4-20)

(3) Pulse and BP

  a) Both are notoriously unreliable parameters in detecting CNS disease or neurologic deterioration. May change late in the course of increased ICP and thus are of limited clinical use.

  b) Cardiac dysrhythmias may be seen with neurologic disorders, particularly with blood in the CSF, after posterior fossa surgery, with increased ICP, or with stroke in certain locations

  c) Tachycardia and hypertension may be seen with injury or compression of the hypothalamus that results in sympathetic nervous system stimulation

■ **TABLE 4-19**
■ ■ **Pupil Abnormalities Associated with Specific Areas of Brain Dysfunction**

Pupil Finding	Related Brain Dysfunction
Small, equal, reactive	Bilateral diencephalic damage that affects the sympathetic innervation originating from the hypothalamus; metabolic dysfunction
Nonreactive, midpositioned	Midbrain damage
Fixed and dilated	Ipsilateral oculomotor (cranial nerve III) compression or injury
Bilateral fixed and dilated	Brain anoxia and ischemia; bilateral cranial nerve III compression
Pinpoint, nonreactive	Pons damage, often from hemorrhage or ischemia that interrupts the sympathetic nervous system pathways
One pupil is smaller that the other, but both reactive to light; associated with ptosis and an inability to sweat on the same side as the smaller pupil (Horner's syndrome)	Interruption of ipsilateral sympathetic innervation that can be caused by a lesion of the anterolateral cervical spinal cord or lateral medulla, damage to the hypothalamus, or occlusion or dissection of the internal carotid artery

    d) Cushing's response occurs when intracranial hypertension causes compression of the medullary vasomotor center. Systolic pressure rises, widens pulse pressure, and may slow pulse.
(4) Pain—the fifth vital sign
    a) Pain that is assessed at regular intervals and treated with the same zeal as abnormalities in other vital signs has a much better chance of being treated effectively (Campbell, 1995)
    b) Key concepts in pain assessment: See Box 4-4

■ **TABLE 4-20**
■ ■ **Respiratory Patterns Associated with Specific Areas of Brain Dysfunction**

Breathing Pattern	Description	Location of Brain Lesion or Type of Dysfunction
Cheyne-Stokes	Regular cycles of respirations that gradually increase in depth to hyperpnea and then decrease in depth to periods of apnea	Usually bilateral lesions deep within the cerebral hemispheres, basal ganglia, or diencephalon; metabolic disorders
Central neurogenic hyperventilation	Deep, rapid respirations	Midbrain, upper pons
Apneustic	Prolonged inspiration followed by a 2- to 3-sec pause; occasionally may alternate with an expiratory pause	Pons
Cluster	Cluster of irregular breaths followed by an apneic period lasting a variable amount of time	Lower pons or upper medulla
Ataxic or irregular	Irregular, unpredictable pattern of shallow and deep respirations and pauses	Medulla

Adapted from McQuillan KA, Mitchell PH: Traumatic brain injuries. In McQuillan KA, Von Rueden KT, Hartsock RL, et al, editors: *Trauma nursing from resuscitation through rehabilitation,* ed 3, St Louis, 2002, Saunders, p 420.

■ **BOX 4-4**
■ **BASIC PAIN ASSESSMENT "PEARLS"**

■ All patients have the right to appropriate assessment and management of pain and should be educated and encouraged to report unrelieved pain.
■ Pain is an individual, subjective sensation. It cannot be proved or disproved.
■ Your attitudes and beliefs about pain can affect the way you treat pain.
■ Pain assessment is conducted and documented as appropriate to the patient's condition.
   1. Include pain intensity, quality, location, pain-related complications, and adverse effects of treatment whenever possible.
   2. Increase assessment frequency during times of inadequately controlled pain.
   3. Obtain a detailed pain assessment, history, and focused physical examination as the patient improves to ensure an accurate diagnosis of pain.
■ Make every effort to obtain the patient's self-report of pain, because this is the most reliable indicator of pain. (Do not assume that a patient cannot provide a self-report without asking.)
   1. Ask simple questions, allow time for response, and repeat or rephrase as needed.
   2. Documenting a simple "yes" or "no" (or nod or shake of head) is acceptable.
■ Assess pain in a patient unable to provide a self-report of pain.
   1. Never assume that a sedated and/or chemically paralyzed patient does not feel pain—medications such as propofol and midazolam do not provide analgesia.
   2. The absence of observable signs does not mean that pain does not exist.
   3. When conditions exist that are known to be painful, assume that pain is present.
■ Reassessment after intervention has taken effect is essential and should include these questions:
   1. How much relief was obtained and how long did it last?
   2. Were there any adverse effects?

    c) Components of pain assessment: See Table 4-21
    d) Adequate pain assessment poses a special challenge in the critically ill patient
    e) Acute pain assessment tools
      1) Pain tools should estimate the severity of pain and accurately reflect changes in pain intensity following interventions
      2) General guidelines for successful use:
        a) Tool should be valid, reliable, and appropriate for the patient's age and cognitive, cultural, developmental, and physical status
        b) Patient and caregivers should be educated on tool use and purpose
        c) Whenever possible, the same tool should be used consistently with a given patient
        d) Whenever possible, a pain tool in the patient's language should be used
      3) Unidimensional tools measure a single element of pain (e.g., intensity). Figure 4-23 shows examples of reliable and valid self-reporting tools for measuring intensity.
        a) Numeric rating scale (NRS)
          i) Either 0 to 5 or 0 to 10 range
          ii) Use horizontally or vertically
          iii) Present verbally or visually

■ **TABLE 4-21**
■ ■ **Components of Pain Assessment**

Component	Sample Questions/Comments
Location and radiation	Where is the pain? Can you point to where you hurt? Does the pain go anywhere else? Consider that there may be more than one location of pain to be assessed
Intensity or severity	Assessed via pain scales, words, gestures See the section on pain assessment in patients who cannot communicate under Patient Assessment
Character or quality	What does the pain "feel" like? Give words to choose from (e.g., sharp, dull, aching, shooting, burning, pins and needles) Description of pain quality helps determine treatment (e.g., neuropathic pain may respond better to adjuvant medications than to opioids)
Timing	When did the pain start? How long did it last? Is it there all the time? Does it come and go?
Alleviating and aggravating factors	What lessens the pain? What makes it worse? Considerations include medications or other remedies, activities, position, foods
Associated factors and symptoms	What else occurs with the pain? Considerations include nausea, vomiting, constipation, confusion, depression
Impact on life and functionality	What can't you do that you'd like to do? What is your expectation of pain relief? Consider the pain's effect on, for example, appetite, sleep, mood, work, home life, hobbies
Relevant medical history	Past surgeries, trauma, coexisting medical conditions, psychiatric illness (e.g., depression) Prior pain experiences Past or current tobacco, drug, or alcohol use Past or present pain management strategies and outcomes (e.g., how much pain relief was obtained, how long did it last) Other medication history

        b) Faces rating scales
          i) Patient selects face
          ii) Often used with other scales
        c) Verbal descriptor scales
          i) Present verbally or visually
          ii) Use words the patient understands
        d) Visual analogue scale (0 to 100): May be difficult for critically ill patients to use
    4) Multidimensional tools measure characteristics and effects of pain on the patient's life. More appropriate with complex pain situations than for critically ill patients. Examples include the following:
        a) Initial Pain Assessment Inventory: Includes a diagram to identify pain location(s)
        b) Brief Pain Inventory: Addresses pain experienced over the preceding 24 hours

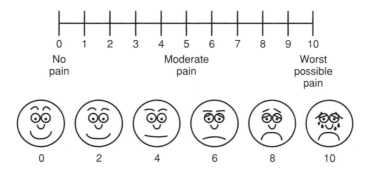

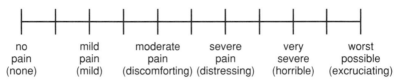

Numerical rating scale (NRS) and Wong-Baker faces scale: Patient indicates number or face that best describes their pain intensity either verbally or by gestures

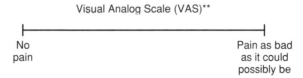

Verbal Descriptor Scale: Patient selects words/phase that best represents their pain intensity

Visual Analog Scale (VAS)**

No pain	Pain as bad as it could possibly be

Visual Analog Scale (VAS): **A 10-cm baseline is recommended
Patient places a mark on the line to represent pain intensity. Measure in millimeters from "no pain" to patient's mark. Score ranges from "0" to "100."

FIGURE 4-23 ■ Pain assessment tools. (Numeric rating scale, Wong-Baker faces scale, and Visual Analog Scale from McCaffery M, Pasero C: *Pain: clinical manual*, ed 2, St Louis, 1999, Mosby, pp 62, 67; faces pain scale modified by McCaffery and Pasero from Whaley LF, Wong DL: *Essentials of pediatric nursing*, St Louis, 1997, Mosby, pp 1215-1216; Verbal Descriptor Scale from Acute Pain Management Guideline Panel: *Acute pain management in adults: operative procedures*, Quick reference guide for clinicians No 1, AHCPR Pub No 92-0019, Rockville, Md, February 1992, Agency for Health Care Policy and Research, Public Health Service, US Department of Health and Human Services, p 116.)

   c) McGill Pain Questionnaire: Looks at sensory, affective, and evaluative dimensions
  f) Pain assessment when the patient cannot communicate
   1) Lack of self-report can lead to undertreatment
   2) When self-report is not possible, assume pain is present based on the presence of a painful condition or procedure (American Pain Society, 2003)
   3) Behavioral and physiologic signs are not always reliable indicators of pain but may be useful to confirm suspicion of pain or evaluate the response to intervention when no alternative exists

        a) Behaviors are often more reliable indicators than physiologic signs

        b) Physiologic signs are temporary, may resolve before pain resolves, and may reflect other phenomena (e.g., anxiety)

     4) Hierarchy of importance of basic measures of pain intensity (criteria are listed in order of reliability) (McCaffery and Pasero, 1999):

        a) Patient's self-report of pain

        b) Pathology (e.g., fractures, incisions)

        c) Behaviors (e.g., grimacing, frowning, wincing) (Table 4-22)

        d) Report of a parent, family member, or other person close to the patient ("proxy pain rating")

        e) Physiologic indices (e.g., increased heart rate, BP) (Table 4-23)

     5) Behavioral pain tools designed for use in critically ill patients require further testing before general use can be recommended (Pasero, 2004a)

        a) If used, evaluate each time a low score is obtained with potentially painful conditions as patients may not be able to demonstrate specific behaviors required for scoring (Pasero, 2004a)

        b) Examples include Behavioral Pain Scale (Payen et al, 2001), Nonverbal Pain Scale (Odhner et al, 2003), Checklist of Nonverbal Pain Indicators (Feldt, 2000)

  b. Monitoring data

     i. ICP monitoring: See specific patient health problems

     ii. Jugular venous oxygen saturation (SjO_2)

       (a) Principle: Assesses the coupling or uncoupling of cerebral oxygen delivery (CBF) and cerebral oxygen consumption (metabolism). Placement of a fiberoptic catheter into the jugular bulb allows for continuous measurement of SjO_2 and intermittent venous blood gas sampling. Reflects a global view of oxygenation in the cerebral hemisphere on the side of catheter placement.

      (b) Clinical uses: May detect episodes of uncoupling between CBF and metabolism indicating cerebral ischemia (CBF is less than the metabolic demand) or hyperemia (CBF exceeds the metabolic demand). Factors that decrease cerebral oxygen supply (i.e., hypoxemia, anemia, insufficient cerebral perfusion) or increase cerebral metabolic demand (e.g., seizures, hyperthermia) lower SjO_2 and can cause ischemia. Factors that increase oxygen supply (i.e., increased CBF, hyperoxia) or reduce cerebral oxygen demand (e.g., large area of cerebral infarction, hypothermia) raise SjO_2 and can cause hyperemia.

       (1) Normal SjO_2 is 55% to 75%; SjO_2 below 55% is indicative of global ischemia and warrants treatment; SjO_2 above 80% indicates hyperemia

       (2) Cerebral extraction of oxygen (CEO_2): Calculated by subtracting SjO_2 from arterial oxygen saturation (SaO_2). Normal = 24% to 40%; lower than 24% indicates hyperemia; higher than 40% indicates cerebral oxygen supply insufficient for demand.

       (3) When venous and arterial blood gas levels are analyzed simultaneously, arteriovenous oxygen difference ($AVDO_2$) can be calculated. Abbreviated formula: $AVDO_2 = 1.34 (SaO_2 - SjO_2)$ hemoglobin/100. Normal $AVDO_2$ is 4.5 to 8.5ml/dl; less than 4.5 ml/dl indicates hyperemia and more than 8.5 ml/dl indicates cerebral oxygen supply insufficient for demand.

■ **TABLE 4-22**
■ ■ **Behaviors Often Associated with Pain in Nonverbal Patients (Pasero, 2004b)**

Category	Behavioral Examples	Comments
Facial expressions	Grimacing, frowning, wincing, wrinkled forehead, eyes either closed or wide open with eyebrows raised, mouth wide open with exposed teeth and tongue, clenched teeth	Grimacing, frowning, and wincing may represent involuntary responses to acute pain and are felt to be valid indicators of acute pain, even in sedated patients (Puntillo, 1997, 2004). Some medical conditions (e.g., Parkinson's disease, stroke, chemical paralysis) may result in distorted or absent facial expressions apart from pain. Eye signals may be used to communicate pain by patients unable to otherwise communicate.
Movement	Restlessness, splinting, guarding, shaking, flailing, fidgeting, rigidity or tenseness, arching, clenching of fists, holding or rubbing of affected area, resistance to movement or care procedures, slow or cautious or no movement, repositioning, rocking, withdrawing	Some patients who are unable to verbally communicate may seek attention to their pain through gestures or other arm and leg movements, or by hitting the bed.
Vocalizations	Verbal complaints of pain, whimpering, crying, groaning, moaning, yelling, screaming, verbal outbursts, protest words (e.g., "Stop," "Don't")	For patients with nonspecific vocalizations (e.g., screaming or yelling) a trial of analgesics should be made rather than relying solely on sedatives and/or anxiolytics.
Other	Agitation, aggression, change in usual activity or behavior, confusion, altered sleep, fatigue	Other conditions besides pain can lead to agitation (e.g., hypoxia, hypercarbia, sepsis).

Summary	All behaviors
	• While self-report of pain is optimal, behaviors may be the only way pain can be communicated in the patient unable to verbalize
	• The degree of behavioral response factors into the degree of pain intensity and distress patients experience (Puntillo et al, 2004)
	• The absence of "pain" behaviors does not mean that the patient is not experiencing pain
		• Pain behaviors are influenced by many factors (e.g., culture, duration of pain, coping skills)
		• Some patients, such as the following, cannot exhibit pain behaviors of any kind:
		  • Sedated or chemically paralyzed patients.
		  • Nonresponsive trauma patients
		  • Comatose patients
		  • Patients sedated for painful procedures
		• Behaviors should be used as only one assessment technique

See chapter text for references.

    (4) Knowledge of uncoupling between cerebral oxygen delivery and demand can prompt implementation of interventions to improve the balance and prevent ischemia or hyperemia (Box 4-5)

  (c) Postprocedure care: After insertion, lateral cervical radiograph confirms location of the catheter tip. Calibrate the continuous Sjo_2 monitor.

■ **TABLE 4-23**
■ ■ **Harmful Effects and Clinical Manifestations of Acute Pain**

Body System	Harmful Effects of Unrelieved Pain	Clinical Manifestations
Endocrine	↑ Catabolic hormones (e.g., adrenocorticotropic hormone, cortisol, catecholamines, antidiuretic and growth hormones, glucagon, renin, angiotensin II, aldosterone); ↓ insulin, testosterone	Alterations in water and electrolyte handling (e.g., decreased urine output, fluid overload, sodium retention, hypokalemia); ↑ demands on various body systems
Metabolic	Gluconeogenesis; glycogenolysis; glucose intolerance; insulin resistance; carbohydrate, fat, and protein catabolism	Hyperglycemia, weight loss, alterations in wound healing, impaired immune function, fever, enhanced tumor development and metastasis
Cardiovascular	Activation of the sympathetic nervous system leading to ↑ cardiac demands; ↓ fibrinolysis Activation of the autonomic nervous system	↑ Heart rate, blood pressure, peripheral vascular resistance, cardiac output, cardiac workload, myocardial oxygen consumption (with possible ischemia, angina and infarction); ↓ blood flow to extremities, hypercoagulability (e.g., ↑ risk for deep venous thrombosis, pulmonary embolism)
	Parasympathetic nervous system activation	↓ Heart rate and blood pressure, atrioventricular block
Respiratory	Alteration in respiratory mechanics: Involuntary spinal reflex response and voluntary reduction of muscle movement in thorax and diaphragm	↑ Respiration rate, ↓ tidal volume, vital capacity, and alveolar ventilation; shunting, hypoxemia, hypercarbia, muscle spasm, grunting noncompliance with ventilator, poor cough, atelectasis, retained secretions, infection
Musculoskeletal	Involuntary reflex motor activity	↑ Muscle tone, spasm, splinting, limitation of movement, rigidity, impaired muscle function (e.g., atrophy, weakness)
Gastrointestinal	↑ Intestinal secretions and smooth muscle sphincter tone; ↓ gastric motility and contractility Activation of the autonomic nervous system	Nausea and vomiting, gastric distention, stasis, ileus, constipation, appetite changes (delayed gastric emptying can also be related to opioids)
Genitourinary	↑ Sphincter activity Activation of the autonomic nervous system	Urinary retention with associated discomfort
Neurologic and skin	Activation of the autonomic nervous system	Dilated pupils, tearing, diaphoresis, pallor, flushing
Cognitive	Negative psychologic and emotional impact	Sleep disturbances, anxiety, depression, confusion

Compiled from Graf C, Puntillo K: Pain in the older adult in the intensive care unit, *Crit Care Clin* 19(4):749-770, 2003; Hamill-Ruth RJ, Marohn ML: Evaluation of pain in the critically ill patient, *Crit Care Clin* 15(1):35-54, 1999; McCaffery M, Pasero C: *Pain: clinical manual,* ed 2, St Louis, 1999, Mosby; Melzack R, Wall PD, editors: *Handbook of pain management,* Edinburgh, 2003, Churchill Livingstone; Pasero C: Pain in the critically ill patient, *J Perianesth Nurs* 18(6):422-425, 2003; and Payen, Olivier, Bosson, et al, 2001.

■ **BOX 4-5**
■ **TREATMENT CONSIDERATIONS FOR IMBALANCE BETWEEN CEREBRAL OXYGEN SUPPLY AND CEREBRAL OXYGEN CONSUMPTION DETECTED WITH Sjo$_2$ MONITORING**

NOTE: Before treating, make sure measured values are accurate.
Ischemia: Cerebral oxygen delivery is insufficient for the cerebral metabolic demand.
- Optimize cerebral perfusion pressure.
- Ensure adequate blood pressure and cardiac output.
- Avoid lowering Paco$_2$ to treat ICP elevations; consider small increases in the Paco$_2$ as tolerated.
- Use other interventions to lower ICP (see Increased Intracranial Pressure under Specific Patient Health Problems).
- Treat factors increasing cerebral metabolic demand (e.g., seizures, fever).
- Ensure adequate oxygenation.

Hyperemia: Cerebral oxygen delivery is excessive for the cerebral metabolic demand.
- Consider lowering Paco$_2$ to reduce ICP if necessary.
- Raise the head of the bed unless contraindicated.

ICP, Intracranial pressure; *Paco$_2$*, partial pressure of arterial carbon dioxide; *Sjo$_2$*, jugular venous oxygen saturation.

Because readings may be inaccurate due to poor catheter position or improper calibration, a strategy for troubleshooting any abnormal value should be established. Potential complications include infection, bleeding, vascular injury, and thrombosis.

  iii. Partial pressure of brain tissue oxygen (Pbto$_2$)
    (a) Principle: Oxygen-sensing probe inserted into brain parenchyma continuously monitors Pbto$_2$ around the tip. Provides data regarding the balance between oxygen delivery to the cerebral extracellular space and oxygen consumption by cerebral tissue.
    (b) Clinical uses: Normal Pbto$_2$ varies depending on the brand of monitor used. Depth and duration of low Pbto$_2$ correlate with a poorer outcome from brain injury. When cerebral hypoxia is recognized, interventions to improve cerebral oxygen delivery and minimize cerebral oxygen consumption can be instituted (Box 4-6). Use of the device may be beneficial for patients with severe traumatic brain injury (TBI), stroke, tumor, or subarachnoid hemorrhage.
    (c) Postprocedure care: Observe for potential complications, including infection, hemorrhage
  iv. Near-infrared cerebral spectroscopy
    (a) Principle: Sensor placed on the scalp emits near-infrared light that penetrates the scalp and skull to measure oxygen saturation in underlying brain tissue
    (b) Clinical uses: Normal values are ill-defined but changes in trends may indicate alterations in regional cerebral oxygen saturation. Measurements may be unreliable due to stray light, sensor disruption, drift, movement artifact, temperature changes, or contamination from extracranial circulation.
    (c) Postprocedure care: No special care
  v. Continuous electroencephalographic (EEG) monitoring
    (a) Principle: Continuously monitors electrical activity of the brain by means of electrodes attached to the scalp

■ **BOX 4-6**
■ **TREATMENT CONSIDERATIONS FOR LOW Pbto$_2$**

IF ICP IS HIGHER THAN 20 mm Hg
1. Implement interventions to minimize ICP and optimize CPP (see Increased Intracranial Pressure under Specific Patient Health Problems).
   ● Avoid lowering Paco$_2$, which may further impair cerebral oxygen delivery. Consider small increases in Paco$_2$ as tolerated based on ICP.
   ● Instead, use other interventions to lower ICP.
2. Ensure a patent airway. (Perform suctioning if necessary.)
3. Increase Flo$_2$ for 5 to 15 minutes.
4. If Pbto$_2$ is unresponsive, try increasing CPP.

IF ICP IS LOWER THAN 20 mm Hg
1. Increase Paco$_2$ to 40 to 45 mm Hg as tolerated based on ICP.
2. Increase Flo$_2$ for 5 to 15 minutes.
3. Evaluate and optimize the patient's hemodynamic and respiratory status.
   ● Ensure a patent airway. (Perform suctioning if necessary.)
   ● Check ventilator settings and manipulate to optimize respiratory gas exchange.
   ● Ensure euvolemia.
   ● Consider transfusion if the hematocrit is lower than 33%.
   ● Implement interventions to optimize cardiac output.
   ● If fluid overload or pulmonary edema is present, treat as prescribed.
4. Ensure normothermia.

CPP, Cerebral perfusion pressure; *Flo$_2$*, fraction of inspired oxygen; *ICP*, intracranial pressure; *Paco$_2$*, partial pressure of carbon dioxide; *Pbto$_2$*, brain tissue partial pressure of oxygen.

    (b) Clinical uses: Identifies the onset of seizures or cerebral ischemia so appropriate interventions can be initiated. Monitors burst activity in patients in drug-induced coma for refractory increased ICP so that the minimal amount of barbiturate or propofol to achieve the desired burst suppression is administered.

    (c) Care during procedure: Move the patient carefully to avoid dislodging the electrodes; EEG readings are influenced by electrical, environmental, movement, and biologic artifacts

  vi. Transcranial Doppler ultrasonography (TCD)

    (a) Principle: Probe positioned over thin areas of the cranium emits a low-frequency pulsed ultrasonic signal to measure the direction and velocity of blood flow through underlying major vessels

    (b) Clinical uses: High velocities correlate with cerebral vasospasm or hyperemia. If middle cerebral artery (MCA) velocity is higher than 120 cm/sec, the ratio of MCA to internal carotid artery (ICA) velocity can be calculated. A ratio of 3 or higher indicates cerebral vasospasm and less than 3 suggests hyperemia. Can detect emboli, stenotic or occluded vessels, and other vascular anomalies. May reveal blood flow alterations indicating ICP elevations. May also be used to evaluate cerebral autoregulation and as a confirmatory test of brain death.

      (1) Advantages: Noninvasive, portable, relatively inexpensive, can be safely repeated often or used continuously to monitor changes

      (2) Disadvantages: Absolute velocities vary depending on many factors—age, hematocrit, Paco$_2$, cardiac output, and the metabolic

activity of the brain tissue supplied by the artery being insonated. Difficult to distinguish anatomic variations of arteries from arterial disease; does not detect bilaterally symmetric disease, long regions of vasoconstriction or stenosis, or distal artery disease.

    (c) Preprocedure and postprocedure care: No specific care required; no known complications

  vii. Continuous CBF monitoring

    (a) Principle: Sensor placed on the surface of the brain continuously measures regional CBF

      (1) Thermal diffusion flowmetry: Temperature variation between two plates on a brain surface sensor provides an inverse measure proportional to CBF

      (2) Laser Doppler flowmetry: Laser Doppler probe positioned on the brain surface or in the parenchyma measures CBF

    (b) Clinical uses: Provides a continuous measure of regional CBF that can be used to evaluate autoregulation and detect local brain ischemia. Can guide therapy to avoid brain ischemia.

    (c) Postprocedure care: Observe for potential complications, including infection or CSF leakage. Troubleshoot abnormal values; data may be unreliable if the probe loses contact with the brain surface or comes in contact with large blood vessels. Alterations in hematocrit, strong external light, or probe movement artifact can influence laser Doppler measurements.

3. **Appraisal of patient characteristics:** Patients with acute, life-threatening neurologic problems enter critical care units with a wide range of clinical characteristics. During their stay, their clinical status may slowly or abruptly improve or deteriorate. Changes in the patient's condition may involve one or all life sustaining functions, and functions can be easy or nearly impossible to monitor with precision. Examples of clinical attributes that the nurse should assess when caring for a patient with an acute neurologic disorder are the following:

  a. Resiliency

    i. Level 1—*Minimally resilient:* A frail, 84-year-old female, hit by a car 10 days earlier, who suffered a complete transection of the spinal cord at the C4-C5 level and has developed respiratory and renal failure

    ii. Level 3—*Moderately resilient:* A 35-year-old woman being treated for Guillain-Barré syndrome who has required ventilator support for the past 7 days. She now has a low-grade fever, elevated white blood cell (WBC) levels, and purulent sputum.

    iii. Level 5—*Highly resilient:* An otherwise healthy, alert, and oriented 17-year-old male complaining of nausea who has been admitted for overnight monitoring following a concussion sustained while playing football

  b. Vulnerability

    i. Level 1—*Highly vulnerable:* A 41-year-old college professor diagnosed with a fast-growing, invasive grade IV glioblastoma 3 months earlier is admitted from the oncology clinic, where he suddenly became unresponsive during a chemotherapy session

    ii. Level 3—*Moderately vulnerable:* A 37-year-old electrician admitted directly from the emergency department following a grand mal seizure preceded by complaints of severe headache and confusion who has been diagnosed with an arteriovenous malformation (AVM). He is awaiting further diagnostic studies and intervention for the lesion.

iii. Level 5—*Minimally vulnerable:* A 23-year-old female rugby player who is alert and oriented 2 days after evacuation of a small epidural hematoma

c. Stability

    i. Level 1—*Minimally stable:* A 32-year-old male who suffered a severe brain injury and bilateral pulmonary contusions 2 days earlier in a motor vehicle crash. He is now having problems with increased ICP above 25 mm Hg that is unresponsive to therapy and respiratory failure requiring increasing ventilator support.

    ii. Level 3—*Moderately stable:* A 50-year-old woman 1 week after a subarachnoid hemorrhage (SAH) and aneurysm clipping who has developed a pronator drift secondary to vasospasm that resolves with hypertensive, hypervolemic therapy

    iii. Level 5—*Highly stable*: A 16-year-old boy who fell off the back of a truck and hit his head, suffering a traumatic SAH. He was unconscious for 15 minutes and confused for 24 hours but is now awake and neurologically intact.

d. Complexity

    i. Level 1—*Highly complex:* A 17-year-old boy who jumped off a third-floor balcony while intoxicated and suffered a C4-C5 subluxation with complete spinal cord injury. He is in neurogenic shock, has a temperature of 93° F (33.9° C), has an ileus, and requires increasing ventilator support.

    ii. Level 3—*Moderately complex:* A 60-year-old diabetic woman with a hemorrhagic hypertensive stroke who develops hydrocephalus

    iii. Level 5—*Minimally complex:* A 40-year-old woman with a 1-cm meningioma resected 2 days earlier who is anxious to go home

e. Resource availability

    i. Level 1—*Few resources:* A 59-year-old homeless man found in a vacant lot with an alcohol level of 320 mg% and an acute on chronic subdural hematoma. Two days after admission, his GCS score is 6 while he is intubated.

    ii. Level 3—*Moderate resources:* A 30-year-old schoolteacher with a small right parietal AVM that hemorrhaged 1 week earlier who is now neurologically intact. She is not married and has no family in the area, but a close friend has been visiting. She is insured and is a candidate for outpatient focused-beam radiation therapy.

    iii. Level 5—*Many resources:* A 35-year-old woman who suffered moderate TBI 5 days earlier and has a right hemiparesis and expressive aphasia that will require in-patient rehabilitation. She is married, has insurance, and has two sisters and parents who live near her.

f. Participation in care

    i. Level 1—*No participation:* A 28-year-old transient worker with no known family in the United States who is comatose and areflexic subsequent to massive head and neck trauma suffered in an automobile crash today

    ii. Level 3—*Moderate level of participation:* A non–English-speaking 76-year-old, newly diagnosed with diabetes, who will be discharged home tomorrow and has moderate expressive dysphasia and right hemiparesis following an ischemic stroke. The patient's primary support person at home is a daughter who works as a nursing assistant and speaks some English.

    iii. Level 5—*Full participation:* A 56-year-old high school teacher who developed acute neurologic deterioration due to infectious meningitis contracted from a student and who is now fully alert and cooperative, recovering rapidly, and planning the details of her home care with the help of her daughter, an agency nurse

g. Participation in decision making

    i. Level 1—*No participation:* A 55-year-old man who had a compressor explode in his face at work 1 week earlier and who has a GCS score of 4 while intubated

    ii. Level 3—*Moderate level of participation:* A 46-year-old woman with an anterior communicating artery aneurysm that ruptured 19 days earlier who has moderate vasospasm and is lethargic but is otherwise neurologically intact

    iii. Level 5—*Full participation:* A 45-year-old college professor who just had surgery for a right hemisphere glioblastoma, has CN VII paresis, and had three seizures but is otherwise neurologically intact. He has asked about experimental research protocols available to him.

h. Predictability

    i. Level 1—*Not predictable:* A 60-year-old woman who is transferred from an outside hospital with an anterior communicating artery aneurysm and grade III SAH suffered 5 days earlier. She is having vasospasm and has developed hydrocephalus. Her aneurysm has not been clipped.

    ii. Level 3—*Moderately predictable:* An 18-year-old high school senior who suffered TBI 3 days earlier and is beginning to localize in response to noxious stimuli. His ICP varies from 10 to 25 mm Hg and is controlled with CSF drainage and sedation.

    iii. Level 5—*Highly predictable:* A 25-year-old woman who suffered a linear skull fracture and brain injury 1 week earlier and is now fully awake, alert, and cooperative

4. Diagnostic studies

  a. Laboratory

    i. Complete blood count (CBC) and differential

    ii. Blood glucose level

    iii. Blood chemistry tests, including osmolality, electrolyte levels

    iv. Clotting profile, including prothrombin time (PT), international normalized ratio (INR), partial thromboplastin time (PTT), d-dimer levels, fibrinogen levels

    v. Arterial blood gas (ABG) levels

    vi. Toxicology screen

    vii. Urinalysis

    viii. CSF analysis: Compare with normal values and request a culture and sensitivity test

  b. Radiologic

    i. Skull series: In the absence of computed tomographic (CT) scans, skull radiographs may be useful in diagnosing skull abnormalities (e.g., fractures, erosion), noting shift of the pineal gland, and detecting intracranial air or abnormal calcifications

    ii. Spine series: Assesses vertebral integrity and alignment to diagnose fractures, dislocations, bony defects, or degenerative processes; CT (Box 4-7) or magnetic resonance imaging (MRI) (Box 4-8 and Table 4-24) often used to further delineate abnormalities

    iii. CT scan (see Box 4-7)

    iv. Perfusion CT (see Box 4-7)

    v. Myelography

      (a) Principle: Radiographic examination of the spinal canal after a radiopaque substance is injected into the subarachnoid space (usually in the lumbar area or occasionally at C1-C2)

■ **BOX 4-7**
■ **COMPUTED TOMOGRAPHIC STUDIES**

COMPUTED TOMOGRAPHY (CT)
TECHNIQUE
- X-ray beam is projected through narrow section of brain or spine; detectors at opposite side measure attenuation of radiation after it passes through tissues. Readings are fed into a computer that derives absorption of x-rays by tissues in path of beam. Computer-generated images are printed as serial thin slices of adjacent anatomy.
- Hyperdense tissue (e.g., bone) absorbs more x-rays and appears whiter on final image. Hypodense features (e.g., air, fluid) absorb fewer x-rays and appear darker.
- Scan may be repeated after patient has received intravenous (IV) contrast agent to delineate vasculature and enhance tissues where there is disruption of blood-brain barrier.

CLINICAL USES
- Brain: Valuable in detection of intracranial hemorrhage, especially subarachnoid hemorrhage, cerebral edema, contusions, hydrocephalus, larger mass lesions, and evidence of probable increased intracranial pressure. Bone windows provide exquisite detail of skull architecture. Limitations include poor visibility of posterior fossa, base of brain and brainstem.
- Spine: Provides clear look at bony structures to better visualize vertebral fractures, dislocations, degenerative changes, canal stenosis, congenital abnormalities, and surgical fixation; may identify mass lesions.
- CT angiogram: Postcontrast CT scan reconstructed to outline cerebral vasculature. Useful in screening for vascular lesions (e.g., aneurysm, arteriovenous malformation). Sometimes helpful in delineating architecture of aneurysm prior to surgical clipping or endovascular intervention.

PREPROCEDURE AND POSTPROCEDURE CARE
- Agitated patients may require sedation to optimize image quality.
- If contrast enhancement used, assess for allergy to contrast medium, secure informed consent. Patients with renal insufficiency are at risk for contrast-induced nephropathy (see Chapter 5 for interventions to reduce risk of contrast-induced nephropathy).

PERFUSION COMPUTED TOMOGRAPHY
TECHNIQUE
- CT scan performed during IV bolus administration of iodinated contrast material
- Computer calculations provide measures of regional cerebral blood volume, mean transit time, and regional cerebral blood flow.

CLINICAL USES
- Used in acute stroke and other cerebrovascular diseases to identify infarcted and marginally perfused areas.

PREPROCEDURE AND POSTPROCEDURE CARE
- Same as for computed tomography.

    (b) Clinical use: To detect spinal cord or nerve root compression; diagnose obstructions to contrast flow (e.g., intervertebral disk herniation, spinal cord tumors or stenosis, vertebral displacement)

    (c) Preprocedure and postprocedure care: Avoid contrast-induced nephropathy. Prior to study, ensure that coagulation parameters are within normal limits; discontinue medications that lower the seizure threshold (e.g., phenothiazides). After the procedure, keep the head of the bed elevated at least 30 to 45 degrees to prevent upward migration of the contrast agent (causes headache and seizures).

      vi. Cerebral angiography

        (a) Principle: Contrast material is injected into the vertebral and carotid arteries to enable radiographic visualization of the intracranial and extracranial vasculature

        (b) Clinical uses: Diagnosis of vascular abnormalities such as aneurysms, AVMs, vasospasm, thrombosis, or occlusion, as well as cerebral vasculitis and vascular tumors. Aids diagnosis of other intracranial abnormalities that cause stretching, displacement, or altered diameter of vessels. Evaluates collateral circulation.

        (c) Preprocedure and postprocedure care: Obtain consent. Patient may be premedicated and should be well hydrated. Avoid contrast-induced nephropathy. BP should be controlled and coagulation parameters within an acceptable range. After the procedure observe for potential complications: Reaction to contrast medium, stroke, vascular damage, thrombosis, seizures, transient or permanent neurologic dysfunction, carotid sinus sensitivity, circulatory insufficiency of the catheterized extremity, bleeding or hematoma at the injection site. Following the application of direct manual pressure, a pressure dressing or ice may be applied to the catheter insertion site.

     vii. Spinal angiography: Used to diagnose the source of bleeding, vessel injuries, and vascular abnormalities (e.g., AVMs) in or around the spinal cord. See the description of cerebral angiography earlier for further information.

    viii. Digital subtraction angiography

        (a) Principle: Fluoroscopic images are taken before and after the intravenous (IV) (occasionally intraarterial) administration of radiographic contrast material; computer digitally subtracts the initial (precontrast) image from the later (postcontrast) image to enhance visualization of cerebral vessels.

        (b) Clinical uses: Aids diagnosis of occlusive vascular disease, vascular abnormalities (e.g., aneurysm, AVM), vessel injury, and tumors. Evaluates vascular surgical repair (e.g., aneurysm clipping). Potentially safer, less invasive, and cheaper, and requires less contrast material than regular angiography.

        (c) Preprocedure and postprocedure care: Patient may require sedation to lie still during study. After the procedure, observe for unlikely potential complications: Reaction to the contrast medium, stroke, hemorrhage, and thrombosis.

      ix. Nuclear medicine studies (Box 4-9)

        (a) Radioisotope brain scan

        (b) Single photon emission tomography (SPECT)

        (c) Positron emission tomography (PET)

  c. Electrophysiologic (Box 4-9)

     i. Electromyography

    ii. Nerve conduction velocity

   iii. EEG

    iv. Evoked potentials

  d. Lumbar puncture

     i. Principle: Needle placed into the subarachnoid space below the conus medullaris, usually at L4-L5 interspace

    ii. Clinical uses

        (a) Obtain CSF for laboratory examination

        (b) Measure or reduce CSF pressure

■ **BOX 4-8**
■ **MAGNETIC RESONANCE IMAGING**

TECHNIQUE
- Magnetic fields and radiofrequency waves create signals that generate an image.
- Factors that contribute to image can be manipulated to emphasize different characteristics of normal and abnormal tissue.
- Gadolinium, a contrast agent, may be used to enhance some lesions.

CLINICAL USES
- Brain: Tissue contrast resolution is superior to that of computed tomography (CT); MRI generally better detects contusions, tumors, infection, edema, subacute and chronic hemorrhage, ischemia or infarction, vascular abnormalities, and degenerative diseases. Better visualizes tissues in posterior fossa, basilar skull, and brainstem; better differentiates gray and white matter. Gadolinium enhances areas of increased vascularity or blood-brain barrier disruption.
- Spine: MRI is far superior to CT in visualizing soft tissues and defining lesions such as cysts, vascular abnormalities, contusions, tumors, edema, hemorrhage, ischemia or infarction of spinal cord, and degenerative processes (e.g., disk disease, stenosis).

PREPROCEDURE AND POSTPROCEDURE CARE
- All metal objects must be removed from patient prior to scanning.
- MRI is contraindicated in patients with metallic implants such as cardiac pacemakers or ferromagnetic aneurysm clips. MRI safety guidelines recommended for other implanted devices must be followed.
- Patient must be able to tolerate removal from metallic life-support devices (i.e., ventilator, intravenous infusion pump) or nonmetallic alternatives may be used during the study.
- Inform patient that he or she will need to lie very still, will be in a small, confined space, and will hear a loud, clunking noise. Patient may need sedation if claustrophobic or agitated.
- No specific postprocedure care or complications.

See Table 4-24 for other MRI technology.

■ **TABLE 4-24**
■ ■ **Some Types of Magnetic Resonance Imaging (MRI) Technology and Their Clinical Uses**

MRI Technology	Clinical Uses
Diffusion-weighted imaging	Detects small movements of water; visualizes acute ischemic lesions and cytotoxic edema
	Enables immediate assessment of stroke-related vasospasm and neurovascular changes
	Differentiates acute from chronic lesions and irreversible from reversible infarction
Fluid-attenuated inversion recovery (FLAIR) imaging	Suppresses signals from certain fluids, such as cerebrospinal fluid, and provides a high signal for brain tissue lesions
	Superior capability in detecting hemorrhage, stroke, infections and white matter lesions that abut the ventricles
Echoplanar imaging	Uses ultrafast imaging technology to assist with diagnosis of quickly evolving disease processes
Functional MRI	Detects changes in the brain's oxygen consumption and blood flow in response to sensory stimuli or performance of a motor activity
	Provides functional data in addition to anatomical information for brain mapping and identifying disease
Magnetic resonance spectroscopy	Provides neurochemical data related to tissue metabolism, including brain pH, levels of metabolites and some neurotransmitters
	May aid in determining tumor malignancy, differentiating tumors from other brain lesions, and locating epileptogenic foci

Continued

Magnetic resonance angiography (MRA)/ magnetic resonance venography (MRV)	Flowing blood affects radiofrequency signals emitted during MRI and these effects are manipulated to create an image of the cerebral and extracranial vasculature; less risk-prone alternative to cerebral angiography, although not as sensitive
	Used for visualizing larger vessels, screening neck vessels for abnormalities (although it typically overemphasizes degree of stenosis), evaluating patency of major veins and venous sinuses, and identifying vascular malformations (e.g., aneurysms)
Diffusion tensor imaging (DTI)	Measures diffusion of water in the brain tissue to enable visualization of anatomic substructures, particularly white matter fiber tracts
	Can detect disruption or damage to white matter tracts from injury/disease

---

■ BOX 4-9
■ NUCLEAR MEDICINE AND ELECTROPHYSIOLOGIC STUDIES

NUCLEAR MEDICINE STUDIES
RADIOISOTOPE BRAIN SCAN
TECHNIQUE
- Radioactive substance introduced into blood prior to brain scanning.
- In some disorders, radioisotope accumulates in abnormal areas of brain, probably owing to blood-brain barrier breakdown or increased vascularity of lesion.

CLINICAL USES
- Used to screen for brain tumors and evaluate cerebrovascular disease, some infectious processes.

PREPROCEDURE AND POSTPROCEDURE CARE
- Radioisotope injected at varying time intervals prior to scanning. Agitated patients may require sedation.

SINGLE PHOTON EMISSION TOMOGRAPHY (SPECT)
PRINCIPLE
- Rotating gamma camera system detects disintegration of single-photon-emitting radioisotopes, such as technetium-99m, thallium-201, iodine-123, or hexamethylpropyleneamine oxime (HMPAO), administered to patient.
- Delineates regional brain perfusion because tracer distribution depends on blood flow.

CLINICAL USES
- Adjunct measurement or a primary modality if other blood flow techniques not available.
- May be used to detect tumors or seizure foci or to determine effects of stroke or brain injury.

PREPROCEDURE AND POSTPROCEDURE CARE
- Radioisotope may be administered at varying times prior to scanning. Patient must lie still during study.

POSITRON EMISSION TOMOGRAPHY (PET)
PRINCIPLE
- Positron-emitting radiopharmaceuticals of C, F, N, or O_2 administered and gamma rays emitted are recorded by pairs of detectors around head.
- Provides high-sensitivity quantitative measurements of regional cerebral blood flow, oxygen metabolism, glucose uptake and metabolism, and blood volume.

CLINICAL USES
- Identifies abnormalities in brain's functional metabolism that precede structural alterations associated with disease.
- Provides information about seizures, tumors, neurodegenerative disease, cerebrovascular disease, and brain injury. Limited availability due to expense of equipment.

PREPROCEDURE AND POSTPROCEDURE CARE
- Patient should take nothing by mouth for prescribed period before testing.
- Study may last over 1 hour and requires patient to lie still.

Continued

■ **BOX 4-9**
■ **NUCLEAR MEDICINE AND ELECTROPHYSIOLOGIC STUDIES—cont'd**

ELECTROPHYSIOLOGIC STUDIES
ELECTROMYOGRAPHY (EMG)
PRINCIPLE

■ Needle electrodes inserted into skeletal muscle record electrical potentials from resting and contracting muscle fibers and display them on oscilloscope.

CLINICAL USES

■ Aids in diagnosis of lower motor neuron disease, neuromuscular junction, and muscle disorders.
■ Differentiates lesions of muscles, peripheral nerves, and anterior horn cells.

PREPROCEDURE AND POSTPROCEDURE CARE

■ No risk to patient, although needle electrodes are uncomfortable.
■ Muscle damage from needle electrodes may elevate creatine phosphokinase level postprocedure.

NERVE CONDUCTION VELOCITY (NCV)
PRINCIPLE

■ Large motor nerve stimulated at two or more locations; response is measured in muscle innervated by that nerve. Nerve conduction velocity and amplitude of muscle response can be determined.
■ Pure sensory fiber may be stimulated and response recorded along course of same nerve.

CLINICAL USE

■ Diagnoses peripheral neuropathies and nerve compression or trauma.

PREPROCEDURE AND POSTPROCEDURE CARE

■ No risk to patient, although needle electrodes are uncomfortable.

ELECTROENCEPHALOGRAPHY (EEG)
PRINCIPLE

■ Electrodes attached to scalp are used to record electrical activity of brain.
■ Amplitude, frequency, and characteristics of brain electrical impulses are evaluated.

CLINICAL USES

■ Most helpful in diagnosis of seizures.
■ May detect changes associated with space-occupying lesions, infectious processes, dementia, drug intoxication, or brain injury.
■ May be used to verify absence of electrocerebral activity to support diagnosis of brain death.

PREPROCEDURE AND POSTPROCEDURE CARE

■ Preprocedure care varies, depending on the institution and type of EEG. Verify whether certain medications should be withheld from patient.
■ Postprocedure: Wash conductive paste from hair. No risks.

EVOKED POTENTIALS (EPs)
PRINCIPLE

■ Electrodes are placed on scalp in locations appropriate for type of evoked response (potential) tested: Brainstem auditory evoked response (BAER), visual evoked response (VER), or somatosensory evoked response (SER).
■ Stimulus is applied (e.g., clicking noise for BAER, strobe light or pattern shift for VER, and electrical stimulation of a peripheral nerve for SER) and evoked responses are measured and recorded by computer, which calculates an average curve. Evoked potential latencies and amplitudes are compared with normal responses and compared for the two sides of the body.

CLINICAL USES

■ Evaluates functional integrity of sensory pathways.
■ BAER is useful in determining brainstem function.

Continued

- VER is useful index of hemispheric function; helps diagnose optic nerve disorders.
- SER may demonstrate lesions of peripheral pathways, spinal cord, or brainstem.
- May aid in detecting lesions, disease, or injury that affects specific sensory path.
- Useful in determining prognosis in severe head injury.
- May be used during intracranial or spinal surgery to monitor patient's response to procedure.

PREPROCEDURE AND POSTPROCEDURE CARE
- No specific care needed.

    (c) Administer medication
    (d) Prepare for other diagnostic studies (e.g., myelography)
  iii. Preprocedure and postprocedure care
    (a) Contraindicated with coagulopathies; extreme caution must be used with increased ICP, because CSF removal may lead to brainstem herniation
    (b) Patients should increase fluid intake and lie flat for a few hours after the procedure
    (c) Potential complications: Infection, headache, backache, temporary voiding difficulties
    (d) Postprocedure CSF leak may require a "blood patch" (small volume of the patient's blood is slowly injected into the epidural space, where it congeals and seals the leak) or in rare cases surgical repair

  e. Brain biopsy
    i. Purpose: Tissue is removed from the brain for histologic evaluation. May be guided by CT scan; stereotactic methods frequently used.
    ii. Clinical uses: Can diagnose tumors, certain degenerative diseases, infections, and inflammatory processes
    iii. Preprocedure and postprocedure care: Ensure that consent is obtained. After the procedure observe for neurologic changes, hemorrhage, and infection.

Patient Care

1. **Inability to establish or maintain a patent airway** secondary to decreased LOC or impaired protective airway reflexes (e.g., gag, cough, swallow): See Chapter 2
2. **Impaired respiratory gas exchange** related to respiratory muscle weakness or paralysis, cerebral pathology, or associated neurologic deficits: See Chapter 2
3. **Myocardial repolarization abnormalities, cardiac arrhythmias** due to ANS disruption or catecholamine release: See Chapter 3
4. **Fluid and electrolyte imbalance associated with intracranial pathology** secondary to inadequate fluid intake, use of diuretics (to treat ICP), ADH imbalance, or onset of cerebral salt wasting
  a. Description of problem: May occur with
    i. Diabetes insipidus: Intracranial pathologic condition affecting hypothalamic or posterior pituitary system can impede or stop the production or secretion of ADH, causing diabetes insipidus (Table 4-25). Also see Chapter 6.
    ii. Syndrome of inappropriate secretion of antidiuretic hormone (SIADH): CNS pathology impairs feedback mechanism responsible for ADH suppression (see Table 4-25 and Chapter 6)
    iii. Cerebral salt wasting: Excessive Na^+ excretion with subsequent diuresis may be associated with acute CNS disease. Thought to be caused, at least in part, by impaired Na^+ reabsorption from the proximal tubules due to an increase in circulating natriuretic peptides (one of which is produced in the brain). Effects of natriuretic factors include vasodilation, natriuresis, diuresis, and suppression of the renin–angiotensin II–aldosterone axis. Brain natriuretic peptide has been found in the hypothalamus; edema or

■ **TABLE 4-25**

■ ■ **Manifestations and Treatment of Neurogenic Diabetes Insipidus, Syndrome of Inappropriate Secretion of Antidiuretic Hormone (SIADH), and Cerebral Salt Wasting**

Parameter	Diabetes Insipidus	SIADH	Cerebral Salt Wasting
Urine specific gravity	Low	Elevated	Elevated
Urine osmolality	Low	Increased	Increased
Urine sodium level	Low in relation to serum	Elevated	Elevated
Serum osmolality	Elevated	Decreased	Decreased
Serum sodium level	Elevated	Decreased	Decreased
Clinical manifestations	Hypovolemia, dehydration Intensive thirst (if mechanism is not impaired) Large volumes of poorly concentrated urine Urine osmolality increase of 9% or more in response to administration of aqueous pitressin	Euvolemia or hypervolemia Usually low urine output, low blood urea nitrogen (BUN) level Muscle cramps, weight gain without edema, lethargy, confusion, personality change, irritability, sluggish deep tendon reflexes, nausea and vomiting, diarrhea, abdominal cramps, fatigue, headache, restlessness Severe signs: Coma, seizures, death	Hypovolemia, dehydration Increased BUN levels, high urine output, net sodium loss
Treatment	Administer fluid to replace urine output and insensible losses Administer exogenous antidiuretic hormone (ADH): • Aqueous pitressin—often used in critical phase • Pitressin tannate in oil • 1-Deamino-8-D-arginine vasopressin (dDAVP, desmopressin) • Nasal lysine vasopressin	Restrict fluids For severe symptoms: • Give hypertonic saline solution • Diurese with furosemide • Give demeclocycline hydrochloride to produce renal resistance to ADH	Replete salt and fluid volume Give fludrocortisone acetate to increase renal tubule sodium reabsorption

Adapted from McQuillan KA, Mitchell PH: Traumatic brain injuries. In McQuillan KA, Von Rueden KT, Hartsock RL, et al, editors: *Trauma nursing from resuscitation through rehabilitation*, ed 3, St Louis, 2002, Saunders, p 445.

infarction of the hypothalamus may trigger its release. Increased sympathetic nervous system activity related to brain injury may also contribute to renal Na^+ excretion (see Table 4-25).

    b. Goals of care

        i. Vital signs and neurologic status remain stable

        ii. Electrolyte levels, osmolality, and intravascular volume are maintained within the desired ranges

    c. Collaborating professionals on health care team

        i. Nurse

        ii. Physician

        iii. Laboratory personnel

    d. Interventions (see also Chapters 5 and 6)

        i. Monitor vital signs, neurologic status, input and output, and hemodynamics at least hourly until condition is stable

        ii. Monitor serum and urine electrolyte levels, osmolality, fluid balance, and daily weight; report abnormal values

        iii. Provide prescribed fluid and electrolyte replacements and pharmacologic agents to correct imbalances (see Table 4-25)

    e. Evaluation of patient care

        i. Vital signs, neurologic status, and fluid and electrolyte balance are maintained within the desired ranges

        ii. Urine output is maintained above 30 ml/hr

5. Infection related to invasive lines, monitoring and therapeutic devices, and traumatic and surgical wounds: See Chapter 9

6. Seizures: See Seizures under Specific Patient Health Problems

7. Potential for gastrointestinal ulceration and bleeding secondary to ANS disruption, stress, lack of enteral nutrition, possible steroid use: See Chapter 8

8. Dysphagia

    a. Description of problem: Dysphagia can occur secondary to dysfunction of the muscles used for mastication and swallowing or to deficits in CN V, VII, IX, X, XI, and XII involved in swallowing. May lead to aspiration and inadequate oral food intake.

    b. Goals of care

        i. Nutritional and fluid intake are adequate

        ii. No aspiration occurs

    c. Collaborating professionals on health care team

        i. Nurse

        ii. Physician

        iii. Speech therapist

        iv. Nutritional specialist

    d. Interventions

        i. Involve a nutrition specialist to identify the patient's caloric needs and the best diet to achieve nutritional goals

        ii. Insure that swallow function is intact prior to starting oral food intake

        iii. If dysphagia is present, have a speech therapist evaluate swallowing and recommend food consistency and feeding techniques to minimize aspiration risk

        iv. Until dysphagia resolves, provide feedings via a nonoral route. In the acute phase, a gastric or postpyloric feeding tube may be used. If dysphagia is likely to persist, a feeding tube may be inserted surgically.

        v. Take precautions to avoid aspiration (also see Chapters 2 and 8)

            (a) Keep suction readily available

      (b) Elevate the head of the bed at least 30 degrees unless contraindicated; discontinue tube feedings if head-down position needed

      (c) Secure the feeding tube to prevent dislodgement

      (d) Regularly assess for proper feeding tube placement

      (e) Evaluate tube feed residuals. If residuals exceed a predetermined volume, withhold tube feedings.

      (f) During oral feeding: Have the patient sit up with the head forward; place food on the unaffected side of the oral cavity; encourage small mouthfuls and thorough chewing; ensure that the mouth is clear of food after each bite; do not leave the patient unattended while the patient is eating

  e. Evaluation of patient care

    i. Patient receives adequate nutrition and hydration

    ii. Aspiration is prevented

9. Pain

  a. Description of problem

    i. Overview

      (a) Pain is a subjective perception consisting of complex sensory, emotional, and cognitive elements

      (b) Because most critically ill patients experience continuous pain related to their condition or treatments, pain management should be a priority

      (c) Despite advances in pain management, the critically ill are at high risk for undertreatment of pain; landmark research (Thunder Project II) describes the importance of providing analgesia before even minor procedures (e.g., turning) (Puntillo, 2001)

    ii. Definitions: See Chapter 10

    iii. Clinical manifestations: Table 4-23 outlines various harmful effects and clinical manifestations of pain (see also Chapter 10); adequate analgesia may lessen the harmful effects of pain

    iv. Factors complicating pain assessment and impeding effective pain management: See Table 4-26

    v. Diagnostic studies

      (a) Imaging studies to outline underlying pathology

      (b) Blood work to identify organ dysfunction(s)

      (c) Electrodiagnostic tests to identify myopathies, some neuropathies

      (d) Nerve blocks to distinguish source or types of pain

  b. Goals of care

    i. Development of potentially harmful far-reaching physical and psychosocial effects of pain are prevented by aggressive and proactive pain management

    ii. Patient comfort and rapid functional recovery are promoted by the achievement of optimal analgesia with the fewest adverse effects

  c. Collaborating professionals on health care team for pain management

    i. Nurses play a pivotal role in coordinating care and achieving effective pain management for patients

    ii. Other disciplines represented can include anesthesia, physical medicine and rehabilitation, neurosurgery, interventional radiology, physical therapy, pain management, pharmacy, psychology, and social and chaplain services

  d. Interventions

    i. Pharmacologic methods

      (a) Choice of an analgesic depends on many factors (e.g., clinical judgment, patient history, type and severity of pain, patient response to interventions)

      (b) Optimal use requires the understanding of a drug's pharmacokinetics (e.g., time to onset, peak effect, duration of action) and pharmacodynamics (e.g., mechanism of action, metabolism, and excretion)

▓ **TABLE 4-26**
▓ ▓ **Factors Complicating Accurate Pain Assessment and Effective Pain Management**

Factor	Issues	Suggestions for Management
IMPAIRED ABILITY TO COMMUNICATE		
Altered level of consciousness, mental status (e.g., agitation, coma, sedation) Sensory deficits	Potential difficulty obtaining pain assessment (e.g., self-report of pain) Failure to recognize pain as a potential cause for agitation	Assume pain is present and treat accordingly Use behaviors and physiologic signs to confirm suspicion of pain Obtain and have patient use glasses or hearing aids as needed
MEDICATION EFFECTS		
Combining of opioids and sedatives	Potential for oversedation	When these agents are given together, less of each medication may achieve desired effect and avoid adverse effects
PHYSIOLOGIC CONDITIONS		
Hemodynamic instability Respiratory instability Weaning from ventilator Head trauma Renal or hepatic impairment	Withholding of opioids related to fear of • Exacerbating hemodynamic or respiratory instability • Delaying extubation • Impairing neurologic assessment Impaired excretion of opioid metabolites can increase opioid adverse effects (e.g., sedation)	Give intravenous fluids and vasopressors as ordered Splinting related to pain can also impair gas exchange Titrate small doses slowly and more often Frequent assessment for opioid adverse effects Consider fentanyl (short acting, less histamine release), nonopioids, epidural opioids, blocks Consider analgesia with Glasgow Coma Scale score higher than 3 (Wisborg and Flaatten, 1999) Use opioids with no clinically relevant metabolites (e.g., hydromorphone, fentanyl) Avoid meperidine; use morphine cautiously
PREEXISTING (CHRONIC) PAIN STATES		
Regular use of pain medications (e.g., opioids, adjuvants)	Potential for undertreatment of pain and development of withdrawal syndrome (signs and symptoms similar to those of pain, such as increased heart rate, restlessness, sleeplessness)	Accept patient's report of pain Higher than "normal" starting dosages of analgesics may be required Continue other routine medications whenever possible

   (c) Three broad categories of analgesics are used in pain management (Tables 4-27, 4-28, and 4-29)
      (1) Nonopioids include acetaminophen and nonsteroidal antiinflammatory drugs (NSAIDs) (see Table 4-27). NSAIDs have limited usefulness in critically ill patients because they have a high adverse effect (AE) profile.

■ **TABLE 4-27**
■ ■ **Nonopioids Commonly Used to Treat Critically Ill Patients**

Overview: A group of analgesics that includes nonsteroidal antiinflammatory drugs (NSAIDs) and acetaminophen (see examples later). Limited use in the critically ill because of adverse effects and limited availability of parenteral formulations. Reduce dosages in the elderly and in those with renal or hepatic insufficiency.

Indications: Acute and chronic pain related to many causes, including surgery, trauma, arthritis, and cancer. May be effective for relief of mild pain when used alone. Both acetaminophen and NSAIDs have analgesic and antipyretic effects; NSAIDs are also effective for inflammatory pain.

Mechanism of action: NSAIDs have both peripheral and central actions. Nonselective NSAIDs inhibit two isoforms of cyclooxygenase (COX-1 and COX-2). Inhibition of COX-1, normally found in tissues (e.g., platelets, gastrointestinal [GI] tract, kidneys), results in well-known adverse effects of NSAIDs (see later). Inhibition of COX-2 decreases inflammation by inhibiting prostaglandin formation. COX-2–selective NSAIDs inhibit COX-2 and do not decrease platelet aggregation. They pose less risk of GI ulceration and bleeding, but no less risk of renal toxicity, compared to nonselective NSAIDs (American Pain Society, 2003). Acetaminophen is believed to cause a central inhibition of prostaglandin, perhaps via a third isoform of COX.

Benefits: Nonopioids provide analgesia without the sedative and respiratory adverse effects of opioids, so their concurrent use allows lower opioid dosages to be given without reducing analgesia (known as "opioid dose–sparing" effect).

Adverse effects (AEs): NSAIDs*: (1) Inhibition of platelet aggregation; (2) adverse GI effects (e.g., ulcerations, bleeding); (3) renal insufficiency and acute renal failure; (4) central nervous system dysfunction (e.g., decreased attention span, headache); and (5) hypersensitivity. Acetaminophen: Can cause severe hepatotoxicity in patients with chronic alcoholism or liver disease and in fasting patients. COX-2–Selective NSAIDs: Risk of renal toxicity similar to that of nonselective NSAIDs.

Examples	Method of Administration	Typical Dosage	Comments
Nonselective NSAIDs (e.g., ibuprofen, ketorolac)	Oral except ketorolac (both oral and parenteral)	Ibuprofen: 200-400 mg q 4-6 hr Ketorolac: 15-30 mg intravenously q 6 hr	Ibuprofen: Limit to 2400 mg/day Ketorolac: Limit to 5 days; may precipitate renal failure in dehydrated patients; do not exceed 60 mg/day in patients >65 yr old or in those with elevated creatinine levels Naproxen: possible increased risk of CV AEs
COX-2 selective NSAIDs (e.g., celecoxib)	Oral	Celecoxib: 200-400 mg q 12-24 hr	Possible increased risk of CV AEs
Salicylates (e.g., aspirin)	Oral, rectal	500-1000 mg q 4-6 hr	Usually avoided in critically ill patients
Acetaminophen	Oral, rectal	500-1000 mg q 4-6 hr	Less risk of GI and renal complications compared to NSAIDs; decrease dosage in patients with chronic alcohol use or liver insufficiency

Data from American Pain Society: Principles of analgesic use in the treatment of acute pain and cancer pain, ed 5, Glenview, IL, 2003, Author; Pasero C, McCaffery M: Multimodal balanced analgesia in the critically ill, *Crit Care Nurs Clin North Am* 13(2):195-206, 2001; and McCaffery M, Pasero C: *Pain: clinical manual,* ed 2, St Louis, 1999, Mosby.

*The cardiovascular effects of various NSAIDs are the subject of ongoing research. Risk is likely increased when NSAIDs are taken in higher than recommended doses and on a long-term basis. Consultation with pharmacy and administration of the lowest effective dose for short-term pain management is recommended in the critically ill.

■ **TABLE 4-28**
■ ■ **Opioids Commonly Used to Treat Critically Ill Patients**

Overview: Foundation of effective pain management in critically ill patients, procedural pain

Indications: Moderate to severe acute and cancer pain, some chronic pain syndromes, procedural pain

Mechanism of action: Bind to opioid receptors (μ, κ, and δ) in the brain, spinal cord, and periphery, inhibiting the release of neurotransmitters (e.g., substance P, glutamate), which blocks transmission of pain impulses

Routes of administration: Oral, parenteral, intraspinal, transdermal, transmucosal; avoid intramuscular route

Adverse effects: Sedation, respiratory depression, nausea, vomiting, mental clouding, pruritus, and urinary retention usually occur with initiation of opioid therapy; however, tolerance develops, usually within a matter of days. Tolerance does not develop to constipation, and regular assessment with prophylactic treatment is required.

Achievement of effective analgesia: Titrate frequent, small, increasing doses to achieve therapeutic effect, then initiate continuous infusion or scheduled boluses to provide steady blood levels. No analgesic ceiling with single-entity opioids.

Management of adverse effects: Most adverse effects are dose related. Initial treatment includes (1) appropriate medications as indicated (e.g., antiemetic); (2) addition of nonopioid, if possible; and (3) reduction in opioid dose. May need to change opioid or route of administration.

Opioid	Method of Administration*	Starting Dosages	Comments
Morphine sulfate Oral formulations Elixirs Immediate release Sustained-release Suppository	Intravenous (IV) loading dose Continuous infusion IV rescue bolus Intraspinal	2.5-5 mg q 10 min prn 1.25-2 mg/hr 1-2 mg q 10 min prn Immediate release/ short acting: 15- 30 mg q 3-4 hr prn Controlled release: 30 mg q 8-12 hr ATC	Active metabolites may cause most adverse effects and accumulate in renal insufficiency Histamine release and vasodilatation can cause hypotension Do NOT crush or break sustained-release tablets 10 mg IV $\approx$ 30 mg PO
Fentanyl Other formulations Transdermal Transmucosal Intraspinal	IV loading (over 2-5 min) Continuous infusion IV bolus (over 2-5 min)	25-50 μg q 10 min prn 10-25 μg/hr 10-25 μg q 10 min prn Transmucosal: 200-400 μg sucked (not chewed) over 15 min	No active metabolites and less histamine release than morphine Good choice with hemodynamic instability or renal insufficiency Risk of chest wall rigidity with rapid large IV doses Transdermal form not for acute pain Fentanyl 25 μg IV $\approx$ morphine 1 mg IV
Hydromorphone Oral, suppository	IV loading dose (over 2-3 min) Continuous infusion IV bolus	0.4-0.8 mg q 10 min prn 0.2-0.4 mg/hr 0.2-0.4 mg q 10 min prn	Metabolites have minimal clinical effect Good alternative in renal insufficiency Hydromorphone IV 1.5 mg $\approx$ morphine 10 mg IV
Oxycodone Elixirs Immediate release	Oral formulation only	Varies Oxycodone starting dosage: 5-10 mg q 4-6 hr	Metabolites have minimal clinical effect Good alternative in renal insufficiency

*Each route has individual onset, peak, and duration of action that will affect dosing intervals.

Continued

■ **TABLE 4-28**
■ ■ **Opioids Commonly Used to Treat Critically Ill Patients—cont'd**

Opioid	Method of Administration	Starting Dosages	Comments
Supplemental analgesia: Acetaminophen with oxycodone Sustained-release		OxyContin: q 12 hr 10-20 mg	Do not crush or break sustained-release tablets
Hydrocodone with acetaminophen	Oral formulation only	5-10 mg q 4-6 hr prn	Combinations come in varying strengths of hydrocodone and acetaminophen; watch daily acetaminophen intake

      (2) Opioids: Primarily μ-agonists, such as morphine, hydromorphone (see Table 4-28)
         a) Duration of action
            1) Most parenteral, immediate-release, and short-acting (oral) formulations can last up to 3 to 4 hours
            2) Controlled release formulation last 8 to 12 hours; should be given "around the clock," not as needed
            3) Oral extended-release formulations last 12 to 24 hours
            4) Transdermal patches last 48 to 96 hours (usually 72 hours)
         b) Use as necessary prior to procedures and before pain gets out of control
      (3) Adjuvants or coanalgesics: Drugs that are analgesic under some conditions, with a primary indication other than pain (e.g., tricyclic antidepressants) (see Table 4-29)
    (d) Multimodal balanced analgesia combines analgesic regimens to reduce the likelihood of adverse effects from a single agent
  ii. Nonpharmacologic methods (see Table 10-4)
e. Evaluation of patient care (see also Chapter 10)
  i. Pain intensity is maintained at a level that allows the patient the best opportunity to heal with the minimum amount of discomfort (usually at or below a rating of 4 on a scale of 10)
  ii. Ongoing assessments appropriate to the critically ill patient identify ineffective pain management and result in revision of the analgesic plan
10. Corneal abrasion secondary to impaired corneal reflex
  a. Description of problem: Impaired corneal reflex caused by CN V, CN VII, or brainstem dysfunction makes the cornea vulnerable to injury
  b. Goals of care: Eyes are protected from corneal injury
  c. Collaborating professionals on health care team
    i. Nurse
    ii. Physician
  d. Interventions
    i. Assess corneas for abrasions, irritation, or drainage
    ii. Cleanse exudate from eyes at least once a shift

TABLE 4-29
Adjuvant Medications Commonly Used to Treat Pain

Category/Example	Mechanism of Action	Indication	Adverse Effects	Comments
Anticonvulsants (e.g., gabapentin, topiramate)	Cell membrane stabilizer, decreases ectopic neuron firing	Shooting or knifelike neuropathic pain (e.g., diabetic or postherpetic neuropathy)	Sedation, mental clouding, dizziness, gastrointestinal upset	Gabapentin usually dosed tid, titrate slowly up to 3600 mg/day until symptoms resolve or adverse effects occur. Reduce dose in renal insufficiency.
Tricyclic antidepressants (e.g., amitriptyline, nortriptyline)	Block reuptake of serotonin and norepinephrine	Continuous burning or hypersensitive neuropathic pain; also migraines, fibromyalgia	Potent anticholinergic effects (e.g., orthostatic hypotension, sedation, constipation, delirium)	Daily dosing (give at night to promote sleep). Analgesic dosages less than antidepressant dosages. Coronary artery disease (conduction abnormalities) is a relative contraindication.
Local anesthetics (e.g., lidocaine 4% spray, 5% patch; EMLA [eutectic mixture of local anesthetics] cream; lidocaine via intravenous, oral, neuraxial route or as nerve block); benzocaine topical lubricant	Block sodium channels to inhibit impulses from damaged neurons	Procedure-related pain (e.g., IV starts, intubation), neuropathic pain (e.g., stump pain, complex regional pain syndrome IV nerve blocks)	Topical administration: Few adverse effects Systemic administration: Dizziness, tremor, paresthesias, seizures	Bupivacaine and ropivacaine also used as regional anesthetic (e.g., nerve blocks, epidural injections, continuous neuraxial analgesia). "Caine" drugs may cause methemoglobinemia EMLA: Onset in 1 hr; lasts 1-2 hr after removal.
Antihistamines (e.g., diphenhydramine, hydroxyzine)	Mild central nervous system depressant	Itching, nausea, anxiety	Mild sedative activity Anticholinergic effects	Carefully monitor for increased sedation levels when used with opioids; no data to support analgesic effect (American Pain Society, 2003). IV hydroxyzine is contraindicated.
Benzodiazepines (e.g., diazepam), lorazepam	Relieve pain by relaxing spasm	Acute anxiety or muscle spasm	Sedation, respiratory depression, risk of dependence	Are not effective analgesics,

Continued

■ TABLE 4-29
■ ■ Adjuvant Medications Commonly Used to Treat Pain—cont'd

Category/Example	Mechanism of Action	Indication	Adverse Effects	Comments
Antispasmodics (e.g., baclofen)	Relaxes spasms and potentiates analgesia by enhancing γ-aminobutyric acid neurotransmitter	Spasm related to muscle injury, fractures; Spasticity; Neuropathic pain	Sedation, risk of dependence	Opioids alone are not effective for muscle spasms; Baclofen can be given orally or intrathecally
Other adjuvants (with general indications for use)	Corticosteroids: For bony, inflammatory, cancer, and neuropathic pain; nausea; mood and appetite stimulation; α_2-adrenergic agonist (e.g., clonidine): For neuropathic pain, chronic headache, withdrawal symptoms; N-methyl-D-aspartate (NMDA) receptor blockers (e.g., ketamine, dextromethorphan): For neuropathic pain; Propanolol: For migraine prophylaxis			

Data from American Pain Society: Principles of analgesic use in the treatment of acute pain and cancer pain, ed 5, Glenview, IL, 2003, Author; National Pharmaceutical Council (NPC): Pain: current understanding of assessment, management, and treatment, 2001, retrieved 2003, from http://www.npcnow.org; McCaffery M, Pasero C: Pain: clinical manual, ed 2, St Louis, 1999, Mosby.

          iii. Apply lubricant to the eyes as prescribed

          iv. Protect the eyes from injury; in some cases, the eyes may be taped closed or protective shields may be applied

    e. Evaluation of patient care: No corneal injury occurs

11. **Inability of the patient to communicate needs effectively**

    a. Description of problem: Barriers to effective communication may include endotracheal (ET) intubation, decreased LOC, expressive or receptive dysphasia, motor speech apraxia, or dysarthria

    b. Goals of care: Effective communication is maintained so the patient's needs can be met

    c. Collaborating professionals on health care team

          i. Nurse

          ii. Speech therapist

    d. Interventions

          i. Collaborate with a speech therapist to assess the patient's comprehension and expression of written and spoken language and to identify the best interventions

          ii. Explain the nature of and reason for communication deficits to the patient and family; encourage patience with communication difficulties

          iii. Speak slowly in a normal tone. Use short phrases. If the patient has a hearing loss, speak to the patient on the unaffected side; repeat or rephrase, as necessary.

          iv. Stand so the patient can see your lip movements and nonverbal expressions. Allow time for the patient to respond.

          v. Use alternative strategies for communicating (e.g., gestures, yes or no questions, pointing, pictures, alphabet board)

          vi. Communicate for short periods to avoid tiring and frustrating the patient; be supportive and understanding of the patient's frustrations

          vii. Involve the family in using effective communication techniques

    e. Evaluation of patient care: Patient effectively communicates needs

12. **Weakness or paralysis of one or more extremities**

    a. Description of problem: Neurologic disorders can decrease muscle strength, control, mass, or endurance. Loss of motor function leaves the patient unable to perform purposeful activities, including repositioning, transfers, and ambulation. Skin breakdown, contractures, and deep venous thrombosis (DVT) may occur as a result. Spasticity, which often occurs in body areas affected by UMN lesions, may also reduce ROM and further impair functional mobility.

    b. Goals of care

          i. Full joint ROM is maintained

          ii. If possible, muscle strength is regained

          iii. Patient demonstrates how to compensate for weakness or paralysis so independence is regained

          iv. Patient exhibits no evidence of complications, such as contractures, skin breakdown, or DVT

          v. Problematic spasticity is controlled

    c. Collaborating professionals on health care team

          i. Physical therapist

          ii. Occupational therapist

          iii. Nurse

          iv. Physician

    d. Interventions

          i. Assess motor strength every shift

  ii. Use pressure-relief devices as appropriate

  iii. Reposition the patient frequently if he or she is not on a rotational bed. Assess skin integrity while turning. Maintain functional anatomic alignment; protect bony prominences; keep head and trunk straight to normalize posture and tone and to encourage symmetry.

  iv. Position hemiplegic patients in opposition to spastic adduction and flexion in the arm and extension in the leg

  v. Position proximal joints (pelvis, shoulders) correctly to reduce tone in extremities

  vi. Follow the recommendations of an occupational therapist and physical therapist on how to move and position the patient, and use splints, braces, and elastic gloves; teach ROM and transfer techniques

  vii. If necessary, administer prescribed antispasmodics (e.g., dantrolene sodium, baclofen, diazepam)

  viii. Perform ROM exercises to joints; progress from passive to active as tolerated. Do not pull on a paretic limb.

  ix. Encourage progressive independent activity as tolerated; encourage movement toward the paretic side

  x. Place items within reach of the unaffected arm

  xi. Involve the family in therapy as appropriate

 e. Evaluation of patient care

  i. Joint mobility is maintained

  ii. If possible, muscle strength is regained

  iii. Patient participates in therapy to strengthen muscles and learns strategies to compensate for motor dysfunction

  iv. Complications of paresis or paralysis are prevented

13. Cognitive deficits

 a. Description of problem: Brain pathology can cause a number of cognitive deficits, including the following:

  i. Disorientation to time, place, person, and situation

  ii. Diminished attention span and problem-solving abilities, impulsiveness, poor judgment, belligerence

  iii. Memory loss and lack of sequential thought (i.e., inability to recall events in the order in which they occurred)

  iv. Inability to follow requests or instructions

  v. Inability to recognize deficits

 b. Goals of care

  i. Patient responds to the environment appropriately

  ii. Patient organizes thoughts and uses appropriate judgment to carry out ADLs with minimal assistance

  iii. Patient is able to compensate for cognitive deficits

  iv. Patient does not injure self

 c. Collaborating professionals on health care team

  i. Nurse

  ii. Physician

  iii. Physical therapist

  iv. Occupational therapist

  v. Speech therapist

 d. Interventions

  i. In an unresponsive patient, increase environmental awareness by providing familiar stimulation to all five senses. Provide only one stimulus at a time for brief periods to avoid sensory overload.

ii. Orient to the environment frequently
   (a) Call the patient by name; tell the patient your name
   (b) Inform the patient about time and location
   (c) Provide tools to help maintain orientation (e.g., calendar, clock, newspapers, radio, television)
   (d) Keep the patient's items in the same place
iii. Establish and maintain a predictable schedule
iv. Provide simple instructions frequently in a calm tone
v. With therapists, teach ADLs using cues and drills
vi. Protect the patient from injury (e.g., use restraints only if necessary, keep side rails up and call light within reach, locate the patient near the nurses' station)
vii. Remove unnecessary or aggravating stimuli; provide prescribed pharmacologic agent(s) to control agitation
viii. Teach and involve the family in care as appropriate

e. Evaluation of patient care
   i. Patient is oriented and responds appropriately to environmental stimuli
   ii. Patient uses adaptive strategies to make appropriate decisions and carry out ADLs with minimal assistance
   iii. Injury is prevented

14. **Situational crisis for the patient** secondary to neurologic deficits causing loss of control and independence, and a change in role: See Chapter 10

15. **Situational crisis for the family** secondary to disruption of the usual family roles, burden of care, and concern about the family member's pathologic condition and deficits: See Chapter 10

SPECIFIC PATIENT HEALTH PROBLEMS

Increased Intracranial Pressure

1. **Pathophysiology**
   a. Nondistensible intracranial cavity is filled to capacity with CSF, intravascular blood, and brain tissue
   b. *Monro-Kellie hypothesis:* If the volume of one of the intracranial constituents increases, a reciprocal decrease in the volume of one or both of the others must occur or ICP will increase
   c. Principal spatial buffers that resist elevations in ICP with volume increases include displacement of CSF from the cranial vault and compression of the low-pressure venous system. Decreased CSF production and increased CSF absorption may also contribute to spatial compensations.
      i. Volume of fluid that can be displaced for spatial compensation is finite; when intracranial volume exceeds the amount of fluid displaced, ICP rises
      ii. Relationship between ICP and volume can be plotted as a pressure-volume curve that depicts the effects of increasing intracranial volume on ICP (Figure 4-24). Flat portion of the curve reflects the phase in which spatial buffers compensate for increases in intracranial volume so there is little change in ICP. *Brain compliance*, a measure of the brain's adaptive capacity, is high at this portion of the curve. Once compensatory mechanisms are exceeded, the curve turns sharply upward, which indicates that small increases in volume then cause significant ICP elevations. At this part of the curve, brain compliance is low. Patient response to changes in intracranial volume depends, in part, on where the patient's condition is on this curve.

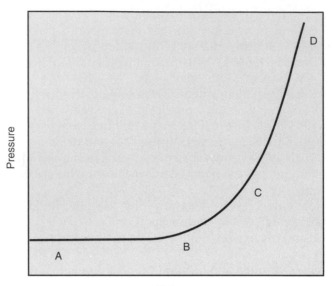

FIGURE 4-24 ■ Pressure-volume curve. From point *A* to point *B*, intracranial pressure (ICP) remains constant with the addition of volume and brain compliance is high. At point *B* brain compliance begins to change and ICP rises slightly. From point *B* to point *C*, compliance is low and ICP rises with increases in intracranial volume. From point *C* to point *D*, small increases in volume cause significant ICP elevations. (From McQuillan KA, Mitchell PH: Traumatic brain injuries. In McQuillan KA, Von Rueden KT, Hartsock RL, et al, editors: *Trauma nursing from resuscitation through rehabilitation*, ed 3, St Louis, 2002, Saunders, p 413.)

    d. As ICP increases and approaches the MAP, CPP decreases. When perfusion pressure falls below a critical point (usually around 40 mm Hg), autoregulation becomes impaired and CBF gradually falls, which leads to cerebral ischemia.

    e. Herniation syndromes: ICP elevations cause displacement of brain structures (Figure 4-25)

       i. *Cingulate* or *subfalcine* herniation: Unilateral cerebral lesion shifts brain tissue laterally across the midline, which causes distortion of the cingulate gyrus under the falx cerebri

      ii. *Uncal* or *lateral transtentorial* herniation: Expanding lesion forces the uncus of the medial temporal lobe over the edge of the tentorium

     iii. *Central transtentorial* herniation: Midline, bilateral, or unilateral cerebral lesions displace one or both hemispheres, the diencephalon, and the midbrain downward through the tentorial notch, which causes midbrain compression; can progress to tonsillar herniation

      iv. *Tonsillar* herniation: Posterior fossa contents, particularly the cerebellar tonsils, are displaced through the foramen magnum, which causes brainstem distortion

2. Etiology and risk factors

    a. Rate and extent of ICP elevation depends on

       i. Amount of volume increase

      ii. Rate of volume change (i.e., the faster volume is added, the greater the rise in ICP)

     iii. Total volume within the intracranial cavity

     iv. Intracranial compliance (i.e., the capacity for compensation)

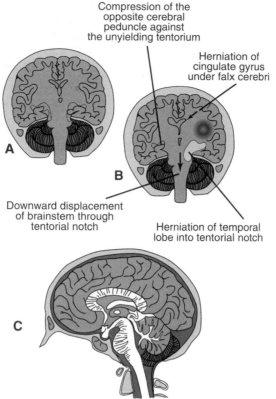

Compression of the
opposite cerebral
peduncle against
the unyielding tentorium

Herniation of
cingulate gyrus
under falx cerebri

A

B

Downward displacement
of brainstem through
tentorial notch

Herniation of temporal
lobe into tentorial notch

C

FIGURE 4-25 ■ Brain herniation. **A,** Normal relationship of intracranial structures. **B,** Shift of intracranial structures. **C,** Downward herniation of the cerebellar tonsils into the foramen magnum. (From Kerr ME: Nursing management intracranial problems. In Lewis SM, Heitkemper MM, Dirksen SR: *Medical surgical nursing assessment and management of clinical problem*, ed 5, St Louis, 2000, Mosby, p 1614.)

   b. Increases in brain volume are caused by
     i. Mass lesions: Any space-occupying lesion
       (a) Hematomas: Subdural, epidural, intracerebral
       (b) Abscesses
       (c) Tumors: May be spherical, well delineated, and encapsulated or diffuse and infiltrating masses. May enlarge due to cell proliferation, necrosis, edema, or hemorrhage. Cause neurologic symptoms due to compression, invasion, or destruction of brain tissue.
    ii. Cytotoxic edema: Intracellular swelling of neurons, glia, and endothelial cells caused by cellular hypoxia or acute hypo-osmolality (water intoxication). Hypoxia depletes cellular ATP and breaks down the ATP-dependent sodium-potassium pump, which leads to intracellular accumulation of Na^+ and water and cellular swelling. Acute hypo-osmolality causes water to move into the cell via osmosis.
   iii. Vasogenic cerebral edema: Direct or hypoxic injury, severe hypertension, endotoxins, or inflammatory mediators break down the blood-brain barrier; this allows osmotically active molecules such as proteins to leak into the interstitium, which draws water from the vascular system and cells into the interstitial space. Seen around contusions, tumors, or abscesses or generalized, as with meningitis or diffuse brain injury.

      iv. Interstitial edema: High intraventricular pressure (e.g., hydrocephalus) causes fluid to extravasate into tissues around the ventricles

   c. Increases in cerebral blood volume (CBV) may be caused by

      i. Venous outflow obstruction

         (a) Head rotation, neck hyperextension or hyperflexion, or tight tracheal tube ties can compress the jugular veins, diminish venous return, and cause venous engorgement

         (b) Thrombus or another venous lesion may block the outflow of intracranial blood

         (c) Raised intrathoracic and/or intraabdominal pressure may impede venous return

      ii. Hyperemia: CBF exceeds metabolic demand

         (a) Increased ICP can reduce CPP and CBF, causing vasodilation, increasing CBV, and further elevating ICP

         (b) Autoregulation may be impaired, globally or regionally, by cerebral injury or insult. When impaired, arterioles passively dilate with elevated arterial BP, increasing CBF and CBV.

         (c) BP that exceeds the limits of autoregulation can increase CBV

         (d) Increased $PaCO_2$ and PaO_2 lower than 60 mm Hg cause cerebral vasodilatation, increasing CBF

         (e) Certain anesthetics (e.g., halothane, nitrous oxide) and other drugs (e.g., nitroprusside, nitroglycerin) cause cerebral vasodilatation, which increases CBV. Use these cautiously with neurosurgical patients.

   d. Increases in CSF volume (hydrocephalus)

      i. Increased production of CSF (an uncommon cause)

      ii. Decreased reabsorption of CSF

         (a) Obstruction of CSF circulation (see Figure 4-11) due to a mass lesion, edema, hemorrhage, or inflammatory process in or near the ventricular system or on the convexity of the brain blocking the subarachnoid space (*noncommunicating hydrocephalus*)

         (b) Impaired reabsorption of CSF from the subarachnoid space into the venous system due to meningeal inflammation or the obstruction of arachnoid villi by debris (e.g., blood cells, infectious matter) (*communicating hydrocephalus*)

3. Signs and symptoms

   a. ICP monitoring data show elevated ICP

   b. Clinical presentation may show little or no change if the cause is a slow, progressive pathologic condition (e.g., slow-growing tumor)

   c. Papilledema may be the initial sign if ICP rises gradually but is a late sign with acute ICP elevations

   d. More commonly, trends in LOC; motor activity; pupillary size, shape, and reactivity; cranial nerve function; and vital signs will indicate possible ICP elevations over time

      i. LOC changes may present as restlessness, agitation, disorientation, or lethargy, which may progress to less responsive or comatose states, or coma may be evident at the outset

      ii. Increased ICP can exert pressure on the motor and sensory nerve tracts, leading to impairment or loss of function, usually on the side contralateral to the compression. Sometimes ipsilateral hemiparesis or hemiplegia is seen if brain tissue is displaced laterally and the contralateral cerebral peduncle is compressed (*Kernohan's notch phenomenon*). See section on motor function under Patient Assessment for a description of other abnormal motor responses.

     iii. Pupil abnormalities are described in Table 4-9. Transtentorial herniation typically compresses the ipsilateral CN III, causing the pupil on the same side to enlarge and have a sluggish or absent direct light reflex. Occasionally, the pupil opposite the side of herniation may dilate if uncal herniation causes contralateral midbrain and CN III compression against the opposite tentorial edge.

     iv. See also section on vital signs under Patient Assessment

  e. Other findings suggesting ICP elevation must be evaluated in light of the history and clinical presentation

     i. Increasing headache, blurred vision, diplopia

     ii. Seizures

     iii. Vomiting: May result from lesions that involve the vestibular nuclei, impinge on the floor of the fourth ventricle, or produce medullary compression

4. Diagnostic study findings

  a. CT scan: Axial CT without contrast shows indications of mass effect and probable increased ICP

     i. Shift of the ventricles and falx away from the mass

     ii. Effacement of the sulci and ventricles

     iii. Compressed or absent basal cisterns

  b. ICP monitoring: Direct measurement of ICP

     i. Indications: Patients with severe TBI (GCS score of ≤8) with abnormal admission CT scan or with normal CT scan but two or more of the following: Age older than 40 years, posturing on one or both sides, systolic BP of less than 90 mm Hg. Physician may determine need for ICP monitoring in patients with TBI with a GCS score higher than 8. May also benefit patients with intracranial hemorrhage, ischemic stroke, infections or tumors, hydrocephalus, or Reye's syndrome.

     ii. ICP monitor placement options: See Table 4-30 and Figure 4-26

     iii. Transducers most commonly used when transmitting ICP: See Table 4-31

     iv. Normal ICP is 0 to 15 mm Hg. Thresholds for treating sustained ICP elevations vary, but 20 to 25 mm Hg is the upper limit beyond which intervention is recommended in patients with TBI. Pressure variations may exist between different intracranial compartments (e.g., supratentorial and infratentorial regions).

     v. ICP waveform is produced by vascular (primarily arterial) pulsations (Figure 4-27). Normal ICP waveform has three characteristic peaks of decreasing amplitude:

       (a) P_1 (percussion wave) has a fairly consistent amplitude

       (b) P_2 (tidal wave) has variable amplitude

       (c) P_3 (dicrotic wave) tapers to baseline

     vi. Different intracranial conditions can alter the waveform configuration. Elevated P2 (P1:P2 ratio is ≥0.8) is thought to reflect reduced brain compliance and impaired autoregulation, which indicates a greater likelihood that the patient's ICP will sustain an exaggerated increase in response to stimuli (e.g., turning, coughing)

5. Goals of care

  a. ICP remains below 20 mm Hg, CPP remains above 60 mm Hg or as ordered, and, if monitored, cerebral oxygenation or CBF remains within the desired range

  b. No complications occur as a result of ICP monitoring

  c. Patient's neurologic status improves

■ **TABLE 4-30**
■ ■ **Placement Options for Intracranial Pressure Monitoring**

Location	Description	Advantages	Disadvantages
Intraventricular (IVC)	A cannula is inserted through the scalp, skull, meninges, and brain tissue into the lateral ventricle (usually the anterior horn in the nondominant hemisphere)	Accurately and reliably measures cerebrospinal fluid (CSF) pressure directly (considered the gold standard for intracranial pressure measurement); excellent waveform; allows for therapeutic drainage of CSF and withdrawal of CSF for analysis	Most difficult to place, especially if the ventricles are small or displaced; highest risk of infection and tissue or vascular injury; inadvertent excessive CSF drainage may occur; may become occluded if there is a large amount of blood in the ventricles
Parenchymal	A probe is placed into the brain parenchyma	Quick and easy to place, not dependent on ventricular size or position; few complications; good waveform; accurate and reliable readings	Does not allow CSF drainage; some risk of infection or vascular damage
Subarachnoid	Tip of a hollow bolt is placed into the subarachnoid space	Quick and easy to insert, not dependent on ventricular size or position; less brain penetration than an IVC or parenchymal monitor	Does not allow CSF drainage; waveform fair; may cause CSF leak from insertion site; easily occluded with debris (e.g., blood clot, brain tissue, bone fragment)
Subdural	A catheter or probe is placed into the subdural space	Easy to insert, not dependent on ventricular size or position; less brain penetration than an IVC or parenchymal monitor	Does not allow CSF drainage; waveform poor; swollen brain may compress the catheter; over time, accuracy and reliability are poor
Epidural	Sensor placed in the epidural space; not commonly used	Quick and easy to insert; least invasive since it lies above the dura mater; few complications	Does not allow CSF drainage; waveform, accuracy, and reliability are poor; indirect ICP measure

6. **Collaborating professionals on health care team**
   a. Nurse, physician, pharmacist, nutritionist, laboratory personnel
   b. Respiratory, physical, speech, and occupational therapists
   c. Case manager or discharge coordinator, social worker, chaplain
7. **Management of patient care**
   a. Anticipated patient trajectory: As the volume in the intracranial compartment is reduced, the patient's ICP will decrease to within normal levels and recovery from the precipitating event will run its course

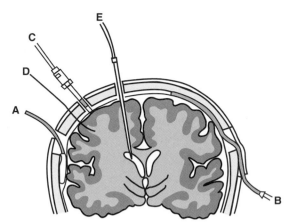

FIGURE 4-26 ■ Coronal section of the brain showing potential sites for placement of intracranial pressure monitoring devices. *A*, Epidural; *B*, subdural; *C*, subarachnoid; *D*, intraparenchymal; *E*, intraventricular. (From McNair ND: Intracranial pressure monitoring. In Clochesy JM, Breu C, Cardin S, et al, editors: *Critical care nursing*, ed 2, Philadelphia, 1996, Saunders, p 296.)

■ **TABLE 4-31**
■ ■ **Transducer Systems Used to Monitor Intracranial Pressure (ICP)**

Transducer	Description	Location Where It Can Be Used	Implications for Practice
External strain gauge (fluid filled)	Uses a static fluid column to transmit pressure from inside the skull to an external strain gauge transducer, which interfaces with a bedside pressure monitor	Intraventricular Subarachnoid Subdural Epidural	Inexpensive; after insertion, system is regularly rezeroed to atmospheric air and recalibrated per hospital protocol; zero-balance if erroneous readings are suspected. Inaccurate measures may result when air, blood clots, or other debris get into the system or from loose connections or kinked tubing. Maintain the external transducer level with the designated anatomic landmark indicating the level of the foramen of Monro (e.g., external auditory meatus, tragus, top of the ear, or the outer canthus of the eye may be used as the reference point). Define and use the same reference point consistently; relevel the transducer after patient position changes.
Fiberoptic transducer tipped	Uses fiberoptics to transmit ICP from a transducer at the tip of the probe; connects to a monitor that provides an analog readout and can be interfaced with a bedside pressure monitor	Intraventricular Parenchymal Subarachnoid Subdural Epidural	Zeroed prior to insertion, then once in place no rezeroing or leveling needed; drift can occur, causing erroneous readings. Do not bend probe to prevent breakage; ensure that bolt connection is tight and that there is no tension on fiberoptic cable to prevent probe dislodgment.

Continued

■ **TABLE 4-31**
■ ■ **Transducer Systems Used to Monitor Intracranial Pressure (ICP)—cont'd**

Transducer	Description	Location Where It Can Be Used	Implications for Practice
Internal microstrain gauge	Electronically transmits ICP measured by a miniature strain-gauge transducer at the tip of the probe; connects to a monitor that provides an analog readout and can be interfaced with a bed-side pressure monitor	Intraventricular Parenchymal Subdural	Zeroed prior to insertion, then once in place no "rezeroing" or leveling needed; drift can occur, causing erroneous readings. Secure probe and avoid excessive kinking to prevent dislodgement and breakage.

   i. Positioning
     (a) Facilitate venous return
       (1) Elevate the head of the bed to a level that minimizes ICP and optimizes CPP (and, if monitored, CBF and oxygenation), usually 30 degrees
       (2) Avoid hyperextension, flexion, or rotation of the head and neck
       (3) Ensure that tracheal tubes ties are not wrapped tightly around the head or neck
       (4) If a cervical collar is used, ensure proper fit and placement
     (b) Avoid sharp hip flexion
     (c) With each patient position change, ensure that the external transducer and intraventricular catheter drainage chamber are appropriately positioned
   ii. Skin care: Provide meticulous care to prevent breakdown in patients with sensory or motor deficits
   iii. Pain management: Short-acting or easily reversible analgesics (e.g., morphine, fentanyl) may be used to control pain and reduce ICP. Give cautiously to patients not on a ventilator; avoid causing hypotension; monitor pain relief.

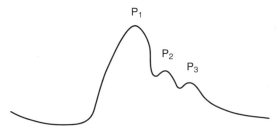

FIGURE 4-27 ■ Components of the intracranial pressure wave. (From McQuillan KA, Mitchell PH: Traumatic brain injuries. In McQuillan KA, Von Rueden KT, Hartsock RL, et al, editors: *Trauma nursing from resuscitation through rehabilitation*, ed 3, St Louis, 2002, Saunders, p 427.)

iv. Infection control: Strict sterile technique must be used during monitor insertion and when accessing the intraventricular catheter system (e.g., to obtain CSF specimens) or zero-balancing an external strain-gauge system. Keep all connections snug; avoid nonessential interruptions. Keep the insertion site dressing dry and intact; change per hospital protocol; use of bactericidal agents at the site is not recommended. Notify the physician if the dressing appears wet with CSF (indicates probable leakage).

v. Transport: Ensure that the ventriculostomy system is properly leveled or turned off to drainage during transport to prevent excessive CSF outflow. Zero-balance external strain-gauge system again after moving the patient.

vi. Discharge planning: Discharge destination (e.g., home, rehabilitation or skilled nursing facility) is determined in large part by the patient's cognitive capabilities and motor or sensory deficits. Educate the family about what the course of the patient's condition is likely to be and what should be expected in the postacute phase of care.

vii. Pharmacology: See Box 4-10

viii. Psychosocial issues: Family presence reduces ICP in some patients. Help alleviate the family's fear and anxiety by providing information and encouraging the use of appropriate coping mechanisms and support systems (see Chapter 10)

ix. Treatments

(a) Noninvasive

(1) Eliminate any unnecessary noxious stimuli that may elevate ICP

(2) Maintain normothermia. Use antipyretic agents and other cooling methods to reduce hyperthermia, which increases CBF approximately 6% for every 1.8° F (1° C) temperature increase and thereby raises ICP

(3) Note the effects of various interventions (e.g., suctioning) on ICP, CPP, and other parameters. If the patient evidences poor brain compliance, provide prescribed sedation prior to performing interventions or space activities to minimize ICP elevations.

(4) Suction only when clinically indicated to avoid excessive ICP elevations; limit the number of suction catheter passes (one or two times); pass the catheter for 10 sec or less; hyperoxygenate with 100% FIO_2 (fraction of inspired oxygen), and hyperinflate with 135% of the tidal volume for four breaths at 20-sec intervals before each catheter pass; may administer sedative, neuromuscular blocking agent, or lidocaine prior to procedure

(5) Hyperventilation causes vasoconstriction, reducing CBF and CBV which lowers ICP. It can reduce CBF and exacerbate cerebral ischemia. Decrease $PaCO_2$, preferably to no lower than 30 mm Hg, only if needed for ICP elevations unresponsive to CSF drainage and sedation. CBF or oxygenation measures can identify when ischemia occurs, so that hyperventilation can be curtailed, or when hyperemia occurs, which indicates that hyperventilation is well tolerated. $PaCO_2$ reduction to less than 30 mm Hg may be used to treat refractory intracranial hypertension.

(6) Maintain normoglycemia. Hypoglycemia or hyperglycemia can worsen cerebral edema and outcome from brain insult.

(7) Decompress the gut and bladder to prevent increased intraabdominal pressure, which can raise ICP

■ **BOX 4-10**
■ **PHARMACOLOGIC MANAGEMENT OF INCREASED INTRACRANIAL PRESSURE (ICP)**

- Supplemental oxygen: To prevent hypoxia and insufficient cerebral oxygen delivery, which can cause or worsen brain ischemia and increased ICP.
- Prescribed fluids: To maintain euvolemic state, normal electrolyte levels, and desired cerebral perfusion pressure (CPP) (usually >60 mm Hg). Typically, isotonic crystalloids (e.g., normal saline, Plasmalyte-A) are administered. Hypotonic and glucose-containing solutions are generally avoided. Colloids, hypertonic saline solutions, and, if indicated, blood products may also be used.
- Vasoactive and inotropic agents: May be used to support blood pressure and CPP once hemodynamic parameters confirm that patient is euvolemic.
- Sedation: Often effective in reducing ICP, particularly in restless or agitated patients. Short-acting or easily reversible agents preferred (e.g., midazolam, propofol). Rule out other physiologic causes of agitation that require different treatment (e.g., hypoxia, electrolyte imbalance). Give cautiously if patient not on ventilator support. Avoid hypotension.
- Neuromuscular blocking agents (e.g., vecuronium, atracurium): May be used to lower ICP if other therapies (e.g., cerebrospinal fluid drainage, sedation) are ineffective and patient is still agitated, has increased muscle tone, or resists ventilator.
- Diuretics: Ensure adequate hydration prior to administration; replace fluids to avoid dehydration and hypotension.
  Mannitol: Osmotic diuretic administered as bolus (0.25 to 1.0 g/kg) to reduce ICP by creating osmotic gradient that pulls fluid from brain tissue into intravascular space; expands plasma volume, which reduces blood viscosity, improves cerebral blood flow (CBF) and oxygen delivery
  Loop diuretics (e.g., furosemide): May lower ICP by reducing sodium and water transport into brain, causing diuresis, and decreasing cerebrospinal fluid production.
- Hypertonic saline solutions: Lower ICP by pulling interstitial fluid from brain tissue into intravascular space, expanding intravascular volume, which improves CBF and oxygen delivery, and perhaps by modifying the injury-induced inflammatory response.
- High-dose barbiturates (commonly pentobarbital) or propofol: To induce therapeutic coma for control of refractory intracranial hypertension. Lower ICP by suppressing cerebral metabolism to decrease CBF and volume, inhibiting free radical–mediated lipid peroxidation, and altering vascular tone.
  Administration: Ensure patient is euvolemic and hemodynamically stable before initiating therapy. Typical loading dosage for pentobarbital is 10 mg/kg intravenously (IV) over 30 minutes, followed by 5 mg/kg/hr for 3 hours, then 1 to 3 mg/kg/hr maintenance. Propofol dosage is 10 μg/kg/min IV, then titration to desired effect.
  Monitoring: Closely monitor hemodynamic status. Vasopressors often required to maintain blood pressure and CPP. Monitor electroencephalogram; titrate pentobarbital or propofol to achieve burst suppression.
  Potential side effects: Hypotension and myocardial depression are of particular concern because they can further compromise CPP and lead to cardiovascular collapse.
- Glucocorticoids: Not recommended for reducing ICP or improving outcome in traumatic brain injury or stroke; may be used to reduce edema and ICP associated with intracranial tumors.
- Lidocaine: Reduces cerebral metabolic rate and suppresses cough reflex to prevent or lower high ICP. Given IV or endotracheally prior to respiratory maneuvers (e.g., intubation, suctioning) to attenuate ICP elevations. Lowers seizure threshold; frequent dosing can cause toxicity.

(8) Avoid the patient's straining, coughing, or using the Valsalva maneuver, which raises ICP via increased intrathoracic pressure and impeding of cerebrovenous outflow

(9) Purposeful touch may help reduce ICP

(b) Invasive

(1) ET intubation and ventilatory support may be required for adequate ventilation

(2) Intracranial monitoring (see ICP Monitoring under Diagnostic Study Findings): Assess neurologic status, ICP, CPP, CBF, and oxygenation parameters and record hourly and when changes occur. Consider all intracranial and extracranial parameters (e.g., vital signs, ABG levels) in treatment decisions (see Boxes 4-5 and 4-6). Notify the physician if parameters remain outside the acceptable range. If the ICP waveform dampens, readings may be inaccurate. Troubleshoot the monitoring system when changes occur in waveform, readings, or drainage; notify the neurosurgeon if the problem cannot be rectified. Secure the monitoring device to the patient to prevent dislodgement.

(3) CSF drainage: Drain continuously or intermittently as ordered; ensure that the air-fluid interface is properly positioned at the prescribed level at or above the foramen of Monro. Close the drainage system to obtain accurate ICP readings. Note the character and volume of drainage at least hourly. Notify the physician if there is no CSF drainage or excessive drainage, or if drainage character changes (e.g., more bloody or cloudy).

(4) Surgical interventions to reduce ICP

a) Removal of a mass lesion, débridement of necrotic brain tissue, resection of a portion of the brain

b) Unilateral or bilateral decompressive craniectomy (i.e., removal of the cranium and opening of the dura) allows room for the edematous brain to control refractory ICP elevations

c) Placement of a ventricular shunt for long-term CSF removal

x. Ethical issues: May consider with the family halting further treatment or withdrawing therapy when the patient has refractory ICP elevations and concurrent findings that indicate a dismal prognosis

b. Potential complications

i. Intracranial infection: Meningitis, ventriculitis, abscess

(a) Mechanism: ICP monitoring devices and surgical interventions provide an entry portal for organisms

(b) Management: See Infection Control under Management of Patient Care earlier and Intracranial Infections: Bacterial Meningitis and Intracranial Infections: Viral Encephalitis later

ii. Hemorrhage at ICP monitor insertion site

(a) Mechanism: Disruption of blood vessels during insertion of ICP monitor

(b) Management: Normalize coagulation parameters before ICP monitor placement. Monitor neurologic status closely before and after insertion; notify the physician of changes. CT scan can identify hemorrhage; surgical evacuation of hematoma may be necessary.

iii. Brain ischemia and death

(a) Mechanism: Uncontrolled intracranial hypertension compromises CPP and CBF leading to brain ischemia; irreversible brain death ensues when

CBF ceases. Criteria for brain death in an adult include unresponsiveness and lack of movement (spinal reflexes may persist); absence of pupillary, oculocephalic, oculovestibular, corneal, cough, and gag reflexes and spontaneous respirations; presence of. a known irreversible cause for coma; body temperature above 90° F (32.2° C); absence of the use of masking neuromuscular or sedative agents; absence of any metabolic or endocrine abnormality. Tests (EEG, angiography, transcranial Doppler ultrasonography, or somatosensory evoked potentials) may be performed to confirm brain death in patients who have one or more components of the clinical examination that cannot be reliably assessed.

    (b) Management: Interventions to minimize ICP and optimize CPP and oxygenation to prevent ischemia. Once brain death occurs, the family should be notified and organ donation considered.

8. Evaluation of patient care

  a. ICP remains below 15 mm Hg and CPP, CBF, and oxygenation remain within the desired range without interventions

  b. No evidence of complications from ICP monitoring is seen

  c. Patient's neurologic status improves

Head Trauma

1. Pathophysiology: Trauma to the head that injures the brain and possibly the overlying scalp and cranium. TBI can be differentiated into primary injury (direct injury to brain tissue and vasculature that occurs at the time of impact) and secondary injury (a cascade of intracellular molecular and biochemical events initiated by the primary insult). Secondary injury occurs over hours to days, worsening the initial injury. Numerous systemic or intracranial complications can initiate or exacerbate secondary brain injury. Brain cells are more vulnerable to these insults in the first few hours and days after injury; their occurrence increases morbidity and mortality.

  a. Molecular and biochemical mechanisms associated with secondary brain injury

    i. Injury depolarizes brain cells and halts aerobic metabolism, which quickly leads to energy depletion

    ii. Ionic fluxes occur (e.g., Na^+, water, Ca^{++} move into cells and K^+ moves out); disruption of calcium homeostasis is thought to trigger numerous pathologic events

    iii. Proteases (i.e., calpains) and lipases are activated and break down cytoskeletal proteins and lipids

    iv. Phospholipases are activated; these break down membranes and lead to free fatty acid accumulation

    v. Production of toxic eicosanoids (i.e., thromboxanes, leukotrienes, prostaglandins) may be triggered

    vi. Conversion to anaerobic metabolism produces acidosis and increased lactate

    vii. Release of excitatory neurotransmitters (e.g., glutamate, aspartate) increases the accumulation of intracellular Ca^{++}

    viii. Excessive free oxygen radicals are produced that damage cell membranes by lipid peroxidation

    ix. Nitric oxide also mediates cell damage related to excitotoxicity and intracellular hypercalcemia

    x. Other mechanisms contribute to delayed cell death after TBI. These may include apoptosis (genetically regulated cell self-destruction) and inflammatory processes.

b. Intracranial insults that can cause secondary brain injury
  i. Intracranial hypertension and factors that elevate ICP (e.g., intracranial hemorrhage or infection, hydrocephalus, brain edema [usually peaks 3 to 5 days after TBI], cerebral hyperemia)
  ii. Seizures—increase cerebral metabolic needs and ICP
  iii. Cerebral vasospasm, loss of cerebral autoregulation, cerebral ischemia
c. Systemic insults that can cause secondary brain injury
  i. Hypotension (systolic BP <90 mm Hg) is associated with doubled mortality rate in patients with severe TBI
  ii. Hypoxia (Pao_2 <60 mm Hg) reduces cerebral oxygenation and causes cerebral vasodilation, which increases ICP
  iii. Hypercapnia causes cerebral vasodilation, which increases ICP; hypocapnia causes vasoconstriction, which contributes to cerebral ischemia
  iv. Hyperthermia increases cerebral metabolic demands
  v. Both hyperglycemia and hypoglycemia have adverse effects
  vi. Acute hypo-osmolality can cause cerebral edema
  vii. Electrolyte disorders, particularly sodium imbalance, can lead to cellular swelling or dehydration
  viii. Systemic inflammatory disorders, anemia, acid-base imbalances have detrimental effects
  ix. Coagulopathy contributes to intracranial hemorrhage
d. Types of head injury: See Box 4-11
2. Etiology and risk factors
  a. Estimated 1.4 million Americans sustain TBIs each year; 230,000 survive and require hospitalization; 80,000 to 90,000 acquire long-term or permanent disabilities and 50,000 die
    i. Males sustain TBI about twice as often as females
    ii. Peak incidence is seen at 15 to 24 years of age; high rate also seen in those over age 75 years
  b. Common causes
    i. Transportation-related crashes involving motor or recreational vehicles, pedestrians, and/or bicycles: Leading cause of TBI; motor vehicle crashes cause most TBIs requiring hospitalization
    ii. Violence: Mostly from firearms
    iii. Falls: Most common cause in those over age 64 years
    iv. Industrial accidents
    v. Sports and leisure activities
  c. Factors that increase the risk for head injury
    i. Alcohol and drug use impairs gross and fine motor skills, reaction time, and judgment. Can confound diagnosis by altering LOC.
    ii. Misuse of or failure to use safety devices (e.g., restraining devices, such as seatbelts, or cycling helmets)
    iii. Medical conditions that cause seizures or reduce LOC, visual acuity, or neuromuscular control
  d. Mechanisms of injury
    i. Skull deformation: Delivery of force directly to the head distorts the skull contour, causing contusion, laceration, and/or hemorrhage beneath the site of contact
    ii. Acceleration-deceleration: Head is thrust quickly forward then backward, which causes straight linear movement of the skull and brain. The brain moves slower than the skull, so the brain is injured as it impacts the sides and rubs against the rough projections of the skull. Compression, tension, and shearing may also injure brain tissue.

■ **BOX 4-11**
■ **TYPES OF HEAD INJURY**

SCALP LACERATIONS
■ Can bleed profusely due to extensive scalp vascularity and poor vessel contractility.
■ Contaminated laceration increases risk of scalp, cranium, or intracranial infection.

SKULL FRACTURES
■ Amount of damage is determined by characteristics (shape, weight, mass), velocity, and momentum of impacting object, direction of force, and thickness of skull at point of contact.
■ Types:
  Linear: Simple break or crack with no displacement of bone. Concern if fracture occurs over a major vascular channel (e.g., temporal region over middle meningeal artery) because laceration can cause intracranial bleeding.
  Depressed: Depression of inner table more than one half thickness of skull; may cause brain contusion, laceration, or hemorrhage.
  Open (compound): Associated with open scalp laceration; increased risk of infection.
  Basilar: At base of skull, most commonly affects anterior and middle fossae; accounts for about 20% of all skull fractures. Most commonly arise from linear fracture that extends to skull base. Potential complications include dural tear (allows cerebrospinal fluid leakage, increases risk of infection), cerebrovascular injury (e.g., internal carotid artery) producing hemorrhage, vessel thrombosis, aneurysm formation or fistula creation, and cranial nerve damage.

FOCAL BRAIN INJURY
■ Contusion: Bruising of brain tissue with associated hemorrhage and edema. Progressive edema formation can create mass effect, cause increased intracranial pressure (ICP) and brain herniation. Can occur anywhere in brain but most often in frontal and temporal lobes where cranial walls, bony projections of skull base, and dural folds restrict movement. Temporal lobe contusions, because of their precarious location near tentorium, warrant special attention because expansion of lesion can cause herniation onto brainstem without warning of ICP elevation. Coup contusions occur at point of impact; contrecoup contusions occur at opposite pole from impact.
■ Epidural hematoma (EDH): Blood accumulation beneath skull and above dura; most often from arterial source. Most commonly associated with temporal bone fracture that lacerates middle meningeal artery. EDH compresses brain yet is associated with little underlying primary brain injury.
■ Subdural hematoma (SDH): Blood accumulation beneath dura, usually due to venous bleeding from torn bridging veins. As SDH expands it compresses brain and increases ICP. Categorized into three groups according to timing of presentation:
  Acute: Often associated with more underlying primary brain injury than EDH; poor prognosis.
  Subacute: Prognosis better than that of acute SDH due to less severe underlying brain injury and lower likelihood of progressing to brainstem compression.
  Chronic: SDH accumulates slowly, likely due to small rebleeds; over 2 to 4 days blood congeals and thickens. After about 2 weeks, clot breaks down and eventually becomes xanthochromic fluid encased by membranes. SDH eventually reabsorbs or becomes calcified.
■ Intracerebral hematoma (ICH): Hemorrhage into brain parenchyma produced by shearing and tensile stresses within brain tissue that result in rupture of intracerebral vessels. Frequently occurs in white matter of frontal and temporal regions, less commonly deep in hemispheres or cerebellum. May be single or multiple, often associated with other intracranial lesions and penetrating injuries. Hypertensive bleed or aneurysm rupture should be ruled out as source if single ICH is present.
■ Subarachnoid hemorrhage (SAH): Bleeding into subarachnoid space. Commonly seen with severe traumatic brain injury; may predispose to hydrocephalus and cerebral vasospasm.
■ Intraventricular hemorrhage (IVH): Bleeding into ventricles; may be associated with extension of SAH or ICH.

Continued

> **DIFFUSE BRAIN INJURY**
> - Most often caused by acceleration-deceleration and rotational forces that create tension, stretching, and shearing of nerve fibers with subsequent failure of conduction.
> - Location, amount, and severity of axonal dysfunction determine clinical severity of injury:
>   *Concussion:* Temporary neurologic dysfunction due to transient conduction impedance.
>   *Diffuse axonal injury (DAI):* Diffuse white matter shearing associated with severe widespread mechanical disruption of axons and neuronal pathways primarily in hemispheres, corpus callosum, diencephalon, and brainstem. Severe DAI often associated with deep intracerebral contusions and diffuse cerebral edema that can raise ICP. It is thought that all head trauma involves varying degrees of histopathologic changes consistent with diffuse axonal disruption with a continuum of clinical responses. Severe DAI has a high mortality; survivors can have profound neurologic deficits.

     iii. Rotation: Acceleration or deceleration causes the brain to move in a non-linear, twisting path. Compressive, stretching, shearing, and tensile strains cause brain and vascular injury, particularly in areas where tissues of different density interface (e.g., gray and white matter, fibrous and cerebral tissue). Rate, extent, and direction of angular acceleration determine the extent of injury.

     iv. Penetrating injuries: Object penetrates the scalp and skull and enters the brain, where it can cause brain contusion, laccration, and/or hemorrhage with subsequent edema and necrosis. Severity of the injury is determined by the velocity, size, shape, direction, and action of the object within the skull, as well as the areas affected. Increases the risk for intracranial infection and posttraumatic seizures.

        (a) Gunshot wounds: Constitute the leading cause of TBI deaths; the mortality rate for such wounds is above 90% in the United States. Two-thirds of firearm-related TBIs are self-inflicted.

           (1) Local parenchymal destruction occurs along the bullet track. Shock waves are transmitted throughout the intracranial vault; a temporary cavity (which may be much larger than missile diameter) forms along the primary bullet track, then collapses within milliseconds, which causes local and remote brain injury.

           (2) If the bullet has insufficient energy to exit the skull, it may ricochet off the inner skull or a dural barrier (e.g., the falx), creating a second and occasionally a third track. Bullet course is highly variable.

           (3) Death results from damage to vital brain structures, extensive tissue destruction, and intracranial hypertension due to cerebral edema and hemorrhage

        (b) Stab wounds: Penetrating object can lacerate the brain parenchyma, cranial nerves, and/or blood vessels

3. Signs and symptoms: See Box 4-12

4. Diagnostic study findings

    a. Laboratory: Abnormal coagulation parameters. Massive brain tissue damage can activate clotting, which results in consumptive coagulopathy.

    b. Radiologic

        i. CT scan: Defines intracranial hematomas, contusions, and occasionally diffuse axonal injury (DAI). Cerebral edema may be seen. Detects shift of intracranial contents as well as effacement of ventricles and basilar cisterns.

■ BOX 4-12
■ SIGNS AND SYMPTOMS OF HEAD TRAUMA

SCALP LACERATIONS
■ Often associated with significant bleeding.

DEPRESSED SKULL FRACTURES
■ Disruption in skull contour; neurologic presentation depends on location and extent of brain injury.

BASILAR SKULL FRACTURES
CEREBROSPINAL FLUID (CSF) LEAK
■ *CSF rhinorrhea* (nasal drainage) seen with anterior fossa fracture with dural tear.
■ *CSF otorrhea* (ear drainage) seen in petrous bone fractures with dural tear and tympanic membrane rupture. If tympanic membrane is intact, CSF can course through eustachian tube into nasopharynx and present as CSF rhinorrhea.
■ Suspect CSF leakage in patients who complain of postnasal drip or salty or sweet taste, or when halo sign (yellowish or clear circle of drainage surrounding blood stain) appears on bed linens or dressings.
■ Most CSF leaks occur immediately after injury but may be delayed; most heal spontaneously in 5 to 7 days.

CRANIAL NERVE (CN) INJURIES
Fracture site and orientation determine which cranial nerves are damaged:
● CN I: Associated with anterior fossa fractures.
● CN V and VI, and particularly CN VII and VIII: Associated with middle fossa fractures
● CN IX, X, XI, and XII: May occur with fractures of posterior fossa involving occipital condyle (rare)

HEMOTYMPANUM, BATTLE'S SIGN, AND RACCOON'S EYES
■ Hemotympanum and Battle's sign (ecchymosis over mastoid bone) indicate middle fossa fracture.
■ Hearing is decreased if CSF is behind tympanic membrane or if tympanic membrane ruptures.
■ "*Raccoon's eyes*" (bilateral periorbital ecchymosis) seen in anterior fossa fractures.

TRAUMATIC BRAIN INJURY
SEVERITY
Severity of head injury is based on Glasgow Coma Scale (GCS) score determined after initial resuscitation; considered reliable predictor of outcome; probability of poor outcome increases as GCS score decreases:
● Mild head injury: GCS score of 13 to 15
● Moderate head injury: GCS score of 9 to 12
● Severe head injury: GCS score of 3 to 8 or deterioration to GCS score of 8 or lower.

DISTINGUISHING TYPES OF BRAIN INJURY
Some types of traumatic brain injury are difficult to distinguish based on clinical presentation alone because multiple kinds of injury often coexist. Neurologic status can deteriorate with time if areas of intracranial hemorrhage and edema expand, intracranial pressure (ICP) rises, or other secondary insults occur. Focal neurologic deficits seen with small localized lesions.

CONTUSIONS
■ Presentation depends on size and location.
■ Focal deficits may progress to signs associated with increased ICP if hemorrhage and edema expand.

INTRACRANIAL HEMATOMAS/HEMORRHAGE
Clinical course varies, depending on location, rate, volume of accumulation, and presence of other intracranial injuries. It is not possible to differentiate type of hematoma based on clinical presentation.

Continued

Epidural Hematoma (EDH)

In as few as one third of patients there is a brief period of unconsciousness followed by a lucid interval and then progressive deterioration of neurologic status. EDH can collect rapidly, and patient's condition can deteriorate precipitously. Irritability and agitation can quickly progress to coma and hemiparesis or hemiplegia to decorticate or decerebrate posturing. Pupil abnormalities (i.e., unilateral fixed and dilated pupil) are often seen. Other symptoms may include headache (usually focal), vomiting, and possibly seizures and late vital sign changes. Posterior fossa EDH, which may have delayed onset, can cause nausea, vomiting, headache, stiff neck, and cardiovascular and respiratory instability.

Subdural Hematoma

Acute: Signs of neurologic deterioration evident within 48 hours. Most patients arrive in coma or deteriorate within hours of injury; in less severe cases patient may be conscious or have a lucid period. Other signs of expanding mass lesion (motor deficits, pupil changes, CN dysfunction, eventually vital sign changes) often seen.

Subacute: Signs of neurologic deterioration and increased ICP are delayed 2 to 14 days after injury.

Chronic: Signs do not develop for 2 weeks or longer after low-impact head injury. Usually occurs in patients with brain atrophy (e.g., elderly, chronic alcoholics). Clinical presentation may include headache, nausea, vomiting, gait disturbance, progressive decline in level of consciousness, seizures, and eventually motor dysfunction and pupil abnormalities.

Intracerebral Hematoma

- Similar to contusions.

Subarachnoid Hemorrhage

See Signs and Symptoms in Intracranial Aneurysms under Specific Patient Health Problems.

CONCUSSION

- Mild concussion causes brief period of confusion without loss of consciousness. Retrograde or posttraumatic amnesia may occur. Repeated mild concussions can have cumulative effects.
- Classic concussion associated with brief loss of consciousness with disorientation and retrograde and posttraumatic amnesia.
- Patient may have persistent complaints of neurologic sequelae such as headaches, visual disturbance, memory problems (particularly short term), short attention span, information-processing problems, behavioral disorders, and dizziness—referred to as *postconcussion syndrome.* No anatomic evidence of injury is noted on computed tomographic scan.

DIFFUSE AXONAL INJURY

- Classified based on clinical presentation and duration of coma, which has an immediate onset:

Mild: Coma lasts 6 to 24 hours with persistent mild to moderate cognitive and neurologic deficits common after emergence from coma. Transient decorticate or decerebrate posturing noted in about one third of patients, but all follow commands within 24 hours.

Moderate: Coma lasts more than 24 hours with mild to severe cognitive, behavioral, memory, and intellectual deficits persisting after emergence from coma. Most patients move purposefully or withdraw, but some exhibit transient decorticate or decerebrate posturing; no prominent signs of brainstem dysfunction.

Severe: Coma lasts days to months. Severe cerebral and neurologic dysfunction is evident (e.g., decorticate and decerebrate posturing). Autonomic dysfunction (i.e., elevated blood pressure, heart rate, and temperature; profuse sweating) seen with diencephalic involvement. Severe residual neurologic deficits are common.

(a) Epidural hematoma (EDH): Appears lens shaped
(b) Subdural hematoma (SDH): Crescent shaped and covers most of the hemisphere
(c) Intracerebral hematoma (ICH): Area of hyperdensity within the parenchyma
(d) Contusions: Heterogeneous areas of hemorrhage and edema
(e) DAI: Suspected if there are small hemorrhages in the deep white matter, corpus callosum, or brainstem; diffuse cerebral edema may be seen; normal in mild cases

ii. Skull radiographs and bone windows of CT scan: May reveal linear, depressed, and basilar skull fractures. Basilar skull fractures may not be seen on plain skull radiographs, but usually are seen on bone windows of CT scans. Air-fluid levels in the sinuses or pneumocephalus may be seen with basilar skull fractures and CSF leaks. Isotopes can be injected into the ventricle or via lumbar puncture to help identify the site of a CSF leak.

iii. Spine radiographs: Cervical spine radiographs are always performed in patients in whom a reliable clinical examination cannot be performed to reveal vertebral fracture or dislocation. Thoracic and lumbar radiographs may also be indicated depending on the mechanism of injury and clinical examination.

iv. Helical CT scan with sagittal reconstruction, MRI, or dynamic flexion-extension films of the cervical spine to rule out spine injury

v. Cerebral angiogram: Performed if vascular injury, vasospasm, or infarction suspected

vi. Transcranial Doppler ultrasonography: May reveal hyperemia, vasospasm, increased ICP, or vascular anomaly

vii. MRI: Although not generally used for diagnostic purposes in TBI, may reveal brain injury not well seen on CT scan (e.g., DAI, brainstem lesions)

5. **Goals of care**
   a. Secondary brain injury is prevented by maintaining adequate CPP (>60 mm Hg) and oxygenation, avoiding brain ischemia, and preventing systemic and neurologic complications
   b. Recovery of neurologic function is optimized
   c. Systemic complications associated with brain injury and neurologic dysfunction (e.g., pulmonary aspiration, fluid and electrolyte imbalance, malnutrition, skin breakdown, contractures, gastrointestinal erosion, DVT) are prevented

6. **Collaborating professionals on health care team:** See Increased Intracranial Pressure

7. **Management of patient care**
   a. Anticipated patient trajectory: Numerous factors influence clinical course and outcome, including the type, location, severity, and extent of the primary injury; the occurrence, frequency, severity, and duration of factors causing secondary brain injury; age; preexisting disease; and associated injuries. Anticipated patient trajectory for increased ICP is also relevant for TBI patients. Other specific needs for patients with acute severe TBI include the following:
      i. Positioning (see also Increased Intracranial Pressure)
         (a) Immobilize the cervical spine with a hard collar until cervical spine injury ruled out
         (b) When a portion of the cranium is removed (e.g., for skull fracture repair, decompressive craniectomy), position the head so there is no compression of the unprotected brain. Once intracranial monitoring devices are removed, apply a protective helmet as indicated.

ii. Skin care: See Increased Intracranial Pressure

iii. Pain management: TBI and associated injuries likely to require analgesia (see Increased Intracranial Pressure)

iv. Nutrition: Maintain normoglycemia. Metabolic expenditure and nitrogen excretion increase after TBI. Nonparalyzed TBI patients should receive nutrition that supplies 140% of their resting metabolic expenditure; paralyzed patients, 100% with 15% of caloric replacement as proteins. When possible, use the enteral route for nutrition. Full caloric replacement should be achieved within 7 days after TBI. (See Dysphagia under Patient Care.)

v. Infection control (see also Increased Intracranial Pressure)
  (a) Ensure adequate débridement and irrigation of contaminated scalp wound prior to closure
  (b) If CSF leak is suspected or confirmed, take precautions to prevent intracranial infection
    (1) Do not put anything into the patient's nose or ears, including tissue, dressings, packing, suction catheters, nasogastric tubes, or nasal cannula
    (2) Place a dry, sterile dressing loosely over the patient's ear or as a mustache dressing to absorb drainage. Note the character and amount of drainage.
    (3) Encourage closure of a dural tear
      a) Instruct the patient not to blow the nose
      b) Prevent the patient from engaging in the Valsalva maneuver or vigorous coughing to avoid further tearing of the dura and increased CSF flow
      c) Maintain a lumbar drain or ventriculostomy to drain CSF
      d) Surgical closure may be required
    (4) Use of prophylactic antibiotics remains controversial
  (c) Administer prescribed prophylactic broad spectrum antibiotics after penetrating TBI

vi. Transport: See Increased Intracranial Pressure

vii. Discharge planning: See Increased Intracranial Pressure

viii. Pharmacology (see also Increased Intracranial Pressure)
  (a) Provide supplemental oxygen; increased FIO_2 may be used for brief periods if the brain tissue oxygen level is low
  (b) Administer prescribed fluids. Typically, isotonic solutions are used and glucose-containing or hypotonic solutions are avoided. Fluid needs should be based on hemodynamic and clinical assessment parameters. Avoid fluid overload, which can exacerbate cerebral edema and respiratory failure.
  (c) Blood and other fluid loss from associated injuries can require large volume and blood product repletion. Hematocrit at or above 30% can help optimize cerebral oxygen delivery. Fresh frozen plasma, platelets, and/or cryoprecipitates may be used to correct coagulopathy.
  (d) Once euvolemia is assured, vasoactive and inotropic agents may be used to support BP so that a CPP above 60 mm Hg is maintained. Be cautious in the administration of sedatives and diuretics to prevent hypotension.
  (e) Interventions directed at brain injury management need not be instituted until after airway, breathing, and circulation are established unless brain herniation or neurologic deterioration not associated with

an extracranial cause is evident. In the latter case, an IV mannitol bolus may be given if the patient is adequately hydrated.

    (f) Administer anticonvulsants as prescribed

ix. Psychosocial issues: See Increased Intracranial Pressure

x. Treatments (see also Increased Intracranial Pressure): Recommended sequence of pharmacologic, noninvasive, and invasive treatments for initial TBI management and treatment of intracranial hypertension are described in Boxes 4-13 and 4-14. Decisions about the use of various interventions may also be influenced by cerebral oxygenation (see Boxes 4-5 and 4-6) or blood flow parameters.

    (a) Noninvasive

        (1) Control blood loss from scalp laceration via direct compression followed eventually by surgical repair

        (2) Maintain normothermia as described under Increased Intracranial Pressure. Therapeutic hypothermia may reduce ICP and risk of death or poor neurologic outcome in severe TBI, but clinical evidence insufficient to recommend routine use.

        (3) Hyperventilation: Can be used during initial resuscitation if the patient demonstrates neurologic deterioration or brain herniation. In the absence of increased ICP, prolonged $Paco_2$ reductions to less than 25 mm Hg and, in first 24 hours after TBI, chronic prophylactic reductions to 35 mm Hg or less should be avoided because cerebral perfusion can be compromised. Brief periods of hyperventilation may be necessary for patients with neurologic deterioration or for longer if ICP elevations are refractory to other therapy. If necessary, first lower $Paco_2$ to 30 to 35 mm Hg; if ICP remains refractory to intervention, then

■ **BOX 4-13**
■ **RECOMMENDED TREATMENT SEQUENCE FOR INITIAL MANAGEMENT OF SEVERE TRAUMATIC BRAIN INJURY**

1. Perform Advanced Trauma Life Support evaluation and emergency diagnostic or therapeutic procedures as indicated.
2. Perform the following interventions:
   - Endotracheal intubation
   - Ventilation to a $Paco_2$ (partial pressure of carbon dioxide) of 35 mm Hg
   - Fluid resuscitation
   - Supplemental oxygen administration
   - Sedation and possibly administration of a short-acting paralytic agent
3. If there is evidence of brain herniation or neurologic deterioration, consider hyperventilation and, if patient is adequately hydrated, bolus administration of mannitol.
4. Take the patient for a computed tomographic (CT) scan of the head.
5. If there is evidence of a surgically treatable lesion on CT scan, move the patient to the operating room for intervention (e.g., removal of a space-occupying lesion).
6. Once operative intervention is complete or if no surgically treatable lesion is present, move the patient to an intensive care unit and monitor and manage intracranial pressure and cerebral perfusion pressure.

Data from Bullock R, Chesnut RM, Clifton G, et al: Guidelines for the management of severe head injury. In Brain Trauma Foundation, American Association of Neurological Surgeons: *Management and prognosis of severe traumatic brain injury*, New York, 2000, Brain Trauma Foundation.

■ **BOX 4-14**
■ **RECOMMENDED TREATMENT PATHWAY FOR INTRACRANIAL HYPERTENSION IN PATIENTS WITH SEVERE TRAUMATIC BRAIN INJURY**

1. Insert intracranial pressure (ICP) monitor and maintain ICP at less than 20 mm Hg and cerebral perfusion pressure at more than 60 mm Hg.
2. Intially treat increasing ICP with general maneuvers such as proper positioning, sedation, seizure prophylaxis, body temperature control, adequate oxygenation, ventilation and volume resuscitation, and possibly pharmacologic paralysis.
3. If intracranial hypertension occurs, treat by draining cerebrospinal fluid if ventriculostomy in place.
4. If intracranial hypertension persists, consider need for repeat head computed tomographic (CT) scan and hyperventilate patient to a $Paco_2$ (partial pressure of carbon dioxide) of 30 to 35 mm Hg.
5. If intracranial hypertension persists, consider need for repeat head CT scan and administer mannitol bolus. (May repeat mannitol administration if patient remains euvolemic with serum osmolarity of less than 320 mOsm/L.)
6. If intracranial hypertension persists, consider need for repeat head CT scan and institute second-tiered therapies, such as
   - High-dose barbiturate coma
   - Hyperventilation to a $Paco_2$ of less than 30 mm Hg, preferably while monitoring effect on cerebral oxygenation or cerebral blood flow
   - Decompressive craniectomy

From Bullock R, Chesnut RM, Clifton G, et al; Guidelines for the management of severe head injury. In Brain Trauma Foundation, American Association of Neurological Surgeons: *Management and prognosis of severe traumatic brain injury*, New York, 2000, Brain Trauma Foundation; and Brain Trauma Foundation, American Association of Neurological Surgeons, Congress of Neurological Surgeons, Joint Section on Neurotrauma and Critical Care: Guidelines for the management of severe traumatic brain injury: cerebral perfusion pressure, 2003, retrieved June 24, 2004, from http://www2.braintrauma.org/guidelines/downloads/btf_guidelines_cpp_u1.pdf.

consider reduction to below 30 mm Hg (see Box 4-13). CBF or oxygenation monitoring recommended if $Paco_2$ is less than 30 mm Hg to detect brain ischemia.
  (b) Invasive
    (1) Patients with severe TBI require ET intubation and ventilatory support
    (2) Repair scalp lacerations within 24 to 48 hours
    (3) Remove space-occupying lesions (e.g., hematoma) as soon as possible
    (4) Unilateral or bilateral decompressive craniectomy (i.e., removal of cranium, opening of dura) allows room for the edematous brain to control refractory ICP elevations
  xi. Ethical issues: See Increased Intracranial Pressure
 b. Potential complications (see also health problems described under Patient Care)
    i. Increased ICP and related complications
      (a) Mechanism: Development of cerebral edema, hyperemia, intracranial hemorrhage, venous outflow obstruction, and posttraumatic hydrocephalus can all increase intracranial volume, which results in intracranial hypertension
      (b) Management: See Increased Intracranial Pressure
    ii. Vasospasm: Most common in patients with severe TBI who have SAH (see complications under Intracranial Aneurysms)

iii. Seizures (see also Seizures section)
(a) Mechanism: Epileptogenic focus created at the time of injury. Early seizures occur within the first 7 days after TBI; late seizures occur at least 7 days following injury. Severity of the TBI directly correlates with the risk for seizures. Other risk factors for late seizures include penetrating head injury, brain contusion, depressed skull fracture, intracranial hemorrhage, prolonged unconsciousness, and early seizures.
(b) Management: Administer prophylactic anticonvulsants (e.g., phenytoin, carbamazepine) for the first 7 days after severe TBI; these agents are not effective in preventing late posttraumatic seizures.
iv. Intracranial infection: See Intracranial Infection: Bacterial Meningitis and Intracranial Infection: Viral Encephalitis

8. **Evaluation of patient care**
   a. ICP, CPP, CBF, and oxygenation remain within the desired range without the need for intervention
   b. Optimal recovery of neurologic function is achieved
   c. Complications are prevented or recognized and effectively managed

Intracranial Aneurysms

1. **Pathophysiology**
   a. Localized dilatation of an artery resulting from weakness of the vessel wall
   b. In adults, 85% occur in the anterior circulation, usually at bifurcations in the anterior circle of Willis. Common sites in the posterior circulation include the basilar artery apex, basilar artery junctions with the adjoining vertebral, anterior inferior cerebellar, and superior cerebellar arteries, and the vertebral and posterior inferior cerebellar artery junction.
   c. Some 10% to 20% of patients have multiple aneurysms
   d. Aneurysm growth is not thoroughly understood but is affected by hemodynamic factors and arterial wall integrity. As the aneurysm enlarges it can compress surrounding nerves and brain tissue, causing neurologic deficits.
   e. Enlargement further weakens the vessel wall, so rupture can occur. Each year, there is a 1% to 2% risk of rupture. Rupture most often causes SAH and less frequently intracerebral, intraventricular (common with anterior communicating artery aneurysms), or subdural hemorrhage.

2. **Etiology and risk factors**
   a. Etiology of most aneurysms is unclear. Although they were once thought due to congenital defects, research indicates that the likely cause is hemodynamically induced degenerative changes.
   b. Familial association in some patients, but causes are not known. Risk of aneurysm-related SAH (aSAH) increases if a first-degree family member has had an aSAH. Risk of aSAH increases with age (highest incidence in 40- to 60-year age group), hypertension, heavy alcohol consumption, amphetamine abuse, use of oral contraceptives, atherosclerosis, and hypercholesterolemia.
   c. Higher risk of aneurysm formation and rupture in association with female gender, ischemic heart disease in women, cigarette smoking, and diseases such as adult polycystic kidney disease and Ehlers-Danlos syndrome
   d. Traumatic aneurysm: Trauma injures the vessel wall
   e. Mycotic aneurysm: Bacterial or fungal infections send septic emboli that attach to the cerebral vessel wall and destroy it
   f. Atherosclerotic aneurysm: Deposition of atheromatous material damages vessel walls, which causes formation of fusiform aneurysms (arterial wall outpouching with no defined aneurysm stem or neck)

3. **Signs and symptoms**
   a. Prior to rupture, most patients are asymptomatic
   b. Large aneurysms may compress nearby brain tissue causing focal neurologic symptoms. Examples of focal symptoms include the following:
      i. Cranial nerve deficits, especially CN III, IV, or VI dysfunction
      ii. Pain behind or above the eye
      iii. Localized headache
   c. Patient usually comes for treatment with signs of intracranial hemorrhage (usually SAH) from aneurysm rupture. Specific signs and symptoms vary with the severity and location of the hemorrhage. Aneurysmal SAH is graded most commonly using the Hunt and Hess scale (Table 4-32). Good outcomes are correlated with Hunt and Hess scores of I to III and worse outcomes with scores of IV and V. (The World Federation of Neurologic Surgeons scale is another tool that may be used to grade aSAH.)
   d. Other signs and symptoms of aSAH
      i. Presenting complaint: "Worst headache of my life"
      ii. Nausea, vomiting, dizziness
      iii. Usually brief loss of consciousness, but may be prolonged if the hemorrhage is large or causes hydrocephalus or brain edema
      iv. Symptoms of meningeal irritation
         (a) *Nuchal rigidity:* Resistance to flexion of the neck
         (b) *Brudzinski's sign:* Adduction and flexion of the legs as the examiner flexes the patient's neck
         (c) *Kernig's sign:* When the patient's hip is flexed and the knee is at a right angle, the examiner's attempts to extend the leg elicit resistance or hamstring pain and spasm
         (d) Headache, photophobia
      v. Cranial nerve deficits (pupillary and eye movement dysfunction)
      vi. Motor deficits (e.g., hemiparesis, decerebrate posturing)
      vii. Alterations in vital signs may be seen
   e. Evidence of ICH or SDH due to rupture (see Head Trauma)
   f. Evidence of stroke syndrome (see Ischemic Stroke, Hemorrhagic Stroke)
   g. Evidence of increased ICP (see Increased Intracranial Pressure)

◼ **TABLE 4-32**
◼ ◼ **Hunt and Hess Classification of Subarachnoid Hemorrhages**

Grade	Description
I	Asymptomatic, or mild headache and slight nuchal rigidity
II	Cranial nerve palsy (e.g., III and VI), moderate to severe headache, nuchal rigidity
III	Mild focal deficit, lethargy, or confusion
IV	Stupor, moderate to severe hemiparesis, early decerebrate rigidity
V	Deep coma, decerebrate rigidity, moribund appearance. Add one grade for serious systemic disease (e.g., hypertension, chronic obstructive pulmonary disease) or severe vasospasm on angiography.

MODIFIED CLASSIFICATION ADDS THE FOLLOWING

0	Unruptured aneurysm
1a	No acute meningeal or brain reaction, but with fixed neurologic deficit

From Hinkle J, Guanci MM, Bowman L, et al: Cerebrovascular events of the nervous system. In Bader MK, Littlejohns LR, editors: *AANN core curriculum for neuroscience nursing,* ed 4, St Louis, 2004, Saunders, p 980.

4. **Diagnostic study findings**
   a. CT scan (initial study of choice) reveals ICH, SDH, intraventricular blood, amount and distribution of SAH, and hydrocephalus. Density of SAH and risk of vasospasm are graded using the Fisher Scale (Table 4-33). Greater density of SAH, especially around the base of the brain, correlates with high incidence and severity of vasospasm.
   b. CT angiogram affords rapid visualization of arterial anatomy, a three-dimensional image that assists in determining the shape of the aneurysm prior to therapeutic intervention
   c. Cerebral angiogram illustrates the size, shape, and location of aneurysms and the presence of vasospasm
   d. MRI reveals evidence of hemorrhage and hydrocephalus but is not the study of choice
   e. MRA may diagnose aneurysms larger than 3 mm
   f. Transcranial Doppler ultrasonography may reveal vasospasm, altered blood flow states, increased ICP, impaired autoregulation, or brain death after aSAH
   g. Lumbar puncture: Performed in patients with suspected SAH for whom there are no evidence of blood on CT scan and no signs of increased ICP. After SAH, the CSF contains red blood cells (RBCs) and appears xanthochromic (yellowish) after centrifuging, which indicates that hemorrhage occurred several hours earlier. CSF protein and WBC counts are elevated. CSF pressure may be elevated.
5. **Goals of care**
   a. Brain ischemia is minimized to optimize neurologic outcomes
   b. Rebleeding, vasospasm, hydrocephalus, increased ICP, seizures, hyponatremia, and cardiac arrhythmias are prevented or, if they occur, are recognized and appropriately managed
   c. Patient and family are prepared for interventions, possible complications, and outcomes
6. **Collaborating professionals on health care team:** See Increased Intracranial Pressure; also interventional radiologist
7. **Management of patient care**
   a. Anticipated patient trajectory: Numerous factors influence the clinical course and outcome, including the location and extent of hemorrhage; the occurrence and severity of complications; age; and preexisting disorders. Anticipated patient trajectory for ICP is also relevant if aneurysm rupture precipitates intracranial hypertension (see Increased Intracranial Pressure). Other acute care needs specific to patients with aneurysms include the following:

■ **TABLE 4-33**
■ ■ **Fisher Grading Scale**

Grade	Blood Seen on Computed Tomographic Scan
0	Unruptured
I	No blood seen on scan
II	Diffuse subarachnoid blood or vertical layers <1 mm thick
III	Dense subarachnoid blood (clot) in the fissures and basal cisterns and/or vertical layers ≥1 mm thick
IV	Intracerebral or intraventricular clot with diffuse or no subarachnoid blood

    i. Positioning: Elevate the head of the bed 30 degrees to promote cerebrovenous outflow

   ii. Skin care: See Increased Intracranial Pressure

 iii. Pain management: Administer prescribed analgesics for headache and surgical incision pain. Short-acting or easily reversible agents preferred. Give cautiously to patients not on ventilator support; avoid hypotension; monitor pain relief.

 iv. Nutrition: Maintain normoglycemia. If LOC or dysphagia precludes oral intake, employ alternative methods of feeding early (see Dysphagia under Patient Care).

  v. Infection control: See Increased Intracranial Pressure if a ventriculostomy tube is placed

 vi. Discharge planning: See Increased Intracranial Pressure

vii. Pharmacology

    (a) Supplemental oxygen to prevent hypoxia and insufficient cerebral oxygen delivery

    (b) Administer prescribed fluids and antihypertensives (e.g., nitroprusside, labetalol) or vasopressors to maintain BP at the desired level; carefully avoid even transient incidents of hypotension. Generally, before aneurysm repair the desired systolic BP is 120 to 150 mm Hg; after repair the desired systolic BP is more than 160 to 200 mm Hg. Goal is to keep CPP above 60 mm Hg. Use measurements from an arterial line, central venous pressure, possibly measurements from a pulmonary artery line to guide therapy.

    (c) Calcium channel blocker (i.e., nimodipine) for vasospasm (see Potential Complications later)

    (d) Sedation may be prescribed to control agitation, which can elevate BP and ICP

    (e) Stool softeners may be prescribed to prevent straining, which can elevate BP and ICP

    (f) Prophylactic anticonvulsants may be prescribed, at least in the acute phase

    (g) Antibiotics may be prescribed for mycotic aneurysm

viii. Psychosocial issue: Intervene to help alleviate the patient's and family's fear and anxiety by providing information and encouraging the use of appropriate coping mechanisms and support systems (see Chapter 10)

 ix. Treatments

    (a) Noninvasive

       (1) SAH patients in poor neurologic and medical condition may be managed medically until status improves

       (2) Prior to aneurysm repair, avoid BP elevations, which increase the risk of rupture: Manage pain; have the patient avoid straining and performing the Valsalva maneuver; provide a private room and quiet environment; limit visitors

       (3) Monitor neurologic status closely and report changes to the physician

    (b) Invasive

       (1) Adequate ventilation may require ET intubation and ventilatory support

       (2) Ventriculostomy tube placed for high-grade SAH (i.e., Hunt and Hess grade of III or higher), hydrocephalus, or increased ICP. Prior to aneurysm repair, slowly drain CSF and avoid overdrainage, which may relieve tamponade on the aneurysm and cause rebleeding.

(3) Cerebral oxygen or blood flow monitor placed to help guide therapy

(4) Surgical or endovascular interventions may be performed to seal off the aneurysm and prevent bleeding or rebleeding. Research demonstrates that performing intervention within the first 24 to 48 hours after rupture improves outcome. Once the aneurysm is obliterated, vasospasm and other complications can be treated more aggressively.

(5) Surgical repair

a) Clipping of the aneurysm neck to obliterate

b) Aneurysms not amenable to clipping may be resected or wrapped to reinforce the vessel wall

(6) Interventional neuroradiologists may insert devices such as coils, detachable balloons, and/or stents to occlude the aneurysm

x. Ethical issues: Halting further treatment or withdrawing current therapy may be considered with the family when diagnostic study findings and neurologic examination indicate a dismal prognosis

b. Potential complications: See Box 4-15; also see health problems under Patient Care

8. **Evaluation of patient care**

a. Patient achieves optimal neurologic outcomes

b. Complications are prevented or are recognized and treated

c. Patient and family are prepared for interventions, possible complications, and outcomes

Arteriovenous Malformations

1. **Pathophysiology:** Abnormal vascular network consisting of one or more direct connections between arteries and veins without an intervening capillary network. May be localized or extensive; most often located in the supratentorial structures; commonly involve the cortex. Affected vessels develop thin walls and become passively enlarged. Seven percent to 17% of patients with AVMs have aneurysms, usually in major feeding arteries. Brain parenchyma between AVM vessels consists of nonfunctional neuroglia. Brain tissue around an AVM may receive insufficient perfusion due to the diversion of blood to the AVM (*vascular steal* phenomenon). High flow volume and increased venous pressure predispose the fragile vessels of the AVM to rupture, most often causing ICH and, less frequently, IVH, SAH, or SDH. Smaller AVMs are more likely to bleed than larger lesions.

2. **Etiology and risk factors**: Congenital lesions caused by an embryonic vascular malformation

3. **Signs and symptoms**: May be caused by mass effect of malformation, inadequate perfusion to adjacent brain tissue, venous hypertension, or hemorrhage from the lesion

a. AVM may be found incidentally during diagnostic tests

b. Most are not symptomatic until the third decade of life

c. Clinical signs and symptoms associated with hemorrhage into the parenchyma (see Hemorrhagic Stroke), subdural space (see Head Trauma), ventricles, or subarachnoid space (see Intracranial Aneurysms) are the most common presentation; other signs and symptoms depend on the extent and location of bleeding

d. Seizures: Second most common presenting sign; more common initial symptom in patients with large AVMs

e. Headache: Recurrent, unresponsive to traditional therapy

■ **BOX 4-15**
■ **POTENTIAL COMPLICATIONS OF INTRACRANIAL ANEURYSMS**

REBLEEDING
MECHANISM
- Most common during first 2 weeks after rupture when aneurysm not repaired.
- Peak incidence in first 24 to 28 hours and at 7 to 10 days after initial subarachnoid hemorrhage (SAH).
- Typically causes sudden severe headache, nausea, vomiting, and neurologic deterioration.
- Associated with significant mortality and morbidity.

MANAGEMENT
- Early surgical or endovascular repair is most effective intervention to prevent rebleed.
- Correct any coagulopathy that may be present.

VASOSPASM
MECHANISM
- Sustained arterial contraction reduces distal cerebral blood flow (CBF) and may cause brain ischemia and infarct.
- Commonly occurs 3 to 14 days after rupture, but may be delayed up to 3 weeks after SAH.
- Incidence and degree are directly related to amount of blood in subarachnoid space.
- Neurologic symptoms may not occur or there may be subtle or dramatic deterioration in neurologic function.
- Signs and symptoms may include the following:
  - Headache, altered level of consciousness, focal neurologic signs (e.g., speech impairment, hemiparesis), seizures; hypotension can worsen ischemia and exacerbate neurologic deficits.
  - Transcranial Doppler ultrasonography, usually done daily for 14 days after SAH, may detect vasospasm (blood flow velocity >120 cm/sec indicates vasospasm, flow velocities >200 cm/sec are diagnostic of severe spasm; ratio of middle cerebral artery velocity to internal carotid artery velocity >3 indicates cerebral vasospasm rather than hyperemia; ratio >6 indicates severe vasospasm).
  - Cerebral angiography used to diagnose or confirm vasospasm.
  - $Pbto_2$ (brain tissue partial pressure of oxygen) or CBF decreases if sensor located in region fed by the spastic vessel.

MANAGEMENT
- Immediately following SAH diagnosis, calcium channel blocker (i.e., nimodipine) is given prophylactically to reduce vasospasm and improve long-term outcomes. Dosage is 60 mg every 4 hours or, if hypotension occurs, 30 mg every 2 hours for 21 days.
- After aneurysm repair, hypervolemia, hemodilution, and hypertension (so-called triple-H therapy) are used to enhance cerebral perfusion. Prior to aneurysm repair a modified version of this intervention may be used. Fluids, vasopressors (e.g., phenylephrine), and inotropic agents (e.g., dobutamine) are used to maintain systolic blood pressure above 160 to about 200 mm Hg but not higher than 240 mm Hg. (Desired systolic blood pressure before aneurysm repair is 120 to 150 mm Hg.) Hemodilution and hypervolemia are accomplished by administration of colloid (e.g., albumin, hetastarch) and isotonic crystalloid solutions.
- Goals are to maintain cerebral perfusion pressure above 60 to 70 mm Hg; pulmonary artery wedge pressure of 10 to 20 mm Hg; central venous pressure of 8 to 12 mm Hg; cardiac index higher than 2.2; and hematocrit below 40% (usual target level is 32% to 38%). Therapeutic goals vary depending on neurologic, pulmonary, and cardiac status. Neurologic, hemodynamic, pulmonary, and fluid and electrolyte status require close monitoring during triple-H therapy so that complications (pulmonary edema, heart failure, myocardial ischemia, stroke, electrolyte imbalance) can be prevented or minimized.
- Endovascular intervention may be used to treat confirmed vasospasm unresponsive to nimodipine or triple-H therapy.

Continued

■ **BOX 4-15**
■ **POTENTIAL COMPLICATIONS OF INTRACRANIAL ANEURYSMS—cont'd**

MANAGEMENT—cont'd
- Balloon angioplasty may be done to enlarge a stenotic vessel.
- A vascular smooth muscle relaxant (e.g., papaverine, verapamil) may be injected into a spastic artery during angiography to relax and dilate the vessel. Effects may be temporary and may cause intracranial pressure (ICP) elevation.

HYDROCEPHALUS
MECHANISM
- Clot formed at rupture site may obstruct flow of cerebrospinal fluid (CSF), and blood in subarachnoid space may obstruct arachnoid villi, impeding reabsorption of CSF.
- Onset may be delayed days or weeks after SAH.
- Symptoms may include diminished level of consciousness, ataxia, headache, blurred vision, diplopia, nausea, vomiting, incontinence and signs of increased ICP

MANAGEMENT
- Initially ventriculostomy tube is placed to drain CSF until ICP is normal and ventricular and subarachnoid spaces are clear of blood. With less acute onset, lumbar drain may be placed to remove CSF.
- Ventricular size is monitored with serial computed tomographic (CT) scans.
- If frequent CSF drainage is required to keep ICP below 20 mm Hg and the ventricular system remains enlarged on CT scan, a ventriculoperitoneal shunt is usually placed.

INCREASED INTRACRANIAL PRESSURE AND RELATED COMPLICATIONS
- Refer to Increased Intracranial Pressure under Specific Patient Health Problems.

SEIZURES
- Refer to Seizures under Specific Patient Health Problems.

HYPONATREMIA
MECHANISM
- Usually secondary to syndrome of inappropriate secretion of antidiuretic hormone or cerebral salt wasting.
- May precede or occur during vasospasm.

MANAGEMENT
- Refer to Fluid and Electrolyte Imbalance under Patient Care; Chapter 5.

CARDIAC ARRHYTHMIAS AND REPOLARIZATION ABNORMALITIES
- Refer to Chapter 3.

MECHANISM
- Associated with SAH; may relate to systemic release of catecholamines.

MANAGEMENT
- Refer to Chapter 3.

f. Pulsatile tinnitus
g. Progressive neurologic deficits; depend on the area of the brain affected
h. Neuropsychiatric behavior: Occurs in about 10% of patients
i. AVMs graded according to the Spetzler-Martin AVM grading scale (Table 4-34). Higher grade of lesion correlates with increased morbidity with surgical intervention.

■ **TABLE 4-34**
■ ■ **Spetzler-Martin Grading Scale for Arteriovenous Malformations**

Feature	Grade
SIZE	
0-3 cm	1
3.1-6.0 cm	2
>6 cm	3
LOCATION*	
Noneloquent	0
Eloquent	1
DEEP VENOUS DRAINAGE	
Not present	0
Present	1

Adapted from Hinkle JL, Guanci MM, Bowman L, et al: Cerebrovascular events of the nervous system. In Bader MK, Littlejohns LR, editors: *AANN core curriculum for neuroscience nursing,* ed 4, St Louis, 2004, Saunders, p 980.
Grade = size + eloquence + venous drainage; that is 1, 2, or 3 + 0 or 1 + 0 or 1.
*Eloquent refers to anatomic areas of the brain known to control important neurologic functions, such as the sensorimotor cortex, thalamus, and brainstem.

4. **Diagnostic study findings**
   a. CT: Noncontrast scan may show areas of calcification in and around the AVM and may detect hemorrhage. Contrast-enhanced scan often shows large tortuous feeding arteries or draining veins.
   b. CT angiography: Reveals composition of the AVM
   c. Cerebral angiography: Most definitive, revealing the anatomy of feeding and draining vessels; the size and location of the AVM; intracranial hemorrhage; and vasospasm
   d. MRI: Identifies AVM location and size; may reveal cerebral edema as well as an old hemorrhage indicated by the presence of hemosiderin
   e. MRA: Reveals the composition of the vessels in the lesion
5. **Goals of care**
   a. AVM is obliterated without hemorrhage or brain tissue injury
   b. Patient's neurologic status remains normal or improves
   c. Complications such as hemorrhage, cerebral edema, hydrocephalus, increased ICP, and seizures are prevented or minimized
   d. Patient and family are prepared for interventions, possible complications, and outcomes
6. **Collaborating professionals on health care team:** See Increased Intracranial Pressure; also interventional radiologist, neuroradiologist
7. **Management of patient care**
   a. Anticipated patient trajectory: Numerous factors influence the clinical course and outcome, including the location, size, and characteristics of the AVM; the occurrence and severity of complications; the effectiveness of interventions to obliterate the lesion; the patient's age; and the presence of comorbidities. If the AVM ruptures, the patient is managed similarly to other patients with intracranial hemorrhage (refer to Head Trauma, Intracranial Aneurysms,

and Hemorrhagic Stroke). Morbidity, mortality, and risk of vasospasm are lower from AVM hemorrhage than from aneurysmal hemorrhage.

  i. Skin care: See Increased Intracranial Pressure
  ii. Pain management and nutrition: See Intracranial Aneurysms
  iii. Discharge planning: See Increased Intracranial Pressure
  iv. Pharmacology
    (a) IV fluids to maintain normovolemia
    (b) Antihypertensives to maintain BP in the desired range
    (c) Anticonvulsants to prevent or treat seizures
  v. Psychosocial issues: See Intracranial Aneurysms
  vi. Treatments: May include conservative management, a single treatment, or a combination of interventions. Choice of treatment depends on AVM size, location, and characteristics; the patient's clinical condition, preexisting comorbidities, and age; and the capabilities of health care providers.
    (a) Noninvasive: Radiosurgery (e.g., gamma knife, proton beam): Uses stereotactically directed radiation to initiate vessel wall inflammation, which causes thickening and eventually thrombosis and obliteration of the AVM vessels. Obliterates or shrinks AVMs up to 3 cm in diameter with little collateral damage to normal brain tissue. AVM is vulnerable to hemorrhage until vessels thrombose (takes 1 to 3 years).
    (b) Invasive
        (1) Craniotomy and microsurgery to resect the AVM: Spetzler-Martin grade 1 and 2 (and some grade 3) lesions usually amenable to surgical resection. Grade 4 to 5 lesions are more complex, have higher treatment-associated morbidity, and therefore may require multifaceted treatment approach.
        (2) Embolization: Flow-directed and flow-assisted microcatheters are navigated through the vasculature to the pathologic area, where a solid or liquid embolic agent is delivered to obliterate some or all of the AVM. May be curative, palliative, or an adjunct to surgery or radiosurgery.
  vii. Ethical issues: See Intracranial Aneurysms
b. Potential complications
  i. Rebleeding
    (a) Mechanism: Slightly increased risk for a year after initial hemorrhage; causes sudden neurologic deterioration
    (b) Management
        (1) Obliterate the AVM; treatment is generally elective unless an ICH or SDH requires urgent intervention
        (2) Maintain BP within the ordered range
        (3) Monitor neurologic status often in the first 24 to 48 hours
  ii. Seizures (see Seizures section): AVM obliteration may reduce the incidence of seizures
  iii. Hydrocephalus
    (a) Mechanism: May occur from SAH, IVH, or compression of the ventricle or aqueduct of Sylvius by the AVM
    (b) Management: See Potential Complications under Intracranial Aneurysms
  iv. Postoperative cerebral edema and hemorrhage
    (a) Mechanism: May result from normal CPP breakthrough as a result of the shunting of high-pressure arterial blood into low-pressure veins. Usually occurs early in the postoperative period; may be complicated

by hypertension. Neurologic deterioration, especially a change in LOC, typically signals onset.

    (b) Management: Monitor BP and neurologic status closely for the first 24 to 48 hours; keep BP within the ordered range

  v. Hemorrhage or ischemia with endovascular therapy

    (a) Mechanism: Vessel rupture or a thromboembolic event may occur during or after an endovascular procedure

    (b) Management

      (1) Administer prescribed heparin therapy to prevent thromboembolism and maintain coagulation within the desired range. If hemorrhage occurs, heparin reversal indicated.

      (2) See Management under Postoperative Cerebral Edema and Hemorrhage Complication for AVMs

  vi. Increased ICP

    (a) Mechanism: Cerebral edema, intracranial hemorrhage, venous outflow obstruction, and hydrocephalus can all increase ICP

    (b) Management: See Increased Intracranial Pressure

8. Evaluation of patient care

  a. AVM is successfully obliterated

  b. Patient's neurologic status remains normal or improves

  c. Complications are prevented or are recognized and minimized

  d. Patient and family are prepared for interventions, possible complications, and outcomes

Ischemic Stroke

1. Pathophysiology: Cerebral artery becomes narrowed or occluded, interrupting CBF and oxygen delivery and causing brain ischemia in that vascular territory. Lack of oxygen halts ATP energy–dependent cell functions, which renders neurons inactive. Depending on the degree of CBF reduction, nonfunctional, ischemic neurons may remain viable and recover function. If the energy supply remains insufficient or is further reduced, numerous intracellular biochemical and molecular cascades are triggered (e.g., ionic shifts; excessive lactic acid production; accumulation of excitatory neurotransmitters; activation of proteases, endonucleases, and phospholipases; increased free radical formation), which produces cytotoxic edema and neuronal death. Area of brain infarction forms surrounded by a marginally perfused dysfunctional but viable ischemic tissue (called the *penumbra*). Tissue in the penumbra is vulnerable to cell death if CBF and oxygen delivery are not quickly restored or if secondary insults occur (e.g., hypoxia, hypotension, metabolic derangements; see Pathophysiology under Head Trauma). Approximately 80% to 85% of all strokes are ischemic. Mechanisms include the following:

  a. Thrombosis (most common cause of stroke)

    i. Atherosclerosis of large cerebral vessels causes injury and plaque formation along the vessel wall. Platelets aggregate with fibrin and a thrombus forms. Progressive vessel narrowing occurs, eventually occluding the vessel or precluding adequate perfusion.

    ii. Plaques may embolize and occlude smaller vessels

  b. Embolus

    i. Emboli may originate from atherosclerotic plaques in the extracranial or large intracranial vessels; a diseased heart; infection; particulate matter, fat, or air that gains access to the vasculature; hypercoagulability; or clots caused by vascular injury

      ii. Emboli usually lodge at arterial bifurcations, where blood flow is the most turbulent and atherosclerotic narrowing is more common. Tiny emboli or fragments may become lodged in smaller vessels.

  c. Small vessel disease (lacunar strokes)

      i. Lipohyalinosis (hyaline-lipid material lines small penetrating arteries, causing vessel wall thickening) and microatheroma occlude small penetrating arteries that perfuse deep cerebral white matter. Affected brain tissue softens and sloughs away, forming a small cavity or lacuna.

      ii. Most prevalent in the basal ganglia, thalamus, and white matter of the pons and internal capsule

      iii. Hypertension is a primary risk factor

  d. Other less common mechanisms: Hematologic diseases, migraine or vasospasm, arteritis, arterial dissection, infection

  e. Cryptogenic: Diagnostic workup fails to identify the stroke origin

2. Etiology and risk factors

  a. Previous stroke or transient ischemic attack (TIA)

  b. Family history of stroke

  c. Age: Risk doubles every 10 years after age 55 years

  d. Gender: Males have a 9% higher incidence than females but over 60% of deaths occur in females

  e. Race: African Americans have a higher incidence of stroke and nearly twice the risk of death compared to white Americans

  f. Hypertension, hypercholesterolemia, diabetes mellitus

  g. Hypercoagulable states such as polycythemia, sickle cell anemia, pregnancy

  h. Vascular inflammatory processes, vasospasm, migraine, cerebral artery atherosclerosis, carotid artery stenosis

  i. Cardiac disease: Atrial fibrillation (most common source of cardioemboli), coronary artery disease, heart failure, valvular disease, myocardial infarction, patent foramen ovale with atrial septal aneurysm, left atrial or ventricular thrombi

  j. Behavioral risk factors: Smoking, heavy alcohol use, illicit drug use, sedentary lifestyle, obesity

  k. Medication history

      i. Oral contraceptive use, especially in women over 30 years of age who smoke

      ii. Nonaspirin NSAIDs: Can interfere with the antiplatelet effects of drugs such as aspirin, clopidogrel, and aspirin with dipyridamole

3. Signs and symptoms

  a. Report of a prior TIA: Ischemic event that results in a reversible, short-lived neurologic deficit (<24 hours but may be only minutes). Deficits are the same as for stroke but are short-lived; the highest risk of stroke is within 24 hours of a TIA, so emergent patient evaluation and treatment for secondary prevention are important to avoid a disabling stroke.

  b. Onset of focal neurologic deficits that correlate with a known vascular territory and persist for over 24 hours

  c. Clinical presentation varies, depending on the area of the brain involved and the extent of injury (Tables 4-35 and 4-36)

  d. Headache present in about 25% of patients

  e. Spontaneous BP elevations are common after acute stroke, although low-normal BP may be seen with stroke affecting the entire anterior circulation or if coronary artery events occur simultaneously

  f. National Institutes of Health Stroke Scale: Routinely used to measure neurologic function after acute ischemic stroke. Scores range from 0 to 42, with

■ **TABLE 4-35**
■ ■ **Signs and Symptoms of Stroke Syndromes Associated with Specific Vessel Involvement**

Occluded Vessel	Signs and Symptoms*
Internal carotid artery	Contralateral face, arm, and leg paralysis and sensory deficits Homonymous hemianopsia (loss of half of field of vision) Transient monocular blindness (amaurosis fugax) due to retinal artery emboli Ipsilateral Horner's syndrome (see Table 4-19) Headache behind ipsilateral eye Dominant hemisphere: Aphasia Nondominant hemisphere: Neglect and/or agnosia
Anterior cerebral artery (ACA)	Motor and sensory deficits in contralateral lower extremity with distal weakness (i.e., foot) worse; impaired gait Possible mild contralateral upper extremity weakness Abulia (slowness to react) Cognitive impairment: Perseveration, amnesia Apraxia Personality changes, flat affect, easy distractibility, lack of initiative Urinary incontinence
Middle cerebral artery (MCA)	Contralateral paralysis and sensory loss in arm with leg spared or with less deficit Contralateral lower face paralysis Homonymous hemianopsia Dominant hemisphere: Aphasia, dyslexia, agraphia (inability to express thoughts in writing), acalculia (inability to do simple math) Nondominant hemisphere: Constructional apraxia (inability to reproduce or complete a drawing, drawing left half incomplete), dressing apraxia (inability to dress self), loss of sense of spatial relationships, autotopagnosia (inability to recognize parts of body)
Vertebral artery	Wallenberg's syndrome (see posterior inferior cerebellar artery, next page) Ipsilateral facial weakness and numbness, facial and eye pain Clumsiness, ataxia, dizziness or vertigo Nystagmus Dysphagia, dysarthria
Basilar artery	Nausea and vomiting Progressive decline in level of consciousness Impaired ocular movement, conjugate gaze paralysis, diplopia Pupillary changes: Pupils miotic (pontine) or large and less light responsive (midbrain) Facial sensory loss; facial, pharyngeal, and lingual muscle weakness Dysarthria, dysphagia Alternating hemiparesis Possible "locked-in syndrome" (no movement except eyelids; consciousness and cortical function, including sensation, are preserved) Dysmetria Ataxia, vertigo Acute deafness
Posterior cerebral artery (PCA)	Manifestations can vary widely: • Homonymous hemianopsia; visual deficits—loss of depth perception, blindness, visual hallucinations • Memory loss • Thalamus involvement: Contralateral sensory loss (all modalities), hemiparesis, intention tremors, spontaneous pain • Cerebral peduncle involvement: Weber's syndrome (contralateral hemiplegia with cranial nerve III palsy)

Continued

■ **TABLE 4-35**
■ ■ **Signs and Symptoms of Stroke Syndromes Associated with Specific Vessel Involvement—cont'd**

Occluded Vessel	Signs and Symptoms*
Posterior inferior cerebellar artery (Wallenberg's syndrome)	Nausea and vomiting Dysphagia, impaired gag reflex and swallowing Dysarthria Nystagmus, diplopia Hiccups Vertigo, ataxia Ipsilateral facial numbness and Horner's syndrome Loss of pain and temperature sensation over contralateral trunk and extremities
Small penetrating arteries (e.g., lenticulostriate branches of ACA and MCA, paramedian branches of basilar artery, thalamoperforate branches of PCA)	Contralateral hemiplegia equally affecting leg, arm, and face without aphasia, visual impairment, or sensory loss Sensory loss in leg, trunk, arm, and face; may be associated with pain without motor loss Dysarthria Clumsiness, ipsilateral ataxia

*Some or all of the deficits may be evident when a particular vessel is occluded; syndromes frequently overlap.

higher scores indicating greater neurologic impairment. Used to determine stroke severity and to guide decisions about thrombolytic use. (Scale available at http://www.ninds.nih.gov/doctors/NIH_Stroke_Scale.pdf.)

4. **Diagnostic study findings**
   a. Laboratory
      i. Serum glucose level, electrolyte levels, CBC, liver and renal function studies, lipid panel, tests for prothrombic states (e.g., levels of protein S, lupus anticoagulant): To assess stroke risk factors, identify imbalances that warrant treatment, and rule out conditions that mimic stroke
      ii. Platelet count, PT, PTT, INR: To check adequacy of coagulation
      iii. Toxicology screen: May identify drug (e.g., cocaine) that precipitated stroke
   b. Radiologic
      i. CT scan without contrast: To exclude hemorrhage or mass lesions as the cause of deficits. Ischemia and infarctions often are not seen for 24 hours or more after the occlusive event, whereas hemorrhage is seen immediately. Ideally the CT scan is done within 25 minutes of the physician's writing the order and is interpreted within 20 minutes of scan completion.
      ii. CT scan with contrast: To rule out lesions mimicking a TIA or stroke
      iii. CT angiography: Helpful to identify acute vascular occlusion and vascular lesions
      iv. Perfusion CT scan: Identifies ischemic stroke, shows area of infarct and penumbra
      v. Cerebral angiography: Reveals vessel abnormalities, occlusion, stenosis, spasm, or displacement

■ **TABLE 4-36**
■ ■ **Signs and Symptoms of Stroke Syndromes Associated with Specific Stroke Location**

Location	Signs and Symptoms
Right (nondominant) hemisphere	Left hemiparesis and sensory loss
	Left visual field deficit
	Right gaze preference
	Dysarthria
	Flat affect
	Spatial perception deficits
	Constructional and dressing apraxia
	Neglect of left side (inattention to objects in the left visual field and to left auditory stimuli)
	Anosognosia (unawareness or denial of deficits on affected side)
Left (dominant) hemisphere	Right hemiparesis and sensory loss
	Right visual field deficit
	Left gaze preference
	Acalculia, agraphia
	Aphasia (expressive, receptive or global)
	Apraxia of left limbs
	Finger agnosia (inability to identify the finger touched)
	Right-left disorientation
Brainstem, cerebellum	Diplopia
	Dysmetria
	Hemiparesis or quadriparesis
	Hemisensory loss or sensory loss in all four limbs and face
	Ocular movement abnormalities
	Acute hearing loss
	Nausea and vomiting, oropharyngeal weakness, dysarthria
	Vertigo, tinnitus, ataxia
	Dysmetria

Adapted from Hinkle JL, Guanci MM, Bowman L, et al: Cerebrovascular events of the nervous system. In Bader MK, Littlejohns LR, editors: *AANN core curriculum for neuroscience nursing*, ed 4, St Louis, 2004, Saunders, p 544.

    vi. MRI: May reveal acute infarction, hemorrhage

   vii. Diffusion-weighted MRI: Detects ischemia from within the first few minutes to 2 weeks

  viii. MRA: Reveals abnormal (occluded, stenosed, atherosclerotic) blood vessels

    ix. PET scan: Provides quantitative values for CBF, CBV, and brain cell metabolism to define infarction size and location; generally not performed in the acute phase after a stroke

     x. SPECT scan: May be used to determine regional and global CBF; generally not used in the acute phase after a stroke

  c. Twelve-lead ECG, continuous ECG monitoring: To detect arrhythmia or cardiac disease contributing to stroke

  d. Lumbar puncture: Done if an SAH is suspected but not seen on CT scan; not used if the patient is a candidate for thrombolytics

  e. Once the patient is stable, additional diagnostic tests to identify the underlying disease that contributed to stroke may be performed

5. Goals of care
   a. Adequate brain perfusion is maintained to minimize ischemia
   b. Optimal recovery of neurologic function occurs
   c. Potential complications are prevented or are recognized and appropriately managed
   d. Patient and family are prepared for interventions, possible complications, and outcomes
6. Collaborating professionals on health care team: See Increased Intracranial Pressure; also possibly interventional radiologist
7. Management of patient care
   a. Anticipated patient trajectory: Patient's clinical course and outcome are influenced by the location and extent of brain ischemia and infarction; the neurologic deficits that result; the occurrence and severity of complications; age; and preexisting health problems. Specific needs for patients with ischemic stroke in the acute care setting include the following:
      i. Positioning
         (a) Keep the head of the bed flat for 24 hours after stroke; then the head can be raised. Get the patient out of bed as early as possible.
         (b) Protect the patient's neglected, paralyzed, or insensate side during positioning
         (c) Position patient items in the unaffected visual field initially; gradually move objects to the affected side and encourage the patient to attend to that side
      ii. Skin care: See Increased Intracranial Pressure
      iii. Pain management: See Increased Intracranial Pressure
      iv. Nutrition: See Intracranial Aneurysms
      v. Transport: When possible, the stroke victim should be rapidly transported to the emergency department for quick assessment and diagnostic studies. If CT scanning is unavailable, the patient's condition should be stabilized and the patient should be transferred to an appropriate facility.
      vi. Discharge planning: See Increased Intracranial Pressure
      vii. Pharmacology: See Box 4-16
      viii. Psychosocial issues (see Intracranial Aneurysms): Depression is common after stroke and if present should be treated with appropriate pharmacotherapy and supportive care. Ensure that the possibility of developing depression is discussed with the patient and family prior to discharge.
      ix. Treatments
         (a) Noninvasive
            (1) Monitor neurologic status closely and report changes to the physician
            (2) Maintain normothermia; use of hypothermia following stroke is under investigation
            (3) Initiate occupational, speech, and physical therapy early
         (b) Invasive
            (1) Intubation and mechanical ventilation may be required for adequate ventilation; avoid $Paco_2$ lower than 35 mm Hg
            (2) Avoid any invasive procedures in patients who are candidates for therapy with tissue plasminogen activator (t-PA). Place a gastric tube or Foley catheter before t-PA is administered.
            (3) CBF or oxygenation monitor may be placed to guide therapy
            (4) Interventional radiology
               a) May be used to deliver thrombolytics to the occlusion site (Box 4-17)

■ **BOX 4-16**
■ **PHARMACOLOGIC THERAPY FOR ISCHEMIC STROKE**

- Supplemental oxygen to maintain adequate systemic and brain tissue oxygenation
- Tissue plasminogen activator (t-PA)
  - Thrombolytic agent that breaks up clot causing vessel occlusion, thereby restoring cerebral blood flow to ischemic tissues and improving neurologic outcome
  - Intravenous (IV) administration considered if within 3 hours of stroke symptom onset and patient meets recommended criteria (see Box 4-16); dose is 0.9 mg/kg to a maximum dose of 90 mg; 10% of dose given over 1 minute and remaining 90% over 1 hour via infusion pump
  - Intraarterial administration may be considered for anterior circulation stroke if within 6 hours of symptom onset; for posterior circulation stroke, typically given up to 8 to 12 hours after symptoms begin but under some circumstances may be given when symptoms have been present even longer; catheter is threaded through the vasculature to the site of the cerebral occlusion, where a small amount of t-PA is delivered; intra-arterial administration not yet approved by the Food and Drug Administration
- Antihypertensives to maintain the blood pressure (BP) within desired range; sublingual calcium channel blockers should not be used; hypotension must be avoided to prevent worsening ischemia!
  - When no thrombolytic agent is used, treatment of hypertension is deferred unless acute myocardial infarction, aortic dissection, hypertensive encephalopathy, or severe left ventricular failure is present or BP exceeds 220 mm Hg systolic, 120 mm Hg diastolic, or mean arterial pressure of 130 mm Hg; use IV labetalol or nitroprusside to achieve BP control
  - For patients who are candidates for thrombolytic administration, systolic BP must be maintained below 185 mm Hg and diastolic below 110 mm Hg to reduce risk of hemorrhage; IV labetalol, nitroprusside, nicardipine, or hydralazine may be used to control BP
- Prescribed IV fluids, isotonic crystalloids without glucose (e.g., normal saline), to maintain hypervolemia or normovolemia
- Vasoactive or inotropic agents if necessary to maintain desired BP
- Insulin as necessary to maintain blood glucose level below 110 mg/dl; hyperglycemia can increase infarct size and cerebral edema
- Antiplatelet agents such as aspirin, clopidogrel (Plavix), and extended-release dipyridamole and aspirin (Aggrenox) to inhibit platelet aggregation and prevent recurrent stroke; initiate once hemorrhage is ruled out in patient not receiving thrombolytics; in patients receiving t-PA, start antiplatelet agent 24 hours after t-PA administration

    b) Angioplasty via balloon inflation at the site of stenosis of a cerebral vessel

    c) Intravascular stenting used with angioplasty to maintain vessel patency

  (5) Surgical interventions to prevent stroke

    a) Carotid endarterectomy removes atherosclerotic plaque and clot from the intraarterial lumen

    b) Extracranial-intracranial bypass: Used selectively to provide collateral circulation for patients with severe major vessel stenosis

  x. Ethical issues: See Intracranial Aneurysms

b. Potential complications: See Box 4-18; also see health problems described under Patient Care

■ **BOX 4-17**
■ **CRITERIA FOR ADMINISTRATION OF THROMBOLYTIC THERAPY**

PATIENT CHARACTERISTICS
- Head computed tomography scan negative for hemorrhage
- Age older than 18 years
- Time of symptom onset less than 3 hours earlier
- No history of intracranial surgery, head trauma, or stroke within past 3 months
- Neurologic signs that are *not* clearing rapidly and spontaneously
- Neurologic signs that are *not* minor and isolated
- No myocardial infarction within the past 3 months
- No gastrointestinal or urinary tract hemorrhage in the previous 21 days
- No major surgery in the previous 14 days
- No arterial puncture at a noncompressible site in the previous 7 days
- No evidence of acute bleeding or acute trauma (fracture) on examination
- No seizure with postictal residual neurologic impairments
- Systolic blood pressure less than 185 mm Hg and diastolic blood pressure less than 110 mm Hg

LABORATORY DATA
- Prothrombin time longer than 15 seconds
- No prolongation of partial thromboplastin time or international normalized ratio less than 1.5
- Platelet count higher than 100,000/mm^3
- Blood glucose level above 50 mg/dl (2.7 mmol/L) and below 400 mg/dl
- Patient *cannot* be lactating or have a positive pregnancy test result

From Hinkle JL, Guanci MM, Bowman L, et al: Cerebrovascular events of the nervous system. In Bader MK, Littlejohns LR, editors: *AANN core curriculum for neuroscience nurses*, St Louis, 2004, Saunders, p 545.

8. Evaluation of patient care
   a. Brain infarct is minimized and ischemia resolves
   b. Optimal neurologic outcome is achieved
   c. Complications are prevented or minimized
   d. Patient and family are prepared for interventions, necessary lifestyle changes, possible complications, and outcomes

Hemorrhagic Stroke

1. Pathophysiology
   a. Rupture of a blood vessel within the cranium. Includes intracerebral hemorrhage (ICH; bleeding into the brain parenchyma), SDH, EDH, intraventricular hemorrhage (IVH), and SAH. SAH most often caused by rupture of an aneurysm or AVM. This section focuses on stroke associated with spontaneous intracerebral hemorrhage.
   b. ICH compresses and irritates cerebral tissues, causing ischemic cellular responses, cerebral edema, intracranial hypertension, and CPP compromise. Functional loss and death of neurons result.
   c. Intracranial hemorrhage associated with hypertension and cerebral amyloid angiopathy usually involves small, deep cortical arteries; most commonly occurs in the basal ganglia, thalamus, cerebellum, or brainstem but may affect more superficial areas of cerebrum
   d. Hemorrhagic strokes account for approximately 15% to 20% of strokes

■ **BOX 4-18**
■ **POTENTIAL COMPLICATIONS OF ISCHEMIC STROKE**

HEMORRHAGE
MECHANISM
- Energy depletion and acidosis in tissue surrounding infarction can allow red blood cell extravasation, creating hemorrhagic infarction.
- Risk is increased if thrombolytics, anticoagulants, or antiplatelet agents given or if severe hypertension occurs.

MANAGEMENT
- Hold anticoagulants and antiplatelet agents for 24 hours after administration of tissue plasminogen activator.
- Monitor vital signs and neurologic status frequently.
  - With thrombolytic therapy: Every 15 minutes for 2 hours, every 30 minutes for 6 hours, hourly for 16 hours, then every 2 to 4 hours
  - Without thrombolytic therapy, hourly for 8 hours, then every 2 hours
- Hold infusion of thrombolytic agent if neurologic condition changes. Report changes to physician and prepare patient for computed tomographic (CT) scan. If CT excludes hemorrhage, may resume thrombolytics per order.
- Monitor for bleeding at puncture sites, sclera, oropharynx, nares, gastrointestinal and genitourinary tracts.
- Maintain blood pressure and coagulation parameters within the desired ranges.
- Monitor coagulation parameters (platelet count, prothrombin time, partial thromboplastin time, international normalized ratio, fibrinogen) and complete blood count.

REPERFUSION INJURY
MECHANISM
- Restoration of perfusion to ischemic tissue causes activation of oxygen free radicals that further injure compromised cells. May occur hours to weeks after initial stroke; new or same stroke symptoms may appear.

MANAGEMENT
- Monitor neurologic status closely after reperfusion is established (e.g., after thrombolytic therapy).

RECURRENT STROKE
MECHANISM
- Most recurrences occur within hours to days of first stroke; highest risk is within first 30 days.

MANAGEMENT
- Identify and treat modifiable risk factors that contribute to stroke
- Administer antiplatelet and antithrombotic therapy as prescribed.
- Provide patient and family education about lifestyle changes needed.

INCREASED INTRACRANIAL PRESSURE
MECHANISM
- Cerebral edema (usually peaks 2 to 5 days after stroke) and intracranial hemorrhage can increase intracranial volume and pressure.

MANAGEMENT
- Refer to Increased Intracranial Pressure under Specific Patient Health Problems.

SEIZURES
- Refer to Seizures under Specific Patient Health Problems.

   2. Etiology and risk factors
      a. Hypertensive vascular disease (most common cause)
      b. Cerebral amyloid angiopathy: β-amyloid protein deposits in small meningeal and cortical blood vessel walls make them more friable
      c. Ischemic stroke with a hemorrhagic conversion; traumatic intracerebral hemorrhage (see Head Trauma)
      d. Vasculitis, vascular brain tumor, venous infarction (e.g., thrombosis in the sagittal sinus)
      e. Use of anticoagulants or platelet aggregation inhibitors; systemic hemorrhagic disorders and diathesis
      f. Use of illicit drugs, particularly cocaine, amphetamines
      g. Increased age; race—young and middle-aged African Americans have a higher incidence than whites of the same age

   3. Signs and symptoms
      a. Sudden, spontaneous onset; may progress in minutes to hours
      b. Specific clinical presentation varies, depending on the location, extent, and rate of bleeding. Symptoms may include severe headache, decreased LOC, nausea and vomiting, ataxia, seizures, hemiplegia or hemiparesis (arm, leg, or both), aphasia, cranial nerve dysfunction, impaired swallowing, and gaze deviations
      c. Table 4-37 shows distinguishing signs and symptoms of hemorrhagic stroke into deep cortical structures

   4. Diagnostic study findings (also see Ischemic Stroke for studies used in generic stroke evaluation)
      a. Laboratory
         i. Clotting profile (platelet count, PT, PTT, INR): To check the adequacy of clotting
         ii. CBC, sedimentation rate: May indicate cause related to infection, inflammation, or malignancy
         iii. Serum glucose and electrolyte levels
         iv. Toxicology screen: To identify drugs that may have precipitated stroke

---

■ **TABLE 4-37**
■ ■ **Distinguishing Signs and Symptoms Associated with Hemorrhagic Stroke**

Deep Cortical Structure	Distinguishing Signs and Symptoms*
Cerebellum	Dizziness
	Vertigo
	Ataxia
	Occipital headache
	Nystagmus, ipsilateral gaze deficit
	Dysarthria
Pons	Contralateral hemiparesis and, with more extensive hemorrhage, quadriparesis and "locked-in" syndrome
	Impaired lateral eye movement
	Small, poorly reactive pupils
	Possible abnormal respiratory patterns (see Table 4-20)
Thalamus	Contralateral hemiparesis and sensory loss, equal in the face, arm, and leg; or hemisensory loss alone
Putamen (often involving the internal capsule)	Contralateral hemiparesis and sensory loss
	Dysarthria

*In addition to these distinguishing features, signs and symptoms of increased intracranial pressure will likely be present.

b. Radiologic
   i. CT scan: Reveals acute hemorrhage size, location, possibly cause (e.g., tumor), complications (e.g., herniation, hydrocephalus)
   ii. MRI: Reveals hemorrhage and areas of edema; may reveal cause
   iii. Studies to rule out vascular lesions, such as CT angiography, MRA, cerebral angiography (refer to Intracranial Aneurysms, Arteriovenous Malformations)
   c. Lumbar puncture: For suspected SAH with no evidence of blood on CT scan and no signs of increased ICP. If hemorrhagic stroke extends into the ventricle or SAH exists, the CSF contains RBCs and appears xanthochromic. CSF protein and WBC levels are elevated. CSF pressure may be elevated.

5. **Goals of care**
   a. Increased ICP is controlled (<20 mm Hg); adequate CPP (>60 mm Hg) and oxygenation are maintained to minimize brain ischemia
   b. Recovery of neurologic functions is optimal
   c. Potential systemic and neurologic complications are prevented or recognized and appropriately managed
   d. Patient and family are prepared for interventions, possible complications, and outcomes

6. **Collaborating professionals on health care team:** See Increased Intracranial Pressure

7. **Management of patient care**
   a. Anticipated patient trajectory: Numerous factors influence the clinical course and outcome, including the location and extent of the hemorrhage, the occurrence and severity of complications; age; and preexisting health problems. Hemorrhagic stroke carries much higher mortality and morbidity than ischemic stroke. Anticipated patient trajectory for increased ICP is relevant for these patients (see Increased Intracranial Pressure). Other needs specific to patients with hemorrhagic stroke in the acute care setting include the following:
      i. Positioning: Maintain the head of the bed at 30 degrees to promote cerebrovenous outflow
      ii. Skin care: See Increased Intracranial Pressure
      iii. Pain management: See Increased Intracranial Pressure
      iv. Nutrition: See Intracranial Aneurysms
      v. Infection control: See Increased Intracranial Pressure if ventriculostomy is performed
      vi. Transport: See Ischemic Stroke
      vii. Discharge planning: See Increased Intracranial Pressure
      viii. Pharmacology
         (a) Provide supplemental oxygen
         (b) Administer prescribed IV fluids, typically isotonic non–glucose-containing solutions
         (c) Administer prescribed antihypertensives; generally IV labetalol or nitroprusside used initially. Typically a systolic BP of 150 to 170 mm Hg and an MAP of less than 130 mm Hg is desired. Avoid hypotension or reduction of MAP by 15% or more of baseline over 24 hours.
         (d) Vasoactive or inotropic agents may be used to maintain BP and CPP
         (e) Fresh frozen plasma, platelets, and/or vitamin K may be used to correct coagulopathy
         (f) Sedation may be prescribed for agitation, which can elevate BP and ICP
      ix. Psychosocial issues: See Ischemic Stroke

     x. Treatments
- (a) Noninvasive: See Ischemic Stroke
- (b) Invasive
  - (1) Intubation and mechanical ventilation may be required for adequate ventilation; avoid $Paco_2$ of less than 35 mm Hg
  - (2) Surgical or stereotactically guided evacuation of the hematoma may be performed to decompress the brain
  - (3) Intraventricular catheter may be necessary to monitor and manage increased ICP
  - (4) Cerebral oxygen or blood flow monitor may be used to guide therapy

     xi. Ethical Issues: See Intracranial Aneurysms

b. Potential complications (see also health problems described under Patient Care)

     i. Increased ICP (see Increased Intracranial Pressure section)

     ii. Hydrocephalus
- (a) Mechanism: Ventricular extension of the bleed can impair CSF flow or reabsorption. Cerebral edema and clot formation can obstruct CSF flow. (See Intracranial Aneurysms for signs and symptoms.)
- (b) Management: See Intracranial Aneurysms

8. Evaluation of patient care

a. Intracranial parameters (e.g., ICP, CPP) remain within the desired range without intervention

b. Brain infarct is minimized and ischemia resolves

c. Optimal recovery of neurologic function is achieved

d. Complications are prevented or minimized

e. Patient and family are prepared for interventions, possible complications, and outcomes

Intracranial Infections

Bacterial Meningitis

1. Pathophysiology: Organisms gain access to the subarachnoid space, CSF, and pia-arachnoid layers of the meninges. Once access is gained, bacteria proliferate because immune defense mechanisms are limited. Bacterial exudate forms in the subarachnoid space and meningeal inflammation occurs, which can obstruct CSF flow. Cerebral capillaries become permeable, which leads to vasogenic edema. Increased ICP results. Progressive involvement may include the following:

a. Vasculitis; ischemia or infarction of neuronal tissue

b. Ependymitis or pyocephalus

c. Petechial hemorrhage within the brain

d. Cranial nerve inflammation

e. Scar tissue formation and fibrotic changes in the arachnoid layer, which contribute to the development of hydrocephalus

f. Subdural hygroma, abscess formation

2. Etiology and risk factors

a. Infecting organisms: Organisms vary with the primary cause. Three organisms account for the majority of bacterial meningitis in adults: *Neisseria meningitides* (meningococcal meningitis); *Haemophilus influenzae,* and *Streptococcus pneumoniae* (pneumococcal meningitis). Other causative bacteria include *Listeria monocytogenes, Mycobacterium tuberculosis,* staphylococci—usually *Staphylococcus aureus* but also *Staphylococcus epidermidis* (most common after neurologic surgery); and gram-negative enteric bacilli (e.g., *Escherichia coli*).

    b. Sources of infection

        i. Neurologic surgery or invasive procedures, monitoring devices; penetrating head injury, basal skull fracture with dural tear

        ii. Otitis media; sinusitis; mastoiditis; osteomyelitis of the skull or vertebrae; dental abscess, recent dental work

        iii. Exposure to infectious organisms (e.g., *N. meningitides*); crowded conditions; infection elsewhere in the body with bacteremia or septic emboli

        iv. IV drug use

    c. Immunosuppression increases susceptibility

3. Signs and symptoms

    a. Headache that becomes progressively worse

    b. General signs of infection: Malaise, fever, tachycardia, chills

    c. Rash: 50% of patients with meningococcal meningitis develop red or purple petechiae progressing to purpura or ecchymosis over the trunk, legs, conjunctiva, and mucous membranes; does not fade when compressed; similar rashes seen with *H. influenzae* and pneumococcal meningitis

    d. Neurologic: Irritability, confusion; progressive decrease in LOC; focal neurologic signs (hemiparesis, hemiplegia), skin hypersensitivity, seizures, cranial nerve deficits

    e. Meningeal irritation: Headache, photophobia, nuchal rigidity, Brudzinski's sign, Kernig's sign

    f. Nausea and vomiting

4. Diagnostic study findings

    a. Laboratory

        i. Cultures: CSF, blood, drainage from sinuses or wounds, nasopharynx, sputum, and rash aspirate to identify causative organism

        ii. Serology tests (e.g., latex agglutination, counterimmunoelectrophoresis, radioimmunoassay, enzyme-linked immunosorbent assay) to identify antibodies or antigens associated with specific disease or organism; polymerase chain reaction detects DNA to identify causative organism

    b. Radiologic

        i. CT scan: Usually normal in acute uncomplicated meningitis; may show meningeal enhancement, hydrocephalus, cerebral edema, cortical infarcts, and cerebral abscesses

        ii. Skull radiographs: May visualize infected sinuses or basilar skull fracture

    c. EEG: May show generalized slow-wave activity over both hemispheres

    d. Lumbar puncture: May be done if no evidence of increased ICP or coagulopathy. If the patient has focal neurologic deficits or increased ICP, a CT scan may be done prior to lumbar puncture. CSF may be obtained from a ventriculostomy. Common CSF findings include the following:

        i. Elevated opening pressure

        ii. Elevated protein level usually seen

        iii. Low glucose content (<40% of serum glucose level) in most cases

        iv. Purulent, turbid appearance

        v. Increased WBCs, primarily polymorphonuclear leukocytes

5. Goals of care

    a. Infection and neurologic deficits resolve

    b. ICP is controlled (<20 mm Hg)

    c. Patient expresses relief from pain

    d. Potential systemic and neurologic complications are avoided or minimized

6. Collaborating professionals on health care team: See Increased Intracranial Pressure; also infectious disease specialist

7. **Management of patient care**
   a. Anticipated patient trajectory: Aggressive treatment, initiated early, may completely resolve signs and symptoms. Amount of brain damage caused by infectious process, resulting neurologic deficits, and incidence and severity of complications will determine the clinical course. Anticipated patient trajectory for increased ICP may also be relevant (see Increased Intracranial Pressure). Other needs specific to patients with intracranial infection in the acute care setting include the following:
      i. Positioning: Raise the head of the bed at least 30 degrees to control headache and ICP
      ii. Skin care: See Increased Intracranial Pressure
      iii. Pain management
         (a) Administer analgesics to treat headache, preferably short-acting or easily reversible agents; give cautiously if the patient is not on ventilator support; avoid inducing hypotension
         (b) Monitor pain relief and neurologic status
         (c) Dim lights to promote rest, relieve photophobia
      iv. Nutrition: See Intracranial Aneurysms
      v. Infection control: Presence of some infectious organisms (e.g., *N. meningitides*) will require patient isolation. Some infections must be reported to state health agencies, federal health agencies, or both.
      vi. Discharge planning: Patient usually discharged home, unless neurologic deficits persist that require rehabilitation or care in a skilled nursing facility
      vii. Pharmacology
         (a) Antibiotics to cover the known or suspected causative organisms at the first suspicion of bacterial meningitis (even before obtaining a CSF sample if lumbar puncture is delayed for any reason). If necessary, antibiotic(s) can be modified after the causative organism is confirmed.
         (b) Dexamethasone (Decadron) may be given prior to or with the first antibiotic dose in children with *H. influenzae* type b meningitis and in adults with suspected or confirmed pneumococcal meningitis. Controversial, particularly for use in children with pneumococcal meningitis and in patients with meningitis due to penicillin- or cephalosporin-resistant strains of *S. pneumoniae*.
         (c) IV fluids (typically isotonic solutions) to maintain euvolemia; if necessary, vasoactive and inotropic agents for cardiovascular support
         (d) Antipyretics to maintain normothermia
         (e) Sedation to treat anxiety and increased ICP
         (f) Anticonvulsants to control seizures
      viii. Treatments
         (a) Noninvasive
            (1) Monitor neurologic status and vital signs frequently
            (2) Institute cooling measures as warranted; avoid patient shivering
         (b) Invasive
            (1) Intubation, mechanical ventilation if needed
            (2) ICP monitor to treat increased ICP
   b. Potential complications (see also health problems described under Patient Care)
      i. Waterhouse-Friderichsen syndrome (adrenal hemorrhage)
         (a) Mechanism: May be seen in fulminating meningococcal meningitis. Results in adrenal insufficiency, subsequent hypotension, respiratory distress, and circulatory collapse.

      (b) Management: Immediate adrenal corticosteroid replacement, supportive therapy

  ii. Disseminated intravascular coagulation

      (a) Mechanism: Associated primarily with meningococcal meningitis

      (b) Management: See Chapter 9

  iii. Brain abscess, subdural effusions, encephalitis

      (a) Mechanism: Extension of bacterial infection into the parenchyma or subdural space

      (b) Management: Antibiotics for brain abscess or encephalitis. Abscess may need surgical decompression.

  iv. Hydrocephalus

      (a) Mechanism: Purulent exudate and meningeal fibrosis in the subarachnoid space can obstruct CSF flow and reabsorption

      (b) Management: See Management of Hydrocephalus in Box 4-1

  v. Increased ICP

      (a) Mechanism: Accumulation of purulent exudates, hydrocephalus, and cerebral edema

      (b) Management: See Increased Intracranial Pressure

  vi. Seizures: See Seizures section

  vii. Fluid and electrolyte imbalance: See the section on fluid and electrolyte imbalances under Patient Care

8. **Evaluation of patient care**

  a. Infection is resolved and ICP is controlled (<20 mm Hg)

  b. Optimal recovery of neurologic function is achieved

  c. Complications are prevented or minimized

Viral Encephalitis

1. **Pathophysiology:** Inflammation of brain tissue caused by viruses that enter the body, colonize, then migrate through the choroid plexus, cerebral capillaries, or along peripheral nerves into the CNS. Viruses attack susceptible neurons, causing brain tissue inflammation and necrosis; may also inflame the meninges.

2. **Etiology and risk factors**

  a. Increased risk with immunosuppression

  b. Caused by viruses such as

    i. Herpes simplex virus (causes most severe and common type of viral encephalitis in adults)

    ii. Enterovirus; cytomegalovirus; measles, mumps, varicella, lymphocytic choriomeningitis viruses; Epstein-Barr virus; rabies virus

    iii. Arboviruses: Borne by arthropods (i.e., mosquito or tic acquires the viral infection after biting an infected host [e.g., horse, bird]; the infected arthropod vector then bites and infects a human). Examples: Eastern equine, Western equine, West Nile, St. Louis, and California encephalitis are all transmitted by mosquitoes. Transmission may also occur via blood transfusion or transplant from an infected donor. Some arboviruses have specific seasonal and geographic prevalence; primarily afflict humans of distinct age groups (e.g., risk of severe neurologic disease with West Nile virus increases significantly in those aged 50 years and older).

3. **Signs and symptoms**

  a. Symptom onset and progression varies with the pathogen and the area of the brain involved

  b. Common findings: Headache, fever, diminished LOC, nuchal rigidity

    c. Possible findings: Cranial nerve dysfunction, focal deficits, aphasia, motor deficits, involuntary movements, ataxia, nystagmus, seizures

    d. Herpes simplex virus: Fever, headache, nausea and vomiting, altered LOC, and seizures develop over days. Frontal and temporal lobe damage from the virus may cause strange behavior, personality changes, hemiparesis, aphasia, temporal lobe seizures, hallucinations, signs of increased ICP, and eventually temporal lobe herniation.

    e. Arthropod-borne encephalitis: Gradual onset of flulike symptoms (e.g., fever, chills, malaise, headache, myalgia, nausea and vomiting). Lymphadenopathy and erythematous rash may also accompany the onset of West Nile virus infection. Then changes in LOC, meningeal signs, seizures, tremors, ataxia, abnormal reflexes, muscle weakness, and possibly motor and cranial nerve deficits appear. West Nile encephalitis may manifest with severe muscle weakness or flaccid paralysis.

4. Diagnostic study findings

    a. Laboratory findings

      i. CSF cultures: To identify the causative organism

      ii. Serologic tests: See Intracranial Infections: Bacterial Meningitis

    b. Radiologic

      i. CT scan: May be normal initially; later may reveal abnormalities in the affected areas

      ii. MRI: Initial studies may be normal; later studies may reveal abnormalities (e.g., hemorrhage, edema) in the affected areas (e.g., inferior frontal and temporal areas with herpes simplex encephalitis; thalamus, midbrain, and other gray matter structures with West Nile encephalitis)

    c. EEG: May show generalized slow-wave activity over both hemispheres. Periodic high-voltage sharp waves in the temporal lobe(s) may be seen with herpes simplex encephalitis.

    d. Lumbar puncture: See Intracranial Infections: Bacterial Meningitis for indications. Findings may initially be normal or may include the following:

      i. Normal or elevated opening pressure

      ii. Elevated protein level

      iii. Normal glucose content

      iv. Increased WBCs, primarily lymphocytes; RBCs present with cerebral hemorrhage

    e. Brain tissue biopsy: Necessary in some cases

5. Goals of care: See Intracranial Infections: Bacterial Meningitis

6. Collaborating professionals on health care team: See Intracranial Infections: Bacterial Meningitis

7. Management of patient care

    a. Anticipated patient trajectory: See patient trajectory for Intracranial Infections: Bacterial Meningitis. Other acute care needs for patients with viral encephalitis include the following:

      i. Positioning. See Intracranial Infections: Bacterial Meningitis

      ii. Skin care: See Increased Intracranial Pressure

      iii. Pain management: See Intracranial Infections: Bacterial Meningitis

      iv. Nutrition: See Intracranial Aneurysms

      v. Infection control: See Intracranial Infections: Bacterial Meningitis

      vi. Discharge planning: See Intracranial Infections: Bacterial Meningitis

      vii. Pharmacology

        (a) Antiviral agents as prescribed (e.g., acyclovir [Zovirax] for treatment of herpes types 1 and 2 and varicella-zoster virus. Early treatment helps reduce mortality and morbidity.

(b) Prescribed IV fluids (typically isotonic solutions) to maintain euvolemia; if necessary, vasoactive and inotropic agents to support cardiovascular function

(c) Prescribed antipyretics to maintain normothermia

(d) Sedation for anxiety and increased ICP

(e) Anticonvulsants to control seizures

    viii. Treatments: See Intracranial Infections: Bacterial Meningitis

b. Potential complications (see also health problems described under Patient Care)

    i. Increased ICP

      (a) Mechanism: Brain inflammation and cerebral edema

      (b) Management: See Increased Intracranial Pressure

    ii. Seizures: See Seizures section

    iii. Fluid and electrolyte imbalance: See Fluid and Electrolyte Imbalance under Patient Care

8. Evaluation of patient care: See Intracranial Infections: Bacterial Meningitis

Guillain-Barré Syndrome

1. Pathophysiology: Acute inflammatory polyneuropathy. Myelin sheath of inflamed and edematous peripheral nerves is destroyed by macrophages and lymphocytes, which causes loss of saltatory conduction. Myelin destruction is patchy. Varied amounts of axonal damage may also worsen outcomes. Remyelination gradually transpires. Four variations of Guillain-Barré syndrome (GBS) exist:

    a. Acute inflammatory demyelinating polyneuropathy (most common)

    b. Acute motor-sensory axonal neuropathy

    c. Acute motor axonal neuropathy without sensory loss

    d. Miller Fisher syndrome: Uncommon, more benign

2. Etiology and risk factors

    a. Exact etiology is unclear; thought to be caused by an autoimmune response, likely to an acute infection

    b. Some 60% to 70% of patients have an infection, usually viral, 1 to 3 weeks before the onset of symptoms; *Campylobacter jejuni* infection is associated with up to 50% of GBS cases

    c. Vaccination may trigger GBS

    d. Surgery and renal transplantation may precede onset

    e. May occur with Hodgkin's disease or systemic lupus erythematous

3. Signs and symptoms

    a. History of acute infection 1 to 3 weeks before symptoms

    b. Acute onset; symptoms progress rapidly over hours to 3 weeks

    c. Progressive symmetrical weakness, usually starting in the legs and ascending to the trunk, arms, and cranial nerves

    d. Ineffective ventilation if the respiratory muscles (especially the diaphragm) are involved

    e. Decreased or lost deep tendon reflexes

    f. Sensory loss usually mild but may be severe or not present; paresthesias common, often affecting the hands and feet

    g. Pain may include dysesthesia, muscle aches, or cramps; back pain often an early symptom

    h. Cranial nerve dysfunction; CN VII most commonly affected

    i. Autonomic dysfunction: BP variation, arrhythmias, ileus, diaphoresis or loss of sweating, urine retention

    j. Miller Fisher syndrome: Ophthalmoplegia, ataxia, areflexia, typically without sensory loss, rarely affecting the respiratory muscles

4. **Diagnostic study findings**
    a. Electromyelography or nerve conduction velocity testing shows slowing or blocked nerve conduction
    b. Lumbar puncture: CSF shows increased protein level; normal or moderate number of mononuclear cells
5. **Goals of care**
    a. Neurologic function returns to normal
    b. Pain is relieved
    c. Complications are prevented or effectively managed
    d. Patient and family are prepared for interventions
6. **Collaborating professionals on health care team:** See Increased Intracranial Pressure
7. **Management of patient care**
    a. Anticipated patient trajectory: Symptoms usually start to subside about 2 weeks after maximal weakness and gradually resolve; most recovery occurs within the first 12 (sometimes to 24) months. Long-term outcome depends on the location and extent of axonal damage; 25% of patients have persistent deficits ranging from fatigue to lower extremity paralysis. Other acute care needs for patients with GBS include the following:
        i. Positioning: Position in good body alignment with the head of the bed raised at least 30 degrees to avoid aspiration; alleviate pressure on vulnerable peripheral nerves
        ii. Skin care: See Increased Intracranial Pressure
        iii. Pain management
            (a) NSAIDs and nonnarcotic analgesics may be tried but are typically ineffective; gabapentin or amitriptyline may be used for neuropathic pain; if narcotics are necessary, give cautiously when the patient is not on a ventilator
            (b) Promote comfort via repositioning or applying warm or cool compresses
        iv. Nutrition: If dysphagia precludes oral intake, employ alternative feeding methods early in the disease course. See recommendations for Dysphagia under Patient Care.
        v. Discharge planning: Discharge destination (e.g., home, rehabilitation center, skilled nursing facility) determined in large part by persisting motor and sensory deficits
        vi. Pharmacology
            (a) Supplemental oxygen as needed to maintain adequate oxygenation
            (b) IV immune globulin (IVIG): 0.4 to 2 g/kg in divided doses over 3 to 5 days to modulate the immune system and neutralize or modify detrimental immune factors
            (c) Anticoagulants for DVT prophylaxis
        vii. Psychosocial issues (see Intracranial Aneurysms): Educate the patient and family regarding the clinical course of GBS and the interventions provided. Reassure that function will likely return. Establish effective means for patient communication. See interventions for Inability of Patient to Communicate Needs Effectively under Patient Care.
        viii. Treatments
            (a) Noninvasive: Monitor neurologic status closely for worsening or resolving deficits
            (b) Invasive
                (1) Therapeutic plasma exchange or plasmapheresis: When IVIG is not used, plasmapheresis may be performed every other day for 10 to 15 days with a total plasma exchange of about 200 to 250 ml/kg per treatment; removes detrimental circulating immune factors.

(2) Intubation may be required to maintain a patent airway, remove secretions, and enable mechanical ventilatory support

b. Potential complications (see also health problems described under Patient Care)

i. Respiratory failure

(a) Mechanism: Weakness of the muscles used for ventilation and secretion clearance; cranial nerve deficits can impair protective airway reflexes; hypoventilation, secretion retention, atelectasis, and pulmonary infection can occur

(b) Management: See Chapter 2

ii. Autonomic dysfunction

(a) Mechanism: Due to ANS involvement; see Signs and Symptoms; may cause death

(b) Management (see also Acute Spinal Cord Injury)

(1) Perform continuous ECG monitoring to detect arrhythmias; monitor BP frequently

(2) Treat arrhythmias, hypertension, or hypotension as appropriate

(3) Sit patient up slowly to prevent orthostatic hypotension

(4) Use a urinary catheter to relieve retention

(5) Gastric tube should be inserted if ileus occurs

iii. Syndrome of inappropriate secretion of antidiuretic hormone: See Fluid and Electrolyte Imbalance under Patient Care and Chapter 6

iv. Sleep deprivation

(a) Mechanism: Pain, autonomic dysfunction, and other factors can disrupt the sleep-wake cycle

(b) Management

(1) Relieve pain and anxiety

(2) Provide uninterrupted time, the patient-desired environment, and prescribed medication to enhance sleep

8. **Evaluation of patient care**

a. Neurologic function returns to normal

b. Complications are prevented or appropriately managed

c. Patient is pain free

Acute Spinal Cord Injury

1. **Pathophysiology**

a. Concussion, compression, contusion, laceration, transection, or ischemia of the spinal cord can be caused by vertebral dislocation, impinging fracture fragments, vascular supply disruption, intervertebral disk rupture, expanding mass lesions, overstretching of neural tissue, or the impact of concussive force. Inflammatory or infectious processes and some tumors may directly damage spinal cord tissue.

b. Not all traumatic spinal cord injury (SCI) occurs at the time of impact (primary injury); over hours to days secondary SCI can develop. Intracellular molecular and biochemical mechanisms leading to secondary SCI are same as those in brain injury. Factors that can trigger or exacerbate secondary SCI include the following:

i. Decreased spinal cord blood flow associated with systemic hypotension, loss of autoregulation, vasospasm, vascular thrombosis, or small vessel compression from expanding hemorrhage or edema

ii. Decreased spinal cord tissue oxygenation related to hypoxia, anemia, or reduced spinal cord perfusion

2. Etiology and risk factors
   a. Trauma
      i. Causes most SCI; usually due to motor vehicle crashes; other causes include falls, interpersonal violence, recreational injuries, and industrial incidents
      ii. About 11,000 new cases of traumatic SCI occur each year; the cervical spine is the most frequently injured
      iii. More than 75% of SCI victims are male
      iv. Mechanisms of injury
         (a) Hyperextension, hyperflexion, rotation, and vertical compression (axial loading) of the spinal column can stretch, tear, or compress the spinal cord; compromise the vasculature of the spinal cord; or cause vertebral fractures, dislocations, or subluxation that impinge on the cord
         (b) Penetrating injury, such as bullet, shrapnel, or stab wounds, may lacerate the cord or associated vasculature, disrupt surrounding bony elements, or cause percussion injury
      v. Chronic conditions such as spondylosis, stenosis of the spinal canal, ossification of the posterior longitudinal ligament, and arthritis increase vulnerability to SCI
   b. Disease processes such as tumors, vascular malformations (e.g., AVM), or infection

3. Signs and symptoms
   a. Spinal column pain or tenderness
   b. Possibly spinal column deformity or discoloration; projectile entry and exit wounds
   c. Transient or permanent impairment or loss of motor, sensory, or autonomic function. Sensory or motor dysfunction typically recognized with assessment of corticospinal tracts (see Table 4-12), spinothalamic tracts, and posterior columns (see Box 4-3).
   d. Classification of SCI by functional loss
      i. Complete SCI: Loss of all motor and sensory function below the level of the lesion
      ii. Incomplete SCI: Varying degrees of motor and/or sensory function preserved below the level of the lesion; indicates that some tracts are spared (Table 4-38)

■ **TABLE 4-38**
■ ■ **Incomplete Spinal Cord Injury (SCI) Syndromes**

Incomplete SCI Syndrome	Associated Type of SCI	Clinical Presentation
Central cord syndrome	Injury and edema in the center of the spinal cord	Greater motor loss in the upper extremities than in the lower limbs; varying sensory loss
Brown-Séquard syndrome	Hemisection of the cord causes injury	Ipsilateral loss of motor, position, and vibratory sense; contralateral loss of pain and temperature perception at and below the SCI
Anterior cord syndrome	Disruption of the blood supply to the anterior two thirds of the spinal cord resulting in cord ischemia	Loss of motor function and pain and temperature sensation below the level of the lesion, with sparing of proprioception, vibration, and light touch sensations
Dorsal column syndrome (rare)	Posterior column injury	Loss of vibration and position sense

    iii. Lesion level correlates with functional loss (Table 4-39)

  e. *Spinal shock:* Immediately or shortly after SCI a state of areflexia with flaccid paralysis, loss of autonomic function, and absence of all sensation below the level of injury can occur; results from sudden withdrawal of predominantly facilitatory influences from higher centers and persistent reflex inhibition below the lesion. Intensity of spinal shock varies; resolves over hours to weeks as evidenced by the return of reflexes below the level of SCI (bulbocavernosus reflex returns first) and the development of spastic paralysis.

  f. Reflexes that involve damaged nerves at the level of the SCI will remain absent even after the resolution of spinal shock

  g. Priapism, a sustained penile erection, may be noted in males with complete SCI due to unopposed parasympathetic nervous system stimulation

  h. Vital sign abnormalities, such as bradycardia, hypotension, and impaired thermoregulation, may be seen and are associated with disruption of the sympathetic nervous system; hypoventilation is caused by loss of respiratory muscle innervation

4. Diagnostic study findings

  a. Radiologic

    i. Three-view spinal series (anteroposterior, lateral, and odontoid views): To identify fractures, subluxations, or the presence of metallic objects (e.g., bullet). All seven cervical vertebrae and the cervicothoracic junction must be visualized. Even with no evidence of fracture or dislocation, there may still be undetected ligamentous disruption that allows vertebrae to move out of alignment, which thereby causes further SCI.

    ii. Flexion and extension views: Lateral cervical spine radiographs of neck flexion and extension done in an awake and cooperative patient to detect vertebral instability; in obtunded patients, dynamic flexion and extension films may be done via fluoroscopy.

    iii. CT: Visualizes bony pathology well—better than MRI; reconstruction of various views aids assessment

    iv. Angiography: May reveal a vascular cause for SCI (e.g., AVM, vessel occlusion); detects vascular injuries associated with cervical SCI, particularly vertebral artery damage

---

■ **TABLE 4-39**
■ ■ **Level of Spinal Cord Injury (SCI) and Associated Motor and Respiratory Muscle Function Loss**

Level of SCI	Motor and Respiratory Muscle Function Loss
C1-C4	Quadriplegia with loss of spontaneous respiratory function
C4, C5	Quadriplegia with possible phrenic nerve involvement
C5, C6	Quadriplegia with gross arm movements; phrenic nerve intact, providing for diaphragmatic breathing
C6, C7	Quadriplegia with biceps intact, diaphragmatic breathing
C7, C8	Quadriplegia with triceps, biceps, and wrist extension intact with some function of intrinsic hand muscles; diaphragmatic breathing
T1-T12	Paraplegia with varying loss of intercostal and abdominal muscle function
Below L1	Cauda equina injury; variable motor and sensory loss in the lower extremities, areflexive bowel and bladder

   v. CT myelography: Shows disk, bony, or mass lesion impingement into the spinal canal; reveals spinal cord or nerve root compression
   vi. MRI: Best at demonstrating soft tissue, ligamentous, and spinal cord pathology
   vii. MRA: To detect vascular injury (see angiography earlier)
  b. Somatosensory evoked potentials: Identify a disruption of the somatosensory pathway that may indicate SCI or disease
  c. CSF analysis: To identify pathologic condition other than trauma (e.g., infection)
5. **Goals of care**
  a. Spinal cord perfusion and oxygen delivery are optimized
  b. Optimal recovery of neurologic function occurs
  c. Patient expresses relief from pain
  d. Complications are prevented or minimized
  e. Patient participates in care to the maximum extent possible
6. **Collaborating professionals on health care team:** See Increased Intracranial Pressure
7. **Management of patient care**
  a. Anticipated patient trajectory: Patient's clinical course and outcome are influenced by the level and extent of SCI; the neurologic deficits that result; the occurrence and severity of complications; age; and preexisting health problems. See Box 4-19 for acute care interventions specific for patients with SCI.
  b. Potential complications: See Box 4-20
8. **Evaluation of patient care**
  a. Optimal recovery of neurologic function is achieved
  b. Patient expresses relief from pain
  c. Complications are prevented or effectively managed
  d. Patient participates in rehabilitation initiatives and in decisions about various aspects of care

Seizures

1. **Pathophysiology**
  a. *Seizures* are paroxysmal episodes of desynchronized and excessive electrical discharges from neurons that result in a sudden transient alteration in brain function
  b. In *status epilepticus,* the brain's excitatory and inhibitory circuits become reconfigured, which allows prolonged or frequently recurring seizures. The longer status epilepticus lasts, the more difficult it is to control.
  c. Seizures increase cerebral metabolic demand and can deplete high-energy phosphates (e.g., ATP), causing failure of energy-dependent functions (e.g., sodium-potassium-ATPase pump)
  d. CBF can increase to three to five times the normal level
  e. Aspiration and trauma may occur during a seizure. Prolonged seizures can cause cerebral edema, neuronal dysfunction and injury, hyperthermia, metabolic derangements, arrhythmias, rhabdomyolysis, and death
  f. Seizures that occur in the acute phase of a neurologic insult can worsen neurologic outcome
2. **Etiology and risk factors** (for seizures in critical care)
  a. Inadequate levels of or withdrawal from anticonvulsant therapy
  b. Acute withdrawal from the chronic use of sedatives or depressants (e.g., alcohol, benzodiazepines, barbiturates)
  c. Drug toxicity or adverse drug reaction
  d. Metabolic disorders (e.g., uremia, hypoglycemia, electrolyte disorders, fever)

■ **BOX 4-19**
■ **ACUTE CARE INTERVENTIONS FOR PATIENTS WITH SPINAL CORD INJURY (SCI)**

POSITIONING
1. Maintain spinal immobilization with prescribed stabilization devices (e.g., cervical collar, brace, halo vest) to prevent movement of bony elements and further injury. Keep head of bed at ordered level; maintain good body alignment.
2. Maintain cervical traction to reduce fracture dislocation and realign spine. Kinetic therapy bed or turning frame may be used to turn patient while maintaining spinal alignment and cervical traction.
3. Once spine is stable, get patient out of bed to a high-backed chair with seat cushion; take care to prevent orthostatic hypotension (i.e., apply elastic stockings, wrap lower extremities with elastic bandages before slowly elevating head).

SKIN CARE
Poor tissue perfusion, sensory loss, immobility, and use of stabilization devices increase risk for skin breakdown.
1. Inspect skin often, especially bony prominences (e.g., heels, sacrum, occiput),
2. Implement pressure reduction efforts: Timely removal of patient from backboard, frequent repositioning, use of specialty cushions and padded collars, and attention to proper fit of stabilization devices.
3. Provide skin care regularly beneath stabilization devices and around pin sites.

PAIN MANAGEMENT
See Pain under Patient Care.
1. Assess pain; administer prescribed analgesics cautiously to patients not on ventilator; avoid hypotension; monitor effectiveness of analgesic therapy.
2. Neuropathic pain often best treated with medication such as gabapentin, carbamazepine, or amitriptyline.

NUTRITION
See Dysphagia under Patient Care. Patient may not tolerate oral or gastric feeding acutely due to ileus, impaired swallowing.
1. Initiate postpyloric feedings; if necessary, use parenteral nutrition.
2. Provide caloric replacement based on energy expenditure measured by indirect calorimetry. Ensure adequate protein to minimize negative nitrogen balance.

TRANSPORT
Maintain immobility of spine during transport.

DISCHARGE PLANNING
1. Once the condition is stabilized, timely movement to a rehabilitation center is desirable.
2. Discharge destination (e.g., home, rehabilitation center, skilled nursing facility, ventilator-dependent unit) determined in large part by motor or sensory deficits.

PHARMACOLOGY
1. Provide supplemental oxygen.
2. Administer prescribed fluids, typically isotonic solutions, to maintain euvolemia.
3. Administer vasoactive and inotropic agents to maintain blood pressure in desired range. *Guidelines for the Management of Acute Cervical Spine and Spinal Cord Injuries* recommends maintaining systolic blood pressure above 90 mm Hg and mean arterial pressure at 85 to 90 mm Hg for first 7 days after SCI.
4. Methylprednisolone (MPSS) may be given within 8 hours of nonpenetrating SCI. Administer loading dose of 30 mg/kg intravenous bolus over 15 minutes, followed by infusion at 5.4 mg/kg/hr for 23 hours. If drug started 5 to 8 hours after injury, a 47-hour continuous infusion is suggested, but may increase risk of steroid-induced complications (e.g., hyperglycemia, infection, gastrointestinal bleed). MPSS thought to offer neuroprotection via a number of mechanisms, although its use in SCI is controversial.

Continued

PHARMACOLOGY—cont'd

5. GM-1 ganglioside may foster neuronal regeneration; suggested as treatment option, although research has not shown significant clinical benefit with its use. After MPSS administration, a 300-mg loading dose of GM-1 ganglioside is given, followed by 100 mg/day for 56 days.
6. Sedation may be prescribed to control anxiety.
7. Stool softeners and stimulant cathartic usually prescribed to prevent constipation.

PSYCHOSOCIAL ISSUES

See Intracranial Aneurysms under Specific Patient Health Problems.

1. Educate patient and family about SCI, surgical interventions, stabilization devices, complication risks and prevention, and importance of participation in self-care and rehabilitation.
2. Depression, grief, and anxiety are common reactions after SCI. Ensure that patient has effective means to summons help and communicate.
3. Offer patient choices when possible to foster patient's sense of control.

TREATMENTS

NONINVASIVE

1. If manually establishing patient's airway, use jaw-thrust or chin-lift technique and minimize neck motion.
2. Perform comprehensive evaluations of motor and sensory function; report deterioration to physician.

INVASIVE

1. Endotracheal intubation may be required; establish while maintaining head and neck alignment. Tracheostomy may be indicated for patients with high SCI.
2. Surgery may be needed to decompress, realign, and/or stabilize the spine.

■ BOX 4-20
■ POTENTIAL COMPLICATIONS OF SPINAL CORD INJURY (SCI)

HYPOVENTILATION AND INEFFECTIVE COUGH

MECHANISM

- SCI above T12 can paralyze muscles involved in respiration (see Table 4-39), reducing maximal inspiratory force and forced vital capacity.
- Functional muscles for respiration may fatigue, which reduces effectiveness of spontaneous ventilation.
- Paralysis of abdominal and intercostal muscles leads to ineffective cough.
- Ineffective cough, decreased vital capacity, and immobility increase risk for atelectasis; together with endotracheal intubation and possible aspiration, increase likelihood of pneumonia.

MANAGEMENT

- Monitor respiratory status, including pulmonary function test results (e.g., vital capacity, tidal volume, negative inspiratory force) and respiratory gas exchange (e.g., pulse oximetry, arterial blood gas levels, end-tidal CO_2) to detect respiratory muscle fatigue and onset of pulmonary complications. Notify physician of respiratory deterioration.
- Noninvasive positive pressure ventilation or intubation and mechanical positive pressure ventilation may be used for inadequate spontaneous ventilation or gas exchange.
- Aggressive pulmonary hygiene (i.e., chest physical therapy, suctioning) should be instituted; bronchoscopy may be used to remove secretions and open airways when routine hygiene maneuvers are ineffective.
- Once patient is stable and able to participate in care, provide manually assisted coughs. An insufflator-exsufflator cough machine may also be used to help clear secretions.
- Apply abdominal binder below costal margin in quadriplegic patients with no abdominal distension; helps to better position diaphragm and improve lung volumes.
- Have patient perform frequent incentive spirometry; teach family to encourage its use.
- Involve physical therapist in respiratory strengthening exercises.

Continued

NEUROGENIC SHOCK
MECHANISM
- SCI at or above T6 (usually complete lesions) causes disconnection of sympathetic nervous system from higher control centers, which results in loss of vascular tone and cardiac accelerator response.
- Vasodilatation results, decreasing venous return and causing hypotension.
- Loss of cardiac accelerator response can lead to bradycardia and possibly junctional rhythm or ventricular escape beats.
- Because vagal nerve remains intact, profound bradycardia and cardiac arrest can occur, sometimes aggravated by fast position changes or suctioning.

MANAGEMENT
- Use hemodynamic parameters and indicators of tissue perfusion to guide fluid replacement and use of inotropic and vasoactive agents. Maintain blood pressure in desired range and ensure adequate tissue perfusion.
- Continuously monitor electrocardiogram; treat symptomatic bradycardia with atropine; pacemaker may be required. Prevent bradycardia by oxygenating well before and after suctioning and avoiding rapid position changes.

POIKILOTHERMIA OR ALTERATION IN THERMOREGULATION
MECHANISM
- Disconnection of sympathetic nervous system from hypothalamic control center causes inability to regulate body temperature, which tends to drift toward ambient room temperature.

MANAGEMENT
- Monitor body temperature frequently.
- Warm or cool patient to maintain normothermia; take precautions to prevent hypothermia and hyperthermia.

ADYNAMIC ILEUS
MECHANISM
- Thought to be triggered by disruption of autonomic innervation to the gastrointestinal tract. Causes abdominal distention, which can interfere with diaphragmatic excursion and increase risk for vomiting and aspiration.

MANAGEMENT
- Inspect abdomen for distention; place gastric tube to decompress bowel.

GASTROINTESTINAL MUCOSAL EROSION AND BLEEDING
See Potential for Gastrointestinal Ulceration and Bleeding under Patient Care; Chapter 8.

URINE RETENTION
MECHANISM
- During spinal shock and after injury to sacral plexus, bladder is atonic and retains urine; may lead to reflux, stone formation, and renal deterioration, and increases risk for urinary tract infection. Manifests with bladder distention and no urine output.

MANAGEMENT
- Indwelling urinary catheter is necessary when spinal shock and hemodynamic instability are present. Once those conditions resolve and fluid intake is limited to 2000 to 2400 ml/day or less, intermittent catheterization should be initiated. Keep urine output at less than 500 ml per catheterization. If patient is able, teach self-catheterization. Monitor patient for urinary tract infection.

WEAKNESS OR PARALYSIS IN ONE OR MORE EXTREMITIES
See Weakness or Paralysis of One or More Extremities under Patient Care.

    e. Neurologic pathologic conditions such as, TBI, CNS infections, brain tumors, cerebral edema, stroke, cerebral anoxia, AVM, increased ICP

3. Signs and symptoms (of seizures commonly seen in critical care)

    a. *Tonic-clonic seizure* (grand mal seizure): Involves the whole body without a focal onset. Loss of consciousness is followed by brief period of muscle rigidity (tonic phase) and then rhythmic muscle jerking (clonic phase). In the tonic phase, apnea may occur momentarily and cyanosis may develop. Hyperventilation may accompany the clonic phase or occur as the seizure terminates. Incontinence, profuse salivation, and diaphoresis are common during the seizure, which usually lasts 1 to 5 minutes. Headache, amnesia for the seizure, confusion, myalgia, and fatigue are common in the postictal phase.

    b. *Myoclonic seizure:* Sudden, brief muscular contractions that may occur singly or repetitively; usually involve the extremities or face, but can be generalized

    c. *Partial seizure:* If the patient remains conscious, the seizure is referred to as a *simple partial seizure;* if loss of consciousness occurs, it is referred to as a *complex partial seizure.* May progress and become generalized. Signs and symptoms relate to the area of the brain affected:

        i. Motor events, such as face twitching or limb jerking

        ii. Automatisms (e.g., lip smacking, fidgeting, blinking): Common with complex partial seizures

        iii. Sensory events: Numbness or tingling; visual, auditory, gustatory, or vertiginous symptoms

        iv. Psychic events (e.g., hallucinations, illusions)

        v. Autonomic events (e.g., diaphoresis, vomiting)

    d. Status epilepticus: Seizures occur for a prolonged period (>5 to 10 minutes) or repetitively without full recovery between ictal episodes. May be generalized convulsive, nonconvulsive (without visible movement), or, less commonly, focal motor seizures.

4. Diagnostic study findings

    a. Laboratory

        i. Electrolyte or metabolic abnormalities (e.g., sodium imbalance, hypomagnesemia, hypoglycemia, hypoxemia) may precipitate or result from seizures

        ii. Serum enzyme levels, particularly creatine phosphokinase levels, elevated after seizures

        iii. Myoglobinuria is common after prolonged seizures

        iv. Other tests (e.g., toxicology screen) may reveal disorders that precipitated the seizure

    b. Radiologic: To determine precipitating or complicating cause

    c. EEG: Identifies seizure activity and localizes the foci

5. Goals of care

    a. Oxygenation and ventilation are maintained

    b. Seizure activity is controlled

    c. No injuries or other complications result from the seizures

    d. No toxic effects are experienced from anticonvulsants

6. Collaborating professionals on health care team

    a. Nurse

    b. Physician, may include neurologist and infectious disease specialist

    c. EEG technician, respiratory therapist

    d. Pharmacist

7. Management of patient care

    a. Anticipated patient trajectory: Seizures are controlled and, if identified, the precipitating factor is effectively treated. Specific needs of patients with seizures may include the following:

    i. Positioning: After seizures, turn the patient on the side to prevent aspiration

    ii. Discharge planning: After seizures and precipitating factors are controlled and metabolic responses to seizure are resolved, the patient can typically be discharged to home. Unresolved neurologic impairment from seizures may require discharge to a rehabilitation center or skilled nursing care facility.

    iii. Pharmacology

        (a) Supplemental oxygen

        (b) Prescribed IV fluids to maintain euvolemia

        (c) Anticonvulsant(s) to control seizures. Monotherapy preferred, but if one anticonvulsant is not effective, another may be added. Monitor and maintain therapeutic plasma levels, observe for toxic effects.

            (1) Benzodiazepines (e.g., lorazepam, midazolam, diazepam) are generally used to control acute seizures. Another anticonvulsant drug (usually phenytoin or fosphenytoin) is given simultaneously to prevent recurrent seizures (Table 4-40).

            (2) Valproic acid or levetiracetam may be added for repeated seizures refractory to phenytoin

            (3) If seizure activity is not halted with these medications in the usual dosages, high-dose pentobarbital, propofol, or midazolam may be used (see Table 4-40)

    iv. Psychosocial issues: Depression and social isolation may occur; ensure provision of counseling and support for dealing with seizures and potentially necessary life changes

    v. Treatments

        (a) Noninvasive

            (1) If the patient has a neurologic disease or injury that puts the person at high risk for seizures, implement seizure precautions: Maintain the bed in a low position with side rails up and padded; ensure that harmful objects are out of reach; keep suction and airway equipment readily available

            (2) Facilitate repeat EEG or provide continuous EEG monitoring to detect subclinical seizures and evaluate the effectiveness of anticonvulsant therapy

            (3) Observe, record, and report seizures, including the body parts involved, the order of involvement, and the nature of movements; eye deviation, nystagmus, and pupil size change; respiratory pattern and function; neurologic status throughout the seizure and postictal phase; the duration of each phase

            (4) Maintain a patent airway; ensure adequate ventilation and circulation during and after a seizure; suction airway as necessary

            (5) Prevent injury during seizures: Stay with the patient; never force anything into the patient's mouth; do not restrain the patient; remove harmful objects from the vicinity; loosen tight clothes; if the patient is out of bed, lower the patient to the floor

            (6) Reorient the patient after the seizure

            (7) Investigate and treat the underlying cause

            (8) Educate the patient and family about seizures, actions to take for another seizure, planned diagnostic tests and interventions, prescribed anticonvulsants

        (b) Invasive: Intubation and ventilator support if necessary

b. Potential complications

    i. Metabolic complications may include acidosis, hypoxemia, hypoglycemia, electrolyte imbalances

■ TABLE 4-40
■■ Anticonvulsants Commonly Used to Treat Status Epilepticus

Drug	Typical Dosage	Onset	Desired Drug Level	Major Adverse Effects
Lorazepam (Ativan)	4 mg (0.1 mg/kg) intravenously (IV) at 2 mg/min; repeat after 10-15 min if seizures persist	Usually around 5 min	Not typically assessed	Sedation; respiratory depression (more common with use of diazepam); may cause hypotension
Diazepam (Valium)	10-20 mg IV at 5 mg/min; can repeat after 10 min if seizures persist	Almost immediate	Not typically assessed	Sedation; respiratory depression, hypotension may occur
Midazolam (Versed)	2-5 mg IV; for refractory seizures, 0.1-0.4 mg/kg/hr IV	1-5 min	Not typically assessed	Sedation, neuromuscular block, respiratory depression and arrest, hypotension
Phenytoin (Dilantin)	15-20 mg/kg IV no faster than 50 mg/min in saline solution; then 300-400 mg/day in divided doses; do not give intramuscularly	30-60 min	10-20 µg/ml; Free level 1-2 µg/ml	Dysrhythmias (e.g., bradycardia); cardiovascular collapse; use cautiously in patients with heart block or Stokes-Adams syndrome; hypotension may occur
Fosphenytoin (Cerebyx)	Dosed as phenytoin equivalents (PE), 20 mg/kg PE IV at 150 mg PE/min; can be given faster than phenytoin IV; may be given intramuscularly; converted to phenytoin; compatible in standard IV solutions, including those with glucose	Conversion to phenytoin half-life is 15 min	Same as for phenytoin (actually assess phenytoin levels)	Same as for phenytoin

Drug	Dosage	Onset	Therapeutic Level	Adverse Effects
Valproic acid (Depakote)	15-60 mg/kg/day IV or by mouth (PO); infuse IV over 60 min (≤20 mg/min)	Peaks in 1-4 hr	50-100 µg/ml	Sedation, tremors, hepatic toxicity, thrombocytopenia, gastrointestinal disturbance, alopecia
Levetiracetam (Keppra)	1000-3000 mg/day PO	Peaks in 1 hr	Not assessed	Sedation, weakness, incoordination, behavioral abnormalities, leukopenia
Phenobarbital (Luminal)	10-20 mg/kg IV at 50-75 mg/min	5-20 min	20-40 µg/ml	Sedation, hypotension, respiratory depression may occur
Pentobarbital (Nembutal)	Loading dose 10 mg/kg IV over 30 min, followed by 5-10 mg/kg/hr for 3 hr, then 1-3 mg/kg/hr infusion	About 1 min	10-50 µg/ml	Hypotension, myocardial and respiratory depression, immune suppression, and CNS depression, which obscures the neurologic examination
Propofol (Diprivan)	10 µg/kg/min IV, then titrated to desired effect	Less than 1 min	Not typically assessed	Hypotension, respiratory depression and arrest; propofol infusion syndrome—metabolic acidosis, cardiac failure, rhabdomyolysis, renal failure

        (a) Mechanism: Seizures cause increased metabolic demands and imbalances

        (b) Management: Identify and correct imbalances

   ii. Cerebral edema, ischemia, and brain dysfunction

        (a) Mechanism: Seizures increase the cerebral metabolic rate; if cerebral oxygen delivery does not keep up with metabolic demand, brain ischemia, edema, neuronal dysfunction, and death can occur. Hyperemia from increased cerebral metabolic rate encourages vasogenic edema.

        (b) Management: Control seizures. Monitor neurologic status. Avoid hypoxia. Optimize cerebral oxygen delivery.

  iii. Increased ICP

        (a) Mechanism: Cerebral edema and hyperemia

        (b) Management: See Increased Intracranial Pressure

  iv. Renal failure

        (a) Mechanism: Myoglobinuria from muscle breakdown during prolonged seizure activity can lead to acute renal failure

        (b) Management: See Chapter 5

   v. Hyperthermia

        (a) Mechanism: Seizures increase the metabolic rate and muscle activity, which elevates body temprature

        (b) Management: Antipyretics, cooling measures as warranted

8. Evaluation of patient care

  a. No evidence of seizure activity is present

  b. There is no injury or neurologic deterioration from seizures

  c. Adverse effects of anticonvulsant therapy are absent or controlled

  d. If possible, the underlying cause of the seizures is effectively treated

  e. Metabolic responses to seizures are resolved

Encephalopathy

1. Pathophysiology: Global mental status dysfunction caused by one or more of the following direct or indirect pathologic conditions affecting the brain: Buildup of toxins, metabolic imbalance, alterations in CBF, changes in the structure or electrical activity of the brain, changes in the supply or utilization of neurotransmitter substances, or other cellular changes that alter neurologic functioning. Encephalopathy is not a disease in itself but results from other systemic or brain disorders.

2. Etiology and risk factors

  a. Numerous disorders in various body systems can lead to encephalopathy, such as severe systemic hypertension, hypoxia, infection, vascular disease, liver or kidney dysfunction, hypoglycemia, hyperglycemia, lead toxicity, concussive brain injury

  b. Systemic diseases are often in their end stage when encephalopathy becomes apparent (e.g., uremic or hepatic encephalopathy)

3. Signs and symptoms

  a. Vary widely, from memory problems to behavioral disorders and depressed LOC; neurologic changes are consistent with the cause of the encephalopathy

  b. Family history: Relevant in degenerative or hereditary disorders that lead to encephalopathy

  c. Social history: May suggest precipitating cause (e.g., chronic alcohol abuse leads to thiamine deficiency and Wernicke's encephalopathy)

  d. Medical history: Consistent with neurologic changes that correlate with the cause of the encephalopathy

4. Diagnostic study findings: Vary, depending on the cause

5. Goals of care

  a. Cause of encephalopathy is resolved

  b. Neurologic status returns to baseline or improves

6. **Collaborating professionals on health care team:** See Increased Intracranial Pressure; also other team members, depending on the cause
7. **Management of patient care:** Relates to the primary cause of encephalopathy
8. **Evaluation of patient care**
   a. Cause of encephalopathy is correctly identified, optimally treated, and, when possible, resolved
   b. Neurologic status returns to baseline or improves

REFERENCES

General

Bader MK, Littlejohns LR, editors: *AANN core curriculum for neuroscience nursing,* ed 4, St Louis, 2004, Saunders.

Barker E: *Neuroscience nursing: a spectrum of care,* ed 2, St Louis, 2002, Mosby.

Geerts WH, Pineo GF, Heit JA, et al: Prevention of venous thromboembolism: the seventh ACCP conference on antithrombotic and thrombolytic therapy, *Chest* 126(3 suppl):338S-400S, 2004.

Hickey JV: *The clinical practice of neurological and neurosurgical nursing,* Philadelphia, 2003, Lippincott Williams & Wilkins.

Sugarman RA: Structure and function of the neurologic system. In McCance KL, Huether SE, editors: *Pathophysiology: the basis for disease in adults and children,* ed 4, St Louis, 2002, Mosby, pp 363-400.

Winn HR, editor: *Youmans neurological surgery,* 5th ed, vols 1-4, Philadelphia, 2004, Saunders.

Physiologic Anatomy

Brodal P: *The central nervous system: structure and function,* New York, 2003, Oxford University Press.

Gilman S, Newman SW: *Manter and Gatz's essentials of microanatomy and neurophysiology,* Philadelphia, 2004, FA Davis.

Paxinos G, Mai JK: *The human nervous system,* ed 2, Boston, 2004, Elsevier Academic Press.

Pick TP, Howden R, editors: *Gray's anotomy,* ed 16, East Molesey, Finland, 2003, Senate.

Slazinski T, Littlejohns LR: Anatomy of the nervous system, In Bader MK, Littlejohns LR, editors: *AANN core curriculum for neuroscience nursing,* ed 4, St Louis, 2004, Saunders, pp 30-86.

Thibodeau GA, Patton KT: *Anatomy and physiology,* ed 5, St Louis, 2003, Mosby.

Patient Care

Conrad SA: Acute upper gastrointestinal bleeding in critically ill patients: causes and treatment modalities, *Crit Care Med* 30(suppl):365-368, 2002.

Danati-Genet PCM, Dubuis J-M, Girardin E, et al: Acute symptomatic hyponatremia and cerebral salt wasting after head injury: an important clinical entity, *J Pediatr Surg* 36:1094-1097, 2001.

Johnson AL, Criddle LM: Pass the salt: indications for and implications of using hypertonic saline, *Crit Care Nurse* 24:36-48, 2004.

Diagnostic Procedures and Assessment

Bader MK, Littlejohns LR, March K: Brain tissue oxygen monitoring in severe brain injury, II, implications for critical care teams and case study, *Crit Care Nurse* 23:29-44, 2003.

Davis AE, Park S, Darwich H, et al: Neurodiagnostic tests. In Bader MK, Littlejohns LR, editors: *AANN core curriculum for neuroscience nursing,* ed 4, St Louis, 2004, Saunders, pp 174-198.

Haselman M, Fox S: Microsensor and microdialysis technology advanced techniques in the management of severe head injury, *Crit Care Nurs Clin North Am* 12:437-446, 2000.

Hobdell EF, Stewart-Amidei C, McNair N, et al: Assessment. In Bader MK, Littlejohns LR, editors: *AANN core curriculum for neuroscience nursing,* ed 4, St Louis, 2004, Saunders, pp 115-173.

Littlejohns LR, Bader MK, March K: Brain tissue oxygen monitoring in severe brain injury, I, research and usefulness in critical care, *Crit Care Nurse* 23:17-25, 2003.

March K: Intracranial pressure monitoring and assessing intracranial compliance in brain injury, *Crit Care Nurs Clin North Am* 12:429-436, 2000.

March K, Wellwood J, Arbour R: Technology. In Bader MK, Littlejohns LR, editors: *AANN core curriculum for neuroscience nursing,* ed 4, St Louis, 2004, Saunders, pp 199-226.

Meixensberger J, Jaeger M, Vath A, et al: Brain tissue oxygen guided treatment supplementing ICP/CPP therapy after traumatic brain injury, *J Neurol Neurosurg Psychiatry* 74:760-764, 2003.

Mulvey JM, Dorsch NWC, Mudaliar Y, et al: Multimodality monitoring in severe traumatic brain injury: the role of brain tissue oxygenation monitoring, *Neurocrit Care* 1:391-402, 2004.

Newberg AB, Alavi A: Neuroimaging in patients with head injury, *Semin Nucl Med* 33:136-147, 2003.

Peerdeman SM, Girbes ARJ, Vandertop WP: Cerebral microdialysis as a new tool for neurometabolic monitoring, *Intensive Care Med* 26:662-669, 2000.

Ricker JH, editor: Advances in neuroimaging: applications to traumatic brain injury, *J Head Trauma Rehabil* 16(2):117-205, 2001.

Spetzler RF, Meyer FB: Vascular and blood flow evaluations. In Winn HR, editor: *Youmans neurological surgery*, ed 5, Philadelphia, 2004, Saunders, pp 1540-1612.

Swanson PD: History and physical examination. In Winn HR, editor: *Youmans neurological surgery*, ed 5, Philadelphia, 2004, Saunders, pp 263-276.

Wedekind C, Hesselmann V, Klug N: Comparison of MRI and electrophysiological studies for detecting brainstem lesions in traumatic brain injury, *Muscle Nerve* 26:270-273, 2002.

Wintermark M, van Melle G, Schnyder P, et al: Admission perfusion CT: prognostic value in patients with severe head trauma, *Radiology* 232:211-220, 2004.

Pain

American Pain Society: *Principles of analgesic use in the treatment of acute pain and cancer pain*, ed 5, Glenview, IL, 2003, Author.

Ardery G, Herr K, Titler M, et al: Assessing and managing acute pain in older adults: a research base to guide practice, *Medsurg Nurs* 12(1):7-18, 2003.

Arnstein P: Comprehensive analysis and management of chronic pain, *Nurs Clin North Am* 38(3):403-417, 2003.

Ballantyne J, Fishman SM, Abdi S, editors: *The Massachusetts General Hospital handbook of pain management*, Philadelphia, 2002, Lippincott Williams & Wilkins.

Blakely WP, Page GG: Pathophysiology of pain in critically ill patients, *Crit Care Nurs Clin North Am* 12(2):167-179, 2001.

Carr DB, Jacox AK, Chapman CR, et al: *Acute pain management in adults: operative procedures*, Quick reference guide for clinicians No 1, AHCPR Pub No 92-0019, Rockville, Md, February 1992, Agency for Health Care Policy and Research, Public Health Service, US Department of Health and Human Services.

Campbell J: Pain: the fifth vital sign, November 11, 1995, retrieved October 20, 2005 from http://www.ampainsoc.org/advocacy/fifth.htm.

Feldt K: The checklist of nonverbal pain indicators (CNPI), *Pain Manag Nurs* 1(1):13-31, 2000.

Graf C, Puntillo K: Pain in the older adult in the intensive care unit, *Crit Care Clin* 19(4):749-770, 2003.

Hall LG, Oyen LJ, Murray MJ: Analgesic agents: pharmacology and application in critical care, *Crit Care Clin* 17(4):899-923, 2001.

Hamill-Ruth RJ, Marohn ML: Evaluation of pain in the critically ill patient, *Crit Care Clin* 15(1):35-54, 1999.

Herr K, Decker S, Bjoro K: Pain in the elderly: State of the art review of tools for assessment of pain in nonverbal older adults, 2004, retrieved June 29, 2004, from http://www.cityofhope.org/prc/elderly.asp.

Joint Commission on Accreditation of Healthcare Organizations: *Comprehensive accreditation manual for hospitals: the official handbook (CAMH)*, Oakbrook Terrace, Ill, 2004, Author.

Kwekkeboom KL, Herr K: Assessment of pain in the critically ill, *Crit Care Nurs Clin North Am* 13(2):181-206, 2001.

McCaffery M, Pasero C: *Pain: clinical manual*, ed 2, St Louis, 1999, Mosby.

Melzack R, Wall PD, editors: *Handbook of pain management*, Edinburgh, 2003, Churchill Livingstone.

Munden J, Eggenberger T, Goldberg KE, et al: *Pain management made incredibly easy*, Philadelphia, 2003, Lippincott Williams & Wilkins.

National Pharmaceutical Council, Inc.: *Pain: current understanding of assessment, management, and treatments*, Reston, Va, 2001 Author.

Odhner M, Wegman D, Freeland N, et al: Assessing pain control in nonverbal critically ill adults: a preliminary study, *Dimens Crit Care Nurs* 22(6):260-267, 2003.

Pasero C: Pain in the critically ill patient, *J Perianesth Nurs* 18(6):422-425, 2003.

Pasero C: *Guideline for developing an institutional pain assessment policy,* Personal e-mail communication, December 14, 2004a.

Pasero C: Personal e-mail communication, December 11-12, 2004b.

Pasero C, McCaffery M: Multimodal balanced analgesia in the critically ill, *Crit Care Nurs Clin North Am* 13(2):195-206, 2001.

Payen JF, Bru O, Bosson JL, et al: Assessing pain in critically ill sedated patients by using a behavioral pain scale, *Crit Care Med* 29(12):2258-2263, 2001.

Puntillo K: Pain assessment and management in the critically ill: wizardry or science? *Am J Crit Care* 12(4):310-316, 2003.

Puntillo KA, Miaskowski C, Kehric K, et al: Relationship between behavioral and physiological indicators of pain, critical care patients' self-reports of pain, and opioid administration, *Crit Care Med* 25(7): 1159-1166, 1997.

Puntillo KA, Morris AB, Thomson CL, et al: Pain behaviors observed during six common procedures: results from Thunder Project II, *Crit Care Med* 32(2):421-427, 2004.

Puntillo KA, White C, Morris AB, et al: Patients' perceptions and responses to procedural pain: results from Thunder Project II, *Am J Crit Care* 10(4):238-251, 2001.

Rakel B, Herr K: Assessment and treatment of postoperative pain in older adults, *J Perianesth Nurs* 19(3):194-208, 2004.

St. Marie B, editor: *ASPMN: core curriculum for pain management nursing,* Philadelphia, 2002, Saunders.

Wisborg T, Flaatten H: Pain management in the pre-hospital emergency medical service environment: on-site and transport. In Rosenberg AD, Grande CM, Bernstein RL, editors: *Pain management and regional anesthesia in trauma,* Philadelphia, 1999, Saunders.

Increased Intracranial Pressure and Head Trauma

Aarabi B, Alden TD, Chesnut RM, et al: Management and prognosis of penetrating brain injury, *J Trauma,* 51(suppl):S1-S43, 2001.

Adelson PD, Bratton SL, Carney NA, et al: Guidelines for the acute medical management of severe traumatic brain injury in infants, children, and adolescents, *Crit Care Med* 31(6 suppl): S417-S491, 2003.

Albanese J, Leone M, Alliez JR, et al: Decompressive craniectomy for severe traumatic brain injury: evaluation of the effects at one year, *Crit Care Med* 31:2535-2538, 2003.

Brain Trauma Foundation, American Association of Neurological Surgeons, Congress of Neurological Surgeons, Joint Section on Neurotrauma and Critical Care: Guidelines for the management of severe traumatic brain injury: cerebral perfusion pressure, 2003, retrieved June 24, 2004, from http://www2.braintrauma.org/guidelines/downloads/btf_guidelines_cpp_u1.pdf.

Bulger EM, Nathens AB, Rivara FP, et al: Management of severe head injury: institutional variations in care and effect on outcome, *Crit Care Med* 30:1870-1876, 2002.

Bullock R, Chesnut RM, Clifton G, et al: Guidelines for the management of severe head injury. In Brain Trauma Foundation, American Association of Neurological Surgeons: *Management and prognosis of severe traumatic brain injury,* New York, 2000, Brain Trauma Foundation.

Fields L, Blackshear C, Mortimer D, et al: *Guide to the care of the patient with intracranial pressure monitoring,* Glenview, Ill, 2004, American Association of Neuroscience Nurses.

Grady MS, Marshall LF: Moderate and severe traumatic brain injury. In Winn HR, editor: *Youmans neurological surgery,* vol 4, part 4, Philadelphia, 2004, Saunders, pp 5083-5296.

Henneman EA, Karras JE Jr: Determining brain death in adults: a guideline for use in critical care, *Crit Care Nurse* 24:50-56, 2004.

Kirkness C, March K: Intracranial pressure management. In Bader MK, Littlejohns LR, editors: *AANN core curriculum for neuroscience nursing,* ed 4, St Louis, 2004, Saunders, 249-267.

Lang EW, Czosnyka M, Mehdorn HM: Tissue oxygen reactivity and cerebral autoregulation after severe traumatic brain injury, *Crit Care Med* 31:267-271, 2003.

March K, Wellwood J, Lovasick DA, et al: Craniocerebral trauma. In Bader MK, Littlejohns LR, editors: *AANN core curriculum for neuroscience nursing,* ed 4, St Louis, 2004, Saunders, 277-334.

McIntyre LA, Fergusson DA, Hebert PC, et al: Prolonged therapeutic hypothermia after traumatic brain injury in adults, *JAMA* 289:2992-2999, 2003.

McQuillan KA, Mitchell PH: Traumatic brain injuries. In McQuillan KA, Von Rueden KT, Hartsock RL, et al, editors: *Trauma nursing from resuscitation through rehabilitation*, ed 3, St Louis, 2002, Saunders, 394-461.

Pilitsis JG, Rengachary SS: Complications of head injury, *Neurol Res* 23:227-236, 2001.

Sullivan J: Positioning of patients with severe traumatic brain injury: research-based practice, *J Neurosci Nurs*, 32:204-209, 2000.

Von Oettingen G, Bergholt B, Gyldensted C, et al: Blood flow and ischemia within traumatic cerebral contusions, *Neurosurgery* 50:781-788, 2002.

Zygun DA, Doig CJ, Aur RN, et al: Progress in clinical neurosciences: therapeutic hypothermia in severe traumatic brain injury, *Can J Neurol Sci* 30:307-313, 2003.

Intracranial Aneurysms

Bederson JB, Awad IA, Wiebers DO, et al: Recommendations for the management of patients with unruptured intracranial aneurysms, *Circulation* 102:2300-2308, 2000.

Bernardini GL, Mayer SA, Kossoff SB, et al: Anticoagulation and induced hypertension after endovascular treatment for ruptured intracranial aneurysms, *Crit Care Med* 29:641-644, 2001.

Cavanagh SJ, Gordon VL: Grading scales used in the management of aneurysmal subarachnoid hemorrhage: a critical review, *J Neurosci Nurs* 34:288-295, 2002.

Dooling E, Winkelman C: Hyponatremia in the patient with subarachnoid hemorrhage, *J Neurosci Nurs* 36:130-135, 2004.

Findlay JM: Cerebral vasospasm. In Winn HR, editor: *Youmans neurological surgery*, ed 5, Philadelphia, 2004, Saunders, pp 1839-1867.

Fisher CM, Kistler JP, Davis JM: Relation of cerebral vasospasm to subarachnoid hemorrhage visualized by computerized tomographic scanning, *Neurosurgery* 6:1-9, 1980.

Hinkle J: The pharmacologic treatment for vasospasm after subarachnoid hemorrhage: a case study, *J Neurosci Nurs* 35:332-335, 2003.

Johnston SC, Higashida RT, Barrow DL, et al: Recommendations for the endovascular treatment of intracranial aneurysms, *Stroke* 33:2536-2544, 2002.

Lanzino G, Guterman LR, Hopkins LN: Endovascular treatment of aneurysms. In Winn HR, editor: *Youmans neurological surgery*, 5th ed, Philadelphia, 2004, Saunders, pp 2057-2078.

LeRoux PD, Winn HR: Surgical decision making for the treatment of cerebral aneurysms. In Winn HR, editor: *Youmans neurological surgery*, 5th ed, Philadelphia, 2004, Saunders, pp 1793-1812.

McDonald RL, Weir B: Perioperative management of subarachnoid hemorrhage. In Winn HR, editor: *Youmans neurological surgery*, 5th ed, Philadelphia, 2004, Saunders, pp 1813-1838.

Oyama K, Criddle L: Vasospasm after aneurysmal subarachnoid hemorrhage, *Crit Care Nurse* 24:58-67, 2004.

Pfohman M, Criddle LM: Epidemiology of intracranial aneurysm and subarachnoid hemorrhage, *J Neurosci Nurs* 33:39-41, 2001.

Sommargren CE: Electrocardiographic abnormalities in patients with subarachnoid hemorrhage, *Am J Crit Care* 11:48-56, 2002.

Spetzler RF, Martin NA: A proposed grading system for arteriovenous malformations, *J Neurosurg* 65:476-483, 1986.

Suarez JI, Qureshi AI, Yahia AB, et al: Symptomatic vasospasm diagnosis after subarachnoid hemorrhage: evaluation of transcranial Doppler ultrasound and cerebral angiographic as related to compromised vascular distribution, *Crit Care Med* 30:1348-1355, 2002.

Wardlaw JM, White PM: The detection and management of unruptured intracranial aneurysms, *Brain* 123:205-221, 2000.

Arteriovenous Malformations

Ogilvy CS, Stieg PE, Awad I, et al: Recommendations for the management of intracranial arteriovenous malformations: a statement for healthcare professionals from a special writing group of the Stroke Council, American Stroke Association, *Circulation* 103:2644-2657, 2001.

Spetzler RF, Meyer FB, editors: True arteriovenous malformations. In Winn HR, editor: *Youmans neurological surgery*, ed 5, Philadelphia, 2004, Saunders, pp 2137-2250.

Stroke

Adams HP, Adams RJ, Brott T, et al: Guidelines for the early management of patients with ischemic stroke: a scientific statement for the Stroke Council of the American Stroke Association, *Stroke* 34:1056-1083, 2003.

Bath P, Chalmers J, Powers W, et al: International Society of Hypertension (ISH): statement on the management of blood pressure in acute stroke, *J Hypertens* 21:665-672, 2003.

Brockington CD, Zivin JA: Acute medical management of ischemic disease and stroke. In Winn HR, editor: *Youmans neurological surgery*, ed 5, Philadelphia, 2004, Saunders, 1495-1502.

Chalmers J, Todd A, Chapman N, et al: International Society of Hypertension (ISH): statement on blood pressure lowering and stroke prevention, *J Hypertens* 21: 651-663, 2003.

Cummins RO, editor: *ACLS provider manual*, ed 2, Dallas, Tex, 2002, American Heart Association.

Hinkle JL, Bowman L: Neuroprotection for ischemic stroke, *J Neurosci Nurs* 35:114-118, 2003.

Hinkle JL, Guanci MM, Bowman L, et al: Cerebrovascular events of the nervous system. In Bader MK, Littlejohns LR, editors: *AANN core curriculum for neuroscience nursing*, ed 4, St Louis, 2004, Saunders, pp 536-585.

National Institute of Neurological Disorders and Stroke: Recommendations for the establishment of primary stroke centers, Sept 30, 2004, retrieved June 20, 2005, from http://www.ninds.nih.gov/disorders/stroke/stroke_center_recommendations_2000.htm.

National Institute of Neurological Disorders and Stroke rt-PA Stroke Study Group: Tissue plasminogen activator for acute ischemic stroke, *N Engl J Med* 333:1581-1587, 1995.

Semplicini A, Maresca A, Boscolo G, et al: Hypertension in acute ischemic stroke: a compensatory mechanism or an additional damaging factor? *Arch Intern Med* 163:211-216, 2003.

Siesjo P, Seisjo BK: Cerebral metabolism and the pathophysiology of ischemic brain damage. In Winn HR, editor: *Youmans neurological surgery*, 5th ed, Philadelphia, 2004, Saunders, pp 117-152.

Singh RVP, Prusmack CJ, Morcos JJ: Spontaneous intracerebral hemorrhage: non-arteriovenous malformation, non-aneurysm. In Winn HR, editor: *Youmans neurological surgery*, ed 5, Philadelphia, 2004, Saunders, pp 1733-1768.

Strege RJ, Lang EW, Stark AM, et al: Cerebral edema leading to decompressive craniectomy: an assessment of the preceding clinical and neuromonitoring trends, *Neurol Res* 25:510-515, 2003.

Intracranial Infections

De Gans J, Van de Beek D: Dexamethasone in adults with bacterial meningitis, *N Engl J Med* 347:1549-1556, 2002.

Gea-Banacloche J, Johnson RT, Bagic A, et al: West Nile virus: pathogenesis and therapeutic options, *Ann Intern Med* 140:545-553, 2004.

Goetz AM, Goldrick BA: West Nile virus: a primer for infection control professionals, *Am J Infect Control* 32:101-105, 2004.

Griffin DE: Encephalitis, myelitis, and neuritis. In Mandell GL, Bennett JE, Dolin R, editors: *Principles and practice of infectious diseases*, ed 6, Philadelphia, 2005, Elsevier, pp 1143-1148.

Lewin JJ, Lapointe M, Ziai WC: Central nervous system infections in the critically ill, *J Pharm Practice* 18:25-41, 2005.

Petersen LR, Marfin AA: West Nile virus: a primer for the clinician, *Ann Intern Med* 137:173-179, 2002.

Southwick FS: *Infectious diseases quick glance*, New York, 2005, McGraw-Hill.

Tunkel AR, Hartman BJ, Kaplan SL, et al: Practice guidelines for the management of bacterial meningitis, *Clin Infect Dis* 39:1267-1284, 2004.

Tunkel AR, Scheld WM: Acute meningitis. In Mandell GL, Bennett JE, Dolin R, editors: *Principles and practice of infectious diseases*, ed 6, Philadelphia, 2005, Elsevier, pp 1083-1126.

Vandemark MV, Lovasik DA, Neatherlin JS, et al: Infectious and autoimmune processes. In Bader MK, Littlejohns LR, editors: *AANN core curriculum for neuroscience nursing*, ed 4, St Louis, 2004, Saunders, pp 619-680.

Guillain-Barré Syndrome

Czaplinski A, Steck AJ: Immune mediated neuropathies: an update on therapeutic strategies, *J Neurol* 251:127-137, 2004.

Dalakas MC: Intravenous immunoglobulin in autoimmune neuromuscular diseases, *JAMA* 291:2367-2375, 2004.

Polak M, Richman J, Lorimer M, et al: Neuromuscular disorders of the nervous system. In Bader MK, Littlejohns LR, editors: *AANN core curriculum for neuroscience nursing*, ed 4, St Louis, 2004, Saunders, pp 757-797.

van Koningsveld R, Schmitz PIM, van der Meche FGA, et al: Effect of methylprednisolone when added to standard treatment with intravenous immunoglobulin for Guillain-Barré syndrome: randomised trial, *Lancet* 363:192-196, 2004.

Spinal Cord Injury

Geisler FH, Coleman WP, Grieco G, et al: The Sygen Study Group: the GM1 ganglioside multi-center acute spinal cord injury study, *Spine* 26(24 suppl):S87-S98, 2001.

Jenkins AL, Vollmer DG, Eichler ME: Cervical spine trauma. In Winn HR, editor: *Youmans neurological surgery*, ed 5, Philadelphia, 2004, Saunders, pp 4885-4914.

Joint Section on Disorders of the Spine and Peripheral Nerves of the American Association of Neurological Surgeons and the Congress of Neurological Surgeons: Guidelines for the management of acute cervical spine and spinal cord injuries, *Neurosurgery* 50(suppl):S1-S199, 2002.

Harrop JS, Sharan AD, Vaccaro AR, et al: The cause of deterioration after acute spinal cervical spinal cord injury, *Spine* 26:340-346, 2001.

Kwon BK, Tetzlaff W, Grauer JN, et al: Pathophysiology and pharmacologic treatment of acute spinal cord injury, *Spine J* 4:451-464, 2004.

Levi ADO: Spine trauma: approach to the patient and diagnostic evaluation. In Winn HR, editor: *Youmans neurological surgery*, ed 5, Philadelphia, 2004, Saunders, pp 4869-4884.

McIlvoy L, Meyer K, McQuillan KA: Traumatic spine injuries. In Bader MK, Littlejohns LR, editors: *AANN core curriculum for neuroscience nursing*, ed 4, St Louis, 2004, Saunders, pp 335-402.

Rabchevsky AG, Smith GM: Therapeutic interventions following mammalian spinal cord injury, *Arch Neurol* 58:721-726, 2001.

Russo-McCourt TA: Spinal cord injuries. In McQuillan KA, Von Rueden KT, Hartsock RL, et al, editors: *Trauma nursing from resuscitation through rehabilitation*, ed 3, St Louis, 2002, Saunders, pp 507-542.

Seizures

Beulow JM, Long L, Rossi AM, et al: Epilepsy. In Bader MK, Littlejohns LR, editors: *AANN core curriculum for neuroscience nursing*, ed 4, St Louis, 2004, Saunders, pp 586-618.

Herman ST: Epilepsy after brain insult: targeting epileptogenesis, *Neurology* 59:S21-S26, 2002.

Mirski MA, Varelas PN: Diagnosis and treatment of seizures in the adult intensive care unit, *Contemporary Crit Care* 1:1-12, 2003.

Encephalopathy

Ames C, Marshall LF: Differential diagnosis of altered states of consciousness. In Winn HR, editor: *Youmans neurological surgery*, ed 5, Philadelphia, 2004, Saunders, pp 277-300.

The Renal System

JUNE L. STARK, RN, BSN, MEd

SYSTEMWIDE ELEMENTS

Physiologic Anatomy

1. **Process of urine formation**

   Urine formation occurs in the renal nephron and involves four processes—filtration, reabsorption, secretion, and excretion

   a. Anatomic structures of the kidney: Most humans are born with two kidneys; a small number are born with one. The kidneys are located in the retroperitoneal space above the waist (Figure 5-1).

   i. Cortical (outermost) layer

   (a) Metabolically active portion of the kidney, where aerobic metabolism occurs and where ammonia and glucose are formed

   (b) Metabolic needs more than satisfactorily met by an abundant oxygen supply

   (c) Contains all glomeruli and portions of the proximal and distal tubules

   ii. Medullary (middle) layer

   (a) Region of active glycolytic metabolism; supplies energy for active transport

   (b) Metabolism demands high oxygen consumption, yet oxygen supply limited

   (c) Plays role in concentration of urine

   (d) Composed of 6 to 10 renal pyramids, formed by collecting ducts and extending into the renal pelvis

   (e) Site of the deepest part of the long loops of Henle and the collecting ducts of the nephron

   iii. Renal sinus, pelvis, and collecting system

   (a) Papillae: Rounded projections of renal tissue located at the apical ends of the renal pyramids positioned with the base facing the cortex and the apices facing the renal pelvis; the apical portion opens into the minor calices

   (b) Corticomedullary junction: Point of division between the cortex and the medulla formed by the base of the pyramids

   (c) Renal lobe: Composed of a pyramid plus the surrounding cortical tissue

   (d) Calix

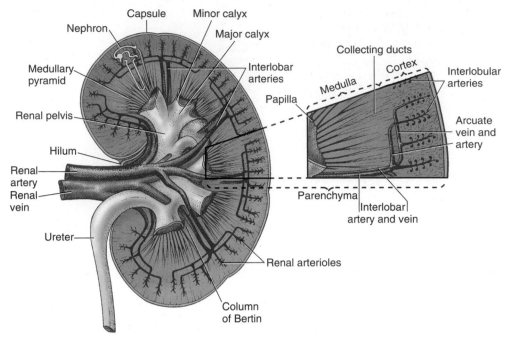

FIGURE 5-1 ■ Major structures of the kidney shown in a diagram of the cut surface of a bisected kidney. (From Brenner BM: *Brenner and Rector's the kidney*, ed 6, Philadelphia, 2000, Saunders.)

> (1) Minor calix wraps around the papilla; receives urine from the collecting duct
> (2) Major calix channels urine from the renal sinus to the renal pelvis
> (3) Urine flows from the renal pelvis to the ureter

iv. Nephron: Anatomic microscopic structure (Figure 5-2)
  (a) Structural and functional unit of the kidney
  (b) Approximately 1 million in each kidney
  (c) Compensates for a significant degree of nephron destruction by
   (1) Filtering a greater solute load
   (2) Hypertrophy of the remaining functional nephrons
  (d) Types of nephrons, based on location and function
   (1) Cortical nephrons located in the outer region of the cortex; contain short loops of Henle with a low capacity for sodium reabsorption
   (2) Juxtamedullary nephrons located in the inner cortex adjacent to the medulla; have long loops of Henle that penetrate deep into the medulla and have a greater capacity for concentration of urine because they are sodium-retaining nephrons
  (e) Functional segments of the nephron
   (1) Renal corpuscle
    a) Bowman's capsule: Specialized portion of the proximal tubule that supports the glomerulus
    b) Glomerulus: Capillary bed with semipermeable membrane
     1) Normally permeable to water, electrolytes, nutrients, wastes; relatively impermeable to large protein molecules, albumin, erythrocytes

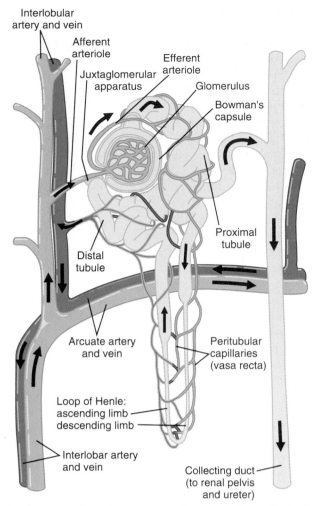

FIGURE 5-2 ■ The functional nephron. (From Guyton AC: *Textbook of medical physiology,* ed 8, Philadelphia, 1996, Saunders.)

2) Composed of three cellular layers: Fenestrated endothelial layer, basement membrane, and epithelium podocyte cells that contribute to characteristic semipermeability of this membrane
3) Characteristics of cellular layers: Endothelial cells contain fenestrations 50 to 100 nm wide, favoring the movement of water and solute; remaining layers are less porous, with openings 1500 nm thick, which may explain the impedance of macromolecules
4) Major factor influencing filtration is molecular size
5) Ionic charge also affects filtration
   a) Electrical potential of the glomerular membrane possesses a negative charge, which favors the passage of positively charged molecules and impedes negatively charged molecules, such as albumin
   b) Loss of membrane electrical potential in glomerular disease is reason for proteinuria

(2) Renal tubules

    a) Segmentally divided into the proximal convoluted tubule, descending loop of Henle, ascending loop of Henle, distal convoluted tubule, and collecting duct

    b) Each segment has a specific cellular structure and function

b. Physiologic processes

    i. Glomerular ultrafiltration is the first step in the formation of urine

        (a) Characteristics of glomerular filtrate

            (1) Normal: Protein-free and red blood cell (RBC)–free, plasmalike substance with a specific gravity (SG) of 1.010. Filtrate contains water, electrolytes, glucose, amino acids, acid-base components, wastes, and other solutes. Pharmaceutical agents can also be included in filtrate.

            (2) Small and middle-sized molecules (up to 60 to 75 kd): Pass freely through the glomerular membrane (i.e., inulin 5 kd, albumin >60 kd)

            (3) Abnormal: Increased permeability of the glomerular membrane allows erythrocytes and protein to be filtered into urine. SG of urine may artificially increase because of the presence of protein or glucose.

            (4) Increased osmotically active substances (glucose, urea): Can cause diuresis

        (b) Filtration is determined by the glomerular pressure and presence of a normal semipermeable glomerular membrane

            (1) Glomerular hydrostatic pressure is 50 mm Hg and favors filtration; this capillary hydrostatic pressure reflects cardiac output

            (2) Colloid osmotic pressure of 25 mm Hg and Bowman's capsule hydrostatic pressure of 10 mm Hg oppose hydrostatic pressure and thus oppose filtration

                a) Colloid osmotic pressure results from oncotic pressure of plasma proteins in the glomerular blood supply

                b) Bowman's capsule pressure reflects renal interstitial pressure

            (3) Net filtration pressure is derived using the following formula:

Glomerular hydrostatic pressure (facilitates):	+50 mm Hg
Colloid osmotic pressure (opposes):	−25 mm Hg
Bowman's capsule pressure (opposes):	−10 mm Hg
Net pressure favoring filtration:	+15 mm Hg

        (c) Glomerular filtration rate (GFR)

            (1) Clinical assessment tool to determine renal function

            (2) Definition: Volume of plasma cleared of a given substance per minute (may be determined by using endogenous creatinine)

            (3) GFR equation

$$GFR = \frac{(U_x \times V)}{P_x}$$

where

    x = a substance freely filtered through the glomerulus and not secreted or reabsorbed by tubules (e.g., creatinine)

    P = plasma concentration of x

    V = urine flow rate (ml/min)

    U = urine concentration of x

            (4) Normal adult GFR: 125 ml/min or 180 L/day

(5) Normal adult urine volume: 1 to 2 L/day, reflecting greater than 99% reabsorption of filtrate

(6) Factors affecting GFR

a) Changes in glomerular hydrostatic pressure

1) Secondary to changes in systemic blood pressure (BP)

2) Caused by variation in afferent or efferent arteriolar tone; increased afferent arteriole resistance decreases GFR; increased efferent arteriole tone increases GFR

b) Alterations in oncotic pressure due to dehydration, hypoproteinemia, or hyperproteinemia

c) Alterations in Bowman's capsule pressure due to urinary tract or nephron destruction, or interstitial edema of kidney

ii. Tubular functions of reabsorption, secretion, and excretion comprise the following steps in urine formation (Figure 5-3):

(a) Conversion of 180 L of plasma filtered per day to 1 to 2 L of excreted urine

(b) Absorption and secretion by two processes:

(1) Passive mechanisms: Solute moves without the expenditure of metabolic energy

a) Diffusion: Solute following either a concentration or an electrical gradient

1) A solute moves from a solution of higher concentration through a semipermeable membrane to a solution of lower concentration

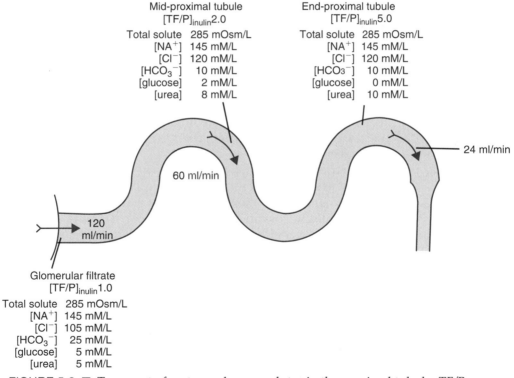

Mid-proximal tubule
$[TF/P]_{inulin}$ 2.0
Total solute 285 mOsm/L
$[NA^+]$ 145 mM/L
$[Cl^-]$ 120 mM/L
$[HCO_3^-]$ 10 mM/L
[glucose] 2 mM/L
[urea] 8 mM/L

End-proximal tubule
$[TF/P]_{inulin}$ 5.0
Total solute 285 mOsm/L
$[NA^+]$ 145 mM/L
$[Cl^-]$ 120 mM/L
$[HCO_3^-]$ 10 mM/L
[glucose] 0 mM/L
[urea] 10 mM/L

24 ml/min

60 ml/min

120 ml/min

Glomerular filtrate
$[TF/P]_{inulin}$ 1.0
Total solute 285 mOsm/L
$[NA^+]$ 145 mM/L
$[Cl^-]$ 105 mM/L
$[HCO_3^-]$ 25 mM/L
[glucose] 5 mM/L
[urea] 5 mM/L

FIGURE 5-3 ■ Transport of water and some solutes in the proximal tubule. *TF/P*, Tubule fluid to plasma ratio. (From Maude DL: *Kidney physiology and kidney disease,* Philadelphia, 1977, Lippincott.)

    2) Selectivity of the membrane's permeability and electrical gradient determine diffusion of the solute

    3) The electrical gradient causes a solute to passively migrate to the oppositely charged compartment (e.g., Na^+, a positive ion, migrates to a negatively charged compartment, whereas Cl^-, a negative ion, moves toward a positively charged compartment)

  b) Osmosis: Water following an osmotic gradient

    1) Water normally moves from an area of low concentration to an area of higher concentration

    2) An osmotic agent, such as sodium or mannitol, normally remains within a single compartment

(2) Active mechanisms:

  a) Ion transport requires energy; adenosine triphosphate [ATP]) permits ions to move *against* the concentration gradient

  b) Maximal tubular transport capacity: Active reabsorption mechanisms in the tubule have limited capacity for reabsorption of certain substances such as glucose. Plasma glucose level of 375 mg/min (transport maximum [Tm]), results in no excretion in urine; plasma glucose level above 375 mg/min results in glucose excretion in urine. Tm for glucose can vary from one nephron to another; as a result, glucose can sometimes spill into the urine at lower serum levels.

(c) Proximal convoluted tubule

  (1) Reabsorbs 60% to 80% of filtrate, which remains isotonic to plasma

  (2) Major function is active reabsorption of sodium chloride (NaCl) with passive reabsorption of water

  (3) Also reabsorbs glucose, amino acids, phosphates (PO_4^{3-}), uric acid, potassium ion (K^+)

  (4) Regulates acid-base balance through reabsorption of carbonic acid (H_2CO_3) and bicarbonate (HCO_3^-) and secretion of hydrogen ions (H^+)

  (5) Secretes K^+, ammonium ion (NH_4^+), organic acids, bases, foreign substances (e.g., drugs)

(d) Loop of Henle

  (1) Variations in length depend on the type of nephron (i.e., juxtamedullary with long loops or cortical with short loops)

  (2) Has two distinct segments

    a) Descending segment, the thin limb, is permeable to water and impermeable to Na^+

    b) Ascending segment, the thick limb, has active NaCl pump and is impermeable to water; target site for loop diuretics

  (3) Major function is concentration or dilution of urine, accomplished by a countercurrent mechanism that maintains hyperosmolar concentration in the interstitium of the renal medulla

(e) Distal convoluted tubule

  (1) Receives hyposmotic (or hypotonic) urine from the ascending loop of Henle

  (2) Major functions

    a) Reabsorption of water, NaCl, and sodium bicarbonate

    b) Secretion of K^+, NH_4^+, and H^+ ions

    c) Regulation of composition, tonicity, and volume

  (3) Water permeability here is controlled by antidiuretic hormone (ADH); Na^+ reabsorption is determined by aldosterone

(f) Collecting duct

(1) Receives urine, which is isotonic to plasma, from the distal convoluted and collecting tubules

(2) Functions with the distal convoluted tubule; affected by ADH and aldosterone

(3) Final urinary adjustments for composition, tonicity, and volume made here before urine enters the renal pelvis and progresses to the ureter and bladder

2. **Renal hemodynamics: Normal blood flow patterns**
   a. Renal vasculature
      i. Specialized arrangement of renal blood vessels reflects interdependence of blood supply with kidney function
      ii. Pathway of blood supply
         (a) Kidney: Aorta→segmented renal arteries→interlobar artery→arcuate artery→interlobular artery→(nephron)→interlobular vein→arcuate vein→interlobar vein→renal vein→inferior vena cava
         (b) Nephron: Afferent arteriole→glomerular capillary→efferent arteriole→peritubular capillary→vasa recta adjacent to tubules→interlobular vein→renal vein→inferior vena cava
      iii. Juxtaglomerular apparatus: Site of renin synthesis
         (a) Specialized cells composed of juxtaglomerular cells and macula densa
            (1) Juxtaglomerular granular cells: Smooth muscle cells containing granules of inactive renin
            (2) Macula densa: Portion of the distal tubule making contact with afferent arterioles of its respective glomerulus
         (b) Responds to arterial BP in afferent and efferent arterioles and to sodium in distal tubule
   b. Renal blood flow (RBF) parameters
      i. Kidney receives 20% to 25% of cardiac output or 1200 ml/min, which translates to flow rate of 4 ml/g/min to the kidney
      ii. Oxygen extraction from renal cells is high, but the amount is not significant enough to account for flow rate; rather, the flow is required to support normal renal function
      iii. RBF is
         (a) Higher in males than in females
         (b) Increased with increasing age (until maturity), in the supine position, and in the afternoon
         (c) Decreased in the elderly, at night, and with exercise
   c. Distribution of RBF
      i. Renal tissue
         (a) Cortex: Metabolically active region, receives most (80%) of the blood supply
         (b) Medulla: Site of anaerobic metabolism, receives 20% of blood supply
      ii. Nephrons: Receive 600 to 650 ml/min of renal plasma flow
   d. Intrarenal autoregulation: General principles
      i. Mean arterial pressure (MAP) is maintained in a range of 80 to 180 mm Hg to prevent large changes in GFR
      ii. Major site of autoregulation is the afferent arteriole
      iii. Increase in the renal arterial pressure causes afferent vasoconstriction; decrease causes efferent vasoconstriction, producing an increased GFR/RBF ratio
      iv. Changes in vascular tone of the efferent arteriole (primarily vasoconstriction) complement efforts to maintain GFR by compensating for reduced blood flow

      v. Autoregulation is essentially absent at an MAP of 70 mm Hg or below

  e. Neural control

      i. Route of nerve supply is along renal blood vessels; renal neurologic intervention is vasoconstrictive

      ii. Hypotension decreases systemic arterial pressure, stimulating the carotid sinus and aortic arch baroreceptors to trigger the sympathetic response (release of epinephrine), which decreases RBF and GFR by vasoconstricting both afferent and efferent arterioles

      iii. Other factors that stimulate increased sympathetic tone are stress, fear, and exercise

      iv. This neuronal effect is not the primary factor in autoregulation; a denervated kidney can be transplanted and still be able to compensate for changes in BP

  f. Hormonal modulation of RBF (see Renal Regulation of Blood Pressure)

      i. Renin-angiotensin system: A mechanism to sustain systemic BP and plasma volume

         (a) Responds to a decreased afferent arteriolar pressure by increasing angiotensin II levels

         (b) Angiotensin II vasoconstricts renal blood vessels, particularly the efferent artery, which reduces RBF but increases GFR

      ii. Renal prostaglandins: Modulate the effects of vasoactive substances, such as angiotensin II, on the kidney by causing vasodilatation

  g. Pharmacologic effects

      i. Epinephrine and norepinephrine: Cause efferent arterioles to vasoconstrict, which leads to a rise in the filtration fraction and a dose-related decrease in RBF

      ii. Dopamine: Pharmacologic action on RBF is dose-related for renal vasodilatation and increased sodium excretion. Generally has a vasodilatory effect on renal vasculature at dosages between 1 and 4 mcg/kg/min intravenously (IV) (optimal dosage, 3 mcg/kg/min); dosages above 10 mcg/kg/min cause renal vasoconstriction, decreasing RBF and GFR. Dopamine therapy has no impact on the prevention of acute tubular necrosis.

      iii. Furosemide and mannitol: Increase GFR initially by increasing blood flow to the kidney and later by decreasing intratubular pressure

      iv. Calcium channel blockers: Relax renal arteriole and ameliorate renal failure related to renal transplantation and nephrotoxicity due to radiocontrast dyes or cyclosporine

      v. Atrial natriuretic factor (atrial natriuretic peptide, or ANP): Improves function in oliguric acute renal failure (ARF), but not preventive

3. Body water regulation

  a. Thirst: Regulator of water intake

      i. Thirst center is located in the anterior hypothalamus

      ii. Neuronal cells are stimulated by intracellular dehydration, which causes sensation of thirst

      iii. Role is maintenance of satiety state (i.e., drinking exact amount of fluid to return body to normal hydration state)

  b. ADH: Sodium osmoreceptor mechanism for control of extracellular fluid (ECF) osmolality and sodium concentration

      i. ADH is synthesized in the paraventricular and supraoptic nuclei of the hypothalamus and travels along the axons of the supraopticohypophysial tract for storage or release from the posterior pituitary. The supraoptic area of the hypothalamus may overlap with the thirst center, providing integration of the thirst mechanism, osmolality detection, and ADH release.

      ii. Release of ADH occurs with the following:
-     (a) Increased serum osmolality stimulates osmoreceptor cells in the hypothalamus that transmit along the neurohypophysial tracts, leading to ADH release from the posterior pituitary; normal serum osmolality is 285 to 295 mOsm/L
-     (b) Volume contraction states reverse the inhibitory effect on ADH release; controlled by stretch receptors in the left atrium that activate the ADH mechanism

      iii. In the presence of ADH, water reabsorption occurs in the distal tubule and collecting ducts, which results in a hypertonic urine, hypotonic medullary interstitium, and eventual correction of contracted ECF

      iv. ADH secretion is inhibited when serum osmolality decreases (water intoxication). When this occurs, the distal tubule and collecting duct become relatively impermeable to water, so that large volumes of hypotonic filtrate are delivered to the collecting duct; this results in dilute urine and excess water loss (compared to extracellular solute concentration), which returns serum osmolality to normal limits.

  c. Countercurrent mechanism of the kidney: Mechanism for the concentration and dilution of urine; adjusts urine osmolality from 50 to 1200 mOsm/L

      i. Isotonic glomerular filtrate leaves the proximal tubule and enters the loop of Henle at 300 mOsm/L

      ii. Descending limb of the loop of Henle is permeable to water only. Water is gradually drawn into the hypertonic medullary interstitium, which gradually increases the osmolality of the filtrate as it becomes dehydrated. At the hairpin turn of the loop, osmolality is dramatically increased by the removal of water and NaCl pump action; osmolality can reach 1000 to 1200 mOsm/L. Concurrently, the medullary interstitium becomes hypotonic.

      iii. Thick ascending limb of the loop of Henle is permeable to NaCl but impermeable to water. The medullary interstitium becomes more hypertonic as its sodium concentration is increased by pumping action at the ascending limb.

      iv. A dilute filtrate reaches the distal tubule. If ADH is absent, dilute filtrate is excreted unchanged, which results in dilute urine with water excretion in excess of solute. If ADH is present, the collecting duct reabsorbs water and concentrated urine is excreted.

4. Electrolyte regulation

  a. Sodium regulation: Normal serum concentration is 136 to 145 mEq/L solute

      i. Na^+ is the major extracellular cation and osmotically active solute. Because variation in body sodium can be associated with an exchange of water between intracellular and extracellular compartments, sodium affects ECF volume.

      ii. Renal reabsorption sites: Normal percentages of reabsorbed filtered sodium
-     (a) Proximal tubule: 65% of filtered Na^+
-     (b) Loop of Henle: 25%
-     (c) Distal tubule: 6%
-     (d) Collecting duct: 2% to 4%

      iii. Major factors that influence Na^+ excretion include GFR, the sympathetic nervous system, aldosterone, the renin-angiotensin-aldosterone system, vasopressin (ADH), and ANP (a peptide hormone that plays a role in regulating and monitoring fluid, electrolyte, and cardiovascular balance)

iv. Sodium reabsorption increases at the renal tubules under the following conditions:

(a) Decreased GFR secondary to renal hypoperfusion (e.g., shock): Less sodium is delivered to the renal tubules, and less is excreted

(b) Secretion of aldosterone (a mineralocorticoid secreted by the adrenal cortex)

(1) Major effects are to increase renal tubular reabsorption of Na^+ and to control selective renal excretion of K^+

(2) Increases Na^+ in ECF, which promotes water reabsorption; at the same time, K^+ is secreted into the distal tubule and collecting duct to be excreted

(3) Regulated by K^+ concentration in the ECF, the renin-angiotensin-aldosterone mechanism, total body sodium, and adrenocorticotropic hormone (ACTH)

(c) ANP action: Causes natriuretic, diuretic, and hypotensive effects secondary to its potent vasodilatory properties; the increased urinary excretion of Na^+ is matched by an accompanying loss of K^+ and PO_4^{3-}

v. Sodium reabsorption decreases at the renal tubules under the following conditions:

(a) Increased GFR (excess ECF volume): Increases renal perfusion and GFR; more sodium is delivered to the renal tubules and more is excreted in urine

(b) Inhibition of aldosterone secretion, which results in renal Na^+ excretion

(c) Secretion of ANP and ADH, administration of diuretics, especially loop-affecting diuretics

b. Potassium regulation: Normal serum concentration is 3.5 to 5.5 mEq/L

i. Potassium is a major intracellular cation (K^+) necessary for the maintenance of osmolality and electroneutrality of cells

ii. Renal transport sites: K^+ is actively reabsorbed in the proximal tubule (60% to 70%) and thick ascending loop (10%); active and passive secretion in the distal tubule and collecting duct maintain the electroneutrality of urine. This electrical gradient is determined primarily by reabsorption of Na^+ from urine.

iii. Factors enhancing K^+ excretion

(a) Increase in cellular potassium via increased exchange with Na^+ (K^+ excreted in urine whereas Na^+ is reabsorbed) or via acute metabolic or respiratory alkalosis (causes movement of K^+ ions into cells)

(b) High-volume tubular flow rates in the distal portion of the nephron: Increase the number of available K^+ ions and thus increase the excretion of potassium

(c) Aldosterone (provides feedback mechanism for maintenance of K^+ in ECF)

(1) Elevation of serum potassium stimulates the secretion of aldosterone

(2) Aldosterone acts on the distal nephrons and collecting ducts, enhancing the retention of Na^+ and excretion of K^+

(3) Excretion of excess K^+ eventually returns levels to normal

(d) Hydrogen ions: Alkalemia (associated decrease in H^+) stimulates K^+ secretion

(e) Diuretics: Loop and thiazide diuretics block NaCl and waste reabsorption, increasing tubular flow and secretion of K^+

  c. Calcium regulation: Normal serum concentration is 8.5 to 10.5 mg/dl or 2.20 to 2.60 mmol/L

    i. Major functions of calcium ions (Ca^{2+}): Generation of cardiac action potential and pacemaker function, contraction of cardiac and vascular smooth muscle, transmission of nerve impulses, blood coagulation, formation of bones and teeth, and maintenance of cellular permeability

    ii. Total serum Ca^{2+}: 40% bound to protein, 50% ionized, and 10% combined with carbonate, phosphate, citrate, and various ions

    iii. Renal transport sites: 98% of filtered Ca^{2+} is reabsorbed. Reabsorptive pathways are similar to those for sodium transport. Most active reabsorption occurs in the proximal tubule. Other sites include the loop (20% to 25%) and the distal tubule (10%).

    iv. Factors influencing Ca^{2+} reabsorption:

      (a) Parathyroid hormone (PTH)

        (1) Decrease in serum calcium stimulates secretion of PTH

        (2) PTH stimulates tubular reabsorption of Ca^{2+} at the distal portion of the nephron, stimulates increased phosphate excretion, and mobilizes calcium and phosphate from bone

      (b) Vitamin D: Calcium absorption from the small intestine depends on the presence of activated vitamin D (1,25-dihydroxycholecalciferol)

        (1) Activation process: Absorption of ultraviolet light converts 7-dehydrocholesterol in skin to cholecalciferol. The liver hydroxylates vitamin D to form 25-hydroxycholecalciferol. The kidney further hydroxylates to the final activated form of vitamin D (1,25-dihydroxycholecalciferol) in the proximal tubule. PTH stimulates this activation process.

        (2) Decreased serum calcium level reduces urinary Ca^{2+} excretion, so activated vitamin D must be available to absorb Ca^{2+} from the small intestine to maintain adequate serum calcium levels

      (c) Corticosteroid effect: Large doses decrease Ca^{2+} absorption in the intestines; may influence the activation of vitamin D in the liver

      (d) Diuretic effect: Diuretics can cause Na^+ and Ca^{2+} excretion. Ultimate effect of reduced serum calcium is decreased excretion. A decrease in total body fluid volume leads to diminished GFR and reduced calcium excretion.

  d. Phosphate regulation: Normal serum concentration is 3.0 to 4.5 mg/dl

    i. About 90% of phosphate is found in bone, 10% in intracellular and extracellular fluid spaces. Phosphates (PO_4^{3-}) play significant role in intracellular energy production and may also influence DNA, RNA, and genetic code information. Phosphates are used by the kidneys to buffer H^+.

    ii. Renal transport sites: Reabsorption of phosphate is an active process that occurs in the proximal tubule and requires Na^+. Factors influencing phosphate excretion include the following:

      (a) PTH secretion: Inhibits phosphate reabsorption (and thus promotes its excretion)

      (b) Alterations in GFR: Increased GFR decreases reabsorption of plasma phosphates and vice versa

  e. Magnesium regulation: Normal serum concentration is 1.5 to 2.2 mEq/L

    i. The magnesium ion (Mg^{2+}) is the second major intracellular cation and is a significant factor in cellular enzyme systems and biochemical reactions

    ii. Mg^{2+} may have a role in the management of acute myocardial infarction (MI), because magnesium administration decreases the mortality rate in

MI by 24% and improves ventricular function by 25%. Benefits may be attributed to magnesium's ability to enhance coronary blood flow, conserve potassium, improve cellular function, and diminish dysrhythmias.

   iii. Renal transport site: The reabsorptive process is similar to that of Ca^{2+} and is linked to Na^+ reabsorption along the renal tubules

   iv. Factors influencing reabsorption include the availability of sodium (Na^+ is necessary for reabsorption) and the availability of PTH (has minimal effect on Mg^{2+} reabsorption)

  f. Chloride regulation: Normal serum concentration is 96 to 106 mEq/L

   i. Renal transport sites: Reabsorbed with Na^+ at all Na^+ absorptive sites in the nephron

   ii. Factors influencing excretion include acidosis (HCO_3^- reabsorbed whereas Cl^- excreted to maintain electrochemical balance) and alkalosis (HCO_3^- excreted as Cl^- reabsorbed)

5. Excretion of metabolic waste products: Excretion is a primary renal function. The kidney excretes more than 200 metabolic waste products. The products measured for interpretation of renal function are blood urea nitrogen (BUN) and serum creatinine.

  a. Urea: Nitrogen waste product of protein metabolism filtered and reabsorbed along the entire nephron

   i. Is an unreliable indicator of GFR, because urea excretion is influenced by

    (a) Urine flow (decrease in urine flow rate may allow for reabsorption of urea)

    (b) Extrarenal factors (e.g., hypoperfusion states or drugs such as corticosteroids)

    (c) Gastrointestinal (GI) bleeding or catabolic states such as fever or infection

    (d) Changes in protein intake or metabolism

   ii. Elevation in BUN level without an associated rise in creatinine level (>25:1 ratio) suggests

    (a) Volume depletion, low renal perfusion pressure

    (b) Severe catabolic process or trauma with massive muscle injury (e.g., burns)

    (c) GI bleeding with blood collection in intestines

   iii. Elevated levels of both BUN and creatinine (at a 10:1 ratio) indicate renal disease

  b. Creatinine: A waste product of muscle metabolism

   i. Amount produced daily is proportional to muscle mass, and production occurs at a constant rate

   ii. Normal kidney excretes creatinine at a rate equal to RBF or GFR

   iii. Creatinine is freely filtered, so its production normally equals its excretion, which makes it a reliable indicator of kidney function

   iv. Elevated serum creatinine level is directly correlated with deterioration in renal function

6. Renal regulation of acid-base balance: The kidneys regulate acid-base balance by minimizing wide variations in body fluid balance in conjunction with retaining or excreting hydrogen ions. Acid-base balance is also regulated by the lungs and the body buffers (serum bicarbonate, blood, and plasma proteins)

  a. Bicarbonate (HCO_3^-) reabsorption

   i. Primarily occurs in the proximal tubule with less in the distal tubule; occurs with reabsorption of Na^+

   ii. Occurs if the filtrate contains more than 28 mEq/L (Tm) as in acidemia, volume contraction

b. Hydrogen ion secretion

    i. Passive secretion occurs in the proximal tubule; active secretion occurs distally in exchange for Na^+

    ii. Acid is buffered by ammonia (NH_3^+) or phosphate (HPO_4^{2-}) before excretion, which provides for hydrogen (H^+) excretion without lowering pH

    iii. H^+ secretion is increased during acidemia and decreased during alkalemia

c. Renal buffers of hydrogen ions

    i. Buffers that are filtered by the glomerulus

        (a) HCO_3^- is completely reabsorbed (up to 28 mEq/L)

        (b) Phosphate (PO_4^{3-}) is secreted and then reacts with hydrogen

        (c) $H^+ + HPO_4^{2-} = H_2PO_4^-$

    ii. Buffers produced by the kidney tubule

        (a) HCO_3^- can be synthesized in the distal tubule when H^+, excreted into urine as HCO_3^-, is delivered by ECF with Na^+. H^+ and HCO_3^- both come from the distal tubule cell as a result of ionization of carbonic acid (H_2CO_3); thus

$$\overset{CA}{H_2CO_3 \rightleftharpoons H^+ + HCO_3^-}$$

    where CA is carbonic anhydrase

        (b) Carbonic acid comes from hydration of carbon dioxide (CO_2) via CA:

$$\overset{CA}{H_2O + CO_2 \rightleftharpoons H_2CO_3}$$

        (c) CO_2 is derived from either cellular metabolism or dissolved CO_2 in venous blood; thus new HCO_3^- can be made in the distal tubule from extraurinary sources

        (d) Complete equation

$$\overset{CA\qquad\quad CA}{H_2O + CO_2 \rightleftharpoons H_2CO_3 \rightleftharpoons H^+ + HCO_3^-}$$

d. Summary of renal responses to acidemia

    i. H^+ secretion is increased at the distal tubule with increased excretion of titratable acids (HPO_4^{2-})

    ii. All HCO_3^- is reabsorbed in the proximal tubule

    iii. Ammonium is produced to accommodate H^+ excretion: $NH_3^+ + H^+ \rightleftharpoons NH_4^+$

    iv. Urinary pH can be as low as 4.5 for excretion of a more acid urine in the presence of acidemia

e. Summary of renal responses to alkalemia

    i. H^+ secretion in the distal tubule is decreased

    ii. Excess HCO_3^- is excreted

    iii. Production of NH_4^+ is decreased

    iv. Urine is alkaline, with a pH over 7

7. Renal regulation of blood pressure: Renal regulation of BP involves five mechanisms:

  a. Maintenance of volume and composition of ECF

    i. Normal plasma volume is essential for control of BP

    ii. Alterations in plasma volume eventually affect BP. Reduction of plasma volume lowers arterial BP, leading to compensation by vasoconstriction. Expansion of plasma volume increases cardiac preload and, in accordance with Starling's curve, raises BP.

  b. Aldosterone–body sodium balance, which determines ECF volume: Aldosterone stimulates renal tubular reabsorption of Na^+ in exchange for excretion of primarily K^+ ions

    c. Renin-angiotensin-aldosterone system: Preserves BP and avoids serious volume reduction

        i. Juxtaglomerular apparatus: Granular cells contain inactivated renin. Factors that trigger juxtaglomerular cells to release renin reflect diminished GFR (e.g., reduced arterial BP in afferent and efferent arterioles, reduced Na^+ content or concentration at distal tubule, sympathetic stimulation of kidneys).

        ii. Renin, an enzyme, is released from juxtaglomerular cells into the afferent arteriole

        iii. On entering the circulation, renin acts on angiotensinogen to split away the vasoactive peptide angiotensin I and convert it to angiotensin II. Requires the presence of angiotensin-converting enzyme (ACE), found primarily in the lung and liver but also in the kidney and all blood vessels. Angiotensin II is a potent systemic vasoconstrictor.

        iv. Circulatory effect of angiotensin II on arterial BP

          (a) Significant peripheral arteriole constriction with moderate venous constriction occurs, which results in the reduction of vascular volume

          (b) Renal arteriolar constriction results in the renal retention of sodium and water; this expands ECF volume, thus increasing arterial BP

        v. Fluid volume response to angiotensin II restores effective circulating volume in the following ways:

          (a) Angiotensin II stimulates aldosterone release, which enhances Na^+ reabsorption

          (b) Vasoconstriction to further decrease GFR leads to Na^+ reabsorption

          (c) The thirst mechanism is stimulated

    d. Renal prostaglandins: Modulating effect

        i. Major renal prostaglandins are prostaglandins E_2, D_2, I_2 (vasodilators) and A_2 (vasoconstrictor)

        ii. Physiologic role is modulation, amplification, and inhibition. Vasoactive substances (angiotensin, norepinephrine, bradykinins) stimulate the synthesis and release of prostaglandins. Prostaglandins modulate the action of the vasoactive substances.

        iii. Prostaglandins diminish arterial BP and increase RBF by arterial vasodilation and inhibition of the distal tubules' response to ADH. Suppressed ADH response leads to sodium and water excretion, which ultimately decreases the effective circulatory volume.

        iv. Pharmacologic prostaglandin inhibitors are the nonsteroidal antiinflammatory drugs (NSAIDs). In cases of compromised renal function avoid the use of NSAIDs (i.e., salicylic acid, ibuprofen [Motrin], indomethacin [Indocin], and naproxen [Naprosyn]).

        v. Loop diuretics stimulate prostaglandin secretion, which leads to vasodilation and decreased preload

    e. Kallikrein-kinin system: Renal kallikreins are proteases that release kinins and are excreted in the urine. Kinins stimulate both the renin-angiotensin and prostaglandin systems, appearing to link renal hemodynamics and fluid-electrolyte excretion.

8. Red blood cell synthesis and maturation

    a. Erythropoietin secretion: Stimulates the production of erythrocytes in the bone marrow and prolongs the life of erythrocytes

    b. Mechanism of erythropoietin synthesis and secretion

        i. Renal cortical interstitial cells produce erythropoietin, a glycosylated, 165-amino-acid protein

  ii. Renal erythropoietin production accounts for 90% of RBC production; the remaining 10% is produced by the liver

  iii. Hypoxia stimulates renal erythropoietin production; the liver is not as responsive to hypoxia and therefore cannot support erythropoiesis in renal failure

 c. Erythropoietin deficiency: Primary cause of anemia in chronic renal failure (CRF); bleeding is the second most common cause

9. Aging kidney

 a. Age-related changes can occur as early as 20 to 40 years of age. Changes include a decrease in tubular length and, at and over age 40 years, a progressive decrease in the percentage of glomeruli. Generally, renal function is diminished by 10% at age 65; may diminish further with aging.

 b. Renal response in the elderly

  i. Decreased renal mass associated with a diminished number of nephrons

  ii. Decreased GFR; diminished RBF secondary to age-related changes in vasculature

  iii. Diminished creatinine production (10 mL/min/1.73 m^2 per decade) and diminished ability to excrete creatinine; therefore, change in serum creatinine level may not be evident. Uric acid levels are slightly increased.

  iv. Decreased serum renin and aldosterone levels reduce the ability to conserve sodium, impair urinary water excretion, and limit urinary concentration

Patient Assessment

1. Nursing history

 a. Patient health history

  i. Previous health problems: Indicate the presence of or predisposition to renal disease

   (a) Kidney and/or urinary tract disease

   (b) Cardiovascular disease

    (1) Hypertension: BP control and treatment may prevent or halt renal damage; hypertension develops in 70% to 80% of patients with advanced renal failure

    (2) Heart failure with diminished renal perfusion

    (3) Atherosclerosis

   (c) Diabetes mellitus: Renal disease caused by vascular disease alterations, infection, or neuropathy

   (d) Immunologic disorders, recent infections (streptococcal)

   (e) Pulmonary disease (Goodpasture's syndrome)

   (f) Allergies, recent blood transfusions (history of incompatibility reaction)

   (g) Other: Toxemia of pregnancy, renal transplantation, anemia, recent surgery, dialysis, exposure to drugs and toxins, renal calculi, azotemia, hematuria, exposure to chemicals or poisons

  ii. History of specific signs and symptoms

   (a) Signs and symptoms of urinary tract disorders

    (1) Dysuria

    (2) Abnormal appearance of urine

     a) Hematuria (grossly bloody)

     b) Pyuria (cloudy)

     c) Biliuria or bilirubinuria (orange)

     d) Myoglobinuria (usually clear; red-brown urine; Hematest positive)

    (3) Urine frequency, urgency, incontinence, hesitancy; nocturia

    (4) Polydipsia

    (5) Patterns of urine output

        a) Normal volume: Approximately 1500 ml/24 hr

        b) Oliguria: Less than 400 ml/24 hr

        c) Anuria: Less than 50 ml to no output over 24 hours

        d) Polyuria: Excessive output exceeding 24-hour intake

        e) Nonoliguria: Normal or excess urine volume in the presence of ARF

    (6) Fever

    (7) Pain in costovertebral angle, flank, or groin

    (8) Pattern of weight gain or loss; dry weight is the ideal weight that minimizes symptomatology for a patient with renal failure as achieved by a dialysis treatment

  b. Family health history: Genetic renal disease accounts for about 30% of azotemia. Genetically transmitted diseases that can cause or precipitate renal disease include the following:

    i. Cardiovascular disease, hypertension

    ii. Diabetes mellitus

    iii. Gout

    iv. Malignancy

    v. Polycystic kidney disease and medullary cystic disease

    vi. Hereditary nephritis (Alport's syndrome)

    vii. Renal calculi

  c. Social history and habits

    i. Social history: Sexual activity prior to renal disease and sexual dysfunction related to renal disease

    ii. Habits

      (a) Dietary habits

        (1) Dietary and fluid restrictions; compliance or noncompliance with these restrictions

        (2) Dietary intake: Number and nutritional value of meals

      (b) Exercise

      (c) Frequency, type, quantity of caffeine, tobacco, alcohol, or illicit drugs

  d. Medication history

    i. Nephrotoxic agents: Radiocontrast dye and antibiotic therapy (tetracyclines, aminoglycosides, gentamicin, amphotericin B)

    ii. Diuretics, antihypertensives

    iii. Cardiac glycosides (digoxin), antiarrhythmic agents

    iv. Electrolyte replacement therapy

    v. Immunosuppressives

      (a) Corticosteroids

      (b) Azathioprine, cyclophosphamide, antithymocyte globulin (ATG), cyclosporine, monoclonal antibody (OKT3), tacrolimus (FK-506)

    vi. Analgesics such as meperidine (Demerol)

2. Nursing examination of patient

  a. Physical examination data

    i. Inspection

      (a) Diminished level of consciousness (lethargy, coma)

      (b) Skin

        (1) Abnormal color: Grayish tinge from anemia, yellowish tinge if retained carotenoids or urochrome pigments in uremia

(2) Capillary integrity: Easily bruised

(3) Skin turgor

(4) Purpura lesions: Present in some forms of renal failure

(c) Eye: Cataracts, periorbital edema

(d) Ear: Nerve deafness (Alport's syndrome)

(e) Edema

(1) Significance depends on amount of water and Na^+ retained

(2) Edema of renal failure often related to hypoalbuminemia

(f) Respiration: May see rate and pattern similar to Kussmaul's respirations

(g) Muscle tremors, weakness, weight loss with uremic syndrome

(h) Tetany: Positive Chvostek's and Trousseau's signs; rarely observed; result from severe hypocalcemia or very rapid correction of acidosis

(i) Asterixis: Indicates progressive uremic state

(1) Ask the patient to face the examiner and raise the upper extremities in a fixed hyperextension position

(2) Palms (fingers separated) must be visible to the examiner

(3) Positive sign—irregular movements of the wrists, flapping movements of the fingers—occurs within 30 seconds

(j) Fatigue: Occurs with activities of daily living and exercise, and at rest

(k) Mobility: Extent and strength with ambulation

(l) Nutritional status

(1) Triceps skinfold thickness (normal is >25 mm for men, >15 mm for women)

(2) Anemia: Pale skin, weakness, shortness of breath

(3) Tolerance of diet: Nausea and vomiting; likes and dislikes

(4) Weight loss

(m) Arteriovenous access: Type, patency, signs of infection

ii. Palpation: To determine size and shape of the kidney and to check for tenderness, cysts, and masses

(a) Right kidney is easier to palpate because it is lower in the abdomen

(b) Palpate the bladder for urinary distention due to obstruction

(c) Palpate the flank area to elicit tenderness or pain

(d) Palpate pulses for a baseline reading and to determine abnormalities

iii. Percussion

(a) At costovertebral angles to elicit pain or tenderness associated with

(1) Pyelonephritis

(2) Calculi

(3) Renal abscess

(4) Intermittent hydronephrosis

(b) At abdomen for the presence of ascites

iv. Auscultation: Listen for aortic and renal artery bruits (heard in flanks or intercostal regions of anterior abdomen)

b. Monitoring data: Intake and output (I&O), hemodynamics, body weight, central venous pressure (CVP) and/or pulmonary artery occlusion pressure to determine relationship between cardiac filling pressures and hydration status; correlate findings with daily weight

3. **Appraisal of patient characteristics:** Patients with acute, life-threatening renal problems come to critical care units with a wide range of biochemical, metabolic, and psychosocial clinical characteristics. During their stay, their clinical status may significantly improve or deteriorate, slowly or abruptly change, involve one or all life-sustaining functions, and be readily or nearly impossible to monitor

with precision. Some attributes of patients with acute renal disorders that the nurse needs to assess are the following:

a. Resiliency

    i. Level 1—*Minimally resilient:* Any patient with end-stage CRF on hemodialysis, who is septic with two other forms of organ failure, such as acute respiratory distress syndrome and cirrhosis

    ii. Level 3—*Moderately resilient:* A 58-year-old patient on postoperative day 3 after uncomplicated coronary artery bypass graft surgery who received prophylactic intravenous therapy intraoperatively to prevent renal involvement but still developed and is recovering from nonoliguric ARF

    iii. Level 5—*Highly resilient:* Any patient with an isolated episode of a prerenal ARF secondary to dehydration with no significant alteration in hemodynamics, receiving hydration

b. Vulnerability

    i. Level 1—*Highly vulnerable:* A 65-year-old male diabetic patient with cardiovascular complications who has rejected his renal transplant and is unable to tolerate hemodialysis

    ii. Level 3—*Moderately vulnerable:* A 24-year-old female with acute postrenal failure from infected renal calculi who is scheduled for surgery today

    iii. Level 5—*Minimally vulnerable:* A 32-year-old single female with a urinary tract infection (UTI)

c. Stability

    i. Level 1—*Minimally stable:* Any cardiogenic shock patient with oliguric ARF on intraaortic balloon pump and continuous renal replacement therapy

    ii. Level 3—*Moderately stable:* An end-stage CRF patient with malignant hypertension whose BP is beginning to respond to a new therapeutic regimen of antihypertensive agents including ACE inhibitors

    iii. Level 5—*Highly stable:* A 36-year-old patient with lupus nephritis in early stages of CRF who requires a protein-restricted diet and is compliant with the medical regimen

d. Complexity

    i. Level 1—*Highly complex:* A 36-year-old elementary school teacher with chronic diabetic renal disease who decided to terminate dialysis treatment and is now in a uremic coma, and whose family does not agree with her decision

    ii. Level 3—*Moderately complex:* A 21-year-old college student who is approaching end-stage renal failure and feels conflicted because two of his younger siblings are a tissue match and are both eager to donate a kidney

    iii. Level 5—*Minimally complex:* A 46-year-old male with CRF who complies with his medical regimen, is dialyzed at home by his supportive wife, and is now admitted for an acute repair of his arteriovenous fistula

e. Resource availability

    i. Level 1—*Few resources:* A 50-year-old Russian immigrant who has been in the United States 2 weeks when it is determined that he requires hemodialysis; he is not insured and is not eligible for state assistance, and his family cannot offer financial support

    ii. Level 3—*Moderate resources:* A middle-aged patient who needs renal transplantation; he has four siblings who offered to donate but none is a tissue match, so he places himself on the cadaveric organ donor list

    iii. Level 5—*Many resources:* Mrs. Jones, a well-respected elementary school nurse for the past 15 years, who has been effectively managing her own continuous ambulatory peritoneal dialysis for 5 years

f. Participation in care
    i. Level 1—*No participation:* A 26-year-old quadriplegic with nephrotoxic acute tubular necrosis (ATN) secondary to carbenicillin administered for an antibiotic-resistant UTI requires 2 weeks of dialysis after which kidney function should return
    ii. Level 3—*Moderate participation:* A blind man with diabetes is taught how to perform his own peritoneal dialysis at night with the assistance of his wife
    iii. Level 5—*Full participation:* A patient who has had a successful renal transplant for the past 3 years makes a practice of visiting local hemodialysis units and teaching the benefits of transplantation as a treatment option
g. Participation in decision making
    i. Level 1—*No participation:* A 70-year-old mentally retarded male patient with advanced chronic kidney disease is approaching the need for dialysis and lives with his 95-year-old mother, who has periods of senility
    ii. Level 3—*Moderate participation:* A 32-year-old female recently diagnosed with renal cancer has a history of admissions for psychosis and is estranged from most of her family except her 29-year-old sister
    iii. Level 5—*Full participation*: After running a marathon, the patient spends a week in the intensive care unit (ICU) recovering from an episode of ARF secondary to rhabdomyolysis; he is surrounded by his family, friends, and representatives from his community, who offer their support during his recovery at home
h. Predictability
    i. Level 1—*Not predictable:* Any critically ill patient who develops ATN after an extensive period of hypotension and experiences repeated episodes of severe dehydration, systemic infection, and exposure to nephrotoxic agents during recovery
    ii. Level 3—*Moderately predictable:* Any critically ill patient who develops contrast media–induced ATN, when renal involvement is identified early and hydration and loop diuretics are administered
    iii. Level 5—*Highly predictable:* A critically ill patient with a relatively uncomplicated condition who develops nonoliguric ATN after a short episode of hypotension, easily reversed, and has an uneventful recovery period

4. **Diagnostic studies**
  a. Laboratory
    i. Blood
      (a) Complete blood count: Reduced hematocrit and hemoglobin levels may reflect bleeding or a lack of erythropoietin
      (b) Serum creatinine: To estimate GFR (normal level, 0.6 to 1.2 mg/dl)
        (1) Creatinine excretion is proportional to its production
        (2) A significant elevation in creatinine level is associated with renal disease and correlates with percentage of nephrons damaged
      (c) BUN: Normal level, 10 to 20 mg/dl (Table 5-1)
        (1) Prerenal problem: Ratio of BUN to serum creatinine equal to or greater than 25:1 suggests extrarenal problem (dehydration, catabolic state). Elevation in both BUN and creatinine results from decreased GFR.
        (2) Renal failure: Caused by nephron damage
      (d) Cystatin C: New test to determine GFR
        (1) Cystatin C is a nonglycosylated basic protein continually produced by nucleated cells

■ **TABLE 5-1**
■ ■ **Interpretation of Blood Urea Nitrogen (BUN) and Serum Creatinine Levels**

Condition	Ratio of BUN to Creatinine	BUN	Serum Creatinine
Normal	20:1	10-20 mg/100 ml	0.6-1.2 mg/100 ml
Prerenal disease	≥25:1	↑	Normal or slight elevation
Renal disease (acute or chronic)	10:1	↑	↑

      (2) Freely filtered by glomeruli, metabolized by tubules
      (3) Serum levels not affected by age, sex, or muscle mass
      (4) More reliable indicator of renal function than creatinine
      (5) Used to detect mild reductions in GFR, especially in renal transplant patients
    (e) Serum chemistry tests (calcium, phosphate, alkaline phosphatase, bilirubin, uric acid, sodium, potassium, chloride, carbon dioxide, magnesium, glucose, cholesterol)
    (f) Baseline arterial blood gas (ABG) levels, clotting profile
    (g) Serum osmolality, total protein and albumin
  ii. Urine
    (a) Visual examination for color and clarity
      (1) Clear and colorless in hyposthenuria
      (2) Cloudy when infection is present
      (3) Foamy when albumin is present
    (b) Osmolality (50 to 1200 mOsm/kg)
    (c) SG: Wide range of normal values (1.003 to 1.030); provides reasonable estimate of urinary osmolality; actually measures density
      (1) Low normal (<1.010): Suspect diabetes insipidus, overhydration, or heart failure
      (2) Above normal (>1.030): Occurs in proteinuria, glycosuria, severe dehydration, presence of x-ray contrast medium
    (d) Creatinine clearance (C_{cr}): 24-hour urine collection
      (1) Purpose: To determine the presence and progression of renal disease, estimate percentage of functioning nephrons, or determine specific medication dosages
      (2) In 24 hours, the following occurs:

$$\frac{(U_{cr} \times V)}{P_{cr}} = C_{cr}$$

    where
    U_{cr} = amount of urinary creatinine excreted
    V = urine volume per minute
    P_{cr} = plasma creatinine level
      (3) In average-size patients, a satisfactory 24-hour urine collection always has approximately 1 g of creatinine, regardless of the degree of renal function
      (4) Cockcroft-Gault formula for estimation of C_{cr}: See Table 5-2
    (e) Culture and sensitivity: Check for infection
    (f) pH (normal range, 4.5 to 8; average value, 6); alkaline urine is frequently seen with infection; in absence of infection, possibly indicates renal tubular acidosis if both alkaline urine and systemic acidosis are present

■ **TABLE 5-2**
■ ■ **Cockcroft-Gault Formula for Estimation of Creatinine Clearance Without Urine Specimen**

Gender	Formula
Male	C_{cr} (in ml/min) = ([140 − age in years] × weight in kg) ÷ (P_{cr} in mg/dl × 72)
Female	C_{cr} (in ml/min) = ([140 − age in years] × weight in kg) ÷ (P_{cr} in mg/dl × 72) × 0.85

C_{cr}, Creatinine clearance; P_{cr}, plasma creatinine level.

(g) Glucose: In urine when renal threshold for glucose exceeded
(h) Acetone: In urine with starvation or diabetic ketoacidosis; a false-positive result can occur in patients taking salicylates
(i) Protein: Expressed quantitatively as 1+ to 4+; diagnostic for the presence of glomerular membrane disease (nephritic syndrome) and allows the detection of myeloma proteins causing renal failure
(j) Spot urine electrolytes
   (1) Measure urinary concentrations of Na^+, K^+, Cl^-
   (2) Screening test for tubular function; assess the kidney's ability to conserve sodium and concentrate urine
(k) Urinary sediment
   (1) Casts: Precipitations of protein in the kidney that take the shape of the tubules in which they are formed
      a) Hyaline casts: Entirely protein; small amounts are normal in urine; if large amounts, suspect significant proteinuria such as albumin or myeloma protein in urine
      b) Erythrocyte casts: Diagnostic for active glomerulonephritis or vasculitis
      c) Leukocyte casts: Indicative of an infectious process and intrarenal inflammation
      d) Granular casts: Small number, possibly the result of degenerating erythrocyte or leukocyte casts indicative of an infectious process or an allergic interstitial nephritis
      e) Fatty casts: Abundant in nephrotic syndrome
      f) Renal tubular casts: Seen in ARF
   (2) Bacteria: Presence determined by Gram stain
   (3) Erythrocytes: Small numbers normal; in abundance during active glomerulonephritis, interstitial nephritis, malignancies, and infection
   (4) Leukocytes: Small numbers normal; present in infection and interstitial nephritis
   (5) Renal epithelial cells: Rarely seen; present in abundance during ATN, nephrotoxic injury, and allergic reaction in the kidney
   (6) Crystals: Seen in diseases of stone formation or following certain intoxications
   (7) Eosinophils: Indicate allergic reaction in the kidney
(l) Nucleomatrix test: Noninvasive, quantitative, painless examination for transitional cell cancer of the bladder

b. Radiologic
   i. Plain abdominal x-ray study: Determines position, shape, and size of the kidney and identifies calcification in the urinary system
   ii. Intravenous pyelography (IVP)
      (a) Visualizes the urinary tract for diagnosing partial obstruction, renovascular hypertension, tumor, cyst, congenital abnormality
      (b) Complications include allergic reaction to dye, dehydration
      (c) Contraindicated in the presence of the following:
         (1) Poor renal function: Dye's dehydrating effect and nephrotoxicity may further compromise function
         (2) Multiple myeloma: IVP dye may precipitate myeloma protein in the kidney
         (3) Pregnancy: Abdominal irradiation should be avoided
         (4) Heart failure: Osmotic effect of dye can compromise cardiac function by expanding vascular volume
         (5) Diabetes mellitus
         (6) Sickle cell anemia: Dye's elevation of renal oncotic pressure can promote renal tissue sickling, infarction
   iii. High-excretion tomography: Indicated when kidneys cannot be readily visualized on IVP
   iv. Renal scan: Determines renal perfusion and function; can provide information about obstructions and renal masses. Radioactive dye is taken up by normal kidney tubule cells. A decrease in uptake indicates hypoperfusion. Often used to assess renal transplants.
   v. Retrograde pyelography: Used to examine upper region of collecting system
   vi. Retrograde urethrography: Used to examine the urethra
   vii. Cystoscopy: Detects bladder or urethral pathology
   viii. Renal arteriography (angiography): Identifies tumors and distinguishes type of renal or renovascular disease. Potential complications can be serious:
      (a) Allergic reaction to dye can cause same complications seen with IVP dye
      (b) Puncture of a peripheral artery, with consequent hematoma, embolism, or thrombus formation, is the greatest technical risk
   ix. Voiding cystourethrography: Identifies abnormalities of lower urinary tract, urethra, bladder to detect reflux and residual urine
   x. Diagnostic ultrasonography: Identifies hydronephrosis, differentiates solid and cystic tumors, localizes cysts or fluid collections
   xi. Computed tomography (CT): Identifies tumors and other pathologic conditions that create variations in body density (e.g., abscess or lymphocele); used in renal trauma to determine reason for acute flank pain
   xii. Magnetic resonance imaging (MRI)
      (a) Provides better tissue characterization than CT; provides direct imaging in several planes for detection of renal cystic disease, inflammatory processes, and renal cell carcinoma
      (b) Detects alterations in blood flow (i.e., slow or absent flow)
      (c) Identifies morphologic changes in renal transplant
   xiii. Magnetic resonance urography: A form of magnetic imaging that offers results similar to those of an IVP, without the use of dye
   xiv. Chest radiography: Identifies pulmonary edema, cardiomegaly, left ventricular hypertrophy, uremic lung, Goodpasture's disease, and infection

   c. Kidney biopsy: The most common invasive diagnostic tool
      i. For renal disease that cannot be definitively diagnosed by other means
      ii. Determines cause and extent of lesions; helpful in planning treatment
      iii. Types of biopsy
         (a) Open: For severe anatomic deformities or if a "deep specimen" is needed for diagnosis; contraindications to open biopsy include bleeding tendency, hydronephrosis, hypertension, cystic disease, and neoplasms
         (b) Closed: A simple percutaneous procedure; used more frequently than open procedure

Patient Care

1. **Overhydration:** A state in which an individual experiences fluid retention and edema because kidneys are unable to excrete excess body water
   a. Description of problem
      i. Intake greater than output
      ii. Weight gain with oliguria or anuria, low SG (≤ 1.015), dilute urine
      iii. Elevated BP, bounding pulses, neck vein distention; elevated CVP, pulmonary artery pressure (PAP), and pulmonary artery occlusive pressure (PAOP), and muffled heart sounds
      iv. Edema: Peripheral, anasarcal, ascitic, periorbital, pulmonary
      v. Dyspnea, orthopnea, crackles on auscultation, pulmonary congestion
      vi. Decreased (diluted) hemoglobin, hematocrit, and electrolyte values
      vii. Anxiety, restlessness, stupor (seen with water intoxication)
   b. Goals of care
      i. Patient maintains dry weight
      ii. BP, CVP, PAP, and PAOP are normal
      iii. Patient is free of edema
      iv. Breath sounds are clear bilaterally
      v. I&O are balanced
   c. Collaborating professionals on health care team
      i. Critical care nurse
      ii. Critical care intensivist or physician
      iii. Nurse practitioner, clinical nurse specialist, or physician assistant
      iv. Case manager
      v. Dietitian
      vi. Nephrology consultant
      vii. Hemodialysis nurse (if dialysis indicated)
   d. Interventions
      i. Identify presence of common causes of fluid volume excess
         (a) Expanded total body water volume secondary to renal failure with oliguria or anuria
         (b) Expanded blood volume due to renal sodium retention
         (c) Lower plasma oncotic pressure due to loss of plasma proteins
         (d) Increased capillary permeability
      ii. Document I&O; compare with daily weight; consider insensible losses—fluid losses via lungs, skin, and bowel (600 to 800 ml/day)
      iii. Assess renal function
         (a) Urine volume, urinalysis, creatinine clearance, and BUN/creatinine ratio
         (b) Spot electrolytes, urine concentration (SG, osmolality)
         (c) 24-hour urine collection for protein evaluation

        iv. Restrict fluids in overhydration associated with impaired renal function, impaired cardiac function, or syndrome of inappropriate secretion of antidiuretic hormone (SIADH)

        v. Administer diuretics (preferably loop) if renal response is a GFR of 25 ml/min or higher

        vi. Consider acute dialysis with ultrafiltration for rapid volume removal

    e. Evaluation of patient care

        i. 24-hour I&O balance is negative or zero

        ii. There is no edema, as evidenced by absence of adventitious breath sounds and hypertension

2. **Dehydration:** A state in which an individual experiences vascular, cellular, or intracellular volume depletion due to active fluid loss. Dehydration may occur in the diuretic phase of ARF or as a result of aggressive diuretic therapy.

    a. Description of problem

        i. Output greater than intake

        ii. Weight loss with elevated SG (≥1.020), concentrated urine, variable urinary output

           (a) Polyuric phase: Large volume of dilute urine with low SG

           (b) Dehydration with normal renal function: Oliguria, concentrated urine with an elevated SG

        iii. Hypotension, increased pulse, decreased CVP

        iv. Thirst, dry skin and mucous membranes, poor skin turgor

        v. Increased body temperature

        vi. Weakness, stupor (seen with severe hypovolemia)

    b. Goals of care

        i. Patient's weight is normal and stable

        ii. Vital signs and hemodynamic parameters are normal

        iii. Fluid balance and urine output are within normal limits (WNL)

    c. Collaborating professionals on health care team: See Overhydration

    d. Interventions

        i. Identify common causes of fluid deficit

           (a) Renal water losses

               (1) Diuretic abuse

               (2) Salt-wasting nephropathies

               (3) Diabetes insipidus (nephrogenic, central)

               (4) Osmotic or postobstruction diuresis

           (b) GI losses

               (1) Diarrhea, vomiting, nasogastric suction

               (2) Fistula and wound drainage

               (3) GI bleeding

           (c) Skin: Insensible losses

           (d) Third-spacing (ECF) phenomena

        ii. Document I&O; compare with daily weight

        iii. Administer fluid therapy

           (a) Fluid challenge to increase RBF and urinary excretion

           (b) Caution for fluid challenge: Monitor for pulmonary edema and renal failure unresponsive to volume expansion (i.e., no increase in urinary output)

           (c) Follow with replacement fluid therapy until volume goal achieved, then proceed to maintenance fluid regimen

        iv. Assess renal function

           (a) Urine volume, creatinine clearance, BUN/creatinine ratio

(b) Urinalysis; urine concentration (SG, urine osmolality), spot electrolytes

(c) 24-hour urine collection for protein evaluation

e. Evaluation of patient care

    i. The 24-hour I&O balance is positive or zero

    ii. Patient has stable, normal weight

    iii. Vital signs and hemodynamic parameters are normal

    iv. Urine volume and SG are normal

3. Malnutrition

a. Description of problem: Malnutrition is associated with increased morbidity in CRF, especially in the presence of hypoalbuminemia. Dietary protein intake is restricted to preserve kidney function in early stages of chronic kidney disease. Protein restriction can contribute to malnutrition.

b. Goals of care

    i. Patient's intake meets nutritional requirements

    ii. Patient maintains stable baseline weight and adequate muscle mass

    iii. Serum protein and albumin, BUN, and creatinine levels are normal

c. Collaborating professionals on health care team: See Overhydration

d. Interventions

    i. Identify cause of inadequate nutritional intake; direct care there

    ii. Teach appetite-enhancing measures

        (a) Provide oral hygiene prior to meals

        (b) Give small, frequent meals

        (c) Identify preferred foods, especially those high in complex carbohydrates and essential amino acids

    iii. Teach the necessary elements of the renal patient's diet

        (a) Essential amino acids, adequate calories, vitamin and iron supplements (folic acid, multivitamins) as warranted

        (b) Adjusted protein and electrolyte intake (Na^+ and K^+) to avoid uremic symptoms and electrolyte imbalances. Excessively diminished protein intake causes use of protein stored in muscles, which leads to body muscle wasting. Providing increased calories can help avoid this situation.

    iv. Monitor pattern of changes in weight and nutritional intake

    v. Assess for noncompliance with dietary instructions

e. Evaluation of patient care

    i. Body weight and muscle mass remain WNL

    ii. Serum protein, albumin, BUN, and creatinine levels are at or approach normal limits

4. Hypertension

a. Description of problem

    i. In renal failure, the hypertensive state (diastolic BP >90 mm Hg, systolic BP >140 mm Hg) is usually created by fluid retention and/or stimulation of the renin-angiotensin mechanism; preexisting hypertension is common

    ii. Clinical findings: See Chapter 3

b. Goals of care (see Chapter 3): Goal in CRF is systolic BP 130 mm Hg or lower and diastolic BP 80 to 85 mm Hg or lower

c. Collaborating professionals on health care team: See Chapter 3

d. Interventions (see Chapter 3): Treatment of hypertension in an aggressive manner with a diuretic, ACE inhibitor, β-blocker, and/or possibly calcium channel blocker has the benefit of slowing the progression of CRF

    i. Administer diuretics, as ordered, to treat edema and hypertension

        (a) General characteristics of diuretics

      (1) Inhibit the active transport of sodium or chloride, resulting in an increase in urine output

      (2) The diuretic effect reduces effective plasma circulating volume, thereby lowering BP

(b) Complications

      (1) Volume depletion

      (2) Hypokalemia, hyponatremia, hypochloremia

      (3) Hyperkalemia, hyperuricemia, azotemia

      (4) Metabolic alkalosis

(c) Types of diuretics: Used as single therapy to treat hypertension or with other antihypertensive agents to enhance their therapeutic effect

      (1) Osmotic diuretic: A nonabsorbable solute (mannitol)

          a) Exerts an osmotic effect, causing water diuresis in excess of NaCl

          b) Side effects: Blurred vision, rhinitis, rebound plasma volume expansion, thirst, urinary retention, and fluid and electrolyte imbalance

      (2) Loop diuretics: The most potent diuretics available (furosemide, indapamide, bumetanide, torsemide, and ethacrynic acid). The primary site of action is the thick segment of the medullary ascending loop of Henle.

          a) Block the reabsorption of NaCl, thus contributing to a large diuresis of isotonic urine; potassium excretion also enhanced

          b) Increase RBF by stimulating increased secretion of prostaglandin, which exerts a vasodilatory effect on renal vasculature leading to reduction in preload

          c) Vasodilatory effect of loop diuretics can be minimized, if the cardiovascular effect is negative, by the administration of ACE inhibitors

          d) Increase GFR even with a decrease in ECF volume, because the tubuloglomerular feedback mechanism is blocked

          e) Side effects: Volume depletion, agranulocytosis, thrombocytopenia, transient deafness, abdominal discomfort, hypokalemia, hypomagnesemia, metabolic alkalosis, and hyperglycemia

          f) Prolonged use without electrolyte replacement results in all other electrolyte imbalances

      (3) Thiazides (hydrochlorothiazide, chlorthalidone, and metolazone)

          a) Sodium reabsorption inhibited in the ascending loop of Henle and the beginning portion of the distal tubule

          b) Increased potassium excretion occurs with a weak carbonic anhydrase inhibitory effect

          c) Side effects: Rashes, leukopenia, thrombocytopenia, hypercalcemia, and acute pancreatitis

      (4) Potassium-sparing diuretics (spironolactone, amiloride, triamterene): Aldosterone inhibitors

          a) Promote Na^+ secretion into the distal tubule and K^+ reabsorption; cause mild diuresis and protect K^+ level

          b) Usually selected for patients receiving digoxin and diuretic therapy who cannot tolerate low serum K^+ levels or when a mild diuretic effect is desirable

          c) Side effects: Hyperkalemia, hyponatremia, headache, rash, nausea, diarrhea, urticaria, and gynecomastia or menstrual disturbances

        (5) Carbonic anhydrase inhibitors (acetazolamide sodium)
           a) Inhibit the enzyme carbonic anhydrase
           b) Increase the excretion of Na^+ by interfering with HCO_3^- reabsorption. Sodium bicarbonate is lost in the urine, which creates a hyperchloremic metabolic acidosis
           c) Are beneficial when an alkaline urine is desirable, such as with metabolic alkalosis
           d) Side effects: Hyperchloremic acidosis, renal calculi, rash, nausea, vomiting, anorexia, diminished renal function
        (6) Other agents: Pharmacologic agents that increase both cardiac output and GFR contribute to diuresis (e.g., xanthines [theophylline, aminophylline] and digoxin)
      (d) General nursing considerations in the administration of diuretics
        (1) Collaborate with the physician to determine the weight and fluid balance desired at the conclusion of diuretic therapy
        (2) Observe for fluid, electrolyte, and acid-base disorders
        (3) Maintain I&O records; correlate with daily weights
        (4) Monitor serum K^+ levels, especially if the patient is taking digoxin (hypokalemia increases risk of digitalis toxicity)
        (5) Administer potent or high doses of diuretics in the early morning or afternoon unless a Foley catheter is in place
        (6) Monitor BP during aggressive diuresis because hypotension can indicate dehydration and impending circulatory collapse
        (7) Advise the patient to report the onset of side effects such as difficulty hearing
        (8) Be aware that a diminished response to diuretics may be related to electrolyte imbalances, particularly hyponatremia, hypochloremia, and hypokalemia
    ii. Administer antihypertensive agents as ordered (see Chapter 3)
  e. Evaluation of patient care: See Chapter 3

5. **Metabolic acidosis:** A condition commonly associated with renal failure caused by the inability of the kidney to excrete hydrogen ions (see Chapter 2)

6. **Anemia:** In renal disease, anemia is related primarily to a lack of erythropoietin synthesis and secretion by the kidney but can also be caused by actual blood loss (e.g., stress ulcer)
  a. Description of problem: See Chapter 7
  b. Goals of care: See Chapter 7
  c. Collaborating professionals on health care team: See Overhydration; include hematology consult if the patient is unresponsive to therapies
  d. Interventions
    i. Identify common causes of anemia associated with renal failure
      (a) Suppression of erythropoietin synthesis and secretion
      (b) Actual blood losses
      (c) Uremic syndrome
    ii. Treat chronic anemia associated with renal failure
      (a) Oral or IV iron unless the patient has excess body iron stores
      (b) Folic acid and pyridoxine (vitamin B_6): Important, especially in dialysis patients, because these are dialyzable vitamins
      (c) Epogen (recombinant human erythropoietin): Stimulates erythrocyte production and prevents the anemia of CRF; effect does not begin until 2 to 6 weeks, with peak results in 3 months after administration; as a result, it is not used in ARF

    e. Evaluation of patient care

        i. Patient maintains acceptable hematocrit level (usually 20% to 24% with traditional therapy and 33% to 36% with epoetin alfa therapy)

        ii. Patient complies with pharmacologic and nutritional supplement therapy regimen

7. Uremic syndrome

    a. Description of problem: Uremic state results from the kidney's inability to excrete toxic waste products; uremic symptoms usually occur at BUN levels above 100 mg/dl or at a GFR below 10 to 15 ml/min (Table 5-3)

    b. Goals of care: BUN level is maintained below 100 mg/dl or at a level that minimizes uremic symptoms

    c. Collaborating professionals on health care team: See Overhydration

    d. Interventions: Based on minimizing azotemia and preventing dehydration

        i. Restrict oral protein intake

        ii. Remove blood if it is present in the GI tract because this is another protein source that can be metabolized to ammonia and urea. These metabolites cannot be handled by diseased kidneys.

        iii. Consider dialysis to maintain BUN level below 100 mg/dl. In each patient, uremic symptoms develop at individual levels of BUN and creatinine. Identify these values, then strive to maintain BUN and creatinine below those levels.

    e. Evaluation of patient care

        i. BUN is below 100 mg/dl

        ii. Uremic symptoms are absent or minimized

8. Infection

    a. Description of problem: Major cause of death in patients with ARF and can seriously compromise patients with CRF (see Chapter 7)

    b. Interventions: See Chapter 7

        i. Keep in mind: Patients with renal failure have an impaired immune response from uremic toxins and reduced phagocytosis by the reticuloendothelial system

        ii. Implement the following precautions

            (a) Obtain a urine specimen for culture on admission: UTI may be asymptomatic

            (b) Prevent introduction of microorganisms; avoid indwelling urinary catheters and unnecessary invasive monitoring procedures

            (c) Use an aseptic technique for urinary and intravenous catheter care

            (d) Maintain the BUN level at 80 to 100 mg/dl or lower to minimize susceptibility to infection

            (e) Implement isolation techniques for hepatitis antigen–positive patients receiving hemodialysis

    c. Evaluation of patient care: See Chapter 7

9. Bone disease—osteomalacia, osteitis fibrosa: Chronic hypocalcemia can precipitate hyperparathyroidism, which leads to the mobilization of calcium from the bone and results in softening of the bone (osteomalacia)

    a. Description of problem

        i. History of chronic hypocalcemia, hyperparathyroidism, or both

        ii. Bone pain, fractures, and radiologic examination of the skull, hands, and feet revealing signs of demineralization

        iii. Activity intolerance with ambulation

    b. Goals of care

        i. Hypocalcemia remains within an asymptomatic range.

        ii. No fractures or bone pain is present.

■ **TABLE 5-3**
■ ■ **Clinical Findings in Uremic Syndrome**

Uremic syndrome affects every organ, producing a constellation of symptoms that can occur in any combination.

System	Findings
Neurologic	Sensorium changes (loss of attention span, lethargy, fatigue, coma)
	Headache
	Peripheral neuropathy
	Tremors
	Uremic seizures
Skin	Pale yellow tinge
	Pruritus
	Dryness
	Ecchymoses
	Edema
	Uremic frost (rare)
Hematologic and immunologic	Bleeding secondary to platelet dysfunction
	Diminished immune response
	Anemia secondary to erythropoietin loss or bleeding
Gastrointestinal	Nausea and/or vomiting
	Anorexia, weight loss
	Stomatitis
	Uremic fctor
	Dysgeusia (metallic, unpleasant taste)
	Gastritis, colitis (rare)
	Constipation
	Carbohydrate intolerance
Metabolic	Carbohydrate intolerance
	Hyperkalemia
	Hyponatremia or hypernatremia
	Hypocalcemia
	Hyperphosphatemia
	Hypermagnesemia
Musculoskeletal	Renal osteodystrophy—soft tissue calcification
	Bone pain
	Diminished mobility with decreased strength and change in gait
	Muscle atrophy and weakness to paralysis
Genitourinary	Flank pain
	Hematuria
	Proteinuria
	Dysuria, urinary frequency, polyuria
	Normal urine volume to oliguria or anuria
	Urinary tract infections
	Sexual dysfunction
Cardiac	Pericarditis
	Heart murmurs
	Increased rate of atherosclerosis
	Hypertension
	Pulse: Normal, bradycardia, or tachycardia secondary to uremia or electrolyte imbalance
	12-Lead electrocardiogram changes consistent with uremic pericarditis, hyperkalemia, or hypocalcemia
	Chest pain—pleuritic, pericardial, or caused by ischemic heart disease
Endocrine	Hyperparathyroidism (secondary)

Continued

■ **TABLE 5-3**
■ ■ **Clinical Findings in Uremic Syndrome—cont'd**

Pulmonary	Pleuritis
	Pulmonary edema
	Deep, rapid respirations; Kussmaul's respirations
	Recent respiratory infections (Goodpasture's syndrome or recent streptococcal infection), antineutrophil cytoplasmic antibody–related or Wegener's granulomatosis
Psychosocial	Altered self-image
	Diminished body image
	Depression to suicidal ideation
Other	Deafness (Alport's syndrome)

    c. Collaborating professionals on health care team: See Overhydration
    d. Interventions: See Electrolyte Imbalances—Calcium Imbalance: Hypocalcemia and Electrolyte Imbalances—Phosphate Imbalance: Hyperphosphatemia later in this chapter
10. **Altered metabolism and excretion of pharmacologic agents related to renal failure**
    a. Description of problem
      i. Kidneys unable to metabolize or excrete pharmacologic agents
      ii. Unusual untoward effects may include enhanced sensitivity to drugs
      iii. Active or toxic metabolites of a medication retained
      iv. Increased azotemia due to elevation in metabolic wastes from drug usage
    b. Goals of care
      i. Patient tolerates pharmacologic therapy with no untoward drug effects
      ii. Prescribed serum drug levels are adequate
    c. Collaborating professionals on health care team: See Overhydration; also Pharmacologist
    d. Interventions
      i. Recognize alterations in the body's use of drugs during renal failure
        (a) Distribution of drugs in a uremic state
          (1) Decreased stores of body fat affect distribution of lipid-soluble drugs
          (2) Low cardiac output states reduce renal metabolism or excretion of drugs
          (3) Acidemia alters tissue uptake of drugs
          (4) Increased body water has a dilutional effect
          (5) Decreased protein binding causes competition by various drugs for tissue binding sites, leading to a higher concentration of unbound drugs
        (b) Uremic effects that can alter drug absorption
          (1) Decreased GI motility and altered gastric pH
          (2) Electrolyte imbalances, which may affect GI tract
          (3) Inability of the kidney to excrete or metabolize drugs
          (4) Diminished protein binding
      ii. Follow general principles for drug administration during renal insufficiency

      (a) Reduce drug dosage

      (b) Increase intervals between doses

      (c) Question orders for nephrotoxic agents (i.e., NSAIDs, meperidine)

      (d) Closely observe patients to recognize toxicity due to drug accumulation

      (e) Report any untoward signs, especially elevated serum creatinine level, so the drug can be reconsidered, reduced in dosage, or discontinued

      (f) Monitor serum drug levels, especially in situations requiring a specific drug concentration (e.g., antibiotics, digoxin, procaine)

      (g) To ensure a more stable serum concentration, administer initial loading doses of drugs that have a long half-life (e.g., digoxin)

   e. Evaluation of patient care: Patient tolerates pharmacologic therapy with no untoward drug effects

11. Ineffective patient and family coping (see also Chapter 10)

   a. Description of problem

      i. Insufficient, ineffective, or compromised support, comfort, assistance, or encouragement, usually by a supportive primary person (family member or close friend). The patient may need to manage adaptive tasks related to the stress of renal failure on the patient and the family.

      ii. Signs of maladaptive patient coping

        (a) Verbalization of the inability to cope or to ask for help

        (b) Inability to meet role expectations and solve problems

        (c) Diminished communication and socialization

        (d) Destructive behavior toward self or others (i.e., suicide attempt)

        (e) Failure to comply with the treatment regimen

     iii. Signs of maladaptive family coping

        (a) Patient communicates concern about the family's response to his or her disease

        (b) Family members demonstrate preoccupation with their own personal reactions—fear, anticipatory grief, guilt, anxiety

        (c) Family has inadequate understanding of the patient's condition, or therapy interferes with effective supportive behaviors

        (d) Family withdraws from communication with the patient or demonstrates overprotective or underprotective behaviors

   b. Goals of care

      i. Patient demonstrates increased functional independence, compliance with treatment regimen, and participation in programs that enhance quality of life (e.g., exercise or rehabilitation program)

      ii. Patient appropriately expresses ideas, feelings, and needs, participates in family activities, and accepts family support, as appropriate

     iii. Patient and family adjust to any necessary role changes

     iv. Patient resumes employment

   c. Collaborating professionals on health care team (see also Overhydration)

      i. Psychiatrist or psychologist

      ii. Social worker

   d. Interventions

      i. Identify common causes of stress in the patient and family

        (a) Life-threatening nature of renal disease

        (b) Inability to perform activities of daily living

        (c) Restrictions caused by a shunt, a fistula, or a Tenckhoff catheter; demands of dialysis schedule and other treatments

        (d) Reversal in family roles, effects on sexual behavior and sexuality, and questions regarding ability to maintain or return to work

  ii. Recognize that psychologic consequences of renal disease and its treatment include denial, depression, and dependency, and that the suicide rate among patients maintained with hemodialysis is believed to be 100 times that of the general population

  iii. Assess the patient's ability to cope with renal disease (see Chapter 10)

  iv. Specific nursing interventions to support adaptation of the patient with renal failure

   (a) Teach the patient about the various treatment alternatives and encourage participation in selection of the treatment method

   (b) Link with support systems

    (1) Visits with successfully adjusted patients

    (2) Support for family members; patients with supportive families tend to have fewer physical complications, survive longer, and adjust more readily

 e. Evaluation of patient care

  i. Patient demonstrates the following:

   (a) Participation in self-care, social and family activities, and use of adaptive coping mechanisms such as functional denial

   (b) Increased self-esteem with acceptance of body image changes

   (c) Cooperation with health care staff and compliance with treatment plan

  ii. Family demonstrates the following:

   (a) Decreased levels of anxiety, adaptive changes in family roles, and appropriate use of health care and community support systems

   (b) Participation in patient care

SPECIFIC PATIENT HEALTH PROBLEMS

Acute Renal Failure

The ARF syndrome affects 5% to 7% of all hospitalized patients and 20% of the critically ill. Oliguria with ARF is associated with a 50% mortality rate in the critically ill and a 50% to 70% mortality rate in trauma or postoperative patients. Nonoliguria with ARF carries a better prognosis and a lower mortality rate of 26%. A mortality rate of 87% is seen in patients with ARF 24 hours after cardiogenic shock due to acute MI. These mortality rates in the critically ill have not improved in the last 45 years, so prevention of ARF remains the best intervention.

1. Pathophysiology

 a. Prerenal conditions

  i. Physiologic states diminish renal perfusion without renal tubular damage

  ii. Effects of diminished kidney perfusion

   (a) Decreased renal arterial pressure

   (b) Decreased afferent arterial pressure (<100 mm Hg), which diminishes forces favoring filtration

 b. Intrarenal conditions

  i. Cortical involvement of vascular, infectious, or immunologic processes

   (a) Causes renal capillary swelling and cellular proliferation, which eventually decrease the GFR

   (b) Edema and cellular debris obstruct the glomeruli, which results in oliguria

  ii. Medullary involvement after prolonged ischemia or hypoperfusion or nephrotoxic injury to the tubular portion of the nephrons (Figure 5-4, *A*)

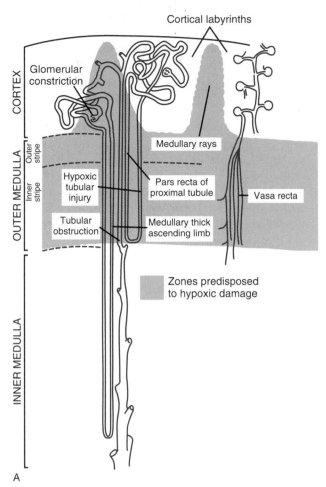

FIGURE 5-4 ■ **A,** Anatomy of intrarenal zones predisposed to hypoxic injury in acute renal failure. (From Heyman SN, Fuch S, Brezis M: The role of indwelling ischemia in ARF, *New Horiz* 3(4):597, 1995.)

Continued, p. 559

(a) Medullary hemodynamics: Hypoperfusion states and oxygen insufficiency disrupt the fine balance between limited oxygen supply and high oxygen consumption in the outer medullary region; may contribute to ARF from hypoxic medullary damage
  (1) Conditions predisposing to hypoperfusion
    a) Presence of endotoxin
    b) Rhabdomyolysis
    c) Hypercalcemia
    d) NSAID use
    e) Exposure to radiologic contrast agents
    f) Antibiotic use (i.e., amphotericin, cyclosporine)
  (2) Pharmacologic agents can also alter medullary hemodynamics, especially if administered in absence of volume depletion (i.e., furosemide, mannitol, dopamine). Other substances suspected of

improving medullary hemodynamics are nitric oxide, which is normally produced by the macula densa to control glomerular blood flow and renin release, and ANP, an endogenous vasodilator.

(b) Tubular necrosis produced as localized damage in patchy pattern (actual necrosis) or in apoptosis as disruption of cellular function (usually in the distal tubules): Extent of the damage differs in nephrotoxic injury, ischemia or hypoperfusion, sepsis-associated states, and multiple organ failure

    (1) Nephrotoxic injury affects the epithelial cellular layer (can regenerate)

    (2) Ischemia and hypoperfusion alter renal tubular cells and damage the tubular basement membrane (cannot regenerate)

        a) Cellular injury may involve several factors: ATP depletion, oxygen free radical formation, loss of epithelial cell polarity, and increased calcium levels; apoptosis causes DNA fragmentation and cytoplasmic condensation

        b) ATP depletion: Begins 30 seconds after the kidney is hypoperfused; normal homeostatic benefits of cellular ATP (preservation of cellular volume, ionic composition, membrane integrity) are lost

        c) Oxidative metabolism produces oxygen free radicals

            1) Because these substances are highly reactive and volatile, intracellular mechanisms (enzyme systems and antioxidants) exist for their rapid breakdown and destruction

            2) Left unopposed, as during ischemic events, these radicals disrupt cellular functioning (e.g., during ischemia, the renal cell is unstable and unable to protect itself from oxygen free radicals, which results in renal cell injury)

        d) Loss of epithelial cell polarity: Ischemia alters the passage of water, electrolytes, and other charged elements through the tubule's epithelial wall, which leads to a concentration defect

        e) Increased calcium levels: Ischemic and hypoperfusion states lead to a rise in intracellular calcium levels that causes renal vasoconstriction and a decrease in GFR

    (3) Systemic inflammatory response syndrome (SIRS): Released endotoxins significantly reduce renal perfusion, and renal vasoactive substances alter renal cellular metabolism and constrict renal vasculature (see Chapter 9)

    (4) Multiorgan dysfunction syndrome results in rapid and progressive deterioration of renal function (see Chapter 9)

(c) Phases of recovery: Classic form of ARF has four phases, whereas nonoliguric form has only three; the nonoliguric phase seems to be synonymous with the diuretic phase, which suggests that nonoliguric ARF reflects less tubular damage so recovery is more rapid

(d) Onset, or initial phase, precedes the actual necrotic injury and correlates with a major alteration in renal hemodynamics

    (1) Associated with a decrease in RBF and GFR

    (2) Most important factor altering RBF is decrease in cardiac output

    (3) Other mechanisms contributing to decreased renal perfusion are increased sympathetic activity and renal vascular resistance

    (4) A consistent increase in cardiac output during this phase will maintain an increase in RBF and protect the patient from impending ARF

(e) Oliguric phase reflects four processes (Figure 5-4, *B*)

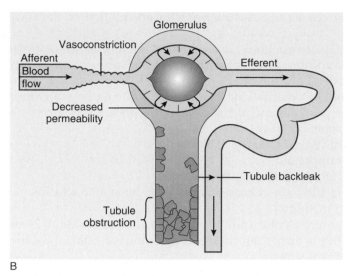

B

FIGURE 5-4—cont'd ■ **B,** Potential mechanisms causing oliguria in patients with acute renal failure. (From Goldman L, Ausiello D, editors: *Cecil textbook of medicine,* ed 22, Philadelphia, 2004, Saunders, p 706.)

    (1) Obstruction of tubules by cellular debris, tubular casts, or tissue swelling

    (2) Reabsorption or back-leak of urine filtration through the damaged tubular epithelium and into circulation

    (3) Tubular cell damage with development of necrotic, patchy areas; the cell leaks ATP and K^+, edema is present, mitochondria are altered, and calcium leaks into the cell

    (4) Renal vasoconstriction continues and may contribute to the decreased GFR

(f) Nonoliguric phase reflects less tubular damage; symptomatology resembles that of the diuretic phase

    (1) Urine output may exceed 1 L/hr

    (2) Solute present in urine at approximately 350 mOsm/L

    (3) Creatinine clearance is as high as 15 ml/min, and Na^+ excretion is low

    (4) Hyperkalemia remains a significant problem

    (5) Phase of short duration; recovery phase reached in 5 to 8 days

(g) Diuretic phase: Signifies that tubular function is returning

    (1) Tubular obstruction relieved, but cellular edema remains as scar tissue forms on necrotic areas

    (2) Large daily urine output, sometimes exceeding 3 L; output due to the osmotic-diuretic effect of elevated BUN level and impaired ability of tubules to conserve Na^+ and water

    (3) Recovery phase

        a) Occurs after gradual improvement of kidney function extending over a 3- to 12-month period

        b) Residual renal impairment in GFR may result, with serum creatinine level remaining higher than previously

    c. Postrenal conditions: Associated with obstruction of the urinary collecting system
        i. Partial obstruction: Can increase renal interstitial pressure, increasing opposing forces of glomerular filtration; result is diminished urine output
        ii. Complete obstruction: Impediment to urine flow accompanies bilateral kidney involvement; the "back-up" pressure of urine compresses the kidneys

2. Etiology and risk factors: See Table 5-4

3. Signs and symptoms
    a. Malaise, fatigue, lethargy, confusion
    b. Twitching and/or weakness secondary to metabolic acidosis
    c. Impaired mobility
    d. Change in urine color and/or volume: Oliguria (<400 ml/24 hr); nonoliguria (excess, dilute urine); anuria (no urine output or <100 ml/24 hr); or hematuria
    e. Cardiac involvement
        i. Dysrhythmias secondary to electrolyte imbalance or heart failure
        ii. Change in pulse rate (either tachycardia or bradycardia)
        iii. Hypertension
        iv. Cardiac friction rub, indicative of pericarditis
    f. Skin changes: Dry skin, edema, pallor, bruising, uremic frost (rare), pruritus
    g. Flank pain
    h. Local or systemic infection presenting with shaking, chills, and fever
    i. Abdominal distention secondary to enlarged bladder, obstruction
    j. Uremic signs and symptoms: See Table 5-3

4. Diagnostic study findings
    a. Laboratory
        i. Prerenal
            (a) Urinalysis
                (1) Urinary sodium level less than 10 mEq/L
                (2) SG greater than 1.020
                (3) Minimal or no proteinuria
                (4) Normal urinary sediment
                (5) Urine osmolality higher than 400 mOsm/kg
            (b) Serum BUN/creatinine ratio higher than 25:1
        ii. Intrarenal—cortical disease
            (a) Urinalysis
                (1) Urinary sodium level less than 10 mEq/L
                (2) SG variable
                (3) Moderate to heavy proteinuria
                (4) Hematuria
                (5) Urinary sediment with erythrocyte casts, leukocytes
                (6) Urine osmolality less than 350 mOsm/kg
            (b) Serum BUN and creatinine levels elevated but remain in 10:1 ratio
        iii. Intrarenal—medullary disease
            (a) Urinalysis
                (1) Urinary sodium level greater than 20 mEq/L
                (2) SG 1.010
                (3) Minimal to moderate proteinuria
                (4) Urinary sediment with numerous renal tubular epithelial cells, tubular casts, and a rare erythrocyte
            (b) Serum BUN and creatinine levels elevated

■ **TABLE 5-4**
■ ■ **Common Causes of Acute Renal Failure**

Type of Renal Failure	Causes
Prerenal failure	Hypovolemia secondary to hemorrhage, gastrointestinal losses, third-spacing phenomena
	Excessive use of diuretics
	Impaired myocardial contractility (such as heart failure, pericardial tamponade)
	Sepsis, such as gram-negative shock with vasodilatation
	Increased renal vascular resistance from anesthesia or surgery
	Bilateral renal vascular obstruction caused by embolism or thrombosis
Intrarenal failure	
Cortical involvement	Acute poststreptococcal glomerulonephritis
	Acute cortical necrosis
	Systemic lupus erythematosus (lupus nephritis)
	Goodpasture's syndrome, antineutrophil cytoplasmic antibody disease such as Wegener's granulomatosis
	Bilateral endocarditis
	Pregnancy (i.e., abruptio placentae and abortion)
	Malignant hypertension
	Human immunodeficiency virus–related nephropathy
Medullary involvement	Nephrotoxic injury: Occurs after exposure to nephrotoxic agents; the effects are accentuated by dehydration, which leads to more extensive tubular damage; nephrotoxic damage may also compound the clinical picture of any type of existing renal deterioration
	• Antibiotics: Aminoglycosides, tetracyclines, penicillins, cephalosporins, pentamidine
	• Antiviral agents: Acyclovir
	• Nonsteroidal antiinflammatory drugs (e.g., ibuprofen)
	• Immunosuppressive drugs: Cyclosporine, tacrolimus
	• Angiotensin-converting enzyme inhibitors (e.g., captopril) or angiotensin II receptor blockers (e.g., losartan)
	• Carbon tetrachloride (found in cleaning agents)
	• Heavy metals: Lead, arsenic, mercury, uranium
	• Pesticides and fungicides
	• Radiocontrast dye (e.g., in angiography or computed tomography)
	• Chemotherapeutic agent toxicity (e.g., cisplatin, uric acid crystals)
	Ischemic injury: During ischemia injury may occur if mean arterial pressure drops below 60 mm Hg for over 40 min; causes include massive hemorrhage, transfusion reaction (tubules are obstructed with hemolyzed erythrocytes), and cardiogenic shock
	Multiple organ dysfunction syndrome: Triggered by the inflammatory or immune response, leading to the progressive deterioration of organs, with the kidneys as a prime target
	Systemic inflammatory response syndrome: Renal injury can result from endotoxins, an inflammatory or immune response, or renal hypoperfusion
Postrenal failure	Ureteral obstruction (e.g., stone, tumor, fibrosis, or clot)
	Abscess
	Prostate hypertrophy
	Crystal deposition (e.g., uric acid, calcium oxalate, acyclovir)

    iv. Postrenal

       (a) Serum BUN and creatinine levels elevated with complete obstruction

       (b) Bacteriologic report showing significant positive results for a specific organism

    v. Special

       (a) Antistreptolysin O titer: To diagnose recent streptococcal infection (may cause poststreptococcal glomerulonephritis)

       (b) Antiglomerular basement membrane titers: To diagnose Goodpasture's syndrome, a devastating disease of pulmonary hemorrhage and renal failure

       (c) Antineutrophil cytoplasmic antibody test for pulmonary and renal failure

       (d) Serum studies for complement components: A fall in complement levels is seen in active complement-mediated glomerulonephritis (e.g., lupus nephritis)

       (e) Serum electrophoresis for immunoglobulin levels: Abnormal proteins (as in multiple myeloma) can damage kidneys

       (f) Hepatitis serologic tests: Hepatitis B and C cause kidney disease

  b. Radiologic: To rule out obstruction as a cause of oliguria or anuria, because immediate treatment may reverse renal failure. Kidney size provides diagnostic information, because small kidneys imply chronic rather than acute renal failure (see Diagnostic Studies under Patient Assessment)

5. Goals of care

  a. ARF is resolved

  b. Normal renal function and urine output resume

6. Collaborating professionals on health care team

  a. Critical care nurse, clinical specialist or physician assistant, case manager, hemodialysis nurse

  b. Physicians: Intensivist, nephrologist (higher mortality when renal consult delayed >48 hours), hematology consult (if blood dyscrasias accompany ARF), vascular surgery consultant

  c. Dietitian

  d. Social worker

  e. Pharmacologist

7. Management of patient care

  a. Anticipated patient trajectory: Patients with ARF experience rapid decline, with recovery from 8 days for nonoliguric ATN and from 2 weeks to 3 months for oliguric ATN. Transfer or discharge varies with the stage of renal recovery. Expect patients with ARF to have needs in numerous areas:

    i. Skin care: Impaired skin integrity due to uremia, malnutrition, immobility

       (a) Assess for uremic effects on skin integrity (Table 5-3)

       (b) Keep skin clean, dry, and intact to prevent infection

       (c) Use aseptic technique during wound care

    ii. Nutrition: ARF is associated with accelerated protein catabolism that contributes to negative nitrogen balance and uncontrollably high BUN levels usually indicative of a hypercatabolic state. Repeated elevations of BUN over 100 mg/dl despite routine dialysis correlate with evidence of rapid muscle wasting and indicate the need for higher levels of protein consumption, together with a continuous form of dialysis.

       (a) Maintain protein intake at a minimum of 0.6 to 0.8 g/kg of body weight; administer higher amounts of protein during hypercatabolism

       (b) Provide total calories of 30 to 35 kcal/kg/day of a carbohydrate and lipid combination while controlling glucose and triglyceride intake

(c) Be aware that hyperalimentation and daily dialysis have been associated with increased survival rates in ARF as well as promotion of renal tubular cell regeneration. Hyperalimentation requirements include consumption of large amounts of both essential and nonessential amino acids.

(d) Give IV glucose and lipid solution to augment caloric and nutritional intake, thereby reducing the need for protein in hypercatabolic states

(e) Maintain fluid restriction by limiting non–electrolyte-containing fluids

(f) Administer water-soluble vitamins. Avoid excessive doses of vitamin C (not exceeding 250 mg/day), which may exacerbate ARF. Be cautious with vitamin A, because excessive intake in the absence of renal excretion can lead to vitamin A toxicity.

(g) Monitor serum protein, albumin, hematocrit, and urea levels and weigh daily to assess the effectiveness of nutritional therapy

iii. Infection control: Uremia increases patient susceptibility to infection

(a) Assess for BUN levels over 80 to 100 mg/dl because these are associated with an increased risk of infection

(b) Monitor for early signs of septic shock (SIRS)

(c) Monitor serum protein and albumin levels, because inadequate levels have an immunosuppressive effect

iv. Discharge planning

(a) Teach patient and family members or significant others the following:

(1) Etiology and course of the disease

(2) Dietary and fluid restriction requirements

(3) Dialysis machine operation, procedure, and schedule

(4) Prospects for recovery

(b) Assess and prepare the home for patient care and, if appropriate, for dialysis

(c) Make the patient and family aware of community resources (e.g., national or local kidney foundation [http://www.kidney.org], local dialysis center)

(d) Assist in patient transition to rehabilitation and/or home care

v. Pharmacology

(a) Use pharmacologic agents with adequate fluid replacement to reestablish or augment RBF. This does not protect the tubules from damage but may limit the extent of damage, creating nonoliguric ATN.

(1) Renal-dose dopamine: No longer the therapy of choice for prevention or treatment. Research (Kellum and Decker, 2001) reveals that dopamine has no benefit in treating ARF. Dopamine may actually compromise the kidney by moving oxygen to the renal medulla; can cause tachycardia and mesenteric ischemia and does not decrease mortality.

(2) Diuretics: Studies (Mehta et al, 2002; Singri, Ahya, and Levin, 2003) question their effectiveness in treating ARF

a) Commonly used agents

1) Traditional diuretics (mannitol, loop diuretics): Used to convert oliguria to nonoliguria

2) Mannitol: Protects the kidney by preventing the buildup of cellular debris, reducing tubular obstruction, and augmenting blood flow. Preserves mitochondrial function via osmotic effect; limits recovery ischemia and free radical production. Administer with caution; may precipitate pulmonary edema.

3) Furosemide (Lasix): Acts as both a diuretic and an augmentor of RBF; maximum dosage should not exceed 4 mg/kg/min

b) Diuresis encourages removal of sloughed tubular cells, eliminating tubular obstruction

c) Volume replacement needs to be a priority before administering diuretics; a trial of diuretics can be attempted but should be limited when effectiveness is in question

d) Monitor and report changes in urine output (onset of oliguria, nonoliguria, or anuria)

e) Obtain urine and blood specimens, analyze results

(b) Metabolism and excretion of pharmacologic agents may be altered in ARF (see Patient Care)

vi. Treatments

(a) Prevention modalities for ARF: Remain the best intervention; preservation of renal function is the desired outcome

(1) Identify patients at higher risk for ARF

a) Hemodynamic instability; blood loss or hypotension in surgical patients

b) Multiple trauma, multiorgan dysfunction syndrome, rhabdomyolysis

c) Systemic and/or renal intravascular hemolysis

d) Receipt of nephrotoxic drugs

(2) Monitor for prerenal or onset stage of ATN (see Diagnostic Study Findings for prerenal failure)

a) Renal hypoperfusion from any cause diminishes the GFR as the MAP drops to 70 mm Hg or below

b) Hypotension can eliminate renal autoregulation

(b) Correct hypotension and/or renal hypoperfusion by fluid administration and/or pharmacologic agents

(1) Fluid administration: The single best modality for reinstating renal perfusion is to increase cardiac output through the administration of fluids, especially in preventing radiocontrast-associated ARF

a) Consider the following fluids: Normal saline, colloids (either albumin or dextran) and/or blood products

b) Monitor patient response to administration of as much as 1 to 2 L normal saline over 2 or more hours; observe for nonresponse to volume expansion or pulmonary edema

(2) Pharmacologic agents: Include calcium channel blockers, ANP

a) Dopamine not proven to be clinically useful

b) Calcium channel blockers vasodilate renal vasculature and augment renal function; found to be useful in ARF secondary to renal transplantation, radiocontrast nephrotoxicity, and cyclosporine use

c) ANP use associated with improvement in oliguric rather than nonoliguric ARF; beneficial in management of heart failure

d) Mucomyst (N-acetylcysteine) beneficial in the prevention of ARF secondary to IV radiocontrast nephrotoxicity; consider 600 mg by mouth twice daily

(c) Determine the need for hemodialysis: Early initiation of any form of dialysis is beneficial for the prevention and management of acute and chronic renal failure

(1) Indications for which hemodialysis remains the initial treatment of choice
  a) ARF
  b) CRF when medications and diet no longer provide effective therapy
  c) Symptomatic uremia (e.g., acidosis, hyperkalemia, pericardial friction rub)
  d) To keep BUN level lower than 100 mg/dl and improve survival rate
(2) Contraindications
  a) Intolerance to systemic heparinization (i.e., heparin-induced thrombocytopenia); consider nonheparin anticoagulant such as lepirudin (Refludan)
  b) Hemodynamic instability: Labile cardiovascular status incompatible with rapid changes in ECF volume
(d) Initiate hemodialysis (Figure 5-5)
  (1) Principles of hemodialysis: Include osmosis (optional), diffusion, and convection-ultrafiltration
   a) Osmosis: Movement of water across a semipermeable membrane from an area of lesser to an area of greater osmolality
   b) Diffusion: Movement of molecules from area of higher to an area of lower concentration

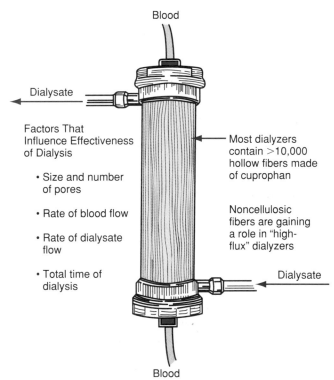

Blood

Dialysate

Factors That
Influence Effectiveness
of Dialysis

• Size and number
  of pores

• Rate of blood flow

• Rate of dialysate
  flow

• Total time of
  dialysis

Most dialyzers
contain >10,000
hollow fibers made
of cuprophan

Noncellulosic
fibers are gaining
a role in "high-
flux" dialyzers

Dialysate

Blood

FIGURE 5-5 ■ Hollow-fiber dialyzer, the most common type in clinical use today. Some use of parallel-plate dialyzers continues, but these dialyzers have almost disappeared from clinical practice. (From Bennett JC, Plum F, editors: *Cecil textbook of medicine*, ed 20, Philadelphia, 1997, Saunders.)

       c) Ultrafiltration and convection: Movement of particles through a semipermeable membrane by hydrostatic pressure

  (2) Hemodynamics: By means of vascular access and a blood pump, about 300 ml of blood travels through an extracorporeal dialyzer, which removes wastes, toxic substances, excess electrolytes, metabolic products, and pharmacologic agents and then returns the blood to the systemic circulation

  (3) Anticoagulation

       a) Prior to the procedure, heparinization is performed to keep blood anticoagulated within the hemodialysis machine (regional heparinization)

       b) For patients without complications, 5000 units heparin is administered to start and 2000 units/hr is given while the patient is on the machine (general heparinization); dosage may be adjusted to meet the needs of the individual patient

       c) Nonheparin hemodialysis is available at some facilities

       d) Patient must be monitored closely for signs of bleeding

  (4) Vascular access for dialysis

       a) Central venous access (i.e., dual-lumen internal jugular, femoral, or subclavian catheter): For emergent dialysis or temporarily after failure of a permanent catheter while awaiting repair or replacement

          1) Blood flow must range from 200 to 500 mL/min to accommodate hemodialysis

          2) Double- or triple-lumen catheter requires the use of a large vein, such as the femoral vein, which limits ambulation and carries the risk of dislodgement, infection, and kinking; other sites include the right or left subclavian and right or left jugular vein

          3) Palpate peripheral pulses in the cannulated extremity

          4) Observe for bleeding or hematoma formation; if it occurs, apply pressure dressing and notify the physician

          5) Properly position the catheter to avoid dislodgment during the dialysis procedure

          6) If the femoral vein catheter is to be maintained after dialysis, connect it to a pressurized IV flow system. Add a low dose of heparin (500 U/L) to the solution. Maintain a secure aseptic dressing to minimize the risk of infection. No standing or ambulation is allowed while the catheter is in place.

          7) On removal of a femoral catheter, apply direct pressure to the puncture site for 5 to 10 minutes (or the time needed to stop the bleeding after dialysis and after the period of heparinization). Complete this procedure with the application of a pressure dressing and a period of bed rest.

       b) Permanent vascular access: An arteriovenous fistula is usually placed in an upper rather than a lower extremity

          1) Surgical procedure with anastomosis of an artery to a vein, or an artificial vascular graft is used

          2) Do not perform venipuncture, start IV therapy, give injections, or take BP with a cuff on the arm with a fistula; post this information on signage above bed

          3) Palpate the thrill or auscultate the bruit to confirm patency

        4) Avoid circumferential dressings and restrictive clothing

        5) Report bleeding, skin discoloration, drainage, and other signs of infection; culture the drainage

        6) For profuse bleeding, apply a pressure dressing

     c) External permanent vascular access: An arteriovenous shunt is rarely selected

        1) Auscultate for the bruit or palpate for the thrill to assess shunt patency

        2) Promptly report any suspicion of clotting (color change of blood, separation of serum from erythrocytes, absence of pulsations in tubing)

        3) Hydrate adequately to minimize clotting

        4) Change the sterile dressing over the shunt at least daily; reinforce the dressing as necessary

        5) Do not perform venipuncture, give IV therapy, give injections, or take BP with a cuff on the shunt arm

        6) Instruct the patient in the care of the shunt site

  (5) Hemodialysis membrane compatibility

  (6) Frequency: ARF may require daily dialysis or a one-time dialysis treatment to resolve an acute problem, such as a hyperkalemic episode

  (7) Complications

     a) Muscle cramps, nausea, vomiting

     b) Bleeding

     c) Infection (e.g., hepatitis C or infection related to catheter placement or skin flora)

     d) Hypertension, anaphylactic reactions

     e) Technical error (dialyzer rupture)

(e) Continuous renal replacement treatment (CRRT)

  (1) Description

     a) Form of dialysis specifically developed for the critically ill, hemodynamically unstable patient

     b) May also be selected when both hemodialysis and peritoneal dialysis are contraindicated

     c) Associated with a shorter length of stay and less resource utilization, but not with lower mortality

  (2) Indications

     a) Conditions of fluid overload or cardiovascular instability requiring a continuous method of fluid removal or compensation for azotemia (e.g., ATN)

     b) Ascites, diuretic-resistant edema, acute pulmonary edema

     c) Post cardiac surgery, recent acute MI

     d) Inability to tolerate the cardiovascular impact of rapid fluid losses associated with hemodialysis or failure of a trial of hemodialysis

  (3) Contraindications: Rare; hematocrit over 45% is a contraindication for manual forms of CRRT (i.e., continuous arteriovenous hemofiltration, continuous arteriovenous hemodialysis)

  (4) Types of CRRT

     a) Slow continuous ultrafiltration (SCUF)

     b) Continuous arteriovenous hemofiltration (CAVH)

     c) Continuous arteriovenous hemodialysis (or hemodiafiltration) (CAVHD)

d) Continuous venovenous hemofiltration (CVVH)

e) Continuous venovenous hemodialysis (CVVHD) or hemodiafiltration (CVVHDF); involves the use of a hollow-fiber hemofilter capable of rapid fluid removal during hypotensive or low blood flow states

(5) Principles: See Principles of Hemodialysis

(6) Anticoagulation

a) Heparin used in SCUF, CAVH, and CAVHD

b) Heparin or trisodium citrate used in CRRT machine forms of CVVH, CVVHD, and CVVHF

c) Trisodium citrate causes binding of serum calcium; therefore, must monitor calcium levels. Calcium administration may be necessary.

(7) Frequency: A continuous dialysis form providing the ability to dialyze 24 hours a day and 7 days a week; the advantage in the critically ill is homeostasis, with avoidance of erratic swings in the levels of toxic substances

(8) Forms of CRRT

a) SCUF and CAVH

1) Use the principle of ultrafiltration, the exchange of primarily plasma water along with particles (e.g., K^+, BUN, creatinine) by convection

2) Exchange rate depends on membrane area, fiber diameter, hematocrit, plasma protein concentration, pressure gradient, and blood flow rate

3) Replacement fluid is administered with CAVH only

b) CAVHD: Incorporates peritoneal dialysis fluid with ultrafiltration, thus combining the principles of diffusion and convection. Peritoneal dialysis fluid administration is regulated by a volumetric pump at 15 ml/min. The dialysis fluid enters the ultrafiltration compartment of the hemofilter and flows in the opposite direction to the blood flow.

c) CVVH: Used more often than CAVH; an adaptation of the previous method. The replacement fluid is often electrolyte or bicarbonate based. Uses a blood pump with a venovenous blood access and administration of replacement fluid. Use of a single venovenous puncture is an advantage over CAVH, which requires arterial and venous punctures. Ultrafiltration is the primary principle involved, and solute is removed by convection. No dialysate is used (Figure 5-6).

d) CVVHD: Uses a blood pump in conjunction with the dialysate flowing countercurrently to the blood for the ultrafiltration, diffusion, and osmotic dialysis effect. No replacement fluid is used.

e) CVVHDF: Similar to CVVHD; uses a blood pump and dialysate flowing countercurrently to remove and replace high volumes of fluid hourly. Solute removal is via both convection and diffusion. Replacement fluid is used.

f) Overview of the method for CRRT

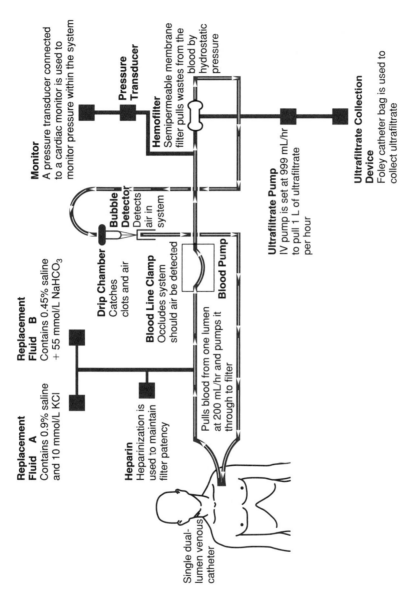

Replacement Fluid A
Contains 0.9% saline and 10 mmol/L KCl

Replacement Fluid B
Contains 0.45% saline + 55 mmol/L NaHCO$_3$

Heparin
Heparinization is used to maintain filter patency

Single dual-lumen venous catheter

Pulls blood from one lumen at 200 mL/hr and pumps it through to filter

Drip Chamber
Catches clots and air

Blood Line Clamp
Occludes system should air be detected

Blood Pump

Bubble Detector
Detects air in system

Monitor
A pressure transducer connected to a cardiac monitor is used to monitor pressure within the system

Pressure Transducer

Hemofilter
Semipermeable membrane filter pulls wastes from the blood by hydrostatic pressure

Ultrafiltrate Pump
IV pump is set at 999 mL/hr to pull 1 L of ultrafiltrate per hour

Ultrafiltrate Collection Device
Foley catheter bag is used to collect ultrafiltrate

FIGURE 5-6 ■ Continuous venovenous hemofiltration. *IV,* Intravenous. (From Clevenger K: Setting up a continuous venovenous hemofiltration educational program, *Crit Care Clin North Am,* 10(2):235-244, 1998.)

1) Prepare the patient: Explain the procedure. Obtain baseline serum analyses, clotting time, blood chemistry analyses, ABG levels, and complete blood count. Administer a loading dose of heparin.
2) Prepare the hemofilter, apply the blood pump if initiating CVVH or CVVHD, and connect to the vascular access properly
3) Attach the peritoneal dialysis fluid infusion if initiating CAVHD
4) Determine the blood flow through the hemofilter and the resulting ultrafiltration rate, and begin fluid replacement therapy
5) Monitor fluid replacement according to the patient's condition and desired rate of filtrate output to prevent circulatory collapse
6) Regulate BP, oncotic pressure, and ultrafiltration compartment to optimize the amount of filtrate (according to the prescribed dialyzing device)
7) Maintain accurate hourly total body I&O records
g) Potential complications include clotting, hypotension, air entry, blood leak

(f) Peritoneal dialysis (PD): Effective in the critically ill for maintaining homeostasis; however, if hemodialysis is contraindicated, CRRT is generally used (CVVH); a combination of PD (for solute removal) and hemodialysis (for ultrafiltration) also effective in ARF (Figure 5-7)

(1) Indications
a) Fluid overload
b) Electrolyte or acid-base imbalance
c) Acute or chronic renal failure
d) Intoxication from dialyzable drugs and poisons
e) Peritonitis or pericarditis
f) Unavailability of vascular access for hemodialysis

(2) Contraindications: Bleeding disorder, abdominal adhesions, recent peritoneal surgery

(3) Principles of PD: Primarily osmosis and diffusion

(4) Description: Dialysate is instilled into the peritoneal cavity through a catheter, allowed to "pool" (usually for a minimum of 30 minutes), then drained. New dialysate is infused, which initiates the next cycle.

(5) Anticoagulation: Minimal amount of heparin required

(6) Frequency: Continuous form of dialysis; dialysis sessions can last 3 to 4 days or longer depending on the needs of the patient

(7) Hemodynamics: No direct impact on hemodynamics

(8) Complications
a) Bladder or bowel perforation secondary to catheter placement
b) Peritonitis, abdominal bleeding
c) Respiratory impairment secondary to increased abdominal size

b. Potential complications
i. Pulmonary edema
(a) Mechanism
(1) Volume overload resulting from volume retention secondary to ARF or excess IV fluids administered to prevent ARF

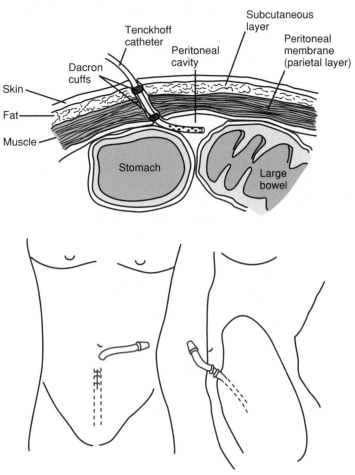

FIGURE 5-7 ■ Permanent peritoneal catheter in place, showing its position with respect to the different layers of the abdominal wall *(top)*, its anteroposterior position *(lower left)*, and the catheter angle with respect to the abdominal wall *(lower right)*. (From Levine DZ: *Care of the renal patient*, ed 3, Philadelphia, 1997, Saunders.)

          (2) Uremic cardiac effects such as left ventricular hypertrophy, uremic pericarditis

      (b) Management: See Chapters 2 and 3

  ii. Uremic pericarditis with effusion

      (a) Mechanism: Uremic toxins on myocardium result in pericarditis with or without pericardial effusion

      (b) Management (see also Chapter 3)

          (1) Daily continuous dialysis to maintain BUN levels below 80 mg/dl

          (2) Consider pericardiocentesis for large effusions over 250 ml

          (3) Pericardiectomy necessary for repeated episodes or those causing cardiac tamponade

 iii. Anemia

      (a) Mechanism: Actual bleeding secondary to primary cause or uremia, septic shock, or SIRS, which is commonly associated with the onset of disseminated intravascular coagulation. Lack of erythropoietin observed at onset of ARF.

    (b) Management (see also Chapter 7)

       (1) Differentiate between anemia due to actual blood loss and that due to lack of erythropoietin

       (2) Administer packed RBCs to maintain hematocrit per physician order

  iv. Electrolyte imbalances

    (a) Mechanism: Inability of kidneys to excrete electrolytes and concentrate urine in ARF

    (b) Management: See later sections on hyperkalemia, hypocalcemia, hyperphosphatemia, and hypermagnesemia, which are the most common imbalances

  v. Metabolic acidosis

    (a) Mechanism: Inability of the kidney to secrete hydrogen ions in urine

    (b) Management (see also Chapter 2)

       (1) Administration of 1 to 3 ampules of sodium bicarbonate mixed in 5% dextrose in water or one half normal saline for a slow drip infusion for acute acidosis; IV push bicarbonate may lead to intracellular acidosis or hypervolemia

       (2) Dialysis to correct or minimize acidosis

  vi. Sleep-pattern disturbance

    (a) Mechanism: During ARF, sleep is interrupted by the intensity of care, critical care environment, sleep apnea, and uremic condition (e.g., tremors, restless leg syndrome). Nursing research reveals an increase in the number of recalled nightmares the night prior to dialysis at the uremic peak, which results in a disturbed sleep pattern. Disruption of sleep interferes with the healing process and quality of life.

    (b) Management

       (1) Obtain a sleep history (i.e., day or night sleeper)

       (2) Organize care to minimize patient interruptions

       (3) Limit noise in the environment

       (4) Provide three to four 90-minute sleep cycles in each 24-hour period

  vii. Altered metabolism and excretion of pharmacologic agents: See Patient Care

8. Evaluation of patient care

  a. Renal perfusion is improved to prevent prerenal failure and ATN

  b. Urine output exceeds 30 ml/hr with normal concentration and volume; balanced 24-hour I&O record coincides with daily weight

  c. Weight is stable, with no evidence of muscle wasting; nutrition is adequate

  d. Electrolyte balance and metabolic acidosis are WNL or minimized at asymptomatic levels

  e. Dialysis is tolerated and corrects or maintains asymptomatic fluid, electrolyte, and acid-base balance

  f. Infection-free skin is dry, clean, and intact with no itching; wound healing is progressing

  g. Patient is free of major anxiety, coping satisfactorily with illness, participating in care, using effective support systems, and not suffering from sleep deprivation

  h. Patient has knowledge of ARF and treatment and is compliant with disease management expectations

Chronic Renal Failure

CRF is a slowly progressive renal disorder culminating in end-stage renal disease (ESRD). The decline in kidney function correlates with the degree of nephron loss.

1. **Pathophysiology:** Systemic changes occur when overall renal function is less than 20% to 25% of normal
   a. The kidney has a unique ability to compensate and preserve homeostasis despite a significant (80%) loss of nephron function. During CRF, injury occurs to the nephrons in a progressive manner. The remaining intact nephrons compensate for loss of functioning nephrons by cellular hypertrophy, which enables these nephrons to accept larger blood volumes for clearances and results in excretion of more solute.
   b. Four stages of CRF: Each stage is associated with a certain degree of nephron loss, which can be correlated with the serum creatinine level
      i. Diminished renal reserve: 50% nephron loss
         (a) Kidney function is mildly reduced, but the excretory and regulatory functions are sufficiently maintained to preserve a normal internal environment; the patient usually is problem free
         (b) The serum creatinine value usually doubles; a normal value of 0.6 mg/dl rises to 1.2 mg/dl, which is still WNL
      ii. Renal insufficiency: 75% nephron loss
         (a) Evidence of impaired renal capacity appears in the form of mild azotemia, slightly impaired urinary concentrating ability, increasing serum phosphorus level, anemia, decreasing serum calcium and bicarbonate levels; hyperkalemia may occur
         (b) Factors that exacerbate renal disease at this stage by increasing nephron damage are infection, dehydration, drugs, cardiac failure, and instability of the primary disease
         (c) Serum creatinine level usually ranges from 4.0 to 9.9 mg/dl
      iii. ESRD: 90% of nephrons damaged; GFR is usually less than 15 ml/min
         (a) Renal function has deteriorated so that persistent abnormalities exist
         (b) Patient requires artificial support to sustain life (dialysis or transplantation)
         (c) Serum creatinine level is 10 mg/dl or higher
      iv. Uremic syndrome: Complete nephron loss
         (a) The body's systemic responses to the buildup of uremic waste products and the results of the failed organ system
         (b) Usually described as the constellation of signs and symptoms exhibited in renal failure
         (c) Symptoms may be avoided or diminished by the initiation of early dialysis treatment or renal transplantation
2. **Etiology and risk factors:** See Table 5-5
3. **Signs and symptoms of uremia:** See Table 5-3
4. **Diagnostic study findings:** See also Diagnostic Studies under Patient Assessment
   a. Laboratory
      i. Urinalysis: The following abnormalities may be the first indicators of renal disease. See later for specific findings for CRF.
         (a) Proteinuria: May exceed 3 g/24 hr in patients with glomerulonephropathies and nephrotic syndrome
         (b) Leukocyte casts and pyuria: Indicate infection in the urinary tract; suspect renal disease when pyuria occurs in conjunction with hematuria, casts, and proteinuria
         (c) Eosinophiluria: May occur in allergic interstitial nephritis
         (d) Epithelial cells: Renal tubular cells with lipid droplets in the cytoplasm suggest nephrotic syndrome; large numbers of these cells are present in glomerulonephritis and pyelonephritis

■ **TABLE 5-5**
■ ■ **Common Causes of Chronic Renal Failure**

Disorder	Underlying Cause
Tubulointerstitial disease or interstitial nephritis	Chronic pyelonephritis (most common cause)
	Analgesic-abuse nephropathy
	Immunologic mechanisms (transplant rejection, allergic response, hypersensitivity)
Glomerulonephropathies	Focal glomerulosclerosis
	Crescentic glomerulonephritis (rapid and progressing)
	Chronic glomerulonephritis
	Systemic lupus erythematosus (lupus nephritis)
	Bacterial endocarditis
Nephrotic syndrome	Glomerular disease
Renal vascular disorders	Systemic vasculitis (i.e., polyarteritis nodosa, hypersensitivity vasculitis)
	Scleroderma
	Coagulopathies such as hemolytic uremic syndrome
	Thromboembolic renal disease
	Sickle cell nephropathy
	Hypertensive nephrosclerosis: Benign, malignant, or accelerated
Renal cancer	Renal cell carcinoma, the most common renal neoplasm

    (e) Casts: Provide important diagnostic clues (see section on casts in Diagnostic Studies under Patient Assessment)

        (1) Mixed leukocyte and erythrocyte casts may be prominent in acute exudative glomerulonephritis

        (2) Fatty casts are seen in glomerular diseases in conjunction with moderate to heavy proteinuria

        (3) Waxy, broad casts are seen in the final stages of renal failure

    (f) Urine osmolality: Varies with the stage of CRF

    (g) Creatinine clearance or GFR

        (1) A decrease of 10 to 50 ml/min or a renal reserve of 25% is associated with the onset of renal insufficiency

        (2) A creatinine clearance of 10 to 15 ml/min is consistent with ESRD

  ii. Serum studies

    (a) Creatinine: An inverse relationship exists between serum creatinine level and GFR, and the stage of CRF

        (1) Diminished renal reserve: A 50% nephron loss is reflected by either a normal creatinine level of 1.4 mg/dl or a twice-normal creatinine level of 2.8 mg/dl

        (2) Renal insufficiency: A 75% nephron loss causes the serum creatinine level to quadruple

        (3) ESRD: A 90% nephron loss correlates with a serum creatinine value of 10 mg/dl or higher

        (4) Uremic syndrome: A creatinine value of 10 mg/dl or higher is maintained by some form of dialysis

    (b) BUN: In CRF, BUN levels above 100 mg/dl are usually associated with uremic symptoms; therefore, BUN level is used to determine the frequency and duration of dialysis treatments

(c) Uric acid: Increased serum levels may suggest gout or gouty nephropathy when the elevation is out of proportion to the degree of renal failure

(d) Serum triglyceride level: May be elevated

(e) Glucose tolerance test: Identifies the presence of carbohydrate intolerance

(f) Serum protein and albumin levels: Decreased values indicate malnutrition associated with a restricted-protein diet, anorexia, or chronic infection

b. Radiologic

   i. IVP

     (a) Small kidneys, or one atrophied and one normal-sized kidney, may indicate bilateral disease; unilateral disease always causes compensatory hypertrophy of the contralateral kidney

     (b) Enlarged kidneys suggest polycystic disease or obstruction

     (c) Scarring and altered calices can suggest chronic pyelonephritis or analgesic nephropathy

   ii. Ultrasonography: Identifies renal parenchymal disease and rules out obstruction; generally lacks the ability to differentiate between renal diseases

   iii. CT: May reveal renal perfusion defects, pyelonephritis, renal cystic disorders, or renal colic

   iv. MRI: Used to diagnose renovascular lesions

   v. Special: Baseline motor nerve conduction velocity studies and long bone x-ray films of the skull, hands, and feet identify the development of uremic neuropathy and bone disease

5. Goals of care

  a. Uremic symptoms are avoided or minimized

  b. Effective renal replacement therapy is provided (e.g., dialysis, renal transplantation)

6. Collaborating professionals on health care team (see also disciplines for ARF)

  a. Cardiologist consult

  b. Renal transplant surgeon

7. Management of patient care

  a. Anticipated patient trajectory: Patients with CRF, especially ESRD, face complex self-care expectations on discharge and the need for lifelong compliance with an intricate health care regimen. Throughout the course of recovery and discharge, patients with CRF may be expected to have needs in the following areas:

   i. Skin care (see Management of Patient Care under Acute Renal Failure)

   ii. Nutrition: Critical element in care; modification of diet in renal disease is implemented during the early stages of CRF for prevention and prolongation of renal health and in ESRD for moderation of uremic symptoms (National Kidney Foundation K/DOQI clinical practice guidelines for nutrition [National Kidney Foundation, 2003])

     (a) General CRF diet: Restricted-protein diet of 0.6 to 0.8 g protein/kg/day with a total caloric intake of 35 mg/kcal/kg body weight and 2 g each of sodium and potassium. High-quality biologic protein (such as eggs, fish, meat) should account for two thirds of daily total protein intake.

     (b) Dietary modifications for CRF: In the early stages of CRF, 0.6 g protein/kg/day plus 0.3 g protein/kg/day of high-quality biologic protein

     (c) Dietary modifications for ESRD: 0.8 g protein/kg/day with a caloric intake of 35 mg/kcal/kg body weight

(d) Adjustments are made to the standard CRF diet depending on the type of dialysis and appetite; in many instances, protein intake is increased
  (1) Hemodialysis or PD: Increased protein requirements. Hemodialysis patients need 1.1 to 1.2 g protein/kg/day; PD patients, 1.3 to 1.4 g protein/kg/day.
  (2) Continuous ambulatory peritoneal dialysis (CAPD): 1.1 to 1.4 g protein/kg/day
  (3) CRRT: Requirements have not been substantiated; however, increased amino acid losses necessitate higher protein supplementation, approximately 1.5 to 2.5 g protein/kg/day
  (4) Diminished appetite: Administer unlimited-protein diet to prevent malnutrition
(e) Be aware that the presence of hypoalbuminemia is associated with increased mortality in CRF
(f) Low BUN value is another predictor of mortality, because it suggests reduced protein intake, reduced muscle mass, chronic illness, and cachexia
(g) Sodium: Restrict to minimize hypertension, thirst, and weight gain
(h) Potassium: Restrict for most hemodialysis patients, but PD patients may not require restriction
(i) Lipids: Hyperlipidemia occurs in 20% to 75% of CRF and dialysis patients
  (1) Most common types
    a) Hypertriglyceridemia
    b) Elevated levels of low-density lipoproteins
    c) Normal or reduced levels of high-density lipoproteins
  (2) Increased risk of atherosclerosis
  (3) Lack of conclusive evidence on treatment. Proponents of treatment can utilize dietary guidelines (e.g., National Cholesterol Education Program and American Heart Association diet).
(j) Vitamins: Water-soluble vitamins (i.e., vitamin B complex and C) are prescribed specifically for dialysis patients

iii. Infection control: Infections are responsible for 15% of the yearly mortality (U.S. Renal Data System, 2003)
  (a) Common infections include peritonitis secondary to PD catheterization and infection at hemodialysis vascular catheter site. Septicemia related to these infections is associated with a high mortality rate.
  (b) Immunocompromise accompanies uremia (see Patient Care)

iv. Discharge planning
  (a) General patient and family teaching: Be aware that the uremia of CRF impairs cognition and memory. In addition, the complexity of the renal replacement therapies demands multiple patient and family teaching sessions. Patient compliance is essential to minimize uremic symptoms as well as to ensure patient safety.
    (1) Assess knowledge related to CRF, treatments, medications
    (2) Assess the effects of uremia on the patient's learning abilities (e.g., decreased attention span and memory, altered cognition)
    (3) Develop a teaching plan including reinforcement, self-care activities, treatment, and compliance expectations
    (4) Instruct the patient and family or significant others about all aspects of CRF
      a) Normal renal function and renal disease state
      b) Management of diet, fluids, medications, skin, rest

c) Avoidance of infection

d) Treatment alternatives and benefits and disadvantages of each; support the patient's and family's decision

(5) Instruct the patient and family about general features and elements of care for dialysis treatments

a) Dynamics of hemodialysis or PD

b) Special diet and fluid allowances

c) Care of the dialysis access

d) Need for weight control

e) Signs and symptoms of complications such as an electrolyte imbalance

f) Transportation to the dialysis center

(b) Outcomes specific to various renal replacement therapies: See Box 5-1

v. Pharmacology (see also Renal Transplantation)

(a) Average CRF patient takes 8 to 10 medications

(b) Impact of CRF on pharmacologic agents: See Patient Care

(c) Compliance necessary to receive optimal effect of pharmacologic therapy; noncompliance is associated with exaggerated uremic symptoms, exacerbation of coexisting disease (i.e., cardiac disease, diabetes, hypertension), and increased morbidity

vi. Psychosocial issues: ESRD and dialysis or transplantation require adaptation and coping; adjustment is difficult and may contribute to depression

(a) Body image disturbance: Results from the effects of uremia, dependency on treatments, and primary illness other than renal disease (see Chapter 10)

(b) Sexual dysfunction: An experience of change in sexual function viewed as unsatisfying, unrewarding, or inadequate; results from uremia, its complications, and/or its treatment (see Chapter 10)

vii. Treatments: Renal replacement therapies include hemodialysis, chronic peritoneal dialysis (CAPD), and renal transplantation. The CRRT form of dialysis is usually reserved for ARF patients but is an option for the CRF patient in the ICU (see Treatments under Acute Renal Failure).

(a) Chronic hemodialysis

(1) Patient usually has hemodialysis treatment 3 times a week (3 to 5 hours per treatment) via a permanent or temporary vascular access

(2) Temporary measure to replace renal function; thus, the patient must be compliant with diet and fluid restrictions

(3) Anticoagulation (heparin) usually required. A minimum heparin dosage can be used for patients at risk (i.e., postoperatively). In rare situations (e.g., patient has coagulopathy), heparin-free hemodialysis may be possible. For heparin-induced thrombocytopenia, use lepirudin or argatroban.

(4) Availability of chronic hemodialysis: Hospital, satellite center, or home performed by a surrogate or the patient

(b) Chronic PD: Follows the same principles and procedures as acute PD; differences relate to the patient's expectations and the use of an automated PD machine

(1) Frequency of treatment varies with the PD approach

a) Hospital based or at home: Usually dialyze 4 times per week for 10 hours

b) Nighttime home PD: Dialyze all night every night

c) CAPD: A continuous form; dialyze 24 hours a day, 7 days a week

■ **BOX 5-1**
■ **OUTCOMES OF RENAL REPLACEMENT THERAPIES**

HEMODIALYSIS
- Circulatory access is maintained.
- Patient has hemodialysis treatment, usually 3 times a week (3 to 5 hours for each treatment).
- Patient complies with rigid diet and fluid restrictions.

HOME HEMODIALYSIS
- Proper environment is available: Adequate space, plumbing, and hygiene.
- Patient demonstrates signs of compliance with the medical regimen and adaptation to the disease process.
- Patient demonstrates ability to physically tolerate dialysis procedure.
- There is evidence of established family support system or acceptance of surrogate dialyzer.
- Patient demonstrates ability to learn technical and aseptic skills.

CHRONIC PERITONEAL DIALYSIS
Follows same principles and procedures as acute peritoneal dialysis; differences relate to patient expectations and use of automated peritoneal dialysis machine.
- Patient expectations for peritoneal dialysis:
  - Maintenance of Tenckhoff catheter
  - Use of aseptic technique throughout the procedure
  - Treatment 3 to 4 times a week for 10 hours each treatment in hospital or 7 days, 4 times per day or every night with cycler
  - Adherence to dietary and fluid restrictions
- Expectations for home peritoneal dialysis:
  - Proper environment: Treatment requires space and storage area for equipment
  - Cardiovascular stability: Not as necessary for home peritoneal dialysis because rapid fluid shifts and dramatic cardiovascular effects are not associated with this treatment
  - Family support systems: Helpful but not essential because most patients use dialysis at night, and the family routine may not be disrupted
  - Cognitive ability: Moderate technological skill is required, but aseptic technique is essential

CONTINUOUS AMBULATORY PERITONEAL DIALYSIS (CAPD)
- Patient demonstrates ability to perform procedure.
- Patient recognizes that exchanges are 4 times a day, 7 days a week. Each exchange is 4 to 8 hours.
- Patient completes a rigorous training program.
- Patient demonstrates proper care of the Tenckhoff catheter.
- Patient adheres to the treatment schedule.
- Patient stores the dialysis equipment appropriately.
- Patient demonstrates measures to avoid complications such as peritonitis, back strain, visceral herniation, obesity, fluid excess.

RENAL TRANSPLANTATION
(See Treatment under Management of Patient Care in Chronic Renal Failure section)
- Patient and family demonstrate knowledge of diet and fluid regimen, signs and symptoms of rejection.
- Patient demonstrates ability to obtain and record daily weight and administer medications.
- Patient reports for frequent clinic and other follow-up outpatient visits.
- Patient adheres to activity limitations and rehabilitation program.

(2) Tenckhoff catheter is permanent access placed surgically

(3) Dietary and fluid restrictions vary

(4) Anticoagulation performed using heparin (low dose)

(c) CRRTs: See Treatment under Acute Renal Failure

(d) Renal transplantation: Promotes primary disease management by minimizing complications, slowing the progression of the primary disease process, and decreasing the mortality rate (Figure 5-8)

  (1) Grafts: Survival rates have improved

    a) Living donor transplants have a longer survival rate than cadaveric transplants

    b) One-year rates are 95% for living grafts and 89% for cadaveric grafts (United Network for Organ Sharing [UNOS])

  (2) Donors: Wait time for cadaveric donation is about 24 months (UNOS). Living donors must have ABO blood type compatibility, maximal compatibility in human leukocyte antigen (HLA) type, acceptable serologic cross-match, and optimal health. Intraperitoneal laparoscopic surgery, a minimally invasive procedure, is a common option for living donors.

  (3) Recipient selection criteria: Begins with the presence of irreversible ESRD; few contraindications exist

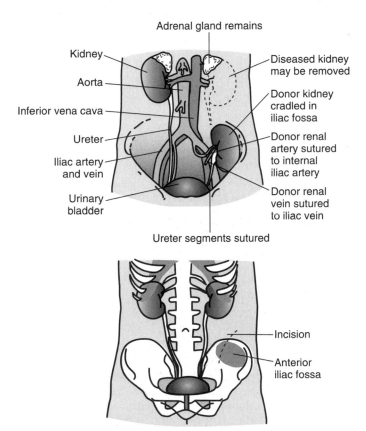

FIGURE 5-8 ■ Kidney transplantation. (From Luckmann J, editor: *Saunders manual of nursing care*, Philadelphia, 1997, Saunders.)

        a) Age no longer a definitive barrier; most programs use 70 years as the upper limit but consider physiologic and individual differences in the decision-making process

        b) No preexisting antibodies (to donor kidney) and/or ABO blood type incompatibility

        c) No preexisting infection

        d) No medical or surgical contraindications

        e) Functioning bladder or urinary tract

        f) No psychosis, severe personality disorder, or history of noncompliance with medical regimen

        g) "Last resort" alternative: Patient may be accepted based on the inability to participate in other treatment alternatives; this may be due to lack of vascular access or physical intolerance of the procedure

(4) Tissue type compatibility

        a) ABO blood typing: To determine blood type compatibility between donor and recipient

        b) HLA typing: Serologic testing for specification of the HLA-A, HLA-B, and HLA-C locus antigen plus lymphocyte-defined typing of the D locus (includes DP, DQ, and DR antigens)

        c) Mixed lymphocyte culture: Reveals degree of difference between the D loci of donor and recipient

        d) Cross-match for preformed antibody (microlymphocytotoxicity cross-match): Presence of preformed antibodies significantly decreases the viability of any graft

(5) Immunocompetent cells: Two kinds of lymphocytes involved in the rejection processes

        a) B lymphocytes: Involved in humoral immunity and are precursors to antibody-producing cells; responsible for hyperacute rejection and partially involved in acute and chronic rejection

        b) T lymphocytes: Implicated in cell-mediated immunity, which is involved in acute and chronic rejection; three types—effectors, helpers, and suppressors

(6) Types of rejection

        a) Hyperacute: Irreversible process; occurs within minutes or hours of surgery

        b) Accelerated: Occurs from the second to fifth day in the immediately postoperative period; physiologic characteristics are similar to those of hyperacute rejection; rarely reversible, involving both humoral and cellular immunity

        c) Acute: Often reversible with high doses of antirejection medication

           1) Occurs most frequently 2 weeks after transplantation but can be seen from the first week postoperatively up to 1 year and beyond

           2) T cells or cellular immunity is the primary mechanism

           3) Antigen leaves the graft and enters the serum, where it is recognized and incorporated into macrophage RNA. With reexposure to antigen, the macrophage releases RNA-antigen complexes into the serum, where plasma lymphocytes man-

ufacture specific antibody. The plasma lymphocytes then travel to the kidney for the immunologic attack.

   d) Chronic: Cannot be reversed; a gradual decline that ultimately leads to organ failure

      1) Usually occurs 1 to 5 years after transplantation

      2) Involves B-cell or humoral response to antibody

      3) A slow, chronic immunologic response, with gradual deterioration of renal tissue; involves primarily the glomerular basement membrane and endothelial layer of the blood vessels

(7) Instruct the patient and family about transplantation as a treatment alternative, including the following:

   a) Survival rates; patient selection criteria; treatment expectations (e.g., antirejection medications); need for frequent clinic visits the first year; and dietary limitations

   b) Benefits: Replacement of renal function, alleviation of most pathophysiologic effects of uremia, and return to many normal life activities

   c) Complications, including rejection; immunosuppressive effects (increased susceptibility to infections, risk of malignancies, esophagitis, peptic ulcer, acute pancreatitis); and surgical complications

(8) Provide preoperative teaching

   a) Need to report to the hospital on request

   b) Expected preoperative workup

   c) Surgical procedure

      1) The kidney is transplanted into the iliac fossa

      2) Revascularization is usually accomplished by anastomosing the renal artery to the hypogastric artery and the renal vein to the external iliac vein (see Figure 5-8)

      3) The ureter is anastomosed to the recipient's ureter at the pelvis of the kidney (ureteropelvic anastomosis), or the donor's ureter can be implanted into the host's bladder (ureteroneocystostomy)

   d) Immediate postoperative recovery period care

(9) Provide postoperative teaching

   a) How to obtain and record daily I&O, temperature, BP, and weight

   b) Antirejection medication and side effects

   c) Need to report signs and symptoms of rejection

      1) Fever

      2) Pain, tenderness, redness, and swelling at the site of the graft

      3) Weight gain

      4) Decreased urine output

      5) Hypertension

   d) Activity limitations in the first 3 months: Avoidance of lifting or strenuous exercise, avoidance of crowds

   e) Need to report signs and symptoms of infection

   f) Knowledge of diet

   g) Schedule of clinic visits

(10) Administer maintenance transplant immunosuppressive therapy as ordered. A single standard of practice for immunosuppressive

therapy has not been agreed upon; various combinations of the following medications may be given:

a) Corticosteroids: Suppress the production of cytotoxic T cells and prevent the production of interleukin-2 (IL-2), which initiates the immunologic response; no agreement on the optimal dosage; begin with a high dosage and taper over the initial few weeks

b) Azathioprine (Imuran): Begin dosing at 2 to 3 mg/kg/day and decrease gradually to 1 mg/kg/day to prevent or deter acute rejection episodes

c) Cyclosporine: To inhibit activated T-cell proliferation and IL-2 production; maintenance dosage 3 to 5 mg/kg/day to be continued for the life of the graft

d) Tacrolimus (similar to cyclosporine): A macrolide antibiotic with immunosuppressive effect; inhibits T-cell receptor signals and IL-2; appears to improve long-term graft survival rate; administer 0.15 mg/day in divided doses

e) Mycophenolate mofetil (MMF): An antimetabolite agent that assists as an intervention for acute rejection; a 50% reduction in acute rejection seen in first year with its use

f) Sirolimus: A macrolide antibiotic; blocks T-cell activation at a phase beyond tacrolimus

g) Cyclophosphamide (Cytoxan): Used when azathioprine is contraindicated to diminish the production of antibodies and initiate the destruction of circulating lymphocytes

(11) Administer antirejection therapy for treatment of acute or accelerated rejection

a) Corticosteroids: IV 500 to 1000 mg/day for a maximum of 5 days, followed by oral corticosteroids

b) Antilymphocyte globulin: To deplete circulating T cells and suppress cell-mediated immunity allograft responses; toxicity includes agranulocytosis and hemolytic response and predisposition to infection

c) OKT3: A murine monoclonal antibody administered over 14 days to suppress or inactivate one or two antigen-recognition sites on T cells (T2 or T3); side effects include respiratory distress, fever, and severe immunosuppression

viii. Ethical issues

(a) Living organ donation: A disparity continues to exist between the number of patients waiting for transplantation and the number of available organs

(b) Donor mortality rate is about 0.03%; rate of serious donor morbidity is 0.23%

b. Potential complications: See Table 5-6

8. Evaluation of patient care

a. No uremic symptoms are present (see Table 5-3)

b. Effective dialysis treatment or successful renal transplantation is accomplished

c. Patient is able to complete the activities of daily living and participate in rehabilitation activities

d. Patient verbalizes achievement and acceptance of a satisfactory level of sexual functioning

e. Patient demonstrates the ability to cope with CRF, renal replacement therapy, and pharmacologic therapy

f. Family members or significant others actively support and participate in the patient's care

■ **TABLE 5-6**
■ ■ **Potential Complications of Chronic Renal Failure**

Potential Complication	Mechanism/Description	Management
Hypervolemia	See Overhydration under Patient Care	See Overhydration under Patient Care
Electrolyte imbalance	Accompanies the inability to concentrate urine; there is risk of imbalance of any electrolyte during ESRD, but the most common imbalances are hyperkalemia, hypocalcemia, and hyperphosphatemia (see sections on specific imbalances)	See section on specific electrolyte imbalance
Metabolic acidosis	See Patient Care	Keep in mind that the dialysis controls metabolic acidosis • Acetate or lactate found in a hemodialysis and peritoneal dialysis bath is to be absorbed into the body and enters the Krebs cycle, where it is converted to bicarbonate; conversion requires the presence of oxygen at the tissue level • Bicarbonate bath: Available with some adjusted hemodialysis machines that dialyze with a bath containing bicarbonate (35 to 36 mEq/L), which obviates the need for the metabolic conversion expected with acetate or lactate
Anemia (see also Patient Care)	Production of erythropoietin is decreased	Assess dosage of epoetin alfa (DNA recombinant–engineered erythropoietin; Epogen, Procrit) on a routine basis, maintaining prescribed HCT value (33% to 36%); dose at approximately 80 to 120 units/kg/wk in 1-3 doses/wk Epoetin alfa is an effective replacement agent for erythropoietin • Takes 3 mo to produce a near-normal HCT associated with a mild to moderate improvement in exercise tolerance and work capacity, increased aerobic performance, and improved oxygen transport • Cardiac output and ejection fraction also improve • Side effects: Increased blood viscosity and HCT may lead to problems such as shortened life of the fistula, hypertension, increased clotting tendencies, limited reuse of dialyzers; these effects are minimized when HCT is maintained in the lower normal range; seizures and hypertension also are potential effects • Darbepoeitin alfa (Aranesp) is a longer-acting erythropoietin substitute than can be used every 2 wk; as effective as epoetin alfa

Continued

■ **TABLE 5-6**
■ ■ **Potential Complications of Chronic Renal Failure—cont'd**

Potential Complication	Mechanism/Description	Management
Uremic syndrome		
Cardiac involvement (major cause of death in ESRD)	Volume-pressure overload results in LV hypertrophy and heart failure CAD—primary CAD is present in about half of hemodialysis patients and is exacerbated in ESRD, especially with dialysis Uremic pericarditis—caused by the accumulation of uremic toxins; may progress to pericardial effusion and, if untreated, cardiac tamponade Symptomatic hyperkalemia—leads to delayed cardiac conduction that may result in asystole Hypertension (essential or nonessential)—underlying cause of ESRD or occurs as a result of ESRD due to hypervolemia, vascular disease	General: See Chapter 3 for heart failure, LV hypertrophy, CAD, hypertension Uremic pericarditis: See Potential Complications under Acute Renal Failure
Pulmonary involvement	Uremic toxins may cause uremic pneumonitis and pleural effusion; in severe cases, fluid overload may mimic clinical picture of ARDS Depressed immunity results in increased susceptibility to infection; increased risk of pneumonia	Initiate frequent dialysis Provide antibiotics as necessary Administer oxygen, provide pulmonary care Monitor progress with ABG analysis and chest radiography

Neurologic involvement (as uremic encephalopathy)	Neurologic presentations include
	• Restless leg syndrome
	• Peripheral neuropathy
	  —"Burning" sensation of the feet progressing to paresthesia and intense pain on the dorsal and ventral surfaces of the feet
	  —Foot drop and diminished muscle strength
	  —Impaired gait and possibly paralysis
	  —Slowing of nerve conduction velocity and a segmental demyelination of the nerves
	• Intellectual and memory impairment
	• Acute postdialysis dementia (i.e., dialysis disequilibrium)
		Intensify dialysis treatments; increase time and/or frequency
		Treat seizures with anticonvulsants
		Administer vitamin replacement therapy, because a deficit may further compromise neurologic function
		Eliminate aluminum hydroxide gels, which are associated with aluminum accumulation and toxicity and are believed to be responsible for dialysis dementia
		Correct electrolyte imbalances (hypocalcemia)
		Orient the patient as necessary

	• Dialysis dementia (rare)—associated with chronic dialysis and long-term exposure to aluminum-containing substances • Seizures • Uremic encephalopathy	
Endocrine and metabolic involvement	Accumulation of uric acid leads to hyperuricemia manifested as gout with joint pain and inflammation, low-grade fever, hypertension Secondary hyperparathyroidism: Combination of hypercalcemia and demineralization of bone with metastatic calcifications Hyperlipidemia: An increase in LDL levels and triglycerides is common in CRF Carbohydrate intolerance: Manifested as moderate levels of hyperglycemia and elevated insulin levels	Initiate dietary therapy for elevated LDL levels; monitor serum lipid profile (total cholesterol, triglycerides, LDL, HDL) Lipid-lowering agents often necessary to lower total LDL to <100 mg/dl High LDL levels may accelerate progression to ESRD Institute dialysis to minimize uremia and improve glucose tolerance Administer allopurinol for gout and monitor uric acid level Administer low-dose corticosteroids to decrease serum lipid levels
Gastrointestinal involvement	Uremic toxins affect gastrointestinal tract, producing • Uremic bowel: Diarrhea or constipation, malabsorption syndrome, weight loss, and fatigue • Peptic ulcer disease: Gastric pain and possibly bleeding	Minimize or alleviate uremia via dialysis Administer a protein-restricted diet Administer zinc to improve taste Use non-magnesium-containing antacids or H_2 blockers (ranitidine) or proton pump inhibitors (omeprazole) for gastrointestinal irritation
Coagulopathy	Platelet adhesiveness is diminished, which is sometimes associated with mild thrombocytopenia Bleeding tendency may be increased, leading to bruising and purpura	Initiate dialysis to minimize the uremic effect on platelet function Give iron and folic acid supplements Testosterone, other androgens may reverse anemia (rarely used)
Musculoskeletal involvement	Hypocalcemia and, if present, secondary hyperparathyroidism may lead to reciprocal hyperphosphatemia Bone pain, impaired growth, and pathologic fractures may occur	Monitor serum calcium level, administer calcium tablets Administer activated vitamin D (1,25-dihydroxychocalciferol) with phosphate-binding therapy
Sexual dysfunction	Amenorrhea, abnormal menstruation, infertility, increased prolactin may occur Diminished testosterone, decreased libido, impotence may be seen	Administer estrogen replacement therapy Assess for zinc deficiency, which may be responsible for male impotence Review current medications (i.e., β-blockers) for contribution to sexual dysfunction Renal transplantation may restore sexual function and fertility Assess for depression and need for an antidepressant

ABG, Arterial blood gas; *ARDS*, acute respiratory distress syndrome; *CAD*, coronary artery disease; *CRF*, chronic renal failure; *ESRD*, end-stage renal disease; *HCT*, hematocrit; *HDL*, high-density lipoprotein; *LDL*, low-density lipoprotein; *LV*, left ventricular.

Electrolyte Imbalances—Potassium Imbalance: Hyperkalemia

The serum potassium level in hyperkalemia is above 5.5 mEq/L

1. **Pathophysiology**
   a. Inability of the kidney tubules to excrete K^+ because of tubular damage, salt depletion, or increased potassium load from injured tissues; or may be induced by drugs such as potassium-sparing diuretics (e.g., spironolactone), which inhibit aldosterone, or amiloride and triamterene, which block the sodium channel and thereby inhibit Na^+ reabsorption and promote K^+ retention
   b. Reduction in K^+ excretion caused by decreased renal perfusion because less Na^+ is available for exchange with K^+ (e.g., in cardiac failure)
   c. Alteration in K^+ release (rhabdomyolysis) or distribution (insulin deficiency)

2. **Etiology and risk factors**
   a. Acute and chronic renal failure or renal disease associated with distal tubule dysfunction (i.e., sickle cell anemia)
   b. Increased cellular destruction with potassium release such as occurs in burns, trauma, crash injuries, severe catabolism, acute acidosis, intravascular hemolysis, rhabdomyolysis, and thrombocytosis
   c. Excessive administration or ingestion of potassium chloride
   d. Adrenal cortical insufficiency: Hypoaldosteronism or Addison's disease
   e. Aldosterone deficiency
   f. Low cardiac output or sodium depletion
   g. Metabolic acidosis: Precipitates the movement of intracellular K^+ to the extracellular space
   h. Certain drugs
      i. Potassium-sparing diuretics, which block Na^+ reabsorption, thereby facilitating K^+ retention
      ii. The antibiotics pentamidine and trimethoprim, which also promote K^+ retention via the same mechanism
      iii. Drugs that inhibit aldosterone production (e.g., ACE inhibitors, NSAIDs, heparin, cyclosporine, tacrolimus) and angiotensin II antagonists (e.g., losartan)
      iv. Drugs that inhibit extrarenal K^+ disposal (nonselective β-blockers, propranolol, nadolol, timolol)
   i. Release of K^+ from injured cells: Seen in cocaine ingestion, rhabdomyolysis, and chemotherapy-induced tumor lysis syndrome

3. **Signs and symptoms:** Detection of electrolyte imbalances is difficult. Suspect imbalances with renal or endocrine disease, with excessive loss of body fluids (e.g., vomiting, diarrhea), in some drug intoxications (e.g., indiscriminate use of electrolyte replacement, hormonal therapy, or vitamins), and with acute changes in mental status (confusion, agitation, coma) (Table 5-7).

4. **Diagnostic study findings**
   a. Laboratory: Serum potassium level exceeds 5.5 mEq/L
   b. Electrocardiogram (ECG): Progressive changes reveal peaked and elevated T waves→widened QRS→prolonged PR interval→flattened or absent P wave and ST segment depression→idioventricular rhythm→asystolic cardiac arrest

5. **Goals of care**
   a. Symptomatic hyperkalemia is eliminated
   b. Cardiac function is restored to WNL for the patient

6. **Collaborating professionals on health care team**
   a. Critical care nurse
   b. Physician or intensivist
   c. Nurse practitioner, clinical nurse specialist, or physician assistant

■ **TABLE 5-7**
■ ■ **Signs and Symptoms of Potassium Imbalance**

System	Hyperkalemia	Hypokalemia
Cardiovascular	Bradycardia Dysrhythmias Hypotension	Diminished, irregular pulses Increased myocardial excitability or irritability Dysrhythmias: Premature atrial contractions, premature ventricular contractions, sinus bradycardia, paroxysmal atrial tachycardia, atrioventricular blocks, atrioventricular or ventricular tachycardia Enhanced digoxin effect to the point of digoxin toxicity
Neurologic	Lethargy Apathy Confusion	Drowsiness to coma, malaise, and confusion Muscle cramping (commonly in calf muscle) Muscular weakness progressing to paralysis
Pulmonary	Deep rapid respiration (Kussmaul's respirations) when hyperkalemia accompanied by acidosis Shallow respirations if muscle paralysis present	Shallow respirations secondary to muscle weakness
Gastrointestinal	Abdominal cramping and diarrhea	Vomiting Paralytic ileus
Musculoskeletal	Irritability to flaccid paralysis and numbness of extremities Fatigue associated with diminished exercise tolerance Diminished mobility to paralysis	Pain in calf similar to that of deep venous thrombosis
Genitourinary	Oliguria	Polyuria

    d. Case manager

    e. Dietitian

    f. Nephrology consult (if cause is associated with renal failure or to advise on treatments)

    g. Cardiologist (for cardiac emergencies)

    h. Endocrinology consult

7. Management of patient care

    a. Anticipated patient trajectory: Patients with acute symptomatic hyperkalemia face a life-threatening condition requiring urgent intervention and resolution. Recovery requires compliance with a treatment plan to prevent repeat episodes. Patients may be expected to have needs in the following areas:

        i. Positioning: Position to promote comfort; hyperkalemia can cause fatigue, muscle irritability, numbness, and flaccid paralysis

        ii. Nutrition: After K$^+$ stabilized to a safe, asymptomatic level, restrict dietary potassium (e.g., orange juice, cola, banana)

        iii. Discharge planning: Include discharge teaching to promote dietary compliance to avoid hyperkalemia

        iv. Pharmacology

      (a) Provide cardiac monitoring before and during pharmacologic therapy; monitor potassium levels frequently

      (b) In emergency situations (e.g., if serum K^+ >6.5 mEq/L or ECG change indicates symptomatic hyperkalemia)

        (1) Administer regular insulin and dextrose IV with β-agonist inhalant to temporarily shift K^+ into cells

          a) Insulin can rapidly lower serum potassium level

          b) Dextrose must accompany insulin; patients who lack endogenous insulin production can experience a paradoxical increase in potassium or hypoglycemia

        (2) Administer a β-agonist (albuterol in a concentrated form) by inhalation; observe drug action in 30 minutes; effect is complementary to the potassium lowering created by insulin

        (3) Use sodium bicarbonate IV when severe metabolic acidosis complicates the hyperkalemia

        (4) Consider IV calcium chloride or calcium gluconate (IV push) to stabilize the cardiac membrane; contraindicated in patients taking digoxin; if no improvement in ECG, can repeat calcium bolus in 3 to 5 minutes

        (5) Essential to follow aforementioned temporary measures with a therapeutic measure to permanently remove potassium from the body (e.g., sodium polystyrene sulfonate [Kayexalate], hemodialysis)

        (6) Kayexalate with sorbitol administered orally or per rectum for the exchange of Na^+ into the intestinal cell and K^+ into the bowel space; when administered in combination with sorbitol, enhances a diarrhea stool for actual K^+ loss

          a) With Kayexalate, Na^+ ion is exchanged 1:1 for a K^+ ion in the bowel cell wall; therefore, assess the amount of sodium retained as well as the potassium loss

          b) Ensure that the Kayexalate and sorbitol mixture is expelled, especially postoperatively, because retained Kayexalate can cause bowel obstruction and perforation

          c) Rectal route of administration is rapid and produces a predictable outcome

    v. Treatment: Hemodialysis is a rapid form of dialysis for serum potassium reduction (see Acute Renal Failure and Chronic Renal Failure)

  b. Potential complications

    i. Cardiac arrhythmia: Bradycardia to asystole

      (a) Mechanism: Hyperkalemia depresses myocardial contractility and conductivity

      (b) Management: Treat hyperkalemia; if warranted, institute cardiopulmonary resuscitation for asystolic cardiac arrest

8. Evaluation of patient care

  a. Serum potassium level is between 3.5 and 5.5 mEq/L or in an asymptomatic range

  b. No cardiac complications of hyperkalemia are present

Electrolyte Imbalances—Potassium Imbalance: Hypokalemia

The serum potassium level in hypokalemia is below 3.5 mEq/L

1. Pathophysiology

  a. Potassium loss exceeding intake

  b. Alkalosis: Stimulates the secretion of K^+ in the distal tubule

  c. Intracellular shifting of K^+

2. **Etiology and risk factors**
   a. Alkalosis: Causes K^+ to shift into the cell
   b. Abnormal GI losses: Nasogastric suction and drainage, laxative abuse, diarrhea, prolonged episode of vomiting
   c. Starvation or malnutrition (including hyperalimentation without adequate potassium replacement)
   d. Diuretic therapy (loop diuretics, thiazides, acetazolamide), renal tubular acidosis
   e. Increased adrenal corticosteroid secretion or corticosteroid therapy
   f. Liver disease
   g. Bartter's syndrome: Hypokalemia, hyponatremia, hypomagnesemia, metabolic alkalosis, and hyperreninemia
   h. Severe stress (K^+ shifts into cells)
3. **Signs and symptoms:** See Table 5-7
4. **Diagnostic study findings**
   a. Laboratory: Serum potassium levels below 3.5 mEq/L
   b. ECG: Depressed ST segments, flat or inverted T wave, presence of U wave, and ventricular dysrhythmias
5. **Goals of care**
   a. Serum potassium level is above 3.5 mEq/L and WNL or within asymptomatic range
   b. Cardiac function is WNL
6. **Collaborating professionals on health care team:** See Electrolyte Imbalances—Potassium Imbalance: Hyperkalemia
7. **Management of patient care**
   a. Anticipated patient trajectory: Patients with acute hypokalemia faces serious cardiac symptomatology that requires immediate resolution in the clinical setting. Recovery and discharge require compliance with a treatment regimen that prevents repeated episodes. Patients may be expected to have needs in the following areas:
      i. Positioning: Place in a position of comfort to minimize muscle cramping and weakness as well as to promote adequate respirations
      ii. Nutrition: Provide foods containing potassium (e.g., orange juice, raisins, milk, green vegetables, etc.)
      iii. Discharge planning: Include discharge teaching to promote sufficient potassium intake and compliance with the dietary regimen
      iv. Pharmacology: Provide cardiac monitoring prior to and during pharmacologic therapy
         (a) Administer oral potassium supplements when indicated; dilute to prevent GI irritation and to facilitate absorption
         (b) Observe for ECG changes and the presence of dysrhythmias
         (c) Monitor serum potassium levels
         (d) Record the amount of urine output and other drainage (gastric aspirate, diarrhea) to aid in calculating total body potassium balance
         (e) Recognize and treat signs of alkalosis
         (f) Administer oral potassium supplements when indicated; dilute to prevent GI irritation and to facilitate absorption
         (g) Never give IV potassium chloride rapidly; large concentrations can precipitate hyperkalemia, producing necrosis of the vessel wall, and possibly inducing ventricular fibrillation. *Never administer an IV push.*
         (h) Determine whether the patient is receiving digitalis or diuretics; correct potassium losses, because these can precipitate digitalis toxicity and decrease the effectiveness of most diuretics

(i) Emergency treatment
(1) Slowly administer IV potassium chloride while the patient is monitored with ECG for dysrhythmias
(2) Monitor for signs and symptoms of hyperkalemia
(3) Maintain a record of serum potassium levels to assess the adequacy of replacement therapy
(j) Follow-up: If the patient is receiving digitalis and diuretics, consider the use of potassium chloride supplements or potassium-sparing diuretics

b. Potential complications
   i. Digoxin toxicity
      (a) Mechanism: Hypokalemia enhances the effect of digoxin
      (b) Management: IV potassium on medication pump with cardiac monitoring
   ii. Dysrhythmias
      (a) Mechanism: Hypokalemia decreases the cardiac threshold, increasing the risk of dysrhythmia
      (b) Management: IV potassium on medication pump with cardiac monitoring

8. **Evaluation of patient care**
   a. Serum potassium levels are above 3.5 mEq/L or within asymptomatic range
   b. No cardiac complications of hypokalemia are present

Electrolyte Imbalances—Sodium Imbalance: Hypernatremia

The serum sodium level in hypernatremia is above 145 mEq/L

1. **Pathophysiology**
   a. Increased ECF volume: Sodium and water retention
   b. Decreased ECF volume: Sodium retention without water retention; greater water loss compared to sodium loss (e.g., diuresis of water without excretion of equal amounts of sodium)

2. **Etiology and risk factors**
   a. Normal kidneys: Lack of ADH or neurohypophyseal insufficiency (e.g., diabetes insipidus, water loss in excess of sodium loss)
      i. Potassium depletion: Creates a concentrating defect in the kidney, causing polyuria
      ii. Hypercalcemia: Polyuria and dehydration
      iii. Drugs (e.g., osmotic diuretics or sodium bicarbonate, or NaCl solution); also mineralocorticoids, laxatives, and antacids
      iv. Excessive adrenocortical secretion
      v. Loss of the thirst mechanism (e.g., in a comatose patient)
      vi. Uncontrolled diabetes mellitus with osmotic diuresis due to hyperglycemia
      vii. Head injury
      viii. Post central nervous system surgery: Causes fluctuation (increase and decrease) in ADH release
   b. Impaired renal function: Inability of renal tubules to respond to ADH (e.g., nephrogenic diabetes insipidus)

3. **Signs and symptoms:** Findings relate to "edematous states" and/or hypoproteinemia (Table 5-8)

4. **Diagnostic study findings**
   a. Serum Na^+ level above 145 mEq/L, elevated hematocrit with volume depletion
   b. Serum osmolality greater than 295 mOsm/L
   c. Urine SG may be greater than 1.030, except in diabetes insipidus, in which SG can be as low as 1.005

■ **TABLE 5-8**
■ ■ **Signs and Symptoms of Sodium Imbalance**

System	Hypernatremia	Hyponatremia
General	Excessive weight gain Dehydration—extreme thirst, fever, decreased urine output, dry mucous membranes	Weight loss or gain Malaise Headache Decreased hematocrit and blood urea nitrogen level (dilutional effect)
Cardiovascular	Weak, thready pulse with increased extracellular fluid (ECF) Tachycardia with decreased ECF often progressing to bradycardia Hypertension with increased ECF Hypotension with or without postural changes with decreased ECF	Rapid pulse with overhydration Hypotension or hypertension Decreased central venous pressure and jugular venous pressure with overhydration
Neurologic	Restlessness Irritability Lethargy Confusion to coma Twitching to seizures Muscle tension	Confusion to coma Muscle weakness
Pulmonary	Labored breathing (dyspnea) associated with pulmonary edema	Dyspnea with crackles Pulmonary edema
Gastrointestinal	Anorexia Edematous tongue	Abdominal cramps Nausea
Musculoskeletal	Muscle weakness	
Integumentary	Dry, flushed skin Dry mucous membranes Pitting edema	Poor skin turgor
Genitourinary	Oliguria or anuria with dehydration Polyuria with osmotic diuresis	Thirst Normal urine output to polyuria Urine sodium level <20 mEq/L

    d. Urine osmolality 800 to 1400 mOsm/L; lower with diabetes insipidus

    e. Urine Na^+ level higher than 40 mEq/L when hypernatremia is due to sodium excess and normal to low value during a water deficit

5. Goals of care

    a. Serum and urine Na^+ levels are in a normal range or in a high, asymptomatic range

    b. Normal fluid status is maintained

6. Collaborating professionals on health care team: See Electrolyte Imbalances—Potassium Imbalance: Hyperkalemia

7. Management of patient care

    a. Anticipated patient trajectory: Patients with hypernatremia are experiencing a hyperosmolar state usually secondary to a serious previously existing condition. Both conditions need to be treated and resolved prior to discharge. Recovery and discharge require compliance with a treatment regimen that prevents repeat episodes. Patients may be expected to have needs in the following areas:

      i. Positioning: Initiate fall prevention protocol if patient exhibits neurologic signs and symptoms

     ii. Skin care

        (a) Dehydration: Hydrate patient and lubricate skin

        (b) Overhydration: Protect bony prominences; change position often

    iii. Nutrition: Dietary and fluid restrictions with restricted sodium; I&O

    iv. Pharmacology: Medication adjustments

        (a) Avoid laxatives and antacids (e.g., sodium bicarbonate) containing high-sodium ingredients

        (b) Utilize diuretics: Promote a greater loss of water than Na^+

        (c) Administer corticosteroids to stimulate reabsorption of Na^+ and excretion of K^+

      v. Treatments

        (a) Monitor serum sodium levels, serum osmolality, urine osmolality, I&O, and body weight

        (b) Perform neurologic assessments and correlate with serum Na^+ levels

        (c) Administer water in excess of sodium if the patient requires volume expansion (5% dextrose in water or 0.45 normal saline or both)

        (d) Avoid rapid correction of sodium level, because this may precipitate acute pulmonary edema or cerebral edema; reduce sodium level gradually by encouraging Na^+ losses via diuretics or administration of fluids

        (e) Determine precipitating factors and treat as ordered

        (f) For patients in renal failure, treat via dialysis

  b. Potential complications

      i. Dyspnea, labored respirations related to pulmonary edema

     ii. Seizures

        (a) Mechanism: Disruption of sodium pump dynamics in cerebral tissues, which leads to electrical instability

        (b) Management: Seizure precautions and correction of hypernatremia

8. Evaluation of patient care

  a. Sodium level is WNL and patient is asymptomatic

  b. Serum osmolality is 280 to 295 mOsm/L

  c. Urine osmolality is within the normal range

  d. Hydration status is normal

Electrolyte Imbalances—Sodium Imbalance: Hyponatremia

The serum sodium level in hyponatremia is below 136 mEq/L

1. Pathophysiology

  a. Excess of water relative to the amount of sodium in the body, producing a dilutional effect on the sodium concentration

  b. Na^+ loss exceeds water loss

2. Etiology and risk factors

  a. Water excess: Excessive water intake without sodium intake; SIADH

  b. Sodium depletion

      i. Abnormal losses via diaphoresis, diuretics, nasogastric suction, diarrhea

     ii. Hyperglycemia (glucose-induced diuresis)

    iii. Salt-losing renal diseases: Interstitial nephritis

    iv. Bartter's syndrome (hyponatremia, hypokalemia, hypomagnesemia, metabolic alkalosis, and hyperreninemia)

  c. Heart failure and cirrhosis of the liver: Decreased cardiac output increases water retention by the kidneys

3. **Signs and symptoms:** Permanent neurologic changes with a serum sodium level below 110 mEq/L (see Table 5-8)
4. **Diagnostic study findings**
   a. Serum Na^+ level below 136 mEq/L and low hematocrit caused by water excess
   b. Urine volume and SG can be normal
   c. Urine Na^+ level less than 20 mEq/L (if due to Na^+ deficit) and normal to elevated (if due to water excess)
   d. Serum osmolality below 280 mOsm/L
5. **Goals of care**
   a. Serum sodium level is WNL or at an asymptomatic level
   b. Normal fluid status is maintained
6. **Collaborating professionals on health care team:** See Electrolyte Imbalances—Potassium Imbalance: Hyperkalemia
7. **Management of patient care**
   a. Anticipated patient trajectory: Patients with hyponatremia experience a hypo-osmolar condition. Recovery requires compliance with a treatment plan that prevents repeat episodes. Patients may be expected to have needs in the following areas:
      i. Skin care: See Electrolyte Imbalances—Sodium Imbalance: Hypernatremia
      ii. Nutrition and fluid balance
         (a) For sodium and water losses: Provide high-sodium diet and adequate fluid intake
         (b) For water intoxication: Restrict fluid intake (limit of 500 ml/day)
         (c) For water intoxication related to SIADH: Restrict water intake, because decreased sodium is due to the inability to excrete water normally
      iii. Pharmacology
         (a) Discontinue medications that cause loss of Na^+ (e.g., diuretics, laxatives)
         (b) Administer NaCl tablets orally as indicated
         (c) Administer diuretics to treat water intoxication
      iv. Treatments
         (a) Monitor neurological signs
         (b) For Na^+ and water losses:
            (1) Replace fluids with normal (0.9%) or hypertonic (3%) saline
            (2) Administer hypertonic saline via an infusion pump; measure serum sodium levels frequently; observe for pulmonary edema; monitor I&O
            (3) Monitor effectiveness of nutrition and other therapies by measuring serum and urine sodium levels and osmolality concentrations
         (c) For water intoxication:
            (1) Restrict fluid intake
            (2) Monitor serum sodium levels to determine whether sodium replacement is indicated
            (3) Do not give normal saline in SIADH; normal saline does not correct the basic cause of SIADH
   b. Potential complications: See Electrolyte Imbalances—Sodium Imbalance: Hypernatremia
8. **Evaluation of patient care**
   a. Sodium levels are WNL or patient is asymptomatic (see Electrolyte Imbalances—Sodium Imbalance: Hypernatremia)
   b. Urinary sodium level is above 30 to 40 mEq/L
   c. Normal hydration status is maintained

Electrolyte Imbalances—Calcium Imbalance: Hypercalcemia

The serum calcium level in hypercalcemia is above 10.5 mg/dl

1. **Pathophysiology**
   a. Increased mobilization of calcium from bone
   b. Increased intestinal reabsorption of calcium ion (Ca^{2+}): May occur with large dietary intake or excessive vitamin D supplementation, or in granulomatous disease (e.g., sarcoidosis)
   c. Altered renal tubular reabsorption of Ca^{2+}
2. **Etiology and risk factors**
   a. Primary hyperparathyroidism: Causes increased tubular reabsorption of Ca^{2+} and Ca^{2+} release from bone
   b. Metastatic carcinoma with "osteolytic lesions" that release calcium into plasma and multiple myeloma
   c. Prolonged bed rest: Causes calcium to be mobilized from the bones, teeth, and intestines
   d. Alkalosis: Increases calcium binding to protein; decreases serum calcium levels
   e. Thyrotoxicosis
   f. Excessive intake of vitamin D: Increases Ca^{2+} reabsorption from intestines
   g. Drugs: Thiazide diuretic therapy inhibits Ca^{2+} excretion
   h. Renal tubular acidosis
3. **Signs and symptoms:** See Table 5-9
4. **Diagnostic study findings**
   a. Laboratory
      i. Serum calcium level: Above 10.5 mg/dl
      ii. Other serum studies: Thyroid-stimulating hormone, PTH, PTH-related peptide, vitamin D levels
      iii. Sulkowitch's urine test for calcium
   b. Radiologic
      i. Nephrocalcinosis: Calcium deposits in renal parenchyma, renal calculi
      ii. Calcium deposits visible on bone films
   c. ECG: Shortening of the ST segment
5. **Goals of care**
   a. Calcium stays WNL or in an asymptomatic range
   b. Cardiac and neurologic function is normal
6. **Collaborating professionals on health care team:** See Electrolyte Imbalances—Potassium Imbalance: Hyperkalemia
7. **Management of patient care**
   a. Anticipated patient trajectory: Clinical course, recovery, and discharge planning for patients with hypercalcemia vary depending on whether the condition is acute or chronic. Patients may be expected to have needs in the following areas:
      i. Nutrition: Restrict dietary calcium (e.g., milk, cheese, yogurt)
      ii. Discharge planning: Teach the patient how to comply with the dietary regimen to avoid hypercalcemia
      iii. Pharmacology
         (a) Administer digitalis cautiously; hypercalcemia enhances the action of digitalis and toxicity can result
         (b) Administer NaCl infusion and diuretics to reduce Ca^{2+} absorption
         (c) Be aware that corticosteroids reduce GI absorption of Ca^{2+}

■ **TABLE 5-9**
■ ■ **Signs and Symptoms of Calcium Imbalance**

System	Hypercalcemia	Hypocalcemia
Cardiovascular	Hypertension (33% of all cases)	Dysrhythmias Irregular pulse
Neurologic	Lethargy Increased fatigue Confusion to coma Subtle personality changes	Lethargy Generalized tonic-clonic seizures
Pulmonary		Labored and shallow breathing Wheezing Bronchospasm when respiratory muscles involved
Gastrointestinal	Anorexia Nausea and vomiting Abdominal pain and constipation	Paralytic ileus with absent bowel sounds Constipation with or without distended abdomen or diarrhea
Renal	Acute or chronic renal failure Renal vascular constriction Polyuria Renal calcium deposits Flank and thigh pain associated with renal calculi	Oliguria or anuria
Musculoskeletal	Hypotonicity and weakness of muscles Pathologic fractures Metastatic calcifications Bone pain	Muscle cramps Muscle tremors Functional and physical limitations on ambulation and exercise Bone pain and fractures

  (d) Institute mithramycin therapy to stimulate bone uptake of calcium
  (e) Consider the administration of bisphosphonates (e.g., pamidronate), calcitonin, or corticosteroids for the treatment of moderate to severe hypercalcemia associated with malignancy to reduce the rate of bone turnover
 iv. Treatments
  (a) Monitor I&O status and renal function parameters
  (b) If the patient is in renal failure, utilize dialysis
  (c) Administer bisphosphonates
 b. Potential complications
  i. Cardiac arrest
   (a) Mechanism: Enhanced digoxin effect, dysrhythmias (particularly atrio-ventricular blocks) may progress to cardiac arrest
   (b) Management: Cardiopulmonary resuscitation
8. Evaluation of patient care
 a. Calcium level is WNL or patient is asymptomatic
 b. Cardiac and neuromuscular function is normal

Electrolyte Imbalances—Calcium Imbalance: Hypocalcemia

The serum calcium level in hypocalcemia is below 8.5 mg/dl

1. **Pathophysiology**
   a. Excessive GI losses of calcium secondary to diarrhea, diuretic use, and increased levels of lipoproteins
   b. Malabsorption syndromes, such as vitamin D deficiency and hypoparathyroidism
2. **Etiology and risk factors**
   a. Hypoparathyroidism or hypomagnesemia (Mg^{2+} needed for effective action of PTH)
   b. CRF
      i. Hyperphosphatemia due to CRF: Potentiates the peripheral deposition of calcium
      ii. Vitamin D deficiency due to CRF, hepatic failure, rickets: Lack of activated vitamin D (1,25-dihydroxycholecalciferol or 25 hydroxycholecalciferol) necessary for Ca^{2+} absorption
   c. Vitamin D resistance: Inability to absorb Ca^{2+} from the intestine; vitamin D mediated
   d. Chronic malabsorption syndrome resulting from magnesium depletion, gastrectomy, high-fat diet (fat impairs Ca^{2+} absorption), small bowel disorder that prevents absorption of vitamin D
   e. Increased thyrocalcitonin: Stimulates osteoblasts to prevent Ca^{2+} entry into serum
   f. Malignancy
      i. Osteoblastic metastasis: Calcium is consumed for abnormal bone synthesis
      ii. Medullary carcinoma of the thyroid: Secretion of thyrocalcitonin is abnormal
   g. Acute pancreatitis: Calcium precipitates in an inflamed pancreas
   h. Hyperphosphatemia: Calcium and phosphate bind together and precipitate in tissues
      i. Cytotoxic drugs (cytolysis of bone)
      ii. Increased oral intake of phosphates
      iii. CRF (decreased excretion of phosphate)
3. **Signs and symptoms:** See Table 5-9
4. **Diagnostic study findings**
   a. Serum calcium level below 8.5 mg/dl
   b. ECG: Prolonged ST segment and QT interval
   c. Trousseau's sign
      i. Apply a BP cuff to the upper arm and inflate
      ii. If carpopedal spasm occurs, the test result is positive
      iii. If no spasm appears in 3 minutes, the test result is negative
      iv. Remove the cuff and tell the patient to hyperventilate (30 times per minute)
      v. Respiratory alkalosis that develops can also produce a carpopedal spasm (a positive result if it occurs)
   d. Chvostek's sign: Tap on the supramandibular portion of the parotid gland; observe for twitches in the upper lip on the side tapped; muscle spasm indicates a positive test result
5. **Goals of care**
   a. Serum calcium level is WNL, and the patient is asymptomatic
   b. There is no evidence of complications from hypocalcemia
6. **Collaborating professionals on health care team:** See Electrolyte Imbalances—Potassium Imbalance: Hyperkalemia

7. Management of patient care
   a. Anticipated patient trajectory: Patients with hypocalcemia face a life-threatening condition requiring urgent pharmacologic intervention. Recovery and discharge focus on preventing repeat episodes. Patients can be expected to have needs in the following areas:
   i. Nutrition
      (a) Assess for a history of starvation, dietary abuse, or malabsorption
      (b) Administer a diet high in calcium
   ii. Discharge planning
      (a) Provide discharge teaching to promote dietary intake of calcium
      (b) Instruct on the warning signs of tetany or seizures
   iii. Pharmacology
      (a) Administer 10% calcium gluconate or calcium chloride slowly IV (1 ml/min) for emergency intervention; monitor for decreased cardiac output, enhanced digitalis effects, and dysrhythmias
      (b) Chronic hypocalcemia necessitates daily oral doses of calcium, usually administered in the range of 1.5 to 3 g/day
      (c) Administer correct vitamin D supplement (1,25-dihydroxycholecalciferol or 25-hydroxycholecalciferol) as ordered
      (d) With phosphate deficiency, replace phosphates before administering calcium; hyperphosphatemia usually accompanies hypocalcemia
   iv. Treatments
      (a) Monitor serum calcium and phosphate levels
      (b) Institute cardiac monitoring; monitor therapeutic effectiveness via Chvostek's and Trousseau's signs plus ECG
      (c) Implement seizure precautions; provide a quiet environment
      (d) Monitor respiratory function; bronchospasm may precipitate respiratory arrest
      (e) In renal failure, utilize dialysis and activated vitamin D
   b. Potential complications
   i. Tetany, seizures
      (a) Seizure precautions
      (b) Calcium bolus at bedside
      (c) Treat cause of hypocalcemia; replace calcium
8. Evaluation of patient care
   a. Patient is asymptomatic, and calcium level is WNL
   b. There is no neuromuscular or cardiac involvement related to hypocalcemia or its treatment

Electrolyte Imbalances—Phosphate Imbalance: Hyperphosphatemia

The serum phosphate level in hyperphosphatemia is above 4.5 mg/dl
1. Pathophysiology
   a. Inability to excrete phosphate (HPO_4^-) via the kidney because of a decrease in GFR to one tenth of normal or because of renal failure
   b. Excessive intake due to diet, or cathartic abuse or drugs (cytotoxic agents)
2. Etiology and risk factors
   a. Acute or chronic renal failure (inability to excrete HPO_4^-)
   b. Hypoparathyroidism: PTH causes hypophosphatemia and lowers body phosphate levels
   c. Cathartic abuse or use of phosphate-containing laxatives or enemas
   d. Use of cytotoxic agents for neoplasms: Serum phosphate level increases as a result of cytolysis
   e. Overadministration of IV or oral phosphates

3. **Signs and symptoms:** Vague symptomatology similar to that of hypocalcemia (Table 5-10)
4. **Diagnostic study findings**
   a. Laboratory: Serum phosphate level higher than 4.5 mg/dl
   b. ECG: Changes comparable with those seen in hypocalcemia
5. **Goals of care**
   a. Phosphate level stays WNL or within a safe asymptomatic range
   b. There are no episodes of tetany or seizures
6. **Collaborating professionals on health care team:** See Electrolyte Imbalances—Potassium Imbalance: Hyperkalemia
7. **Management of patient care**
   a. Anticipated patient trajectory: Patients with hyperphosphatemia differ in clinical course depending on whether it is an acute or chronic problem. Recovery and discharge focus on preventing repeat episodes. Patients may be expected to have needs in the following areas:
      i. Nutrition: If hypocalcemia accompanies hyperphosphatemia, administer a diet high in calcium and low in phosphorus
      ii. Discharge planning
         (a) Provide discharge teaching to promote dietary compliance to avoid hyperphosphatemia (e.g., compliance with use of HPO_4^- binders)
         (b) Instruct on the warning signs of seizures
      iii. Pharmacology
         (a) Administer phosphate binders, which act on the intestines to limit phosphate absorption, thereby reducing the serum phosphate level (e.g., calcium carbonate)
         (b) Administer acetazolamide to increase urinary phosphate excretion via the normal kidney
         (c) Monitor serum phosphate and calcium levels to determine the effectiveness of therapy
      iv. Treatment: Institute dialysis for rapid correction of hyperphosphatemia
   b. Potential complications: See Electrolyte Imbalances—Calcium Imbalance: Hypocalcemia
8. **Evaluation of patient care**
   a. Serum phosphate level is WNL
   b. No neuromuscular symptomatology related to phosphate level is present

---

■ **TABLE 5-10**
■ ■ **Signs and Symptoms of Phosphate Imbalance**

System	Hyperphosphatemia	Hypophosphatemia
General	Vague, like those of hypocalcemia	Vague
Other	Seizures Muscle cramping Joint pain Pruritus	Fatigue Confusion and malaise Lack of appetite, changes in weight Muscle weakness and wasting with or without impaired ambulation Dyspnea Tachycardia Hypotension Decreased urine output

Electrolyte Imbalances—Phosphate Imbalance: Hypophosphatemia

The serum phosphate level in hypophosphatemia is below 3.0 mg/L

1. **Pathophysiology**
   a. Increased cell uptake to form sugar phosphates: Occurs during hyperventilation or glucose administration
   b. Decreased phosphate absorption from the bowel
   c. Renal phosphate wasting (loss of proximal tubular function): Seen in Fanconi's syndrome and vitamin D–resistant rickets
2. **Etiology and risk factors**
   a. Inadequate phosphate intake (seen in chronic alcoholism)
   b. Chronic phosphate depletion: Occurs in osteomalacia and rickets
   c. Long-term hyperalimentation without adequate phosphate replacement; glucose phosphorylation uses phosphate and can lead to phosphate depletion if no replacement is available
   d. Hyperparathyroidism: Causes renal phosphaturia
   e. Malabsorption syndrome
   f. Abuse or overadministration of phosphate-binding gels
   g. Fanconi's syndrome: Loss of phosphates in urine leading to osteomalacia (adults)
3. **Signs and symptoms:** Vague presentation (Table 5-10)
4. **Diagnostic study findings**
   a. Laboratory
      i. Serum phosphate level below 3.0 mg/dl, low serum alkaline pyrophosphate level, and high serum pyrophosphate level
      ii. Hypercalcemia and hypophosphatemia: Indicators of acute phosphate depletion in hyperparathyroidism; PTH increases the serum calcium level by promoting the release of Ca^{2+} from bone and decreases serum phosphate level by promoting excretion of HPO_4^- into urine
   b. Radiologic: Skeletal abnormalities resembling osteomalacia (i.e., pseudofractures characterized by thickened periosteum and new bone formation over what appears to be an incomplete fracture)
5. **Goals of care**
   a. Serum phosphate level is in an asymptomatic range
   b. No neuromuscular signs of hypophosphatemia are present
6. **Collaborating professionals on health care team:** See Electrolyte Imbalances—Potassium Imbalance: Hyperkalemia
7. **Management of patient care**
   a. Anticipated patient trajectory: Patients with hypophosphatemia differ in their clinical course depending on whether the condition is acute or chronic. The treatment regimen aims to prevent repeat episodes. Patients may have needs in the following areas:
      i. Nutrition: If hypercalcemia accompanies hypophosphatemia, use a calcium-restricted diet
      ii. Discharge planning
         (a) Provide teaching to promote the proper use of phosphate binders
         (b) Instruct on the warning signs of seizures; numbness and tingling around the month can occur immediately prior to a seizure
      iii. Treatments
         (a) Treat the primary cause of hypophosphatemia
         (b) Monitor phosphate and calcium levels
         (c) Administer oral phosphate (potassium phosphate) or IV phosphorus
         (d) Dialysis is an option in renal failure for acute episodes and/or for maintenance once the imbalance is corrected

    b. Potential complications: See Electrolyte Imbalances—Calcium Imbalance: Hypocalcemia

8. Evaluation of patient care
    a. Phosphate level is within an asymptomatic range
    b. No neuromuscular involvement is present

Electrolyte Imbalances—Magnesium Imbalance: Hypermagnesemia

The serum magnesium level in hypermagnesemia is above 2.5 mEq/L
1. Pathophysiology
    a. Mg^{2+} regulates nerve and muscle tone by preventing their activation by Ca^{2+}. Elevated level of Mg^{2+} can lead to excessive relaxation of nerves and muscles, including the myocardium and respiratory muscles.
    b. Magnesium is required for more than 300 enzymes to work, including those involved in protein, fat, and carbohydrate metabolism. Elevated Mg^{2+} levels can disrupt numerous metabolic interactions.
2. Etiology and risk factors
    a. Renal failure: Decreases excretion of Mg^{2+}
    b. Adrenal insufficiency
    c. Excessive intake or administration of Mg^{2+}-containing antacid gels or laxatives
    d. Acidotic states (e.g., diabetic ketoacidosis)
3. Signs and symptoms: Vague presentation (Table 5-11)
4. Diagnostic study findings
    a. Laboratory: Serum magnesium level over 2.5 mEq/L
    b. ECG: Peaked T wave similar to that seen in hyperkalemia
5. Goals of care
    a. Serum magnesium level is WNL
    b. There is no neuromuscular or cardiac involvement
6. Collaborating professionals on health care team: See Electrolyte Imbalances—Potassium Imbalance: Hyperkalemia
7. Management of patient care
    a. Anticipated patient trajectory: Patients with acute hypermagnesemia have a clinical course complicated by dramatic shifts in neurologic status. Emergent

---

■ **TABLE 5-11**
■ ■ **Signs and Symptoms of Magnesium Imbalance**

System	Hypermagnesemia	Hypomagnesemia
General	Lethargy to coma	Dizziness
	Fatigue	Lethargy
	Muscle weakness with or without loss of deep tendon reflexes	Confusion to psychosis
		Muscle weakness or tremors to tetany
	Bradycardia	Seizures
	Decreased respiration to apnea	Irregular pulse
	Hypotension secondary to depressed myocardial contractility, may lead to cardiac arrest	Dysrhythmias
		Enhanced digitalis effect
		Normal to decreased blood pressure
		Positive Chvostek's sign
		Positive Trousseau's sign

therapies are followed by preventive measures prior to discharge. Patients may have needs in the following areas:

    i. Nutrition: Eliminate or avoid magnesium-containing nutritional supplements (e.g., total parenteral nutrition, tube feeding, or oral protein drinks)

    ii. Discharge planning: Teach dietary and pharmacologic restrictions

    iii. Pharmacology

        (a) Teach the patient to avoid medications containing magnesium (e.g., laxatives, antacids)

        (b) If renal function is normal, administer diuretics or induce diuresis with saline to encourage magnesium loss

        (c) Consider calcium gluconate administration to minimize symptoms of increased magnesium

    iv. Treatments

        (a) Determine the primary cause of hypermagnesemia and intervene

        (b) Consider dialysis if excesses are due to renal failure

        (c) Monitor ECG and neurologic signs

        (d) Monitor serum magnesium levels

  b. Potential complications: See Electrolyte Imbalances—Potassium Imbalance: Hyperkalemia

8. Evaluation of patient care

  a. Magnesium levels are WNL or patient is asymptomatic

  b. There is no evidence of neuromuscular or cardiac complications

Electrolyte Imbalances—Magnesium Imbalance: Hypomagnesemia

The serum level in hypomagnesemia is below 1.5 mEq/L

1. Pathophysiology

  a. Decreased intake, diminished intestinal reabsorption, or excess losses of magnesium in urine, wounds, or extracellular drainage

  b. Diminishes ability to relax muscular and neural tone

  c. Disrupts numerous physiologic and metabolic enzyme reactions

2. Etiology and risk factors

  a. Starvation, malabsorption syndrome, hypocalcemia, prolonged hyperalimentation without adequate Mg^{2+} replacement; excessive fistula or GI losses of Mg^{2+} (e.g., severe diarrhea, nasogastric suction) without sufficient replacement

  b. Bartter's syndrome

  c. Excessive diuretic therapy or excessive corticosteroid administration

  d. Chronic alcoholism

  e. Alkalotic states (in some instances)

  f. Hypocalcemia, hypoparathyroidism, hyperaldosteronism, hyperthyroidism

  g. Drugs: Cisplatin, cyclosporine, amphotericin, gentamycin

  h. Acute or chronic pancreatitis

3. Signs and symptoms: Vague presentation (Table 5-11)

4. Diagnostic study findings

  a. Laboratory: Serum magnesium levels below 1.5 mEq/L

  b. ECG: Flat or inverted T waves, possible ST segment depression, and prolonged QT interval

5. Goals of care

  a. Serum magnesium level returns to normal

  b. There are no significant cardiac or neuromuscular symptoms

6. Collaborating professionals on health care team: See Electrolyte Imbalances—Potassium Imbalance: Hyperkalemia

7. Management of patient care
  a. Anticipated patient trajectory: Patients with acute hypomagnesemia can experience serious neuromuscular symptoms. Emergent therapies are followed by a preventive regimen. Patients may be expected to have needs in the following areas:
    i. Nutrition
      (a) Provide magnesium-containing supplements (e.g., seafood, green vegetables, whole grains, nuts)
      (b) Observe for coexisting electrolyte imbalances (e.g., hypocalcemia)
    ii. Discharge planning
      (a) Teach dietary measures to increase magnesium intake
      (b) Teach diuretic regimen
    iii. Pharmacology
      (a) Administer magnesium sulfate 50% intramuscularly or IV; in acute MI, IV infusion rates vary, and the dose of magnesium may range from 33 to 91.6 mmol
      (b) Calcium gluconate may be given when replacing with large boluses of magnesium, because calcium retards the effects of a sudden reversal to hypermagnesemia
      (c) If hypokalemia occurs simultaneously with hypomagnesemia, correct the magnesium deficit first
      (d) Be aware that hypomagnesemia enhances digitalis toxicity
    iv. Treatments
      (a) Establish seizure precautions
      (b) Correct alkalosis if present
      (c) Monitor ECG changes
      (d) Monitor serum magnesium levels
  b. Potential complications: See Electrolyte Imbalances—Potassium Imbalance: Hypokalemia
8. Evaluation of patient care
  a. Level of magnesium is in an asymptomatic range
  b. There are no significant cardiac or neuromuscular symptoms

Renal Trauma

Renal trauma occurs most often in men aged 20 to 40 years
1. Pathophysiology: Renal trauma may result from the combination of an applied force and the hydrostatic pressure generated within this liquid-containing organ, the kidney. Injury occurs more frequently to the kidneys than to any other structure in the genitourinary tract. Renal tissue trauma may be associated with the types of injury described in the following items.
  a. Disruption of the renal system caused by
    i. Nonpenetrating injuries (blunt trauma): 80% to 90% of all renal injuries
    ii. Penetrating injuries: 10% to 20% of all renal injuries
  b. Classifications of renal injury according to severity
    i. Contusions: Constitute about 85% of all renal injuries (e.g., subcapsular hematomas, minor cortical lacerations); renal collecting system not involved
    ii. Lacerations: Deep renal parenchyma injury (10% of renal injuries), usually associated with bleeding in the renal capsule; damage can also involve the renal collecting system
    iii. Fractures: Extensive lacerations at various sites in the renal parenchyma, with collecting system damage and extravasation of urine

iv. Vascular or pedicle injuries: Renal arterial intima tears or vessel disruptions; renal arterial tears cause blood collections between the intima and the intact media, usually leading to thrombosis, sometimes of the entire vessel's length

v. High-velocity trauma: May result in fistula, hemorrhage, infection, necrosis

2. **Etiology and risk factors**
   a. Nonpenetrating renal injuries
      i. Vehicular crash (e.g., impact with dashboard, steering wheel)
      ii. Impact to the abdomen or flank associated with an assault or a sports injury
      iii. Accidents involving sudden deceleration or acceleration (e.g., pedestrian-vehicular accident, fall from significant height) typically precipitate vascular injuries
   b. Penetrating renal injuries: Associated with a high incidence of intraperitoneal visceral injury, hemorrhage, fistulas, and infections
      i. Gunshot wounds (responsible for 95% of penetrating urethral injuries), stab wounds
      ii. Vehicular crashes, industrial accidents, impalements, and the like

3. **Signs and symptoms:** See Box 5-2

4. **Diagnostic study findings**
   a. Laboratory
      i. Serum
         (a) BUN elevation indicates a catabolic process or a hypovolemic state. Elevation of both BUN and creatinine indicates significant renal injury.
         (b) Hematocrit and hemoglobin: A decrease indicates hemorrhage; origin must be determined
         (c) Electrolytes: Variety of results may occur. Potassium level is usually elevated due to leakage from cellular injury, acidosis, or catabolism. Other electrolyte values may be decreased if electrolyte loss occurs through a wound or fistula.

■ BOX 5-2
■ SIGNS AND SYMPTOMS OF RENAL TRAUMA

- Pain or tenderness in
  - Flank
  - Upper quadrant of abdomen
  - Ribs and/or pelvis (must rule out pelvic fracture)
  - Costovertebral angle
- Asymmetry of abdomen and/or flanks
- Flank mass; retroperitoneal bleeding
- Hematoma over the posterior aspect of the eleventh or twelfth rib or flank area
- Hematuria (gross or microscopic)—a common sign in renal injury; degree of hematuria does not correlate with extent of injury
- Ecchymosis if site of entrance wound is lateral abdomen or flank area
- Blood clots obstructing urinary collection system
- Bleeding or ecchymosis on external genitalia, perineum, and urethral meatus
- Crepitation or contusion in flank

    ii. Urine

      (a) Volume: May be diminished if significant renal damage, obstruction, or hypovolemia present

      (b) Urinalysis: Erythrocytes and protein may be present, but renal trauma can still exist without this response

      (c) Hematuria: Gross or microscopic; negative findings allow the exclusion of a penetrating genitourinary injury with 90% confidence

  b. Radiologic

    i. Plain film of the abdomen

      (a) Rib fractures over the kidney

      (b) Obliteration of a renal or psoas shadow

      (c) Displacement of the bowel

    ii. High-dose infusion pyelography: To establish the status of both the uninvolved and the involved kidney. Results suggestive of renal injury are the following:

      (a) Delayed excretion of dye

      (b) Renal outline enlargement

      (c) Diminished concentration of contrast medium level in renal parenchyma; outlines the collecting system and ureters

      (d) If the patient is in shock, a radiologic examination should include only the first two studies

    iii. Tomography: Particularly helpful when a nonpenetrating injury is suspected; establishes the location and extent of renal parenchymal damage with an 80% to 95% accuracy. To perform this examination, a systolic BP above 90 mm Hg must be maintained.

    iv. Ultrasonography: Has minimal value for nonpenetrating injury; can determine renal parenchymal injury and locate a hematoma

    v. Renal scan: Used to evaluate RBF and possible parenchymal injury

    vi. Retrograde pyelography: Provides minimal information and can contaminate the trauma victim

    vii. Renal angiography: A more precise diagnostic tool when injury not clearly defined by other radiologic studies (e.g., continuous bleeding impairs visualization or causes extravasation of contrast medium)

    viii. CT: Provides a precise means for determining the extent of an injury

  c. Surgical exploration: Usually indicated for all hematomas; allows the immediate repair of major lacerations

5. Goals of care

  a. Hemostasis is reestablished by the replacement of fluid and blood volume

  b. Vital signs are stable, and ABG levels are acceptable

  c. Renal function is reestablished and maintained

6. Collaborating professionals on health care team: See Electrolyte Imbalances—Potassium Imbalance: Hyperkalemia

7. Management of patient care

  a. Anticipated patient trajectory: Clinical course of renal trauma patients is affected by the nature and extent of concurrent injury to one or more organ systems, complications, comorbidities, rehabilitative potential, and degree of support from patients' families or significant others. Patients with renal trauma may be expected to have needs in the following areas:

    i. Skin care: Wound management

      (a) Control bleeding

      (b) Determine fluid volume loss

      (c) Provide wound care as warranted; apply sterile dressings

(d) Observe for signs of infection—redness, swelling, pus, complaints of pain, numbness or coolness; with evidence of infection, consider topical or IV antibiotic

ii. Pain management
   (a) Assess and document objective and subjective complaints of pain
   (b) Collaborate with the physician and pain management team to establish pharmacologic and nonpharmacologic approaches for pain relief
   (c) Evaluate the effectiveness of pain control, including patient expression of relief

iii. Nutrition
   (a) Identify the route for nutritional supplements and fluid replacement (e.g., oral, nasogastric, feeding tube, IV)
   (b) Provide adequate calories, protein, vitamins, minerals, and nutrients to promote wound healing and protein sparing, and prevent rhabdomyolysis

iv. Infection control
   (a) Consider the need for tetanus toxoid
   (b) Obtain a urine sample for culture and sensitivity testing upon emergency department admission
   (c) Administer antibiotics as ordered
   (d) Use an aseptic and sterile technique as appropriate (e.g., in wound care)

v. Transport: High-risk situations requiring consideration for early transfer include the following:
   (a) Open pelvic injury with or without renal injury
   (b) Pelvic ring injury: Unstable fracture
   (c) Pelvic fracture associated with shock, and uncontrolled hemorrhage

vi. Discharge planning
   (a) Rehabilitation (e.g., at a facility or with support at home)
   (b) Family or significant other support system
   (c) Wound care: Nature and frequency
   (d) Pain management

vii. Psychosocial issues
   (a) Traumatic stress syndrome; provide posttraumatic stress support, if warranted
   (b) Implement measures to reduce anxiety, stress, and fear in the patient and family

viii. Treatment: Surgical intervention may be necessary for a shattered kidney (nephrectomy), vascular injuries with a falling hematocrit, deep renal lacerations (controversial), pulsatile or expanding hematomas, or urinary extravasation

b. Potential complications
   i. Hemorrhage
      (a) Mechanism: Intraabdominal and bladder injuries are associated with a high risk of major blood loss due to the sites of major vascular channels
      (b) Management: See Chapters 3 and 9
   ii. Extravasation of urine
      (a) Mechanism: Puncture, tear, or laceration to the kidney, ureter, bladder, and/or urethra
      (b) Management
         (1) Early recognition
         (2) Urinary catheterization

a) Increased resistance during catheter insertion warrants radiologic examination; catheters should never be forced because obstruction suggests trauma or hematoma
b) Extravasated urine contributes to infection (i.e., peritonitis); temperature must be monitored closely
c) Adequate hydration should be provided to sustain urine output
d) Patency of the catheter should be maintained; constant irrigation may be prescribed

    (3) Surgical intervention (when indicated)
    (4) Effective pain management

iii. Systemic complications
  (a) Other early complications
    (1) Ileus
    (2) Sepsis, shock
    (3) Impairment or loss of renal function
    (4) Perinephric or renal abscess, fistula formation
  (b) Late complications may include
    (1) Hypertension
    (2) Hydronephrosis
    (3) Chronic pyelonephritis
    (4) Calculus formation
    (5) Intrarenal calcification
  (c) Management
    (1) Stabilize a patient who is in shock during the initial period (see Chapters 3 and 9)
    (2) Stabilize a patient with minor renal injury
     a) Maintain bed rest, administer analgesics as needed
     b) Monitor hematocrit and hemoglobin levels
     c) Monitor for hematuria; have the patient ambulate once the urine is clear of gross hematuria
     d) Measure vital signs and report any sudden changes
     e) Administer broad-spectrum antibiotics as prescribed
     f) Be aware that renal tissue heals from a minor injury within 4 to 6 weeks
    (3) Stabilize a patient with major renal injury
     a) Administer fluids based on precise I&O records; provide adequate nutrition
     b) Monitor vital signs; hypertension may be a sign of constricting parenchymal fibrosis
     c) Obtain urine for culture and sensitivity testing, check for hematuria
     d) Obtain hematocrit, hemoglobin, electrolyte, BUN, and creatinine values
     e) Provide preventive pulmonary maintenance therapies
     f) Administer broad-spectrum antibiotics as prescribed; the renal parenchyma is susceptible to infection due to hematuria, ischemia, and urinary extravasation
     g) Maintain the patency of the Penrose drain (usually placed in the renal fossa to extrude liquefying hematoma)
     h) Provide analgesics
     i) Have the patient ambulate on the first postoperative day

8. **Evaluation of patient care**
   a. Patient is hemodynamically stable with normal circulating blood volume and renal function
   b. Complications such as hemorrhage, urine extravasation, infection, rhabdomyolysis, ileus, and hypertension are absent
   c. Nutrition is adequate to promote protein sparing
   d. There is evidence of the healing of injuries and the renal and urinary tract is intact and functional
   e. Laboratory findings confirm the maintenance of a fluid, electrolyte, and acid-base balance

REFERENCES

Physiologic Anatomy

Brenner BM: *Brenner and Rector's the kidney*, ed 6, Philadelphia, 2000, Saunders.

Massry SG, Glassuck RS: *Textbook of nephrology*, Philadelphia, 2000, Lippincott Williams & Wilkins.

Nissenson AR: *Dialysis therapy*, ed 3, Philadelphia, 2000, Harley and Belfens.

Pfettscher SA: Renal anatomy and physiology. In Bucher L, Melander S, editors: *Critical care nursing*, Philadelphia, 1999, Saunders.

Schrier RW: *Diseases of the kidney and urinary tract*, ed 7, Philadelphia, 2002, Lippincott Williams & Wilkins.

Tanagho EA, McArich JW: *Smith's general urology*, New York, 2000, Lange Medical Books/McGraw-Hill.

Walsh PC, Retie AR, Vaughan ED, et al: *Campbell's urology*, ed 7, Philadelphia, 2002, Saunders.

Patient Assessment

Krau SD: Selecting and managing fluid therapy: colloids versus crystalloids, *Crit Care Nurs Clin North Am* 10(4):401, 1998.

Luckey AE, Parsa CJ: Fluid and electrolysis in the aged, *Arch Surg* 138(10):1055-1060, 2003.

Proceedings of the 34th course on advances in nephrology and dialysis, *J Nephrol* 16(suppl 7):S1-69, 2002.

Sherman DS, Fish DN, Tertelbaum I: Assessing renal function in cirrhotic patients: problem and pitfalls, *Am J Kidney Dis* 41:269, 2003.

Sloan RS: Renal assessment. In Bucher L, Melander S, editors: *Critical care nursing*, Philadelphia, 1999, Saunders.

Stark J: Interpretation of BUN and serum creatinine: an interactive exercise, *Crit Care Nurs Clin North Am* 10(4):491, 1998a.

Stark J: The interrelation between renal and cardiac function, *Crit Care Nurs Clin North Am* 10(4):411, 1998b.

Toto KH: Fluid balance assessment, *Crit Care Nurs Clin North Am* 10(4):383, 1998.

Acute Renal Failure

Bellomo R, Runco C: *Atlas of hemofiltration*, Philadelphia, 2002, Saunders.

Craig M: Applications in continuous venous to venous hemofiltration: interactive case studies in the adult patient, *Crit Care Nurs Clin North Am* 10(2):209, 1998.

Criddle L: Rhabdomyolysis: pathophysiology, recognition and management, *Crit Care Nurse* 23(6):14, 2003.

Debaveye YA, Vanden Berghe GH: Is there still a place for dopamine in the modern ICU? *Anesth Analg* 98(2):461-468, 2004.

Dirkes SM: Continuous renal replacement therapy: dialytic therapy for acute renal failure in intensive care, *Nephrol Nurs J* 27(6):501-512, 2000.

Harbarth S, Pestotnik S, Lloyd J, et al: The epidemiology of nephrotoxicity associated with conventional amphotericin B therapy, *Am J Med* 111:528, 2001.

Kay J, Chow WH, Chan TM, et al: Acetylcysterine for prevention of acute deterioration of renal function following elective coronary angioplasty and intervention: a randomized controlled trial, *JAMA* 289:553, 2003.

Kear T: Renal therapy: continuous renal replacement therapy in the critical care unit, *Adv Nurses* 4(2):20, 2004.

Kellum J, Decker J: Use of dopamine in acute renal failure: a meta-analysis, *Crit Care Med* 29(8):1526-1531, 2001.

Lameire N, Vanholder R, Van Biesen W: Loop diuretics for patients with acute renal failure: helpful or harmful? *JAMA* 288:2599, 2002.

Lassnigg A, Donner E, Grubhofer G, et al: Lack of renoprotective effects of dopamine and furosemide during cardiac surgery, *J Am Soc Nephrol* 11:97, 2000.

Liu Y, Coresh JA, Eustace JC, et al: Association between cholesterol level and mortality in dialysis patients: rule of inflammation and malnutrition, *JAMA* 291(4):451, 2004.

McAlpine L: CAVH: Principles and practical applications, *Crit Care Nurs Clin North Am* 10(2):179, 1998a.

McAlpine L: CAVHD: Transitioning from CAVH, *Crit Care Nurs Clin North Am* 10(2): 197, 1998b.

Mehta R, McDonald B, Gabbai F, et al: A randomized clinical trial of continuous versus intermittent dialysis for acute renal failure, *Kidney Int* 60:1154, 2001.

Mehta R, Pascual M, Soroko S, et al: Diuretics mortality and non-recovery of renal failure, *JAMA* 288:2547, 2002.

Molitoris BA, Finn WF: *Acute renal failure,* Philadelphia, 2001, Saunders.

Mueller C, Buerkle G, Buetner H, et al: Prevention of contrast media–associated nephropathy, *Arch Intern Med* 162:329, 2002.

O'Neill C: Sonographic evaluation of renal failure, *Am J Kidney Dis* 35:1021, 2000.

Politoski G, Mayer B, Davy T, et al: Continuous renal replacement therapy: a natural perspective AACN/NKF, *Crit Care Nurs Clin North Am* 10(2):171, 1998.

Safirstein R: The pathophysiology of acute renal failure. In Greenberg A, editor: *Primer on kidney diseases,* ed 2, National Kidney Foundation, New York, 1998, Academic Press.

Singri N, Ahya SN, Levin ML: Acute renal failure, *JAMA* 289(6):747, 2003.

Stark J: Acute renal failure: focus on advances in acute tubular necrosis, *Crit Care Nurs Clin North Am* 10(2):159, 1998.

Stark J, Melander S: Acute renal failure. In Bucher L, Melander S, editors: *Critical care nursing,* Philadelphia, 1999, Saunders.

Tepel M, Vander Giet M, Schwartzfeld C, et al: Prevention of radiographic-contrast–induced reduction in renal function by acetylcysteine, *N Engl J Med* 343:180, 2000.

Thompson EJ, King SL: Acetylcysteine and fenoldopam: promising new approaches for preventing effects of contrast nephrotoxicity, *Crit Care Nurse* 23(3):39, 2003.

Chronic Renal Failure

Baer CL: Care of the critically ill chronic renal failure patient, *Crit Care Clin North Am* 10(4): 433, 1998a.

Baer CL: Ethical decision making: models for the dialysis dependent patient, *Crit Care Clin North Am* 10(2):255, 1998b.

Chatterjee PK, Thiemermann C: Emerging drugs for renal failure, *Expert Opin Emerg Drugs* 8(3):389-435, 2003.

Cherton GM: A 43-year-old woman with chronic renal insufficiency, *JAMA* 291(10): 1252, 2004.

Coles GA, Topley N: Long term peritoneal membrane changes, *Adv Ren Replace Ther* 7:289, 2000.

Conlon PJ, Kovalik E, Schumm D, et al: Normalization of hematocrit in hemodialysis patients with cardiac disease does not increase blood pressure, *Ren Fail* 22:435-444, 2000.

Corwin HL, Gettinger A, Rodriquez RU, et al: Efficiency of recombinant human erythropoietin in the critically ill patient: a randomized double blind, placebo-controlled trial, *Crit Care Med* 27:2346-2350, 1999.

Eknoyan G, Beck GJ, Cheung AK, et al: Effect of dialysis dose and membrane flux in maintenance hemodialysis, *N Engl J Med* 347:2010-2019, 2002.

Goodman WG: Medical management of secondary hyperparathyroidism in chronic renal failure, *Nephrol Dial Transplant* 18(suppl 3):2-8, 2003.

Kanik JA, Young BS, Lew NL, et al: Cardiac arrest and sudden death in dialysis units, *Kidney Int* 60:350, 2001.

Liu Y, Caresh J, Longeneckers JC, et al: Association between cholesterol level and mortality in dialysis patients: role of inflammation and malnutrition, *JAMA* 291(4):451, 2004.

Longnecker JC, Coresh J, Powe NR, et al: Traditional cardiovascular disease risk factors in dialysis patients compared with the general population: the CHOICE Study, *J Am Soc Nephrol* 13:1918, 2002.

Lowrie EG: Acute-phase inflammatory process contributes to malnutrition, anemia and possibly other abnormalities in dialysis patients, *Am J Kidney Dis* 32:S105-S112, 1998.

Medicare Payment Advisory Commission: *Report to the Congress: blood safety in hospitals and medicare inpatient payments,* Washington, DC, December 2001, Medicare Payment Advisory Commission.

Miller PE, Tolwani A, Luscy CP, et al: Predictors of adequacy of arteriovenous fistulas in hemodialysis patients, *Kidney Int* 56:275-280, 1999.

Muramoto O: Recent developments in medical care of Jehovah's witnesses, *West J Med* 170:297-301, 1999.

National Kidney Foundation: K/DOQI clinical practice guidelines for managing dyslipidemias in chronic kidney disease, *Am J Kidney Dis* 41(4 suppl 3):522-559, 2003.

US Renal Data System: *USRDS 2003 annual report,* Bethesda, MD, 2003, National Institutes of Health, National Institute of Diabetes and Digestive and Kidney Disease.

Vanholder R: The uremic syndrome. In Greenberg A, editor: *Primer on kidney disease,* ed 2, National Kidney Foundation, New York, 1998, Academic Press.

Renal Transplantation

Cetingok M, Winsett RP, Hathaway DK: A comparative study of quality of life among the age group of kidney transplant recipients, *Prog Transplant* 14(1):33-38, 2004.

Goel M, Flechner SM, Zhoul L, et al: The influence of various maintenance immunosuppressive drugs on lymphocele formation and treatment after kidney transplantation, *J Urol* 171(5):1788-1792, 2004.

Hardinger KL, Park JM, Schnitzler MA, et al: Pharmacokinetics of tacrolimus in kidney transplant recipients: twice daily versus once daily dosing, *Am J Transplant* 4(4):621, 2004.

Johnson EM, Remucal MJ, Gillingham KJ, et al: Complications and risks of living donor nephrectomy, *Transplantation* 64:1124-1128, 1997.

Kasiske BL: The evaluation of prospective renal transplant recipients. In Greenberg A, editor: *Primer on kidney diseases,* ed 2, National Kidney Foundation, New York, 1998, Academic Press.

Lorber MI: What's new in general surgery: transplantation, *J Am Col Surg* 198(3):424-430, 2004.

Paul LC, de Fijter JH: Cyclosporine-induced renal dysfunction, *Transplant Proc* 36:224S, 2004.

Pietrzyk M, Hoffman U, Kramer BK: Chronic allograft nephropathy, *N Engl J Med* 350(12):1254, 2004.

Rodriguez DS, Jankowska-Gan G, Haynes LD, et al: Immune regulations and graft survival in kidney transplant recipients are both enhanced by human leukocyte antigen matching, *Am J Transplant* 4(4):537, 2004.

Sandrini S, Setti G, Bossini N, et al: Experience with cyclosporine, *Transplant Proc* 36(2 suppl):152S, 2004.

United Network for Organ Sharing. (UNOS): Annual report of the US Organ Procurement and Transplant Network and the Scientific Registry of Transplant Recipients, 2004, http://unos.org.

Vagmordur MC, Sevmis S, Emiroglu R, et al: Tacrolimus conversion in kidney transplant recipients: analysis of 107 patients, *Transplant Proc* 36(1):144, 2004.

Electrolyte Imbalances

Abraham S, Bhavan B, Lee L, et al: Upper gastrointestinal tract injury in patients receiving Kayexalate (sodium polystyrene sulfonate) in sorbitol: clinical, endoscopic and histopathologic findings, *Am J Surg Pathol* 25:637, 2001.

Akizawa T, Kamimura M, Mizobuchi M, et al: Management of secondary hyperparathyroidism of dialysis patients, *Nephrology* 8(suppl 2):S53, 2003.

Ariyan CE, Susa JA: Assessment and management of patients with abnormal calcium, *Crit Care Med* 32(4):S146, 2004.

Armstrong LE: Exertional hyponatremia, *J Sports Sci* 22(1):144, 2004.

Babatin DM, Lee SS: Vasopressin antagonists and dilutional hyponatremia, *Can J Gastroenterol* 18(2):117, 2004.

Chmielewski CM: Hyperkalemic emergencies: mechanisms, manifestations and management, *Crit Care Clin North Am* 10(4):449, 1998.

Dickerson RN: Hyperkalemia in the patient receiving specialized nutrition support, *JPEN J Parenter Enteral Nutr* 28(2):124, 2004.

Gould KA, Stark J: Quick resource for electrolyte imbalance, *Crit Care Clin North Am* 10(4):477, 1998.

Hajjar I, Graves JW: Hyponatremia in older women, *J Clin Hypertens* 6(1):37, 2004.

Hsieh M: Recommendations for treatment of hyponatremia at endurance events, *Sports Med* 34(4):231, 2004.

Hsu CY, Cherton GM: Elevations of serum phosphorus and potassium in mild to moderate chronic renal insufficiency, *Nephrol Dial Transplant* 17:419, 2002.

Katapodis KP, Kolious EL, Andrikos EK, et al: Magnesium homeostasis in patient undergoing continuous ambulatory peritoneal dialysis: role of dialysate magnesium concentration, *Artif Organs* 27(9):853-857, 2003.

Malinoski DJ, Slater MS, Mullins RJ: Crush injury and rhabdomyolysis, *Crit Care Clin* 20(1):171, 2004.

Miltiadons G, Mikhailidis DP, Elisaf M: Acid-base and electrolyte abnormalities observed in patient receiving cardiovascular drugs, *J Cardiovasc Pharmacol Ther* 8(4): 267, 2003.

Rivard AL, Raup RM, Berlman GJ: Sodium polystyrene sulfonate used to reduce the potassium content of a higher protein internal formula: a quantitative analysis, *JPEN J Parenter Enteral Nutr* 28(2):76, 2004.

Sirken G, Raja R, Garcus J, et al: Contrast-induced translocational hyponatremia and hyperkalemia in advanced kidney disease, *Am J Kidney Dis* 43(2):E31, 2004.

Stark J: A comprehensive analysis of the fluid and electrolytes system: an interactive system, *Crit Care Clin North Am* 10(4):471, 1998.

Uribarri J, Prabhakas S, Kahn T: Hyponatremia in peritoneal dialysis patients, *Clin Nephrol* 61(1):54, 2004.

Yeates KE, Singer M, Morton AR: Salt and water: a simple approach to hyponatremia, *CMAJ* 170(3):365, 2004.

Renal Trauma

Abraham E, Andrews P, Antonelli M, et al: Year in review in intensive care medicine: 2003. II. Brain injury, hemodynamics, gastrointestinal tract, renal failure, metabolism, trauma, and postoperative, *Intensive Care Med* 30(7):1266-1275, 2004.

Brown CV, Rhee P, Chan L, et al: Preventing renal failure in patients with rhabdomyolysis: do bicarbonate and mannitol make a difference? *J Trauma* 56(6):1191-1196, 2004.

Bschleipfer T, Kallieris D, Hallscheidt P, et al: Validity of computerized tomography in blunt renal trauma, *J Urol* 170(6):2475-2479, 2003.

Chan LN: Nutritional support in ARF, *Curr Opin Clin Nutr Metab Care* 7(2):207-212, 2004.

Channing DA: Blunt renal trauma—blessing in disguise? *J Urol* 170(1):332-333, 2003.

Goldman SM, Sandler CM: Urogenital trauma: imaging upper GU trauma, *Eur J Radiol* 50(1):84-95, 2004.

Lameire NH, DeVriese AS, Vanholder R: Prevention and non-dialytic treatment of ARF, *Curr Opin Crit Care* 9(6):481-490, 2003.

Malinoski DJ, Slater MS, Mullins RJ: Crush injury and rhabdomyolysis, *Crit Care Clin* 20(1):171-192, 2004.

Novak A: Abdominal, genitourinary and pelvic trauma. In Sheehy SB, Blansfield JS, Davis DM, et al, editors: *Manual of clinical trauma care*, ed 3, Philadelphia, 1999, Mosby.

Schrier RW: *Disease of the kidney and urinary tract*, ed 7, Philadelphia, 2002, Lippincott Williams & Wilkins.

Schrier RW: *Renal and electrolyte disorders*, ed 6, Philadelphia, 2003, Lippincott Williams & Wilkins.

Slone DS: Nutritional support of the critically-ill and injured patient, *Crit Care Clin* 20(1):135-157, 2004.

Tanagho EA, McAninch JW: *Smith's general urology*, New York, 2004, McGraw-Hill.

Thomsen TW, Brown DF, Nadel ES: Blunt renal trauma, *J Emerg Med* 26(3):331-337, 2004.

The Endocrine System

KIM LITWACK, PhD, RN, CFNP, FAAN

SYSTEMWIDE ELEMENTS

Physiologic Anatomy

1. **Definition of a hormone**
   a. Hormones are molecules that are synthesized and secreted by specialized cells and released into the blood, exerting biochemical effects on target cells away from the site of origin
   b. Hormones control metabolism, transport of substances across cell membranes, fluid and electrolyte balance, growth and development, adaptation, and reproduction
2. **Chemically categorized by physiologic action**
   a. Peptide or protein hormones: Vasopressin (antidiuretic hormone [ADH]) thyrotropin-releasing hormone (TRH), insulin, growth hormone (somatotropin [GH]), follicle-stimulating hormone (FSH), luteinizing hormone (LH), corticotropin (adrenocorticotropic hormone [ACTH]), calcitonin
   b. Steroids: Glucocorticoids (cortisol), mineralocorticoids (aldosterone), estradiol, progesterone, testosterone
   c. Amines and amino acid derivatives: Norepinephrine, epinephrine, triiodothyronine (T_3), thyroxine (T_4)
3. **Hormone receptors**
   a. Specificity of hormone action is determined by the presence of a specific hormone receptor on or in the target cell
      i. Protein hormones react with receptors on the cell surface
      ii. Steroid hormones react with receptors inside the cell
   b. Receptors distinguish hormones from each other and translate the hormonal signal into a cellular response
   c. The hormone-receptor complex initiates intracellular events that lead to the biologic effects of the hormone acting on the target cell
4. **Mechanisms of hormone action**
   a. Activation of cyclic adenosine monophosphate (cAMP): Thyrotropin (thyroid-stimulating hormone [TSH]), ACTH, parathyroid hormone (PTH), and ADH
   b. Activation of genes: Steroid hormones and gonadal hormones
5. **Feedback control of hormone production** (Figure 6-1)
   a. Feedback control can be positive (low levels of hormone stimulate the release of its controlling hormone) or negative (high levels of hormone inhibit the release of its controlling hormone)

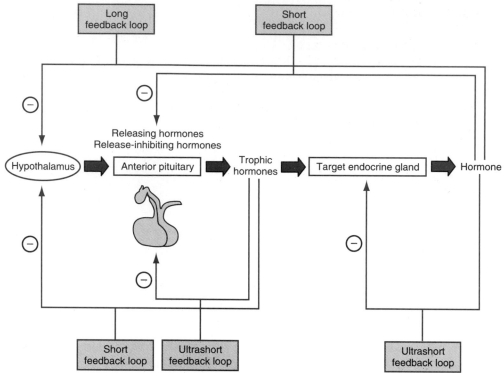

FIGURE 6-1 ■ Negative feedback in the hypothalamic-pituitary axis. Three levels of negative feedback regulate secretion in the hypothalamic-pituitary axis. In the *long feedback loop*, circulating levels of the target endocrine gland hormone influence hypothalamic secretion of releasing and release-inhibiting hormones. In a *short feedback loop*, levels of target gland hormones or tropic hormones feed back to the anterior pituitary or hypothalamus, respectively. In an *ultrashort feedback loop*, hormone levels signal the gland from which they were secreted. (From Hansen M: *Pathophysiology: foundations of disease and clinical intervention*, Philadelphia, 1998, Saunders, p. 802.)

   b. Feedback control systems allow self-regulation and prevent hormonal over-production

Pituitary Gland

1. **Location:** Base of the skull in the sphenoid bone; connected to the hypothalamus by the pituitary stalk (infundibulum), which links the nervous and endocrine systems
2. **Composition**
   a. Anterior lobe (adenohypophysis—75% of gland): Hormones are controlled by hypothalamic releasing or inhibiting hormones in response to stimuli received in the central nervous system
   b. Posterior lobe (neurohypophysis—25% of gland)
      i. Hormones are controlled by nerve fibers originating in the hypothalamus and terminating in the posterior pituitary gland
      ii. Hormones are synthesized in the hypothalamus, stored in the posterior pituitary, and released after activation of the cell bodies in the nerve tract

3. **Anterior pituitary hormones**
   a. GH
      i. Regulation of secretion
         (a) Stimulation: GH-releasing hormone (GRH) in response to physical and/or emotional stress, starvation, hypoglycemia, other protein-depleted states
         (b) Inhibition: Somatostatin from the hypothalamus, postprandial hyperglycemia, and pharmacologic doses of corticosteroids
      ii. Physiologic activity
         (a) Increases rate of protein synthesis
         (b) Increases lipolysis
         (c) Decreases protein catabolism
         (d) Decreases carbohydrate use
         (e) Stimulates bone and cartilage growth
         (f) Works with insulin, thyroid hormones, and sex steroids to promote growth
      iii. Disorders resulting from dysfunction: Not of significance in critical care
         (a) Excess: Gigantism (prepubertal), acromegaly (postpubertal)
         (b) Deficiency: Dwarfism (prepubertal)
   b. ACTH
      i. Regulation of secretion
         (a) Stimulation: Corticotropin-releasing hormone (CRH) in response to physical or emotional stress, trauma, hypoglycemia, hypoxia, surgery, decreased plasma cortisol levels
         (b) Inhibition: Increased plasma cortisol levels exert negative feedback on CRH and thus ACTH; stress can overcome this negative feedback
      ii. Physiologic activity: Production and release of adrenocortical hormones (glucocorticoids, adrenal androgens, and mineralocorticoids)
      iii. Disorders resulting from dysfunction
         (a) Excess: Cushing's disease
         (b) Deficiency: Adrenal insufficiency (chronic), adrenal crisis (acute)
   c. TSH
      i. Regulation of secretion
         (a) Stimulation: TRH in response to low concentration of thyroid hormones
         (b) Inhibition: Somatostatin from the hypothalamus, increased thyroid hormone levels
      ii. Physiologic activity
         (a) Increases synthesis of thyroid hormones
         (b) Releases stored thyroid hormones
         (c) Stimulates iodide uptake into thyroid cells
         (d) Increases size, number, and secretory activities of thyroid cells
      iii. Disorders resulting from dysfunction: See Thyroid Gland
   d. Other anterior pituitary hormones under hypothalamic control
      i. LH
      ii. FSH
      iii. Prolactin
4. **Posterior pituitary hormones**
   a. ADH
      i. Regulation of secretion
         (a) Stimulation: Increase in plasma osmolality, hypoxia, reduction in blood volume or blood pressure
         (b) Inhibition: Decrease in plasma osmolality

    ii. Physiologic activity
       (a) Increases water permeability in renal collecting duct epithelial cells, thereby controlling extracellular fluid osmolality
       (b) In pharmacologic amounts, constricts arterioles to increase blood pressure
    iii. Disorders resulting from dysfunction
       (a) Primary: Pituitary dysfunction (syndrome of inappropriate ADH secretion [SIADH])
       (b) Secondary: Renal dysfunction (diabetes insipidus)
  b. Oxytocin
    i. Dilatation of the cervix and stimulation of the vagina, lower segment of the uterus, and nipple causes reflex release of oxytocin
    ii. Oxytocin stimulates uterine contractions and milk ejection during lactation

Thyroid Gland

1. Location: Immediately below the larynx laterally and anterior to the trachea
2. Composition: Two lobes connected by an isthmus
  a. Follicular cells: Produce T_3 (20%) and T_4 (80%); T_4 converted in periphery to T_3
  b. Parafollicular cells (C cells): Produce thyrocalcitonin
3. Regulation of secretion (thyroid hormones)
  a. Stimulation: TSH stimulates thyroid hormone release, which is regulated by TRH from the hypothalamus; decreased levels of thyroid hormones stimulate the release of TSH and TRH
  b. Inhibition: Elevated levels of thyroid hormones inhibit TSH and TRH
4. Physiologic activity
  a. Increases the metabolic activity of cells, which results in increased oxygen consumption, increased rate of chemical reactions, and heat production
  b. Stimulates carbohydrate, fat, and protein metabolism
  c. Works with insulin, GH, and sex steroids to promote growth
  d. Critical for fetal neural and skeletal system development (intrauterine hypothyroidism causes cretinism)
  e. Positive chronotropic and inotropic effects on the heart
  f. Required for a normal hypoxic and hypercapnic drive in respiratory centers
  g. Increases erythropoiesis
  h. Increases metabolism and clearance of steroid hormone and insulin
5. Disorders resulting from dysfunction
  a. Thyroid enlargement (goiter)
  b. Excess: Hyperthyroidism (chronic), thyroid storm (acute)
  c. Deficiency: Hypothyroidism (chronic), myxedema coma (acute)
6. Thyrocalcitonin (calcitonin)
  a. Regulation of secretion
    i. Stimulation: Increase in calcium levels
    ii. Inhibition: Decrease in calcium levels
  b. Physiologic activity
    i. Decreases blood calcium levels by inhibiting calcium mobilization from bone and decreasing calcium resorption in the kidney
    ii. Decreases phosphate levels by inhibiting bone remodeling and by increasing phosphate loss in urine

Parathyroid Glands

1. Location: Four glands on the posterior surface of the thyroid gland
2. Composition: Chief cells release PTH

3. **Regulation of secretion**
   a. Stimulation: Decrease in serum calcium level
   b. Inhibition: Increase in serum levels of calcium and vitamin D metabolites, hypermagnesemia, and hypomagnesemia
4. **Physiologic activity**
   a. Kidney
      i. Increases renal tubular reabsorption of calcium and magnesium
      ii. Decreases renal tubular reabsorption of phosphate and bicarbonate
      iii. Stimulates the formation of the fat-soluble form of vitamin D
   b. Gastrointestinal tract: Increases calcium absorption
   c. Bone: Larger amounts increase calcium reabsorption
5. **Disorders resulting from dysfunction**
   a. Excess: Hypercalcemia (not significant in critical care)
   b. Deficiency: Hypoparathyroidism leads to hypocalcemia (in critical care, most hypocalcemia is due to renal disease, not hypoparathyroidism)

Adrenal Glands

1. **Location:** Retroperitoneal, superior to the kidney
2. **Composition:** Two separate endocrine tissues that produce distinct hormones
   a. Cortex (90% of gland) produces aldosterone, glucocorticoids, and adrenal androgens
   b. Medulla (10% of gland) produces catecholamines
3. **Cortical hormones**
   a. Glucocorticoids (cortisol is the major hormone)
      i. Regulation of secretion
         (a) Stimulation: ACTH (diurnal variation—increased 1 hour after awakening, incidence of myocardial infarction increased in the morning)
         (b) Inhibition: Cortisol exerts negative feedback on the anterior pituitary and hypothalamus
      ii. Physiologic activity
         (a) Carbohydrate metabolism
            (1) Increases gluconeogenesis
            (2) Decreases glucose uptake in muscle and adipose tissue (insulin-antagonistic effect)
         (b) Protein metabolism
            (1) Decreases protein stores and protein synthesis in all cells except liver cells
            (2) Increases protein catabolism
            (3) Promotes gluconeogenesis
         (c) Promotes lipolysis
         (d) Increases tissue responsiveness to other hormones, such as glucagon and the catecholamines
         (e) Antiinflammatory effects
            (1) Decreased migration of inflammatory cells to sites of injury
            (2) Inhibition of production and/or activity of vasoactive substances
            (3) Prevention of immune response to tissue antigens released by injury
      iii. Disorders resulting from dysfunction
         (a) Excess: Cushing's syndrome
         (b) Deficiency: Adrenal insufficiency (common in the intensive care unit), adrenal crisis (acute)
   b. Mineralocorticoids (aldosterone is the major hormone)
      i. Regulation of secretion

(a) Stimulation: Renin-angiotensin system as well as hyponatremia, hyperkalemia, and ACTH

(b) Inhibition: Hypokalemia, sodium loading, and increased plasma volume

ii. Physiologic activity

(a) Increases sodium reabsorption, indirectly increasing extracellular fluid volume

(b) Increases potassium excretion

iii. Disorders resulting from dysfunction

(a) Excess: Primary aldosteronism, characterized by potassium depletion, extracellular fluid volume expansion, and nephrosclerotic hypertension

(b) Deficiency: Adrenal insufficiency (chronic), adrenal crisis (acute)

(c) Adrenal androgens: Not of significance in critical care

4. **Medullary hormones:** Epinephrine and norepinephrine

   a. Regulation of secretion: Stimulated by fear, anxiety, pain, trauma, fluid loss, hemorrhage, extremes in temperature, surgery, hypoxia, hypoglycemia, hypokalemia, hypernatremia, hypotension

   b. Physiologic activity (Table 6-1)

      i. Fight or flight (stress) response

      ii. Critical in the recovery from insulin-induced hypoglycemia

      iii. Major insulin antagonists

   c. Disorders resulting from dysfunction

      i. Excess: Pheochromocytoma; tumor produces epinephrine and/or norepinephrine, causing hypertension

      ii. Deficiency: Persons with an intact sympathetic nervous system manifest no clinically significant disability

Pancreas

1. **Location:** Lies transversely behind the peritoneum and stomach

2. **Composition:** Exocrine and endocrine components. Endocrine functions originate from the islet cells, which constitute less than 2% of the total pancreatic volume; 65% of the islet cells are beta cells, which produce insulin. Glucagon is produced by the alpha cells; somatostatin and gastrin are produced by the delta cells.

■ **TABLE 6-1**
■ ■ **Adrenergic Responses of Selected Organs**

Organ	Receptor Type	Effect
Heart		
Sinoatrial node	β_1	Inotropic effect (↑ rate)
Atrioventricular node	β_1	↑ Automaticity and conduction speed
Ventricle	β_1	↑ Automaticity, conduction speed, and contractility
Arterioles	α	Vasoconstriction
	β_2	Vasodilation
Kidney	β	↑ Renin release
Lung: Bronchial muscle	β_2	Relaxation (dilatation)
Liver	α, β	↑ Glycogenolysis
Pancreas	α	↓ Insulin and glucagon release
	β	↑ Insulin and glucagon release
Uterus	α	Contraction
	β_2	Relaxation

3. **Insulin**
   a. Regulation of secretion
      i. Stimulation: Increases in blood glucose, gastrin, secretin, cholecystokinin, and gastrointestinal hormone levels, and β-adrenergic stimulation
      ii. Inhibition: α-adrenergic effects of somatostatin, catecholamines, and drugs, including diazoxide, phenytoin, and vinblastine
   b. Physiologic activity
      i. Carbohydrate metabolism
         (a) Increases glucose transport across the cell membrane in muscle and fat
         (b) Increases glycogenesis
         (c) Inhibits gluconeogenesis
      ii. Protein metabolism
         (a) Increases amino acid transport across the cell membrane
         (b) Increases protein synthesis
         (c) Decreases protein catabolism
      iii. Fat metabolism
         (a) Increases triglyceride synthesis
         (b) Increases fatty acid transport across the cell membrane
         (c) Inhibits lipolysis
      iv. Works with thyroid hormones, the sex steroids, and GH to promote growth
   c. Disorders resulting from dysfunction
      i. Excess: Hypoglycemia
      ii. Deficiency: Diabetes mellitus
         (a) Type 1: Absolute deficiency of insulin due to islet cell antibodies; genetic link, autoimmune disorder
         (b) Type 2: Relative deficiency of insulin caused by decreased sensitivity of receptors to insulin, decreased production, premature destruction of insulin or receptors, and/or hyperinsulinemia; polygenetic etiologies, dietary link
4. **Glucagon**
   a. Regulation of secretion
      i. Stimulation: Hypoglycemia, catecholamines, gastrointestinal hormones, and glucocorticoids
      ii. Inhibition: Hyperglycemia and somatostatin
   b. Physiologic activity
      i. Increases blood glucose via glycogenolysis and gluconeogenesis
      ii. Increases lipolysis
      iii. Increases amino acid transport to the liver and the conversion of amino acids to glucose precursors
      iv. Is a major insulin-antagonistic hormone
      v. Critical hormone in the recovery from insulin-induced hypoglycemia
   c. Deficient glucagon production is thought to play a role in defective glucose counterregulation in insulin-induced hypoglycemia in type 1 diabetes mellitus
   d. Available as a pharmacologic agent to correct insulin-induced hypoglycemia (all diabetics should have a readily available source)
5. **Somatostatin**
   a. Present in islet cells, the hypothalamus, and the gastrointestinal tract
   b. Physiologic activity: Inhibits the secretion of insulin, glucagon, GH, TSH, and gastrointestinal hormones (gastrin, secretin)

Gonadal Hormones (Testosterone, Estrogen, Progesterone)

Not significant in critical care

PATIENT ASSESSMENT

1. **Nursing history**
   a. Patient health history
      i. Presence of pathophysiologic processes that can result in endocrine dysfunction
         (a) Adrenal gland hypoperfusion
         (b) Infection, inflammation, autoimmune processes
         (c) Neoplasms and exposure to the chemotherapeutic agents and radiotherapy used to treat the neoplasms
         (d) Infiltrative disorders
         (e) Acquired immunodeficiency syndrome (AIDS)
      ii. Pregnancy, postpartum state
      iii. Presence of preexisting chronic endocrine disorder (diagnosed or undiagnosed)
      iv. Poor compliance with pharmacologic therapy for a preexisting endocrine disorder
      v. Presence of an unrelated critical illness in a patient with a preexisting chronic endocrine disorder
      vi. Positive family history of an endocrine disorder
      vii. Use of systemic steroids
      viii. Indicators of altered health patterns
         (a) Cognition and perception
            (1) Personality changes, lethargy, emotional lability, attention span deficit, memory impairment
            (2) Visual disturbances
            (3) Changes in level of consciousness
            (4) Depression, paranoia, delusions, delirium
            (5) Verbalizations that indicate lack of knowledge or misconceptions regarding self-care management
         (b) Nutrition and metabolism
            (1) Change in weight (increase or decrease)
            (2) Nausea, anorexia, vomiting
            (3) Polydipsia
            (4) Heat or cold intolerance
            (5) Edema
         (c) Elimination
            (1) Diarrhea or constipation
            (2) Polyuria, anuria, oliguria, nocturia
            (3) Excessive perspiration
         (d) Activity and exercise
            (1) Fatigue, weakness
            (2) Impairment in performance of the activities of daily living
         (e) Sleep and rest: Restlessness, inadequate sleep
         (f) Sexual function
            (1) Menstrual irregularities
            (2) Impotence
            (3) Decreased libido
            (4) Infertility
         (g) Roles and relationships
            (1) Discord in previously stable relationships
            (2) Physical and emotional inability to engage in usual role activity

(h) Coping and stress tolerance
  (1) Inability to cope
  (2) History of a past or present psychiatric disorder
(i) Health perception and health management: Evidence of noncompliance with the prescribed medical regimen
  b. Family history: Endocrine disorders in other family members
  c. Social history
  i. Elderly persons may be at special risk for the development of an endocrine crisis because of changes associated with aging and a diminished thirst mechanism
  ii. Economically disadvantaged persons may be at risk for the development of an endocrine crisis because many of the regimens for treating chronic endocrine disorders are costly and necessitate regular medical follow-up
  iii. Teenagers with poor compliance with a prescribed medical regimen, particularly diabetic patients, are at increased risk of crisis
  d. Medication history
  i. Use of pharmacologic agents to treat chronic endocrine disorders
  ii. Use of pharmacologic agents that may stimulate or inhibit hormone release, or interfere with hormone action at target tissue
  iii. Exposure to radiographic contrast dyes
2. **Nursing examination of patient**
  a. Physical examination data
  i. Inspection
    (a) Excessive or diminutive stature
    (b) Fat distribution in relation to gender and maturational level
    (c) Mobility, tremor, hyperkinesis
    (d) Scars, especially in the neck area
    (e) Hair distribution and texture relative to gender and maturational level
    (f) Edema
    (g) Goiter
    (h) Seizure activity
    (i) Presence of medical alert identification
    (j) Hydration status of oral cavity
    (k) Periorbital edema, ptosis, eye protrusion, stare, dry eyes
    (l) Unusual pigmentation, temperature, turgor, striae, or thinning of the skin
  ii. Palpation: Enlarged or nodular thyroid gland, often painful
  iii. Percussion: Abnormal deep tendon reflexes (may be hyperreflexic or hyporeflexic)
  iv. Auscultation
    (a) Neck: Bruits over the thyroid gland
    (b) Heart: Distant heart sounds, third heart sound (due to pericardial effusion, heart failure)
    (c) Blood pressure: Hypotension, hypertension
    (d) Heart rate and rhythm disturbances
    (e) Altered respiratory pattern
    (f) Altered bowel sounds
    (g) Pericardial and/or pleural friction rub (due to effusion)
  b. Monitoring data
  i. Pulse oximetry
  ii. Electrocardiography
  iii. Blood pressure monitoring

    iv. Temperature monitoring

    v. Electrolyte analysis

    vi. Arterial blood gas (ABG) analysis

    vii. Hormonal assays

3. Appraisal of patient characteristics

  a. Resiliency

    i. Level 1—*Minimally resilient*: 88-year-old female admitted in a diabetic coma with concomitant antibiotic-resistant bacterial pneumonia

    ii. Level 3—*Moderately resilient*: 14-year-old male admitted in diabetic ketoacidosis following an episode of the flu; no other medical conditions

    iii. Level 5—*Highly resilient*: 57-year-old man with a blood glucose level of 50 mg/dl who reports feeling sweaty, agitated, and slightly disoriented following 3 days of vomiting with the flu

  b. Vulnerability

    i. Level 1—*Highly vulnerable*: 79-year-old male with a history of myocardial infarction and subsequent congestive heart failure who develops diabetes insipidus following head trauma after a motor vehicle accident; fluid replacement causes cardiac deterioration

    ii. Level 3—*Moderately vulnerable*: 49-year-old female who develops nephrogenic diabetes insipidus following repeated episodes of pyelonephritis with scarring

    iii. Level 5—*Minimally vulnerable*: 44-year-old male following transsphenoidal removal of a pituitary tumor who develops diabetes insipidus but remains hemodynamically stable and responds immediately to administration of vasopressin

  c. Stability

    i. Level 1—*Minimally stable*: 38-year-old female who attempts suicide by ingestion of excessive amounts of thyroid hormone; arrives at the unit with severe tachycardia, hypotension, and a temperature of 105° F (40.6° C), in a coma

    ii. Level 3—*Moderately stable*: 44-year-old female who comes for treatment with tachycardia and a blood pressure of 90/60 mm Hg after restarting thyroid hormone therapy with a new formulation

    iii. Level 5—*Highly stable*: 32-year-old female with hyperthyroidism as evidenced by abnormal laboratory test results who responds well to propranolol and propylthiouracil and who is scheduled for thyroidectomy

  d. Complexity

    i. Level 1—*Highly complex*: 88-year-old female admitted in hyperosmolar, nonketotic coma. Patient has a history of malnutrition and chronic obstructive pulmonary disease. She lives alone, has mobility impairments, and has no family nearby. Has Medicare insurance only.

    ii. Level 3—*Moderately complex*: 44-year-old male admitted in diabetic ketoacidosis following inability to obtain insulin. Patient recently became unemployed and lost health insurance and prescription coverage.

    iii. Level 5—*Minimally complex*: 79-year-old male with newly diagnosed diabetes who has a blood glucose level of 200 mg/dl and a hemoglobin A_{1C} fraction of 8.6%. Patient shows cardiovascular and neurologic stability. Has good family support and insurance. Is well educated.

  e. Resource availability

    i. Level 1—*Few resources*: Patient with newly diagnosed diabetes who has no insurance and no family, is unemployed, is new to the area, and is homeless

ii. Level 3—*Moderate resources*: Patient with newly diagnosed diabetes who has Medicare coverage and a niece who lives an hour away and who currently resides in an assisted living facility

iii. Level 5—*Many resources*: Patient with newly diagnosed diabetes who has insurance and prescription coverage. Patient is well educated and has strong family support. Independent in care and finances.

f. Participation in care

i. Level 1—*No participation*: 48-year-old female admitted in myxedema coma following thyroidectomy. Patient did not start thyroid replacement therapy after surgery. No family nearby.

ii. Level 3—*Moderate level of participation*: 68-year-old female admitted with bradycardia, anemia, and fatigue who confesses to having stopped thyroid hormone replacement therapy because she couldn't afford to visit her physician for a new prescription

iii. Level 5—*Full participation*: A 14-year-old male who is treated successfully for diabetic ketoacidosis and who, with his family, requests assistance in learning more about his disease and its management

g. Participation in decision making

i. Level 1—*No participation*: Fiftyish homeless male admitted in diabetic ketoacidosis. Patient is alcoholic with a history of mental health problems requiring hospitalization. No known family.

ii. Level 3—*Moderate participation*: 78-year-old patient with newly diagnosed diabetes who has a history of prostate cancer. Has a sister who is also diabetic. Asks for information to access home nursing care for assistance.

iii. Level 5—*Full level of participation*: 44-year-old patient admitted in addisonian crisis. Patient has durable power of attorney for health care and living will. Patient's family is present with the patient and fully knowledgeable about the disease. Family provides history and treatment authorization, and will be available to aid in care after discharge.

h. Predictability

i. Level 1—*Not predictable*: 44-year-old patient with brittle diabetes admitted in diabetic ketoacidosis for the fourth time this year. Poorly compliant with the medical regimen, smokes; chronic obstructive pulmonary disease has been newly diagnosed.

ii. Level 3—*Moderately predictable*: 32-year-old diabetic patient admitted in diabetic ketoacidosis. Responds well to administration of insulin and fluids. Aware that her triggers for diabetic ketoacidosis are infection, particularly bladder infections, and the flu.

iii. Level 5—*Highly predictable*: 88-year-old female admitted from a nursing home in hyperosmolar, nonketotic coma following dehydration caused by the flu. Responds well to rehydration and insulin.

4. Diagnostic studies

a. Laboratory: Blood and urine

i. Electrolyte levels

ii. Glucose, ketoacid, blood urea nitrogen, cholesterol, creatinine, serum creatine phosphokinase levels

iii. Plasma osmolality, hematocrit, white blood cell count with differential

iv. ABG levels

v. Specific hormone assays

vi. Urine specific gravity, osmolality, pH

b. Radiologic (to identify precipitating factor)

i. Radiography (skull, chest, abdomen)

  ii. Scans (thyroid, pancreas)
  iii. Computed axial tomography
  iv. Magnetic resonance imaging
  v. Arteriography
  vi. Bone mineral densitometry
c. Other
  i. Electrocardiography
  ii. Visual field testing
  iii. Temperature monitoring

PATIENT CARE

1. **Fluid volume deficit (hypovolemia)**
   a. Description of problem
     i. Dry skin and mucous membranes, decreased skin turgor
     ii. Hypertension, orthostasis, tachycardia
     iii. Hypernatremia
     iv. Weight loss
     v. Polyuria
     vi. Negative intake and output (I&O) balance
   b. Goals of care
     i. Fluid and electrolyte balance are achieved and maintained
     ii. Cardiovascular stability is maintained
   c. Collaborating professionals on health care team
     i. Nurse
     ii. Physician
   d. Interventions
     i. Administer fluids and hormone therapy as prescribed
     ii. Monitor and document I&O, electrolyte levels, vital signs, central venous pressure, urine specific gravity, weight, laboratory test results on flow sheet
     iii. Provide oral care and skin care
   e. Evaluation of patient care
     i. Fluids, electrolytes, and I&O in balance
     ii. Cardiovascular stability
     iii. No skin or mucous membrane breakdown
2. **Fluid volume excess (hypervolemia)**
   a. Description of problem
     i. Intake exceeding output
     ii. Weight gain
     iii. Third heart sound
     iv. Pulmonary congestion and dyspnea
     v. Deterioration of mental status
     vi. Hemodilution
     vii. Abnormal electrolyte values
     viii. Edema
   b. Goals of care: Fluid and electrolyte balance is achieved and maintained
   c. Collaborating professionals on health care team
     i. Nurse
     ii. Physician
     iii. Respiratory therapist

    d. Interventions

        i. Monitor I&O, electrolyte levels

        ii. Use flow sheet to document I&O, vital signs, central venous pressure, urine specific gravity, weight, laboratory test results

        iii. Identify patients at risk for fluid overload

        iv. Monitor pulmonary status and function

        v. Administer prescribed diuretics

    e. Evaluation of patient care

        i. I&O and electrolytes in balance

        ii. Cardiovascular and pulmonary stability

        iii. ABG levels and pulse oximetry within normal limits

3. Altered carbohydrate, fat, and/or protein metabolism

    a. Description of problem

        i. Hyperglycemia with or without ketosis

        ii. Decreased serum albumin level

        iii. Weight loss of 10% to 20%

        iv. Generalized fatigue and weakness

    b. Goals of care

        i. Body weight normalizes and stabilizes

        ii. No evidence of ketosis is present

        iii. Nitrogen balance is positive

        iv. Serum albumin level is within normal limits

    c. Collaborating professionals on health care team

        i. Nurse

        ii. Physician

        iii. Dietitian

    d. Interventions

        i. Provide sufficient calories and vitamins

        ii. Administer hormone or antihormone therapy as prescribed

        iii. Monitor ABG, serum albumin, electrolyte levels

    e. Evaluation of patient care

        i. Stable body weight

        ii. No ketosis

        iii. Normal serum albumin level

4. Need for patient and family education and discharge planning

    a. Description of problem

        i. Lack of knowledge or skills may seriously compromise self-care

        ii. Patient and/or family is unable to explain or follow instructions correctly

        iii. Patient and/or family raises questions and requests information

    b. Goals of care: Patient demonstrates knowledge and skills needed for providing self-care and contacting health care resources

    c. Collaborating professionals on health care team

        i. Nurse, clinical nurse specialist, nurse practitioner

        ii. Physician

        iii. Diabetes educator

        iv. Dietitian

        v. Care manager

    d. Interventions

        i. Assess patient and family knowledge of the health disorder and the required self-care

        ii. Provide appropriate information about the health disorder and self-care

    iii. Provide an opportunity for the patient and family to demonstrate needed skills

    iv. Provide appropriate resources for additional information and support

  e. Evaluation of patient care: Ability of the patient and family to explain and demonstrate optimal self-care management

SPECIFIC PATIENT HEALTH PROBLEMS

Diabetes Insipidus

1. **Pathophysiology:** Occurs when any organic lesion or chemical substance (e.g., alcohol) affecting the hypothalamus or posterior pituitary interferes with ADH synthesis and transport or release. Deficiency results in the inability to conserve water and the excretion of large amounts of dilute urine.

2. **Etiology and risk factors**
   a. Central or neurogenic diabetes insipidus (ADH sensitive)
      i. Idiopathic (30%): Autoimmune (common), familial (rare)
      ii. Trauma: Injury to hypothalamus or pituitary trauma (most common cause of polyuria after neurosurgery)
      iii. Craniopharyngioma, pituitary tumor
      iv. Infections: Meningitis, encephalitis
      v. Vascular disorder: Aneurysm
      vi. Infiltrative disorders (histiocytosis X, sarcoidosis)
      vii. Malignancy (lung cancer, leukemia, lymphoma)
      viii. History of an impaired thirst mechanism or a state in which the patient is confused, incapacitated, or otherwise unable to secure fluids
   b. Nephrogenic diabetes insipidus (ADH insensitive): Most common forms are the following:
      i. Renal: Polycystic kidneys, pyelonephritis, congenital disorder
      ii. Multisystem disorders: Multiple myeloma, amyloidosis
      iii. Familial
   c. Pharmacologic agents: Ethanol, lithium, glyburide, and phenytoin inhibit ADH secretion and action
   d. Insufficient exogenous ADH in a person with diabetes insipidus

3. **Signs and symptoms**
   a. Polydipsia
   b. Polyuria (5 to 20 L/24 hr)
   c. Decreased skin turgor, dry mucous membranes
   d. Fatigue
   e. Tachycardia; hypotension if the patient has become dehydrated

4. **Diagnostic study findings**
   a. Elevated plasma osmolality (>295 mOsm/kg), decreased urine osmolality (<500 mOsm/kg; can be as low as 30 mOsm/kg)
   b. Hypernatremia
   c. Low urine specific gravity (1.001 to 1.005)
   d. Water deprivation test: With adequate stimulus for ADH release (simple dehydration), the kidneys cannot concentrate urine. Differentiates psychogenic polydipsia from diabetes insipidus; no response occurs in either neurogenic or nephrogenic diabetes insipidus.
   e. ADH test: To demonstrate that the kidneys can concentrate urine with exogenous ADH. Corrects central diabetes insipidus; no response in nephrogenic diabetes insipidus
   f. Low plasma ADH levels in patients with central diabetes insipidus

5. **Goals of care**
   a. Tissue hypoperfusion is prevented
   b. Fluid and electrolyte balance is maintained
6. **Collaborating professionals on health care team**
   a. Nurse
   b. Physician
7. **Management of patient care**
   a. Anticipated patient trajectory: Patients with diabetes insipidus may experience the spontaneous resolution of symptoms or require lifetime medication. The success of pharmacologic therapy depends solely on patient compliance. Throughout their course of recovery and discharge, patients with diabetes insipidus may be expected to have needs in the following areas:
      i. Pharmacology
         (a) Administer hormone replacement for central diabetes insipidus
            (1) Aqueous pitressin (intravenous [IV] or subcutaneous [SQ])
            (2) Lysine vasopressin (nasal)
            (3) Desmopressin acetate (DDAVP)
         (b) Administer pharmacologic agents for nephrogenic diabetes insipidus
            (1) Chlorpropamide: Stimulates ADH release and promotes renal response to ADH
            (2) Thiazide diuretics: Promote concentration of urine, improving specific gravity and urine osmolality
      ii. Discharge planning
         (a) Medication instruction
         (b) Signs and symptoms to report
      iii. Treatments
         (a) Monitor I&O, urine specific gravity, and osmolality
         (b) Monitor serum osmolality
   b. Potential complications
      i. Dehydration
         (a) Mechanism: Secondary to fluid loss
         (b) Management: Fluid and hormone replacement
      ii. Hypoperfusion
         (a) Mechanism: From decreased intravascular volume
         (b) Management: Restoration of circulatory volume via fluid and hormone replacement
      iii. Electrolyte imbalance
         (a) Mechanism: Secondary to fluid loss
         (b) Management: Restoration of circulating volume
8. **Evaluation of patient care**
   a. Normalization of fluid balance
   b. Electrolyte levels within normal limits
   c. Patient's understanding of the purpose and dosing of medications

Syndrome of Inappropriate Antidiuretic Hormone Secretion (SIADH)

1. **Pathophysiology:** Syndrome characterized by plasma hypotonicity and hyponatremia that result from aberrant secretion of ADH, which in turn is caused by the failure of the negative feedback system. Dysfunction results in water intoxication.
2. **Etiology and risk factors**
   a. Central nervous system disorders
      i. Trauma: Skull fracture, subdural hematoma, subarachnoid hemorrhage, cerebral contusion, post neurosurgery

ii. Neoplasms

iii. Infections: Meningitis, encephalitis, brain abscess, Guillain-Barré syndrome, AIDS

iv. Vascular disorders: Aneurysm, cerebral vascular accident

b. Stimulation of ADH release via hypoxia and/or low left atrial filling pressure

 i. Pulmonary infections

 ii. Asthma

 iii. Heart failure

 iv. Positive pressure ventilation

c. Pharmacologic agents: Either increase ADH secretion or potentiate its action

 i. Cancer chemotherapeutic agents: Cyclophosphamide, vincristine

 ii. Chlorpropamide, acetaminophen, amitriptyline, thiazide diuretics, carbamazepine, pentamidine

d. Excessive exogenous ADH therapy

e. Ectopic ADH production associated with bronchogenic, prostatic, or pancreatic cancers and with leukemia

3. **Signs and symptoms**

a. Nausea, vomiting

b. Confusion, impaired memory

c. Muscle twitching or seizure activity, delayed deep tendon reflexes

4. **Diagnostic study findings**

a. Hyponatremia

b. Decreased plasma osmolality

c. Elevated urine sodium level and osmolality

d. Elevated plasma ADH levels

5. **Goals of care**

a. Fluid balance is restored

b. Patient safety is ensured

6. **Collaborating professionals on health care team**

a. Nurse

b. Physician, consulting physician

7. **Management of patient care**

a. Anticipated patient trajectory: If the underlying cause of SIADH is treated, the symptoms will resolve. If the precipitating cause cannot be removed or treated, the patient will require ongoing electrolyte monitoring throughout recovery and discharge. Patients with SIADH may be expected to have needs in the following areas:

 i. Pharmacology: Fluid therapy based on urine output plus insensible losses

 ii. Treatments

   (a) Monitor electrolyte levels, osmolality, weight

   (b) Initiate seizure and injury precautions

b. Potential complications

 i. Fluid overload and congestive heart failure

   (a) Mechanism: Secondary to excess ADH secretion

   (b) Management: Administration of diuretics and inotropic support

 ii. Electrolyte imbalance

   (a) Mechanism: Secondary to fluid overload

   (b) Management: Monitor electrolyte levels during and with administration of diuretics

 iii. Seizures

   (a) Mechanism: Secondary to sodium and osmolality alterations

   (b) Management: Restore fluid balance; protect the patient

8. **Evaluation of patient care**
   a. Normalization of fluid and electrolyte balances
   b. Absence of seizures
   c. Absence of injury

Thyrotoxicosis (Thyroid Storm)

1. **Pathophysiology:** Life-threatening augmentation of the signs and symptoms of hyperthyroidism; rare, because hyperthyroidism in most patients is well controlled by antithyroid drug therapy
2. **Etiology and risk factors**
   a. Surgical procedures or trauma of any kind
   b. Infection
   c. Poor compliance with antithyroid therapy (rare)
   d. Past or present use of methimazole or propylthiouracil, with disruption of established medication regimen; use of antiarrhythmic agents
   e. Diabetic ketoacidosis, eclampsia, postpartum state
3. **Signs and symptoms**
   a. Confusion, overt psychosis, coma
   b. Warm, moist, flushed, soft skin; hyperthermia (105° F [40.6° C]). Diagnosis is confirmed by high fever and altered mental status in a severely ill hyperthyroid patient.
   c. Severe tachycardia, third heart sound, irregular pulse (especially in an otherwise young and healthy person), hypotension, shock
   d. Adventitious breath sounds caused by pulmonary edema
   e. Hyperkinesis and tremor, restlessness and agitation, hyperreflexia
   f. Weakness, fatigue
   g. Nausea, abdominal pain, hepatomegaly
   h. Eyelid lag, retracted eyelids, stare, exophthalmos, irritated eyes
   i. Alopecia
   j. Goiter: Diffuse or multinodular, nontender, audible bruits
4. **Diagnostic study findings**
   a. Elevated total and free T_3 and T_4 levels and reduced TSH level (TSH level may remain normal if the precipitating event was a viral infection)
   b. Elevated hepatic aminotransferase level; hyperbilirubinemia common
   c. Elevated levels of alkaline phosphatase and creatine phosphokinase
5. **Goals of care**
   a. Vital signs, including temperature, are stable
   b. Cardiac, renal, and neurologic status is intact
6. **Collaborating professionals on health care team**
   a. Nurse
   b. Physician, consulting physician
7. **Management of patient care**
   a. Anticipated patient trajectory: Once cardiovascular stability is restored and the patient is stabilized, definitive management will include thyroidectomy or pharmacologic termination of thyroid function. These treatments will render the patient hypothyroid, which requires lifelong thyroid hormone replacement. Throughout their recovery and discharge, patients with thyrotoxicosis may be expected to have needs in the following areas:
      i. Pharmacology
         (a) Administer β-adrenergic antagonists (propranolol) IV or by mouth (PO)
         (b) Administer antithyroid medications

(1) Propylthiouracil, methimazole, or carbimazole

(2) Ipodate sodium

(c) Administer antipyretics: Salicylates inhibit T_4 and T_3 binding, increasing levels of T_4 and T_3; do not use

(d) Administer antibiotics if the precipitating event was an infection

ii. Treatments

(a) Perform frequent cardiovascular, respiratory, and neurologic assessments

(b) Monitor I&O and daily weights

(c) Institute cooling measures; avoid causing shivering

b. Potential complications

i. Cardiac arrest

(a) Mechanism: Secondary to elevated T_3 and T_4 levels, and hyperthermia

(b) Management: Cardiopulmonary resuscitation (CPR)

ii. Heart failure

(a) Mechanism: Secondary to severe tachycardia

(b) Management: Inotropic support; IV administration of β-adrenergic antagonists

iii. Hypoxemia and hypercarbia

(a) Mechanism: Due to pulmonary edema

(b) Management: Oxygen therapy, pulse oximetry, monitoring of ABG levels, intubation, and mechanical ventilation, if needed

iv. Hyperthermia

(a) Mechanism: Accelerated metabolism due to excess thyroid hormones

(b) Management: Institute cooling; administer antipyretics

v. Hypermetabolism

(a) Mechanism: Secondary to excess thyroid hormones

(b) Management: Administer β-adrenergic antagonists and antithyroid agents

vi. Insufficient caloric intake

(a) Mechanism: Secondary to hypermetabolism

(b) Management: Provide nutritional support to achieve a positive nitrogen balance

8. Evaluation of patient care

a. Stable vital signs, including arterial oxygen saturation (SaO_2)

b. Normal temperature

c. Clear breath sounds

d. No dysrhythmias

e. Initiation of definitive antithyroid therapy

f. Resolution of infection if present

Myxedema Coma

1. Pathophysiology: Life-threatening emergency resulting from extreme hypothyroidism. Often occurs in the presence of concurrent illness but may manifest as the initial findings in hypothyroidism. May also be due to noncompliance with the thyroid replacement therapy regimen, especially in the elderly living alone.

2. Etiology and risk factors

a. Decompensation of a preexisting hypothyroid state after infection; trauma; exposure to cold; administration of tranquilizers, barbiturates, and narcotics; or other physical stress. Preexisting hypothyroidism may result from

i. Autoimmune or idiopathic condition (most common cause)

ii. Destruction of the thyroid gland after radioactive iodine therapy for hyperthyroidism

      iii. Chronic thyroiditis

      iv. Thyroidectomy

      v. Dysfunction within the hypothalamic-pituitary axis (hypophysectomy, pituitary irradiation, pituitary infarction)

  b. Insufficient provision of exogenous thyroid hormone (e.g., a hypothyroid patient who discontinues replacement therapy, a critically ill patient who has preexisting hypothyroidism but does not receive continued replacement therapy while hospitalized)

  c. Family history of Graves' disease, Hashimoto's thyroiditis, or type 1 diabetes mellitus

  d. Lithium carbonate: Blocks thyroid hormone synthesis and release; can cause hypothyroidism

3. Signs and symptoms

  a. Nonpitting edema of the feet and hands; periorbital edema

  b. Macroglossia

  c. Loss of the eyebrows and scalp hair; cool, rough, dry skin

  d. Goiter may not be palpable because of atrophy, prior radiation, or prior surgery

  e. Delayed deep tendon reflexes, especially the relaxation phase

  f. Slow, shallow respirations

  g. Bradycardia

  h. Blood pressure inconclusive

  i. Hypothermia (91° to 95° F [32.8° to 35.0° C])

  j. Exaggerated response to sedatives

4. Diagnostic study findings

  a. Hyponatremia

  b. Respiratory acidosis, hypoxemia

  c. Hypoglycemia

  d. Enlarged cardiac outline, pleural and pericardial effusions on radiograph

  e. Electrocardiogram (ECG): Sinus bradycardia, T-wave depression, ST changes, prolonged RT and QT intervals

  f. Low free T_4, T_3 resin uptake, increased TSH level

  g. Anemia (25% of patients)

  h. High cholesterol level, hyperlipoproteinemia

  i. Because of the potential for concurrent adrenal insufficiency, a rapid ACTH stimulation test should be performed for patients with myxedema

5. Goals of care

  a. Pulmonary, cardiovascular, and neurologic function are normalized

  b. Temperature is normalized

6. Collaborating professionals on health care team

  a. Nurse

  b. Physician, consulting physician

  c. Respiratory therapist

7. Management of patient care

  a. Anticipated patient trajectory: Once their condition is stabilized, patients will require lifelong thyroid hormone replacement and compliance with the medical regimen to prevent reoccurrence. Throughout their clinical course, patients with myxedema coma may be expected to have needs in the following areas:

    i. Pharmacology

      (a) Administer thyroid hormone replacement IV

      (b) Administer glucocorticoids as needed. *Note:* Thyroid replacement therapy may aggravate preexisting adrenal insufficiency.

    ii. Treatments
        (a) Institute rewarming; monitor temperature
        (b) Monitor vital signs, neurologic status, peripheral perfusion
        (c) Prevent infection
            (1) Patient incapable of responding with fever
            (2) Susceptibility to infection increased

  b. Potential complications
    i. Severe hypercapnia and hypoxemia
        (a) Mechanism: Profound hypothyroidism causes reduced central ventilatory drive and respiratory muscle weakness
        (b) Management: Initiate endotracheal intubation and mechanical ventilation for hypercapnic respiratory failure
    ii. Adverse drug reactions
        (a) Mechanism: Decreased metabolic rate slows drug turnover and degradation
        (b) Management: Avoid agents that further decrease respiratory drive

8. Evaluation of patient care
  a. Stable vital signs, including temperature and SaO_2
  b. Normalized thyroid function test results when the patient is taking thyroid replacement hormones

Hypoparathyroidism and Hyperparathyroidism

1. Pathophysiology: Parathyroid gland dysfunction or production of a tumor-derived PTH-related peptide is associated with disturbances in calcium and phosphorus balance and bone metabolism. See Chapter 5 for further discussion of the pathophysiology of calcium and phosphorus imbalances.

2. Etiology and risk factors
  a. Hyperparathyroidism (hypercalcemia)
    i. Primary hyperparathyroidism: Increased secretion of PTH resulting from a benign neoplasm or adenoma (80% of cases)
    ii. Secondary hyperparathyroidism: Compensatory response to hypocalcemia caused by chronic renal failure, osteomalacia, or intestinal malabsorption syndromes
    iii. Humoral hypercalcemia of malignancy: Squamous cell carcinomas of the lung, head, and neck; hypernephroma; ovarian cancers secrete a PTH-like peptide
  b. Hypoparathyroidism: Inadequate PTH with hypocalcemia
    i. Congenital absence of parathyroid glands
    ii. Parathyroidectomy or damage to the parathyroid glands during thyroidectomy or radical neck surgery
    iii. Autoimmune disorder
    iv. Hypomagnesemia: Interferes with PTH secretion

3. Signs and symptoms: See Chapter 5

4. Diagnostic study findings: Include measurement of intact PTH levels, vitamin D levels, and levels of total and ionic calcium, phosphorus, magnesium, and urinary cAMP

5. Goals of care: See Chapter 5

6. Collaborating professionals on health care team: See Chapter 5

7. Management of patient care (see also Chapter 5)
  a. Hypercalcemia
    i. Acute hypercalcemia: Interventions include hydration and administration of furosemide

    ii. Humoral hypercalcemia of malignancy: Treatment may include administration of calcitonin, glucocorticoids, diphosphonates, or mithramycin and diuretics

  b. Hypocalcemia: Interventions include administration of calcium, vitamin D, magnesium

Acute Adrenal Insufficiency (Addisonian Crisis)

1. **Pathophysiology:** Deficiency of cortisol production with electrolyte and fluid abnormalities that result in life-threatening cardiovascular collapse
2. **Etiology and risk factors**
   a. Acute injury to or infection of the adrenal glands
   b. Critical illness in a patient with chronic adrenal insufficiency
   c. Abrupt cessation of corticosteroid therapy
   d. Current or past corticosteroid use of 20 mg of hydrocortisone or its equivalent for longer than 7 to 10 days has the potential for suppressing the hypothalamic-pituitary-adrenal axis. Recovery may take 2 to 12 months or longer.
   e. Adrenal hemorrhage may occur with anticoagulant therapy
   f. Ketoconazole and etomidate can interfere with steroid biosynthesis
   g. Rifampin increases the metabolic clearance rate of corticosteroids
   h. Often seen in patients with human immunodeficiency virus infection
3. **Signs and symptoms**
   a. Confusion, altered mental status
   b. Vomiting
   c. Petechiae
   d. Hyperpigmentation (chronic insufficiency): "Bronze diabetes"
   e. Tachycardia, severe hypotension, vascular collapse
4. **Diagnostic study findings**
   a. Hyponatremia, hyperkalemia, hypercalcemia
   b. Hypoglycemia (more severe in children than in adults)
   c. Azotemia
   d. Eosinophilia
   e. Fever
   f. ACTH stimulation test will confirm the diagnosis
5. **Goals of care**
   a. Blood pressure and tissue perfusion are maintained
   b. Cortisol levels are restored
6. **Collaborating professionals on health care team**
   a. Nurse
   b. Physician, consulting physician
   c. Respiratory therapist
7. **Management of patient care**
   a. Anticipated patient trajectory: If the precipitating event is avoidable (e.g., abrupt withdrawal of steroid use), symptoms will not recur. Any patient requiring continued steroid use will need close monitoring; physiologic stress (illness, surgery) may require increased dosage or cause inadvertent discontinuation of steroid use. Abrupt withdrawal or unmet increased demand will increase symptoms throughout the course of recovery and discharge. Patients with acute adrenal insufficiency may be expected to have needs in the following areas:
      i. Pharmacology
         (a) Rapid administration of IV fluids and electrolytes (usually 0.9% NaCl)
         (b) Hormone replacement

(1) Glucocorticoid (hydrocortisone)

(2) Mineralocorticoid (fludrocortisone)

   ii. Treatments: Monitor heart rate and rhythm

 b. Potential complications

   i. Cardiovascular collapse

     (a) Mechanism: Related to ACTH deficiency

     (b) Management: CPR, inotropic support, fluid administration

8. Evaluation of patient care

 a. Stable vital signs

 b. Electrolyte and fluid balance parameters within normal limits

 c. Normal cortisol levels

Diabetic Ketoacidosis

1. Pathophysiology: Diabetic ketoacidosis (DKA) is the most serious metabolic complication of insulin-dependent, or type 1, diabetes mellitus. DKA is a state of insulin deficiency combined with an increase in the level of insulin-antagonistic hormones (glucagons, cortisol, catecholamines, and GH). The result is altered metabolism of carbohydrate, fat, and protein (Figure 6-2) and hyperglycemia.

 a. Decreased insulin level with gluconeogenesis and increased insulin resistance result in exaggerated hepatic glucose production

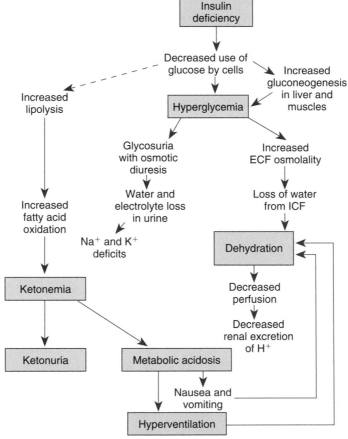

FIGURE 6-2 ■ Pathophysiology of acidosis in diabetes mellitus. *ECF,* Extracellular fluid; *ICF,* intracellular fluid. (From Hockenberry M: *Wong's nursing care of infants and children,* ed 7, St Louis, 2003, Mosby, p. 1735.)

    b. Ketosis and metabolic acidosis result from increased synthesis of ketones and lactic acidosis

    c. Fluid and electrolyte imbalance and osmotic diuresis are caused by glycosuria; accompanied by loss of sodium, potassium, and chloride

    d. Altered mental status results from hyperosmolality, cellular dehydration, acidosis, and possibly impaired oxygen dissociation, because glycosylated hemoglobin binds oxygen more tightly

2. Etiology and risk factors

    a. Diagnosed diabetes mellitus

        i. Insufficient exogenous insulin: Dose missed or insufficient for needs

        ii. Infection or trauma

        iii. Poor compliance with established self-care regimen

            (a) Alcohol or drug use

            (b) Educational deficits

            (c) Psychosocial distress or disease

            (d) Adolescence

        iv. Medication side effects

            (a) Glucocorticoids increase gluconeogenesis

            (b) Thiazide diuretics, diazoxide, and phenytoin decrease insulin resistance

    b. Undiagnosed diabetes mellitus: Positive family history of diabetes

3. Signs and symptoms

    a. Blurred vision, diminished level of consciousness

    b. Nausea, abdominal cramping, vomiting

    c. Polyphagia, polyuria, polydipsia

    d. Fatigue, weakness

    e. Muscle cramps

    f. Decreased skin turgor, dry mucous membranes

    g. Fruity odor to breath (ketosis)

    h. Tachycardia, orthostatic hypotension

    i. Tachypnea, Kussmaul's respirations

4. Diagnostic study findings

    a. Elevated plasma and urine glucose levels: Plasma glucose level above 250 mg/dl; presence of glucose in urine (normal = no trace)

    b. Metabolic acidosis: Arterial pH less than 7.3; serum HCO_3^- less than 18 mEq/dl

    c. Positive results for serum and urine ketones

    d. Azotemia

    e. Anion gap: $Na^+ - (Cl^- + HCO_3^-) > 10$ (other formulas may be used)

    f. ECG: May reflect hypokalemia, although serum potassium level may be normal or elevated; flat T waves

    g. Hypocalcemia in 30% of patients

    h. Hyperosmolality

5. Goals of care

    a. Acid-base balance is restored

    b. Blood glucose level is normalized and maintained

    c. Fluid balance is restored

    d. Any infection, if present, is resolved

6. Collaborating professionals on health care team

    a. Nurse

    b. Physician, consulting physician

    c. Diabetes educator or diabetes case manager

    d. Dietitian

7. **Management of patient care**
   a. Anticipated patient trajectory: DKA can reoccur easily in diabetic patients if medication compliance, diet, and sick-day management are not well understood. Reoccurrence is most common in teens and patients with newly diagnosed diabetes. Patients with DKA may have needs in the following areas:
      i. Discharge planning
         (a) For patients with newly diagnosed diabetes: Education about the disease, pathophysiology, and self-care management
         (b) For patients with previously diagnosed diabetes: Education about the self-care regimen, compliance, and sick-day management
      ii. Pharmacology
         (a) Administer IV fluids to correct dehydration based on *corrected* sodium
            (1) Corrected Na^+ = Measured serum Na^+ + {[(Serum glucose in mg/dl − 100)/100] × 1.6}
            (2) 0.9% NaCl is recommended if the corrected Na^+ level is low
            (3) 0.45% NaCl is recommended if the corrected Na^+ level is normal or high
            (4) 5% dextrose added to prevent hypoglycemia when the glucose level is less than 250 mg/dl
         (b) Administer regular insulin via IV bolus then continuous drip
            (1) Change to SQ insulin 1 to 2 hours before stopping the drip to prevent the recurrence of ketosis and accelerated hyperglycemia
            (2) Monitor the serum glucose level hourly
            (3) Measure urine ketone levels (insulin infusion may be stopped if the patient stops excreting ketones)
            (4) Insulin infusion is usually stopped when the serum glucose level is less than 250 mg/dl
         (c) Administer sodium bicarbonate if the pH is less than 7.0
            (1) Goal is cerebral and myocardial protection
            (2) Monitor ABG levels
         (d) Administer antibiotics if infection is present
      iii. Psychosocial issues
         (a) For patients with newly diagnosed diabetes: Major lifestyle changes required
         (b) For patients with preexisting diabetes: Must address noncompliance and poor compliance with the medical regimen
      iv. Treatments
         (a) Assess respiratory and neurologic status (a decline may signal cerebral edema)
         (b) Monitor electrolyte levels while acidosis and volume deficits are being corrected (K^+, Na^+, PO_4^-)
         (c) Monitor liver enzyme levels
         (d) Record I&O, daily weights
   b. Potential complications
      i. Metabolic acidosis
         (a) Mechanism: Ketosis secondary to insulin deficiency and stress hormone excess
         (b) Management: Administration of insulin and sodium bicarbonate as needed
      ii. Hyperglycemia
         (a) Mechanism: Secondary to insulin deficiency, ketosis, stress hormone excess, infection

(b) Management: Insulin administration with reduction of serum glucose levels at rates not to exceed 100 mg/dl/hr

iii. Dehydration

(a) Mechanism: Due to osmotic diuresis induced by hyperglycemia; deficit worsened by vomiting and/or inadequate oral intake

(b) Management: Fluid replacement

iv. Hypoglycemia

(a) Mechanism: Secondary to insulin therapy and a decrease in levels of circulating insulin-antagonist hormones (blood glucose level <50 mg/dl); hypoglycemia can precipitate dysrhythmias, extend infarcts

(b) Management: Requires administration of a rapid-acting carbohydrate, 50% dextrose IV or glucose-containing solution orally if consciousness is not depressed

8. **Evaluation of patient care**

a. Acid-base and potassium levels within normal limits

b. Normal anion gap

c. Blood glucose level stabilized at 150 to 200 mg/dl with no episodes of hypoglycemia

d. Absence of ketosis

e. Restoration of fluid balance as evidenced by I&O, laboratory values, and cardiovascular stability

f. Resolution of any infection

g. If the diabetes is newly diagnosed, referral of the patient for diabetic management teaching

h. If the diabetes is preexisting, ability of the patient to identify precipitating factors and to modify self-care management as needed

Hyperglycemic, Hyperosmolar Nonketotic Coma (Hyperglycemic, Nonacidotic Diabetic Coma)

1. **Pathophysiology:** Life-threatening hyperglycemic emergency accompanied by hyperosmolality, severe dehydration, and alterations in neurologic status without ketosis. Pathophysiologic processes (Figure 6-3) include the following:

a. Relative insulin deficiency that impairs glucose transport across the cell membrane. There may be sufficient insulin present to inhibit lipolysis or ketogenesis in the liver but not enough to control hyperglycemia. Not uncommon for some ketosis to be present, but pH is rarely lower than 7.3.

b. Hyperosmolality resulting from hyperglycemia and hypernatremia may impair insulin secretion, promote insulin resistance, and inhibit free fatty acid release from adipose tissue

c. Fluid shifts from intracellular to extracellular space to offset hyperosmolality

d. Osmotic diuresis caused by hyperglycemia results in extracellular fluid volume depletion; fluid deficits usually are greater than those seen in DKA

e. Severe electrolyte losses (sodium, chloride, phosphate, magnesium, potassium) occur with osmotic diuresis

f. Volume depletion compromises glomerular filtration, diminishing urinary escape of glucose

g. Coma results from cellular dehydration

2. **Etiology and risk factors**

a. Inadequate insulin secretion and/or action (newly diagnosed type 2, or non–insulin-dependent, diabetes)

b. Advanced age and severe dehydration (majority of patients)

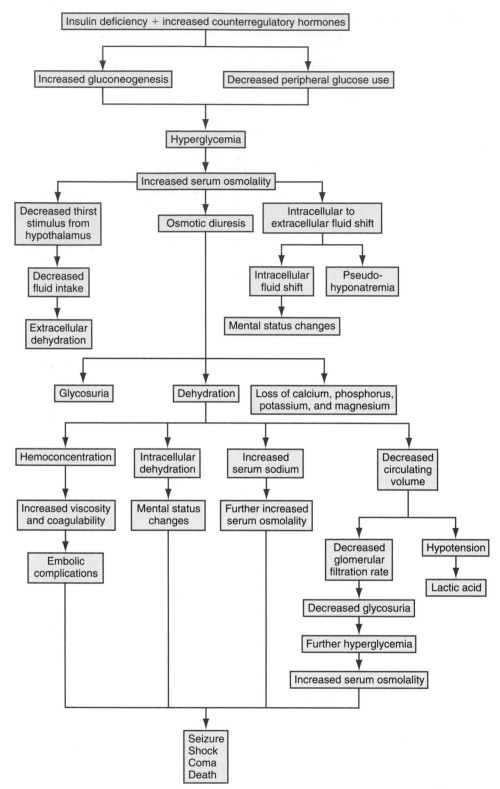

FIGURE 6-3 ■ Hyperosmolar, hyperglycemic nonketotic syndrome. (From Jakubauskas K: Hyperosmolar hyperglycemic nonketotic coma, *AACN News*, pp 14–17, May 2001.)

    c. Concomitant illness that increases glucose production or contributes to dehydration, including sepsis, pancreatitis, stroke, uremia, burns, myocardial infarction, and gastrointestinal hemorrhage

    d. Lack of ready access to fluids or inability to recognize or express the need for fluids

    e. Use of insulin or oral hypoglycemic, disruption of an established medication regimen

    f. Use of medications known to elevate glucose levels and/or resist insulin action, including corticosteroids, thiazide diuretics, phenytoin, sympathomimetics

    g. Preadmission medication regimen that suggests cardiovascular or renal disease; crisis is more common in late-middle-aged patients and in elderly patients with preexisting renal or cardiovascular disease

3. **Signs and symptoms**

    a. Lethargy, fatigue, coma

    b. Polydipsia, polyuria, polyphagia

    c. Flushed skin and dry mucous membranes

    d. Tachycardia, hypotension

    e. Shallow, rapid respirations

4. **Diagnostic study findings**

    a. Severely elevated glucose levels (>1000 mg/dl)

    b. No ketosis

    c. Sodium and potassium levels vary with the state of hydration; often severely depleted as a result of osmotic diuresis; hypokalemia necessitates potassium replacement

    d. Plasma hyperosmolality (>330 mOsm/kg)

    e. Acidosis, if present, usually caused by lactic acid or renal dysfunction

5. **Goals of care**

    a. Dehydration is corrected

    b. Hyperglycemia is corrected

    c. Peripheral tissue perfusion is restored

6. **Collaborating professionals on health care team**

    a. Nurse

    b. Physician, consulting physician

    c. Diabetes educator

    d. Home care coordinator or discharge planner

7. **Management of patient care**

    a. Anticipated patient trajectory: Hyperglycemic, hyperosmolar nonketotic coma (HHNKC) can develop rapidly in an elderly patient with type 2 diabetes who becomes ill and then dehydrated. These patients will require aggressive sick-day management to prevent recurrence. Throughout their course of recovery and discharge, patients with HHNKC may be expected to have needs in the following areas:

        i. Pharmacology

           (a) Fluid replacement with 0.9% NaCl

           (b) IV insulin via infusion to correct hyperglycemia

        ii. Treatments

           (a) Hourly serum glucose monitoring

           (b) Strict management and recording of I&O

    b. Potential complications

        i. Heart failure

           (a) Mechanism: Many of these patients are elderly or have preexisting heart disease. Rapid fluid replacement to treat severe fluid deficits may result in heart failure. The patient may require placement of a central venous catheter or pulmonary artery catheter.

(b) Management: Provide inotropic support, administer diuretics, oxygen

ii. Hypoglycemia

(a) Mechanism: As hyperglycemia resolves, the serum glucose level must be closely monitored to avoid hypoglycemia

(b) Management: Stop insulin administration; give IV glucose if the patient is conscious or PO glucose (orange juice) if tolerated

iii. Thromboembolic event

(a) Mechanism: Dehydration causes diminished tissue perfusion, hyperviscosity, and increased platelet activity, and thereby increases the risk of thrombus formation

(b) Management

(1) Assess for decreased pulses, pallor in extremities, decreased blood pressure

(2) Assess for and report localized redness, swelling, tenderness, or increased warmth

(3) Replace fluids

(4) Have the patient perform active or passive range-of-motion exercises

8. **Evaluation of patient care**

a. Blood pressure stable at baseline

b. No evidence of heart failure (edema, crackles, weight gain)

c. Maintenance of blood glucose levels within normal limits

d. No evidence of thrombus formation or embolization

e. Correction of the underlying cause that precipitated the crisis

Hypoglycemic Episode

1. **Pathophysiology:** Decrease in serum glucose level to 50 mg/dl or below. Glucose production (feeding and/or liver gluconeogenesis) lags behind glucose use. May be caused by decreased clearance of insulin or oral hypoglycemia agents or by drug interactions.

2. **Etiology and risk factors**

a. Insulin therapy

i. Insulin dose greater than the body's current needs

ii. Sudden rotation of injection sites from a hypertrophied area to one with unimpaired absorption

iii. Interruption of enteral tube feedings

b. Oral hypoglycemic therapy, especially with sulfonylurea agents

c. Insufficient caloric consumption—a meal or snack missed or delayed or intake compromised due to nausea, vomiting, or anorexia

d. Strenuous physical exercise that is not compensated by increased food intake or decreased dose of insulin

e. Potentiation of hypoglycemic medications

i. Renal insufficiency (decreased creatinine clearance)

ii. Use of medications that potentiate the action of the sulfonylureas (phenylbutazone, large doses of salicylates, sulfonamides)

f. Excessive alcohol intake, which inhibits gluconeogenesis

g. Decreased requirements for exogenous insulin resulting from

i. Recovery from physiologic stress, which decreases the levels of insulin-antagonistic hormones and thus decreases the need for insulin

      ii. Weight loss, which decreases insulin resistance

      iii. Immediate postpartum period: Sudden reduction in antiinsulin effects of placental hormones

      iv. Decrease in steroid dose

    h. Use of pentamidine to treat *Pneumocystis carinii* infection, which is associated with pancreatic islet cell necrosis with resultant acute increase in insulin release

    i. Presence of other health problems (e.g., severe liver disease, pancreatic islet cell tumor)

    j. Use of regular insulin can be associated with a rapid fall in glucose levels and may prompt more adrenomedullary symptoms. Use of intermediate-acting insulins or continuous insulin infusion devices may result in a more gradual drop in plasma glucose level and thus may produce central nervous system symptoms (neuroglycopenia).

    k. Patients taking β-adrenergic blocking agents (e.g., propranolol) may not exhibit adrenomedullary symptoms; the use of β-adrenergic blocking agents can also impair recovery from hypoglycemia by inhibiting glycogenolysis

3. Signs and symptoms

    a. Headache, fatigue, irritability

    b. Pallor

    c. Hunger

4. Diagnostic study findings: Serum glucose levels lower than 50 mg/dl

5. Goals of care: Hypoglycemia and its sequelae are corrected

6. Collaborating professionals on health care team

    a. Nurse

    b. Physician

    c. Diabetes educator

7. Management of patient care

    a. Anticipated patient trajectory: Hypoglycemia is a potential complication with a high likelihood of recurrence in patients in whom diabetes has been newly diagnosed or in whom an insulin-food-activity balance either has not been achieved or has been disrupted. Throughout their recovery and discharge, patients with hypoglycemia may be expected to have needs in the following areas:

      i. Pharmacology

        (a) Administer oral or IV glucose

          (1) Remeasure serum glucose level 20 to 30 minutes after treatment

          (2) Readminister glucose, if needed

          (3) Discontinue insulin infusion if present

    b. Potential complications

      i. Seizures

        (a) Mechanism: Due to hypoglycemia

        (b) Management: Administer IV glucose; protect the patient from injury

      ii. Dysrhythmias

        (a) Mechanism: Secondary to hypoglycemia; important to note that hypoglycemia has the potential to extend infarcts

        (b) Management: Administer oral or IV glucose and antiarrhythmic agent per advanced cardiac life support (ACLS) protocols

8. Evaluation of patient care

    a. Maintenance of serum glucose level at 80 to 110 mg/dl

    b. No subjective or objective evidence of hypoglycemia

    c. Patient use of medical alert identification indicating diabetes mellitus

REFERENCES

Physiologic Anatomy

Berne R, Levy M, Koeppen B, Stanton B: *Physiology*, ed 5, St Louis, 2003, Mosby, chaps 45–51.

Larsen P, Kronenberg H, Melmed S, Polonsky K: *Williams textbook of endocrinology*, ed 10, Philadelphia, 2003, Saunders.

LiVolsi V, Asa S: *Endocrine pathology*, Edinburgh, 2002, Churchill Livingstone.

Patient Assessment

Dirksen S, Lewis S, Collier I: *Clinical companion to medical-surgical nursing*, ed 3, St Louis, 2004, Mosby.

Diabetes Insipidus

Bichet DG: Nephrogenic diabetes insipidus, *Am J Med* 105:431–442, 1998.

Diabetes Insipidus Foundation: Welcome to the water world of diabetes insipidus: "a different diabetes!", 2003, retrieved May 17, 2005, from http://www.diabetesinsipidus.org.

Knoers N, Monnens LL: Nephrogenic diabetes insipidus, *Semin Nephrol* 19:344–352, 1999.

Morello J, Bichet DG: Nephrogenic diabetes insipidus, *Annu Rev Physiol* 63:607–630, 2001.

Syndrome of Inappropriate Antidiuretic Hormone Secretion

Adroque HJ, Madias NE: Hyponatremia, *N Engl J Med* 342:1581–1589, 2000.

Martin AJ: Hyponatremia, *N Engl J Med* 343(12):886, 2000.

Terpstra TL: Syndrome of inappropriate antidiuretic hormone secretion: recognition and management, *Medsurg Nurs* 9(2): 61–70, 2000.

Thyrotoxicosis, Myxedema Coma

Cooper DS: Hyperthyroidism, *Lancet* 362 (9382):459–468, 2003.

Diez JJ: Hyperthyroidism in patients older than 55 years: an analysis of the etiology and management, *Gerontology* 49(5):316–323, 2003.

Fliers E, Wiersinga W: Myxedema coma, *Rev Endocr Metab Disord* 4(2):137–141, 2003.

Franklyn J: Thyrotoxicosis, *Clin Med* 3(1): 11–15, 2003.

Holcomb SS: Thyroid diseases: a primer for the critical care nurse, *Dimens Crit Care Nurs* 21(4):127–133, 2002.

Roffi M, Cattaneo F, Topol EJ: Thyrotoxicosis and the cardiovascular system: subtle but serious effects, *Cleve Clin J Med* 70(1):57–63, 2003.

Sarlis NJ, Gourgiotis L: Thyroid emergencies, *Rev Endocr Metab Disord* 4(2):129–136, 2003.

Hypoparathyroidism and Hyperparathyroidism

Levine MA, Germain-Lee E, Jan DeBeur S: Genetic basis for resistance to parathyroid hormone, *Horm Res* 60(suppl 3):87–95, 2003.

Sosa JA, Udelsman R: New directions in the treatment of patients with primary hyperparathyroidism, *Curr Probl Surg* 40(12): 812–849, 2003.

Thakker RV: Genetic development in hypoparathyroidism, *Lancet* 357(9261):974–976, 2001.

Acute Adrenal Insufficiency

Arlt W, Allolio B: Adrenal insufficiency, *Lancet* 361(19372):1881–1893, 2003.

Bloomfield R, MacMillan M, Noble DW: Corticosteroid insufficiency in acutely ill patients, *N Engl J Med* 348(21):2157–2159, 2003.

Nieman LK: Dynamic evaluation of adrenal hypofunction, *J Endocrinol Invest* 26(7 suppl): 74–82, 2003.

Marik PE, Zalooga GP: Adrenal insufficiency in the critically ill: a new look at an old problem, *Chest* 122(5):1784–1796, 2002.

Diabetic Ketoacidosis; Hyperglycemic, Hyperosmolar Nonketotic Coma; Hypoglycemia

American Diabetes Association: Position statement: hyperglycemic crisis in patients with diabetes mellitus, *Diabetes Care* 25(suppl 1):S100–S108, 2002.

Buse J: Evolution in the American Diabetes Association Standards of Care, *Clin Diabetes* (21):24–26, 2003.

Herbel G, Boyle PJ: Hypoglycemia: pathophysiology and treatment, *Endocrinol Metab Clin North Am* 29(4):725–743, 2000.

Kaufman FR: Type I diabetes mellitus, *Pediatr Rev* 24(9):291–300, 2003.

Neu A, Willasch A, Ehehalt S, et al: Ketoacidosis at onset of type 1 diabetes mellitus in children: frequency and clinical presentation, *Pediatr Diabetes* 4(2):77–81, 2003.

White NH: Management of diabetic ketoacidosis, *Rev Endocr Metab Disord* 4(4):343–353, 2003.

Hematologic and Immunologic Systems

DENNIS J. CHEEK, RN, PhD, FAHA
MARY A. HALL, RN, MSN

SYSTEMWIDE ELEMENTS

Physiologic Anatomy

1. **Hematologic system**
   a. Anatomic structures
      i. Bone marrow
         (a) Spongy center of the bones where the hematologic and immunologic cell lines originate and mature before being released into the circulation
         (b) Present throughout the bones of the body, although the majority of the cells are produced in the vertebrae, ribs, sternum, pelvis, and proximal epiphyses of the femur and humerus
      ii. Liver
         (a) Located in the upper right quadrant of the abdomen in the peritoneal space below the diaphragm and under the rib cage. The liver receives 27% of the resting cardiac output—approximately 1350 ml of blood flow each minute—via the hepatic artery and portal vein.
         (b) Synthesizes various plasma proteins, including clotting factors and albumin. In addition, the liver clears damaged and nonfunctioning red blood cells (RBCs), or erythrocytes, from circulation.
   b. Components: See Table 7-1 and Figure 7-1
   c. Functions: See Table 7-2 and Figure 7-2
2. **Immunologic system**
   a. Anatomic structures
      i. Bone marrow (see preceding description)
      ii. Thymus
         (a) The thymus is a bilobed lymphoid organ located in the mediastinum below the thyroid. Early in life, lymphocytes released from the bone marrow migrate to the thymus, where they mature into T cells before being released into the circulation.
         (b) During fetal development and throughout the first 2 years of life, the thymus grows rapidly. After puberty the thymus slowly involutes as the circulating, long-lived T-cell population is maximized.
      iii. The lymph system is a separate vessel system that collects plasma and leukocytes that are not returned to the circulatory system from the tissue capillary beds. This lymph fluid is filtered and returned to the circulatory system, so that appropriate tissue fluid pressures are maintained and edema

■ **TABLE 7-1**
■ ■ **Components of the Hematologic System**

Component	Description
Pluripotent stem cell	The pluripotent stem cell is a self-renewing cell from which all the differentiated bone marrow cell lines derive.
	Various developmental cell lineages can be identified in the bone marrow before the mature cells are released into the circulation (Figure 7-1).
Red blood cells (RBCs)	RBCs are biconcave disk-shaped cells enveloped with a tough, flexible membrane.
	Erythropoiesis, or the production of RBCs, occurs in the bone marrow, where the pluripotent stem cell gives rise to the erythrocyte lineage, as shown in Figure 7-1. Erythropoiesis is regulated by the glycoprotein erythropoietin, which is produced primarily by the kidneys. In response to decreased oxygen levels in the blood, the kidney produces more erythropoietin, which acts on the bone marrow to increase and accelerate erythropoiesis. Iron, cobalamin (vitamin B_{12}), and folic acid are all needed for RBC production.
	RBCs have a life span of approximately 120 days, at the end of which they are filtered out of circulation by the spleen and liver. Iron released from the heme is transported by transferrin back to the bone marrow, where it is recycled to make new RBCs. The porphyrin ring of the heme is reduced to bilirubin and eliminated as bile through the intestine.
	Genetically determined antigens are located on the RBC cell membrane. The major antigens are designated A and B. On the basis of the presence or absence of these two antigens, four major blood groups are defined. Persons without a given antigen will form a naturally occurring antibody against the absent antigen shortly after birth. Rh is another type of RBC antigen that is different from A and B antigens. Persons without the Rh antigen (known as *Rh-negative* persons) form antibody against Rh only when exposed to Rh-positive blood.
	Rh-negative persons can be exposed to the Rh antigen if they receive Rh-positive blood through transfusion. An Rh-negative woman can be exposed to the Rh antigen if she delivers an Rh-positive baby.
Platelets (thrombocytes)	Platelets are nonnucleated cell fragments of megakaryocytes produced in the bone marrow (see Figure 7-1).
	Platelets activate the blood clotting system by going to sites of blood vessel or tissue injury, forming a platelet plug, and releasing cytokines that recruit more platelets and the clotting factors to the injury site.
	The life span of a platelet is approximately 10 days.
Clotting factors	Clotting factors are proteins and other substances, numbered I to XIII, that form a fibrin matrix at sites of blood vessel or tissue injury. Factors commonly referred to include the following:
	• Factor I, also known as *fibrinogen*
	• Factor II, also known as *prothrombin*
	• Factor III, also known as *tissue thromboplastin* or *tissue factor*
	• Factor IV, which is *calcium*
	• Factor V, also known as *AC-globulin*
	• Factor VII, also known as *prothrombin conversion accelerator* or *proconvertin*
	• Factor VIII, also known as *antihemophilic factor*
	• Factor IX, also known as *Christmas factor*
	• Factor X, also known as *Stuart-Prower factor*
	• Factor XI, also known as *thromboplastin antecedent factor*
	• Factor XII, also known as *Hageman factor*
	• Factor XIII, also known as *fibrin-stabilizing factor*
Plasma	Plasma is the straw-colored fluid that carries the blood components through the circulatory system and is made up primarily of water, proteins (albumin, globulins, and fibrinogen), small amounts of nutrients, electrolytes, hormones, enzymes, and metabolites. Serum is plasma without clotting factors.

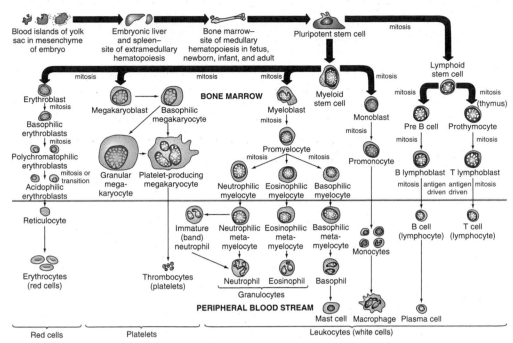

FIGURE 7-1 ■ Maturation of cells in the hematologic and immunologic systems. (From Copstead LC, Banasik JL: *Pathophysiology*, ed 3, St Louis, 2005, Mosby, p 324.)

is prevented. Lymph fluid is propelled along the system by the normal contraction of skeletal muscles.

(a) Lymph fluid is a pale yellow liquid made up of plasma, leukocytes, enzymes, and antibodies; it lacks clotting factors and thus coagulates very slowly

(b) Lymphatic capillaries and vessels are a network of open-ended tubes with one-way valves that collect lymph fluid from the tissues and eventually return it to the venous system via both the right lymphatic duct, which drains into the right subclavian vein, and the thoracic duct, which drains into the left subclavian vein

(c) Lymph nodes are small, flat, bean-shaped patches of tissue located along the length of the lymphatic system that filter microorganisms from the lymph fluid before it is returned to the bloodstream

    (1) Lymph nodes can become swollen with white blood cells (WBCs), or leukocytes, that are responding to invading microorganisms if an infectious process is occurring in the area drained by the lymph node

    (2) Lymph nodes can also become swollen with metastatic cancer cells that have migrated away from the primary site and become trapped in the network of the lymph node

  iv. The spleen is a lymphoid organ located in the upper left quadrant of the abdomen that clears damaged or nonfunctioning RBCs and filters antigens from the blood for evaluation by lymphocytes

b. Components: See Tables 7-3, 7-4, and 7-5, and Figure 7-3

c. Functions: See Table 7-6

■ **TABLE 7-2**
■ ■ **Functions of the Hematologic System**

Function	Description
Oxygenation	The red blood cells (RBCs) transport oxygen from the lungs to the tissues and carry carbon dioxide from the tissues to the lungs for excretion.
	Hemoglobin in the RBCs combines with oxygen, carbon dioxide, and nitric oxide. As hemoglobin transfers oxygen to the tissue, it also sheds small amounts of nitric oxide.
	The affinity of hemoglobin for oxygen and the mechanism by which oxygen is bound to hemoglobin in the lungs and released in the tissues is best described by the oxyhemoglobin dissociation curve (see Chapter 2).
Hemostasis	**Vascular constriction**
	Vessel spasm is initiated by endothelial cell injury caused by local and humoral mechanisms such as the release of the vasoconstrictor thromboxane A_2 from the cells and platelets as well as local myogenic contraction. The value of the vascular constriction is to reduce the blood flow and allow platelets to adhere to the exposed surfaces.
	Platelet plug
	1. Platelets then degranulate, releasing serotonin, histamine, von Willebrand factor, adenosine diphosphate, fibrinogen, and thromboxane from cell vesicles into the surrounding environment, which constricts the blood vessel further to minimize blood loss and recruits more platelets and clotting factors to the area. The coagulation cascade is initiated through mechanisms dependent on phospholipids in the platelet membrane.
	2. The platelets form an initial, unstable platelet plug.
	Coagulation
	1. At the same time the platelet plug is forming, the coagulation pathway is initiated.
	2. Two primary mechanisms activate the coagulation pathway (see Figure 7-2).
	a. The extrinsic pathway is activated after tissue trauma when factor III released from the damaged tissues comes in contact with factor VII (proconvertin) circulating in the blood.
	b. The intrinsic pathway is activated after endothelial damage when factor XII (Hageman factor) circulating in the blood comes in contact with subendothelial substances such as collagen exposed by vascular injury.
	c. Division of the coagulation process into strictly defined extrinsic and intrinsic pathways has been modified because the cascade theory has been revised. These revisions include the fact that factor VIIa of the extrinsic pathway can directly activate factor IX of the intrinsic pathway and that factor VII can be activated by factors XIIa, IXa, Xa, and thrombin (see Figure 7-2).
	3. At each step in each pathway, an inactive proenzyme is converted into an active enzyme by proteolytic cleavage. Calcium, coenzymes, or phospholipids are required for some of the reactions to proceed.
	4. The activation of the pathway results in the conversion of factor I (fibrinogen) to factor Ia (fibrin), which forms a fibrin clot; in the presence of factor XIIIa, a stabilized fibrin clot is formed.
	5. The final step of hemostasis is clot retraction, in which the formed clot expels serum. Fibrin strands shorten; become denser and stronger, approximating the edges of the injured vessel; and seal the site of injury.
	Limiting and focusing of hemostasis to sites of blood vessel damage
	1. Platelet aggregation and the coagulation cascade are normally initiated only when blood comes in contact with nonvascular tissues, which thus localizes hemostasis to sites of injury.

Continued

2. As the clot extends to areas where the blood vessel is intact, antithrombin III, a plasma protein normally circulating in the blood, inactivates thrombin. Heparin greatly improves the activity of antithrombin III.

3. The fibrin clot is eventually removed by an enzyme called *plasmin*. Damaged endothelial cells secrete a protein that converts the inactive form of plasmin, plasminogen, to its active form so that degradation of the fibrin clot can begin. Like antithrombin III, plasminogen normally circulates freely in the blood. As the fibrin clot is degraded, fibrin split products can be detected in the blood.

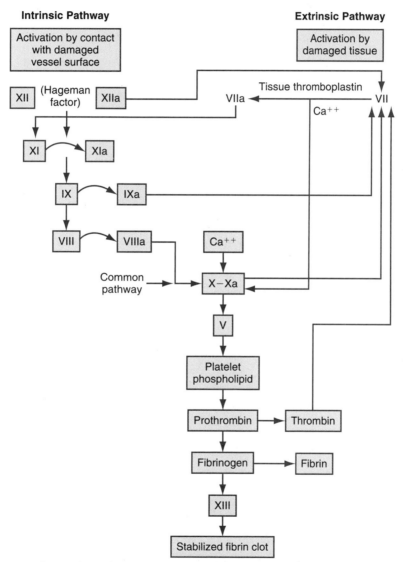

FIGURE 7-2 ■ Intrinsic and extrinsic coagulation cascades. (From McCance KL, Huether SE: *Pathophysiology: the biologic basis for disease in adults and children,* St Louis, 2002, Mosby.)

■ **TABLE 7-3**
■ ■ **Components of the Immunologic System**

Component	Description
Pluripotent stem cell	See description in Table 7-1.
White blood cells (WBCs)	WBCs circulate throughout the body, detecting and destroying bacteria, viruses, fungi, parasites, and other proteins identified as foreign to the body. The pluripotent stem cell gives rise to all WBC lineages. The different WBCs mature primarily in the bone marrow before being released into circulation (Figure 7-1). The average life span of a WBC in circulation is 12 hr.

Granulocytes or myeloid series of leukocytes

1. Neutrophils
   - Because these cells are segmented polymorphonuclear neutrophils, they are also known as *segs, PMNs, polys,* or *neuts.* Because these cells are also granulocytes, they are also known as *grans.*
   - Neutrophils are the most numerous of the WBCs. They are efficient phagocytic cells that are able to migrate through endothelial cells to sites of microbial invasion.
   - Neutrophils are often destroyed during phagocytosis. Pus is the accumulation of cellular debris from the destruction of microorganisms and neutrophils at the site of infection.
2. Monocytes
   - Monocytes and macrophages compose the mononuclear phagocyte system (MPS).
   - Monocytes are released from the bone marrow into the peripheral circulation, where they mature. When they enter the tissue, they become highly efficient phagocytic macrophages.
   - Some macrophages move throughout the body, whereas others stay in one particular tissue and are named according to where they reside. For example, Kupffer cells are liver macrophages, Langerhans cells are skin macrophages, alveolar macrophages are lung macrophages, mesangial cells are kidney macrophages, and microglial cells are central nervous system macrophages.
   - Unlike neutrophils, which are often destroyed during phagocytosis, macrophages can phagocytose many foreign antigens, surviving months to years.
3. Eosinophils
   - Eosinophils are motile phagocytic cells that combat infection with multicellular parasites. They are also associated with allergic reactions and other inflammatory processes.
4. Basophils
   - Basophils are nonphagocytic cells that attract immunoglobulin E (IgE) antibodies to their cell membranes. When the IgE binds antigen, the basophils release histamine, bradykinin, serotonin, heparin, and slowly reacting substances of anaphylaxis, triggering a massive inflammatory response.
   - Basophils are involved in various inflammatory conditions.
5. Mast cells
   - Mast cells, like basophils, attract IgE antibodies to their cell membranes. Also like basophils, mast cells release histamine, bradykinin, serotonin, heparin, and slowly reacting substances of anaphylaxis when the IgE binds antigen, triggering a massive inflammatory response.
   - Mast cells and basophils differentiate along separate pathways. Basophils circulate in the blood and survive only days, whereas mast cells are located in the tissue and live weeks or months.
   - IgE-mediated mast cell degranulation is responsible for type I hypersensitivity reactions.

Continued

6. Lymphocytes
   - B cells or B lymphocytes
     a) B cells manufacture and express antigen-binding proteins called *immunoglobulins* on their cell membranes.
     b) When the B-cell immunoglobulin binds a particular antigen, the cell is stimulated to differentiate into two separate cells called *plasma cells* and *memory B cells*.
        1) Plasma cells are antibody factories that immediately produce and secrete large amounts of antibody to bind to the antigen.
        2) Memory B cells go into a resting state but can be quickly reactivated to produce plasma cells and antibody if exposed to the same antigen in the future.
     c) Antibodies are secreted protein immunoglobulins that can bind to more of the same antigen. There are five major types of antibodies:
        1) Immunoglobulin M (IgM) is the first immunoglobulin to be secreted during the primary immune response to an antigen.
        2) Immunoglobulin G (IgG) is secreted during the secondary immune response and is more specific to a particular antigen.
        3) Immunoglobulin A (IgA) is present in secretions such as mucus and breast milk.
        4) Immunoglobulin E (IgE) attaches to the cell membranes of basophils and mast cells. When IgE binds to antigen, it triggers the cell to release histamine.
        5) Immunoglobulin D (IgD) is found primarily on the cell membrane of B lymphocytes and serves as an antigen receptor for initiating the differentiation of B cells.
   - T cells or T lymphocytes
     a) T cells mature in the thymus and recognize antigen in association with cell membrane proteins. The cell membrane proteins are known as *major histocompatibility complexes* (MHCs). There are two classes of MHC proteins (I and II) that work with different T cells as part of the immune system. Class I MHC proteins are found on all cells, whereas class II MHC proteins are found on B cells and macrophages.
     b) Helper T cells (T_H), also called *CD4 cells* because they display the membrane glycoprotein antigen CD4, recognize class II MHC molecules on the cell surface of B cells and macrophages. In response to recognition of a foreign antigen–MHC II complex, T_H cells secrete hormones, called *cytokines*, that activate other components of the immune system (see also Acquired Immunity in Table 7-6).
     c) Cytotoxic T cells (T_C), also called *CD8 cells* because they display the membrane glycoprotein CD8, recognize class I MHC molecules on the surface of cells. In response to recognition of a foreign antigen–MCH I complex, T_C cells secrete cytotoxic substances that directly destroy the cell (see also Acquired Immunity in Table 7-6).
   - Natural killer (NK) cells are a type of null (neither T nor B) lymphocyte. NK cells do not express antigen-binding receptors but do have cytotoxic capabilities against bacteria-infected and virus-infected cells as well as against tumor cells.

Complement	Complement is a group of more than 20 serum proteins, designated C1 to C9, B, and D, that act through an enzymatic cascade against invading pathogens. These proteins act sequentially and in concert to lyse microorganisms and/or infected cells.
Cytokines	Cytokines are protein hormones secreted by cells to signal other cells and play an important role in mediating the process of inflammation. As can be seen in Table 7-4, cytokines can be released from both immune and nonimmune cell types and be either proinflammatory or antiinflammatory depending on the response.

Continued

■ **TABLE 7-3**
■ ■ **Components of the Immunologic System—cont'd**

Component	Description
Eicosanoids	Eicosanoids such as prostaglandins, prostacyclin, thromboxanes, leukotrienes and hydroxyeicosatetraenoic acid (HETE) and *cis*-epoxyeicosatrienoic acid (EET) are short-lived compounds that signal cells in a paracrine fashion, some of which are listed in Table 7-5. Many commonly prescribed drugs, such as aspirin and other nonsteroidal antiinflammatory agents, inhibit eicosanoid production but, in the process, affect other physiologic processes dependent on eicosanoid regulation (Figure 7-3).

■ **TABLE 7-4**
■ ■ **Examples of Cytokines**

Cytokine	Source	Major Activities/Comments
IL-1	IL-1α: Macrophages, endothelial cells, and fibroblasts; IL-1β: NK cells, macrophages, and monocytes	Generic name for two different proteins, IL-1α and IL-1β, which are regulatory and inflammatory cytokines. Important in up- and down-regulation of acute inflammation. IL-1 is associated with bone formation, appetite regulation, and fever induction.
IL-2	Primarily from activated helper T cells	IL-2 autocrine activity $\rightarrow$ differentiation of antigen-specific cells. Paracrine activity $\rightarrow$ stimulation of B cells and NK cells.
IL-3	T cells	Enhances production of a variety of hematopoietic precursor cells, mast cells, basophils, and NK cells. Regulates differentiation and growth of many cell types.
IL-4	T cells	Stimulates proliferation of activated B and T cells, enhances the production of specific immunoglobulin subclasses, and increases cytotoxic activity of lymphocytes.
IL-5	Eosinophils, NK cells, T cells, and mast cells	Has key role in coordinating inflammatory process originating with eosinophils.
IL-6	Fibroblasts, synoviocytes, adipocytes, osteoblasts, endothelial cells, cerebral cortex neurons, neutrophils, monocytes, and eosinophils	This is the archetypal pleiotropic cytokine as evidenced by the variety of names originally given to it (e.g., interferon-$\beta2$, hepatocyte-stimulating factor, and cytotoxic T-cell differentiation factor). Has both proinflammatory and antiinflammatory action. Modulates bone resorption and induces activation of plasma cells.
IL-7	Stromal cells	Pleiotropic in regulation of helper T cells. Necessary for T-cell memory. Early B- and T-cell differentiation.
IL-8	Monocytes, lymphocytes	Chemotactic for neutrophils and basophils.
IL-9	T helper cells	Pleiotropic cytokine involved in allergic response and mast cell response.
IL-10	T cells, monocytes, and macrophages	Pleiotropic immunosuppressive and immunostimulatory cytokine. Inhibits IL-2 synthesis in helper T cells. Inhibits cytokine synthesis in monocytes. Stimulates IL-3 and IL-4 production.
IL-11	Bone marrow stroma	Involved in lymphopoiesis, thrombopoiesis, and myelopoiesis.
IL-12	Antigen-presenting cells, monocytes	Stimulates T and NK cells. Regulates cell-mediated immunity. Induces the production of interferon γ.

Continued

IL-13	T cells	IL-13 and IL-4 are pleiotropic immunoregulatory cytokines. Induces vascular cell adhesion molecule-1 on endothelial cells. Inhibits the proinflammatory gene expression of IL-1, TNF, and IL-6.
IL-14	T cells	Enhances proliferation of activated B cells, inhibits immunoglobulin synthesis, and is involved in B-cell memory.
IL-15	Monocytes, epithelial cells	Stimulates T-cell proliferation.
IL-16	Mast cells, lymphocytes	Chemotactic for monocytes and eosinophils.
IFN-α	T cells, B cells, monocytes, macrophages, and fibroblasts	Antiviral. Stimulates macrophages and NK cell activity. Has antitumor properties.
IFN-β	Mast cells	Antiviral—similar activity to IFN-α.
IFN-γ	T, NK cells	Involved in regulation of immune and inflammatory responses. Weak antiviral activity. Increases the antiviral and antitumor action of IFN-α and IFN-β. Activates macrophages.
TGF-β	Macrophages, lymphocytes, dendritic cells	TGF-β belongs to a family of TGF proteins. Pleiotropic immunoregulatory functions. Autocrine and paracrine function controls differentiation, proliferation, and level of activation of immune cells. Chemotactic for leukocytes during inflammatory response and inhibits the same cells once activated.
TNF-α	Monocytes, macrophages, T cells, B cells, fibroblasts, neutrophils, NK cells, LAK cells, endothelial cells	Paracrine and endocrine mediator of inflammation and immune system functions. B cell, T cell, macrophage, and neutrophil activity. Regulates growth and differentiation of a wide variety of cells types. Kills tumors.
TNF-β	T cells, B cells	Similar to TNF-β. Inflammation, tumor killing, and enhancement of phagocytosis.

From Rankin JA: Biological mediators of acute inflammation, *AACN Clin Issues* 15(1):6, 2004.
IFN, Interferon; *IL*, interleukin; *LAK*, lymphocyte-activated killer; *NK*, natural killer; *TGF*, transforming growth factor; *TNF*, tumor necrosis factor.

▓ TABLE 7-5
▓ ▓ Functions of Eicosanoids

Eicosanoid	Function
Prostaglandins	Cardiovascular: Vasodilation
	Pulmonary: Constriction of airways
	Gastrointestinal: Maintenance of mucosal barrier
	Endocrine: Temperature elevation
	Renal: Renin release, regulation of renal blood flow
	Genitourinary: Uterine contraction
	Hematologic: Antiplatelet aggregation
	Immunologic: Inflammatory response
Thromboxanes	Cardiovascular: Vasoconstriction
	Hematologic: Platelet aggregation
Leukotrienes	Pulmonary: Bronchial smooth muscle contraction
	Immunologic: Inflammatory response
Epoxygenase products (HETE and EET)	Vascular: HETE, potent vasoconstriction; EET, vasodilation and angiogenesis

Data from Boron W, Boulpaep EL: *Medical physiology*, Philadelphia, 2003, Saunders.
EET, *Cis*-epoxyeicosatrienoic acid; *HETE*, hydroxyeicosatetraenoic acid.

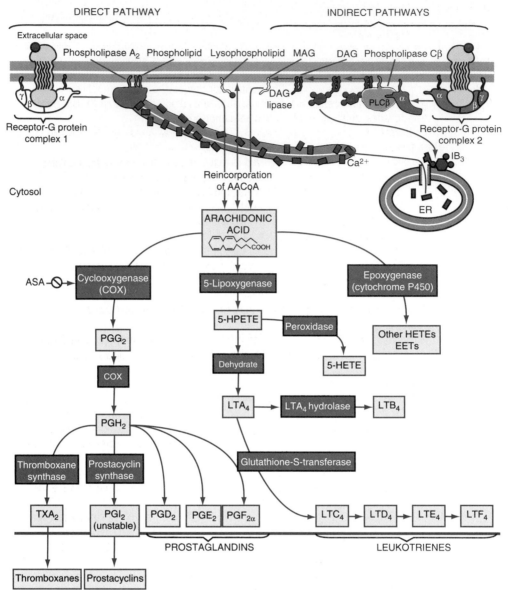

FIGURE 7-3 ■ Eicosanoid production. *AACoA,* Acetoacetyl coenzyme A; *ASA,* acetylsalicylic acid; *DAG,* diacylglycerol; *ER,* endoplasmic reticulum; *EET, cis*-epoxyeicosatrienoic acid; *HETE,* hydroxyeicosatetraenoic acid; *5-HETE,* 5-hydroxyeicosatetraenoic acid; *5-HPETE,* 5-hydroperoxyeicosatetraenoic acid; *IP₃,* inositol 1,4,5-triphosphate; *LTA₄, LTB₄, LTC₄, LTD₄, LTE₄, LTF₄,* leukotriene A₄, B₄ C₄, D₄, E₄, F₄; *MAG,* monoacylglycerol; *PGD₂, PGE₂, PGF₂ₐ, PGG₂, PGH₂, PGI₂,* prostaglandin D₂, E₂, F₂, G₂, H₂, I₂; *PLCβ,* phospholipase Cβ; *TXA₂,* thromboxane A₂. (From Boron W, Boulpaep EL: *Medical physiology,* Philadelphia, 2003, Saunders.)

■ **TABLE 7-6**
■ ■ **Functions of the Immunologic System**

Function	Description

Innate immunity	**Anatomic and physiologic barriers**
	1. Mechanical barrier of the skin and mucosa
	2. Acid pH on the skin and in the stomach
	3. Flushing or mechanical removal of pathogens (e.g., bladder emptying, gastrointestinal motility, coughing and sneezing, ciliary activity)
	4. Mucous secretions (e.g., saliva, tears) that contain enzymes and immunoglobulin A
	Inflammation
	1. The hallmarks of inflammation are rubor (erythema), tumor (edema), calor (heat), and dolor (pain) that occur as a result of the following:
	  a. Vasodilation of the capillary bed in the affected area
	  b. Increased capillary permeability, which allows fluid and immune competent cells into the area
	  c. An influx of phagocytic cells to attack microorganisms
	2. The eicosanoids thromboxane and leukotriene are potent mediators of inflammation that increase the migration of inflammatory cells to the area and increase capillary permeability.
	Phagocytosis
	1. Neutrophils and macrophages are capable of ingesting and digesting antigens such as microorganisms, dead cells, and cellular debris.
	2. Inside the phagocytic cell, lysozymes break down antigens, recycling usable products and displaying antigenic protein pieces on their class II major histocompatibility complex (MHC) molecule for evaluation by T cells.
	Complement pathway
	1. The classical complement pathway is the major effector of the humoral branch of the immune response. The trigger for the classical pathway is either immunoglobulin G or immunoglobulin M (IgM) bound to antigen. Binding of antibody to antigen exposes a site on the antibody that is a binding site for the first complement component, C1. The alternative complement pathway does not require antibody for activation. A variety of antigens such as bacteria lipopolysaccharide and components of viruses and other pathogens have the ability to activate this pathway.
	2. The complement pathway acts against invading pathogens by inducing inflammation, attracting neutrophils and monocytes, promoting phagocytosis, and building a membrane attack complex (MAC), which makes a hole in the microorganism's cell membrane and thereby kills it.

Acquired immunity	**Humoral or antibody-mediated immunity** is aimed primarily at extracellular microorganisms and is also responsible for immediate hypersensitivity reactions.
	1. Immunoglobulins on B cells bind antigen on the cell surface. The B cells internally process the antigen-antibody complex, redisplaying the antigen on the B cell's surface on a class II MHC molecule.
	2. A helper T CD4 cell then binds the antigen displayed on the class II MHC molecule of the B cell and, recognizing it as foreign, secretes cytokines that stimulate the B cell to both secrete IgM and differentiate into antibody-secreting plasma cells and memory B cells.
	3. When antibody binds to an antigen, it does not actually destroy the antigen, but it facilitates its neutralization, elimination, or destruction in the following ways:
	  a. Neutralization or binding of the antigen so that the function of the antigen is disrupted until the antigen can be phagocytized
	  b. Opsonization or coating of the invading microorganism so that it can be easily recognized as foreign and phagocytized
	  c. Activation of complement, which lyses the invader's cell membrane

Continued

■ **TABLE 7-6**
■ ■ **Functions of the Immunologic System—cont'd**

Function	Description
	Cell-mediated or T-cell immunity is aimed primarily at intracellular microorganisms, viruses, and cancer and is also responsible for delayed hypersensitivity reactions and transplanted tissue rejection. When cytotoxic T (T_C) CD8 cells recognize foreign antigen on a cell's surface on class I MHC molecules, the T_C cell secretes cytotoxic substances that destroy the foreign cell. This is particularly important in eliminating virus-infected cells, tumor cells, and cells of a transplanted tissue graft.
Tolerance	In addition to recognizing foreign antigens and initiating an immunologic response, the immune system must also be able to recognize its own proteins and not mount an immune response against self.
	This process of self-recognition occurs as part of normal neonatal growth and development.
	Autoimmune diseases occur when there is a breakdown of tolerance in which the immune system identifies its own proteins as foreign and inappropriately mounts a response to destroy these self proteins.
	Examples of autoimmune diseases include systemic lupus erythematosus, rheumatoid arthritis, acute rheumatic fever, Graves' disease, Hashimoto's thyroiditis, and type 1 diabetes mellitus.
Hypersensitivity reactions	Hypersensitivity reactions, or allergies, are exaggerated immune responses that can be uncomfortable and potentially harmful to the individual.
	There are four types of hypersensitivity reactions, classified according to the time between the exposure and the reaction, the immune mechanism involved, and the site of reaction.
	Hypersensitivity reactions to drugs, or drug allergies, are one of many possible adverse drug reactions. Drug-induced hypersensitivity reactions can be any of the four types of hypersensitivity reaction. See Anaphylactic Hypersensitivity Reactions under Patient Health Problems in text.

Patient Assessment

1. Nursing history
   a. Patient health history
       i. Many times a hematologic or immunologic problem is identified when the patent seeks medical attention for some other reason
       ii. Elements of the medical history indicating a potential or existing hematologic or immunologic problem include the following:
           (a) Recent, recurrent, or chronic infections
           (b) Cancer or prior treatment for cancer
           (c) Human immunodeficiency virus (HIV) infection
           (d) Liver disorder
           (e) Kidney disorder
           (f) Malabsorption disorder
           (g) Any prolonged bleeding or delayed healing with prior surgeries and/or dental extractions
           (h) Receipt of a blood transfusion
           (i) Splenectomy
           (j) Placement of a prosthetic heart valve
           (k) Placement of an indwelling venous access device, which indicates that the patient needed long-term venous access

    iii. Review of systems with the patient and/or family for signs and symptoms

      (a) General: Fatigue, weakness, lethargy, malaise, fever, chills, night sweats, dyspnea, restlessness, apprehension, pain, altered mental status, vertigo, dizziness, confusion

      (b) Skin: Pruritus, change in skin color, rash, unusual bruising, ulcers or other lesions

      (c) Head and neck: Headache, change in vision, sinus pain, epistaxis, gingival bleeding, sore throat, pain with swallowing, enlarged lymph nodes

      (d) Respiratory: Cough, hemoptysis, dyspnea, orthopnea

      (e) Cardiovascular: Palpitations, dizziness with position changes

      (f) Gastrointestinal: Change in eating habits, anorexia, abdominal fullness, nausea, vomiting, hematemesis, change in bowel habits, hematochezia, melena, pain with defecation, change in weight

      (g) Genitourinary: Hematuria, pain with urination, menorrhagia, enlarged inguinal lymph nodes

      (h) Musculoskeletal: Swelling of joints, tenderness or pain in the bones or joints

      (i) Endocrine: Heat or cold intolerance

b. Family history indicating a potential hematologic or immunologic problem: Hemophilia, sickle cell anemia, cancer, or death of a relative at a young age for reasons other than trauma

c. Social history and habits that may assist with the diagnosis and treatment of the underlying condition, including the following:

    i. Any unusual or excessive exposure to chemicals (e.g., gasoline, benzene, solvents, glues, paints, varnishes) or radiation (e.g., x-rays) at work or in pursuit of a hobby

    ii. Any unusual dietary preferences, pica

    iii. Excessive alcohol consumption

    iv. Sexual preference, number of partners, history of sexually transmitted diseases, current contraceptive method, use of safe sex practices

    v. Intravenous (IV) drug use

d. Medication history

    i. Current medications or a recent change in medication may suggest an underlying hematologic or immunologic problem. Always ask about over-the-counter medication use, because many of these preparations contain aspirin or nonsteroidal antiinflammatory drugs (NSAIDs).

    ii. Many medications used to treat nonhematologic and nonimmunologic problems can affect the hematologic and immunologic systems; examples of these drugs are the following:

      (a) Analgesics and antiinflammatory drugs

        (1) Aspirin and aspirin-containing drugs, such as

          a) Oxycodone and aspirin (Percodan)

          b) Bismuth subsalicylate (Pepto-Bismol)

        (2) NSAIDs, such as

          a) Ibuprofen (Motrin)

          b) Indomethacin (Indocin)

          c) Ketoprofen (Orudis)

          d) Ketorolac (Toradol)

          e) Sulindac (Clinoril)

        (3) Steroids, such as

          a) Dexamethasone (Decadron)

          b) Prednisone

(b) Antibiotics, such as
   (1) Chloramphenicol (Chloromycetin)
   (2) Isoniazid (INH)
   (3) Paraaminosalicylic acid (PAS)
   (4) Penicillin
   (5) Streptomycin
   (6) Trimethoprim-sulfamethoxazole (TMP-SMX, Bactrim, Septra)
   (7) Zidovudine (AZT, Retrovir)
(c) Anticoagulants, such as
   (1) Heparin
   (2) Warfarin (Coumadin)
(d) Anticonvulsants, such as
   (1) Carbamazepine (Tegretol)
   (2) Phenytoin (Dilantin)
(e) Antidiabetic agents, such as chlorpropamide
(f) Antineoplastic chemotherapy agents, such as
   (1) Cyclophosphamide (Cytoxan)
   (2) Cytosine arabinoside (ara-C)
   (3) Daunorubicin (daunomycin)
   (4) Doxorubicin (Adriamycin)
   (5) Etoposide (VP-16)
   (6) Hydroxyurea (Hydrea)
   (7) Methotrexate
   (8) Nitrogen mustard
   (9) Paclitaxel (Taxol)
   (10) Vinblastine (Velban)
(g) Antipsychotic agents, such as clozapine (Clozaril)
(h) Antirheumatic agents, such as
   (1) Gold
   (2) Methotrexate
(i) Cardiovascular agents, such as
   (1) Digoxin
   (2) Methyldopa (Aldomet)
   (3) Procainamide (Pronestyl)
   (4) Quinidine sulfate
(j) Diuretics, such as chlorothiazide (Diuril)
(k) Hormones, such as
   (1) Estrogens
   (2) Androgens
(l) Immunosuppressives, such as
   (1) Azathioprine (Imuran)
   (2) Cyclophosphamide
   (3) Cyclosporine
   (4) Methotrexate
   (5) Vincristine (Oncovin)
(m) Oral contraceptives
2. Nursing examination of patient
  a. Physical examination data
    i. Inspection
     (a) Temperature: Exceeds 101° F (38.3° C)
     (b) Skin: Pallor, jaundice, flushing, rash, petechiae, purpura, ecchymoses, hematomas, urticaria, integrity

(c) Head and neck: Integrity of mucosal membranes, tongue appearance (e.g., smooth, coated), conjunctival bleeding

(d) Chest: Shortness of breath, hemoptysis

(e) Abdomen: Vomiting, hematemesis, hematuria, diarrhea, melena

(f) Musculoskeletal system: Swelling of joints

ii. Palpation and percussion

(a) Skin: Warm to touch

(b) Neck: Enlarged lymph nodes

(c) Abdomen: Hepatomegaly, splenomegaly, enlarged lymph nodes in the axilla or groin

(d) Musculoskeletal system: Pain on palpation

iii. Auscultation

(a) Tachycardia

(b) Hypotension

(c) Orthostatic changes (pulse increases 20 beats/min and blood pressure decreases 20 mm Hg when the patient moves from lying to sitting or standing)

(d) Tachypnea

(e) Crackles, rhonchi

(f) Decreased breath sounds

b. Monitoring data

i. Fatigue related to hypoxemia

ii. Pulse oximetry

iii. Skin color

iv. Skin turgor as an indicator of dehydration

v. Overt and covert bleeding

vi. Acute or persistent pain

vii. Exposure to infection or disease

viii. Body temperature

ix. Development of unusual cancers

3. **Appraisal of patient characteristics:** Patients needing acute or life-saving care for hematologic disorders or for immunologic compromise come to critical care units as a result of their comorbidities or primary complications. The need for critical care may be brief or extended with quick to no recovery. Many hematologic and immunologic disorders are incurable. Occasionally, the focus is anticipated end-of-life care, although in no case is one able to predict with any certainty. Some patient characteristics that the nurse needs to assess for this population are the following:

a. Resiliency

i. Level 1—*Minimally resilient:* A frail 27-year-old young man with acquired immunodeficiency syndrome (AIDS) dementia, severe stomatitis, and chronic diarrhea, who is unresponsive to antiretroviral therapy

ii. Level 3—*Moderately resilient:* A 55-year-old woman with newly diagnosed acute lymphocytic leukemia following her second bone marrow transplant due to failed engraftment of the original donor stem cells

iii. Level 5—*Highly resilient:* An 18-year-old man with a hemoglobin level of 8.0 g/dl recovering from a hypovolemic hemorrhage related to a table saw accident at his family's farm

b. Vulnerability

i. Level 1—*Highly vulnerable:* A 45-year-old man with acute myelogenous leukemia who is neutropenic and has a lung abscess and thrombocytopenia

       ii. Level 3—*Moderately vulnerable:* A 36-year-old man, who is otherwise healthy, experiencing a type I hypersensitivity reaction to poison ivy hidden in the brush he was removing

      iii. Level 5—*Minimally vulnerable:* A petite 40-year-old woman with vitamin B_{12} deficiency anemia and alcoholism

  c. Stability

       i. Level 1—*Minimally stable:* A 78-year-old widowed retired Air Force colonel who develops a viral pneumonia and confusion on the second day after admission for induction chemotherapy for acute lymphocytic leukemia

      ii. Level 3—*Moderately stable:* A 59-year-old housewife diagnosed with thrombocytopenia who has a platelet count of $60,000/mm^3$

      iii. Level 5—*Highly stable:* A 28-year-old professor with lymphoma recovering in contact isolation from a methicillin-resistant *Staphylococcus aureus* toenail infection

  d. Complexity

       i. Level 1—*Highly complex:* A 48-year-old mother of four who develops disseminated intravascular coagulation (DIC) after a bilateral mastectomy and transversus rectus abdominis myocutaneous (TRAM) flap surgical reconstruction

      ii. Level 3—*Moderately complex:* A 19-year-old man with a diagnosed HIV infection that he wishes to be kept confidential from his parents and siblings

      iii. Level 5—*Minimally complex:* A 35-year-old accountant in whom autoimmune thrombocytopenic purpura (ATP) is diagnosed following a prolonged case of the flu

  e. Resource availability

       i. Level 1—*Few resources:* A 47-year-old housekeeper with rheumatoid arthritis who provides the sole income for a family of six and receives a diagnosis of leukemia

      ii. Level 3—*Moderate resources:* A 32-year-old Spanish-speaking migrant worker who contracted hepatitis C after a blood transfusion and has a bilingual sister who is a United States citizen and a social worker

      iii. Level 5—*Many resources:* A 49-year-old chief executive officer of a major computer software company who is hospitalized for maintenance chemotherapy

  f. Participation in care

       i. Level 1—*No participation:* An obese 26-year-old woman in anaphylactic shock with pulmonary edema and oral intubation

      ii. Level 3—*Moderate level of participation:* A 67-year-old salesman who is learning about home care for a Hickman catheter

      iii. Level 5—*Full participation:* A 32-year-old woman with AIDS who is compliant with antiretroviral therapy, exercise, and diet recommendations

  g. Participation in decision making

       i. Level 1—*No participation:* A 30-year-old children's tennis coach who chooses to let God's will be done after the physician team decides not to render further treatment for advanced cancer of the thoracic spine

      ii. Level 3—*Moderate level of participation:* A 56-year-old Mediterranean man who defers to his wife for decisions about treating his blood disorder

      iii. Level 5—*Full participation:* A 37-year-old kindergarten teacher who asks to know platelet counts before consenting to each platelet transfusion

  h. Predictability

       i. Level 1—*Not predictable:* An elegant 82-year-old grandmother with newly diagnosed chronic myelocytic leukemia

ii. Level 3—*Moderately predictable:* A 29-year-old day care worker receiving a second bone marrow transplant (BMT) after complete engraftment of the primary BMT stem cells

iii. Level 5—*Highly predictable:* A 27-year-old man with cognitive and behavioral challenges from AIDS dementia

4. **Diagnostic studies**
   a. Laboratory: See Table 7-7 for normal values
      i. Blood: See Table 7-8
      ii. Sputum culture: Detects and identifies microorganisms in the sputum
      iii. Urine tests
         (a) Urinalysis can detect gross amounts of blood or protein in the urine
         (b) Urine cultures detect and identify microorganisms in the urine
         (c) Urine protein electrophoresis determines the levels of proteins excreted in the urine, particularly the levels of immunoglobulins
      iv. Stool occult blood test (Hemoccult): Detects microscopic amounts of blood in the stool
   b. Radiologic
      i. Spleen ultrasonography is used to estimate the size of the spleen
      ii. In a liver-spleen scan, a radioactive tracer is used to evaluate the size as well as the function of the liver and spleen
      iii. In a gallium scan, a radioactive tracer is used to detect the presence of malignant tissue, particularly malignant lymphoid tissues
      iv. In a lymphangiogram, contrast dye is used to radiologically visualize the lymph system, particularly the size and architecture of lymph nodes
   c. Biopsy
      i. Bone marrow biopsy includes aspiration of bone marrow fluid and removal of a needle core biopsy sample of the bone marrow tissue for pathologic examination
      ii. In a lymph node biopsy, one or more lymph nodes are removed for pathologic examination
   d. Skin tests: Barometers of immune functioning, pointing out hyposensitivities or hypersensitivities to a particular antigen. Examples of allergens used in skin testing are allergenic extracts (e.g., dust, pollen, animal dander); purified protein derivative (PPD) for tuberculin skin tests; mumps virus; *Candida albicans*; and skin fungi.

Patient Care

1. **Susceptibility to infection**
   a. Description of problem
      i. Immune compromise and/or coagulopathy increases patient risk for opportunistic and host infections
      ii. Clinical findings include reports of fever, chills, night sweats, sore throat, cough, malaise, pain with swallowing, pain with urination, pain with defecation, diarrhea, reddened areas, sore areas, and swollen areas (these symptoms may not be present if the patient is neutropenic and unable to mount a WBC response); flushing, lethargy, skin warm to touch; abnormal vital signs—temperature exceeding 101° F (38.3° C), hypotension, tachycardia; WBC count lower than 1500/mm^3, absolute neutrophil count (ANC) lower than 500/mm^3
   b. Goals of care
      i. Vital signs within normal limits for the patient
      ii. Absence of signs or symptoms of active infection

Laboratory Test	Reference Values	Description
(White blood cell (WBC) count	4500-10,000/mm^3	Total number of leukocytes
Differential WBC:		Part of CBC; indicates distribution of five types of leukocytes
Neutrophils	2500-7000/mm^3	
Segments	2500-6500/mm^3	
Bands	0-500/mm^3	
Monocytes	200-600/mm^3	
Basophils	40-100/mm^3	
Eosinophils	100-300/mm^3	
Lymphocytes	1700-3500/mm^3	
Red blood cell (RBC) indices:		Erythrocyte indicators for anemia
RBC count		
Men	4.6-6.0 million/mm^3	
Women	4.0-5.0 million/mm^3	
Mean corpuscular volume (MCV)	80-98 mm^3	Indicates size of RBC
Mean corpuscular hemoglobin (MCH)	27-31 pg	Indicates weight of hemoglobin in RBC
Mean corpuscular hemoglobin concentration (MCHC)	32%-36%	Hemoglobin per volume RBC
RBC distribution width (RDW)	11.5-14.5 Coulter S	Size (width) difference of RBCs
Hemoglobin (Hb) level		Iron composition of RBC for oxygen-carrying capability
Men	13.5-17 g/dl	
Women	11.2-115 g/dl	
Hematocrit (HCT) of blood		Measure of the percentage of the total blood volume that is made up by RBCs
Men	40%-54%	
Women	36%-46%	
Panic value	<15% and >60%	
Reticulocyte count	0.5%-1.5%	Indicator of bone marrow activity
Erythrocyte sedimentation rate		Rate at which erythrocytes settle (sediment) in unclotted blood
Men	0-9 mm/hr (Wintrobe method)	
Women	0-15 mm/hr (Wintrobe method)	
Serum ferritin level		An indicator of protein stores of iron in the tissues, where 1 ng/ml ferritin = 8 mg stored iron
Men	15-445 ng/ml	
Women	10-235 ng/ml	
Postmenopausal	15-310 ng/ml	
Total iron-binding capacity (TIBC)	250-450 mg/dl	Total (maximum) iron-binding capacity of transferrin for transport of iron to marrow for hemoglobin synthesis
Platelet count (PLT)	150,000-400,000/mm^3	Measure of thrombocytes available for coagulation of blood
Fibrin split products (FSP)	2-10 mg/ml	Indicator of fibrin degradation products acting as anticoagulant in continuous bleeding associated with hemorrhage
Clotting times		Measures clotting factor ability
Prothrombin time (PT)	10-13 sec	
Partial thromboplastin time (PTT)	60-70 sec	Detects deficiencies in clotting factors
International normalized ratio (INR)	2.5-3.5	Standard for warfarin-sensitive PT

Data from Kee JL: *Laboratory diagnostic tests with nursing implications*, ed 5, Stamford, Conn, 1999, Appleton & Lange.

■ **TABLE 7-8**
■ ■ **Blood Studies**

Study	Abbreviation	Comments
Complete blood count with differential	CBC	The total white blood cell (WBC) count measures the total number of WBCs found in 1 mm^3 of blood The differential measures the contribution that each type of WBC (neutrophils, monocytes, basophils, eosinophils, and lymphocytes) makes to the total WBC count A "shift to the right" on a CBC indicates that only a small percentage of the WBCs are neutrophils. The lower the neutrophil count, the greater the patient's risk of infection. To calculate the absolute neutrophil count (ANC), multiply the percentage of neutrophils indicated on the differential of the CBC by the total number of WBCs. A "shift to the left" on a CBC indicates that a large percentage of the WBCs are neutrophils. This usually implies that the bone marrow has been stimulated to produce more neutrophils to fight a severe infection.
Red blood cell count	RBC	Total number of RBCs found in 1 mm^3 of blood
Hemoglobin count	Hb	A measure of the amount of hemoglobin in 1 dl of blood and an indicator of the blood's oxygen-carrying capacity
Hematocrit	HCT	Percentage of RBCs in a volume of whole blood
Mean corpuscular volume	MCV	Average size (volume) of RBCs
Mean corpuscular hemoglobin concentration	MCHC	Average concentration of hemoglobin in the RBCs
Mean corpuscular hemoglobin	MCH	Average amount of hemoglobin per RBC
Platelet count		Total number of platelets per 1 mm^3 of blood
Reticulocyte count		Number or percentage of immature RBCs in the peripheral circulation
Erythrocyte sedimentation rate	ESR, or sed rate	Rate at which RBCs settle out of anticoagulated whole blood sample over a specified period of time. The ESR can be elevated in inflammatory conditions or anemia. ESR is best used for assessment of response to treatment, rather than as a diagnostic test.
Serum iron level		Amount of iron in serum
Total iron-binding capacity	TIBC	Reflects the body's ability to transport available iron
Ferritin level		A rough measure of the body's iron stores and a good indicator of the body's iron storage status
Bleeding time		The primary phase of hemostasis: How long it takes platelets to adhere to the broken blood vessel and form the platelet plug; a rough gauge of platelet function
Thrombin time	TT	Time it takes thrombin (factor IIa) to convert fibrinogen (factor I) to fibrin (factor Ia); it is markedly prolonged by the presence of heparin
Prothrombin time	PT	Clotting ability of the extrinsic coagulation cascade (factor VII) and the common pathway (factor X [Stuart-Prower factor], factor V [proaccelerin or AC-globulin], factor II [prothrombin], and factor I [fibrinogen]). PT is used to monitor warfarin (Coumadin) therapy.

Continued

▨ **TABLE 7-8**
▨ ▨ **Blood Studies—cont'd**

Study	Abbreviation	Comments
Partial thrombo-plastin time	PTT	A more sensitive measure of the clotting ability and a test of the common pathway (factor X [Stuart-Prower factor], factor V [proaccelerin], factor II [prothrombin], and factor I [fibrinogen]). PTT is used to monitor heparin therapy.
International normalized ratio	INR	A comparative rating of PT ratios in which the measured PT is adjusted by the International Reference Thromboplastin. It is a uniform way of monitoring warfarin therapy.
Fibrin split products	FSP	The levels of fibrin degradation products
D-dimers level		Also reflects levels of fibrin degradation products but is a more specific test for disseminated intravascular coagulation because D-dimers are specific for fibrinolysis
Fibrinogen level		Blood level of fibrinogen (factor I)
Serum bilirubin level		Amounts of the various types of bilirubin in the blood; bilirubin is produced during the breakdown of hemoglobin in RBCs
		Conjugated or direct bilirubin circulates freely in the blood until it is cleared by the liver and excreted in bile; an increase in conjugated bilirubin level is indicative of a dysfunction or blockage of the liver
		Unconjugated or indirect bilirubin is protein bound; an increase in unconjugated bilirubin often is evidence of increased RBC destruction
		Total bilirubin level is a measure of both conjugated and unconjugated bilirubin
Serum protein electrophoresis	SPEP	Determines the levels of serum proteins in blood, particularly levels of immunoglobulins
Coombs' test		The direct Coombs' test detects the presence of antibody on the RBC membrane
		The indirect Coombs test detects antibody in the serum
T-cell count		Reflects the levels of T-cells in the blood
Human immuno-deficiency virus (HIV)		Include the enzyme-linked immunosorbent assay (ELISA) and the Western blot. Both of these tests are used to detect the presence of antibody to HIV. The Western blot is a more specific and sensitive test.
Blood and tissue typing		Blood typing detects ABO and Rh antigens present on RBCs and is necessary for compatibility testing before blood product transfusion
		A more specific blood typing test detects human leukocyte antigens (HLAs) and is necessary for compatibility testing before some types of tissue transplantation (e.g., bone marrow transplantation)
Blood culture		Detects and identifies microorganisms in the blood

      iii. Maintenance of the WBC count within an acceptable range
      iv. Patient's and family's verbalization of an understanding of the underlying pathology and infection prevention
   c. Collaborating professionals on health care team
      i. Nurse
      ii. Pharmacist

      iii Physician

      iv. Radiologist

      v. Laboratory technician

      vi. Blood bank specialist

   d. Interventions: See Table 7-9

   e. Evaluation of patient care

      i. Absence of fever

      ii. Maintenance of an ANC exceeding $1000/mm^3$

      iii. Ability of the patient and family to describe how to reduce the patient's risk of infection

2. Increased risk for hemorrhage

   a. Description of problem

      i. Disease and/or treatment creates an altered state of protection against bleeding

      ii. Clinical findings include reports of unusual bruising, prolonged bleeding, hematemesis, hemoptysis, hematochezia, melena, hematuria, menorrhagia

   b. Goals of care

      i. No evidence of spontaneous bleeding

      ii. Maintenance of platelet counts and levels of clotting factors within an acceptable range

      iii. Patient's and family's verbalization of an understanding of the underlying pathology and bleeding precautions

---

■ **TABLE 7-9**
■ ■ **Leukocyte Intervention Activity Bundle**

Root cause	**Protection from infection:** A proliferation of immature leukocytes or a chemotherapy-induced neutropenic state creates immunocompromise leading to a high alteration in patient's ability to fight infection.
Interventions to protect against and detect infection	1. Assess daily absolute neutrophil count, white blood cell count and differential for abnormal granulocyte levels.
	2. Bathe or assist the patient with bathing daily, because normal flora pose highest risk for infection.
	3. Inspect skin and mucous membranes every 4 hr for areas of redness or wound formation.
	4. Assess each invasive site (intravenous line, Hickman catheter, peripherally inserted central catheter, nasogastric tube, gastrostomy tube, Foley catheter, etc.) twice a shift for signs of portal infection.
	5. Obtain cultures immediately from any new sites with suspicious drainage.
	6. Administer antibiotics on schedule and as prescribed.
	7. Monitor and supplement nutritional intake of vitamins, proteins, and fats.
	8. Monitor, encourage, and supplement free water intake.
	9. Anticipate daily chest radiography for patients prone to pneumonia.
	10. Encourage deep breathing and coughing and change of position every 2-4 hr.
	11. Place fresh flower and plant gifts for patients outside of patient area, yet within patient's sight.
	12. Ensure that all persons entering room are free of communicable disease.
	13. Ensure that all persons entering room observe contact and neutropenic precautions.
	14. Recommend private rooms for all patients at risk of infection.

From Schneider S: Interventions for hematologic problems. In Ignatavicius DD, Workman ML, editors: *Medical-surgical nursing: critical thinking for collaborative care*, ed 4, Philadelphia, 2002, Saunders.

    c. Collaborating professionals on health care team
        i. Nurse
        ii. Pharmacist
        iii. Physician
        iv. Laboratory technician
        v. Blood bank specialist
    d. Interventions: See Table 7-10
    e. Evaluation of patient care
        i. No evidence of spontaneous bleeding
        ii. Maintenance of a platelet count of more than $50,000/mm^3$ and prothrombin time (PT) and partial thromboplastin time (PTT) within prescribed ranges
        iii. Ability of the patient and family to describe how to reduce the patient's risk of bleeding

▨ TABLE 7-10
▨ ▨ Erythrocyte Intervention Activity Bundle

Root causes	**Monitor oxygen transport:** Alterations in hemoglobin due to anemic states or profuse bleeding cause a lack of sufficient oxygen binding and oxygen-carrying capability, potentially leading to respiratory compromise and tissue ischemia.
	Precautions for bleeding: A proliferation of immature erythrocytes or a severe lack of platelets from idiopathic or induced thrombocytopenia prevents clot formation and induces bleeding.
Interventions to prevent and detect hypoxia	1. Monitor pulse oximetry every 2-4 hr or more often as indicated. 2. Assess ferritin and hemoglobin levels daily to predict oxygen-carrying capability. 3. Assess circumoral area and the nailbeds of fingers and toes every 4 hr for cyanosis. 4. Monitor for changes in mental status and difficulty breathing every 2-4 hr. 5. Administer prophylactic supplemental oxygen and/or hematopoietic growth factors as prescribed. 6. See Interventions to Protect Against and Detect Infection in Table 7-9.
Interventions to prevent hemorrhage	1. Monitor daily hematocrit, hemoglobin level, clotting times, and platelet counts. 2. Monitor temperature, heart rate, breathing pattern, and blood pressure every 2-4 hr and with every episode of bleeding. 3. Check expectorant, residuals from feedings, urine, and feces for frank blood. 4. Administer platelets, fresh frozen plasma, or clotting factors as prescribed using proper method. 5. Administer stool softeners, vitamin K supplements, and synthetic platelet aggregates as ordered. 6. Avoid administration of nonsteroidal antiinflammatory drugs and anticoagulants. 7. Protect patient from injury, constipation, falls, and trauma at all times. 8. Avoid damage to rectal mucosa; avoid intramuscular, subcutaneous, and venous or arterial cannulation. 9. Use a soft toothette for oral care and an electric razor for shaving. 10. Instruct patient and family on risks and signs of bleeding. 11. Encourage patient to eat green leafy vegetables and fruits high in vitamin K.

From Schneider S: Interventions for hematologic problems. In Ignatavicius DD, Workman ML, editors: *Medical-surgical nursing: critical thinking for collaborative care*, ed 4, Philadelphia, 2002, Saunders.

3. **Impaired respiratory gas transport:** See Chapter 2
   a. Interventions: See Table 7-10
4. **Impaired fluid volume regulation** (see also Chapter 5)
   a. Description of problem
      i. Fever, vomiting, diarrhea, hemorrhage, and shock deplete body fluid volume
      ii. Clinical findings include reports of thirst, sweating, vomiting, polyuria, diarrhea, lightheadedness; pallor, mucosal dryness, loss of skin turgor, decreased venous filling; abnormal vital signs—fever, tachycardia, hypotension, changes in orthostatic vital signs; decreased urine output and concentrated urine with a specific gravity exceeding 1.020; altered mental status
   b. Goals of care
      i. Absence of dehydration, hypovolemia, and shock
      ii. Urine output greater than 30 ml/hr
   c. Collaborating professionals on health care team
      i. Nurse
      ii. Pharmacist
      iii. Physician
      iv. Blood bank specialist
   d. Interventions: See Table 7-11
      i. Administer IV fluids and blood products as prescribed
         (a) Transfuse blood products (Table 7-12)
         (b) Keep in mind special considerations related to blood product administration (Table 7-13 and Box 7-1)
      ii. Treat underlying condition as prescribed
      iii. Encourage oral fluid intake as the patient's condition allows
      iv. Monitor fluid balance with recording of intake and output and daily weights

---

▨ TABLE 7-11
▨ ▨ Dehydration Intervention Activity Bundle

Root cause	**Fluid volume deficit:** Nausea, vomiting, diarrhea, loss of appetite, loss of insensible water due to fever, and bleeding tendencies result in chronic phases of dehydration.
Interventions to prevent and detect dehydration	1. Monitor daily serum chemistry values for sodium, potassium, and chloride.
	2. Monitor daily serum renal panel values, arterial blood gas levels, and liver panel values as indicated.
	3. Determine patient's self-report of activities and interventions that contribute to fluid losses.
	4. Monitor temperature, heart rate, breathing pattern, and blood pressure every 4 hr.
	5. Assess daily LOC, skin turgor, appetite, and number, character, color, and frequency of emesis, diarrhea, urine, and bleeding.
	6. Assess and manage treatable contributing factors (food odors or appearance, flavor, preference and availability of oral fluids, antiemetic choice, medication side effects, room temperature, air currents in room).
	7. Administer prophylactic antiemetics as indicated.
	8. Administer supplemental or maintenance intravenous fluids as ordered.
	9. See Interventions to Prevent Hemorrhage in Table 7-10.

From Schneider S: Interventions for hematologic problems. In Ignatavicius DD, Workman ML, editors: *Medical-surgical nursing: critical thinking for collaborative care,* ed 4, Philadelphia, 2002, Saunders.
LOC, Level of consciousness.

■ **TABLE 7-12**
■ ■ **Indications for Treatment with Blood Components**

Component	Volume	Infusion Time	Indications
Packed red blood cells (PRBCs)	200-250 ml	2-4 hr	Anemia; hemoglobin level <6 g/dl, 6-10 g/dl, depending on symptoms
Washed red blood cells (white blood cell–poor PRBCs)	200 ml	2-4 hr	History of allergic transfusion reactions; bone marrow transplant clients
Platelets			
Pooled	Approximately 300 ml	15-30 min	Thrombocytopenia, platelet count <20,000/mm^3; clients who are actively bleeding with a platelet count <80,000/mm^3
Single donor	200 ml	30 min	History of febrile or allergic reactions
Fresh frozen plasma	200 ml	15-30 min	Deficiency in plasma coagulation factors; prothrombin or partial thromboplastin time 1.5 times normal
Cryoprecipitate	10-20 ml/U	15-30 min	Hemophilia VIII or von Willebrand's disease; fibrinogen levels <100 mg/dl
White blood cells	400 ml	1 hr	Sepsis, neutropenic infection not responding to antibiotic therapy

From Schneider S: Interventions for clients with hematologic problems. In Ignatavicius DD, Workman ML, editors: *Medical-surgical nursing: critical thinking for collaborative care,* ed 4, Philadelphia, 2002, Saunders, chap 40.

    e. Evaluation of patient care
        i. Maintenance of vital signs within normal limits; when the patient moves from lying to sitting or standing, change in pulse and blood pressure of no more than 20 points
        ii. Patient urine output exceeding 30 ml/hr
        iii. Near equality in patient's 24-hour intake and output
        iv. Stability of patient's weight
5. Fatigue
    a. Description of problem
        i. Potential for activity intolerance related to disease or the treatment of disease
        ii. Clinical findings include reports of fatigue, weakness, malaise, inability to sleep, and inability to concentrate; changes in vital signs with activity
    b. Goals of care
        i. Vital signs within normal limits for the patient
        ii. Patient's ability to accomplish the activities of daily living without tachycardia or hypotension
        iii. Patient's report of a reduction in fatigue
        iv. Patient's ability to concentrate and socialize normally
    c. Collaborating professionals on health care team
        i. Nurse
        ii. Pharmacist
        iii. Physician
        iv. Psychologist
    d. Interventions: See Table 7-14
    e. Evaluation of patient care
        i. Pulse increase of no more than 20 beats/min with nonaerobic activity and return to baseline within 5 minutes of stopping the activity

■ TABLE 7-13
■ ■ Types of Blood Transfusion Reaction

Reaction	Mechanism	Signs and Symptoms	Time of Occurrence	Treatment
Hemolytic	Type II antigen-complement reaction to transfusion of ABO- or Rh-incompatible blood	Fever, chills, headache, chest pain, low back pain, tachypnea, tachycardia, disseminated intravascular coagulation (DIC) or circulatory collapse	Immediately or may not occur until subsequent units have been transfused	Stop the transfusion; notify the physician and blood bank immediately; provide supportive therapy to maintain blood pressure and urine output
Allergic-urticaric-anaphylactic	Type I hypersensitivity to plasma proteins	Urticaria, wheezing, dyspnea, hypotension	Within 30 min of transfusion, but may also be up to 24 hr	Temporarily stop the transfusion; notify the physician and blood bank; be prepared to administer antihistamines or epinephrine orally or intramuscularly; use washed red blood cells (RBCs)
Febrile	Antibody to donor leukocyte	Fever, chills, tachycardia, tachypnea, hypotension	Within 30-90 min of the start of the transfusion	Administer antipyretics, white blood cell–poor RBCs, or single-donor human leukocyte antigen–matched platelets
Bacterial	Blood contaminated with gram-negative organisms (endotoxin producing)	Fever, chills, tachycardia, shock, DIC, renal failure	Within 30 min of the start of the transfusion	Stop the transfusion; notify the physician and blood bank; give high-dose antibiotics, steroids, and blood pressure support
Circulatory overload	Transfusion administered too quickly	Restlessness, confusion, dyspnea, bounding pulse, hypertension	Anytime during the transfusion	Slow the transfusion; provide supportive therapy and monitor

Data from Hankins J, Lonsway RAW, Hedrick D, et al: *Infusion therapy in clinical practice*, ed 2, St Louis, 2001, Saunders; and Ignatavicius DD, Workman ML, editors: *Medical-surgical nursing: critical thinking for collaborative care*, ed 4, Philadelphia, 2002, Saunders.

■ **BOX 7-1**
■ **CONSIDERATIONS IN ADMINISTERING BLOOD PRODUCTS**

1. **Alloimmunization** is a state in which the patient develops antibodies against human leukocyte antigen (HLA), granulocyte-specific antigens, red blood cell (RBC)–specific antigens, or platelet-specific antigens after repeated blood product transfusions. As a result, the transfused cells are destroyed and the transfusion is ineffective in correcting the patient's blood counts. Platelet destruction related to HLA antibodies accounts for 95% of cases of alloimmunization in patients who fail to respond to platelet transfusions. HLA matching and platelet cross-matching are two options for patients with alloimmunization. For both of these options, nearly 2 days can be required to provide a proper match.

2. **Pathogen contamination of blood products** has been reduced due to better screening of donors, viral nucleic acid testing of donor blood, purification of plasma and plasma-derived products, and recombinant factor concentrate production technology. Current estimated risk of transmission of viruses ranges from 0.5 to 7.0 per million transfusions. However, 1 in 500 to 2000 platelet transfusions has bacterial contamination. Consideration should be given to the rate at which new blood-borne pathogens are identified and the inability to outpace growth with appropriate screening tests. Pathogen inactivation technologies are actively being studied.

3. **Irradiation of blood products** incapacitates lymphocytes, with approximately 2500 rads of gamma radiation thus reducing the incidence of cytomegalovirus (CMV) infection, alloimmunization, and transfusion-associated graft-versus-host disease (GVHD). Cryoprecipitate and fresh frozen plasma are lymphocyte free and need not be irradiated. Irradiation of blood is beneficial for immunocompromised patients at risk for GVHD, hematopoietic stem cell donors, and transplant patients, and in cases of cellular (T-cell) immunodeficiency, intrauterine transfusion, transfusions from family members, matched platelet transfusions, Hodgkin's disease, neonatal exchange transfusions, acute myelogenous leukemia, acute lymphocytic leukemia, and lymphoma.

4. **CMV-negative blood products** are necessary for patients who need a bone marrow transplant and who have never been exposed to CMV. A CMV infection during transplantation could be life-threatening. Use of CMV-negative blood products benefits premature infants or infants younger than 4 weeks of age, fetuses undergoing intrauterine transfusions, and any CMV-negative patient who is pregnant, potentially a transplant candidate, about to undergo splenectomy, or has acquired immunodeficiency syndrome, human immunodeficiency virus infection, or a congenital immune deficiency.

5. **Leukocyte-reduced (LR) blood products** reduce the risk of developing a nonhemolytic transfusion reaction, alloimmunization, or GVHD, and potentially prevent the transmission of CMV. When administering LR blood products, be sure to use an appropriate blood filter at the bedside to trap the cellular debris accumulated since the original filtration process. Leukocyte reduction benefits patients with a history of more than one nonhemolytic febrile transfusion reaction, immunocompromised patients at risk for CMV, and patients who will potentially receive multiple transfusions and are at an increased risk for alloimmunization.

6. **Washing of blood** removes proteins, electrolytes, antibodies, and glycerol (from frozen RBCs) that could trigger severe reactions in some recipients. To wash blood, 0.9% normal saline is added to the unit and mixed, the mixture is centrifuged, and the saline is removed. Washing of blood benefits patients receiving RBCs frozen in glycerol and patients exhibiting severe hypersensitivity to donor plasma components such as immunoglobulin A or B.

7. **Blood substitutes** (hemoglobin solutions and perfluorocarbon emulsions) are currently under investigation, but common adverse effects have been identified. Increased systemic and pulmonary vascular resistance leading to a decreased cardiac index and impaired oxygen delivery is the primary adverse effect associated with hemoglobin solutions. Cell-free hemoglobin acts as a nitric oxide scavenger. Perfluorocarbon emulsions can immerse in water, are chemically inert, and are not metabolized in vivo. Both types of blood substitute have a half-life of hours to days versus a half-life of weeks for an RBC. The dark red color of blood substitutes makes ABO typing a challenge. Blood substitutes may be useful as a bridge to transfusion in patients difficult to transfuse.

Data from Fitzpatrick L: When to administer modified blood products, *Nursing* 32(5):36-42, 2002; Fung M, Triulzi D: Pathogen inactivation of blood products, *Transfusion Medicine Update,* Issue 2, 2002, retrieved May 28, 2004, from the Institute for Transfusion Medicine website: http://www.itxmdiagnostics.com/tmu2002/issue7.htm; Nester T: Blood substitutes, *Transfusion Medicine Update,* December 2000, retrieved May 28, 2004, from the Institute for Transfusion Medicine website: http://www.itxmdiagnostics.com/tmu2000/tmu12-2000.htm; and Sepulveda J: Alloimmunization from transfusions, Dec 21, 2001, retrieved May 28, 2004, from http://www.emedicine.com/med/topic107.htm.

■ **TABLE 7-14**
■ ■ **Fatigue Intervention Activity Bundle**

Root cause	**Energy expenditure/energy resource variant:** Chronic neutropenia and thrombocytopenia, chemotherapy, radiation therapy, and side effects contribute to patient expressions of weariness and lack of ability to perform independent functions.
Interventions for fatigue	1. Determine the patient's or family's and/or significant other's perception of the causes of fatigue.
	2. Assess and manage treatable contributing factors (pain, emotional distress, sleep disturbances, anemia, hypoxia, organ dysfunction, infection, and fluid and electrolyte imbalances).
	3. Provide a diet high in vitamin C for stress.
	4. When feasible, provide aromas of cooking (bread or cookies baking, soup) to stimulate appetite and motivate the patient to expend the energy required to walk to the kitchen, as possible.
	5. Encourage scheduled aerobic exercise to combat cancer fatigue.
	6. Cluster care and limit the number of interruptions during scheduled rest periods.
	7. Provide stress management and a calm environment to promote relaxation.
	8. Make distractions (music, games, videos, books, magazines, humor, socialization) available.
	9. Establish an on-site or on-unit library to make learning resources available to technical personnel.
	10. Assess the energy needed for an activity and gauge expenditure of the patient's energy resources.
	11. Schedule activities at times of peak energy in order to conserve energy for priority activities.
	12. Reassure the patient that treatment-related fatigue does not directly indicate disease progression.
	13. See Interventions to Protect Against and Detect Infection in Table 7-9.
	14. See Interventions to Prevent and Detect Dehydration in Table 7-11.
	15. See Interventions to Prevent and Detect Hypoxia in Table 7-10.
	16. See Interventions to Prevent Hemorrhage in Table 7-10.

From Schneider S: Interventions for clients with hematologic problems. In Ignatavicius DD, Workman ML, editors: *Medical-surgical nursing: critical thinking for collaborative care,* ed 4, Philadelphia, 2002, Saunders; and National Comprehensive Cancer Network: Practice guidelines for cancer related fatigue, 2003, retrieved May 24, 2004, from http://www.nccn.org.

    ii. Patient's statement that the level of fatigue experienced in performing the activities of daily living is manageable

SPECIFIC PATIENT HEALTH PROBLEMS

Anemia

1. **Pathophysiology**
   a. Anemia is a reduction in the number of RBCs, the quantity of hemoglobin, or the volume of RBCs. Because the main function of RBCs is oxygenation, anemia results in varying degrees of hypoxia. The body compensates for anemia by increasing cardiac output and respiratory rate, by redistributing blood to sustain blood supply to the brain and heart through a reduction in blood supply to the skin, gut, and kidneys, and by increasing the kidney's production of erythropoietin to stimulate erythropoiesis.

b. Acute blood loss, such as with arterial rupture, dramatically changes the body's hemodynamic status and necessitates emergency intervention. With chronic blood loss occurring over weeks or months, such as in slow gastrointestinal bleeding or menorrhagia, the body has time to compensate, and thus the symptoms of chronic blood loss may be more insidious. Although patients with chronic anemia are not usually admitted to the critical care unit, chronic anemia can complicate other medical conditions that do necessitate treatment in a critical care setting.

2. **Etiology and risk factors**
   a. Inadequate RBC production
      i. Aplastic anemia
      ii. Chronic inflammatory disease (e.g., rheumatoid arthritis, chronic osteomyelitis)
      iii. End-stage renal disease
      iv. Bone marrow infiltration with malignant cells
      v. Current or recent treatment with antineoplastic chemotherapy
      vi. History of radiation therapy to bones where blood cells are made (i.e., vertebrae, ribs, skull, pelvis, femur, or humerus)
      vii. Bone marrow transplantation
      viii. Dietary deficiencies, particularly in iron, cobalamine (B_{12}), or folate
      ix. Certain drugs (e.g., zidovudine)
   b. Increased RBC destruction
      i. Immune mediated
         (a) Autoimmune hemolytic anemia
         (b) Cytotoxic hypersensitivity reaction (e.g., drug-induced)
      ii. RBC membrane defects (e.g., hereditary spherocytosis)
      iii. Hemoglobin defects
         (a) Sickle cell anemia is an autosomal recessive genetic disorder found primarily in persons of African descent that results from substitution of the amino acid valine for glutamic acid at position 6 of the β-globin protein; this substitution leads to the production of defective hemoglobin, hemoglobin S (HbS). The deoxygenation of HbS leads to distortion of the RBC into the classic sickle cell shape.
         (b) The major consequence of the sickle cell shape is that RBCs are less able to deform and thus obstruct the microcirculation. Sickle-shaped RBCs have a life span of 10 to 20 days (vs. 120 for nonsickled RBCs) and hemolyze rapidly.
         (c) Clinical manifestations of sickle cell anemia are commonly divided into vasoocclusive, hematologic, and infectious crises
            (1) Vasoocclusive crisis occurs when the microcirculation is occluded by sickled RBCs, which causes ischemic injury to the organ perfused; pain is the most frequent complaint
            (2) Hematologic crisis is manifested by sudden exacerbation of anemia with a corresponding drop in hemoglobin level
            (3) Infectious crisis is due to a compromised immune system that is susceptible to common infectious agents such as *Haemophilus influenzae, Streptococcus pneumoniae, Mycoplasma pneumoniae, Salmonella typhimurium, S. aureus,* and *Escherichia coli*
         (d) Treatment for patients with sickle cell anemia includes rest, hydration, supplemental oxygen, analgesia, antibiotic therapy, and blood transfusion as needed
      iv. Mechanical (e.g., trauma from prosthetic heart valves)

   c. Major blood loss
3. **Signs and symptoms**
   a. Symptoms: Fatigue; dyspnea, especially with exertion; shortness of breath; possible bone pain if the bone marrow is infiltrated with malignant cells; altered mental status (e.g., dizziness, especially when changing position from lying down to sitting or standing; inability to concentrate; confusion)
   b. Signs: Pallor, possibly jaundice; possible hepatosplenomegaly with liver disease and some types of malignant disease, tenderness of the liver and spleen with palpation and percussion; tachycardia, hypotension, and orthostatic changes in vital signs
4. **Diagnostic study findings**
   a. Laboratory
      i. Urine: Can test positive for blood
      ii. Stool: Can test positive for blood
      iii. Blood
         (a) Hemoglobin level of less than 7 g/dl, hematocrit (HCT) of less than 21%
         (b) Other findings vary with the cause of anemia and can include increased reticulocyte count, decreased serum iron level, increased or decreased total iron-binding capacity, decreased ferritin level, increased indirect bilirubin level, positive Coombs' test result
   b. Radiologic: Gastrointestinal series may be obtained to detect the source of bleeding
   c. Biopsy: Bone marrow biopsy may be performed to evaluate bone marrow production of RBCs or detect the presence of bone marrow infiltration with malignant cells
   d. Endoscopy: To detect the source of bleeding
5. **Goals of care**
   a. Adequate gas exchange
   b. Absence of dehydration due to bleeding
   c. Tolerable level of fatigue
6. **Collaborating professionals on health care team**
   a. Nurse
   b. Blood bank specialist
   c. Pharmacist
   d. Physician
7. **Management of patient care**
   a. Anticipated patient trajectory: Patients with anemia can have an acute event related to loss of RBCs due to hemorrhage or a chronic disorder related to inadequate production of RBCs and/or hemoglobin. Throughout their course of recovery and discharge, patients with anemia may be expected to have needs in the following areas:
      i. Positioning: High Fowler's position for shortness of breath
      ii. Nutrition: Diet or feeding supplement with iron, vitamin B_{12}, and folate may need to be considered
      iii. Pharmacology: Patient may need education on taking oral iron preparations with food to prevent peptic ulcers and on treating constipation as a primary side effect
      iv. Treatment: Invasive treatment with whole blood or packed RBCs
   b. Potential complications
      i. Shortness of breath
         (a) Mechanism: Due to diminished oxygen-carrying capacity

(b) Management: Place the patient in a position of comfort to ease the work of breathing; oxygen administration and transfusion of packed RBCs may be required
  ii. Weakness and fatigue
    (a) Mechanism: Inadequate circulating hemoglobin decreases oxygen availability to cells, creating decreased energy stores in the body
    (b) Management: Conserve the patient's energy by assisting with nutrition and the activities of daily living, passive range-of-motion exercises; consider providing supplemental oxygen if the patient is out of bed to a chair or is ambulating
8. **Evaluation of patient care**
   a. Absence of dyspnea
   b. Pink skin color, skin warm to the touch
   c. Heart rate of 60 to 100 beats/min
   d. Hemoglobin level higher than 7 g/dl, HCT higher than 21%

Disseminated Intravascular Coagulation

1. **Pathophysiology**
   a. DIC is a hypercoagulable state that occurs when the normal coagulation cascade is overstimulated; this results in simultaneous thrombosis and hemorrhage. DIC is always secondary to another pathologic process.
   b. Coagulation takes place normally, but it occurs at so many sites in the body that the normal inhibitory mechanisms are overwhelmed. Eventually all available platelets and clotting factors are depleted, and systemic uncontrolled hemorrhage results.
2. **Etiology and risk factors**
   a. Shock
   b. Major trauma, crush injuries, burns
   c. Malignancy
   d. Acute tumor lysis syndrome (see Acute Leukemia)
   e. Obstetric complications, such as abruptio placentae or fetal demise
   f. Sepsis
3. **Signs and symptoms**
   a. Symptoms: Diagnosis of DIC is based on a constellation of findings, including the sudden onset of a bleeding disorder without a prior history of bleeding or blood coagulation abnormalities
   b. Signs: Occurrence of spontaneous bleeding for no obvious reason, a preceding or concurrent pathologic process that is known to precipitate DIC, petechiae, purpura, ecchymoses, hematomas, epistaxis, conjunctival bleeding, spontaneous and/or uncontrollable hemorrhage from multiple unrelated sites, such as sites of venipuncture, tubes, drains, lines, incisions, and wounds
4. **Diagnostic study findings**
   a. Blood: Prolonged PT, decreased fibrinogen level, increased level of fibrin split products, increased levels of D-dimers, and prolonged PTT
   b. Radiologic: Findings are usually noncontributory except to identify the underlying pathologic process
5. **Goals of care**
   a. Optimal oxygen delivery
   b. Reversal of the clotting mechanism
   c. Replacement of coagulation components
   d. Prevention of clinical sequelae, such as hypovolemic shock, cardiac arrest, organ damage, and limb loss

6. **Collaborating professionals on health care team**
   a. Nurse
   b. Blood bank specialist
   c. Pharmacist
   d. Physician
7. **Management of patient care**
   a. Anticipated patient trajectory: Patients with DIC are in a life-threatening clinical situation secondary to overstimulation of the coagulation cascade. Because primary disorders such as sepsis, shock, crushing injury, burns, acute respiratory distress syndrome, or obstetrical complications precipitate DIC, death results in over half of the cases. The best treatment is prevention. Throughout their recovery, patients may be expected to have needs in the following areas:
      i. Pharmacology: Patient and family may need education on clotting mechanisms, coagulation components, and oxygen delivery
      ii. Psychosocial issues: Patient and/or family may need chaplain or social service support in the event of death, organ failure, loss of limbs, or alteration in self-concept related to compartment syndrome, petechiae, and bruising
      iii. Treatments: Oxygen therapy, mechanical ventilation, blood product transfusion, and infusion of anticlotting agents
   b. Potential complications
      i. Hypovolemic shock
         (a) Mechanism: Thrombocytopenia creates bleeding that is difficult to control
         (b) Management: Monitor the patient for a systolic blood pressure of less than 90 mm Hg, heart rate of over 100 beats/min, anxiety, unresponsiveness, diaphoresis, urine output of less than 0.5 ml/kg/hr, platelet count of less than $50,000/mm^3$, PTT of longer than 40 seconds, and visible uncontrolled bleeding; anticipate transfusions of platelets, fresh frozen plasma, and/or cryoprecipitate
      ii. Multiple organ dysfunction syndrome
         (a) Mechanism: Microvascular thrombus formation causes tissue ischemia and necrosis in solid organs and peripheral circulation
         (b) Management: See Chapter 9
8. **Evaluation of patient care**
   a. Determination of the cause of DIC and treatment of the cause
   b. Avoidance of hypovolemia and anoxia due to hemorrhage
   c. Preservation of life and limbs

Thrombocytopenia

1. **Pathophysiology:** The number of platelets available to assist with coagulation is inadequate, which puts the patient at increased risk of hemorrhage. In various hematologic malignancies such as leukemia and lymphoma, the cancerous cells crowd out normal cell lines in the bone marrow, which results in thrombocytopenia as well as neutropenia and anemia. Management includes treating the underlying malignancy with antineoplastic chemotherapy, which can itself also cause pancytopenia. Treatment of either solid tumor or hematologic malignancies with antineoplastic chemotherapy is a major cause of thrombocytopenia. Chemotherapy indiscriminately targets rapidly dividing cells in the bone marrow, including megakaryocytes. Thrombocytopenia can be expected to appear 10 to 14 days after chemotherapeutic treatment; it lasts until the bone marrow is able to replenish its megakaryocyte pool.

2. Etiology and risk factors
   a. Decreased platelet production
   i. Bone marrow infiltration with malignant cells (e.g., leukemia, multiple myeloma, malignant metastases)
   ii. Current or recent treatment with antineoplastic agents
   iii. History of radiation therapy to the bones in which blood cells are made
   iv. Bone marrow aplasia
   b. Increased platelet destruction
   i. DIC: See Disseminated Intravascular Coagulation section
   ii. Antibody mediated
   (a) Immune thrombocytopenic purpura (ITP)
   (1) Agents known to induce ITP include sulfonamides, thiazide diuretics, chlorpropamide, quinidine, and gold
   (2) Patients with HIV infection are at increased risk for development of ITP
   (b) Heparin-induced thrombocytopenia and thrombosis
   (c) Alloimmunization after multiple platelet transfusions
   iii. Thrombotic thrombocytopenic purpura (TTP) or hemolytic uremic syndrome (HUS) (see Hypercoagulable Disorders)
   iv. Sepsis
   c. Sequestration of platelets in the spleen (e.g., with liver disease and portal hypertension)
   d. Massive transfusion of RBCs over a short period of time, which can lead to a dilutional thrombocytopenia
3. Signs and symptoms
   a. Symptom: Unexplained bleeding
   b. Signs: Pallor, petechiae, purpura, ecchymoses; oozing of blood from venipuncture sites, conjunctival bleeding; bleeding from the oropharynx, gastrointestinal tract, or genitourinary tract and splenomegaly may be present
4. Diagnostic study findings
   a. Laboratory
   i. Urine: Can test positive for blood
   ii. Stool: Can test positive for blood
   iii. Blood
   (a) Platelet count is lower than $50,000/mm^3$
   (b) Both hemoglobin level and HCT are usually decreased as a result of blood loss
   b. Radiologic: Spleen ultrasonography or liver-spleen scan to determine the size of the spleen
   c. Bone marrow biopsy to determine whether adequate numbers of platelets are being made in the bone marrow
5. Goals of care
   a. Absence of hemorrhage
   b. Prevention of injury
6. Collaborating professionals on health care team
   a. Nurse
   b. Blood bank specialist
   c. Pharmacist
   d. Physician
7. Management of patient care
   a. Anticipated patient trajectory: Children with thrombocytopenia usually develop symptoms after a viral infection, and the disorder resolves spontaneously in 90% of cases. Adult ITP and ATP is not as well understood; only

10% to 20% of adult patients experience a spontaneous remission. Patients may be expected to have needs in the following areas:

    i. Positioning: Handle with care due to ease of bruising

    ii. Transport: May need supplies for spontaneous nose bleeding or oral bleeding; inform team members of risk for bruising

    iii. Discharge planning: Patient and family may need education about home environmental risks for injury that may precipitate spontaneous bleeding, need to seek health care for monitoring of platelet counts or if bleeding occurs, and effects of steroid therapy

  b. Potential complications

    i. Bleeding

      (a) Mechanism: Platelet count lower than $50,000/mm^3$

      (b) Management: Treatment for ITP can include administration of steroids, IV administration of immunoglobulin, platelet transfusion, splenectomy, and immunosuppressive therapy

8. Evaluation of patient care

  a. Absence of clinical or spontaneous bleeding

  b. Platelet count above $50,000/mm^3$

  c. Absence of bruising related to injury

Hypercoagulable Disorders

1. Pathophysiology

  a. Hypercoagulable disorders occur when the normal mechanisms of hemostasis involving platelets and clotting factors are disrupted, which results in uncontrolled or inappropriate clotting. Paradoxically, a secondary bleeding disorder develops in many of these patients when their reserves of platelets and clotting factors are depleted.

  b. Venous thromboses result from activation of the coagulation cascade caused by venous stasis, ischemia, or infarction. Arterial emboli result when a venous thrombus breaks away from its site of origin and migrates into the arterial vascular system. Pulmonary embolus, myocardial infarction, and thrombotic cerebrovascular accidents can be caused by arterial emboli. Patients are often admitted to critical care units for hemodynamic and neurologic support as well as for thrombolytic therapy with streptokinase, urokinase, or tissue plasminogen activator. Anticoagulation therapy puts these patients at risk for bleeding, although they have an underlying hypercoagulable disorder.

  c. TTP appears to be an exaggerated immunologic response to vessel injury that results in extensive thrombus formation and decreased blood flow to the affected site. These patients are critically ill; fever, thrombocytopenia, hemolytic anemia, renal impairment, and neurologic symptoms develop. HUS appears to be a variant of TTP that is seen more commonly in children. Patients with HUS tend to have more severe renal impairment, but fewer neurologic signs and symptoms, than do patients with TTP.

  d. DIC is another hypercoagulable disorder (see Disseminated Intravascular Coagulation)

2. Etiology and risk factors

  a. Changes in blood flow (e.g., deep vein thrombosis)

  b. Changes in circulating blood coagulation factors (e.g., TTP)

  c. Changes in the vessel wall

3. Signs and symptoms

  a. Symptoms: Tenderness or pain with palpation

  b. Signs: Unexplained bleeding, sudden painful swelling of one extremity, and other signs may be present, depending on the organ system involved; temperature exceeding 101° F (38.3° C), petechiae, purpura, ecchymoses, hematomas; circumference of one extremity different from that of the other corresponding extremity; changes in vital signs; with an arterial thrombosis, decreased blood flow in one extremity may be detected by Doppler ultrasonography

4. **Diagnostic study findings**
   a. Laboratory
      i. With venous stasis, laboratory values may be normal until anticoagulation therapy begins
      ii. With TTP, RBC levels are decreased; reticulocyte count, bilirubin level, and lactate dehydrogenase levels are increased; fragmented RBCs are seen on peripheral smear
   b. Radiologic: Angiography or venography can indicate vessel blockage
5. **Goals of care**
   a. Prevention of ischemic injury
   b. Prevention of dehydration
   c. Absence of hemorrhage
   d. Restoration of homeostatic coagulation
6. **Collaborating professionals on health care team**
   a. Transfusion specialist
   b. Blood bank specialist
   c. Pharmacist
   d. Nurse
   e. Physician
7. **Management of patient care**
   a. Anticipated patient trajectory: Full recovery from the complications of hypercoagulopathies, such as deep venous thrombosis, polycythemia, and temporary hyperviscosity of blood, can reasonably be expected when the patient is given early thrombolytic therapy combined with watchful collaborative care. Hypercoagulable disorders complicated by comorbidities, poor response to thrombolytics or collaborative care, and septicemia, however, may lead to loss of limbs due to ischemia or life-threatening DIC. Patients may be expected to have needs in the following areas:
      i. Positioning: Care in handling the patient due to the ease of bruising and propensity to create an embolus
      ii. Skin care: Prevention of complications of immobility and prolonged bed rest, which could lead to tissue alterations and ischemia
      iii. Pain management: Patient-controlled analgesia for deep venous thrombosis, joint swelling
      iv. Treatments: Thrombolytic therapy and potential blood product administration
   b. Potential complications
      i. Bleeding
         (a) Mechanism: Platelet count lower than 50,000/mm^3
         (b) Management: Clotting factor replacement and platelet transfusion, administration of antithrombolytics
8. **Evaluation of patient care**
   a. Absence of clinical or spontaneous bleeding
   b. Platelet count higher than 50,000/mm^3
   c. Absence of bruising related to injury
   d. Pain management

Neutropenia

1. **Pathophysiology**
   a. Occurs when the total number of neutrophils is abnormally low and puts the patient at increased risk of infection. The longer the patient is neutropenic, the greater the chance of infection. Patients are often admitted to critical care units with a diagnosis such as sepsis or acute leukemia that is complicated by neutropenia.
   b. The most common sites of infection seen in neutropenic patients are the lung (pneumonia), blood (septicemia), skin, urinary tract, and gastrointestinal tract (mucositis, esophagitis, perirectal lesions). The major infectious gram-negative bacilli include *Klebsiella pneumoniae* and *E. coli*. The major infectious gram-positive cocci include *S. aureus*, *Enterococcus*, and *Staphylococcus epidermidis*. Because affected patients do not have adequate numbers of WBCs to mount an immunologic response, the classical signs of infection may be absent. Fever may be the only sign of infection.

2. **Etiology and risk factors**
   a. Decreased neutrophil production
      i. Bone marrow infiltration with malignant cells
      ii. Recent history of antineoplastic chemotherapy, especially if high-dose chemotherapy was administered as part of bone marrow transplantation
      iii. Any history of radiation therapy to bones in which blood cells are made
      iv. Use of certain drugs (e.g., zidovudine, clozapine)
      v. Autoimmune disorder (e.g., systemic lupus erythematosus, rheumatoid arthritis)
   b. Increased neutrophil use: Overwhelming sepsis

3. **Signs and symptoms**
   a. Symptoms: Malaise; reports of fever, chills, and night sweats; sore throat; dyspnea; shortness of breath; abdominal pain, sinus pain, headache; confusion; pain with swallowing, urination, or defecation
   b. Signs: Cough, diarrhea, temperature exceeding 101° F (38.3° C), loss of integrity of skin and mucous membranes (especially at IV and central venous catheter sites), lymphadenopathy, tachycardia, hypotension, crackles, and rhonchi

4. **Diagnostic study findings**
   a. Laboratory: ANC lower than 500/microliter
   b. Radiologic: Findings are usually noncontributory to the diagnosis of neutropenia, but studies may be indicated to identify the source of infection secondary to neutropenia
   c. Bone marrow biopsy

5. **Goals of care:** Absence of infection

6. **Collaborating professionals on health care team**
   a. Nurse
   b. Blood bank specialist
   c. Pharmacist
   d. Physician

7. **Management of patient care**
   a. Anticipated patient trajectory: Mortality rate is 18% to 40% in the first 48 hours for patients with an ANC lower than 500/microliter. The goal of therapy is to support the patient until his or her own WBCs are available to fight infection.
   b. Potential complications
      i. Infection resulting in febrile episodes

        (a) Mechanism: Low WBC availability decreases the ability to fight infection

        (b) Management: Protect the patient from sources of community or nosocomial infection, institute neutropenic precautions (Table 7-9)

8. **Evaluation of patient care:** Protection successful in avoiding infectious processes

Acute Leukemia

1. **Pathophysiology**
   a. Leukemia is a cancer of the WBCs. There are many different types of leukemia, each based on which WBC lineage is affected and how quickly the leukemic clone multiples. Acute nonlymphocytic leukemia (ANLL), also called acute myelogenous leukemia (AML), is a cancer of the granulocyte cell line (Figure 7-1) affecting primarily adults. Acute lymphocytic leukemia (ALL) is a cancer of the lymphocyte cell line (Figure 7-1) affecting primarily children. The leukemic cells themselves are nonfunctional. They crowd out the normal bone marrow cells and thereby induce pancytopenia, manifested as anemia, neutropenia, and thrombocytopenia.
   b. Patients with leukemia are usually treated on oncology wards, but two complications of leukemia, overwhelming sepsis and acute tumor lysis syndrome, bring patients to critical care units for hemodynamic support and close observation

2. **Etiology and risk factors**
   a. Largely unknown, probably multifactorial
   b. Excessive radiation exposure
   c. Previous exposure to certain chemicals (e.g., benzene)
   d. Previous exposure to certain drugs (e.g., alkylating chemotherapy agents)
   e. Chromosomal abnormalities (e.g., as in Down syndrome)

3. **Signs and symptoms**
   a. Symptoms: Fatigue, malaise, bone pain, headache; reports of fever, chills, night sweats
   b. Signs: Pallor, petechial rash, easy bruising, weight loss, temperature exceeding 101° F (38.3° C), flushing, lethargy, petechiae, purpura, ecchymosis, hematomas, possible lymphadenopathy, possible hepatomegaly, possible splenomegaly, tachycardia, and hypotension

4. **Diagnostic study findings**
   a. Laboratory
      i. Total WBC count is very high or very low with primarily immature blast cells seen on the differential
      ii. Low RBC and platelet counts are usually also seen because these cell lines are crowded out of bone marrow by leukemic cells
      iii. In acute tumor lysis syndrome, uric acid levels exceed 7.2 mg/dl, potassium levels exceed 5.3 mg/dl, PO_4 levels exceeds 4.5 mg/dl, and calcium level is less than 8.6 mg/dl
   b. Bone marrow biopsy is usually performed to help with the diagnosis and guide treatment

5. **Goals of care**
   a. Protection against infections
   b. Protection against injury from bleeding
   c. Pain management
   d. Adequate nutrition
   e. Minimization of fear and anxiety
   f. Maintenance of family processes

6. **Collaborating professionals on health care team**
   a. Nurse
   b. Blood bank specialist
   c. Pharmacist
   d. Physician
7. **Management of patient care**
   a. Anticipated patient trajectory: Patient trajectory depends on demographic factors, type of WBC affected, and the maturational pathway from which the abnormal cells arise. Deaths from leukemia account for 4% of cancer deaths in the United States. During the course of treatment to discharge, patients with leukemia may be expected to have needs in the following areas:
      i. Pain management: Increased work of the bone marrow causes pain in both ALL and AML
      ii. Nutrition: Nausea, vomiting, and diarrhea may indicate a need to manage dietary intake with supplements
      iii. Infection control: Because 80% of infections are due to the patient's own endogenous flora, daily and frequent bath care with an oral examination every 4 hours is essential
      iv. Transport: During induction chemotherapy, a patient in profound neutropenia must be protected from infection
      v. Discharge planning: Information on prognosis, availability of leukemia support groups, and treatment protocol needs to be shared with the family and patient prior to discharge
      vi. Pharmacology: Patient and family may need education about chemotherapy, radiation therapy, and the physiologic markers for leukemia
      vii. Psychosocial issues: Social service support for the patient and family may be indicated when the patient's stay is prolonged (4 to 8 weeks) during induction or consolidation chemotherapy; provision of therapeutic distractions from pain, alopecia, nausea and vomiting, and fatigue can be challenging
      viii. Treatments: Chemotherapy, radiation, IV antibiotics, transfusions, bone marrow transplantation
   b. Potential complications
      i. Sepsis
         (a) Mechanism: The acute leukemias are initially treated with high-dose chemotherapy, called *induction therapy*, to induce bone marrow hypoplasia and allow normal cells to repopulate the bone marrow; the patient's ability to fight off infection is reduced until this repopulation is complete
         (b) Management: Monitor for persistent hypotension and hypoperfusion despite adequate fluid resuscitation, IV antibiotic therapy, and contact and neutropenic precautions
      ii. Tumor lysis syndrome
         (a) Mechanism: Tumor cell destruction creates a metabolic imbalance with rapid serum uptake of intracellular potassium, phosphorus, and nucleic acids
         (b) Management: In anticipation of the possibility of acute tumor lysis syndrome, medical management should include aggressive IV hydration, alkalinization of the urine, and allopurinol administration before chemotherapy is initiated. After chemotherapy is started, blood electrolyte levels should be monitored frequently and adjustments to the plan of care rapidly implemented as indicated. Hemodialysis may be

necessary to prevent acute tumor lysis syndrome even with aggressive management. For patients with WBC counts exceeding 100,000/mm^3, leukapheresis may be performed to remove the leukemic WBCs from the circulation before chemotherapy is initiated. This reduces the risk of acute tumor lysis syndrome.

8. **Evaluation of patient care**
   a. Absence of septic shock
   b. Renal function and serum electrolyte levels within normal limits
   c. Absence of hemorrhage
   d. Adequate pain management
   e. Adequate nutrition

Bone Marrow Transplantation and Peripheral Blood Stem Cell Transplantation

1. **Pathophysiology**
   a. Bone marrow transplantation (BMT) and peripheral blood stem cell transplantation (PBSCT) are procedures performed to reconstitute the hematologic and immunologic systems after patients with malignancies receive dosages of chemotherapy and radiation therapy high enough to permanently kill the bone marrow. BMT is also used in patients with aplastic anemia in an attempt to repopulate the marrow. Harvested marrow or peripheral stem cells are infused into the patient intravenously. Through their innate homing mechanism, the cells travel to the bone marrow and reestablish normal hematopoiesis.
   b. Types of transplant
      i. In allogeneic BMT, bone marrow from a human leukocyte antigen (HLA)–matched donor is used. Overall, there is a 25% chance that a sibling of a patient needing a BMT will be an HLA match. The chances of finding an HLA-matched unrelated donor (MUD) for a MUD allogeneric transplant are much smaller.
      ii. In autologous BMT, or bone marrow rescue, bone marrow from the patient is harvested and preserved before chemotherapy is initiated; the harvested bone marrow is infused after treatment. Using the patient's own bone marrow eliminates the risk of rejection and graft-versus-host disease (GVHD); however, the risk of cancer recurrence is higher. This type of BMT is the best option for patients with a solid tumor who require high doses of chemotherapy and radiation therapy but who have healthy bone marrow that can be harvested before treatment and returned after therapy. Patients with hematologic malignancies can have their bone marrow harvested during remission, purged of malignant cells, and then returned after high-dose therapy.
      iii. In PBSCT, the patient's bone marrow is stimulated with colony-stimulating factors, and then the patient's peripheral stem cells are harvested through repeated phereses. After chemotherapy and radiation therapy treatment, the patient's stem cells are reinfused, as in BMT. As with autologous BMT, the risks of rejection and GVHD are eliminated. In addition, stem cells reengraft more quickly than bone marrow, which reduces the length of neutropenia and risk of infection. Often, PBSCT is performed concurrently with autologous BMT.
2. **Etiology and risk factors** (i.e., indications for BMT or PBSCT)
   a. Administration of dosages of chemotherapy and radiation to treat a malignancy that are toxic to bone marrow
   b. Genetic defect (e.g., severe combined immunodeficiency disease)
   c. Aplastic syndromes (e.g., aplastic anemia, agranulocytosis)

3. **Signs and symptoms during transplantation**
   a. Symptoms: Malaise, fatigue, weakness, lethargy, reports of chills and night sweats, sore throat, dyspnea, shortness of breath, sinus pain, headache, confusion; pain with swallowing, urination, or defecation
   b. Signs: Petechial rash, cough, diarrhea, temperature exceeding 101° F (38.3° C), pallor, jaundice, petechiae, rash, weight changes, loss of integrity of skin and mucous membranes; bleeding from the oropharynx, gastrointestinal tract, or genitourinary tract; hepatomegaly, tachycardia, hypotension, crackles, rhonchi, hyperactive bowel sounds

4. **Diagnostic study findings**
   a. Laboratory
      i. WBC count, HCT, hemoglobin level, and platelet count all can be expected to be low
      ii. With renal insufficiency, increased creatinine levels and electrolyte abnormalities
      iii. Increased bilirubin level, increased liver enzyme levels, prolonged PT, and prolonged PTT
   b. Biopsy: Definitive diagnosis of the complications of transplantation often requires a tissue biopsy; however, biopsy is often contraindicated because of coagulopathies

5. **Goals of care**
   a. Absence of infection
   b. Absence of hemorrhage related to disease or treatment
   c. Absence of fluid volume deficit due to fever, diarrhea, hemorrhage, or shock
   d. Adequate renal functioning
   e. Adequate pain management

6. **Collaborating professionals on health care team**
   a. Nurse
   b. Blood bank specialist
   c. Pharmacist
   d. Physician
   e. Transplant surgery team

7. **Management of patient care**
   a. Anticipated patient trajectory: BMT or PBSCT places a client at considerable risk of death from infection
   b. Potential complications
      i. Pancytopenia
         (a) Mechanism: Conditioning chemotherapy and radiation prior to BMT obliterates the patient's own marrow
         (b) Management: Targeted at side effects of conditioning therapy, including profound nausea and vomiting, mucositis, capillary leak syndrome, diarrhea, and bone marrow suppression
      ii. Failure to engraft
         (a) Mechanism: Failure of transfused peripheral stem cells and marrow cells to take up residence engrafted to recipient's bones
         (b) Management: Repeat transfusion of peripheral stem cells to prevent certain death
      iii. GVHD
         (a) Mechanism: Immunocompetent cells of donated marrow mount an autoimmune response against the recipient's tissue
         (b) Management: Treatment includes administration of immunosuppressive drugs to suppress the transplanted T lymphocytes (with antithymocyte globulin or murine monoclonal antibody to CD3), cyclosporine,

and low-dose methotrexate, and hemodynamic support (see also Transplant Rejection)

    iv. Veno-occlusive disease

      (a) Mechanism: Occlusion of hepatic circulation by clotting and phlebitis

      (b) Management: Supportive treatment with fluid resuscitation and assessment of increased girth, hepatomegaly, ascites, or weight gain

    v. Sepsis

      (a) Mechanism: Pancytopenia obliterates the patient's own ability to fight off infection

      (b) Management: Prophylactic use of the antifungal drug fluconazole decreases the incidence of *C. albicans* infection in BMT patients; prophylactic treatment with acyclovir can decrease the incidence of reactivation of herpes simplex virus and cytomegalovirus in seropositive BMT patients

8. **Evaluation of patient care**

    a. No evidence of sepsis

    b. Absence of community and hospital-associated infection

    c. No evidence of hemorrhage

    d. Urine output above 30 ml/hr

    e. Pain managed or absent

    f. Ability of the patient to express anxieties and fears

Transplant Rejection

1. **Pathophysiology**

    a. When tissue from one person is transplanted into another person, the immune system of the recipient can recognize the transplanted tissue, or allograft, as foreign. Rejections occur through various mechanisms:

      i. Type III, Arthus-type hypersensitivity reaction in the blood vessels of the graft immediately after transplantation

      ii. Cytotoxic T lymphocytes (T_C) can directly attack the allograft, which results in acute transplant rejection and occurs within days of the transplantation

      iii. B lymphocytes can make antibodies against the allograft; these activate the complement pathways and attract platelets. Fibrin accumulates on the transplanted tissue, causing ischemia. In this way the allograft is slowly rejected over many months to years.

    b. HLA matching of donor to recipient before transplantation is an attempt to choose a donor whose antigens match the recipient's as closely as possible so that the recipient's immune system is not triggered to attack the allograft after the transplantation procedure

    c. Allogeneic BMT is fundamentally different from solid organ transplantation. In allogeneic BMT, the immune system itself is being transplanted into a new host. Therefore, it may attack any tissue in the new host, resulting in GVHD (see Bone Marrow Transplantation and Peripheral Blood Stem Cell Transplantation). Because GVHD is usually a limited (albeit serious) problem, the majority of patients undergoing allogeneic BMT can eventually discontinue immunosuppressive therapy. In patients receiving solid organ transplants, the host's own immune system attacks the donated organ, so recipients must receive lifelong immunosuppressive therapy.

2. **Etiology and risk factors:** Activation of the immune response against transplanted tissue

3. **Signs and symptoms**
   a. Symptoms: Malaise, poor appetite, myalgia, tenderness of the allograft
   b. Signs: Swelling of the allograft, temperature exceeding 101° F (38.3° C)
4. **Diagnostic study findings:** Specific to the organ transplanted
5. **Goals of care**
   a. Nonproliferation of immunocompetent cells
   b. Suppression of the activity of helper T cells (T_H) and T_C cells
   c. Engraftment of donor tissue or organ
6. **Collaborating professionals on health care team**
   a. Nurse
   b. Blood bank specialist
   c. Pharmacist
   d. Physician
   e. Transplant surgery team
7. **Management of patient care**
   a. Anticipated patient trajectory: Hyperacute rejection and graft failure can occur immediately following transplantation; acute rejection can occur weeks to months later; chronic rejection can progress over a period of several years
   b. Potential complications
      i. Proliferation of immunocompetent cells
         (a) Mechanism: Antigens on transplanted tissue cells are immediately recognized as nonself and rejection of donor tissue occurs
         (b) Management: Immunosuppression (see Immunosuppression section)
8. **Evaluation of patient care**
   a. Immunosuppression
   b. Engraftment of donor tissue or organ

Immunosuppression

1. **Pathophysiology**
   a. Immunosuppression occurs when some defect in the immunologic system puts the patient at increased risk for infection. The longer the patient is immunosuppressed, the greater the risk of infection. Neutropenia is one form of immunosuppression (see Neutropenia). Although there are primary forms of immune dysfunction, patients are more often admitted to critical care units with immunosuppression as a complication of an underlying disease.
   b. Various drugs prescribed to suppress one part of the immune system have untoward effects on other parts of the hematologic and immunologic systems. After organ transplantation, various drugs are used to suppress the immune system and prevent transplant rejection. These drugs act primarily on B cells and T cells and suppress not only the immunologic response to the allograft but also the patient's ability to fight bacteria, viruses, fungi, and parasites.
2. **Etiology and risk factors**
   a. Drug induced
      i. Steroids
      ii. Azathioprine (Imuran)
      iii. Cyclosporine
      iv. History of antineoplastic chemotherapy, especially in high doses as is administered for BMT
   b. Genetic (e.g., severe combined immunodeficiency disease)
   c. Decreased neutrophil production (see Neutropenia)
   d. HIV infection (see HIV Infection)
3. **Signs and symptoms:** See Neutropenia

4. **Diagnostic study findings**: Laboratory cultures give positive results for unusual or opportunistic organisms (e.g., *Pneumocystis carinii*)
5. **Goals of care:** See Neutropenia and Table 7-9
6. **Collaborating professionals on health care team:** See Neutropenia
7. **Management of patient care:** See Neutropenia and Table 7-9
8. **Evaluation of patient care:** See Neutropenia and Table 7-9

HIV Infection

1. **Pathophysiology**
   a. HIV type 1, previously known as human T-lymphotropic virus type 3 (HTLV-3), is a retrovirus that infects cells expressing CD4 on their cell membranes, primarily T_H lymphocytes and macrophages. The HIV copies its RNA into the host cell's DNA and then remains quiescent until the host cell is activated to mount an immunologic response. Activation of the host CD4 cells also initiates replication and production of the HIV RNA, which is released into the circulation. This newly made HIV then infects other cells expressing CD4.
   b. Disease course
      i. The initial stage of HIV infection last 4 to 8 weeks. High levels of virus are in the blood. The patient experiences generalized flulike symptoms.
      ii. The virus then enters a latent stage in which it is inactive in infected, resting CD4 cells, replicating only when the host cell is activated for an immune response. Levels of virus are high in the lymph nodes, where CD4 cells reside, but low in the blood. T_C cells, which express CD8 and so are not infected by HIV, and B cells attempt to destroy the CD4 cells harboring the virus. However, the T_C cells and B cells are crippled without adequate T_H support. This latent stage lasts on the average between 2 and 12 years, during which time the patient is asymptomatic. During this time, the number of CD4 cells declines.
      iii. During the third stage of HIV infection, the patient begins to experience opportunistic infections. Levels of CD4 cells are usually below $500/mm^3$ and declining, whereas levels of virus in the blood are increasing. This stage can last 2 to 3 years.
      iv. Once the CD4 cell levels drop below $200/mm^3$, the patient is considered to have AIDS. Virus levels in the blood are high. This stage ends in death, usually within 1 year.
2. **Etiology and risk factors:** HIV is transmitted via intimate sexual contact, contaminated needles or contaminated blood products, from mother to fetus, and from mother to breast-feeding infant
3. **Signs and symptoms**
   a. Symptoms and history: Fatigue, night sweats, sore throat, dyspnea, shortness of breath, pain, history of frequent infections, social history of IV drug abuse with shared needles, history of unprotected sexual contact with persons possibly infected with HIV, history of blood transfusion
   b. Signs: Weight loss, diarrhea, temperature exceeding 101° F (38.3° C), loss of integrity of skin and mucous membranes, possible cachexia, possible lymphadenopathy, tachycardia, hypotension, crackles, and rhonchi
4. **Diagnostic study findings**
   a. Laboratory
      i. Western blot test result that is positive for HIV (NOTE: Enzyme-linked immunosorbent assay [ELISA] is a less expensive screening test for HIV antibody. If the ELISA result is positive, a Western blot test should be performed to confirm the findings, because false-positive results do occur with ELISA.)

    ii. CD4 lymphocyte counts that are lower than $500/mm^3$

    iii. Nonreactive results on skin test panel

    iv. Infection with unusual or opportunistic organisms (e.g., *P. carinii*)

  b. Radiologic: Infiltrates on chest radiograph

5. Goals of care

  a. Education about prevention of the spread of HIV infection

  b. Maintenance of universal precautions

  c. Containment of associated opportunistic diseases

  d. Ability of the patient to express fear, grief, and social isolation

6. Collaborating disciplines

  a. Nurse

  b. Chaplain

  c. Social worker

  d. Physician

  e. Pharmacist

  f. Psychiatrist

7. Management of patient care

  a. Anticipated patient trajectory: The time from initial HIV infection to the development of AIDS ranges from months to years depending on demographic characteristics, lifestyle, and interventional factors. Progression to death accelerates with the development of multiple opportunistic infections. Throughout their course of clinical care and discharge, patients may be expected to have needs in the following areas:

    i. Nutrition: Avoid fatty foods if chronic diarrhea is present, avoid fruits with peels, maintain good hydration, maintain high protein consumption, encourage consumption of foods that the patient likes, assess for oral lesions and hygiene

    ii. Infection control: Education of the patient and the family or significant others may be key in decreasing the spread of infection by sexual contact, IV needle use, and maternal-child transmission; health care workers must use universal precautions

    iii. Pharmacology: Education for the patient and the family or significant others may be warranted to describe antiretroviral therapy, prophylactic treatment for opportunistic infections, and use of hematopoiesis-stimulating factors

    iv. Psychosocial issues: There is no cure for HIV infection or AIDS; therefore, individual coping ability should be explored

    v. Ethical issues: Presence of HIV infection or AIDS raises the concern of intentional spread of infection

  b. Potential complications

    i. AIDS dementia complex

      (a) Mechanism: HIV invasion of the central nervous system, which occurs in 70% of cases

      (b) Management: Initiation of fall precautions and support for cognitive, motor, or behavioral impairment

    ii. Opportunistic infections

      (a) Mechanism: Suppression of immune responses resulting from infection with HIV

      (b) Management: Antiretroviral therapy with zidovudine, didanosine (ddI, Videx), zalcitabine (ddC, Hivid), or stavudine (d4T, Zerit); prophylactic antibiotic therapy with trimethoprim-sulfamethoxazole, aerosolized pentamidine (Pentam), and/or other agents; antiretroviral therapy with agents with HIV-1 protease inhibitors such as saquinavir (Invirase), indinavir (Crixivan), nelfinavir (Viracept), and/or ritonavir (Norvir)

8. **Evaluation of patient management**
   a. Controlled infective state
   b. Ability of the patient to express fears, anxiety, and grief
   c. Low number and severity of opportunistic infections

Anaphylactic Hypersensitivity Reactions

1. **Pathophysiology**
   a. There are four types of hypersensitivity reaction, classified according to the time between the exposure and the reaction, the immune mechanism involved, and the site of the reaction
      i. *Type I* immediate hypersensitivity reactions are mediated by immunoglobulin E (IgE) in reaction to common allergens such as dust, pollen, animal dander, insect sting, some foods, and various drugs. These reactions can be local, resulting in local swelling and discomfort, or systemic, resulting in anaphylaxis and possibly in death if not recognized and treated promptly.
      ii. *Type II* immediate hypersensitivity reactions are mediated by antibody and complement. These reactions can occur with a mismatched blood transfusion or as a response to various drugs.
      iii. *Type III* immediate hypersensitivity reactions result in tissue damage caused by precipitation of antigen-antibody immune complexes. These reactions can occur with serum sickness or in response to various drugs.
      iv. *Type IV* delayed hypersensitivity reactions result from migration of immune cells to the site of exposure days after the exposure to the antigen. These reactions can occur in contact dermatitis, measles rash, or tuberculin skin testing or in response to various drugs. Transplanted graft rejection is a type IV hypersensitivity reaction.
   b. After a first, sensitizing exposure to a specific allergen, such as an insect sting, in which abnormally large amounts of IgE antibodies are made, subsequent exposures to the same allergen trigger an exaggerated antibody reaction. When the patient comes in contact with the antigen a second time, IgE triggers the release of histamine, heparin, and other cytokines (see Table 7-4) from mast cells, causing bronchiole constriction, peripheral vasoconstriction, and increased vascular permeability, which quickly progress to airway obstruction, pulmonary edema, peripheral edema, hypovolemia, hypotension, shock, and circulatory collapse.

2. **Etiology and risk factors**
   a. Drugs (e.g., penicillin, local anesthetics, vaccines, contrast dye)
   b. Insect stings
   c. Foods (e.g., shellfish, milk, eggs, fish, wheat)

3. **Signs and symptoms**
   a. Symptoms: Apprehension, dyspnea, restlessness
   b. Signs: Urticaria, facial edema, tachypnea, stridor, cyanosis, tachycardia, hypotension, wheezing

4. **Diagnostic study findings:** Usually noncontributory to the diagnosis of anaphylaxis

5. **Goals of care**
   a. Patent airway, maintenance of breathing and circulation
   b. Absence of hypovolemia due to shock
   c. Stable hemodynamic state

6. **Collaborating professionals on health care team**
   a. Nurse
   b. Pharmacist
   c. Physician
   d. Respiratory therapist
7. **Management of patient care**
   a. Anticipated patient trajectory: Patients experiencing an anaphylactic hypersensitivity or anaphylactoid event differ in their clinical course depending on age, medical history, number of prior exposures, and the extent of prior reactions. Throughout their course of recovery, airway and circulatory compromise or collapse may threaten life. Mild hypersensitivity reactions with localized symptoms can be prevented from becoming acute if pharmacologic management is immediate. Patients may be expected to have needs in the following areas:
      i. Positioning: Use a chin lift in the supine position or high Fowler's position to provide a patent airway
      ii. Transport: Maintain a patent airway, circulatory support, and cervical neck traction until the patient is hemodynamically stable
      iii. Discharge planning: Patient education may be required to reinforce the importance of wearing a medic alert bracelet, the home use of epinephrine, the need to contact health care personnel immediately at the onset of a hypersensitivity reaction, and the importance of avoiding allergens
   b. Potential complications
      i. Cardiopulmonary arrest
         (a) Mechanism: Antibody response to allergen results in vasodilation and bronchoconstriction
         (b) Management: Cardiopulmonary resuscitation, administration of corticosteroids (IV Solu-Cortef or Solu-Medrol) and histamine blockers (diphenhydramine [Benadryl], 25 to 50 mg; epinephrine, 0.2 to 0.5 ml subcutaneously or 0.5 ml of 1:1000 IV)
      ii. Respiratory compromise
         (a) Mechanism: Histamine release creates interstitial edema and potential bronchoconstriction resulting in pulmonary edema
         (b) Management: Administration of corticosteroids, histamine blockers, and supplemental oxygen
8. **Evaluation of patient care**
   a. Patent airway with uncompromised breathing
   b. Absence of circulatory collapse or compromise
   c. Controlled local clinical manifestations, such as hives or urticaria

REFERENCES

Physiologic Anatomy

Guyton AC, Hall JE: *Textbook of medical physiology,* ed 10, Philadelphia, 2000, Saunders.

Janeway CA Jr, Travers P: *Immunobiology,* ed 3, New York, 1997, Garland.

McCance KL, Huether SE: *Pathophysiology: the biologic basis for disease in adults and children,* ed 4, St Louis, 2002, Mosby.

McMahon TJ, Exton Stone A, Bonaventura J, et al: Functional coupling of oxygen binding and vasoactivity in S-nitrosohemoglobin, *J Biol Chem* 275:16738-16745, 2000.

Metcalf D: Cellular hematopoiesis in the twentieth century, *Semin Hematol* 36(4 suppl 7):5-12, 1999.

Porth CM: *Pathophysiology: concepts of altered health status,* ed 6, Philadelphia, 2002, Lippincott Williams & Wilkins.

Patient Assessment

Deglin JH, Vallerand AH: *Davis drug guide for nurses,* ed 8, Philadelphia, 2003, FA Davis.

Hankins J, Lonsway RAW, Hedrick D, et al: *Infusion therapy in clinical practice,* ed 2, St Louis, 2001, Saunders.

Ignatavicius DD, Workman ML, editors: *Medical-surgical nursing: critical thinking for collaborative care,* ed 4, Philadelphia, 2002, Saunders.

Kee JL: *Laboratory and diagnostic tests with nursing implications,* ed 5, Stamford, Conn, 1999, Appleton & Lange.

Pagana KD, Pagana TJ: *Mosby's diagnostic and laboratory test reference,* ed 6, St Louis, 2003, Mosby.

Wilson BA, Shannon MT, Stang CL: *Nurse's drug guide,* Upper Saddle River, NJ, 2004, Prentice Hall.

Specific Patient Health Problems
Anemia

Cook LS: A simple case of anemia: pathophysiology of a common symptom, *J Intraven Nurs* 23(5):271-281, 2000.

Goram AL: Factors and predictors of response with epoetin alfa for chemotherapy-related anemia, *J Pharm Technol* 16(6): 227-235, 2000.

Loney M, Chernecky C: Anemia, *Oncol Nurs Forum* 27(6):951-966, 2000.

Ludwig H, Strasser K: Symptomatology of anemia, *Semin Oncol* 28(2 suppl 8):7-14, 2001.

Pearl RG, Pohlman A: Understanding and managing anemia in critically ill patients, *Crit Care Nurse* (suppl):1-16, 2002.

Sobrero A, Puglisi F, Guglielmi A, et al: Fatigue: a main component of anemia symptomatology, *Semin Oncol* 28(2 suppl 8):15-18, 2001.

Taher A, Kazzi Z: Anemia, sickle cell, January 5, 2005, retrieved July 12, 2004, from http://www.emedicine.com/emerg/topic26.htm.

Volberding P: Consensus statement: anemia in HIV infection: Current trends, treatment options, and practice strategies, *Clin Ther* 22(9):1004-1020, 2000.

Disseminated Intravascular Coagulation

Dice RD: Intraoperative disseminated intravenous coagulopathy, *Crit Care Nurs Clin North Am* 12(2):175-179, 2000.

Levi M: Pathogenesis and treatment of disseminated intravascular coagulation in the septic patient, *J Crit Care* 16(4):167-177, 2001.

Levi M, de Jonge E: Current management of disseminated intravascular coagulation, *Hosp Pract (Off Ed)* 35(8):59-66, 92, 2000.

Maxson JH: Management of disseminated intravascular coagulation, *Crit Care Nurs Clin North Am* 12(3):341-352, 2000.

Stillwell SB, editor: *Mosby's critical care nursing reference,* St Louis, 2002, Mosby.

Thrombocytopenia

Ansani NT: Heparin-induced thrombocytopenia and thrombosis: a review of pharmacologic therapy, *J Pharm Technol* 17(5): 189-197, 2001.

Argatroban is a new option for patients with heparin-induced thrombocytopenia, *Drugs Ther Perspect* 17(19):1-4, 2001.

Deitcher SR: Heparin-induced thrombocytopenia: pathogenesis, management, and prevention, *Formulary* 36(1):26-28, 30, 39-41, 2001.

Doyle B, Porter DL: Thrombocytopenia, *AACN Clin Issues* 8(3):469-480, 1997.

Fukuyama SN, Itano J: Thrombocytopenia secondary to myelosuppression, *Am J Nurs* (suppl):5-8, 34-36, 1999.

Horrell CJ, Rothman J: The etiology of thrombocytopenia, *Dimens Crit Care Nurs* 20(4):10-16, 2001.

Nguyen TN, Gal P, Ransom JL, et al: Lepirudin use in a neonate with heparin-induced thrombocytopenia, *Ann Pharmacother* 37(2):229-233, 2003.

Todisco M, Casaccia P, Rossi N: Severe bleeding symptoms in refractory idiopathic thrombocytopenic purpura: a case successfully treated with melatonin, *Am J Ther* 10(2):135-136, 2003.

Hypercoagulable Disorders

Dickey TL: The hypercoagulable state as a risk factor for venous thromboembolism, part I, *J Am Acad Physician Assist* 15(11):28-30, 32, 35, 2002.

Gardner J: Factor V Leiden with deep venous thrombosis, *Clin Lab Sci* 16(1):6-9, 2003.

Lapointe LA, Von Rueden KT: Coagulopathies in trauma patients, *AACN Clin Issues* 13(2):192-203, 2002.

Meissner MH, Chandler WL, Elliott JS: Venous thromboembolism in trauma: a local manifestation of systemic hypercoagulability? *J Trauma Injury Infect Crit Care* 54(2):224-231, 2003.

Mulroy JF, De Jong MJ: Syndromes of hypercoagulability: protein C and protein S deficiencies in acutely ill adults, *Am J Nurs* 103(5):Critical Care Extra, 64KK, 64MM, 64OO, 2003.

Neufeld EJ: Coagulation disorders and treatment strategies, *Hematol Oncol Clin North Am* 12(6):ix-x, 1141-1144, 1998.

Subar M: Clinical evaluation of hypercoagulable states, *Clin Geriatr Med* 17(1):57-70, 2001.

Spero JA: Venous thromboembolism and hypercoagulability, *Top Emerg Med* 22(3):9-22, 2000.

van Cott EM, Laposata M: Your lab focus: overview. Algorithms for hypercoagulation testing, *Lab Med* 34(3):216-220, 222, 2003.

Neutropenia

Asumang A, Criswell J: Neutropenic patients, *Care Crit Ill* 14(6):195-198, 1998.

Bow EJ: Management of the febrile neutropenic cancer patient: lessons from 40 years of study, *Clin Microbiol Infect* 11(suppl 5):24-29, 2005.

Burney KY: Tips for timely management of febrile neutropenia, *Oncol Nurs Forum* 27(4):617-618, 2000.

Corey L, Boeckh M: Persistent fever in patients with neutropenia, *N Engl J Med* 346(4):222-224, 2002.

Freifeld AG, Walsh TJ, Pizzo PA: Infections in the cancer patient. In DeVita VT, Hellman S, Rosenberg SA, editors: *Cancer: principles and practice of oncology*, ed 5, Philadelphia, 1997, Lippincott, pp 2659-2704.

Klastersky J, Paesmans M, Rubenstein EB, et al: The Multinational Association for Supportive Care in Cancer Risk Index: a multinational scoring system for identifying low-risk febrile neutropenic cancer patients, *J Clin Oncol* 18(16):3038-3051, 2000.

Mutnick AH, Kirby JT, Jones RN: CANCER Resistance Surveillance Program: initial results from hematology-oncology centers in North America, *Ann Pharmacother* 37(1):47-56, 2003.

Reigle BS, Dienger MJ: Sepsis and treatment-induced immunosuppression in the patient with cancer: tables/charts, *Crit Care Nurs Clin North Am* 15(1):109-118, 2003.

Santolaya ME, Alvarez AM, Becker A, et al: Prospective, multicenter evaluation of risk factors associated with invasive bacterial infection in children with cancer, neutropenia, and fever, *J Clin Oncol* 19(14):3415-3421, 2001.

Soni S, Radel E: Neutropenia: striking a balance between caution and alarm, *Contemp Pediatr* 19(8):77-78, 82-85, 2002.

Wilson BJ: Dietary recommendations for neutropenic patients, *Semin Oncol Nurs* 18(1):44-49, 2002.

Acute Leukemia

Devine H, DeMeyer E: Hematopoietic cell transplantation in the treatment of leukemia, *Semin Oncol Nurs* 19(2):118-132, 2003.

Dietz-Lovett K: An overview of acute and chronic leukemias, *Dev Support Cancer Care* 2(3):66-72, 103-105, 1998.

Mackey HT, Klemm P: Leukemia: aggressive therapies predispose patients to a host of side effects, *Am J Nurs* (suppl):27-31, 52-54, 2000.

Medoff E: Oncology today: new horizons: leukemia, *RN* 63(9):42-46, 49-50, 2000.

Murphy-Ende K, Chernecky C: Assessing adults with leukemia, *Nurse Pract* 27(11): 49, 52-56, 59-60, 2002.

Rodak BF, Leclair SJ: The new WHO nomenclature: introduction and myeloid neoplasms, *Lab Sci* 15(1):44-54, 60-63, 2002.

Scheinberg DA, Maslak P, Weiss M: Acute leukemias. In DeVita VT, Hellman S, Rosenberg SA, editors: *Cancer: principles and practice of oncology*, ed 5, Philadelphia, 1997, Lippincott, pp 2293-2321.

Shannon-Dorcy K, Wolfe V: Decision-making in the diagnosis and treatment of leukemia, *Semin Oncol Nurs* 19(2):142-149, 2003.

Warrell RP: Metabolic emergencies. In DeVita VT, Hellman S, Rosenberg SA, editors: *Cancer: principles and practice of oncology*, ed 5, Philadelphia, 1997, Lippincott, pp 2486-2500.

Wujcik D: Molecular biology of leukemia, *Semin Oncol Nurs* 19(2):83-89, 2003.

Yoder LH: Diseases treated with blood cell transplants, *Semin Oncol Nurs* 13(3):164-171, 1997.

Bone Marrow Transplantation and Peripheral Blood Stem Cell Transplantation

Buchsel PC, Leum EW, Randolph SR: Delayed complications of bone marrow transplantation: an update, *Oncol Nurs Forum* 23(8):1267-1291, 1996.

Campos de Carvalho E, Goncalves PG, Bontempo APM, et al: Interpersonal needs expressed by patients during bone marrow transplantation, *Cancer Nurs* 23(6): 462-467, 2000.

Centers for Disease Control and Prevention, Infectious Disease Society of America, American Society of Blood and Marrow Transplantation: Guidelines for preventing opportunistic infections among hematopoietic stem cell transplant recipients, *MMWR Recomm Rep* 49(RR-10):1-95, 97-125, CE1-7, 2000.

Cohen MZ, Ley CD: Bone marrow transplantation: the battle for hope in the face of fear, *Oncol Nurs Forum* 27(3):473-480, 2000.

Farquhar C, Basser R, Marjoribanks J, et al: High dose chemotherapy and autologous bone marrow or stem cell transplantation versus conventional chemotherapy for women with early poor prognosis breast cancer, *Cochrane Database of Systematic Reviews* Issue 1, Art No: CD003139. DOI: 10.1002/14651858.CD003139, 2003.

Fife BL, Huster GA, Cornetta KG, et al: Longitudinal study of adaptation to the stress of bone marrow transplantation, *J Clin Oncol* 18(7):1539-1549, 2000.

Hacker ED: Quantitative measurement of quality of life in adult patients undergoing bone marrow transplant or peripheral blood stem cell transplant: a decade in review, *Oncol Nurs Forum* 30(4):613-631, 2003.

Hematopoietic stem cell therapy, *Hematol Oncol Clin North Am* 13(5):xi-xii, 889-1112, 1999.

Hematopoietic stem cell transplantation, *Curr Opin Hematol* 9(6):477-508, 2002.

Keller C, Thieszen S: Researchers extending potential for stem cell transplants, *Blood Marrow Transplant Newsl* 14(1):2, 4, 2003.

Maloy BJ: Hematopoiesis, stem cells, and transplantation: what have we learned for the new millennium? *J Intraven Nurs* 23(5): 298-303, 2000.

Maningo J: Peripheral blood stem cell transplant: easier than getting blood from a bone, *Nursing* 32(12):52-55, 2002.

Marena C, Zecca M, Carenini ML, et al: Incidence of, and risk factors for, nosocomial infections among hematopoietic stem cell transplantation recipients, with impact on procedure-related mortality, *Infect Control Hosp Epidemiol* 22(8):510-517, 2001.

Middleton R: Changing treatment options in bone marrow transplantation, *Transplant Nurses J* 8(2):8-13, 1999.

Myer SA, Oliva J: Severe aplastic anemia and allogeneic hematopoietic stem cell transplantation, *AACN Clin Issues* 13(2):169-191, 2002.

Olver WJ, James SA, Lennard A, et al: Nosocomial transmission of *Saccharomyces cerevisiae* in bone marrow transplant patients, *J Hosp Infect* 52(4):268-272, 2002.

Rebellato LM, Dobbs LJ Jr: Haploidentical transplantation: importance of histocompatibility testing and chimerism studies in allogeneic bone marrow/stem cell transplantation, *J Infus Nurs* 24(5):311-318, 2001.

Schmit-Pokorny K, Franco T, Frappier B, et al: The cooperative care model: an innovative approach to deliver blood and marrow stem cell transplant care, *Clin J Oncol Nurs* 7(5 pt 1):509-514, 556, 542-543, 2003.

Schneider S: Interventions for clients with hematologic problems. In Ignatavicius DD, Workman ML: *Medical-surgical nursing: critical thinking for collaborative care*, ed 4, Philadelphia, 2002, Saunders, pp 853-856.

Serody JS, Shea TC: Prevention of infections in bone marrow transplant recipients, *Infect Dis Clin North Am* 11(2):459-477, 1997.

Shivnan J, Shelton BK, Onners BK: Bone marrow transplantation: issues for critical care nurses, *AACN Clin Issues* 7(1):95-108, 179-180, 1996.

Yeager KA, Webster J, Crain M, et al: Implementation of an oral care standard for leukemia and transplantation patients, *Cancer Nurs* 23(1):40-48, 2000.

Transplant Rejection

Giuliano KK, Sims TW: Transplant issues: infections and immunosuppressant drugs, *Dimens Crit Care Nurs* 18(2):16-19, 1999.

Lake K: Acute rejection: prevention, diagnosis and management, *Dis Manag Digest* 4(4):4-5, 14-15, 2000.

Morris RE: New immunosuppressive molecules for control of organ transplant rejection. In Williams BAH, Sandiford-Guttenbeil DM, editors: *Trends in organ transplantation*, New York, 1996, Springer, pp 83-94.

NIH tests ways to prevent transplant rejection, *Diabetes Dateline*, pp 1-4, Winter 1999-2000.

O'Donnell M, Parmenter KL: Transplant medications, *Crit Care Nurs Clin North Am* 8(3):253-271, 1996.

Poole P, Greer E: Immunosuppression in transplantation: a new millennium in care, *Crit Care Nurs Clin North Am* 12(3):315-321, 2000.

Immunosuppression

Bush WW: Overview of transplantation immunology and the pharmacotherapy of adult solid organ transplant recipients: focus on immunosuppression, *AACN Clin Issues* 10(2):253-269, 304-306, 1999.

Cohen SM: Current immunosuppression in liver transplantation, *Am J Ther* 9(2):119-125, 2002.

Huizinga R: Update in immunosuppression, *Nephrol Nurs J* 29(3):261-267, 2002.

Immunosuppressive therapies: an overview, *Dis Manag Digest* 4(5):2-3, 14-15, 2000.

Poole P, Greer E: Immunosuppression in transplantation: a new millennium in care, *Crit Care Nurs Clin North Am* 12(3):315-321, 2000.

Reigle BS, Dienger MJ: Sepsis and treatment-induced immunosuppression in the patient with cancer, *Crit Care Nurs Clin North Am* 15(1):109-118, 2003.

Wahrenberger A: Pharmacologic immunosuppression: cure or curse? *Crit Care Nurs Q* 17(4):27-36, 1995.

HIV Infection

Abel E, Painter L: Factors that influence adherence to HIV medications: perceptions of women and health care providers, *J Assoc Nurses AIDS Care* 14(4):61-69, 2003.

Drug resistance guide being pondered by CDC: as HIV drug resistance rises, surveillance needed, *AIDS Alert* 18(11):146-147, 2003.

Ferri RS, Adinolfi A, Orsi AJ, et al: Treatment of anemia in patients with HIV infection, part 2: guidelines for management of anemia, *J Assoc Nurses AIDS Care* 13(1):50-59, 2002.

Goldschmidt RH, Dong BJ: Treatment of AIDS and HIV-related conditions: 2001, *J Am Board Fam Pract* 14(4):283-309, 2001.

Jones SG: Nursing practice for HIV/AIDS fever care: a descriptive study, *J Assoc Nurses AIDS Care* 9(5):53-60, 1998.

Anaphylactic Type I Hypersensitivity Reactions

Brazil E, MacNamara AF: "Not so immediate" hypersensitivity: the danger of biphasic anaphylactic reactions, *J Accid Emerg Med* 15(4):252-253, 1998.

Carr BW, Burke C: Outpatient chemotherapy: hypersensitivity and anaphylaxis: oncology nurses must know how to respond quickly and correctly, *Am J Nurs* (suppl):27-30, 49-50, 2001.

Carroll P: Anaphylaxis, *RN* 64(12):45-50, 2001.

Green LC: Anaphylactic shock and its implication for nurses, *Accid Emerg Nurs* 6(2):103-105, 1998.

Jurewicz MA: Anaphylaxis: when the body overreacts, *Nursing* 30(7):58-61, 2000.

Fatigue

Dimeo F, Rumberger BG, Keul J: Aerobic exercise as therapy for cancer fatigue, *Clin J Am Coll Sports Med* 30(4):475-478, 1998.

Mock V, Dow KH, Meares CJ, et al: Effects of exercise on fatigue, physical functioning, and emotional distress during radiation therapy for breast cancer, *Oncol Nurs Forum* 24(6):991-1000, 1997.

National Comprehensive Cancer Network: NCCN clinical practice guidelines in oncology, retrieved June 1, 2004, from http://www.nccn.org/physician_gls/f_guidelines.html.

Porock D, Kristjanson LJ, Tinnelly K, et al: An exercise intervention for advanced cancer patients experiencing fatigue: a pilot study, *J Palliat Care* 16(3):30-36, 2000.

Schneider S: Interventions for hematologic problems. In Ignatavicius DD, Workman ML, editors: *Medical-surgical nursing: critical thinking for collaborative care,* ed 4, Philadelphia, 2002, Saunders.

The Gastrointestinal System

PATRICIA RADOVICH, RN, MSN, CNS, FCCM

SYSTEMWIDE ELEMENTS

Physiologic Anatomy

1. **Upper gastrointestinal (GI) tract** (Figure 8-1)
   a. Mouth and accessory organs
      i. Lips, gums and teeth, and inner structures of the cheeks, tongue, hard and soft palate, and salivary glands
      ii. Chewing prepares food by softening and moving it around, mixing it with saliva, and forming a bolus
      iii. Skeletal muscles for chewing are coordinated by cranial nerves V, VII, IX, X, XI, XII
      iv. Saliva aids in swallowing; approximately 570 ml/day of saliva is secreted. Submandibular, parotid, and sublingual salivary glands along with minor salivary glands in the oral mucosa secrete mixed saliva, which is 99% water and 1% solids, and includes electrolytes and organic protein molecules.
   b. Pharynx
      i. Extends from the cricoid cartilage to the level of the sixth cervical vertebra
      ii. Swallowing receptors are stimulated by the autonomic nervous system when a food bolus moves toward the back of the mouth. The motor impulses to swallow are transmitted via cranial nerves V, IX, X, and XII.
   c. Esophagus
      i. Transports food from the mouth to the stomach and prevents retrograde movement of the stomach contents
      ii. Collapsible tube about 25 cm long that lies posterior to the trachea and the heart
         (a) Begins at the level of the sixth cervical vertebra and extends through the mediastinum and diaphragm to the level of the first thoracic vertebra, where it attaches to the stomach below the level of the diaphragm
         (b) Upper portion of the esophagus is striated skeletal muscle, which is gradually replaced by smooth muscle so that the lower third of the esophagus is totally smooth muscle
         (c) Motor and sensory impulses for swallowing and food passage derive from the vagus nerve. Lower esophagus also innervated by splanchnic and sympathetic neurons. Food moves by the strong muscular

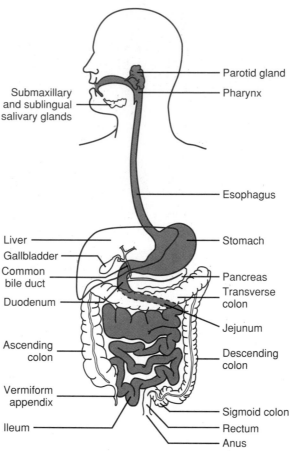

FIGURE 8-1 ■ Digestive tract of the human being. (From Westfall UE, Heitkemper M: Gastrointestinal physiology. In Clochesy JM, Breu C, Cardin S, et al, editors: *Critical care nursing,* ed 2, Philadelphia, 1996, Saunders, p 979.)

contraction of peristalsis and by gravity. In the absence of gravity, nutrients transported by muscular contractions.
(d) Sphincters: Hypopharyngeal (proximal) prevents air from entering the esophagus during inspiration; gastroesophageal (distal) prevents gastric reflux into the esophagus

iii. Blood supply
(a) Arterial supply: Celiac trunk includes the gastric, pyloric, right, and left gastroepiploic arteries
(b) Venous drainage: Splanchnic bed drains the entire GI tract; gastric vein drains the stomach and esophagus
(c) Direct drainage into the azygous and hemiazygous veins of the mediastinum; all of these then drain into the portal vein

d. Stomach
i. Food storage reservoir and site of the start of the digestive process. Normal capacity is 1000 to 1500 ml but can hold up to 6000 ml.
ii. Layers of the stomach and intestinal wall (Figure 8-2)
(a) Mucosa: Cells produce mucus that lubricates and protects the inner surface. These cells are replaced every 4 to 5 days. This layer receives the majority of the blood supply of the stomach.

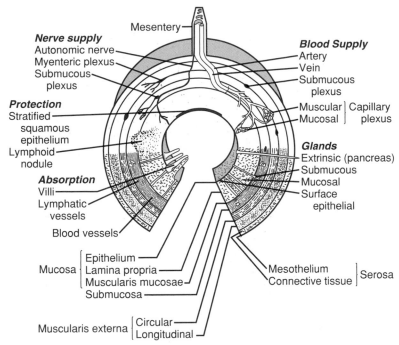

FIGURE 8-2 ■ Layers of the intestinal wall. Histology of the gastrointestinal tract, stomach through large intestine. (From Kinney MR, Dunbar S, Brooks-Brunn J, et al, editors: *AACN clinical reference for critical care nursing*, St Louis, 1998, Mosby, p 982.)

(1) Epithelium: Contains the gastric, cardiac, fundic, and pyloric glands
  a) Gastric cells: Contain microvilli that monitor intragastric pH
  b) Cardiac glands: Secrete alkaline mucus, a lubricant that continually bathes and protects the epithelial lining from autodigestion
  c) Fundic glands
    1) Chief cells: Secrete pepsinogen, an inactive form of pepsin, in response to food ingestion; in its active form, pepsin digests proteins
    2) Parietal cells secrete hydrochloric acid, which lowers pH and kills bacteria, and intrinsic factor, a glycoprotein necessary for vitamin B_{12} absorption
(2) Lamina propria: Contains lymphocytes; site of gut immunologic response
(3) Muscularis mucosae: Contains thin smooth muscle layer
(b) Submucosa: Contains connective tissue and elastic fibers, blood vessels, nerves, lymphatic vessels, and structures responsible for secreting digestive enzymes
(c) Circular and longitudinal smooth muscle layers: Continue the modification of food into a liquid consistency and move it along the GI tract. Movements are tonic and rhythmic, occurring every 20 seconds. Electrical activity is constantly present in the smooth muscle layers.
(d) Serosa: Outermost layer

    iii. Gastric hormones

      (a) Gastrin

        (1) Hormone secreted in response to distention of antrum or fundus by food

        (2) Stimulates secretion of hydrochloric acid by the parietal cells and secretion of pepsin by chief cells

        (3) Increases gastric blood flow

      (b) Histamine: Hormone secreted by mast cells in the presence of food that is critical to the regulation of gastric acid secretions

        (1) Stimulates gastric acid and pepsin secretion

        (2) Initiates contraction of the gallbladder

        (3) Relaxes sphincter of Oddi

        (4) Increases GI motility

   iv. Gastric secretion

      (a) Approximately 1500 to 3000 ml is secreted daily and mixes with food entering the stomach

      (b) Phases of gastric secretion

        (1) Cephalic phase: Fibers of the vagus nerve stimulate the stomach to secrete gastrin (from the antrum) and hydrochloric acid

        (2) Gastric phase: Vasovagal reflexes stimulate the parasympathetic system to increase the secretion of gastrin

   v. Gastric emptying

      (a) Is proportional to the volume of material in the stomach

      (b) Depends on the character of the ingested material: Liquids, digestible solids, fats, indigestible solids

      (c) Factors accelerating gastric emptying: Large volume of liquids; anger; insulin

      (d) Factors inhibiting gastric emptying: Fat, protein, starch, sadness, duodenal hormones

      (e) Vomiting

        (1) Coordinated by the vomiting center in the medulla in response to afferent impulses from various regions of the body

        (2) Stimuli that induce vomiting: Tactile stimulation to the back of the throat, increased intracranial pressure (ICP), intense pain, dizziness, anxiety

        (3) Autonomic nervous system discharge may precede vomiting: Sweating, increased heart rate, increased salivation, nausea, muscular force by the diaphragm and abdomen

   vi. Blood supply

      (a) Arterial: Celiac artery flows into the right gastric artery, left gastric artery, gastroduodenal artery, and finally into the right gastroepiploic artery; the splenic artery flows into the left gastroepiploic artery

      (b) Venous drainage: Splanchnic bed drains the entire GI tract, the gastric vein drains the stomach and esophagus; both vessels drain into the portal vein

  vii. Innervation

      (a) Intrinsic nervous system (intramural neurons) within the wall of the GI tract is independent of central nervous system controls

        (1) Myenteric (Auerbach's) plexus: Located between the circular and longitudinal muscles; stimulation increases muscle tone, contractions, velocity, and excitation of the digestive tract

(2) Submucosal (Meissner's) plexus: Located between the circular and submucosal layers; influences secretions of the digestive tract; contains secretomotor and enteric vasodilator neurons

(b) Extrinsic system: Via the central nervous system, parasympathetic system, and sympathetic system

(1) Parasympathetic: Fibers arise from the medulla and spinal segments (i.e., vagus nerves)

a) Cranial segments: Transmission via the vagus nerve; innervate the stomach, pancreas, and first half of the small intestine

b) Sacral segments: Innervate the distal half of the large intestine, sigmoid, rectum, and anus

c) Enhances function of the intrinsic nervous system and the secretion of acetylcholine

d) Increases glandular secretion and muscle tone; decreases sphincter tone

(2) Sympathetic: Motor and sensory fibers arise from the thoracic and lumbar segments; distribution is via the sympathetic ganglia (i.e., celiac plexus)

a) Fibers run alongside blood vessels and secrete norepinephrine

b) Inhibit GI activity by acting on smooth muscle

2. **Middle GI tract: Small intestine**
   a. Approximately 5 m long; extends from the pylorus to the ileocecal valve
   b. Consists of three divisions: Duodenum, jejunum, ileum
   c. Primary function is absorption of nutrients
   d. Layers of the intestinal wall (Figure 8-2)
      i. Mucosa: Innermost layer; receives the majority of the blood supply; the predominant site of nutrient absorption
         (a) Epithelium: Covered with villi and microvilli that increase the surface area of the small intestine several hundred times; contain glands, crypts of Lieberkühn (intestinal glands) that secrete approximately 2 L of fluid every 24 hours and goblet cells that secrete mucus
         (b) Lamina propria: Contains lymphocytes; site of gut immunologic responsiveness
         (c) Muscularis mucosae: Contains thin smooth muscle
      ii. Submucosa: Contains loose connective tissue and elastic fibers, blood vessels, lymphatic vessels, and nerves
      iii. Muscularis: Muscle layer; function is involuntary and involved in motility
      iv. Serosa: Outermost layer; protects and suspends intestine within the abdominal cavity
   e. Peristalsis: Propulsive movements that move the intestinal contents toward the anus. Approximately 3 to 5 hours is necessary for passage through the entire small intestine.
   f. Blood supply
      i. Arterial: Derived from the celiac artery (first portion of the duodenum) and the superior mesenteric arteries (remainder of the duodenum, jejunum, ileum, cecum)
      ii. Venous drainage: Splanchnic bed drains the entire GI tract
         (a) Superior mesenteric vein: Drains the small intestine and the ascending and transverse colon
         (b) Inferior mesenteric vein: Drains the sigmoid colon and rectum
   g. Innervation: Same as for stomach
   h. Small intestine digestive enzymes not secreted, but integral components of the mucosa

     i. Bile and pancreatic enzymes are secreted into the duodenum

     ii. In the jejunum and the ileum, food is digested and absorbed

     iii. Up to 3000 ml/day of digestive enzymes (e.g., lipase, amylase, maltase, and lactase)

     iv. pH is approximately 7.0

i. Intestinal hormones

     i. Secretin: Secreted by the mucosa of the duodenum in response to acidic gastric juice from the stomach and to alcohol ingestion

         (a) Augments the action of cholecystokinin (CCK)

         (b) Stimulates release of the alkaline component of pancreatic juice and the secretion of water

         (c) Increases the bile secretion rate

         (d) Decreases the motility of most of the GI tract

     ii. CCK: Secreted by the mucosa of the jejunum in response to the presence of fat, protein, and acidic contents in the intestine

         (a) Increases contractility and emptying of the gallbladder and blocks the increased gastric motility caused by gastrin

         (b) Stimulates secretion of pancreatic digestive enzymes, bicarbonate, and insulin

     iii. Gastric inhibitory peptide (GIP): Secreted by the mucosa of the upper portion of the small intestine in response to the presence of carbohydrates and fat in the intestine; inhibits gastric acid secretion and motility, slowing the rate of gastric emptying

     iv. Vasoactive intestinal peptide: Secreted throughout the gut in response to acidic gastric juice in the duodenum

         (a) Main effects are similar to those of secretin

         (b) Stimulates the secretion of intestinal juices to decrease the acidity of chyme and inhibits gastric secretion

     v. Somatostatin: Secreted throughout the intestine in response to vagal stimulation, ingestion of food, and release of CCK, GIP, glucagon, and secretin

         (a) Inhibits the secretion of saliva, gastric acid, pepsin, intrinsic factor, and pancreatic enzymes

         (b) Inhibits gastric motility, gallbladder contraction, intestinal motility, and blood flow to the liver and intestine

         (c) Inhibits the secretion of insulin and growth hormone

     vi. Serotonin: Secreted throughout the intestine in response to vagal stimulation, increased luminal pressure, and the presence of acid or fat in the duodenum; inhibits gastric acid secretion and mucin production

j. Functions: Almost all absorption occurs in the small intestine via four mechanisms: Active transport, passive diffusion, facilitated diffusion, and nonionic transport

     i. Vitamins are absorbed primarily in the intestine by passive diffusion, except for the fat-soluble vitamins, which require bile salts for absorption, and vitamin B_{12}, which requires intrinsic factor

     ii. Water absorption: Approximately 8 L of water per day is absorbed by the small intestine

     iii. Electrolyte absorption: Most occurs in the proximal small intestine

     iv. Iron absorption: Absorbed in the ferrous form in the duodenum

         (a) Facilitated by ascorbic acid

         (b) Increases in states of iron deficiency

     v. Carbohydrate absorption: Complex carbohydrates are broken down into monosaccharides or basic sugars (fructose, glucose, galactose) by specific enzymes (e.g., amylase, maltase)

    vi. Protein absorption: Protein is broken down into amino acids and small peptides; essential amino acids are lysine, phenylalanine, isoleucine, valine, methionine, leucine, threonine, and tryptophan

    vii. Fat absorption

3. Lower GI tract

  a. Colon

    i. Approximately 6.5 cm in diameter and 1.5 m long; extends from terminal ileum at the ileocecal valve to the rectum

    ii. Ileocecal valve: Prevents return of feces from the cecum into the ileum

  b. Divisions of the colon

    i. Cecum: Blind pouch to which the appendix is attached; about 2.5 cm from the ileocecal valve

    ii. Ascending colon: Extends from the cecum to the lower border of the liver, where it forms the right hepatic flexure

    iii. Transverse colon: Crosses the upper half the abdominal cavity, curving downward at the lower end of the spleen at the left colonic (splenic) flexure anterior to the small intestine

    iv. Descending colon: Extends from the splenic flexure to the sigmoid colon

    v. Sigmoid colon: S-shaped curve extending from the descending colon to the rectum

    vi. Rectum: Extends from the sigmoid colon to the anus

  c. Layers of the large intestine wall (Figure 8-2): No villi and no secretion of digestive enzymes. Layers similar to those of the middle GI tract with exceptions:

    i. Epithelial surface contains cells that absorb water and electrolytes

    ii. Crypts covered by epithelial cells that produce mucus

  d. Blood supply (Figure 8-3)

    i. Arterial supply

      (a) Superior mesenteric artery supplies the ascending colon and part of the transverse colon

      (b) Inferior mesenteric artery feeds the transverse colon, sigmoid colon, and upper rectum

      (c) Hypogastric arteries give rise to the middle and inferior rectal and hemorrhoidal arteries

      (d) Rectal arteries, which arise from the internal iliac arteries, supply the distal rectum

    ii. Venous drainage

      (a) Superior mesenteric vein drains the ascending colon and part of the transverse colon

      (b) Inferior mesenteric vein drains the transverse colon, sigmoid colon, and rectum

      (c) Internal iliac vein

  e. Colonic functions

    i. Absorption of water and electrolytes: Approximately 500 ml of chyme (the byproduct of digestion) enters the colon per day and, of this, 400 ml of water and electrolytes are reabsorbed

    ii. Breakdown of cellulose by enteric bacteria

    iii. Synthesis of vitamins (folic acid, vitamin K, riboflavin, nicotinic acid) by enteric bacteria

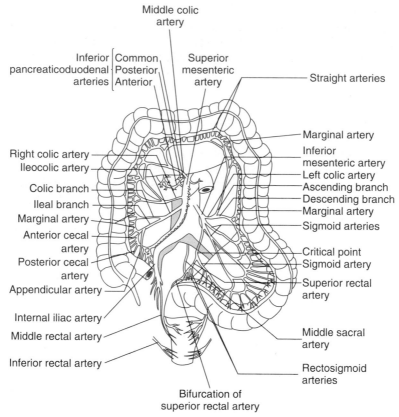

FIGURE 8-3 ■ Arterial and venous blood supplies to the primary and accessory organs of the alimentary canal. (From Ruppert SD, Englert DM: Patients with gastrointestinal bleeding. In Clochesy JM, Breau C, Cardin S, et al, editors: *Critical care nursing,* ed 2, Philadelphia, 1996, Saunders, p 1028.)

    iv. Storage of fecal mass until it can be expelled from the body
       (a) Takes approximately 18 hours from the time food enters the colon until the intestinal contents reach the distal portion of the colon
       (b) Time from ingestion of food to defecation of the residue may be 24 hours or longer
   v. Motility
       (a) Peristalsis: Propulsive movements that push GI contents toward the anus
       (b) Haustral churning is the major type of movement in the colon
       (c) Factors that enhance motility: Bacterial enterotoxins, viral infections of the gut, regional enteritis, ulcerative colitis, increased bile salts, osmotic overload, laxatives
       (d) Factors that inhibit motility: Low-bulk diet, parenteral nutrition, bed rest, dehydration, ileus, fasting, drugs
       (e) Poor motility causes more absorption, and the development of hard feces in the transverse colon causes constipation
       (f) Aging causes a reduction in peristalsis and decreased GI motility throughout the GI system
  f. Innervation: Same as for the stomach and small intestine

g. Gut defenses

   i. The gut encounters a variety of potentially harmful substances daily; these can include natural toxins in food, insecticides, preservatives, chemical waste products, and airborne particulate matter that is swallowed.

   ii. Mechanisms exist within the GI tract to protect the integrity of the gut and thus the individual

  iii. Fluid and cellular layers

     (a) Aqueous layer: Stationary layer immediately adjacent to the microvillus border of the enterocytes; consists of acids, digestive enzymes, and bacteria depending on the location in GI lumen

     (b) Mucosal barrier: Physical and chemical barriers that protect the wall of the gut from harmful substances. Surfaces of the stomach, intestine, biliary and pancreatic ducts, and gallbladder have cells that synthesize and release mucus.

     (c) Epithelial cells: Tight junctions between cells regulated by hormones and cytokines make them relatively impervious to large molecules and bacteria; rapid proliferation of cells minimizes the adherence of flora. The level of permeability varies within the various segments of the GI tract.

     (d) Mucus-bicarbonate barrier: Forms a layer of alkalinity between the epithelium and luminal acids that neutralizes the pH and protects against surface shear

  iv. Motility: Prevents bacteria in the distal small intestine from migrating proximally into the sterile parts of the upper GI system

     (a) Stomach

        (1) Expulsion of toxic substances as a result of stimulation of the vomiting center in the medulla

        (2) Barrier against the reflux of duodenal contents back into the stomach

     (b) Colon: Moves pathogens and potential carcinogens out of the body

   v. Gut immunity: Necessary because the gut is a reservoir of potentially pathogenic bacteria

     (a) B lymphocytes that bear surface immunoglobulin A (IgA) or synthesize secretory IgA that prevents antigens from binding to mucous cells

     (b) Macrophages in the lamina propria

        (1) Gut-associated lymphoid tissue in the submucosa (lamina propria or Peyer's patches) of the GI tract

        (2) Glutamine is the primary fuel of the gut and maintains the gut mucosal barrier

  vi. Gastric acid: Intragastric pH below 4.0 is essential

     (a) Protects the stomach from ingested bacteria and other harmful substances

     (b) Prevents bacteria from entering the intestine

 vii. Commensal bacteria: Natural gut flora are stable and protective in a healthy person by competing with pathogenic species for nutrients and attachment sites, and produce inhibitory substances against pathogenic species

     (a) Stomach, duodenum, and jejunum are sterile

     (b) Ileum contains aerobic and anaerobic bacteria: Dietary intake is a major factor in determining intestinal flora

     (c) Large intestine contains large numbers of aerobic and anaerobic bacteria, and smaller numbers of yeast and fungi

 viii. Impaired gut barrier function facilitates bacterial translocation, which is the egress of bacteria and/or their toxins across the mucosal barrier and into the lymphatic vessels and portal circulation

4. Accessory organs of digestion (Figure 8-4)
  a. Liver
    i. Largest solid organ, weighing approximately 3 lb (1500 g), located in the right upper quadrant, beneath the diaphragm
    ii. Consists of three lobes divided into eight independent segments, each of which has its own vascular inflow, outflow, and biliary drainage. Because of this division into self-contained units, each can be resected without damaging those remaining.
      (a) Right lobe: Anterior (segments V and VIII) and posterior (segments VI and VII)
      (b) Left lobe: Medial (segment IV) and lateral (segments II and III); the left lobe extends across the midline into the left upper quadrant
      (c) Caudate lobe (segment I)
    iii. Microscopically the liver consists of functional units called *lobules* composed of portal triads in which the bile ducts, hepatocytes, and artery are located. The portal triads are then bounded by sinusoids and a central vein. A cross section of a classic lobule or acinus is hexagonal.
    iv. Blood supply (Figure 8-5): Derived from both a vein and an artery
      (a) 25% of cardiac output flows through the liver per minute
      (b) Portal vein (after draining the mesenteric veins and pancreatic and splenic veins) and hepatic artery (off the aorta via the celiac trunk) enter the liver at the porta hepatis or hilum (a horizontal fissure in the liver, containing blood and lymph vessels, nerves, and the hepatic ducts)
      (c) 75% is supplied by the portal vein; each segment receives a branch of the portal vein and 25% is supplied by the hepatic artery

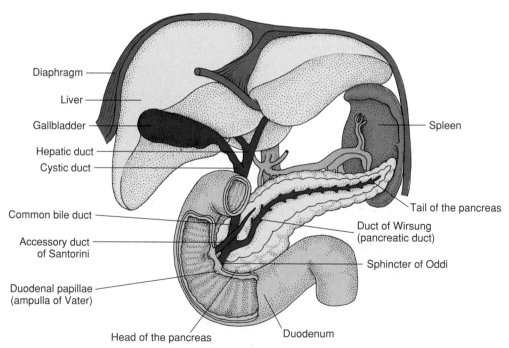

FIGURE 8-4 ■ Anatomy of the liver and biliary tract. (From Westfall UE, Heitkemper M: Gastrointestinal physiology. In Clochesy JM, Breau C, Cardin S, et al, editors: *Critical care nursing,* ed 2, Philadelphia, 1996, Saunders. p 992.)

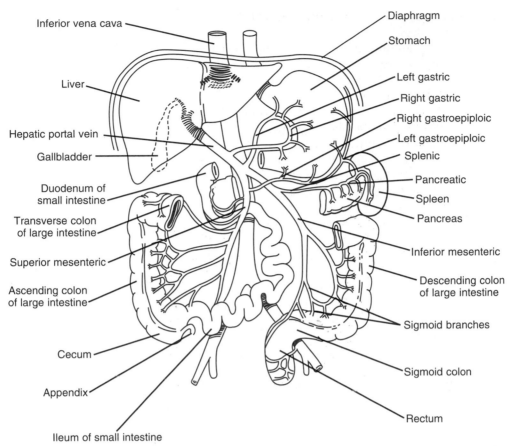

FIGURE 8-5 ■ Hepatic portal circulation. (From Totora GJ, Anagnostakos NP: *Principles of anatomy and physiology,* ed 4, New York, 1984, Harper & Row, p 510.)

(d) Small branches of each of these vessels enter the acinus at the portal triad (an area in the liver consisting of the portal vein, branches of the hepatic artery, and tributaries to the bile duct

(e) Functionally, the liver can be divided into three zones, based on oxygen supply. Zone 1 encircles the portal tracts where the oxygenated blood from hepatic arteries enters. Zone 3 is located around the central veins, where oxygenation is poor. Zone 2 is located in between.

(f) Blood from both the portal vein and the hepatic artery mixes together in the hepatic sinusoids and then flows through the sinusoids to the hepatic venules (zone 3) through the central veins, branches of the hepatic vein

(g) Sinusoids
   (1) Found between plates (layers) of hepatocytes; have a porous lining with fenestrations that allows nutrients in the blood plasma to wash freely over exposed surfaces (the spaces of Disse)
   (2) Sinusoidal lining consists of endothelial cells, Kupffer cells, perisinusoidal fat-storing cells, and pit cells.

(h) Venous drainage: Begins in the central veins in the center of the lobules; central veins empty into the hepatic veins, which empty into the inferior vena cava

v. Biliary duct system for draining bile

(a) Begins at the sinusoidal level as bile canaliculi, which branch into ductules, intralobular bile ducts, and larger intrahepatic ducts

(b) Intrahepatic ducts come together at the porta hepatis to form the common hepatic duct, which becomes the common bile duct after joining with the cystic duct and drains into the duodenum

vi. Physiology: The liver is a metabolically complex organ with interrelated digestive, metabolic, exocrine, hematologic, and excretory functions. The many functions it performs are interwoven; each lobe is an independent functional unit, so that up to 80% of the liver can be destroyed and it will regenerate.

(a) Digestive functions: Plays a role in the synthesis, metabolism, and transport of carbohydrates, fats, and proteins

(1) Carbohydrates: Maintains normal serum glucose levels by

a) Glycogen storage: Approximately 900 kcal of glycogen reserves are stored in the adult liver

b) Glycogenesis: Conversion of excess carbohydrates to glycogen for storage in the liver as a metabolic reserve

c) Glycogenolysis: Conversion of large stores of glycogen in muscles and liver to glucose

d) Gluconeogenesis: Manufacture of glucose from noncarbohydrate substrate (fat, fatty acids, glycerol, amino acids)

(2) Fats

a) Bile secretion for fat digestion plays a role in fat and lipid synthesis, metabolism, and transport

b) Principal site of synthesis and degradation of lipids (cholesterol, phospholipids, lipoprotein): Produces approximately 1000 mg of cholesterol per day

c) Exogenous lipoprotein metabolism

d) Endogenous lipoprotein metabolism: Major lipoprotein synthesized by the liver is very-low-density lipoprotein (VLDL); one third of VLDL remnants are converted to low-density lipoprotein (LDL)

1) Direct removal of VLDL remnants

2) Removal of 75% of LDL remnants by LDL receptors in the liver

e) Conversion of excess carbohydrate to triglyceride, which is stored as adipose tissue

f) Conversion of triglyceride to glycerol and fatty acids for energy

g) Storage of triglyceride and fat-soluble vitamins (A, D, E, and K)

h) Storage of fats, cholesterol, proteins, vitamin B_{12}, and minerals

(3) Protein

a) Production of plasma proteins (albumin, prealbumin, transferrin, clotting factors, haptoglobin, ceruloplasmin, α_1-antitrypsin, complement, α-fetoprotein)

b) Deamination: Metabolism of amino acids

c) Transamination: Conversion of amino acids to ammonia, conversion of ammonia to urea for urinary excretion

(b) Endocrine functions: Metabolism of glucocorticoids, mineralocorticoids, hormones

(c) Exocrine functions

(1) Excretion of bile pigment

(2) Excretion of cholesterol

(3) Urea synthesis

(4) Detoxification of drugs and foreign substances

(d) Hematologic functions: Synthesis of bilirubin, coagulation factors

(e) Excretory functions

(1) Detoxifies and eliminates drugs, hormones, and toxic substances

(2) Produces and secretes 600 to 1000 ml/day of bile

(3) Stores vitamin B_{12}, copper, and iron

(4) Filters blood via Kupffer cells (macrophages) that reside in the liver sinusoids

b. Gallbladder: Pear-shaped saclike organ that serves as a reservoir for bile

i. Attached to the inferior surface of the liver in the area that divides the right and left lobes (gallbladder fossa)

ii. Approximately 7 to 10 cm long; holds and concentrates approximately 30 ml of bile

iii. Blood supply: Arterial blood supply is from the cystic artery; venous drainage is via a network of small veins.

iv. Innervation: Splanchnic nerve, right branch of the vagus nerve

v. Cystic duct attaches the gallbladder to the common hepatic duct

(a) Union of the cystic duct and the common hepatic duct forms the common bile duct

(b) Common bile duct either joins the pancreatic duct outside the duodenum or forms a common channel through the duodenal wall at the ampulla of Vater

(c) Intraduodenal segment of the common bile duct and the ampulla is the sphincter of Oddi

vi. Presence of CCK in the blood (in response to chyme in the duodenum)

(a) Facilitates delivery of bile to the duodenum

(b) Contracts the gallbladder

(c) Relaxes the sphincter of Oddi

vii. Bile is composed of water, bile salts, and bile pigments

(a) Bile salts are responsible for the absorption and emulsification of fat and fat-soluble vitamins

(b) Bile pigments: High in cholesterol and phospholipids, give feces a brown color

(c) Bilirubin is the major bile pigment; it is a breakdown product of hemoglobin metabolism from senescent red blood cells

(d) Serum bilirubin

(1) Total: Indirect bilirubin plus direct bilirubin; when total bilirubin level is elevated and the cause is unknown, indirect and direct bilirubin fractions can be measured

(2) Indirect (unconjugated): Bilirubin bound to albumin before it binds to glucuronic acid; fat soluble. Causes of elevation of indirect bilirubin concentration in serum include the following:

a) Any hemolytic process (e.g., ABO mismatch in blood transfusion, β-hemolytic streptococcal infection)

b) Gilbert's syndrome, a common disorder characterized by a mild, chronic fluctuating increase in the level of unconjugated bilirubin

c) Inherited deficiency of bilirubin, which results in variations of the Crigler-Najjar syndrome

d) Diffuse hepatocellular necrosis

(3) Direct (conjugated): Bilirubin bound to glucuronic acid, water soluble; concentration elevates with biliary tract obstruction (except cystic duct), diffuse biliary tract damage, acute cellular rejection after liver transplantation. Causes of elevation of direct bilirubin concentration in serum include the following:

a) Bile duct obstruction (e.g., stones, tumor, biliary stricture after liver transplantation)

b) Cholecystitis

c) Necrosis of the bile duct (e.g., hepatic artery thrombosis)

d) Autoimmune diseases of biliary stasis (e.g., primary biliary cirrhosis, primary sclerosing cholangitis)

e) Inherited disorders of conjugated bilirubin excretion (e.g., Dubin-Johnson syndrome, Rotor's syndrome)

c. Pancreas: Soft, flattened gland with a lobular structure but without an external capsule

i. 12 to 20 cm long, located in the retroperitoneal area

ii. Head lies in the C-shaped curve of the duodenum at the level of the body of L2

iii. Body extends horizontally behind the stomach

iv. Tail is contiguous with the spleen, lying between the two layers of the peritoneum that form the lienorenal ligament at the level of the body of L1

v. Blood supply

(a) Arterial blood supplies from the celiac axis, which divides into the common hepatic, splenic, and left gastric arteries and the superior mesenteric artery

(b) Venous drainage via the portal vein, which is formed by the joining together of the superior mesenteric and splenic veins

vi. Innervation

(a) Sympathetic efferent innervations via the greater, lesser, and least splanchnic nerves have an inhibitory function

(b) Parasympathetic innervation via the vagal nerves, which stimulate exocrine secretion

vii. Duct of Wirsung: Main pancreatic duct whose terminal end, the sphincter of Oddi in the ampulla of Vater, empties into the duodenum; shares the sphincter of Oddi with the common bile duct

viii. Duct of Santorini: Accessory pancreatic duct (present in 40% to 70% of persons) that lies anterior and opens into the second part of the duodenum proximal to the duct of Wirsung

ix. Pancreatic secretions: Consist of aqueous and enzymatic components

(a) Aqueous component

(1) Approximately 1 L of fluid per day is secreted

(2) Ductule cells secrete water and bicarbonate

(b) Enzymatic component

(1) Acinar cells (part of the exocrine function of the pancreas) secrete the pancreatic enzymes

(2) Amylase (for digestion of starches) and lipase (for digestion of fats) are secreted as active enzymes

(3) Pancreatic proteases are secreted as inactive precursors and are converted to active enzymes in the lumen of the small intestine (for digestion of proteins)

x. Food in the intestine stimulates the secretion of enzymes. Changes in the proportions of various nutrients in the diet result in changes in the proportions of enzymes in the pancreatic secretions. Adaptation of the pancreatic secretions is accomplished by hormones that operate at the level of gene expression:

- (a) GIP and secretin increase the expression of the lipase gene
- (b) CCK increases the expression of the protease genes
- (c) In diabetic individuals, insulin regulates the expression of the amylase gene; however, how amylase expression is normally regulated in nondiabetic individuals is unknown
- (d) Certain conditions decrease pancreatic secretion: Pancreatitis, cystic fibrosis, tumors, and protein deficiency

xi. Endocrine cells found in the islets of Langerhans
- (a) Alpha cells secrete glucagon, which is responsible for glycogenolysis and gluconeogenesis
- (b) Beta cells secrete insulin, which facilitates the use of glucose by tissues
- (c) Delta cells secrete somatostatin, which inhibits the secretion of insulin, glucagon, and growth hormone
- (d) Polypeptide cells are associated with the hypermotility of the GI tract and diarrhea

Patient Assessment

1. Nursing history
- **a.** Patient health history
    - **i.** Chief complaint
    - **ii.** History of present illness
    - **iii.** Past medical conditions (e.g., neurologic conditions, cirrhosis, diabetes), eating disorders, or communicable diseases (e.g., viral hepatitis, jaundice)
    - **iv.** Surgical history (e.g., appendectomy, gastric bypass)
    - **v.** Allergies
        - (a) Food allergies, intolerances (e.g., lactase deficiency causes lactose intolerance)
        - (b) Drug allergies
    - **vi.** Pain: Location, duration, character, severity, alleviating and aggravating factors, relationship to changes in eating, bowel habits, or position
    - **vii.** Oral health status: Teeth, gums, tongue, pharynx
    - **viii.** Nausea or vomiting: Duration, alleviating and aggravating factors, description of vomitus (undigested food, unrecognizable digested product, blood—bright red or resembling coffee grounds), timing, and relationship to pain
    - **ix.** Loss of appetite (loss of desire or interest in food), duration, association with other symptoms
    - **x.** Dysphagia: Difficulty in swallowing, types of foods and/or liquids causing difficulty
    - **xi.** Heartburn (dyspepsia, reflux): Duration, alleviating and aggravating factors
    - **xii.** Fecal elimination: Diarrhea or constipation, color of stools, presence of blood (black, maroon, or bright red color); clay-colored stool—absence of bile pigment as a result of biliary obstruction or advanced cirrhosis
    - **xiii.** Urinary elimination: Color of urine; dark (tea-colored) urine—acute hepatocellular necrosis or severe biliary obstruction
    - **xiv.** Fatigue, weakness
    - **xv.** Easy bruising or bleeding

      xvi. Fever, night sweats

     xvii. Muscle wasting, atrophy: Wasting of the muscle over the temporal bones in the face or the thenar muscle of the thumb

    xviii. Weight loss or weight gain, obesity

      xix. Eating disorders

  b. Family history

      i. Carcinoma, liver disease, pancreatitis, peptic ulcer disease

     ii. Diabetes mellitus, anemia, tuberculosis

    iii. Inflammatory bowel disease: Crohn's disease, ulcerative colitis

    iv. Obesity

  c. Social history

      i. Substance abuse: Tobacco use, alcohol use, drug use

     ii. Sexual history: Heterosexual, homosexual relationships; involvement with prostitutes

    iii. Place of birth, travel history

    iv. History of tattoos, piercings

  d. Medication history (all medications evaluated but specifically herbal supplements, vitamins, anabolic steroids, motility agents, antacids, histamine or proton pump inhibitors, anticholinergics, antibiotics, antidiarrheals, laxatives, enemas, narcotics, sedatives, barbiturates, stimulants, antihypertensives, diuretics, anticoagulants, analgesics, nonsteroidal, steroids, chemotherapy agents)

2. Nursing examination of patient

  a. Physical examination data

    i. Inspection

      (a) Anatomic landmarks are used to locate and describe normal and abnormal assessment findings

        (1) Xiphoid process, subcostal margins, costovertebral angle

        (2) Abdominal quadrants (Figure 8-6), midline of abdomen

        (3) Umbilicus, rectus abdominus muscle

        (4) Anterior superior iliac spine, symphysis pubis, inguinal ligament

        (5) Flanks

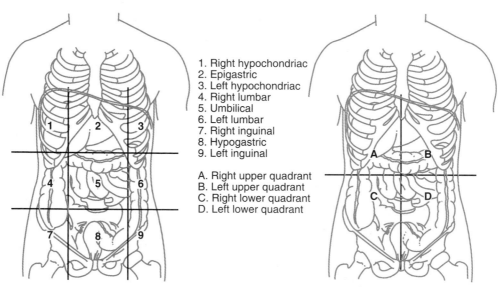

FIGURE 8-6 ■ Regions and quadrants of the abdomen. (From Wright JE, Shelton BK: *Desk reference for critical care nursing,* Boston, 1993, Jones & Bartlett, p 854.)

(b) General appearance: Physical signs of altered nutritional status (e.g., cachexia, obesity)

(c) Oral cavity: Gingivitis, lesions (e.g., herpes simplex, *Candida albicans*, leukoplakia), ability to swallow, presence of odors (e.g., ketones, fetor, alcohol)

(d) Abdominal profile: Evaluate with the patient lying supine on the examination table or bed

   (1) Symmetry, size (girth), and contour of the abdomen from the costal margins to the symphysis pubis (flat, rounded, scaphoid, protuberant)

   a) Abdominal distention can be due to fluid, fat, flatus, fetus, feces, malignancies, nonmalignant tumors

   b) Asymmetry can be due to these causes as well as to obstructions, cysts, or scoliosis

   (2) Condition of umbilicus (protruding; nodular; inverted; with calculus, ecchymoses, or drainage)

   (3) Caput medusa: Engorged abdominal veins around the umbilicus are seen in patients with portal hypertension or obstruction of the superior or inferior vena cava

   (4) Collateral vessels that come to the skin surface and traverse the abdomen: Seen in obesity and ascites

   (5) Masses, visible peristalsis or pulsations

   (6) Striae, ecchymoses, hematomas, scars, wounds, stomas, hernias, engorged veins, diastasis recti, fistulas, tubes, or drains

   (7) Spider angiomas: Found above the umbilicus on the anterior and posterior thorax, head, neck, and arms

   (8) Jaundice: Evident in skin and sclerae

ii. Auscultation: Performed in all quadrants before percussion and palpation to note location and characteristics of bowel and other sounds

   (a) Normal bowel sounds: Low-pitched, continuous gurgles heard in abdominal quadrants

   (b) Abnormal bowel sounds

   (1) Factors related to hypoactive or absent sounds: Peritonitis, paralytic ileus, anesthesia, inflammation, electrolyte imbalance, gastric or intraabdominal bleeding, pneumonia, both mechanical and nonmechanical obstruction

   (2) Factors related to hyperactive sounds: Hyperkalemia, gastroenteritis, gastric or esophageal bleeding, diarrhea, laxative use, mechanical obstruction

   (c) Bruit: Denotes increased turbulence or significant dilatation

   (1) Aortic bruit can be heard 2 to 3 cm above the umbilicus in the epigastric area and denotes partial aortic occlusion

   (2) Hepatic bruit can be heard over the liver and may indicate primary liver cancer, alcoholic hepatitis, or vascular liver metastases

   (3) Renal artery bruit can be heard to the left and/or right of midline in the epigastric areas in renal artery stenosis

   (4) Iliac artery bruit can be heard in the left and/or right inguinal areas

   (5) Venous hum or murmur heard over the liver denotes liver disease such as alcoholic hepatitis, hemangiomas, or dilated periumbilical circulation

   (6) Friction rub over the spleen denotes inflammation or infarction of the spleen

          (7) Peritoneal friction rub indicates peritoneal irritation

          (8) Hepatic friction rub over the liver can be heard in cases of abscess and various types of hepatitis (e.g., syphilitic)

  iii. Percussion

     (a) Percussion notes or tones

        (1) Tympany is noted when percussing air-filled organs such as the stomach

        (2) Resonance is noted when striking air-filled lungs

        (3) Dullness is noted over solid organs such as the liver or spleen

     (b) Percussion to evaluate the sizes of the liver and spleen

        (1) Liver size can be estimated by percussing from the right clavicle straight down the right midclavicular line to detect changes in percussion tones

           a) Beginning at the midclavicular line below the umbilicus, percuss for the lower edge of the liver. Over the bowel, the percussion tone is tympanic and transitions to dull, which denotes the lower edge of the liver.

           b) At the level of the fifth intercostal space, percuss downward. The percussion tone transitions from the resonance of the lung tissue to dull, which denotes the upper edge of the liver.

           c) Distance between the upper and lower edges of the liver at the midclavicular line is normally about 12 cm. A span of greater than 12 cm or less than 6 cm is abnormal. Gas in the colon, pregnancy, or tumors can impair accurate assessment of the liver span.

        (2) Spleen can be percussed (dull tones) only if grossly enlarged (e.g., portal hypertension) at the left midclavicular line below the left costal margin. To determine the presence of masses or abnormal fluid (ascites) and air collections:

           a) Collections can be confirmed by shifting dullness (fluid remains dependent with changes in position)

           b) Fluid waves can be elicited by placing the hands on either side of the abdomen, then tapping one hand against the abdomen and feeling the wave transmitted to the opposite hand

           c) Difference between fluid and fat can be determined by placing the hands on either side of the abdomen, having an assistant place his or her hand on the midline, and then pressing downward with one hand. Transmission of fat waves will be halted by the center hand, whereas fluid waves will continue toward the opposite hand.

  iv. Palpation

     (a) Light and deep palpation are done to determine the tone of the abdominal wall (relaxed, tense, rigid), areas of tenderness or pain, and the presence and characteristics of masses. Light palpation is done prior to deep palpation to determine areas of tenderness or resistance (guarding); observe the patient's face for nonverbal signs of discomfort.

     (b) Visceral tenderness: Dull, poorly localized (e.g., bowel obstruction)

     (c) Somatic tenderness: Sharp, well localized (e.g., late appendicitis, capsular stretching of the swollen liver)

     (d) Rebound tenderness: Occurs when palpation is suddenly withdrawn; associated with peritonitis

(e) Contralateral tenderness: Tenderness on the side opposite palpation (e.g., early appendicitis)

(f) Referred tenderness: Tenderness in an area distant from the source (e.g., right shoulder blade pain referred from the gallbladder)

(g) Murphy's sign: Severe right upper quadrant tenderness elicited on deep palpation under the right costal margin, exacerbated by deep inspiration and associated with cholecystitis

(h) To determine liver size: Palpate at the patient's right side

(1) Right flank area is supported with the left hand and the fingertips of the right hand are slid under the right costal margin, using firm pressure

(2) Fingertips are advanced as the patient inhales deeply and the liver edge moves 1 to 3 cm downward

(3) Fingertips are held steady as the patient exhales and inhales again, and the smooth (normal) edge of the liver may be felt moving past the fingertips

(4) The liver is not normally palpated more than 1 to 2 cm below the right costal margin (in cases of alcoholic liver disease or fatty liver disease, the liver may be enlarged with the margins projecting down into the abdomen 4 to 5 cm)

(i) To determine spleen size: Palpate from the patient's right side

(1) Left flank area is supported with the right hand and the fingertips of the left hand are slid under the left costal margin, using firm pressure

(2) Fingertips are advanced as the patient inhales deeply and the spleen edge moves 1 to 3 cm downward

(3) Fingertips are held steady as the patient exhales and inhales again, and the smooth (normal) edge of the spleen may be felt moving past the fingertips

(4) The spleen is not normally palpable, except in cases of enlargement or inferior displacement

b. Monitoring data

i. Heart rate, blood pressure, intake and output

ii. Daily weights, calorie counts or dietary intake notations

iii. Estimation of metabolic expenditures

3. **Appraisal of patient characteristics:** Patients in critical care units with acute GI problems have conditions that vary in complexity. During their hospitalization their clinical status may move along the continuum of care from improvement to deterioration in a nonlinear fashion. This potential for gradual or abrupt changes in clinical condition with possibly life-altering effects creates barriers in the ability to monitor life sustaining functions with precision. Clinical attributes of patients with acute GI disorders that the nurse needs to assess include the following:

a. Resiliency

i. Level 1—*Minimally resilient:* A 24-year-old female college student admitted in fulminant liver failure due to autoimmune hepatitis with encephalopathy, coagulopathy, and acute renal failure

ii. Level 3—*Moderately resilient:* A 68-year-old male accountant with a ruptured appendix who develops sepsis and acute renal failure

iii. Level 5—*Highly resilient:* A 16-year-old male high school student with blunt abdominal trauma after a motor vehicle accident. He was wearing a seatbelt and the vehicle air bags deployed.

   b. Vulnerability

      i. Level 1—*Highly vulnerable:* A 45-year-old female diagnosed with cirrhosis and spontaneous bacterial peritonitis who experiences an esophageal variceal hemorrhage during hospitalization

      ii. Level 3—*Moderately vulnerable:* A 56-year-old attorney with acute pancreatitis, high fever, and positive blood culture results, which indicate septicemia

      iii. Level 5—*Minimally vulnerable:* A 24-year-old Chinese male with acute hepatitis B viremia

   c. Stability

      i. Level 1—*Minimally stable:* An 84-year-old male who came to the emergency department with a ruptured aortic aneurysm and develops a bowel ischemia following surgery to repair his aorta

      ii. Level 3—*Moderately stable:* A 62-year-old newly retired male with colon cancer who is undergoing chemotherapy after tumor resection

      iii. Level 5—*Highly stable:* A 45-year-old homemaker who has undergone a cholecystectomy for gallstones and had no prior health problems

   d. Complexity

      i. Level 1—*Highly complex:* A 36-year-old grocery store clerk with cirrhosis and newly diagnosed liver cancer who is listed for liver transplantation shortly after separating from his wife and moving back in with his parents

      ii. Level 3—*Moderately complex:* An 18-year-old male who suffered abdominal trauma in a motor vehicle accident that killed his girlfriend

      iii. Level 5—*Minimally complex:* A 34-year-old married mechanic after small bowel resection for Crohn's disease

   e. Resource availability

      i. Level 1—*Few resources:* An illiterate 78-year-old widower with no children who has a small bowel obstruction due to cancer and has minimal income, has no transportation, and cannot afford his medications or insurance copayment

      ii. Level 3—*Moderate resources:* A 48-year-old field worker with cirrhosis with decompensations of encephalopathy and ascites who has a 17-year-old son. He has medical and Supplemental Security Income disability benefits that will cover the cost of medications.

      iii. Level 5—*Many resources:* A 58-year-old college professor, who is married with three grown children who live locally and who has chronic hepatitis C cirrhosis

   f. Participation in care

      i. Level 1—*No participation:* A 51-year-old migrant field worker with no known family in the United States who has encephalopathy from fulminant liver failure due to exposure to agricultural chemicals

      ii. Level 3—*Moderate level of participation:* A 68-year-old widow being discharged following an upper GI bleed from a peptic ulcer. She underwent gastric resection and her primary caregiver will be her daughter.

      iii. Level 5—*Full participation:* A 25-year-old secretary with a mild episode of pancreatitis, recovering without complications and planning her follow-up care with her husband and a good family friend who is a nurse

   g. Participation in decision making

      i. Level 1—*No participation:* A 98-year-old female with Alzheimer's disease who has no family and who has been in a motor vehicle accident with severe abdominal injuries, renal failure, and sepsis

      ii. Level 3—*Moderate level of participation:* A 45-year-old businessman, married with two young children, who has esophageal cancer and is undergoing esophageal resection followed by chemotherapy. The patient and his wife are overwhelmed by the changes in their lives and unsure of what the treatment options and posthospitalization issues are.

   iii. Level 5—*Full participation:* A 34-year-old tennis coach with severe gastroenteritis that resolved after 2 days in the hospital who is planning to continue his recovery using vacation time

h. Predictability

   i. Level 1—*Not predictable:* A 43-year-old health food store manager who suddenly develops jaundice, elevated liver enzyme levels, and encephalopathy with no prior history or risk factors for liver disease

   ii. Level 3—*Moderately predictable:* A 34-year-old Vietnamese general manager with jaundice, abnormal liver test results, malaise, and hepatosplenomegaly after returning from a trip to South America

   iii. Level 5—*Highly predictable:* A 40-year-old store manager who recently underwent liver transplantation and is progressing well toward discharge

4. Diagnostic studies

  a. Laboratory

    i. Complete blood count (CBC)

    ii. Serum electrolyte, glucose, blood urea nitrogen (BUN), creatinine, calcium, magnesium, ammonia, and cholesterol levels

   iii. Liver function tests: Total protein, albumin, serum alanine aminotransferase (ALT; formerly serum glutamate pyruvate transaminase [SGPT]), aspartate aminotransferase (AST; formerly serum glutamic-oxaloacetic transaminase [SGOT]), alkaline phosphatase, lactate dehydrogenase, γ- glutamyl transferase (GGT) levels

   iv. Serum bilirubin level: Total, indirect, direct

    v. Ceruloplasmin level

   vi. Serum amylase, lipase, cholinesterase levels

  vii. Prothrombin time (PT), international normalized ratio (INR)

 viii. Level of α-fetoprotein, a tumor marker used to diagnose liver cancer; level of carbohydrate antigen 19-9 (CA 19-9), a tumor marker used for the diagnosis of pancreatic or hepatobiliary cancer

   ix. Carcinoembryonic antigen level

    x. Levels of smooth muscle antibody (SMA), antimitochondrial antibody (AMA), antinuclear antibody (ANA), antineutrophil cytoplasmic antibody (ANCA), and anti–liver-kidney microsomal antibody (anti-LKM antibody), an assay used to diagnose autoimmune disorders

   xi. Fasting lipid levels

   xii. Hepatitis serologic testing (hepatitis A, B, C)

  xiii. Blood cultures (if an infectious process is suspected or with new onset of ascites or abdominal pain)

  xiv. Urine: Amylase, lipase, and bilirubin levels; culture and sensitivity testing; urinalysis; microalbumin level

   xv. Nutritional parameters

     (a) Total iron-binding capacity, serum iron level, ferritin level

     (b) Serum transferrin, prealbumin, retinol-binding protein levels

     (c) 24-hour urine urea nitrogen, creatinine, sodium levels

  xvi. Stool: Occult blood, fat, protein, ova and parasites, cultures

  b. Radiologic

    i. Abdominal flat-plate radiography: To visualize the position, size, and structure of the abdominal contents, truncal skeleton, and soft tissues of the abdominal wall. Dilated bowel loops, free air, fluid accumulations, and intramural bowel gas can be identified on plain radiographic films.

ii. Upper GI series: Contrast is used to visualize the position, contours, and size of the entire upper GI tract (especially the stomach and duodenum); to detect ulcers, tumors, strictures, and obstructions. Barium swallow is used to examine swallowing, motility, and emptying in the esophagus.

iii. Small bowel follow-through: To visualize the small bowel from the ligament of Treitz to the ileocecal valve to detect ulcers, tumors, diverticula, polyps, and inflammatory bowel disease

iv. Lower GI series: Barium enema is used to visualize the position, contours, and size of the entire lower GI tract; to detect ulcers, tumors, strictures, obstructions, polyps, inflammatory bowel disease, and diverticula; and to evaluate melena after inconclusive upper GI series

v. Esophagogastroduodenoscopy (EGD) or upper endoscopy: Visualization and photography of the esophagus, stomach, and proximal duodenum by means of an endoscope

   (a) To detect obstruction, strictures, ulcers, or tumors

   (b) To evaluate melena, hematemesis, heme-positive nasogastric drainage, dysphagia, odynophagia, dyspepsia, nausea, vomiting, or unexplained abdominal pain

   (c) To perform biopsy and obtain brush cytology and culture specimens; to place stents; to remove foreign bodies; to place feeding tubes; or to control bleeding

vi. Flexible sigmoidoscopy: Visualization and photography of the rectum, sigmoid colon, and descending colon up to 65 cm by means of a flexible sigmoidoscope or colonoscope

   (a) To detect inflammatory disease, tumors, obstruction, strictures, and polyps

   (b) To evaluate unexplained chronic diarrhea or pain, lower GI bleeding

   (c) To perform biopsy, obtain specimens for brush cytology studies, perform polypectomy, and obtain culture specimens; to remove foreign bodies; and to control bleeding

vii. Colonoscopy: Visualization and photography of the colon from the rectum to the ileocecal valve by means of a colonoscope

   (a) To detect polyps, strictures, obstruction, tumors, or inflammatory disease

   (b) To evaluate lower GI bleeding, unexplained chronic abdominal pain, unexplained iron-deficiency anemia, or changes in bowel patterns

   (c) To perform biopsy, obtain specimens for brush cytology studies, perform polypectomy, and obtain culture specimens; to remove foreign bodies; and to control bleeding

viii. Endoscopic retrograde cholangiopancreatography (ERCP): Visualization and photography of the biliary and/or pancreatic ducts by means of a flexible (fiberoptic) endoscope

   (a) To detect tumors, bile duct stones, obstruction, and pancreatitis

   (b) To evaluate jaundice, elevated levels on liver tests, and chronic unexplained abdominal pain

   (c) To perform biopsy and obtain specimens for brush cytology studies and cultures; to place stents; or to remove stones

ix. Angiography: Selective catheterization of the visceral arterial system and portal venous system, to reveal vessel sizes, patency, and flow rates of the vessels as well as the direction of the blood flow

x. Cholangiography: Radiopaque dye is used to enhance the radiograph and allow visualization of the gallbladder and bile ducts

xi. Computed tomography (CT) of the abdomen: Can be done with or without intravenous, oral, or rectal contrast

(a) To visualize the gallbladder, liver, pancreas, spleen, loops of the small and large intestine, extrahepatic bile ducts, and portal vein

(b) To determine the presence of vascular problems, infection, tumors, and pancreatic pseudocyst

(c) Use of contrast-enhanced images allows for improved visualization of tumors, vascularity of masses, and differences within bowel loops

xii. Positron emission tomography (PET): Use of radioisotopes (carbon, oxygen, nitrogen, and fluorine, and some metals like copper and gallium and their decay products) to reveal physiologic function, not anatomic structure. It is used to evaluate for colorectal, liver, pancreatic, and neuroendocrine diseases.

xiii. Magnetic resonance imaging (MRI)

(a) Same applications as CT with a greater potential for tissue characterization and a greater ability to diagnose and characterize diffuse liver and pancreatic disease

(b) Can also detect arterial and venous blood flow, vessel patency, bile ducts, and the presence of strictures within the ducts

(c) Less effective than CT for evaluating disorders of the bowel because the movement of the intestine degrades MRI images

xiv. Ultrasonography of the abdomen: To visualize the sizes and echotextures of the gallbladder, liver, pancreas, and spleen; to determine the presence or absence of disease (fatty infiltration, cirrhosis), the cause of masses (cysts, abscesses, tumors), and the presence of foreign bodies (gallstones); to evaluate the bile ducts and accumulation of fluids; and to determine the direction of blood flow, the development of collateral vessels, and vessel patency.

c. Other testing

i. Biopsy: Needle or forceps aspiration of tissue from the esophagus, stomach, duodenum, colon, rectum, or liver or soft tissues masses for histologic analysis

ii. Abdominal paracentesis: Withdrawal of peritoneal fluid for diagnostic purposes or symptomatic relief by means of a large-bore needle

iii. Peritoneoscopy (laparoscopy): Examination of the structures and organs within the abdominal cavity by means of a laparoscope

iv. Gastric lavage: Insertion of a gastric tube through the nose or mouth to examine the gastric contents or secretions for occult blood or pH

v. Schilling's test: Vitamin B_{12} absorption test to determine whether vitamin B_{12} absorption is defective and if the cause is intrinsic factor deficiency. Oral radioactively labeled vitamin B_{12} and intrinsic factor, and intramuscular nonradioactive vitamin B_{12} are administered, and 24- to 48-hour urine excretion is measured.

Patient Care

1. **Inability to establish or maintain a patent airway**

a. Description of problem: With acute hemorrhage or encephalopathy there may be an inability to maintain the airway due to altered levels of consciousness or possible aspiration due to vomiting. Clinical findings may include altered rate and depth of respirations, decreased oxygen saturation, dyspnea or tachypnea, and cyanosis.

b. Goals of care: Reestablish and maintain a patent airway

c. Collaborating professionals on health care team: Physician, nurse, anesthesiologist, respiratory therapist, radiologist

d. Interventions: See Chapter 2

     e. Evaluation of patient care: Patent airway and no signs of aspiration

2. Fluid volume deficit

     a. Description of problem: Associated with hemorrhage, GI fluid and blood losses, third-spacing, or sepsis. Clinical findings may include the following:

          i. Anxiety or diminished mental status

          ii. Tachycardia; decreased pulse pressure, cardiac output, and cardiac index

          iii. Orthostatic hypotension progressing to profound hypotension

          iv. Oliguria, anuria

          v. Decreased hemoglobin level, hematocrit, and platelet count; increased INR; hematemesis or melena

          vi. Elevated BUN, creatinine, lactate levels

          vii. Metabolic acidosis

     b. Goals of care: Restore normal circulating fluid volume

     c. Collaborating professionals on health care team: Physician, nurse, laboratory technician, pharmacist, blood bank personnel

     d. Interventions: See Chapters 3 and 5

     e. Evaluation of patient care: Restoration of adequate circulating volume as evidenced by vital signs, cardiac filling pressures, serum electrolyte and lactate levels, urine output, and oxygen delivery

3. Electrolyte and/or acid-base imbalances

     a. Description of problem: May be related to hemorrhage, GI losses, third-spacing, sepsis, or renal failure (see Chapters 2 and 5 for specific clinical findings)

     b. Goals of care: Restore and maintain electrolyte balance and normalize pH

     c. Collaborating professionals on health care team: Physician, nurse, pharmacist, laboratory technician, respiratory therapist

     d. Interventions: See Chapters 2 and 5

     e. Evaluation of patient care: Maintenance of normal values for serum electrolytes, lactate, and arterial blood gases

4. Impaired nutrition

     a. Description of problem: May be associated with inadequate intake, anorexia (intake less than body requirements) due to nausea, vomiting, diarrhea, reduced absorption, or increased metabolic needs

     b. Goals of care: Ensure that minimum daily requirements for both calories and nutrients are met

     c. Collaborating professionals on health care team: Physician, dietitian, total parenteral nutrition team, pharmacist

     d. Interventions

          i. Perform accurate monitoring and recording of patient weight; monitoring of intake and output, including calorie count

          ii. Assess bowel sounds and for signs of malabsorption or obstruction

          iii. Complete a comprehensive nutritional assessment, including increases in energy requirements

          iv. Administer oral and/or parenteral nutritional support and monitor the patency of feeding tubes if used

          v. Monitor for complications of central venous catheters if used

          vi. Monitor patient response to and tolerance of the nutritional regimen (e.g., electrolyte balance, hydration, hypoglycemia or hyperglycemia)

     e. Evaluation of patient care

          i. Meeting of the nutrient and caloric needs of the body as evidenced by lean muscle weight gain

          ii. Enhancement of immune response

          iii. Minimization of negative nitrogen balance

SPECIFIC PATIENT HEALTH PROBLEMS

Acute Abdomen

1. **Pathophysiology:** Condition of complex etiology characterized by the sudden onset of abdominal pain, associated with inflammation of the peritoneal cavity and usually necessitating emergency surgical intervention
2. **Etiology and risk factors**
   a. Perforated or ruptured viscus (esophagus, stomach, liver, pancreas, gallbladder, bile duct, bowel, appendix, or diverticulum) caused by erosion, technical error during surgery or other procedure, foreign body, trauma, or infection
   b. Perforated or ruptured blood vessel as in peptic ulcer disease, abdominal aortic aneurysm, tumor, or trauma
   c. Bowel ischemia: Decrease in blood flow or tissue perfusion that can be acute or chronic, occlusive or nonocclusive
      i. Arterial occlusion (embolus or thrombus)
      ii. Venous occlusion (hypercoagulable state, trauma)
      iii. Nonocclusive (cardiopulmonary bypass, vasoconstrictive medication, dehydration, shock, or congestive heart failure)
   d. Bowel obstruction: Blockage of the forward flow of intestinal contents
      i. Classification: Acute, subacute, chronic, or intermittent (only acute obstruction leads to infarction or strangulation)
      ii. Extent: Partial, complete
      iii. Location
         (a) Intrinsic: Originates within the lumen of the intestine
         (b) Extrinsic: Originates outside the lumen of the intestine
      iv. Effects on the intestine
         (a) Simple: Does not occlude blood supply
         (b) Strangulated: Occludes blood supply
         (c) Closed loop: Obstruction at each end of an intestinal segment
      v. Causal factors
         (a) Mechanical (gallstones, tumor, impactions, foreign bodies, inflammatory bowel diseases, adhesions, volvulus, intussusception)
         (b) Functional (paralytic ileus after abdominal surgery or caused by electrolyte imbalances, peritonitis, spinal fractures, megacolon, ischemia, pancreatitis)
         (c) Infection (abscess, sepsis)
         (d) Extraabdominal cause (cirrhosis, altered host response)
3. **Signs and symptoms**
   a. Persistent severe abdominal pain, referred pain
   b. Nausea, vomiting, reflux, or anorexia
   c. Alteration in bowel patterns
   d. Abdominal distention; hyperactive or hypoactive bowel sounds
   e. Guarding of the abdomen, rebound tenderness
   f. Fever, pallor, tachypnea
   g. Dehydration
   h. Evidence of blunt or penetrating trauma
   i. Fecal odor of gastric drainage
4. **Diagnostic study findings:** Differential diagnosis is complex
   a. Laboratory
      i. Elevated white blood cell (WBC) count with a shift to the left: Elevated segmented neutrophil and basophil counts, increased numbers of bands (immature neutrophils)

    ii. Elevated alkaline phosphatase level

    iii. Findings consistent with a diagnosis of pancreatitis; elevated serum amylase, lipase levels

    iv. Findings consistent with hemorrhage

    v. Arterial blood gas levels: Metabolic acidosis

    vi. Blood and body fluid culture results positive for infectious organisms

  b. Radiologic

    i. Abdominal flat-plate radiography: Alteration in the position, size, or structure of abdominal contents; free air or free fluid in the abdomen

    ii. Abdominal ultrasonography: Masses (cysts, abscesses, tumors), foreign bodies (gallstones), infarction

    iii. Cholangiography: Cholangitis

    iv. ERCP: Biliary or pancreatic stones, obstruction of ducts

    v. Arteriography: Bleeding, infarction

    vi. Abdominal CT or MRI: Vascular problems, infection, masses, or pancreatic pseudocyst

  c. EGD: Bleeding from peptic ulcer, esophageal tear

  d. Flexible sigmoidoscopy or colonoscopy: Lower GI ulceration, perforation, bleeding, abscess, ischemia

  e. Abdominal paracentesis: Blood, bile, pus, urine, or feces in abdominal cavity

  f. Peritoneoscopy (laparoscopy): Bleeding, perforation, rupture, abscess, ischemia

5. Goals of care

  a. Restore hemodynamic equilibrium and fluid balance

  b. Restore electrolyte balances

  c. Restore optimal GI function

  d. Minimize other organ dysfunction and damage

  e. Provide pain relief

  f. Eliminate any infectious process

6. Collaborating professionals on health care team: Physician, nurse, dietitian, respiratory therapist, pharmacist, radiologist or technician, consultant (e.g., hepatologist, infectious disease specialist)

7. Management of patient care

  a. Anticipated patient trajectory: Patients with an acute abdomen can differ greatly in their clinical course and status at discharge, depending on factors such as age and preexisting conditions. Throughout their course of recovery and discharge, patients with an acute abdomen may be expected to have needs in the following areas:

    i. Positioning: As the patient's condition and comfort dictate

    ii. Skin care: Postoperative wound care and pressure relief are required, because the patient is susceptible to skin breakdown from diarrhea, fistula formation, wound drainage, dehydration, hypotension, and malnutrition

    iii. Pain management: Hypotension makes pain management more complex; however, dosage reduction and nonpharmacologic techniques may be effective. Frequent reassessment and gradual titration of medication required. (See discussion of pain in Chapters 4 and 10.)

    iv. Nutrition: Nutritional needs will be increased because of increased metabolic needs. There will have been a reduction in intake prior to surgery because of the acute condition. Postoperatively the reduction in intake will continue in the face of increased metabolic demands of surgery, fever, wound healing, and complications such as infection. Cause of the condition and the caloric requirements will determine how these metabolic needs are met (enteral or parenteral route).

v. Infection control: Patients with blunt or penetrating trauma, infection, or pancreatitis will have an increased risk of infectious complications secondary to the ruptured viscus or translocation of bacteria. Vigilance is required to identify signs and symptoms of an infectious process early and initiate treatment promptly.

vi. Transport: Patient will undergo a variety of diagnostic tests and procedures, which will require that the patient be maintained in a mobile environment. Monitoring of various tubes, drains, and catheters is required in addition to monitoring of vitals signs.

vii. Discharge planning: Patient may need assistance at home for dressings, intravenous antibiotics, wound care, parenteral or enteral nutrition. Physical therapy may also be required.

viii. Pharmacology: Patients will be receiving a complex variety of medications postoperatively (antibiotics, insulin, narcotics, anxiolytics, vasopressors, inotropic agents, proton pump inhibitors, diuretics, cathartics)

ix. Psychosocial issues: Due to the acute nature of the illness, the family may be unprepared for role changes and financial issues. There may be significant alteration in body image and/or resumption of prior roles in the family.

x. Treatments: Postoperatively the patient can receive noninvasive treatments (motility agents) as well as invasive treatments (additional surgery)

xi. Ethical issues: Living will, durable power of attorney for health care, refusal of treatment, consent for treatment

  b. Potential complications

    i. Sepsis

      (a) Mechanism: Translocation of bacteria through the lumen of an ischemic GI tract, abscess, invasive monitoring lines

      (b) Management: See Chapter 9

    ii. Myocardial infarction

      (a) Mechanism: Myocardial ischemia secondary to reduced preload

      (b) Management: See Chapter 3

    iii. Dehydration

      (a) Mechanism: Hemorrhage, third-spacing, nausea, vomiting, diarrhea, intraoperative losses

      (b) Management: See Chapter 5

    iv. Renal insufficiency

      (a) Mechanism: Reduction in mean arterial pressure, infection, hypotension, nephrotoxic drugs, hepatorenal syndrome

      (b) Management: See Chapter 5

    v. Fistula formation or abscesses

      (a) Mechanism: Pancreatic enzymes or perforation of bowel

      (b) Management

        (1) Wound care to minimize fluid collections and abscesses

        (2) Administration of antibiotics to prevent or minimize complications

8. Evaluation of patient care

  a. Hemodynamic stability

  b. Fluid, electrolyte, nitrogen, and acid-base balance

  c. Freedom from pain

  d. Absence of infection

  e. Absence of complications

Acute (Fulminant) Liver Failure

1. **Pathophysiology**
   a. Clinical syndrome defined as the development of hepatic encephalopathy within 8 weeks of symptoms or within 2 weeks of the onset of jaundice
   b. Occurs in individuals with a history of normal liver function and is characterized by massive hepatocellular necrosis as evidenced by a raised serum alanine transaminase level; prolonged coagulation and hypoglycemia can also occur
   c. Except in cases of acute fulminant liver failure caused by acetaminophen toxicity, the mortality rate is 80% to 100% without liver transplantation

2. **Etiology and risk factors**
   a. Viral hepatitis: Acute hepatitis A and B
   b. Autoimmune hepatitis
   c. Acetaminophen toxicity: Liver failure from intentional overdose and unintentional therapeutic misadventure has a better prognosis than that resulting from other causes
   d. Hepatotoxic drugs or substances
   e. Mushroom poisoning (e.g., due to *Amanita phalloides*, *Amanita verna*, and *Amanita venosa*; Galerina autumnalis, Galerina marginata, and Galerina venenata; *Gyromitra* species)
   f. Viral infections: Herpesvirus family, especially in immunocompromised patients
   g. Acute Wilson's disease, acute Budd-Chiari syndrome
   h. Veno-occlusive disease and graft-versus-host disease after bone marrow transplantation
   i. Reye's syndrome

3. **Signs and symptoms**
   a. Prodromal symptoms (vague, flulike symptoms), fever
   b. Jaundice
   c. Hyperventilation, respiratory alkalosis
   d. Hepatic encephalopathy (confusion): Rapid progression to hepatic coma
   e. Profound coagulopathy and hypoglycemia
   f. Hepatorenal syndrome
   g. Sepsis, metabolic acidosis
   h. Intracranial hypertension
   i. Hyperdynamic circulation
   j. Systolic ejection murmur
   k. Eventual cardiovascular collapse
   l. Liver is enlarged during the acute inflammatory stage, then becomes atrophied as hepatocellular necrosis progresses

4. **Diagnostic study findings**
   a. Laboratory
      i. Increased levels of AST, ALT, and, to a lesser degree, alkaline phosphatase and GGT. Severe elevations followed by a progression back to normal that may be misinterpreted as improvement in the patient's status but is not a favorable sign if it occurs in the setting of increasing PT, INR, and bilirubin levels; indicates near-complete hepatocellular necrosis.
      ii. Increased serum bilirubin, creatinine, BUN levels
      iii. Prolonged PT and INR
      iv. Levels of factors V and VII less than 20% of normal (poor prognostic sign)
      v. Decreased serum glucose level, hemoglobin level, and hematocrit
      vi. Increased serum lactate level, serum ammonia level, and WBC count
      vii. Positive results on cultures of body fluids

        viii. Positive results on hepatitis serologic testing or tests for autoimmune markers depending on cause

        ix. Positive urine toxicology screen results

        x. Positive stool guaiac test results

  b. Radiologic

      i. Chest radiograph: Bilateral infiltrates or evidence of aspiration pneumonitis

      ii. CT scan of the head: Normal until very late in the process

      iii. Cerebral perfusion scan may show decreased or absent flow late in the process; performed before liver transplantation to rule out brain death

  c. Pressure measurement

      i. Increased ICP, increased mean arterial pressure, normal cerebral perfusion pressure (early signs)

      ii. Increased ICP, normal or decreased mean arterial pressure, decreased cerebral perfusion pressure (late signs)

5. Goals of care

  a. Optimize liver function

  b. Stabilize for liver transplantation if appropriate

  c. Monitor and treat complications

6. Collaborating professionals on health care team: Physician, nurse, pharmacist, laboratory technician, respiratory therapist, consultant

7. Management of patient care

  a. Anticipated patient trajectory: Very unstable with long recovery. Liver transplantation may be necessary when progression of liver failure continues; this requires either a graft from a living donor or a cadaveric liver. Patients may be expected to have needs in the following areas:

      i. Positioning: Head of bed raised 30 degrees for treatment of increased ICP

      ii. Skin care: Itching can be severe with the onset of jaundice; scratching is unconscious, which results in excoriations; in patients with prolonged coagulation times, this can result in hematoma formation

      iii. Pain management: Difficult due to liver failure. Pain is rare because encephalopathy inhibits the reception of transmitted pain impulses. Consultation with a hepatologist necessary if pain medication required.

      iv. Nutrition: Metabolic rate can be increased; fluid balance is a problem with renal failure. Special enteral and parenteral solutions required due to liver and renal dysfunction.

      v. Infection control: Immobility, altered level of consciousness, invasive lines, and depressed immune system results in increased risk of infection

      vi. Transport: Monitor for changes in ICP; mobile environment increases the risk of infection

      vii. Discharge planning: Recovery is long, and the patient and family will need assistance with home care, rehabilitation, medications, office visits

      viii. Pharmacology: Patient will be taking a complex regimen of medications, and alternative choices (shorter-acting drugs or drugs with shorter half-lives) and dosing patterns (every 12 hours instead of every 6 or 8 hours) will be required due to liver dysfunction

      ix. Psychosocial issues: Acuity of the situation will have a profound impact on the family and increase stress

      x. Treatments

        (a) Noninvasive: Medications

        (b) Invasive: Surgery, endoscopy with esophageal variceal ligation or sclerosis, colonoscopy with cauterization, angiography with embolization

    xi. Ethical issues: Cause of the liver disease can affect the potential for liver transplantation and may lead to a discussion regarding end-of-life issues

  b. Potential complications

    i. Infection or sepsis

      (a) Mechanism: Depressed immune system and breaks in the skin barrier due to monitoring needs; altered level of consciousness and risk of aspiration

      (b) Management: See Chapter 9

    ii. Brainstem herniation (most common cause of death in fulminant liver failure) or intracranial hemorrhage

      (a) Mechanism: Increased coagulation times increase the risk of intracranial bleeding and pulmonary hemorrhage; increased risk of hypoxia, which increases the risk of cerebral edema

      (b) Management: See Chapter 4

   iii. Renal failure

      (a) Mechanism: Progression of liver failure may lead to renal failure (hepatorenal syndrome)

      (b) Management: See Chapter 5

   iv. Respiratory failure

      (a) Mechanism: Pulmonary edema, hemorrhage, pneumonia, altered mental status

      (b) Management: See Chapter 2

    v. Liver transplantation

      (a) Treatment option for fulminant liver failure and end-stage liver disease, and certain cases of hepatoma

      (b) Liver disease may reoccur in the transplanted liver

      (c) Currently approximately 20,000 patients need liver transplantation; however, only about 6000 are done per year

        (1) Cadaveric (deceased) donor

          a) Donor declared brain dead

          b) Either entire liver or split liver can be used

          c) Donor and recipient are matched by blood group, age, size

        (2) Living donor

          a) Donor provides 60% of his or her liver

          b) Donor between the ages of 21 and 45 years in most cases

          c) Recipient usually in healthier condition than those receiving cadaveric organs due to the ability to transplant earlier in the disease course

          d) During the early postoperative period the patient requires monitoring for primary nonfunction of the new liver, monitoring for improvement in mentation and levels of coagulation factors, and monitoring for infection

8. Evaluation of patient care: Normalization of liver functions, neurologic function, renal function, and vital signs

Chronic Liver Failure: Decompensated Cirrhosis

1. Pathophysiology

  a. Cirrhosis is a chronic and usually slowly progressive disease of the liver involving the diffuse formation of connective tissue (fibrosis), nodular regeneration of the liver after necrosis, and chronic inflammation

  b. Changes are often irreversible

  c. Once the diagnosis of cirrhosis has been made, there is generally a 5- to 10-year period prior to decompensation

2. Etiology and risk factors
  a. Alcoholism (Laënnec's cirrhosis): Development of cirrhosis preceded by a reversible stage of alcoholic hepatitis
  b. Postnecrotic cirrhosis
    i. Viral hepatitis (chronic active hepatitis B, C, F, or G
    ii. Drug or toxin induced (prescription drugs, herbs, heavy metals)
    iii. Autoimmune hepatitis
  c. Autoimmune diseases of biliary stasis (primary biliary cirrhosis, primary sclerosing cholangitis)
  d. Inborn errors of liver metabolism: Wilson's disease (copper metabolism), hemochromatosis (iron metabolism), α_1-antitrypsin deficiency
  e. Nonalcoholic fatty liver disease, associated with obesity, hyperlipidemia, protein-calorie malnutrition, diabetes mellitus, chronic corticosteroid use, jejunoileal bypass, short bowel syndrome
  f. Hepatic vein thrombosis (Budd-Chiari syndrome)
  g. Right-sided heart failure: Cardiac cirrhosis

3. Signs and symptoms
  a. Fatigue, alteration in sleep pattern: Insomnia, day-night reversal
  b. Pruritus
  c. Muscle wasting, weight loss
  d. Abdominal distention with ascites
  e. Anemia, hematomas, ecchymoses
  f. Clay-colored stools
  g. Fetor hepaticus: Musty breath, poor dentition
  h. Altered mental status, asterixis
  i. Visible stigmata of liver disease: Jaundice, temporal and upper body muscle wasting, parotid enlargement, spider angiomas, palmar erythema, leukonychia, possible clubbing of the fingers, testicular atrophy, gynecomastia in males, striae, the development of abdominal wall collaterals, caput medusae
  j. Umbilical hernia, incisional hernia, splenomegaly
  k. Hyperdynamic circulation: Increased heart rate, systolic ejection murmur
  l. Possible decrease in lung sounds in the bases because of pleural effusions
  m. Hepatic bruit (hepatoma or alcoholic hepatitis superimposed on cirrhosis)

4. Diagnostic study findings
  a. Laboratory: Depend on the cause and stage of disease
    i. ALT, AST, alkaline phosphatase, GGT levels: Not usually markedly elevated in advanced cirrhosis but depends on the cause of the liver disease
    ii. Bilirubin level: Elevated in advanced cirrhosis except in diseases of biliary stasis, in which it is elevated early in the disease
    iii. PT, INR: Prolonged PT and increased INR; the most sensitive index of synthetic liver function in a readily available laboratory test
    iv. Platelet count: May be decreased due to splenomegaly
    v. Blood ammonia level: May be elevated (may be affected by a variety of factors not related to liver disease)
    vi. Hemoglobin level, hematocrit: Decreased
    vii. BUN, creatinine levels: Decreased until hepatorenal syndrome occurs
    viii. Serum sodium level: Decreased (at times critically)
    ix. Hepatitis serologic findings: Variable
    x. Ascitic fluid: WBC increased absolute neutrophil count, culture results positive for a specific organism

   b. Radiologic
      i. CT: Liver volume decreased, spleen volume increased, possible presence of ascites or tumor
      ii. MRI, magnetic resonance venography, magnetic resonance arteriography, magnetic resonance cholangiopancreatography: To evaluate organs, vessels, bile ducts for abnormalities (portal vein thrombosis, liver cancer)
      iii. Abdominal ultrasonography: To determine liver and spleen sizes, portal vein patency, presence of hepatoma, bile duct dilatation, presence of small amounts of ascites
   c. ERCP: May show dilated bile ducts or beading (narrowing) of ducts
   d. Upper GI endoscopy: Reveals esophageal, gastric, and/or duodenal varices
   e. Abdominal paracentesis if ascites present: To test fluid for infection (important)
   f. Liver biopsy: For staging of inflammation and fibrosis
5. Goals of care
   a. Optimize remaining liver function
   b. Stabilize decompensations
6. Collaborating professionals on health care team: Physician, nurse, dietitian, laboratory technician, physical therapist, consultant (hepatologist, gastroenterologist, surgeon)
7. Management of patient care
   a. Anticipated patient trajectory: Patient with chronic liver failure may plateau prior to decompensation then deteriorate rapidly. Patients may be expected to have needs in the following areas:
      i. Positioning: Development of orthostatic hypotension dictates the need for slow, deliberate movements to prevent dizziness and falls. Patient with encephalopathy may not be able to coordinate thoughts and movements.
      ii. Skin care: Skin will be very dry, and there will be an increase in bruising due to reduction of the platelet count and levels of coagulation factors
      iii. Pain management: See Acute (Fulminant) Liver Failure
      iv. Nutrition: Ascites may cause early satiety; low zinc levels in liver disease may result in diminished taste or metallic taste; patients develop severe muscle wasting and malnutrition
      v. Infection control: Depressed immune system increases the risk of infection; presence of ascites creates the risk of peritonitis
      vi. Transport: Mobile environment increases the risk of infection; ascites creates the risk for spontaneous bacterial peritonitis
      vii. Discharge planning: Recovery periods are short and rehospitalization can be frequent as the patient decompensates. Family and patient will need assistance with home care, rehabilitation, medications, office visits.
      viii. Pharmacology: See Acute (Fulminant) Liver Failure
      ix. Psychosocial issues: Chronicity of the situation will have a profound impact on the family unit and increase stress. Depression can occur in both the patient and primary caregiver.
      x. Treatments: See Acute (Fulminant) Liver Failure
      xi. Ethical issues: Lack of available organs and prolonged hospitalizations increase the risk of sepsis, which prevents transplantation and leads to discussions of withdrawal of life support
   b. Potential complications
      i. Portal hypertension
         (a) Mechanism
            (1) Increased hydrostatic pressure (higher than 10 mm Hg) within the portal venous system as a result of disruption of the normal liver

architecture, which increases the resistance to blood flow into and out of the liver (25% of the cardiac output per minute)

  (2) Development of esophageal varices and gastroesophageal variceal bleeding

  (3) Splenomegaly: Increased size and congestion of the spleen as a result of portal hypertension, with backward venous congestion via the splenic vein, which results in pancytopenia (anemia, leukopenia, thrombocytopenia)

 (b) Management

  (1) Restriction on the amount of weight to be lifted (no more than 40 lb)

  (2) Frequent monitoring for consequential cytopenia

  (3) Use of β-blockers or scheduled endoscopic treatments

  (4) Sarfeh shunts may be used for refractory bleeding

  (5) Transjugular intrahepatic portosystemic stents may be used for refractory bleeding

ii. Ascites

 (a) Mechanism: Caused by transudation of fluid from the liver surface as a result of portal and lymphatic hypertension and increased membrane permeability, which lead to increased hydrostatic pressure and decreased oncotic pressure in the portal venous system, characterized by a rise in hepatic sinusoidal pressure, excess hepatic lymph, and hypoalbuminemia

 (b) Management

  (1) Low-sodium diet, use of diuretics

  (2) Accurate intake and output measurements

  (3) Monitoring for refractory conditions (increasing ascites with increasing creatinine level)

  (4) Transjugular intrahepatic portosystemic stents may be used for refractory ascites

iii. Spontaneous bacterial peritonitis

 (a) Mechanism: Result of the translocation of bacteria from GI lumens to the ascitic fluid

 (b) Management

  (1) Paracentesis to verify primary versus secondary peritonitis

  (2) Administration of antibiotics

  (3) Adjustment of diuretic therapy

iv. Malnutrition

 (a) Mechanism: Reduced caloric intake, reduced synthesis of albumin by the liver, increased caloric needs

 (b) Management

  (1) Nutritional supplements

  (2) Enteral feedings

  (3) Parenteral nutrition

v. Hepatic encephalopathy

 (a) Mechanism

  (1) Neuropsychiatric syndrome that develops when nitrogenous and other potentially toxic compounds arising from gut flora accumulate as a result of impaired transformation and elimination

  (2) Four grades of alteration of mentation (Table 8-1)

 (b) Management

  (1) Neurologic monitoring for altered level of consciousness (see Chapter 4)

TABLE 8-1
Clinical Assessment of Hepatic Encephalopathy

	Grade I	Grade II	Grade III	Grade IV
Level of consciousness	Awake	Decreased, but opens eyes spontaneously	Somnolent to semistuporous but arousable to verbal and painful stimuli; does not open eyes spontaneously	Comatose; no response to pain
Orientation	Total orientation with trivial lack of awareness then progression to disorientation	Minimal disorientation to time and place progressing to severe confusion	Complete disorientation when aroused	Coma
Intellectual functions	Mental clouding; slowness in answering questions; impaired handwriting; subtle changes in intellectual function; impaired performance on addition takes; decrease in psychometric test scores	Amnesia for past events; impaired performance on subtraction tasks; decrease in psychometric. test scores	Inability to perform computations	Coma
Behavior	Forgetfulness, restlessness, irritability, untidiness, apathy, disobedience	Subtle personality changes, inappropriate behavior, decreased inhibitions	Lethargy; bizarre behavior (e.g., unprovoked rage)	Coma
Mood	Euphoria, anxiety, depression, crying	Lethargy or apathy, paranoia	Increased apathy	Coma
Neuromuscular function	Muscular incoordination, tremors, yawning, insomnia	Hypoactive reflexes, asterixis, ataxia, slurred speech	Inability to cooperate; nystagmus and Babinski's sign	Coma

HEPATIC ENCEPHALOPATHY TYPES

A: Encephalopathy associated with acute liver failure
B: Encephalopathy associated with portal-systemic bypass and/or intrinsic hepatocellular disease
C: Encephalopathy associated with cirrhosis and portal hypertension or portal systemic shunts
Subcategory of type C
   Episodic hepatic encephalopathy subdivisions: Precipitated, spontaneous, recurrent
   Persistent hepatic encephalopathy subdivisions: Mild, severe, treatment-dependent
   Minimal hepatic encephalopathy

From Ferenci P, Lockwood A, Mullen K, et al: Hepatic encephalopathy—definition, nomenclature, diagnosis, and quantification: final report of the working party at the 11th World Congresses of Gastroenterology, Vienna 1998, *Hepatology* 35:716-721, 2002.

(2) Administration of lactulose to enhance GI motility

(3) Maintenance of airway

    vi. Pulmonary complications

       (a) Mechanism: Variety of pulmonary conditions develop as a result of hypoxemia, increased intrapulmonary vascular shunting, and changes in intrapleural and intraabdominal pressures; for example, pleural effusions, hepatopulmonary syndrome (pulmonary capillary vasodilation and intrapulmonary shunts)

       (b) Management: See Chapter 2

    vii. Hepatorenal syndrome

       (a) Mechanism: "Functional" form of acute renal failure that occurs in patients with advanced end-stage liver disease, resulting from decreased effective circulating plasma volume and the release of mediators of vasoconstriction, which cause diversion of renal blood flow

       (b) Management: See Chapter 5

    viii. Infection or sepsis

       (a) Mechanism: Depressed immune system and breaks in the skin barrier due to monitoring needs; altered level of consciousness and risk of aspiration

       (b) Management: See Chapter 9

8. Evaluation of patient care: Optimization of liver function, neurologic function, vital signs, renal function

Acute Pancreatitis

1. Pathophysiology

  a. Overview: Inflammation of the pancreas results when activated pancreatic proteases digest pancreatic tissue itself. Pancreatic secretions build up, and trypsin accumulates and activates the other pancreatic proteases. Normal defense mechanisms are overwhelmed, which results in pancreatic tissue autodigestion.

  b. Classification of pancreatitis

    i. Acute pancreatitis: Single episode characterized by abdominal pain and elevated levels of enzymes (amylase, lipase) with inflammation of the pancreas, which returns to normal after resolution of the episode

       (a) 80% of cases are related to biliary stones or alcohol use

       (b) Mild pancreatitis does not have other organ damage or complications and recovery is uneventful. Severe pancreatitis is characterized by impaired pancreatic function and systemic complications; recovery prone to complications.

    ii. Recurrent chronic pancreatitis: Progressive destruction of the acinar cells as a result of persistent inflammation

       (a) Classification of chronic pancreatitis: Lithogenic (chronic calcifying stones), obstructive, inflammatory, or fibrotic

       (b) Cause can be alcohol use, malnutrition, or idiopathic causes

  c. Regardless of the initiating mechanism, acinar cell injury occurs with activation of pancreatic proenzymes to their active forms, which results in autodigestion of the pancreas

  d. Three processes contribute to the initiation of pancreatitis

    i. Obstruction of the pancreatic duct

    ii. Pancreatic ischemia

    iii. Premature activation of zymogens (inactive digestive enzymes), leading to premature release of active pancreatic enzymes, which begin autodigestion of the pancreas

(a) Release of cytokines (platelet-activating factor, tumor necrosis factor, interleukin-1), which damage the pancreas

(b) Release of kinins, which creates capillary wall permeability

(c) Pancreatic and peripancreatic edema with loss of up to 6 L of fluid into the interstitial space

(d) Release and activation of systemic inflammatory mediators (cytokines), including complement, kinins, histamine, prostaglandin, clotting factors; results in systemic effects, including systemic inflammatory response syndrome (SIRS)

(e) End results include increased vascular permeability, vasodilation, vascular stasis, and microthrombosis, with significant effects on other organ systems

   e. Forms of acute pancreatitis

   i. Mild, edematous (interstitial pancreatitis): Accounts for 95% of cases; mortality rate is 5%; edematous pancreas with minimal or no necrotic damage; gross architecture is preserved

   ii. Severe, hemorrhagic (necrotizing pancreatitis): Accounts for 5% of cases; mortality rate is 50%

   iii. Extensive peripancreatic tissue necrosis and hemorrhage. There is necrosis of fat throughout the abdomen. Retroperitoneal hemorrhage caused by tissue necrosis or erosion of a pseudocyst into the vascular structure, vascular inflammation, and thrombus may occur.

2. **Etiology and risk factors**

   a. Alcoholism

   b. Obstruction of the pancreatic ducts

   i. Gallstones (biliary, pancreatic)

   ii. Structural abnormalities (duodenum-ampulla, bile ducts, pancreatic duct)

   iii. Tumor

   iv. Inflammation, infection

   v. Edema

   c. Complication of abdominal surgery or diagnostic procedure (e.g., ERCP)

   d. Abdominal trauma: Blunt or penetrating

   e. Drug toxicity: Cyclosporine, corticosteroids, azathioprine, thiazides, sulfonamides, tetracycline, estrogens

   f. Familial hyperlipidemia

   g. Chronic hyperparathyroidism, hypercalcemia

   h. Infection: *Mycoplasma, Streptococcus, Salmonella,* Paramyxovirus (mumps), cytomegalovirus, echovirus, Epstein-Barr virus, coxsackievirus, hepatitis virus

   i. Shock

3. **Signs and symptoms**

   a. Vary from a mild, almost asymptomatic case to a fulminant condition of massive pancreatic necrosis

   b. Abdominal pain manifested in 95% of cases

   i. Epigastric or right upper quadrant pain is knifelike and twisting in nature; begins suddenly and reaches the apex quickly; may radiate to all abdominal quadrants and the lumbar area; associated with nausea and vomiting, low-grade fever

   ii. Diminished bowel sounds, tenderness on palpation

   c. Visceral tenderness

   i. Initial tenderness is diffuse, caused by capsular distention and release of kinins

  ii. May cause the patient to double over, with a facial expression of pain, nausea, vomiting, pallor, diaphoresis

 d. Somatic tenderness: Extrapancreatic involvement (peritoneal, retroperitoneal)

  i. Sharp, well localized, yet can be diffuse

  ii. Accompanied by nausea, vomiting, rigid abdomen, rebound tenderness

  iii. Standard dosages of analgesics may be ineffective for pain relief

 e. Low-grade fever

 f. Diaphoresis

 g. Anorexia, vomiting, diarrhea

 h. Dehydration

 i. Abdominal distention

 j. Jaundice; dark, foamy urine

 k. Steatorrhea: Bulky, pale, foul-smelling stools

 l. Cullen's sign: Bluish discoloration of the periumbilical area

 m. Turner's sign: Bluish discoloration of the flanks

 n. Peritoneal lavage reveals blood in the peritoneal cavity ("beef broth" tap)

 o. Hypoactive or absent bowel sounds

 p. Rebound tenderness

4. Diagnostic study findings

 a. Laboratory

  i. Elevated serum amylase level that peaks between 4 and 24 hours after the onset of pancreatitis and returns to normal within 4 days; the degree of elevation does not necessarily correlate with the severity of the illness. Not a sensitive test unless done early after the onset of signs and symptoms.

  ii. Elevated serum lipase level: Stays elevated longer than does serum amylase level

  iii. Elevated urine amylase and lipase levels: In patients with good renal function, these are better indexes of pancreatic damage than are serum levels

  iv. Decreased serum ionized calcium level (less than 2.0 mg/dl): Calcium binds to areas of fat necrosis

  v. Intermittently elevated serum glucose level: Indicates beta-cell involvement

  vi. Presence of C-reactive protein

  vii. Increased trypsin level

  viii. Elevated WBC count and serum bilirubin, BUN, triglyceride levels

  ix. Elevated serum AST, ALT, lactate dehydrogenase, alkaline phosphatase levels

  x. Decreased albumin level

  xi. Elevated or decreased hematocrit

 b. Radiologic

  i. Abdominal plain film: Presence of dilated duodenum (sentinel loop) or transverse colon

  ii. CT: Evidence of pancreatic inflammation, pseudocyst, abscess, obstruction of the pancreatic duct, peripancreatic and retroperitoneal necrosis

  iii. MRI: Similar to CT in identifying inflammation; also identifies areas of poor perfusion and debris in fluid collections

  iv. Ultrasonography: Evidence of diffuse pancreatic enlargement, pseudocyst, or abscess, or presence of gallstones, bile duct dilatation

 c. ERCP: Not accurate for the diagnosis of acute pancreatitis but can provide evidence of biliary or pancreatic stones. Early ERCP with sphincterotomy and stone extraction may ameliorate the course of biliary pancreatitis.

5. **Goals of care**
   a. Optimize pancreatic function
   b. Minimize complications
6. **Collaborating professionals on health care team:** Physician, nurse, dietitian, laboratory technician, physical therapist, consultant (gastroenterologist, surgeon), pain management team
7. **Management of patient care**
   a. Anticipated patient trajectory: May be variable, with improvements, plateaus, decompensations, then rapid deterioration. Relapses may occur after weeks of improvements. Patients may be expected to have needs in the following areas:
      i. Positioning: For patient comfort
      ii. Skin care: Prevention of excoriation due to fistula drainage; keep clean and dry
      iii. Pain management: Essential, as there can be severe pain affecting multiple other organ systems. Consultation with a pain management team is necessary, because certain narcotics will affect the pancreatic sphincters.
      iv. Nutrition: Patient will need to be on nothing-by-mouth (NPO) status initially, sometimes for weeks, which necessitates the use of total parenteral nutrition (TPN) or lower elemental enteral feedings
      v. Infection control: Depressed immune system increases the risk of infection. Pain may lead to shallow respirations and atelectasis or pneumonia. Pleural effusions may become infected.
      vi. Transport: Frequent diagnostic testing increases the risk of infection and catheter dislodgement
      vii. Discharge planning: Recovery periods are prolonged and rehospitalizations occur; patient will need assistance with home care, rehabilitation, medications, frequent office visits
      viii. Pharmacology: Patient will be taking a complex regimen of medications, and alternative drug choices and dosing patterns will be necessary due to the potential for liver and kidney dysfunction
      ix. Psychosocial issues: Chronicity of the illness will increase the stress on the family unit. Depression may occur in both the patient and primary caregiver.
      x. Treatments
         (a) Noninvasive: Medications
         (b) Invasive: Surgery
      xi. Ethical issues: Need for ongoing care with the use of multiple resources over very long periods, withdrawal of life support due to inability to prevent or resolve multiple organ failure
   b. Potential complications
      i. Local complications: Wound infections and skin breakdown in the area of wounds, incisions, and fistulas
         (a) Mechanism: Pancreatic enzymes autodigest body tissues they contact, which leads to fistula formation, and increased skin breakdown
         (b) Management
            (1) Keep skin clean and dry
            (2) Use ostomy bags or drains to minimize drainage contact with skin
      ii. Hypovolemia
         (a) Mechanism: Massive third-spacing of fluids may result in fluid collections, necrosis, pseudocysts, abscesses, fistulas, intestinal obstruction
         (b) Management: See Chapter 5
      iii. SIRS and sepsis

(a) Mechanism: Can develop when peripancreatic or ascitic fluid collections become infected and spread through areas of necrosis

(b) Management: See Chapter 9

iv. Multiple organ dysfunction syndrome (MODS)

(a) Mechanism: Result of sepsis in the setting of an abscess or necrotizing pancreatitis

(b) Management: See Chapter 9

v. Adult respiratory distress syndrome (ARDS)

(a) Mechanism: Respiratory failure in the setting of sepsis, which leads to increased VQ mismatch, decreased compliance

(b) Management: See Chapter 2

vi. Acute renal tubular necrosis, acute renal failure

(a) Mechanism: Hypotension, inadequate preload, use of nephrotoxic antibiotics, vasoconstriction from vasoactive medications

(b) Management: See Chapter 5

vii. Disseminated intravascular coagulation

(a) Mechanism: Due to sepsis, hypotension, elevated cytokine levels

(b) Management: See Chapter 7

viii. Pain

(a) Mechanism: Pancreatitis is usually described by patients as the worse pain they have ever had. This can be due to gallstones or to the inflammation of the tissues where autodigestion is occurring.

(b) Management (see also the discussion of pain in Chapters 4 and 10): Administration of analgesics and use of nonpharmacologic pain treatments (distraction, imagery)

8. **Evaluation of patient care**

   a. Normalization of pancreatic functions, vital signs, digestive function

   b. Relief of pain

Gastrointestinal Bleeding

1. **Pathophysiology**

   a. Peptic ulcer disease

   i. Both duodenal and gastric ulcers are classified as peptic ulcers. The mucosal lining of the stomach and duodenum is digested by pepsin and acid, which causes ulcerations, due to either an imbalance between acid and pepsin production or the loss of the protective factors of bicarbonate, mucus, and cell renewal in the affected mucosa.

   ii. In duodenal ulcers there is an oversecretion of acid. In gastric ulcers there is a reduction in the gastric mucosal barrier caused by decreased mucosal blood flow, altered cellular renewal, reduction in mucus secretion, bacterial infection, or damaging agents.

   iii. Infection with *Helicobacter pylori*, a bacterium, contributes to the development of gastric ulcers; a high incidence of colonization with *H. pylori* is found in people with gastric ulcers.

   b. Variceal bleeding: 50% of patients with alcoholic cirrhosis develop esophageal varices within 2 years of their diagnosis. Esophageal variceal hemorrhage accounts for one third of deaths in patients with cirrhosis and portal hypertension. The mortality rate is 30% to 50% for each episode of bleeding.

   i. Portal circulation is high flow (approximately 1100 ml/min) with low pressure (about 7 mm Hg); an increase in resistance (either intrahepatic or extrahepatic) to blood flow in this system results in portal hypertension

      ii. Spontaneous rupture and bleeding occur when the portosystemic gradient is higher than 12 mm Hg, which causes the formation of varices in collateral venous channels between the portal and systemic circulation

      iii. Varices in the distal esophagus and at the esophagogastric junction are the most prone to bleeding; however; varices can also form in the peritoneum, retroperitoneum, and throughout the GI tract, including the rectum (Figure 8-7).

  c. Other causes of upper GI bleeding

      i. Mallory-Weiss syndrome: Tear in the mucosa or submucosa at the gastro-esophageal junction. Tear is usually longitudinal, caused by forceful or prolonged vomiting; 75% of cases occur in males with a history of excessive alcohol ingestion or salicylate use.

      ii. Esophagitis

      iii. Stress ulcers (gastric, duodenal): Extremely common in critically ill patients; associated with sepsis, shock, burns, trauma, acute head injuries, renal failure, hepatic failure, ARDS, mechanical ventilation, and major operative procedures; characterized by mucosal ischemia that leads to alterations which result in the loss of protective functions

  d. Causes of lower GI bleeding

      i. Crohn's disease: Less common, usually due to deep ulceration in the colon

      ii. Ulcerative colitis: Can cause exsanguination due to diffuse ulceration

      iii. Colitis resulting from ischemia, radiation, chemotherapy

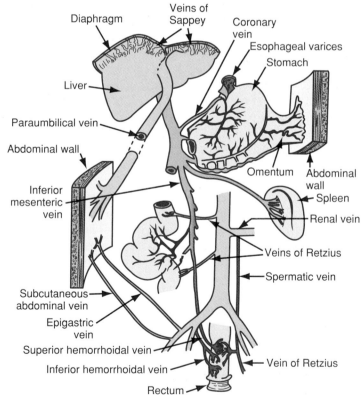

FIGURE 8-7 ■ Collateral circulation in the liver. (From Krumberger JM: Gastrointestinal disorders. In Kinney MR, Packa DR, Dunbar SB, editors: *AACN's clinical reference for critical-care nursing,* St Louis, 1993, Mosby, p 1149.)

    iv. Diverticula: Most common cause of acute massive colonic blood loss

    v. Intestinal polyps: Intermittent or occult bleeding

    vi. Angiodysplasia (arteriovenous malformation of the mucosa): Common cause of chronic or intermittent low-grade bleeding in aged patients

    vii. Hemorrhoids

2. Etiology and risk factors

  a. Gastric ulcers associated with decreased tissue resistance; three to four times more common in men; associated with malignancy; may lead to nonhealing ulcer in stomach

  b. Duodenal ulcers associated with increased hydrochloric acid level

    i. Most frequent sites are the pylorus and the first portion of the duodenum

    ii. Can occur at any age; common among young adults

    iii. Seem to have a seasonal trend, with higher incidence in the spring and fall

    iv. Pharmacologic agents may play a role: Salicylates, indomethacin, phenylbutazone, nonsteroidal antiinflammatory drugs (NSAIDs), corticosteroids, antineoplastic agents, vasopressors, reserpine

    v. Caffeine use, alcohol abuse, cigarette smoking

    vi. Familial tendency

  c. Variceal bleeding is associated with portal hypertension

    i. Prehepatic (presinusoidal) factors in which the wedge hepatic venous pressure is less than the portal pressure: Portal vein thrombosis due to the presence of cirrhosis, hepatoma, umbilical vein catheterization in infancy, or hypercoagulable state

    ii. Intrahepatic (sinusoidal) factors in which the wedge hepatic venous pressure is increased and equals the portal pressure: Postnecrotic cirrhosis (e.g., chronic active hepatitis and cirrhosis), alcoholic cirrhosis

    iii. Posthepatic (postsinusoidal) factors in which the site of obstruction to flow is distal to the sinusoids: Hepatic vein thrombosis (e.g., Budd-Chiari syndrome), veno-occlusive disease after bone marrow transplantation

    iv. Diseases causing portal hypertension: Splenomegaly or splenic vein thrombosis not due to liver disease; fulminant hepatitis; cirrhosis of various causes; metastatic carcinoma; diseases of the hepatic venules, veins, or inferior vena cava; cardiac diseases

3. Signs and symptoms

  a. Ulcers

    i. Epigastric pain with bleeding: Heartburn; with duodenal ulcers, pain is relieved by food; pain stops when bleeding begins

    ii. Nausea, vomiting

    iii. Hematemesis (blood is bright red or resembles coffee grounds)

    iv. Melena

    v. Weight loss

    vi. Abdominal tenderness, guarding

    vii. Hyperactive bowel sounds

    viii. Orthostatic hypotension

    ix. Narrow pulse pressure

  b. Esophageal varices

    i. Sudden onset of hematemesis (may be projectile): Coffee-ground vomitus or bright red blood

    ii. Coagulopathy: Prolonged PT, increased INR, decreased platelet count

    iii. Hyperdynamic circulation: Increased cardiac output, decreased systemic vascular resistance, systolic ejection murmur

      iv. Hemodynamic changes: Decreased pulse pressure, orthostatic hypotension, tachycardia

      v. Increased minute ventilation

      vi. Lethargy, malaise

      vii. Pale skin and/or mucous membranes

4. Diagnostic study findings

  a. Laboratory

      i. Hemoglobin level, hematocrit: Decreased; true extent of blood loss may not be immediately apparent

      ii. BUN level: May be elevated

      iii. PT, INR: Prolonged PT, increased INR

      iv. Albumin: May be decreased

      v. Platelet count: May be decreased in cirrhosis

      vi. Blood tests or stomach biopsy: To detect colonization by *H. pylori*

      vii. Guaiac testing of nasogastric drainage and stool for occult blood

  b. Radiologic

      i. Upright chest radiography or upright and lateral abdominal radiography: Shows free air under the diaphragm with perforated, bleeding ulcers

      ii. Upper GI series: To localize an ulcer

      iii. Selective mesenteric angiography: To localize the site of bleeding when endoscopy cannot be performed

      iv. Upper GI endoscopy: To reveal the location of an ulcer, rule out other causes of bleeding

        (a) Differential diagnosis for variceal bleeding is complex and includes peptic ulcer disease, gastritis, Mallory-Weiss tear of the esophagus, and Boerhaave's syndrome, among others

        (b) Definitive identification is made by endoscopic examination of the esophagus, stomach, and duodenum and/or colonoscopy

        (c) During endoscopy it is possible to grade and classify esophageal, gastric, and/or duodenal varices according to size, location, and risk factors

      v. Superior mesenteric artery arteriography: To measure hepatic vein pressure gradient and to image the portal and hepatic venous systems

      vi. Angiography: To evaluate blood flow, identify the source of bleeding; can be used to embolize a vessel

      vii. CT: To document cirrhosis, identify the presence of collateral circulation, and rule out hepatoma

      viii. Doppler ultrasonography: To evaluate patency of and flow in the portal vein and hepatic veins

  c. Nasogastric intubation: To obtain gastric aspirate

5. Goals of care

  a. Minimize blood loss; replenish losses

  b. Optimize hemodynamic status

  c. Restore circulating blood volume

  d. Provide pain relief

6. Collaborating professionals on health care team: Physician, nurse, dietitian, laboratory technician, consultant (gastroenterologist, surgeon)

7. Management of patient care

  a. Anticipated patient trajectory: Once bleeding is halted, rapid stabilization is possible. If it is difficult to halt the hemorrhage, then the patient course is more problematic. Patients may be expected to have needs in the following areas:

      i. Positioning: Head of the bed raised to prevent aspiration; the patient may need to lie on the side to minimize the risk of aspiration

    ii. Skin care: Prevention of breakdown due to lower GI bleeding or decreased skin perfusion due to shock, keep clean and dry

   iii. Pain management: Gastric ulcer pain may be sharp or dull and may worsen with food consumption. Proton pump inhibitors and pain medication may reduce the discomfort as the ulcer heals. Aspirin and other NSAIDs should be avoided because they may worsen the condition. Pain management is individualized depending on comorbidities (encephalopathy, renal failure).

   iv. Nutrition: Patient will need to be on NPO status due to bleeding; depending on the duration and cause; the use of TPN or lower elemental enteral feedings may be necessary

    v. Infection control: Depressed immune system increases the risk of infection if surgery is performed; risk of aspiration is significant

   vi. Transport: A significant amount of the treatment can be done at the bedside, which will minimize the need for transport

  vii. Discharge planning: Recovery periods may be either short or prolonged, depending on the cause of the bleeding and comorbidities; this may be a new diagnosis requiring increased patient and family education

 viii. Pharmacology: Patients will be taking few medications unless infection ensues. Most medications will be related to treatment of the primary cause of the bleeding and prevention of complications. If shock is prolonged, dosing will need to be altered for liver or kidney dysfunction.

   ix. Psychosocial issues: Acute nature of the situation will have a profound impact on the family unit and increase stress

    x. Treatments

      (a) Noninvasive: Medications

      (b) Invasive: Surgery, variceal ligation or cautery via endoscopy, cautery via colonoscopy, embolization via angiography

   xi. Ethical issues: Blood replacement (against some religious views), advance directives

b. Potential complications

    i. Hypovolemia

      (a) Mechanism: Can occur as a result of massive third-spacing of fluids or hemorrhage

      (b) Management

        (1) Third-spacing: Rapid replacement of fluids

        (2) Hemorrhaging: Administration of blood products, use of a Minnesota tube

        (3) Either third-spacing or hemorrhaging: Use of vasoactive medications; accurate and rapid recording of intake and output

        (4) GI surgery for gastric ulcers or refractory variceal bleeding

    ii. Aspiration

      (a) Mechanism: Vomiting of blood or GI contents, hypotension, or encephalopathy prevents the ability to protect the airway and can result in aspiration, which may lead to bacterial pneumonia

      (b) Management: See Chapter 2

   iii. MODS

      (a) Mechanism: Severe hypotension, reduced oxygen delivery, hypoxia

      (b) Management: See Chapter 9

   iv. ARDS, respiratory failure

      (a) Mechanism: VQ mismatch, acidosis, increased ventilatory pressures, aspiration

      (b) Management: See Chapter 2

   v. Acute renal tubular necrosis, acute renal failure
   - (a) Mechanism: Prolonged hypotension, use of vasoactive medications or nephrotoxic antibiotics
   - (b) Management: See Chapter 5
8. **Evaluation of patient care**
   a. Normalization of GI functions, neurologic function, vital signs, and renal function
   b. Cessation or control of GI bleeding

Carcinoma of the Gastrointestinal Tract

1. **Pathophysiology**
   a. Esophageal carcinoma: About 15% of esophageal cancers occur in the upper third of the esophagus, 40% are in the middle third, and 45% are in the lower third
   b. Gastric neoplasms
      i. Second most common cancer in the world
      ii. Most common type of neoplasm is primary carcinoma beginning in the mucosal glands
      iii. Malignant neoplasms: 85% of stomach cancers are adenocarcinomas; 15% are lymphomas or leiomyosarcomas
      iv. Gastric adenocarcinomas may be either diffuse or tubular
   c. Neoplasms of the colon and rectum
      i. Most are due to malignant conversion of an adenomatous (polyp) lesion and take years to develop
      ii. Most tumors are adenocarcinomas (most common) or adenomas
      iii. Slightly more than half are found in the descending or distal colon; one fourth are in the cecum and ascending colon
2. **Etiology and risk factors**
   a. Squamous cell esophageal cancer
      i. Most common type of esophageal cancer with multifactorial etiology
      ii. Incidence increases over age 40 years
      iii. Precipitating factors
         - (a) Excess alcohol consumption, cigarette smoking, opiate smoking
         - (b) Ingestion of nitrites, lye
         - (c) Consumption of dry rations or rough foods without adequate fluid intake
         - (d) Barrett's esophagus
         - (e) Insufficient intake of vitamins A, C, E, B_{12}, riboflavin, folic acid
         - (f) Gastroesophageal reflux: Persistent heartburn and acid regurgitation. Some people have gastroesophageal reflux disease without heartburn. Instead, they experience pain in the chest, hoarseness in the morning, or trouble swallowing.
   b. Gastric cancer
      i. Adenocarcinomas account for 95% of gastric cancers
      ii. Affects mostly white males over 50 years of age and persons of lower socioeconomic status
   c. Colorectal cancer: Risk factors
      i. Alcohol use, acromegaly
      ii. Colorectal polyps, metastatic neoplasm in other organ(s)
      iii. Irradiation for gynecologic cancers
      iv. Diet high in animal fat, low in fiber, low in selenium
      v. Pernicious anemia

    d. Neoplasms of the liver

        i. Primary liver cancer is the most common type of liver cancer. It is rare in the United States and more prevalent in the Pacific Rim and Africa.

        ii. Incidence increases with age; most cases occur in individuals 50 to 70 years of age; a male predominance is seen

        iii. Most neoplasms originate in the parenchymal cells; sarcomas and angiosarcomas form in connective tissue

        iv. Hemangioendotheliomas are tumors of blood vessels in the liver

        v. Commonly associated with cirrhosis, especially when of viral origin

    e. Neoplasms of the hepatobiliary tract

    f. Adenocarcinoma of the extrahepatic ducts: Seen predominantly in 50- to 70-year-old men

3. Signs and symptoms

    a. Esophageal cancer

        i. Progressive dysphagia, odynophagia, weight loss over a short time

        ii. Anorexia, regurgitation or vomiting, aspiration pneumonia

        iii. Pain radiating to the chest and/or back

        iv. Cough, hoarseness

    b. Gastric cancer

        i. Heartburn, epigastric pain, and odorous breath

        ii. Belching, bloating, early satiety, postprandial fullness

        iii. Dysphagia, dyspepsia, vomiting, weight loss

        iv. Blood in the stool, frank bleeding, pernicious anemia

    c. Colorectal cancer

        i. Left colon: Abdominal distention, pain, vomiting, constipation, cramps, bright red blood in the stool

        ii. Right colon: Pain, palpable mass in the right lower quadrant, anemia, brick-red blood in the stool

        iii. Proximal colon: Iron deficiency

        iv. Sigmoid colon: Hematochezia

        v. Rectum: Bright red blood coating the stool

        vi. Change in bowel habits: Constipation, diarrhea, smaller-diameter stools

    d. Liver cancer

        i. Hepatomegaly, splenomegaly, ascites, abdominal pain

        ii. Jaundice, fever, weight loss

    e. Hepatobiliary cancer

        i. Hepatomegaly, biliary obstruction, painless jaundice, pruritus, white stools

        ii. Weight loss

        iii. Vague localized pain in the right upper quadrant

4. Diagnostic study findings

    a. Laboratory

        i. Elevated levels of carcinoembryonic antigen, α-fetoprotein, and CA 19-9

        ii. Decreased hemoglobin and glucose levels

        iii. Increased red cell mass, alkaline phosphatase level, serum calcium level

        iv. Positive result on stool guaiac test

    b. Radiographic

        i. Upper GI studies reveal "linitis plastica" (leather bottle stomach) with gastric neoplasms

        ii. Barium swallow testing, ultrasonography, bone scan, chest CT or MRI, abdominal CT or MRI

    c. Esophagogastroduodenoscopy, sigmoidoscopy, or colonoscopy: Biopsy specimen obtained during procedure tests shows carcinoma; used for staging and classification

    d. Digital rectal examination: Yields positive findings for blood

5. Goals of care

    a. Immediately recognize and treat GI bleeding

    b. Reverse anemia with administration of blood products or recombinant erythropoietin

    c. Prevent malnutrition through nutritional support

    d. Minimize GI distress and the side effects of treatments (nausea, vomiting, diarrhea)

    e. Control pain

    f. Provide emotional and psychosocial support to the patient and family

6. Collaborating professionals on health care team: Physician, nurse, dietitian, laboratory technician, consultant (gastroenterologist, surgeon, oncologist, pain specialist)

7. Management of patient care

    a. Anticipated patient trajectory: Once the diagnosis is made, stabilization is dependent on treatment options. Patients may be expected to have needs in the following areas:

        i. Positioning: Head of the bed raised to minimize reflux

        ii. Skin care: Prevention of breakdown due to treatment, nutritional deficits, diarrhea, weight loss

        iii. Pain management: Pain management is individualized depending on the symptoms, the cause of the disease, and treatment options; use of a pain management team is optimal

        iv. Nutrition: Patient's nutritional needs depend on the location of the cancer and the treatment. Nutritional counseling assists in maintaining weight and optimizing wound healing. Supplements, enteral feedings, TPN may all be employed.

        v. Infection control: Depressed immune system, loss of integrity of the GI system, and treatment options increase the risk of infection

        vi. Discharge planning: Recovery after surgical interventions is short; however, chemotherapy or radiation therapy may create the need for home health care. Frequent rehospitalization due to complications or progression of the disease. If a new diagnosis, increased patient and family education will be required. Palliative care and hospice care are the only options for some patients.

        vii. Pharmacology: Patient will be taking a complex regimen of medications; monitoring for food and drug interactions is needed

        viii. Psychosocial issues: Fears of pain and death, and financial and family impact need to be addressed

        ix. Ethical issues: Advance directives, palliative care

        x. Treatments

            (a) Medications, radiation, or chemotherapy

            (b) Surgery (single or recurrent): A variety of surgical options now exist for patients with carcinoma of the GI tract

                (1) Esophagogastrectomy

                    a) Indication: Esophageal cancer

                    b) Description

                        1) Removes the lower esophagus containing the cancer, the upper portion of the stomach at the gastroesophageal junction, and adjacent lymph nodes

                        2) Remaining portions of the esophagus and stomach are anastomosed to enable food to pass into stomach

                    c) Potential complications

      1) Anastomotic leak

      2) Paralyzed vocal cord

      3) Chylothorax

      4) Gastroparesis

(2) Gastrectomy: Subtotal or total with either duodenostomy (Billroth I) or Roux-en-Y (Billroth II)

  a) Indication: Gastric cancer

  b) Description

      1) Depending on the location of the cancer, either a total gastrectomy (entire stomach removed) or subtotal gastrectomy (distal esophagus and portion of the stomach removed) with resection of adjacent lymph nodes

      2) Remaining portions of the esophagus and stomach are anastomosed to a jejunal loop with a free duodenal limb

  c) Potential complications

      1) Anastomotic leak (more likely with paraaortic lymph node dissection [D4] than with conventional lymph node dissection [D2])

      2) Evisceration

      3) Hemorrhage

      4) Cardiac failure, dysrhythmias

      5) Infection—wound or respiratory

      6) Malnutrition; ileus

  b. Potential complications

    i. Hypovolemia (see prior coverage)

    ii. Malnutrition (see prior coverage)

    iii. Acute liver or renal failure (see prior coverage and Chapter 5)

8. Evaluation of patient care

  a. Optimization of GI function, vital signs, renal function

  b. Weight stabilization or weight gain

  c. Early identification and treatment of other system dysfunction (e.g., renal, hepatic)

Neoplasms of the Pancreas

Diagnosed in 29,000 patients annually in the United States. Pancreatic cancer is the fifth leading cause of cancer deaths among Americans.

1. Pathophysiology: Most pancreatic cancers begin in the pancreatic ducts. Ninety-five percent begin in the exocrine pancreas, five percent in the endocrine pancreas. Can metastasize to lymph nodes, liver, lungs, or peritoneum.

2. Etiology and risk factors

  a. Cigarette smoking: Heavy smokers are two to three times more likely to develop the disease

  b. African American race, male gender, age over 60 years

  c. Chronic pancreatitis, long-standing diabetes mellitus, obesity

  d. Genetic mutation of a gene on chromosome band 9p21k

3. Signs and symptoms

  a. Initial symptoms are often insidious and exist for months prior to diagnosis

  b. Jaundice

  c. Clay-colored stools due to the lack of conjugated bilirubin

  d. Dark, tea-colored urine due to increased excretion of bilirubin

  e. Weight loss

    f. Pain: Gnawing, visceral type radiating at times from the epigastric area to the back. Usually improves by bending or sitting forward.

4. Diagnostic study findings

    a. Laboratory: Elevated liver enzyme, amylase, lipase levels; decreased hemoglobin level

    b. Radiologic

        i. CT and MRI: Show alteration, thickening of pancreatic tissues

        ii. Ultrasonography: Pancreatic mass

5. Goals of care

    a. Optimize nutritional status

    b. Provide systemic or local pain control

    c. Manage side effects of treatment (e.g., nausea, mouth sores)

    d. Provide assistance for the patient and family in dealing with the prognosis, since all treatment for this cancer is palliative, not curative

6. Collaborating professionals on health care team: Physician, nurse, clergy, dietitian, laboratory technician, consultant (GI specialist, surgeon, oncologist, pain management team)

7. Management of patient care

    a. Anticipated patient trajectory: After the diagnosis is made, patient treatment can be curative only when the cancer is found early (prior to metastasis). Treatment may involve surgery, chemotherapy, or radiation therapy, or if the patient and family prefer, palliative or hospice care, rather than aggressive treatment. Patients may be expected to have needs in the following areas:

        i. Positioning: For comfort

        ii. Skin care: Prevention of breakdown

        iii. Pain management: Very important because this pain can be excruciating; alterative therapies like acupuncture and massage may help

        iv. Nutrition: Consumption of chilled foods with little odor may help, as will avoidance of greasy or spicy foods, because these stimulate the release of pancreatic enzymes. High-calorie supplements or special recipes may be used. If caloric intake cannot be maintained, TPN or lower elemental enteral feedings may be used.

        v. Infection control: Depressed immune system increases the risk of infection

        vi. Discharge planning: Home care, palliative care, or hospice care depending on the needs and wishes of the patient and family

        vii. Pharmacology: Patient may be on a complex chemotherapy regimen and other medications for pain control, nausea, diarrhea, and GI motility. Vigilance needed for drug-drug or drug-food interactions.

        viii. Psychosocial issues: Acute nature of the situation will have a profound impact on the family unit and increases stress. Crisis intervention and planning will be needed.

        ix. Ethical issues: Advance directives, nature and extent of care desired, code status

        x. Treatments: Surgery—pancreaticoduodenectomy (Whipple's procedure)

            (a) Indications: Pancreatic cancer

            (b) Description: Antrum of the stomach (spared in some cases), the head of the pancreas, a portion of the duodenum, blood vessels, and lymph nodes are removed

            (c) Potential complications

                (1) Pancreatic fistula

                (2) Intraabdominal abscess

                (3) Delayed gastric emptying

   b. Potential complications

   i. Hypovolemia (see prior coverage and Chapter 3)
  ii. Malnutrition (see prior coverage)
  iii. Acute liver or renal dysfunction (see prior coverage and Chapter 5)
8. Evaluation of patient care
 a. Optimization of weight, weight gain
 b. Allowance for the grieving process and patient-family closure
 c. Control of pain

Hepatitis

1. Pathophysiology: Acute inflammation of the entire liver, characterized on biopsy specimens by centrilobular necrosis and infiltration of the portal tracts by leukocytes. May be a multisystem infection involving many organs: Regional lymphadenopathy, splenomegaly, ulceration of the GI tract, acute pancreatitis, myocarditis, serum sickness, vasculitis, and nephritis.

2. Etiology and risk factors
 a. Causes may be viral, drug related, or autoimmune
 b. Less acute forms can produce subacute hepatic necrosis or cholestatic liver disease, or can silently progress to cirrhosis
 c. Multiple viruses cause hepatitis in humans
   i. Hepatitis A virus infection (formerly called infectious hepatitis)
   (a) RNA virus infection that occurs sporadically or endemically
   (b) Fecal-oral transmission; can also be transmitted by ingestion of raw or undercooked shellfish contaminated by sewage dumped into the ocean
   (c) Usually self-limiting
  ii. Hepatitis B virus infection (formerly called serum hepatitis)
   (a) In infected individuals, DNA virus is present in all body secretions
   (b) Transmission
    (1) Mother-to-neonate vertical transmission
    (2) Homosexual and heterosexual transmission
    (3) Parenteral transmission (intravenous drug abuse, transfusion of blood or blood products, hemodialysis, exposure to contaminated equipment, body piercings, razors)
   (c) Associated with hepatitis delta virus (hepatitis D virus, an RNA virus), a small RNA particle that is unable to replicate on its own but is capable of infection when in the presence of hepatitis B virus (hepatitis B surface antigen needed)
  iii. Hepatitis C virus infection (formerly called non-A, non-B hepatitis)
   (a) RNA virus
   (b) Transmission
    (1) Parenteral transmission (intravenous drug abuse, nasal cocaine use, transfusion of blood or blood products, hemodialysis, body piercings, razors, toothbrush sharing, acupuncture, health care exposure)
    (2) Sexual and maternal: Low frequency of transmission to neonate (5% to 12% risk of vertical transmission)
    (3) Accounts for more than 90% of posttransfusion hepatitis
  iv. Hepatitis D virus infection
   (a) Single-stranded RNA virus
   (b) Worldwide distribution
   (c) Requires presence of hepatitis B virus to establish infection
   (d) Transmitted parenterally and as a coinfection with hepatitis B; may lead to fulminant hepatitis
   v. Hepatitis E virus infection
   (a) RNA virus

  (b) Epidemiology and clinical course similar to those of hepatitis A
  (c) Most prevalent among young adults
  vi. All viruses in the herpesvirus family (herpes simplex, cytomegalovirus, Epstein-Barr virus, varicella-zoster virus)
d. Autoimmune hepatitis
  i. Idiopathic hepatitis characterized by chronic inflammation and plasma cells in liver tissue, autoantibodies, and increased serum globulin levels
  ii. Predominance in women aged 30 to 45 years
  iii. Associated with four antibodies: ANA, anti–smooth muscle antibodies (ASMA), ANCA, anti-LKM
e. Drug-related hepatitis
  i. Form of drug allergy in which the immune response is directed toward the liver cells, causing necrosis that affects a particular region of the liver lobule (e.g., acetaminophen causes centrilobular necrosis)
  ii. Severe reaction produces diffuse necrosis and/or cholestasis
  iii. Prognosis is variable
f. Categories (or types) of hepatitis
  i. Acute hepatitis: Acute onset of inflammation, usually self-limiting
  ii. Acute fulminant hepatitis
  iii. Asymptomatic carrier state (viral hepatitis)
    (a) Infected person is unable to clear hepatitis antigen because of ineffective cellular immunity
    (b) Carrier is able to transmit hepatitis to others but suffers no liver damage
  iv. Chronic hepatitis
    (a) Hepatitis antigen, chronic liver inflammation, and viral replication persist for at least 6 months
    (b) Progressive liver damage may develop into cirrhosis

3. **Signs and symptoms**
a. Anicteric (not jaundiced) cases: Usually asymptomatic except for flulike symptoms; occasionally hepatomegaly, splenomegaly, and lymphadenopathy may occur
b. Icteric cases (small proportion of cases)
  i. Prodromal period associated with not feeling well: Malaise, fatigue
  ii. Symptoms subside with the onset of jaundice
  iii. Among smokers and drinkers, loss of the desire to smoke or drink
  iv. Dark urine, followed by lightening of the urine
  v. Fever, nausea, vomiting, diarrhea
  vi. Hepatomegaly, splenomegaly

4. **Diagnostic study findings**
a. Laboratory
  i. Increased WBC count, serum total bilirubin level
  ii. Increased levels of ALT, AST, and, to a lesser degree, alkaline phosphatase and GGT
  iii. Positive results on hepatitis serologic testing (Table 8-2)
  iv. Presence of autoimmune markers: ANA, ASMA, ANCA, anti-LKM
b. Radiologic: Ultrasonography may show hepatomegaly or splenomegaly, or give normal results

5. **Goals of care**
a. Minimize symptoms
b. Optimize liver function and functional status
c. Restore physical and mental energy

TABLE 8-2
Serologic Testing for Viral Hepatitis

Serologic Test	Description and Purpose
HEPATITIS A VIRUS (HAV)	
HAV total antibody	Presence in serum confers lifelong immunity
HAV IgM	Level rises early during infection (detectable at 3-4 wk after exposure and just before liver test values become elevated); indicates acute infection; returns to normal in approximately 8 wk
HAV IgG	Level rises slowly during infection (detectable at 6-12 wk after exposure and persists for more than 10 yr after infection)
HEPATITIS B VIRUS (HBV)	
HBsAg	HBV *surface* antigen; most commonly used marker for HBV infection; detectable within 30 days of exposure and persists up to 3 mo after jaundice appears unless a carrier state develops, in which case it will persist longer; presence in serum (seropositivity) indicates active HBV infection
Anti-HBs	Antibody to HBsAg; presence in serum (seropositivity) indicates HBV immunity due to HBV infection or vaccination; detectable 4-12 wk after HBsAg disappears
HBeAg	HBV *e* antigen; found only in sera positive for HBsAg; presence in serum (seropositivity) indicates high titer of HBV (extensive viral replication) and increased infectiousness (ongoing viral replication); detectable 4-6 wk after exposure; persistence of this marker in blood predicts development of chronic HBV infection
HBcAg	HBV *core* antigen; not detectable in serum, detectable only in hepatocytes
Anti-HBc (total)	Antibody to HBcAg; detectable 3-12 wk after exposure during what is referred to as the "window phase" (after HBsAg disappears but before antibody to HBsAg appears)
HBV DNA	HBV DNA detected by process of nucleic acid hybridization
PCR for HBV DNA	Test detects polymerase-containing virions; PCR process amplifies DNA in blood so that it is easily detected; very sensitive test
HEPATITIS C VIRUS (HCV)	
HCVAb	Antibody to HCV; presence in serum (seropositivity) is diagnostic for chronic infection only; absence (seronegativity) does not exclude the diagnosis of HCV infection; false-positive results may occur
HCV RNA	HCV RNA detected by process of nucleic acid hybridization; presence in serum is diagnostic of viremia in acute or chronic HCV hepatitis; test also used to monitor response to interferon-α therapy
HCV genotype	Test identifies six different genotypes and several subtypes of the virus; used to determine appropriate treatment options and durations
PCR for HCV RNA	Detects polymerase-containing virions; PCR process amplifies RNA in blood so that it is easily detected; very sensitive test
bDNA	Quantitative test of HCV RNA for determining amount of virus; research assay not yet licensed by the Food and Drug Administration

Continued

TABLE 8-2
Serologic Testing for Viral Hepatitis—cont'd

Serologic Test	Description and Purpose
HEPATITIS D VIRUS (HDV; HEPATITIS DELTA VIRUS)	
HDAg (total)	HDV antigen; detectable only concurrently with HBV infection
HDV IgM	Level rises early in infection; if persistent, may indicate chronic infection
HDV IgG	Level rises slowly during infection; persists for life
HDVAb	Antibody to HDV; detectable only concurrently with HBV infection
HDV RNA	Detected by process of nucleic acid hybridization
HEPATITIS E VIRUS (HEV)	
PCR for HEV RNA	Detects polymerase-containing virions; PCR process amplifies RNA in blood so that it is easily detected; very sensitive test

From Pagana KD, Pagana TM: *Mosby's manual of diagnostic and laboratory tests*, ed 2, St Louis, 2002, Mosby.
IgG, Immunoglobulin G; *IgM*, immunoglobulin M; *PCR*, polymerase chain reaction test.

6. **Collaborating professionals on health care team**: Physician, nurse, dietitian, laboratory technician, consultant (hepatologist)
7. **Management of patient care**
   a. Anticipated patient trajectory: Can be a slow recovery with symptomatic irritations; however, some will progress to fulminant liver failure or cirrhosis. Patients may be expected to have needs in the following areas:
      i. Skin care: Prevention of breakdown due to pruritus caused by deposition of bile salts, dryness, itching
      ii. Pain management: Avoid acetaminophen as well as aspirin and other NSAIDs in severe cases of hepatitis
      iii. Nutrition: If disease is severe, nutritional supplements may be required
      iv. Discharge planning: Recovery periods occur after prolonged illness without relapse. If the disease is fulminant, the hospital course may vary from long hospitalization to liver transplantation.
      v. Pharmacology: Caution required with medications because of decreased liver function and possible renal impairment
      vi. Psychosocial issues: In the acute or chronic state, the psychosocial issues may involve body image and intimacy issues (fear of transmission); however, the acute nature of fulminant hepatitis will have a profound impact on the family unit and increase stress. If this is a new condition, there may be significant educational needs and complex treatment decisions.
      vii. Treatments: Medications, transplantation
      viii. Ethical issues: Social stigma related to disease etiology
   b. Potential complications
      i. Cirrhosis (see Chronic Liver Failure)
      ii. Ascites (see Chronic Liver Failure)
      iii. Encephalopathy (see prior coverage and Chapter 4)
      iv. Increased ICP (see Chapter 4)
      v. Liver failure (see Acute [Fulminant] Liver Failure)
      vi. Infection or sepsis (see Chapter 9)
      vii. Renal failure (see Chapter 4)
      viii. Liver cancer (see prior coverage)
      ix. Malnutrition (see prior coverage)
8. **Evaluation of patient care**
   a. Normalization of liver function, neurologic function, vital signs, renal function
   b. Increased mental and physical energy

Abdominal Trauma

1. **Pathophysiology**
   a. Liver is the most commonly injured organ in the body regardless of the cause of the trauma
   b. Injuries occurring from the nipple line to the midthigh are considered abdominal trauma and often involve injury to multiple organs
2. **Etiology and risk factors**
   a. Penetrating abdominal trauma
      i. Knife (stab) wounds; injury with a sharp metal or wooden objects; impalement on a sharp object
      ii. Gunshot wounds: Visceral injury possible, even when the bullet does not penetrate the abdomen; caused by blast effect; caliber of bullet important
   b. Blunt abdominal trauma
      i. Moving vehicular crashes: Most common cause; failure to wear a seatbelt, seatbelt-related injuries, steering wheel–related injuries

    ii. Acceleration-deceleration injuries in passengers and pedestrians, ejection from a vehicle, falls

    iii. Physical violence: Punch, kick, use of a blunt object, rape, sports injury, crush injury

3. Signs and symptoms

  a. Pallor, orthostatic hypotension, decreased pulse pressure, abdominal bruit, diminished or absent femoral pulses

  b. Respiratory difficulty, diminished or absent breath sounds

  c. Increased abdominal girth, entrance and exit wounds, impalement by foreign object

  d. Abdominal tenderness, pain with guarding, rebound tenderness

  e. Dullness on percussion suggests fluid in the abdomen; hyperresonance indicates a perforated viscus

  f. Marbled appearance of the abdomen

  g. Cullen's sign: Bluish discoloration of the periumbilical area

  h. Turner's sign: Bluish discoloration of the flanks

  i. Coopernail's sign: Bruising of the scrotum or labia

  j. Peritoneal lavage: Reveals blood ("beef broth" tap), urine, bile, or feces in the peritoneal cavity

4. Diagnostic study findings

  a. Laboratory

    i. Decreased hemoglobin level, hematocrit

    ii. Increased serum amylase level

    iii. Increased WBC count

    iv. Hematuria

    v. Stool guaiac test result positive for occult blood

  b. Radiologic

    i. Abdominal radiograph: Loss of psoas shadow indicating retroperitoneal bleeding, free air in the abdomen, location of a bullet

    ii. Chest radiograph: Fractured ribs

    iii. Arteriogram: May show vascular injuries

    iv. Liver and spleen scan

    v. Intravenous pyelogram if blood in urine

    vi. Abdominal or pelvic CT scan: Hematoperitoneum, retroperitoneal hematoma, liver or spleen fracture, ruptured viscus

5. Goals of care

  a. Minimize blood loss

  b. Optimize hemodynamic status

  c. Prevent infection

  d. Stabilize concomitant injuries

6. Collaborating professionals on health care team: Physician, nurse, dietitian, laboratory technician, physical therapist, respiratory therapy, radiologist, consultant (gastroenterologist, surgeon, hematologist)

7. Management of patient care

  a. Anticipated patient trajectory: Once bleeding or perforation is resolved, rapid stabilization is possible. If it is difficult to halt the hemorrhage or if there was significant spillage of gastric contents, more complications may ensue and patient course is more problematic. Patients may be expected to have needs in the following areas:

    i. Positioning: Head of the bed raised to prevent aspiration and optimize ventilation and pain reduction

      ii. Skin care: Prevention of breakdown caused by decreased skin perfusion due to shock, multiple incisions, GI drainage; keep clean and dry

     iii. Pain management: Pain management must be individualized

     iv. Nutrition: Patient will need to be on NPO status if surgery is considered or performed; TPN or lower elemental enteral feedings may be needed

      v. Infection control: Risk of peritonitis or sepsis is significant

     vi. Transport: Significant amount of transport can occur with increased risk to the client in the form of infection, tube or catheter dislodgement

    vii. Discharge planning: Recovery may be short or prolonged, depending on the nature and extent of injuries and the development of complications

   viii. Pharmacology: Patient will be taking a variety of medications depending on the injuries incurred

     ix. Psychosocial issues: There will be a profound impact on the family unit and increased stress because of the sudden and unanticipated nature of the trauma. In severe cases, there may be body image issues as well as grieving over loss of function. Significant educational deficits and lifestyle changes may need to be addressed depending on the outcome of the injuries and rehabilitation needs.

      x. Ethical issues: Blood replacement (against some religious views), advance directives

  b. Potential complications

      i. Hypovolemia (see prior coverage)

     ii. Infection or sepsis (see prior coverage and Chapter 9)

    iii. Malnutrition (see prior coverage)

    iv. MODS (see Chapter 9)

     v. ARDS, respiratory failure (see Chapter 2)

    vi. Acute renal tubular necrosis, acute renal failure (see Chapter 5)

8. Evaluation of patient care

  a. Normalization of body functions, neurologic function, vital signs

  b. Progression to rehabilitation

Inflammatory Bowel Disease

1. Pathophysiology

  a. Crohn's disease

      i. Chronic transmural inflammation of the digestive tract that can involve one or more areas of any portion of the GI tract from the mouth to the anus

     ii. Ileum, colon, perianal area most common sites of inflammation

    iii. Extraintestinal organs may be affected

    iv. Incurable condition associated with relapses and remissions

     v. Inflammation begins in the intestinal mucosa and spreads inward and outward to involve the mucosa and serosa. Bowel becomes congested, thickened, and rigid, with adhesions. Edema and thickening of the muscularis mucosae may narrow the lumen of the involved colon.

    vi. Fistulas, abscesses, and perforation may occur

  b. Ulcerative colitis

      i. Idiopathic inflammation involving the mucosa of the colon

     ii. Inflammation is continuous and circumferential; begins in the rectum and progresses proximally toward the cecum

    iii. Inflammation begins at the base of the crypts of Lieberkühn; small erosions form and coalesce into ulcers, followed by abscess formation, necrosis, and ragged ulcerations of the mucosa

2. **Etiology and risk factors**
   a. Crohn's disease
      i. Cigarette smoking, NSAID use
      ii. Exact etiology unknown; possible causes include bacterial, viral, allergic, autoimmune, and hereditary factors
      iii. Prevalence equal in men and women; most common age at onset is 10 to 30 years
      iv. Other concurrent autoimmune disorders common
      v. Familial predisposition
      vi. Increased suppressor T-cell activity and alterations in IgA production
   b. Ulcerative colitis
      i. Etiology unknown: Genetic, infectious, and immunologic factors suspected
      ii. Other concurrent autoimmune disorders common
      iii. Prevalence higher among women, especially those of Jewish descent; onset usually between 10 and 40 years of age
3. **Signs and symptoms**
   a. Crohn's disease
      i. Pain: Initially, a constant right-sided pain that mimics appendicitis; later, crampy abdominal pain most often associated with eating
      ii. Meals omitted to avoid pain; weight loss, malnutrition, cachexia
      iii. Nausea and vomiting, watery diarrhea, steatorrhea, anal excoriation or fistula
      iv. Arthralgias, malaise, fever
      v. Aphthous ulcers of the lips and mouth
      vi. Vitamin B_{12} deficiency (when the ileum is involved)
      vii. Metabolic bone disease
   b. Ulcerative colitis
      i. Sensation of rectal urgency
      ii. Crampy abdominal pain and tenderness, hypertympanic abdomen
      iii. Bloody, purulent, watery diarrhea: Up to 30 stools per day
      iv. Weight loss, cachexia, orthostasis
      v. Vomiting, dehydration, fever
      vi. Extracolonic manifestations such as anemia, arthritis, hepatic dysfunction
4. **Diagnostic study findings**
   a. Crohn's disease
      i. Laboratory
         (a) Decreased hemoglobin level, hematocrit, potassium level, serum albumin level
         (b) Increased WBC count, alkaline phosphatase level
         (c) Occult blood in stool
      ii. Radiologic: "String sign" (irregular narrowing of the distal ileum) on abdominal radiograph
      iii. Sigmoidoscopy: Inflammation of the intestinal mucosa and surrounding musculature, as well as longitudinal and transverse ulcers (cobblestoning) and stenosis of the intestinal lumen
      iv. Colonoscopy: To determine the extent of disease
      v. Rectal biopsy: Inflammation of the intestinal mucosa and surrounding musculature
   b. Ulcerative colitis
      i. Laboratory
         (a) Decreased hemoglobin level, hematocrit, potassium level, serum albumin level

(b) Increased WBC count, alkaline phosphatase level

(c) Occult blood in stool

    ii. Radiologic: Abdominal radiograph reveals crypt abscess, mucosal ulcerations, dilated loops of bowel

    iii. Proctosigmoidoscopy: Shows diffuse erythema, mucosal inflammation, loss of vascular network, mucosal bleeding

5. **Goals of care**

  a. Crohn's disease

    i. Optimize GI function

    ii. Restore and maintain nutritional status

    iii. Relieve symptoms

  b. Ulcerative colitis

    i. Minimize complications

    ii. Restore and maintain nutritional status

    iii. Optimize colon function

6. **Collaborating professionals on health care team**: Physician, nurse, dietitian, laboratory technician, consultant (gastroenterologist, surgeon)

7. **Management of patient care** (for both Crohn's disease and ulcerative colitis)

  a. Anticipated patient trajectory: These are chronic condition with exacerbations. Patients may be expected to have needs in the following areas:

    i. Positioning: Position of comfort; usually the head of the bed is raised

    ii. Skin care: Prevention of breakdown due to diarrhea; keep clean and dry

    iii. Pain management: Will be individualized; antidiarrheal agents and anticholinergics to ease cramping

    iv. Nutrition: Each patient will have variations in nutritional intake; high-fiber, low-sugar diet and adjustment for food allergies such milk or yeast allergies

    v. Infection control: Perforation or ulceration risk

    vi. Discharge planning: Chronicity of these conditions may result in frequent rehospitalizations for exacerbations

    vii. Pharmacology: Patients will be taking a variety of medications to control symptoms, such as antidiarrheal agents, anticholinergics, vitamin supplements

    viii. Psychosocial issues: Chronic nature of these diseases and their impact on the patient's social structure may lead to isolation and may significantly affect the family unit and increase stress

    ix. Ethical issues: Advance directives

  b. Potential complications

    i. Crohn's disease

      (a) Acute complications

        (1) Toxic megacolon (loss of contractility and massive dilatation of colon)

        (2) GI hemorrhage

        (3) Perforation of the ileum

        (4) Bowel obstruction

      (b) Chronic complications

        (1) Rheumatoid arthritis

        (2) Sclerosing cholangitis

        (3) Urinary calculi

        (4) Iron-deficiency anemia

    ii. Ulcerative colitis

      (a) Toxic megacolon: Associated with fulminant disease

      (b) Friable colon

(c) Increased risk of colon cancer

(d) SIRS and sepsis: Can develop if the colon perforates

   iii. Management

     (a) Crohn's disease

      (1) Monitor for infections or peritonitis

      (2) Check the stool for pus, blood

      (3) Keep an accurate record of intake and output to optimize nutritional status

      (4) Optimize bowel function; minimize episodes of diarrhea, abdominal pain

      (5) Administer medications as ordered

     (b) Ulcerative colitis

      (1) Monitor for exacerbation of symptoms

      (2) Keep accurate intake and output measurements

      (3) Monitor electrolyte, hemoglobin levels

      (4) Optimize nutritional status

      (5) Administer medications as ordered

8. Evaluation of patient care: Optimization of GI functions

REFERENCES

Physiologic Anatomy

Crissinger KD, Granger DN: Gastrointestinal blood flow. In Yamada T, editor: *Textbook of gastroenterology*, ed 3, vol 1, Philadelphia, 1999, Lippincott Williams & Wilkins.

Del Valle J, Todisco A: Gastric secretion. In Yamada T, editor: *Textbook of gastroenterology*, ed 3, vol 1, Philadelphia, 1999, Lippincott Williams & Wilkins.

Furness JB, Bornstein JC, Kunze WAA, et al: The enteric nervous system and its extrinsic connections. In Yamada T, editor: *Textbook of gastroenterology*, ed 3, vol 1, Philadelphia, 1999, Lippincott Williams & Wilkins.

Kikhorn MJ: Advances in treatment of gastrointestinal disorders. In Copstead LC, Banasik JL, editors: *Pathophysiology: biological and behavioral perspectives*, Philadelphia, 2000, Saunders.

Krumberger JM: Gastrointestinal clinical physiology. In Kinney MR, Dunbar S, Brooks-Brunn J, et al, editors: *AACN clinical reference for critical care nursing*, St Louis, 1998, Mosby.

Nauntofte B, Jensen JL: Salivary secretion. In Yamada T, editor: *Textbook of gastroenterology*, ed 3, vol 1, Philadelphia, 1999, Lippincott Williams & Wilkins.

Watkins PB: The barrier function of the gut. In Yamada T, editor: *Textbook of gastroenterology*, ed 3, vol 1, Philadelphia, 1999, Lippincott Williams & Wilkins.

Patient Assessment

DeGowin RL, Brown DD, Christensen J: *DeGowin and DeGowin's diagnostic examination*, ed 6, New York, 1994, McGraw-Hill.

Estes ME: *Health assessment and physical examination*, ed 2, Albany, NY, 2002, Delmar/Thomson Learning.

Acute Abdomen

Chan FK, Leung WK: Peptic ulcer disease, *Lancet* 360:933–942, 2002.

Johnson LR: Secretion. In Johnson LR, editor: *Essential medical physiology*, ed 3, Amsterdam, 2003, Elsevier Academic Press.

Krumberger JM, Hammer B: Gastrointestinal disorders. In Kinney MR, Dunbar SB, Brooks-Brunn J, et al, editors: *AACN clinical reference for critical-care nursing*, St Louis, 1998, Mosby.

Levenson D, Fromm H: Medical management of gallbladder disease. In Zakim D, Boyer TD, editors: *Hepatology: a textbook of liver disease*, ed 3, vol II, Philadelphia, 1996, Saunders.

Acute (Fulminant) Liver Failure

Ferenci P, Lockwood A, Mullen K, et al: Hepatic encephalopathy—definition, nomenclature, diagnosis, and quantification: final report of the working party at the 11th World Congresses of Gastroenterology, Vienna 1998, *Hepatology* 35:716–721, 2002.

Hayes PC, Simpson KJ: Approach to the patient with fulminant (acute) liver failure. In Yamada T, editor: *Textbook of gastroenterology*, ed 4, vol 2, Philadelphia, 2003, Lippincott Williams & Wilkins.

Krige JE, Bechingham IJ: Portal hypertension—2. Ascites, encephalopathy, and other conditions, *BMJ* 322:416–419, 2001.

Krumberger JM, Hammer B: Gastrointestinal disorders. In Kinney MR, Dunbar SB, Brooks-Brunn J, et al, editors: *AACN clinical reference for critical-care nursing*, St Louis, 1998, Mosby.

Levenson D, Fromm H: Medical management of gallbladder disease. In Zakim D, Boyer TD, editors: *Hepatology: a textbook of liver disease*, ed 3, vol II, Philadelphia, 1996, Saunders.

Luketic VA: Management of portal hypertension after variceal hemorrhage. In Sanyal AJ, editor: *Clinics in liver disease*, Philadelphia, 2001, Saunders.

Radovich PA: Portal vein thrombosis and liver disease, *J Vasc Nurs* 18:1–5, 2000.

Radovich PA: Use of transjugular intrahepatic portosystemic shunt in liver disease, *J Vasc Nurs* 18:83–87, 2000.

Riley TR, Bhatti AM: Preventive strategies in chronic liver disease. Part II: cirrhosis, *Am Fam Physician* 64:1735–1741, 2001.

Riodan SM, Williams R: Treatment of hepatic encephalopathy, *J Hepatol* 337:473–479, 1997.

Chronic Liver Failure: Decompensated Cirrhosis

Butterworth RF: Complications of cirrhosis III: hepatic encephalopathy, *J Hepatol* 32:171–180, 2000.

Clark JM, Diehl AM: Nonalcoholic fatty liver disease: an underrecognized cause of cryptogenic cirrhosis, *JAMA* 289:3000, 2003.

Dove LM, Wright TL: Chronic viral hepatitis. In Friedman LS, Keefe EB, editors: *Handbook of liver disease*, Philadelphia, 2002, Elsevier Science.

Ferenci P, Lockwood A, Mullen K, et al: Hepatic encephalopathy—definition, nomenclature, diagnosis, and quantification: final report of the working party at the 11th World Congresses of Gastroenterology, Vienna 1998, *Hepatology* 35:716–721, 2002.

Habib A, Bond WM, Heuman DM: Long-term management of cirrhosis: appropriate supportive care is both critical and difficult, *Postgrad Med* 109:101–108, 2001.

Radovich PA: Portal vein thrombosis and liver disease, *J Vasc Nurs* 18:1–5, 2000.

Radovich PA: Use of transjugular intrahepatic portosystemic shunt in liver disease, *J Vasc Nurs* 18:83–87, 2000.

Riley TR, Bhatti AM: Preventive strategies in chronic liver disease. Part II: cirrhosis, *Am Fam Physician* 64:1735–1741, 2001.

Riodan SM, Williams, R: Treatment of hepatic encephalopathy, *J Hepatol* 337:473–479, 1997.

Acute Pancreatitis

Hennessy K: Patients with acute pancreatitis. In Clochesy JM, Breau C, Cardin S, et al, editors: *Critical care nursing*, ed 2, Philadelphia, 1996, Saunders.

Indar AA, Beckingham IJ: Acute cholecystitis, *BMJ* 325:639–644, 2002.

Johnson LR: Secretion. In Johnson LR, editor: *Essential medical physiology*, ed 3, Amsterdam, 2003, Elsevier Academic Press.

Kelly D, Skidmore S: Hepatitis C-Z: recent advances, *Arch Dis Child* 86:339–344, 2002.

Owyang C: Chronic pancreatitis. In Yamada T, editor: *Textbook of gastroenterology*, ed 3, Philadelphia, 1999, Lippincott Williams & Wilkins.

Topazian M, Gorelick FS: Acute pancreatitis. In Yamada T, editor: *Textbook of gastroenterology*, ed 3, Philadelphia, 1999, Lippincott Williams & Wilkins.

Gastrointestinal Bleeding

Elta GH: Approach to the patient with gross gastrointestinal bleeding. In Yamada T, editor: *Textbook of gastroenterology*, ed 4, vol 2, Philadelphia, 2003, Lippincott Williams & Wilkins.

Escorsell A, Garcia-Pagan JC, Bosch J: Assessment of portal hypertension in humans. In Sanyal AJ, editor: *Clinics in liver disease*, Philadelphia, 2001, Saunders.

Farrell RJ, Mazen A, LaMont JT: Is successful triage of patients with upper-gastrointestinal bleeding possible without endoscopy? *Lancet* 356:1289–1290, 2000.

Krige JE, Beckingham IJ: Portal hypertension—2. Ascites, encephalopathy, and other conditions, *BMJ* 322:416–419, 2001.

Luketic VA: Management of portal hypertension after variceal hemorrhage. In Sanyal AJ, editor: *Clinics in liver disease*, Philadelphia, 2001, Saunders.

Molina E, Reddy KR: Noncirrhotic causes of portal hypertension. In Sanyal AJ, editor: *Clinics in liver disease*, Philadelphia, 2001, Saunders.

Simeone DM, Mulholland MW: Pancreas: anatomy and structural anomalies. In Yamada T, editor: *Textbook of gastroenterology*, ed 4, vol 2, Philadelphia, 2003, Lippincott Williams & Wilkins.

Zervos EE, Goode SE, Rosemurgy AS: Small-diameter H-graft portacaval shunt reduces portal flow yet maintains effective hepatic blood flow, *Am Surg* 64:7176, 1998.

Carcinoma of the Gastrointestinal Tract

Alexander GA: Association of *Helicobacter pylori* infection with gastric cancer, *Mil Med* 165:21–27, 2000.

Bonnin-Scaon S, Lafon P, Chasseigne G, et al: Learning the relationship between smoking, drinking alcohol and the risk of esophageal cancer, *Health Educ Res* 17:415–424, 2002.

Brooks-Brunn J: Esophageal cancer: an overview, *Medsurg Nurs* 9:248–255, 2000.

Demeter P, Visy KV, Gyulai N, et al: Severity of gastroesophageal reflux disease influences daytime somnolence: a clinical study of 134 patients who underwent upper panendoscopy, *World J Gastroenterol* 10:1798–1801, 2004.

Forman D, Goodman KJ: The epidemiology of stomach cancer: correlating the past with the present, *BMJ* 320:1682–1684, 2000.

Henteleff JJ, Darling G: GERD as a risk factor for esophageal cancer, *Can J Surg* 46:208–210, 2003.

Il-Serag HB, Peterson NJ, Carter J, et al: Gastroesophageal reflux among different racial groups in the United States, *Gastroenterology* 126:1692–1699, 2004.

Shaheen N, Ransohoff DF: Gastroesophageal reflux, Barrett esophagus, and esophageal cancer: scientific review, *JAMA* 287:1972–1981, 2002.

Shaheen N, Ransohoff DF: Gastroesophageal reflux, Barrett esophagus, and esophageal cancer: clinical applications, *JAMA* 287:1972–1981, 2002.

Todd KE, Gloor B, Rhber HA: Pancreatic adenocarcinoma. In Yamada T, editor: *Textbook of gastroenterology*, ed 3, Philadelphia, 1999, Lippincott Williams & Wilkins.

Gastrointestinal Surgery

Headrick JR, Nichols FC 3rd, Miller DL, et al: High-grade esophageal dysplasia: long-term survival and quality of life after esophagectomy, *Ann Thorac Surg* 73:1697–1702, 2002.

Isozaki H, Okajima K, Ichinona T, et al: Risk factors of esophagojejunal anastomotic leakage after total gastrectomy for gastric cancer, *Hepatogastroenterology* 44:1509–1512, 1997.

Mitsuru S, Hitoshi K, Takeshi S, et al: Management of complications after gastrectomy with extended lymphadenectomy, *Surg Oncol* 9:31–34, 2000.

Nemes R, Curca T, Paraliov T, et al: The esophagogastric junction cancer: diagnosis and surgical treatment challenges, *Rom J Gastroenterol* 12:193–197, 2003.

Newbury L, Dolan K, Hatzifotis M, et al: Calcium and vitamin D depletion and elevated parathyroid hormone following biliopancreatic diversion, *Obes Surg* 13:893–895, 2003.

Rizl NP, Bach PB, Schrag D, et al: The impact of complications on outcomes after resection for esophageal and gastroesophageal junction carcinoma, *J Am Coll Surg* 198:42–50, 2004.

Roviello F, Marrelli D, De Stefano A, et al: Complications after surgery for gastric cancer in patients aged 80 years and over, *Jpn J Clin Oncol* 28:116–122, 1998.

Spector NM, Hicks FD, Pickleman J: Quality of life and symptoms after surgery for gastroesophageal cancer: a pilot study, *Gastroenterol Nurs* 25:120–125, 2002.

Velanovich V: Esophagogastrectomy without pyloroplasty, *Dis Esophagus* 16:243–245, 2003.

Woodward BG: Bariatric surgery options, *Crit Care Nurs Q* 26:89–100, 2003.

Yu J, Turner MA, Cho SR, et al: Normal anatomy and complications after gastric bypass surgery: helical CT findings, *Radiology* 231:753–760, 2004.

Hepatitis

Czaja AJ: Autoimmune hepatitis. In Friedman LS, Keefe EB, editors: *Handbook of liver disease*, Philadelphia, 2002, Elsevier Science.

Dove LM, Wright TL: Chronic viral hepatitis. In Friedman LS, Keefe EB, editors: *Handbook of liver disease*, Philadelphia, 2002, Elsevier Science.

Smith SL: Patients with liver dysfunction. In Clochesy JM, Breau C, Cardin S, et al, editors: *Critical care nursing*, ed 2, Philadelphia, 1996, Saunders.

Abdominal Trauma

Border JR, editor: *Blunt multiple trauma: comprehensive pathophysiology and care*. New York, 1990, Marcel Dekker.

Greenfield LJ, editor: *Complications in surgery and trauma*, ed 2, Philadelphia, 1990, Lippincott.

Johnson LR: Secretion. In Johnson LR, editor: *Essential medical physiology*, ed 3, Amsterdam, 2003, Elsevier Academic Press.

Metheny N: Achieving successful nasogastric tube placements in emergency situations, *Am J Crit Care*, 9(5):303–304, 306, 2000.

Metheny NA, Steward BJ, Smith L, et al: pH and concentrations of pepsin and trypsin in feeding tube aspirates as predictors of tube placement, *JPEN J Parenter Enteral Nutr* 21:279–286, 1997.

Scaletta TA, Schaider JJ: *Emergent management of trauma*, Boston, 2001, McGraw-Hill.

Urden LD, Stacy KM, Lough ME, editors: Thelan's critical care nursing: diagnosis and management, St Louis, 2002, Mosby.

Inflammatory Bowel Disease

Somers SC, Lembo A: Irritable bowel syndrome: evaluation and treatment. *Gastroenterol Clin* 32:507–529, 2003.

Stenson WF: Inflammatory bowel disease. In Yamada T, editor: *Textbook of gastroenterology*, ed 3, Philadelphia, 1999, Lippincott Williams & Wilkins.

Multisystem

MARILYN SAWYER SOMMERS, RN, PhD, FAAN
PAMELA J. BOLTON, RN, MS, ACNP, CCNS, CCRN, PCCN

Systemic Inflammatory Response Syndrome and Septic Shock

SYSTEMWIDE ELEMENTS

Physiologic Anatomy

1. **Definitions**[*]
   a. *Systemic inflammatory response syndrome (SIRS)*: Systemic inflammatory response to a variety of severe clinical insults (such as pancreatitis, ischemia or reperfusion, multiple trauma and tissue injury, hemorrhagic shock, and immune-mediated organ injury) in the absence of infection (Figure 9-1). Response is manifested by two or more of the following conditions:
      i. Temperature above 100.4° F (38° C) or below 96.8° F (36° C)
      ii. Heart rate above 90 beats/min
      iii. Respiratory rate above 20 breaths/min or arterial partial pressure of carbon dioxide ($Paco_2$) below 32 mm Hg
      iv. White blood cell (WBC) count above 12,000/mm³ or below 4000/mm³, or more than 10% immature (band) forms
   b. *Infection*: Microbial phenomenon characterized by an inflammatory response to the presence of microorganisms or the invasion of normally sterile host tissue by organisms
   c. *Bacteremia*: Presence of viable bacteria in the blood
   d. *Sepsis*: Bacterial infection of the blood
      i. In 2002, the PIRO model was developed as a tool to diagnose and track the progression of sepsis
         (a) *P*: Predisposition for individual patients to respond to infection in different ways
         (b) *I*: Infection
         (c) *R*: Response to inflammation
         (d) *O*: Organ dysfunction
      ii. Sepsis may be a complication following burns, surgery, or illness
      iii. Sepsis is associated with a generalized inflammatory response that often leads to abnormal clotting and bleeding in the presence of infection

---

[*]Accepted definitions by Bone, Balk, Cerra, and colleagues (1992) with modifications made by the Society of Critical Care Medicine in 2002.

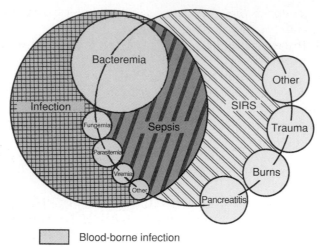

Blood-borne infection

FIGURE 9-1 ■ Interrelationship between systemic inflammatory response syndrome (SIRS), sepsis, and infection. (From Bone RC, Balk RA, Cerra FB, et al: Definitions for sepsis and organ failure and guidelines for the use of innovative therapies in sepsis, *Chest* 101:1645, 1992.)

      iv. This condition is manifested by the presence of two or more of the four conditions that define SIRS (see earlier)
  e. *Severe sepsis*: Sepsis associated with organ dysfunction. Associated signs and symptoms include chills, tachypnea, unexplained alterations in mental status, tachycardia, altered WBC count, decreased platelet count, elevated numbers of immature neutrophils, decreased skin perfusion, decreased urine output, skin mottling, poor capillary refill, hypoglycemia, and petechiae.
  f. *Septic shock*: Sepsis-induced state with hypotension despite adequate volume resuscitation along with perfusion abnormalities that may include, but are not limited to, lactic acidosis, oliguria, and acute alterations in mental status. Frequently, patients have cardiovascular system failure as evidenced by hypotension and reduced perfusion to vital organs. Patients receiving inotropic or vasopressor agents may not be hypotensive at the time that perfusion abnormalities are measured.
  g. *Multiple organ dysfunction syndrome (MODS)*: Presence of progressive physiologic dysfunction in two or more organ systems after an acute threat to systemic homeostasis
2. Epidemiology
  a. Sepsis is the tenth leading cause of death in the United States
    i. Sepsis is the leading cause of death in intensive care units (ICUs)
    ii. Sepsis develops in more than 750,000 people annually, with 2000 new cases per day in the United States
    iii. Approximately 40% of patients with sepsis develop septic shock
  b. Mortality rates in the United States: Approximately 215,000 people die each year of either septic shock or bacteremia
    i. Sepsis due to gram-negative organisms carries a mortality rate of 20% to 50%
    ii. Severe sepsis carries a mortality rate of 28% to 50% or higher and is present in 6.3% of all patients admitted to the ICU
  c. Health care costs of severe sepsis exceed $17 billion annually

3. **Influences of gender on the response to sepsis:** Gender-based differences exist in the response to infection and sepsis
   a. Females: Estrogen may enhance immune function to the extent of inducing autoimmune disease
      i. Estrogen provides a protective effect in the presence of sepsis
      ii. Monocytes produce more interleukin (IL)-1, cause chemotaxis and phagocytosis
   b. Males: Testosterone suppresses immune function, placing males at risk for worse outcomes; androgens depress the immune response
   c. Once sepsis or septic shock develops, there is no difference in the mortality rate between males and females
4. **Cellular pathophysiology**
   a. Many experts agree that, prior to the development of SIRS, a physiologic insult occurs. The insult may take the form of an infection, traumatic injury, surgical incision, burn injury, or pancreatitis. The initial physiologic response to the insult is the development of a proinflammatory state characterized by the expression of multiple mediators in an effort to limit damage from the insult (Figure 9-2).
   b. Gram-positive bacteria are responsible for approximately 50% of infections resulting in sepsis; gram-negative bacteria account for approximately 25%; 15% of the infections are due to a mix of gram-positive and gram-negative organisms; fungal pathogens account for 5% to 10% of the infections
   c. When phagocytic cells destroy bacteria, a cascade of events follows. Sequence of events varies depending on whether gram-negative or gram-positive organisms are involved.
   d. All gram-negative bacteria have a common group of molecules in the outer membrane, referred to as lipopolysaccharide (LPS) or endotoxin
      i. LPS is composed of lipid A and a polysaccharide core linked to an "O-polysaccharide" side chain of repeating sugars
         (a) Lipid A and the polysaccharide core are identical or nearly identical in most gram-negative bacteria
         (b) O-polysaccharide varies for each specific gram-negative organism

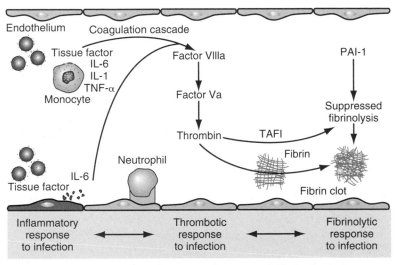

FIGURE 9-2 ■ Inflammation, coagulation, and impaired fibrinolysis in severe sepsis. *IL*, Interleukin; *PAI*, plasminogen activator inhibitor; *TAFI*, thrombin activatable fibrinolysis inhibitor; *TNF*, tumor necrosis factor. (From Ahrens T, Vollman K: Severe sepsis management: are we doing enough?, *Crit Care Nurse Suppl* 23(5):2-16, 2003.)

    ii. LPS (in particular, lipid A) interacts with the body's immune system to produce a septic state

    iii. LPS binds to a circulating LPS-binding protein to form a complex in the blood

        (a) Complex can then bind to a macrophage membrane receptor (CD14), which presents LPS to a signal-transducing receptor in the cell membrane

        (b) Binding triggers the production of mediators known as *cytokines* (soluble molecules released from cells of the immune system whose function is to signal to other cells) (Table 9-1); the proinflammatory cytokine activity attracts further macrophages and monocytes, which results in a repetitive cycle

  e. Components of the gram-positive bacteria cell wall, such as lipoteichoic acid or peptidoglycan, bind to receptors to stimulate cytokine release; bacterial components stimulate the coagulation and complement cascades

  f. Regardless of the inciting pathogen, the cytokines involved in the massive inflammatory reaction known as SIRS may lead to multiple organ dysfunction and are similar to those released in septic shock

  g. Consequences of cytokine production

    i. Systemic vasodilation with decreased afterload and hypotension

    ii. Increased capillary permeability with decreased preload, third-spacing, and interstitial edema

    iii. Relative hypovolemia

    iv. Decreased tissue oxygen extraction

    v. Platelet aggregation, fibrin deposits, and activation of a clotting cascade, leading to microcirculatory coagulation, maldistribution of blood flow, and tissue hypoxia

    vi. Multiple organ dysfunction

  h. Cytokine regulation

    i. Proinflammatory cytokine production and an inflammatory process are normally strongly repressed by the antiinflammatory compensatory response mechanisms

    ii. SIRS and septic shock develop when homeostasis is disrupted and are associated with overproduction of proinflammatory cytokines

  i. Cytokine cascade: Triggering actions of LPS not fully understood; bacterial products stimulate the production of cytokines by macrophages and monocytes

    i. Cytokine release begins with the release of tumor necrosis factor-α (TNF-α) followed by the release of IL-1 and IL-6

    ii. TNF-α and IL-1 cause a variety of physiologic effects; interferon-γ, released from natural killer cells in response to TNF and bacterial products, amplifies the functions of IL-1 and TNF-α

        (a) Increased temperature set point, which causes fever or may cause hypothermia

        (b) Decreased systemic vascular resistance and increased capillary permeability

        (c) Increased release of leukocytes from the bone marrow

    iii. IL-6 is released from T cells and monocytes after tissue injury and may inhibit the release of other cytokines (TNF-α, IL-1); IL-6 stimulates the liver to release chemical mediators known as *acute-phase proteins* (i.e., C-reactive protein [CRP])

        (a) CRP levels increase in tissue-damaging infections

■ **TABLE 9-1**
■ ■ **Response to Cytokine and Mediator Release in Systemic Inflammatory Response Syndrome**

Cytokine/Mediator/Precursor	Release	Response
ARACHIDONIC ACID METABOLITES		
Arachidonic acid is one of the nutritional essential fatty acids of the body; present in the cell membrane; accounts for 5% to 15% of fatty acids in phospholipids	Arachidonic acid gives rise to mediators during interactions with three enzymes: cyclo-oxygenase and peroxidase (cyclooxygenase pathway) and lipoxygenase (lipoxygenase pathway) Arachidonic acid gives rise to eicosanoids (physiologically active compounds known as prostaglandins, thromboxanes, and leukotrienes)	See prostaglandins, thromboxane A_2, and leukotrienes
BRADYKININ		
Vasoactive peptide generated by the contact (kallikrein-kinin) system Proinflammatory	Bacterial product Product of the Hageman factor (factor XII), clotting factor XI, prekallikrein, and high-molecular-weight kinlnogen TNF-α and IL-1 activate Hageman factor, which stimulates release	Vasodilation, hypotension Increased vessel permeability
HISTAMINE		
Vasoactive amine	C5a of complement cascade binds to mast cells and triggers release	Increased vessel permeability of postcapillary venules Pulmonary vasoconstriction
Proinflammatory	Also released from basophil granules	Vasodilation of capillaries and venules
INTERLEUKINS Generic term for cytokines produced by leukocytes; name derived from function: Communicates (inter) among white blood cells (leukins); affect the growth and differentiation of immune system cells IL-1		
Proinflammatory	Bacterial products stimulate the release of IL-1 from macrophages, monocytes, lymphocytes, neutrophils, and endothelial cells Similar to TNF-α; has a synergistic effect Increases in concentration as a "second wave" to TNF-α	Production of other cytokines (TNF-α, IL-6, IL-8, PAF, leukotrienes, thromboxane, prostaglandins) Activation of T and B cells with B-cell growth and immunoglobulin production Vasodilation, hypotension Increased vessel permeability Fever, sleep, anorexia Myocardial depression, hypercoagulability, and ACTH release

Continued

■ **TABLE 9-1**
■ ■ **Cellular Response to Cytokine and Mediator Release in Systemic Inflammatory Response Syndrome—cont'd**

Cytokine/Mediator/ Precursor	Release	Cellular Response
INTERLEUKIN FAMILY—cont'd		
IL-6		
Proinflammatory and antiinflammatory	Released early in sepsis by activated T cells, antigen-presenting cells, monocytes, and macrophages in the presence of bacterial antigens, TNF-α, and IL-1	Fever Cortisol production Decreased IL-1 and TNF-α production Activation of T and B cells; B-cell growth and immunoglobulin production Hepatic synthesis of acute-phase proteins, such as C-reactive protein
IL-8 (NEUTROPHIL-ACTIVATING FACTOR)		
Proinflammatory	Produced under the influence of TNF-α and IL-1 by macrophages and endothelial cells C5a, bacterial products, IL-1, and TNF-α stimulate the production of IL-8	May be involved in mediating local organ dysfunction Chemoattraction for neutrophils and T cells to participate in inflammatory response; stimulation of cell oxidative burst, degranulation, and release of proteases Tissue damage, cell aggregation Increased vessel permeability
IL-10		
Antiinflammatory	Released by T cells, B cells, and macrophages Produced late in the activation process; stimulated by LPS (endotoxin)	Inhibition of the release of TNF-α and IL-1 from activated T lymphocytes Deactivation of macrophages by suppression of the production of reactive oxygen intermediates Promotion of B-cell production of immunoglobulins
INTERFERONS		
IFN-α		
Antiviral cytokine Proinflammatory Soluble factor that interferes with viral replication when applied to uninfected cells	Released from white blood cells to target uninfected cells	Chills and fever Sickness symptoms: Fatigue, myalgia T-cell proliferation Antiviral effect
IFN-β		
Antiviral cytokine Proinflammatory Soluble factor that interferes with viral replication when applied to uninfected cells	Released from fibroblasts to target uninfected cells	T-cell proliferation Antiviral effect

Continued

IFN-γ Antiviral cytokine Proinflammatory	Released from natural killer cells and T cells in response to TNF-α and IL-1 Targets unaffected cells, macrophages, proliferating B cells, and inflammatory cells	Enhanced release and amplified actions of TNF-α and IL-1 Increased number of TNF-α receptors on macrophages, which makes them more sensitive to TNF-α effects Antiviral effect Differentiation of immunoglobulin synthesis Activation of natural killer cells
LEUKOTRIENES Metabolites of arachidonic acid Proinflammatory	PLA$_2$ is an enzyme secreted during shock and in response to TNF-α, IL-1, IL-8, and complement PLA$_2$ triggers the release of fatty acids, such as arachidonic acid, from many body cells, which leads to the production of leukotrienes Leukotrienes are produced from neutrophils, monocytes, and eosinophils	Tissue inflammation, vessel damage, and increased permeability of vessels, which occur as a result of the production of superoxide PMN accumulation and activation due to chemotactic properties Renal, pulmonary, and coronary vasoconstriction Reduced cardiac contractility
MONOCYTE CHEMOATTRACTANT PROTEIN-1 Amino acid polypeptide Chemotactic agent Proinflammatory	Bacterial products, activated complement, and cytokines activate PMNs, monocytes, and endothelial cells to produce MCP-1	Attraction and activation of monocytes and macrophages due to its chemotactic properties Oxidative burst from cells, which increases metabolism and degranulation Release of proteases with resultant vessel damage and increased vessel permeability
NITRIC OXIDE Free radical molecule Molecule synthesized by NOS, thought to be endothelium-derived relaxant factor Proinflammatory	Two forms of NOS: (1) an inducible form (iNOS), whose production is stimulated by LPS and cytokines; (2) a constitutive (or endothelial) form (cNOS), normally produced in the vascular endothelium cNOS is continuously produced by the endothelium near vascular smooth muscle cells and inhibits leukocyte and platelet adhesion iNOS is released from many body cells in response to LPS, cytokines, and activated mediators	Smooth muscle relaxation, vasodilation, hypotension (*Note*: iNOS has a greater potential to produce pathologic hypotension than does cNOS) Depressed myocardial function Mitochondrial respiration inhibition Increased capillary permeability Increased leukocyte adhesion

Continued

■ **TABLE 9-1**
■ ■ **Cellular Response to Cytokine and Mediator Release in Systemic Inflammatory Response Syndrome—cont'd**

Cytokine/Mediator/ Precursor	Release	Cellular Response
PLATELET-ACTIVATING FACTOR Lipophilic organic mediator Phospholipid produced by a variety of cells, including activated mast cells, platelets, endothelium, basophils, and leukocytes Proinflammatory	PLA_2 enzymes, found in most cells, are secreted during shock and in response to LPS, TNF-α, IL-1, IL-8, complement, and other cytokines PLA_2 triggers the release of lipid mediators, including PAF, from many body cells	Activation of neutrophils and eosinophils Inflammation of many body tissues: Nerves, GI tract, cartilage, and blood vessels Increased permeability of vessels; decreased myocardial contractility; vasodilation; hypotension; bronchoconstriction Platelet aggregation Prostaglandin synthesis
PROSTAGLANDINS Metabolites of arachidonic acid produced in the cyclooxygenase pathway	PLA_2 enzymes are found in most cells and are secreted during shock in response to TNF-α, IL-1, IL-6 and complement; PLA_2 causes the release of arachidonic acid from the cell membrane, which leads to the production of prostaglandins; several types are produced: PGD_2, PGE_2, and PGI_2 prostacyclin	Chemoattraction Vasodilation Fever PGD_2 is produced by connective tissue mast cells and leads to vasodilation and bronchial constriction PGI_2 inhibits platelet aggregation PGE_2 inhibits T-cell and B-cell proliferation, inhibits immunoglobulin synthesis
THROMBOXANE A$_2$ Metabolite of arachidonic acid produced in the cyclooxygenase pathway Proinflammatory	PLA_2 enzymes, found in most cells, are secreted during shock and in response to LPS (endotoxins), TNF-α, IL-1, IL-6, PAF, and complement PLA_2 causes release of arachidonic acid from the cell membrane, which leads to the production of thromboxane A_2 Thromboxane A_2 is synthesized by platelets	Inflammation Platelet aggregation; increased WBC adherence Increased vascular permeability Vasoconstriction in the pulmonary circulation
TUMOR NECROSIS FACTOR-α Polypeptide secretory product of the monocyte-macrophage system Proinflammatory	Released from activated macrophages in response to endotoxins, IL-1, and IL-2 Plasma levels rise immediately after administration of endotoxin, before fever or stress hormone levels increase	Increased formation of oxygen radicals; injury to lungs, GI tract, and kidney injury Recruitment and activation of neutrophils, macrophages, lymphocytes

Continued

Increased cytokine production
(IL-1, IL-6, IL-8, PAF); mediation
and replication of all effects of LPS;
stimulation of arachidonic acid
metabolism and production of
leukotrienes, thromboxane,
prostaglandins, and further
production of TNF-α

Initial hyperglycemia followed by
hypoglycemia; hypotension,
metabolic acidosis, coagulopathy

Fever, increased oxygen
consumption, sleep, anorexia

Increased capillary permeability,
vasodilation, microvascular
constriction, noncardiac pulmonary edema

Activation of the coagulation cascade

Activation of NOS to produce nitric
oxide

TNF-β also produced with
similar effects

ACTH, Adrenocorticotropic hormone; *GI*, gastrointestinal; *IFN*, interferon; *IL*, interleukin; *LPS*, lipopolysaccharide (endotoxin); *MCP-1*, monocyte chemoattractant protein-1; *NOS*, nitric oxide synthase; *PAF*, platelet-activating factor; *PG*, prostaglandin; *PLA$_2$*, phospholipase A$_2$; *PMNs*, polymorphonuclear cells; *TNF*, tumor necrosis factor; *WBC*, white blood cell.

(1) CRP binds to the C-polysaccharide cell wall complement found in bacteria and fungi

(2) Complement system is activated following the binding of CRP to the cell wall component, which leads to a complement-mediated increase in phagocytosis

(b) Increased serum concentrations of CRP are associated with sepsis and death

iv. Effects of cytokines are mediated at target tissues by nitric oxide, arachidonic acid metabolites (prostaglandins, eicosanoids, platelet-activating factor), and lipoxygenase derivatives

v. TNF-α and IL-1 stimulate the production of other cytokines, which leads to a cascade effect with complex amplification and modulation (upregulation and downregulation)

(a) IL-8 induces chemotaxis of activated polymorphonuclear leukocytes and acts as an inflammatory mediator, which leads to tissue damage

(b) TNF-α and IL-1 activate the coagulation cascade

(1) Bacterial products, TNF-α, and IL-1 induce intravascular coagulation and fibrin deposits

(2) Thromboplastin (factor III) and factor VIII activate the extrinsic coagulation pathway

(3) Factor XII (Hageman factor) activates the intrinsic coagulation pathway

(c) TNF-α and IL-1 activate the complement cascade by factor XII and bacterial products

(1) C5a component (one of more than 20 proteins involved in the complement cascade) is a vasoactive anaphylatoxin that binds to macrophages and monocytes

(2) Complement stimulates an oxidative burst

(3) Complement causes the release of oxygen radicals and proteases that damage cells, particularly type II pneumonocytes in the lungs

(4) Complement enhances adherence to the endothelium with degranulation (emptying out granules with digestive substances) and aggregation (clumping), which leads to microvasculature damage

(5) C5a binds to mast cells, basophils, and platelets; causes the release of histamine, serotonin, prostaglandins, and leukotrienes; results in vessel dilation, increased blood flow, increased capillary permeability, and increased plasma leakage

(6) C5a leads to the release of more TNF-α, IL-1, and IL-8

(d) TNF-α and IL-1 activate the kinin cascade with the production of bradykinin

(1) Potent vasodilation

(2) Increased vascular permeability

5. **Role of microbial translocation:** Controversial theory in humans; describes the passage of microbes such as normal bacterial flora of the gut or of microbial products across an injured intestinal mucosal wall from the gut lumen to the mesenteric lymph nodes, other organs, and blood stream; may be a major contributor to the development of the septic cascade

   a. Common enteric organisms: *Enterococcus, Escherichia coli, Clostridium perfringens, Enterobacter cloacae*

   b. Conditions thought to increase gut permeability and microbial translocation

   i. Mucosal ischemia and mucosal hypoperfusion caused by shock or mesenteric vasoconstriction from intense sympathetic nervous system (SNS) stimulation

   ii. Immunoglobulin A deficit associated with total parenteral nutrition, thermal injury, glucocorticoid administration, and endotoxin release

   iii. Glutamine and fiber deficiencies

   iv. Alteration of normal flora

   c. Conditions that contribute to microbial translocation include obstructive jaundice, burns, endotoxemia, hemorrhage, immunosuppression, malnutrition, ischemia, reperfusion injury, total parenteral nutrition, and antibiotic therapy

6. **Etiology and risk factors**

   a. Most common sites of origin of bacteremia and sepsis

   i. Respiratory tract

   ii. Intraabdominal and pelvic sites

   iii. Urinary tract

   iv. Skin

   v. Intravascular catheters

   b. Most common organisms in hospitalized patients: Gram-negative aerobes

   i. *E. coli*

   ii. *Klebsiella* and *Citrobacter* species

   iii. *Pseudomonas aeruginosa*

   c. Other gram-negative aerobes: *Enterobacter* and *Proteus*

   d. Infections with gram-positive organism are becoming more common because these organisms are associated with use of intravascular catheters and invasive devices. Most common aerobic organisms are the following:

   i. *Staphylococcus aureus*

      ii. Coagulase-negative staphylococci

      iii. *Streptococcus pyogenes*

      iv. *Streptococcus pneumoniae*

      v. Less common organisms

         (a) Methicillin-resistant *S. aureus*

         (b) Oxacillin-resistant *S. aureus*

         (c) Vancomycin-resistant *Enterococci*

  e. Other organisms

      i. Viruses, protozoa, parasites

      ii. Fungi, such as *Candida albicans*

      iii. Anaerobic organisms: *Clostridium, Bacteroides fragilis*

  f. Predisposing factors for the development of bacteremia or sepsis

      i. Extremes of age: Elderly and very young

      ii. Granulocytopenia

      iii. Prior antimicrobial therapy

      iv. Severe burn injury, recent trauma, recent surgical procedures, and invasive procedures

      v. Functional asplenia

      vi. Immunosuppression: Infection with human immunodeficiency virus (HIV), chemotherapy, corticosteroids, and bone marrow suppression

      vii. Malnutrition and total parenteral nutrition

      viii. Alcohol use and abuse; abuse of other drugs

      ix. Prolonged ICU stay

         (a) Endotracheal intubation longer than 48 hours (aspiration of pharyngeal secretions, contaminated respiratory equipment)

         (b) Ventilator-associated pneumonia

            (1) Most important cause of infections acquired in the ICU

            (2) Leading cause of death from nosocomial infections

            (3) Higher mortality than community-acquired pneumonia

            (4) Etiology different from that of community-acquired pneumonia

Patient Assessment

1. Nursing history

  a. Patient health history: Significant past medical and surgical history, with a review of all major systems and the identification of recent invasive procedures and recent travel history

      i. History of chronic disease (diabetes mellitus; alcoholism; and liver, heart, and renal failure) places the patient at risk

      ii. Acute illness: Trauma, burns, cholelithiasis, intestinal obstruction, pancreatitis, appendicitis, peritonitis, diverticulitis

      iii. Wounds

  b. Family health history: Chronic disease or infections

  c. Social history: Significant others, ability of the patient and significant others to manage stress, financial obligations of the patient and significant others, and parenting responsibilities of the patient

  d. Medication history, especially medications with immunosuppressive properties (chemotherapeutic drugs, corticosteroids) and antibiotics

  e. Nutritional history, with a special focus on the causes of primary malnutrition (anorexia nervosa, alcohol abuse) and secondary malnutrition (iatrogenic malnutrition, surgical malnutrition)

2. Nursing examination of patient

  a. Physical examination data

    i. Inspection: Clinical presentation may vary, depending on the patient's underlying health and organ function

      (a) Acute distress with anxiety, restlessness, confusion, and disorientation progressing to unresponsiveness

      (b) Flushed, warm, dry skin or pale, cold, mottled skin (particularly in the elderly), decreased capillary refill; shaking chills and shivering in some patients

      (c) Tachypnea and dyspnea

      (d) Decreased urinary output; significant edema or positive fluid balance

      (e) Petechiae, purpura

    ii. Palpation

      (a) Tachycardia with rapid, weak, and thready peripheral pulses. Initially, pulses may be bounding and rapid with a hyperdynamic state.

      (b) Warm skin (elderly may present with cool skin rather than hyperthermia)

      (c) Abdominal distension

    iii. Percussion: Dullness over areas of consolidation

    iv. Auscultation

      (a) Pulmonary crackles from interstitial pulmonary edema; wheezing without a history of bronchospastic airway disease

      (b) Hypotension, narrowed or widened pulse pressure

      (c) Absence of bowel sounds; may progress to paralytic ileus

b. Monitoring data

    i. Core temperature: Above 100.4° F (38° C) or below 96.8° F (36° C)

    ii. Heart rate above 90 beats/min

    iii. Respiratory rate: Higher than 30 breaths/min

    iv. Blood pressure (BP): Below 90 mm Hg systolic or

      (a) Fall in systolic BP of more than 40 mm Hg

      (b) Diastolic BP below 70 mm Hg

    v. Pain is the fifth vital sign (see Multisystem Trauma)

    vi. Hemodynamic variables

      (a) Cardiac index: More than 3.5 L/min/m^2; may be low in elderly patients and those with underlying cardiac disorders, or in those in the stagnant phase of septic shock

      (b) Systemic vascular resistance: Below 900 dynes/sec/cm^{-5}

      (c) Pulmonary artery wedge pressure (PAWP): Normal to low; below 6 mm Hg

      (d) Oxygen delivery and consumption: Variable, but often decreased as septic shock progresses; oxygen extraction below 20% of oxygen delivery (normally 20% to 25%)

        (1) Experts suggest that the designations of "warm shock" and "cold shock" be abandoned and that the extent of tissue perfusion be used to determine the extent of shock

        (2) If derived hemodynamic variables (such as oxygen delivery and consumption) are not available, lactate levels or base deficit can be used (see Diagnostic Studies)

3. Appraisal of patient characteristics: A 55-year-old male factory worker is admitted to the hospital with perforated colonic diverticula. He complains of a 2-day history of fever (102° F [38.9° C]), nausea, vomiting, distended abdomen, and abdominal pain, which worsened over the last 6 hours. Patient takes albuterol and metaproterenol for asthma and recently started taking oral steroids for an acute asthma attack. Wife reports that the patient has had a severe cough with production of green sputum and was not taking antibiotics. After diagnosis via computerized tomographic (CT) scan, the patient is taken to the operating room to undergo a Hartmann procedure. Antibiotics, intravenous (IV) fluids, and mechanical ventilation were initiated within 1 hour of admission directly to the ICU. Hemodynamic values are consistent with a hyperdynamic state and WBC count of 10,000/mm^3. Family members are at the bedside and provide much support for the patient. They have arranged for assistance with medical technology from a neighbor who works as a critical care registered nurse.

a. Resiliency (level 3—*moderately resilient*): Patient comes to the hospital with SIRS and sepsis; demonstrates strong reserves and the ability to mount an immune response as manifested by fever and hyperdynamic state; is maintaining stable vital signs; the WBC count must be followed to verify his ability to maintain an immune response despite the recent initiation of oral steroid therapy

b. Vulnerability (level 1—*highly vulnerable*): Patient has had definitive resuscitation and treatment for an infectious-inflammatory process, but with the recent history of a productive cough is highly prone to hospital-associated infections

c. Stability (level 3—*moderately stable*): Patient is hemodynamically stable, yet in a hyperdynamic state with a requirement for large volume replacement; stability potential would be limited with the removal of interventions

d. Complexity (level 1—*highly complex*): Based on acute onset, multiple intensive therapies; preexisting symptoms of probable respiratory infection; altered body image due to surgical incision; need for strong family support

e. Resource availability (level 5—*many resources*): Financial resources readily available from stable employment and benefit package; the patient's knowledge is limited, but he has a neighbor with 20 years' experience as a critical care nurse and extended family readily available to assist with his care

f. Participation in care (level 5—*full participation*): As previously

g. Participation in decision making (level 3—*moderate level of participation*): Yet to be determined for this patient; the family has the ability to seek assistance from the neighbor

h. Predictability (level 3—*moderately predictable*): Based on symptom onset and presentation for intervention, and age

4. **Diagnostic studies**
    a. Laboratory
        i. Arterial blood gas (ABG) levels
            (a) Respiratory alkalosis with Paco$_2$ below 32 mm Hg attempting to compensate for metabolic acidosis, with pH below 7.35 and decreased HCO$_3$
            (b) Late: Respiratory acidosis with Paco$_2$ above 45 mm Hg
            (c) Progressive intrapulmonary shunt, with an increasing fraction of inspired oxygen (FIo$_2$) needed to maintain arterial partial pressure of oxygen (Pao$_2$) at 70 mm Hg and oxygen saturation by pulse oximetry above 92%
        ii. Mixed venous blood gas levels, arterial lactate level, base deficit
            (a) Increasing hemoglobin saturation of mixed venous blood (S$\bar{v}$o$_2$) above 80% as tissues are unable to extract delivered oxygen
            (b) Increasing arterial lactate level (>2 mEq/L) as cells use anaerobic rather than aerobic pathways for metabolism
            (c) Base deficit more negative than −5
        iii. Complete blood count (CBC) and differential: Either increased (>12,000/mm^3) or decreased (<4000/mm^3) or above 10% immature (band) forms
        iv. Serum glucose levels: Elevated from the stress response
        v. Blood cultures and antibiotic sensitivities

        (a) Identify causative organisms; blood culture results are positive in only 50% of septic patients for uncertain reasons (bacteremia may be intermittent)

        (b) Urine, sputum, and wound cultures to correlate with blood cultures

   vi. Elevated blood urea nitrogen (BUN) and creatinine levels

   vii. Coagulation studies: May show elevations in prothrombin time (PT) and partial thromboplastin time (PTT); decreased fibrinogen level and increased level of fibrin split products

   viii. Decreased platelet levels

   ix. Decreased CRP and elevated procalcitonin levels

   x. Elevated serum enzyme levels, indicating liver or cardiac impairment

Patient Care

1. **Infection and exaggerated inflammatory process**
   a. Description of problem
      i. Exaggerated or "malignant" inflammation
      ii. Inadequate primary defenses (broken skin, traumatized tissues) and secondary defenses (immunosuppression), invasive procedures, and/or malnutrition
      iii. Defining characteristics: See definition of SIRS
   b. Goals of care
      i. WBC count is 4000 to 12,000/mm^3
      ii. Temperature is 96.8° to 100.4° F (36° to 38° C)
      iii. Heart rate is 60 to 100 beats/min
      iv. Respiratory rate 12 to 20 breaths/min
   c. Collaborating professionals on health care team: Registered nurse, medical/surgical attending physician, respiratory therapist, pharmacist, dietitian, infectious disease specialist, pastoral counselor
   d. Interventions
      i. Administer antimicrobial agents on time
      ii. Monitor antibiotic levels, particularly aminoglycoside levels, for renal and ototoxic effects
      iii. Monitor for reaction to antibiotics
         (a) Superinfection: Infection with organisms such as *C. albicans* is usually controlled by normal body flora
         (b) Allergy: Rash and anaphylactic shock
         (c) Resistance: Reemergence of symptoms of fever, purulence, and increased WBC count
      iv. Monitor compliance with unit infection control protocols, as recommended by the Centers for Disease Control and Prevention
         (a) Hand washing
         (b) Dressing changes
         (c) Wound isolation
         (d) Catheter and tubing changes
         (e) Use of maximum barrier precautions during catheter insertions
      v. Drotrecogin alfa (activated) is recombinant human activated protein C; indicated for the treatment of severe sepsis in adult patients with a high risk of mortality
         (a) Evaluate all patients for possible drotrecogin alfa (activated) therapy if receiving an antibiotic and vasopressor
         (b) Drug properties: Antithrombotic, antiinflammatory, and profibrinolytic

(c) Continuous intravenous infusion at a dose of 24 mcg/kg/hr for a total of 96 hours

(d) Side effect: Bleeding; if it occurs, the physician should be notified immediately

(e) Discontinue administration of the drug 2 hours before a surgical procedure and restart once adequate hemostasis is achieved (usually within 12 hours after the procedure)

vi. Corticosteroids may be administered to decrease inflammation, improve vessel reactivity to vasopressor agents, decrease the time the patient requires vasopressors, and improve patient outcome

(a) An adrenocorticotropic hormone (ACTH) test should precede therapy. Treatment should be continued only in patients with corticosteroid insufficiency (randomly measured cortisol level of 15 mcg/dl or less, peak cortisol level of 20 mcg/dl or less, or a cortisol increment of 9 mcg/dl or less).

(b) Dosage: Hydrocortisone 200 to 300 mg IV and fludrocortisone 50 mcg orally daily may be given for 1 week from the onset of shock (defined by vasopressor requirement)

vii. Provide twice-a-day brushing of the teeth, oral cleansing every 2 hours, and suctioning above the endotracheal tube

viii. Assist with treatments to limit the nidus of infection

(a) Removal of necrotic tissue

(b) Débridement of burned tissue

(c) Drainage of abscesses

ix. Stabilize fractures promptly to limit tissue damage and inflammation

x. Maintain strong rapport with the family and provide frequent updates and education, because the course of this disease is often unpredictable

e. Evaluation of patient care

i. No clinical manifestations of SIRS are evident

ii. Culture and sensitivity test results are negative

2. **Maldistribution of blood flow** (renal, cerebral, cardiopulmonary, gastrointestinal, peripheral)

a. Description of problem

i. Hyperdynamic state with increased cardiac output and index is the usual presentation

ii. Subsequently, hypovolemia develops

iii. Arterial lactate levels begin to increase

iv. Inability of the tissues to use oxygen; $S\bar{v}O_2$ above 80%; oxygen extraction ratio below 20%

v. Decreased urine output

vi. Decreased gastric mucosal pH showing cellular acidosis

vii. Diminished bowel sounds and/or paralytic ileus

viii. Excessive microvascular coagulation and impaired fibrinolysis

ix. Decreased systemic vascular resistance and hypotension (systolic BP below 90 mm Hg)

x. Changes in the sensorium (restlessness, anxiety, and disorientation progressing to unresponsiveness)

b. Goals of care

i. Oxygen delivery and consumption are normal or supranormal

ii. $S\bar{v}O_2$ is 65% to 75%, and oxygen extraction ratio is improved (>20%)

iii. Arterial lactate levels are normal

iv. Urine output is at least 1 ml/kg/hr

     v. Systolic BP is above 90 mm Hg, and systemic vascular resistance is normal

    vi. Bowel sounds are present and there is no abdominal distention

   vii. Sensorium is clear; the patient is oriented to time, place, and person

  c. Collaborating professionals on health care team: See Infection and Exaggerated Inflammatory Process

  d. Interventions

     i. Monitor hemodynamic parameters and $S\bar{v}O_2$ along with derived parameters, such as systemic vascular resistance, oxygen delivery, and oxygen consumption

    ii. Be prepared to administer fluid resuscitation

      (a) Suggested possible end point is a PAWP of 12 mm Hg but it varies, depending on the patient's underlying condition

      (b) Type of fluid to be used (colloid versus crystalloid) is controversial; blood transfusion may be needed if the hemoglobin level is less than 10 mg/dl

   iii. See interventions for hypovolemic shock

   iv. Be prepared to administer vasoactive medications as needed if fluid resuscitation fails to maintain BP and organ perfusion

      (a) Combined inotropic agent and vasopressor may be used

        (1) Norepinephrine, 1 to 30 mcg/min

        (2) Phenylephrine, 40 to 180 mcg/min

        (3) Vasopressin, 0.01 to 0.04 units/min; appropriate in patients requiring high-dose vasopressors

        (4) Dopamine (6 to 25 mcg/kg/min) and epinephrine (1 to 10 mcg/min) may also be used; may induce or exacerbate tachycardia

      (b) Early goal-directed therapy (EGDT); involves maximizing cardiac preload, afterload, and contractility to balance oxygen delivery with demand (Rivers, Nguyen, Havstad, et al, 2001)

        (1) Patient monitoring is necessary with arterial line and central venous oxygen saturation ($ScVO_2$)

        (2) Goal of patient therapy: Central venous pressure (CVP) of 8 to 12 mm Hg, maintained with 500-ml crystalloid bolus every 30 minutes; mean arterial pressure between 65 and 90 mm Hg, maintained with vasoactive agents; $ScVO_2$ of 70% or higher, maintained with transfusion of red cells to sustain a hematocrit of 30% or higher and inotropic agents. Goal is to complete resuscitation within 6 hours of diagnosing sepsis.

        (3) Among septic patients receiving EGDT, in-hospital mortality was reduced by 34% and hospital length of stay declined by 3.8 days

     v. Monitor for symptoms of diminished visceral perfusion

      (a) Decreased or absent bowel sounds

      (b) Elevated serum amylase level

      (c) Decreased platelet count

    vi. Avoid Trendelenburg's position, which may impair gas exchange and decrease cerebral perfusion

   vii. Maximize oxygen delivery and utilization; minimize oxygen demand

      (a) Control hyperthermia

        (1) Use tepid baths or a cooling blanket

        (2) Prevent chills and shivering

        (3) Remove extra blankets

        (4) Use antipyretic agents other than aspirin to reduce fever

(b) Reduce the work of breathing with mechanical ventilation, as appropriate; work with physicians to sedate and paralyze the patient, as needed, to maintain adequate ventilation and gas exchange

viii. Limit patient activity; maintain a restful environment; provide uninterrupted rest; maintain family visitations as appropriate

ix. Manage pain, anxiety, and restlessness with medications and nursing interventions

x. Administer medications if appropriate to modify mediators (Table 9-2)

e. Evaluation of patient care

i. Hemodynamic parameters and vital signs are within normal limits

ii. $S\bar{v}O_2$ is 65% to 75%; the oxygen extraction ratio is 20% to 25%

iii. Arterial lactate level and base deficit are normal

iv. Peripheral pulses are present and equal bilaterally

v. Urine output is at least 1 ml/kg/hr

vi. Sensorium is clear

3. **Impaired oxygenation and ventilation:** See Chapter 2

■ TABLE 9-2
■ ■ New Concepts and Implications for Future Treatment of Sepsis

Therapy	Rationale/Target(s)
ANTIBACTERIALS	
Antiendotoxin antibodies	To bind to endotoxin and neutralize its effects
Antilipid A antibodies	
Lipopolysaccharide analogues	
Lipopolysaccharide removal	
ANTIINFLAMMATORY AND IMMUNOMODULATING ADJUNCTIVE THERAPIES	
Corticosteroids	To decrease neutrophil adhesion and levels of
Immunoglobulins	tumor necrosis factor (TNF)
Interferon-γ	
Pentoxifylline	
PROINFLAMMATORY CYTOKINE INHIBITORS*	
	To inhibit specific mediators and their effects:
Anti-TNF antibodies	TNF
Interleukin-1 receptor antagonist	Interleukin-1
Phospholipase A_2 inhibitor	Phospholipase A_2
Ibuprofen	Cyclooxygenase
Dazoxiben, ketoconazole	Thromboxane
Platelet-activating factor antagonists	Platelet-activating factor
Platelet-activating factor acetylhydrolase	Platelet-activating factor
N-acetylcysteine, selenium	Oxygen free radicals
N-methyl-L-arginine	Nitric oxide
Bradykinin antagonist	Bradykinin
Antithrombin III	To correct coagulopathy and improve microvascular
Tissue factor pathway inhibitor	perfusion
Activated protein C	
Colony-stimulating factor	To increase synthesis and function of white blood cells in response to infection

*Much is unknown about the need to modify the action of cytokines. Although current investigators are considering the usefulness of these medications to treat septic shock in humans and animals, many remain investigational.

4. **Altered thermoregulation**
    a. Description of problem
        i. Related to the body's response to infection and the inflammatory process
        ii. Core temperature below 96.8° F (36° C) or above 100.4° F (38° C)
        iii. Flushed, warm skin or pale, cool skin
        iv. Increased or decreased metabolic rate
    b. Goals of care
        i. Core temperature is between 96.8° and 100.4° F (36° and 38° C)
        ii. Skin is warm and dry
    c. Collaborating professionals on health care team: See Infection and Exaggerated Inflammatory Process
    d. Interventions
        i. Monitor core temperature hourly
            (a) Pulmonary artery (PA) thermistor is the instrument of choice
            (b) If no PA catheter is in place, use the rectal, urinary bladder, esophageal, or tympanic route
        ii. After the source of increased or decreased temperature is identified, maintain normothermia by the use of antipyretic medication as prescribed; avoid aspirin products
        iii. Use tepid baths or a cooling blanket to reduce hyperthermia
            (a) Monitor core temperature at all times to reduce the risk of hypothermia
            (b) Do not decrease temperature too rapidly, because this may lead to shaking chills
            (c) Reposition frequently, and check for tissue breakdown if a cooling blanket is used
        iv. Use warming blankets and a warmed ambient temperature to manage hypothermia
    e. Evaluation of patient care: Normothermia is achieved
5. **Catabolic state resulting in malnutrition**
    a. Description of problem
        i. Increased body temperature
        ii. Increased body metabolism
        iii. Decreased intake of nutrients
        iv. Loss of body weight
    b. Goals of care
        i. Stable body weight as appropriate for gender and body frame
        ii. Nitrogen balance is positive
        iii. Muscle mass is adequate
    c. Collaborating professionals on health care team: See Infection and Exaggerated Inflammatory Process
    d. Interventions: See Chapter 8
        i. Initiate enteral feedings within 48 hours to limit gastrointestinal microbial translocation
        ii. Establish caloric requirements based on body size and degree of hypermetabolism; 20 to 25 kcal/kg/day is average
        iii. Maintain glucose level at 80 to 110 mg/dl because hyperglycemia is associated with a poor prognosis
        iv. Provide family/significant others with distinct goals for nutritional support
    e. Evaluation of patient care
        i. Serum albumin level is above 3.5 g/dl
        ii. Body weight is within 2 kg of normal
        iii. There is no evidence of electrolyte or vitamin imbalances

Multiple Organ Dysfunction Syndrome

SYSTEMWIDE ELEMENTS

Physiologic Anatomy

1. **Definition** developed by a consensus conference and reported in Bone, Balk, and Cerra, et al (1992): Multiple organ dysfunction syndrome (MODS) is the presence of altered organ function in an acutely ill patient such that homeostasis cannot be maintained without intervention. Other terms used are the following:
   a. Multiple system organ failure (MSOF)
   b. Progressive systems failure
2. **History of treatment of organ failure**
   a. Single organ failure
      i. World War I: Profound hypotension with injury led to cardiovascular failure and shock. Results:
         (a) Recognition of the need for aggressive volume replacement in hemorrhagic shock
         (b) Storage of plasma and whole blood by blood banks to be used in volume resuscitation
      ii. World War II and Korean War: Resuscitation of war casualties to a preselected BP improved the number of patients who survived the initial insult, only to die from renal failure
         (a) BP end point was not sufficient; rather, volume loading with salt solutions was needed in addition to administration of blood products
         (b) Concept of the "third space" evolved
         (c) When urine output was used to monitor the adequacy of shock resuscitation, the frequency of renal failure was reduced
      iii. Viet Nam conflict: Pulmonary failure ("shock lung") became a limiting organ system failure
         (a) Pulmonary failure was attributed to shock and overly aggressive fluid resuscitation
         (b) Result: Development of high-technology pulmonary support
   b. Advanced technology led to the ability to support patients during critical illness; consequence of that support is the emergence of MODS
3. **Epidemiology**
   a. MODS develops in 15% of all patients admitted to the ICU
   b. MODS occurs in 20% to 47% of patients with multiple trauma
      i. Infection is the leading cause of MODS after trauma
      ii. Inadequate early resuscitation accounts for 50% of MODS cases
   c. MODS is responsible for up to 80% of all ICU deaths
   d. Mortality rates have remained stable at approximately 70% to 80% for the past 25 years in spite of advances in critical care practice
   e. Death rates increase as the number of involved organs increases
      i. When two organ systems are involved, mortality rates are approximately 60%
      ii. When four or more organ systems are involved, mortality is nearly 100%
   f. MODS results in ICU costs of more than $100,000 per patient and approximately $500,000 per survivor
4. **Sequence of organ failure:** Patients do not necessarily follow the prototype pattern; sequence depends on the reserve of each organ system
   a. Begins with low-grade fever, tachycardia, and dyspnea with the appearance of infiltrates on chest radiographs; normal renal and liver test results

    b. Generally, during the first week, dyspnea progresses until the patient undergoes endotracheal intubation and mechanical ventilation is required; the patient maintains hemodynamic stability with compensatory mechanisms; hyperglycemia (in the absence of diabetes or pancreatitis), hyperlactatemia, and increased urea nitrogen excretion (>15 g/day) develop

    c. Days 7 to 10, bilirubin level increases, approaching 10 mg/dl; serum creatinine level begins to rise; the hyperdynamic state becomes pronounced; positive culture results are seen; impaired wound healing begins; fluid resuscitation and inotropic support are required

    d. Compensatory mechanisms begin to fail during days 14 to 21; the patient becomes hemodynamically unstable despite aggressive intervention; renal dysfunction worsens, so that dialysis is required

    e. Death often occurs within 21 to 28 days after the initial insult

5. Theories of pathogenesis: All or some of the following hypotheses may be relevant simultaneously (see Figure 9-2):

    a. Infection and host septic response

        i. Hypothesis: Organ dysfunction develops due to the direct effect of one or more microbial toxins

        ii. In the presence of no identified infection and no reversal of the syndrome with treatment, it is suggested that infection may be a cause of organ dysfunction, yet not the fundamental mechanism

    b. Two-hit hypothesis: Initial assault (i.e., trauma, infection) primes the host; the patient is then presented with a second modest insult that produces a markedly exaggerated host response

        i. Less severely injured patients enter a less intense state of SIRS but are vulnerable to secondary inflammation that amplifies SIRS

        ii. Complications: Increasing organ failure, secondary infection, or repeated surgery

    c. Complexity theory: A system (body), composed of multiple parts, normally interacts with purpose and order

        i. Purpose and order take precedence in the healthy environment

        ii. Loss of intrinsic variability is the hallmark of the complexity theory and is an indicator of a failing or diseased system prone to the development of MODS

    d. Macrophage-cytokine hypothesis: Excessive or prolonged stimulation of macrophages and neutrophils leads to the production of cytokines (see Systemic Inflammatory Response Syndrome Septic Shock) and other products, which results in harmful cellular and systemic effects

        i. Cytokines: IL-1, IL-6, IL-8, TNF, and interferon-γ

        ii. Site of infection is unnecessary for the development of MODS; up to 30% of patients who die of MODS have no infection

    e. Microcirculatory hypothesis: Failure of oxygen delivery to keep up with oxygen consumption results in tissue ischemia and organ dysfunction

        i. Ischemia leads to damage of the vascular endothelium

        ii. Endothelial cell surface adhesion molecules and the interaction between the endothelium and cytokines lead to tissue injury

        iii. Tissue injury from ischemia-reperfusion occurs because of oxygen radical formation

        iv. Decreased ability of red blood cells (RBCs) to deform themselves because of peroxidation of the lipid membrane leads to the inability of RBCs to move through the circulation

    f. Gastrointestinal dyshomeostasis hypothesis: Gut acts as a reservoir for bacteria and endotoxin, which cause and perpetuate the development of MODS (see the discussion of microbial translocation under Systemic Inflammatory Response Syndrome Septic Shock)

6. **Organ failure:** Progressive deterioration of two or more organs over a brief period
   a. Pulmonary: Acute respiratory distress syndrome (ARDS)
      i. Unexplained hypoxemia with suspected sepsis (PaO_2/FIO_2 <175 to 250 mm Hg)
      ii. Bilateral pulmonary infiltrates on a frontal chest radiograph along with PAWP below 18 mm Hg
      iii. Deterioration of ABG parameters from the baseline
   b. Hepatobiliary
      i. Elevation of liver function enzymes to more than twice the normal level
      ii. Serum bilirubin level above 2 mg/dl
      iii. Decreased albumin level
      iv. PT elevated to twice the normal time
   c. Gastrointestinal
      i. Intolerance of gastric feeding for longer than 5 days; paralytic ileus
      ii. Gastrointestinal bleeding
   d. Renal (not prerenal)
      i. Oliguria with urine output below 0.5 ml/kg/hr
      ii. Increase in serum creatinine level to 2 to 3 mg/dl with urine sodium level below 40 mmol/L in a patient with normal baseline renal function
      iii. Increase in serum creatinine level of 2 mg/dl in a patient with chronic renal failure
   e. Central nervous system (CNS)
      i. Glasgow Coma Scale score below 15 when previously normal or decreased by 1
      ii. Acute change in mental status (confusion, agitation, lethargy, psychosis)
   f. Coagulation and hematologic
      i. Confirmatory test results for disseminated intravascular coagulation (DIC): Level of fibrin degradation products above 1:40 or of D-dimers above 2 mcg/ml
      ii. Thrombocytopenia or a fall in the platelet count by 25%
      iii. Elevated PTT to more than 125% of normal
      iv. Clinical evidence of bleeding
   g. Cardiovascular
      i. Decreased ejection fraction with persistent capillary leak consistent with altered CVP and PAWP
      ii. Tachycardia and hypotension
7. **Quantification of organ failure:** May be measured with two MODS outcome prediction scores
   a. Marshall, Cook, Christou, et al (1995) developed the Multiple Organ Dysfunction Score, which is a reliable physiologic measure of dysfunction in six organ systems (respiratory, renal, hepatic, cardiovascular, hematologic, neurologic); the Multiple Organ Dysfunction Score correlates with the risk of mortality
      i. Score of 9 to 12: Mortality rate of 25%
      ii. Score of 13 to 16: Mortality rate of 50%
      iii. Score of 17 to 20: Mortality rate of 75%
   b. Sequential Organ Failure Assessment (SOFA) score (Table 9-3)
      i. This predictive tool evaluates dysfunction in the respiratory, renal, hepatic, cardiovascular, hematologic, and neurologic systems

■ **TABLE 9-3**
■ ■ **Sequential Organ Failure Assessment (SOFA)**

Organ System and Assessment	Score				
	0	1	2	3	4
Respiratory: Pao_2/Flo_2 (mm Hg)	>400	≤400	≤300	≤200*	≤100*
Renal: Creatinine level (mg/dl) or urine output	<1.2	1.2-1.9	2.0-3.4	3.5-4.9 or <500 ml/day	≥5.0 or <200 ml/day
Hepatic: Bilirubin level (mg/dl)	<1.2	1.2-1.9	2.0-5.9	6.0-11.9	≥12.0
Cardiovascular: Hypotension	No hypotension	MAP <70 mm Hg	Dopamine >5 or dobutamine (any dose)†	Dopamine >5 or epinephrine ≤0.1 or norepinephrine ≤0.1†	Dopamine >15 or epinephrine >0.1 or norepinephrine >0.1†
Hematologic: Platelet count ($×1000/mm^3$)	>150	≤150	≤100	≤50	≤20
Neurologic: Glasgow Coma Scale score	15	13-14	10-12	6-9	<6

From Vincent JL, Moreno R, Takala J, et al: The SOFA (sepsis-related organ failure assessment) score to describe organ dysfunction/failure, *Intensive Care Med* 22:707–710, 1996.
Flo₂, Fraction of inspired oxygen; *Pao₂*, arterial partial pressure of oxygen.
*With ventilatory support.
†Adrenergic agents administered for at least 1 hr (doses given are in mcg/kg/min).

    ii. SOFA score is a reliable outcome predictor for organ failure
  c. When Bota, Melot, Ferreira, et al (2002) compared the Multiple Organ Dysfunction Score with the SOFA score, they found that the SOFA therapy-related cardiovascular score was a superior predictor of dysfunction
8. **Etiology and risk factors**
  a. Predisposition
    i. Chronic diseases and preexisting organ dysfunction: Diabetes mellitus, angina pectoris, myocardial infarction, heart failure, chronic obstructive pulmonary disease, acute and chronic renal failure, liver failure, pancreatitis, and HIV infection
    ii. Immunosuppressive therapy: Use of corticosteroids or drugs with immunosuppressive properties
    iii. Extremes of age: The elderly and the very young
    iv. Malnutrition, alcohol use, and alcoholism
    v. Cancer
    vi. Severe trauma: Extensive tissue damage; presence of necrotic tissue; persistent inflammation; hemodynamic instability, inadequate tissue perfusion, and acidosis; hemorrhagic shock and multiple transfusions; burns;

inadequate fluid resuscitation; and infection (*Note:* MODS is rarely associated with infection in trauma patients despite a high rate of SIRS)

    vii. Sepsis

  b. Etiology (see also Systemic Inflammatory Response Syndrome and Septic Shock)

    i. Normal integrated inflammatory immune response continues unchecked, releasing cellular mediators that cause organ dysfunction

    ii. Clinical and cellular events leading to MODS

      (a) Inflammation: Pancreatitis and retained necrotic tissue

      (b) Hypoperfusion: Shock and trauma

      (c) Infection: Endotoxemia

Patient Assessment

1. Nursing history

  a. Patient health history: Past medical and surgical history, with special emphasis on sepsis, shock, trauma, recent surgical procedures, recent infections, and preexisting organ compromise

  b. Social history: See Systemic Inflammatory Response Syndrome and Septic Shock

  c. Medication history, with particular attention to drugs that cause immunosuppression

    i. Use of corticosteroids

    ii. Use of immunosuppressive drugs following organ transplantation

    iii. Use of antimicrobial agents

  d. Nutritional status of patient (including dietary intake, alcohol use, use of enteral or parenteral nutrition, and normal body weight)

2. Nursing examination of patient

  a. Physical examination data

    i. Assessment findings depend on the organ system involved

      (a) Pulmonary failure (ARDS): See Chapter 2

      (b) Hepatobiliary failure: See Chapter 8

      (c) Gastrointestinal failure

        (1) Paralytic ileus: Abdominal distention, absent bowel sounds, inability to tolerate enteral feeding, nausea, and vomiting

        (2) Gastrointestinal bleeding (see Chapter 8)

      (d) Intrarenal acute renal failure: See Chapter 5

      (e) CNS failure

        (1) Acute change in mental status (confusion, agitation, lethargy)

        (2) Glasgow Coma Scale score below 15 when previously normal or decreased by 1

      (f) DIC (see Chapter 7)

    ii. Inspection: Findings vary across the continuum of organ failure

      (a) Clinical presentation may vary, depending on the patient's underlying health, the degree of organ dysfunction, the number of organs involved, and the progression of time

      (b) Acute distress with anxiety, restlessness, confusion, irritability, and disorientation progressing to unresponsiveness and prostration

      (c) Tachypnea, increased work of breathing, intercostal retractions, nasal flaring, and dyspnea

      (d) Tachycardia; cardiac dysrhythmias

      (e) Decreased urinary output despite adequate intake

      (f) Interstitial edema

      (g) Bleeding from orifices, old puncture wounds, and mucous membranes; bruising

      (h) Asterixis (late); jaundiced skin

   iii. Palpation: Findings vary across the continuum of organ failure

      (a) Vocal fremitus: Increased because of increased density from pulmonary edema

      (b) Rapid, weak, and thready peripheral pulses

      (c) Distended abdomen, enlarged liver

   iv. Percussion: Findings vary across the continuum of organ failure

      (a) Dullness over areas of consolidation, pleural effusion

      (b) Hepatomegaly

   v. Auscultation: Findings vary across the continuum of organ failure

      (a) Pulmonary crackles from interstitial pulmonary edema; wheezing without a history of bronchospastic airway disease; bronchovesicular breath sounds as consolidation worsens

      (b) Narrowed pulse pressure and variable BP

      (c) Absent bowel sounds

      (d) Pericardial friction rub (late)

      (e) Reduced lung expansion

  b. Monitoring data: Vital signs—see definitions section under Systemic Inflammatory Response Syndrome and Septic Shock. Note that vital signs vary, depending on the nature of the underlying disorder and the organ systems involved.

3. Appraisal of patient characteristics: A 65-year-old retired female who lives alone with no immediate family comes to the hospital with diaphoresis, shortness of breath, and bilateral lower extremity edema. Her medical history includes the presence of diabetes mellitus type 2 since age 45 years, renal insufficiency (not requiring dialysis), two episodes of myocardial infarction, and hypertension. Diagnostic test results include a brain natriuretic peptide level of 3000 pg/ml and a chest radiograph consistent with moderate cardiomegaly and bilateral pleural effusions. The physician orders 4 L oxygen by nasal cannula, diuretic therapy, and admission for telemetry. Echocardiogram reveals an ejection fraction of 30%. Within 3 days, the patient's BUN and creatinine levels elevate to 110 mg/dl and 7.3 mg/dl, respectively, which necessitates hemodialysis. Insulin administration on a sliding scale is instituted for hyperglycemia. Patient requires multiple interventions to stabilize her newly diagnosed heart failure and acute renal failure.

  a. Resiliency (level 1—*minimally resilient*): Patient presents with new-onset heart failure (HF) and demonstrates minimal reserves—inability to respond adequately to elevated glucose level or fluid overload. Her compensatory mechanisms have failed because her renal and endocrine systems are unable to compensate.

  b. Vulnerability (level 3—*moderately vulnerable*): Patient can undergo dialysis to reduce fluid overload, can receive exogenous insulin to control glucose levels, and can be provided with continuous IV medications to improve her cardiac function

  c. Stability (level 3—*moderately stable*): Patient is able to maintain a steady state with improvement of glucose level and HF symptoms with dialysis

  d. Complexity (level 1—*highly complex*): Multiple system dysfunction involving multiple complex therapies

  e. Resource availability (level 1—*few resources*): Patient lives alone, has no immediate family, and has no support systems; has a limited knowledge of her complex medical problems; has a fixed monthly income

  f. Participation in care (level 3—*moderate participation*): Patient will require assistance with transportation to dialysis and clinic appointments

  g. Participation in decision making (level 5—*full participation*): There is no support, but the patient is compliant and follows the regimen without difficulty

  h. Predictability (level 3—*moderately predictable*): HF is highly predictable but is complicated by the patient's multiple medical problems and age

4. **Diagnostic studies:** See Systemic Inflammatory Response Syndrome and Septic Shock

Patient Care

1. **Infection and exaggerated inflammatory process:** See Systemic Inflammatory Response Syndrome and Septic Shock

2. **Maldistribution of blood flow (renal, cerebral, cardiopulmonary, gastrointestinal, peripheral):** See Septic Shock

3. **Impaired oxygenation and ventilation:** See Chapter 2

4. **Altered state of consciousness:** See Systemic Inflammatory Response Syndrome and Septic Shock; see Chapter 4

5. **Coagulopathy:** See Chapter 7

6. **Altered thermoregulation:** See Systemic Inflammatory Response Syndrome and Septic Shock

7. **Catabolic states resulting in malnutrition:** See Systemic Inflammatory Response Syndrome and Septic Shock

8. **Impaired clearance of metabolic wastes:** See Systemic Inflammatory Response Syndrome and Septic Shock

9. **Alteration in coping by patient and family during a situational crisis of a critical illness and knowledge deficit:** See Chapter 10

Multisystem Trauma

SYSTEMWIDE ELEMENTS

Physiologic Anatomy

1. **Definitions**
   a. Injury: Physical harm or damage to the body resulting from an exchange, usually acute, of mechanical, chemical, thermal, or other environmental energy that exceeds the body's tolerance
   b. Unintentional injury: Accidental harm or damage to the body resulting from sudden, unplanned traumatic events such as motor vehicle crashes, burns, drowning, exposure to poisons, falls, explosions, electrical accidents, firearm injuries
   c. Intentional injury: Harm or damage to the body resulting from planned or premeditated injurious acts, for example, assaults (beatings, gunshot wounds, stab wounds), homicides, and suicides

2. **Epidemiology**
   a. Injury remains the leading cause of death in people aged 1 to 37 years
   b. Injury is the fourth leading cause of death for all age groups, following heart disease, cancer, and stroke (Figure 9-3)
   c. In 2000, approximately 97,900 deaths resulted from unintentional injury (Table 9-4)
   d. Approximately 55,000 intentional deaths (particularly suicides and homicides) occur each year; homicide rates are on the rise in many states

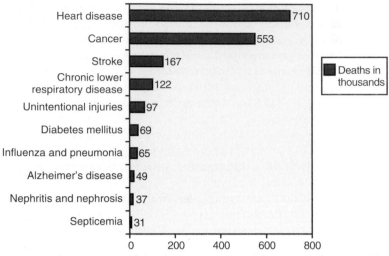

FIGURE 9-3 ■ Leading causes of death among United States residents of all ages. (Data from National Safety Council: *Injury facts*, Itasca, Ill, 2003, Author.)

3. **Physiologic response to injury**
   a. Stress response
      i. Initial stress response known as the "ebb phase" begins 12 to 24 hours after injury; initiated by tissue injury, acute blood loss, shock, hypoxia, acidosis, and hypothermia as well as feelings of pain, anxiety, and fear
      ii. SNS: Afferent nerve signals reach the brain following the presentation of stimuli. Stimulation of the splanchnic nerves occurs, which leads to the release of epinephrine, norepinephrine, cortisol, and growth hormone into the circulation.
         (a) Increase in heart rate and contractility, vasoconstriction, and BP
         (b) Increase in minute ventilation
         (c) Prolonged and excessive stimulation leads to severe and uneven arteriolar vasoconstriction, reduced microcirculatory blood flow, and impaired delivery of oxygen and nutrients to tissues

■ **TABLE 9-4**
■ ■ **Deaths Caused by Unintentional Injury in 2000**

Classification	Number of Deaths	Change from 1999
Motor vehicle crashes	43,354	+2.0%
Falls	13,322	+1.0%
Poisoning	12,757	+4.5%
Choking	4,313	+10.0%
Drowning	3,482	−1.0%
Fires, flames	3,377	+1.0%
Mechanical suffocation	1,335	−17.0%
Natural heat or cold	1,043	−13.0%
Total unintentional deaths	97,900	0%

Data from National Safety Council: *Injury facts*, Itasca, Ill, 2002, Author; and National Safety Council: *Injury facts*, Itasca, Ill, 2003, Author.

        (1) In the absence of hypovolemia, redistribution of intravascular volume from the venous capacitance vessels leads to increased central blood volume and increased intraluminal capillary pressure

        (2) Loss of intravascular volume due to increased capillary permeability leads to intravascular hypovolemia, hypoperfusion, and edema

    (d) Following restoration of the fluid balance, the body develops a hyperdynamic state or "flow phase" to compensate for oxygen debt

        (1) This phase may last for weeks; the degree and duration of the hypermetabolic response depend on the injured tissue mass, loss of barriers to infection, degree of malnutrition, age, gender, and preinjury health status

        (2) Inability to achieve and maintain a hyperdynamic state (high cardiac index, oxygen delivery, and oxygen consumption) is associated with higher mortality rates

iii. Hypothalamic-pituitary-adrenal secretions: Adrenal secretion of corticosteroids is regulated by both the hypothalamus and pituitary

    (a) Stimuli: Fear, pain, hypotension, hypovolemia, tissue injury

    (b) Effects of corticosteroid secretion: Sodium retention, insulin resistance, hyperglycemia, gluconeogenesis, lipolysis, protein catabolism, ketogenesis, and enhancement of the catabolic effects of TNF-α, IL-1, and IL-6

iv. Protein synthesis is modified to enhance immune function

    (a) Increase in the synthesis of acute-phase proteins (i.e., CRP)

    (b) Decrease in the synthesis of other proteins (i.e., albumin, skeletal muscle, transferrin)

    (c) These physiologic effects occur in an effort to increase energy, which is needed to heal massive tissue injury

v. Antidiuretic hormone (ADH) release: Loss of blood volume is sensed by atrial receptors, and hypotension is sensed by pressure receptors in the carotid sinus, aortic arch, and pulmonary artery

    (a) Receptors communicate with neurons in the hypothalamus, which synapse with cells in the posterior pituitary gland

    (b) Posterior pituitary gland releases ADH, which leads to vasoconstriction and water retention

vi. Renin-angiotensin release: Renin is released from the juxtaglomerular cells when renal blood flow is diminished or when they are stimulated by the SNS. Renin catalyzes a reaction that leads to vasoconstriction, aldosterone stimulation, and decreased sodium and water excretion.

vii. Endogenous opioids: Released from the pituitary gland as part of an initial stress response to decrease pain, inhibit feedback of pituitary activation, decrease ACTH release, and increase insulin release; may decrease immune response

viii. Coagulopathy: From excessive bleeding, massive blood transfusions, hypothermia, and inflammatory response

ix. Locally produced mediators

    (a) Endothelial disruption leads to activation of Hageman factor (factor XII), which activates other systems

        (1) Coagulation cascade, leading to clotting and fibrinolysis

        (2) Complement cascade, initiating inflammation and increased capillary permeability

        (3) Kinin and plasmin systems

(b) Activation of arachidonic acid metabolism leads to activation of other mediators
  (1) Prostaglandins: Vasoconstriction and platelet aggregation
  (2) Leukotrienes: Mediator of vascular tone and inflammation
  (3) Platelet-activating factor: Stimulates platelet and neutrophil activation, which leads to microvascular thrombosis at the site of injury
  (4) Activation of cytokine cascades: TNF-α, IL-1, IL-6, and IL-8
(c) Oxygen radicals: Released from ischemic tissues on reperfusion and activated by localized circulating immune effector cells, which leads to further tissue injury

b. Psychologic response (varies with the circumstances): Fear, withdrawal, anger, hostility, anxiety, depression, regression, intrusion or avoidance, and hyperarousal

c. Metabolic derangements
  i. Edema: Prolonged trauma and stress lead to an influx of sodium and water from the intravascular space into the interstitial space, which results in intravascular fluid volume deficit and interstitial edema; increased capillary permeability from circulating mediators increases edema
  ii. Increased cardiac output: Heart rate and contractility increase as a result of the stress response; when bleeding is controlled and the fluid volume is replaced, hyperdynamic circulation occurs; the patient may not exhibit the response of tachycardia in the presence of certain medications (i.e., β-adrenergic and calcium channel blockers)
  iii. Impaired oxygen transport: Altered microcirculation due to vasoconstriction at the tissue level leads to decreased tissue perfusion
  iv. Hypermetabolism: Oxygen consumption increases to supranormal levels 10% to 25% above the baseline. Extent of the increase depends on the severity of the injury.
  v. Altered protein metabolism: Total body catabolism is increased, particularly within the skeletal muscles, which results in a loss of lean body mass. Hepatic synthesis of proteins increases. Growth hormone induces potent anabolic effects to incorporate amino acids into proteins.
  vi. Altered glucose metabolism: Glucose level increases because of stress hormones; insulin resistance occurs; glycogen stores are converted to glucose
  vii. Altered fat metabolism: Lipids in the form of stored fuel are broken down into fatty acids for energy
  viii. Leukocytosis: Increased number of granulocytes, which occurs even without infection; increased degranulation

4. **Etiology and risk factors**
  a. Factors associated with trauma
    i. Physical
      (a) Age: Elderly and very young are at risk
        (1) Patients older than 75 years of age fare worse after trauma than younger patients
          a) Injury is more severe because of increased body fragility, blunted compensatory mechanisms, and the presence of underlying organ dysfunction, with decreased organ reserve
          b) Risk for trauma is higher because of poor vision, weak lower extremities, unsteady gait, and impaired balance
        (2) Very young (<5 years) have higher mortality rates than children aged 6 to 14 years

    (b) Gender and the incidence of trauma: More males than females are injured; in 2002, 65% of unintentional injuries occurred in males, 35% in females; risk from trauma is 2.5 times higher in males than in females
       (1) Pregnancy affects injury severity and outcome
       (2) Females more at risk for domestic violence
       (3) Mortality in trauma is not affected by gender after appropriate stratification for injury severity, age, admission parameters, and preexisting disease
    (c) Ethnicity
       (1) Teenaged African American males are tenfold more likely to die as a result of homicide than are European American males of the same age
       (2) Native Americans have the highest rate of unintentional injury; Asian Americans have the lowest
    (d) Type of injury: Blunt versus penetrating
    (e) Preinjury health status: Preexisting organ dysfunction or conditions such as diabetes mellitus, chronic obstructive pulmonary disease, atherosclerotic heart disease, hypertension, and cystic kidney disease increase susceptibility to injury and impair the response to injury
  ii. Environmental factors: Speed limits, legal drinking age, mandatory helmet laws, availability of guns, residence near water, residence in cold climates
    (a) Unintentional injury rates are highest in rural areas
    (b) Intentional injury rates are highest in urban areas
 iii. Socioeconomic factors: Working in a high-risk occupation (construction, heavy industry), living in a high-crime area, living in a poorly maintained home, and membership in a gang; the lower the income, the higher the death rate in African Americans and whites
  iv. Personality and psychologic-neurologic factors: Risk-taking behaviors, antisocial behavior, mental illness, depression, poor judgment, and previous head injury
   v. Use of alcohol and other drugs: Approximately half of all trauma patients have a history of alcohol or substance use; use of alcohol and other drugs places the patient at risk for injury
    (a) Decreased level of alertness; impaired motor function, coordination, and balance; increased reaction time
    (b) Impaired judgment, perception, and cognitive ability; increased risk-taking behavior and feeling of invulnerability among adolescents; increased violent behavior; reduced inhibitions
    (c) Increased physiologic fragility; injury may be severe, and recovery may be slower
  vi. Temporal factors
    (a) Time of day: Death rate from motor vehicle crashes highest between 10 PM and 4 AM
    (b) Day of the week
       (1) Weekends, with a Saturday peak, are the most common times for deaths from motor vehicle crashes, pedestrian accidents, drowning, and homicides
       (2) Suicide rate is highest on Mondays
       (3) Occupational injury rates are highest on Mondays and Fridays
b. Mechanisms of injury

    i. Blunt injury: Trauma that occurs without communication to the outside environment; common causes are motor vehicle crashes and falls. Caused by a combination of forces:

      (a) Acceleration: Change in the rate of velocity or speed of a moving body; as velocity increases, so does tissue damage

      (b) Deceleration: Decrease in the velocity of a moving object; acceleration-deceleration forces are a common cause of blunt injury

      (c) Shearing: Structures slip relative to each other because of forces across a plane

      (d) Crushing and compression: Squeezing, stretching, or inward pressure; hollow organs (stomach, bowel, urinary bladder) are less likely to rupture (except in a seatbelt injury) than are solid organs (liver, spleen), which are less compressible

   ii. Penetrating injury: Trauma that occurs from the motion of foreign objects that enter into tissue, causing direct damage from entry or indirect damage because of the tissue deformation associated with energy transference into the surrounding tissues

      (a) Gunshot wounds

        (1) Energy of a missile is dissipated into the tissues. When the missile enters the body, a permanent cavity is formed that distorts, stretches, and compresses the surrounding tissues (Figure 9-4).

        (2) Blast effect (muzzle blast): Cavity from a gunshot wound produces damage to structures not in the direct path of the missile

        (3) High-velocity missiles cause extensive cavitation and significant tissue destruction. Low-velocity missiles have limited cavitation potential and result in less tissue destruction.

        (4) Extent of the injury is proportional to the amount of kinetic energy lost by the missile: $K = [\text{mass} \times (V1^2 - V2^2)]/2$, where K = kinetic energy, $V1$ = impact velocity, and $V2$ = velocity after impact

        (5) Tissue yaw: Amount of tumbling and movement of the nose of the missile; the more yaw, the more damage (Figure 9-5)

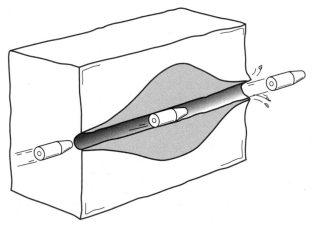

FIGURE 9-4 ■ Formation of temporary *(shaded region)* and permanent *(white region)* cavities during injury from a bullet. The temporary cavity is a localized area of blunt trauma; the permanent cavity occurs with crushing, stretching, and breaking of the elastic bonds of tissue along the wound tract of the bullet. (From Hinkle J, Betz S: Gunshot injuries, *AACN Clin Issues* 6:178, 1995. Illustration by Jef Dirig.)

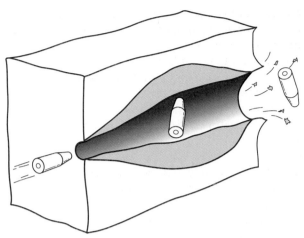

FIGURE 9-5 ■ Tumbling is the action of forward rotation around the center of mass, similar to a somersault action. Yawing is the deviation or deflection of a bullet's nose in the longitudinal axis from a straight line. The more tumbling and yawing, the more tissue destruction. (From Hinkle J, Betz S: Gunshot injuries, *AACN Clin Issues* 6:179, 1995. Illustration by Jef Dirig.)

      (b) Stab wounds: Follow a more predictable pattern than gunshot wounds and may involve less tissue destruction unless vital organs or vessels are lacerated

      (c) Impalement: Usually a low-velocity injury that occurs in motor vehicle crashes, with falls, and after being hit by falling or flying objects

      (d) Avulsion and degloving: Tearing away of tissue, which results in full-thickness skin loss; occurs when the skin is sliced by a sharp object or when a person is thrown from a moving vehicle

Patient Assessment

1. **Nursing history**
   a. Source: Patient, family, partner, significant other, prehospital personnel, or bystander
   b. Mechanism of injury
      i. Motor vehicle crashes
         (a) Restrained, unrestrained, or airbag; helmet use (motorcycle)
         (b) Driver or passenger; location in vehicle; ejection from the vehicle
         (c) Type of vehicle; speed of the vehicle
         (d) Direction and force of the collision, rollover crash
      ii. Falls
         (a) Setting and context (e.g., slipping on ice, falling from a balcony during a party)
         (b) Angle and height of the fall; the risk for serious injury is increased for falls from a height above 10 ft; type of impact surface; landing position
      iii. Gunshot wound
         (a) Type of weapon (rifle, handgun, shotgun); caliber of the weapon
         (b) Velocity of the bullet; range at which the weapon was fired; position of the assailant
         (c) Intentional or unintentional

        (d) If self-inflicted, hand dominance

        (e) Estimated depth of penetration; entry site; angle of entry, exit site; angle of exit

     iv. Stab wound

        (a) Type of weapon; size and length of blade

        (b) Intentional or unintentional

        (c) If self-inflicted, hand dominance

        (d) Estimated depth of penetration; entry site; angle of entry

  c. Description of the event

     i. Location and time

     ii. People involved and their disposition

     iii. Context (e.g., during an argument, while at a party, during work, or while driving home)

  d. Alcohol and substance use involvement

  e. Past health history: AMPLE

     i. *A:* Allergies

     ii. *M:* Medications

        (a) Prescription and over-the-counter drugs

        (b) Herbal and natural substances

        (c) Tetanus immunization

     iii. *P:* Past illnesses (medical and surgical)

     iv. *L:* Last meal (time, quantity, type)

     v. *E:* Events preceding the injury

  f. Social history

     i. Partner, spouse, house mates, roommates, significant others, contact person, dependents, children, parents, guardians

     ii. Education; occupation; financial considerations, ability to maintain income, and insurance coverage

     iii. Religion

  g. Other

     i. Height, weight

     ii. Last menstrual period, potential for pregnancy

2. Nursing examination of patient

  a. Physical examination data

     i. Primary survey: Rapid assessment (30 sec to 2 min) that simultaneously identifies and manages life-threatening injuries: ABCD (Emergency Nurses Association, 2000)

        (a) *A:* Airway—maintain a patent airway. *Note:* Stabilizing the cervical spine (via cervical collar, manual stabilization, taping) is mandatory during airway assessments and interventions.

          (1) Assessment: Airway is open

            a) Patient speaks or makes appropriate sounds

            b) No foreign material visible in the mouth

            c) Look, listen, and feel for exhaled breath

          (2) If the airway is obstructed, expect some of the following signs:

            a) Inability to speak or make sounds

            b) Substernal and intercostal retractions

            c) No air exchange

            d) Stridor (inspiratory, expiratory)

            e) Nasal flaring (children, infants)

            f) Restlessness and confusion, progressing rapidly to unresponsiveness

(3) Emergency interventions during the primary survey (*Note:* Maintain alignment of the cervical spine *at all times*):
  a) Chin lift or jaw thrust
  b) Suction
  c) Artificial airway: Orotracheal or nasotracheal intubation preferred
  d) Cricothyroidotomy: When other means of airway maintenance are not possible or are contraindicated

(b) *B:* Breathing—maintain adequate breathing
  (1) Assessment: Spontaneous, regular respirations of at least 10 breaths/min with equal, bilateral chest expansion and audible breath sounds
  (2) If breathing is compromised, expect
    a) Respiratory rate less than 10 or more than 29 breaths/min (adults)
    b) Difficult or labored breathing; intercostal or substernal retractions
    c) Decreased or absent breath sounds
    d) Asymmetric or paradoxical chest expansion
    e) Changes in color (pallor, duskiness, cyanosis)
    f) Tracheal deviation
    g) Restlessness, confusion, anxiety, and disorientation, progressing to unresponsiveness
  (3) Emergency interventions during the primary survey
    a) Manual resuscitator bag with bag-valve-mask and oxygen therapy
    b) Other options as needed in emergencies
      1) Needle or tube thoracostomy
      2) Covering of sucking chest wounds with a three-sided occlusive dressing
      3) Intubation and mechanical ventilation

(c) *C:* Circulation—maintain adequate circulation. *Note:* In early circulatory compromise, few clinical signs may occur.
  (1) Assessment: Easily palpable carotid pulse, with 50 to 120 beats/min; the patient is awake and answering questions appropriately; capillary refill in less than 2 seconds; no external, uncontrolled bleeding
  (2) If circulation is compromised (late), expect
    a) Decreased level of consciousness
    b) Cold, damp skin; delayed capillary refill (>3 seconds)
    c) Absent, weak, thready, and rapid (>120 beats/min) or slow (< 50 beats/min) pulse
    d) Overt or covert uncontrolled bleeding
    e) Hypotension (systolic BP <90 mm Hg), a late sign, generally occurs with a loss of more than 30% of circulating vascular volume
      1) If a radial pulse is present, BP is approximately 80 mm Hg
      2) In the absence of a radial pulse, a femoral pulse equates to a minimum BP of 70 mm Hg
      3) In the absence of radial and femoral pulses, a carotid pulse equates to a minimum BP of 60 mm Hg
  (3) Emergency interventions during the primary survey
    a) Control of external hemorrhage with direct pressure or a pneumatic antishock garment; this is a controversial measure, but it may decrease hemorrhage with lower-extremity or pelvic fracture
    b) Parenteral fluid resuscitation with crystalloid or blood products (after two 2-L fluid boluses)

      c) Consider autotransfusion if a large amount of blood has been lost

      d) Vasoactive medications only after fluid deficit is managed

  (d) *D:* Disability—monitor the level of consciousness

    (1) Assessment: A (alert), V (verbal), P (pain), U (unresponsive)

      a) *A:* Speak to the patient; score as A if the patient is alert and responsive

      b) *V:* If the patient responds to verbal stimuli, score as V

      c) *P:* If the patient does not respond to verbal stimuli but responds to a painful stimulus, score as P

      d) *U:* If the patient is unresponsive and does not respond to a painful stimulus, score as U

    (2) If mental status is compromised, expect

      a) Decreased alertness; unresponsiveness to verbal and tactile stimulation

      b) Pupils unequal in size or responsiveness; fixed and dilated pupils

      c) Ipsilateral or bilateral deficits in motor response; extremity rigidity

    (3) Emergency interventions during the primary survey

      a) Maintain and protect the airway; maintain breathing and circulation

      b) Initiate emergency measures to control increased intracranial pressure (see Chapter 4)

      c) Protect the patient from self-harm

ii. Secondary survey: *E* though *I* mnemonic; complete head-to-toe physical examination begun as soon as the primary survey and emergency life-saving interventions are accomplished. *Note:* Ongoing trauma resuscitation continues during the secondary survey as needed (Emergency Nurses Association, 2000).

  (a) *E:* Exposure; completely undress the patient to perform a thorough visual examination

    (1) Entry wounds that appear "minor" may be associated with extensive internal injury

    (2) Until the cervical spine is found to be free of injury, log-roll the patient carefully onto the side to maintain spinal alignment

    (3) Cover the patient as soon as possible to prevent hypothermia and initiate rewarming measures (see Hypothermia)

  (b) *F: F*ull set of vital signs, *F*ive interventions, *F*acilitate family presence

    (1) Measure full set of vital signs including BP, pulse rate, respiratory rate, and temperature

    (2) Five interventions consist of pulse oximetry, insertion of an indwelling urinary catheter, insertion of a nasogastric tube, ordering of laboratory studies, evaluation of laboratory values

    (3) Assess the family's understanding of the patient's condition, facilitate visiting and support of the patient, and use the family to assist in meeting the patient's emotional and spiritual needs

  (c) *G: G*ive comfort through administration of analgesia, positioning, and verbal reassurance.

  (d) *H: H*istory and *H*ead-to-toe assessment

    (1) Mnemonic MIVT may be used in obtaining prehospital information: *M*echanism of injury, *I*njuries sustained, *V*ital signs, and *T*reatment

       (2) Complete, systematic head-to-toe assessment should be completed
- **iii.** Tertiary survey: Complete head-to-toe reexamination of the patient immediately before ambulation or after the patient regains consciousness to identify missed injuries; often occurs days after initial injury and resuscitation
- **iv.** Inspection
  - (a) Abrasions, ecchymoses, swelling, and skin lacerations may indicate involvement of underlying structures or mechanism of injury. *Note:* Absence of external injury does not rule out the possibility of severe underlying injury.
  - (b) Unusual drainage may indicate injury to internal structures
    - (1) Otorrhea, rhinorrhea, and blood from the nose or ears may indicate a basilar skull fracture
    - (2) Blood at the urinary meatus may indicate a lower urinary tract injury or a pelvic fracture
  - (c) Inspect for protruding bone fragments or viscera
  - (d) Note a deformity or dislocation of the extremities
  - (e) Locate the entry and exit wounds of penetrating injuries. Do not remove impaled objects until a surgeon is present and ready for an operative procedure (or the injury may be worsened).
- **v.** Palpation: Abnormal findings
  - (a) Skull depressions and deformities; facial deformity
  - (b) Deformity or abnormal movement of the bony thorax; presence of subcutaneous emphysema
  - (c) Abdominal guarding, tenderness, and rigidity
  - (d) Pelvic fractures: Palpate for instability over the iliac crests and the symphysis pubis
  - (e) Deformities and point tenderness of extremities and spine
  - (f) Absence of peripheral pulses
- **vi.** Percussion: Note dullness over blood-filled collections or internal hematomas
- **vii.** Auscultation of the heart and lungs for adventitious sounds and of the gastrointestinal tract for hypoactivity or hyperactivity
- **b.** Monitoring data
  - **i.** Vital signs: Widely variable depending on catecholamine response, the severity of the injury, and medication administration; serial measurement of vital signs is essential to detect changes in the patient's condition
    - (a) Respiratory rate
      - (1) Ideal: 12 to 20 breaths/min
      - (2) Typical following trauma: Tachypnea; absence of tachypnea following major trauma suggests CNS injury or significant substance use (alcohol, opioids, and others)
    - (b) Heart rate
      - (1) Ideal: 60 to 100 beats/min
      - (2) Typical following trauma: Tachycardia
        - a) β-adrenergic and calcium channel blockers may decrease heart rate responsiveness to trauma
        - b) Some patients maintain a normal heart rate despite the loss of large amounts of blood (particularly during pregnancy)
        - c) Some patients with blunt cardiac trauma may have a decreased heart rate or irregular heart rhythm because of cardiac dysrhythmias
        - d) Well-conditioned athletes have slow heart rates

(c) BP
   (1) Ideal: Systolic pressure above 90 mm Hg
   (2) Typical following trauma: Variable, depending on blood loss and age
      a) Young adults tend to remain normotensive until major blood loss occurs
      b) Older adults may have more limited compensatory mechanisms and may be less able to tolerate volume deficits
      c) Alcohol intoxication may lead to hypotension or hypertension
(d) Temperature
   (1) Ideal: Core temperature above 98.6° F (37° C)
   (2) Typical following trauma: Decreased core temperature (95° to 98.6° F [35° to 37° C]) is most common, but hypothermia (<95° F [35° C]) may occur (see Hypothermia)
(e) Pain is the fifth vital sign; pain is what the patient perceives it to be
   (1) Assessment of pain
      a) Mechanism of pain
      b) Location of pain
      c) Quality and characteristics of pain
      d) Intensity of pain
      e) Aggravating and associated factors
   (2) Treatment is based on the type of pain
      a) Somatic pain is often treated with topical therapies, nonsteroidal antiinflammatory drugs, acetaminophen, opioids, and local anesthetics
      b) Visceral pain is commonly treated with nonsteroidal antiinflammatory drugs, opioids, and intraspinal local anesthetic agents
      c) Neuropathic pain is better treated with anticonvulsants or antidepressants but may respond to opioid therapies
   (3) Reassessment should be completed following the treatment of pain and with each vital sign evaluation
   (4) Requirements for pain relief are variable and unpredictable for each individual patient. Frequent and ongoing attention must be given to monitoring, treating, and individualizing treatment of the patient's pain.

3. **Appraisal of patient characteristics:** A 31-year-old female driver wearing a seatbelt was t-boned on the driver's side by a utility truck. She arrives at the emergency department awake and frightened. Prehospital care providers state that, at the scene, the patient did not lose consciousness, had stable vital signs, denied shortness of breath, complained of abdominal pain, and reported that she was 20 weeks pregnant. Focused abdominal sonography for trauma (FAST) shows a "small" amount of abdominal fluid and considerable blood in the left side of the chest. A tube thoracostomy collects 1.5 L of blood. During surgery, the patient develops hemodynamic instability. Significant blood loss is controlled by ligation of the gastric artery. Postoperatively, the patient is taken to the ICU for aggressive resuscitation and rewarming. An obstetrical consult determines that the fetus was nonviable and it is subsequently expelled. The patient is returned to the operating room for abdominal closure. She requires aggressive resuscitation and critical care over the next 10 days and is transferred to progressive care on day 12. A psychiatrist is consulted because the patient is having a difficult time coping with the loss of her baby. This was the patient's third pregnancy in the last 5 years and was preceded by two spontaneous abortions. The patient's parents

and boyfriend provide a great deal of support for her. The legal firm at which the patient is an attorney holds her position open and she returns to work within 5 months of her automobile crash.

    a. Resiliency (level 5—*highly resilient*): Based on age and rapid positive response to resuscitation and definitive care

    b. Vulnerability (level 1—*highly vulnerable*): Patient is highly susceptible to ongoing hemodynamic instability and fetal demise

    c. Stability (level 3—*moderately stable*): Patient exhibits an excellent response to therapies with improved hemodynamic stability

    d. Complexity (level 1—*highly complex*): Status of the patient and fetus are highly intricate and potentially complex

    e. Resource availability (level 5—*many resources*): Patient is employed as an attorney and has excellent benefits; has strong support from her family and significant other

    f. Participation in care (level 5—*full participation*): Family is highly supportive and very active in addressing patient care and needs

    g. Participation in decision making (level 5—*full participation*): Family is very much involved in patient care decisions while the patient is unconscious; once the patient is awake, alert, and oriented, she is actively involved in her care and recovery

    h. Predictability (level 1—*not predictable*): Initial course unpredictable due to the severity of the condition and the high mortality associated with vascular injury

4. Diagnostic studies

    a. Laboratory

        i. CBC: Reflects the amount of blood lost but may take more than 2 hours to show a decrease in hematocrit with slow bleeding

            (a) Marked drop in hemoglobin level and hematocrit after fluid resuscitation with crystalloids due to dilution and mobilization of fluid during the recovery phase

            (b) Leukocytosis with a "shift to the left," which reflects the release of immature cells in response to either trauma or infection

            (c) Platelets: Need to be replaced to stem additional bleeding if below $50,000/mm^3$

        ii. Blood typing and cross-matching: To determine the presence of antigens to ensure compatible blood transfusions

        iii. Blood chemistry panel: To determine levels of glucose (usually elevated from stress response and decreased peripheral utilization of insulin), magnesium (may be decreased from loss in urine), and ionized calcium (often decreased because of the use of citrate in blood transfusions)

            (a) Baseline levels of BUN and creatinine, and liver function tests to determine the response to injury

            (b) Baseline electrolyte levels

        iv. Arterial lactate levels: To determine the adequacy of tissue oxygen extraction and to warn of impending organ failure

        v. Arterial and venous blood gas levels: To determine the adequacy of ventilation, oxygen delivery, and oxygen consumption

            (a) Acidosis may be seen with tissue perfusion deficits; hypoxemia may be seen with hypoventilation

            (b) Arterial oxygenation may be monitored noninvasively with pulse oximetry

            (c) Base deficit may occur because of perfusion deficits and metabolic acidosis

        vi. Urine and blood toxicologic tests

      (a) Blood alcohol concentration: Legal intoxication level in most states is 100 mg/dl

      (b) Routine urine toxicologic screens for commonly abused substances in the given community

    vii. Urinalysis: To determine the presence of blood, bacteria, ketones, glucose, myoglobin, and bilirubin

    viii. Other blood studies: Amylase and coagulation studies

    ix. Pregnancy test: Performed for girls (12 to 17 years of age) and women of childbearing age; if the patient is verbal, consider the need for a test based on sexual history

  b. Radiologic

    i. Radiographic studies are used to locate fractures, abnormal air or fluid collections, and foreign objects such as bullets

      (a) Indicate the position of major organs

      (b) In multiple trauma, views of the cervical spine, chest, abdomen, pelvis, and extremities are necessary

    ii. FAST is a noninvasive ultrasonographic study of four abdominal compartments (subxiphoid, left upper, right upper, and suprapubic region) to detect intraabdominal injuries and cardiac tamponade; it is not intended to replace CT

    iii. CT: Detects the presence of soft tissue injury, hematomas, fractures, and tissue swelling; definitive examination when FAST results are equivocal

    iv. Intravenous pyelography, cystography, and retrograde urethrography: For renal or lower urinary tract injury

    v. Magnetic resonance imaging, angiography, ultrasonography, echocardiography

  c. Electrocardiography (ECG)

  d. Diagnostic peritoneal lavage (DPL) may be used to determine the extent of an abdominal injury or bleeding. Use of DPL may be helpful in patients with blunt trauma with an unstable condition when a solid or hollow organ injury is suspected. DPL has largely been replaced by sophisticated imaging techniques.

Patient Care

1. Impaired oxygenation and ventilation: See Chapter 2

  a. Additional interventions

    i. Maintain cervical spine alignment during airway management until cervical spine injury is ruled out

    ii. Do not use the nasotracheal route for intubation if the patient has facial or basilar skull fractures (to avoid possible penetration of cribriform plate and iatrogenic brain injury)

    iii. Suspect airway compromise in intoxicated patients

2. Intravascular volume depletion: See Chapter 3

  a. Additional interventions

    i. Warm all fluids to body temperature, if possible, to prevent hypothermia

    ii. Use short, large-bore peripheral IV catheters or large-bore trauma catheters at multiple sites for rapid volume resuscitation

      (a) Avoid stopcocks, which slow infusion

      (b) Avoid long lengths of tubing, which increase resistance to flow

    iii. Administer pressurized fluids rapidly using a rapid volume infuser or pressure bag

      iv. Monitor for hypocalcemia and coagulopathy if multiple blood transfusions are needed

      v. Anticipate the need for immediate transfer to the operating room in cases of intravascular volume depletion and hemodynamic instability

        (a) Definitive operative repair versus damage-control surgery

          (1) Extensive, definitive surgical repair may result in complications (triad of death) and poor patient outcomes

            a) Hypothermia

            b) Acidosis

            c) Coagulopathy

          (2) To reduce these complications and the resultant mortality, damage-control surgery or a staged laparotomy has been implemented; sacrifices the completeness of immediate repair. Repair accomplished in three stages:

            a) First stage: Operative repair of life-threatening injuries only

            b) Second stage: Patient transport to the ICU for aggressive rewarming, ongoing resuscitation, and attainment of hemodynamic stability

            c) Third stage: Within 24 to 48 hours after the initial operation, the patient returns to the operating room for definitive repair of intraabdominal injuries

        (b) Use of the three-stage approach has improved patient outcomes and allows for the stabilization of hemodynamics, correction of coagulopathy, rewarming, and optimization of pulmonary function

3. Altered thermoregulation: See Hypothermia

4. Infection and exaggerated inflammatory process: See Chapter 7

5. Impaired fibrinolysis system: See Chapter 7

6. Pain: See Chapters 4 and 10

7. Catabolic state resulting in malnutrition: See Systemic Inflammatory Response Syndrome and Septic Shock; Chapter 8

8. Posttraumatic stress disorder

  a. Description of problem: Reexperiencing of a traumatic event, psychic or emotional numbness, difficulty in interpersonal relationships, or substance use

  b. Goals of care

    i. Patient verbalizes appropriate coping behaviors

    ii. Patient does not abuse alcohol or other substances

    iii. Patient resumes daily activities to his or her maximum capability

  c. Collaborating professionals on health care team: Registered nurse, medical-surgical attending physician, social worker, pastoral counselor

  d. Interventions

    i. Discuss the patient's memories of the traumatic event and his or her emotional response

    ii. Be honest about the level of recovery to baseline, preinjury status

    iii. Make the appropriate referrals if the patient demonstrates ineffective coping or substance abuse

    iv. Explain the role of the family in the support of the patient with posttraumatic stress disorder

  e. Evaluation of patient care

    i. Patient demonstrates coping skills

    ii. Patient resumes activities appropriate for level of functioning after rehabilitation

Burns

SYSTEMWIDE ELEMENTS

Physiologic Anatomy

1. **Definitions**
   a. Burn: Tissue injury due to the coagulation of cellular proteins as a result of heat produced by thermal, chemical, electrical, or radiation energy; degree of coagulation depends on the following:
      i. Temperature of the injuring agent
      ii. Duration of exposure to the injuring agent
      iii. Area exposed to the injuring agent
      iv. Special considerations: The young and the elderly may experience more severe burns because their skin is thinner and more vulnerable
   b. Extent of thermal injury: Total surface area of the injured tissue (Figure 9-6)
   c. Depth of thermal injury: Extent of the injury through the layers (thicknesses) of skin (Figures 9-7 and 9-8)
      i. Zone of hyperemia
         (a) Outer zone of minimal injury; heals rapidly
         (b) Tissue is red (hyperemic) but blanches and refills with pressure
         (c) No cell death
      ii. Zone of stasis: Represents cellular damage of variable degree due to the decreased blood flow
         (a) Middle zone of injury, the cells of which can either recover or become necrotic over the initial 24 hours following injury
         (b) Tissue is red but does not blanch with pressure
         (c) Recovery depends on prompt, adequate resuscitation to correct hypovolemia and restore blood flow
      iii. Zone of coagulation
         (a) Area of injury where the temperature reached at least 113° F (45° C)
         (b) Protein coagulation and cell death
         (c) Tissue is black, gray, or khaki to white and does not blanch with pressure

2. **Epidemiology**
   a. Third leading cause of death from unintentional injury in the United States; infection is the leading cause of death among hospitalized patients with burns
   b. Approximately 2 million to 2.5 million Americans experience burns serious enough to require medical care each year
   c. Approximately 70,000 people require hospitalization for burns each year
   d. Approximately 12,000 people die each year from burns
   e. 66% of burn fatalities are in those at the ends of the life span
      i. Children younger than age 11 years and the elderly older than age 60 years constitute 22% of all those with burn injuries and account for 40% of all fire fatalities
      ii. Aging process makes older adults less able to respond to conventional therapy. Underlying organ dysfunction leads to a diminished compensatory response to burn injury and greater potential to develop MODS.

3. **Influences of gender on response to burns**
   a. Males are more commonly involved in serious burn injuries
   b. Males have a higher mortality rate than females after burns involving more than 30% of the total body surface area

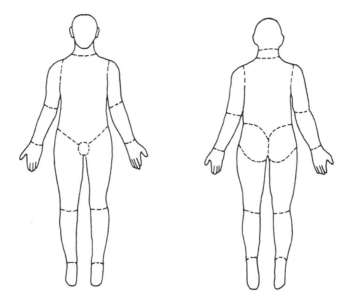

Lund and Browder chart								
Area	**Age (yr)**					**%**	**%**	**%**
	0–1	**1–4**	**5–9**	**10–15**	**Adult**	**2**	**3**	**Total**
Head	19	17	13	10	7			
Neck	2	2	2	2	2			
Ant. Trunk	13	17	13	13	13			
Post. Trunk	13	13	13	13	13			
R. Buttock	$2\frac{1}{2}$	$2\frac{1}{2}$	$2\frac{1}{2}$	$2\frac{1}{2}$	$2\frac{1}{2}$			
L. Buttock	$2\frac{1}{2}$	$2\frac{1}{2}$	$2\frac{1}{2}$	$2\frac{1}{2}$	$2\frac{1}{2}$			
Genitalia	1	1	1	1	1			
R.U. Arm	4	4	4	4	4			
L. U. Arm	4	4	4	4	4			
R.L. Arm	3	3	3	3	3			
L.L. Arm	3	3	3	3	3			
R. Hand	$2\frac{1}{2}$	$2\frac{1}{2}$	$2\frac{1}{2}$	$2\frac{1}{2}$	$2\frac{1}{2}$			
L. Hand	$2\frac{1}{2}$	$2\frac{1}{2}$	$2\frac{1}{2}$	$2\frac{1}{2}$	$2\frac{1}{2}$			
R. Thigh	$5\frac{1}{2}$	$6\frac{1}{2}$	$8\frac{1}{2}$	$8\frac{1}{2}$	$9\frac{1}{2}$			
L. Thigh	$5\frac{1}{2}$	$6\frac{1}{2}$	$8\frac{1}{2}$	$8\frac{1}{2}$	$9\frac{1}{2}$			
R. Leg	5	5	$5\frac{1}{2}$	6	7			
L. Leg	5	5	$5\frac{1}{2}$	6	7			
R. Foot	$3\frac{1}{2}$	$3\frac{1}{2}$	$3\frac{1}{2}$	$3\frac{1}{2}$	$3\frac{1}{2}$			
L. Foot	$3\frac{1}{2}$	$3\frac{1}{2}$	$3\frac{1}{2}$	$3\frac{1}{2}$	$3\frac{1}{2}$			
					Total			

FIGURE 9-6 ■ The Lund and Browder chart is used to assess and graphically document size and depth of the burn wound. (From Wiegand DJL-M, Carlson KK: *AACN procedure manual for critical care*, ed 5, Philadelphia, 2005, Saunders, p 1055.)

    c. Females between the ages of 30 and 59 years have an increased adjusted risk of death compared to men in the same age group, regardless of burn severity and size (O'Keefe, Hunt, and Purdue, 2001)

    d. There are no gender-related differences in mortality among young patients or elderly patients (O'Keefe et al, 2001)

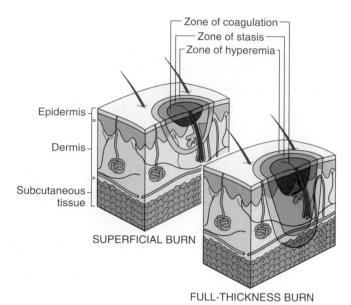

FIGURE 9-7 ■ Concentric zones of hyperemia, stasis, and coagulation within a burn.

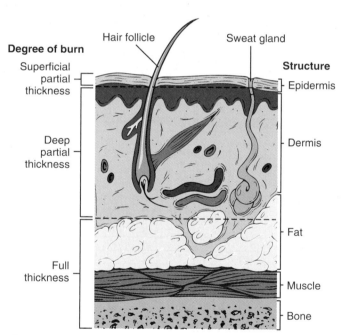

FIGURE 9-8 ■ Cross section of human skin demonstrating burn classification by depth.

4. **Cellular pathophysiology:** Cellular injury occurs when tissues are exposed to an energy source (thermal, chemical, electrical, radiation); responses are both local and systemic
   a. Local response: Coagulation of cellular proteins, which leads to irreversible cell injury with local production of complement, histamine, and oxygen free radicals

      i. Activation of complement (particularly C5a) and histamine release lead to increased vascular permeability

         (a) C5a attracts neutrophils to the area

         (b) Neutrophil activation leads to a respiratory burst with increased metabolism and production of oxygen free radicals

     ii. Creation of oxygen free radicals (by-products formed during oxidative processes; independent molecules with positive or negative charges) such as superoxide or hydroxyl; produce tissue injury

         (a) Attach to electrons from cell lipids and proteins to alter the integrity of the cell membrane and endothelium in the microvascular circulation, which leads to edema

            (1) Pulmonary vascular injury, pulmonary interstitial edema, and intraalveolar hemorrhage

            (2) RBC lysis and intravascular hemolysis

         (b) Alter the structure of DNA and prevent the repair of the genetic code; may lead to total cell destruction

b. Systemic response: Initiation of SIRS with the release of mediators (see Systemic Inflammatory Response Syndrome and Septic Shock and Table 9-1 for a list of mediators and cytokines)

      i. Burn injury causes the release of vasoactive substances, such as histamine, prostaglandins, interleukins, arachidonic acid metabolites, bradykinin, and serotonin

     ii. Some experts suggest that bacterial translocation may occur (see Systemic Inflammatory Response Syndrome and Septic Shock)

    iii. Stress hormones are produced: Release of cortisol, glucagon, and epinephrine

c. Consequences of local and systemic responses

      i. Fluid shift from blood into the interstitial and intracellular spaces as the injured tissue releases mediators that cause increased vascular permeability

         (a) Systemic response occurs when the burn covers 20% or more of the total body surface area

         (b) Sodium-rich fluid and plasma proteins are lost into the interstitium; most evident in the first 12 hours after injury

            (1) Decreased capillary oncotic pressure

            (2) Increased interstitial oncotic pressure

         (c) Tissue edema is often associated with airway instability, respiratory failure, limb ischemia, and compartment syndromes (increased pressure within an anatomic compartment that compromises the perfusion, viability, and function of the associated tissues)

         (d) Usually leads to hemoconcentration, increased hematocrit, and increased blood viscosity

     ii. Decreased intravascular volume; decreased blood flow to the skin, kidneys, and the gastrointestinal tract

         (a) Compensatory increase in systemic vascular resistance

         (b) Decreased cardiac output

         (c) Further decrease in organ perfusion

    iii. Uncorrected response

         (a) Hypovolemic shock

         (b) Anaerobic metabolism: Metabolic acidosis develops; decreased adenosine triphosphate to fuel the sodium-potassium pump, which results in increased intracellular sodium and water, and decreased intracellular potassium, magnesium, and phosphate

(c) Hyperkalemia from cellular lysis and as a complication of metabolic acidosis

(d) Delayed resuscitation increases the risk for the development of abdominal compartment syndrome; patient presentation consists of abdominal distension, declining urine output, hypotension, and decreasing pulmonary compliance

iv. Burn hypermetabolism: Increased oxygen consumption, negative nitrogen and potassium balance, excessive muscle wasting, glucose intolerance, hyperinsulinemia, insulin resistance, sodium retention, and peripheral leukocytosis

v. Specific changes in organ systems other than the skin

(a) Immune: SIRS

(b) Neurologic: Mental status changes (agitation, confusion) may occur in the presence of hypoxia or hypovolemia

(c) Cardiovascular

(1) Initial: Tachycardia, increased BP, decreased cardiac output, and hypovolemia. BP can be a relatively insensitive indicator of moderate fluid changes because catecholamine release raises BP and thereby masks the signs of inadequate organ and tissue perfusion.

(2) After 24 hours: Increased cardiac output from hypermetabolism

(d) Pulmonary

(1) Pulmonary hypertension; vascular and perivascular inflammation

(2) Microvascular leak with interstitial pulmonary edema (ARDS) and ventilation-perfusion mismatch

(3) Changes with smoke inhalation (Table 9-5)

(e) Gastrointestinal

(1) Delayed peristalsis and possible development of ileus due to SNS response

(2) Decreased albumin production

(f) Renal

(1) Decreased renal perfusion and ischemic injury

(2) Myoglobinuria from muscle damage, leading to obstructed renal tubules

5. **Classification of burn injury**

a. American Burn Association classification: See Table 9-6

b. Classification by depth

i. Superficial partial-thickness (formerly first-degree) burns

(a) Skin layer: Epidermal

(b) Appearance: Pink to red without blistering but there may be slight edema; blanching with pressure

(c) Discomfort: Uncomfortable to touch, but discomfort decreases as burn heals; itchy

(d) Healing: 3 to 5 days without scarring

ii. Moderate partial-thickness (formerly second-degree) burns

(a) Skin layer: Superficial dermal

(b) Appearance: Red or mottled and pink with blistering; skin moist and weeping; blanching with pressure

(c) Discomfort: Very painful

(d) Healing: Less than 3 weeks

iii. Deep partial-thickness (formerly second-degree) burns

(a) Skin layer: Deep dermal

■ **TABLE 9-5**
Chemical, Inhalational, and Electrical Injuries

Severity	Description	Reaction	Findings	Management
CHEMICAL				
Severity of injury depends on	Tissue injury and destruction from necrotizing substances	Cellular dehydration	Burning	Remove chemical from body contact; brush off chemical powders
1. Strength or concentration of chemical	1. *Strong acids (desiccants):* Sulfuric and muriatic acid, hydrofluoric acid	Denaturation	Discoloration	Flush chemical from wound with large amounts of saline or water for at least 15 min; flush eyes for 30 min
2. Length of contact	2. *Alkalis:* Lime (cement), ammonia, caustics (sodium hydroxide, potassium hydroxide)	Oxidation	Tissue degeneration; injury to skin and underlying structures continues until chemical is removed or inactivated	Remove all clothing and discard
3. Quantity of chemical	3. *Corrosives:* Phenol, lye, white phosphorus	Chemical coagulation of protein	Localized pain and edema	Do not rub skin; blot or brush off with a washcloth
4. Extent of tissue penetration	4. *Oxidizing agents:* Chromic acid, potassium permanganate	Precipitation of chemical compounds in cell	Systemic effects depend on substance	Cover all burned areas with dry sterile dressings until appropriate burn care is instituted
5. Mode of chemical's action	5. *Vesicants:* Dimethyl sulfoxide, chemical warfare agents (gases)	Protoplasmic poisoning	Alkali injuries cause marked edema and fluid loss	
	6. *Protoplasmic poisons:* Formic acid, tannic acid, hydrochloric acid			

Continued

■ **TABLE 9-5**
Chemical, Inhalational, and Electrical Injuries—cont'd

Severity	Description	Reaction	Findings	Management
INHALATIONAL				
Inhalation of hot air, steam, or noxious chemicals causes thermal damage, asphyxiation, and irritation to the respiratory tract	Carbon monoxide inhalation	Carbon monoxide is produced by incomplete burning of materials; displaces oxygen from hemoglobin because hemoglobin has a 200 times higher affinity for carbon monoxide than for oxygen	Cherry-red skin Hypoxia leading to anoxia Elevated carboxyhemoglobin (COHb) level: Normal is 5% for nonsmokers and less than 10% for smokers Exposure levels of 30% to 40% or more COHb cause significant neurologic effects (syncope, severe headache, visual disturbances) Xenon-ventilation-perfusion scan may be used to detect inhalation injury in lower airways and terminal bronchioles	Administer warmed, humidified 100% oxygen Determine COHb level Administer bronchodilators Provide for postural drainage Perform intubation, mechanical ventilation, and bronchoscopy as appropriate Hyperbaric oxygenation therapy is controversial; may be considered if COHb >25% and patient is hemodynamically stable (accelerates dissociation of COHb from hemoglobin)
	Inhalation above glottis: Hot air, steam, smoke (injury usually thermally produced)	Mucosal burns of oropharynx and larynx Injury and swelling	Redness, blistering, edema Risk for upper airway obstruction Facial burns, singed hair, circumoral or neck burns Sooty or gray mucus Smoky breath Hoarseness or stridor, dyspnea	Remove patient from smoky or toxic environment Maintain patent airway Provide humidified oxygen Elevate head of bed

Inhalation below glottis (injury usually chemically instead of thermally produced)	Exposure to toxic fumes or smoke leads to acute respiratory distress syndrome (ARDS) Toxins damage type II pneumocytes and decrease surfactant production Epithelial sloughing with bronchitis occurs 6 to 72 hr after burn injury	Respiratory distress Dyspnea Decreased lung compliance Severe hypoxemia Ventilation, perfusion imbalances	See Chapter 2 for ARDS
ELECTRICAL Severity of injury depends on 1. *Amperage:* Amount of electric current 2. *Voltage:* Measure of force of flow of current 3. *Type of current:* Alternating or direct 4. *Duration of contact:* Longer contact causes more injury 5. *Surface area of contact:* Larger surface area causes greater injury 6. *Tissue resistance:* High resistance (skin, bone, fat) versus low resistance (blood vessels, nerves, organs) 7. *Current's course in body*	Injury caused by intense heat generated from electrical current or lightning Coagulation necrosis Direct damage to nerves and vessels Tissue anoxia and cell death Asphyxiation caused by tetany of muscles of respiration or respiratory arrest Long bone or vertebral fractures from tetanic contractions of muscles Muscle destruction	White, charred skin; leathery skin Odor of burned skin Decreased or absent pain Cardiac dysrhythmias (ventricular fibrillation, asystole) Entrance and exit wounds with degree of damage greater than is visible Contraction of skeletal muscles Changes in vision, seizure activity, paralysis	Patient should be removed by trained personnel Turn off electrical source Initiate basic life support to maintain airway, breathing, and circulation Administer humidified oxygen Monitor cardiac rhythm Cover entry and exit wounds with dry sterile dressings

■ **TABLE 9-6**
■ ■ **American Burn Association Burn Classification**

| Degree of Injury | Partial Thickness | | Full Thickness | Considerations |
	Adults	Children	Adults and Children	
Minor	<15%	<10%	<2%	Does not include burns to special areas, such as eyes, ears, face, hands, feet, or perineum Does not include people at high risk (people at extremes of age, those with inhalation injury or electrical injury, those with complex injuries, those with chronic illnesses) Can be treated on an outpatient basis
Moderate	15%–25%	10%–20%	<10%	Excludes special area burns as earlier Excludes high-risk patients as earlier Can be treated on an outpatient or inpatient basis, depending on severity and location
Major	>25%	>20%	>10%	Includes special area burns as earlier Includes high-risk patients as earlier Should be treated at specialized burn unit or burn center

Data from Johnson JY: Burns. In Swearingen PL, Keen JH, editors: *Manual of critical care nursing: nursing interventions and collaborative management*, ed 4, St Louis, 2001, Mosby.

(b) Appearance: Pink to pale ivory; wound may be dry with blisters or bullae; no blanching with pressure
(c) Discomfort: Pain response varies from severe to minimal
(d) Healing: Usually 3 to 6 weeks
iv. Full-thickness (formerly third-degree) burns
(a) Skin layer: Injury extends beneath the dermal layer to fat, muscle, and bone
(b) Appearance: White or red to brown or black; no blistering; with or without thrombosed vessels; dry, leathery, and hard; depressed if the underlying muscle is damaged
(c) Discomfort: Pain to superficial pinprick is absent, but deep aching pain occurs
(d) Healing: Longer than 1 month with grafting required
6. **Etiology and risk factors**
a. Factors associated with burns
i. Physical factors
(a) Age: Incidence highest in the elderly patient and in children younger than 2 years of age; children 2 to 5 years of age are also at risk
(1) Elderly (>65 years of age) may have poor vision, are at risk for overmedication, may have poor living conditions, or may smoke while using oxygen
(2) Very young patients (<5 years of age) lack an understanding of the consequences of their behavior, such as playing with fire or matches

        (b) Type of burn: Thermal, electrical, chemical, radiation

        (c) Preburn health status: Preexisting organ dysfunction or conditions (e.g., diabetes mellitus, chronic obstructive lung disease, heart failure, hypertension, renal insufficiency or failure) impair compensatory responses to burns

    ii. Environmental factors

        (a) Presence of fire escapes, smoke alarms, sprinkler systems, firewalls, fire extinguishers

        (b) Compliance with federal regulations on combustible and flammable products (nightclothes, plastic in airplanes)

   iii. Socioeconomic factors

        (a) Working in a high-risk occupation: Firefighters, construction workers, roofers, chemical workers, paving contractors, electricians or electrical line workers

        (b) Living in a poorly maintained home

        (c) Living in areas where arson is a problem

    iv. Personality and psychologic factors: Risk-taking behaviors, antisocial behavior, mental illness, depression, poor judgment, inadequate child care, geriatric abuse or neglect

        (a) Burns are sometimes associated with physical abuse (cigarette burns, burns from curling irons, scaldings)

        (b) Burns may occur when young children are inadequately supervised

           (1) Playing with matches or lighters

           (2) Setting of fireworks

           (3) Kitchen accidents: Boiling water, stoves

           (4) Bathroom accidents: Hot water in a bathtub

        (c) Burn may be a suicide gesture or attempt

    v. Alcohol and other drugs of abuse (see Multisystem Trauma): People who use alcohol often smoke; intoxication increases the risk for burns

    vi. Temporal factors

        (a) Most deaths from house fires occur during the winter

        (b) Injuries from fireworks and barbecue grills occur during the summer

b. Causes

    i. Thermal: Contact with flames or hot objects

        (a) House fires are responsible for 75% of all burn deaths, but most of these deaths are due to smoke inhalation or carbon monoxide poisoning

           (1) Causes of house fires: Cigarette smoking, malfunctioning heaters, propane tanks, electrical wiring

           (2) Only 5% of all burn victims have a thermal injury from house fires

        (b) Clothing ignition: Contact with flames

           (1) Responsible for 5% of all burn deaths (up to 75% in the elderly population)

           (2) Second leading cause of hospitalization, but rates are decreasing because of legislation requiring nonflammable clothing

    ii. Scalds: Contact with hot liquids or steam

        (a) Responsible for 3% of all burn deaths and 30% of burn hospital admissions

        (b) Often caused by hot water in bathtubs and showers and spillage of hot coffee

        (c) Children under age 4 years are most often affected

        (d) Elderly are susceptible because of fragile, thin skin

    iii. Chemical: Contact with caustic or toxic chemicals, leading to coagulation of tissue protein, precipitation of chemical compounds in cells, cellular dehydration, and protoplasmic poisoning

        (a) Home: Cleaning agents

        (b) Industry: Explosions and contact with chemicals

        (c) Chemical agents

            (1) Oxidizing agents: Cause tissue oxidation (e.g., potassium permanganate)

            (2) Corrosive agents: Cause tissue denaturation (loss of normal properties of cellular proteins) (e.g., phenol, lye, white phosphorus)

            (3) Desiccants: Cause severe cellular dehydration (e.g., sulfuric acid)

            (4) Vesicants: Cause blistering (e.g., dimethyl sulfoxide, poisonous gases used in warfare)

            (5) Protoplasmic poisons: Cause cellular coagulation (e.g., acetic acid, tannic acid, oxalic acid)

  iv. Electrical: Contact with an electrical current or flash caused by electrical arcing

        (a) Cause approximately 1000 deaths per year

        (b) Most common in summer: Lightning; electrocution in homes, on farms, or in industrial locations

        (c) Household: Hair dryers and wall sockets

        (d) Industrial: Electrical transmission lines

        (e) Toddlers at risk for biting on electrical cords or putting objects into electrical outlets

  v. Radiation: Exposure to ionizing radiation (alpha and beta particles, gamma rays, X-rays), either inadvertent or due to a catastrophic disaster or accident

        (a) Long-term biologic effect, which results in chronic health concerns

        (b) Intracellular destruction of DNA, loss of genetic information

        (c) Acute injury symptoms similar to the early symptoms of thermal injury (pain, swelling, redness, tissue ischemia); several weeks may pass before symptoms appear

Patient Assessment

1. Nursing history

  a. Complete description of the burn injury

    i. Time: Delay of treatment may result in a minor or moderate burn's becoming a major injury

    ii. Location: Closed-space injuries are related to smoke inhalation

    iii. Context or situation: Falling asleep while smoking; pulling boiling water off a stove; occupational exposure

    iv. Burning agent, temperature of agent, length of exposure; determine if an odor or visible airborne substance was present, as well as the quality and intensity of the odor or visible substance

    v. Actions of witnesses

  b. Suspicion of physical abuse: If abuse is suspected, obtain in-depth information. Factors that raise suspicion include the following:

    i. Delay in seeking treatment

    ii. Burns not consistent with the reported history

    iii. Bruising at different stages of healing

    iv. Reports of the burn differ among household members

    v. History of previous injury

    c. Past medical and surgical health history, with particular emphasis on organ malfunction: Heart failure, hypertension, chronic obstructive pulmonary disease, diabetes mellitus, and renal failure

    d. Substance use and abuse: Detailed history of smoking, use of alcohol and other drugs of abuse

    e. Family and social history: Household members and relationships; household and child care responsibilities; occupation, education, and job status; financial situation and insurance coverage; religion

    f. Allergies, current medications

2. Nursing examination of patient

    a. Physical examination data

      i. Primary survey: Rapid assessment (30 seconds to 2 minutes) that simultaneously identifies and manages life-threatening injuries

        (a) ABCDEF (See Multisystem Trauma for assessments and interventions): *A*irway; *B*reathing; *C*irculation; and *D*isability; *E*xposure, evaluation, and emergency, life-saving interventions; and *F*luid resuscitation

        (b) Interventions that should take place for exposure

          (1) Remove burning clothing to stop further injury and inspect all skin surfaces

          (2) Cover the patient with dry sterile dressings to prevent heat loss; wet dressings compromise an already impaired temperature regulation, and the lower temperature further complicates resuscitation efforts

      ii. Burn-specific secondary survey: This survey compliments the trauma secondary survey and includes a complete head-to-toe assessment to identify accompanying traumatic injuries, such as fractures, internal hemorrhage, and head injury; details of this survey include neurologic, otolaryngologic, chest, cardiac, abdomen, genitourinary, and extremity assessments, and radiography and laboratory studies (discussed later); usually takes place in an intensive care or burn unit. *Note:* Ongoing resuscitation continues during the secondary survey as needed.

        (a) Neurologic: Assess for significant anoxic or carbon monoxide injury, address pain and anxiety; a decreased level of consciousness may also be related to drugs, alcohol, pain medications, hypoxia, or hypotension

        (b) Otolaryngologic and ophthalmologic: Evaluate the external ear and cornea for injury; fluorescein staining may be needed to detect subtle eye injury

        (c) Chest: Ensure adequate oxygenation and ventilation; treat bronchospasm with bronchodilators; if circumferential chest burns are present, an escharotomy may be required to adequately ventilate; suspect inhalation injury if one or more of the following are present: Odor of smoke, burns of the intraoral cavity, cough, hoarseness, expiratory wheezes, chest pain, shortness of breath, singed nasal hair, circumoral burns, and blackened, carbonaceous sputum

        (d) Abdomen: Evaluate torso compliance to exclude abdominal compartment syndrome; hallmarks of compartment syndrome are the inability to ventilate and decreasing urine output despite aggressive resuscitation

        (e) Genitourinary: Considerations include attention to the foreskin following catheter insertion to prevent the development of paraphimosis with edema of the soft tissue

(f) Extremities: Monitoring of perfusion is paramount; early identification of the loss of perfusion, sensation, and/or movement is vital to detecting compartment syndrome

(g) Miscellaneous: Determine the presence of electrical or chemical injury, ascertain tetanus immune status, and evaluate whether abuse is a possibility

iii. Inspection of the burn: See classification by depth

(a) Location: Severity is increased for burns on the hands, face, eyes, ears, feet, and genitalia

(b) Appearance: Color, consistency, and changes in vessels

(c) Depth: Severity depends on the intensity and duration of the exposure

(d) Extent: Percentage of the body surface area involved; severity depends on the intensity and duration of exposure

(e) Considerations

(1) Check for current entry and exit sites for electrical burns. There may be small entry and exit sites but large areas of injury lying underneath the skin ("iceberg effect"). Internal damage may not be evident for hours or days.

(2) Monitor for increased swelling and edema, which may lead to airway obstruction or compartment syndrome

(3) Depth and severity of a burn may not be evident until several days after the initial injury

iv. Palpation, percussion, and auscultation of body systems to monitor for multisystem effects of an injury and inflammatory response (see Multiple Organ Dysfunction Syndrome and Multisystem Trauma)

b. Monitoring data

i. Vital signs: Widely variable depending on the catecholamine stress response, burn severity, and medication therapy

(a) Serial measurement of vital signs: Essential to monitor the response to burns and to interventions

(b) Respiratory rate

(1) Ideal: 12 to 20 breaths/min

(2) Typical following major burns: Tachypnea

(3) Absence of tachypnea following a major burn indicates CNS suppression (due to alcohol or other drugs of abuse) or injury, airway obstruction, and restricted chest excursion from injured skin

a) Monitor for edema of neck and airway

b) Monitor for circumferential eschar formation around the neck or chest

c) Monitor for signs of obstruction: Stridor, hoarseness, restlessness, behavior changes, and decreased level of consciousness

(c) Heart rate

(1) Ideal: 60 to 100 beats/min

(2) Typical following burn: Tachycardia

a) Well-conditioned athletes and patients taking β-adrenergic or calcium channel blockers have slow heart rates

b) Electrical burns may lead to dysrhythmias (ventricular fibrillation, asystole)

c) Patient may have decreased or absent peripheral pulses or delayed capillary refill

(d) BP

(1) Ideal: Systolic pressure above 90 mm Hg

(2) Typical following burns: Variable, depending on fluid loss and the patient's age, but hypotension often present

(3) Young adults may maintain BP in spite of significant fluid losses

(4) Older adults have less compensatory mechanisms and less tolerance for fluid deficits

(5) Alcohol intoxication may lead to either hypotension or hypertension

(e) Temperature

(1) Ideal: Core temperature above 98.6° F (37° C)

(2) Typical following burns: Decreased core temperature of 95° to 98.6° F (35° to 37° C) because of exposure or loss of heat from open wounds

(3) Hyperthermia may develop because of increased tissue metabolism and infection

(f) Pain: See Systemic Inflammatory Response Syndrome and Septic Shock

(g) Hemodynamics and urinary output: Generally a PA catheter is not used during initial burn resuscitation; urine output is more commonly used to determine the success of fluid resuscitation; the PA catheter may be used if there is failure to resuscitate

(1) Ideal: Urine output above 1 ml/kg/hour

(2) Typical following burns: Decreased urine output

3. **Appraisal of patient characteristics:** An 82-year-old female who lives alone in an apartment falls asleep while watching television. Her cat leaps onto the mantle, knocking a burning candle into the live Christmas tree, which ignites. Neighbors notice smoke coming from the window and call 911, but are unable to enter the apartment. Within 5 minutes of their arrival, firefighters rescue the patient. The patient suffers burns over 60% of her body (40% partial thickness, 20% full thickness) and severe smoke inhalation. Prehospital care providers intubate the patient and begin transport to a regional burn center. During transport, the patient is difficult to oxygenate and ventilate, hemodynamically unstable, and unconscious. Her family soon arrives at the hospital and offers strong support for the patient. Following a conference with the attending physician, the family verbalizes an understanding of the patient's critical status and the gravity of the situation. The patient succumbs to her injuries within 24 hours of her arrival at the hospital.

   a. Resiliency (level 1—*minimally resilient*): Based on age, extent of injury

   b. Vulnerability (level 1—*highly vulnerable*): Integrity of the pulmonary and integumentary system is destroyed

   c. Stability (level 1—*minimally stable*): Patient is hemodynamically unstable, requiring aggressive, ongoing life-sustaining support (aggressive fluid resuscitation, pressure-control ventilation, thermal control, vasopressors)

   d. Complexity (level 1—*highly complex*): Based on multisystem insult, advanced age

   e. Resource availability (level 5—*many resources*): Patient has strong support from a well-educated family, Medicare and supplemental insurance coverage

   f. Participation in care (level 1—*no participation* for patient): Based on the severity of the patient's condition and the rapidity of her decline; the family is having difficulty coping with the situation; the daughter is especially overwhelmed with guilt because the patient was supposed to move in with her within the next 2 months; if the patient had already relocated, this event might have been avoided

   g. Participation in decision making (level 5—*full participation*): Family shows an understanding of the criticality of the event and the probable poor patient outcome

    h. Predictability (level 5—*highly predictable*): Based on known high morbidity and mortality rates given the patient's advanced age and burn severity

4. Diagnostic studies

  a. Laboratory

    i. ABG levels

      (a) Respiratory alkalosis with a Pa_{CO_2} below 35 mm Hg may occur early because of tachypnea

      (b) Metabolic acidemia with a pH below 7.34 occurs after major burns

        (1) pH usually returns to normal with the correction of fluid deficit and the correction of low cardiac output states

        (2) Base deficit is typical

      (c) Metabolic acidosis also occurs with topical application of mafenide acetate (Sulfamylon) over a large burn

      (d) In severe burns and inhalation injuries, a progressive increase in the fraction of inspired oxygen is needed to maintain Pa_{O_2} and arterial oxygen saturation (Sa_{O_2})

    ii. Carboxyhemoglobin (COHb) level: More than 10% is diagnostic of carbon monoxide poisoning (see Table 9-5). Absence of COHb does not rule out inhalation injury.

    iii. CBC and differential

      (a) Postburn period is associated with leukocytosis (increased WBC count, as high as 30,000/mm^3; usually resolves in 48 hours)

      (b) Leukopenia may occur as a side effect of topical treatment with silver sulfadiazine or due to SIRS

      (c) Local heat may lead to RBC destruction; however, usually increased hematocrit due to hemoconcentration and "third-spacing" occurs

      (d) Thrombocytopenia may occur during the first 72 hours as a result of dilution and some microvascular thromboses

    iv. Nutritional parameters

      (a) Serum glucose levels: Elevated from the stress response

      (b) Total protein and albumin levels: Decreased because of protein loss from increased vascular permeability

    v. Electrolyte levels

      (a) Hyperkalemia due to tissue destruction, RBC hemolysis, and increased intracellular sodium concentration from osmotic changes

      (b) Sodium imbalance

        (1) Hypernatremia resulting from intravascular fluid loss and hemoconcentration

        (2) Hyponatremia resulting from sodium loss and hemodilution

    vi. Coagulation studies: Elevations in PT and PTT during the first 3 days after burn injury because of the leakage of clotting factors from the intravascular space

    vii. Blood alcohol level and drug toxic screen to identify

      (a) Circumstances of the burn injury

      (b) Risk of withdrawal

      (c) Complications of substance use

    viii. BUN level often is elevated because of increased tissue and RBC destruction and dehydration; creatinine level is normal unless acute renal failure is occurring

    ix. Wound specimen cultures and wound biopsy as ordered to isolate infectious source

b. Radiologic

    i. Chest radiograph may be normal early in the patient's course; bilateral patchy infiltrates suggest developing pneumonitis

    ii. Helical CT may be useful for patients with possible blunt injuries of the head, neck, chest, abdomen, or pelvis

c. Laryngoscopy (with upper airway involvement) and/or bronchoscopy (with lower airway involvement) may be necessary in suspected cases of inhalation injury

Patient Care

1. **Potential for airway compromise:** See Chapter 2

  a. Description of problem: Secretions and obstruction from airway edema

  b. Additional interventions

    i. Monitor for carbonaceous sputum, hoarseness, and stridor

    ii. Maintain the airway with an oral or nasal airway or jaw lift and chin thrust. *Note:* Keep the patient's head in a neutral position until the cervical spine has been determined to be without injury, or maintain intubation as needed.

2. **Impaired oxygenation and ventilation:** See Chapter 2 and additional interventions in Table 9-5

  a. Description of problem: Inflammatory process, decreased lung expansion, tracheobronchial obstruction, and alveolar-capillary membrane changes

  b. Additional interventions

    i. Institute low-volume ventilation (5 to 8 ml/kg)

    ii. Institute intravenous pain control measures rapidly

    iii. Avoid overly aggressive fluid resuscitation, which can lead to increasing pulmonary and peripheral edema

    iv. Monitor for the formation of inelastic eschar on the upper chest and neck, which impedes adequate respiratory excursion

    v. Monitor intraabdominal pressures if intraabdominal hypertension is suspected in the presence of decreasing pulmonary compliance

3. **Intravascular volume depletion:** See Chapter 3

  a. Additional interventions (Table 9-7)

    i. Control any bleeding with pressure

    ii. Use large-bore peripheral catheters or central trauma catheters to initiate rapid fluid resuscitation

    iii. Use an accepted formula to calculate fluid replacement needs

      (a) Do not overresuscitate with fluids

      (b) Use hourly urinary output values to guide fluid replacement, with a goal of more than 1 ml/kg/hr of urinary output

4. **Infection and exaggerated inflammatory process:** See Chapter 7

5. **Inadequate primary defenses:** See Chapter 7

  a. Additional interventions

    i. Administer tetanus toxoid as prescribed

    ii. Initial débridement: Wash the surface of the wound with a mild soap or antiseptic solution

    iii. Débride the devitalized tissue

    iv. Cover the wound with antibacterial agents and absorbent gauze

    v. Maintain hand-washing and isolation techniques as appropriate

6. **Altered thermoregulation:** See Systemic Inflammatory Response Syndrome and Septic Shock and Hypothermia

■ **TABLE 9-7**
■ ■ **Phases of Burn Care Management**

Phase	Goals	Management Considerations

EMERGENT
Resuscitative phase:
  Lasts 48-72 hr after injury or until diuresis takes place
	Maintain airway, breathing, and circulation
	Maintain excretory function
	Preserve joint function and mobility
	Prevent complications
	Preserve self-concept
		1. Endotracheal intubation and mechanical ventilation if needed
		2. Fluid resuscitation (formulas vary)
		  a. Standard formula is usually a balanced salt solution, such as lactated Ringer's solution or normal saline: (4 ml) × (% burn) equals volume per 24 hr; 50% is given in first 8 hr, 25% in second 8 hr, and 25% in third 8 hr
		  b. Electrolyte replacement based on laboratory results
		3. Intravenous medication for pain and anxiety management
		4. Wound care and ongoing débridement
		  a. Wash burn surface with mild soap; rinse; apply appropriate topical antimicrobial (silver sulfadiazine, aqueous 0.5% silver nitrate, and 5% or 11.1% mafenide acetate cream); cover wounds with sterile dry sheets
		  b. Immerse minor burns in normal saline solution at 131° F (55° C)
		5. Nutritional support (often enteral by nasoduodenal route)

ACUTE/WOUND COVERAGE *Acute phase:* Characterized by eschar separation; lasts until spontaneous healing of burn wound occurs or until grafts are in place (variable time period lasting weeks to months)	Perform early excision of eschar and grafting Provide wound coverage; may use allograft if autograft is not available Prevent complications (sepsis, cardiovascular collapse)	1. Maintenance of hydration and electrolyte balance (monitor for decreased potassium and sodium) 2. Wound cleansing with bedside shower or shower tables 3. Ongoing débridement followed by topical application of antimicrobial agents (silver sulfadiazine, mafenide acetate, silver nitrate) 4. Skin grafting 5. Ongoing pain management, emotional support, nutritional support, occupational and physical therapy
CONVALESCENT/REHABILITATIVE Time period for inpatient rehabilitation	Promote return (functionally and cosmetically) to usual roles and responsibilities Support patient in adapting emotionally to burn injury Encourage maximum function of body parts	Ongoing pain management, emotional support, nutritional support, occupational and physical therapy, speech therapy if needed

7. **Exposure**
   a. Additional interventions
      i. Do not cover large burns with saline-soaked dressings, which lower core temperature
      ii. If the patient is hypothermic, maintain a warm ambient temperature; keep the patient covered
      iii. Limit traffic into the patient's room to prevent drafts
8. **Catabolic state resulting in malnutrition and hyperglycemia:** See Systemic Inflammatory Response Syndrome and Septic Shock; Chapter 8
   a. Additional interventions: Initiate glycemic control with intensive insulin therapy
9. **Altered tissue perfusion (peripheral):** See Chapter 3
10. **Fluid shifts**
    a. Additional interventions
       i. Remove constricting jewelry to limit tissue hypoperfusion
       ii. Monitor for the need of escharotomy (incision is made through an encircling eschar to release constricted tissue) or fasciotomy
          (a) Check peripheral pulses hourly and as needed, with a Doppler ultrasonographic examination if necessary
          (b) Notify the physician if capillary refill time is longer than 3 seconds or if numbness and tingling of the extremities or dusky extremities are present
11. **Altered patient and family coping:** See Chapter 10
    a. Additional interventions: If the patient is not being cared for in a burn center and is in need of transfer, explain the reasoning and support the family in the transport process

Hypothermia

SYSTEMWIDE ELEMENTS

Physiologic Anatomy

1. **Temperature regulation**
   a. Core temperature, the temperature of the deep tissues of the body, ranges between 97° and 99.5° F (36.1° and 37.5° C)
   b. Normal core temperature remains relatively constant, with a range of ±1° F (±0.6° C) during periods of health
   c. Body temperature is regulated by neural feedback mechanisms operating through temperature-regulating centers in the hypothalamus
      i. Anterior hypothalamic-preoptic area of the brain has large numbers of heat-sensitive neurons along with one third as many cold-sensitive neurons
      ii. Heat-sensitive neurons increase their rate of firing as the temperature rises, whereas cold-sensitive neurons increase their firing as the temperature drops
      iii. Temperature receptors to detect cold exist in the skin and deep tissues (spinal cord, abdominal viscera, great veins) and are thought to protect the body from low temperatures
      iv. Signals from peripheral receptors and temperature sensory signals from the anterior hypothalamic-preoptic area stimulate the posterior hypothalamus to control heat-producing and heat-conserving reactions
      v. When the body is too cold, the posterior hypothalamus control system institutes physiologic reactions

(a) Skin vasoconstriction caused by the stimulation of posterior hypothalamus SNS centers

(b) Piloerection ("goose flesh" or hairs standing on end): SNS stimulation causes arrector pili muscles attached to the hair follicles to contract

(c) Increased heat production by metabolic systems

(1) Shivering

a) Primary motor center for shivering is located in the dorsomedial portion of the posterior hypothalamus; this center is excited by cold signals from the skin and spinal cord when the body temperature falls below a critical value

b) Signals increase the tone of skeletal muscles; when the tone reaches a critical level, shivering begins, which increases body heat production to four times the normal level

(2) SNS stimulation: Chemical thermogenesis (production of heat) occurs with an increased release of norepinephrine and epinephrine, which raises the rate of cellular metabolism and heat production by 10% to 15%

(3) Thyroxine secretion

a) Hypothermia causes the release of thyrotropin-releasing hormone from the hypothalamus

b) Further stimulation of the release of thyroid-stimulating hormone and subsequent thyroxine production occur

c) Thyroxine causes chemical thermogenesis, but changes require several weeks because of the need for the thyroid gland to hypertrophy

d. Temperature set point in the hypothalamus

i. Core temperature of 98.8° F (37.1° C) is considered the set point; that is, all temperature control mechanisms continually attempt to bring the body temperature back to this level

ii. At temperatures above this level, the rate of heat loss is greater than the rate of heat production

iii. At temperatures below this level, the rate of heat production is greater than the rate of heat loss

e. Thermoneutral zone

i. Ambient temperature at which the basal rate of thermogenesis is sufficient to offset continuing heat loss; that is, 82.4° F (28° C)

ii. When the ambient temperature is below this point, the body increases heat production by combustion

2. **Physiology of hypothermia**

a. Definition: Core temperature below 95° F (35° C) (Table 9-8)

b. Once the body temperature falls below 93.2° F (34° C), the hypothalamus has an impaired ability to regulate temperature. At temperatures of 85° F (29.4° C) and below, the hypothalamus can no longer regulate temperature at all.

i. Failure is due partly to a loss of the ability to generate chemical heat production

ii. Failure also is due to sleepiness, progressing to coma, which depresses heat control mechanisms and shivering mechanisms

c. Once the body temperature falls below 77° F (25° C), ventricular fibrillation, asystole, and death occur

d. Mechanisms of heat loss

i. Radiation: Transfer of heat from warmer to cooler areas through the air without direct contact

■ **TABLE 9-8**
■ ■ **Classification of Hypothermia*†**

Classification	Range	Accompanying Physiologic Changes
Mild	<95°-89.6° F (<35°-32° C)	Relatively safe zone with depression of cerebral metabolism, confusion, faulty judgment, and amnesia; tachycardia, increased blood pressure, and increased cardiac output leading to progressive bradycardia and vasoconstriction; tachypnea progressing to decreased minute volume and bronchospasm; diuresis; increased preshivering muscle tone followed by shivering; paralytic ileus
Moderate	<89.6°-82.4° F (<32°-28.0° C)	Decreased level of consciousness, pupil dilation, hallucinations; decrease in pulse and cardiac output, prolonged systole, increased atrial and ventricular dysrhythmias, conduction disturbances, Osborne wave (hypothermic hump—secondary deflection in QRS in medial and lateral precordial leads and inferior leads, related to delayed ventricular depolarization and early ventricular repolarization, acidosis, and myocardial anoxia) on electrocardiogram; coagulopathies; hypoventilation, decreased carbon dioxide production, decreased oxygen consumption, absence of protective airway reflexes; decreased renal blood flow; hyporeflexia, diminished shivering, rigidity
Severe	<82.4°-68° F (<28°-20° C)	Decreased cerebral blood flow, coma; decreased cardiac output, hypotension, bradycardia, ventricular fibrillation; pulmonary edema, apnea; oliguria; 80% decrease in basal metabolism; decreased nerve conduction velocity, peripheral areflexia, hyperkalemia
Profound	<68°-57.2° F (<20°-14° C)	Asystole, isoelectric electroencephalogram, cell death
Deep	<57.2° F (<14° C)	Incompatible with life unless therapeutically induced

Data from Collins J: Hypothermia, *Practitioner* 239:22-26, 1995; American Heart Association, International Liaison Committee on Resuscitation: Guidelines 2000 for cardiopulmonary resuscitation and emergency cardiovascular care, *Circulation* 102(8 suppl):I229-I232, 2000; Danzl DF, Pozos RS: Accidental hypothermia, *N Engl J Med* 331:1756-1760, 1994; Fritsch DE: Hypothermia in the trauma patient, *AACN Clin Issues* 6:196-211, 1995; Gentilello LM: Advances in the management of hypothermia, *Surg Clin North Am* 75:243-256, 1995; Humbli EH, Demling RH: Hypothermia and cold-related injuries. In Ayers SM, editor: *Textbook of critical care*, ed 3, Philadelphia, 1995, Saunders; and Mecchem CC: Hypothermia and hyperthermia. In Lanken PN, Hanson CW, Manaker S, *The intensive care unit manual*, Philadelphia, 2001, Saunders.
*Multiple trauma is complicated by hypothermia. Some sources consider mild hypothermia for trauma patients to be a temperature of <96.8°-93.2° F (<36°-34° C), moderate hypothermia to be a temperature of <93.2°-89.6° F (<34°-32° C), and severe hypothermia to be a temperature of <89.6° F (<32° C).
†Advanced Cardiac Life Support guidelines classify mild hypothermia as 93.2°-96.8° F (34°-36° C), moderate hypothermia as 86°-93.2° F (30°-34° C), and severe hypothermia as <86° F (<30° C).

    (a) Normal radiation mechanism accounts for as much as 55% to 65% of the total heat loss in humans
    (b) Depends on the amount of skin exposed to the environment and the degree of vasodilation or vasoconstriction
    (c) Heat loss by radiation is limited by clothing and by warming of the environment
  ii. Conduction: Transfer of heat by direct contact with cool objects; accounts for approximately 15% of the body's heat loss
    (a) Heat loss is increased when the body is in contact with water, the ground, or metal

(b) Heat loss by conduction is limited by placing the body in contact with a poor heat conductor, such as wool

iii. Convection: Heat loss caused by the movement of gases or liquids over the skin (wind, fans, drafts). Liquids decrease the temperature internally or externally when the body is in contact with wet linens or during baths, irrigations, and blood transfusions.

iv. Evaporation: Transfer of heat from moist skin or mucous membranes into the atmosphere; accounts for approximately 30% of the heat loss

(a) Heat loss by evaporation is decreased if the skin is covered, but it increases with open wounds, wet skin, and increased respirations

(b) Evaporation increases in conditions of low humidity, high environmental temperature, and increased air flow

3. **Etiology and risk factors**

a. Predisposing factors

i. Environmental: Skin exposure, wet clothing, low outside temperature, and air movement (wind, drafts)

ii. Extremes of age: Infancy (<2 years), advanced age (>70 years)

iii. Disease states that decrease metabolism: Hypothyroidism, hypoadrenalism, malnutrition, hypoglycemia, circulatory shock, water intoxication

iv. Cutaneous disruptions: Wounds, burns

v. Hospital-associated causes: Exposure during an examination, fluid resuscitation, blood transfusion, immobilization, or surgery

vi. Medications and other substances: Alcohol, phenothiazines, hypnotics, anxiolytics, antidepressants, narcotics, neuromuscular blocking agents, anesthesia, oral hypoglycemics

b. Types of hypothermia

i. Accidental hypothermia: When an otherwise healthy person experiences overwhelming environmental cold. Examples: Outdoor accidents (associated with hiking, mountaineering, or skiing), cold water immersion, sleeping outdoors in winter (particularly by homeless people), multiple trauma leading to exposure to cold environmental conditions, falls, and immobilization indoors (particularly in the elderly).

ii. Primary hypothermia: Associated with an inherent defect of CNS control of thermoregulation. Examples: Diencephalic epilepsy, cerebrovascular accidents, head injuries, neoplasms, and degenerative diseases.

iii. Secondary hypothermia: Associated with an underlying disease process, multiple trauma, mental illness, a severe infection, and medication or substance use or abuse; can also be a type of accidental hypothermia

(a) Diseases: Hypothyroidism, hypopituitarism, malnutrition, myocardial infarction, vascular insufficiency, pancreatitis, uremia, and carcinoma

(b) Multiple trauma: Hypovolemic shock, burns, and near drowning

(c) Mental illness: Dementia, self-neglect

(d) Infection: Bacterial, viral, parasitic

(e) Medication and substance use as mentioned previously

iv. Induced hypothermia (IH): Controlled lowering of the core temperature for therapeutic reasons

(a) Mild to moderate IH: 89.6° to 93.2° F (32° to 34° C)

(b) Routinely used during operative procedures to reduce tissue oxygen and nutrient demands

(c) Optimal patient population

(1) Patients with anoxic neurologic injury

(2) Patients with major stroke

(3) Patients with traumatic brain injury

(d) Physiology
    (1) Following ischemic insult and reperfusion of the brain, IH acts by decreasing glutamate, glycerol, lactate, and pyruvate concentrations in the infarct area where tissue is at risk; these excitotoxic substances overstimulate neurons in the area of ischemic damage
    (2) IH decreases the adhesion of neutrophils in the ischemic tissue
    (3) Decrease in temperature by 1.8° F (1° C) results in a 6% to 7% decrease in cerebral metabolic rate
    (4) Oxygen supply to ischemic areas of the brain improves when blood flow increases subsequent to reduction of metabolic rate
    (5) Two additional potential benefits (mechanisms for these changes are unknown)
        a) Intracranial pressure is decreased with IH
        b) May act as an anticonvulsant

Patient Assessment

1. **Nursing history**
   a. Patient health history
      i. Current history of exposure or trauma, including the length of time of exposure and ambient or outdoor temperature
      ii. Significant past medical and surgical history, with a review of all major systems and of past traumatic injuries
   b. Relevant family history
   c. Social history
      (a) Living situation: Older people who live alone on limited incomes are at high risk for hypothermia during the winter or after falling
      (b) Alcohol use: Daily and weekly patterns
      (c) Outdoor activities, hobbies, and occupations
      (d) Relationships with significant others
      (e) Nutrition, daily patterns of eating, and ability to afford adequate nutrition
   d. Medication history: Prescribed and over-the-counter medications, particularly phenothiazines, hypnotics, anxiolytics, and antidepressants
2. **Nursing examination of patient** (see also Multisystem Trauma for guidelines on primary and secondary surveys)
   a. Physical examination data
      i. Inspection
      (a) Respiratory: Assess the adequacy of the airway and breathing. Expect tachypnea progressing to bradypnea, hypoventilation, and apnea; the more severe the hypothermia, the more depressed the respiratory drive and the higher the risk for inadequate maintenance of the airway and breathing.
      (b) Circulatory: Pallor and increased bleeding tendencies
      (c) Neurologic: Confusion, anxiety, and apathy progressing to a decreased level of consciousness, pupil dilation, and coma
      (d) Musculoskeletal: Increased preshivering muscle tone progressing to shivering and then rigidity
      (e) Renal: Cold-induced diuresis progressing to oliguria
      (f) Skin: Piloerection
      (g) Terminal burrowing behavior: Paradoxical reaction of severely hypothermic patients who undress and find a position of protection because of vasodilation and feelings of warmth

(1) Final mechanism of protection, with slowly developing lethal hypothermia

(2) Autonomous process of the brainstem; triggered in final, lethal hypothermia

  ii. Palpation

    (a) Circulatory: Weak, rapid pulses progressing to a slow or absent pulse, diminished capillary blanching, and cold skin

    (b) Gastrointestinal: Distention from paralytic ileus

    (c) Musculoskeletal: As shivering diminishes at lower temperatures, hyporeflexia occurs, followed by rigidity and finally peripheral areflexia

  iii. Percussion

    (a) Gastrointestinal: Increased tympany accompanied by upper abdominal distention indicates paralytic ileus

    (b) Respiratory: With severe hypothermia, dullness may indicate lung congestion and pulmonary edema

  iv. Auscultation

    (a) Circulatory: Rapid heart rate progressing to slow and then absent heart sounds; hypertension progressing to hypotension and an absence of BP

    (b) Respiratory: Decreased air flow, diminished or absent breath sounds, and crackles and gurgles from pulmonary congestion and pulmonary edema

    (c) Gastrointestinal: Diminished bowel sounds progressing to absent bowel sounds

b. Monitoring data

  i. Vital signs: Core temperature determines extent of hypothermia. *Note:* Measure core temperature with a PA thermistor if available; if no PA catheter is in place, use a rectal, urinary bladder, esophageal, or tympanic route. A difference of 1.8° to 3.6° F (1° to 2° C) may be found between esophageal, PA, rectal, and bladder temperature measurements. Whichever method is chosen should be used consistently to enhance precision.

    (a) Mild hypothermia is usually accompanied by

      (1) Tachycardia

      (2) Increased BP and cardiac output

      (3) Increased respirations

    (b) Moderate hypothermia is associated with

      (1) Bradycardia

      (2) Hypotension

      (3) Decreased cardiac output

    (c) Severe and profound hypothermia is associated with

      (1) Ventricular dysrhythmias

      (2) Asystole

      (3) Apnea

  ii. Pain: See Systemic Inflammatory Response Syndrome and Septic Shock

3. Appraisal of patient characteristics: A 26-year-old male driver who was not wearing a seatbelt is witnessed to have lost control of his automobile on a curve, which resulted in the car's being driven into an icy pond. A bystander pulls the victim out of the car after notifying emergency medical services. Emergency personnel arrive within 5 minutes of the motor vehicle accident. It is winter with an atmospheric temperature of 32° F (0° C). On the patient's admission to the emergency department, his core temperature is 92° F (33.3° C). Vital signs on admission are as follows: Heart rate, 70 beats/min; BP 100/60 mm Hg; respirations controlled by mechanical ventilation. Trauma laboratory testing reveals positive results on toxicology screens for amphetamines, barbiturates, and cocaine. Initial identified injuries include a frontal laceration and contusion diagnosed by CT of the head. Additional recognized injuries are fractures of right ribs 4, 5, and 6 with an associated hemothorax; grade II liver laceration; right complex humerus fracture; and right tibia-fibula fracture. Patient's long history of drug abuse has led to alienation from his family.

a. Resiliency (level 5—*highly resilient*): Based on age and minimal injury

b. Vulnerability (level 3—*moderately vulnerable*): Patient is hypothermic and recreational drugs are identified in the patient's system

c. Stability (level 3—*moderately stable*): Patient exhibits intermittent premature ventricular contractions and bradycardia

d. Complexity (level 1—*highly complex*): Patient has been in drug rehabilitation several times without resolution of his abuse problem

e. Resource availability (level 1—*few resources*): Patient is unemployed; has no health care resources and no automobile insurance; and is alienated from his family due to drug use

f. Participation in care (level 3—*moderate participation*): Depends on whether the patient will realize the extent of his problem and gain assistance in resolving issues

g. Participation in decision making (level 1—*no participation*): Patient confused, with loss of inhibitions and without knowledge of his surroundings; no family present

h. Predictability (level 1—*not predictable*): Depends on the patient's neurologic outcome

4. **Diagnostic studies**
   a. Laboratory
      i. ABG and derived hemodynamic parameters: Hypoxemia, hypocapnia progressing to hypercapnia, metabolic acidosis, and decreased oxygen delivery and consumption
      ii. Hematocrit: Increases approximately 2% for every 1.8° F (1° C) decrease in body temperature
      iii. Coagulation profile: PT and PTT may appear to be normal in spite of coagulopathies because tests are performed at 98.6° F (37° C) in the laboratory. At lower temperatures, decreased fibrinogen levels and thrombocytopenia may occur.
      iv. Serum electrolyte levels: Hypothermia masks ECG changes associated with hyperkalemia. Hyperkalemia and hyponatremia may occur with damage to the sodium–potassium–adenosine triphosphatase pump.
      v. Blood ethanol level: Blood or urine toxicity screen to detect the presence of alcohol or other drugs of abuse
      vi. BUN and creatinine levels: Elevated as renal function deteriorates
      vii. Urine myoglobin level: Elevated due to muscle damage from excessive shivering (rhabdomyolysis)
   b. ECG: Tachycardia progressing to bradycardia, atrial and ventricular dysrhythmias, asystole; conduction disturbances with prolonged PR, QRS, and QT intervals. At temperatures above 84.2° F (29° C), an Osborn or J wave (hypothermic hump) develops; secondary deflection in the QRS is best seen in medial and lateral precordial leads and inferior leads; hypothermia can simulate changes consistent with acute myocardial infarction or ischemia and can obscure expected ECG findings associated with hyperkalemia.

Patient Care

1. **Hypothermia**
   a. Description of problem: Decrease in body temperature caused by patient exposure to cold, inadequate clothing, evaporation from skin, or inactivity; core temperature below 95° F (35° C), shivering, cold skin, pallor, delayed capillary refill, tachycardia progressing to bradycardia, hypertension progressing to hypotension, piloerection
   b. Goals of care: Core temperature is 98.6° F (37° C) within 24 hours
   c. Collaborating professionals on health care team: Registered nurse, medical-surgical attending physician, respiratory therapist
   d. Interventions
      i. Institute passive rewarming (relies on endogenous heat generation and ambient temperature to increase the core body temperature slowly at a rate of 0.9° to 3.6° F [0.5° to 2°] C/hour) until normothermia is restored
         (a) Remove the patient from a cold environment
         (b) Remove wet clothing
         (c) Increase the ambient room temperature
         (d) Decrease the air flow in the room
         (e) Cover the patient with blankets; cover the patient's head
         (f) Passive rewarming is reserved for relatively healthy, mildly hypothermic (temperature >89.6° F [32° C]), and hemodynamically stable patients
      ii. Institute active rewarming using both external and internal methods (Table 9-9)
      iii. Monitor for afterdrop (decrease in core temperature of up to 3.6° F [2° C]) after internal active rewarming is discontinued. Occurs when blood circulates to peripheral tissues, recools, and returns to the body's core.
      iv. Monitor for rewarming shock (vascular collapse due to decreased cardiac output, hypotension, cardiac dysrhythmias); consequence of warming the periphery before the core
         (a) When the periphery is warmed before the core, cold, hyperkalemic, lactate-rich blood is shunted to the core of the body, which leads to shock
         (b) Limit rewarming to 3.6° F (2° C)/hr to decrease the risk of rewarming shock
      v. Teach preventive strategies to at-risk patients and staff caring for them
         (a) Limit exposure to cold temperatures
         (b) Maximize body coverage
         (c) Monitor the intake of cold or room-temperature fluids
   e. Evaluation of patient care
      i. Core temperature is 98.6° F (37° C)
      ii. Patient has no complications of rewarming (afterdrop, bleeding tendencies, or burns)

2. **Alcohol and drug intoxication**
   a. Description of problem: Core temperature below 95° F (35° C) with evidence of hypotension and alcohol or drug intoxication (assessment findings depend on the toxic substance—see Table 9-10; Toxin Ingestion)
   b. Goals of care
      i. Temperature returns to 98.6° F (37° C) within 24 hours
      ii. Patient experiences no symptoms of alcohol or substance withdrawal
   c. Collaborating professionals on health care team: See Infection and Exaggerated Inflammatory Process in the Patient Care section under Systemic Inflammatory Response Syndrome and Septic Shock

■ TABLE 9-9
■ ■ Interventions for Active Rewarming

Type of Rewarming	Intervention	Rationale and Discussion
ACTIVE EXTERNAL		
Use of a heat source outside the patient's body to raise the core body temperature; used in patients with temperatures between 89.6° F (32° C) and 93.2° F (34° C) and as an adjunct to active internal rewarming for temperatures <89.6° F (<32° C) Advantages: Works quickly, is inexpensive and readily available Disadvantage: Rewarms the periphery before the core	Fluid-circulating heating blanket	Heating blankets placed below the patient are in contact with the occiput, shoulder, presacral region, and heels, only 20%-30% of the body surface; place the blanket on top of the patient because the patient loses most heat through radiation and convection to the overlying air Warms by decreasing heat loss from radiation and convection Disadvantage: Burns at pressure points
	Convective air blanket	Creates an environment of 109.4° F (43° C) to prevent further heat loss into the environment through convection Blanket must cover a substantial portion of the patient's body (neck to toes) and borders must be fastened tightly Radiant blanket that increases the insulating capacity of standard blanket coverage
	Aluminum space blanket	Blanket must be wrapped closely around the patient with an additional standard blanket on top to minimize convective and conductive heat loss Patient's head must be covered with reflective material to decrease radiant heat loss
	Radiant warmer	Produces intense local heat close to the skin Disadvantage: May cause burns if there is not enough local circulation to carry heat away from the skin
ACTIVE INTERNAL		
Use of a heat source inside the patient's body to raise the core body temperature; used in the hospital for patients with core temperatures of <89.6° F (<32° C)	Airway rewarming	Humidified, warmed gases (107.6°-114.8° F [42°-46° C]) are often provided through an endotracheal tube via mechanical ventilation or through warmed gas delivered via a mask With airway rewarming, only a modest core temperature rise is achieved and an afterdrop occurs until body temperature begins to equilibrate with the surroundings
	Body cavity lavage	Irrigation of body cavities (peritoneal, pleural, mediastinal, bladder) with warmed solution raises body temperature an average of 3.6° F (2° C)/hr Gastric or colonic irrigations may also be used Potassium-free solution is used to prevent hyperkalemia

Continued

TABLE 9-9

Interventions for Active Rewarming—cont'd

Type of Rewarming	Intervention	Rationale and Discussion
ACTIVE INTERNAL—cont'd		

	Warm intravenous infusions	Disadvantages:
		   Peritoneal lavage may not be an option for patients with abdominal trauma or abdominal surgeries
		   Mediastinal lavage is associated with high morbidity because of the need for a median sternotomy
		   Infection is a risk
		Infusion of prewarmed fluids (109.4° F [43° C]) and blood products (98.6° F [37° C]) prevents further heat loss and helps correct hypothermia
		Methods to warm fluid include warm water baths, microwave device (treatment is controversial; do not use for blood products or dextrose-containing solutions), fluid warmers (may provide a flow too slow to correct fluid deficit), and rapid volume infusers
		Disadvantages:
		   Fluids must be used rapidly or will lose heat to the environment
		   If blood is warmed to a temperature >104° F (>40° C), cells will hemolyze
		   If the flow is too slow, the patient will be underresuscitated for hypovolemia
		Considerable expertise is needed to manage the techniques

	Extracorporeal circulatory rewarming	Continuous venovenous or arteriovenous rewarming uses the arterial (femoral) and venous (femoral or subclavian) pressure difference to create circulation through a heparin-bonded tubing circuit to a countercurrent fluid warmer
		Increases core temperature approximately 7.2° F (4° C)/hr
		Other techniques include extracorporeal venovenous rewarming and cardiopulmonary bypass
		Disadvantages:
		   Bleeding tendencies from heparin
		   High cost
		   Need for expertise in operation of high-technology equipment

■ **TABLE 9-10**
■ ■ **Symptoms and Toxic Ranges for Commonly Ingested Toxic Substances**

Substance	Therapeutic Level	Toxic Level	Vital Signs	Symptoms	Diagnostic Findings
Acetaminophen	10-20 mcg/ml	>150 mcg/ml at 4 hr; fatal hepatic necrosis can occur with 30-60 regular-strength tablets (10-20 g)	Normal (early), hypotension may be present	Anorexia, nausea, vomiting, diaphoresis, and malaise, followed by right upper quadrant abdominal pain and tenderness, bleeding	Abnormal results on liver function tests: AST, ALT, bilirubin levels, PT
Amphetamines	None	Varies by compound	β- and α-adrenergic toxidrome: Hypotension, tachycardia; hyperthermia, tachypnea	β- and α-adrenergic toxidrome: Mydriasis, diaphoresis, dry mucous membranes; hyperactivity, agitation, psychosis, paranoia, headache, hyperreactive reflexes, tremor, seizures, hyperactive bowel sounds, flushing	Increased CK levels: Rhabdomyolysis (from hyperthermia or agitation) ECG: Dysrhythmias; acidosis
Anticholinergics	Varies by compound	Varies by compound	Hallucinogenic toxidrome: Hyperthermia, labile blood pressure, circulatory collapse, tachycardia	Hallucinogenic toxidrome: Hallucinations, psychosis, panic, mydriasis Variable, ranging from anxiety, agitation, confusion, hyperactivity, seizures, and delirium to lethargy, decreased mental status, and coma	ECG: Tachycardia
Arsenic	<100 mcg/day	>100 mcg/day	Hypotension and tachycardia	Nausea, vomiting, abdominal pain, difficulty swallowing, diarrhea, dehydration	Elevated BUN and creatinine levels; ECG: Tachycardia and other dysrhythmias

Continued

■ **TABLE 9-10**
■ **Symptoms and Toxic Ranges for Commonly Ingested Toxic Substances—cont'd**

Substance	Therapeutic Level	Toxic Level	Vital Signs	Symptoms	Diagnostic Findings
Barbiturates (phenobarbital)	10-25 mcg/ml	>30 mcg/ml	Hypothermia, hypotension, and bradypnea progressing to apnea; bradycardia	Sedative-hypnotic toxidrome: Stupor and coma, confusion, slurred speech, apnea; ataxia, decreased reflexes, coma, blisters (bullae)	Hypercapnia; ECG: Tachycardia; hypoglycemia
Benzodiazepines (diazepam)	300-400 ng/ml	Unknown	With parenteral but not oral doses: Hypotension and bradypnea progressing to apnea	Sedative-hypnotic toxidrome: Stupor and coma, confusion, slurred speech, apnea; weakness, headache, and vertigo; diminished or absent bowel sounds, nausea, diarrhea, decreased reflexes	Hypercapnia (mild with oral doses)
Carbamazepine	6-12 mcg/ml	>15 mcg/ml	Hypotension, hypothermia, bradypnea, tachycardia	CNS stimulation, hallucinations, seizures, mydriasis, nystagmus	ECG: Tachycardia; leukopenia
Cocaine	None	Variable	β- and α-adrenergic toxidrome: Hypertension, tachycardia; hyperthermia, tachypnea to apnea	β- and α-adrenergic toxidrome: Mydriasis, diaphoresis, dry mucous membranes; hyperactivity, restlessness, anxiety, agitation, delirium, headache, nausea, vomiting, chest pain, seizures, coma	Increased CK levels; ECG: Tachycardia, ventricular fibrillation, ventricular tachycardia; acidosis
Cyclic antidepressants	Varies by compound	Varies by compound	Hypotension, tachycardia, bradypnea	Lethargy, confusion, dizziness, somnolence, seizures, coma	ECG: Prolonged QRS, dysrhythmias such as bundle branch blocks, torsades de pointes

Substance	Therapeutic level	Toxic level	Cardiovascular effects	Signs and symptoms	Laboratory findings
Cyanide	<1 mcg/ml	Blood level >0.5 mg/L Oral: 200 mg potassium cyanide; airborne: Immediately fatal at >270 ppm and life threatening at 110 ppm for 30 min	Variable but may follow pattern: First, hypertension and bradycardia; second, hypotension and tachycardia; third, hypotension and bradycardia; bradypnea and apnea	Smell of bitter almonds, anxiety, agitation, lethargy, headache, seizures, abdominal pain, vomiting, cherry-red color or cyanosis	ECG: Variable; acidosis with elevated lactate levels
Digoxin	0.8-2 ng/ml	>2.5 ng/ml	Hypotension, bradycardia, or tachycardia	Patient may be asymptomatic; nausea, vomiting, anorexia, visual changes (colored lights, blurred vision)	Hyperkalemia; ECG: Heart block, tachydysrhythmias, bradydysrhythmias
Ethanol	None	50-100 mg/dl	Bradycardia or tachycardia; hypertension or hypotension; hypothermia; tachypnea leading to apnea	Sedative-hypnotic toxidrome: Stupor and coma, confusion, slurred speech, apnea; agitation, released inhibitions progressing to depressed mental status, nausea, vomiting, ataxia, poor motor coordination, poor decision-making ability	Respiratory alkalosis progressing to respiratory acidosis; hyperosmolarity of blood
Ethylene glycol (antifreeze)	None	50-100 mg/dl	Hypertension, tachycardia, tachypnea	Decreased mental status, lethargy, seizures, slurred speech, coma; abdominal pain, nausea, vomiting	Hypoglycemia, metabolic acidosis, hypocalcemia, calcium oxalate crystals in urine
Iron	<100 mcg/dl	350 mcg/dl	Hypotension, tachycardia	Five stages of iron poisoning: Stage I—GI symptoms; stage II—GI symptoms improve; stage III—shock and acidosis; stage IV—hepatic necrosis; stage V—bowel obstruction	Hyperglycemia, leukocytosis, metabolic acidosis, and blood in stool and vomitus

Continued

■ TABLE 9-10
■ ■ Symptoms and Toxic Ranges for Commonly Ingested Toxic Substances—cont'd

Substance	Therapeutic Level	Toxic Level	Vital Signs	Symptoms	Diagnostic Findings
Isoniazid	3-5 mcg/ml 1 to 2 hr after dose	Variable	Tachycardia, hypotension, and hyperthermia	*Note:* One of the most common causes of drug-induced seizures in the United States; nausea, vomiting, dizziness, ataxia, hyperreflexia, slurred speech; hallucinations, seizures, coma, oliguria	Metabolic acidosis, hyperglycemia, leukocytosis, and eosinophilia; EEG monitoring may detect seizures
Isopropyl alcohol (rubbing alcohol)	None	Variable	Hypotension, bradypnea, and hypothermia	Ataxia, areflexia, dizziness, headache, muscle weakness, abdominal pain and cramping, gastritis, hematemesis, poor peripheral tissue perfusion	Ketones (in blood and urine) without acid-base disorder, hyperosmolarity of blood
Lead	<10 mcg/dl	>10 mcg/dl	Hypertension and tachycardia	Anorexia, constipation, abdominal pain, vomiting, lethargy, fatigue, hyper-activity, ataxia, seizures, coma, numbness and tingling of extremities	Anemia, abdominal radiographic changes, increased urinary coproporphyrin levels, hemolysis, proteinuria
Lithium	0.6-1.2 mEq/L	>2 mEq/L	Hypotension (late)	Weakness, fatigue, tremor, muscle twitching, ataxia, slurred speech, confusion, restlessness, hyperreflexia, stupor, coma, diuresis, dehydration, diarrhea	ECG: Prolonged QT interval, ST segment, and T wave abnormalities; if diabetes insipidus occurs: Increased serum osmolarity and decreased urine osmolarity

Continued

Mercury	<10 mcg/L	>35 mcg/L	Hypotension (late), tachypnea (inhaled mercury)	Tremor, ataxia, paresthesias, tunnel vision, dyspnea, increased salivation, diarrhea, abdominal pain	Proteinuria, increased BUN and creatinine levels
Methanol (antifreeze)	None	Variable	Hypotension, tachypnea, temperature variations	Visual disturbances, blindness, blurred vision, dimmed vision (snowstorm), inebriation, headache, dizziness, seizures, coma, nausea, vomiting, abdominal pain	Metabolic acidosis, hyperosmolarity, hypophosphatemia, elevated CK and amylase levels
Opioids	None	Variable	Narcotic toxidrome: Hypotension, bradycardia, hypothermia, bradypnea	Sedative-hypnotic toxidrome: Stupor and coma, confusion, slurred speech, apnea; narcotic toxidrome: Altered mental status, miosis, decreased bowel sounds; seizures, ataxia, nausea, vomiting, hyporeflexia	Hypercapnia
Phencyclidine (PCP)	None	None	β- and α-adrenergic toxidrome: Hypertension, tachycardia, tachypnea, hyperthermia	β- and α-adrenergic toxidrome: Mydriasis, diaphoresis, dry mucous membranes; range of neurologic behaviors: From calm and unresponsive to excited, paranoid behavior; tremor; hyperactivity; myoclonic or dystonic movements; blank stare, dysconjugate gaze, nystagmus, blurred vision, miosis	Leukocytosis, hyperkalemia, metabolic acidosis; elevated CK, LDH, and AST levels; ketonuria, myoglobinuria, EEG changes

■ **TABLE 9-10**
■ **Symptoms and Toxic Ranges for Commonly Ingested Toxic Substances—cont'd**

Substance	Therapeutic Level	Toxic Level	Vital Signs	Symptoms	Diagnostic Findings
Phenothiazines	Variable	Variable	Hypotension, tachycardia, temperature variations	Memory deficits, confusion, dizziness, lethargy progressing to coma, decreased bowel sounds, miosis or mydriasis	ECG: Heart block, supraventricular and ventricular tachycardias, QRS duration >0.12 sec, or QT >0.5 sec
Salicylates	15-30 mg/dl	>30 mg/dl	Uncoupling of oxidative phosphorylation toxidrome: Tachycardia; hyperthermia, tachypnea	Uncoupling of oxidative phosphorylation toxidrome: Metabolic acidosis; tinnitus, diminished hearing, vertigo, agitation, hyperactivity, stupor, coma, increased bleeding tendencies, diaphoresis, nausea, vomiting	Increased anion gap, mixed acid-base disturbances with metabolic acidosis, prolonged PT, hypoglycemia or hyperglycemia
Sedatives	Variable	Variable	Hypotension, hypothermia, bradypnea progressing to apnea, bradycardia	Sedative-hypnotic toxidrome: Stupor and coma, confusion, slurred speech, apnea; ataxia, incoordination, paradoxical excitement, skin bullae	Hypercapnia
Theophylline	8-20 mcg/ml	>20 mcg/ml	β-adrenergic toxidrome: Hypotension, tachycardia; tachypnea	β-adrenergic toxidrome: Tremor; hyperactivity, confusion, restlessness, agitation, seizures, nausea, vomiting	Hypokalemia; ECG: Tachycardias; metabolic acidosis, respiratory alkalosis, leukocytosis, hyperglycemia, elevated CK levels with seizures

ALT, Alanine aminotransferase; *AST,* aspartate aminotransferase; *BUN,* blood urea nitrogen; *CK,* creatinine phosphokinase; *CNS,* central nervous system; *ECG,* electrocardiogram; *EEG,* electroencephalogram; *GI,* gastrointestinal; *LDH,* lactic dehydrogenase; *ppm,* parts per million; *PT,* prothrombin time.

d. Interventions
  i. Institute rewarming techniques described previously
  ii. Monitor blood alcohol concentration to determine the degree of alcohol intoxication. Blood alcohol concentration of 100 mg/dl or higher indicates legal intoxication in most states.
    (a) Alcohol impairs thermoregulation by diminishing shivering, decreasing cold perception, and suppressing the hypothalamus
    (b) Monitor for hypotension related to depression of the vasomotor center and vasodilation
    (c) Malnourished or alcoholic patients should receive thiamine intravenously during rewarming to limit the risk of neurologic impairment from thiamine deficiency
    (d) Institute alcohol and substance abuse assessment and appropriate therapeutic strategies to limit substance use and abuse in the future
e. Evaluation of patient care
  i. Core temperature is 98.6° F (37° C)
  ii. Patient has no complications of alcohol or substance abuse withdrawal

3. Altered state of consciousness: See Chapters 2 and 4
  a. Additional interventions
    i. Decreased mental status that accompanies hypothermia may result in airway obstruction from the patient's tongue
    ii. Endotracheal intubation can be managed safely in most hypothermic patients without inducing cardiac dysrhythmias
    iii. Use care during airway management to immobilize the cervical spine until cervical spine injury, which may accompany hypothermia, is ruled out

4. Altered oxygenation and ventilation: See Chapter 2
  a. Additional interventions
    i. Monitor respirations; a respiratory rate of 4 breaths/min or more may be sufficient for a hypothermic patient with adequate airway protection
    ii. Increase the usual time to determine breathlessness to up to 45 seconds before initiating cardiopulmonary resuscitation (CPR), because the presence of breathing may be difficult to detect in hypothermic patients
    iii. Administer warm (107.6° to 114.8° F [42° to 46° C]), humidified oxygen

5. Altered hemodynamics: See Chapter 3
  a. Additional interventions
    i. Handle hypothermic patients gently to prevent stimulation of an irritable myocardium, which may lead to lethal ventricular dysrhythmias
      (a) Physical manipulation during endotracheal or nasotracheal intubation may precipitate ventricular fibrillation; intubate only when essential to maintain the airway
      (b) Temporary transvenous pacemaker and PA catheter insertion may precipitate ventricular fibrillation and should be avoided unless essential
    ii. Move and maintain the patient in a horizontal position to avoid aggravating hypotension and to prevent orthostasis
    iii. Increase the usual time to determine pulselessness to up to 45 seconds before initiating CPR, because the presence of a pulse may be difficult to detect in hypothermic patients
    iv. Consider using IV fluids other than lactated Ringer's solution to support circulation because the hypothermic liver may have trouble metabolizing the lactate in the solution
    v. Consider withholding potassium-containing solutions to prevent hyperkalemia

    vi. Attempt defibrillation at 200, 300, and 360 J (up to a total of only three shocks) until the patient's temperature exceeds 86° F (30° C); then attempt defibrillation again

    vii. Use IV vasoactive medications cautiously because toxicities may occur during rewarming. Increase the interval between medication doses (longer than the intervals recommended by the American Heart Association's Advanced Cardiac Life Support standards). Note the following:

        (a) Bradydysrhythmias may be atropine resistant; slow heart rates are usually not corrected with medications or pacemakers unless the rhythm persists after rewarming

        (b) As long as the temperature is below 86° F (30° C), after three defibrillations, medications are withheld until the patient's temperature exceeds 86° F (30° C)

        (c) Lidocaine and procainamide are often ineffective in cases of hypothermia complicated by ventricular fibrillation; bretylium may be more useful

        (d) If inotropic support is needed, dopamine or dobutamine is less likely than epinephrine or levarterenol to cause ventricular dysrhythmias

Toxin Exposure

SYSTEMWIDE ELEMENTS

Physiologic Anatomy

1. Definitions

    a. Toxicology: Study of adverse effects of chemicals on living organisms

    b. Toxicant: Any poison

    c. Absorption: Extent and rate of substance movement from outside the body to an intravascular compartment (blood). Factors affecting absorption include the following:

        i. Route: Subcutaneous, oral, intravenous, cutaneous, inhaled, intranasal, intramuscular, rectal, ocular

        ii. Bioavailability: Solubility, molecular weight, dissolution rate, presence of adsorbent substances, gastric emptying time, intestinal motility, spontaneous vomiting, tissue perfusion, metabolism

    d. Distribution: Way in which a substance disseminates throughout the body. Factors affecting distribution include the following:

        i. Tissue perfusion

        ii. pH

        iii. Protein and tissue binding

        iv. Lipid solubility

    e. Clearance: Measurement of the body's ability to eliminate a substance from blood or plasma over time

        i. Expressed as the volume of blood or plasma completely cleared of a drug per unit of time

        ii. Elimination results from several processes

            (a) Metabolic processes, renal excretion, respiratory excretion, and excretion in sweat

            (b) Chelation: Combining of metallic ions with molecular ring structures so that the ion is held by chemical bonds from each of the participating rings

            (c) Binding to activated charcoal

(d) Extracorporeal drug removal through processes such as hemodialysis and hemoperfusion

f. Median lethal dose (LD_{50}): Concentration of a drug that is lethal in 50% of the population

2. **Epidemiology**

 a. There are between 4 million and 5 million cases of exposures to poisons in the United States annually

 b. Approximately 2 million exposures to potential poisons are reported to poison control centers each year

 c. Approximately 0.5% of poisoned individuals suffer life-threatening effects, major disabilities, or death

 d. 1153 fatalities reported to poison control centers in 2002 were the result of poison

 e. Of the 2.3 million poison exposures in 2002, approximately 181,894 (7.6%) were the result of suicidal intent; 629 of the total 1153 fatalities were the result of suicide poisoning

3. **Physiologic response to toxins:** If the concentration of a chemical in tissues does not exceed a critical level, the effects of toxin ingestion are usually reversible

 a. Local toxicity: Effects that occur at the site of first contact between a biologic system and a toxicant

 b. Systemic toxicity: Effects that occur after the absorption and distribution of a toxicant

 i. Most toxins affect one or two organs predominantly, but a target organ for toxicity is not always the place where a substance accumulates

 ii. CNS is involved most frequently, followed by the cardiovascular system, blood and hematopoietic organs, visceral organs (liver, kidney, lung), and skin

 iii. Muscle and bone are least often affected

 c. Physiologic effect of a toxicant depends on the particular nature of the poison (Table 9-10)

4. **Etiology and risk factors**

 a. Common substances

 i. Analgesics and cleaning substances are the two substances most frequently involved in accidental human poison exposure reported to poison control centers (Table 9-11)

 ii. Analgesics are a category of substances with the largest number of deaths from poisoning reported to poison control centers (Table 9-12)

 iii. Local community trends dictate the epidemiology of toxin ingestion by substance abusers for recreational use. Common drugs of abuse include the following:

 (a) Cocaine

 (b) Heroin

 (c) Methamphetamine

 (d) Inhalants

 b. Designer drugs (Table 9-13)

 i. Active compounds synthesized for legitimate and illicit use

 ii. Most are analogues of phenylethylamine, fentanyl, meperidine, and phencyclidine

 c. Factors associated with poisoning

 i. Physical factors

 (a) Life-span considerations

 (1) In 2002, children younger than 6 years of age accounted for 52% of poisoning incidents but only 2.7% of deaths reported to poison control centers

■ **TABLE 9-11**
■ ■ **Ten Most Common Substances in Human Poison Exposure**

Rank	Substance	% of Total
1	Analgesics	10.8
2	Cleaning substances	9.5
3	Cosmetics and personal care products	9.2
4	Foreign bodies	5.0
5	Sedatives, hypnotics, antipsychotics	4.7
6	Topicals	4.4
7	Cough and cold preparations	4.2
8	Antidepressants	4.2
9	Bites, envenomations	4.1
10	Pesticides	4.0

Data from Watson WA, Litovitz TL, Rodgers GC, et al: 2002 annual report of the American Association of Poison Control Centers Toxic Exposure Surveillance System, *Am J Emerg Med* 21:353–421, 2003.

(2) People 19 years of age and older accounted for 90% of poison fatalities
  (b) Gender
    (1) Among children younger than 13 years of age, boys are more likely to be affected than girls
    (2) Teenagers and adults ingesting toxins are more likely to be female than male
    (3) Females account for 60% of cases of intentional toxin ingestion
  (c) Mode of ingestion
    (1) Inhaled and IV routes are usually more rapid-acting than oral routes
    (2) "Body packing": Swallowing of containers, condoms, balloons, or plastic bags filled with illegal drugs for the purpose of smuggling; drugs are carefully packaged to prevent absorption

■ **TABLE 9-12**
■ ■ **Ten Most Common Causes of Lethal Poison Ingestion**

Rank for All People	Substance
1	Analgesics
2	Sedatives, hypnotics, psychotics
3	Antidepressants
4	Stimulants and street drugs
5	Alcohols
6	Chemicals
7	Anticonvulsants
8	Gases and fumes
9	Antihistamines
10	Muscle relaxants

Data from Watson WA, Litovitz TL, Rodgers GC, et al: 2002 annual report of the American Association of Poison Control Centers Toxic Exposure Surveillance System, *Am J Emerg Med* 21:353–421, 2003.

■ **TABLE 9-13**
■ ■ **Designer Drugs**

Street Name	Chemical Name	Characteristics
AMPHETAMINES		
Serenity, tranquility, peace	4-Methyl-2, 5-dimethoxyamphetamine	2-3 mg causes euphoria 5 mg causes sympathetic nervous system stimulation and hallucinations
Ecstasy, "E," Adam, XTC	3,4-Methylenedi- oxymethamphetamine	Euphoria, empathy Nausea, anorexia, anxiety Insomnia, sympathetic nervous system stimulation Enhanced pleasure, heightened sexuality, expanded consciousness, extraversion
Love drug	3,4-Methylenedioxyamphetamine	Relaxation, sensory distortion Agitation, hallucinations
FENTANYL		
China white	α-Methyl fentanyl	Signs of opioid toxicity Lethargy to coma
MEPERIDINE		
New heroin, synthetic heroin	1-Methyl-4 phenyl-4 propionoxypiperidine and N-methyl-4-phenyl-2,3,5, 6-tetrahydropyridine	Euphoria similar to that produced by heroin Parkinson-like syndromes

        a) Individual transporting a substance is known as a "mule"
        b) This practice is more dangerous when a person ingests drugs in an unplanned and hurried manner to conceal evidence ("body stuffing"). Deaths have occurred in cocaine body stuffers when a package reaches the alkaline milieu of the small intestine and the contents burst, causing cardiopulmonary arrest.
    ii. Environmental factors
        (a) About 92% of poison exposures are in the home
        (b) About 2% of poison exposures are in the workplace
  d. Reason for and incidence of exposure (Watson, Litovitz, and Rodgers, 2003): 63% of poison exposures are classified as general (undefined, or not related to one of the causes in the following list). Other types of exposure include the following:
    i. Environmental (2.7% of total): Any passive, nonoccupational exposure resulting from the contamination of air, water, or soil
    ii. Occupational (1.5% of total): Exposure that occurs as a direct result of being in the workplace or on the job
    iii. Therapeutic error (8.1% of total): Unintentional deviation from a proper therapeutic regimen that results in use of the wrong dosage, incorrect route, or wrong substance
    iv. Unintentional misuse (3.8% of total): Improper or incorrect use of non-pharmaceutical substances
    v. Bite or sting (3.8% of total): Animal bites and stings

      vi. Food poisoning (1.8%): Suspected or confirmed ingestion of contaminated food

     vii. Suspected suicide (7.6% of total): Exposure resulting from inappropriate use of substances for reasons that are suspected to be self-destructive

   viii. Intentional misuse (1.7% of total): Improper use of a substance for reasons other than pursuit of a psychotropic effect

Patient Assessment

1. **Nursing history**
   a. Source: Patient, family, partner, significant other, prehospital personnel, or bystander
   b. Description of the event
      i. Location and time
      ii. Substances involved
         (a) Where a substance is routinely kept
         (b) Type of container: Ask for a pill container if available, but many people carry multiple medications in one container. The container label may lead to inaccurate conclusions about a substance ingested.
         (c) Volume or number of substances in a container
         (d) Amount ingested
         (e) Patient's symptoms after ingestion
         (f) Home first aid or prehospital treatment
      iii. Body packing or body stuffing: If the patient was confronted by police for illegal substance use or transport, suspect hurried substance ingestion
   c. Regular pattern of alcohol and substance use
      i. Suspect polydrug use in substance users and abusers, which is far more common than single drug or alcohol use
      ii. Attempt to obtain collateral reports of substance use patterns from significant others
   d. Past health history: AMPLE
      i. *Allergies*
      ii. *Medications*
         (a) Prescription and over-the-counter drugs
         (b) Herbal and natural substances
         (c) Tetanus immunization
      iii. *Past illnesses (medical and surgical)*
      iv. *Last meal (time, quantity, type)*
      v. *Events preceding ingestion*
   e. Social history
      i. Partner, spouse, house mates, roommates, significant others, or contact person
      ii. Occupation and education
      iii. Dependents, children
      iv. Religion
      v. Financial considerations: Ability to maintain income and insurance coverage
   f. Other
      i. Height, weight
      ii. Last menstrual period and potential for pregnancy
2. **Nursing examination of patient**
   a. Physical examination data
      i. Primary survey: Rapid assessment (30 seconds to 2 minutes) that simultaneously identifies and manages life-threatening injuries: ABCDE

      (a) *Airway*: Maintain a patent airway. *Note:* Stabilizing the cervical spine (via cervical collar, foam blocks, rolled sheets, manual stabilization, taping) is mandatory during airway assessment and interventions if injury accompanies toxin ingestion.

      (b) *Breathing*: Maintain adequate breathing

      (c) *Circulation*: Maintain adequate circulation

      (d) *Disability*: Monitor the level of consciousness

      (e) *Exposure*: Completely undress the patient to perform a thorough visual examination

      (f) Early consultation with a poison control center is essential when the ABCDE survey has been completed

   ii. Secondary survey: Complete physical examination is begun as soon as the primary survey and emergency life-saving interventions are completed

      (a) If the patient is suspected of body stuffing or body packing, monitor for cardiovascular compromise in intensive care

      (b) Use a nonjudgmental and honest approach to evaluate symptoms and obtain a precise count of the number of bags ingested

  iii. Inspection

      (a) Inspect all areas of the skin and mucous membranes for needle marks or abscesses

      (b) Know the practices of the substance-abusing population to identify signs and symptoms of unusual routes of administration

      (c) Note the symptom complex of a specific type of poisoning (toxidrome) (Mokhlesi, Leiken, and Murray, 2003b)

  iv. Palpation, percussion, and auscultation techniques depend on the substances involved

      (a) Assess for multiple trauma

      (b) Assess for hypothermia

  b. Monitoring data

    i. Vital signs are widely variable, depending on the toxic compound (see Table 9-10)

    ii. Pain: See Systemic Inflammatory Response Syndrome and Septic Shock

3. Appraisal of patient characteristics: The mother of a 19-year-old male finds him unconscious after the manager at the restaurant where he is employed calls her to ask why her son did not report to work at 9 AM that day. The mother has returned home to find her son unconscious on his bed with an empty Tylenol regular strength bottle and 12 empty beer cans on the floor. She calls 911 for transport and tells the emergency department physician that she had taken two Tylenol caplets the night before and had noted that the 75-caplet, 325-mg/caplet bottle was less than one fourth full. The patient had been fighting with his girlfriend after discovering that she was 10 weeks pregnant. The girlfriend wanted to abort the fetus, and the patient was adamantly against terminating the pregnancy. His girlfriend, on arrival at the hospital, tells the medical team that he had threatened suicide but had not identified a plan. The patient is moaning incomprehensible words in the emergency department. It is determined that he had consumed between 6000 and 8000 mg of regular strength Tylenol and a 12-pack of beer. Because the alcohol level is 220 mg/dl and the Tylenol level is 160 mg/kg, *N*-acetylcysteine is administered. The patient is taken to the ICU for ongoing monitoring, and suicide precautions are initiated. Within 6 days, the patient's hepatic enzyme levels decrease, which reflects improved liver function. He is then transferred to the psychiatry unit, where he admits that he is concerned not only about his girlfriend's pregnancy, but also about his lack of medical insurance and limited financial resources. The psychiatrist notes that the patient's progress is very slow. At discharge, the patient's mother agrees to let her son's girlfriend move in with them and to assist with the pregnancy and financial support over the next few months.

    a. Resiliency (level 1—*minimally resilient*): Patient comes to the emergency room with an inability to cope with a stressful situation; the patient demonstrates weak reserves

    b. Vulnerability (level 1—*highly vulnerable*): Patient admits the desire to commit suicide and demonstrates a possible attempt, although no definitive plan was made

    c. Stability (level 3—*moderately stable*): Patient is hemodynamically stable with decreasing liver function test values; the patient will require ongoing monitoring to determine if further intervention will be necessary

    d. Complexity (level 1—*highly complex*): Complex patient–family–significant other dynamics; stability of the relationship between the patient and his girlfriend is suspect; family support may be limited over the next few months

    e. Resource availability (level 3—*moderate resources*): Financial resources are limited, but the patient's mother will at least temporarily provide residence and emotional support for the patient and his girlfriend; the patient is employed but has no medical coverage

    f. Participation in care (level 5—*full participation*): Patient is actively participating in his medical and psychiatric recovery; his girlfriend and mother are visiting often and participating in therapy as needed

    g. Participation in decision making (level 5—*full participation*): Currently, both the patient and his support system are actively involved in his care and decision making

    h. Predictability (level 3—*moderately predictable*): Based on the severity of the suicide attempt and limited resource availability

4. Diagnostic studies: Do not delay treatment while awaiting results

    a. Laboratory

        i. Urine, blood (rarely, gastric contents for toxicologic screen); acetaminophen level indicated in all patients with suspected intentional overdose

        ii. CBC

        iii. Serum electrolytes and glucose levels, renal function, PT and PTT

        iv. Liver function tests

        v. BUN, creatinine levels

        vi. ABG levels

        vii. Pregnancy test: Performed for all girls 12 to 17 years of age and women of childbearing age

    b. Chest radiograph

    c. ECG

Patient Care

1. Potential for compromised airway: See Chapter 2

2. Impaired oxygenation and ventilation: See Chapter 2

    a. Additional nursing interventions

        i. Determine whether respirations are adequate

            (a) Adult: 5 to 10 ml/kg/breath at a rate of 12 to 18 breaths/min (100 ml/kg/min)

            (b) Child older than 5 years of age: "adequate" rate increases to 20 breaths/min

        ii. If respirations are not deemed adequate, hyperventilate with bag-valve-mask and 100% oxygen followed by intubation

       iii. 100% oxygen may be considered an antidote for carbon monoxide poisoning while COHb results are awaited (do not rely on PaO_2 or SaO_2 determinations for carbon monoxide poisoning)

3. Ingestion of poison or toxic substance (Figure 9-9)

  a. Description of problem

    i. Self-report or collateral report by significant others of toxin ingestion

    ii. Impaired airway, breathing, and circulation

    iii. Decreased mental status

    iv. Nausea, vomiting, diarrhea

    v. Hypothermia or hyperthermia

  b. Goals of care

    i. Airway, breathing, and circulation are adequate

    ii. Toxic substance is removed or eliminated, or its effects reversed

    iii. Preingestion level of consciousness is restored

    iv. Organ function is preserved

    v. Normothermia is attained and maintained

  c. Collaborating professionals on health care team: Registered nurse, emergency medicine and internal medicine attending physician, respiratory therapist, pharmacist, social worker, psychiatrist (as needed)

  d. Interventions (see also Tables 9-8 and 9-9)

    i. Monitor core temperature with a rectal or PA catheter thermistor, if available, and manage hypothermia and hyperthermia

    ii. Monitor cardiac rhythm and manage dysrhythmias and hypovolemia with IV crystalloids

    iii. In all comatose adult and adolescent patients, even those without pinpoint pupils, be prepared to give the following drugs if they are prescribed (keeping in mind that routine use of these drugs is not recommended):

      (a) Dextrose, 100 ml IV 50% in water (50 g dextrose), to rule out hypoglycemia as a cause for coma (except in patients known to be hyperglycemic)

        (1) Hypoglycemia may result from exposure to insulin, oral hypoglycemic agents, ethanol, and salicylates

        (2) If the blood glucose level can be determined rapidly, administer hypertonic dextrose only to patients with a blood glucose level below 60 mg/dl

        (3) If the glucose level cannot be determined rapidly, consider hypertonic dextrose for patients with altered consciousness and nonfocal neurologic examination results

      (b) Thiamine, 100 mg IV, to prevent precipitation of Wernicke-Korsakoff syndrome

        (1) Routine use is warranted

        (2) Administer at the same time as hypertonic dextrose

      (c) Naloxone, 2 mg IV, intramuscularly, or endotracheally, to antagonize narcotics

        (1) Use smaller doses (0.1 or 0.2 mg) for opioid-dependent patients who are not apneic to avoid withdrawal symptoms

        (2) Use routinely for patients with CNS or respiratory depression who have a low likelihood of opioid addiction and polydrug addiction

        (3) Administer routinely to patients with respiratory rates below 12 breaths/min

        (4) Half-life is 30 minutes; symptoms may recur after then, which indicates a need for continuous infusion

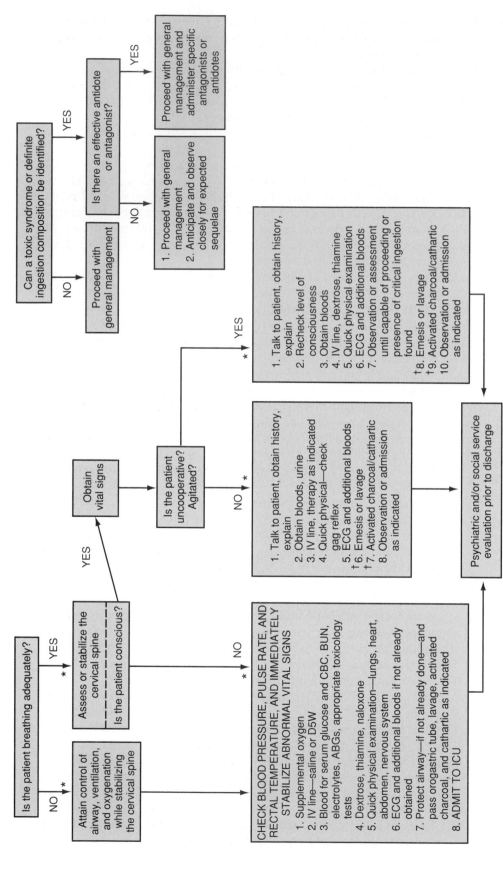

FIGURE 9-9 ■ Generic pathway explaining management of the poisoned or overdosed patients without specific toxic symptoms. The asterisks refer to the smaller algorithm, which reminds the clinician to consider antidotal intervention when appropriate throughout toxicologic care. †If indicated. *ABG,* Arterial blood gas; *BUN,* blood urea nitrogen; *CBC,* complete blood count; *D5W,* 5% dextrose in water; *ECG,* electrocardiogram; *ICU,* intensive care unit; *IV,* intravenous. (From Goldfrank LR, Flomenbaum NE, Lewin NA, et al: *Toxicologic emergencies,* 5th ed, Norwalk, Conn, 1994, Appleton & Lange, pp 28-29.)

   (d) Do not administer physostigmine, analeptics (amphetamines, caffeine), or flumazenil routinely until the toxicant is identified and use of these drugs is warranted

iv. Provide an antidote (Table 9-14): If no antidote is available, maintain vital functions, remove the toxic substance, and limit the absorption of any remaining substance

v. General management strategies for decontamination

   (a) Orogastric lavage: Elimination of unabsorbed toxins; usually performed in the emergency department

      (1) Indications: Generally accepted for use instead of emesis in comatose patients *except* in cases of ingestion of a caustic agent (chemical injury, including ingestion of acetic acid [permanent wave solution], ammonia [cleaning agents], phosphorus [matches, fireworks], benzalkonium chloride [detergents], oxalic acid [disinfectants, bleach], formaldehyde, iodine [antiseptics], and sulfuric acid [batteries, drain cleaners]).

      (2) Management of caustic agent ingestion:
         a) Intubate if needed
         b) Examine for splash injuries to skin or eyes
         c) If there are no signs of visceral perforation and the patient can swallow, dilute the toxicant with cool milk or tap water
         d) Do not give emetics or perform gastric lavage

      (3) Procedure
         a) Intubate to protect the airway if appropriate
         b) For gastric lavage, use a No. 36 to 40 orogastric French tube, which is large enough to be able to remove particulate matter
         c) Pass the tube orally to limit epistaxis and trauma to the nasal mucosa
         d) If necessary, use the oral airway to prevent the patient from biting the tube
         e) Verify tube placement in the stomach, place the patient in the left lateral decubitus position with the head lower than the feet, attach the lavage funnel to the end of the orogastric tube, and administer 150 to 200 ml (to adults) of tap water or normal saline. In some protocols, a catheter-tipped syringe is used to irrigate and withdraw fluid until the fluid is clear.
         f) Allow the tube to drain by gravity
         g) Monitor for complications: Aspiration, esophageal or gastric perforation, and laryngospasm

      (4) Other contraindications to lavage
         a) Hemorrhagic diathesis, ingestion of nontoxic substances, ingestion of sharp materials or drug packets
         b) Orogastric lavage is not routinely recommended in the management of poisoning unless a potentially life-threatening amount of poison has been consumed

   (b) Emetics: Ipecac is no longer used routinely as a poison treatment intervention in the home or emergency department. At home, the first intervention should be to contact the local poison control center. The administration of syrup of ipecac should occur only if poison control personnel or an emergency department physician recommends it.

      (1) Dose: 15 ml of syrup with 16 to 21 mg of cephaeline and emetine at a ratio of 1:1 to 2.1:1; mix with warm water

■ **TABLE 9-14**
■ ■ **Management Considerations for Ingestion of Toxic Substances**

Substance	Antidote	Management
Acetaminophen	NAC (Mucomyst); loading: 140 mg/kg PO; maintenance: 70 mg/kg PO every 4 hr for 17 doses. Dilute dose of NAC 1:4 in chilled soft drink or juice.	Perform gastric emptying if less than 1 hr since ingestion. Give activated charcoal if less than 4 hr since ingestion. Use NAC if levels are toxic even if ingestion was over 24 hr earlier. Repeat dose if patient vomits within 1 hr. If vomiting persists, use nasogastric decompression and metoclopramide.
Amphetamines	None	Consider administration of 100 ml 50% glucose (if warranted after fingerstick glucose testing) and 100 mg thiamine IV. Give activated charcoal with a cathartic for oral ingestion. Supportive therapy: Administer benzodiazepines (for agitation or seizures), external cooling (for hyperthermia), phentolamine (for hypertension), IV hydration (to replace fluid losses and prevent myoglobin damage in renal tubules), esmolol or propranolol for tachyarrhythmias. Keep patient in a cool, quiet room. Implement hemodialysis for patients with acute renal failure, acidosis, and hyperkalemia, but do not use it to remove drug.
Arsenic	None	Give chelating agents, such as British anti-Lewisite, D-penicillamine, and dimercaptosuccinic acid. *Note: These drugs have many side effects.* Support circulation with crystalloids and pressor agents as needed. Administer blood if GI hemorrhage occurs. Treat ventricular dysrhythmia with lidocaine and defibrillation. Monitor for seizure activity. Orogastric lavage may be used if patient comes for treatment shortly after ingestion; do not use charcoal; initiate hemodialysis for renal dysfunction and clearance of arsenic.
Barbiturates	None	Administer sodium bicarbonate to enhance elimination of phenobarbital only. GI evacuation: Lavage with large-bore orogastric tube followed by MDAC therapy; charcoal hemoperfusion for severe poisoning. Consider giving adults with altered mental status 100 ml dextrose 50% (if warranted after fingerstick glucose testing), 2 mg naloxone, and 100 mg thiamine. Withdrawal symptoms may lead to vomiting and risk for aspiration; maintain patient in left lateral position.
Benzodiazepines	Flumazenil; *use caution*—severe withdrawal risk exists	GI evacuation: Lavage with large-bore orogastric tube followed by MDAC therapy. Consider giving adults with altered mental status 100 ml dextrose 50% (if warranted after fingerstick glucose testing), 2 mg naloxone, and 100 mg thiamine.

Continued

Carbamazepine	None	GI evacuation: Lavage with large-bore orogastric tube followed by MDAC therapy.
		Implement whole bowel irrigation if medication is enteric coated.
		Give cathartics.
		Monitor for seizures.
		Wide complex tachycardia may respond to sodium bicarbonate bolus therapy.
Cocaine	None	Consider administration of 100 ml 50% glucose (if warranted after fingerstick glucose testing) and 100 mg thiamine IV.
		Administer high-flow oxygen immediately.
		For oral ingestion, irrigate through a large-bore orogastric tube, with MDAC and a single dose of cathartic; use whole bowel irrigation for body packers.
		Supportive therapy: Administer benzodiazepines (for sedation); vasodilators (for hypertension); nitrates, phentolamine, and calcium channel blockers (for myocardial ischemia); aspirin, heparin, opioids, and possibly thrombolytic therapy (for myocardial infarction); lidocaine, sodium bicarbonate, or propranolol (for ventricular dysrhythmias).
		Provide cooling for hyperthermia, a quiet environment, and reassurance.
		Monitor for seizures.
Cyanide	Amyl nitrate, crushed into gauze and inhaled (may be placed over intake valve of manual resuscitator bag or between oxygen source and endotracheal tube); sodium nitrate 3% 10 ml IV over 4 min; sodium thiosulfate 25% 50 ml IV; hydroxocobalamin 4–5 g IV as one-time dose	Administer 100% oxygen.
		Administer crystalloids and vasopressors for hypotension.
		Give sodium bicarbonate to correct acidosis.
		Administer amyl nitrate (patient should inhale while nurse prepares sodium nitrate), sodium nitrate, and sodium thiosulfate; all drugs are needed in combination for synergistic effects and are prepared as a cyanide kit.
		Suspect cyanide poisoning with any serious smoke inhalation injury.
		Perform orogastric lavage followed by MDAC therapy for acute ingestions.
Cyclic antide- pressants	Sodium bicarbonate	Administer sodium bicarbonate to prevent and treat dysrhythmias, and lidocaine to treat ventricular arrhythmias.
		Give MDAC therapy without orogastric lavage.
		Consider giving adults with altered mental status 100 ml dextrose 50% (if warranted after fingerstick glucose testing), 2 mg naloxone, and 100 mg thiamine.
		Withdrawal symptoms may lead to vomiting and risk for aspiration; maintain patient in left lateral position.
		Monitor heart rhythm continuously.
		Administer sodium bicarbonate, and consider hyperventilation to keep pH at 7.50-7.55.
		Correct hypotension with crystalloids and norepinephrine if needed; avoid dopamine, which may increase dysrhythmias and may not correct hypotension because catecholamine stores have been depleted by overdose.

Continued

Substance	Antidote	Management
Ethanol (acute intoxication)	None	Never assume that decreased mental status is a reflection of intoxication alone, because alcohol intoxication is often associated with traumatic injuries; threshold for CT of the head should be low. Treat recent ingestion (within 1 hr) with gastric lavage and activated charcoal in severely intoxicated patients. Perform fingerstick glucose test and administer 50 ml 50% glucose if indicated. Administer 100 mg thiamine IV. Consider magnesium and potassium administration to counteract electrolyte depletion, often seen in chronic alcoholics. Supportive therapy: Administer multivitamins with folate (for nutrition), blood products (for coagulopathies), benzodiazepines (for withdrawal).
Ethylene glycol (antifreeze) and methanol	None	Administer ethanol 100–150 mg/dl IV to prevent formation of toxic metabolites by competitive inhibition; maintain blood alcohol level of 100–150 mg/dl. Maintain normal pH with sodium bicarbonate administration. Maintain hydration. Consider hemodialysis as an option. Administer thiamine 100 mg IV and pyridoxine 50 mg every 6 hr. Administer benzodiazepines for seizures. Replace calcium.
Isoniazid (INH)	Control seizures with pyridoxine 1 g for every gram of INH ingested (give 1 g over 2-3 min) along with diazepam and lorazepam.	Phenytoin is ineffective and is not recommended. Implement peritoneal dialysis, hemodialysis, and hemoperfusion.
Isopropyl alcohol (rubbing alcohol)	None	Provide supportive treatment, with attention to cardiorespiratory problems. Controversial: Activated charcoal lavage used early in the overdose; hemodialysis for patients with high levels (400–500 mg/dl).
Lithium	None	GI evacuation: Use lavage with large-bore orogastric tube; sodium polystyrene sulfonate binds to lithium and decreases absorption. Administer normal saline to enhance elimination. Implement hemodialysis. Monitor for seizures.
Opioids	Naloxone 2 mg (may be repeated, up to a total of 10 mg); if opioid dependence is suspected, give 0.1-0.2 mg naloxone; *duration of action of most opioids exceeds duration of action of naloxone* (repeated doses may be necessary).	Monitor for opioid withdrawal in dependent patients: Vomiting, abdominal pain, agitation, diaphoresis, pilo erection; aspiration of stomach contents is a risk for comatose patients. *Note:* Higher doses may be needed to reverse effects of propoxyphene, pentazocine, methadone, and fentanyl. Position patient to limit risk of aspiration, since vomiting is a consequence of withdrawal.

Continued

Phencyclidine (PCP)	None	Administer MDAC, cathartic (sorbitol, magnesium citrate). Supportive therapy: Treat hypertension with nitroprusside, benzodiazepines (for agitation); IV hydration, diuretics, mannitol (to limit damage from rhabdomyolysis); cooling blanket (for hyperthermia).
Phenothiazines	None	GI evacuation: Lavage with large-bore orogastric tube, followed by MDAC, cathartic (sorbitol, magnesium citrate). Implement cardiac monitoring.
Salicylates	None	GI evacuation: Perform lavage with large-bore orogastric tube, followed by MDAC, cathartic. Cooling: Provide hypothermia blanket, ice packs, and a cool environment. Provide alkalization of urine with sodium bicarbonate. Implement hemodialysis. Monitor for and treat hypokalemia.
Theophylline	None	Implement charcoal hemoperfusion or hemodialysis. GI evacuation: Perform lavage with large-bore orogastric tube, followed by MDAC, cathartic. Implement cardiac monitoring.

CT, Computed tomography; *GI,* gastrointestinal; *IV,* intravenous; *MDAC,* multiple-dose activated charcoal; *NAC, N*-acetylcysteine; *PO,* by mouth.

(2) Causes vomiting by local activation of peripheral sensory receptors in the gastrointestinal tract and central stimulation of the chemoreceptor trigger in the central vomiting center of the brain

(3) Vomiting usually begins in 20 minutes, occurs at least three times, and lasts about 30 to 60 minutes

(4) Considerations

  a) Do not give with milk, which may slow action

  b) May be inactivated by activated charcoal

  c) In the emergency department, gastric decontamination is preferable if gastric emptying is required

  d) Toxicity: Protracted vomiting, diarrhea, seizures, cardiac toxicity, and neuromuscular weakness

(c) Activated charcoal: May be administered alone or after several liters of gastric lavage produces a clear effluent; administer as a slurry

(1) Dose: 1 g/kg of body weight or 10:1 ratio of activated charcoal to drug (whichever is greater); mix with water or a cathartic via a tube or orally

(2) Often given with a cathartic at an appropriate dose; premixed solutions are available; do not use multiple-dose cathartics

  a) Magnesium citrate, magnesium sulfate, sorbitol

  b) Contraindications to cathartic use: Trivial toxin ingestion in children, adynamic ileus, diarrhea, abdominal trauma, intestinal obstruction, renal failure

(3) Composition

  a) Produced from destructive distillation of organic materials such as wood and petroleum; treated at high temperatures to increase its ability to adsorb toxins

   b) Adsorption relies on external pore size and internal surface area; adsorbs (attracts) by ionic binding and molecular forces
   c) Adsorption begins 1 minute after administration
  (4) Administer activated charcoal if within 1 to 2 hours after ingestion; benefit is negligible if administered more than 4 hours after ingestion; administer in cases of multiple ingestants where gastric emptying may occur; activated charcoal may absorb N-acetylcysteine, which is also given to protect the liver from toxic levels of acetaminophen; however, the amount absorbed is clinically insignificant
  (5) May be given in multiple doses every 1 to 4 hours, but do not repeat the cathartic dose; discontinue after the first charcoal stool
  (6) Other uses: Overdose of digitalis, phenobarbital, carbamazepine, phenytoin, theophylline, salicylate, propoxyphene, cyclic antidepressants, isoniazid, amphetamines, cocaine, amitriptyline, phenylbutazone
  (7) Not useful for overdose of alcohol, caustic agents, iron, or lithium
  (8) Hazards: Diarrhea, constipation, vomiting, aspiration, intestinal obstruction, reduction of therapeutic levels of prescribed drugs
 (d) Whole-bowel irrigation: Polyethylene glycol and electrolytes for oral solution
  (1) Dose: 2 L/hr orally or by nasogastric tube for 4 to 6 hours until the effluent is clear
  (2) Clears the entire gastrointestinal tract without inducing emesis or causing a fluid and electrolyte disturbance
  (3) Indications: Ingestion of sustained-release drugs, slowly dissolving agents (iron tablets, paint chips), "crack" vials, drug packets (cocaine, heroin) for smuggling purposes
  (4) Complications: Rectal itching, vomiting
  (5) Contraindications: Ileus, obstruction, perforation, gastrointestinal bleeding, or ingestion of quickly absorbing drugs, liquids, parenterally administered drugs, or caustic agents
 (e) Hemodialysis, hemoperfusion, and hemofiltration (Table 9-15)
  (1) Hemodialysis is usually performed for 4 to 6 hours in poisoned patients
  (2) Hemodialysis also corrects metabolic acid-base disturbances, hyperkalemia, and fluid overload
  (3) Hemoperfusion is better than hemodialysis for clearing the blood of substances that bind to plasma proteins
  (4) Cartridge needs to be changed every 6 hours because its adsorptive capacity decreases
  (5) Hemofiltration is mostly experimental; dialysis is generally used
   a) Hemofiltration can remove larger molecules, such as aminoglycoside antibiotics
   b) Can be used after the other two techniques to prevent a rebound of toxin levels
  (6) Hypotension makes all three techniques difficult to apply
 vi. Treatment for body stuffing and body packing
 (a) If the patient becomes symptomatic while in police custody, suspect body stuffing unless proven otherwise
 (b) Treatment is controversial and should be guided by the poison control center; some possibilities include metoclopramide, oral activated charcoal, polyethylene glycol and electrolyte solutions, surgical intervention, and laparotomy

■ TABLE 9-15
■ ■ Hemodialysis and Hemoperfusion

Technique	Characteristics	Toxic Compounds
HEMODIALYSIS		
Toxic compounds diffuse down the concentration gradient through semi-permeable membrane from blood into dialysis solution.	Low molecular weight (<500 d) Water soluble Low volume of distribution (<1 L/kg) Poor protein binding (<70%–80%) Low body clearance (<4 ml/min/kg)	Bromide Ethylene glycol Lithium Methanol Salicylate Chloral hydrate Ethanol
HEMOPERFUSION		
Blood is pumped through a cartridge containing activated charcoal and/or carbon, which absorbs toxin.	High molecular weight Low volume of distribution Not limited by protein binding (as is hemodialysis) Low body clearance (<4 ml/min/kg)	Carbamazepine Phenobarbital Phenytoin Theophylline Procainamide

    e. Evaluation of patient care

       i. Patent airway, regular breathing, and adequate circulation are maintained

       ii. Toxic substance is removed or its effects are reversed

       iii. Preingestion level of consciousness is restored

       iv. Patient's temperature is 96.8° to 100.4° F (36° to 38° C)

4. Diminished self concept: See Chapter 10

    a. Additional interventions

       i. Make appropriate referrals to a social worker or psychiatric clinical nurse specialist

       ii. Monitor the environment for items that could be used for self-inflicted injury

       iii. Implement suicide precautions if appropriate

REFERENCES

Systemic Inflammatory Response Syndrome and Septic Shock

Ahrens T, Vollman K: Severe sepsis management: are we doing enough? *Crit Care Nurse* 23(5 suppl):2–17, 2003.

Aird WC: Vascular bed-specific hemostasis: role of endothelium in sepsis pathogenesis, *Crit Care Med* 29:S28–S35, 2001.

American Association of Critical-Care Nurses: Identification and management of the patient with severe sepsis, *AACN Critical Care Publication,* 1–155, 2002.

Angus DC, Wax RS: Epidemiology of sepsis: an update, *Crit Care Med* 29:S109–S116, 2001.

Annane D, Sebille V, Charpentier C, et al: Effect of treatment with low doses of hydrocortisone and fludrocortisone on mortality in patients with septic shock, *JAMA* 288:862–871, 2002.

Anne D, Cavaillon J: Corticosteroids in sepsis: from Bench to bedside? *Shock* 20:197–207, 2003.

Balk RA: Severe sepsis and septic shock: definitions, epidemiology, and clinical manifestations, *Crit Care Clin* 16:179–192, 2000.

Balk RA: Steroids for septic shock: back from the dead? *Chest* 123:490S–499S, 2003.

Beery TA: Sex differences in infection and sepsis, *Crit Care Nurs Clin North Am* 15:55–62, 2003.

Bernard GR: Drotrecogin alfa (activated) (recombinant human activated protein C) for the treatment of severe sepsis, *Crit Care Med* 31:S85–S93, 2003.

Bernard GR, Vincent J, Laterre P, et al: Efficacy and safety of recombinant human activated protein C for severe sepsis, *N Engl J Med* 344:699–709, 2001.

Bochud P, Calandra T: Pathogenesis of sepsis: new concepts and implications for future treatment, *BMJ* 326:262–266, 2003.

Bone RC, Balk RA, Cerra FB, et al: Definitions for sepsis and organ failure and guidelines for the use of innovative therapies in sepsis, *Chest* 101:1644–1655, 1992.

Cooper MS, Stewart PM: Corticosteroid insufficiency in acutely ill patients, *N Engl J Med* 348:727–734, 2003.

Dellinger RP: Cardiovascular management of septic shock, *Crit Care Med* 31:946–955, 2003.

Ely ES, Kleinpell R, Goyette RE: Advances in the understanding of clinical manifestations and therapy of severe sepsis: an update for critical care nurses, *Am J Crit Care* 12:120–135, 2003.

Esmon CT: Protein C anticoagulant pathway and its role in controlling microvascular thrombosis and inflammation, *Crit Care Med* 29:S48–S51, 2001.

Felblinger DM: Malnutrition, infection, and sepsis in acute and chronic illness, *Crit Care Nurs Clin North Am* 15:71–78, 2003.

Fisher CJ, Yan SB: Protein C levels as a prognostic indicator of outcome in sepsis and related diseases, *Crit Care Med* 28:S49–S56, 2000.

Griffiths RD: Nutrition support in critically ill septic patients, *Curr Opin Clin Nutr Metab Care* 6:203–210, 2003.

Guven H, Altintop L, Baydin A, et al: Diagnostic value of procalcitonin levels as an early indicator of sepsis, *Am J Emerg Med* 20:202–206, 2002.

Holmes CL, Patel BM, Russell JA, et al: Physiology of vasopressin relevant to management of septic shock, *Chest* 120:989–1002, 2001.

Kleinpell RM: Advances in treating patients with severe sepsis: role of drotrecogin alfa (activated), *Crit Care Nurse* 23:16–29, 2003.

Kleinpell RM: The role of the critical care nurse in the assessment and management of the patient with severe sepsis, *Crit Care Nurs Clin North Am* 1:27–34, 2003.

Levy MM, Fink MP, Marshall JC, et al: 2001 SCCM/ESICM/ACCP/ATS/SIS International Sepsis Definitions Conference, *Crit Care Med* 31:1250–1256, 2003.

Levy MM, Vincent JL: Sepsis: pathophysiologic insights and current management. In *Proceedings of the 2002 Society of Critical Care Medicine/European Society of Intensive Care Medicine summer conference,* 2002.

Martin GS, Mannino DM, Eaton S, et al: The epidemiology of sepsis in the United States from 1979 through 2000, *N Engl J Med* 348:1546–1554, 2003.

Mathiak G, Neville LF, Grass G: Targeting the coagulation cascade in sepsis: did we find the "magic bullet"? *Crit Care Med* 31:310–311, 2003.

Munford RS: Sepsis and septic shock. In Braunwald E, Fauci AS, Kasper DL, et al, editors: *Harrison's principles of internal medicine,* ed 5, New York, 2001, McGraw-Hill.

O'Grady NP, Alexander M, Dellinger E, et al: Guidelines for the prevention of intravascular catheter-related infections, Centers for Disease Control and Prevention, *MMWR Recomm Rep* 51:1–29, 2002.

Patel BM, Chittock DR, Russell JA, et al: Beneficial effects of short-term vasopressin infusion during severe septic shock, *Anesthesiology* 96:576–582, 2002.

Pearl RG, Pohlman A: Understanding and managing anemia in critically ill patients, *Crit Care Nurse* suppl:1–16, Dec 2002.

Rivers E, Nguyen B, Havstad S, et al: Early goal-directed therapy in the treatment of severe sepsis and septic shock, *N Engl J Med* 345:1368–1377, 2001.

Ruokenen E, Parviainen I, Uusaro A: Treatment of impaired perfusion in septic shock, *Ann Med* 34:590–597, 2002.

Shafazand S, Weinacker AB: Blood cultures in the critical care unit: improving utilization and yield, *Chest* 132:1727–1736, 2002.

Sommers MS: The cellular basis of septic shock, *Crit Care Nurs Clin North Am* 15:13–25, 2003.

Van den Berghe G, Wouters P, Weekers F, et al: Intensive insulin therapy in critically ill patients, *N Engl J Med* 345:1359–1367, 2001.

Vincent J, Abraham E, Annane D: Reducing mortality in sepsis: new directions, *Crit Care* 6:S1–S18, 2002.

Waxman K: Physiologic response to injury. In Grenvik A, Ayres SM, Holbrook PR, et al, editors: *Textbook of critical care,* ed 4, Philadelphia, 2000, Saunders.

Yan SB, Helterbrand JD, Hartman DL, et al: Low levels of protein C are associated with poor outcomes in severe sepsis, *Chest* 120: 915–922, 2001.

Young LS: Sepsis syndrome. In Mandell GL, Bennett JE, Dolin R, editors: *Mandell, Douglas, and Bennett's principles and practice of infectious diseases*, ed 5, Philadelphia, 2000, Churchill Livingstone.

Multiple Organ Dysfunction Syndrome

Aiboshi J, Moore EE, Clesia DJ, et al: Blood transfusion and the two-insult model of post-injury multiple organ failure, *Shock* 15:302–306, 2001.

Bota DP, Melot C, Ferreira FL, et al: The multiple organ dysfunction score (MODS) versus the sequential organ failure assessment (SOFA) score in outcome prediction, *Intensive Care Med* 28:1619–1624, 2002.

Charalambos AG, Lekkou A, Papageorgiou O, et al: Clinical prognostic markers in patients with severe sepsis: a prospective analysis of 139 consecutive cases, *J Infect* 47:301–306, 2003.

Durham RM: Multiple organ failure in trauma patients, *J Trauma* 55:608–616, 2003.

Kaplan L, Bailey H: Systemic inflammatory response syndrome, *eMedicine,* Oct 2001.

Khadaroo RG, Marshall JC: ARDS and the multiple organ dysfunction syndrome: common mechanisms of a common systemic process, *Crit Care Clin* 18:127–141, 2002.

Kleinpell RM: The role of the critical care nurse in the assessment and management of the patient with severe sepsis, *Crit Care Nurs Clin North Am* 15:27–34, 2003.

Lee CC, Marill KA, Carter WA, et al: A current concept of trauma-induced multiorgan failure, *Ann Emerg Med* 38:170–176, 2001.

Levy MM, Fink MP, Marshall JC, et al: 2001 S C C M / E S I C M / A C C P / A T S / S I S International Sepsis Definitions Conference, *Crit Care Med* 31:1250–1256, 2003.

Marshall JC: Inflammation, coagulopathy, and the pathogenesis of multiple organ dysfunction syndrome, *Crit Care Med* 29:S99–S106, 2001.

Marshall JC: Multiple organ dysfunction syndrome. In Wilmore DW, Chung LY, Harken AH, et al, editors: *ACS surgery: principles and practice*, Danbury, Conn: WebMD Professional Publishing, 2003.

Marshall JC, Cook DJ, Christou NV, et al: Multiple organ dysfunction score: a reliable descriptor of a complex clinical outcome, *Crit Care Med* 23:1638–1657, 1995.

Moss M, Burnham EL: Chronic alcohol abuse, acute respiratory distress syndrome, and multiple organ dysfunction, *Crit Care Med* 31:S207–S212, 2003.

Nimah M, Brilli RJ: Coagulation dysfunction in sepsis and multiple organ system failure, *Crit Care Clin* 19:441–458, 2003.

Pettila V, Pettila M, Sarna S, et al: Comparison of multiple organ dysfunction scores in the prediction of hospital mortality in the critically ill, *Crit Care Med* 30:1705–1711, 2002.

Schuster DP, Kozlowski JK, McCarthy T: Effect of endotoxin on oleic acid lung injury does not depend on priming, *J Appl Physiol* 91:2047–2054, 2001.

Sharma S, Eschun G: Multisystem organ failure of sepsis, *eMedicine,* Feb 2003.

Turki M, Parsons PE: Acute respiratory distress syndrome. In Parsons PE, Wiener-Kronish JP: *Critical care secrets*, ed 3, Philadelphia, 2003, Hanley & Belfus.

Ueno H, Hirasawa H, Oda S, et al: Coagulation/fibrinolysis abnormality and vascular endothelial damage in the pathogenesis of thrombocytopenic multiple organ failure, *Crit Care Med* 30:2242–2248, 2002.

Vary T, McLean B, VonRueden KT: Shock and multiple organ dysfunction syndrome. In McQuillan KA, VonRueden KT, Hartsock RL, et al: *Trauma nursing from resuscitation through rehabilitation*, ed 3, Philadelphia, 2002, Saunders.

Vincent JL, Moreno R, Takala J, et al: The SOFA (sepsis-related organ failure assessment) score to describe organ dysfunction/failure, *Intensive Care Med* 22:707–710, 1996.

Waxman K: Physiologic response to injury. In Grenvik A, Ayres SM, Holbrook PR, et al, editors: *Textbook of critical care*, ed 4, Philadelphia, 2000, Saunders.

Widrich J, Gropper MA: Sepsis syndrome. In Parsons PE, Wiener-Kronish JP: *Critical care secrets*, ed 3, Philadelphia, 2003, Hanley & Belfus.

Multisystem Trauma

Atwell S: Trauma in the elderly. In McQuillan KA, VonRueden KT, Hartsock RL, et al: *Trauma nursing from resuscitation through rehabilitation*, ed 3, Philadelphia, 2002, Saunders.

Beachley M: Evolution of the trauma cycle. In McQuillan KA, VonRueden KT, Hartsock RL, et al: *Trauma nursing from resuscitation through rehabilitation,* ed 3, Philadelphia, 2002, Saunders.

Centers for Disease Control and Prevention: Injury fact book 2001–2002, http://www.cdc.gov/ncipc/fact_book/, November 14, 2001.

Demetriades D: Technology-driven triage of abdominal trauma: the emerging era of nonoperative management, *Ann Rev Med* 54:1–15, 2003.

Drummond JC, Petrovitch CT: The massively bleeding patient, *Anesthesiol Clin North Am* 19:633–649, 2001.

Eastern Association for the Surgery of Trauma Practice Management Guidelines Work Group: *Practice management guidelines for the evaluation of blunt abdominal trauma,* Allentown, Penn, 2001, Eastern Association for the Surgery of Trauma.

Eastern Association for the Surgery of Trauma Practice Management Guidelines Work Group: *Practice management guidelines for geriatric trauma,* Allentown, Penn, 2001, Eastern Association for the Surgery of Trauma.

Emergency Nurses Association: *Trauma nursing core course: provider manual,* ed 5, Des Plaines, IL, 2000, Author.

Emergency Nurses Association: *Course in advanced trauma nursing—II: a conceptual approach to injury and illness,* ed 2, Dubuque, Iowa, 2003, Kendall/Hunt Publishing Company.

Farrar JA: Psychosocial impact of trauma. In McQuillan KA, VonRueden KT, Hartsock RL, et al: *Trauma nursing from resuscitation through rehabilitation,* ed 3, Philadelphia, 2002, Saunders.

Fleming AW, Linder JE: Traumatic injuries. In Yoshikawa TT, Norman DC, editors: *Acute emergencies and critical care of the geriatric patient,* New York, 2000, Marcel Dekker.

Gannon CJ, Napolitano LM, Pasquale M, et al: A statewide population-based study of gender differences in trauma: validation of a prior single-institution study, *J Am Coll Surg* 195:11–18, 2002.

Grossman MD: When is an elder old? Effect of preexisting conditions on mortality in geriatric trauma, *J Trauma* 52:242–246, 2002.

Hinkle J, Betz S: Gunshot injuries, *AACN Clin Issues* 6:175–186, 1995.

Jehle DV, Stiller G, Wagner D: Sensitivity in detecting free intraperitoneal fluid with the pelvic views of the FAST exam, *Am J Emerg Med* 21:476–478, 2003.

Kouraklis G: Damage control surgery: an alternative approach for the management of critically injured patients, *Surg Today* 32: 195–202, 2002.

Loiselle JM: The adolescent trauma patient, *Clin Pediatr Emerg Med* 4:4–11, 2003.

McMahon DJ, Shapiro MB, Kauder DR: The injured elderly in the trauma intensive care unit, *Surg Clin North Am* 80:1005–1019, 2000.

McNelis J, Marini CP, Jurkiewica A: Prolonged lactate clearance is associated with increased mortality in the surgical intensive care unit, *Am J Surg* 182:481–485, 2001.

Montonye JM: Abdominal injuries. In McQuillan KA, VonRueden KT, Hartsock RL, et al: *Trauma nursing from resuscitation through rehabilitation,* ed 3, Philadelphia, 2002, Saunders.

National Safety Council: *Injury facts,* Itasca, Ill, 2002, Author.

National Safety Council: *Injury facts,* Itasca, Ill, 2003, Author.

Orlinsky M, Shoemaker W, Reis ED, et al: Current controversies in shock and resuscitation, *Surg Clin North Am* 81:1217–1262, 2001.

Shin H, Hu S, Yang C, et al: Alcohol intoxication increases morbidity in drivers involved in motor vehicle accidents, *Am J Emerg Med* 21:91–94, 2003.

Shoenberger JM, Houpt JC, Swadron SP: Occult trauma in high-risk populations, *Emerg Med Clin North Am* 21:1145–1152, 2003.

Sommers MS, Dyehouse JM, Howe SR, et al: Attribution of injury to alcohol involvement in young adults seriously injured in alcohol-related motor vehicle crashes, *Am J Crit Care* 9:28–35, 2000.

Stanek GS, Klein C: Metabolic and nutritional management of the trauma patient. In McQuillan KA, VonRueden KT, Hartsock RL, et al: *Trauma nursing from resuscitation through rehabilitation,* ed 3, Philadelphia, 2002, Saunders.

Weigelt JA, Klein JD: Mechanism of injury. In McQuillan KA, VonRueden KT, Hartsock RL, et al: *Trauma nursing from resuscitation through rehabilitation,* ed 3, Philadelphia, 2002, Saunders.

Burns

Acute Respiratory Distress Syndrome Network: Ventilation with lower tidal volumes as compared with traditional tidal volumes for acute lung injury and the acute respiratory distress syndrome, *N Engl J Med* 342:1301–1308, 2000.

Alson R: Thermal burns, *eMedicine*, 2003.

American Burn Association: Practice guidelines for burn care, *J Burn Care Rehabil* suppl:1S–69S, May-June 2001.

Bayley EW, Turcke SA: *A comprehensive curriculum for trauma nursing*, Boston, 1992, Jones & Bartlett.

Borgeson D, Liotta EA: Electrical burns, *eMedicine*, 2002.

Branas B, Gomez-Bajo GJ, Rodriguez FL, et al: Hypothermia and burns: a meta-analysis, *Ann Burns Fire Dis* 2:1–6, 2003.

Edlich RF, Farinholt HA: Thermal burns, *eMedicine*, 2003.

Flynn MB: Burn injuries. In McQuillan KA, VonRueden KT, Hartsock RL, et al: *Trauma nursing from resuscitation through rehabilitation*, ed 3, Philadelphia, 2002, Saunders.

Gore DC, Chinkes D, Heggers J, et al: Association of hyperglycemia with increased mortality after severe burn injury, *J Trauma* 51:540–544, 2001.

Kumar P: Fluid resuscitation for burns: a double edge weapon, *Burns* 23:258–265, 2002.

LaBorde P, Willis J: Burns. In Sole ML, Lamborn ML, Hartshorn JC: *Introduction to critical care nursing*, ed 3, Philadelphia, 2001, Saunders.

Lafferty KA: Smoke inhalation, *eMedicine*, 2001.

Lund CC, Browder NC: The estimation of areas of burns, *Surg Gynecol Obstet* 79:353, 1944.

Murphy KD, Lee JO, Herndon DN: Current pharmacotherapy for the treatment of severe burns, *Expert Opin Pharmacother* 4:369–384, 2003.

O'Keefe GE, Hunt JL, Purdue GF: An evaluation of risk factors for mortality after burn trauma and the identification of gender-dependent difference in outcomes, *J Am Coll Surg* 192:153–160, 2001.

Rabinowitz PM, Siegel MD: Acute inhalation injury, *Clin Chest Med* 23:707–715, 2002.

Reagan B, Staiano-Coico L, LaBruna A, et al: The effects of burn blister fluid on cultured keratinocytes, *J Trauma* 40:361–367, 1996.

Sadowski D: Burns. In Sommers MS, Johnson S, editors: *Davis's manual of nursing therapeutics for disease and disorders*, Philadelphia, 1997, FA Davis.

Saffle JR: What's new in general surgery: burns and metabolism, *J Am Coll Surg* 196: 267–289, 2003.

Schiller WR: Burn care and inhalation injury. In Grenvik A, Ayres SM, Holbrook PR, et al, editors: *Textbook of critical care*, ed 4, Philadelphia, 2000, Saunders.

Schwarz K, Dulchavsky S: Burn wound infections, *eMedicine*, 2002.

Sheridan R: Specific therapies for inhalation injury, *Crit Care Med* 30:718–719, 2002.

Sheridan RL: Burns, *Crit Care Med* 30: S500–S514, 2002.

Sheridan RL, Tompkins RG: What's new in burns and metabolism, *J Am Coll Surg* 198: 243–263, 2004.

Van den Berghe G, Wouters PJ, Bouillon R, et al: Outcome benefit of intensive insulin therapy in the critically ill: insulin dose versus glycemic control, *Crit Care Med* 31:359–366, 2003.

Van den Berghe G, Wouters P, Weekers F, et al: Intensive insulin therapy in the critically ill patients, *N Engl J Med* 345:1359–1367, 2001.

Vindenes H, Ulvestad E, Bjerknes R: Increased levels of circulating interleukin-8 in patients with large burns: relation to burn size and sepsis, *J Trauma* 39:635–640, 1995.

Hypothermia

American Heart Association, International Liaison Committee on Resuscitation (ILCOR): Guidelines 2000 for cardiopulmonary resuscitation and emergency cardiovascular care, *Circulation* 102(8 suppl): I229–I232, 2000.

Bernard SA, Buist M: Induced hypothermia in critical care medicine: a review, *Crit Care Med* 31:2041–2051, 2003.

Biem J, Koehncke N, Dosman J: Out of the cold: management of hypothermia and frostbite, *Can Med Assoc J* 168:305–311, 2003.

Cohen S, Hayes JS, Tordella T, et al: Thermal efficiency of prewarmed cotton, reflective and forced warm air inflatable blankets in trauma patients, *Int J Trauma Nurs* 8:4–8, 2002.

Collins J: Hypothermia, *Practitioner* 239: 22–26, 1995.

Corneli HM: Hot topics in cold medicine: controversies in accidental hypothermia, *Clin Pediatr Emerg Med* 2:179–191, 2001.

Danzl DF: Hypothermia and frostbite. In Braunwald E, Fauci AS, Kasper DL, et al, editors: *Harrison's principles of internal medicine*, ed 5, New York, 2001, McGraw-Hill.

Danzl DF, Pozos RS: Accidental hypothermia, *N Engl J Med* 331:1756–1760, 1994.

Drummond JC, Petrovitch CT: The massively bleeding patient, *Anesthesiol Clin North Am* 19:633–649, 2001.

Fritsch DE: Hypothermia in the trauma patient, *AACN Clin Issues* 6:196–211, 1995.

Gentilello LM: Advances in the management of hypothermia, *Surg Clin North Am* 75:243–256, 1995.

Heimbach D, Jurkovich GJ, Gentilello LM: Accidental hypothermia. In Grenvik A, Ayres SM, Holbrook PR, et al, editors: *Textbook of critical care*, ed 4, Philadelphia, 2000, Saunders.

Humbli EH, Demling RH: Hypothermia and cold-related injuries. In Ayers SM, editor: *Textbook of critical care*, ed 3, Philadelphia, 1995, Saunders.

Inamasu J, Ichikizaki K: Mild hypothermia in neurologic emergency: an update, *Ann Emerg Med* 40:220–230, 2002.

Kudoh A, Takase H, Takazawa T: Chronic treatment with antidepressants decreases intraoperative core hypothermia, *Anesth Anal* 97:275–279, 2003.

Mattu A, Brady WJ, Perron AD: Electrocardiographic manifestations of hypothermia, *Am J Emerg Med* 20:314–326, 2002.

Mecchem CC: Hypothermia and hyperthermia. In Lanken PN, Hanson CW, Manaker S, *The intensive care unit manual*, Philadelphia, 2001, Saunders.

Muszkat M, Durst RM, Yehuda A: Factors associated with mortality among elderly patients with hypothermia, *Am J Med* 113:234–237, 2002.

Olsen TS, Weber UJ, Kammersgaard LP: Therapeutic hypothermia for acute stroke, *Lancet Neurol* 2:410–416, 2003.

Petrone P, Kuncir E, Asensio JA: Surgical management and strategies in the treatment of hypothermia and cold injury, *Emerg Med Clin North Am* 21:1165, 2003.

Phillips TG: Hypothermia, *eMedicine*, 2001.

Sessler DI: Complications and treatment of mild hypothermia, *Anesthesiology* 95:531–543, 2001.

Toxin Exposure

Albertson TE, Dawson A, Latorre FD, et al: TOX-ACLS: toxicologic-oriented advanced cardiac life support, *Ann Emerg Med* 37:S78–S90, 2001.

Chiang WK: Mercury. In Ford MD, Delaney KA, Ling LJ, et al, editors: *Clinical toxicology*, ed 1, Philadelphia, 2001, Saunders.

Ford MD, McMartin K: Ethylene glycol and methanol. In Ford MD, Delaney KA, Ling LJ, et al, editors: *Clinical toxicology*, ed 1, Philadelphia, 2001, Saunders.

Goldfrank LR, Flomenbaum NE, Lewin NA, et al: *Toxicologic emergencies*, ed 5, Norwalk, Conn, 1994, Appleton & Lange.

Henry GC, Haynes S: Isoniazid and other antituberculous drugs. In Ford MD, Delaney KA, Ling LJ, et al, editors: *Clinical toxicology*, ed 1, Philadelphia, 2001, Saunders.

Hryhorczuk D, Eng J: Arsenic. In Ford MD, Delaney KA, Ling LJ, et al, editors: *Clinical toxicology*, ed 1, Philadelphia, 2001, Saunders.

Kalant H: The pharmacology and toxicology of "ecstasy" (MDMA) and related drugs, *Can Med Assoc J* 165:917–928, 2001.

Kleinschmidt KC, Wainscott M, Ford MD: Opioids. In Ford MD, Delaney KA, Ling LJ, et al, editors: *Clinical toxicology*, ed 1, Philadelphia, 2001, Saunders.

Kosnett MJ: Lead. In Ford MD, Delaney KA, Ling LJ, et al, editors: *Clinical toxicology*, ed 1, Philadelphia, 2001, Saunders.

Liegelt EL: Sedative hypnotics. In Ford MD, Delaney KA, Ling LJ, et al, editors: *Clinical toxicology*, ed 1, Philadelphia, 2001, Saunders.

Linden CH: Digitalis glycosides. In Ford MD, Delaney KA, Ling LJ, et al, editors: *Clinical toxicology*, ed 1, Philadelphia, 2001, Saunders.

Linden C, Burns MJ: Illnesses due to poisons, drug overdosage, and envenomation. In Braunwald E, Fauci AS, Kasper DL, et al, editors: *Harrison's principles of internal medicine*, ed 5, New York, 2001, McGraw-Hill.

McKinney PE, Birnbaum K: Carbamazepine. In Ford MD, Delaney KA, Ling LJ, et al, editors: *Clinical toxicology*, ed 1, Philadelphia, 2001, Saunders.

Mokhlesi B, Leiken JB, Murray P, et al: Adult toxicology in critical care. Part I: general approach to the intoxicated patient, *Chest* 123:577–592, 2003a.

Mokhlesi B, Leiken JB, Murray P, et al: Adult toxicology in critical care. Part II: specific poisonings, *Chest* 123:897–922, 2003b.

National Safety Council: *National Safety Council: injury facts*, Itasca, Ill, 2002, Author.

National Safety Council: *National Safety Council: injury facts*, Itasca, Ill, 2003, Author.

Ordog GJ, Wasserberger J: Medical toxicology in critical care medicine. In Grenvik A, Ayres SM, Holbrook PR, et al, editors: *Textbook of critical care*, ed 4, Philadelphia, 2000, Saunders.

Otten EJ, Prybys KM, Gesell LB: Ethanol. In Ford MD, Delaney KA, Ling LJ, et al, editors: *Clinical toxicology,* ed 1, Philadelphia, 2001, Saunders.

Tenenbein M: Iron. In Ford MD, Delaney KA, Ling LJ, et al, editors: *Clinical toxicology,* ed 1, Philadelphia, 2001, Saunders.

Traub SJ, Su M, Hoffman RS, et al: Use of pharmaceutical promotility agents in the treatment of body packers, *Am J Emerg Med* 21:511–512, 2003.

Watson WA, Litovitz TL, Rodgers GC, et al: 2002 annual report of the American Association of Poison Control Centers Toxic Exposure Surveillance System, *Am J Emerg Med* 21:353–421, 2003.

Watson WA, Rose SR: Pharmacokinetics and toxicokinetics. In Ford MD, Delaney KA, Ling LJ, et al, editors: *Clinical toxicology,* ed 1, Philadelphia, 2001, Saunders.

Williams LC, Keyes C: Psychoactive drugs. In Ford MD, Delaney KA, Ling LJ, et al, editors: *Clinical toxicology,* ed 1, Philadelphia, 2001, Saunders.

Zimmerman JL: Poisonings and overdoses in the intensive care unit: general and specific management issues, *Crit Care Med* 31: 2794, 2003.

Psychosocial Aspects of Critical Care

ELIZABETH A. HENNEMAN, RN, PhD, CCNS
JAN MARIE BELDEN, MSN, APRN, BC, FNP (Contributor for content related to pain)

SYSTEMWIDE ELEMENTS

Psychosocial Considerations

1. **Scope of critical care nursing practice**
   a. "The scope of practice for acute and critical care nursing is defined by the dynamic interaction of the acutely and critically ill patient, the acute or critical care nurse and the health care environment" (American Association of Critical-Care Nurses [AACN], 2000, p. 2) (Figure 10-1)
   b. Critical illness is a crisis for both the patient and family members. This crisis situation can present numerous, oftentimes complex psychosocial issues and problems that require the expertise of the critical care nurse working collaboratively with the multidisciplinary team. The crisis of a critical illness may be superimposed on other chronic stressors (e.g., addiction).
   c. Needs or characteristics of the patient and family influence and drive the characteristics or competencies of the critical care nurse (AACN, 2003)
   d. Challenges of meeting psychosocial needs
      i. Other conflicting priorities such as addressing the physiologic instability of the patient may preclude or inhibit nurses from meeting the psychosocial needs of the patient and family
      ii. Psychosocial needs often involve family members (an aspect unique to psychosocial needs in contrast to physiologic needs); for example, issues such as grief and loss, and powerlessness may pertain more to the family than to the patient in some situations (e.g., brain-dead patient)
      iii. Value systems in critical care units often emphasize performing nursing tasks over attending to the psychosocial needs of the patient and family
      iv. Meeting psychosocial needs demands a coordinated, multidisciplinary approach to care
      v. Critical care environment is often a barrier to effectively meeting psychosocial needs
      vi. Growing evidence supports an interrelationship between psychosocial and physiologic problems (e.g., stress and immunity)
   e. Patient
      i. Critically ill patients share some common, predicable psychosocial needs (e.g., the need for reassurance and support)
      ii. Specific patient psychosocial needs vary depending on patient and family characteristics and the patient's status on the health-to-illness continuum

849

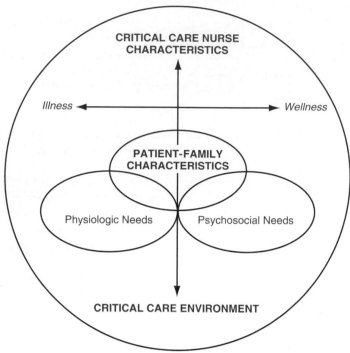

FIGURE 10-1 ■ Complexity of the psychosocial needs of critically ill patients and their families.

      iii. The more compromised the patient, the more complex the patient's needs

      iv. Critically ill patients' psychosocial needs are based on patient characteristics, including resiliency, vulnerability, stability, complexity, resource availability, participation in care and decision making, and the predictability of the illness (AACN, 2003; Hardin and Kaplow, 2005)

      v. Patient characteristics and needs influence family members' needs and psychosocial issues

   f. Family

      i. Definition of family

         (a) Traditional: "A group of two or more people who reside together and who are related by birth, marriage, or adoption" (US Bureau of the Census, 2000)

         (b) Contemporary: "Group of people who love and care for each other" (Seligmann, 1990)

         (c) As the patient defines it

      ii. Families of critically ill patients share a variety of predictable psychosocial needs

      iii. Specific psychosocial needs of family members vary depending on patient characteristics, family characteristics, and the patient's status on the health-to-illness continuum (e.g., cultural diversity issues)

      iv. Predicable needs of family members of critically ill patients include the following:

         (a) To obtain information

         (b) To receive support and reassurance

         (c) To be with the patient

    g. Critical care nurse

        i. Critical care nurse characteristics influence the extent to which patient and family psychosocial needs are met

        ii. Continuum of nursing characteristics includes clinical judgment, advocacy and moral agency, caring practices, collaboration, systems thinking, response to diversity, clinical inquiry, and facilitation of learning (Hardin and Kaplow, 2005)

    h. Critical care team

        i. Members of the critical care team include the nurse, physician, respiratory therapist, social worker, clergy, physical therapist, occupational and speech therapist, others as needed

        ii. Psychosocial needs of the patient and family are met through the collaborative efforts of a multidisciplinary team; each member brings a unique perspective and specific expertise to the shared plan of care and patient goals

    i. Critical care environment (interaction among elements—hence complexity)

        i. High-technology, fast-paced environment presents challenges to meeting psychosocial needs

        ii. Physical environment: Noise, lights, lack of privacy, odors, drafts, and hot or cold rooms are sources of environmental stress

2. Common elements

    a. Life cycle

        i. Patients and family members come to critical care units at all phases of the life cycle

        ii. Growth and development of the patient and family members influence psychosocial needs, response to critical illness, and behaviors (e.g., body image changes may present serious psychologic stressors to young adults)

        iii. Erikson's eight stages of the life cycle: See Table 10-1

    b. Needs of the patient

        i. Maslow categorized needs in terms of a hierarchy

            (a) Physiologic requirements

            (b) Safety and security

            (c) Love and sense of belonging

            (d) Self-esteem

            (e) Self-actualization

        ii. Basic needs must be satisfied before higher-level needs can be met

        iii. Needs change throughout the life cycle

        iv. Critical illness may require refocusing on the achievement of basic needs

    c. Family issues

        i. Family system theories

            (a) Derived from general system theory—a method of viewing systems that are composed of related parts that interact together as a whole

            (b) Can be used by critical care nurses to understand family cultural patterns and dynamics, including communication patterns, power, economics, and interaction. Also helps give insight into dysfunctional family relationships (Satir, 1967).

        ii. Family systems

            (a) Groups of individuals bonded together by their interests

            (b) Community whose members nurture and support one another

            (c) Members have a set of rules, roles, power structure, forms of communication, and styles of problem solving that allow tasks to be accomplished effectively

■ **TABLE 10-1**
■ ■ **Erikson's Eight Stages of the Life Cycle**

Stage*	Developmental Tasks	Approach
ACQUISITION OF HOPE		
Trust versus mistrust (0–2 yr)	Incorporative stage by oral, tactual, and visual senses Needs are met; sense of trust of self and others develops Mother figure important	Provide oral gratification. Provide soft touch, cuddling. Use gentle voice. Provide safe, warm environment. Physical and emotional safety: Enable mother to stay with patient. Supply special toys and blanket. Be a consistent care provider.
ACQUISITION OF WILL		
Autonomy versus shame (2–3 yr)	Muscle system maturation Coordination of holding on and letting go Beginning of autonomous will Self-control without loss of self-esteem Illness may be seen as shameful and/or dirty or bad	Use gentle firmness and reassurance by word and act. Talk to patient before performing procedures. Enhance self-esteem. Foster autonomy and self-reliance. Take time to explain in simple terms; use touch and gentle words.
ACQUISITION OF PURPOSE		
Initiative versus guilt (3–6 yr)	Becomes part of family relationships: *I am a person*, but what kind of person? Identifies with parents Social circles widen; makes friends Has enough language skills to understand and *misunderstand* Imagination increases to point of frightening self Child psychomotor skills, mental curiosity, social nature intrude on how child thinks Curious about sexuality Early sense of responsibility and conscience	Satisfy curiosity with simple and practical information. Provide comfort when patient has bad dreams (loss of life, limb). Dispel fantasies; encourage questions. Answer within patient's understanding. Make patient a partner in treatment, within patient's limits. Enable family to visit or stay with patient. Be a consistent provider.
ACQUISITION OF COMPETENCE		
Industry versus inferiority (6–12 yr)	Active period of socialization Period of learning: *I am what I learn* Balance between *what I want to do* and *what I am told to do* If child is too rigid, develops overly strict sense of duty, which restricts socialization and creativity Needs to work and learn to feel good about self Wants to be recognized by doing things well Needs time for self and others	Respect patient's need for privacy. Provide balance of social time and alone time. Let patient help with care. Teach about what is going on around area. Use gentle firmness. Engage in conversation about school activities, sports, classes, hobbies. Engage in active listening. Recognize importance of respect and dignity. Recognize importance of friends' communicating and visiting.

Continued

ACQUISITION OF FIDELITY

Identity versus role confusion (13–20 yr)

Searches for self, *new self emerging*, with physical growth and development of secondary sex characteristics

Takes very seriously how he or she thinks others see him or her, in comparison with what he or she feels about self

Needs to incorporate new changes and old roles and skills into a person that fits with image of today

Identity equals how he or she thinks others see him or her

Identity diffusion is confusion between what person thinks others see and what person believes about self

Use name of patient.

Recognize that peers are important and have a powerful influence on patient's identity.

Foster decision making by patient within safety parameters.

Encourage patient to believe that he or she is part of the treatment process.

Encourage patient to talk about plans and dreams, what he or she wants to do.

Recognize importance of personal grooming.

Focus on strengths.

Provide information to patient.

Make patient's input part of treatment process.

ACQUISITION OF LOVE

Intimacy versus isolation (21–45 yr)

Increased importance of human closeness

Work and study for life's role

Interpersonal intimacy with another adult

Endless talking about what one feels, what others seem to feel, expectations and hopes

If intimacy not accomplished, will isolate self and lack spontaneity

Recognize importance of patient's family.

Allow involvement of significant others.

Encourage patient to talk about plans of life, what he or she does and hopes to accomplish.

Make patient's input part of treatment planning.

Share information, involve family.

Talk about children, work, hobbies.

Communicate openly and honestly about patient's condition.

ACQUISITION OF CARE

Generativity versus stagnation (45–65 yr)

Individuals combine their personalities and energies in producing fulfilling relationships, possibly common offspring, creativity, job fulfillment

Believes in self; enhanced self-esteem and self-concept allows for closeness of relationships

When unable to develop relationships, become self-absorbed or withdrawn

Show respect and concern.

Recognize patient's need to be involved in treatment along with significant others.

Provide information to patient and family.

Engage in information sharing.

Even if patient is unconscious, talk to him or her.

Explain what is happening.

ACQUISITION OF WISDOM

Ego integrity versus despair (≥65 yr)

Acceptance of one's own life as significant and others' as important

Feels responsible for own life, *I accept what I am* (responsible for own life), life has dignity and love

Emotional integration provides the strength to deal with life as it is *right now*

Treat with respect and dignity.

Address as Mr./Mrs./Ms. or by title.

Involve patient in treatment planning.

Encourage expressions of life experiences.

Recognize that significant others are very important in the decision-making process.

Provide control of pain to enhance dignity and *clarity of mind*.

*Ages are approximate and should be considered only as a guide.

   (d) Critical illness alters rules, roles, power, and so on, in the family, which creates stress and the need for adaptation to a new environment and situation
   (e) Influenced by cultural factors, spiritual support
  iii. Caregiver issues
   (a) Caregivers, including family members and nursing staff, are exposed to environmental stressors; may lead to role strain
   (b) Can lead to exhaustion if not recognized and managed effectively
 d. Critical care environment
  i. Can directly affect the ability to meet a patient's needs, including the need for rest and sleep (e.g., lack of doors on patient rooms, fluorescent overbed lighting, etc.).
  ii. Staff awareness and behaviors also can have a profound effect on modifying environmental influences that affect the patient.
  iii. Unusual patterns of light and noise, together with the constant activity of a critical care unit, alter the patient's biologic rhythms and may negatively affect patient outcomes (Jastremski and Harvey, 1998)
  iv. Environmental factors may lead to sensory overstimulation or sensory deprivation
   (a) Noise: Sources of noise include staff conversations, alarms, and equipment. Critically ill patients have reported the sound of human voices outside the room to be the most disturbing sound (Topf, Bookman, and Armand, 1996). Adverse effects of noise include increased adrenaline levels, diminished immune function, and decreased pain tolerance (Grumet, 1993; Pope, 1995).
   (b) Lights: Ceiling lights and glare disturb patients
  v. Strategies for creating a healing environment: See Box 10-1
 e. Stress

■ **BOX 10-1**
■ **STRATEGIES FOR CREATING A HEALING ENVIRONMENT**

- Provide the patient with reassurance that the patient is being closely watched and that you are available to meet the patient's needs.
- Create a personalized space for the patient, keep the patient's personal items (such as eyeglasses) within reach, and display cherished items (such as family pictures).
- Ensure privacy and dignity (e.g., close curtains and doors and talk quietly during sensitive conversations).
- Provide information about caregivers (e.g., write the names of nurses and other caregivers on a dry-erase board in the room).
- Use dimmers to adjust the brightness of lights.
- Adjust the curtains to block out bright lights.
- Provide natural light and outside views when possible.
- Use incandescent lighting if possible.
- Decrease sensory deprivation by allowing family visitation, surrounding the patient with familiar items, providing radio or television, etc., according to the patient's desires.
- Use music therapy, which provides comforting background noise and helps manage stress, anxiety, and pain.

      i. Definition: Condition that exists in an organism when it encounters stimuli (Selye, 1974)

     ii. Critical illness is a stressful situation. Directed interventions by the nurse can lessen stress and/or the impact of stress on the patient and family. Nursing presence and the anticipation of patient needs have been reported to be associated with less stressful critical care experiences (Holland, Cason, and Prater, 1997; Pettigrew, 1990).

    iii. Selye (1974) identified two types of stress

       (a) Eustress: Condition that exists in an organism when it meets with non-threatening stimuli

       (b) Distress: Condition that exists in an organism when it meets with noxious stimuli

    iv. Common psychologic stressors for critically ill patients and their families

       (a) Powerlessness (lack of control)

       (b) Sleep deprivation

       (c) Grief and loss

       (d) Sensory overload or deprivation

       (e) Pain

     v. Response to stress

       (a) Noxious psychosocial stimuli can overwhelm the body's compensatory ability to maintain homeostasis and can elicit a stress response

       (b) Major neural response to a stressful stimulus is activation of the sympathetic nervous system

       (c) Relationship between psychologic stress and health: Psychoneuro-immunologic research has identified a relationship between stress and immune function (i.e., an increased stress response is associated with decreased immunity) (Caine, 2003)

Patient and Family Psychosocial Assessment

1. Nursing history

  a. Patient history

      i. Identify preexisting psychiatric, psychologic, and social problems

     ii. Identify preillness coping mechanisms

    iii. Identify sources of support (e.g., family, friends, spiritual support, pets)

    iv. Identify patient proxy, living will, durable power of attorney, and so on

  b. Family history: Family assessment data obtained on admission or as soon as possible

      i. Health care proxy or family spokesperson

     ii. Contact information (e.g., home and cell phone numbers, pager numbers)

    iii. Diversity issues (culture, language, etc.) that affect the patient and family

    iv. Coping strategies

     v. Family caregivers

    vi. Support systems (family, friends, church group, other spiritual support)

    vii. Special family needs (e.g., young children, handicaps, etc.)

   viii. Family concerns regarding this hospitalization

    ix. Best time for family to visit the patient

     x. Preferred method of meeting and communicating with intensive care unit (ICU) team members (e.g., participation in scheduled ICU rounds, scheduled evening meetings, phone calls)

2. Nursing examination of patient

  a. Physical examination

   b. Cognitive assessment (e.g., ability to concentrate, level of judgment, presence of confusion)

   c. Behavioral assessment (sleep patterns, level of agitation, interaction with family and staff)

   d. Review of findings from other diagnostic studies (e.g., computed tomographic [CT] scan, electroencephalogram [EEG], etc.)

3. Appraisal of patient characteristics: Almost all patients with a critical illness experience some psychosocial issues during the course of their illness. However, each patient and family is unique and brings a unique set of characteristics to the care situation (Hardin and Kaplow, 2005). Examples of characteristics of patients and family that the nurses need to assess include the following:

   a. Resiliency

     i. Level 1—*Minimally resilient:* A 52-year-old divorced woman who has attempted suicide via drug overdose on three previous occasions is admitted with a nonlethal self-inflicted gunshot wound to the head

     ii. Level 3—*Moderately resilient:* A 23-year-old man with a 9-year history of "problem drinking," stabilized after chest trauma suffered in an alcohol-related automobile accident, is being prepared for transfer to a military hospital where he will receive extended treatment for alcohol abuse

     iii. Level 5—*Highly resilient:* A healthy 21-year-old female college student with a 3.9 grade point average comes to the emergency department exhibiting multiple abrasions and unruly, belligerent, and delirious behavior after attending her first "spring breakout celebration," which included drinking, some drug experimenting, and falling off the roof of a moving car

   b. Vulnerability

     i. Level 1—*Highly vulnerable:* A malnourished 9-year-old child who has been a victim of child abuse since birth is recovering from his most recent "fall down the stairs" and is scheduled for discharge home the next day

     ii. Level 3—*Moderately vulnerable:* An extremely overweight 37-year-old woman admits to feeling "even more depressed" following her unsuccessful suicide attempt. Numerous diets, pills, and plans have not worked, and her primary physician relates that she does not meet the criteria for surgical treatment of morbid obesity.

     iii. Level 5—*Minimally vulnerable:* A 44-year-old single father, admitted for monitoring overnight subsequent to an automobile crash in which he was cited for aggressive driving, relates that since his recent divorce, he occasionally has had episodes when his anger quickly escalates to violent behaviors. He fears "taking it out" on his two sons.

   c. Stability

     i. Level 1—*Minimally stable:* A 65-year-old woman develops acute respiratory distress syndrome following the ingestion of an alkali solution during an attempted suicide

     ii. Level 3—*Moderately stable:* A 50-year-old male with a history of drinking four beers a day is admitted to the ICU for an initial episode of gastrointestinal bleeding secondary to a duodenal ulcer. He is receiving benzodiazepines to prevent delirium tremens from acute alcohol withdrawal.

     iii. Level 5—*Highly stable:* A 25-year-old female is admitted to the ICU from the emergency department, to which she was brought by friends who could not wake her after a night of heavy drinking. She is now awake and alert.

d. Complexity

   i. Level 1—*Highly complex:* An 89-year-old man is experiencing liver failure secondary to the ingestion of 200 acetaminophen tablets following the death of his wife. Patient has multiple medical problems, including lung cancer. He stated in his suicide note that he "is tired" and wants to be with his wife. Family is adamant that everything be done to save his life.

   ii. Level 3—*Moderately complex:* A 60-year-old patient with amyotrophic lateral sclerosis develops acute respiratory failure while in the ICU. Patient has already stated he does not desire mechanical ventilation to prolong life. Family is supportive of the patient's wishes.

   iii. Level 5—*Minimally complex:* A 50-year-old woman in the ICU for the management of gastrointestinal bleeding secondary to nonsteroidal antiinflammatory use develops delirium after receiving sedatives

e. Resource availability

   i. Level 1—*Few resources:* A 40-year-old homeless man is admitted to the ICU after attempted suicide by gunshot to the head. No patient identification is available.

   ii. Level 3—*Moderate resources:* An 83-year-old woman is admitted from a local nursing home to the ICU with possible urosepsis. Patient's family has been paying out of pocket for the nursing home but says "the money is almost gone."

   iii. Level 5—*Many resources:* A 60-year-old computer executive develops delirium tremens 4 days after undergoing elective hip surgery. Family is very supportive and confident the patient would be concerned if he realized how his drinking (three to four glasses of wine per day) had affected him. Patient has excellent insurance coverage for both inpatient care and outpatient substance abuse treatment.

f. Participation in care

   i. Level 1—*No participation:* An 85-year-old male patient underwent a complicated aortic aneurysm repair 3 days earlier. Patient has a 10-year history of dementia and is now experiencing delirium. He is intubated and unable to communicate with the staff.

   ii. Level 3—*Moderate level of participation:* A 35-year-old man, who sustained a head injury after falling out of a tree while intoxicated, is now regaining consciousness and is asking for some water

   iii. Level 5—*Full participation:* A 70-year-old man is admitted to the ICU following extensive abdominal surgery. He asks the nurse for more pain medication so that he can "sit up more and take some deep breaths" like his preoperative instructions directed.

g. Participation in decision making

   i. Level 1—*No participation:* The mother of an 18-year-old brain-dead patient collapses when approached about organ donation. She asks the patient's doctor to make all the necessary decisions.

   ii. Level 3—*Moderate level of participation:* The wife of a 67-year-old man who requires a tracheostomy for long-term airway management following a suicide attempt requests multiple consults from other pulmonary services

   iii. Level 5—*Full participation:* A 65-year-old patient with cancer and chronic pain asks to be removed from the ventilator and be "allowed to die with dignity"

h. Predictability

   i. Level 1—*Not predictable:* A 75-year-old woman with ovarian cancer is admitted after ingesting one-half of a bottle of acetaminophen to "stop the pain"

    ii. Level 3—*Moderately predictable:* A 60-year-old patent with acute respiratory failure develops delirium secondary to a combination of hypoxemia and electrolyte imbalances

    iii. Level 5—*Highly predictable:* A 20-year-old patient is admitted with altered consciousness after drinking at a college fraternity party

4. **Diagnostic studies**
  a. Laboratory studies
  b. EEG
  c. Cerebral blood flow studies

Psychosocial Care Issues

1. **Interdependence**—Many of the psychosocial issues and concerns of the critically ill patient are interdependent. For example, inadequately managed pain may lead to feelings of powerlessness, anxiety, and depression that, in turn, heighten the patient's perception of pain (Figure 10-2).

2. **Powerlessness**
  a. Description of problem
    i. Perceived lack of control over the outcome of a specific situation. The ability of an event to engender a sense of powerlessness is influenced by the individual's self-esteem and self-concept and where the individual is in the life cycle.
    ii. Critically ill patients lose their ability to control even the most basic of functions, including the ability to communicate, to breath on their own, and to control bladder and bowel function. Depending on the philosophy and organization of the critical care environment, they may also lose the ability to participate in decision making about their own health care and future.
  b. Goals of care
    i. Patient communicates needs and wishes verbally or nonverbally
    ii. Patient (and family as appropriate) participates in decision making regarding the plan of care
    iii. Patient and family members do not demonstrate signs of dysfunction associated with powerlessness, such as the following:
      (a) Withdrawal

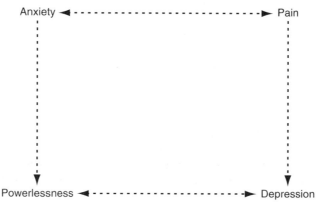

FIGURE 10-2 ■ Relationship between psychosocial needs and problems during a critical illness.

(b) Aggressive behavior

(c) Demanding behavior

(d) Excessive repetition of the same questions

(e) Placing of unrealistic demands on the staff

(f) Blaming of the staff for the patient's condition

iv. Patient participates in decision making regarding daily care activities (e.g., timing of bath, sleep, visiting hours)

c. Collaborating professionals on health care team

i. Nurse

ii. Physician

iii. Respiratory therapist

iv. Physical therapist

v. Social worker

vi. Clergy

vii. Case manager

d. Interventions

i. Promote patient-nurse communication

(a) This intervention presents significant challenges, particularly if the patient is intubated or speaks a language other than English (or the predominant language at the facility)

(b) Methods of communication should be based on patient preferences and abilities. Common communication techniques for use with intubated patients include lip reading, picture or alphabet boards, pen or pencil and paper, and computer.

(c) Utilize available interpreter services for non–English speaking patients and family members

(d) Enlist help from family members and volunteers in the communication process

ii. Involve the patient and family in the care planning process and decision making

(a) Ask the patient (or health care proxy) what level of involvement he or she would like in the care planning process

(b) Encourage the patient and family members to keep a record of questions and concerns

(c) Provide the patient, proxy, or a family member with daily (or more frequent) updates regarding the patient's status and care plan

iii. Encourage the patient and family members to meet with spiritual support persons if they would find this helpful

iv. Prepare the patient for procedures: Explain what will be happening, when it will happen, and how the patient will be affected

e. Evaluation of patient care: Patient and family are active participants in care planning and delivery (to the extent possible)

3. **Sleep deprivation**

a. Description of problem: Sleep deprivation in the critically ill patient involves a decrease in the amount, consistency, and/or quality of sleep that occurs in a 24-hour period. Sleep fragmentation occurs when the patient fails to complete a 90-minute average sleep cycle that includes both rapid eye movement and non–rapid eye movement sleep (Gawlinski and Hamwi, 1999).

b. Goals of care

i. Patient has at least two 90-minute periods of sleep in a 24-hour period

ii. Patient states that he or she feels rested

      iii. Patient does not demonstrate signs and symptoms of sleep deprivation, including the following:

        (a) Altered mental status (e.g., confusion, delusions)

        (b) Decreased alertness

        (c) Irritability

        (d) Aggressive behavior

        (e) Restlessness

        (f) Anxiety

        (g) Exhaustion

  c. Collaborating professionals on health care team

      i. Nurse

      ii. Physician

      iii. Pharmacist

      iv. Respiratory therapist

  d. Interventions

      i. Attempt to provide at least two 90-minute periods of uninterrupted sleep in a 24-hour period

      ii. Cluster activities so that the patient is allowed periods of rest

      iii. Prioritize activities to allow a stable patient to have periods without unnecessary, frequent assessments

      iv. Decrease the noise level to promote sleep

      v. Decrease overhead lighting to promote sleep

      vi. Provide adequate pain relief

      vii. Teach the patient and family relaxation techniques to promote rest and sleep

      viii. Administer pharmacologic agents as needed to promote sleep (e.g., benzodiazepines, diphenhydramine). *Note:* Long-term use of benzodiazepines can abolish stage IV sleep.

      ix. Consult with a pharmacist regarding the best drug choices for promoting sleep, particularly for high-risk populations such as the elderly

  e. Evaluation of patient care

      i. Patient does not demonstrate signs or symptoms of sleep deprivation

      ii. Patient states that he or she feels rested

4. Grief and loss

  a. Description of problem: The grief reaction is the emotional response to a loss in which something valued is changed or altered so that it no longer has its previously valued traits (Gawlinski and Hamwi, 1999)

      i. Grief can be experienced during a critical illness by both the patient and family members

      ii. Grief may result from loss (or potential loss) of health, body image, role, and financial security

      iii. Family members experience grief related to a patient's death or in anticipation of death or potential death

      iv. Degree of grief experienced is related to the meaning of the loss to the individual, the adequacy of coping responses, and the availability of support systems

      v. Expressions of grief have wide variation and are culturally determined

  b. Goals of care

      i. Patient and family express feelings of grief and loss (if they choose)

      ii. Patient and family are able to state the prognosis and current plan of care

  c. Collaborating professionals on health care team

      i. Nurse

      ii. Clergy

      iii. Social worker

      iv. Physician

   d. Interventions

      i. Appreciate cultural variation in expressions of grief

      ii. Allow the patient and family members to express grief in their own way

      iii. Provide privacy for family members and patients

      iv. Provide ongoing, honest information to the patient and family regarding the patient's illness and expected recovery

      v. Provide the patient and family with teaching regarding the normal grief response

   e. Evaluation of patient care: Patient and family express grief in a culturally appropriate way

5. Sensory overload or deprivation: See Box 10-1

SPECIFIC PATIENT HEALTH PROBLEMS

Anxiety

1. Definition: Anxiety is the apprehensive anticipation of future danger or misfortune accompanied by a feeling of dysphoria or somatic symptoms of tension. Focus of anticipated danger may be internal or external (American Psychiatric Association [APA], 2000).

2. Etiology and risk factors: Results from multiple sources in the ICU, including the following:

   a. Unstable physiologic status (e.g., hypoxemia with shortness of breath)

   b. Pain

   c. Fear of the unknown

   d. Procedures

   e. Separation from family and support system

   f. Underlying psychiatric disorder (including panic disorders, phobias, and post-traumatic stress disorder)

3. Signs and symptoms: See Box 10-2

4. Diagnostic study findings

   a. When behavioral manifestations of anxiety are present, possible physiologic causes (e.g., hypoxemia and hypoglycemia) must be ruled out

   b. Toxicologic screen: To assess for possible drug-induced anxiety

   c. Mental status examination: Findings may be abnormal with severe anxiety

5. Collaborative diagnoses of patient needs: Minimize anxiety for the patient and family by preparing them for potentially anxiety-producing situations

6. Goals of care

   a. Patient does not demonstrate signs or symptoms of anxiety (e.g., no tachypnea, tachycardia, muscle tension)

   b. Patient communicates that he or she is not anxious

7. Management of patient care

   a. Anticipated patient trajectory: With reassurance, support, and pharmacologic therapy as needed, anxiety can be minimized

      i. Treatments

         (a) Nonpharmacologic

            (1) Reassure the patient and give explanations about the patient's condition and treatment plan

■ **BOX 10-2**
■ **CLINICAL MANIFESTATIONS OF ANXIETY**

COGNITIVE
- Apprehension
- Difficulty concentrating
- Hypervigilance
- Impaired judgment
- Self-consciousness
- Worry

BEHAVIORAL
- Easy fatigue
- Fidgeting
- Refusal of medical treatment
- Restlessness
- Sleep disturbances
- Unrealistic demands for attention

PHYSIOLOGIC
- CARDIAC
- Chest pain
- Dysrhythmias
- Increased blood pressure
- Palpitations
- Tachycardia

RESPIRATORY
- Choking sensation
- Shortness of breath
- Tachypnea

NEUROMUSCULAR
- Dilated pupils
- Dizziness
- Light-headedness
- Muscle and motor tension
- Tremors

GASTROINTESTINAL
- Anorexia
- Nausea
- Vomiting

GENITOURINARY
- Frequency
- Urgency

    (2) Ask the patient to discuss fears and worries
    (3) Assure the patient that adequate sedation and pain medication will be provided during painful procedures
    (4) Allow family members to stay with the patient as much as possible to provide support
    (5) Use music therapy
    (6) Use pet therapy if available
  (b) Pharmacologic
    (1) Benzodiazepines
    (2) Sedatives and hypnotics
    (3) Pain medication (as needed)
 ii. Discharge planning
  (a) Teach the patient and family methods of anxiety reduction (e.g., imagery, distraction)
  (b) Patient may require post-ICU follow-up (psychiatric and/or social services) for unresolved anxiety issues
  (c) Patient may require follow-up teaching regarding pharmacologic and nonpharmacologic interventions to treat anxiety

Pain

1. Description
  a. Pain is an individual, subjective, and complex biopsychosocial process whose existence cannot be proved or disproved. Unrelieved pain is a major psychologic and physiologic stressor for patients.

b. Pain is "whatever the person says it is, existing whenever he says it does" (McCaffery, 1968)

c. Pain is "an unpleasant sensory and emotional experience" (Mersky, 1979)

    i. Amount of tissue damage is not the only predictor of when and how pain is experienced (Koestler and Doleys, 2002)

    ii. Other factors influence the response to the cognitive integration of pain (e.g., age, gender, culture, beliefs, mood, previous pain experiences, current diagnosis and situation, amount of perceived control over the situation)

    iii. Negative impact of pain on one's quality of life can include suffering, fear, anxiety, depression, and hopelessness (Cullen, Greiner, Titler, et al, 2001; Graf and Puntillo, 2003; Hamill-Ruth and Marohn, 1999)

d. In critical care patient populations, pain is often undertreated and represents one of patients' greatest worries (Lang, 1999)

2. Etiology and risk factors

  a. Acute conditions

    i. Surgical events (e.g., incisions; presence of drains, tubes, orthopedic hardware)

    ii. Traumatic injuries (e.g., fractures, lacerations)

    iii. Medical conditions (e.g., pancreatitis, ulcerative colitis, migraine headache)

    iv. Psychologic conditions (e.g., anxiety), which can increase pain perception, prolong the pain experience, and lower the pain threshold (Koestler and Doleys, 2002)

  b. Procedures (e.g., turning; suctioning; placement or removal of catheters, tubes, or drains; paracentesis)

  c. Immobility

  d. Preexisting chronic pain conditions

    i. Musculoskeletal conditions (e.g., arthritis, low back pain, fibromyalgia)

    ii. Other conditions (e.g., cancer, stroke, diabetic neuropathy)

  e. Pain can also be perceived without the current presence of a physiologically unpleasant stimulus (Koestler and Doleys, 2002)

3. Signs and symptoms

  a. See Chapter 4 for physiologic aspects of pain

  b. Most reliable indicator of pain is the patient's self report (Acute Pain Management Guideline Panel, 1992)

  c. Other important points related to manifestations of pain include the following:

    i. Patients in pain often demonstrate one or more behavioral signs or indicators of pain intensity (see Table 4-22)

    ii. When patients are unable to respond or self-report pain, behavioral indicators may be used (Pasero, 2003). Due to the individuality of pain expression, these indicators may be absent despite the presence of severe pain, which may cause clinicians to conclude erroneously that pain is not present (American Pain Society [APS], 2003).

    iii. When conditions known to be painful exist, assume that pain is present and proceed with appropriate treatment (APS, 2003; Graf and Puntillo, 2003)

    iv. Several barriers and misconceptions about pain hinder effective pain management (Table 10-2), including the clinician's personal values and beliefs, and confusion about addiction, tolerance, and physical dependence with regard to pain medications. See Table 10-3 for distinctions in these terms as they relate to pain and opioid use.

■ **TABLE 10-2**
■ ■ **Barriers to Pain Management in the Critically Ill Patient**

Barrier	Comment
Pain management often is not a priority because of life-threatening illness or other physiologic conditions.	Patients have the right to effective pain management, and every effort should be made to include analgesia in the treatment plan.
Cultural beliefs about pain (e.g., pain builds character, pain is a sign of weakness or a form of punishment) may affect pain management.	Provide education about harmful effects of pain, benefits of effective pain management, and need to report the effectiveness of pain management.
Lack of knowledge about the process of pain (see Chapter 4) • Individuality of a patient's pain response • Failure to accept a patient's self-report of pain • Harmful effects of pain	Meaning and expression of pain vary among patients. Self-report is the single most reliable indicator of pain (patient is the authority on his or her pain, not you). Pain is not an acceptable consequence of surgery or trauma. Unrelieved pain can lead to life-threatening complications, delayed healing, increased length of hospital stay, and development of future pain issues.
Lack of knowledge about pharmacology of opioids (see Chapter 4) • Exaggerated fear of opioid-induced adverse effects, especially respiratory depression • Ignorance of onset, peak, duration of action, equianalgesia	Respiratory depression is preventable in most cases by slow opioid titration and decrease of dosage when increased sedation occurs. Physicians often underprescribe opioids and nurses often administer the lowest prescribed dose, which contributes to the undertreatment of pain.
Exaggerated fears related to addiction (see Table 10-3) • Fear of creating addiction or causing relapse in a patient with a history of addiction • Fear of being lied to about the severity of pain in order to obtain drugs to support an existing addiction	When opioids are used for pain relief, the addiction rate is less than 1% (McCaffery and Pasero, pp 50–51). Patients with chronic pain often are knowledgeable about which analgesics and dosages they need to relieve their pain. This is not always a sign of addiction.
Inability to communicate (see Chapter 4) • Language barrier or aphasia • Mechanical ventilation • Use of neuromuscular blocking agents, sedatives • Other conditions (e.g., delirium, coma)	Use translators as indicated. Assume pain is present based on physical findings (e.g., trauma, surgery, procedures) and treat with analgesics.
Noisy and chaotic critical care environment	Sleep deprivation, anxiety, and lack of control can negatively affect the patient's perception of, response to, and tolerance of pain.

    d. Practitioners must accept and respond to patient reports of pain

    e. Decrease in or elimination of a pain behavior following an analgesia intervention can indicate a reduction in pain and reflect an ongoing need for analgesia (Hamill-Ruth and Marohn, 1999; McCaffery and Pasero, 1999)

4. Diagnostic study findings

    a. "Pain is described by the person experiencing it; it doesn't have to be diagnosed any other way" (Puntillo, 1995)

■ **TABLE 10-3**
■ ■ **Definitions Related to the Use of Opioids in the Treatment of Pain**

Term	Definition	Comment
Addiction	Chronic, neurobiologic disease Persistent pattern of compulsive and dysfunctional opioid use characterized by an impaired control over drug use, continued use despite harm, use for effect other than pain relief, and craving	When opioids are used for pain relief, the incidence of addiction is less than 1%. Patients with addictive disease are at high risk for undertreatment of pain and have the right to receive quality pain management. Be prepared to titrate opioids and benzodiazepines to dosages higher than usual based on assessment findings (e.g., pain, side effects, mood).
Physical dependence	Physiologic state of reliance on an opioid, evidenced by withdrawal symptoms if the opioid is abruptly stopped or an opioid antagonist is given Does not, in and of itself, imply addiction	Signs and symptoms of withdrawal include lacrimation, rhinorrhea, pupil dilation, yawning, tremor, gooseflesh, insomnia, diarrhea, vomiting, irritability, elevated blood pressure, muscle cramps, dysphoria.
Tolerance	State of adaptation characterized by the need for increasing or more frequent doses of medication to maintain an effect Does not, in and of itself, imply addiction	Tolerance occurs to both the analgesic and adverse effects of opioids (except constipation).
Pain tolerance	Point at which an increasing intensity of a stimulus is felt as painful	Individual, influenced by many factors (e.g., endorphin levels)
Pain threshold	Duration or intensity of pain that a person is willing to endure	Individual, influenced by many factors (e.g., energy level, past pain experiences)

Data and definitions compiled from American Academy of Pain Medicine, American Pain Society, American Society of Addiction Medicine: *Consensus document: Definitions related to the use of opioids for the treatment of pain*, Glenview, Ill, 2001, American Academy of Pain Medicine. Available at http://www.asam.org/ppol/paindef.htm; American Society of Pain Management Nurses: *ASPMN position statement: pain management in patients with addictive disease*, Pensacola, Fla, 2002, Author; and McCaffery M, Pasero C: *Pain: clinical manual*, ed 2, St Louis, 1999, Mosby.

    b. Diagnostic studies may supplement, but should not replace, a comprehensive physical examination and history (National Pharmaceutical Council, 2001)

    c. Diagnostic studies can help to accurately identify the causes for pain; however, the absence of positive study findings should not be used to deny the existence of pain

    d. While diagnostic studies are in progress, treatment of pain should be initiated. It is rarely justified to defer analgesia until a diagnosis is made (APS, 2003; Pace and Burke, 1996).

5. Goals of care

    a. Pain, including procedural pain, is consistently controlled at or below the patient's stated comfort level (e.g., a pain score of 2 to 3 on a scale of 0 to 10)

b. In a patient unable to provide a self-report of pain, there is a marked decrease or absence of pain behaviors following pharmacologic intervention

c. Patient demonstrates a decrease in anxiety and other psychologic effects of unrelieved pain

d. Patient is able to comfortably perform or participate in activities necessary for recovery

e. Patient experiences increased periods of uninterrupted sleep

f. Medication adverse effects are avoided or managed

g. Length of hospital stay is not extended because of poorly managed pain

h. Patient is satisfied with pain management

6. **Management of patient care**

a. Joint Commission on Accreditation of Healthcare Organizations (JCAHO, 2004) pain management standards include the following:

i. "Patients have the right to pain management" (RI.2.160)

ii. "When pain is identified, the patient is assessed and treated by the hospital or referred for treatment" (PC.8.10)

b. Anticipated patient trajectory

i. Assessment

(a) Perform thorough history taking (including a pain history), physical examination, and pain assessment

(b) Identify the underlying cause whenever possible

(c) Identify any previously effective methods of coping with and relieving pain

ii. Treatments

(a) Nonpharmacologic methods

(1) May be used to supplement, but not replace, analgesic medications. Table 10-4 provides an overview of these therapies.

(2) There is a lack of conclusive scientific evidence to support the efficacy of their use for pain management

a) Results are unpredictable

b) Many do not relieve pain; some may only make pain more tolerable for brief intervals

c) Patients must be willing and physically and mentally able to try them

(3) No universally accepted categorizations or definitions of these methods exist. Broad categories include the following:

a) Cutaneous stimulation and physical modalities

b) Cognitive and behavioral modalities

c) Complementary and alternative medicine

(4) Use of these methods in the critically ill patient is limited due to the severity of the patient's illness and other demands on the nurse's time

(b) Pharmacologic methods (see also Chapter 4)

(1) Analgesics are the mainstay of treatment for acute and cancer pain, and some chronic noncancer pain

(2) Three classes of analgesic are nonopioids, opioids, and coanalgesics (adjuvants)

iii. Discharge planning: Patient and family teaching regarding the following:

(a) Appropriate use of pain scales or other methods to be used to assess pain

■ TABLE 10-4
■ ■ Nonpharmacologic Approaches to Pain Management in the Critically Ill Patient*

Examples	Indications	Presumed Mechanism of Pain Reduction	Comments
CUTANEOUS STIMULATION†			
Superficial heat • Hot packs • Hot water bottles • Heating pads • Chemical gel packs Superficial cold • Ice packs • Towels soaked in ice water Gel packs	Joint and muscle pain, spasm, and stiffness, as from surgery Trauma Arthritis Acute low back pain Itching Heat preferred for thrombophlebitis Cold preferred for acute trauma and migraine pain; avoid in peripheral vascular disease	Activation of large myelinated primary afferent fibers may modify response of spinal cord to noxious stimuli May decrease muscle spasm, sensitivity to pain Heat may increase elastic properties of muscles Cold may cause local numbing	May apply at pain site or distal, proximal, or contralateral to pain Avoid both heat and cold over radiation-therapy sites Skin must be protected to avoid tissue damage Cold often more effective and long-lasting than heat
Massage	Stress, anxiety Muscle tension, spasm, pain Immobility	May inhibit transmission of painful stimuli Relaxes muscles	May be acceptable form of touch to convey care and concern Family can be involved
Transcutaneous electrical nerve stimulation (TENS)	Acute surgical, musculoskeletal, neuropathic pain	May inhibit transmission of painful stimuli	Avoid if patient has on-demand pacemaker
Vibration	Muscle, joint and neuropathic pain Avoid in thrombo-phlebitis, headaches	Paresthesia or numbness over site	May change pain from sharp to dull Can be substituted for TENS
PHYSICAL†			
• Mobilization • Range-of-motion exercises • Physical therapy • Repositioning	Prolonged immobility and decreased function	Relieves muscle tension Keeps joints and ligaments flexible	Helps decrease loss of function, strength
• Immobilization	Some postoperative conditions, fractures	Relieves muscle tension Keeps joints and ligaments flexible	Maintains joints in position of maximum function
COGNITIVE-BEHAVIORAL			
• Distraction • Television • Reading • Visiting • Imagery • Music, singing • Humor	Mild to moderate pain of brief duration, such as procedural pain	In general, thought to interfere with neural perception of pain in the brain Refocuses or directs attention away from painful stimuli	Pain awareness may be increased after distraction, so patient may need analgesia to rest

Continued

■ **TABLE 10-4**
■ ■ **Nonpharmacologic Approaches to Pain Management in the Critically Ill Patient*—cont'd**

Examples	Indications	Presumed Mechanism of Pain Reduction	Comments
COGNITIVE-BEHAVIORAL—cont'd			
Relaxation • Deep or rhythmic breathing • Progressive muscle relaxation • Imagery • Massage • Music • Repetition of word or phrase	Muscle tension Anxiety, stress Acute or chronic pain	May be related to reduction in muscle tension, distress, and anxiety	May not "look" like patient is in pain Teach and use as coping skill for stress reduction Dim light and noise reduction promote relaxation
Education • Pain-management concepts	Any pain condition Throughout shift	Reduces stress, anxiety Increases sense of control	Teach patient, family, significant other
COMPLEMENTARY AND ALTERNATIVE MEDICINE (CAM) MODALITIES			
Prayer Meditation Biofeedback Hypnosis Aromatherapy Yoga Therapeutic touch Reflexology Acupuncture Herbs Vitamins	Mainly chronic pain conditions Same methods for acute pain, such as prayer or massage	Promote balance, harmony, and healing by interaction of mind, body, and spirit	Overlap exists between CAM and other nonpharmacologic approaches

*In most clinical situations, these approaches should be used in addition to analgesics.
†Physician order may be required.

   (b) Effective pain management concepts and options (e.g., pain medications and the difference between addiction, physical dependence, and tolerance)
   (c) Pain management as an important part of patient care
   (d) Responsibility of the patient to report ineffective pain relief and concerns regarding the pain management plan
   iv. Useful pain management resources: See pain section in the reference list

Delirium (Acute Confusional State)

1. **Definition:** Clinical state associated with a disturbance of consciousness that is accompanied by a change in cognition that cannot be accounted for by a preexisting or evolving dementia. Delirium develops over a short time (hours to days) and fluctuates during the course of a day (APA, 2000). Delirium is often a temporary condition.

2. **Etiology and risk factors**
    a. Incidence (rates)
        i. 50% of the critically ill experience delirium (Gawlinski and Hamwi, 1999)
        ii. 80% of terminally ill develop delirium near death
    b. Delirium due to a general medical condition
        i. Hypoxia
        ii. Hypercapnia
        iii. Metabolic acidosis
        iv. Heart, kidney, liver failure
        v. Hyperthyroidism or hypothyroidism
        vi. Hyperparathyroidism
        vii. Cerebrovascular accident, transient ischemic attack
        viii. Concussion
        ix. Postictal state
        x. Electrolyte imbalances (hyperkalemia, hypokalemia)
        xi. Hyperglycemia or hypoglycemia
        xii. Alcohol or drug withdrawal
        xiii. Infection
        xiv. Pain
    c. Substance-induced delirium (due to a medication, toxin exposure, drug abuse)
        i. Anesthetics (emergence delirium [Burns, 2003])
        ii. Analgesics
        iii. Sedatives (e.g., benzodiazepines)
        iv. Antiemetics
        v. Cardiac medications (e.g., antihypertensives, digoxin)
        vi. Steroids
        vii. Anticholinergics
        viii. Delirium due to multiple causes
        ix. Other (i.e., not able to be specified)
3. **Signs and symptoms**
    a. Cognitive
        i. Diminished attention span
        ii. Reduced ability to focus
        iii. Disorientation to person, place, time
        iv. Confusion over daily events
        v. Hallucinations (visual are more common)
        vi. Abnormal results on a mental status examination (i.e., Folstein Mini-Mental State Examination)
    b. Behavioral: May vary markedly from patient to patient
        i. Excessive restlessness
        ii. Sluggishness and lethargy
        iii. Inappropriate behavior
        iv. Irritability
        v. Picking or groping at bed linens, gown
        vi. Attempting to get out of bed (when unsafe)
        vii. Crying out, screaming, moaning, muttering
        viii. Personality changes
        ix. Changes in affect
    c. Physiologic
        i. Tremors (alcohol withdrawal)
        ii. Seizures (alcohol withdrawal)

4. **Diagnostic study findings:** Dependent on the underlying problem (e.g., may have abnormal electrolyte levels, CT scan, etc.)
5. **Collaborative diagnoses of patient needs**
   a. Assess for possible factors that could contribute to delirium
   b. Decrease the use of medications that could contribute to delirium
6. **Goals of care**
   a. Patient is oriented to person, time and place
   b. Patient does not demonstrate signs or symptoms of anxiety, fear, and confusion
   c. Patient responds to simple, concrete questions
7. **Management of patient care**
   a. Anticipated patient trajectory: With treatment of the underlying cause of delirium, the problem can be managed and eliminated
      i. Treatments
         (a) Nonpharmacologic
            (1) Assess for delirium (e.g., Confusion Assessment Method–ICU) (Inouye, Van Dyke, Alessi, 1990; Truman and Ely, 2003)
            (2) Provide for adequate rest and sleep
            (3) Review medication list with the physician and discontinue suspect medications
            (4) Monitor and manage electrolyte and acid-base disorders
            (5) Consult a psychiatrist if delirium does not resolve with standard management
            (6) Use restraints only as needed for patient safety
            (7) Explain to family members the nature of delirium and why it occurs. Stress the temporary nature of the condition in hospitalized patients.
            (8) Give family members updates on patient management and progress (e.g., findings related to the underlying cause of the delirium)
            (9) Reassure the family that the patient is not in control or responsible for his or her behaviors
         (b) Pharmacologic: Avoid additional drugs unless needed for patient, family, or staff safety
            (1) Antipsychotic (e.g., haloperidol)
            (2) Benzodiazepine (in combination with an antipsychotic). *Note:* Benzodiazepines may worsen delirium, especially in the elderly. Use the smallest dosage possible.
      ii. Discharge planning
         (a) No specific needs anticipated related to delirium
         (b) May require follow-up with primary care provider

Depression

1. **Definition:** Mood state characterized by feeling of sadness, lowered self-esteem, and pessimistic thinking and guilt (Gawlinski and Hamwi, 1999). Depressive episodes and depressive disorders are psychiatric diagnoses given to patients based on specific criteria (e.g., etiology, length of depression) (APA, 2000).
2. **Etiology and risk factors**
   a. Incidence in the medically ill ranges from 6% to 72% (APA, 2000)
   b. Causes of depression
      i. Psychodynamic
         (a) Illness progression
         (b) Fear and anxiety regarding the illness and the outcome of the illness

          (c) Illness-related regime

          (d) Reaction to loss and deprivation

          (e) Partial or complete loss of self-esteem

      ii. Cognitive: Patient's beliefs (thoughts such as "It's all my fault") may lead to depression

      iii. Biochemical

          (a) Neurotransmitter imbalance

          (b) Thyroid dysfunction

          (c) Hypocalcemia or hypercalcemia

          (d) Medications (e.g., antihypertensives, thiazides, spironolactone, β-blockers, digoxin [at toxic levels], steroids, benzodiazepines, cocaine withdrawal, alcohol)

    iv. Social

          (a) Lack of social support

          (b) Abandonment or isolation

    v. Other

          (a) Lack of sleep

          (b) Chronic or acute unmanaged pain

3. Signs and symptoms

  a. Cognitive

    i. Decreased ability to concentrate

    ii. Difficulty making decisions

  b. Behavioral

    i. Psychomotor agitation

    ii. Abnormal sleep patterns

    iii. Apparent sadness (tears, furrowed brow, downturned corners of the mouth, lack of eye contact)

    iv. Fatigue

    v. Recurrent thoughts of death

4. Diagnostic study findings

  a. Diagnosis based on history and clinical examination (i.e., cognitive and behavioral changes)

  b. Diagnostic test results may be abnormal if there is an underlying physiologic problem contributing to the depression (e.g., digoxin toxicity)

  c. Mini-mental status examination to rule out delirium (delirium may be confused with depression)

  d. EEG: Sleep EEG abnormalities may be present in up to 90% of inpatients during a major depressive episode (APA, 2000)

5. Collaborative diagnoses of patient needs

  a. Allow the patient to participate in goal setting with the ICU team

  b. Treat manageable symptoms such as pain and anxiety that may contribute to depression

  c. Review the plan of care with the patient and stress areas of improvement as appropriate

  d. Allow the patient control over the environment as much as possible

  e. Assist the patient in understanding the biochemical nature of depression (when appropriate)

6. Goals of care

  a. Patient verbalizes concerns about his or her medical condition, treatment plan, and so on, that led to feelings of depression

  b. Patient is able to describe the presumed cause and management of depression for his or her particular situation

    c. Patient is able to describe his or her role in the plan of care

    d. Patient sets realistic goals with the health care team regarding the plan of care

7. Management of patient care

    a. Anticipated patient trajectory: With counseling, ongoing support from family and friends, and, when indicated, pharmacologic therapy, patients with depression can resume and maintain normal lives

      i. Treatments

        (a) Nonpharmacologic

          (1) Assist in performing a differential diagnosis: Grief reaction, mood disorder, organic brain syndrome, delirium, dementia, metabolic conditions presenting as depression (e.g., hypercapnia, metabolic acidosis, uremia)

          (2) Discuss the treatment plan and progress with the patient—engage the patient in care planning as appropriate

          (3) Discuss concerns over possible or actual depressed state

          (4) Acknowledge that a depressed mood can be normal during or following a serious illness

          (5) Provide a mechanism to increase social support (family support, social services)

          (6) Attend to any suicidal ideation (is the patient a threat to self or others?)

          (7) Secure a psychiatric referral as appropriate

        (b) Pharmacologic: Antidepressants (e.g., tricyclics, selective serotonin reuptake inhibitors)

      ii. Discharge planning

        (a) Provide information to the patient and family about depression and available treatments

        (b) Discuss pharmacologic therapy, including mode of action, benefits, and side effects

        (c) Patient may require follow-up evaluation and teaching on pharmacologic and nonpharmacologic treatments for depression

Alcohol Withdrawal

1. Definition: Presence of a characteristic withdrawal syndrome that develops after the cessation of (or reduction in) heavy and prolonged alcohol use

2. Etiology and risk factors: Abrupt cessation of alcohol use in persons with a physical dependence

3. Signs and symptoms (12 to 48 hours after cessation of alcohol intake): Withdrawal syndrome includes two or more symptoms of autonomic hyperactivity (e.g., sweating, pulse >100 beats/min, insomnia, agitation) (APA, 2000)

    a. Mild to moderate dependency

      i. Agitation

      ii. Anxiety

      iii. Tremors

      iv. Nausea and vomiting

      v. Weakness

      vi. Diaphoresis

      vii. Hallucinations

    b. Delirium tremens (48 to 72 hours after cessation of alcohol intake)

      i. Anxiety attacks

      ii. Sleeplessness

iii. Disorientation

iv. Confusion

v. Cognitive impairment

vi. Delirium

vii. Tachycardia

viii. Fever

ix. Grand mal seizure

4. **Diagnostic study findings**

   a. Blood alcohol level: Elevated on admission

   b. Liver function studies: Values may be elevated

   c. Clinical Institute Withdrawal Assessment for Alcohol (CIWA-Ar) (Sullivan, Sykora, Schneiderman, et al, 1989) or Clinical Institute Withdrawal Assessment for Alcohol *DSM-IV* version (CIWA-AD) (Sellers, Sullivan, and Somer, 1991) to quantify the severity of withdrawal and guide collaborative diagnoses of patient needs

5. **Goals of care**

   a. Patient does not demonstrate signs or symptoms of withdrawal (e.g., seizures, agitation, irritability) that affect patient, family, and staff safety

   b. Patient states negative effects of alcohol on body systems (e.g., liver failure)

6. **Management of patient care**

   a. Anticipated patient trajectory: With aggressive pharmacologic and nonpharmacologic management, patients undergoing acute alcohol withdrawal should recover without incident. Life-long counseling and support (e.g., Alcoholics Anonymous) is needed for patients with an alcohol addiction.

      i. Treatments

         (a) Nonpharmacologic

            (1) Protect the patient, family, and staff from harm (e.g., use padded bed rails)

            (2) Use a nonthreatening, supportive manner with the patient

            (3) Engage the patient in short, directed conversations

            (4) Decrease stimulation that could precipitate aggressive or violent behaviors

         (b) Pharmacologic

            (1) Administer medications to a patient who is at risk for withdrawal or who demonstrates withdrawal behaviors

            (2) Benzodiazepines (give based on results of CIWA-Ar or Severity Assessment Scale)

            (3) Adjunctive pharmacologic treatment (e.g., thiamine, folate, multivitamins)

      ii. Discharge planning

         (a) Patient referral to Alcoholics Anonymous for current and future management

         (b) Referral of family members to Al-Anon or Alateen

      iii. Ethical issues: Staff may have ethical issues or conflicts caring for patients whose health problems they perceive to be "self-inflicted"

Aggression and Violence

1. **Definition:** Aggression is forceful physical or verbal behavior that may or may not cause harm to others. Violence is the ultimate maladaptive coping response and is the acting out of aggression that results in injury to others or destruction of property (Gawlinski and Hamwi, 1999).

2. **Etiology and risk factors:** Violence in the critical care setting may be triggered by the accumulation of stress in patients or family members who have

feelings of desperation and who lack coping skills and/or resources to resolve a situation by other means. Aggression and violence can be present with the following:

    a. Personality disorders

    b. Organic illness

    c. Psychiatric illness

    d. Substance abuse or withdrawal

3. **Signs and symptoms**

    a. Cognitive

        i. Inability to think clearly and rationally

        ii. Paranoia

    b. Behavioral

        i. Anger, yelling, use of profanity

        ii. Agitation

        iii. Pacing (family member)

        iv. Verbal threats

        v. Striking, pushing, kicking of staff

    c. Physiologic

        i. Tachycardia

        ii. Tachypnea

        iii. Increased blood pressure

        iv. Increased muscle tension

4. **Diagnostic study findings**

    a. Mental status examination: To help rule out organic brain disease

    b. Laboratory tests: To rule out metabolic problems

    c. Drug screens: May reveal toxic drug levels, high blood alcohol levels

5. **Collaborative diagnoses of patient needs**

    a. Protect patient, family, and staff from injury

    b. Provide the patient and family members with support and information early in the ICU stay

    c. Attend to aggressive behavior rapidly and definitively

    d. Be proactive in using appropriate resources (e.g., social services, security)

6. **Goals of care:** Patient does not demonstrate aggressive or violent behaviors toward self or others

7. **Management of patient care**

    a. Anticipated patient trajectory: With ongoing support and counseling, patients exhibiting aggressive and/or violent behaviors have the potential to modify these behaviors and live normal lives

        i. Treatments

            (a) Nonpharmacologic

                (1) Review medication list and discontinue suspect medications

                (2) Identify and remove other possible causes or stimuli that precipitate aggressive or violent behaviors (e.g., argumentative, challenging family members)

                (3) Involve social service personnel early in the patient's stay, particularly in high-risk situations (e.g., known alcohol abuse in family members)

                (4) Patient issues

                    a) Verbal, chemical, and physical restraints may be required to relieve symptoms and maintain safety

                    b) Use of physical restraints requires a plan, and explanation of their use to the patient and family, daily renewal of the restraint order, close monitoring, and use of alternative methods of restraint as appropriate

    (5) Patient and family member issues

      a) Speak in a calm, soft, noncondescending manner

      b) Allow the patient and family member to ventilate verbally without interruption

      c) Focus on the particular incident at hand

      d) Place clear limits on what will and will not be tolerated—outline the consequences of aggressive or violent behavior

      e) Do not attempt to educate the patient and family about aggression and violence during the aggressive or violent episode

      f) Obtain psychiatric consultation as needed

  (b) Pharmacologic

    (1) Anxiolytics

    (2) Neuroleptics (i.e., haloperidol)

  ii. Discharge planning

    (a) Discuss strategies for avoiding aggression or violence in the future

    (b) Post-ICU support and psychiatric follow-up may be required

    (c) Refer the individual to anger management classes

Suicide

1. **Definition:** A suicide attempt is the actual implementation of a self-injurious act with the express purpose of ending one's life (Keltner, Schwecke, and Bostrom, 2003). Patients coming to a critical care setting have often been unsuccessful in their suicide attempt and are admitted for actual or potential medical problems (e.g., respiratory depression, liver failure following acetaminophen overdose). A patient who has attempted suicide may be admitted to the ICU to determine if the person meets the criteria for brain death.

2. **Etiology and risk factors**
   a. Self-destructive behaviors resulting from a perceived, overwhelming threat to oneself
   b. Important differential diagnoses include
      i. Unintentional drug overdose or other injury (i.e., gunshot) related to altered mental status, cognitive impairment, or physical handicap (visual impairment)
      ii. Elder or spousal abuse

3. **Signs and symptoms:** May vary markedly depending on the type and extent of the injury present and the time that has elapsed since the injury
   a. Cognitive and behavioral
      i. Altered level of consciousness and orientation
      ii. Severe anxiety (if conscious)
      iii. Severe depression (if conscious)
      iv. Marked disorientation or confusion
   b. Physiologic (related to the agent used in the suicide attempt, the extent of injury and the time that has elapsed)
      i. Drug overdose
         (a) Tachycardia (amphetamines)
         (b) Bradycardia (digitalis)
         (c) Tachypnea (salicylates)
         (d) Bradypnea (barbiturates, opiates)
         (e) Dilated pupils (amphetamines)
         (f) Constricted pupils (opiates)

      ii. Trauma (gunshot wounds, stabbing, auto "accident")

        (a) Cardiovascular involvement: Hypotension, shock

        (b) Pulmonary involvement: Pneumothorax, lung contusions

4. Diagnostic study findings

  a. Related to the method of attempted suicide

    i. Elevated liver enzyme levels: Acetaminophen overdose

    ii. Abnormal CT scan: Gunshot wound to the head

    iii. Abnormal arterial blood gas levels

      (a) Metabolic acidosis: Salicylate, methanol overdose

      (b) Respiratory acidosis: Barbiturate, benzodiazepine, and/or opiate overdose

      (c) Respiratory alkalosis: Lower doses of salicylates

    iv. Electrolyte abnormalities: Hyperkalemia with digitalis overdose

    v. Abnormal coagulation results (increased international normalized ratio and prothrombin time): Warfarin overdose

    vi. Hypoglycemia: Insulin overdose

    vii. Drug screens: Urine and blood

5. Collaborative diagnoses of patient needs

  a. Provide a safe environment for the patient, family, and staff

  b. Demonstrate trust, respect, and acceptance of the patient

6. Goals of care

  a. Patient discusses suicidal thoughts with health care team

  b. Patient verbalizes the need for help

  c. Patient verbalizes needs and concerns

  d. Patient verbalizes positive feelings about self

  e. Patient verbalizes desire to recover

  f. Patient is future oriented

7. Management of patient care (see Box 10-3 for more information related to the nursing care of the suicidal patient)

  a. Anticipated patient trajectory: Outcomes for patients who have attempted suicide vary significantly depending on the mechanism and extent of injury. Many suicidal patients can live normal lives if they receive counseling and support.

    i. Treatments (will be specific to the mechanism of injury)

      (a) Stabilize the airway, breathing, and circulation

      (b) Institute specific treatment related to toxin ingestion, wounds (e.g., gastric lavage for drug overdose when indicated). Consult the poison control center or POISINDEX® (Thomson Micromedex) when relevant.

      (c) Assess the patient's risk for future suicide attempts

      (d) If the patient is at continued risk for a suicide attempt, provide for protection from injury (e.g., constant observation, restraints). See JCAHO standards for the use of physical restraints (http://www.JCAHO.org).

      (e) Once the patient's condition has stabilized, allow for opportunities to discuss the attempted suicide and the patient's feelings (e.g., hopelessness, anger, shame, sadness) in a private setting

      (f) Obtain a mental health consultation (patient's private psychiatrist, or staff psychiatrist or advanced practice nurse)

      (g) Facilitate visits from the patient/family support system (friends, clergy)

      (h) Allow family members to verbalize their feelings and concerns related to the suicide or attempted suicide

■ **BOX 10-3**
■ **CHARACTERISTICS OF SUICIDAL PATIENTS**

The acute crisis period or high-lethality time is of short duration; it can be counted in hours or days.
Suicidal patients are usually ambivalent about dying. At the same time that they plan suicide, they have fantasies of rescue.
People who commit suicide may have talked about it or may not have talked about it.
Suicidal persons usually give clues about their intentions.
Suicidal behavior has no racial, social, religious, cultural, or economic boundaries.
Suicide has no characteristic genetic qualities; however, its incidence is higher in families in which there have been previous suicides.
Suicidal behavior does not necessarily mean that the person is mentally ill; in some cases, suicide is viewed as a logical last step by someone who is overwhelmed by stress.
Most important, directly asking a person about suicidal intent will not cause suicide.

    ii. Discharge planning
      (a) Varies depending on patient factors (e.g., physical and psychologic state) and family and social support systems
      (b) Provide information on a 24-hour suicide prevention hotline
      (c) Provide phone numbers and websites for illness-specific support services (e.g., http://www.americanheart.org; http://www.americancancersociety.org; http://www.multiplesclerosis.org)
    iii. Ethical issues: Attempted assisted suicide by the patient and family in cases of terminal disease or unbearable chronic condition (see Chapter 1)

Dying Process and Death

1. **Description:** Process of dying in the critical care setting can take many forms. Patient may die suddenly as a result of the injury or condition, after a protracted illness, after the withdrawal of life support, or as a result of brain death.
   a. Care of patients and family members during or following the dying process is heavily influenced by the circumstances surrounding the patient's death
   b. Kübler-Ross described five psychologic stages of the dying process (Table 10-5)
     i. Denial or isolation
     ii. Anger, rage, envy, resentment
     iii. Bargaining
     iv. Depression
     v. Acceptance
2. **Signs and symptoms**
   a. Clinical death: Cardiopulmonary arrest
   b. Brain death: Lack of brainstem function
     i. Loss of spontaneous respiratory effort (i.e., failed apnea test)
     ii. Loss of cough and/or gag reflex
     iii. Loss of oculocephalic reflex (doll's eyes phenomenon is seen)
     iv. Loss of caloric response following instillation of ice water against the tympanic membrane
3. **Diagnostic study findings:** Most commonly used in the diagnosis of brain death. Studies include EEG, cerebral blood flow studies.
4. **Collaborative diagnoses of patient needs**
   a. Ensure that the patient does not experience discomfort (pain, shortness of breath, etc.) or anxiety during the dying process

■ **TABLE 10-5**
■ ■ **Kübler-Ross Stages of Grieving and Suggested Nursing Interventions**

Stage of Grieving	Nursing Interventions
Denial	Because denial operates protectively in a person on the verge of crisis, it is important for the nurse to respond to dying patients by • Listening to find out their perceptions of their situation. • Showing acceptance whenever they are found to be in the dying process. • Not encouraging false beliefs. • Attempting to understand why they are behaving as they are.
Anger	Allow patients to express their feelings to you and to ask, "Why me?" Remember, you need not attempt to answer that unanswerable question. • The anger that patients are expressing is not directed at you personally but, rather, toward what you represent (continued life) and toward their own painful situation.
Bargaining	Find out what kind of help patients need to complete their unfinished business. • Try to make time just to be with dying persons and to listen.
Depression	Avoid interrupting the grieving process. • Support patients in their grief. • Share your feelings of sadness appropriately, if you feel sad.
Acceptance	During this stage, the issue of letting go of a dying person arises. Show your support by • Not deserting the patient or family. • Respecting their acceptance of death. • Assisting the family with letting go of someone whom they love by listening and by intervening in areas in which family members feel they need help. Other interventions for comfort and dignity include • Adequate medication for control of pain. • Frequent mouth care. • Positioning for comfort. • Allowing family members to visit more frequently when the patient desires closer contact with loved ones. • Supporting the family's involvement in providing comfort measures for the dying person.

  b. Ensure that family members' needs to be with the patient, receive reassurance and support, and have hope for a peaceful death are met
5. **Goals of care**
  a. Patient and family members openly discuss fears and concerns regarding the dying process
  b. Patient rates pain as within the goal range (determined by the patient)
  c. Patient does not complain of shortness of breath
  d. Brain death: Family members recognize the brain-dead patient as legally dead and do not confuse brain death with a vegetative state
6. **Management of patient care** (see Table 10-5 for more information on caring for the dying patient)
  a. Anticipated patient trajectory: A peaceful death, in the manner desired by the patient and family, is the expected outcome
    i. Treatments
      (a) Nonpharmacologic
        (1) Ensure that do-not-resuscitate orders are written when appropriate
        (2) Allow the patient and family members to discuss fears and concerns regarding the dying process

(3) Allow the patient and family members time to be alone (if desired)
(4) Use nonpharmacologic methods of pain relief (see Pain)
(5) Determine cultural preferences related to the dying process and postmortem care
(6) Assist the dying person and his or her family members to validate their feelings (e.g., anger, pain)
(7) Acknowledge the grieving that accompanies the dying process
(8) Help the patient and family to prepare for the dying process by describing possible symptoms and how they can be treated
(9) Explain the role of pain medication—to relieve pain versus hasten dying
(10) Determine the patient's and family's desires for spiritual support and assist in obtaining support (notify clergy, etc.)
(11) Assist with the withdrawal of life support (e.g., extubation); use guidelines for the withdrawal process (http://www.american-heart.org)
(12) Allow family members to be present if they choose
(13) Provide for patient comfort (e.g., mouth care, positioning, suctioning)
  (b) Pharmacologic
    (1) Pain medication
    (2) Sedatives
    (3) Oxygen therapy
    (4) Diuretics and other agents as needed for patient comfort
  ii. Discharge planning: Bereavement support services for the family after the patient's death

REFERENCES

Psychosocial—General References

American Association of Critical-Care Nurses: *Standards for acute and critical care nursing practice,* Aliso Viejo, Calif, 2000, Author.

American Association of Critical-Care Nurses: *The synergy model of certified practice,* Aliso Viejo, Calif, 2003, Author.

American Psychiatric Association: *Diagnostic and statistical manual of mental disorders (DSM-IV-TR),* ed 4, text rev, Washington, DC, 2000, Author.

Biondi M, Kotzalidis GD: Human psychoneuroimmunology today, *J Clin Lab Anal* 4:22–38, 1990.

Caine RM: Psychological influences in critical care: perspectives from psychoneuroimmunology, *Crit Care Nurse* 23(2):60–70, 2003.

Caine RM, Ter-Bagdasarian L: Early identification and management of critical incident stress, *Crit Care Nurse* 23(1):59–65, 2003.

Carlson VR, Mroz I: Barriers to effective patient care. In Grenvik A, Ayres SM, Holbrook PR, et al, editors: *Textbook of critical care,* ed 4, Philadelphia, 2000, Saunders.

Curley MAQ: Patient-nurse synergy: optimizing patients' outcome, *Am J Crit Care* 7:64–72, 1998.

Erikson E: *Childhood and society,* ed 2, New York, 1963, WW Norton.

Erikson E: *Identity, youth and crisis,* New York, 1968, WW Norton.

Fortinash KM, Holoday-Worret PA: *Psychiatric nursing care plans,* ed 3, St Louis, 1999, Mosby.

Grumet GW: Pandemonium in the modern hospital, *N Engl J Med* 328:433–437, 1993.

Hardin SR, Kaplow R, editors: *Synergy for clinical excellence: the AACN synergy model for patient care,* Boston, 2005, Jones and Bartlett.

Holland C, Cason CL, Prater LR: Patient's recollections of critical care, *Dimens Crit Care Nurs* 16:132-141, 1997.

Jastremski CA, Harvey M: Making changes to improve the intensive care unit experience for patients and their families, *New Horiz* 6(1):99–109, 1998.

Keltner NL, Schwecke LH, Bostrom CE: *Psychiatric nursing,* ed 4, St Louis, 2003, Mosby.

Maslow AH: *Toward a psychology of being,* Princeton, NJ, 1968, Van Nostrand.

Mullen JE: The synergy model in practice: the synergy model as a framework for nursing rounds, *Crit Care Nurse* 22:66–68, 2002.

Pettigrew J: Intensive nursing care: the ministry of presence, *Crit Care Clin North Am* 2:503–508, 1990.

Pope DS: Music, noise, and the human voice in the nurse-patient environment, *Image* 27:291–295, 1995.

Satir V: *Conjoint family therapy*, Palo Alto, Calif, 1967, Science & Behavior Books.

Schrader KA: Stress and immunity after traumatic injury: the mind-body link, *AACN Clin Issues* 3:351–358, 1996.

Seligmann J: Variation on a theme, *Newsweek* 114:38, 1990.

Selye H: *Stress without distress*, Philadelphia, 1974, Lippincott.

Solomon GF: Psychoneuroimmunology: interactions between the central nervous system and immune system, *J Neurosci Res* 18:1–9, 1987.

Topf M, Bookman M, Armand D: Effects of critical care unit noise on the subjective quality of sleep, *J Adv Nurs* 24:545–551, 1996.

Urban N: Patient and family responses to the critical care environment. In Kinney MR, Dunbar SB, Brooks-Brunn J, et al, editors: *AACN clinical reference for critical-care nursing*, ed 4, St Louis, 1998, Mosby.

US Bureau of the Census: *Uses for questions on the Census 2000 forms*, 2000, retrieved September 26, 2005, from http://census.gov/dmd/www/content.htm.

Patient Care

Andrews M, Boyle J: *Transcultural concepts in nursing*, ed 4, Philadelphia, 2003, Lippincott Williams & Wilkins.

Arbour R: Sedation and pain management in critically ill adults, *Crit Care Nurse* 20(5):39–56, 2000.

Beers MH, Berkow R: *The Merck manual of diagnosis and therapy*, ed 17, Whitehouse Station, NJ, 1999, Merck.

Carpenito-Moyet LJ: *Nursing diagnosis: application to clinical practice*, ed 10, Philadelphia, 2004, Lippincott Williams & Wilkins.

Chlan L, Tracy MF: Music therapy in critical care: indications and guidelines for intervention, *Crit Care Nurse* 19(3):35–41, 1999.

Cullen L, Titler M, Drahozal R: Protocols for practice: family and pet visitation in the critical care unit, *Crit Care Nurse* 19(3):84–87, 1999.

Gawlinski A, Hamwi D, editors: *Acute care nurse practitioner: clinical curriculum and certification review*, Philadelphia, 1999, Saunders.

Gerdner LA, Buckwalter KC: Music therapy. In Bulechek GM, McCloskey JC, editors: *Nursing interventions: effective nursing treatments*, ed 3, Philadelphia, 1999, Saunders.

Giuliano KK, Bloniasz E, Bell J: Implementation of a pet visitation program in critical care, *Crit Care Nurse* 19(3):43–50, 1999.

Henneman EA, Cardin S: Family-centered critical care: a practical approach for making it happen, *Crit Care Nurse* 22(6):12–19, 2002.

Leske JS: Needs of relatives of critically ill patients: a follow-up, *Heart Lung* 15:189–193, 1986.

Stuart GW, Sundeen S: *Principles and practice of psychiatric nursing*, ed 6, St Louis, 2002, Mosby.

Tullmann DF, Dracup K: Creating a healing environment for elders: complimentary and alternative therapies, *AACN Clin Issues* 11:34–50, 2000.

Anxiety

Bally K, Campbell D, Chesnick K, et al: Effects of patient-controlled music therapy during coronary angiography on procedural pain and anxiety distress syndrome, *Crit Care Nurse* 23(2):50–51, 2003.

Keegan L: Protocols for practice: applying research at the bedside. Alternatives and complimentary modalities for managing stress and anxiety, *Crit Care Nurse* 20:93–96, 2000.

Simon NM, Pollack MH, Labbate LA, et al: Recognition and treatment of anxiety in the intensive care unit patient. In Irwin RS, Rippe JM, editors: *Intensive care medicine*, ed 5, Philadelphia, 2003, Lippincott.

Wong HLC, Lopez-Nahas V, Molassiotis A: Effect of music therapy on anxiety in ventilator dependent patients, *Heart Lung* 30:376–387, 2001.

Pain

Acute Pain Management Guideline Panel: *Acute pain management in adults: operative procedures*, Quick reference guide for clinicians No 1, AHCPR Pub No 92–0019, Rockville, Md, February 1992, Agency for Health Care Policy and Research, Public Health Service, US Department of Health and Human Services.

American Academy of Pain Medicine, American Pain Society, American Society of Addiction Medicine: *Consensus document: Definitions related to the use of opioids for the treatment of pain*, Glenview, Ill, 2001, American Academy of Pain Medicine. Available at http://www.asam.org/ppol/paindef.htm.

American Geriatrics Society: The management of pain in older persons: AGS panel on chronic pain in older persons, *J Am Geriatr Soc* 46(5):635–651, 1998.

American Pain Society: *Principles of analgesic use in the treatment of acute pain and cancer pain*, ed 5, Glenview, Ill, 2003, Author.

American Society of Pain Management Nurses: *ASPMN position statement: pain management in patients with addictive disease*, Pensacola, Fla, 2002, Author.

Ardery G, Herr K, Titler M, et al: Assessing and managing acute pain in older adults: a research base to guide practice, *Medsurg Nurs* 12(1):7–18, 2003.

Acute Pain Management Guideline Panel: *Acute pain management: operative or medical procedures and trauma,* Clinical practice guideline No 1, AHCPR Pub No 92–0032, Rockville, Md, 1992, Agency for Health Care Policy and Research, Public Health Service, US Department of Health and Human Services.

Cullen L, Greiner J, Titler MG: Pain management in the culture of critical care, *Crit Care Nurs Clin North Am* 13(2):151–166, 2001.

Dalton JA, Coyne P: Cognitive-behavioral therapy: tailored to the individual, *Nurs Clin North Am* 38(3):465–476, 2003.

Graf C, Puntillo K: Pain in the older adult in the intensive care unit, *Crit Care Clin* 19(4):749–770, 2003.

Hamill-Ruth RJ, Marohn ML: Evaluation of pain in the critically ill patient, *Crit Care Clin* 15(1):35–54, 1999.

Jacobi J, Fraser GL, Coursin BD, et al: Clinical practice guidelines for the sustained use of sedatives and analgesics in the critically ill adult, *Crit Care Med* 30(1):119–141, 2002.

Joint Commission on Accreditation of Healthcare Organizations: *Comprehensive accreditation manual for hospitals (CAMH): the official handbook*, Oakbrook Terrace, Ill, 2004, Author.

Kanner R, editor: *Pain management secrets*, ed 2, Philadelphia, 2003, Hanley & Belfus.

Koestler AJ, Doleys DM: The psychology of pain. In Tollison CD, Satterthwaite JR, Tollison JW, editors: *Practical pain management*, Philadelphia, 2002, Lippincott Williams & Wilkins.

Lang JD Jr: Pain: a prelude, *Crit Care Clin* 15(1):1–16, 1999.

Loeser JC, Butler SH, Chapman CR, et al, editors: *Bonica's management of pain,* ed 3, Baltimore, 2001, Lippincott Williams & Wilkins.

McCaffery M: *Nursing practice theories related to cognition, bodily pain, and man-environment interactions,* Los Angeles, 1968, University of California at Los Angeles Student's Store.

McCaffery M, Pasero C: *Pain: clinical manual,* ed 2, St Louis, 1999, Mosby.

Mersky H: Classification of chronic pain: description of chronic pain syndromes and definitions of pain terms, *Pain* 3(suppl): S217, 1979.

Munden J, Eggenberger T, Goldberg KE, et al, editors: *Pain management made incredibly easy,* Philadelphia, 2003, Lippincott Williams & Wilkins.

National Pharmaceutical Council, Inc.: *Pain: current understanding of assessment, management, and treatments,* Reston, Va, 2001, Author.

Pace S, Burke T: Intravenous morphine for early pain relief in patients with acute abdominal pain, *Acad Emerg Med* 3(12): 1086–1092, 1996.

Pasero C: Pain in the critically ill patient, *J Perianesth Nurs* 18(6):422–425, 2003.

Puntillo K: Pain: assessment, treatment and the coming thunder, interview by Michael Villaire, *Crit Care Nurse* 15(6):75–81, 1995.

Puntillo KA, Morris AB, Thompson CL, et al: Pain behaviors observed during six common procedures: results from Thunder Project II, *Crit Care Med* 32(2):421–427, 2004.

Puntillo KA, White C, Morris AB, et al: Patients' perceptions and responses to procedural pain: results from Thunder Project II, *Am J Crit Care* 10(4):238–251, 2001.

Rakel B, Barr JO: Physical modalities in chronic pain management, *Nurs Clin North Am* 38(3):477–494, 2003.

Snyder M, Wieland J: Complementary and alternative therapies: what is their place in the management of chronic pain? *Nurs Clin North Am* 38(3):495–508, 2003.

St. Marie B, editor: *ASPMN: core curriculum for pain management nursing*, Philadelphia, 2002, Saunders.

Titler MG, Rakel BA: Nonpharmacologic treatment of pain, *Crit Care Nurs Clin North Am* 13(2):221–232, 2001.

Websites

Agency for Healthcare Research and Quality: http://www.ahrq.gov

American Academy of Pain Management: http://www.aapainmanage.org

American Academy of Pain Medicine: http://www.painmed.org

American Pain Society: http://www.ampainsoc.org

American Society for Pain Management Nursing: http://www.aspmn.org

American Society of PeriAnesthesia Nurses: http://www.aspan.org

American Society of Regional Anesthesia and Pain Medicine: http://www.asra.com

International Association for the Study of Pain: http://www.iasp-pain.org

Joint Commission on Accreditation of Healthcare Organizations: http://www.jcaho.org

Medscape: http://www.medscape.com

Oncology Nursing Society: http://www.ons.org

Pain/Palliative Care Resource Center: http://www.cityofhope.org/prc/

Delirium (Acute Confusional State)

Burns SM: Delirium during emergence from anesthesia: a case study, *Crit Care Nurse* 23(1):66–69, 2003.

Inouye SK, Van Dyke CH, Alessi CA, et al: Clarifying confusion: the confusion assessment method, *Ann Intern Med* 112:941–948, 1990.

Truman B, Ely EW: Monitoring delirium in critically ill patients: using the confusion assessment method for the intensive care unit, *Crit Care Nurse* 23(2):25–36, 2003.

Depression

American Psychiatric Association: *Diagnostic and statistical manual of mental disorders*, ed 4, Washington DC, 2000, Author.

Alcohol Withdrawal

Schumacher L: Identifying patients "at risk" for alcoholic withdrawal syndrome and a treatment protocol, *J Neurosci Nurs* 32:158–163, 2000.

Sellers EM, Sullivan JT, Somer G: Characterization of DSM-III-R criteria for uncomplicated alcohol withdrawal provides an empirical basis for DSM-IV, *Arch Gen Psychiatry* 48:442–447, 1991.

Sommers MS, Dyehouse JM, Howe SR, et al: Nurse, I only had a couple of beers: validity of self-reported drinking before serious vehicular injury, *Am J Crit Care* 11:106–114, 2002.

Sullivan JT, Sykora K, Schneiderman J, et al: Assessment of alcohol withdrawal: the revised clinical institute withdrawal assessment for alcohol scale (CIWA-Ar), *Br J Addict* 84:1353–1357, 1989.

Website

Alcoholics Anonymous: http://www.alcoholics-anonymous.org

Suicide

Cummins RO: *Advanced Cardiac Life Support provider manual*, Dallas, Tex, 2001, American Heart Association.

Simons M: Patient contracting. In Bulechek GM, McCloskey JC, editors: *Nursing interventions: effective nursing treatments*, ed 3, Philadelphia, 1999, Saunders.

Website

American Association of Poison Control Centers: http://www.aapcc.org

Dying Process and Death

Chapple HS: Changing the game in the intensive care unit: letting nature take its course, *Crit Care Nurse* 19(3):25–34, 1999.

Cummins RO: *Advanced Cardiac Life Support provider manual*, Dallas, Tex, 2001, American Heart Association.

Kübler-Ross E: *On death and dying*, New York, 1969, Macmillan.

Myers TA, Eichhorn DJ, Guzzetta CE, et al: Family presence during invasive procedures and resuscitation: the experience of family members, nurses, and physicians, *Am J Nurs* 100:32–42, 2000.

Websites

American Cancer Society: http://www.cancer.org.

American Heart Association: http://www.americanheart.org.

Critical Care Patients with Special Needs

Bariatric Patients: SUSAN GALLAGHER, RN, MSN, CNS, PhD
Geriatric Patients: GINETTE A. PEPPER, PhD, RN, FAAN
High-Risk Obstetric Patients: AMY A. NICHOLS, RN, CNS, EdD
Patient Transport: RENEE HOLLERAN, RN, PhD, CEN, CCRN, CFRN, FAEN
Pediatric Patients: NANCY BLAKE, RN, MN, CCRN, CNAA
Sedation in Critically Ill Patients: JAN ODOM-FORREN, MS, RN, CPAN, FAAN

Bariatric Patients

INTRODUCTION

1. **Description:** Obesity is a multifaceted condition of excess stores of body fat
2. **Etiology:** Complex and multifactorial
   a. Causes may include behavioral, genetic, metabolic, biochemical, cultural, and psychosocial factors
   b. Diet, appetite control, ethnicity, and sedentary lifestyle are contributing factors
3. **Definitions** (American Society of Bariatric Surgery)
   a. *Body mass index* (BMI): Ratio of weight (in kilograms) to the square of height (in meters)
      i. Most common and widely accepted means of measuring and expressing the degree of excess weight or obesity
      ii. Significantly correlated with total body fat content; caution needed when interpreting BMI in children and in adults with edema, ascites, pregnancy, or highly developed muscles because elevated BMI does not accurately reflect excess adiposity in such cases
      iii. Normal: BMI of 18.5 to 24.9
      iv. Overweight: BMI of 25 to 29
      v. Obese
         (a) Grade I: BMI of 30 to 34
         (b) Grade II: BMI of 35 to 39
         (c) Grade III: BMI of 40 or higher
   b. *Overweight:* Excess body weight compared to established standards (e.g., National Center for Health Statistics defines overweight as a BMI of ≥ 27.8 in men and ≥ 27.3 in women). Excess weight may come from muscle, bone, fat, and/or water.
   c. *Obesity:* BMI of 30 or higher
      i. Refers to an abnormal proportion of body fat
      ii. Individual may be overweight without being obese (e.g., body builder); however, many people are both

    d. *Morbid obesity*
       i. Lifelong, progressive, life-threatening, genetics-related, multifactorial disease
      ii. Excess fat storage with multiple comorbidities
    e. *Bariatrics* (from the Greek *baros* for "weight"): Health care related to the treatment of obesity and associated conditions

4. Prevalence
    a. Recent estimates suggest that more than 67% of U.S. adults are overweight (Goulenok, Monchi, and Chiche, 2004)
    b. Among Americans aged 26 to 75 years, 10% to 25% are obese and more than 3% to 10% are morbidly obese, which reflects an increase of more than 25% over the past three decades irrespective of age, gender, ethnicity, socioeconomic status, or race
    c. Worldwide problem in both developed and developing countries

5. Pathophysiology of obesity: Physiologic sequelae of excess body weight adversely affect most body systems (Table 11-1)

6. Clinical significance to critical care nursing
    a. Recent evidence suggests that high BMI may be an independent prognostic risk factor for mortality in intensive care unit (ICU) patients
    b. Obesity is directly and indirectly associated with a wide spectrum of serious health disorders (see Table 11-1) that may accompany, underlie, and complicate whatever caused the patient to be admitted into a critical care unit
    c. When obese patients are hospitalized, they pose a number of additional challenges to health care facilities and staff
       i. Increased risk for all complications related to the immobility imposed by their size (i.e., skin breakdown, cardiac deconditioning, atelectasis, deep venous thrombosis, muscle atrophy, urinary stasis, constipation, bone demineralization)
      ii. Likelihood of longer length of stay than nonobese
    iii. Vulnerability to care issues more or less unique to this population
       (a) Technical difficulties with common procedures such as endotracheal intubation, weaning from mechanical ventilation, positioning, weighing, and ambulation
       (b) Challenges in establishing vascular access, managing fluid balance, and determining nutritional requirements
       (c) Altered pharmacokinetics for some drugs due to differences in metabolism, protein binding, distribution, and clearance in obese persons, which leads to uncertain effects
       (d) Inability to use some diagnostic tests due to size or weight limits
       (e) Lack of availability of equipment, supplies, or additional staff that optimal care might suggest

NURSING CARE OF THE CRITICALLY ILL BARIATRIC PATIENT

1. Pulmonary complications
    a. Obesity hypoventilation syndrome (also known as Pickwickian syndrome)
       i. Definition: Oxygenation decreases as BMI increases, likely due to elevated intraabdominal pressure in which mass and weight compress the thoracic cavity and limit diaphragmatic excursion. Chronic CO_2 retention leads to hypercapnia, respiratory acidosis, and dependence on hypoxia for ventilatory drive.

■ **TABLE 11-1**
■ ■ **Pathophysiology and Potential Health Problems Associated with Obesity**

System	Major Pathophysiologic Sequelae	Potential Health Problems
Pulmonary	Limited diaphragmatic excursion leads to ↓ vital capacity, functional residual capacity, total lung capacity ↓ Alveolar ventilation, shunting ↓ Expiratory reserve volume ↓ Thoracic and pulmonary compliance ↑ Work of breathing Alveolar collapse Small airway closure, asthma ↓ Respiratory drive, chronic CO_2 retention Risk for central or obstructive sleep apnea Risk for difficult intubation	↑ Respiratory rate, shallow breaths Ventilation/perfusion mismatching Hypoxemia, respiratory acidosis Difficulty weaning from ventilator Obstructive sleep apnea Obesity hypoventilation syndrome ↑ Risk of pneumonia, aspiration
Cardiovascular	Possible chronic hypoxemia, polycythemia, and pulmonary hypertension due to sleep apnea ↑ Left ventricular mass, hypertrophy, dilatation ↑ Total blood volume due to accumulated adipose tissue, which increases stroke volume and cardiac output ↑ Cardiac deconditioning	Right and left heart failure Systemic arterial hypertension Myocardial infarct, stroke Chronic venous insufficiency, deep vein thrombosis, pulmonary embolism
Endocrine	↑ Metabolic requirements of excess adipose tissue ↑ Insulin resistance Stress of critical illness may deplete protein rather than glucose stores	Type 2 diabetes mellitus; need for monitoring and managing serum glucose levels Hyperlipidemia Gallbladder disease, gallstones
Gastrointestinal	↑ Intraabdominal pressure ↑ Gastric volumes ↑ Nutritional requirements affected by mobilization of protein rather than lipid stores for ↑ energy needs Hypermetabolism associated with critical illness may lead to malnutrition and depleted protein reserves	↑ Gastroesophageal reflux ↑ Risk of aspiration pneumonia (enteral feeding route preferred) ↑ Constipation ↑ Pancreatitis
Immune	Protein-energy malnutrition that may coexist with obesity can impair cell-mediated immunity, phagocyte function, complement system, and antibody concentrations Obesity is associated with an impaired immune response	↑ Impaired healing, wound infection ↑ Skin breakdown, pressure ulcers ↑ Risk for some types of cancers[8] ↓ Resistance ↓ Phagocytosis
Musculoskeletal	↑ Joint trauma due to weight bearing Impaired, low, or no mobility ↑ Pain with movement ↑ Disuse atrophy of musculature	Osteoarthritis of hips, hands, back, knees Rheumatoid arthritis
Genitourinary	↑ Intraabdominal pressure ↑ Estrogen levels	↓ Fertility ↑ Incontinence ↑ Menstrual disturbance

Continued

■ **TABLE 11-1**
■ ■ **Pathophysiology and Potential Health Problems Associated with Obesity—cont'd**

System	Major Pathophysiologic Sequelae	Potential Health Problems
Psychosocial	Possible low self-esteem, negative body image due to social stigma of obesity ↑ Perceived or actual social rejection or lack of compassionate care from health care staff ↑ Anxiety, self-induced social isolation	Depression Lack of cooperation with or participation in care Possible limited support system

    ii. Related to obstructive sleep apnea, characterized by drowsiness, narcosis, daytime napping, difficulty sleeping at night, fatigue, hypersomnolence, depression, right heart failure, and further weight gain

    iii. Incidence of respiratory complications has a direct relationship to BMI, especially among those over 350 lb

    iv. Risk factors include male gender, middle age, mild sedation, BMI over 30

    v. Intervention: Noninvasive positive pressure ventilation can be tried; however, mechanical ventilation must be readily available

  b. Respiratory failure

    i. Obese patients are at risk for respiratory failure due to their high oxygen consumption, decreased functional residual capacity (FRC) (which decreases exponentially with increased BMI), decreased expiratory reserve volume, and decreased total lung capacity

    ii. FRC may fall into the range of closing capacity, which leads to small airway closure, ventilation/perfusion mismatch, arterial hypoxemia, and limited oxygen reserve

    iii. Obese patients often experience diaphragmatic fatigue. Pressure-supported ventilation alone or with backup allows resting of the diaphragm.

    iv. Interventions

      (a) Mechanical ventilation initiated with a tidal volume (V_T) of 5 to 7 ml/kg, based on ideal (not actual) body weight, then titrated to the patient's ventilator mechanics

      (b) Placement in reverse Trendelenburg's position at 45 degrees may improve respiratory mechanics, maximize lung function, and increase successful ventilation or weaning. Supine position leads to decreased compliance and increased airway resistance.

      (c) Placement in the prone position can improve FRC, compliance, and oxygenation. Placing a morbidly obese patient in the prone position is difficult but not impossible; hydraulic lifts help. Positive caregiver attitude and preplanning are essential.

    v. Airway management requires securing of the airway, intubation, secretion control, use of special equipment, and proper positioning

      (a) Assess risk factors for airway placement

        (1) Obesity

        (2) Short or thick neck

        (3) Facial edema

        (4) Swollen or thick tongue

        (5) Receding mandible

        (6) Protruding or missing maxillary incisors

        (7) Irregular jaw movement

(8) Unusually small or large mandible

(9) Erratic head or neck movement

(10) Upper incisor prominence

(b) Measure the distance from the sternal notch to the tip of the chin in the neutral and maximally extended positions (extension should increase by 5 cm)

(c) Intubation may be challenging, with difficulty in visualizing landmarks. The Combitube is an esophageal-tracheal double-lumen airway recognized by the American Heart Association and the American Association of Anesthesiologists as an alternative to the endotracheal tube for use in obese patients.

    vi. Failure to control tracheostomy secretions leads to skin breakdown, odor, and threat to a patent airway. For patients with a thick, short neck and excessive parapharyngeal fat deposits, tracheostomy surgery can be difficult, because the trachea may be buried deep in tissues. Wound is managed like any other open wound: Nonadhesive, absorbent, ¼-inch foam dressing is used to absorb excess drainage, protect the wound, and prevent injury from adhesives. Tracheostomy ties should be longer and wider to prevent trauma within skin folds.

    vii. Equipment should be tailored to best serve patient and caregiver needs

  c. Pneumonia (see also Chapter 2)

    i. Most common cause of death from hospital-associated infection, with a prevalence of 5 to 10 per 1000 admissions. Incidence is fourfold higher in intubated, mechanically ventilated patients, because of decreased V_T, decreased mucociliary transport, increased atelectasis, and infectious complications, which lead to increased morbidity and mortality.

    ii. Interventions

(a) Literature suggests that the widely accepted standard of care calling for repositioning every 2 hours is seldom met; even when it is included in the hospital-mandated protocol, the standard is met only 50% of the time in critical care settings (Krishnagopalan, Johnson, and Low, 2002)

(b) Until pneumonia resolves, wound healing usually plateaus or deteriorates. Use of full-body lateral rotation therapy may reduce interface pressures, promote pulmonary function, and provide therapeutic positioning. Value of rotation therapy when used to prevent physical hazards of immobility and to manage difficulties with repositioning must be determined.

  d. Pulmonary embolism (PE) (see also Chapter 2)

    i. Risk factors in obesity

(a) Prolonged immobility

(b) Venous stasis

(c) Polycythemia (associated with obesity hypoventilation syndrome)

(d) Increased intraabdominal pressure (increased pressure on deep veins)

(e) Venous thrombosis (deep vein thrombosis incidence is twice as high in the obese)

(f) Increased incidence of PE with BMI above 29

    ii. Bariatric surgery is associated with a 2.4% to 4.5% incidence of PE

    iii. Interventions: See Chapter 2

2. Potential skin integrity complications: Pressure ulcers

  a. Result from pressure, friction, and/or shear; often related to insufficient frequency of and/or ineffective repositioning of the very obese patient as well as the presence of multiple overlapping skin folds that can foster the growth of bacteria or yeast

b. Contributing factors include moisture, dehydration, and malnutrition
c. Staging depends on the depth of damage to underlying tissue
d. Obese patients are at risk for atypical pressure ulcers caused by pressure within skin folds related to tubes, catheters, or an ill-fitting chair or wheelchair
   i. Pressure within skin folds can be sufficient to cause skin breakdown; tubes and catheters burrow into skin folds and further erode the skin surface
   ii. Pressure from side rails or armrests not designed to accommodate a larger person can cause pressure ulcers on the patient's hips
   iii. Interventions
      (a) Use equipment properly sized for the patient
      (b) Place and secure tubes so the patient does not rest on them
      (c) Reposition (including tubes, lines, catheters) at least every 2 hours
      (d) In patients with a large abdominal panniculus, it too must be repositioned to prevent ulceration beneath the panniculus. Alert patients can help lift the panniculus; dependent or unconscious patients can be turned onto the side to aid the nurse in lifting it.
e. Rotation therapy can afford effective and timely repositioning for very large patients who otherwise pose a considerable challenge to frequent turning. Even when rotation therapy is used, precautions must be taken to prevent friction and shear by using correct pressure settings, using an appropriately sized surface, and monitoring skin integrity frequently.
3. **Other potential complications related to obesity:** See Table 11-1

CARE OF THE MORBIDLY OBESE BARIATRIC SURGERY PATIENT

1. **Surgical options**
   a. Restrictive procedures
      i. Roux-en-Y gastric bypass: Bypasses the duodenum and some portion of the jejunum; most frequently performed open procedure
      ii. Adjustable gastric banding
      iii. Vertical banded gastroplasty
   b. Malabsorptive procedures
      i. Biliopancreatic diversion
      ii. Duodenal switch (variant of biliopancreatic diversion)
   c. Combination restrictive and malabsorptive procedures
2. **Potential postoperative surgical problems** (beyond usual surgical risks such as bleeding, infection, emboli, aspiration, etc.), especially for open abdominal (vs. laparoscopic) procedures, for the morbidly obese and for those with underlying cardiopulmonary disorders
   a. Complications of restrictive procedures
      i. Gastric perforation or tearing
      ii. Esophagitis, gastritis, peritonitis
      iii. Band slippage, strictures, partial or complete bowel obstruction
   b. Complications of malabsorptive procedures
      i. Gastric, duodenal, or distal anastomosis leaks
      ii. Fistula formation, peritonitis, sepsis
      iii. Incisional hernia, wound infection
      iv. Diarrhea, abdominal cramping

RELATED BARIATRIC CARE ISSUES

1. **Caregiver issues**
   a. Potential for physical injury
      i. Increasing incidence, cost, and number of back injury claims associated with patient care. More than half of strains and sprains are attributed to manual lifting. Manual lifting and transferring of patients are among the most frequent causes of nursing-related injuries.
      ii. Lack of appropriate equipment and/or staff support at the facility
   b. Greater complexity: Nursing care becomes increasingly more complicated and problematic as the size and weight of the patient population increase
   c. Attitudes toward obese patients may include and communicate a negative bias
2. **Bariatric equipment issues**
   a. Standard hospital equipment, such as chairs or bed frames, may pose safety risks for obese patients and their caregivers
   b. Equipment specially designed for obese patients can improve quality of care, reduce length of stay, and make care easier and safer by reducing work-related back injuries among caregivers and lowering the risk of patient injury
   c. Heavy-duty walkers (for patients weighing 300 to 1000 lb) and heavy-duty beds, lifts, and wheelchairs that support up to 1000 lb are available to facilitate mobilization of very large patients. Preplanning with vendors is important.
3. **Policy issues**
   a. Policy makers, insurance carriers, health care facilities, and clinicians all need to use standardized measurements and definitions when developing policies, procedures, and protocols for critically ill bariatric patients
   b. Bariatric patient criteria (e.g., actual weight, width at widest point, or BMI) should determine which health care professionals and resources are needed in patient care to prevent complications and improve outcomes
      i. Institutional policies and procedures must be available to obtain transport, transfer, and patient care devices
      ii. Criteria-based protocols for the use of bariatric devices are designed to ensure more appropriate, timely, and cost-sensitive use of equipment
      iii. Performance improvement teams can help develop and implement policies and identify resources for bariatric equipment needs
   c. Health care professionals on the bariatric care team (physical therapist occupational therapist, or respiratory therapist; internist; bariatric surgeon; dietitian; bariatric clinical nurse specialist; wound, ostomy, and continence nurse; pharmacologist; home care coordinator; equipment vendors) need to be interested in improving critical care for the obese patient

Geriatric Patients

AGE-RELATED BIOLOGIC AND BEHAVIORAL DIFFERENCES

1. **Biologic and behavioral differences between older adults and younger adults** require modification of nursing care
2. **Age-related changes derive from three sources,** according to Sloane's rule of thirds (1992):
   a. One-third are related to disease processes that are more common in older adults

b. One-third are related to disuse and inactivity, which increase with age

c. One-third result from the aging process and occur in virtually all people who live long enough. These changes aggravate diseases and the changes associated with disuse.

3. **Normal age-related changes and implications for nursing care** are summarized in Table 11-2

AGE-RELATED CHANGES IN MEDICATION ACTION

1. **Adverse drug reactions are more** common in older adults than young adults (Routledge, Mahony, and Woodhouse, 2003)

   a. General rate of adverse drug reactions in the community is 6.7%

   b. Rate for elderly adults in hospitals is 20%

2. **Major reason older adults have more adverse drug reactions** is that they have more diseases and take more medications, but age-related changes in drug pharmacokinetics also contribute. The most clinically significant pharmacokinetic changes in old age include the following (Pepper, 2004; Turnheim, 2003):

   a. Absorption of drugs shows few age-related changes, although decreased gastric acid alters the dissolution of some drugs (e.g., enteric-coated tablets dissolve faster and may cause irritation)

   b. Distribution of drugs is altered by changes in body composition. Greater fat mass increases the storage and half-life of lipid-soluble drugs (e.g., psychotropic drugs). Highly protein-bound drugs (>90% bound) are more likely to be involved in drug interactions.

   c. Metabolism of high-clearance drugs (those that are avidly metabolized) is decreased due to decreased liver blood flow

      i. If a drug reference indicates that a drug undergoes first-pass metabolism, it has a high hepatic clearance

      ii. Effects of agents with high hepatic clearance should be assessed carefully to detect toxicity, especially if an elderly patient is not prescribed a dose lower than the typical adult dose

   d. Excretion of drugs that are eliminated unchanged or as active metabolites by the kidneys is markedly impaired with aging

      i. Use the Cockcroft-Gault formula to estimate creatinine clearance (C_{cr}) (Semla, Beizer, and Higbee, 2005):

         (a) For men (where IBW = ideal body weight and S_{cr} = serum creatinine):

$$\text{Estimated } C_{cr} = \frac{(140 - \text{age}) \times (\text{IBW in kg})}{(72 \times S_{cr})}$$

         (b) For women: Multiply the previous formula by 0.85

      ii. Adjust according to the dosing in the package insert or a drug reference for the estimated creatinine clearance

3. **Drug interaction** is another important factor in adverse drug reactions in older adults, primarily due to the number of drugs taken. The most significant drug interactions include the following:

   a. Drugs that decrease gastric acid production (e.g., H2-blockers, proton pump inhibitors, antacids) may alter the absorption of oral drugs

   b. Concurrent use of two drugs highly bound (>90%) to plasma albumin will increase the effect of one or both drugs, especially if drug elimination is impaired by age or disease. Use a current drug handbook for data on the degree of protein binding.

■ **TABLE 11-2**
■ ■ **Normal Changes with Aging**

Organ/Function	Normal Age-Related Changes	Implications
NEUROSENSORY		
Vision	Decrease in peripheral vision, color discrimination, pupil size and response time, tear production, lens accommodation Yellowing and opacifying of lens Thinning and yellowing of conjunctiva	Increase lighting levels. Eliminate glare. Avoid blue-green contrasts in written materials. Increase time to accommodate to darkness and close vision. Provide artificial tears as needed. Provide access to reading glasses.
Hearing	Ossification of middle ear structures Degeneration of cerumen glands, tympanic membrane, cochlea, otic nerve Loss of speech discrimination, especially sibilant consonants Possible increased confusion due to poor hearing	Remove accumulated wax that intensifies hearing loss. Minimize background noise that impairs speech discrimination. Assume position to promote lip reading (face in the light, hands away from the mouth). Ensure that hearing aid is functional and used.
Taste and smell	Degeneration of taste buds Increased threshold for taste Smell declines more than any other sense	Use patient's preferred seasoning to help increase food intake.
Proprioception, balance, and gait	Slowed kinesthetic reflexes and increased postural sway, which increase fall risk Altered gait patterns Decreased deep tendon reflexes	Provide handrails and assistive devices. Ensure an uncluttered environment. Provide prosthetics for other senses (hearing and vision).
Sleep patterns	Low sleep efficiency (time asleep/time in bed), more awakenings, less stage 4 sleep	Be aware that daytime sleepiness may increase fall risk. Investigate insomnia for treatable causes.
Tactile	Skin changes and nerve loss decrease tactile sensitivity, especially of fingertips, palms, and lower body.	Use caution with heating pads, ice, pressure, and immobility because damage may occur without the awareness of the patient.
PSYCHOEMOTIONAL		
Cognition	Decrease in neurons, brain mass, and levels of certain neurotransmitters Slowed central processing, depression, decreased vocabulary, benign forgetfulness (not dementia)	Present stimuli individually and at a slow pace. Allow time for response. Regularly assess cognition and depression with standardized measurement tools. Provide environmental cues for memory.
CARDIORESPIRATORY		
Heart	Increased mass (causes benign fourth heart sound) Decreased coronary blood flow, contractility, cardiac output, stroke volume, cardiac reserve, pulse rate Systolic murmurs (>50% of older adults)	Adjust assessment to accommodate altered response patterns: Heart rate slower to accelerate and slower to return to baseline Pulse is less responsive to fever, blood loss, anxiety.

Continued

■ **TABLE 11-2**
■ ■ **Normal Changes with Aging—cont'd**

Organ/Function	Normal Age-Related Changes	Implications
CARDIORESPIRATORY—cont'd		
Lungs	Weaker chest wall muscles and increased anterior-posterior diameter	Consider susceptibility to hypoxia and pneumonia in assessments.
	Decreased chest compliance, chemoreceptor response, expiratory flow, vital capacity, cough response, ventilation at lung bases	
Vasculature	Decreased baroreflex, elasticity, blood flow	Do not decrease blood pressure rapidly, as this can compromise blood flow to brain and vital organs.
	Increased circulation time, systolic hypertension, atherosclerosis	Do not draw blood from a sclerosed vein.
GENITOURINARY		
Kidneys	Decline in all aspects of renal function; decreased renal reserve	Use measured or age-adjusted calculated estimate of creatinine clearance to determine renal function. (See Cockcroft-Gault formula in Age-Related Changes in Medication Action.)
	Function may decline markedly with stress	
	Due to decreased muscle mass, serum creatinine is poor indicator of renal function	Ensure adequate hydration.
Micturition	Prostatic hypertrophy in males	Consider obstruction as a reason for low urine output, especially in males taking anticholinergic drugs.
	Decreased perineal muscle tone and spastic detrusor, which may cause urgency or incontinence in women	Assess for incontinence history and provide pads as needed.
GASTROINTESTINAL		
Secretions	Decreased saliva, hydrochloric acid (approximately 40% of older adults are achlorhydric), digestive enzymes	Elevate head after meals to promote esophageal emptying.
		Provide frequent, small meals.
	Impaired vitamin and nutrient absorption	Provide multivitamin therapy with B vitamins and fat-soluble vitamins (A, D, E, K).
		Recognize higher risk for infections.
Motility and sphincters	Slowed peristalsis, which increases constipation	Provide dietary bulk and fluids to reduce constipation.
	Decreased tone of internal anal sphincter, which may lead to fecal incontinence	Respond rapidly to toileting requests.
MUSCULOSKELETAL		
Bones	Decrease of 1-3 inches from maximum height	Reported height may overestimate actual height, so measure height for body mass index or dosage calculations.
	Bones smaller, more fragile	Use hip protectors to reduce fracture risk.
Muscle and soft tissue	Decreased muscle mass (reduces strength, balance, and glucose tolerance) and subcutaneous fat (impairs temperature control)	Implement measures to decrease fall risk.
		Provide warm environment due to cold sensitivity.
	Crosslinking of cartilage, which increases stiffness	Basal temperature is lower, so "normal" temperature may represent fever.

Continued

OTHER

Endocrine	Increased insulin concentration; decreased insulin receptor sensitivity	Assess for evidence of decreased glucose tolerance.
Integumentary	Slow cell replacement, loss of elasticity, dryness, thinning of skin Decreased subcutaneous fat and nerve density	Avoid bathing with drying soaps. Handle extremities with palms (not fingertips) because tissue is friable.
Immunologic	Decreased T-cell function and cell-mediated immunity Decreased antibody response to foreign antigens, but increased autoimmune response	Ensure that vaccinations are current.
Hematologic	Slight decrease in hemoglobin level, iron level, hematocrit, T-cell count, white cell count Slight increase in erythrocyte sedimentation rate	If changes are more than slight, evaluate for treatable conditions.
Blood chemistry	Slight decreases in levels of albumin, B_{12}, thyroid hormones Slight increase in creatinine, potassium, cholesterol levels	If changes are more than slight, evaluate for treatable conditions.

Compiled from Beers MH, Jones TV, Berkwits M, et al: *The Merck manual of health and aging,* Whitehouse Station, NJ, 2004, Merck Research Laboratories; Ebersole P, Hess P, Luggen AS: *Toward healthy aging,* ed 6, St Louis, 2004, Mosby; Kane RL, Ouslander JG, Abrass IB: *Essentials of clinical geriatrics,* ed 5, New York, 2004, McGraw-Hill; and Timeras PS, editor: *Physiological basis of aging and geriatrics,* ed 3, Boca Raton, Fla, 2003, CRC Press.

c. Drugs that induce or inhibit cytochrome P450 (CYP) enzymes can cause drug toxicity. Use a reference source that is frequently updated, such as Drug-Interactions.com (2005). CYP inhibition is the most significant drug interaction–related cause of adverse drug effects in elderly patients.

d. Drugs whose output is affected by urine pH (quinidine, amphetamines, ephedrine, phenobarbital) or that undergo tubular secretion (probenecid, cimetidine, omeprazole) can interact with and contribute to the toxicity of drugs like methotrexate, procainamide, acyclovir, nitrofurantoin, and cisplatin (Karyekar, Eddington, Briglia, et al, 2004)

4. **Nonadherence to the drug regimen and prescribing error,** in addition to physiologic and pharmacologic factors, may contribute to adverse drug reactions

a. Nonadherence with the prescribed drug regimen is a common cause of hospitalization among the elderly, although many comply closely with the regimen for prescribed medications (Beijer and de Blaey, 2002)

i. Teaching patients about medications as they are administered in the hospital may improve knowledge and result in better adherence (Barat, Andreason, and Damsgaard, 2001)

ii. At a minimum, the name and purpose of the medication should be stated at the time of administration if the patient is awake and cognitively intact

b. Often there is no accurate list of a patient's medications during transitions (from home to hospital; from unit to unit in the hospital), which are times of high risk for prescription and transcription error

i. Elderly patients are more likely to have errors in the medication list (Bedell, Jabbour, and Goldberg, 2000)

       ii. Joint Commission on Accreditation of Healthcare Organizations (JCAHO, 2005) recommends the reconciliation of medication lists at transitions to promote accuracy in medication regimens (Pronost, Weast, and Schwarz, 2003)

    c. Expert consensus panels have identified medications to avoid prescribing for older adults; the guidelines regarding potentially inappropriate medication use are called the Beers criteria (Fick et al, 2003)

COMMON GERIATRIC SYNDROMES

1. **Geriatric syndromes** are broad categories of signs and symptoms that may have a variety of contributing factors, including normal aging changes, multiple diagnoses, and adverse effects of therapeutic interventions. Syndromes are a major focus of nursing research and best practice guidelines.
2. **SPICES** is a tool for assessing major geriatric syndromes (Wallace and Fulmer, 1998). Pain is another important geriatric syndrome.
   a. S: Sleep disorders
   b. P: Problems with eating or feeding
   c. I: Incontinence
   d. C: Confusion
   e. E: Evidence of falls
   f. S: Skin breakdown
3. **Nutritional and hydration disorders**
   a. Older adults with multiple illnesses are at risk for malnutrition (Lawrence and Amella, 2004). Risk factors for decreased muscle mass, poor immune function, and poor outcomes include underweight (BMI <19) and overweight (BMI >26).
   b. Mini Nutritional Assessment (MNA) is a quick, noninvasive screening and assessment tool to identify older adults at risk of malnutrition (Nestlé Nutrition, 2005). Seek nutritional team consultation for at-risk elderly.
   c. Assess hydration status using a dehydration risk appraisal checklist. If no parenteral fluids are being administered, consider shortening the nothing-by-mouth time before diagnostic tests (2 hours) and replenish fluids as soon as tests are completed (Mentes, 2004).
4. **Confusion**
   a. "Geriatric triad" includes three conditions that can cause confusion: Delirium, depression, and dementia
   b. Delirium is an acute, reversible, life-threatening syndrome characterized by fluctuating alteration in mental status, inattention, and altered level of consciousness. Stereotypy (repetitive behaviors such as picking at the bedding) may be present. It is a cognitive reaction to a physiologic state.
      i. Prevalence is up to 25% of the hospitalized elderly and up to 65% of postoperative elderly patients older than 70 years of age (Beers, 2005). Increases the risk for death or poor outcome.
      ii. Mnemonic DELIRIUM summarizes the most common causes:
         (a) D: Drug use
         (b) E: Electrolyte imbalance
         (c) L: Lack of drugs (withdrawal)
         (d) I: Infection
         (e) R: Reduced sensory input
         (f) I: Intracranial events (stroke, meningitis)
         (g) U: Urinary incontinence and fecal impaction
         (h) M: Myocardial infarction

      iii. Confusion Assessment Method is used to differentiate delirium from dementia and other conditions (Inouye, van Dyck, Alessi, et al, 1990)

      iv. Having a family member or sitter present until the physical condition is resolved reassures the patient

  c. Dementia is a chronic, irreversible, progressive condition with insidious onset that is characterized by memory and thinking deficits involving orientation, visuospatial skills, language, judgment, concentration, and the ability to sequence tasks

      i. Present in about one third of the hospitalized elderly but undiagnosed in many. Often dementia is uncovered by the stress of hospitalization (Mezey and Maslow, 2004). Unrecognized dementia increases the risk for delirium (Fick and Foreman, 2000).

      ii. Question the family or identify behaviors to detect dementia (Mezey and Maslow, 2004)

  d. Depression is common in older adults, affecting up to 43% of older adults in acute care. Can be reversed if detected early. Untreated depression can lead to cognitive impairment, physical debilitation, and suicide (Kurlowicz, 1999).

      i. Assess for depression using a standardized scale

      ii. Refer for pharmacologic treatment and psychotherapy

5. Fall syndrome

  a. Incidence and severity of falls is higher among hospitalized patients than among the community-dwelling elderly. Injury rate for hospital falls is 10% to 25%. Injuries associated with falls account for 6% of medical expenses for older adults (American Geriatric Society, 2001).

  b. Risk for falls is multifactorial. JCAHO 2005 goals require facilities to assess and periodically reassess patients' risk for fall. Validated risk assessment tools are the Morse Falls Scale (Morse, Morse, and Tylko, 1989) and the Fall Assessment Tool (Farmer, 2000; Hollinger and Patterson, 1992).

  c. Implement standardized and individualized fall prevention program (Resnick, 2003)

6. Pain

  a. Pain management principles are the same as for other age groups

      i. Manage persistent pain with around-the-clock or long-acting medication

      ii. Provide medication as needed for breakthrough pain

  b. Regular assessment for pain is imperative. Cognitively impaired older adults can give reliable reports of whether they currently have pain. Pain scale most commonly preferred by older adults is a verbal descriptor scale, rather than a visual analogue, face, or numerical scale.

  c. Due to age-related changes in pharmacokinetics, older adults do not tolerate some analgesics (Ferrell, 2004; McCaffery and Pasero, 1999):

      i. Propoxyphene-containing drugs carry an excess risk of central nervous system (CNS) adverse effects with limited analgesic benefit

      ii. Meperidine has a toxic metabolite that accumulates in older adults due to decreased renal function, which results in irritability or even seizures. Avoid repeated dosing if used at all.

      iii. Mixed agonist-antagonist analgesics should be avoided in older adults due to their unreliable efficacy and cognitive and cardiovascular effects

      iv. Nonsteroidal antiinflammatory drugs (NSAIDs) such as ibuprofen carry a high risk of gastrointestinal adverse effects with prolonged or regular use. Cyclooxygenase-2 inhibitors (e.g., celecoxib) carry a cardiovascular risk.

      v. Regular dosages of acetaminophen are preferred for osteoarthritis, but the total dose should not exceed 4 g/day. Some older adults have experienced hepatic damage at 3 g/day, so the minimum effective daily dose should be used.

vi. Long-acting opioids (e.g., methadone) and amitriptyline (Elavil) should be avoided due to potential adverse effects

END-OF-LIFE CARE

1. **Advance directives:** Legal in every state, but laws vary widely (Warm and Weismann, 2000)
   a. There are two types of advance directive:
      i. Living will: Written document that specifies a person's wishes regarding medical care if the person becomes unable to communicate at the end of life
      ii. Health care power of attorney, also called the durable power of attorney for health care or health care agent: Appoints someone to make decisions if the patient is unable to communicate. A financial power of attorney is different and does not permit the holder to make health care decisions.
   b. Nurses can help patients understand advance directives (Douglas and Brown, 2002)
      i. Advance directives do not mean "do not treat," but specify how to treat
      ii. Patient can rescind a health care power of attorney as long as he or she has decision-making capacity
      iii. No professional providing health care to the patient can be the health care agent
2. **Syndrome of imminent death** (Weisman, 2000)
   a. Progresses through three stages over 24 hours to 2 weeks
      i. Early stage: Either hypoactive or hyperactive delirium or increasing sleepiness, bed bound
      ii. Middle stage: Further decline in mental status; pooled oral secretions from loss of swallowing reflex results in "death rattle"; fever is common
      iii. Late stage: Coma; altered respiratory pattern—either fast (as high as 40 breaths/min) or slow; cold extremities
   b. Confirm treatment goals with the family when the syndrome is recognized. Discuss the removal of treatments that do not contribute to comfort. Scopolamine may be used to dry secretions (decrease death rattle) and morphine may be used to control rapid respirations (goal is 10 to 15 breaths/min). Provide meticulous mouth and skin care.

High-Risk Obstetric Patients

PHYSIOLOGIC CHANGES IN PREGNANCY

During pregnancy, nearly every body system undergoes adaptations that protect the growing fetus and prepare the mother for delivery. Some changes appear early and continue throughout gestation; others occur later. Tables 11-3, 11-4, and 11-5 summarize some of the most significant normal changes that critical care nurses need to keep in mind. Box 11-1 defines some common obstetric abbreviations that may be encountered in obstetric patients' charts.

▨ **TABLE 11-3**
▨ ▨ **Normal Physiologic Changes in Pregnancy**

System	Changes
Cardiovascular	Between 10th and 12th weeks of pregnancy, blood volume starts to rise, peaking at 40% to 50% above baseline at 32nd to 34th weeks, then declining slightly by 40th week. Systemic vascular resistance decreases, which causes blood to pool in lower extremities and often results in orthostatic hypotension.
	Midpregnancy, systolic blood pressure falls 3-5 mm Hg, as diastolic declines 5-10 mm Hg.
	During last half of pregnancy, decrease in colloid osmotic pressure shifts fluid into the extravascular space, which causes lower-extremity edema.
	Between 14th and 20th weeks, pulse slowly rises 10-15 beats/min to a new rate that persists to term.
	Cardiac output increases by 30% to 50%.
Pulmonary	Diaphragm may rise up to 4 cm even before enlarging uterus exerts much upward pressure. After 24th week, thoracic breathing replaces abdominal breathing and mild dyspnea is common. Higher estrogen levels cause nasal mucosa to swell, which makes nasal stuffiness and nosebleeds common.
	As oxygen requirements increase, rising estrogen levels relax costal ligaments so the chest can expand. This permits deeper breathing, which allows minute respiratory volume to increase by 26%, while respiratory rate increases only about 2 breaths/min. This hyperventilation decreases alveolar CO_2 concentration and is reflected in arterial blood gas levels as compensated respiratory alkalosis (pH, 7.40-7.45; partial pressure of oxygen [Pao_2], 100-110 mm Hg; arterial partial pressure of carbon dioxide [$Paco_2$], 25-30 mm Hg; bicarbonate [HCO_3] level, 17-22 mEq/L). The alkalotic state facilitates the diffusion of nutrients to and wastes from the fetus through the placenta.
Renal	To compensate for the drop in alveolar CO_2 concentration, the kidneys excrete additional HCO_3. During the second trimester, renal plasma flow and glomerular filtration rate (GFR) increase 35% and 50%, respectively, but both drop late in pregnancy. In response to hormonal changes, an enlarging uterus, and increased blood volume, ureters dilate and elongate, which leads to urinary stasis.
	Because of the increased GFR, serum levels of blood urea nitrogen, creatinine, and uric acid are lower, and patients may require higher or more frequent doses of some drugs to maintain therapeutic levels.
Gastrointestinal	Progesterone relaxes smooth muscle, which causes progressive gastric reflux as the uterus enlarges.
	Intestinal transit time increases, which allows better absorption of nutrients but also causes constipation.
Reproductive	The uterus enlarges to about 20 times its normal size to hold the fetus, placenta, and amniotic fluid. After the 12th week of pregnancy, it grows out of the pelvis and into the abdominal cavity.
	After 16 weeks, the supine position may cause the uterus to compress the vena cava and iliac veins, which decreases blood flow to the uterus and lower extremities; the left lateral position is recommended.
Hematologic	Hemoglobin level and hematocrit are slightly lower in the second trimester (the "physiologic anemia" of pregnancy) because of a rise in plasma that is disproportionate to that of red blood cells. A hemoglobin level of 10-13 g/dl and a hematocrit of 32% to 39% are considered normal during this time.
	Because white blood cell (WBC) levels respond to physiologic stress, WBC counts rise to between 10,000 and 12,000/mm³ during pregnancy and up to 25,000/mm³ during labor. Platelet counts stay within the normal range. A falling platelet count could signal trouble. Platelet counts below 130,000/mm³ might indicate disseminated intravascular coagulation, and platelet counts below 100,000/mm³ could signal HELLP syndrome, an extension of pregnancy-induced hypertension characterized by **h**emolysis, **e**levated **l**iver enzyme **l**evels, and **l**owered **p**latelet counts.

■ **TABLE 11-4**
■ ■ **Changes in Physiologic Parameters in Pregnancy**

System Changed	Increased	Decreased
Cardiovascular	Blood volume Cardiac output Uterine blood flow Heart rate Myocardial size	Systemic vascular resistance Pulmonary vascular resistance Colloid osmotic pressure
Hematologic	Plasma volume Red blood cells Clotting factors Fibrinogen White blood cells Sedimentation rate	Serum osmolarity Albumin
Respiratory	Diaphragm elevation Oxygen compensation pH, partial pressure of oxygen (Po_2) Minute ventilation	Residual capacity Oxygen reserve Bicarbonate level Partial pressure of carbon dioxide (Pco_2)
Renal	Urine output Plasma flow Glomerular filtration rate	Specific gravity
Gastrointestinal	Alkaline phosphatase level Absorption Risk of aspiration	Motility Tone
Endocrine	Basal metabolic rate Body temperature Hypertrophic pituitary Insulin resistance	
Electrocardiogram	Q wave in lead III and aVF Flattened or inverted T waves Premature atrial contractions Systolic ejection murmur	

■ **TABLE 11-5**
■ ■ **Comparison of Hemodynamic Profiles in Pregnant and Nonpregnant Women**

Hemodynamic Parameter	Pregnant	Nonpregnant
Cardiac output (L/min)	6.2	4.3
Central venous pressure (mm Hg)	3.7	3.6
Colloid osmotic pressure (mm Hg)	18	20.8
Heart rate (beats/min)	83	71
Left ventricular stroke index (ml/beat)	48	41
Mean arterial pressure (mm Hg)	90	86
Pulmonary capillary wedge pressure (mm Hg)	7.5	6.3
Pulmonary vascular resistance (dyne/sec/cm^{-5})	78	119
Systemic vascular resistance (dyne/sec/cm^{-5})	1210	1530

■ **BOX 11-1**
■ **GLOSSARY OF OBSTETRIC TERMS**

This list of common obstetric abbreviations can aid in interpreting the patient's chart and prenatal record.

BOWI	Bag of waters intact
EDC	Estimated date of confinement (same as EDD)
EDD	Estimated date of delivery
EFM	External fetal monitoring
EGA	Estimated gestational age
FHR	Fetal heart rate
G	Gravida (number of pregnancies)
+GFM	Gross fetal movement present
IUP	Intrauterine pregnancy
LMP	Last menstrual period
P	Parity (number of live births)
PIH	Pregnancy-induced hypertension
PROM	Premature rupture of membranes (rupture not followed by labor within an hour)
PPROM	Preterm premature rupture of membranes
ROM	Rupture of membranes
US	Ultrasonography

POSTPARTUM HEMORRHAGE

1. **One of the leading causes of maternal morbidity and mortality,** contributing to 30% of obstetric deaths. Definitions include subjective assessments of blood loss greater than standard norms, a 10% decline in hematocrit, and need for blood transfusion.
   a. Average blood loss for vaginal delivery, cesarean section, and cesarean hysterectomy is 500, 1000, and 1500 ml, respectively
   b. Management requires understanding normal delivery blood loss, the physiologic response to and common causes of postpartum hemorrhage, and appropriate interventions
2. **Physiologic response to postpartum hemorrhage**
   a. Pregnant patients adapt more effectively to blood loss due to increased red blood cell (RBC) mass, plasma volume, and cardiac output
   b. Early during hemorrhage, systemic vascular resistance rises to maintain blood pressure and perfusion of vital organs. If bleeding continues, vasoconstriction affords less support, which results in drops in blood pressure, cardiac output, and end-organ perfusion. Table 11-6 classifies the physiologic responses that occur at various stages of postpartum hemorrhage.
3. **Etiologic factors:** Distinguished by the timing of the hemorrhage
   a. Early postpartum hemorrhage (within 24 hours of delivery)
      i. Uterine atony
      ii. Lower genital tract lacerations
      iii. Lower urinary tract lacerations
      iv. Retained placental fragments
      v. Uterine rupture

■ **TABLE 11-6**
■ ■ **Postpartum Hemorrhage Classification and Physiologic Response**

Hemorrhage Class	Acute Blood Loss (ml)	% Lost	Physiologic Response
1	900	15	Asymptomatic
2	1200-1500	20	Tachycardia, tachypnea, narrowed pulse pressure, orthostatic hypotension
3	1800-2100	30-35	Worsening tachycardia, worsening tachypnea, hypotension, cool extremities
4	>2400	40	Shock, oliguria or anuria

From Gary D: Postpartum hemorrhage, *New Manage Options* 45(2):335, 2002.

  b. Late postpartum hemorrhage (24 hours to 6 weeks after delivery)
   i. Infection
   ii. Retained placental fragments
4. **Patient assessment**
  a. History of precipitous or prolonged stages of labor, overstretching of the uterus, administration of medications (e.g., magnesium sulfate for pregnancy-induced hypertension), past placental retention, use of forceps or other intravaginal manipulations
  b. Related to blood loss
   i. Draw blood for possible cross-matching and baseline laboratory values: Hemoglobin level, hematocrit, platelet count, fibrinogen level, prothrombin time, partial thromboplastin time
   ii. Estimate the volume of blood loss
   iii. Identify the cause of the hemorrhage
    (a) *Uterine atony:* Boggy, large uterus, clots, bleeding
    (b) *Lacerations:* Firm uterus, bright red blood, steady stream of unclotted blood
    (c) *Hematoma:* Firm uterus, bright red blood, extreme perineal-pelvic pain, unexplained tachycardia
    (d) *Retained placental fragments:* Placenta not delivered intact, uterus remains large, absence of pain, bright red blood
5. **Patient care specific to obstetric patients** (see Chapter 3 for hemorrhagic shock interventions)
  a. Assess the fundus: Determine the level of firmness and the placement of the fundus
  b. Include estimates of the amount of lochia in intake and output assessments
  c. Administer prescribed uterotonic medications, which are the basis of drug therapy for postpartum hemorrhage. Table 11-7 lists available pharmacologic therapies for hemorrhage.
  d. Select an appropriate time for mother-baby interaction
6. **Evaluation: Desired patient outcomes include the following:**
  a. Fundus firm, midline, and at the umbilicus or below
  b. Lochia red, moderate in amount, unclotted
  c. Vital signs normal, intake and output satisfactory
  d. Support and information provided by caregivers to the patient and family
  e. Family supportive to the patient

■ TABLE 11-7
■ ■ Medications for Postpartum Hemorrhage

Agent	Dose	Route	Dosing Frequency	Side Effects	Contraindications
Oxytocin (Pitocin)	10-80 units in 1000 ml of crystalloid solution	First line: IV Second line: IM or IU	Continuous	Nausea, emesis, water intoxication	None
Methylergoncvine (Methergine)	0.2 mg	First line: IM Second line: IU	Every 2-4 hr	Hypertension, hypotension, nausea, emesis	Hypertension, preeclampsia
Prostaglandin F$_2$ (Hemabate)	0.25 mg	First line: IM Second line: IU	Every 15-90 min 8 doses maximum	Nausea, emesis, diarrhea, flushing, chills	Active cardiac, pulmonary, renal, or hepatic disease
Prostaglandin E$_2$ (Dinoprostone)	20 mg	PR	Every 2 hr	Nausea, emesis, diarrhea, flushing, headache	Hypotension
Misoprostol (Cytotec)	600-1000 mcg	First line: PR Second line: PO	Single dose	Nausea, emesis, diarrhea, fever, chills	None

From Dildy GA: Postpartum hemorrhage: new management options, *Clin Obstet Gynecol* 4(2):330-344, 2002.
IM, Intramuscular; *IV,* intravenous; *IU,* intrauterine; *PO,* by mouth; *PR,* per rectum.

HYPERTENSIVE DISORDERS OF PREGNANCY

Hypertensive disorders, the most common medical complications of pregnancy, affect 5% to 10% of pregnancies. About 30% of cases are due to chronic hypertension and 70% are due to gestational hypertension, or preeclampsia. Spectrum of the disorder ranges from mildly elevated blood pressure with minimal clinical significance to severe hypertension and multiorgan dysfunction.

1. **Definitions:** Hypertension is defined as systolic blood pressure 30 mm Hg above baseline and diastolic blood pressure 15 mm Hg above baseline. In pregnancy, abnormal proteinuria is 300 mg protein or more in 24 hours.
2. **Classification of hypertensive states in pregnancy**
   a. Gestational hypertension: Occurs in the second half of pregnancy or the first 24 hours postpartum
      i. Mild: Systolic less than 160 mm Hg or diastolic less than 110 mm Hg, plus proteinuria less than 1+ on dipstick and less than 5 g in 24 hours
      ii. Severe: Systolic more than 160 mm Hg or diastolic more than 110 mm Hg, plus proteinuria of more than 5 g in 24 hours
   b. Preeclampsia, or pregnancy-induced hypertension (PIH): Occurs at more than 20 weeks' gestation
      i. Mild: Mild hypertension and mild proteinuria
      ii. Severe: Severe hypertension and proteinuria with other symptoms including headache, visual changes, epigastric or right upper quadrant pain, and shortness of breath. May also include thrombocytopenia, pulmonary edema, and oliguria (< 500 ml in 24 hours).
   c. HELLP syndrome
      i. Occurs in 15% to 20% of patients with severe preeclampsia or eclampsia
      ii. Symptoms of HELLP syndrome (three characteristic abnormalities): *H*emolysis, *e*levated *l*iver enzymes, *l*ow *p*latelet count (blood pressure may be normal)
3. **Pathophysiology**
   a. Characterized by vasoconstriction, hemoconcentration, and possible ischemic changes in the placenta, kidney, liver, and brain
   b. Intense vasoconstriction due to dysfunction of the normal interactions of vasodilatory and vasoconstrictive substances
   c. Thrombocytopenia: Platelet count lower than 100,000/mm^3
   d. Decreased renal perfusion and reduced glomerular filtration rate
   e. Hepatic system: Mildly elevated liver enzyme levels, subcapsular hematomas, or hepatic rupture
   f. CNS: Eclamptic convulsions
   g. HELLP syndrome
      i. Chronic vasoconstriction that occurs in PIH causes fibrin deposits in hepatic sinusoids, which obstruct hepatic blood flow and alter liver function
      ii. Liver swells, stretching Glisson's capsule and producing epigastric and right upper abdominal quadrant pain
      iii. Hemorrhagic periportal necrosis, subcapsular hemorrhages, and spontaneous liver rupture may occur in extreme cases. Serum liver enzyme levels rise, with aspartate aminotransferase values of 60 IU or higher (normal ≥35 IU). Jaundice and acute hepatic failure may occur.
      iv. Maternal hypoglycemia is a serious prognostic indicator
      v. Risk of developing DIC is compounded: Patients with severe HELLP syndrome (all three abnormalities) are at greater risk for developing DIC than

patients with partial HELLP syndrome (one or two clotting abnormalities). Despite treatment, the syndrome can escalate into DIC because the production of many clotting factors is increased in pregnancy (Table 11-9). With DIC, the clinical picture is hemorrhage and shock (see Chapter 7).

4. **Etiologic factors:** Specific cause of preeclampsia is unknown (Box 11-2 lists common risk factors)

5. **Patient assessment:** Systematic assessments are critical to patient management; frequency is dictated by the patient's condition and response to therapy
   a. Nursing history: Medical history, past pregnancies, current pregnancy
   b. Nursing examination of patient
      i. Frequent monitoring for signs of cardiac decompensation (see Chapter 3), pulmonary edema (see Chapter 2), and renal failure (see Chapter 5)
      ii. Hourly monitoring (deep tendon reflexes, clonus, level of consciousness) for signs of increasing CNS irritability, increasing intracranial pressure, and magnesium sulfate toxicity
      iii. If the patient is antepartum, examination for fetal status and signs of placental abruption or decreased uteroplacental perfusion
         (a) Assess for uterine activity, hypertonicity, hypercontractility
         (b) Assess fetal movements, baseline fetal heart rate and variability
   c. Psychosocial and family assessment
   d. Laboratory tests
      i. Monitor RBC count, platelet count, hemoglobin level, hematocrit, coagulation profile (for hemolysis); assess for coagulation defects (increased factor VIII activity, platelet aggregation), decreased oxygen-carrying capacity, hemoconcentration or thrombocytopenia
      ii. Measure serum creatinine, uric acid, blood urea nitrogen (BUN), and alkaline phosphatase levels
      iii. Order liver function tests to check for elevated lactate dehydrogenase, serum glutamic-oxaloacetic transaminase, and serum glutamic-pyruvic transaminase levels

6. **Patient care** (Table 11-8)
   a. Only cure for PIH (regardless of gestational age) is delivery
   b. Goal is to end the pregnancy with the fewest adverse effects to the mother and fetus
   c. Additional management decisions may include the use of an arterial and/or pulmonary artery line for patients with severe PIH in the following situations:
      i. Oliguria unresponsive to fluid challenge
      ii. Pulmonary edema
      iii. Hypertensive crisis refractory to conventional therapy

---

BOX 11-2
MOST COMMON RISK FACTORS FOR PREGNANCY-INDUCED HYPERTENSION

- First pregnancy or pregnancy of new genetic makeup (e.g., same mother, different father)
- Multiple gestation
- Preexisting medical conditions (i.e., diabetes, vascular disease, hypertension, or renal disease)
- Maternal age <18 or >35 years
- Maternal weight <100 lb or obesity prior to pregnancy
- African American ethnicity
- Family history of pregnancy-induced hypertension
- Low socioeconomic status
- Late entry into or no prenatal care

■ TABLE 11-8
■ ■ **Pharmacologic Therapies for Pregnancy-Induced Hypertension**

Drug	Uses	Action	Dosage	Maternal Side Effects	Fetal Side Effects
Magnesium sulfate	Primary	Anticonvulsant	Loading dose: 4-6 g IV over 15-30 min Maintenance dose: 2-3 g per IV infusion	CNS depression Flushing Nausea Vomiting Headache Respiratory depression Cardiac arrest	Decreased variability in fetal heart rate Slower extrauterine life transition
Hydralazine	Primary or secondary	Antihypertensive	5-10 mg IV bolus q 20 min to total dose of 30-40 mg	Rebound hypotension Tachycardia Headache	Tachycardia Uteroplacental insufficiency with subsequent tachycardia and late decelerations
Labetalol	Secondary	Antihypertensive	Progressive by increasing doses, 20, 40, 80 mg every 10-15 min to a total dose of 300 mg	Increased uteroplacental perfusion Decreased uterine vascular resistance Contraindicated in women with history of asthma and first-degree heart block Less rebound hypotension	Fetal and neonatal bradycardia, hypotension, and hypoglycemia
Nifedipine	Tertiary	Antihypertensive	10 mg PO, repeated after 30 min	Rebound hypertension Exacerbation of effect if magnesium sulfate on board	Fetal safety not established
Nitroglycerin	Use with caution	Antihypertensive	Initial IV infusion rate of 5 mcg, titrated to desired response by doubling dose every 5 min	Hypotension Tachycardia Nausea Vomiting Pallor Sweating Headache	Fetal response dependent on maternal response
Calcium gluconate	Antagonist	Antidote for magnesium toxicity	1 g prefilled cartridge-needle unit (Carpuject) slow IV push	Cardiac dysrhythmias if given too fast	

CNS, Central nervous system; *IV,* intravenous; *PO,* by mouth.

    iv. Cerebral edema
    v. Disseminated intravascular coagulation (DIC)
    vi. Multisystem organ failure
  d. Nursing care requires accurate and astute patient assessments, strict regulation of input and output, urinary catheterization with a urometer, and comprehensive knowledge of pharmacologic therapies, management regimens, and possible complications
  e. Specific to HELLP
    i. Patients who progress from HELLP to DIC need transfusions of fresh frozen plasma, platelets, cryoprecipitate, and packed RBCs. Hypotension is treated with vasopressors (e.g., dopamine). Until the patient's condition is stabilized, the patient requires close monitoring in the ICU.
    ii. Critical care nurses need to know what the signs of trouble are and how to handle complications
      (a) Focus on maintaining adequate organ perfusion and watching for signs of fluid overload, bleeding, and thrombosis
      (b) Administer volume replacement based on the patient's hemodynamic values
      (c) Monitor blood pressure every 5 to 15 minutes while titrating vasopressors; keep mean arterial pressure at 60 mm Hg or higher
      (d) Regularly assess peripheral pulses, perfusion, and heart rate and rhythm; check intravenous (IV) and puncture sites for bleeding
      (e) Administer supplemental oxygen; assess breath sounds at least every 30 minutes; respiratory difficulty could indicate fluid overload or adult respiratory distress syndrome
      (f) Monitor arterial blood gas concentrations and lactate, electrolyte, BUN, and creatinine levels

---

TABLE 11-9
Comparison of HELLP Syndrome and Disseminated Intravascular Coagulation (DIC)

	HELLP Syndrome	DIC
Signs and symptoms	Nausea with or without vomiting Epigastric pain or pain in right upper abdominal quadrant Hypertension varying from mild to severe Malaise	Obvious signs of bleeding, such as hematuria or hematoma development at venipuncture sites, hemorrhage in the conjunctiva, and petechiae
Laboratory blood values	Increased aminotransferase, bilirubin, hemoglobin levels, and increased hematocrit Decreased platelet count	Elevated levels of fibrin degradation products, prothrombin time, and stimulated partial thromboplastin time
Treatment	Delivery of the fetus if the outcome of the mother or fetus is endangered Platelet administration if the cell count is <20,000/mm³ Monitoring of liver function Observation for organ systems dysfunction	Volume blood and clotting factor replacement Removal of the underlying precipitating factor to reverse the DIC Support for organ systems dysfunction

From Bridges EJ, Womble S, Wallace M, et al: Hemodynamic monitoring in high-risk obstetrics patients: I. Expected hemodynamic changes during pregnancy, *Crit Care Nurse* 23:53-62, 2003.
*HELLP, H*emolysis, *e*levated *l*iver enzyme levels, and *l*ow *p*latelet count.

(g) Watch for signs of acute tubular necrosis (e.g., decreased urinary output, increased BUN and creatinine levels, electrolyte abnormalities, metabolic acidosis)

(h) Check urine output hourly until stable, then check every 2 hours

(i) Assess vaginal discharge, bleeding at incision sites, and level of consciousness hourly while the patient's condition is unstable and every 2 hours once stable

(j) Assess bowel sounds every 2 hours, and monitor the patient for signs of returning gut motility. Initiate an oral diet as tolerated.

(k) Continue to monitor deep tendon reflexes; watch for clonus and signs of CNS irritability. Seizures can occur up to 48 hours after delivery, so maintain seizure precautions.

AMNIOTIC FLUID EMBOLISM

1. **Pathophysiology:** Amniotic fluid is normally contained within the uterus, sealed off from the maternal circulation by the amniotic sac. Amniotic fluid embolism (AFE) occurs when this barrier is broken and, possibly under a pressure gradient, amniotic fluid enters the maternal venous system via the endocervical veins, placental site (if the placenta is separated), or uterine trauma site. Release of amniotic fluid containing vasoactive substances leads to pulmonary arterial spasm. Pulmonary hypertension, pulmonary capillary injury, hypoxia, hypotension, and cor pulmonale with left ventricular failure may result.

2. **Etiology and risk factors:** Predisposing factors for AFE include placental abruption, uterine overdistension, fetal death, trauma, tumultuous or oxytocin-stimulated labor, multiparity, advanced maternal age, and rupture of membranes

3. **Patient assessment:** AFE is clinically a biphasic process with the initial alterations involving central hemodynamics and oxygenation
   a. Respiratory: Severe cyanosis, dyspnea, tachypnea, pink frothy sputum
   b. Cardiovascular: Hypotension, shock, and dysrhythmias, but no chest pain
   c. CNS: Extreme anxiety, apprehension, and convulsions

4. **Patient care**
   a. Once a presumptive diagnosis is made, supportive measures must be initiated
   b. With cardiac arrest, resuscitation follows standard advanced cardiac life support (ACLS) protocols for obstetric patients
   c. AFE should be managed in the ICU. Critical care nurses without obstetric expertise may become anxious when caring for pregnant patients; however, the initial priorities of care are the same as for any emergency: Maintenance of the airway, breathing, and circulation. The major difference in obstetric emergencies is the need to care for two patients.
   d. Continuous fetal monitoring for signs of compromise should be performed by an obstetric nurse with expertise in electronic fetal monitoring
   e. To ensure optimal uterine perfusion, the mother's hips should be displaced to the left (which prevents the gravid uterus from compressing the inferior vena cava and decreasing venous return)
   f. Oxygenation
      i. Administer oxygen at a concentration of 100%
      ii. If a more aggressive approach is needed, provide endotracheal intubation and mechanical ventilation using a high fraction of inspired oxygen (FIO_2)

(>60%) and positive end-expiratory pressure (typically started at 5 cm H_2O with 2- to 3-cm increments) until arterial partial pressure of oxygen (PaO_2) is satisfactory

   iii. Goal is to maintain PaO_2 above 60 mm Hg and arterial oxygen saturation at 90% or higher

g. Circulation

   i. Position flat or in slight Trendelenburg's position to improve venous return and CNS perfusion

   ii. Provide fluid therapy, pharmacologic agents, electrocardiographic (ECG) monitoring to detect and treat arrhythmias

   iii. Placement of a pulmonary artery catheter is highly recommended for monitoring cardiac output, central venous pressure, and pulmonary artery pressure and for direct access for blood samples

   iv. Volume replacement with isotonic crystalloids is first-line therapy for maintaining blood pressure and avoiding overhydration in those predisposed to pulmonary edema

   v. Maintain systolic blood pressure at 90 mm Hg or higher and acceptable organ perfusion (urinary output ≥ 25 ml/hr)

h. Fetal considerations: In some instances, AFE does not occur until after delivery. When AFE occurs before or during delivery, however, the fetus is in grave danger from the outset due to maternal cardiopulmonary crisis. Therefore, as soon as the mother's condition is stabilized, delivery of a viable infant should be expedited. If resuscitation of the mother is futile, emergency bedside cesarean delivery may be necessary to save the infant.

Patient Transport

DEFINITIONS

1. *Inter*facility critical care transport involves the conveyance of a critically ill or injured patient from a scene or from one clinical facility to another when the patient's condition warrants care commensurate with the scope of practice of a specialty-trained transport nurse or physician
2. *Intra*facility critical care transport involves the transfer of a critically ill or injured patient from one diagnostic, treatment or inpatient area within the hospital to another

MEMBERS OF THE CRITICAL CARE TRANSPORT TEAM

1. **Interfacility transport team**
   a. Medical team must, at a minimum, include a specialty-trained physician or registered nurse (RN) as the primary care provider
      i. At least one team member must be a registered transport nurse
      ii. Program should be accredited by the Commission on Accreditation of Medical Transport Systems (CAMTS). (Refer to http://www.camts.org for a list of accredited programs.)
   b. Physician or RN may be designated as the primary care provider if the following criteria are met:
      i. Adequate and appropriate personnel are available to provide full coverage with physicians and RNs who are primarily assigned to the medical trans-

port service and who are readily available within the response time determined

    ii. Individual designated as the primary care provider has the appropriate state licensure

2. Intrafacility transport team

    a. Personnel able to anticipate, assess, and intervene effectively if the patient experiences problems during transport. Patient whose condition is unstable or who requires a specific type of monitoring should be accompanied by staff competent in managing the instability and in interpreting and intervening appropriately based on the monitoring data. Level of care that the patient requires should be maintained in any area of the hospital. Although the CAMTS identifies staff competencies required for patient transport between hospital facilities, some of the same principles apply to staff who comprise intrahospital transfer teams.

    b. RN with critical care or emergency experience and ACLS certification or its equivalent (Pediatric Advanced Life Support or Neonatal Resuscitation Program certification, or the equivalent, for an RN caring for neonatal or pediatric patients)

    c. Physician familiar with the patient or with the care provided on the patient's unit

    d. Respiratory therapist if the patient is on a ventilator

    e. Technician or certified nursing assistant to assist with moving or safely monitoring equipment

INDICATIONS FOR TRANSPORT

1. Interfacility: There is no universal algorithm that identifies indications for transport. Numerous associations have guidelines that recommend when a patient should be transported (see References). General indications for transport include the following:

    a. Illness or injury cannot be appropriately managed at the referring facility

    b. Diagnostic test, procedure, or treatment is not available at the referring facility

    c. State or local regulations dictate that a particular type of patient (e.g., pediatric or trauma patient) must be cared for at a specific facility

    d. Patient or family requests the transfer and transport

2. Intrafacility

    a. Transfer to perform a required diagnostic test or therapeutic procedure that cannot be handled within the unit (e.g., computed tomography, magnetic resonance imaging, cardiac catheterization)

    b. Transfer to another critical care unit or to a monitored bed

    c. Transfer to an operative suite

MODES OF INTERFACILITY TRANSPORT

1. Air transport

    a. Advantages

        i. Time saving

        ii. Air medical transport teams are generally educated and competent in advanced and critical care life support

        iii. Aircraft (especially rotary-wing aircraft) may be able to access environments that ground vehicles cannot

    b. Disadvantages

        i. Physiologic impact of flight stressors such as altitude and noise

        ii. Weather restrictions

        iii. Space and weight limitations

        iv. Fear of flying

2. Ground transport

    a. Advantages

        i. Ground vehicles can travel in inclement weather

        ii. Space allows for more personnel and equipment

        iii. More readily available

    b. Disadvantages

        i. Time consuming

        ii. Traffic and road conditions can impede transport

RISKS AND STRESSES OF TRANSPORT

1. All types of patient transport

    a. Physiologic instability during transport (e.g., inadequate stabilization of the patient's airway, breathing, and circulation; unstable cardiac rhythm)

    b. Potential for further injury or death when the patient is moved

    c. Inadequate patient assessment and/or monitoring during transport

    d. Lack of equipment, medications, or supplies required for care or resuscitation

    e. Equipment that malfunctions or is ill suited to the patient's age, condition, or size

    f. Rapid, disorganized transport due to lack of a team leader or to ineffective leadership

    g. Inadequately trained transport personnel

    h. Unavailability or lack of readiness of treatment area personnel to perform the procedure

2. Interfacility transport

    a. Risks of transport

        i. Possibility of transport vehicle crash

        ii. Long distances between treatment areas

        iii. Loss of the effects of sedation or anesthesia during the transport

        iv. Delayed patient arrival due to mechanical failure of the transport vehicle, traffic problems, or bad weather

    b. Stresses of air transport

        i. Barometric pressure changes

            (a) May cause *dysbarism* (body gas expansion) and barotrauma (tissue damage)

            (b) Trapped gases may affect the following:

                (1) Patient condition (e.g., gas expansion may lead to tension pneumothorax or cause abdominal pain)

                (2) Equipment (e.g., high altitude may slow IV flow rate)

        ii. Hypoxia: Decreased oxygen at high altitude

            (a) *Hypoxic hypoxia*—due to reduced FIO_2 or some condition that interferes with the diffusion of oxygen from the alveoli into the systemic circulation

            (b) *Hypemic hypoxia*—due to reduced oxygen-carrying capacity caused by conditions such as anemia, blood loss, carbon monoxide poisoning

      (c) *Stagnant hypoxia*—caused by conditions such as shock, acute myocardial infarction, or heart failure, which slow the transport of oxygen to tissues

      (d) *Histotoxic hypoxia*—due to interference with the tissue utilization of available oxygen caused by agents such as alcohol or narcotics, or poisons such as cyanide

  c. Stresses of air and ground transport

    i. Noise: Can range from 100 to 120 dB

      (a) May come from sources such as rotor blades, engines, sirens, or cabin noises from equipment or loud voice communications

      (b) May make it difficult to hear physiologic sounds (heart, breath, Korotkoff sounds) and equipment alarms, and to communicate verbally with the patient

    ii. Temperature: Thermal changes (heat or cold) may be related to the following:

      (a) External factors

        (1) Ambient temperature outside the transport vehicle

        (2) Vehicle's inability to maintain a comfortable environment

        (3) Altitude—temperature decreases as altitude and barometric pressure increase

      (b) Internal factors: Patient may not be able to maintain body temperature due to illness, injury, or medications, particularly neuromuscular blocking (NMB) agents

    iii. Vibration

      (a) Sources vary with the mode of transport

        (1) Ground: Road conditions

        (2) Fixed-wing aircraft: Air turbulence, especially at lower altitudes

        (3) Rotary-wing aircraft: Transition from main or tail rotors

      (b) Can cause symptoms of mild startle reaction, including increased heart, respiratory, and metabolic rates

    iv. Motion (acceleration, turning or banking, gravitational forces, visual field motion)

      (a) May lead to motion sickness, vomiting, disorientation, fear

      (b) Sunlight flickering through the main rotors of rotary-wing aircraft can cause *flicker vertigo*, nausea, disorientation; covering the eyes may help prevent this

3. Intrafacility transport

  a. Insufficient number of staff accompanying the patient

  b. Inadequate transport team staff mix to meet the patient's needs during transport

  c. Unanticipated delays related to elevator or electrical power failure

  d. Lack of communication between the originating and receiving areas regarding the transport

OVERRIDING PRIORITIES IN PATIENT TRANSPORT

1. Paramount determinants in decisions regarding patient transfer and transport

  a. Health, well-being, and safety of the patient require the following:

    i. Securing of the patient for transport

    ii. Securing of all equipment and supplies

    iii. Possible restraint of the patient to avoid harm to self or others, via one or more of the following means: Pharmacologic restraint (e.g., NMB agents), pharmacologic sedation, physical restraint

  b. Health, well-being, and safety of the transport team require the following:

       i. Physical restraint of team members during takeoffs, landings, ground vehicle movement

      ii. Training to ensure competence of all transport team members

     iii. Training of all who use the transport service

        (a) Method for setting up a landing area

        (b) Safety at the helicopter pad and in approaching aircraft, ground vehicle safety

2. **Safety of the patient and transport team** may require refusal to transport due to
   a. Weather restrictions
   b. Maintenance issues: Unsafe maintenance of an aircraft or ground vehicle (e.g., vehicles not properly inspected according to the manufacturer's recommendations or state or federal regulations)
   c. "Program shopping": One program or facility refuses the transport due to weather and the referring entity attempts to find another program to undertake the transport despite unsafe weather conditions

PREPARATION FOR TRANSPORT

1. **Select the appropriate transport service:** Determined by the needs of the patient to be transported
   a. Basic life support team
   b. Advanced life support team
   c. Critical care transport team
   d. Specialty team (e.g., neonatal, pediatric, perfusion, respiratory care)
2. **Select the equipment for transport:** Desired attributes (see Warren et al., 2004, for equipment suggested by the American College of Critical Care Medicine)
   a. Indicated by the patient's illness or injury
   b. Adapted for the transport setting
   c. Able to be safely restrained in the transport vehicle
   d. Lightweight and portable
   e. Redundant, multifunction (e.g., noninvasive and invasive blood pressure monitoring, end-tidal CO_2 and pulse oximetry)
   f. Easy to clean and maintain
   g. Sufficient battery life for transport with backup power source
   h. Able to withstand the stresses of transport, including vibration, temperature changes, accidental dropping, use by multiple persons
3. **Secure equipment and supplies for transport**
   a. Following items are suggested for inclusion:
          i. Monitor, defibrillator, external pacemaker
         ii. Pulse oximeter and end-tidal CO_2 monitor
        iii. Advanced airway equipment (age appropriate)
        iv. Transport ventilator or bag-valve device
         v. Portable suction devices
        vi. Adequate portable oxygen
       vii. Emergency medications (for ACLS, NMB, sedation, analgesia)
       viii. IV supplies: Fluids, needles, start kits (in case IV is lost during transport), infusion pumps
        ix. Any other device or medication the patient may require to maintain vital functions
   b. Ensure that the equipment and supplies are adequate to last for transport to the diagnostic or treatment area, for completion of the procedure, and, when warranted, for the return of the patient to the unit

4. **Assess and prepare the patient for transport**
   a Airway
      i. Rapid primary survey with immediate interventions to secure and maintain a patent airway
      ii. Assessment of the patency of any in-place airway device such as an endotracheal tube
   b. Ventilation
      i. Determine if altitude may place the patient at risk (e.g., a patient with thoracic trauma may need a chest tube for transport)
      ii. Ventilator-dependent patient should be given a trial run using the transport team's equipment
      iii. In general, all patients are given oxygen during transport
   c. Circulation
      i. Control of bleeding
      ii. Establishment and maintenance of venous access
      iii. Insertion of other invasive lines as indicated
      iv. Anticipation of IV fluid and medication needs
      v. Securing of the necessary circulatory support equipment (e.g., intraaortic balloon pump, left ventricular assist device)
   d. Gastric function
      i. Altitude can increase the risk of vomiting; determine whether a nasogastric tube should be inserted to prevent aspiration
      ii. Motion can cause nausea and vomiting; administer prophylactic antiemetics, as ordered
   e. Splinting: To prevent further injury and enhance patient comfort
   f. Pain
      i. Estimate the patient's probable needs for analgesia
      ii. Determine whether the patient has received an NMB agent; if so, plan to closely monitor the need for analgesia and/or sedation
   g. Wound care: Perform an initial appraisal; reinforce for transport if indicated
   h. Safety: Assess the potential of the patient to harm self or the transport team; restrain if necessary
5. **Notify the receiving unit or procedure area**
   a. Time the unit or area should expect the patient to arrive
   b. Equipment the patient will be using
   c. Equipment that will be required to maintain the patient during the procedure
6. **Prepare the family for interfacility transport**
   a. Always allow the family to see the patient before transport
   b. Explain to the family why the patient must be transferred
   c. Identify who will be caring for their family member during transport
   d. Provide directions to the receiving facility
   e. Remind the family to follow all traffic laws while in transit to the receiving facility
7. **Other interventions recommended before intrafacility transport**
   a. Suction the endotracheal tube or other airway device, as indicated
   b. Attach the patient to the transport ventilator; assess tolerance before leaving the unit
   c. Ensure the patency and flow rate of IV sites and medications
   d. Assess the patient's neurologic status
   e. Administer sedatives, analgesics, and any other medications that may be required during the transport. Remember that movement can cause the patient severe pain and anxiety.

f. Ensure that patients who require monitoring equipment will continue to be monitored during transport whenever possible (e.g., via wireless or battery-powered equipment)
g. Explain the need for transport to the patient and family
h. Ensure that adequate personnel are available to safely move the patient
i. If there is a procedure nurse, notify the nurse with a report that includes patient diagnosis, current medications and treatments, and planned interventions or procedures

PATIENT CARE DURING TRANSPORT

1. **Patient access:** Team members are positioned so they can assess and manage the patient
2. **Management of care**
   a. Airway equipment, including suction device, is readily accessible
   b. All IV lines are visible; at least one is accessible for medication administration
   c. All intake and output (urinary, gastric, chest tube, other), as well as responses to IV infusions and medications, are monitored
   d. All tubes and drainage systems are secured to reduce the possibility of dislodgement
   e. All transport monitors and equipment are placed within the team's line of sight. Visible alarms should be used.
   f. If the patient requires chemical or physical restraint for safe transport, ensure that the patient receives adequate sedation, analgesia, and environmental control
   g. Team needs to keep in mind that movement, noise, temperature changes, and fear can increase the patient's pain and make its management more challenging
3. **Documentation of care**
   a. Interfacility transport
      i. Continuity of care requires maintaining a complete and accurate record of care from the referring facility to the transport team to the receiving facility
      ii. Information needed by the receiving facility includes the following, for example:
         (a) Patient's age, chief complaint or admitting diagnoses, interventions provided, and the patient's response
         (b) Reason(s) for transport, the patient's status during transport
   b. Intrafacility transport
      i. Indications and authorization for transport
      ii. Preparation and baseline vital signs, assessment prior to transport
      iii. Patient care during transport

LEGAL AND ETHICAL ISSUES RELATED TO TRANSPORT

1. **Emergency Medical Treatment and Active Labor Act (EMTALA)**
   a. All patients who come to an emergency department should be medically screened to determine whether a medical emergency is present
   b. Condition of a patient with a medical emergency must be stabilized within the capabilities of the emergency department
   c. If the patient must be transported for care, the receiving hospital must accept the patient, if a bed and personnel are available

  d. Referring hospital must send all copies of medical records, diagnostic studies, informed consent documents, and physician transfer certifications

  e. Patient must be transported by qualified personnel, with appropriate equipment, and via the most suitable mode of transport

2. **Consent for transport**

  a. Explanation of the need for transport

  b. Explanation of the risks and benefits of transport

  c. Signed transfer form

3. **Written policies and procedures**

  a. Must include the indications for transport, facilities to which patients may be referred, and procedure for preparing patients for transfer and transport

  b. Should specify whether a family member may or may not accompany the transport team

4. **Documentation**

  a. Quality improvement parameters

  b. Regulations of the Health Insurance Portability and Accountability Act (HIPAA): Appropriate use of patient information to improve care

5. **Decision to transport or not to transport**

  a. No-transport decisions: Transport team needs established policies for "no transport" or the ability to consult with medical directors when making this decision

  b. Family consultation: When possible, the patient's family should be included in decisions not to transport

  c. Cardiopulmonary arrest

   i. Patients who have had a cardiopulmonary arrest must be carefully assessed to determine the benefits of transport, because the effectiveness of cardiopulmonary resuscitation (CPR) is compromised during transport

   ii. In addition, the transport team may be placed at risk by not being adequately restrained while performing CPR, by sustaining needle sticks when administering drugs during CPR, and by being exposed to blood or body fluids during CPR

  d. Advance directives

  e. Do-not-resuscitate orders

  f. Refusal of transport by the patient, family, or others

Pediatric Patients

1. **Children—a unique population:** Children are not small adults. Differences in size, anatomy, and developmental level result in unique responses to illness and technical challenges. Nurses who care for children in an adult critical care area need basic competency in developmental care, which involves first identifying the child's developmental level and then planning care around that level. This section provides an overview of assessments, developmental levels, and anatomical differences that may influence nursing care of the critically ill child.

2. **Guidelines for assessment of children**

  a. Whenever possible, allow the parents to hold and be with their child

  b. Before touching a child, measure vital signs and complete visual assessments. Children may cry or become frightened, so that assessment findings are altered.

  c. Speak in terms the child can understand based on developmental level

  d. Allow the child to touch and play with medical equipment (e.g., stethoscope) used for assessment

e. Whenever possible, offer the child choices. For example, does the child want the IV line in the hand or the arm?

f. Offer positive reinforcement and give rewards, whenever possible

g. With a mature child, work together with the child to plan his or her care

h. Always tell the truth. Building a trusting relationship requires this. If something is going to hurt, do not tell the child that it won't.

i. Listen to the parents. They are the ones who know the child best and can more readily discern subtle changes in the child's condition.

3. **Developmental levels**

a. Infant (ages 0 to 1 year)

   i. Fear separation from caregivers. Allow the parents to be at the bedside as much as possible.

   ii. Touch is very important. Allow the parents to hold the child; if that is not possible, encourage the parents to stroke and touch the child.

   iii. Infants like to be swaddled. Keep their hands and arms at midline.

   iv. Infants fear strangers. Insofar as possible, provide consistent caregivers.

   v. Infants fear pain and may cry when approached, anticipating that something may hurt. Use analgesics as needed.

   vi. As infants get older, they will grab at medical equipment within their reach. Although therapeutic play is beneficial and usually safe, it is important to keep dangerous items out of reach.

   vii. Infants need comfort measures. Encourage the parents to bring the child's favorite blanket or crib toy to the hospital. Hold the child awhile after procedures are completed.

   viii. Infants have a need for deep sleep. Insofar as possible, cluster procedures and care to maximize periods of uninterrupted sleep.

   ix. Because infants are not able to tell caregivers what is wrong, additional tests may be necessary to reach a diagnosis

   x. Presence of strong visual and auditory stimuli may increase stress to infants, so lights and noise should be minimized to promote rest

   xi. Restraints should be used only to keep a child safe

   xii. Bronchiolitis due to respiratory syncytial virus frequently causes apnea and may require intubation

   xiii. Diagnoses most frequently seen in this age group are sepsis, congenital heart disease, hypoglycemia, and bronchiolitis

b. Toddler (ages 1 to 3 years)

   i. Toddlers fear separation from their caregivers. Allow caregivers to remain at the bedside as long as feasible.

   ii. Toddlers frequently use the word *no* to gain control and autonomy. Toddlers need to be offered choices when these exist. That does not mean that they can refuse necessary care, but, for example, they can decide which arm to use for drawing blood.

   iii. Toddlers have an intense fear of mutilation as well as a magical imagination. They may fixate on having adhesive strips over all needle sticks because they fear their blood could come out through those holes. For these reasons, caregivers need to use concrete terms and incorporate play when preparing toddlers for procedures.

   iv. Toddlers have a strong sense of curiosity. Caregivers need to perform a complete safety check of the environment to ensure that they cannot delve into anything that might harm them.

   v. Toddlers take things very literally, so explanations need to be in simple terms to avoid creating unwarranted fears and misinterpretation

vi. Toddlers need their normal routines followed whenever these can be preserved. Parents can identify routines important to their child.

vii. Toddlers need to be told the truth to develop trust in caregivers

viii. Toddlers do not understand the concept of time, so they do not distinguish between 2 hours and 2 weeks. As a result, 2 days might be better described as "two wake-ups."

ix. Diagnoses most commonly seen in this age level are head trauma, near drowning, accidental ingestion of harmful substances, asthma, and seizures

c. Preschooler (ages 3 to 5 years)

i. Preschoolers are offended by lies and lose trust in adults rapidly, so do not say that something will not hurt if it will

ii. Preschoolers have great imaginations. The truth (no matter how bleak) in simple words is often less frightening than what they are imagining. This also needs to be remembered when dealing with the critically ill child's siblings.

iii. Preschoolers share toddlers' fears of bodily harm and mutilation. They may also fear that they are in the hospital because they have done something wrong or "bad."

iv. Preschoolers are afraid of the dark and of being alone. Adjusted lighting and familiar faces nearby can help allay these fears.

v. Preschoolers fear the unknown and want to be in control of the environment. Their developing sense of self can be supported by always preparing them for procedures, by explaining what will happen in simple terms, by incorporating play into this preparation, and by allowing them to ask questions.

vi. Preschoolers may be able to help in some of their own care

vii. As with toddlers, preschoolers do not fully understand the concept of time, except for familiar distinctions such as "lunchtime"

viii. When hospitalized, preschoolers may regress to behaviors such as thumb sucking or bed wetting

ix. Preschoolers can easily misinterpret conversations and unfamiliar terms. Staff can minimize this problem by avoiding discussions about the child's condition in locations where they might be overheard.

x. Diagnoses most often seen among preschoolers are trauma and dehydration related to influenza

d. School-aged child (ages 5 to 12 years)

i. School-aged children are concrete, operational thinkers

ii. They need to be prepared in advance for procedures, using body diagrams or models to explain what is going to happen

iii. Encourage these children to ask questions. They understand cause and effect relationships, so treatments or medications can be explained in terms of how these help them to recover.

iv. They fear loss of control, so provide choices when possible

v. They fear mutilation and understand that death is final

vi. Privacy can be extremely important. They understand that their bodies are different and do not want others to see them undressed.

vii. They want to help, to be involved; enlist their participation in care

viii. Friends are very important in their lives. Letters from friends, family, and classmates are encouraged.

ix. Diagnoses most often seen for this age group are arteriovenous malformation and trauma

   e. Adolescent (ages 12 to 21 years)

   i. When communicating with adolescents, it is important to be straightforward, scrupulously honest, and nonjudgmental to establish trust. Unless they feel trust, they will not be open, honest, or cooperative with caregivers; they need to know that caregivers are on their side.

   ii. Exerting independence is important to adolescents, who may be noncompliant with care to express this need

   iii. It is important to involve adolescents in decision making that affects their care so they can maintain a sense of control

   iv. Adolescents require advance preparation for events related to their care

   v. Body image is highly important. Disfiguring conditions or injuries can be especially traumatic and demand considerable therapeutic intervention.

   vi. Privacy, modesty, confidentiality, and acceptance as a person are priorities to adolescents that caregivers must respect

   vii. Adolescent "acting-out" behaviors may reflect relationship problems with parents, peers, or girlfriends or boyfriends that may be difficult for others to see or fully appreciate

   viii. It is important to ask about drug, alcohol, and tobacco use. Adolescents may not volunteer this information, and such use could impede their care.

   ix. Diagnoses most often encountered among adolescents are trauma and intentional ingestion of substances

4. Anatomical differences between children and adults

   a. General differences

   i. Children have a higher center of gravity, so are more prone to falls

   ii. They have a relatively larger head and weaker neck muscles. In a car crash or long distance fall, the head may act like a missile and propel the body with greater velocity and subsequently greater force on impact and whiplash.

   iii. Infants are especially vulnerable to head trauma because of their thin craniums and open fontanelles (until about 18 months of age)

   iv. They have lax ligaments and can have spinal cord injury without radiographic abnormality

   v. Their bones and ligaments are more pliable. In chest trauma, ribs may not be fractured, yet underlying organs can be damaged.

   vi. Motor skills may not be fully developed, which makes them more vulnerable to falls and injury

   vii. Normal ranges of vital signs differ by age (Table 11-10)

   b. Respiratory differences

   i. Infants are obligate nose breathers; they can have trouble breathing if their nares are blocked by mucus or a nasogastric tube

   ii. In children the tongue is disproportionately larger and can occlude the airway

   iii. Airway cartilage is soft, particularly in the larynx. Care must be taken to avoid hyperextension and hyperflexion of the neck, because either could cause airway occlusion.

   iv. Larynx is higher and more anterior, which makes children more prone to aspiration or airway obstruction. It can also make intubation more difficult.

   v. Tracheal diameter is proportional to body size. As a result, small degrees of swelling can occlude the airway of a small infant (Figure 11-1).

   vi. In children younger than 8 years of age, the cricoid cartilage is the narrowest portion of the trachea. An inappropriately large endotracheal tube could cause tracheal swelling and damage.

■ TABLE 11-10
■ ■ Vital Signs by Age

Age	Heart Rate (beats /min)	Respiratory Rate (breaths/min)	Systolic Blood Pressure (mm Hg)	Cardiac Output (L/min)
Infant	100-160	30-60	87-105	1.0-1.3
Toddler	80-110	24-40	95-105	1.5-2.0
Preschooler	70-110	22-34	95-105	2.3-2.75
School-aged child	65-110	18-30	97-112	3.8-4.0
Adolescent	60-90	12-16	112-128	6.0

vii. Tracheal length is shorter, so there is a risk of intubating the right mainstem bronchus

viii. Diaphragm is positioned more horizontally. Children use diaphragmatic breathing for ventilation, so air in the stomach can raise the diaphragm and compromise lung capacity.

ix. Chest wall is more pliable in children. They could have underlying organ damage in trauma that may be missed because of lack of obvious external injury.

c. Cardiovascular differences

   i. Differences in pediatric heart rate and blood pressure are important to note (see Table 11-10)

   ii. Children increase their cardiac output primarily by increasing their heart rate. Vasoconstriction may be seen, but only when fluid loss is great. Decreased blood pressure can be a very late sign of shock.

   iii. Blood volume depends on the size of the child

   iv. Children compensate extremely well by maintaining blood pressure. When a child's blood pressure begins to fall, the end is near.

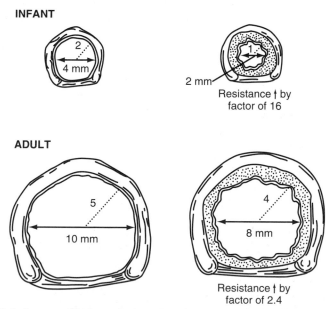

FIGURE 11-1 Adult versus infant airway size. (From Hazinski MF: *Nursing care of the critically ill child*, ed 2, St Louis, 1992, Mosby, p 11.)

   d. Thermoregulatory differences
       i. Children, especially infants, have a large surface area–to–volume ratio and less subcutaneous tissue. As a result, they lose heat to the environment more readily and are more susceptible to poisoning by chemicals that can be absorbed through the skin.
       ii. Cold stress is important to avoid because it can cause significant energy and oxygen consumption, increased metabolism, and hypoglycemia
   e. Neurologic differences
       i. Skull of the infant or young child is thin and offers little protection to the brain
       ii. Children are more prone to head injuries because the head diameter is relatively larger than that of adults
       iii. In children, head trauma is more often associated with hemorrhage related to shear forces and intracranial swelling
       iv. Glasgow Coma Scale assessments are modified for infants and children (Table 11-11)
   f. Abdominal differences
       i. Children have a protruding abdomen, which may help protect them from major pelvic injuries
       ii. Organs injured most often in children are the liver and spleen
       iii. Abdominal muscles are thinner and weaker, and afford less protection to underlying organs
       iv. Pelvis is more anterior, and thus more vulnerable to impact, than in the adult
5. Summary: Children are not just small adults. When they are admitted to an adult ICU, critical care nurses need to plan and provide care based on the physiologic and psychologic attributes summarized here. It is important that nurses have some basic competency in caring for children. The eight patient characteristics in the Synergy Model are different in children depending on their developmental stage because they do not have the ability to care for themselves. When nurses have the basic competencies to care for children and they understand children's characteristics, optimal patient outcomes can result.

■ **TABLE 11-11**
■ ■ **Modified Glasgow Coma Scale for Infants and Children**

	Child	Infant	Score
Eye opening	Spontaneous	Spontaneous	4
	To verbal stimuli	To verbal stimuli	3
	To pain only	To pain only	2
	No response	No response	1
Verbal response	Oriented, appropriate	Coos and babbles	5
	Confused	Irritable cries	4
	Inappropriate words	Cries to pain	3
	Incomprehensible words or nonspecific sounds	Moans to pain	2
	No response	No response	1
Motor response	Obeys commands	Moves spontaneously	6
	Localizes pain stimulus	Withdraws to touch	5
	Withdraws to pain	Withdraws to pain	4
	Flexion to pain	Decorticate posturing	3
	Extension to pain	Decerebrate posturing	2
	No response	No response	1

Sedation in Critically Ill Patients

GENERAL CONSIDERATIONS

1. **Concerns with sedation**
   a. Assessment of the patient's level of anxiety, agitation, and sedation, and response to sedative medication
   b. Altered response to drugs due to underlying medical conditions
   c. Tolerance to medication due to prior experience with the drug or the length of time it was received
   d. Delayed emergence
      i. Overdose of sedative due to individual variability or drug interaction
      ii. Delayed elimination due to comorbidities, age, liver or kidney dysfunction
   e. Withdrawal symptoms: May cause agitation or confusion
      i. From drugs the patient was previously taking
      ii. From sudden cessation of sedative or opioid use, which can cause a return of agitation; early symptoms of opioid withdrawal include salivation, yawning, diarrhea
   f. Drug interactions of sedatives with other medications the patient is receiving
2. **Balancing of sedation**
   a. Effects of undersedation
      i. Anxiety, agitation, increased metabolic demand
      ii. Tachycardia, hypertension, myocardial ischemia, dysrhythmias
      iii. Wound disruption, patient injury
      iv. Recall or awareness, need for paralytics
   b. Effects of oversedation
      i. Delayed emergence, delayed weaning from ventilator
      ii. Pressure injury, venous stasis, muscle atrophy
      iii. Increased tests, ICU and/or hospital length of stay, costs
   c. Indications for sedation in the ICU
      i. Anxiety (Park, Coursin, Ely, et al, 2001)—feelings of nervousness, apprehension, or fear
      ii. Agitation (McGaffigan, 2002)—a more extreme form of excessive, uncontrolled, or irrational activity commonly associated with increased muscle tone and increased catecholamine levels
      iii. Delirium (Bixby and Picard, 2005)—characterized by confusion, disordered speech, and hallucinations; an acute, reversible organic mental syndrome
      iv. Pain—from injuries, surgery, trauma, procedures, preexisting conditions, and so on
3. **Plan for patient comfort**
   a. Overall plan
      i. Set treatment goals
      ii. Use quantitative tools to assess sedation and pain
      iii. Choose the right drug or combination of drugs; reevaluate the need for sedation
      iv. Treat withdrawal
   b. Pain management
      i. Before sedating, rule out the need for analgesia and treat reversible physiologic causes
      ii. When the patient can communicate, assess via a quantitative scale; use the patient's report of pain as the basis for treatment

      iii. When the patient is unable to communicate, assess via subjective criteria (e.g., facial expressions, posturing, vital signs)

4. Assessment of sedation

    a. Establish a sedation goal and ensure that it is regularly redefined and documented

    b. Use a validated sedation assessment scale, a subjective measure

    c. Keep in mind that sedation scales do not assess anxiety, pain, or sedation in paralyzed patients

    d. Sedation scales in current use: See Table 11-12

      i. Ramsay scale

      ii. Riker Sedation-Agitation Scale (SAS)

      iii. Motor Activity Assessment Scale (MAAS)

      iv. Richmond Agitation-Sedation Scale

      v. Other scales: Luer scale; Shelly scale; COMFORT scale (tested only in children); Vancouver Interaction and Calmness Scale (VICS)—scores up to 30 for interaction (communication) and up to 30 for calmness (calm to pulling at lines); Faces Anxiety Scale

      vi. New sedation assessment scale under development (including validity and reliability testing) by Abbott, American Association of Critical-Care Nurses, and the Saint Thomas Health Systems Expert Panel (DeJong MJ: Personal communication, October 11, 2004)

    e. Objective measures of assessment

      i. Vital signs, such as blood pressure and heart rate—not specific or sensitive

      ii. Electroencephalography (EEG), auditory evoked potentials

      iii. Lower esophageal contractility

      iv. Bispectral index monitor (BIS)

        (a) Measures effects of sedatives on the brain and consciousness

        (b) Consists of a single sensor with several electrodes attached to the forehead

        (c) BIS value (0 to 100) is an empirical, statistically derived number that correlates with the hypnotic level of the patient

          (1) BIS value above 95 indicates full consciousness

          (2) BIS value below 60 indicates reduced likelihood of consciousness

          (3) BIS value of 0 indicates isoelectric EEG

        (d) Useful with deeply comatose patients or those under NMB; scores may be artificially elevated by muscle-based electrical activity in patients not under NMB

        (e) BIS monitoring not completely validated as useful in the ICU, but may be a promising tool in the future

5. Pharmacology

    a. Benzodiazepines: Produce amnesia, hypnosis, and anxiolysis, but not analgesia

      i. Midazolam

        (a) Recommended for short-term use only because it causes unpredictable awakening when infusions continue longer than 48 to 72 hours

        (b) Midazolam or diazepam should be used for rapid sedation of the acutely agitated

        (c) Onset of action after IV dose, 2 to 5 minutes; half-life, 3 to 11 hours

      ii. Lorazepam

        (a) Recommended for sedation of most patients via intermittent or continuous IV

        (b) Onset of action after IV dose, 2 to 5 minutes; half-life, 8 to 15 hours

■ **TABLE 11-12**
■ ■ **Sedation Assessment Scales for Adult Patients**

Ramsay Scale	Sedation-Agitation Scale	Motor Activity Assessment Scale	Richmond Agitation-Sedation Scale
6 No response	1 Unarousable (minimal or no response to noxious stimuli, does not communicate or follow commands)	0 Unresponsive (does not move in response to noxious stimuli)	−5 Unresponsive (no response to voice or physical stimulation)
5 Patient asleep with a sluggish response to a light glabellar tap	2 Very sedated (arouses to physical stimuli but does not communicate or follow commands, may move spontaneously)	1 Responsive only to noxious stimuli (opens eyes or raises eyebrows or turns head toward stimulus or moves limb in response to noxious stimulus)	−4 Deep sedation (no response to voice, but any movement to physical stimulation)
4 Patient asleep with a brisk response to a light glabellar tap	3 Sedated (difficult to arouse, awakens to verbal stimuli or gentle shaking but drifts off again, follows simple commands)	2 Responsive to touch or name (opens eyes or raises eyebrows or turns head toward stimulus or moves limb when touched or when name is loudly spoken)	−3 Moderate sedation (any movement, but no eye contact to voice)
3 Patient responds to commands only	4 Calm and cooperative (calm, awakens easily, follows commands)	3 Calm and cooperative (no external stimulus is required to elicit purposeful movement and patient follows commands)	−2 Light sedation (brief, <10 sec awakening with eye contact to voice)
2 Patient cooperative, oriented, and tranquil	5 Agitated (anxious or mildly agitated, attempts to sit up, calms down to verbal instructions)	4 Restless and cooperative (no external stimulus is required to elicit movement and patient is picking at sheets or tubes or uncovering self and and follows commands)	−1 Drowsy (not fully alert, but has sustained, >10 sec awakening with eye contact to voice)
1 Patient anxious or agitated or both	6 Very agitated (does not calm, despite frequent verbal reminding of limits; requires physical restraints; bites endotracheal tube)	5 Agitated (no external stimulus is required to elicit movement and patient is attempting to sit up or moves limbs out of bed and does not consistently follow commands)	0 Alert and calm

Continued

| 7 Dangerous agitation (pulling at endotracheal tube, trying to remove catheter, climbing over bed rail, striking at staff, thrashing from side to side) | 6 Dangerously agitated, uncooperative (no external stimulus is required to elicit movement and patient is pulling at tubes or catheters or thrashing from side to side or striking at staff or trying to climb out of bed and does not calm down when asked) | 1 Restless (anxious or apprehensive but movements are not aggressive or vigorous) 2 Agitated (frequent nonpurposeful movement or patient-ventilator dyssynchrony) 3 Very agitated (pulls on or removes tubes or catheters or shows aggressive behavior toward staff) 4 Combative (overly combative or violent, immediate danger to staff) |

From Consensus conference on sedation assessment: a collaborative venture by Abbott Laboratories, American Association of Critical-Care Nurses, and Saint Thomas Health System, *Crit Care Nurse* 24(2):35, 2004. Data from Ramsay MA, Savege TM, Simpson BR, et al: Controlled sedation with alphaxalone-alphadolone, *BMJ* 2:656-659, 1974; Devlin JW, Boleski G, Mlynarek M, et al: Motor Activity Assessment Scale: a valid and reliable sedation scale for use with mechanically ventilated patients in an adult surgical intensive care unit, *Crit Care Med* 27:1271-1275, 1999; Riker RR, Fraser GL, Cox PM: Continuous infusion of haloperidol controls agitation in critically ill patients, *Crit Care Med* 22:433-440, 1994; Sessler CN, Gosnet MS, Grap MJ, et al: The Richmond Agitation-Sedation Scale: validity and reliability in adult intensive care unit patients, *Am J Respir Crit Care Med* 166:1338-1344, 2002; Ely EW, Truman B, Shintani A, et al: Monitoring sedation status over time in ICU patients: reliability and validity of the Richmond Agitation-Sedation Scale (RASS), *JAMA* 22:2983-2991, 2003.

   iii. Diazepam

      (a) Very irritating to the vein; can cause phlebitis when administered IV

      (b) Onset of action after IV dose, 2 to 5 minutes; half-life, 20 to 120 hours

  b. Propofol: Produces hypnosis, anxiolysis, less amnesia than benzodiazepines, no analgesia

     i. IV sedative-hypnotic general anesthetic; approved for sedation of intubated adults on mechanical ventilation in the ICU

     ii. Rapid onset of action (1 to 2 min); short persistence of action once discontinued; half-life, 26 to 32 hours

    iii. Preferred sedative when rapid awakening is important

    iv. Can elevate triglyceride levels; monitor after 2 days of infusion

     v. Add total caloric intake from lipids contained in medication in nutritional support orders

    vi. Requires *strict aseptic* technique for administration because it contains absolutely *no* preservative

  c. Opioids: Provide analgesia and anxiolysis

     i. Recommended for IV use in the critically ill: Fentanyl, hydromorphone, morphine

    ii. Scheduled doses or continuous infusion preferred over "as needed." Patient-controlled analgesia can be used if the patient is able to understand and operate the equipment

        iii. NSAIDs or acetaminophen may be used as adjuncts to opioids. Ketorolac use should be limited to a maximum of 5 days.

   d. α_2-Agonists: Provide hypnosis, anxiolysis, and analgesia, but no amnesia

      i. Clonidine

        (a) Inhibits norepinephrine release from central and peripheral presynaptic junctions

        (b) Enables use of lower dosages of opiates to achieve comfort

        (c) Thought to have analgesic actions

      ii. Dexmedetomidine

        (a) Selective α_2-agonist that inhibits the release of norepinephrine

        (b) Has sedative and analgesic effects without causing respiratory depression

        (c) Patients remain sedated when not disturbed, but arouse easily with gentle stimulation

        (d) Approved for short-term use (<24 hours)

        (e) May produce transient elevations in blood pressure, bradycardia, and hypotension

6. Nonpharmacologic methods to decrease anxiety

   a. Reorientation and validation of anxiety

   b. Use of cards with phrases to aid communication with intubated patients unable to speak

   c. Soft lighting, restful music, pleasant room design and color, pictures from home

   d. Music therapy, massage, therapeutic touch, pet therapy, liberal visitation

7. Delirium

   a. Fluctuating mental status, disorganized thinking, altered level of consciousness, with or without agitation

   b. Assessment of delirium

      i. Gold standard: Clinical history and examination

      ii. Bedside scale: Confusion Assessment Method for the ICU (CAM-ICU)

        (a) Involves observation for the onset of changes in mental status or level of consciousness, inattention, disorganized thinking

        (b) Can be completed in 2 minutes

   c. Pharmacologic treatment for delirium: Neuroleptic agents

      i. Chlorpromazine—not routinely used in critical care patients

      ii. Haloperidol

        (a) Preferred agent for use in the ICU

        (b) Monitor for ECG changes (QT prolongation, dysrhythmias)

8. Other considerations

   a. Sleep promotion is imperative for patients in the ICU, although those on high dosages of sedatives demonstrate atypical sleep patterns

   b. Sedative dose should be titrated with the end point defined and administration interrupted daily to reassess the patient and minimize the effects of prolonged sedative use

   c. Withdrawal effects can occur if opioids, benzodiazepines, or propofol is used for longer than 7 days

   d. Use of sedation guidelines, an algorithm, or a protocol is recommended (Figure 11-2)

9. Competency of the RN administering sedatives (these requirements are equally applicable to nurses administering procedural sedation)

   a. Receipt of specialized instruction related to the use of sedatives and analgesics

   b. Possession of the following required competencies (Synergy Model—nursing competencies based on patient needs):

BIDMC CRITICAL CARE GUIDELINE FOR SEDATION AND ANALGESIA

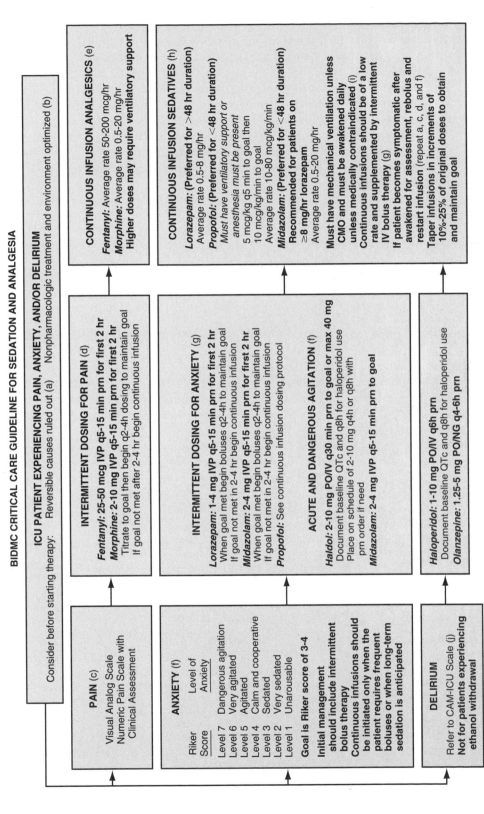

ICU PATIENT EXPERIENCING PAIN, ANXIETY, AND/OR DELIRIUM

Consider before starting therapy: Reversible causes ruled out (a)   Nonpharmacologic treatment and environment optimized (b)

PAIN (c)

Visual Analog Scale
Numeric Pain Scale with
Clinical Assessment

ANXIETY (f)

Riker   Level of
Score   Anxiety

Level 7   Dangerous agitation
Level 6   Very agitated
Level 5   Agitated
Level 4   Calm and cooperative
Level 3   Sedated
Level 2   Very sedated
Level 1   Unarousable

Goal is Riker score of 3-4

**Initial management
should include intermittent
bolus therapy**

**Continuous infusions should
be initiated only when the
patient requires frequent
boluses or when long-term
sedation is anticipated**

DELIRIUM

Refer to CAM-ICU Scale (j)
**Not for patients experiencing
ethanol withdrawal**

INTERMITTENT DOSING FOR PAIN (d)

Fentanyl: 25-50 mcg IVP q5-15 min prn for first 2 hr
Morphine: 2-10 mg IVP q5-15 min prn for first 2 hr
Titrate to goal then begin q2-4h dosing to maintain goal
If goal not met after 2-4 hr begin continuous infusion

INTERMITTENT DOSING FOR ANXIETY (g)

Lorazepam: 1-4 mg IVP q5-15 min prn for first 2 hr
When goal met begin boluses q2-4h to maintain goal
If goal not met in 2-4 hr begin continuous infusion
Midazolam: 2-4 mg IVP q5-15 min prn for first 2 hr
When goal met begin boluses q2-4h to maintain goal
If goal not met in 2-4 hr begin continuous infusion
Propofol: See continuous infusion dosing protocol

ACUTE AND DANGEROUS AGITATION (f)

Haldol: 2-10 mg PO/IV q30 min prn to goal or max 40 mg
Place baseline QTc and q8h for haloperidol use
Place on schedule of 2-10 mg q4h or q8h with
prn order if need
Midazolam: 2-4 mg IVP q5-15 min prn to goal

Haloperidol: 1-10 mg PO/IV q6h prn
Document baseline QTc and q8h for haloperidol use
Olanzepine: 1.25-5 mg PO/NG q4-6h prn

CONTINUOUS INFUSION ANALGESICS (e)

Fentanyl: Average rate 50-200 mcg/hr
Morphine: Average rate 0.5-20 mg/hr
Higher doses may require ventilatory support

CONTINUOUS INFUSION SEDATIVES (h)

Lorazepam: (Preferred for >48 hr duration)
Average rate 0.5-8 mg/hr
Propofol: (Preferred for <48 hr duration)
Must† have ventilatory support or
anesthesia must be present
5 mcg/kg q5 min to goal then
10 mcg/kg/min to goal
Average rate 10-80 mcg/kg/min
Midazolam: (Preferred for <48 hr duration)
Recommended for patients on
≥8 mg/hr lorazepam
Average rate 0.5-20 mg/hr

Must have mechanical ventilation unless
CMO and must be awakened daily
unless medically contraindicated (i)
Continuous infusions should be of a low
rate and supplemented by intermittent
IV bolus therapy (g)
If patient becomes symptomatic after
awakened for assessment, rebolus and
restart infusion (repeat a, c, and f)
Taper infusions in increments of
10%-25% of original doses to obtain
and maintain goal

FIGURE 11-2 Beth Israel Deaconess Medical Center (BIDMC) algorithm for sedation and analgesia. *CAM-ICU,* Confusion Assessment Method for the Intensive Care Unit; *CMO,* comfort measures only; *ICU,* intensive care unit; *IV,* intravenous; *IVP,* intravenous push; *max,* maximum; *NG,* nasogastric tube; *PO,* by mouth; *pts,* patients; *vent,* ventilator.

  i. Knowledge of the relevant anatomy, physiology, pharmacology, recognition and management of cardiac dysrhythmias, CPR procedures
  ii. Ability to assess total patient care requirements
  iii. Ability to apply principles of respiratory physiology and oxygen transport and uptake, and to use oxygen delivery devices to maintain and/or restore a patent airway
  iv. Ability to anticipate and recognize all of the following potential complications and to institute nursing interventions in accordance with existing orders, protocols, or guidelines
    (a) Pulmonary: Respiratory depression, hypoxemia, hypercapnia, respiratory obstruction, laryngospasm, bronchospasm
    (b) Cardiovascular: Cardiac dysrhythmias, hypertension, hypotension
    (c) Allergic reaction
  v. Knowledge of the legal ramifications for nurses administering sedatives and analgesics

PROCEDURAL SEDATION AND ANALGESIA FOR THE PATIENT IN THE INTENSIVE CARE UNIT

1. **Definitions**
   a. *Minimal sedation:* Drug-induced state in which response to a verbal command is normal. Cognitive function and coordination may be impaired, but ventilatory and cardiovascular functions are unaltered.
   b. *Moderate (conscious) sedation:* Drug-induced depression of consciousness in which the patient gives a purposeful response to verbal commands alone or to verbal commands accompanied by light tactile stimulation. Spontaneous ventilation is adequate; no interventions are required to maintain a patent airway. Cardiovascular function is usually maintained.
   c. *Deep sedation:* Drug-induced depression of consciousness in which the patient cannot be easily aroused but responds purposefully following repeated or painful stimulation. Assistance may be required to maintain a patent airway and to independently maintain ventilatory function. Spontaneous ventilation may be inadequate, but cardiovascular function is usually maintained.
2. **Moderate sedation and analgesia procedures and guidelines**
   a. Should assure the comfort and safety of patients undergoing sedation and analgesia
   b. Should establish standardized guidelines for the administration of sedatives
   c. Should ensure that qualified, competent staff provide care for patients undergoing procedures requiring sedation and can rescue patients who reach a deeper level of sedation than intended
3. **Indications and contraindications for procedural sedation**
   a. Procedural sedation is indicated for patients needing moderate (conscious) sedation for invasive, manipulative, or constraining procedures
   b. Procedural sedation is *not* appropriate for managing pain or anxiety in the terminally ill, in patients on ventilators, or in those who require seizure control
4. **Practice issues**
   a. State board of nursing (SBN) position statements: Some SBNs have specific position statements on the issue of sedation and analgesia; some rely on decision trees; others do not address this practice. Know your SBN's stance on the issue.
   b. National position statements
      i. American Nurses Association position statement: Available at http://www.ana.org/readroom/position/joint/jtsedate.htm

    ii. Position statements of specialty organizations

       (a) American Association of Critical-Care Nurses: Available at http://www.aacn.org/AACN/pubpolcy. nsf/vwdoc/MainPublicPolicy

       (b) American Society of Anesthesiologists (ASA): Available at http://www.asahq.org/publicationsAndServices/sedation1017.pdf

       (c) American Association of Nurse Anesthetists (AANA): Available at http://www.aana.com/practice/qualified.asp and http://www.aana.com/practice/conscious.asp

   iii. Position statements on the use of anesthetic agents (e.g., propofol) for moderate sedation

       (a) Some SBNs specifically say it is not within the RN's scope of practice; others say it is within the scope of practice; others have not addressed the issue

       (b) Controversial issue. Do not confuse with the appropriate use of propofol for the sedation of patients on mechanical ventilation.

       (c) AANA and ASA have a joint position statement saying that it is not appropriate for a non–anesthesia provider to administer an anesthetic agent for moderate sedation. (See http://www.asahq.org/news/propofolstatement.htm or http://www.aana.com/news/2004/news050504_joint.asp.)

       (d) American College of Gastroenterology, American Gastroenterological Association, and American Society for Gastrointestinal Endoscopy have a joint position statement saying that, under certain conditions, it is appropriate for a non–anesthesia provider to administer an anesthetic agent for moderate sedation. (See http://www.gastro.org/wmspage.cfm?parm1=371.)

       (e) Know the position of your SBN and your hospital policy and procedure

5. Preprocedural assessment

  a. History

    i. Abnormalities of major organ systems

    ii. Adverse experience with sedation-analgesia or general anesthesia

    iii. History of smoking, alcohol use, drug use

    iv. History of a condition associated with increased risk in maintaining the airway: Snoring, stridor, sleep apnea, advanced rheumatoid arthritis, Down syndrome

    v. Current medications, including over-the-counter or herbal products; drug allergies

    vi. Time of last oral intake

  b. Physical examination—focused on the heart and lungs

    i. Physical airway examination

       (a) Significant obesity

       (b) Short neck or limited extension of the neck

       (c) Small mouth opening, dental appliances, nonvisible uvula, micrognathia, trismus, significant malocclusion

    ii. Baseline vital signs and oxygen saturation

    iii. Pregnancy status if the patient is a female of childbearing age

    iv. Pain assessment

    v. Confirmation of the individual as the correct patient using two methods of identification

  c. Preprocedural preparation

    i. Educate the patient and family or significant other

    ii. Obtain informed consent. Discuss the benefits, risks, and limitations of, as well as alternatives for, sedation and analgesia. Informed consent is given to a physician, but the nurse can ensure that the presence of a signed consent form is documented.

iii. Start an IV line

iv. Immediately prior to commencing sedation, verify that the patient and the procedure are the correct ones

v. Immediately prior to commencing the procedure, measure vital signs and oxygen saturation level

6. **Intraprocedural monitoring of patients**
   a. Basic assessments
      i. Level of consciousness
      ii. Ventilation and oxygenation: Respiratory rate, bilateral ventilation (using a stethoscope), oxygen saturation via pulse oximeter
      iii. Heart rate and rhythm: ECG monitor
      iv. Blood pressure: Noninvasive continuous blood pressure monitor
      v. Vital signs: Document every 5 minutes during the procedure
      vi. Report significant variations to the physician immediately (i.e., abnormal vital signs, nasal flaring, grunting, retractions, wheezing, dyspnea, apnea, flaccid muscle tone, inability to arouse the patient, mottling or cyanosis)
   b. Other nursing responsibilities
      i. Monitor the response to medications
      ii. Monitor the IV site and intake
      iii. Ensure the patient's dignity, privacy, and comfort
      iv. Act as patient liaison with the physician
   c. RNs responsible for patient monitoring should have no other duties that would take them from the patient's bedside

7. **Postprocedural monitoring of patients**
   a. Standard of nursing care postprocedure is the same as that for patients who recover in the postanesthesia care unit
   b. Continued observation and monitoring (via a validated scale and objective measurements) are required until the patient has recovered from the sedation-analgesia; then care is resumed as before

8. **Emergency equipment**
   a. Supplemental oxygen, suction apparatus, appropriately sized airways, positive pressure device, reversal medication in room where sedation is performed
   b. Defibrillator immediately available

9. **Pharmacology for procedures** (see also Pharmacology under General Consideration)
   a. Benzodiazepines: Midazolam, diazepam
   b. Opioids: Fentanyl, morphine, meperidine
   c. NSAIDs: Toradol (may be given intramuscularly or IV), ibuprofen, naproxen when the patient is able to take medications orally
   d. Reversal agents: Naloxone, flumazenil
   e. Medication administration: Titrate all medications to effect (decreases risks and increases patient comfort)

10. **Special conditions**
    a. Patients at increased risk for developing complications (e.g., patients at extremes of age; those with severe cardiac, pulmonary, hepatic, or renal disease; pregnant patients; those who abuse drugs or alcohol) may need preprocedural consultation with an appropriate specialist
    b. For severely compromised or medically unstable patients, an anesthesia provider may need to administer sedation

REFERENCES

Bariatric Patients

American Society for Bariatric Surgery: Guidelines of the American Society for Bariatric Surgery, retrieved July 20, 2005, from http://www.obesity-online.com/guidelines_ASBS.htm.

Begany T: ICU management of the morbidly obese, *Pulm Rev Com* 7(4):1-5, 2002.

Burns SM, Egloff MB, Ryan B, et al: Effect of body position on spontaneous respiratory rate and tidal volume in patients with obesity, abdominal distension and ascites, *Am J Crit Care* 3:102-106, 1994.

Charney W, Hudson A, editors: *Back injury among healthcare workers*, Boca Raton, Fla, 2004, CRC Press.

Gallagher S: Obesity and the skin in the critical care setting, *Crit Care Nurs* 25(1):69-75, 2002.

Gallagher S: Panniculectomy: not just a tummy tuck, *Nursing* 34(12):58-64, 2003.

Gallagher S: Bariatrics: mobility, considering safety, patient safety, and caregiver injury. In Charney W, Hudson A, editors: *Back injury among healthcare workers*, Boca Raton, Fla, 2004, CRC Press.

Gallagher S: Issues of caregiver injury: addressing the needs of a changing population, *Bariatric Times* 2005;2(1):1-5.

Gallagher S, Arzouman J, Lacovara J, et al: Criteria-based protocols and the obese patient: planning care for a high-risk population, *Ostomy Wound Manage* 50(5):32-44, 2004.

Gallagher S, Langlois C, Spacht D, et al: Preplanning with protocols for skin and wound care in obese patients, *Adv Skin Wound Care* 17(8):436-443, 2004.

Garza SF: Bariatric weight loss surgery: patient education, preparation, and follow-up, *Crit Care Nurs Q* 26(2):101-104, 2003.

Goulenok C, Monchi M, Chiche JD, et al: Influence of overweight in ICU morality, *Chest* 125:1441-1445, 2004.

Hahler B: Morbid obesity: a nursing care challenge, *Medsurg Nurs* 11(2):85-90, 2002.

Kramer KL, Gallagher S: WOC nurses as advocates for patients who are morbidly obese: a case study promoting the use of bariatric beds, *J Wound Ostomy Continence Nurs* 31(6):379-387, 2004.

Krishnagopalan S, Johnson EW, Low LL, et al: Body positioning of intensive care patients: clinical practice versus standards, *Crit Care Med* 30(11):2588-2592, 2002.

Marik P: The obese patient in the ICU, *Chest* 113:492-498, 1998.

Marrone O, Bonsignore MR: Pulmonary hemodynamics in obstructive sleep apnea, *Sleep Med Rev* 6:175-193, 2002.

National Heart, Lung, and Blood Institute: Clinical guidelines on the identification, evaluation, and treatment of overweight and obesity in adults, retrieved July 20, 2005, from http://www.nhlbi.nih.gov/guidelines/obesity/ob_home.htm.

National Institute of Diabetes and Digestive and Kidney Diseases: Gastrointestinal surgery for severe obesity, December 2004, retrieved July 20, 2005, from http://win.niddk.nih.gov/publications/gastric.htm.

Owens TM: Morbid obesity: the disease and its comorbidities, *Crit Care Nursing* 26(2):162-165, 2003.

Sussman C, Bates-Jensen B: *Wound care: a collaborative practice manual for physical therapists and nurses,* Gaithersburg, Md, 1998, Aspen.

Websites

American Obesity Association: http://www.obesity.org

American Society for Bariatric Surgery: http://www.asbs.org

American Society of Bariatric Physicians: http://www.asbp.org

Eating Disorders Awareness and Prevention, Inc.: http://www.edap.org

National Institutes of Health Obesity Research Task Force: http://obesityresearch.nih.gov/

North American Association for the Study of Obesity: http://www.naaso.org

Obesity Care: http://www.obesitycare.com

Obesity Help: http://www.obesityhelp.com

Weight Control Information Network: *WIN Notes,* newsletter for health professionals: http://win.niddk.nih.gov/notes/index.htm

Geriatric Patients
Normal Age-Related Changes and Implications for Nursing Care

Beers MH, Jones TV, Berkwits M, et al: *The Merck manual of health and aging,* Whitehouse Station, NJ, 2004, Merck Research Laboratories.

Ebersole P, Hess P, Luggen AS: *Toward healthy aging,* ed 6, St Louis, 2004, Mosby.

Kane RL, Ouslander JG, Abrass IB: *Essentials of clinical geriatrics*, ed 5, New York, 2004, McGraw-Hill.

Sloane PD: Normal aging. In Ham RJ, Sloane PD, editors: *Primary care geriatrics: a case-based approach*, ed 3, St Louis, 1992, Mosby.

Timeras PS, editor: *Physiological basis of aging and geriatrics*, ed 3, Boca Raton, Fla, 2003, CRC Press.

Age-Related Changes in Medication Action

Barat I, Andreason F, Damsgaard S: Drug therapy and the elderly: what doctors believe and patients actually do, *Br J Clin Pharmacol* 51:615-620, 2001.

Bedell SR, Jabbour S, Goldberg R: Discrepancies in the use of medications: their extent and predictors in outpatient practice, *Arch Intern Med* 160:2129-2134, 2000.

Beijer HJ, de Blaey CJ: Hospitalizations caused by adverse drug reactions (ADR): a meta-analysis of observational studies, *Pharm World Sci* 24:46-54, 2002.

Drug-Interactions.com: Drug interactions table (cytochrome P450), retrieved May 2, 2005, from http://medicine.iupui.edu/flockhart/table.htm.

Fick DM, Cooper JW, Wade WE, et al: Updating the Beers criteria for potentially inappropriate medication use in older adults: results of a US Consensus Panel of Experts, *Arch Intern Med* 163:2716-2724, 2003.

Joint Commission on Accreditation of Healthcare Organizations: 2005 Hospitals' national patient safety goals, retrieved July 20, 2005, from http://www.jcaho.org/accredited+organizations/patient+safety/05+npsg/05_npsg_hap.htm.

Karyekar CS, Eddington ND, Briglia A, et al: Renal interaction between itraconazole and cimetidine, *J Clin Pharmacol* 44, 919-927, 2004.

Pepper GA: 2004 Pharmacokinetics and pharmacodynamics. In Younglin EQ, Swain KJ, Kissinger KF, et al: *Pharmacotherapeutics: a primary care clinical guide,* ed 2, Newark, NJ, 2004, Prentice Hall, pp 8-45.

Pronost P, Weast B, Schwarz WM, et al: Medication reconciliation: a practical tool to reduce the risk of medication errors, *J Crit Care* 18(4):201-205, 2003.

Routledge PA, Mahony MS, Woodhouse KW: Adverse drug reactions in elderly patients, *Br J Clin Pharmacol* 57:121-126, 2003.

Semla TP, Beizer JL, Higbee MD: *Geriatric dosage handbook*, ed 9, Cleveland, 2005, Lexi-Comp.

Turnheim K: When drug therapy gets old: pharmacokinetics and pharmacodynamics in the elderly, *Exp Gerontol* 38(8):843-853, 2003.

Geriatric Syndromes

American Geriatric Society: Guideline for the prevention of falls in older persons, *J Am Gerontol Soc* 49(5):665-672, 2001.

Beers MB: *The Merck manual of geriatrics*, ed 3, Whitehouse Station, 2005, Merck.

Farmer BC: Fall risk assessment, *Try This* 1(8):1-2, 2000. Available at http://www.hartfordign.org/publications/trythis/issue08.pdf.

Ferrell BA: Pain management, *Clin Geriatr Med* 16(4):853-874, 2004.

Fick D, Foreman M: Consequences of not recognizing delirium superimposed on dementia in hospitalized elderly individuals, *J Gerontol Nurs* 26:130-140, 2000.

Hollinger L, Patterson RA: Fall prevention program for the acute care setting. In Funk SG, Tornquist EM, Champagne RA, et al, editors: *Key aspects of elder care: managing falls, incontinence, and cognitive impairment,* New York, 1992, Springer Publishing Co.

Kurlowicz L: The geriatric depression scale (GDS), *Try This* 1(4):1-2, 1999. Available at http://www.hartfordign.org/publications/trythis/issue04.pdf.

Inouye S, van Dyck C, Alessi C, et al: Clarifying confusion: the Confusion Assessment Method, *Ann Intern Med* 113(12):941-948, 1990. Instrument available at http://www.hartfordign.org/publications/trythis/issue13.pdf.

Lawrence JF, Amella EJ: Assessing nutrition in older adults, *Try This* 9:1-2, 2004. Available at http://www.hartfordign.org/publications/trythis/issue_9.pdf.

McCaffery M, Pasero C: *Pain: clinical manual*, ed 2, St Louis, 1999, Mosby.

Mentes JC: Hydration management, Iowa City, Feb 2004, University of Iowa Gerontological Nursing Interventions Research Center, Research Dissemination Core. Available at http://www.guidelines.gov.

Mezey M, Maslow K: Recognition of dementia in hospitalized older adults, *Try This* 1(5):1-2, 2004. Available at http://www.hartfordign.org/publications/trythis/finRecog.pdf.

Morse JM, Morse RM, Tylko SJ: Development of a scale to identify the fall-prone patient, *Can J Aging* 8(4):366-367, 1989. Scale available at http://www.nursing.upenn.edu/centers/hcgne/gero_tips/pdf_files/Morse_Fall_scale.htm.

Nestlé Nutrition: MNA Mini Nutritional Assessment, 2005, retrieved July 20, 2005, from http://www.mna-elderly.com.

Resnick B: Preventing falls in acute care. In Mezey M, Fulmer T, Abraham I, et al, editors: *Geriatric nursing protocols for best practice*, ed 2, New York, 2003, Springer Publishing Co. Available at http://www.guidelines.gov.

Wallace M, Fulmer T: Fulmer SPICES: an overall assessment tool of older adults, *Try This* 1(1):1-2, 1998.

End-of-Life Care

Douglas R, Brown HN: Patient attitudes toward advanced directives, *J Nurs Scholarsh* 31(1):61-65, 2002.

Warm E, Weisman D: Fast Fact and Concept #012: Myths about advanced directives, 2000, retrieved July 20, 2005, from End of Life/Palliative Education Resource Center website: http://www.eperc.mcw.edu/fastFact/ff_012.htm.

Weissman D: Fast Fact and Concept #003: Syndrome of imminent death, 2000, retrieved July 20, 2005, from End of Life/Palliative Education Resource Center website: http://www.eperc.mcw.edu/fastFact/ff_003.htm.

High-Risk Obstetric Patients

Baker R: Hemorrhage in obstetrics, *Obstet Gynecol Annu* 6:295, 1977.

Bastien JL, Graves JR, Bailey S: Atypical presentation of amniotic fluid embolism, *Anesth Analg* 87:124-126, 1998.

Chronic hypertension in pregnancy, *ACOG Pract Bull*, No 29, July 2001.

Cochrane Collaboration Group: The Cochrane pregnancy and childbirth database, 1998.

Diagnosis and management of preeclampsia and eclampsia, *ACOG Pract Bull*, No 33, Jan 2002.

Dildy GA, Cotton DB: Trauma, shock, and critical care obstetrics. In Reece EA, Hobbins JC, Mahoney MJ, et al, editors: *Medicine of the fetus and mother*, Philadelphia, 1992, Lippincott, pp 883-924.

Duley L, Henderson-Smart DJ: Drugs for treatment of very high blood pressure during pregnancy. In *The Cochrane Database of Systematic Reviews*, Issue 4, Chichester, UK, 2002, John Wiley & Sons, DOI: 10.1002/14651858.CD001449.

Locksmith GJ: Amniotic fluid embolism, *Obstet Gynecol Clin North Am* 26:435-444, 1999.

Magee LA, Ornstein MP, von Dadelszen P: Fortnightly review: management of hypertension in pregnancy, *BMJ* 318:1332-1336, 1999.

Martin PS, Leaton MB: Emergency: amniotic fluid embolism [published correction in *Am J Nurs* 101(5):14, 2001], *Am J Nurs* 101(3):43-44, 2001.

Repke JT, Power ML, Holzman GB, et al: Hypertension in pregnancy and preeclampsia: knowledge and clinical practice among obstetrician-gynecologists, *J Reprod Med* 47:472-476, 2002.

Robinson JN, Norwitz ER, Repke JT: Antihypertensive use during pregnancy. In Yankowitz J, Niebyl JR, editors: *Drug therapy in pregnancy*, Philadelphia, 2001, Lippincott Williams & Wilkins.

Sibai BM: Diagnosis and management of gestational hypertension and preeclampsia, *Obstet Gynecol* 102:181-192, 2003.

Thomson AJ, Greer IA: Non-haemorrhagic obstetric shock, *Ballières Best Pract Res Clin Obstet Gynaecol* 14:19-41, 2000.

von Dadelszen P, Ornstein MP, Bull SB, et al: Fall in mean arterial pressure and fetal growth restriction in pregnancy hypertension: a meta-analysis, *Lancet* 355:87-92, 2000.

Weiner CP: The obstetric patient and disseminated intravascular coagulation, *Clin Perinatol* 13:705-717, 1986.

Yankowitz J: Fetal effects of drugs commonly used in critical care. In Dildy GA, Belfort MA, Saade GR, et al, editors: *Critical care obstetrics*, Malden, Mass, 2004, Blackwell Science, Chap 43.

Patient Transport
Indications and Equipment for Transport

Air and Surface Transport Nurses Association: *Transport nurse advanced trauma course (TNATC)*, Denver, 2002, Author.

American Academy of Pediatrics: *Guidelines for air and ground transport of neonatal and pediatric patients*, Elk Grove Village, Ill, 1999, Author.

American College of Emergency Physicians: Guidelines for transfer and transport of injured or ill persons, *Ann Emerg Med* 3:337, 1990.

American College of Surgeons: *Indications for transfer of the injured patient*, Chicago, Ill, 2005, Advanced Trauma Life Support.

Association of Air Medical Services: *Guidelines for air medical crew education*, Dubuque, Ia, 2004, Kendall/Hunt.

Holleran RS, editor: *Air and surface patient transport: principles and practice*, ed 3, St Louis, 2003, Mosby.

Holleran RS: *Mosby's emergency and transport nursing examination review*, ed 4, St Louis, 2005, Mosby.

Warren J, Fromm RE, Orr R, et al: Guidelines for the inter- and intrahospital transport of critically ill patients, *Crit Care Med* 32(1): 256-262, 2004.

Transport Standards

Arndt K, editor: *Standards for critical care and specialty rotor-wing transport*, Denver, 2003, Air and Surface Transport Nurses Association.

Holleran R, Rhoades C: Ask the experts: transferring patients, *Crit Care Nurse* 25(1): 58-59, 2005.

James S, editor: *Standards for critical care and specialty ground transport*, Denver, 2002, Air and Surface Transport Nurses Association.

Intrafacility Transport

Emergency Nurses Association: *Trauma nursing core course*, Des Plaines, Ill, 2000, Author.

Gavin-Fought S, Nemeth L: Intrahospital transport: a framework for assessment, *Crit Care Nurs Q* 15:87-90, 1992.

Pediatric Patients

American Heart Association: *Pediatric advanced life support*, Dallas, Tex, 2002, Author.

Curley M, Maloney-Harmon P: *Critical care nursing of infants and children*, ed 2, Philadelphia, Saunders, 2001.

Emergency Nurses Association: *Emergency nursing pediatric certification*, ed 3, Des Plaines, Ill, 2004, Author.

Emergency Nurses Association: *Trauma nursing core course*, ed 5, Des Plaines, Ill, 2004, Author.

Hazinski MF: *Nursing care of the critically ill child*, ed 2, St Louis, 1992, Mosby.

Hazinski MF: *Manual of pediatric critical care*, St Louis, 1999, Mosby.

Maloney-Harmon P, Czerwinski S: *Nursing care of the pediatric trauma patient*, St Louis, 2003, Saunders.

Newberry L, editor: *Sheehy's emergency nursing principles and practices*, 5 ed, St Louis, 2003, Mosby.

Slota M: *AACN core curriculum for pediatric critical care*, Philadelphia, 1998, Saunders.

Wong DB, Hess C, Karspiser C: *Wong and Whaley's clinical manual of pediatric nursing*, 5 ed, St Louis, 2000, Mosby.

Sedation in Critically Ill Patients

Abbott/American Association of Critical-Care Nurses/Saint Thomas Health System Sedation Expert Panel Members: Consensus conference on sedation assessment: a collaborative venture, *Crit Care Nurse* 24(2): 33-40, 2004.

Ambuel B, Hamlett KW, Marx CM, et al: Assessing distress in pediatric intensive care environments: the COMFORT scale, *J Pediatr Psychol* 17:95-109, 1992.

American Society of Anesthesiologists Task Force on Sedation and Analgesia by Non-Anesthesiologists: Practice guidelines for sedation and analgesia by non-anesthesiologists, *Anesthesiology* 96:1004-1017, 2002.

Ball J: Assessing the adequacy of sedation: why and how, *Minerva Anestesiol* 68:245-247, 2002.

Bixby M, Picard K: Sedation in the mechanically ventilated patient. In Odom-Forren J, Watson D, editors: *Practical guide to moderate sedation/analgesia*, 2nd ed, St Louis, 2005, Mosby.

Carrasco G: Instruments for monitoring intensive care unit sedation, *Crit Care* 4(4): 217-225, 2000.

De Lemos J, Tweeddale M, Chittock D, et al: Measuring quality of sedation in adult mechanically ventilated critically ill patients: the Vancouver Interaction and Calmness Scale, *J Clin Epidemiol* 53:908-919, 2000.

Devlin JW, Boleski G, Mlynarek M, et al: Motor Activity Assessment Scale: A valid and reliable sedation scale for use with mechanically ventilated patients in an adult surgical intensive care unit, *Crit Care Med* 27:1271-1275, 1999.

Jacobi J, Fraser GL, Coursin DB, et al: Clinical practice guidelines for the sustained use of sedatives and analgesics in the critically ill adult, *Crit Care Med* 30(1): 119-141, 2002.

Kost M: Moderate sedation/analgesia. In American Society of PeriAnesthesia Nurses, Quinn DMD, Schick L: *Perianesthesia nursing core curriculum: preoperative, phase I and phase II PACU nursing,* Philadelphia, 2004, Saunders, pp 432-443.

Luer J: Sedation and chemical relaxation in critical pulmonary illness: suggestions for patient assessment and drug monitoring, *AACN Clin Issues* 6(2):333-343, 1995.

McGaffigan PA: Advancing sedation assessment to promote patient comfort, *Crit Care Nurse* 22(1 suppl):29-36, 2002, retrieved September 2004 from http://www.aacn.org/pdfLibra.NSF/Files/McGaffigan_Ccn_Feb02S/$file/McGaffiganCareerGd.pdf.

McKinley S, Stein-Parbury J, Cheheinabi A, et al: Assessment of anxiety in intensive care patients by using the Faces Anxiety Scale, *Am J Crit Care* 13:146-152, 2004.

Odom J: Conscious sedation/analgesia. In Burden N, Quinn DMD, O'Brien D, et al, editors: *Ambulatory surgical nursing,* ed 2, Philadelphia, 2000, Saunders.

Odom-Forren J, Watson D, editors: *Practical guide to moderate sedation/analgesia,* ed 2, St Louis, 2005, Mosby.

Park G, Coursin D, Ely EW, et al: Balancing sedation and analgesia in the critically ill, *Crit Care Clin* 17(4):1015-1027, 2001.

Ramsay MA, Savege TM, Simpson BR, et al: Controlled sedation with alphaxalone-alphadolone, *Br Med J* 2:656-659, 1974.

Riker RR, Picard JT, Fraser GL: Prospective evaluation of the Sedation-Agitation Scale for adult critically ill patients, *Crit Care Med* 27:1325-1329, 1999.

Shelly M: Assessing sedation, *Care Crit Ill* 10(3):118-121, 1994.

Voluntary Hospitals of America: Sedation in critical care: the latest approaches and guidelines (video teleconference), Irving, Tex, March 5, 2002, Author.

White SK, Hollett JK, Dress JP, et al: A renaissance in critical care nursing: technological advances and sedation strategies, *Crit Care Nurse* 21(5 suppl):1-14, 2001, retrieved September 2004 from http://www.aacn.org/pdfLibra.NSF/Files/ZENECA%20SUPPLMT/$file/ZENECA%20SUPPLMT.PGS.pdf.

Index

Page numbers followed by *f* indicate figures; *t*, tables; *b*, boxes.

THE AMERICAN AGE

Other Books by Walter LaFeber:

The American Search for Opportunity, 1865–1913
Inevitable Revolutions: The United States in Central America, *2nd edition*
The Panama Canal: The Crisis in Historical Perspective, *2nd edition*
The Third Cold War
The American Century: A History of the United States since the 1890's
   (with Richard Polenberg and Nancy Woloch), *4th edition*
America, Russia, and the Cold War, 1945–1992
John Quincy Adams and American Continental Empire
The New Empire: An Interpretation of American Expansion, 1860–1898

THE AMERICAN AGE

United States Foreign Policy
at Home and Abroad

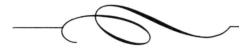

WALTER LAFEBER

Second Edition

1750 to the Present

W · W · NORTON & COMPANY · NEW YORK · LONDON

This book is dedicated to Michael Kammen, Larry Moore, Mary Beth Norton, Richard Polenberg, and Joel Silbey for being, over the years, friends, colleagues, and co-teachers of the U.S. Survey Course.

The text of this book is composed in Linotype Walbaum,
with display type set in Walbaum.
Composition and manufacturing by The Maple-Vail Book Manufacturing Group.
Book design by Antonina Krass

Second Edition

The poems "Dusty" and "Dear Smitty" from *Shrapnel in the Heart* by Laura Palmer copyright © 1987 by Laura Palmer. Reprinted by permission of Random House, Inc.

Library of Congress Cataloging in Publication Data
LaFeber, Walter.
   The American age : United States foreign policy at home and abroad /
Walter LaFeber. — 2nd ed.
      p.   cm.
   Includes bibliographical references and index.
   1. United States—Foreign relations.   I. Title.
E183.7.L27   1994
327.73—dc20   93-14460

One Vol: ISBN 0-393-96474-4 (pa)
Vol 1: ISBN 0-393-96475-2 (pa)
Vol 2: ISBN 0-393-96476-0 (pa)

W. W. Norton & Company, Inc., 500 Fifth Avenue, New York, N.Y. 10110
W. W. Norton & Company Ltd., 10 Coptic Street, London WC1A 1PU

2 3 4 5 6 7 8 9 0

Contents

3 | The First, the Last: John Quincy Adams and the Monroe Doctrine (1815–1828)   71

4 | The Amphibious Expansion of a Sixty-Five-Hundred-Thousand-Horsepower Steam Engine (1828–1850)   94

5 | The Climax of Early U.S. Foreign Policy: The Civil War (1850–1865)   130

19 | Back to the Future: The Carter-Reagan Years (1977–1988) 680

List of Maps

Preface to the Second Edition

Since the first edition of this book appeared in 1989, we and our world have gone through changes that are not merely memorable, but historic—the kinds of changes that occur only several times a century. Because of these transformations, and also because this book was fortunate in the kind of interest shown by teachers and scholarly reviewers, this new edition analyzes the 1989–1993 watershed in some detail while strengthening the features that students and teachers found useful in the first edition. Four additions are especially important:

- The end of the Soviet empire, the U.S. response as the sole remaining superpower, and Bill Clinton's election are discussed not only from the American perspective, but from other perspectives as well.
- The pre-1900 sections have been enlarged. *The American Age* was written especially for courses in the post-1914 history of U.S. foreign relations. It has been a pleasant surprise to learn that pre-1900 material is receiving increased attention in classrooms, and that teachers have found the book's early chapters useful—but they want more detail. So new discussions and graphics have been added, especially on the Jeffersonian era, the 1830s–1840s, and 1890s. (Perhaps one reason for the interest in the pre–World War I era is that it so eerily, and sometimes frighteningly, resembles the 1989–1993 years with their ethnic violence, disruptions in the Balkans and eastern Europe, the rise of a vigorous Japan and a united Germany, and the appearance of radically new—and politically disruptive—technology and communications.)
- Materials have been used from newly opened files and fresh research to rewrite the book's sections on the outbreak of the cold war, the causes of the Korean War, the Cuban missile crisis, and President Richard Nixon's policies and personality.
- Additional references are made to motion pictures and television, and new graphics of films have been used. Readers liked the book's use of these references, and the new material has been added in the belief that films do reflect large concerns of Americans and their foreign policies. (Sometimes this reflection is badly distorted and

dangerously misleading, even while being influential.) Television has increasingly shaped U.S. foreign-policy choices, not least in the Central American upheavals, the Persian Gulf War, and Somalia.

Virtually every chapter has had revisions and / or additions. All the bibliographies, especially the General Bibliography at the end of the book, are updated. For those interested in a more specific listing, the following are some of the topics discussed on the new pages: the beginnings of the secretary of state's office; Daniel Webster's Whig policies; the *Caroline* and *Creole* affairs, and the Maine boundary dispute; women's key role in the anti-imperialist movement after 1898; a new interpretation that frames the 1880s to 1913 era; the 1900–1913 revolutionary outbreaks in Latin America and Asia, with attention to the Chinese upheaval; the role of motion pictures in the 1915–1917 debates and again (with *Sergeant York*) in 1941; Truman's decisions to use the atomic bomb and to delay before accepting Japan's surrender; newly opened Soviet materials giving Moscow's perspective on the Marshall Plan and the Klaus Fuchs spy case; Stalin's and Mao's roles in the Korean War; John F. Kennedy's approach to the possibility of bombing China's nuclear facilities; Kennedy's views on Vietnam and the views of Oliver Stone's film, *JFK;* the post-1948 roots of U.S. policies on South Africa; the Chilean crises of 1973 and the film *Missing;* Reagan, Gorbachev, and breakthrough agreements; the end of the cold war, a growing disorder, and David Lynch's world on television and in films, 1989–1993.

In addition to the friends thanked in the Acknowledgments of the first edition, I am greatly indebted to Robert Beisner, Barton Bernstein, Tim Borstelmann, Philip Brenner, Kenton Clymer, Warren Cohen, Michael Doyle, Robert Hannigan, Alan Kraut, Fumiaki Kubo, Julius Milmeister, Martin Sklar, and Evan Stewart, as well as several outside readers, who provided criticism and materials for this edition. I am especially grateful to Steve Forman, History Editor of W. W. Norton's College Division, to Bonnie Hall and Kate Brewster, editorial assistants, and to a most helpful copy editor, Sandy Lifland, all of whom improved this edition considerably; and to long-time friends Ed Barber and Gerry McCauley. Lizann Rogovoy and Bob Rouse provided indispensable research help. Above all, I thank the students and teachers, as well as the general readers, who have used *The American Age* and found it helpful in understanding United States foreign policy.

Walter LaFeber
Spring 1993

Preface to the First Edition

This book has been written to provide a relatively brief (and, I hope, readable) overview of post-1750 U.S. foreign relations. Chapters' lengths increase markedly after 1890. The pre-1890 sections, however, include the material needed to understand the first century of those foreign relations; all or part of those chapters can be used as introductory assignments in a one-semester post-1890 class.

The title is taken seriously. As Professor Thomas A. Bailey once observed, the United States was a world power at the birth of its independence in 1776. Then, if not before, the American age began because the country already ranked with the great European nations in terms of territory, population, economic strength, and natural resources, not to mention ambition. This survey tries to develop several themes that tie 250 years together, make sense of them, and give students and teachers starting points for discussion. The most obvious theme is the landed and commercial expansion that drove the nation outward between 1750 and the 1940s. Then, resembling other living things that age, the country's power began a relative decline after the mid-1950s. Americans have yet to understand and come to terms with the causes and consequences of that decline, although presidents from Kennedy through Reagan have, in varying ways, shaped their policies so that the country could adjust to this new world.

The book's second theme is the steady centralization of power at home, especially in the executive branch of government after 1890. This centralization occurred not merely because of the normal quest of human beings for power, but also because the foreign policies that Americans have desired since the nineteenth century are most effectively carried out by a strong presidency. There are no recurring cycles in this book, only the long rise and the relative decline of U.S. power, and the steady accretion of authority by presidents because of the way Americans have wanted to exercise that power. U.S. diplomatic history has often been written as if constitutional questions ceased to be important after 1865; this volume tries in small part to rectify that neglect.

A third theme is "isolationism," which means in U.S. history not withdrawal from world affairs (a people does not conquer a continent and become the world's greatest power by withdrawal or by assuming it enjoys "free security"), but maintaining a maximum amount of freedom of action. Americans who have professed to believe in individualism at home not surprisingly have often professed the same abroad.

A fourth theme is the importance of the transitional 1850-to-1914 era, a time when Americans' attitudes toward democracy, the Monroe Doctrine, the Constitution, and, especially, revolution underwent profound change and ushered in modern U.S. foreign policy. It is perhaps the great irony—and dilemma—of the nation's experience that it became a great power and wanted either to preserve the political *status quo* or only gradually to effect change precisely when the world began to erupt in revolution. This book tries to note some of the results of that irony and dilemma.

Finally, in the belief that how Americans act at home reveals much about how they act abroad, the analysis often focuses on domestic events (including films and sports). Social and diplomatic history have too seldom been wedded; parts of this account attempt in a minor way to start, at least, the courtship.

THE AMERICAN AGE

If I should not be thought too presumptuous I would beg leave to add what is my idea of the qualifications necessary for an American foreign minister in general. . . .

In the first place, he should have an education in classical learning and in the knowledge of general history, ancient and modern, and particularly the history of France, England, Holland, and America. He should be well versed in the principles of ethics, of the law of nature and nations, of legislation and government, of the Civil Roman law, of the laws of England and the United States, of the public law of Europe and in the letters, memoirs, and histories of those great men who have heretofore shone in the diplomatic order and conducted the affairs of nations and the world. He should be of an age to possess a maturity of judgment, arising from experience in business. He should be active, attentive, and industrious, and, above all, he should possess an upright heart and an independent spirit, and should be one who decidedly makes the interest of his country, not the policy of any other nation nor his own private ambition or interest, or those of his family, friends, and connexions, the rule of his conduct.

—JOHN ADAMS (1783)

Domestic issues can only lose elections, but foreign policy issues can kill us all.

—PRESIDENT JOHN F. KENNEDY (1962)

1

The Roots of American Foreign Policy (1492–1789)

The Beginnings: Gold, God, and Paradise

William Seward, a fascinating scholar and New York backroom politician as well as Abraham Lincoln's secretary of state during the Civil War, once called the story of American development "the most important secular event in the history of the human race."[1] Seward might well have been correct. Americans, however, have viewed their secular, or more earthly, successes (such as making money) as part of a higher purpose. This view goes back to the origins of their country. Portuguese explorer Vasco da Gama needed few words to explain why a new world was discovered in the late fifteenth century: "We come in search of Christians and spices."

Mission and money or, as some historians prefer to phrase it, idealism and self-interest have for nearly five hundred years been the reasons Americans have given for their successes. From their beginnings, they have justified developing a continent and then much of the globe simply by saying they were spreading the principles of civilization as well as making profit. They have had no problem seeing their prosperity—indeed, their rise from a sparsely settled continent to the world's superpower—as part of a Higher Purpose or, as it was known during much of their history, a Manifest Destiny.

The most spectacular chance taker of his time said it directly. "Gold is most excellent, Gold is treasure," Christopher Columbus observed, "and he who possesses it does all he wishes to in this world, and succeeds in helping souls into paradise." Columbus was the original self-made man in America. As historian Edward Bourne observes: "His hopes, his illusions, his vanity and love of money, his devotion to by-gone ideals, his keen and sensitive observation of the natural world, his lack of practical power in dealing with literary evidence, his practical abilities as a navigator, his tenacity of purpose and boldness of execution, his lack of fidelity as a husband and a lover, his family pride,"[2] all mark Columbus as an appropriate figure to start the story of America's place in the world.

Columbus is also a useful symbol and starting point in American foreign policy for another reason: he founded empires by going westward. Again, nature, perhaps even the supernatural, seemed to be guiding Americans. They simply had to follow the sun. "We held it ever certain," the explorer Cabeza de Vaca declared in 1535, "that going toward the sunset we would find what we desired." Two centuries later, George Berkeley captured this vision in his famous poem that has the line "Westward the course of empire takes its way."

ON THE PROSPECT OF PLANTING ARTS AND LEARNING IN AMERICA

The Muse, disgusted at an age and clime
   Barren of every glorious theme,
In distant lands now waits a better time,
   Producing subjects worthy fame:

In happy climes where from the genial sun
   And virgin earth such scenes ensue,
The force of art by nature seems outdone,
   And fancied beauties by the true:

In happy climes, the seat of innocence,
   Where nature guides and virtue rules,
Where men shall not impose for truth and sense
   The pedantry of courts and schools:

There shall be sung another golden age,
   The rise of empire and of arts,
The good and great inspiring epic rage,
   The wisest heads and noblest hearts.

Not such as Europe breeds in her decay;
  Such as she bred when fresh and young,
When heavenly flame did animate her clay,
  By future poets shall be sung.

Westward the course of empire takes its way;
  The four first acts already past,
A fifth shall close the drama with the day;
  Time's noblest offspring is the last.

Berkeley set out a great theme in Americans' foreign policy as they settled a continent by crossing from the Atlantic to the Pacific, moved across the Pacific Ocean to become a great world power for the first time in 1900, and then fought three major wars on the Asian mainland in the twentieth century. This westward movement has shaped much of the nation's best literature (the novels of Mark Twain and Willa Cather, and Robert Penn Warren's *All the King's Men* come to mind), as it has U.S. foreign policy.

[handwritten margin note: westward movement]

Another key theme of American diplomacy also appeared during the era of discovery: the country's prosperity and success, sometimes its very existence, have depended on events thousands of miles away. The birth of Americans as a separate people came out of fourteenth- and fifteenth-century events. Religious crusades, scientific discoveries, attempts to find new routes to Asia so expensive Italian middlemen could be avoided—all led Portugal and Spain to undertake the expeditions that climaxed in the discovery of the New World. The Spanish finally built a three-century-old empire because they had succeeded in consolidating power at home (sometimes brutally, as expelling or enslaving Moors and some 100,000 Jews who would not join the Roman Catholic church) and seizing the money needed to pay for Columbus's voyages. This centralized power then set about discovering and colonizing parts of North America and most of South America, exploring the Pacific, circling the globe, and introducing the first black slaves into the New World as early as 1502, a full century before the British brought such slaves to their colonies. Aside from their "Christianizing" the New World's inhabitants, Spain so violently extracted gold and valuable minerals that Native Americans ("Indians") and black slaves who worked in the mines died in large numbers.

The political events in Spain and the economic opportunities in America combined to revolutionize world trade. From their beginnings, Americans formed part of a world economic system. Nor could they successfully isolate themselves from the upheavals of Europe. On the other hand, they also were pivotal in reshaping the globe's politics and economics. Their wealth and labor allowed Spain and then England and Holland to replace Italian and German cities as the world's trade centers. Furs, tobacco, sugar, and fish from North America replaced Asia's spices as the most valuable products in Europe's trade.

There is also another theme that links the five hundred years of America's relations with the rest of the world: the effect on those relations of new technology and scientific discoveries. Columbus depended on fresh calculations that indicated the world was round, not flat. He proved those calculations correct by using the latest compasses, astrolabe, and elaborate tables that measured longitude. From these first voyages of discovery through the Yankee clipper ship that conquered world trade, the Colt .44 revolver that conquered the West, the airplane that conquered distance, the atomic bomb, and the multistage rocket that conquered space, American foreign policy cannot be understood apart from the technology that transformed the world and made diplomacy ever more complex—and dangerous. Those technological conquests also help us to understand why Americans have too often believed that crises in foreign affairs might well be solved through new scientific breakthroughs.

The early quests for wealth, personal salvation, westward empire, control of the world's centers of political and economic power, and supremacy in technology led to both the settlement of America and its rise as the globe's superpower.

THE CITY ON A HILL—AND ON THE WATER

Throughout the 1500s, England watched Spain and Portugal explore the New World. But the British also shared in the profits by looting Spanish ships that carried precious metals back to Europe. England's settlements, however, failed disastrously until 1606–1607, when a group of wealthy investors established Jamestown, Virginia. Jamestown's founding and survival could be traced to its economic role in international trade. The founders were looking for the river system that supposedly provided entry into the fabled markets of Asia. They hoped that the James River might be such a system. Some 10,000 miles short of their goal, the settlers quickly discovered that they had to find an export crop to pay for their food and other imports from the home country. They tried silk and sassafras, but unfortunately neither was habit-forming. Then John Rolfe experimented in 1612 with Indian tobacco. In 1614, two barrels of cured tobacco left for England. Four years later, tobacco was a rage in Europe. Virginia shipped nearly 50,000 pounds abroad annually. The "hellish, devilish, and damned tobacco," as English critics called it, provided the settlement's lifeline to the world.[3]

Thus, hardly had America been settled than it transformed Europe's trade and personal habits. But tobacco also forced Virginia's foreign relations into surprising avenues. As growers discovered the profitability of importing black slaves to tend the fields, new trade routes extended southward to Africa. Westward the Virginians began seizing fresh land to replace the soil worn out by as few as three tobacco crops. The "hellish" weed had both locked America into Africa's history and had driven the settlers westward toward the sun—and the Native Americans.

To the north, another group of English men and women settled at Massachusetts Bay in 1630. Their leader, John Winthrop, uttered words that resounded nearly four hundred years later, when he urged the devout separatists: ["We must consider that we shall be as a city upon a hill, the eyes of all people are upon us."] Those are among the most famous words in American history and have been quoted repeatedly—from the founders in the 1780s to President Ronald Reagan in the 1980s—to define the U.S. mission in the world. Much less quoted are Winthrop's warnings in that famous utterance. "The care of the public must oversway all private respects," and "Wee must be knitt together in this work as one man." Or again: "Wee [should] be willing to abridge ourselves of superfluities for the supply of others' necessities."[4] Those words have been less popular in American history.

Indeed, from the start, the opportunities of foreign trade and landed expansion destroyed Winthrop's hope that "the city upon a hill" would be "knitt together . . . as one man." The city on a hill was actually a city on an ocean.[5] It had open to it world trade, especially the export of the famous Boston cod, which was exploited by adventurous individualists who cared more about profit margins than about Puritan restraints. From the start, fish were vital to American foreign relations because they brought in much-needed hard money (gold and silver) from Europe. The fisheries of the North Atlantic were the equivalent of the gold mines in South America—and the fish even reproduced. Moreover, one devout observer wrote at the time of settlement that the fisheries were so bleak that sailors would be tempted by neither "wine nor women."[6] It seemed a perfect combination of gold and God. No wonder that, as we shall see, three generations of the famous Adams family of Massachusetts devoted much of their distinguished diplomatic careers to keeping the fisheries in American hands. But the fisheries and other trade also shaped early foreign relations in another way: New Englanders invested their growing profits in western lands and thus pushed settlement toward the sunset until it collided with Native Americans and with Frenchmen who were settling Canada and exploring the Great Lakes region.

These first American foreign relations did nothing less than change American society. As one scholar has noted, the possibility of making fortunes in overseas trade and western territories made settlers "more interested in saving dollars than souls, more concerned with good land than compact villages, more excited about individual wealth than group welfare."[7] From their beginnings, Americans have never been able to separate their foreign relations from the way they carry on their lives at home.

THE FIRST AMERICANS

The settlers did not discover a vacant East Coast. For the next 350 years they did not move over an empty continent. A central theme of American diplomatic history must be the clash between the European settlers and the Native Americans between 1620 and 1890. That clash led the settlers to fight wars of conquest, create a unique military machine. to wage war, and nearly exterminate the Indian tribes.

Probably 8.5 to 10 million Native Americans populated all of North America in 1492. The first American immigrants had arrived well before the Europeans—in about 30,000 B.C. With as many as 600 different societies and over 200 languages, they had developed complex civilizations that carefully preserved—even as they lived from—the rivers, woods, land, and wild animals. By the time settlements of whites appeared in Virginia and Massachusetts, many Native Americans had already disappeared because of lack of immunity to the explorers' diseases, especially smallpox and measles which ravaged many tribes.

At the beginning of settlement, the Indians provided the food and agricultural know-how that allowed many of the whites to survive. But the Native Americans gradually began to fear the Europeans' growing numbers and different culture. Moreover, they were inflamed by internal divisions and fears of neighboring tribes. In 1622, on Good Friday, the Powhatans suddenly attacked and destroyed one-quarter of Virginia's white population. Thus began a series of wars between whites and Native Americans that soaked the rest of colonial history in blood. With British help and at great cost, the settlers not only won most of the conflicts, but virtually wiped out such tribes as the powerful Pequots in New England. The Indians had long been independent, were deeply divided among themselves, and could not cooperate in waging war. Some were easily bought off with money or European goods. Many even served as guides or raiders for the whites against other tribes. Although usually superior fighters individually, Native Americans did not fight for long periods with the intensity of the whites, nor—although they were highly skilled in making weapons—did they learn in the early decades how to make gunpowder.[8]

The settlers quickly drew several lessons from these seventeenth-century encounters. They developed a racism that provided an excuse to remove or kill Indians who blocked landed expansion. Native American cultures were not individualistic, Christian, or even monotheistic. It was, therefore, easy for the great Puritan divine, Cotton Mather, to believe that "Probably the Devil decoyed" the Indians to America "in hopes that the gospel of the Lord Jesus Christ would never come here to destroy or disturb his absolute empire over them."[9] The "noble savage" idea fascinated those in faraway British and French coffee shops, but it never interested American leaders such as Mather. The whites also learned that exploiting the environment—that is, destroying woods and killing large numbers of fur-bearing animals—not only was profitable for their overseas trade, but severely weakened the Native Americans. As colonial population grew, so many animals were killed and so many fields were cleared that the climate in North America changed.[10]

Finally, the settlers discovered from the Indian wars that they had to break with the European tradition of a professional army. Instead, they gave weapons to all able-bodied male settlers, who farmed part-time and fought part-time. Thus was born the militia system that formed the backbone for the American military over the next several centuries. Thus were also born the tactics for "Indian fighting"—guerrilla-type warfare instead of the traditional European armies-in-mass that slaughtered each other on open battlefields. These new tactics shaped U.S. military strategy in wars from the American Revolution through the interventions in the Caribbean–Central American region in the 1920s.

THE AMERICAN "MULTIPLICATION TABLE" AND THE EUROPEAN POWER STRUGGLE

The settlers sharply honed those military tactics in the century before 1776. The Indian wars diminished slightly by 1700, but the colonials then turned their rifles on other Europeans. From the beginning of their history, Americans lived not in any splendid isolation, far from the turmoil and corruption of the Europe many had hoped to escape. They instead had to live in settlements that were surrounded by great and ambitious European powers. France controlled the St. Lawrence River region through eastern Canada and down the Great Lakes to the Mississippi River. The French explorer La Salle had claimed Louisiana (that is, nearly all the vast lands whose rivers emptied into the Mississippi) as early as 1682. To the south, Spain moved out of Florida and consolidated its hold on the Caribbean region.

Perhaps the three great empires (British, French, and Spanish) might have lived at peace in the New World through much of the eighteenth century except for an incredible development: the American "multiplication table." This "table" referred to the high birth rate of colonials that produced families of five to ten children even as infant mortality rates dropped. The term itself was coined much later, in the 1840s by Representative Andrew Kennedy of Indiana. Kennedy told the House of Representatives that "our people are spreading out with the aid of the American multiplication table." He elaborated: "Go to the West and see a young man with his mate of eighteen; after a lapse of thirty years, visit him again, and instead of two, you will find twenty-two. That is what I call the American multiplication table."[11]

One result of the American "multiplication table" was almost continual war with France and Spain between 1689 and 1763. These struggles in the New World formed part of a larger European conflict among the three great imperial nations. But the wars also showed how Americans—whether they liked it or not—were part of European power politics even as they moved into the forests and fertile lands beyond the Appalachian Mountains. They could not separate their destiny from the destiny of those they had left behind in Europe. Their own imperial ambitions were not small. In 1745, William Shirley, the restless, imaginative governor of Massachusetts, captured the French fortress at Louisbourg in eastern Canada. He then set his sights on conquering the rest of Canada and all the French holdings in the Mississippi region. London officials, however, infuriated Shirley by making peace with the French (those hated Roman Catholics to the north) and restoring Louisbourg as part of an overall peace settlement.

Shirley and other colonial leaders impatiently waited for another opportunity they knew would soon arise. In the early 1750s, it happened. British settlers established forts in the central part of present-day Ohio. In 1752, the French retaliated by seizing a key fortress in the region. England's Indian allies swung over to support the French.

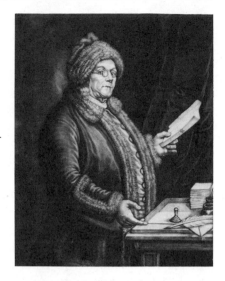

Benjamin Franklin (1706–1790), man of the world and Pennsylvania politician, colonial postmaster general, author of wise advice for a growing nation in Poor Richard's Almanack, *and member of the Continental Congress and the 1787 Constitutional Convention. He was also the original U.S. diplomat who combined worldly knowledge with the ability to play the New World "primitive" to charm both the salons as well as the foreign ministry in Paris in order to negotiate the crucial alliance with France.*

The Native Americans were coming to see that the French, who wanted the Indians' trade and Roman Catholic souls but not their territory, posed less danger than did the land-hungry British settlers. Virginia sent out a twenty-one-year-old surveyor-soldier, George Washington, to negotiate with the French. When talks failed, Washington attacked the French around the key strategic position of present-day Pittsburgh. Thus began the Seven Years' War—or the Great War for Empire, as it later became known. The struggle transformed the political face of North America and led directly to the American Revolution.

Benjamin Franklin and the Problems of a Rising People

The conflict also brought Benjamin Franklin to the world stage. The first American diplomat, Franklin's life illustrated the ambition and intelligence of the settlers. His career also demonstrated how Americans created a landed empire, then broke with England so that they could themselves run and profit from that empire.

Born in 1706 as the tenth child of Josiah and Abiah Folger Franklin in Boston, Franklin, at the age of seventeen, fought with his family and moved to Philadelphia. There he became a printer, accumulating both personal wealth (especially with his *Poor Richard's Almanack*) and political power. Franklin paraded as an ordinary man, but his travels and contacts with leading figures in colonial life gave him unique knowledge about America. He set up profitable printing companies in Antigua, Connecticut, and New York. In that sense, Franklin was perhaps America's first multinational corporation.

In 1751, Franklin, drawing on his research and knowledge of colonial life, published a pamphlet that remains crucial for understanding American foreign policy. *Observations Concerning the Increase of Mankind* began with careful calculations showing that Americans were doubling their population approximately every twenty years. This unbelievable figure, Franklin argued, had far-reaching consequences. First, it meant that additional land would soon be needed for settlement or else the colonies would be dammed up and become stagnant. Second, it meant that Britain should help find the land because Britain's manufacturers and merchants would enjoy a most profitable market in the new settlements. Finally, it became apparent that finding the necessary room meant war against the French and their Indian allies.[12] Franklin seemed to welcome that conclusion.

In his 1751 pamphlet, Franklin thus helped explain the causes of both the Great War for Empire and the American Revolution. When the struggle began in 1754, Franklin immediately focused on the problem that henceforth haunted American officials: How could they govern the tremendous expanse of land they hoped to conquer? He answered with the Albany Plan of 1754, a scheme that concentrated power in a central colonial agency that could effectively deal with Native Americans and fight the French. Neither the British Crown nor the thirteen colonial governments, however, would surrender power to the agency, so Franklin's idea died. It was thirty-three years ahead of its time and the Constitutional Convention.

In 1757, the Pennsylvanian sailed to London to serve as the colony's official representative. British military victories over France led to heated discussions over peace terms. The major question was whether London should take the rich French sugar island of Guadeloupe in the Caribbean or the largely empty expanse of Canada. Franklin had no doubt. Using his 1751 pamphlet as a weapon, he argued that the population explosion and the resulting sales for British manufacturers dictated seizing Canada. But his argument did not go unchallenged. A British pamphleteer, William Burke, warned that if Franklin's advice were followed and the French were expelled, the Americans would rush into the vast region and become uncontrollable. Burke also touched a nerve that remained sensitive for the next two hundred years of American diplomacy. Noting Franklin's argument that "security" required removing the French from Canada, Burke argued that "to desire the enemy's whole country on no other principle but that otherwise you cannot secure your own, is turning the idea of mere defense into the most dangerous of all principles. It is leaving no medium between safety and conquest. It is to suppose yourself never safe, whilst your neighbor enjoys any security."[13]

Franklin won the argument. In 1763, the British took Canada and all the land that stretched southward and westward to the Mississippi River. Spain, a French ally, received Louisiana territory from Paris in return for agreeing to an immediate peace. The Spanish gave East and West Florida to England in exchange for Cuba, which the British navy had seized. France's long career as a New World power was over. But Burke had the last word: "What the consequences will be to have a numerous, hardy, independent people [loose in the Canadian wilderness]" he left to the reader's imagination.

Humiliated French officials plotted revenge for their losses in 1763. Delighted colonials prepared to find their fortunes by following the sun.

THE ROAD TO REVOLUTION (1763–1775)

But the colonials instead crashed into boundaries set by the British Empire. The empire's theory had for a century been "mercantilist"— that is, Great Britain had the right to operate the colonies for its own profit; in return, London protected the colonials from outsiders. Such was the theory. In reality, the colonials acted independently and largely protected themselves. By 1700, probably half of Boston's trade was illegal because it was with the French West Indies instead of with British merchants, as London's mercantile laws required. Few in London or Boston cared. Profits from the French trade went to London to pay for British goods. Prime Minister Sir Robert Walpole nicely, if insensitively, described colonial policy before the 1754 war as "Let sleeping dogs lie." But the dogs did not sleep. Merchants, settlers, and colonial legislators did as they pleased until they came to believe that they were the equal of London's Parliament in running colonial affairs.

From 1763 to 1765, Parliament decided to pay for the costs of the 1754–1763 war by taxing the colonies. London merchants, moreover, demanded that the illegal trade with France be stopped. The Stamp Act, taxing colonial newspapers and mail, raised the revenue. Other acts clamped down on smuggling. Americans responded with the revolutionary doctrine that they had been self-governing since the first

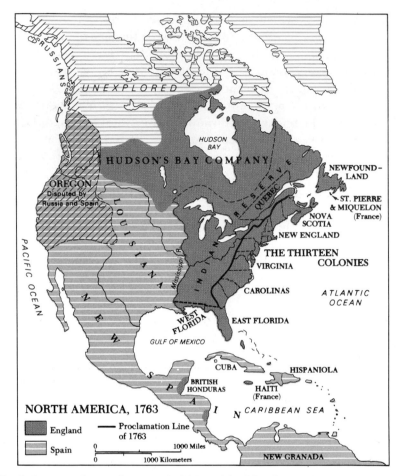

North America, during the war of 1754 to 1763 (The Great War for Empire), after the British drove the French from Canada and as the thirteen colonies started down the road to revolution.

settlements and that, consequently, Parliament had no right to regulate each colony's trade. Americans refused to import British goods. London officials dismissed the claim of self-government. They and the British merchants, however, could not dismiss the nonimportation policy. As trade declined, Parliament finally repealed most of the 1764–1765 acts. But it then tried to raise revenue more subtly—such as imposing a tax on tea. In late 1773, the colonials, led by a deeply religious revolutionary, Samuel Adams, dumped large amounts of tea in

Boston Harbor. The infuriated British lashed back with the Intolerable Acts (as the colonials termed them) of 1774: Boston port was closed, political power in Massachusetts was largely switched from the colonials to appointed British officials, and—in a related move that made Protestant land speculators of Massachusetts and Virginia furious— Canada's boundaries were extended to the Ohio River. The colonials could no longer follow the sun without running into the Roman Catholic Canadians who were now loyal to Great Britain.

Colonial legislatures convened a Continental Congress to discuss retaliation. Americans had suddenly learned that their foreign policy and individual freedoms were closely related. London's claim to regulate foreign trade struck at the heart of their political independence, which they had long taken for granted. The *Georgia Gazette* urged support in the South for the far-off Bostonians in 1774 by arguing that if the British claim to "have a right or power to put a duty on my tea," they "have an equal right to put a duty on my bread, and why not on my breath, why not on my daylight and smoke, why not on everything?"[14] The South also shared another grievance with the North. In 1763, the British had declared a "Proclamation Line" that prohibited colonials from settling west of the Appalachian Mountains. The purpose was to regulate settlement and avoid Indian wars. Treaties with Native Americans allowed some expansion after 1770, but the Quebec Act closed the door again in 1774. The door closed, moreover, just as frustrated Americans were turning westward to find the trade and profit that the British denied them in the French West Indies.

Colonial leaders concluded that they could no longer find help in London. British politics changed rapidly in the 1760s as new factions, created in part from profits from the colonies, moved to control Parliament. London's politics, as Franklin described it from the scene, were most corrupt: "This whole venal nation is now at market," he wrote in 1768.[15] Decent colonials had little hope for relief from such an indecent system. Such sentiments were returned by Londoners, who considered the colonials grasping and ungrateful. As England's most famous literary figure put it, "Sir, [Americans] are a race of convicts and ought to be thankful for anything we allow them short of hanging." Dr. Samuel Johnson continued: "You know I am willing to love all mankind, except an American."[16]

The links of British colonial policy were now being pulled apart from both sides of the Atlantic. Foreign-policy issues (trade, westward expansion) were in the middle of this pulling and hauling.

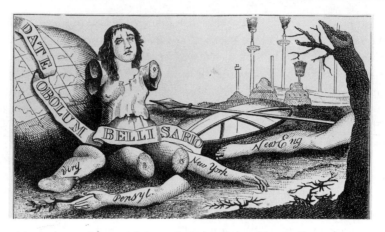

This 1774 cartoon of a woeful Great Britain, shorn of her badly needed colonial limbs, was by Benjamin Franklin. In addition to his other many talents, Franklin was one of the first important American political cartoonists. His view of the former British Empire (two years before the Revolution actually began) is indicated by the "Date Obolum Bellisario"—or "Give a Farthing to Belisarius," who was a general in Ancient Rome after the Roman Empire collapsed.

THE FOREIGN POLICY OF INDEPENDENCE (1776)

By early 1776, many of the 2.5 million white Americans thought of themselves as a separate people. As early as ten years before, a shrewd British observer told his nephew in North America that "you [in the colonies] wish to be an Empire by itself."[17] But revolution against the world's greatest power was not trivial. According to one British legal source, a convicted traitor was to be hanged and taken down while alive, then his entrails were to be removed and burned, his head to be chopped off, and his body divided into four parts.[18]

Despite the long shadows of British gallows, the First Continental Congress met in September 1774 to bring together twelve colonies and discuss the Intolerable Acts. The delegates pledged not to import or consume British goods until the acts were repealed. But the British were now determined to enforce their own law. They also ordered their troops to seize the powder and arms of the colonials at Concord, Massachusetts. On April 19, 1775, British forces and American militia clashed at Lexington and Concord. A Second Continental Congress, more radical than the first, convened. It learned that early military operations had gone badly. But Franklin, ever upbeat, urged his fellow rebels to consider the glories of the American "multiplication table":

"Britain, at the expense of three millions [pounds], has killed 150 Yankees this campaign, which is twenty thousand pounds a head. During
the same time 60,000 children have been born in America."[19]

The rebels nevertheless rapidly needed other kinds of help as well.
The Congress established a five-member Secret Committee of Correspondence to find allies abroad. Independence required an active, successful foreign policy. The committee marked the beginning of the later
Department of State. Its members included Franklin and John Jay of
New York. The committee sent three agents abroad to seek help,
including the first official U.S. diplomat, Silas Deane of Connecticut,
who was to sound out the French foreign minister, Charles Gravier,
Count de Vergennes, about political aid and arms purchases. France
had already decided to make a secret loan of $2 million to the colo-
nials. Vergennes, who had been thirsting for revenge against the British since France's 1763 defeat, sent a secret agent to contact rebel leaders
in late 1775, then moved to isolate Great Britain by forming alliances
with Spain, Austria, and Prussia. The Dutch, whose ambitious traders
clashed with British naval power, also helped by sending gunpowder
and rifles badly needed by the colonial militias.

The Congress meanwhile decided to invade and annex Canada. It
was one of the more amazing and disastrous decisions in American
diplomatic history. Many colonials had lusted after Canada, and a
number wanted to teach Roman Catholics a lesson. Resources for the
invasion were scarce, but as Richard Henry Lee of Virginia put it in
late 1775, "We must have that country with us this winter cost what it
will."[20] The Congress, whose members had long damned Canadians,
now switched tactics and begged the "fellow sufferers" to join the Revolution. When the Canadians refused, General Richard Montgomery's
army moved from upper New York toward Montreal. Another force,
commanded by General Benedict Arnold, marched on Quebec. Neither army reached its objective. Winter weather forced Montgomery's
"half-naked" troops to retreat and join Arnold. Montgomery died, and
Arnold was wounded in a brave but useless attack on Quebec on New
Year's Eve. Arnold later distinguished himself in October 1776 by brilliantly blocking the British invasion from Canada. It was a significant
but anticlimactic victory, given the original American desire of annexing their "fellow sufferers" in Canada.

Defeats in the north and second thoughts in the Congress threatened the Revolution. Then, in January 1776, appeared *Common Sense*,
an incendiary, skillfully written pamphlet by Thomas Paine, whom
Franklin had sent to America after Paine was fired from the British

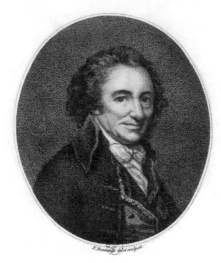

Thomas Paine (1737–1809), born in England and author of Common Sense, *the incendiary pamphlet that helped push Americans to revolution. After serving as secretary of the Committee on Foreign Affairs, Paine moved to France, where he defended the French Revolution. He then returned to the United States but made the mistakes of attacking organized religion and criticizing George Washington. He lived out his life in poverty.*

government for demanding higher wages. *Common Sense* revitalized the revolutionary cause. Moreover, it directly stated themes that dominated U.S. foreign policy over much of the next two hundred years. Paine attacked the British king, George III, as an "ass" and disdained remaining subject to Great Britain: "There is something absurd, in supposing a continent to be perpetually governed by an island. In no instance hath nature made the satellite larger than its primary planet." The new United States had a higher calling: "The cause of America is in a great measure the cause of all mankind." As historian Reginald Horsman notes, Paine helped Americans "convince themselves that what was good for America was good for the world."[21]

How did Paine plan to achieve independence? By using trade as a diplomatic lever. Thus appeared one of the assumptions in U.S. history that Great Britain (and later Russia, Japan, Communist China, Cuba, and South Africa) could be tamed because, as Paine phrased it, American products "are the necessaries of life, and will always have a market while eating is the custom of Europe." Victory, moreover, could be won without political alliances. Because all Europe needed U.S. goods, "we ought to form no partial connection with any part of it. It is the true interest of America to steer clear of European contentions." Paine thus made a famous statement of U.S. "isolationism"—that Americans should maintain maximum freedom of action to protect their interests, which were distinct from, and purer than, Europe's.

Paine's pamphlet was electrifying not because it said much that was new, but because he so skillfully expressed the views of many revolutionaries. The timing was perfect. It appeared as the Congress faced its most fateful decisions on independence. Moreover, in those days Americans read. Literacy rates ran as high as 95 percent among white males in some states and was probably the highest in the world. (In the 1980s, by comparison, the United States ranked forty-ninth among 158 nations in rate of literacy.[22]) The 500,000 copies of *Common Sense* printed in 1776 are equivalent to 25 million copies in the 1990s, given the difference in population size. High literacy and a successful (and orderly) revolution coincided in American history.

French help, Paine's writing, and Britain's inability to score crushing military victories finally gave the Congress the courage to open American ports in April 1776 to the entire world. America had broken free of British mercantile laws. Two months later, Richard Henry Lee resolved that "these United Colonies are, and of right ought to be, free and independent states." He then proposed the necessary measure for independence: "That it is expedient forthwith to take the most effectual measures for forming foreign alliances." On July 2, the Congress accepted Thomas Jefferson's draft of the Declaration of Independence, but only after it was heavily rewritten. Even then, John Dickinson of Pennsylvania launched an attack to defeat the Declaration. He warned that Americans could never conquer and govern an empire that stretched beyond the Appalachian Mountains. He feared that the country would come apart in twenty or thirty years and believed that the Hudson River was "a proper boundary" for America's western limit. He warned that if Americans allied with France to win that empire, they would only exchange British for even more intolerable French masters.[23] Dickinson's arguments were prophetic, but Lee and John Adams had the votes. The United States declared its independence.

THE FRENCH TRAP

Two weeks later, John Adams gave the Congress his draft of a Model Treaty for alliances. It repeated some of Paine's principles but translated them into diplomatic tactics that shaped U.S. foreign policy long after 1776:

> What Connection may We safely form with [France]? 1st. No Political Connection. Submit to none of her Authority—receive no Governors, or officers from her. 2nd. No Military Connection. Receive no troops from her. 3rd. Only a Commercial Connection, i.e., make a Treaty to receive

her Ships into our Ports. Let her engage to receive our Ships into her
Ports—furnish Us with Arms, Cannon, Salt, Petre, Powder, Duck, Steel.[24]

Adams thus expected France to provide full economic aid and wage
war with Great Britain in return for no political payoff except the possible breakup of the British Empire. He also expected France to treat
Americans as commercial equals and help them conquer parts of North
America, including the rich fisheries of Newfoundland, while France
kept its hands off North American territory.[25] Congress accepted Adams's
dreams. It was doubtful that France would accept. The doubt grew as
Lord Howe's British troops won a major victory on Long Island that
nearly destroyed the American army under the command of General
George Washington. U.S. trade slowed, tobacco piled up on southern
docks. New England fishermen could not ply their trade because of
British warships.

In late December 1776, a frightened Congress remodeled the Model
Treaty. It offered France islands in the West Indies. If the French brought
into the war their Spanish allies, Spain (which most Americans despised
because it was Roman Catholic as well as in control of the immense
empire of Louisiana) could have the Floridas. Americans prepared to
pay a price, even bargain away some of their possible empire, for help
in obtaining independence. Paine's and Adams's belief in the power
of mere commercial ties had been proven wrong. The Congress dispatched Franklin to France, John Adams to Holland, and John Jay to
Spain to obtain alliances and money.

In France, Franklin described himself as "very plainly dress'd" among
"the Powder'd Heads of Paris." He was, however, hardly the "noble
savage" he liked to portray. In historian Tadashi Aruga's words, the
shrewd Franklin did nothing less than "call in the Old World to liberate the New World from the Old World."[26] The word *diplomacy* comes
from the Greek word for a message that is folded so that its contents
cannot be read. In that sense, Franklin superbly practiced diplomacy,
for the "noble savage" was more devious and sophisticated than he
seemed. The French once even caught him trying to collect one loan
from them twice. The twentieth-century poet, William Carlos Williams, summarized Franklin's achievements by writing, "He played
with lightning and the French Court."[27] Franklin did so, moreover,
despite his age (he was seventy-two in 1778); difficult ocean voyages;
a bad case of gout; the desertion of his beloved son, William, to Great
Britain; and a private secretary (Edward Bancroft) who, unknown to
Franklin, was a British spy.

When the Philadelphian landed in Paris late in 1776, the cause seemed lost. British armies were poised to take Philadelphia and Albany, while the U.S. Treasury was nearly empty. Franklin's great test arose in late 1777, when news arrived of the U.S. victory in October over General John Burgoyne's British army at Saratoga, New York. The French became worried, moreover, when British officials approached Franklin about possible reconciliation, talks that the American imaginatively enlarged upon for his French friends. Vergennes decided it was time to make a formal treaty. He and Franklin signed the deal on February 6, 1778. The commercial provisions provided for reciprocity, much as Adams's Model Treaty had requested. But the political provisions did not resemble Adams's scheme. Each nation pledged military cooperation. The United States had to guarantee French control of certain West Indian islands and promise not to sign a separate peace with the British. The Americans even had to pledge to remain France's partner "forever." Franklin had nevertheless played it well. "My dear papa," a beautiful French woman wrote him, why do people criticize "the sweet habit I have taken of sitting on your lap, and your habit of soliciting from me what I always refuse?" But Franklin had also been using the wife to form a friendship with her husband—who became a key agent for selling weapons to Washington's armies.[28]

No sooner did France promise to help, however, than Vergennes instructed his agents in the New World to keep the United States as small and weak as possible. If the Americans grew powerful, he feared, they would conquer the West Indies, then "advance to the Southern Continent of America . . . and in the end not leave a foot of that Hemisphere in the possession of any European power."[29] He had, moreover, finally convinced Spain to join the war effort. The Spanish cared most about reconquering Gibraltar from the British and seizing more land in the New World—not about helping Americans become independent. Thus, France held contradictory treaty obligations: to the Americans to fight until independence was won, but to the Spanish to fight until Gibraltar was won.

When Jay arrived in Madrid to obtain more Spanish help, he was snubbed and infuriated. Spain's officials had no desire to create an independent American giant on the boundaries of their New World empire. Adams fared better in Holland. He received financial and commercial help—indeed, so much that the British finally turned and destroyed much of Holland's fleet while sacking valuable Dutch islands in the West Indies. After those disasters, Dutch help was necessarily limited.

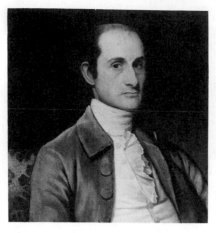

John Jay (1745–1829), a well-to-do gentleman lawyer in New York, was U.S. minister to Spain when he helped negotiate the 1783 peace treaty with Great Britain. For that he was honored, but was damned and hanged in effigy when he negotiated another treaty with the British twelve years later.

By 1779–1780, the Continental Congress seemed to be a slave to Vergennes. Its sad state was not due solely to the number of American politicians on the French payroll—although in Lawrence Kaplan's words, that payroll "was long, illustrious, and well-padded"[30]—but because U.S. survival seemed to depend on French help. The currency was so worthless that Washington complained "that a wagon-load of money will scarcely purchase a wagon-load of provisions." For a moment, the Congress hoped to get help from Catherine the Great of Russia. She worked with Vergennes to set up a League of Armed Neutrality to lay low England's commercial power. But she did so for Russian, not American, interests—she hated revolutionaries. When Francis Dana arrived as the first U.S. minister to Russia in 1781, he found the reception as frigid and desolate as the Russian winter. After two years of failure, Dana finally trudged back home.

But the news reaching the Congress was not all bad. Americans helped themselves in 1778–1779, when George Rogers Clark and his Kentucky militia braved a Midwest winter to surprise and capture key British posts in Wabash River country (the later states of Indiana and Illinois). The United States then signed its first treaty with an Indian tribe, the Delaware, who promised to help U.S. forces. In western New York, General John Sullivan attacked Indians who, with British aid, had massacred several settlements of whites. In 1779, Sullivan's troops virtually destroyed the great Iroquois nation that comprised many tribes. These victories, especially Clark's, helped establish the U.S. claim to the transappalachian West that the British, to the surprise of many, recognized in the 1783 peace treaty.

In the East, Washington's armies marked time in 1779–1780. The

---

CHRONOLOGY: 1774–1778

September 1774	First Continental Congress meets; twelve colonies represented.
October 1774	Colonies protest Quebec Act by pledging not to import British goods.
May 1775	Second Continental Congress meets; more radical membership than First.
August 1775	King George III declares colonies in rebellion.
November 1775	Secret Committees of Correspondence established.
December 1775	French secret agent arrives in America as King George III cuts off all trade into the colonies.
Winter 1775–1776	American attempt to conquer Canada fails disastrously.
January 1776	Thomas Paine publishes *Common Sense*.
March 1776	Continental Congress sends Silas Deane to France.
April 1776	Continental Congress opens American ports to the world.
May 1776	King Louis XVI of France accepts Vergennes's argument to aid Americans.
June 1776	Richard Henry Lee proposes resolutions to declare independence, form a confederation, and make foreign alliances.
July 2, 1776	Continental Congress accepts Declaration of Independence.
July 18, 1776	John Adams presents Model Treaty.
August 1776	General Howe leads British army into New York.
December 1776	Continental Congress revises Model Treaty's provisions; Benjamin Franklin arrives in France as U.S. representative.
December 1777	News of U.S. victory at Saratoga in October arrives in Paris.
December 1777– January 1778	British approach Franklin to discuss reconciliation.
February 6, 1778	U.S. and France sign treaties of alliance in Paris.

British decided to concentrate their forces in the South, where the largest number of pro-British Americans (the Loyalists) lived. The growing threat to the South between 1779 and 1781 led frightened Virginians to strengthen the new nation's government by ceding to it lands north of the Ohio River claimed by Virginia. Since 1776, the states had haggled bitterly over the question of western lands. Some of the landless states refused to ratify the Articles of Confederation, which formed the national government, until the wealthier landed states, such as Virginia, gave up their western claims. Now the logjam was broken, and all thirteen states prepared to join hands under a common constitution. But even under the Articles, the government would have little real power. Most important, the critical right to tax and regulate commerce remained in the hands of each state. The currency's value continued to sink.

In 1780, a nervous Congress instructed Franklin to surrender U.S. rights to the Mississippi River, if necessary, to obtain quick French and Spanish help. Jay, whose short-fused temper had already exploded in his dealings with the Spanish, and Franklin refused to follow instructions. The visionary but pragmatic Pennsylvanian wrote that he would rather buy more U.S. rights to the Mississippi, even at "a great price . . . than sell a Drop of its Waters. A Neighbour might as well ask me to sell my Street Door."[31]

After months of U.S. begging, the French fitted out 6 ships and 5,000 troops for warfare. This fleet was large enough to help save the colonies, but not large enough to conquer more land for the Americans. Before the French fleet could arrive in mid-1780, the British won a major battle at Charleston and prepared to move north to trap Washington's forces. But British General Lord Cornwallis's troops suffered heavy losses at the hands of Generals Nathanael Greene and Daniel Morgan at Guilford Courthouse, North Carolina, on March 15, 1781. Cornwallis withdrew to Yorktown, Virginia, to await orders for marching north. Washington's troops and the French army of Comte de Rochambeau had planned to attack New York, but when the French fleet drove British ships from Yorktown, the two commanders swung south and defeated Cornwallis's bottled-up forces on October 19, 1781.

Yorktown was the Revolution's decisive campaign. In the months that followed, a new British government under Lord Shelburne came to power. Shelburne reversed London's position of not recognizing American independence. He shrewdly understood that granting independence did not mean U.S. dependence on France. To the contrary, the double bait of independence and British trade could lure Americans back under England's control. For his part, Franklin initially demanded that, in return for peace, the British give the United States most of their holdings in North America, including Canada. Shelburne abruptly dismissed that demand, and the two sides sat down to hammer out more realistic terms. The boundaries of an independent United States were to be the Great Lakes on the North, the Mississippi on the west, and the thirty-first parallel on the south. Americans received rights to fish the rich Newfoundland banks. In return, the United States promised not to hinder the British from collecting millions of dollars of debts owed by colonials to London and Scottish merchants, and to help restore the property of perhaps 200,000 Loyalists who had left the country to join the British side. The Mississippi was to be open to both the British and Americans.

The U.S. negotiators (Franklin, Jay, Adams, and Henry Laurens) agreed to the terms on November 30, 1782. The first three negotiators (especially Jay) handled the talks, and their major problem was whether to obey the Congress's instructions to deal away the Mississippi, if necessary. Another complication was the promise of 1778 not to make peace without Vergennes's participation. Franklin had no intention of obeying such instructions and promises. And when he asked for Jay's opinion, the angry New Yorker said that if they conflicted with U.S. interests, "I would break them like this"—and he snapped the stem of his clay pipe.[32] Vergennes, who actually had little choice in the matter, allowed the talks to go on because they gave him an excuse not to prolong the war simply for Spain's sake. The Spanish were insisting on fighting until they regained Gibraltar. A major British naval victory finally destroyed that dream, and Spain—bought off by the promise that it could have the Louisiana Territory—allowed Vergennes to make peace.

Bittersweet Results of Peace

That the Americans ended the conflict with their independence and a large landed territory is remarkable. That they did so with so little bloodshed and class conflict is astonishing. Unlike the great revolutions that later struck France, Mexico, China, and Russia, the American Revolution did not become radical and kill off the class that started the revolt. John Adams led the revolutionaries in 1776 and insisted that maintaining order would be "the most difficult and dangerous Part" for Americans in "this Mighty Contest."[33] Adams and his colleagues, however, maintained not only order, but, remarkably, their own political power.

In this sense, the American Revolution was not revolutionary at all. Instead, it was the first modern anticolonial war. With rich opportunities for landed settlement and money-making, and having decades of experience in the art of self-government, Americans just wanted the

British to get out of the way. The legacy of this experience turned out to be momentous for U.S. foreign policy. Henceforth, Americans smiled on anticolonial wars but frowned on revolution—unless it resembled their own. Given their own unique history, no other revolution could be the same.

TO THE CONSTITUTION: "WHAT WILL RENDER US RESPECTABLE ABROAD?"

In September 1783, Franklin penned the famous phrase "There never was a good war or a bad peace." [34] But having won independence through war by 1783, Americans nearly lost it in peacetime within three years. Shelburne had been correct: the United States needed British markets and goods. Lord Sheffield's widely read pamphlet of 1784, *Observations on the Commerce of the United States*, laid out British policy. Because the United States depended on British trade, Sheffield argued, London could demand tough terms. It especially could do so because under the Articles of Confederation, the thirteen states were too weak and decentralized to fight back with a united policy. Parliament consequently decreed that U.S. ships could not trade with the British West Indies, certain goods could be carried only on British ships, and Canadian-U.S. trade would be severely limited. John Adams angrily condemned Parliament as "a parcel of sots" for passing such rules, but the British were succeeding in making Americans into mere providers of raw materials for British factories and then buyers of the finished British goods carried on British ships.

In 1783, the United States bought three times the amount of goods from the British that it sold to them. Prices fell, money grew scarce. Depression rocked the country between 1783 and 1786. Unpaid, disgruntled soldiers threatened rebellion until Washington personally intervened in 1783 with a resounding speech that condemned anyone "who wickedly attempts to open the floodgates of civil discord and deluge our rising empire in blood." [35] Searching desperately for economic help, the United States signed commercial treaties with France, Holland, Sweden, Prussia, and Morocco, but even combined they could not equal England's ability to provide markets and capital. In 1784, Boston investors fitted out the *Empress of China* for the first U.S. venture to exploit the legendary markets of Asia. It was a scene that would be repeated in such later postwar depressions as the 1820s, 1840s, 1890s,

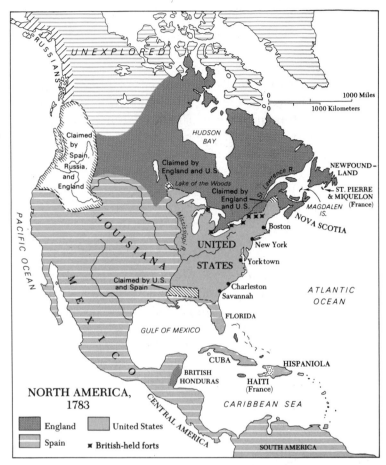

The United States in 1783, newly independent but surrounded by the navies and landed possessions of the great European powers.

and 1970s. Discovering the huge demand for ginseng, which the Chinese considered a stimulant for sexual activity, the first U.S. voyages carried over the herb, brought back tea, and made enormous profits. But the narrow, undeveloped China market—whose trade the Chinese tightly regulated so that they endured only slight personal contact with those they called the less civilized "New People"—could not replace British purchases.

The only solution was a unified, strong U.S. government able to discriminate against British goods and ships until London officials would open the West Indies and allow U.S. ships more rights. But such discrimination was impossible under the Articles of Confederation, which gave each state the right to control its own commerce. The British simply played off state against state.

This foreign-policy failure soon produced political crisis. In frontier Massachusetts, money virtually disappeared. Debtors, threatened with the loss of their land, organized under Daniel Shays to gain control of the courts through military force. The Massachusetts governor managed to put down Shays's Rebellion in 1786, but the effects of this near-revolution rippled as far away as Virginia. Washington, Jefferson (now U.S. minister to France), and James Madison all viewed Shays as the dangerous product of a bankrupt foreign policy. Other sections of the West seemed almost out of control as war veterans and other settlers rushed into the Ohio River territory. In 1779, Kentucky had about 200 white settlers. Six years later it contained 30,000. These Americans needed money and credit. They also needed protection against both Indians and the Spanish agents who sought to seduce them into Spain's empire—an empire that encircled Kentucky from the Mississippi around to the Floridas. George Washington visited the West, then warned that "the western settlers . . . stand as it were upon a pivot; the touch of a feather would turn them any way."[36] The individual states, however, could not coordinate an effective policy to deal with the Indians and Spain. In the background loomed British power. London officials refused to evacuate the northwest forts at Niagara, Detroit, and Oswego until the Americans settled their pre-1776 debt. British agents exploited the fur trade and encouraged Native Americans to drive back the settlers.

Washington's "rising empire" was fragmenting. The danger reached a peak when, in 1784, the Spanish sealed the Mississippi trade at New Orleans. Americans in Kentucky country suddenly faced the choice of losing their trade or joining the Spanish Empire. Spain then sent the smooth Don Diego de Gardoqui to strike a deal with the U.S. secretary of foreign affairs, John Jay. Spain knew that Americans needed markets and specie (gold and silver). Gardoqui offered new trade opportunities in Spain and its Canary Islands in return for Spanish control of the Mississippi for thirty years. An agonized Jay decided to accept. He concluded that Americans needed markets immediately. Anyway, he reasoned, the American multiplication table would soon swarm over the river to take possession of the trans-Mississippi. But Jay had chosen eastern merchant interests over western landed-commercial interests. The West rose in fury. The Congress accepted the Jay-Gardoqui Treaty 7 states to 5, but under the Articles of Confederation, 9 states were

James Madison (1751–1836), born in Virginia, educated at Princeton, deeply schooled in both the politics of a new nation and the political theory of the Western world. As the "Father of the Constitution," a founder of the American political party system, secretary of state between 1801 and 1809, and then president (1809–1817), the soft-spoken Virginian was perhaps the country's greatest political thinker, but also one of its least successful presidents.

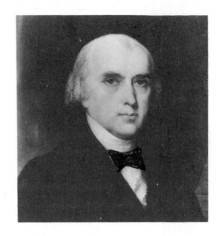

needed to ratify a treaty. Thus, the West and South effectively blocked it. Westerners threatened to join the British in Canada and then, they warned the Congress, "Farewell, *a long farewell* to all *your* boasted greatness, [for we] will be able to conquer you."[37]

Jay and other nationalists tried to amend the Articles to give the Congress new power to deal with Spain, but under the Articles of Confederation any amendments required unanimous consent of the states. One state (usually Rhode Island or New York, whose trade prospered) could block Jay. In Virginia, Madison grew concerned about the growing crisis. Thirty-five years old in 1786, educated at Princeton (where he finished in three years by sleeping only two to five hours a night), and a young but powerful member of the Congress in 1781–1782, Madison knew intimately both national politics and political theory. Indeed, he remains the best and most influential political theorist the United States has produced. By late 1786, he had reached certain conclusions with which such friends as Washington, Jefferson, Jay, and Alexander Hamilton of New York agreed.

How, Madison asked, could America hope to survive? Only by having the power to retaliate against England and Spain. How could such power be obtained? "Only by harmony in the measures of the States," Madison responded. How could such harmony be obtained? Only by allowing a "reasonable majority" of states to make policy for all, instead of allowing a single state (such as Rhode Island) to block effective action. As Madison summarized the problem, "In fact most of our political evils may be traced to our commercial ones, as most of our moral [evils can be traced] to our political."[38] Radical change was needed. Madison and his friends led a drive to have the states meet in Philadelphia.

Publicly, they indicated that they only intended to amend the Articles. But in reality, they intended to establish a new form of government, one that would allow the United States to survive in the brutal world of clashing empires.

THE "GRAND MACHINE" OF THE CONSTITUTION

During six months of secret debate in an intensely hot Philadelphia summer, the convention's delegates wrote a constitution that transformed the nation's ability to handle foreign-policy problems. First, under Madison's urging, the delegates gave Congress the power to regulate trade and pass commercial measures by a mere majority vote (not the two-thirds required by the Articles). Southerners, afraid that the more populous North could outvote and thus control their tobacco and cotton trade, fought the proposal. Madison observed "that the real difference of interests lay not between the large and small but between the N[orthern] and Southn. States. The institution of slavery and its consequences formed the line" between the two sections.[39] In one of the convention's major compromises, the South agreed that a mere majority vote could pass trade measures; in return, the North accepted the continuation of the slave trade until at least 1808.

Second, treaties with other nations could be made lawful when the president proposed them and "two-thirds of the Senators present concur." This provision not only protected the South and West against another Jay-Gardoqui treaty, but it also created a stronger central government because only the senators "present" had to agree. States could no longer threaten to kill treaties simply by not attending Congress, as some did before 1787. This provision also applied to treaties made with Indian tribes, whom the whites usually considered separate nations.

Third, a single-person executive, the president, was created. It had no counterpart in the Articles of Confederation. Congress, however, had the ultimate power: the appropriation of funds for the executive's use. The executive was to be "Commander in Chief of the Army and Navy," could negotiate treaties for Senate consideration, and might nominate ambassadors and "other public Ministers" with "the advice and consent" of the Senate. The Constitution thus established a new agency to conduct day-to-day foreign policy.

Fourth, Congress received an amazing series of powers that it could exercise through a mere majority vote. Congress, not the states, could now "regulate Commerce with foreign Nations, and among the several

States, and with the Indian Tribes." It could do so, moreover, through its new "Power To lay and collect Taxes, Duties, Imposts and Excises." Of equal importance, the convention, acting on Madison's proposal, gave Congress the sole power to "declare" war. The 1787 convention clearly did not want the president to have the power to "make" war without Congress "declaring" it first. As Jefferson later observed, it was only right that the power to involve the nation in conflict should be taken from those in the executive "who are to spend" and given to those in Congress "who are to pay." The delegates, moreover, viewed the president's right to repel sudden attacks as only a necessary exception to the general rule.[40]

Congress received the power to rule all territory outside state control. In another meeting also held in 1787, members of the old Confederation Congress drew up the Ordinance of 1787 that specified a three-stage process through which a territory (such as Kentucky or Ohio in the 1780s) would have to pass to become a state. To ensure that the frontiersmen and -women behaved themselves, the ordinance gave Congress virtual dictatorial power in the first stage so that the territory could be run as a colony. After 1787, a new Congress had the money and ability to operate the ordinance and keep the restless West under control. Overall, the founders clearly wanted Congress to make general laws and rules for foreign policy. The president was to carry out these measures and conduct detailed diplomacy.

Finally, Madison provided a brilliant political theory on which these powers rested. He argued that the national government could be given great powers to defend the United States against other empires (such as the British and Spanish), but also protect individual freedom within America. This seemingly impossible job could be done, he believed, by placing checks and balances within the government itself. As he nicely phrased it, "Ambition must be made to counter ambition." Thus, the states retained significant authority to counter the national government. Thus, three branches of the federal government—the executive, Congress, and the Supreme Court—checked each other. Thus, the two parts of Congress itself, the House and the Senate, checked one another. With these devices and the vast powers in the hands of the new government, Madison felt that he and the other founders had solved a 2,500-year-old problem that the greatest minds—Aristotle, Montesquieu, Hume—had believed could not be solved: how to maintain a just and democratic system over an area as vast as the United States. Aristotle and the others had feared that selfish, individual interests would tear apart a large empire and lead to either anarchy or dictatorship.

Madison disagreed. He believed that dangerous "factions" could be neutralized by spreading them across a vast territory and then having the new government—with its federalism and its checks and balances—rule the territory.[41] Madison thus reversed the beliefs that had governed political theory. In doing so, he explained the new constitutional system and justified the creation of a new American Empire stretching over vast distances.

GREAT LOSERS: THE ANTIFEDERALISTS

The detailed proceedings of the Constitutional Convention remained secret until the 1830s, but Madison publicly outlined his reasoning that undergirded the new government in *The Federalist*, a series of eighty-five essays, written with Jay and Hamilton and published anonymously in 1787–1788. The essays were needed because "Antifederalists" were determined to kill the Constitution in the ratifying conventions that each state convened to accept or reject the document.

The Antifederalists powerfully argued that Aristotle was right: republics must be small so that rulers and other dangerous factions could be closely watched. Other critics warned that the president would be of "the most dangerous kind too—an *elective* King." Elbridge Gerry of Massachusetts had quit the convention in disgust because he feared the new Congress could "raise armies and money without limit." Such power would ruin the people's liberties. Gerry was furious that Madison and Hamilton had succeeded in creating such centralized power and then had the nerve to call themselves "Federalists." Gerry suggested it would be more accurate to call the two sides "rats and antirats."[42]

The pivotal battle occurred in Virginia, where Madison's group opposed Governor Patrick Henry's. Head of a strong state machine, Henry did not want to surrender his powers. He was a talented politician and orator. (A poll in 1958 revealed that Henry's "Give me liberty or give me death" had become the second best-known quote in American history. Only "Come up and see me sometime," seductively uttered by movie actress Mae West, was more famous.)[43] Henry charged that the new government would sell out the transappalachian region, suppress liberty within the states, glorify the few who controlled the national government, and destroy the Articles of Confederation, which had pulled the country through the war. Madison responded that the Articles made up a "contemptible system," disdained by the world's powers. He then struck at the core of the problem: Americans had to govern themselves better at home so that they could protect themselves abroad. Madison summarized this in a classic phrase: "Does [Henry] distinguish between what will render us secure and happy at home, and what will render us respectable abroad? If we be free and happy at home, we shall be respectable abroad."[44]

Successful foreign policy, Madison argued, grew from the inside out. But Americans could survive as a people only if they could effectively fight the other great world empires. The United States has never been isolated or outside the world's political struggles. It was born in the middle of those conflicts, and its great problem was—and has always been—how to survive those struggles while maintaining individual liberty at home. Madison believed that he and his colleagues had gone far in solving that central problem. They devised a system that Franklin termed "the grand machine." Madison defeated Henry in the Virginia ratifying convention because of the promise of that "machine," because George Washington threw his great prestige back of the Constitution, and because the Federalists shrewdly agreed to add a bill of rights that would explicitly protect certain personal and state rights.

The Antifederalists lost the argument. They nevertheless raised the pivotal questions that plagued Americans over the next two hundred years. The more immediate problem, however, was to see whether the "machine" would work and the "course of empire" continue to move westward.

NOTES

1. William H. Seward, *Life and Public Services of John Quincy Adams* (Auburn, N.Y., 1849), p. 362.
2. Edward G. Bourne, *Spain in America, 1450–1580* (New York, 1904), pp. 82–88.
3. D. A. Farnie, "The Commercial Empire of the Atlantic, 1607–1783," *The Economic History Review*, 2d ser., 15 (December 1962): 205–208.
4. The quote and useful analysis are in Samuel Eliot Morison, *Builders of the Bay Colony* (Boston, 1930), pp. 73–74.
5. Daniel Boorstin, *The Americans: The National Experience* (New York, 1965), p. 3.
6. Louis B. Wright, *The Dream of Prosperity in Colonial America* (New York, 1965), pp. 27–29.
7. Harold U. Faulkner, *Economic History of the United States* (New York, 1937), p. 93.
8. Allan R. Millett and Peter Maslowski, *For the Common Defense: A Military History of the United States of America* (New York, 1984), pp. 2, 9–18.

9. William T. Hagan, *The Indian in American History* (Washington, D.C., 1971), p. 8; Frederic E. Hoxie, "The Indians versus the Textbooks," *American Historical Association Perspectives* 23 (April 1985): 18–22.

10. Pauline Maier, "Second Thoughts on Our First Century," *New York Times Book Review*, 7 July 1985, p. 20.

11. Thomas R. Hietala, *Manifest Design: Anxious Aggrandizement in Late Jacksonian America* (Ithaca, N.Y., 1985), p. 111; an earlier citation is in Thomas A. Bailey's *A Diplomatic History of the American People*, 7th ed. (New York, 1964), p. 224.

12. Benjamin Franklin, *Observations Concerning the Increase of Mankind . . .*, in *The Papers of Benjamin Franklin*, ed. Leonard W. Labaree *et al.* (New Haven, 1959–), IV, pp. 233–234.

13. Franklin's Canada pamphlet is in *The Writings of Benjamin Franklin*, ed. Albert Henry Smyth, 10 vols. (New York, 1905), IV, pp. 55–57; Burke's argument can be found in Gerald Stourzh, *Benjamin Franklin and American Foreign Policy* (Chicago, 1954), pp. 70–74.

14. *New York Times*, 4 July 1976, p. F2; a key analysis of Sam Adams and these events is in William Appleman Williams, *The Contours of American History* (Cleveland, 1961), p. 112.

15. Benjamin Franklin to William Franklin, 13 March 1768, in *The Writings*, ed. Smyth, V, p. 117. A fine analysis of this crucial change in British politics is in Michael Kammen, *Rope of Sand* (Ithaca, N.Y., 1968), esp. pp. 314–318.

16. *Boswell's Life of Johnson*, ed. R. W. Chapman (New York, 1953), pp. 590, 876, 946.

17. Richard Van Alstyne, *Empire and Independence* (New York, 1976), p. 28.

18. Curtis P. Nettels, "The Origins of the Union and of the States," *Proceedings of the Massachusetts Historical Society* 72 (1957–1960), p. 71.

19. Benjamin Franklin to Joseph Priestly, October 1775, in *The Writings*, ed. Smyth, VI, p. 430.

20. Richard Henry Lee to George Washington, 26 September 1775 and 22 October 1775, in *The Letters of Richard Henry Lee*, ed. James C. Ballagh, 2 vols. (New York, 1911–1914), esp. I, p. 153.

21. Reginald Horsman, *The Diplomacy of the New Republic, 1776–1815* (Arlington Heights, Ill., 1985), p. 7; Thomas Paine, *Common Sense* (New York, 1942), pp. 23, 26–27, 31–32.

22. See Neil Postman's review of Jonathan Kozol's *Illiterate America* in *Washington Post Book World*, 31 March 1985, p. 5.

23. J. H. Powell, ed., "Speech of John Dickinson," *Pennsylvania Magazine of History and Biography* 65 (October 1941): 458–481.

24. John Adams, *Diary and Autobiography*, ed. Lyman H. Butterfield *et al.*, 4 vols. (Cambridge, Mass., 1961), II, p. 236.

25. Worthington C. Ford, ed., *Journals of the Continental Congress* (Washington, D.C., 1906), V, pp. 768–778.

26. Tadashi Aruga, "Revolutionary Diplomacy and the Franco-American Treaties of 1778," *Japanese Journal of American Studies* no. 2 (1985): 60. The Franklin quotes are in Benjamin Franklin to Mrs. Thompson, 8 February 1777, in *The Writings*, ed. Smyth, VII, p. 26.

27. William Carlos Williams, *In the American Grain* (New York, 1957), p. 153.

28. Recounted in *New York Times*, 3 January 1987, p. 11; the "forever" clause and the

treaties themselves are conveniently found in *The Record of American Diplomacy*, ed. Ruhl J. Bartlett, 4th ed. (New York, 1964), pp. 24–27.

29. Van Alstyne, pp. 92–93.
30. *The American Revolution and "A Candid World,"* ed. Lawrence Kaplan (Kent, Ohio, 1977), p. 141.
31. Benjamin Franklin to John Jay, 2 October 1780, in *The Writings*, ed. Smyth, VIII, pp. 143–144.
32. Robert Calhoon, *Revolutionary America: An Interpretive Overview* (New York, 1976), p. 153.
33. John R. Howe, *The Changing Political Thought of John Adams* (Princeton, 1966), pp. 8–9.
34. Benjamin Franklin to Josiah Quincy, 11 September 1783, in *The Writings*, ed. Smyth, IX, p. 96.
35. Richard Van Alstyne, *The Rising American Empire* (Chicago, 1960), esp. pp. 1–20.
36. Merrill Jensen, *The New Nation* (New York, 1950), p. 171. The best overview now is Frederick W. Marks III, *Independence on Trial: Foreign Affairs and the Making of the Constitution* (Baton Rouge, 1973, 1986).
37. *The Revolutionary Diplomatic Correspondence of the United States*, ed. Francis Wharton, 6 vols. (Washington, D.C., 1889), VI, pp. 223–224.
38. James Madison to James Monroe, 7 August 1785, in *The Writings of James Madison*, ed. Gaillard Hunt, 9 vols. (New York, 1901), II, pp. 155–157, 228–229; Irving Brant, *James Madison*, 6 vols. (Indianapolis, 1944–1961), III, pp. 55–56.
39. *The Records of the Federal Convention of 1787*, ed. Max Farrand, 4 vols. (New Haven, 1937), II, pp. 9–10. I am greatly indebted here to Professor Diane Clemens of the University of California, Berkeley, who is preparing a major monograph (to be published by Oxford University Press) on executive powers.
40. Abraham Sofaer, *War, Foreign Affairs, and Constitutional Power* (Cambridge, Mass., 1976), pp. 31–32.
41. *The Federalist*, ed. Clinton Rossiter (New York, 1961), p. 325; Sofaer, pp. 42–43.
42. Merrill Jensen, *The American Revolution within America* (New York, 1974), pp. 213–214; *The Anti-Federalist Papers*, ed. Morton Borden (East Lansing, Mich., 1965), esp. pp. 27–28, 37–39, 213; *Records of the Federal Convention*, ed. Farrand, II, p. 633.
43. Bernard Mayo, *Myths and Men* (Athens, Ga., 1959), pp. 1–24, has the poll and a good analysis of Henry.
44. *The Writings of James Madison*, ed. Hunt, V, p. 146.

For Further Reading

Most of the bibliographical references given in these sections specify post-1980 publications. For pre-1981 materials, no textbook can hope to compare with *Guide to American Foreign Relations since 1700*, ed. Richard Dean Burns (1983), which, with three indexes and more than 1,200 pages of references, is the necessary starting place for any student who wants to read more on the first three centuries of U.S. foreign policy. See also the notes to this chapter and the General Bibliography at the end of this book.

A stimulating account, much influenced by the U.S. experience in Vietnam during the 1960s and the 1970s, is Robert W. Tucker and David C. Hendrickson, *The Fall of the First British Empire: Origins of the War of American Independence* (1982), which should be used with Alison Gilbert Olson, *Making The Empire Work: London and American Interest Groups 1690–1790* (1992). Of special importance on the development of the American view of empire are Douglas Edward Leach, *Roots of Conflict: British Armed Forces and Colonial Americans, 1677–1763* (1966), and Francis Jennings, *Empire of Fortune* (1988), on the Seven Years' War. For a "realist" perspective, see the readable essays in Norman Graebner, *Foundations of American Foreign Policy* (1986), especially those on Franklin and Adams. Jonathan Dull has written on the first American diplomat in "Benjamin Franklin and the Nature of American Diplomacy," *International History Review* 5 (August 1983) and in "Franklin the Diplomat: The French Mission," *Transactions of the American Philosophical Society* 72, pt. 1 (1982) and has examined the larger picture in *A Diplomacy of the American Revolution* (1985). A fascinating account of Silas Deane's escapades is in James West Davidson and Mark H. Lytle, *After the Fact* (1982), and of an opponent of the Declaration of Independence in Milton E. Flower, *John Dickinson* (1983), while Louis W. Potts delves into U.S.-French diplomacy in *Arthur Lee: A Virtuous Revolutionary* (1981), and Lynne Withey presents a fresh perspective on the Revolution and its diplomacy in *Dearest Friend: A Life of Abigail Adams* (1981), as does Edith B. Gelles, *Portia: The World of Abigail Adams* (1992).

Encounters with Native Americans are covered in important essays in *The American Indian and the Problem of History*, ed. Calvin Martin (1986), from the Indians' viewpoint. Superb accounts have opened new perspectives on the military experience: *Arms at Rest*, ed. Joan R. Challinor and Robert L. Beisner (1987), especially the essays by Harold D. Langley and James A. Field, Jr., on the pre-1815 years; *Arms and Independence*, ed. Ronald Hoffman and Peter J. Albert (1984), especially the Royster, Higgenbotham, and Buel essays on foreign-policy aspects; Reginald C. Stuart, *War and American Thought: From the Revolution to the Monroe Doctrine* (1982); and Lawrence D. Cress, "Republican Liberty and National Security: American Military Policy as an Ideological Problem, 1783 to 1789," *William and Mary Quarterly* 38 (January 1981). George Washington deserves a special place: Don Higginbotham's excellent *George Washington and the American Military Tradition* (1985); Edmund S. Morgan's succinct *The Genius of George Washington* (1980); and *The Papers of George Washington: Revolutionary War Series*, Vol. I: *June–September 1775*, ed. Philander D. Chase (1985), with more volumes scheduled to appear soon.

Special topics are well handled in *Diplomacy and Revolution: The Franco-American Alliance of 1778*, ed. Ronald Hoffman and Peter J. Albert (1981); Lawrence S. Kaplan, "The Treaty of Paris, 1783: A Historiographical Challenge," *International History Review* 5 (August 1983); and the key sources in *The United States and Russia: The Beginning of Relations, 1765–1815*, ed. Nina N. Bashkina, Nikolai N. Bolkhovitinov, *et al.* (1980). On the years 1783 to 1789, begin with Frederick W. Marks III, *Independence on Trial*, 2d ed. (1986), which sees foreign policy as the major reason for the 1787 convention. Note *Beyond Confederation: Origins of the Constitution and American National Identity*, ed. Richard Beeman, Stephen Botein, and Edward C. Carter II (1987). A deserved examination of the "losers" is given in *The Anti-Federalist: An Abridgment of the Seven-Volume Set of the Complete Anti-Federalist*, ed. Herbert J. Storing (1985), and of the "winners" in *The Papers of James Madison*, ed. Robert A. Rutland *et al.* (1973, 1975), whose volumes are now up to the 1793–1795 years. Marks, *Independence on Trial*, has a useful bibliography on the foreign-policy implications of the decisions leading to the adoption of the Constitution. See also the important perspective in Jonathan Marshall, "Empire or Liberty: The Antifederalists and Foreign Policy, 1787–1788," *Journal of Libertarian Studies* 4 (Summer 1980).

2

A Second Struggle for Independence and Union (1789–1815)

Americans were doubly blessed at the time of their independence. They had before them a vast, fertile territory that strained even the pioneers' wild imagination. A Pennsylvanian proudly wrote that the trees were taller, the soil richer than anywhere else in the world, while the Mississippi was "the prince of rivers, in comparison of whom the Nile is but a rivulet, and the Danube a mere ditch."[1] But Americans were also given a unique federal form of government by founders who were unique. The generation that gave Americans their independence and Constitution was the only generation in U.S. history that combined the nation's political leaders and its intellectual leaders in the same people.[2] The theoretical and the practical met, fortunately for Americans, at the moment their Constitution was written.

But even James Madison, the "father of the Constitution," as he later became known, was unsure whether the first government under the new laws could survive. "We are in a wilderness without a single footstep to guide us," he wrote to Jefferson in 1789. Madison quickly learned that the survival of individual freedom at home was related to the course of policy abroad. As he observed in the late 1790s, "The management of foreign relations appears to be the most susceptible of abuse of all the trusts committed to government."[3] Between 1789 and 1814, the United States struggled both to survive within the world of

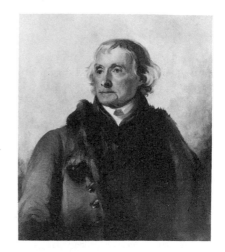

Thomas Jefferson (1743–1826) wrote the original draft of the Declaration of Independence, served as governor of Virginia and U.S. minister to France, became the nation's first secretary of state under the new Constitution, and, as president, bought the Louisiana Purchase in 1803. He hoped to obtain the rest of North America in 1812, when he unfortunately thought that conquering Canada would be a mere matter of marching.

the titanic Napoleonic Wars, and to keep alive the union that had been formed in 1787–1788.

There was irony here. The person who was to run foreign policy for the new system was originally entitled "secretary for foreign affairs," but it turned out that the official seemed to have so little to do in the late 1780s that the job was renamed "secretary of state" and given the responsibility of guarding the nation's Great Seal, publishing laws, and taking the census. Thomas Jefferson thought so little of the position that he wanted to remain in Paris rather than join Washington's cabinet. But the Virginian finally accepted the post that paid $3,500 annually and had a staff of five for copying and translating messages. The War and Treasury departments were much larger and also worked in rather stately buildings, while the original State Department building was a small house on Broadway in New York City, where Washington's first government gathered before moving to Philadelphia in 1790.[4] But the irony was that the State Department, for all its lack of glamor, was to be the very center of the debate over the next quarter-century on whether the new nation, surrounded by great empires, could conduct a foreign policy that would allow the survival of the constitutional experiment. As was to be the case so often over the next several centuries, American domestic politics were crucial, but foreign policies involved matters of life and death.

THE FRAMEWORK: THE UNITED STATES (1789–1814)

When John Quincy Adams traveled as U.S. minister to Prussia in the mid-1790s, he had to wait outside the Berlin city gates while an officer tried to discover if a place called the United States actually existed. No such uncertainty was found in the Western Hemisphere. With astounding speed, Americans moved to conquer the land and commerce of the New World. The "multiplication table" continued to double the population approximately every twenty-two years. In Connecticut (the seedbed for populating much of New York and the Midwest), couples could brag of a dozen children, five times that number of grandchildren, and two hundred to three hundred great-grandchildren.[5] In the South, onrushing population put great pressure on Native Americans and the relatively few Spaniards who tried to hold on to the vast territories of Florida and the trans-Mississippi.

Not only the Constitution, but literature and technology shaped the nation. Noah Webster, an ardent nationalist (and Federalist), wrote his famous speller, reader, and dictionary to make Americans aware and proud of their distinct language, as well as to make them literate. Soon after the steam engine began to revolutionize British industries, it started replacing animal and human muscle in America. John Fitch may have been ugly, bad-mannered, and a wife deserter, but he also ran a newly invented steamboat on the river in Philadelphia, where the founders could see it in 1787. By 1790, the vessel was coming into regular use. Three years later, Eli Whitney perfected the cotton gin, which separated fiber from seed with such speed that the new machine fastened a cotton culture on the South. Cotton exports rocketed from 2 million pounds in 1794 to 18 million pounds in 1800 to 128 million pounds by 1820.[6] In 1798, Whitney devised the radical process of making rifles rapidly and cheaply out of interchangeable parts in an assembly-line process. American expansion was increasingly linked to its people's genius for machinery and technology.

Native Americans felt the brunt of this expansionism. Since many had fought alongside the British between 1775 and 1782, the settlers had no qualms about pushing them aside after the Revolution. The Indians fought effectively against the badly organized Americans. The new Constitution, however, gave the government the needed authority to raise armies, oversee settlement, and make treaties with the tribes. With this new power came a new philosophy: instead of being destroyed, the Indians were to be "civilized" and made to act like white farmers.

Thomas Jefferson best exemplified this approach. As president in 1808, he told a group of Indians that they should become small capitalist landowners. Then "you will mix with us by marriage. Your blood will run in our veins and will spread with us over this great land." If they did not follow his advice, Jefferson later commented, the alternative was not pretty: "They will relapse into barbarism and misery . . . and we shall be obliged to drive them, with the beasts of the forests into the Stony [Rocky] Mountains."[7]

The region between the Appalachian Mountains and the Mississippi (an area bordering the British Empire on the north and the Spanish Empire on the south and west) was becoming extremely productive, politically complex, and quickly populated. By 1795, Tennessee exported cast iron as well as whiskey and bacon. The West was not being filled by idyllic, self-sufficient Daniel Boones, but by settlers whose multiplying commercial interests produced so many farm and manufacturing goods that they thought of themselves as part of an international trading network. As the new Constitution took effect, moreover, Europe lost much of its ability to feed itself. The quarter-century agony of the French Revolution and Napoleonic Wars began. U.S. farm prices rose as foreign markets blotted up American cotton, tobacco, grain, meat, and fish. In the North as well as in the plantation South, as a Philadelphia orator put it, "the Star-bespangled Genius of America . . . points to agriculture as the stable Foundation of this rising mighty Empire."[8]

U.S. exports leaped from $19 million in 1791 to $108 million in 1807. But the country remained a debtor as imports shot up from $19 million in 1791 to $138 million in 1807. The debt was often paid for by the success of U.S. merchants and shipowners. They not only carried American trade, but the trade of others—especially the commerce generated by the rich British and French West Indies. As the European wars grew bloodier, this trade grew greater and the U.S. traders grew richer even as they became in reality parts of the British or French empires rather than the American system. As these traders came to care more about European than U.S. interests, they caused major problems for Washington officials between 1805 and 1814. Indeed, some northeastern merchants almost destroyed the new Union in 1814. But in the earlier years, they acted as a cutting edge for the expansion of American power in some unusual places. For example, they helped undermine Spain's control of Latin America by dominating the Spanish-American carrying trade.

The Yankees also targeted Russia's colonies in Alaska and the present American Northwest until they monopolized the rich fur trade between Alaska and China. That trade produced as much as 500 percent annual profit. In historian Howard Kushner's words, the supposedly Russian-controlled areas actually "depended on Yankee traders" for both supplies and exports.[9] The Russian tsar Alexander I tried to retaliate by giving a trading monopoly to John Jacob Astor's American fur company, which, the tsar hoped, would undercut other Americans and allow him to control Astor. Alexander next sent a mission into California to take over the San Francisco region so food from the area could replace supplies provided by Americans. Neither policy worked. By 1820, the Yankees were handsomely, if illegally, growing rich from the Russian Empire. A Bostonian, Captain Robert Gray, in 1792 found the magnificent river that he named after his ship, the *Columbia*. Gray's discovery gave the United States strong claim to the vast Oregon territory. Other American traders exploited the coasts for furs and, in three-year expeditions, grew rich selling them to China. They sometimes stopped for rest in Hawaii, thus giving them an early interest in those strategic islands as well. Before it was ten years old, the new United States was becoming a power in the Pacific region.

Americans also were proving that they could govern their growing continental empire. Shays-type rebellions were no longer to be tolerated. When William Blount (a leading politician in Tennessee) and James Wilkinson (a well-known scoundrel and schemer) renewed earlier plots to sell parts of the new West to Spain, Washington used his power simply to buy Blount and Wilkinson by giving them political jobs and military commissions. Washington became the central figure who held together the nation's domestic and foreign affairs. The first president set many of the precedents that later chief executives had to follow. He had "neither the quickness nor the brilliance of genius," the British minister reported to London, perhaps because of "his natural shyness and reserve." But, the minister granted, the president had "sound sense and . . . excellent judgement."[10] Jefferson noted that Washington was tall, "his deportment easy, erect, and noble; the best horseman of his age."[11] His long military career, the leadership of the revolutionary forces, and his service as chair of the Constitutional Convention gave him unequaled experience. He knew the West intimately, largely as a result of his own extensive land speculation. The first president believed that the Constitution's success depended not only on its words, but on its citizens' character. "A good general government," he wrote to one of his several intimate women admirers, "without good morals and good habits, will not make us a happy People."[12]

Jefferson agreed about the need for good morals, but he had fewer doubts than Washington. In designing a national seal, Jefferson suggested that it show the children of Israel led by a pillar of light from the heavens. He was confident that Americans were the new chosen people of God. Returning from France in 1790 to become the first secretary of state under the Constitution, his confidence was put to the test.

CHOSEN PEOPLE, THE BRITISH EMPIRE, AND THE FRENCH REVOLUTION

Washington understood his most important foreign-policy problem: "That we avoid errors in our system of policy respecting Great Britain."[13] The British continued to hold forts on U.S. territory and encouraged Indians to oppose American settlement. London also tightened its control on U.S. trade. To break that control, Madison rose in the first session of the First Congress to propose a series of measures that would utilize the new powers of the Constitution as a club to smash the British hold. His approach was direct: threaten other nations with commercial retaliation unless they treated American trade fairly. As the Virginian phrased it, "We possess natural advantages which no other nation does; we can, therefore, with justice, stipulate for a reciprocity in commerce. The way to obtain this is by discrimination."[14] Congress passed bills levying tonnage duties eight times higher on foreign vessels than on U.S. ships in American ports, and also imposed import taxes on foreign goods entering the country. Americans wanted freer trade, but they were prepared to play rough mercantilist trading games if necessary.

Madison nevertheless wanted more. He sought to favor French trade (because France bought more than it sold to Americans) and discriminate against the British. His proposals quickly encountered opposition from Secretary of the Treasury Alexander Hamilton. The illegitimate son of a Scottish merchant, at twenty Hamilton had been a brilliant pamphleteer for the Revolution and at twenty-six a hero at Yorktown. After practicing law and marrying into a powerful New York family, he had joined Madison to push through the Constitution. Only thirty-four in 1789 (Madison was thirty-eight), Hamilton split with the Virginian and Jefferson over foreign policy. The Treasury secretary put together a program that gave the new nation sound, centralized finances. His program promised to pay the large national debt and to establish a national bank to oversee the country's economy. But these schemes required a great deal of money, and those sums had to come from land sales or import taxes on goods that were mostly British. Hamilton, therefore, feared any measure that threatened Great Britain and that might lead to a cutting off of British capital or, worse, another devastating conflict. Thus, he opposed Madison's every attempt to get tough with the British. He even worked secretly with the British minister to undercut Madison's influence.

Jefferson and Madison were furious. Hamilton is "panic-struck if we refuse our breeches to every kick which Gr. Brit. may choose to give us," Jefferson fumed.[15] Nor did it lessen the Virginians' fear when Jefferson told Hamilton that the leading men in history were Francis Bacon, Isaac Newton, and John Locke, only to have the secretary of the Treasury reply dryly that he personally preferred Caesar.

In 1790, a cabinet crisis erupted when Spanish naval officers stupidly seized British ships in Nootka Sound off the northwest coast. London quickly planned to retaliate by marching troops from Canada to conquer Spanish lands along the Caribbean, a march that would take the troops through the Mississippi Valley. The British could end by surrounding the new nation on all four sides. Jefferson advised Washington that the British must never be allowed to make that march. Hamilton, however, warned that nothing should be done to alienate Great Britain, and, he added, it would help to have the Spanish thrown off the continent. Before Washington had to take action, however, the Spanish wisely apologized for the ship seizures, and the crisis passed.

It was quickly replaced by an even graver problem. In 1789, the French Revolution had begun. By 1793, it became an international struggle as France declared war on England, Holland, and Austria. Jefferson sympathized with the French. They seemed to be following the example of 1776. Madison was less starry-eyed about the upheaval, but for his own reasons he also favored the French. A great opportunity opened for U.S. commerce. As Jefferson phrased it, the United States wanted no part of the Europeans' problems except "we have only to pray that their soldiers may eat a great deal."[16] Hamilton agreed.

But the two men sharply divided over U.S. obligations to France under the 1778 alliance, a pact that remained in effect between the two nations, even though the 1778 governments had changed. Hamilton argued that U.S. national interests rose above any vague obligations under the treaty. Washington took his advice and issued a Neutrality Proclamation. Madison blasted the president's announcement for disregarding U.S. "duties to France," ignoring "the cause of liberty," and—of special concern—exercising a power that Madison believed belonged to Congress: the power to declare neutrality could also decide whether and against whom the United States might declare war.[17] But Washington stuck to his policy and established a constitutional precedent that claimed important power for the president. Nor did it help Jefferson when a new French minister, Edmond Charles Genêt, arrived and immediately began breaking U.S. laws by fitting out French privateers in U.S. ports to seize British ships. He then enlisted American boys to fight in France. Washington refused to deal with "Citizen" Genêt. As the Frenchman grew unpopular, Jefferson "saw the necessity of quitting a wreck which could not but sink all who should cling to it."

The French Revolution soon got out of hand. Dr. J. I. Guillotin's device for separating heads from bodies worked more frequently until King Louis XVI became a victim. After Genêt's supporters in Paris fell to a more radical faction, even he recoiled at the thought of returning. (He married into a wealthy American family and lived in the United States for the rest of his life.) Jefferson was sickened. The French were not following the moderate example of 1776. Two centuries later, one can see that the French Revolution, not the American, was more the model for such great upheavals as those in Russia, China, Iran, and Vietnam. As the British foreign minister Lord Grenville sniffed to an American in 1798, "None but Englishmen and their Descendents know how to make a Revolution." That belief became a central assumption in U.S. diplomacy.

In 1793–1794, Madison pushed his campaign to destroy British control of U.S. commerce. He received help from the British themselves in late 1793, when they seized 250 U.S. vessels that were carrying goods between France and the West Indies. Madison arose in the House of Representatives in March 1794 and bitterly attacked the action. He observed that the British sold the United States twice as much as they bought, while the French bought seven times more than they sold to the United States. It was time to cut British trade and shipping until London officials treated Americans fairly. Madison gained support from many who were outraged by the ship seizures. As Hamilton's program seemed about to collapse, the Treasury secretary brilliantly gained time and undercut Madison by convincing Washington to send Chief Justice John Jay to London to negotiate a settlement in order to avert possible war with the British.

A TURN: FROM JAY TO X Y Z

Jay had one high card to play: he could threaten to join the new League of Armed Neutrality formed by several European nations to check British naval power. Hamilton, however, undercut his own diplomat by secretly telling London that the United States had no intention of joining the league. This deviousness left Jay to sign a treaty that sharply limited U.S.–West Indian trade. The pact gave Americans nothing on the issues of neutral rights (such as the valued U.S. principle that "free ships make free goods"), or impressment (the hated British practice of seizing their own—and sometimes American—citizens from U.S. ships on the grounds that they had deserted His Majesty's fleet). The British repeated their 1783 pledge that the Mississippi was opened to both nations. On the other hand, the British did agree to leave the northwest forts, and they opened Great Britain and the British East Indies to U.S. merchants. American trade with Asia consequently boomed. By 1801, Yankee ships carried 70 percent of all foreign trade with India.

But even this opportunity did not stop anti-Jay riots from erupting throughout the East. Mobs in Philadelphia threatened Vice-President John Adams's house and stoned the windows of the British minister's office. Americans were incensed at the limits placed on the West Indies trade. Westerners threatened to leave the Union if the British used the treaty to try to control the Mississippi. Madison was deeply angered. He argued that the House of Representatives had an equal right with the Senate to act on the treaty because the House had to appropriate money to put treaties into effect. Washington set another crucial constitutional precedent by invoking executive privilege and refusing to release the documents of the Jay mission. Then he denied that anything more than a two-thirds vote of the Senate was needed to ratify treaties. The president faced down the House, but his growing concern was over those he called "the restless and impetuous spirits of Kentucky," who threatened in the West to take matters into their own hands.

Since 1789, he had tried to protect the settlers from Indian attacks that were at least winked at by the British. In 1791, about a hundred miles north of Cincinnati, the Miami chief Little Turtle inflicted one of the worst defeats in history on a U.S. military force. Nine hundred whites were killed. The rest broke and ran. In 1793–1794, Washington finally placed General "Mad Anthony" Wayne in command of 3,000 men. After careful preparation, Wayne defeated the Shawnee in 1794 at the Battle of Fallen Timbers in the Ohio territory. The general leveled every Indian settlement he could reach, built forts (including Fort Wayne, now in Indiana), and opened the region to settlement.

Washington then enjoyed another well-timed success. The Spanish had joined Great Britain against France in 1793, but within a year they were ready to rejoin their traditional ally in Paris. To do so, however, created the danger that the British would retaliate by sweeping down on Spanish possessions in America. Those possessions were indeed already slipping away. Several years earlier, Spain had tried to seduce American settlers by encouraging them to settle in the Floridas. Jefferson was elated that the doors would be open: "We may complain of this seduction of our inhabitants just enough to make [the Spanish] believe it very wise policy for them & confirm them in it."[18] By 1794, Spain had lost control of most of those settlers and much of the Indian trade. When Madrid ordered the situation to be brought under control, a beleaguered Spanish official responded: "You cannot lock up an open field." Beset in both Europe and America, the Spanish were ready to talk. Washington sent Thomas Pinckney to Madrid. In late 1795, he signed a pact that pledged mutual cooperation to stop Indian attacks in the South and, most important, to open Spanish-held New Orleans to tax-free use for three years to the hundreds of thousands of Americans whose prosperity now depended on Mississippi trade.

The Pinckney Treaty was a godsend to Washington. In it, Spain promised the West the use of the Mississippi just as the Jay Treaty gave the East's merchants peace with the British fleet. Moreover, those who continued to oppose the Jay Treaty in Congress were quickly sobered by threats of losing the Union. New Jersey, for one, said it would dissociate itself from the South if the Jay pact were not ratified. As one Federalist wrote, "The conversation of a separation is taking place in almost every company."[19] Washington also threw his immense prestige behind Jay's agreement. The Senate barely accepted it by a 20-to-10 vote. Madison complained that "banks, the British merchants, the insurance companies" had won through bribery and threats. More accurately, however, the new nation had been saved in 1795–1796 by "Mad Anthony" Wayne, Pinckney, and Washington.

Americans now made a major turn. U.S.-British relations rapidly improved, while the French—embittered that the United States would accept the Jay Treaty but not honor the 1778 alliance—turned against Washington's administration. The French minister to Philadelphia, Pierre Adet, first tried to block the Jay Treaty, then worked vigorously to have Jefferson win the 1796 presidential election over Federalist candidate John Adams. That interference influenced Washington to

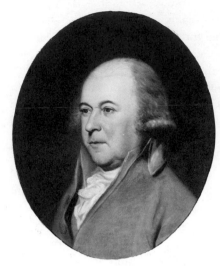

John Adams (1735–1826) was dour, brilliant, a leader of the revolutionary movement, and a co-negotiator of the 1783 peace treaty. The nation's first vice-president, then president (1797–1801), he demonstrated courage and skill in making peace instead of war with France in 1799–1800 and, as a result, decisively lost re-election in 1800.

issue (in a newspaper) his Farewell Address that warned Americans against tying themselves to the fortunes of any "foreign influence." In words that have not lost their importance nearly two hundred years later, the president observed that "the nation which indulges toward another an habitual hatred or an habitual fondness is in some degree a slave." If such "slavery" could be avoided, he held out a magnificent vision: the growth of their power until Americans could virtually do whatever they wished. The Farewell Address remains significant because it argued that if Americans were restrained in the 1790s, they would have to suffer few restraints later. Of equal importance, the Farewell Address remains the major statement of the need for American freedom of action, a central theme in the first two centuries of U.S. foreign policy.[20]

Adams won the election, but Jefferson's triumph would have produced much the same foreign policy, Adet believed:

> [Jefferson, Adet reported to Paris,] seeks to draw near to us because he fears us less than England; but tomorrow he might change his opinion about us if England should cease to inspire his fear. . . . Jefferson, I say, is an American, and as such, he cannot sincerely be our friend. An American is the born enemy of all the peoples of Europe.[21]

John Adams led a rapidly developing but still primitive country—so primitive that when his wife Abigail took a coach from Philadelphia to join him in the new capital city of Washington, she became lost in the wilderness south of Baltimore. "You find nothing but a forest and woods on the way," she complained. But the city's location revealed great insight into the country's future, because it had been placed on the Potomac River in the belief that the waterway was to become a major route westward.[22]

With usual American sensitivity to events beyond the mountains, Adams quickly heard of Spanish and French plots to win over the distant settlements. George Rogers Clark, hero of the American Revolution, even became involved in some of the schemes, despite—or because of—a severe drinking problem. The president seized the initiative by sending three diplomats to France for talks. They were to terminate the 1778 alliance, make the French promise to behave in the West, and win France's recognition of wide-ranging U.S. trading rights. Three French agents, code-named "X," "Y," and "Z," countered with simpler proposals: Adams must apologize for his past criticism of the French, then give Paris a large loan as well as a $250,000 bribe to grease the negotiations. They also expected help in the ongoing war against the British. An astounded Adams broke off the talks. The cry was born, "Millions for Defense, but not one Cent for Tribute!"

The president had to fight a two-front struggle. An "undeclared war" broke out with France, which seized more U.S. ships between 1797 and 1800 than did the greater British fleet. On the home front, Hamilton, now a powerful lawyer in New York City, worked through his informants in Adams's cabinet to seize the opportunity and strike at the crumbling Spanish Empire in the South and West—preferably with British help. Adams and Hamilton, despite being fellow Federalists, had become bitter political enemies. Their personalities clashed, and the president strongly disagreed with Hamilton's pro-British views. Closer to Madison on the trade question, Adams wanted a vigorous, independent U.S. commerce. He called Hamilton "the bastard brat of a Scots peddler." Hamilton, in turn, had tried to block Adams's victory in 1796. Now Hamilton not only hoped to break ties with France, but personally to lead an army that would conquer the Floridas and trans-Mississippi—and even "take a squint at Mexico." Adams, who knew about Hamilton's admiration for Caesar, concluded that "this man is stark mad or I am."

Meanwhile, the Federalists pushed the Alien and Sedition Acts through Congress. These measures gave the government power to arrest aliens as well as newspaper editors who were suspected of being pro-French. In reality, the Federalists used the acts to persecute Jeffersonians. Not for the last time in American history was the threat of conflict abroad used to justify a witch hunt at home. Jefferson and Madison responded with resolutions passed in the Virginia and Kentucky state

legislatures. These measures defied the two acts and implied that disunion would occur if the Federalists did not retreat.

The danger thus arose of both a full-scale war with France and a
constitutional crisis at home. Adams commissioned three fighting ships
and established the United States Navy Department to oversee operations. George Logan, a Pennsylvania Quaker, took it upon himself to
sail to France and work out a peace settlement. His mission failed, and
the Federalists passed the Logan Act, which made it illegal for any
private citizen to negotiate with a foreign government. (In the 1960s
through 1980s, the government threatened to invoke the law—for
example, against actress Jane Fonda, who traveled to Vietnam—but
the law was not applied.)

As U.S.-French relations reached a critical point, Adams took a
politically dangerous but statesmanlike step. He overruled Hamilton
and dispatched a peace mission to Paris. The president believed that
France posed less of a danger ("There is no more prospect of seeing a
French army here, than there is in heaven," Adams thought) than did
Hamilton. Adams worried more about the probability of becoming
involved in the Napoleonic Wars and the possibility of a severed Union.
The French were now ready to deal. They needed U.S. trade, especially after the British fleet had nearly destroyed their navy. The Convention of 1800 ended the 1778 alliance. In return, the United States
agreed to assume claims against France (although these were never
fully honored). Each side agreed to grant the other most-favored-nation
rights in trade and—not surprisingly—declared that neutrals (such as
the United States) should have extensive rights to trade during wartime.

The United States thus ended the last European alliance it would
have for nearly a century and a half. The experience had been bitter.
The costs even touched the possibility of disunion. In 1801, Jefferson
recalled how the western and eastern states had preserved the new
constitutional system by balancing each other in the Jay Treaty and
undeclared war crises. He concluded that those experiences provided
"a new proof of the falsehood of Montesquieu's doctrine, that a republic can be preserved in only a small territory. The reverse is the truth.
Had our territory been even a third only of what it is, we were gone."[23]

JEFFERSON AND LOUISIANA

To the astonishment of many, the United States managed a peaceful
transition of power in the 1800 election from Adams's Federalists to

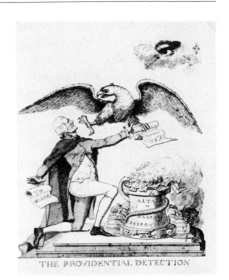

THE PROVIDENTIAL DETECTION

"The Providential Detection" is a superb American graphic drawn for the bitter 1800 election fight by an artist who clearly hated Jefferson and his supposed ties to revolutionary France. As the Virginian kneels at the burning altar of French "despotism," a powerful (and beautifully sketched) American eagle stops Jefferson from throwing the Constitution into the flames. Note the all-seeing eye (in the upper right corner) watching out for the United States.

Jefferson's Republicans. The campaign had been brutal. The pro-Adams president of Yale, Timothy Dwight, warned that if Jefferson won, "we may see the Bible cast into a bonfire, the vessels of the sacramental supper borne by an ass in public procession," and "our wives and daughters the victims of legal prostitution." The reality was less exciting. Historian William Stinchcombe has noted that Adams was actually beaten by the backlash against the Federalist war scare—"the greatly increased defense spending, particularly on the army, and the notorious Alien and Sedition Acts," which Jefferson turned to his political advantage. The news of peace with France arrived too late to save Adams. In any case, years later he wrote that "I desire no other inscription on my gravestone than: 'here lies John Adams, who took upon himself the responsibility of peace with France in 1800.' " The new president moved quickly to build a consensus. "We are all Republicans, we are all Federalists," he declared in his 1801 inaugural address.[24]

He appointed his close friend James Madison secretary of state. Their foreign-policy assumptions were few but direct. As Jefferson wrote in 1801, American expansion should be thought of as virtually unlimited:

> However our present situation may restrain us within our own limits, it is impossible not to look forward to distant times, when our rapid multiplication will expand itself beyond those limits, and cover the whole northern, if not the southern continent, with a people speaking the same language, governed in similar forms, and by similar laws; nor can we contemplate with satisfaction blot or mixture on that surface.[25]

To achieve these goals, Americans had to protect their freedom of action: "Peace, commerce, and honest friendship with all nations, entangling alliances with none," as he announced in his inaugural address. In a rephrase of Paine's *Common Sense* and Washington's Farewell Address, Jefferson told a friend that "we have a perfect horror of everything connecting ourselves with the politics of Europe," but because Americans are "daily growing stronger," if they can have a few more years to build their power, they can tell others how the United States must be treated, "and we will say it."[26] Power abroad, as Madison had told Patrick Henry in 1788 (see p. 35), depended on effective rule at home. In this sense, Jefferson became the first chief executive to manage Congress through well-disciplined party leaders who followed the president's wishes. His foreign policies were often effective because he was able to whip Congress into line to support them. Jefferson successfully centralized power in the new Executive Mansion.[27]

Nor was Jefferson reluctant to build and use military power. However, he kept a sense of proportion. He never believed that the young United States could build a navy to challenge the British fleet, but he built a small flotilla of gunboats to fight the Barbary States between 1801 and 1805. Operating out of the North African Islamic states of Tripoli, Algiers, Tunis, and Morocco, the raiders demanded large tributes from ships plying the Mediterranean or the ships would be seized and sailors brutalized. Washington and Adams had paid tribute to these robbers. Jefferson refused and sent four warships to protect U.S. commerce. One ship ran aground, and Tripoli seized the crew. It was the first overseas hostage crisis in American history.

Jefferson went to war. Scoring several sensational victories on both sea and land, the president nevertheless had to pay $60,000 to obtain Tripoli's pledge not to capture other U.S. ships. During the War of 1812, the plundering of U.S. ships began again, but in 1815 President Madison dispatched a small fleet that forced the Barbary States to retreat. The U.S. Navy then leased a port on the island of Majorca in the Mediterranean so it could move quickly against future plundering. The American war with Barbary, however, was over.[28]

These characteristics of Jefferson's foreign policy—expansionism, freedom of action, centralization of power, and the willingness to use force in selected situations—appeared in his greatest triumph, the purchase of Louisiana in 1803. But the affair could have been a diplomatic catastrophe. Jefferson and Madison found themselves facing a crisis in 1801 when they learned that the weakened Spanish had finally

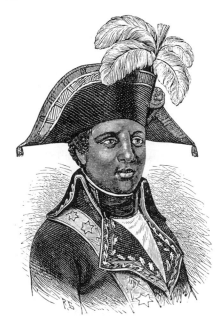

Toussaint L'Ouverture (1743–1803), the black revolutionary who led the fight to drive the French from Haiti, inadvertently helped the United States to purchase the Louisiana Territory from France.

surrendered to Napoleon's demands and sold him the Louisiana Territory. His war with Great Britain had stopped (temporarily, it soon turned out), and Napoleon turned to developing a New World empire. He especially wanted to find a food supply in Louisiana for the black slaves who produced highly profitable sugar crops in Haiti and Santo Domingo. In 1802, the crisis intensified when Spanish officials (who still controlled New Orleans) suddenly shut off the Mississippi to U.S. trade. Madison had long understood that whoever controlled that great river controlled the rapidly multiplying Americans settling in the West: "The Mississippi is to them everything," he wrote privately in late 1802. "It is the Hudson, the Delaware, the Potomac, and all the navigable rivers of the Atlantic States formed into one stream."[29]

In 1802, Jefferson and Madison devised a brilliant series of policies that finally forced Napoleon to sell not only New Orleans (the primary American objective), but most of the immense area between the Mississippi and the Rocky Mountains. First, Madison sent secret help to black revolutionaries, led by Toussaint L'Ouverture, who were fighting to overthrow French rule in Haiti. The secretary of state knew that without the sugar island of which Haiti was a part, Napoleon would not need Louisiana as a granary. The French finally captured Toussaint. But his followers fought on, and their successes—together with malaria, which devastated the French troops—led Napoleon to blurt out in frustration in early 1803, "Damn sugar, damn coffee, damn colonies."

Second, Jefferson used his Indian policy to pressure the French. Having long hoped to "civilize" the Native Americans, Jefferson suddenly ordered the removal of tribes into the trans-Mississippi region. This order forced Napoleon to worry about them, while turning the Midwest into a secure all-white base from which Jefferson could attack New Orleans. The greatest historian of the Jeffersonian era, Henry Adams, graphically summarized the effect on the Native Americans: "No acid ever worked more mechanically on a vegetable fibre than the white man acted on the Indian. As the line of American settlements approached, the nearest Indian tribes withered away."[30] Some tribes, however, finally fought bitterly in 1810–1811 before retreating.

Third, the president obtained authority from Congress to build 15 gunboats and raise 80,000 men for an assault on the lower Mississippi. Napoleon learned of this in early April 1803, just as he was pondering the failure of a large French force to sail to the New World because a late winter had frozen over European ports. Since Jefferson had sent James Monroe and Edward Livingston to purchase New Orleans and the Floridas for $10 million, they were in Paris (where Livingston was the U.S. minister) when Napoleon decided to unload all of his mainland holdings. About to start the war against Great Britain once more, he needed freedom from New World malaria, slave revolts, and possible war with the United States, as well as the money the sale would bring. He asked, and Jefferson finally agreed to pay, $15 million for all of Louisiana. Luck had helped give Jefferson and Madison the opportunity, but they had seized upon it to double the size of the United States.[31]

But the crisis was not over. Nothing in the Constitution provided for such an acquisition. When Louisiana developed into numerous new states, the balance of political power and the nature of American society could be radically changed. Federalists in New England were especially fearful. "We rush like a comet into infinite space," proclaimed Fisher Ames of Massachusetts. "Our country is too big for union, too sordid for patriotism, too democratic for liberty." Ames and other Federalists began planning to pull New England out of the Union. They apparently received encouragement from, of all people, Aaron Burr, vice-president of the United States. By 1803–1804, Burr and Jefferson had become bitter political enemies. The Ames Federalists, however, remained a small, if dangerous, minority. More representative was his-

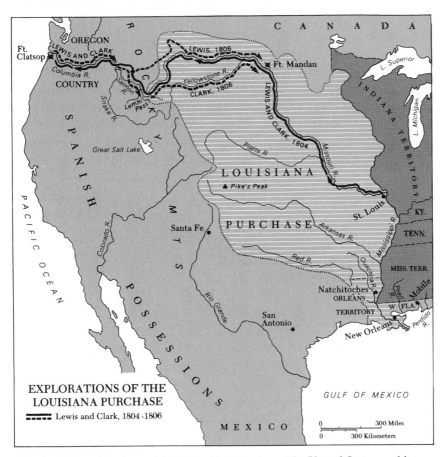

EXPLORATIONS OF THE
LOUISIANA PURCHASE
▰▰▰▰ Lewis and Clark, 1804-1806

The Louisiana Purchase of 1803 doubled the size of the United States and later provided thirteen of the fifty states. The map also shows exploration that led to further settlement and expansion. When Napoleon sold the territory and was told that the boundaries were vague, he observed, correctly, that he supposed the Americans would make the most of vague territorial claims.

torian David Ramsay's oration of 1804 on the theme "What territory can be too large for a people, who multiply with such unequalled rapidity?"[32]

With that kind of support, Jefferson construed the Constitution liberally and assumed the United States could acquire and rule large new areas. He received backing from Gouverneur Morris, who had written a draft of the Constitution for the convention's debates in 1787. Morris pointed to Article IV, Section 3: "New States may be admitted . . . into this Union. . . . The Congress shall have Power to dispose of and make all needful Rules and Regulations respecting the Territory or other

Property belonging to the United States." In 1803, Morris added, "I always thought that when we should acquire Canada and Louisiana it would be proper to govern them as provinces and allow them no voice in our Councils."[33] Jefferson followed Morris's advice. He had little hope that the Indians, French, Spaniards, Creoles, and runaway Americans who had fled to New Orleans (often to escape a U.S. jail) were capable of self-government. Consequently, he obtained legislation that allowed him to rule Louisiana as a virtual dictator until it was peopled by responsible Anglo-Saxons. Meanwhile, order and security were to be maintained through force, if necessary.[34]

Thus, strong national power secured Louisiana. But arguments over who was to exert this power did lead to civil war in 1861, although not in the way Ames had envisioned. Meanwhile, Jefferson and Madison so disregarded Federalist fears that from 1804 to 1806 they tried through diplomacy, bribery, and covert pressures to pry the Floridas out of Spanish hands. These efforts stalled, especially as the two men suddenly faced a major conflict with the British Empire on the Atlantic sea lanes.

THE SECOND WAR FOR INDEPENDENCE AND UNION

In 1805, prospering U.S. trade with both warring nations, Great Britain and France, came under attack from British author Sir James Stephen, who, in his *War in Disguise; or, The Frauds of the Neutral Flags*, argued that England should use its naval superiority to stop U.S. trade that aided Napoleon. That same year, British courts issued the *Essex* decision. It declared illegal and subject to seizure those U.S. ships that picked up goods in the French West Indies, off-loaded them briefly in the United States so that they would appear to be American goods, and then carried them to France. As the British began seizing U.S. ships, Napoleon retaliated by announcing a blockade of Great Britain, a blockade he could not enforce. Any ship entering European ports after stops in England, he declared, would be seized.

After "fattening upon the follies" of the Old World, as Jefferson had phrased it, Americans were becoming victims trapped between the two European giants. In a brilliant pamphlet of 1806, Madison attacked the new British regulations and warned that "all history" proved that war results from "commercial rivalships" of nations. He and Jefferson tried to counter not with military force, but with a Nonimportation Act of 1806 that threatened to exclude imports, especially British, until the Europeans promised to respect U.S. neutral rights. In compiling the list of excluded goods, however, the two men made a frightening discovery: Americans were more dependent on British textiles, iron, and steel than the British were on American goods. Jefferson believed that he could not afford to exclude those badly needed products. U.S. economic power was turning out to be quite different than Paine, Madison, and others had assumed it would be.

While he delayed putting the Nonimportation Act into effect, Jefferson confronted a more immediate problem. Great Britain had intensified its impressment searches of deserters from its fleet. Tens of thousands of British sailors had escaped from the poor pay, unspeakable food and conditions, and brutality (lashings were frequent) at a moment when England was locked into a battle to the death with Napoleon. A large number—perhaps as many as eight out of every ten men seized—were Americans who were then impressed into the dangers of British service. In June 1807, a British warship, the *Leopard*, boarded the U.S. ship *Chesapeake* just ten miles off Chesapeake Bay, killed three Americans, wounded eighteen, then carried off four men, of whom only one was a British citizen. Americans demanded revenge. At this moment, Jefferson could have taken a near-united nation into war against Great Britain. He realized, however, his relative military weakness and believed that economic pressure could force the British to behave. In November 1807, London announced orders in council tightening control over neutral shipping. Napoleon responded with a similar decree affecting ships dealing with the British.

When the president raised the possibility of war, his able secretary of the Treasury Albert Gallatin warned that the British could "land at Annapolis, march to [Washington]," and return to England before Jefferson could even raise a militia to fight. Meanwhile, as Federalist senator John Quincy Adams noted, the British orders struck "at the very root of our independence."[35] Jefferson finally responded with an Embargo Act that closed U.S. ports and made exports illegal. Unintentionally, the president helped the British, who could handle their own commerce, by cutting off French trade. He also infuriated American merchants and producers of exports, whose survival depended on trade. When smuggling intensified, Jefferson made arbitrary arrests and seizures of goods. As historian Burton Spivak argues, Jefferson faced a terrible choice between his belief in democratic ideals and his belief in the commercial destiny of Americans.[36] The president's political party as well as his ideals were threatened. In 1808, Madison won the Executive Mansion, but the Federalists, using the embargo as a whip against him, tripled their 1804 electoral vote.

Leaving office in early 1809, Jefferson proudly told his successor that, with Louisiana and after Florida, Cuba, and Canada were annexed, the United States would be "such an empire for liberty as [the world] has never surveyed since the creation; and I am persuaded no constitution was ever before so well calculated as ours for extensive empire and self-government."[37] Both his vision and his confidence in the Constitution, however, were to be tested in the next five years.

Jefferson, under strong congressional pressure, was forced to end the embargo as he left office. Congress replaced it with the Nonintercourse Act of 1809 that prohibited both British and French ships and goods from U.S. ports but pledged to restore normal commerce with any country that repealed its restrictions on American trade. When this measure brought no good result, Congress, in 1810, passed Macon's Bill Number 2, which reopened U.S. ports to all peaceful commerce but promised commercial nonintercourse against one country (for example, Great Britain), if the other (France) repealed its anti-U.S. trade laws. It was a law heaven-sent to a manipulator like Napoleon. He declared the restrictions lifted, then added conditions that meant that they were not lifted at all. A desperate, if suspicious, Madison foolishly accepted the emperor's assurance and cut off trade with England in early 1811. The British were furious, Madison humiliated, once Napoleon's scheme became clear. U.S. economic pressures were not working.

As early as 1809, the president had wondered whether war might be the only real alternative; by 1811, it was his firm conviction. He was not alone. The South and West were emerging from a severe three-year economic depression caused, in the view of the brilliant young South Carolina congressman John Calhoun, not by Madison's actions, but by "foreign injustice" committed by the British, who aimed to enslave Americans again into a "colonial state." The sharp decline of southern cotton exports from 93 million pounds in 1809 to 62 million pounds in 1811 allowed Calhoun to conclude that if the British continued to control U.S. trade, "the independence of this nation is lost. . . . This is the second struggle for our liberty."[38] The young Speaker of the House of Representatives in 1811–1812, Henry Clay of Kentucky, loudly agreed. Born in Virginia, trained in the law as well as in the dueling ritual and the gambling and drinking halls of frontier Kentucky, the tall, dynamic thirty-four-year-old Clay was rightly described by one political oppo-

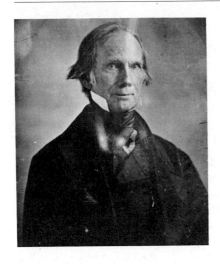

Henry Clay (1777–1852) was born in Virginia and became a plantation owner in Kentucky. A power in the House of Representatives (1811–1825), he led the war hawks into the War of 1812. Later, as a U.S. senator, he championed commercial expansion and, as "the Great Pacificator," helped craft the compromises of 1820 and 1850 that temporarily preserved the Union from the strain of expansionism.

nent as "bold, aspiring, presumptuous, with a rough overbearing eloquence."[39] Running the House with a firm hand and working closely with Madison, Clay and Calhoun led a group of "War Hawks" elected in 1810 who were determined to force the British to behave.

Their determination turned to fury when news arrived in Washington during late November 1811 that a battle with Indians at Tippecanoe in Indiana territory resulted in the deaths of sixty-eight white men, including some well known to Clay and other war hawks. Evidence also arrived that the British had incited the Indians.[40] War hawks wore black armbands and charged London with "inciting the savages to murder." In truth, territorial governor William Henry Harrison's sharp practices had cheated the Native Americans of most of Indiana for a few dollars. Led by two great leaders, Tecumseh (a statesman and orator who preached that all land belonged to all Indians) and his brother Tenskwatawa the Prophet, the Native Americans had warned Harrison that they wanted no part of the white man's version of private property. "Sell a country!" Tecumseh exclaimed. "Why not sell the air, the clouds and the great sea, as well as the earth? Did not the Great Spirit make them all for the use of his children?"[41] Tecumseh hoped to avoid war—at least until he organized tribes as far south as Florida. But when Harrison marched close to the Prophet's town, the Winnebago tribe attacked. Suffering fewer casualties than Harrison's forces, the Native Americans nevertheless retreated, meanwhile scalping isolated white settlers on the way.

The war hawks and Madison prepared for battle. The president took the opportunity to order a secret operation to seize West Florida from

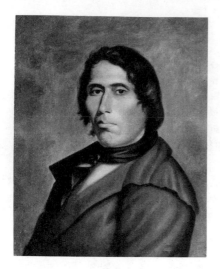

Tecumseh (1768–1813), a Shawnee leader who tried to stop the expansionism of the whites by allying Indian tribes from the Great Lakes to Florida. When the War of 1812 erupted, he fought with the British and was killed at the Battle of the Thames in Canada during the autumn of 1813.

the Spanish. He organized a coup, after which the plotters asked for U.S. annexation. The president nicely reasoned that the seizure was necessary to prevent the British from taking the area first. West Florida formally became a part of the Union in 1811. Madison then tried to repeat the operation in East Florida. That attempt, however, became an embarrassment when his secret agents botched the scheme. The president and Congress nevertheless declared in 1811 that henceforth they would not tolerate the transfer of New World territory owned by a foreign power to another foreign country. This "nontransfer principle" later became a part of the Monroe Doctrine.

Madison next named fellow Virginian James Monroe, who had close ties with the West, to replace Robert Smith as secretary of state. Smith, a Marylander, came from a mercantile group that hated Madison's economic policies. Moving toward war, the president then proposed to build a larger navy. But that measure lost 62 to 59 in the House. Clay and Calhoun voted for it, but every westerner except Clay voted "nay" on the grounds that the bill would, in the words of a Kentucky journal, "give an overwhelming influence to the commercial interest" in eastern cities. It was an odd way to prepare for war against the world's greatest naval power. The West, however, along with Madison and Jefferson, thought that the war would actually be decided beyond the Appalachians, especially in an invasion of Canada.

On June 1, 1812, Madison sent his war message to Congress. He charged the British with impressment, spilling "American blood" within American territory (a reference to the *Chesapeake* affair), "pretended blockades" and orders in council that allowed the British to have "plundered" U.S. shipping, and the "warfare just renewed by the savages" in the West. In reality, since 1807, the British had seized only 389 U.S. ships, while Napoleon had taken at least 460. But those numbers did not move Madison. The British threatened U.S. interests globally because of their naval power, their avowed competition for markets in such newly opening areas as Latin America (a region now breaking away from Spain), and their ties to the Native Americans. The House voted for war 79 to 49, the Senate 19 to 13. Voting was along party lines. The pro-war vote stretched through all geographical sections, including the coastal cities, whose merchants worked closely with British mercantile interests. Some of these merchants apparently preferred war to continued halfway measures such as embargoes. (Moreover, once war began, many of them grew rich smuggling and supplying British forces.) There can be no doubt, however, that, in the words of historian Ronald Hatzenbuehler, it was Madison, Monroe, and Clay who were "primarily responsible for directing war preparations."[42]

In July 1812, Americans were stunned to learn that on June 16 the British had repealed their orders in council. An economic depression, demands from British merchants, and a change in government in London led to the repeal. Historians have since speculated whether, if a transatlantic telegraph had existed in 1812 to speed the news of the repeal, the war would have been avoided. Probably not, for the impressment and Indian issues remained. The opportunity to conquer Canada was irresistible. Madison refused to reconsider the war declaration. Since 1789, he had determined to free U.S. commerce from British control. Now he had a chance to do it.

FROM NEAR-CATASTROPHE TO NEAR-VICTORY

No sane American hoped for victory on the high seas (the British fleet had three fighting *ships* for every U.S. *cannon*).[43] Instead, Madison hoped to take advantage of Great Britain's preoccupation with Napoleon and believed that Canada could be seized as a hostage (as well as turned into a future U.S. state).

However, when U.S. forces drove into Canada, they were met by determined resistance—which included many Loyalists who had left the United States during the Revolution—and suffered a series of humiliating defeats. Tecumseh, in late 1812, seized the opportunity to unite tribes and join the British to capture both Detroit and an entire

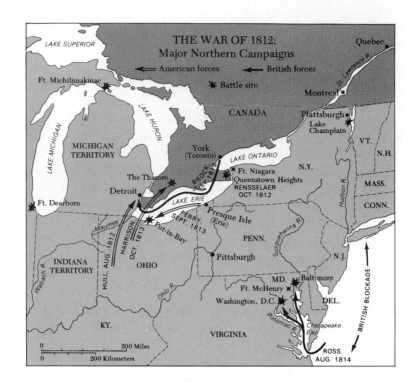

THE WAR OF 1812:
Major Northern Campaigns

← American forces ← British forces

✴ Battle site

LAKE SUPERIOR

Quebec

Ft. Michilimackinac

CANADA

Montreal

Plattsburgh
Lake
Champlain

LAKE HURON

MICHIGAN
TERRITORY

LAKE MICHIGAN

York
(Toronto)

LAKE ONTARIO

VT.

N.H.

BROCK, JULY 1812

Ft. Niagara
Queenstown Heights
RENSSELAER
OCT. 1812

N.Y.

MASS.

Hudson R.

The Thames

Detroit

CONN.

Ft. Dearborn

LAKE ERIE

Presque Isle
(Erie)

PERRY
SEPT. 1813

Put-in-Bay

Maumee R.

HARRISON, OCT. 1813

HULL, AUG. 1812

PENN.

Susquehanna R.

INDIANA
TERRITORY

OHIO

Pittsburgh

N.J.

Wabash R.

Ohio R.

MD.

Baltimore

Ft. McHenry

Washington, D.C.

DEL.

BRITISH BLOCKADE

KY.

VIRGINIA

Potomac R.

Chesapeake
Bay

0   200 Miles

0   200 Kilometers

ROSS,
AUG. 1814

St. Lawrence R.

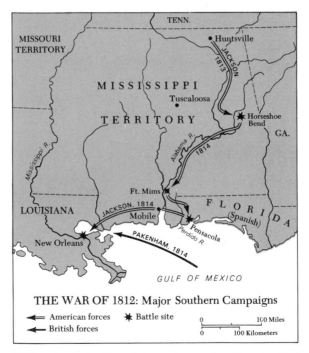

TENN.

MISSOURI
TERRITORY

Huntsville

JACKSON
1813

MISSISSIPPI

Tuscaloosa

TERRITORY

Horseshoe
Bend

GA.

Alabama R.

1814

Mississippi R.

Ft. Mims

FLORIDA
(Spanish)

LOUISIANA

JACKSON, 1814

Mobile

Pensacola

Perdido R.

New Orleans

PAKENHAM, 1814

GULF OF MEXICO

THE WAR OF 1812: Major Southern Campaigns

← American forces ✴ Battle site

← British forces

0   100 Miles

0   100 Kilometers

The War of 1812, which the United States lost on land but finally battled the British to a draw because of U.S. victories on the lakes and rivers.

American army. The Potawatomi tribe took the occasion to massacre everyone at Fort Dearborn (now Chicago). William Henry Harrison finally killed Tecumseh in 1813 after a series of brilliant U.S. naval victories on the Great Lakes sealed off British aid and isolated the Indian leader. Harrison held the Old Northwest, but Canada could not be conquered.

In the South, General Andrew Jackson of Tennessee, aided by Cherokees, defeated Creek Indians (the "Red Sticks") and then dictated a peace that opened much of Alabama to whites. Jackson was suddenly a national hero. He soon became a household word in January 1815, when his troops squashed a British invasion at the Battle of New Orleans. That triumph helped propel Jackson to the White House in 1828, although it occurred two weeks after the peace treaty was signed in Europe.

Otherwise, the war was notable because it nearly destroyed the new constitutional government. British ships controlled the coast. Their troops landed in Washington, burned the city in 1814, and forced James and Dolley Madison to escape into the hills across the Potomac River. Even Calhoun was dispirited: "Our executive officers are most incompetent men. . . . We are literally boren [*sic*] down under the effects of errors and mismanagement."[44] New England's (especially Boston's) merchants openly traded with, and loaned money to, Great Britain. In late 1814, some of these New Englanders met at Hartford, Connecticut, and threatened to leave the Union unless constitutional amendments gave them veto power over such issues as commercial questions and the admission of new western states into the Union. Only the peace treaty negotiated at Ghent, Belgium, in late 1814 ended this threat of possible secession.

Actually, within two weeks after war began, Madison had sought peace talks. By late 1813, the British were ready to deal: the wars with Napoleon seemed to be ending, so impressment could be stopped. London military officials had no stomach for dispatching the huge, costly force and fighting the long war required to conquer the United States. Sharp changes in Europe's diplomatic situation demanded British attention as well. As historian Donald Hickey summarizes, the British wanted peace because "of the lack of military progress in America [especially on the Great Lakes], unfavorable diplomatic developments in Europe, and domestic discontent over taxes."[45] The distinguished U.S. diplomatic team consisted of Henry Clay, John Quincy Adams, and Albert Gallatin (Jefferson's brilliant former secretary of the Treasury, who spent much of his time keeping peace between the ram-

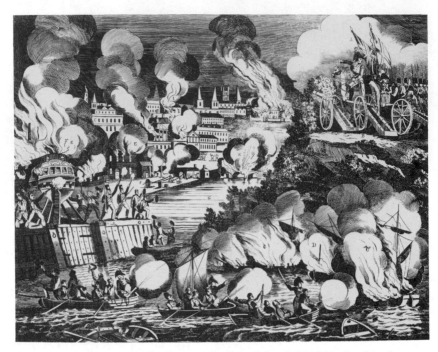

As part of their major land offensive, the British landed in Maryland in August 1814, then marched on and burned the capital at Washington, D.C. President and Dolley Madison fled the city, and then a tornado hit the capital to complete the destruction. The British were finally beaten at Baltimore, and peace terms were signed in December 1814.

bunctious Clay and the dour Adams). They stopped a British demand for the annexation of Maine and parts of New York. The two sides then worked out the Treaty of Ghent (or the Peace of Christmas Eve). Both countries simply accepted the prewar territorial boundaries. Nothing was included about neutral rights.

Given the disastrous military situation around Washington and the disastrous political situation in New England, the United States won a remarkable diplomatic victory. The War of 1812 would be remembered less for Madison's embarrassed rush from a burning capital than for producing "The Star Spangled Banner," Uncle Sam (an actual person who provided supplies to beleaguered U.S. troops), and Jackson's postwar triumph at New Orleans. Because of the end of the Napoleonic Wars in Europe, impressment and orders in council no longer troubled relations. Hartford Federalists and their demands evaporated in the warm light of peace.

But it had been a brush with tragedy. The Jay Treaty, the X Y Z affair, the Alien and Sedition Acts, New England's anger over political power moving toward Louisiana, and Hartford's last-gasp attempt to remain within the rich British trading system even if it meant leaving the American one—all had threatened to destroy the Union. The nation had survived—if barely—and Americans were free for the first time since their independence forty years before to turn west and seize the incredible opportunities of a continental empire. It was to be a turn, however, that again nearly destroyed their Union in civil war.

NOTES

1. Merrill Jensen, *The New Nation* (New York, 1950), pp. 88–92.
2. Edmund S. Morgan, "The American Revolution Considered as an Intellectual Movement," in *Paths of American Thought*, ed. Morton White and A. M. Schlesinger (Boston, 1963), pp. 32–33.
3. Richard B. Morris, *Seven Who Shaped Our Destiny* (New York, 1973), p. 1; Arthur M. Schlesinger, Jr., *The Imperial Presidency* (Boston, 1973), p. 15.
4. Bradford Perkins, *From Sea to Sea, 1776–1865*, in *The Cambridge History of U.S. Foreign Relations*, ed. Warren Cohen (New York, 1993), ch. III.
5. Rowland A. Berthoff, *An Unsettled People* (New York, 1971), pp. 136–137.
6. U.S. Bureau of the Census, *Historical Statistics of the United States: Colonial Times to 1957* (Washington, D.C., 1960), p. 547.
7. Reginald Horsman, "American Indian Policy and the Origins of Manifest Destiny," *University of Birmingham Historical Journal* 11, no. 2 (1968): 131–134.
8. Joyce Appleby, "Commercial Farming and the 'Agrarian Myth' in the Early Republic," *Journal of American History* 68 (March 1982): 840–841.
9. See Howard Kushner's review of N. N. Bashkina *et al.*, *The United States and Russia* in *Journal of American History* 68 (June 1981): 125; Irby C. Nichols, Jr., "The Russian Ukase and the Monroe Doctrine: A Re-evaluation," *Pacific Historical Review* 36 (February 1967): 13–26.
10. Bradford Perkins, *The First Rapprochement: England and the United States, 1795–1805* (Philadelphia, 1955), p. 24.
11. Saul Padover, *Jefferson* (New York, 1942), p. 182.
12. *Washington Post*, 22 February 1985, p. E1; Marcus Cunliffe, *George Washington, Man and Monument* (Boston, 1958), p. 129.
13. Arthur B. Darling, *Our Rising Empire, 1763–1803* (New Haven, 1940), p. 130.
14. Irving Brant, *James Madison*, 6 vols. (Indianapolis, 1944–1961), III, pp. 246–254.
15. William P. Cresson, *James Monroe* (Chapel Hill, N.C., 1946), pp. 120–121.
16. J. Fred Rippy and Angie Debo, *The Historical Background of the American Policy of Isolation* (Northampton, Mass., 1924), pp. 148–149.
17. Brant, III, pp. 375, 382.
18. Joseph E. Charles, *The Origins of the American Party System* (New York, 1961), p. 85.

19. *Ibid.*, p. 113.
20. Burton I. Kaufman, "Washington's Farewell Address: A Statement of Empire," in *Washington's Farewell Address: The View from the Twentieth Century*, ed. Burton I. Kaufman (Chicago, 1969), a fine selection; Victor Hugo Paltsits's *Washington's Farewell Address* (New York, 1935) remains the best study that includes the various drafts.
21. The quote and an analysis are in Samuel Flagg Bemis, "The Farewell Address: A Foreign Policy of Independence," *American Historical Review* 39 (January 1934): 267.
22. Alfred Kazin, "In Washington," *New York Review of Books*, 29 May 1986, pp. 11–12.
23. Thomas Jefferson to Nathaniel Niles, 22 March 1801, in *The Writings of Jefferson*, ed. Paul Leicester Ford, 10 vols. (New York, 1892–1899), IX, p. 221.
24. William Stinchcombe, *The XYZ Affair* (Westport, Conn., 1980), p. 129; Albert Jay Nock, *Jefferson* (Washington, D.C., 1926), pp. 237–239; Perkins, *From Sea to Sea*, ch. IV.
25. Thomas Jefferson to James Monroe, 24 November 1801, in *The Writings of Thomas Jefferson*, ed. Andrew A. Libscomb, 20 vols. (Washington, D.C., 1903), X, p. 296.
26. Thomas Jefferson to William Short, 3 October 1801, in *The Writings*, ed. Ford, VIII, p. 98.
27. Good discussions of Jefferson's use of presidential powers are Abraham D. Sofaer, *War, Foreign Affairs, and Constitutional Power: The Origins* (Cambridge, Mass., 1976), pp. 167–227, and Robert M. Johnstone, Jr., *Jefferson and the Presidency* (Ithaca, N.Y., 1978); on Madison's role, Richard E. Ellis, *The Jeffersonian Crisis* (New York, 1971), pp. 236–237.
28. An interesting post-1979 perspective is Forrest McDonald, "The Hostage Crisis of 1803," *Washington Post*, 20 May 1980, p. A19; also Reginald Horsman, *The Diplomacy of the New Republic, 1776–1815* (Arlington Heights, Ill., 1986), pp. 84–86.
29. James Madison to Thomas Pinckney, 27 November 1802, in *The Writings of James Madison*, ed. Gaillard Hunt, 9 vols. (New York, 1901), VI, p. 462.
30. Henry Adams, *History of the United States during the Administrations of Jefferson and Madison*, 9 vols. (New York, 1889–1891), VI, 69.
31. The best account is Alexander DeConde, *This Affair of Louisiana* (New York, 1976); see also E. Wilson Lyon, *Louisiana in French Diplomacy, 1759–1804* (Norman, Okla., 1934), pp. 195–202; James Madison to Edward Livingston, 18 January 1803, in *The Writings*, ed. Hunt, VII, p. 7.
32. William H. Goetzmann, *When the Eagle Screamed* (New York, 1966), p. 9; Julian P. Boyd, "Thomas Jefferson's 'Empire of Liberty,'" *Virginia Quarterly Review* 24 (Autumn 1948): 553.
33. Drew McCoy, *The Elusive Republic* (Chapel Hill, N.C., 1980), p. 203; Gouverneur Morris to Robert Livingston, 4 December 1803, quoted in *Congressional Record*, 55th Cong., 3d sess., 19 December 1898, p. 294.
34. James Madison to Robert R. Livingston, 31 January 1804, in *The Writings*, ed. Hunt, VII, pp. 114–116. Jefferson's constitutional problems set historical precedents and are examined in Walter LaFeber, "An Expansionist's Dilemma," *Constitution* 5 (Fall 1993):5–13.
35. Gilbert Chinard, *Thomas Jefferson . . .* (Boston, 1926), pp. 420–421.
36. Bradford Perkins, *Prologue to War: England and the United States, 1805–1812* (Berkeley, 1961), p. 77; Paul A. Varg, *Foreign Policies of the Founding Fathers* (East Lansing,

Mich., 1963), pp. 190–192; Burton Spivak's *Jefferson's English Crisis* (Charlottesville, Va., 1984) is a fine analysis.

37. Boyd's "Thomas Jefferson's 'Empire of Liberty' " gives the context.

38. John Calhoun's reply to John Randolph, 12 December 1811 and defense of 29 November, House Foreign Affairs Report, in *John Calhoun, Papers*, ed. Robert L. Meriwether (Columbia, S.C., 1959–), I, p. 83; Perkins, pp. 434–435; U.S. Bureau of the Census, *Historical Statistics of the United States . . .* , p. 547. Madison's aggressive policies were pushed by a small but powerful group labeled "the militants of 1809" by Reginald C. Stuart in his important article "James Madison and the Militants," *Diplomatic History* 6 (Spring 1982): 145–167.

39. Edmund Quincy, *Life of Josiah Quincy* (Boston, 1868), p. 255.

40. Henry Clay to ____, 18 June 1812, in *The Papers of Henry Clay*, ed. James F. Hopkins (Lexington, Ky., 1959–), I, p. 674.

41. Angie Debo, *A History of the Indians of the United States* (Norman, Okla., 1970), pp. 90–93.

42. Ronald L. Hatzenbuehler, "The War Hawks and the Question of Congressional Leadership in 1812," *Pacific Historical Review* 45 (February 1976): 1–22; the best book-length study on the subject is now J. C. A. Stagg, *Mr. Madison's War . . .* (Princeton, 1983).

43. Brant, VI, p. 39.

44. John Calhoun to Dr. James MacBride, 25 December 1812, in *Papers*, ed. Meriwether, I, p. 146.

45. Donald R. Hickey, "American Trade Restrictions during the War of 1812," *Journal of American History* 68 (December 1981): 517–538.

For Further Reading

In addition to the notes to this chapter, most of whose references are not repeated here, consult the General Bibliography at the end of this volume. For pre-1981 materials, one must examine *Guide to American Foreign Relations since 1700*, ed. Richard Dean Burns (1983). The best recent overview with excellent bibliography is Bradford Perkins, *From Sea to Sea, 1776–1865*, in *The Cambridge History of U.S. Foreign Relations*, ed. Warren Cohen (1993). A brilliant examination of the context is *Capitalism and a New Social Order: The Republican Vision of the 1790s* by Joyce Appleby (1984), especially important for commercial policies. Other accounts examining the framework of the era are *The American and European Revolutions, 1776–1848*, ed. Jaroslaw Pelenski (1980), conference papers on comparative aspects; Peggy K. Liss, *Atlantic Empires: The Network of Trade and Revolution 1713–1826* (1983), key on post-1800 Western Hemisphere relationships; Javier Cuenca Esteban, "Trends and Cycles in U.S. Trade with Spain and the Spanish Empire, 1790–1819," *Journal of Economic History* 44 (June 1984); Daniel C. Lang, *Foreign Policy in the Early Republic: The Law of Nations and the Balance of Power* (1986); Dorothy V. Jones, *License for Empire* (1982), beautifully arguing that post-1776 Indian policy was a form of "containment"; Reginald Horsman, *Race and Manifest Destiny: The Origins of American Racial Anglo-Saxonism* (1981), indispensable; Ralph Ketcham, *Presidents above Party: The First American Presidency, 1789–1829* (1984); and Steven Watts's superb *The Republic Reborn . . . 1790–1820* (1987).

For the 1790s specifically, a succinct treatment is Frank T. Reuter, *Trials and Triumphs: George Washington's Foreign Policy* (1982); Jacob E. Cooke's biography, *Alexander Hamilton* (1982); Paul D. Nelson, *Anthony Wayne: Soldier of the Early Republic* (1985), on both the military and Indian campaigns. Lawrence Kaplan is a leading scholar of the era, as is demonstrated in his *"Entangling Alliances with None": American Foreign Policy in the Age of Jefferson* (1987); and a useful essay is Burton Spivak, "Thomas Jefferson . . . ," in *Traditions and Values: American Diplomacy, 1790–1865*, ed. Norman Graebner (1985), as is Spencer C. Tucker, "Mr. Jefferson's Gunboat Navy," *American Neptune* 43 (April 1983). A new overview is Robert W. Tucker and David C. Hendrickson, *Empire of Liberty: The Statecraft of Thomas Jefferson* (1990). And for the most colorful—and dangerous—opponent to Jefferson, see *Political Correspondence and Public Papers of Aaron Burr*, ed. Mary-Jo Ryan and Joanne Wood Ryan, 2 vols. (1983). The 1807 debacle is examined in several centuries of context in Richard J. Ellings's *Embargoes and World Power* (1985), while Clifford L. Egan's *Neither Peace nor War; Franco-American Relations, 1803–1812* (1983) provides important counterpoint; J. C. A. Stagg, *Mr. Madison's War* (1983), superbly examines Canada and the West Indian trade as causes of the 1812 war, but within the entire 1783–1830 framework; Ronald L. Hatzenbuehler and Robert L. Ivie, *Congress Declares War* (1983), skillfully dissects congressional voting behavior; Robert Rutland, "James Madison . . . ," in *Traditions and Values*, ed. Graebner, is by a leading scholar who is also the lead editor of *The Papers of James Madison, Presidential Series* (1984–   ); C. Edward Skeen, *John Armstrong, Jr., 1758–1843* (1981), has important material on French diplomacy and the mismanagement of the 1812 war; Lawrence D. Cress, *Citizens in Arms* (1982), has written a superb social history of the 1812 conflict. An excellent account of expansionism is *Astoria and Empire* by James P. Ronda (1990), on the U.S.-British rivalry on the Pacific to 1812. For extensive recent sources, consult Dwight L. Smith *The War of 1812: An Annotated Bibliography* (1985).

3

The First, the Last: John Quincy Adams and the Monroe Doctrine (1815–1828)

Windmills, Clipper Ships, and Good Feelings

Soon after the peace of 1814, Lord Castlereagh, the British foreign minister, shrewdly observed that Americans won their wars not on the battlefield but "in the bedchamber." He could have made much the same observation about how Americans won much of the North American continent between 1815 and 1850. Freed of European quarrels for the first time in their history, Americans burst westward. Sixteen states existed in 1800, but there were twenty-four by 1824. As early as 1820, as many people lived in the new states formed after 1789 as had inhabited the original thirteen states before the Revolution. These new states formed the springboard for the drive across the continent.

The doubling of the population every twenty to twenty-five years fueled the search for new land, as did basic changes in the economy. Since their early history, Americans had prospered from the carrying and re-export trade—that is, carrying anyone's goods (not just American products) in the efficient ships that worked out of such ports as Salem, Boston, New York, Philadelphia, Alexandria, and Charleston. The profits had grown so fat in carrying British goods worldwide that between 1807 and 1814 some New England merchants cooperated more with London's laws than with Jefferson's and Madison's wishes. After 1815, these merchants began to disappear. With peace, British ships were free to carry British goods.

The U.S. merchant, moreover, found a more profitable investment in a new home-grown industrial complex. That complex remained in its infancy until the Civil War, but a major first step was taken in 1813–1815 when a group of wealthy merchants established the Waltham textile works. For the first time, this factory efficiently brought under one roof the various processes of spinning and weaving. Waltham's profits soon demonstrated that Americans could begin to compete with British manufacturers. But that success came much later. Between 1815 and 1819, the British dumped so many goods on the United States that Americans suffered a severe economic panic in 1819. New Englanders demanded a tariff wall to protect them from the dumping. By 1820, about $50 million was invested in U.S. manufacturing. (By 1860, that figure was to amount to $1 billion.)

These twists and turns of the 1815-to-1820 economy bankrupted many Americans, who then moved west to find their fortune. The country seemed to be in perpetual motion as people flooded over the Appalachians and the Mississippi. A German visitor wondered how Americans could survive while acting as if they were always "tied to the wing of a windmill." Events occurred so rapidly, he said, that "ten years in America are like a century in Spain."[1] One of those broken by the 1819 panic was Moses Austin, an Illinois lead miner. Austin decided to start anew by leading a small band of Americans into Mexico's province of Texas. Thus began the U.S. conquest of the region. Other victims of the economy turned farther west to search out land and trading opportunities in Oregon, although the 1837 depression sent the major flood of settlers into the Northwest. By 1825, American geography texts showed Texas already having closer ties with the United States than with Mexico. By 1834, a widely used geography primer already showed Texas, California, and Oregon as parts of the United States, even though they were not to be annexed for a decade or more.[2]

Not that everyone moving west had given up on the carrying trade. Indeed, the U.S. merchant fleet was entering its greatest era. These years ushered in the period of the magnificent Yankee clipper ship, admired on the world's oceans. As early as 1820, U.S. consuls watched over American interests in such exotic spots as French Mauritius, Java, the Philippines, and Hawaii. Treaties to protect Americans were signed in the 1820s with Tahiti and Hawaii. In the 1830s, the first official U.S. diplomat to Asia, Edmund Roberts, sailed west to the Far East and made treaties with Siam (later Thailand) and Zanzibar.[3] The U.S. ships that explored these corners of the globe carried not British (or French) goods, but American exports. They also transported to Europe the cotton and tobacco grown on the South's slave plantations. Cotton allowed Americans to dominate European markets and obtain the capital needed to buy new lands and build needed roads and canals. Between 1815 and 1860, cotton accounted for more than half the value of all U.S. exports. Its importance began to slide after 1840, when western grain crops started to capture foreign markets.[4] But by then, the system was fixed: the Northeast possessed much of the nation's capital, ships, and manufacturing, while the South was wedded to cotton and the slave labor that produced it.

Thus, precisely at the moment U.S. landed expansion accelerated westward, two systems—a northern free-labor industrial and commercial complex, and a southern slave-agricultural complex—began to struggle over which system would control the course of the nation's foreign policy. The struggle demonstrated again how domestic developments molded foreign policy, and how foreign policy, in turn, influenced the everyday lives of Americans—until the Civil War that the foreign policy helped bring about took 600,000 of those lives.

That horror was in the future. Between 1815 and 1825, optimism, not fear, guided U.S. expansion. For example, in an 1824 cabinet meeting, President James Monroe declared that he was afraid that the distant Oregon settlements would become a separate nation. Instantly, his secretary of state, John Quincy Adams, and secretary of war, John Calhoun, disagreed. Although Adams hated slavery and Calhoun justified it, both fully agreed, in Adams's words, that the Constitution's federal system "would be found practicable upon a territory as extensive as this continent."[5] Oregon might be three thousand miles away and claimed by the Russian and British empires, but these men had no doubt about the future. The nation was entering the 1815-to-1860 era of "manifest destiny"—that is, the belief that God had created North America for exactly the kind of white farmers and merchants that the American settlers happened to be.

They had such confidence despite (or was it because of?) the virtual disappearance of political parties by 1820. As the Federalists committed political suicide at the 1814 Hartford Convention, James Monroe managed to establish one major party, the Jeffersonian Democrat-Republican, that removed much of the two-party competition. The nation headed into the so-called "era of good feelings." The name was most misleading. Even if formal political-party competition had disappeared, factions and individuals attacked each other so bitterly inside Monroe's cabinet and in Congress that at times the government came to a halt. Monroe nevertheless bragged that with his one general party

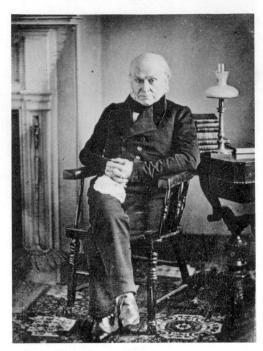

John Quincy Adams (1767–1848) became the nation's greatest secretary of state because of his vast experience (minister to Russia, the Netherlands, and Prussia, as well as U.S. senator from Massachusetts), education, intelligence, and sense of history. He was also possessed by a discipline and an intensity that clearly appear in this photograph.

in control, the nation's government had "approached . . . perfection; that in respect to it we have no essential improvement to make."[6] Such beliefs also generated confidence in their manifest destiny as Americans moved west and across the oceans. The "era of good feelings" also made possible virtual miracles: the re-election of Monroe in 1820 to a second term with only one electoral vote opposing him, and—more significantly—the rise to power of John Quincy Adams.

ADAMS

The years 1816 to 1824 marked one of the most successful eras in American diplomatic history. Without doubt, John Quincy Adams remains the nation's greatest secretary of state because of his accomplishments during those years.

No one was ever better trained to guide the nation's foreign policy.

Born in 1767, he was the son of two of the most talented Americans, Abigail and John Adams. At the age of eleven, he traveled with his father to Europe and in his teens served as secretary to the first U.S. mission to Russia. Meanwhile, he mastered five languages, French literature, ancient as well as modern history, European and American theater, and began to learn the often-fatal intricacies of Europe's power politics. From both his father and mother, he inherited a strong American nationalism, intense suspicion of British politics, and stern Calvinist discipline. The nationalism appeared when he won election from Massachusetts to the U.S. Senate in 1802, after returning from serving as U.S. minister to the Netherlands and Berlin. Although representing a strong Federalist state, Adams supported Jefferson's and Madison's purchase of Louisiana and the embargo. For such political treason, the Federalists threw Adams out of office. Madison named him minister to Russia in 1809. In St. Petersburg, his dislike of Great Britain was not hidden. As an English observer vividly described Adams in 1812:

> Of all the men whom it was ever my lot to accost and to waste civilities upon, [Adams] was the most doggedly and systematically repulsive. With a vinegar aspect, cotton in his leathern ears, and hatred to England in his heart, he sat in the frivolous assemblies of Petersburg like a bull-dog among spaniels; and many were the times that I drew monosyllables and grim smiles from him and tried in vain to mitigate his venom.[7]

Adams's view of England was not in doubt, but his personality was more complex than this observer wanted to admit. Adams loved parties and was an expert on wines. He also loved the theater, so much so that at age fourteen he decided he must leave actresses alone if he were to discipline himself to be a statesman. In 1795, he had such a fine time in London that he wrote in his diary, "There is something so fascinating in the women I meet in this country that it is not well for me. I am obliged immediately to leave it."[8] At age thirty, he married the talented Louisa Catherine Johnson. Her spouse's dedication to protecting U.S. interests carried her into a special kind of hell. She suffered twelve pregnancies, with eight ending in miscarriages, as she followed her husband throughout Europe and the United States. Louisa buried their only daughter in Russia, where her husband took the family without consulting his wife.[9] One son later committed suicide.

Throughout, John Quincy Adams never doubted his country's destiny. In a cabinet meeting, one of Monroe's advisers declared that Americans must not be so openly ambitious, because the British were criticizing U.S. expansionism. Adams shot back that nothing should be done: "Nothing we could say or do would remove this impression until the world shall be familiarized with the idea of considering our proper dominion to be the continent of North America." It would only be a matter of time before the "law of nature" led to the annexation of Spain's holdings in the south, and Canada in the north. Until Europeans understood "that the United States and North America are identical," the secretary of state lectured the cabinet, any denial of U.S. ambition "will have no other effect than to convince them that we add to our ambition hypocrisy."[10]

He could utter such spread-eagle, manifest-destiny statements, but Adams never believed that Americans would always be on God's side regardless of what they did. When he heard that naval hero Stephen Decatur had cried the famous words "Our country, right or wrong," Adams disagreed. "May our country be always successful," his version went, "but whether successful or otherwise always right. I disclaim as unsound all patriotism incompatible with the principles of eternal justice."[11] His faith in "eternal justice" was strong, although Adams's religious beliefs were complex. He did believe that the Creator worked according to fixed, scientific laws and that with discipline and education these laws could be discovered. Thus, Adams arose each morning at 5:00 A.M. to read the Bible for an hour in the belief that because God had especially blessed the United States, the proper course of U.S. foreign policy could be discovered by studying God's word.[12] And, thus, he wrote the historic and still used *Report on Weights and Measures* that provided scientific standards for the use of—and to tie together— the continent. Adams wrote the *Report* during his busiest days as secretary of state by arising an hour or two earlier each morning—that is, 3:00 A.M.

Adams studied diplomacy as carefully as he studied his science and Latin. He understood the first principle: the greatest threat to the United States came from the British, for they occupied Canada, could control the seas, and were moving to dominate the newly independent Latin American states that were breaking away from Spain. But there was a second principle: if the British could be contained in Canada, over the long run the American "multiplication table" and U.S. commercial ambition would occupy and control the rest of the continent and, perhaps, such choice Latin American areas as Cuba. The key to his policy was containment, a policy famous in dealing with the Soviet Union after World War II, but which Adams brilliantly created to block the British 125 years earlier. A third principle was his understanding that the Americans and British had certain common interests that he could exploit. Most important was London's interest in having the Spanish Empire break up so that London merchants could develop Latin American markets. The United States also wanted Spain out of the New World. Thus, Adams saw that the powerful British fleet would actually protect U.S. interests by keeping Spain and other Old World powers out of Latin America—without Americans having to pay for it. To reap such benefits, however, he understood that Great Britain and the United States had to be at peace. It was a well-conceived diplomatic strategy that soon gained historic victories.

Setting the Stage

Adams helped ensure peace with Great Britain by overseeing two agreements, the first signed by Acting Secretary of State Richard Rush. The Rush-Bagot pact of 1817 was an executive agreement made between the U.S. and British governments that demilitarized the Great Lakes and helped prevent accidental clashes along the U.S.-Canadian border. Many Canadians were not pleased. Having been invaded twice by the United States within forty years, they preferred to keep their defenses fully armed. When they pulled their cannons off the Great Lakes, they nevertheless kept them aimed at the Americans. London officials, however, wanted no border outbreaks. They had enough problems in Europe and Latin America. Consequently, they sacrificed Canadian wishes to make a deal with the United States. It was not the last time they would sacrifice Canadian interests. The Rush-Bagot deal was historically important for another reason. Instead of submitting it to the Senate as a treaty that would require a two-thirds vote for ratification, Monroe put it into effect by merely announcing it to Congress in his annual message. The usual straight-arrow Monroe, however, knew he was stretching his constitutional powers, so he asked Congress whether the executive was constitutionally competent to put such a pact into effect. The Senate never gave a direct reply, but it did approve this "agreement" without voting on it as a treaty. Thus the major constitutional precedent was set that allowed presidents to make such agreements with other governments without asking for Senate ratification. By the mid-twentieth century, such "executive agreements" were to replace treaties as the most numerous form of agreements with other nations.[13]

A second historic pact with the British was the Convention of 1818.

Adams obtained the perpetual U.S. right to fish along the Newfoundland coast, settled outstanding disputes over slaves that the British had taken from southern states, and opened new opportunities for each nation in the other's commerce. More important, Adams established the forty-ninth parallel as the U.S.-Canadian boundary from Lake of the Woods to the Rockies. This boundary shut the British off from northern access to the Mississippi River. He thus unknowingly obtained most of the present states of Idaho, Montana, and North Dakota, as well as parts of the incredibly rich Mesabi iron-ore range that was to help create the U.S. steel industry sixty years later. Finally, and of equal importance, the convention provided that the disputed region of Oregon would remain "free and open" to both nations. Adams believed the provision would allow the American population explosion to seize Oregon peacefully.

He next tried to open the British West Indies to U.S. trade. After Adams threatened economic retaliation against London shipping, the British opened several ports. But Adams wanted more. He demanded that the British charge a U.S. ship no higher tariff than they charged their own vessels. That demand was too much. London officials closed the West Indies to teach Adams (now president) a lesson, and it was left to Adams's hated political opponent, Andrew Jackson, to use diplomatic politeness and regain access again in 1830.

The West Indies episode revealed Adams's belligerence and ambition. He assessed himself in 1817 as "a man of reserved, cold, austere, and forbidding manners; my political adversaries say a gloomy misanthropist, and my personal enemies, an unsocial savage." A friend was more complimentary: "Mr. Adams is in person short, thick, and fat . . . and neither very agreeable nor very repulsive. . . . He is regular in his habits, and moral and temperate in his life."[14] By 1821, Spanish officials doubtless thought Adams's own view was more accurate.

THE TRANSCONTINENTAL TREATY

With the British contained, Adams, in 1818, began negotiations to obtain East Florida from Spain. The Spanish Empire was gasping its last breath in most of Latin America, but its minister to Washington, Luís de Onís y Gonzalez, used every diplomatic trick he knew to stall the U.S. advance. "I have seen slippery diplomats . . . ," Adams complained, "but Onís is the first man I have ever met with who made it a point of honor to pass for more of a swindler than he was."[15]

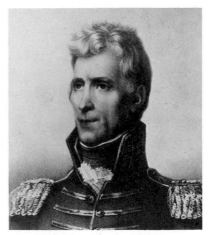

Andrew Jackson (1767–1845) gave his name to an entire age (the Jacksonian Age of the 1820s to the 1850s) and, after becoming president in 1828, had a bitter personal feud with John Quincy Adams. But in 1818–1820, the two men were the perfect pair for American expansionism—General Jackson as the ruthless frontier fighter who seized key parts of Florida, Adams as the tough diplomat who parlayed Jackson's victory into a treaty that gave the United States not only Florida, but a continent.

In 1817–1818, drama in Florida radically changed the context of the Adams-Onís talks. Monroe had ordered General Andrew Jackson to the Florida border to stop attacks by the Seminole Indians on the advancing white settlements. Jackson, who was seldom moderate when dealing with Indians or the British, decided to attack the problem's root. He marched into East Florida, destroyed Indian villages, captured and promptly hanged two British citizens who he claimed were egging on the tribes against Americans, and took the region for the United States. Monroe and most of his cabinet were horrified. Hanging British citizens could cause the second burning of Washington in just five years. Adams alone defended Jackson. The secretary of state argued that London would not retaliate because the two British subjects were in the wrong. Besides, England wanted no war with the United States. Adams wrote a blistering public paper condemning the two victims and the Seminoles. As historian Richard Drinnon notes, the paper "was a virtuoso performance that added luster and reach to the theme of merciless savages and outside agitators."[16] Adams carried the day. The cabinet decided to support Jackson, who had become, after all, enormously popular for killing Englishmen and Indians at New Orleans and now East Florida.

Adams put it to Onís directly: if Spain did not give up Florida immediately, "Spain would not have the possession of Florida to give us." The British had refused to move against Jackson. The Spanish were isolated. The secretary of state now demanded more. Negotiating the 1818 convention had reopened Adams's long interest in Oregon and the Pacific coast. He asked for Spain's claims to that region. Onís

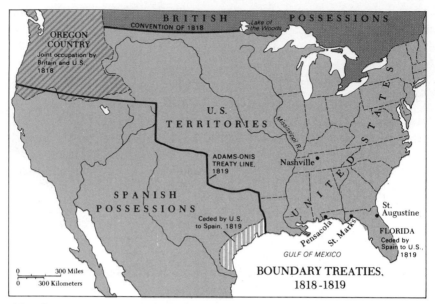

*After three years of negotiations, Adams obtained a treaty continental in scope
but whose boundaries turned out to be vague—so vague that Americans could
later use them in the Texas region to make further landed claims.*

responded by asking for Adams's promise not to recognize the Latin
American nations that were rebelling against Spain, and for the U.S.
recognition that Spain owned Texas. Adams flatly refused to make the
promise. He also objected to giving up rights to Texas; but on this
issue, the Monroe cabinet overruled him. Thus, the deal was struck:
Spain turned over Florida and its rights to the Pacific coast in return
for the United States dropping certain monetary claims against Spain
and recognizing Spanish claims to Texas. For virtually no money and
the surrender of no actual U.S. interest, Adams obtained all of Florida
and the first U.S. formal rights to the Pacific coast. When the Senate
finally ratified the Transcontinental Treaty in 1821, Adams bragged in
his diary that he had first proposed the Pacific-coast part of the pact
and had almost single-handedly carried the talks through to victory.
The treaty, he observed, "forms a great epocha in our history."[17]

OPENING "A GREAT TRAGIC VOLUME"—AND JULY 4, 1821

It was ominous that at the same moment Adams was expanding the
United States to the Caribbean in the south and to the Pacific in the

west, he and the country suddenly had to confront the deadly issue of
slavery. Adams quickly understood that it was the issue that could destroy
the Union he was creating.

The struggle began in 1819, when Missouri applied for admission to
the nation as a slave state. Northerners responded by proposing to
exclude slavery from all the former Louisiana Purchase Territory, of
which Missouri was a part. Southerners condemned the proposal for
bottling up their own expansion of cotton lands. The slave system
depended on continual expansion, not least because without the possibility of shipping young slaves west, southerners in the older states
could find themselves (as one warned) "dammed up in a land of slaves."
Congressional business stalled as the debate grew bitter. Adams initially paid little attention to it, but he came to see that slavery threatened the future of U.S. foreign policy. He had always believed that
God intended Americans to rule all of North America as a land of
freedom, but by 1820 he concluded, "The greatest danger of this Union
was the overgrown extent of its territory, combining with the slavery
question." Even Adams now wanted neither Texas nor Florida unless
slavery was excluded from them. He understood earlier than most that

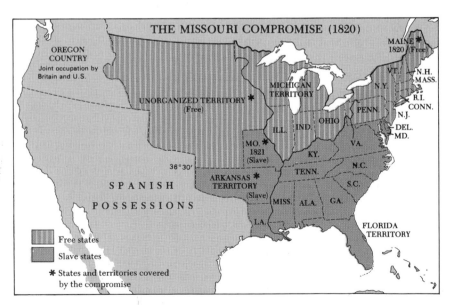

*The furor and sectional bitterness that led to the great debate of 1819–1820
were not quieted by the 1820 Missouri Compromise, but only blunted until further expansion in the 1840s resurrected the issue of slave expansionism and led
to the Civil War.*

American expansion could no longer be discussed without having to decide whether slave or free states would benefit from expansion. In this respect, he confided to his diary, the Missouri debate "is a mere preamble—a title-page to a great tragic volume."[18] In 1820, Congress struck a compromise: Missouri entered as a slave state, Maine a free state—thus maintaining the balance—and slavery was prohibited in northern Louisiana Territory but allowed in the southern. Adams doubted that the compromise would settle the problem.

For the first time, Adams began seriously to wonder whether God was blessing or condemning the United States. He began rethinking his nation's and his own ambitions. Adams wanted quiet and no more debates over slavery. He certainly wanted no wars for conquest to the south that could enlarge slave territory and increase the power of the South. Adams's views clashed with those of Henry Clay, the powerful Kentucky senator who was openly challenging Adams and Jackson for the presidency in 1824. Clay pushed to recognize the new Latin American nations, regardless of relations with Spain. The Kentuckian even urged helping the revolutionaries "by all means short of actual war." Adams condemned immediate recognition. It could destroy his deal with Onís. He believed, moreover, that the United States had little in common with the monarchical Roman Catholic governments appearing to the south. Adams had no illusion they were following the example of 1776. The great South American liberator, Simón Bolívar, actually agreed with Adams. Bolívar admired how North Americans made their "weak and complicated" Constitution work. But he thought that applying the political, civil, and religious system of the "English-American" to the "Spanish-American" was an impossibility.[19]

Adams was especially afraid that any U.S. involvement, even in supposed wars for liberty and independence, could destroy the United States. In an address on July 4, 1821, Adams answered Clay by warning—in words that would be repeatedly quoted 150 years later by those opposing the U.S. war in Vietnam—about certain American commitments:

> Wherever the standard of freedom and independence has been or shall be unfurled, there will her [the United States'] heart, her benedictions, and her prayers be. But she goes not abroad in search of monsters to destroy. She is the well-wisher to the freedom and independence of all. She is the champion and vindicator only of her own. . . . She well knows that by once enlisting under other banners than her own, were they even the banners of foreign independence, she would involve herself beyond the power of extrication, in all the wars of interest and intrigue, of individual avarice,

envy, and ambition, which assume the colors and usurp the standard of freedom. The fundamental maxims of her policy would insensibly change from *liberty* to *force*. . . . She might become the dictatress of the world. She would no longer be the ruler of her own spirit.[20]

Adams continued to oppose recognition of new Latin American nations, but in 1822 Monroe overruled him. The president wanted to reap the economic benefits of recognizing the new governments before the British. Adams gave in but made it clear that the United States recognized only governments that controlled their country and that promised to respect that country's international obligations (such as protecting U.S. citizens). No moral approval, he emphasized, was involved. Adams's recognition policy (which followed Jefferson's policy set in 1793) was followed by all future presidents until Woodrow Wilson changed it nearly ninety years later.

THE MONROE DOCTRINE

In his annual message to Congress in December 1823, Monroe climaxed six years of successful foreign policy by announcing a historic set of principles. Later (after 1844) called "the Monroe Doctrine," the message was largely shaped by Adams. It summarized the secretary of state's containment policy in the Western Hemisphere. The message told Europeans to stay out of American developments, thus leaving the United States as potentially the strongest power in the hemisphere. Moreover, as Adams had long since realized, a delicious part of the policy was that the British, for their own interests, would actually keep other Europeans out of the New World while the United States developed its own strength.

The belief that the Americas were for Americans had deep roots. It at least went back to Paine's *Common Sense* (see p. 19). But more immediate events triggered the 1823 declaration. One was the rapid development of U.S. trade with Latin America that gave Washington officials good reason for preventing the reconquest of South America by Spain or her European friends, especially France and Russia. U.S. exports to Latin America rose from $6.7 million in 1816 to nearly $8 million in 1821, despite a slump caused by the 1819 economic panic. Latin America took 13 percent of U.S. exports, and if the Spanish could be kept out—and British economic competition cut out—the Southern

Hemisphere promised to be a rich market for North American producers.

In 1821, the problem of possible European intervention moved closer to home. The Russian tsar, Alexander I, notified the world that in order to protect his claims stretching from the Aleutians and Alaska down to San Francisco, all land north of 51 degrees latitude would be sealed off, and no non-Russian ship was to be allowed within 100 miles of the northwest coasts. The tsar thus directly excluded both U.S. claims to parts of the Northwest that Adams obtained from Spain, and the right of American merchants to trade in the vast region. The United States and Great Britain protested. Adams bluntly told the Russians in July 1823 that "the American continents are no longer subjects for *any* new European colonial establishments."[21] Nor would the secretary of state recognize the 100-mile limit. He passionately believed that U.S. merchants should be able to buy and sell wherever they wished. Adams condemned European colonialism not only because it politically sealed off pieces of land, but also because it closed down trade. He had already told the British government in late 1822 of his feelings about these central issues: "The whole system of modern colonization is an abuse of government and it is time that it should come to an end." He had aimed that barrage specifically against London's claim to Oregon.

These problems of trade and Russian-British ambitions arose in an explosive political atmosphere. In 1821, the Greeks had revolted against the brutalities of Turkish control. Americans jumped to the conclusion that it was 1776 again. They raised thousands of dollars (especially among idealistic college students who knew their Greek), and such names as Syracuse and Athens came into vogue as city names. Monroe searched for a way to help the Greeks but was cut short by Adams, who warned that it was a European quarrel over which the United States had no control. When Adams received a request for a personal contribution to help Greece, he flatly refused. Not only would such a contribution break U.S. neutrality, he replied, but "we had objects of distress to relieve at home more than sufficient to absorb all my capacities of contribution."[22] He was practicing what he had preached in his July 4, 1821, address.

The shrewd British foreign secretary, George Canning, carefully watched Adams's performance. Although he disliked being lectured about his country's colonialism, Canning understood that U.S. and British interests coincided. Both nations wanted Spain, France, and Russia out of the New World. British merchants were busily profiting from trade with the newly independent Latin Americans. Canning,

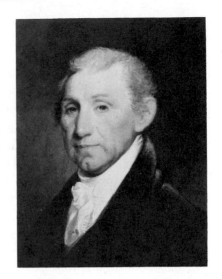

*James Monroe (1758–1831), although
president between 1817 and 1825, was
not so much the author of the Monroe
Doctrine (1823) as was his secretary of
state, John Quincy Adams. But Monroe
had been an early and a successful U.S.
diplomat himself. The Virginian had
helped negotiate the Louisiana Purchase while serving in Paris during
1803 and was Madison's secretary of
state between 1811 and 1817 as well as
secretary of war part of that time.*

moreover, wanted the Quadruple Alliance, led by the tsar and including other European monarchies who opposed British foreign policies,
to gain no dramatic victory by restoring Latin America to Spain. He,
therefore, sent a most attractive offer to Adams: the United States could
make a joint announcement with the world's greatest power, Great
Britain, that no more colonial rule would be allowed in Latin America.
Both nations would then show their own good faith by promising to
take no more territory in the region.

Flattered, Monroe asked Jefferson and Madison for advice. Both
former presidents recommended accepting Canning's offer. Adams,
however, single-handedly stopped the move for the joint declaration.
He saw that the second part of the deal (a mutual promise to take no
more territory) would prevent the United States from someday annexing Texas and Cuba. He had no doubt that both areas were to become
parts of his country, although not necessarily through armed conquest.
As he instructed the U.S. minister to Spain in April 1823:

> There are laws of political as well of physical gravitation; and if an apple
> severed by the tempest from its native tree cannot choose but fall to the
> ground, Cuba, forcibly disjoined from its own unnatural connection with
> Spain, and incapable of self-support, can gravitate only towards the North
> American Union, which by the same law of nature cannot cast her off
> from its bosom.[23]

Nature's will, the secretary of state argued, must not be blocked by
the pledge suggested by Canning. Adams, moreover, had long argued

that any such deal was unnecessary because the British would keep out other Europeans anyway. Nor did he want to join the British so openly against Russia. It was in the U.S. interest to play off those two European powers in the Northwest, to neutralize both, and then to move in itself. Adams thus convinced Monroe to announce the policy by himself and maintain complete freedom of action: "It would be more candid, as well as more dignified . . . , than to come in as a cock-boat in the wake of the British man-of-war."[24]

In his annual address to Congress on December 2, 1823, the president announced the Monroe Doctrine's substance in three principles. First, he reviewed the exchanges with the tsar, exchanges which had been friendly. The Russians were willing to discuss their claims in the Northwest. Making no threats, Monroe issued the noncolonization principle that Adams had carefully crafted: "The American continents . . . are henceforth not to be considered as subjects for future colonization by any European powers." Historian Edward Crapol has discovered a letter of 1831 in which Adams stated that this principle was aimed not only at Russia, but was "a warning to Great Britain herself."[25] All the Europeans were to be contained—then expelled.

Next, Monroe discussed the Greek crisis, then used it to introduce the doctrine's second principle: the so-called two-spheres policy. But in declaring that the affairs of the Old and New Worlds should not become entangled (or what some historians have called a policy of "isolationism"), Monroe carefully chose his words: "In the wars of the European powers in matters relating to themselves we have never taken any part, nor does it comport with our policy to do so." The president—note—did not say that the United States would remain out of all foreign quarrels, only those involving "matters relating" solely to Europeans. He and Adams fully understood that as a budding world power, U.S. interests might have to become involved in European quarrels—as in 1812–1814.

Third, Monroe announced a general hands-off policy: "We should consider any attempt on [the Europeans'] part to extend their system to any portion of this hemisphere as dangerous to our peace and safety." The president quickly added that "with the existing colonies or dependencies of any European power we have not interfered and shall not interfere." But no further European expansion or influence could be tolerated. These phrases were directed against Spanish and French hopes of restoring Spain's influence in Latin America, but they could also be applied to British activities in the Northwest.

Although supposedly aimed at the Russians, the Spanish, and the

French, Adams's policies, in historian Ernest May's phrase, were "particularly hard on the British."[26] London officials posed the greatest threat to the United States, especially to continued American landed and commercial expansion. Monroe's 1823 message took that expansion for granted—indeed, it was viewed as a requirement for the country's survival. In a rephrase of Madison's argument in *The Federalist* Numbers 10 and 14 (see p. 34), Monroe recounted proudly the American population explosion and the creation of new states:

> It is manifest that by enlarging the basis of our system and increasing the number of States the system itself has been greatly strengthened in both its branches. Consolidation [that is, centralized government] and disunion have thereby been rendered equally impracticable. Each government [the states and the national], confiding in its own strength, has less to apprehend from the other.[27]

Adams must have read those words with mixed emotions. He fully understood after the Missouri Compromise debate of 1820 that continued expansion might not render disunion "impracticable," but instead bring on fresh threats of disunion.

The Monroe Doctrine set up the ground rules for the great game of empire that was to be played in the New World. European colonization was to stop, European influence to be contained. The Old World and the New World were to be increasingly separated, unless U.S. interests forced it to become involved in Old World struggles. Especially notable was the Adams-Monroe view of Latin American revolution. The two officials did not praise it for being in the U.S. tradition, for it was not. They nevertheless refused to interfere in those revolutions, nor did the two men hope to guide the outbreaks (or, as Adams put it in his 1821 speech, to go abroad "in search of monsters to destroy"). Monroe demanded that Europe follow this example.

Meanwhile, the Latin Americans were to be on their own. When they soon made five direct requests to Washington for U.S. guarantees of their independence, the North Americans refused to act. France sent a fleet to make demands of Haiti, and in 1833 the British seized the Malvinas (Falkland Islands) over Argentina's protests, but the United States did nothing. The Monroe Doctrine's importance for North America was immediate, especially in the Northwest; but for Latin America, its impact was to be felt in the more distant future.

It had been a remarkable eight years in American foreign policy: settlement of explosive Canadian boundary questions, the contain-

ment of the world's greatest power, annexing Florida, the first claims
to the Pacific coast, and the announcement of the Monroe Doctrine
principles. If he had not been overruled by the president, Adams might
also have successfully laid claim to Texas, and not only annexed another
empire, but averted the Texas question that helped push the United
States into civil war. Remarkably, Adams had accomplished all this
with brains, not brawn, for the United States military power paled in
comparison with the British. Historian William Earl Weeks has noted
that "the gap between relative power and relative accomplishment is
the true measure of statesmanship. Surely no other statesman in
American history accomplished as much as Adams did with so little
economic and military power."[28]

GREAT LOSERS: ADAMS THE PRESIDENT

During the 1817–1825 "era of good feelings," Adams acted without
having to worry too much about an opposing political party sniping at
him. But an absence of parties did not mean an absence of politics.
Quite the contrary. Without the controls and understood procedures of
a political-party system, politics turned individualistic and vicious. As
historian Joel Silbey has argued, the American democratic system
worked best when two strong institutional political parties competed
against each other in that system, and worked worst when those parties
were weak.[29] The Monroe administration proved Silbey's argument.
While Adams conducted his brilliant, lone-wolf diplomacy, Monroe
accomplished little at home. Nor could the president control the personal ambitions and hatreds that tore his administration apart. Adams
was even accused (falsely) of appearing in church barefoot and tie-
less.[30] (It was true, however, that the secretary of state regularly swam
nude in the Potomac River.)

In this political confusion, Adams outmaneuvered three other opponents to win the presidency in 1824. Andrew Jackson obtained the
largest number of popular votes, but because no candidate won a majority
of electoral ballots the decision was thrown into the House of Representatives, as the Constitution provides. At a crucial moment, Henry
Clay threw his support to Adams, who then triumphed. Clay's action
was not unnatural: he disliked Jackson personally and agreed with
Adams's strong nationalist program for creating roads, canals, and a
higher tariff. The new president, however, then made Clay secretary
of state. Jacksonians cried that they had been victimized by a "corrupt

bargain." No such "bargain" has been documented by historians, but obviously Adams and Clay understood each other. The accusation, in any case, destroyed whatever chance the new president might have had to pass his political program or win re-election in 1828. Clay and Adams were ruthlessly attacked by the brilliant and eccentric John Randolph of Virginia, a long-time power in Congress. When Randolph called the two men a combination of "the puritan with the blackleg," Clay challenged him to a duel. In the famous encounter on the Virginia side of the Potomac in April 1826, Clay's second shot pierced Randolph's coat, while the Virginian fired in the air. (Critics claimed that Randolph took pains to wear an extra-large coat that day.) Randolph so hated Clay that when the Virginian died in 1833 he ordered that he be buried with his face to the West—so he could keep his eyes on Henry Clay.

With this kind of political dirt flying around him, Adams had little chance of realizing his great dream: uniting and developing the empire he had acquired as secretary of state. His presidency is important because it marked the last attempt by a chief executive to tie North and South together through a nationally supervised program of roads, tariffs, canals, and with such scientific projects as a national university, naval academy, and exploring expeditions. Adams saw what most failed to see: that the nation was sharply dividing along the lines of a free-labor, rapidly growing North and West that were commercial, wheat-growing, and increasingly industrial, and a slave South that was becoming locked into a one- or two-crop economy and could not keep up with the North's population gains. As he became president, however, Americans were fanning out across a continent, states were rewriting constitutions to decentralize and democratize their politics, and Jacksonians were accusing Adams of wanting to centralize power because "all Adamses are monarchists." Andrew Jackson rode this democratic wave into the presidency in 1828. Believing in the centralization of Madison, Hamilton, and John Adams, John Quincy Adams was, in this sense, the last important figure of the revolutionary generation. He was also largely isolated. Nor did his dislike of mass democracy and his lack of talent and sensitivity for public politics help him.

While he did uncomfortably live at the Executive Mansion, Adams's major foreign-policy problem arose in 1826, when delegates from newly independent Latin America planned to meet in Panama to discuss cooperation and mutual protection. They invited the United States to participate. At first, Adams was not enthusiastic. He feared the delegates wanted to involve the United States in their revolutions. When he was assured that the Panama congress planned to discuss other topics, the president agreed to send delegates, but only to work for more liberal trade, for an agreement to the noncolonization principle announced in the Monroe Doctrine, and—most interestingly—for the end of an "exclusive" (that is, Roman Catholic) church that he believed held back religious liberty. Secretary of State Clay, long an advocate of North-South cooperation, wanted to embody these principles in what he called "good neighborhood" treaties. The U.S. Congress, however, refused to appropriate money to send the two delegates. Southerners feared that Adams secretly planned to use the conference to oppose the slave trade and work with black revolutionaries in Haiti. Adams finally laid these worries to rest, but it was too late. While the debate roared on, one of the two delegates had died. The other never reached the meeting. The episode revealed not only the deep divisions between North and South America, but also within U.S. politics.[31]

In 1825–1827, Adams unsuccessfully attempted to acquire Texas. He believed that the area could be annexed as a free territory. Within ten years, as Texans became independent and slaveholding, Adams turned violently against any plans for annexation. In 1826, he also renewed the joint-occupation pledge with England in regard to Oregon territory. In doing so, he beat back proposals that would have surrendered U.S. claims to fine harbors in the present state of Washington. The renewal was Adams's only major achievement as president. The nation's greatest secretary of state, he was also one of its least successful presidents.

Defeated overwhelmingly in 1828, Adams despised his conqueror. When Adams's own alma mater gave Jackson an honorary degree in 1833, he refused to attend "to see my darling Harvard disgrace herself by conferring a Doctor's degree upon a barbarian and savage who could scarce spell his own name."[32] Adams at first decided to retire, "as much as a nun taking the veil." But he missed Washington and was determined to fight, alone if necessary, against the Jacksonians. Ralph Waldo Emerson caught him perfectly at this point: "He is no literary old gentleman, but a bruiser, and he loves the melee."[33] Elected by his home district in 1830, Adams spent the last seventeen years of his life in the House of Representatives fighting for the rights of free speech of antislave groups and working tirelessly against expansion of any slave territory. "Old Man Eloquent," as he was called, died on the floor of the House in 1848 as he attacked the U.S. attempt to conquer much of Mexico. He had long since concluded that because Jackson had defeated his national programs of 1825 to 1828, the Union was doomed to split between North and South.

Poet Walt Whitman wrote in 1848 that "John Quincy Adams was a virtuous man—a learned man—and had singularly enlarged diplomatic knowledge; but he was not a man of the People."[34] More than a century later, however, a superb historian of the era, Bradford Perkins, concluded that Adams's "new American generation vindicated the aspirations of their fathers in 1776."[35] No greater compliment could be paid to the statecraft of 1817 to 1828.

NOTES

1. Marvin Meyers, *The Jacksonian Persuasion* (Stanford, 1957), pp. 122–127.
2. Laurence M. Hauptmann, "Westward the Course of Empire: Geography Schoolbooks and Manifest Destiny, 1783–1893," *The Historian* 40 (May 1978): 430–431.
3. William H. Goetzmann, *When the Eagle Screamed* (New York, 1966), pp. 95–96.
4. Douglass C. North, *Growth and Welfare in the American Past* (Englewood Cliffs, N.J., 1966), ch. VI.
5. *Memoirs of John Quincy Adams*, ed. Charles Francis Adams, 12 vols. (Philadelphia, 1874–1877), VI, pp. 250–251.
6. Richard Hofstadter, *The Idea of a Party System . . . 1780–1840* (Berkeley, 1969), pp. 192–197.
7. George Dangerfield, *The Era of Good Feelings* (New York, 1952), p. 7.
8. Samuel Flagg Bemis, *John Quincy Adams and the Foundations of American Foreign Policy* (New York, 1949), p. 8.
9. Jack Shepherd, *Cannibals of the Heart: A Personal Biography of Louisa Catherine and John Quincy Adams* (New York, 1981), is especially useful on this relationship.
10. *Memoirs of John Quincy Adams*, ed. Adams, IV, pp. 438–439.
11. John Quincy Adams to John Adams, 1 August 1816, in *The Writings of John Quincy Adams*, ed. Worthington C. Ford, 7 vols. (New York, 1913–1917), VI, p. 61.
12. Henry Adams, *The Degradation of the Democratic Dogma* (New York, 1919), pp. 28–31.
13. Frederick Merk, *The Oregon Question* (Cambridge, Mass., 1967), pp. 122–124; Bradford Perkins, *From Sea to Sea, 1776–1865*, in *The Cambridge History of U.S. Foreign Relations*, ed. Warren Cohen (New York, 1993), ch. III.
14. Quoted in *Writings of Adams*, ed. Ford, VI, p. 519n; Bemis, p. 253.
15. On Onís, 7 August 1821, in *Writings of Adams*, ed. Ford, VII, p. 167.
16. Richard Drinnon, *Facing West: The Metaphysics of Indian-Hating and Empire-Building* (Minneapolis, 1980), pp. 108–111.
17. *Memoirs of John Quincy Adams*, ed. Adams, IV, p. 275.
18. *Ibid.*, IV, pp. 502–503, 524–525, 530, 531; V, pp. 3–12, 68.
19. *Selected Writings of Bolívar, vol. I: 1810–1822*, ed. Harold A. Bierck, Jr. (New York, 1951), p. 179.
20. The text is in *John Quincy Adams and American Continental Empire*, ed. Walter LaFeber (Chicago, 1965), pp. 42–46. Italics in original.

21. *Memoirs of John Quincy Adams*, ed. Adams, VI, pp. 157, 163.
22. *Ibid.*, VI, pp. 324–325.
23. John Quincy Adams to Hugh Nelson, 28 April 1823, in *Writings of Adams*, ed. Ford, VII, pp. 372–373.
24. *Memoirs of John Quincy Adams*, ed. Adams, VI, p. 179.
25. Edward P. Crapol, "John Quincy Adams and the Monroe Doctrine: Some New Evidence," *Pacific Historical Review* 48 (August 1979): 414.
26. Ernest May, *The Making of the Monroe Doctrine* (Cambridge, Mass., 1975), pp. 181–182.
27. *A Compilation of the Messages and Papers of the Presidents, 1789–1897*, ed. James D. Richardson, 10 vols. (Washington, D.C., 1900), II, pp. 219–220.
28. William Earl Weeks, "New Directions in the Study of Early American Foreign Relations," *Diplomatic History* 17 (Winter 1993): 88–89; William Earl Weeks, *John Quincy Adams and American Global Empire* (Lexington, Ky., 1992), especially its discussion of the 1819–1821 treaty talks; Kenneth M. Coleman, "The Political Mythology of the Monroe Doctrine," in *Latin America, the United States and the Inter-American System*, ed. John D. Martz and Lars Schoultz (Boulder, Col., 1980), pp. 98–99. There is a good overview from the French perspective and an interesting thesis about the split between official and public opinion in Réne Rémond, *Les États-Unis devant l'opinion française, 1815–1852*, 2 vols. (Paris, 1962), II, pp. 606–611. For the quite different U.S. policy on the Malvinas in 1982, see p. 706.
29. Joel H. Silbey, *The Partisan Imperative* (New York, 1985 and 1987), especially chs. III and IV.
30. James Sterling Young, *The Washington Community* (New York, 1966), pp. 186–188, 236–238.
31. *Compilation of the Messages and Papers of the Presidents*, ed. Richardson, II, p. 319; an excellent survey is Andrew R. L. Clayton, "The Debate over the Panama Congress and the Origins of the Second American Party System," *The Historian* 47 (February 1985): 219–238; also Bemis, pp. 537–561.
32. Samuel Flagg Bemis, *John Quincy Adams and the Union* (New York, 1956), p. 250.
33. Gore Vidal, *Matters of Fact and of Fiction* (New York, 1979), p. 169.
34. Walt Whitman, *The People and John Quincy Adams* (Berkeley Heights, N.J., 1961), p. 17.
35. Bradford Perkins, *Castlereagh and Adams* (Berkeley, 1964), p. 347.

FOR FURTHER READING

Consult the notes to this chapter and the General Bibliography at the end of this book; most of those references are not repeated here. Most important, begin with *Guide to American Foreign Relations since 1700*, ed. Richard Dean Burns (1983), whose thoroughness in listing pre-1981 materials cannot be matched by any textbook.

In addition to the Weeks, Dangerfield, North, May, and—above all—Bemis and Perkins volumes listed in the notes, the following provide important interpretations and superb contexts for understanding this era of Adams: Ronald E. Seavoy, *The Origins of* the *American Business Corporation, 1784–1855* (1982), good on the interchange between economics and politics; the essays on the 1815-to-1861 era in William H. Becker and Samuel F. Wells, Jr., *Economics and World Power: An Assessment of American Diplomacy since 1789* (1984); Ralph Ketcham, *Presidents above Party* (1984), which discusses the political framework; and Peter D. Hall, *The Organization of American Culture, 1700–1900* (1982), which stresses how the northeastern elites maintained their power through the new corporation.

Harry Ammon, Monroe's leading biographer, summarizes his views in "James Monroe and the Persistence of Republican Virtue," in *Traditions and Values: American Diplomacy, 1790–1865*, ed. Norman Graebner (1985); and in the same volume Graebner analyzes "John Quincy Adams and the Federalist Tradition." The sad, sometimes comic, and most instructive story is told in Mary Hargreaves, *The Presidency of John Quincy Adams* (1985); while the key Latin American view is examined in David Bushnell, "Simon Bolívar and the United States: A Study in Ambivalence," *Air Force University Review* 37 (July–August 1986); and there is overlapping material on Adams's nemesis in John M. Belohlavek, *"Let the Eagle Soar!": The Foreign Policy of Andrew Jackson* (1985). Especially revealing is Vivien Green Fryd, *Art and Empire: The Politics of Ethnicity in the U.S. Capitol, 1815–1860* (1992).

4

The Amphibious Expansion of a Sixty-Five-Hundred-Thousand-Horsepower Steam Engine (1828–1850)

THE CONTEXT: MANIFEST DESTINY AND RAILROADS IN RUSSIA

During the 1830s, increasing numbers of Americans moved into Texas and Oregon. In the 1840s, these two areas plus one-third of Mexico were annexed to the United States. The nation's territory increased by more than 50 percent to about three million square miles. At the same time, the amphibious Americans, who were moving on sea as well as land, sealed their first formal trade and diplomatic agreements with China. Henry David Thoreau, the philosopher of Walden Pond, observed Americans spreading out over continents and ocean as if "we have the Saint Vitus dance." Half a century later, at the height of British power, Lord Salisbury advised students who wished to understand England's history to use very large maps. The same advice could have been given in the 1830s and 1840s to observers of American history.

These decades mark the zenith of U.S. Manifest Destiny. The term appeared, appropriately, in mid-1845, when a Democratic editor, John

L. O'Sullivan of New York, summarized the feelings of most Americans: any European attempt to prevent the U.S. annexation of Texas was an act against God, for opposition might check "the fulfillment of our manifest destiny to overspread the continent allotted by Providence for the free development of our yearly multiplying millions."[1] Two years later, Secretary of the Treasury Robert J. Walker explained both history and the American future by declaring in a government report that "a higher than any earthly power" had guided American expansion and "still guards and directs our destiny, impels us onward, and has selected our great and happy country as a model and ultimate centre of attraction for all the nations of the world."[2]

But there also existed a darker side to Manifest Destiny. O'Sullivan's newspaper, the *Democratic Review*, warned in 1848 that Americans had no choice: "A State must always be on the increase or the decrease," for this was "the law of movement."[3] Expand or die became the shadowy underside of American thinking, especially as the population continued to double each generation and as millions of immigrants— including those driven out in the late 1840s by Irish famine and German revolutions—flooded into American cities. The threat perhaps appeared most dangerous to the South's slaveholders. They demanded more land to replace worn-out soil in southeastern states, to provide more room for blacks who were outnumbering whites in the older states, and to increase representation in Congress so that the South could breathlessly try to keep up with rampaging northern growth. O'Sullivan himself, although from the North, ended his career by supporting the South's attempts to seize new lands in the Caribbean. He finally declared himself proslavery, claimed that in the Civil War the South fought for "American liberty," and urged American blacks to erect a monument to the first slave trader.[4]

O'Sullivan and the other Manifest Destiny faithful believed that God had given them a special sign of His favor in the 1830s and 1840s. At the moment the United States grew by half, it also began to experience a transportation and communication revolution. That revolution enabled Americans to tie their vast land together with links undreamed of just a generation earlier. If Americans believed in the supernatural aspect of Manifest Destiny, they could also trust in the hard realities—the iron and steel—that made Manifest Destiny possible. Editor Thomas Ritchie noted in 1847 that James Madison had believed that the United States, under the new Constitution, could expand indefinitely, but not even Madison understood how new inventions made expansion possible. The railroad, new ships, the "magnetic telegraph had not entered into the dreams of the most enthusiastic philosophers." In 1844, just five days after a telegraph sent the first message, its inventor, Samuel F. B. Morse, received in Washington the news, via wireless from a partner in Baltimore, that James K. Polk had received the Democrats' presidential nomination. Polk's war with Mexico was the first American conflict covered by war correspondents. They used telegraph and pony express to speed reports published in the new "penny press" that quickly reached tens of millions of Americans.[5]

U.S. engineers even supervised 30,000 Russians building railroads in the tsar's empire. In 1847, an overinspired author prophesied the results when U.S. know-how encountered Europe's downtrodden:

> Who knows but in a few years the now Russian serf may stand a free man at his own cottage door, and as he beholds the locomotive fleeting past, will take off his cap . . . and bless God that the mechanics of Washington's land were permitted to scatter the seeds of social freedom in benighted Russia.[6]

Asa Whitney, who had made his fortune in the China trade, lobbied in the 1840s for a transcontinental American railroad that would attain two historic objectives at once: link together the sections of the United States and enable U.S. producers to ship their products cheaply so that they could capture Asian markets. The railroad, Whitney believed, would "revolutionize the entire commerce of the world; placing us directly in the centre of all." He preached that the American Empire need not go the way of all past empires that were now dust: "They had not the press, nor the compass, nor the steam-engine."[7] Whitney and other believers, led by Democratic senator Stephen A. Douglas from Illinois, soon obtained federal funds to build railways, but southerners—content with their waterways and fearful that the new iron horse would most benefit northern merchants—prevented building the transcontinental railway system until they left the Union in 1861.

The pull of Manifest Destiny and new technology was so strong that, O'Sullivan argued, Americans would never have to kill for conquest: "It will never be the forcible subjugator of other countries."[8] Poet Walt Whitman phrased it best as he caught the new power and confidence of an expanding, industrializing America:

> While the foreign press . . . is pouring out ridicule on this Republic and her chosen ones—Yankeedoodledom is going ahead with the resistless energy of a sixty-five-hundred-thousand-horsepower steam engine! It is

carrying everything before it South and West, and may one day put the Canadas and Russian America in its fob pocket! Whether it does these things in a conventionally "genteel" style or not, isn't the thing: but that it will tenderly regard human life, property and rights, whatever step it takes, there is no doubt.[9]

John Winthrop's seventeenth-century dream of an American community of virtue was giving way to a fragmented, spread-out society that cared more about wealth than virtue and more for individual freedom than community. During this era, the acute French observer, Alexis de Tocqueville, studied America and coined the word "individualism" for the first time. Tocqueville feared that unless it were controlled, individualism would isolate Americans and lead to the destruction of their society and freedom.[10] The remarkable limited liability company, or the corporation, developed at this time. Many states happily issued charters to individuals, which gave them the right to raise money through public sale of stock to build railways, and telegraph and steamship lines.

Two forces tried to pull Americans back and keep them under some control. The first was a new political party system that grew from the grass roots in the 1820s and 1830s. It cut across state lines to bring Americans together.[11] The Democratic party of Jackson and Polk believed in a passive federal government that largely left the states and individuals to conduct their own affairs. The Democrats thus favored low tariffs, a decentralized Treasury system, and state-built internal improvements. In foreign policy, their party contained such ardent landed expansionists as Polk, Douglas, and Walker. It also included many who favored mercantile expansion, especially if it came at the expense of the British, whom the Democrats—notably the growing number of their Irish members—feared and despised. The Whig party leadership, on the other hand, tended to come from commercial, manufacturing, and wealthier slaveholding classes. These groups wanted government support as they tried to create an orderly, regulated society at home and to find more overseas markets. They worked for higher tariffs, and national banking and internal improvement systems. In foreign policy, Whigs lined up consistently against landed expansion. They were afraid that its inevitable warfare and unpredictability could pull apart American society. But they did favor mercantile expansion. Whigs feared any conflict with the British that might upset their trade routes.

Leading Whigs included Daniel Webster and Henry Clay. Webster embodied Whig foreign-policy principles in the 1840s. The political power of mercantile, industrializing Massachusetts, he also acted as the U.S. agent for the Baring Brothers banking house of London. The Barings financed much of the new U.S. merchant fleet and manufacturing complex. They had even lent the money for the Louisiana Purchase. Always in need of cash, Webster naturally wanted no wars with the British, nor did he and Clay want to lose the cotton markets and Whig votes in the South that might result from such a war. They led in forging political compromises, especially in 1850, that kept the Union together. Moreover, it was Webster who sent the historic U.S. mission to China in 1842–1844, which formally opened that country to Americans, and it was Webster who was responsible for opening Japan to the West in the 1850s. For all their caution, concern for pocketbook commercial issues, and desire for quiet, however, not even Whigs were immune to certain virulent forms of Manifest Destiny that were sweeping through the United States. They, like most Americans then and long after, strongly believed that Manifest Destiny would bring the blessings of American democracy to many other peoples. "Do we deceive ourselves," Webster proclaimed in 1832, "or is it true that at this moment that love of liberty and that understanding of its true principles which are flying over the whole earth, as on the wings of all the winds, are really and truly of American origin?"[12] Nature seemed to be spreading the "principles" of American democracy as nature's winds spread the smell of sweet blossoms.

Nature, however, received considerable help from an increasingly powerful presidency. The Jacksonian era's political system contributed much to the development of the modern presidency, especially as democracy spread and popular votes for the president gained importance over the old, elitist electoral-college system. Elections focused more and more on the presidential vote. A shrewd winner, in turn, could dominate both his party and Congress, especially on foreign-policy questions. Jackson and Polk, both masters of the new politics, became such powerful chief executives that they could ram through their foreign policies despite strong congressional opposition.

The U.S. system thus began to resemble an hourglass: large at the top with a strong presidency, large at the bottom with an expanding population and state powers, but narrow in the middle where congressional and federal powers were located. The question became whether that slim middle could hold the hourglass together, especially as expansionism and Manifest Destiny exerted tremendous pressure on the system.

REMOVING NATIVE AMERICANS

After the War of 1812, the government's policy toward the Indians changed for the worse. Jefferson had hoped that they could be turned into farmers and assimilated into white society. After 1815, Native Americans were not to be assimilated, but removed—if necessary, by force—to unwanted lands beyond the Mississippi. The warfare of 1811 to 1814 shaped the new policy, but so did the belief of Clay, Jackson, and others that Indians could not be "civilized." As Jackson declared in 1830, "What good man would prefer a country covered with forests and ranged by a few thousand savages to our extensive Republic, studded with cities, towns, and prosperous farms . . . , occupied by more than 12,000,000 happy people, and filled with all the blessings of liberty, civilization, and religion?"[13]

During the 1820s and 1830s, the five great Indian tribes in the South were forced to move westward. The Choctaws went into Oklahoma territory. After brief resistance, the Creeks' men were put in chains by Alabama forces and moved to Oklahoma with neither weapons nor cooking utensils. The Chickasaws moved out peacefully, but the Seminoles hid in the Florida Everglades until the U.S. Army used bloodhounds to track them down. Forty percent of the Seminole population died in that struggle and in the final march west.

Most notable was Cherokee resistance. The Cherokees lived, unluckily, in an area of Georgia where gold was discovered. In 1830, state authorities began evicting the Indians. Jackson fully supported Georgia. The Cherokees, however, took their case to the United States Supreme Court. In the famous *Cherokee Nation* decision of 1831, Chief Justice John Marshall ruled that an Indian tribe was not a "foreign state." But it was "a distinct political society," and tribes were "domestic dependent nations." The next year, the Court ruled that U.S. law and the Constitution, not state law, controlled Indian-white relations. Jackson, however, refused to carry out the decision. The president allegedly declared, "John Marshall has made his decision; now let him enforce it." Georgia, then the U.S. Army, arrested and sent the Indians on a terrifying forced march. One observer estimated that 4,000 of the 18,000 Cherokees forced out after 1835 died on the journey westward.[14]

In the North, the Native Americans were also driven across the Mississippi. After being cheated by a fraudulent treaty, the Sauk and Fox tribes fought back in the short-lived Black Hawk War of 1831–1832.

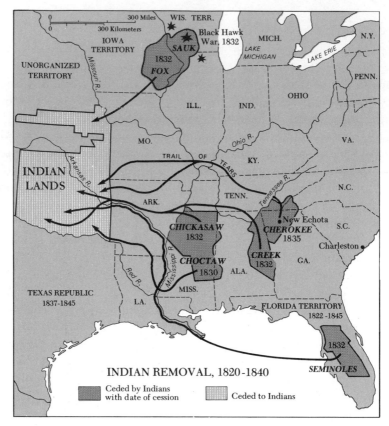

While the U.S. government steadily expanded the national boundaries after 1800, it also used force to remove large numbers of Native Americans from their lands. U.S. foreign policy and policy toward American Indians have been closely related.

That conflict is better remembered because of a young, nervous Illinois militiaman, Abraham Lincoln, who served patrol duty. Otherwise, the tribes moved out peacefully, if unwillingly. The removals confirmed the whites' view that the Indians were inferior, could be brutalized whenever necessary, and were not under the protection of the national government but were at the mercy of local authorities. These views could be transferred to other peoples. As the United States prepared to annex parts of Mexico, O'Sullivan's *Democratic Review* declared, "The Mexican race now see, in the fate of the aborigines of the north, their own inevitable destiny." The *New York Evening Post* neatly combined Manifest Destiny and Indian policy to justify the killing: "Providence has so ordained it. . . . The Mexicans are aboriginal

Indians, and they must share the destiny of their race."[15] The Indian
removals and wars of the 1830s provided racial beliefs and battlefield
experience that helped prepare Americans for their war of 1846–1848.

THE ROAD TO CHINA

American expansion moved on both land and sea. It thus reflected the
needs of both agrarians who sought new lands, and producers (both
agrarian and industrial) and merchants who required foreign markets.
U.S. officials had to take such needs into account. Polk, for example,
carefully tried to balance his policies for landed and overseas expansion. Often the two nicely meshed, as in the drive for Oregon and California. But above all, the history of the 1830s and 1840s shows how
Americans thought of Asia not as the Far East (which was a British
term), but the Far West, the natural extension of their movement across
the continent.

The maritime wing of U.S. expansionism rapidly gained momentum
in the 1830s. In 1832, growing U.S. trade with the western Pacific led
Jackson to send Edmund Roberts to make commercial treaties with
Siam, Southeast Asia, and Japan. Roberts succeeded in Siam and
Muscat, but failed at Hue—not the last time U.S. diplomacy was to
have problems in the area later known as Vietnam. He died before
reaching Japan. In 1839, President Martin Van Buren played to mercantile interests by ordering Captain Charles Wilkes to explore the
Pacific. Wilkes gave the nation its first claim to Antarctica (which he
was the first also to recognize as a separate continent) and the strategic
port of Pago Pago in Samoa. As historian Thomas McCormick observes,
the Wilkes mission of 1839–1842 helped make the United States "the
most knowledgeable power in the world as far as the great Pacific basin
was concerned."[16]

Americans also staked out claims to the way station of Hawaii. U.S.
traders and missionaries had been settling on the beautiful islands for
more than a generation. The settlements created replicas of Protestant
Boston society, even to the extent of restricting native and Roman
Catholic religious practices. When British and Canadian claims
threatened the newcomers, President John Tyler publicly warned in
December 1842 that non–United States governments were to keep their
hands off the islands. It marked the first time that Hawaii was brought
under a Monroe Doctrine–type of policy.

The double column of U.S. traders and missionaries also marched into the much larger arena of China during these years. The United States had no formal treaties with the Chinese but instead depended on, and cooperated with, British power—even to the point of working with English traders to develop the highly profitable opium traffic. Chinese called the Americans "second chop Englishmen."[17] U.S. exports of furs, ginseng, and—of all things—ice chopped from ponds around Boston were exchanged for imports of tea, hides, and gunnysacks. Nevertheless, of the fifty-five foreign firms in the great trading city of Canton in 1836, only nine were American. U.S. businessmen had difficulty understanding the Orient's customs. In one story, an ignorant trader learned to his distress that he was eating not a "quack quack," but a "bow-wow-wow."[18] Even missionaries, who adjusted to strange ways better than most merchants, met major problems. Between 1814, when the first Chinese was baptized in a Protestant ceremony, and 1839, the dozen Protestant missions (of which seven were American) each averaged less than one convert per year.[19]

Missionaries and traders alike began to push for formal U.S. treaties so that they could better compete for their China markets. Then, between 1839 and 1842, the Chinese and British engaged in the Opium War. The conflict resulted from European demands for continued use of Canton as part of the rich, illegal opium trade. When the British won those rights in the 1842 Treaty of Nanking, they also seized Hong Kong, opened four other Chinese ports to the West, and assumed power over China's ability to fix tariff and customs rates. The Americans now realized that they had to win equal trading privileges on their own.

Their new interest in Asia also resulted from internal U.S. pressure. The intense economic depression of 1837–1841 severely struck merchants and New England–southern textile manufacturers. In 1842, President Tyler flatly declared that "the greatest evil which we have to encounter is a surplus of production beyond the home demand, which seeks, and with difficulty finds, a partial market in other regions."[20] The president's Whig administration, led by Secretary of State Daniel Webster, appointed Caleb Cushing as the first U.S. minister to China. Cushing came from an old Massachusetts merchant family. Tyler's quaint personal letter to the emperor of China began: "I hope your health is good. . . . The Chinese are numerous. You have millions and millions of subjects. . . . The Chinese love to trade with our people, and to sell them tea and silk, for which our people pay silver, and sometimes other articles. But if the Chinese and the Americans will trade, there should be rules."

Webster then laid down the rules. These were incorporated in the

1844 Treaty of Wangxia (i.e., Wanghia). The United States received most-favored-nation status in China's trade—that is, it automatically received any trade rights the Chinese gave others (such as the British). Americans also received extraterritorial rights, meaning that all U.S. citizens and their property were to be free of Chinese law and instead regulated and protected by U.S. officials and law. The British and Americans congratulated themselves for forcing extraterritoriality out of the Chinese. In truth, the practice had begun with medieval China's decision to let foreign "barbarians" and their queer ways stay to themselves so that they would not disturb the superior Chinese civilization.

Americans, ignorant of that nation's traditions and convinced of their own unselfish desire to help the Chinese, entered into a "special relationship." That relationship rested for the next century on most-favored-nation and extraterritorial privileges. Later in the nineteenth century, it would become known as the "open door" and would be defined in the 1890s by Secretary of State John Hay as "a fair field and no favor" for all the nations involved in trying to exploit the China market. The open-door policy attempted to protect China from European or Japanese colonization so all of it would be open to U.S. traders. Americans soon prided themselves as being the only anti-imperialists who dealt with the Middle Kingdom. The Chinese quickly sensed this misplaced self-satisfaction. They played off Americans against the other foreign nations in an attempt to keep all of them at bay.

U.S. trade developed well after the Treaty of Wangxia. So did the work of Roman Catholic and Protestant missionaries. They became interpreters for U.S. diplomats and merchants, the cutting edge of American influence that penetrated the nation's interior, and, in all, the eyes and ears through which most Americans saw and heard about China. The emperor continued to fight Christianity. The vast and bloody Taiping Rebellion of 1850–1864, in which perhaps as many as 20 million people died, was aimed at destroying foreign influences as well as the Manchu dynasty. But the missionaries remained. They soon justified the use of force to bring the Chinese to God. One popular book, *Hand of God in American History*, argued that "war is the sledgehammer of Providence" to open China to "the family of nations and the benign influence of Christianity."[21] Thus, when France and Great Britain made war on China in 1857–1858 to obtain new trade rights, Americans refused to join the conflict. In 1858, however, they signed with China the Treaty of Tianjin (i.e., Tientsin) that gave them the spoils won by the Europeans. Nearly all of China was opened to U.S. trade, the emperor finally accepted Western diplomats at his capital of

Beijing (i.e., Peking), and he now had to tolerate openly the work of the missionaries. The Wangxia and Tianjin treaties formed the legal and diplomatic base on which U.S.-China relations rested for the next ninety years.

Texas, Maria Child, and James K. Polk

The Americans' movement into China between 1830 and 1860 coincided with their annexation of the immense Pacific-coast strip that stretched from Oregon territory to San Diego. China, like California and Oregon, formed part of the great westward movement that shaped and shook American society during the mid-nineteenth century. But it was the Texas question that triggered the U.S. seizure of the West Coast during the climactic years 1844 to 1848.

The three hundred American families led by Moses Austin into Texas during 1819–1821 had become 15,000 Americans by 1830. The Mexican province turned into another part of the American frontier as immigrants, lured by the possibility of obtaining 4,400 acres of land for a mere $200, flocked in to find their fortune. In addition to accepting Mexican citizenship, Mexico required the settlers to be Roman Catholic and have no slaves. The Americans ignored the last two rules. In 1830, Mexico City officials realized that Texas was being swamped by the multiplying Americans, some of whom ranked among the most uncontrollable gunslingers on the frontier. Santa Anna, who ruled Mexico, finally abolished all state legislatures, centralized power in Mexico City, and moved an army into Texas to control the settlers. Instead of obeying, the Texans replayed 1775–1776: they demanded full restoration of their rights, set up Committees of Correspondence to coordinate resistance, and finally, in 1836, declared their independence. Texas won a short, bloody war. The new government was helped by thousands of Americans who rushed in for glory, action, and land. Some of the emigrants died when the Texas garrison at the Alamo was wiped out in early 1836, but others helped win the pivotal battle of San Jacinto. Meanwhile, Stephen Austin, Moses' son, borrowed most of his funds from the United States to fight the war.

President Andrew Jackson soon recognized Texas independence. He wanted to annex the country, but he and his successor, Martin Van Buren, knew that the time was not ripe. Annexation could lead to an unpopular U.S. war with Mexico. Moreover, after the 1837 depression struck, Americans concentrated on their economic problems at home.

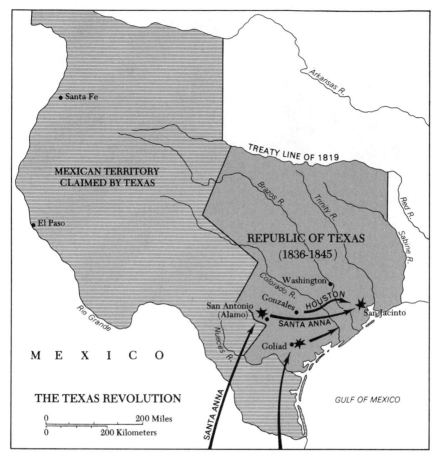

The Texas revolution of 1836 not only ended Mexico's rule of the region, but helped trigger the massive U.S. expansionism of the 1840s. Texas was indepen-dent between 1836 and 1845, when, amid bitter debate, it joined the Union as the twenty-eighth state.

Most important, any move to take Texas triggered a vicious debate within the United States. Annexation would mean that the South had a vast new area for slavery. John Quincy Adams led the opposition in Congress, but he enjoyed support from the rising antislave movement.

Anti-Texas voices reverberated throughout the North. None was clearer than Lydia Maria Child's. By the 1830s, this remarkable woman was a widely read novelist and publisher of the first children's maga-zine in the United States. She concluded that women's rights could be won only in a society that first repudiated black slavery. In 1833, she published *An Appeal in Favor of That Class of Americans Called Afri-*

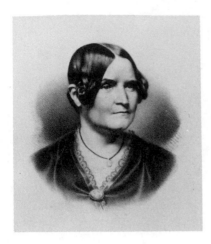

Lydia Maria Child (1802–1880) was a pioneer in publishing and women's rights, then but made a special mark on U.S. diplomatic history as a vigorous opponent of American—especially slave—expansion.

cans, apparently the first book by a white American to call for immediate emancipation of the slaves. It also laid out the explosive argument that slaveowners controlled the U.S. government. The *Appeal* angered many of Child's readers and nearly bankrupted her. Child did not retreat. When the wife of a Virginia senator argued that southern women helped slave women, especially during childbirth, Child shot back that in the North, "after we have helped the mothers, *we do not sell the babies.*" In the words of historian Edward Crapol, "For more than forty years as writer, petitioner, organizer, pamphleteer, and editor, she fought slavery, sought racial and sexual equality, and decried [what she called] 'the insane rage for annexation in this country.' "[22] Child, Adams, and other antislave advocates stalled the Texas annexation movement until early 1844. Then, President Tyler and his new secretary of state, John Calhoun, pushed for a Senate vote on the issue. Calhoun publicly used proslavery arguments to justify annexation. Needing a two-thirds vote of approval, the treaty went down to an overwhelming 35-to-16 defeat in June 1844.

Within eleven months, however, the United States annexed Texas and was about to declare war on Mexico. The remarkable turnaround was brought about by James K. Polk. One of the most successful presidents in achieving his goals, especially in foreign policy, Polk is usually rated by historians as one of the half-dozen "great" presidents. Born in North Carolina in 1795, Polk soon moved to frontier Tennessee. When he was seventeen years old, Polk was strapped to a table, given a large amount of whiskey, and then suffered through a gallstone operation that broke his health. Unable to farm and fascinated by books, he went to the University of North Carolina, where he won honors in mathematics and classics. He studied law, entered politics, and was elected to the House of Representatives. Polk quickly made his reputation as a Jacksonian who opposed nearly everything John Quincy Adams stood for. The Tennessean attacked "consolidation" of government, ideas favoring national universities or internal improvements, "expensive and unnecessary foreign missions," and "European etiquette."[23] Polk showed little interest in political theory or history. Adams caustically remarked that Polk had "no wit, no literature . . . , no philosophy," but Adams had to grant that Polk possessed immense determination and will. He also was blessed with uncommon political instinct. His ability as an open-air orator won him the title "Napoleon of the stump." In 1839, he became governor of Tennessee. In 1841 and 1843, however, he was defeated in the governor's race. But in 1844, he was elected president of the United States.

That this first "dark horse" candidate in American history won the presidency owed much to Texas and the power of Manifest Destiny. As the Texas issue heated up in early 1844, the two leading presidential candidates, Democrat Martin Van Buren of New York and Whig Henry Clay of Kentucky, publicly declared they did not want to annex Texas. Both preferred the issue to die down so that they could discuss less dangerous, but politically attractive, issues such as tariff and banks. Polk, however, came out for annexation. Already close to Andrew Jackson, who, with his dying breath, now worked to take Texas, Polk won support from powerful politicians in the South and West who wanted a spread-eagle foreign policy. These operators manipulated the Democratic nominating convention's rules and, when it deadlocked,

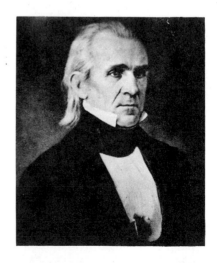

James K. Polk (1795–1849) of Tennessee (shown in an early daguerrotype by Mathew Brady) is often considered one of the strongest of all presidents. Polk added more land to the nation than any president except Jefferson. But the Tennessean also presided over a disintegrating political party system that had helped hold the Union together, and his foreign policy was a cause of the Civil War.

pushed Polk forward as a compromise candidate. The nominee's platform called for strict construction of the Constitution, but also "the re-occupation of Oregon and the re-annexation of Texas at the earliest practicable period." (The "re-" prefixes alluded to the Democrats' mistaken claim that John Quincy Adams had happily given away U.S. claims to Texas and Oregon in the 1820s.) The 1844 campaign was close and bitterly fought. One Whig claimed that Polk's supporters called Whig candidate Clay such awful names that one could conclude "he was more suitable as a candidate for the penitentiary than President of the United States."[24] The Whigs returned the name-calling in kind, but Polk won by a paper-thin margin.

John Tyler, the outgoing president, decided to leave his mark on history by annexing Texas not through the usual constitutional method of a two-thirds Senate vote (which remained unobtainable), but through the unusual tactic of a joint resolution that required only a majority of the House and Senate. The House passed the measure. The Senate, however, balked when several powerful members feared that claims over the vague Texas-Mexico boundary would lead to war. Polk, preparing for his inauguration, won these key votes by apparently promising to send a mission to negotiate the boundary issue peacefully. The Senate then voted for annexation 27 to 25. Texas became part of the Union on December 29, 1845, as Tyler set a constitutional precedent by acquiring empire through a simple majority of both houses. But Polk then somehow neglected to settle the boundary issue. He instead attempted to use it and other claims to force Mexico to sell California. Although weak and divided, the Mexican government refused to deal on Polk's terms. Meanwhile, the new president alienated pivotal Democrats, including Van Buren, with his appointments and positions on domestic issues. Even Vice-President George Dallas became angry: Polk's "most devoted friends [complained] . . . with bitter grief and shame, of his crooked politics. His defeats, they said, gave them less pain than his intrigues."[25]

WEBSTER, POLK, AND LOOKING JOHN BULL IN THE EYE

After his election as president in 1968, Richard Nixon told his speech-writers to study James Polk's 1845 inaugural address, because the Tennessean, in Nixon's words, promised to be "president of all the people."[26] Regardless of their promises, however, both Polk and Nixon soon came to preside over a nation tragically divided by their foreign

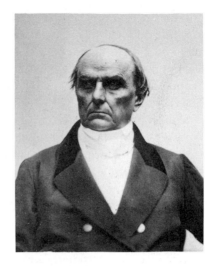

Daniel Webster (1782–1852) was elected to Congress from New Hampshire at age twenty-nine, and in 1827 became a senator from Massachusetts. For the next quarter-century, he, along with Henry Clay, embodied Whig foreign policy that emphasized commercial expansion (especially in Asia); peace with Great Britain; and the 1850 Compromise that, temporarily saved the Union. Historian Kenneth Shewmaker concludes that the Webster-Ashburton Treaty of 1842 not only "possibly averted a third Anglo-American war, it laid the basis for a rapprochement with England that has endured to the present." (Daniel Webster: The Complete Man *[Hanover, N.H., 1990], p. xxiii.)*

policies. In Polk's case, that division began with Texas and nearly exploded into war with Great Britain over Oregon.

Polk's (and the Democratic party's) sometime recklessness in twisting the British Lion's tail can be better understood by comparing his policy with the Whig party's approach fashioned by Daniel Webster just a few years before in the early 1840s. A host of U.S.-British confrontations were erupting, but Webster—who, as a good Whig wanted peaceful commercial expansion, no clashes with the world's great economic power (Great Britain), and no jarring political debates that would threaten the Union—took a distinctly different approach to these confrontations than did Polk.

The crises began in 1837 when some Canadians rebelled against British rule. Ever willing to help their neighbors in such efforts, a few Americans used the vessel *Caroline* to send supplies to the small band of revolutionaries. Pro-British Canadians attacked the *Caroline* in U.S. waters, killed a U.S. citizen, and spectacularly sunk the boat in flames just above Niagara Falls. Outraged Americans south of the border prepared for war, in part by exhibiting in Buffalo, New York, the body of their slain countryman (his "pale forehead mangled by the pistol ball, and his locks matted with his blood!" according to one hard-breathing New York newspaper). President Martin Van Buren cooled passions by sending General Winfield Scott, who warned that any attack on Canada would have to be "over my body."

The issue festered for two years until 1840, when a Canadian, Alexander McLeod, made the serious mistake of drinking too much in a

Buffalo tavern and then bragging that he had done the killing in the *Caroline* raid. He was immediately jailed on charges of arson and murder. The British demanded McLeod's release on the grounds that he had not been near the *Caroline* and, anyway, the attack had been ordered by the government in Canada and was not the act of a single man. As New Yorkers (and other anti-British voices) angrily demanded McLeod's execution, Webster became secretary of state in early 1841. Publicly, Webster took a hard line. Privately, he worked with New York to free the prisoner before another clash broke out. The jury finally freed McLeod for the good reason that he had proven he had been miles away from the *Caroline* on the night of the attack. Webster and his good friend, Lord Ashburton, the British minister to the United States, then tied up loose ends. Ashburton essentially apologized for the *Caroline* attack, and Webster apologized for McLeod's long detention. The secretary of state also had Congress pass a law in 1842 that henceforth brought under federal (not state) jurisdiction any foreigners charged with criminal acts who were acting under orders of their government.

Having solved the international problems caused by drunkards in Buffalo, Webster and Ashburton then had to contend with a more serious crisis: slavery. In 1839, slaves aboard the Spanish slave ship, the *Amistad*, mutinied and tried to force their white captives to take them back to Africa. Instead, the whites steered the ship north until, finally, a U.S. ship captured the *Amistad* off Long Island. Abolitionists instantly demanded freedom for the Africans. In 1841 the Supreme Court indeed granted their freedom on the grounds that the *Amistad* had broken treaties between Great Britain and Spain that prohibited the slave trade. The Spanish, in turn, demanded indemnity in cash. Webster flatly refused, and the Africans returned to their home in 1842.

The slave-trade question refused to go away. In late 1841, slaves took over a U.S. ship, the *Creole*, sailing from Virginia to New Orleans, and piloted it to the British possession of Nassau. There officials freed the slaves on the grounds that the king had ended slavery in all his possessions a decade earlier. Webster bitterly opposed slavery, but as secretary of state he had to listen to southern slaveholders who warned that the *Creole* mutiny could not be allowed to stand without either punishment or indemnity (or, preferably, both). Again Webster and Ashburton worked out a solution. The British did not return the Africans, but they did promise no future interference with U.S. vessels driven into British ports by "accident or by violence." In 1853, a claims commission awarded the United States $110,000 for the property in humans lost in the *Creole* affair.

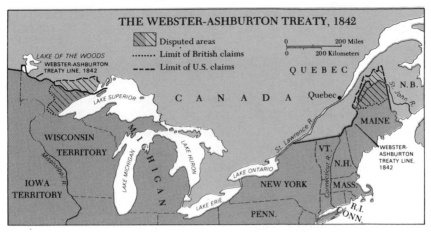

THE WEBSTER-ASHBURTON TREATY, 1842

Disputed areas

0 .... Limit of British claims

0 ---- Limit of U.S. claims

200 Miles

200 Kilometers

LAKE OF THE WOODS
WEBSTER-ASHBURTON
TREATY LINE, 1842

LAKE SUPERIOR

C A N A D A

QUEBEC

Quebec

N.B.

St. John R.

MAINE

WISCONSIN
TERRITORY

St. Lawrence R.

St. Lawrence R.

VT.

N.H.

WEBSTER-
ASHBURTON
TREATY LINE,
1842

LAKE HURON

LAKE MICHIGAN

M I C H I G A N

Mississippi R.

IOWA
TERRITORY

LAKE ONTARIO

NEW YORK

Connecticut R.

MASS.

LAKE ERIE

PENN.

R.I.

CONN.

*The Webster-Ashburton Treaty of 1842 settled the disputed boundaries of Maine
(although not to the satisfaction of everyone in Maine) and gave the United
States land between Lake Superior and Lake of the Woods, on which were later
found the rich Mesabi iron deposits—a base for the nation's iron and steel
industries several generations later.*

Webster and Ashburton had narrowly avoided two potential catastrophes in the *Caroline* and *Creole* affairs. Perhaps their success was not too surprising since Ashburton had married an American woman and was head of the great banking institution, the House of Baring (his family name had been Alexander Baring), which poured money into U.S. investments—and which over the years had paid handsomely for legal advice from Daniel Webster. The two men understood each other perfectly. But that understanding was strained to a near-breaking point in the most dangerous U.S.-British problem of the early 1840s: an argument over the boundary between Maine and Canada. That boundary had been fuzzy ever since the 1783 peace treaty (see pp. 26–27) failed to make clear which country owned some 12,000 square miles of highly strategic and rich (especially because of lumber) territory. Webster secretly held two old maps that seemed to put most of the land inside Canada. He kept these from his good friend, Ashburton, while using secret funds controlled by President John Tyler to send an agent to Maine and explain to the local citizens why a compromise was necessary with the British. That compromise was worked out between Webster and Ashburton in July 1842. The sixty-seven-year-old British aristocrat was ready to deal—in part to escape the "oven," as he accurately called summertime Washington, D.C.

The United States received about 7,000 of the disputed 12,000 square miles, and also obtained territory in New York, Vermont, and in the Lake Superior region (an area soon discovered to have rich iron-ore deposits). Webster then told Ashburton of the old maps upholding much of the British claim. The minister was not unhappy; he valued good relations with the United States over the acreage (and Canadians) in question. But his British critics unleashed a blistering attack on Ashburton's diplomacy—only, in a melodramatic turn in a series of U.S.-British melodramas—to have *another* map suddenly turn up in London that upheld the most extreme U.S. claim to the territory. Thus, Ashburton's high reputation as a diplomat was preserved. So which of these various maps was correct? Which nation deserved some of the richest lumber and mineral resources in the Western Hemisphere? The answer, as historian Howard Jones suggests, is that "no map was both authentic and valid" because they either had not been used at Paris in 1783 or boundary questions had been delayed, to be decided later. But the Webster-Ashburton Treaty was both a tribute to the skill of the two negotiators and a signal that differences between Americans and the British no longer had to be resolved with war.[27]

Unfortunately, that historic lesson was almost lost on President Polk in 1845–1846. Granted, the stakes in his struggle with the British were enormous. The Oregon contest was fought over an empire that contained nearly half a million square miles—or an area larger than France, Germany, and Hungary combined. U.S. merchants dominated the region's commerce. Word had spread rapidly after one shipowner had traded several dollars of trinkets to Indians for $20,000 worth of otter pelts. The Native Americans soon called all white men "Bostons" because every white person seemed to come from the Massachusetts port.[28] Few permanent white settlers lived in Oregon by 1830, but that changed rapidly after missionaries came to believe that the Indians wanted to learn about Christianity. With Samuel Parker and the intrepid Marcus and Narcissa Whitman in the foreground, during 1835–1836 the missionaries followed a pathway along the Oregon Trail out of Independence, Missouri. They moved their wagon trains through plains and desert, across the Rockies, and then down into the lush Willamette Valley. The economic troubles of 1837–1841 also pushed out-of-luck farmers along the Oregon Trail. In 1845, some 3,000 Americans arrived in Oregon to double the white population. The new technologies, moreover, were now cutting distances. If you had represented Oregon in the U.S. Congress before the mid-1840s, you would have had to spend about twenty-five weeks going to Washington and another twenty-five weeks returning home, leaving about two weeks to spend in the capital. After the mid-1840s, the railroad, telegraph, and steamship rapidly reduced travel time.

At first, Polk handled the growing problem with the British over Oregon carefully and wisely. In mid-1845 he offered the king's minister to Washington, Richard Pakenham, a deal that divided the Oregon territory along the forty-ninth parallel. The proposal placed both banks of the Columbia River in U.S. territory, even though no American settlements existed north of the great waterway. Faced with a grave political crisis in London at that moment, the British government would probably have accepted Polk's offer just to resolve the distant Oregon question. But Pakenham foolishly rejected the deal without consulting London. Polk, angry and believing that the British had now put themselves at a disadvantage, then demanded all the land to the northernmost U.S. claim, 54°40'. The British flatly rejected the demand. They were not about to surrender much of their northwestern territory and virtually all of the region's best harbors.

Polk received vibrant support from Democrats in the Midwest, where land hunger and faith in God-directed expansionism was strongest. The cry of "Fifty-four forty or fight" soon resounded, encouraged by John L. O'Sullivan, who at this point coined the term "manifest destiny." Northern and many southern Whigs, however, wanted no war with their best customers in England. The U.S. Army, which numbered only 6,000 in 1830 (and one-quarter of those deserted within the year), had grown to 11,000 by the early 1840s, but it was both highly undependable and too small to fight the British Empire in such a faraway place. With Americans divided and his military unprepared, Polk nevertheless whipped up feelings over Oregon. In his annual message of December 1845, he resurrected the Monroe Doctrine (which had slept peacefully and largely forgotten since 1823). He used it to warn Great Britain that "no future European colony or dominion shall with our consent be planted or established on any part of the North American continent."

The president then urged Congress to terminate the 1827 joint-occupation agreement that had regulated Oregon affairs. When a timid congressman expressed the fear that this meant war, Polk retorted "that the only way to treat John Bull was to look him straight in the eye." Behind those overly defiant words was Polk's belief that the British needed U.S. trade—notably cotton (especially since the British Parliament was just then committing itself to a radically new free-trade policy). "We hold England by a cotton string," a Virginia Democrat bragged.[29]

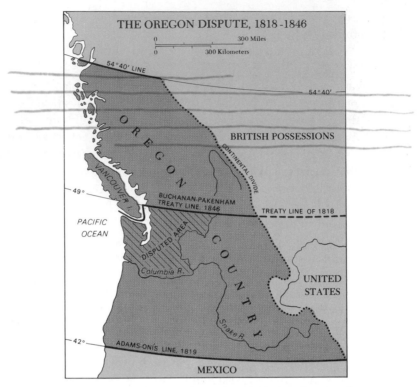

The disputed northwest region and the 1819 and 1846 settlements that preserved peace with Great Britain, and also preserved the U.S. hold on invaluable land and ports.

 The "string" proved to be more fragile than John Bull's eye. The British told Polk that they would not retreat beyond the forty-ninth parallel. They next mobilized thirty warships for possible action. Polk, a devout Presbyterian who seldom conducted business on the Sabbath, quickly called a cabinet meeting on Sunday to discuss the crises. Already facing a war with Mexico, he decided to send the Oregon issue to the Senate for resolution. This decision shifted responsibility, and the president no doubt assumed that the Senate, with Webster (now returned to represent Massachusetts) and Calhoun in the lead, would accept the forty-ninth-parallel compromise. Webster gloated that the Oregon treaty reversed the Constitution's procedure: "Here is a treaty negotiated by the Senate, and only agreed to by the President." Polk had nevertheless turned possible war and his own humiliation into a victory. The United States obtained the Oregon territory, including both banks of the Columbia River. The agreement came none too soon, for the president had meanwhile maneuvered the country into war with Mexico.

The "Fire-Brand in the Body": The Mexican War and Slavery

In his inaugural address of 1845, Polk stressed that U.S. expansionism meant extending "the dominions of peace. . . . The world has nothing to fear from military ambition in our Government. . . . Our Government can not be otherwise than pacific." Within fifteen months, Polk took the country into a war for conquest. The reason was his determination to obtain California.

Americans had sailed along California's coast for generations. As early as 1829, they controlled its cattle-hide and provision exchanges as surely as they monopolized Russian America's trade to the north. Richard Henry Dana's famous account, *Two Years before the Mast*, popularized the romance of the California coast. By 1845, about a thousand Americans, many pushed out by the 1837 panic, had trekked across the continent to settle the region. There was, however, no popular cry to annex California in 1845. The settlers were outnumbered by at least 7,000 Spanish and Mexican natives. Most Americans knew or cared little about the area. The issue of California never arose in the 1844 presidential campaign. Only Polk seemed to care, but he cared a great deal.

An astute politician, the Tennessean wanted California not only for its land, but especially for its fine ports. Owning the harbors of San Francisco and San Diego could magnificently enhance the mushrooming U.S. trade in the Pacific and—as Polk fully appreciated—greatly please American merchants. The president, moreover, suspected that the British were using their financial control over Mexico's debt to force the Mexicans to sell, or at least to mortgage, their province of California to London financiers. It was for that reason, as he privately told a friend, that "in reasserting Mr. Monroe's doctrine [in the 1845 message] I had California and the fine bay of San Francisco as much in view as Oregon."[30]

In late 1845, Polk sent John Slidell (a U.S. congressman and influential lawyer from New Orleans) to make Mexico a series of offers, including one of $25 million and the U.S. assumption of its claims against the Mexicans in return for much of California, New Mexico

Chronology, 1844–1848

June 1844	Secretary of State John Calhoun's treaty for annexing Texas overwhelmingly defeated 35–16 in Senate.
November 1844	James K. Polk wins presidential race over Henry Clay.
February 1845	Polk secretly makes deal with Senate leaders for Texas.
March 1, 1845	President John Tyler signs joint resolution to annex Texas.
March 4, 1845	Polk inaugurated.
July 1845	Polk proposes division of Oregon at 49°; British minister rejects proposal without submitting it to his superiors in London.
October 1845	Polk sends Thomas O. Larkin to stir up demands in California for annexation.
November 1845–March 1846	Polk sends John Slidell to Mexico to obtain California and New Mexico. Slidell mission fails.
December 1845	Polk revives Monroe Doctrine to demand the "whole" of Oregon.
January 1846	Polk sends General Zachary Taylor's troops into disputed territory of Rio Grande.
February 1846	Rise of "Manifest Destiny" and "Fifty-Four-Forty-or-Fight" cries in Congress over Oregon issue.
May 8, 1846	Polk learns of Slidell mission's failure; prepares for war.
May 9, 1846	Polk learns that Mexican forces attacked Taylor's troops in disputed territory.
May 11, 1846	Polk sends war message to Congress.
June 1846	Treaty with Great Britain to settle Oregon passes Senate.
July 1846	Walker tariff, lowering rates significantly, passes Congress.
August 8, 1846	David Wilmot proposes the Wilmot Proviso in House.
August 18, 1846	U.S. Army occupies Sante Fe.
February 1847	After bitter debate, House passes Wilmot Proviso; Senate kills it.
September 1847	General Winfield Scott's forces capture Mexico City.
January 1848	Discovery of gold sets off California gold rush.
February 1848	Nicholas Trist signs Treaty of Guadalupe Hidalgo to end war.
November 1848	Zachary Taylor wins presidency over two candidates of divided Democratic party.

territory, and the Rio Grande as the Texas-Mexico boundary. To the Mexico City government, this was but one more in a continual stream of political crises. It refused to deal with Slidell, nor could it have negotiated Polk's terms without falling from power. A change in early 1846 brought an even more ardent anti-U.S. regime into office. Polk turned to other alternatives. He had earlier instructed the U.S. consul in California, Thomas O. Larkin, to watch for both British activities and any opportunity to start a revolt against Mexican rule. Larkin could find no opportunity to play the role of Thomas Jefferson in California. But in June 1846, American settlers in the Sacramento area took advantage of the looming U.S.-Mexican war to declare their own independent "Bear Flag" state. The Republic of California survived less than a month, for, by July 1846, Polk was embarked on his main policy: conquest of all of California by force.

The president's policy was both simple and devious. He slowly squeezed Mexico militarily until it struck back. He then misrepresented the evidence for the attack to obtain Congress's declaration of war. In July 1845, ten months before war began, Polk instructed the U.S. military commander in Texas, Zachary Taylor, to move across the Nueces River into territory (between the Nueces and the Rio Grande) that was hotly disputed between Texas and Mexico. In January 1846, the president told Taylor to encamp on the Rio Grande itself. In April, the Mexican army demanded that Taylor move back. He responded by blockading the Mexicans and threatening them with starvation. On April 24, they tried to break the blockade, and blood was spilled. Back in Washington, Polk was becoming frustrated by Mexico's refusal to deal with Slidell. On May 9, he and his cabinet decided to settle the claims against Mexico and block British influence by declaring war. Later that day, Polk received word of the attack on Taylor's forces.

The president immediately sent a war message to Congress that was as historically inaccurate as it was politically potent. "The cup of forbearance had been exhausted" even before the news of the fighting arrived in Washington, Polk declared. "But now . . . Mexico . . . has invaded our territory and shed American blood upon the American soil." Doubting Whigs, even some Democrats, demanded evidence. The key documents, Polk's followers responded, were at the printer's and not available. Besides, they added, Congress should trust the president. The House of Representatives voted for war 174 to 14 (with John Quincy Adams in the small minority, as usual). In the Senate, John Calhoun—who now had acquired Texas for the South and wanted no war for Mexican territory that probably could not support slavery—and

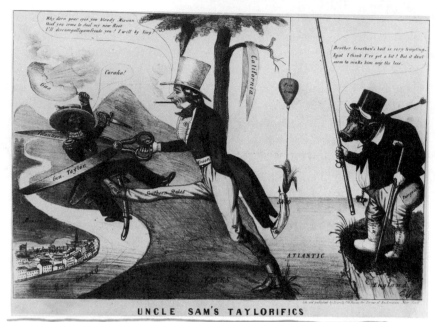

UNCLE SAM'S TAYLORIFICS

E. W. Clay's 1846 cartoon is a classic example of good American graphic art as well as of rampant American Manifest Destiny and anti-British feelings in 1846. The "Union," or an early "Uncle Sam" figure, is cutting up Mexico for trying to steal his "boot" of Texas. Note the early "John Bull" figure of the British Empire fishing for all of Oregon while Uncle Sam's back is turned.

a few others tried to slow down the rush to battle. They failed. The war declaration passed 40 to 2, with Calhoun abstaining.[31]

Polk finally had his war, but he also faced a terrible dilemma. He had called the war merely a defensive response to a Mexican attack, but in reality he wanted a war for conquest. Such a war could require high and politically unpopular expenses, as well as a large army that would have to be paid for by an already suspicious Congress. He discovered, moreover, that his two top military commanders, Generals Winfield Scott and Zachary Taylor, were both Whigs. If they covered themselves with glory, they could become leading presidential nominees. Polk had already declared that he would not be a candidate in the 1848 race, but he coldly disliked Whigs (whom he often condemned as "Federalists") and especially feared Scott and Taylor.

The two generals made real the president's nightmare. Attacking across the Rio Grande, Taylor won a series of victories at Monterey and Buena Vista, although at Buena Vista, Taylor's 5,000 troops had been surprised by a 20,000-man Mexican force. At Monterey, the

Americans won despite the absence of one of their top officers, who had taken a strong laxative the night before. (Nevertheless, Congress later gave the officer a jeweled sword for his "gallantry at Monterey.")[32] Meanwhile, Scott landed at Vera Cruz in a brilliant amphibious operation, for which he had designed the first landing crafts in U.S. military history. He then began a march toward Mexico City that no less an authority than the Duke of Wellington (conqueror of Napoleon) said could not be done. In a careful campaign that kept his casualties low, Scott reached Mexico City in late summer 1847 and prepared to wait for the government's surrender. He had even avoided costly battles with the Mexican army in the hope that patience would bring about a political settlement.

Polk had neither the time nor the temperament for such a campaign. As soon as war was declared, he asked Congress for $2 million to purchase peace (and California) from Mexico. His request set off an

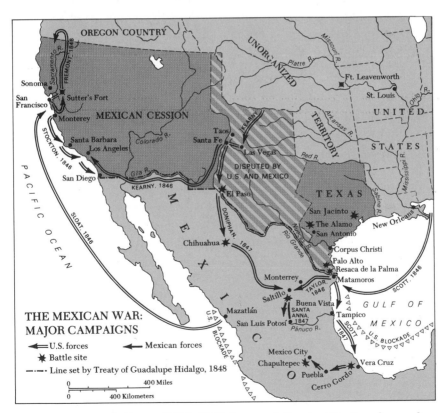

The U.S. war with Mexico (1846–1848) increased American territory by nearly 50 percent, gained valuable California ports, and helped lead to the Civil War.

explosion that reverberated for the next twenty years. When he asked Congress to legislate the funds, Democrats—who had become angered by Polk's political appointments and proslavery foreign policy in Texas—attached an amendment to the legislation that became known as the Wilmot Proviso. It was named after a Pennsylvania Democrat, David Wilmot, who belonged to Van Buren's Free Soil wing of the party. The proviso required that the money not be used to purchase any territory that would allow slavery. Democrats and Whigs from the South immediately condemned the measure. In the House vote, Polk's Democratic party splintered, but the proviso passed. Fifty-two northern free-state Democrats supported, and all fifty southern Democrats opposed, the measure. The Senate, where free- and slave-state representation was in balance, prevented the Wilmot Proviso from becoming law. Nevertheless, everyone involved understood that a political monster had appeared, one that could not be easily killed.

Polk could not understand what he had done. He denied that the great domestic issue had anything to do with foreign policy: slavery "was purely a domestic question" and "not a foreign question." In reality, of course, slavery had everything to do with foreign policy. Expansion, the central theme of the American experience since 1607, now raised the possibility of one side—either slave or nonslave—controlling vast new territories and, thus, soon controlling the government itself. Polk did see that "the slavery question . . . is a fire-brand in the body,"[33] but he also believed that because slavery could not exist on the poor soils of northern Mexico, Congress was raising the issue simply to embarrass him. The president proposed to settle the rising argument by extending the 1820 Missouri Compromise line of 36°30′ to the Pacific. But that compromise was no longer adequate. It could leave the vast Mexican territories south of the line open to slavery. Foreign policy and domestic concerns were so intertwined that each now threatened to strangle the other.

Congress quarreled and Democrats split while Whig generals triumphed. Those were not the results for which Polk had bargained. Despite the battlefield victories, however, Mexico refused to surrender. By the summer of 1847, even John L. O'Sullivan had doubts about Manifest Destiny: "I am afraid it was not God that got us into the war, but that He may get us out of it is the constant prayer of yours very truly."[34] The president finally decided to send Nicholas Trist to discuss peace with the Mexicans. A State Department clerk, Trist had mostly made his political fortune by marrying Thomas Jefferson's favorite granddaughter. He believed ardently in Manifest Destiny but now feared that the war threatened to destroy the Union. Trist wanted a quick peace. His early talks with Mexico, however, collapsed. Polk began to wonder whether Trist wanted peace so badly that he might even be willing to give up claims to much of California to achieve it. Almost as bad, the president learned that Trist and Scott had become fast friends. Polk told the diplomat to return immediately.

Mexico's refusal to surrender then produced another crisis for the president. An "All-Mexico" movement appeared. It demanded that U.S. claims and loss of life could only be satisfied by seizing the entire country. The movement had its most feverish supporters among northern Democrats, both among the sensationalistic press in cities such as New York and the agrarian–Manifest Destiny expansionists of the Midwest. Polk fueled the All-Mexico drive by leaving open the possibility of more war and more conquest if Mexico did not immediately give him what he wanted. As the All-Mexico mania intensified, however, Trist killed it in a single stroke. He ignored Polk's orders to return after he heard that Mexico might be prepared to discuss peace terms. Scott's plan to wait out his opponents had finally worked. Trist obtained all that Polk had originally demanded: California, New Mexico, and the Rio Grande boundary.

Infuriated that Trist had disobeyed his order to return, Polk nevertheless had little choice but to accept the peace treaty of Guadalupe Hidalgo. It was either accepting what he had initially wanted or facing a profound political crisis generated by the All-Mexico and Wilmot Proviso zealots. Polk chose peace. After all, as he told Congress on July 6, 1848, California and the New Mexico territory "constitute of themselves a country large enough for a great empire."

Two Near-Misses and a Near-Settlement

Polk had apparently learned little from the experience. His passion for expansion and his inability to understand the links between domestic and foreign policy forced him to face two more potential crises.

In April 1848, Yucatán—a province of Mexico—asked for U.S. aid against an Indian revolt. Yucatán also asked Spain and Great Britain for aid. Polk immediately requested permission from Congress to intervene. Waving once again the Monroe Doctrine, he warned that the United States would occupy Yucatán before allowing it to come under European influence. Americans were tired of hearing about Mexico, none more so than John Calhoun. The South Carolina sena-

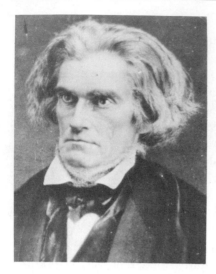

John C. Calhoun (1782–1850) of South Carolina defended slavery and slave expansionism almost literally until his dying breath. But Calhoun disliked the War with Mexico and bitterly fought Polk's attempt to use the Monroe Doctrine as a tool to obtain more territory.

tor unleashed an attack on the request that not only finally killed the plan, but raised fundamental questions for Americans in the future.

Calhoun, who had been in Monroe's cabinet in 1823, denied that the original doctrine had anything to do with occupying such places as Mexico. It only said that North America would keep its hands off Latin American problems and expected Europeans to do the same. The South Carolinian observed that if the United States occupied Yucatán, a most dangerous precedent would be established: other Latin American countries (such as Yucatán) will have obtained the power "to make us a party to all their wars" on their terms and according to their own, not United States', interests. "We shall be forever involved in wars" to save Latin Americans from themselves, Calhoun warned. It was one of the most powerful attacks ever made on the Monroe Doctrine. Fortunately for both Polk and Calhoun, Yucatán resolved its problem, and Polk withdrew the request.[35]

Even though the debate had been an embarrassment, Polk next set his sights on Cuba. In May 1848, John L. O'Sullivan and Democratic senator Stephen A. Douglas from Illinois privately urged Polk to buy Cuba from Spain. Americans had long coveted the island. In 1848, moreover, France had freed its West Indian slaves. England had freed its bondsmen in 1833. Cuba now remained as the major slave society in the Caribbean. American slaveholders believed that the island had to be saved from the building pressure for emancipation. They were joined by northern merchants who profited from Cuban routes and even from the secret, but highly lucrative, trade in black men and women—a trade that had been outlawed forty years before. Cuba exemplified slavery at its worst. About 324,000 slaves and 425,000 whites lived on the island, bound together in a decaying and brutal system.

Polk nevertheless pushed for annexation. He believed that it would ease the fears of southerners who felt that they were becoming a minority section. The island, moreover, "would speedily be Americanized [with whites] as Louisiana had been," as Secretary of State James Buchanan phrased it. Perhaps nothing could have more aroused and divided American society in 1848 than a debate over Cuban annexation. Fortunately, Polk's plan never reached that point. Despite U.S. pressure, Spain refused to sell. Buchanan had used the occasion, however, to warn Spain that Cuba must never pass into the hands of any other power.

Polk's proposals on Yucatán and Cuba occurred amid a wild U.S. political scene. In mid-1848, the Democrats split. The regular party nominated Lewis Cass of Michigan, a zealot for Manifest Destiny who had fought to take Texas and opposed the Wilmot Proviso. Antislave Democrats quit the convention and nominated Martin Van Buren of New York on the Free Soil ticket. The Whigs countered with Zachary Taylor. The Mexican War hero was such a strong believer in traditional values that he acknowledged his nomination late because the notification letter arrived with postage due and he refused to pay it. After Taylor won and assumed the presidency, he moved to settle the central question of how to govern the vast territory conquered by Polk.

In one of the great debates in U.S. history, the Compromise of 1850 was hammered out in the Senate. A dying Calhoun warned that "the cords which bind these states together" were snapping under "the agitation of the slavery question." He intimated the need for constitutional amendments to protect the rights of slaveholders in the new territories. But the aged Henry Clay and Daniel Webster carried the day for the more moderate forces. They argued that local conditions and climate should settle the issue. The final compromise, therefore, brought in California as a free state (as its inhabitants desired). It allowed citizens in New Mexico and Utah territories to work out their own policy on the slave question. This approach became known as popular sovereignty. The slave trade (but not slavery) was finally abolished in the District of Columbia, where humans had been traded for cash and crops in the shadows of U.S. government buildings for half a century. In return, the federal government promised, in a Fugitive Slave Law, to help southerners capture and return runaway slaves. This "businessman's peace," as the compromise was called, postponed the war over the Union for ten years.

MANIFEST DESTINY IN CENTRAL AMERICA

The Senate also passed another historic measure in 1850: the Clayton-Bulwer Treaty gave Americans their first formal right to realize a dream of centuries—an isthmian canal in Central America to link the Atlantic and the Pacific. The treaty was an appropriate act with which to climax the U.S. trade and territorial conquest of the 1840s.

Until this time, Great Britain dominated Central American affairs. Growing U.S. interest in Asian trade, the annexation of Oregon and California, then the dramatic discovery of gold in California during 1848 transformed the Central American power balance. Adventurers and entrepreneurs from the United States profited from turning the region into a passageway for Americans who traveled from the East to the West Coast or to the far Pacific. Newly arrived Americans discovered that the British controlled several strategic areas on the Atlantic-coast side of a possible canal (the Mosquito Coast in Nicaragua, and Belize, bordered by Guatemala) and had been eying the Panamanian area of New Granada. U.S. diplomats neatly played on the fears of the Latin Americans to checkmate the British. The U.S. minister to New Granada, Benjamin Bidlack, signed a treaty in 1846 that gave the United States transit rights across Panama. In return, the United States guaranteed transit rights in the area for other parties. The Senate, realizing that this deal amounted to an entangling alliance, delayed ratification until 1848. The Bidlack pact enabled Americans to build the first transcontinental railway (of 48 miles) in Panama during the 1850s and provided the excuse, in 1903, for Theodore Roosevelt's seizure of Panama to build the present canal. Nicaragua and Honduras, also fearful of British imperialism, next signed treaties giving the United States transit rights. The Americans and British were on a collision course.

To avoid possible war, British minister Sir Henry Bulwer and Secretary of State John Clayton worked out a pact providing that (1) neither nation would build an isthmian canal in Central America without the consent or cooperation of the other, (2) neither would fortify or found new colonies in the area, and (3) if a canal were built, both powers would guarantee its neutrality. It was a handsome victory for Zachary Taylor's administration. The British had recognized the United

States as an equal in Central America. Whigs were delighted with both the isthmian rights and the dodging of war with Great Britain. Democrats, led by Stephen A. Douglas, not surprisingly condemned the treaty for compromising with the hated John Bull.

THE LEGACIES OF MANIFEST DESTINY AND JAMES K. POLK

The importance of 1840s expansionism in American history goes far beyond the new influence in Central America or even the conquest of the million-square-mile empire in the West. Ralph Waldo Emerson compared the Mexican War to a dose of arsenic for the Union. The military hero of the Civil War, General Ulysses S. Grant, recalled in his memoirs that he had "bitterly opposed" invading Mexico and wanted to obtain the southwest territory through peaceful means. "The Southern rebellion [the Civil War] was largely the outgrowth of the Mexican War," Grant believed.[36] More than a century later, historian Thomas Hietala would look back over Polk's systematic expansionism and conclude that it "was not manifest destiny. It was manifest design."[37]

Polk also left another historic legacy. The way in which he led the United States into the Mexican War set precedents for later powerful chief executives—indeed, provided an early preview of the so-called "imperial presidency" of the twentieth century. Abraham Lincoln, then a young Illinois Whig strongly opposed to Polk's policies toward Mexico, attacked these new presidential powers in a now-famous letter written to a friend in 1848:

> Allow the President to invade a neighboring nation, whenever *he* shall deem it necessary to repel an invasion, and you allow him to do so, *whenever he may choose to say* he deems it necessary for such purpose—and you allow him to make war at pleasure. Study to see if you can fix *any limit* to his power in this respect, after you have given him so much as you propose. . . . You may say to him, "I see no probability of the British invading us" but he will say to you, "be silent; I see it, if you don't."
>
> The provision of the Constitution giving the war-making power to Congress, was dictated, as I understand it, by the following reasons. Kings had always been involving and impoverishing their people in wars, pretending generally, if not always, that the good of the people was the object. This, our Convention [of 1787] understood to be the most oppressive of all Kingly oppressions; and they resolved to so frame the Constitution that *no one* man should hold the power of bringing this oppression upon us.[38]

Polk never lived to see the Civil War that his own use of presidential power had helped bring about. As chief executive, he worked long hours to supervise every act of his administration. While other officers fled Washington's summer heat, the president remained. Polk grew to believe, moreover, that his administration was the victim of petty politics and the presidential ambitions of others. "I now predict that no President of the U.S. of either party will ever again be re-elected" to a second term, he said.[39] The self-discipline and the politics and passions of U.S. foreign policy killed him. Within four months of leaving the presidency, Polk died at the age of fifty-four.

NOTES

1. Julius W. Pratt, "The Ideology of American Expansion," in *Essays in Honor of William E. Dodd*, ed. Avery Craven (Chicago, 1935), p. 343.
2. *Ibid.*, p. 342.
3. Albert K. Weinberg, *Manifest Destiny* (Baltimore, 1935), pp. 192–223.
4. Arthur M. Schlesinger, Jr., *The Age of Jackson* (Boston, 1945), pp. 496–497.
5. The Ritchie quote is in Thomas R. Hietala, *Manifest Design: Anxious Aggrandizement in Late Jacksonian America* (Ithaca, 1985), p. 198; good background can be found in John Holenberg, *Foreign Correspondents: The Great Reporters and Their Times* (New York, 1964), pp. 28–29.
6. Leo Marx, *The Machine in the Garden* (New York, 1964), is a superb analysis.
7. Charles Vevier, "American Continentalism: An Idea of Expansion, 1845–1910," *American Historical Review* 65 (January 1960): 324–327, a small classic; Hietala, pp. 198–199.
8. Frederick Merk, *Manifest Destiny and Mission in American History: A Reinterpretation* (New York, 1963), pp. 107–108.
9. Walt Whitman, *The Gathering of the Forces*, 2 vols. (New York, 1920), I, pp. 32–33.
10. "What's So Bad about Feeling Good?" *Public Opinion* 8 (April/May 1985): 3, is an update and evaluation of Tocqueville's insight.
11. Joel H. Silbey, "The Election of 1836," in *History of American Presidential Elections, 1789–1968*, ed. Arthur M. Schlesinger, Jr., 4 vols. (New York, 1971), I, pp. 577–583, 598–599; *The American Party System*, ed. William N. Chambers and William Dean Burnham (New York, 1975), p. 112.
12. Robert W. Tucker and David C. Hendrickson, *The Imperial Temptation* (New York, 1992), p. 173.
13. Reginald Horsman, "American Indian Policy and the Origins of Manifest Destiny," *University of Birmingham Historical Journal* 11, no. 2 (1968): 138.
14. Angie Debo, *A History of the Indians of the United States* (Norman, Okla., 1970), pp. 101–111.

15. Pratt, p. 344.
16. Thomas McCormick, "Liberal Capitalism . . . ," in Lloyd Gardner *et al., Creation of the American Empire,* 2d ed. (Chicago, 1976), pp. 120, 130.
17. Stuart C. Miller, "The American Trader's Image of China, 1785–1840," *Pacific Historical Review* 36 (November 1967): 381.
18. Mira Wilkins, *The Emergence of Multinational Enterprise: American Business Abroad from the Colonial Era to 1914* (Cambridge, Mass., 1970), p. 9; Miller, 384–385.
19. Peter W. Fay, "The Protestant Mission and the Opium War," *Pacific Historical Review* 40 (May 1971): 145–149.
20. Hietala, pp. 60–63.
21. John R. Bodo, *The Protestant Clergy and Public Issues, 1812–1848* (Princeton, 1954), pp. 230–231.
22. Edward P. Crapol, "Lydia Maria Child: Abolitionist Critic of American Foreign Policy," in *Women and American Foreign Policy,* ed. Edward P. Crapol (Westport, Conn., 1987), pp. 1–18, and Crapol's superb essay, "The Foreign Policy of Antislavery, 1833–1846," in *Redefining the Past: Essays in Diplomatic History in Honor of William Appleman Williams,* ed. Lloyd C. Gardner (Corvallis, Ore., 1986).
23. Charles G. Sellers, *James K. Polk, Jacksonian: 1795–1843* (Princeton, 1957), p. 112.
24. James T. Hathaway, *Incidents in the Campaign of 1844* (New Haven, 1905), p. 26.
25. Norman A. Graebner, "James K. Polk," in *America's Ten Greatest Presidents,* ed. Morton Borden (Chicago, 1961), p. 135.
26. William Safire, "Second Inaugural Address," *New York Times,* 14 January 1985, p. A19.
27. Howard Jones, "Daniel Webster, the Diplomatist," in *Daniel Webster: "The Completest Man,"* ed. Kenneth E. Shewmaker (Hanover, N.H., 1990), pp. 204–218, provides an especially good summary of these episodes; Howard Jones, *To the Webster-Ashburton Treaty: A Study in Anglo-American Relations, 1783–1843* (Chapel Hill, N.C., 1977), is excellent on the background and standard on the negotiations, especially pp. 88–102; Howard Jones, *Mutiny on the Amistad* (New York, 1987), tells the story of the mutiny by the slaves and negotiations for their freedom, especially pp. 204–219 on Webster.
28. Ray Allen Billington, *Westward Expansion* (New York, 1949), pp. 509–511.
29. *The Diary of James K. Polk during His Presidency,* ed. Milo M. Quaife, 4 vols. (Chicago, 1910), I, p. 155; Hietala, p. 74.
30. *Diary of Polk,* ed. Quaife, I, p. 71.
31. Charles Sellers, *James K. Polk, Continentalist: 1843–1846* (Princeton, 1966), pp. 416–421, has a good account of the debate and Polk's springing of the war declaration preamble on Congress.
32. *Parade Magazine,* 8 April 1984, p. 17.
33. *Diary of Polk,* ed. Quaife, II, pp. 289, 305.
34. Frederick Merk, *The Monroe Doctrine and American Expansion, 1843–1849* (New York, 1966), p. 253.
35. *Ibid.,* p. 231; Dexter Perkins, *The Monroe Doctrine, 1826–1867* (Baltimore, 1933), pp. 182–183.
36. Gore Vidal, *Matters of Fact and of Fiction* (New York, 1977), p. 179, for context.
37. Hietala, ch. II, has a good discussion.
38. *The Political Thought of Lincoln,* ed. Richard N. Current (Indianapolis, 1967), pp.

43–44. Lincoln, of course, used those presidential powers to the utmost just thirteen years later.

39. *Diary of Polk*, ed. Quaife, II, p. 314.

FOR FURTHER READING

Consult the notes of this chapter and the General Bibliography at the end of this book (most of whose references are not repeated below), but especially note *Guide to American Foreign Relations since 1700*, ed. Richard Dean Burns (1983), light-years ahead of anything else on pre-1981 sources and helpfully organized as well.

A sweeping cultural overview on Manifest Destiny is Vivien Green Fryd's *Art and Empire: Ethnicity in the U.S. Capitol, 1815–1860* (1992). The earlier years are covered in Robert Remini's prize-winning biography *Andrew Jackson and the Course of American Empire* (1981) and in John H. Schroeder's fine *Shaping a Maritime Empire* (1985), which covers the U.S. Navy's activities from the 1830s to the Civil War. Four superb books make westward expansion come alive: Sandra L. Myres, *Westering Women and the Frontier Experience, 1800–1915* (1982), and Annette Kolodny, *The Land before Her: Fantasy and Experience of the American Frontiers, 1630–1860* (1984), Julie Ray Jeffrey, *Converting the West: A Biography of Narcissa Whitman* (1991), which are vivid on the horrors that confronted women in the westward trek; and Bill Gilbert, *Westering Man: The Life of Joseph Walker* (1983).

The best and most complete overview remains David M. Pletcher, *The Diplomacy of Annexation: Texas, Oregon, and the Mexican War* (1973), with excellent sources noted; specific areas are well covered in Wilbur D. Jones, *The American Problem in British Diplomacy, 1841–1861* (1985); Michael H. Hunt's pathbreaking *The Making of a Special Relationship: The United States and China to 1914* (1983); Curtis T. Henson, Jr., *Commissioners and Commodores: The East India Squadron and American Diplomacy in China* (1982); and the readable Arthur P. Dudden, *The American Pacific* (1992); while key figures are analyzed in Frederic A. Greenhut, "Edmund Roberts: Early American Diplomat," *Manuscripts* 35 (Fall 1983), and in three superb works by Kenneth Shewmaker: "Daniel Webster and American Conservatism," in *Traditions and Values: American Diplomacy, 1790–1855*, ed. Norman Graebner (1985); "Forging the 'Great Chain': Daniel Webster and the Origins of American Foreign Policy toward East Asia and the Pacific, 1841–1852," *American Philosophical Society* 129 (September 1985); and *The Papers of Daniel Webster: Diplomatic Papers* (1983–), of which Shewmaker is chief editor. The South's leading figure tells his story in *The Papers of John C. Calhoun*, ed. Clyde N. Wilson *et al.* which, by 1991, had reached 1844 documents and Calhoun's more intense involvement in foreign policy; and John Niven, *John C. Calhoun and The Price of Union: A Biography* (1992). Deborah Pickman Clifford, *Crusader for Freedom: A Life of Lydia Maria Child* (1991), is an important biography.

On the Mexican War, aside from the Pletcher volume (and its bibliographical references) noted above, the following are important: Paul H. Bergeron, *The Presidency of James K. Polk* (1987); Carlos Bosch Garcia, "The Mexican War," in *Diplomatic Claims: Latin American Historians View the United States*, trans. and ed. Warren Dean (1985), an important Latin American perspective; Neal Harlow, *California Conquered: War and Peace on the Pacific, 1846–1850* (1982); Ernest M. Lander, Jr., *Reluctant Imperialists: Calhoun, the South Carolinians, and the Mexican War* (1984); four essays on the 1840s in *Foundations of American Foreign Policy*, ed. Norman Graebner (1986); and two works by Graebner himself: "The Mexican War: A Study in Causation," *Pacific Historical Review* 49 (August 1980), and the reprint of his 1955 book, *Empire on the Pacific* (1983), with an important interpretation and an updated bibliography.

Especially useful is Norman E. Tutorow, *The Mexican-American War, an Annotated Bibliography* (1981).

5

The Climax of Early U.S. Foreign Policy: The Civil War (1850–1865)

FOREIGN POLICY AS A CAUSE OF THE CIVIL WAR

American expansion accelerated after 1815. It seemed out of control by 1850. The new Democratic president, Franklin Pierce, candidly declared in his 1853 inaugural address that "my administration will not be controlled by any timid forebodings of evil from expansion." Pierce had been elected on a platform that embodied Manifest Destiny. It termed the Mexican War "just and necessary." George Sanders, a Kentucky politician, caught perfectly the spirit of the age: Americans "are booted and spurred, and are panting for conquest."[1]

The Civil War logically climaxed post-1815 expansionism and the fragmentation of the United States. But it was also part of larger changes in the Western world. Europe endured an era of revolution between 1789 and 1850. Modern industrial capitalism and middle-class society were born amid the rubble of old classes overwhelmed by the new forces. This birth, moreover, was made more painful because large numbers of common people became active political participants for the first time, both in the United States and in western Europe. Many of these people were also caught up in mass migrations that shocked and transformed many parts of the world.[2] The United States especially experienced the astonishing effects of the immigration. Between 1820 and 1840, about 700,000 newcomers entered the country; but between 1840 and 1860, some 4.2 million flooded over eastern cities and western lands. In Europe, communism first began to appear as a movement to be reckoned with; in the United States, the first important labor unions emerged. The United States could not escape the crosscurrents that rocked the Western world.

Amid this rapid change and the promise of indefinite expansion in the post-1815 era, two factions emerged in the United States to struggle over the question of who would control the foreign policies and benefit from the expansion. They were the same two that James Madison had observed were the main opponents in the 1787 Constitutional Convention: the slave and the nonslave states (see p. 32). Since 1787, the Union had been kept in precarious balance by equally dividing the new territories between the two. After 1850, however, the balance began to disappear when California entered the Union and the free states gained a majority in the U.S. Senate. The North, with its much larger population, already could control the House of Representatives. In addition, the North was becoming wealthier faster than the South. By 1859, the value of the former's manufacturing alone was ten times greater than that of the latter's cotton. People discussed King Cotton, but the real rulers were iron, leather, and wheat. Per-capita income in the industrial Northeast was double that of the South.

Power created power. Railroad mileage in New England and the Midwest outstripped the South's. Western farmers were linked to the Northeast's merchants by bands of iron. The new rail system neutralized the Mississippi and other north-south waterways. Chicago, nonexistent in 1800, became a railroad hub and saw its population jump from 30,000 in 1850 to 110,000 in 1860—an amount larger than the South's Charleston, Memphis, Mobile, and Atlanta combined. Southerners found themselves trapped in a one-crop slave economy. They were dependent on northeastern bankers and shippers. They were at the mercy of world cotton markets over which they had little control. They lived in the middle of a growing black population that had already set off slave revolts. They were unable to increase the number of white or immigrant inhabitants to keep pace with the North. And now they were in a minority in both houses of Congress.

These developments directly shaped U.S. foreign policy: southerners believed that the survival of their society relied on acquiring new land. Cuba and Central America were the areas most frequently targeted. Only expansion could give the South new soil to replace worn-out land in the older states. Only expansion could give southerners hope to bal-

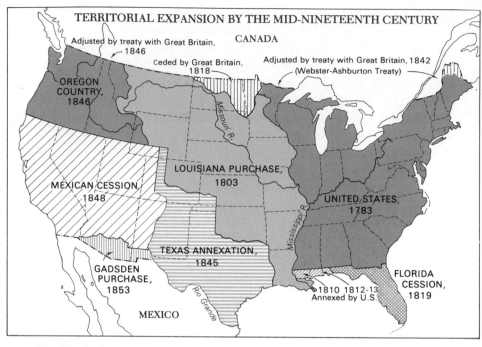

The United States in the 1850s, after expansion rounded out the continental boundaries and just before the Civil War nearly tore it in half.

ance once again the North's power in Congress. Northerners, for their part, had no intention of losing their newly found power. And northern farmers certainly had no intention of allowing the South to block them from settling their free-labor system in new territories.

In the 1850s, therefore, two explosive forces collided. A great debate erupted over the direction of American expansion. In 1860, the election of Abraham Lincoln (a free-soil Republican who gained fame and income as a sharp lawyer for the new railroads) convinced the South that it had finally lost control of U.S. foreign policy. It could no longer hope to obtain fresh lands for slavery, cotton, and political power. So the southerners left the Union. The bloodiest event in their history demonstrated how Americans could not escape the intimate relationship between their foreign and domestic affairs.

YOUNG AMERICA: SOUTH, NORTH, AND AT HOME

More than a century later, it is difficult to recapture the ferocity, even violence, with which Americans conducted this foreign-policy debate in the 1850s. In the Democratic party, an extreme group, Young America, used popular racist arguments to put down those who urged restraint ("the old fogies") and instead insisted on "sympathy for the liberals of Europe, the expansion of the American republic southward and westward, and the grasping of the magnificent purse of the commerce of the Pacific." Young America's leading politician, Stephen A. Douglas of Illinois, believed his country too great to have silly "disputes about boundaries" or to "suffer mere 'red lines' on maps." Douglas and his friends condemned their "unnatural mother," Great Britain, for trying to contain U.S. expansion.[3] Young America's idea was to expand both north and south, then worry about the political problems later—although some, such as Douglas, believed that the problem of which section was to govern the newly acquired regions could be resolved through "popular sovereignty," that is, allowing the settlers to decide whether they wanted a slave or free society.

Young America was more than rhetoric and bombast. Its favorite presidential candidate in 1852, Franklin Pierce of New Hampshire, won the election and promptly gave diplomatic posts to the group's members. The appointments included minister to France (John Mason of Virginia) and minister to Spain (Pierre Soulé of Louisiana). Young America, however, then ran into a series of difficulties. Expanding southward meant dealing with black and other nonwhite races in Cuba and Latin America, an encounter that most Americans hoped to avoid. In 1854, for example, a crisis arose when Spain illegally seized a U.S. ship. Then rumors flew that the Spanish were about to free the slaves in Cuba. The Pierce administration used the opportunity to order Soulé

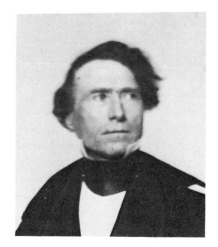

Franklin Pierce (1804–1869) from New Hampshire had never made a mark as a member of Congress or the Senate, and was even accused of being the sad "hero of many a well-fought bottle." But his expansionism, identification with the Young America movement, and hatred of abolitionists surprisingly gained him the Democratic party's nomination, then the presidency in 1853. Over the next four years, the expansionism of this untalented man further dragged the nation down the path toward civil war.

to buy Cuba for $130 million. If Spain refused, the minister was to plan "to detach" Cuba from Spain.

Soulé, Mason, and James Buchanan (U.S. minister to Great Britain) met in Ostend, Belgium, to coordinate their moves. The three were not the calmest of diplomats (Soulé had already shot the French minister in Madrid during a duel after someone in the French Embassy had publicly commented on Mrs. Soulé's breasts). The ministers now sent a secret message to Washington—the Ostend Manifesto—that urged "wresting Cuba from Spain" if the island could not be purchased. Both Europeans and northerners in the United States instantly condemned the "manifesto." Pierce beat a hasty retreat. The clumsiness of Young America deepened free-soilers' suspicions of a slave-power conspiracy to control U.S. foreign policy. The episode and the reaction to it also ruined any chance to annex Cuba during the 1850s.

Another setback to Young America occurred in the North. Few believed that Canada could simply be seized; after all, it was owned by the world's greatest power. But Canadians were growing restless under British rule. They especially wanted more trade with the growing market to their south. In 1854, the United States made a significant reciprocity agreement by signing the Marcy-Elgin Treaty. (Trade reciprocity means lowering U.S. tariffs to a nation in return for that country making reciprocal, or similar, concessions.) Young Americans viewed the treaty as a first step toward annexation of Canada. In reality, however, the pact helped quiet Canadian unrest. The British also promised Canada greater independence, and in 1867 Canada gained control over many of its own affairs.

Ardent expansionists suffered a major setback at home between 1854 and 1857. Douglas brought a bill before Congress to organize Nebraska Territory into two states, Kansas and Nebraska, where a key section of the proposed transcontinental railroad was to be built. Southerners refused to support Douglas unless the Missouri Compromise of 1820 (which prohibited slavery north of 36°30′) was explicitly repealed. Douglas successfully worked for the repeal of the prohibition. All of Kansas-Nebraska opened to slaveowners. Free-soilers were furious. They used the North's superiority in money and population to flood the region with antislave advocates. Violence erupted. As the southern part of the territory became known as "bleeding Kansas," free-soilers turned bitterly against Douglas and his idea of popular sovereignty. But so did many slaveholders who now realized that they could no longer compete with the North's power.

Both sides began to demand government guarantees and protection for their own cause. Popular sovereignty became discredited. When Douglas insisted on retaining the idea, southern Democrats, who wanted Washington to protect slavery in all territories, disavowed him. The Democratic party split in 1857–1858. An adhesive that had kept the Union together, the two-party system (which contained in each party both northerners and southerners), now became a three-party system: northern Democrats, southern states-rights Democrats, and the new Republican party. Political affiliations began to divide more and more along sectional lines.

No longer could Americans conquer new lands and assume that the question of who was to control the area could be worked out peacefully and democratically. Now foreign-policy expansionism could mean war at home in the form of a "bleeding Kansas." But Americans were not about to stop doing what they had been doing for centuries. They continued to try to carry out a vigorous expansionist foreign policy. Three case studies—the first involving Japan, the second revolving around the ambitions of William Henry Seward, and the third focusing on Central America—are especially revealing. The first two give a glimpse into the future. The third attempted to recreate a past that, as southerners and Young America boosters learned to their sorrow, was not to be repeated.

WHIGS AND ASIA

In 1850, Millard Fillmore moved up to the presidency after Zachary Taylor's sudden death. Fillmore appointed Daniel Webster as secretary of state. The nation was still recovering from the bitter 1850 Compromise debate (see p. 123), and Webster set out to use bombastic pronouncements (but little action) on foreign policy as a means of making Americans proud and bringing them back together. A superb opportunity arose after Hungary revolted against Austria. Tsarist Russia, Austria's conservative ally, quickly smashed the rebellion and restored the monarchy. When Austria discovered that the United States had planned to recognize the revolutionaries, it shot off a strong protest to Washington. Webster responded with the so-called Hülsemann letter (sent to Austria's chargé in Washington, Chevalier Hülsemann) in which he told Austria in grand terms how Americans would support freedom anywhere they pleased. For good measure, Webster added that compared with the United States, Austria was nothing more than "a patch on the earth's surface." As historian Kenneth Shewmaker observes, the Hülsemann letter was a "classic example of tailoring foreign policy to the needs of domestic politics."[4]

Webster and the Whigs also stirred hearts when they loudly welcomed Louis Kossuth, the Hungarian revolutionary leader, to the United States in 1851. Kossuth, however, mistakenly believed that when Webster and other Americans praised his revolution, they also were offering to help it directly. No U.S. political leader, especially among Whigs, considered challenging the Russian use of force in Hungary. As historian Donald S. Spencer has shown, Young America Democrats more strongly supported Kossuth's cause than did the Whigs, but not even these Democrats offered their bodies to ensure that Hungary could enjoy the blessings of 1776.[5] The disillusioned Kossuth left the United States in 1852 virtually unnoticed.

Other than fine, if empty, declarations, the Whigs offered one other outlet for expansionist-minded Americans in the 1850s: the promise of new opportunities in Asia. China had been opened to Americans by the last Whig administration. Webster now focused on Japan. As the London *Times* understood, once Americans took San Francisco, "the course lies straight and obvious to Polynesia, the Philippines . . . and China, and it is not extravagant to suppose that the merchants of this future emporium may open the commerce of Japan."[6] The commerce had largely been closed to the West. U.S. businessmen, as well as politicians such as John Quincy Adams, had long believed that it was against the laws of nature for countries to close themselves off from commerce and "civilization." "We do not admit the right of a nation of people to exclude themselves and their country from intercourse with the rest of the world," declared a group of U.S. merchants who eyed the Japanese market.[7] Hating iron curtains and colonial powers that shut them out of some markets, Americans have long looked at trade as a natural and an inalienable right. Japan needed to be opened as well to protect shipwrecked U.S. sailors. They had often been brutally treated when washed up on Japanese shores.

But above all was the lure of profit—a profit that came from the new technology of steamships and the growing trade they carried to and from Asian ports. President Fillmore's May 10, 1851, letter to the Japanese emporor (a letter written by Webster) stressed the importance of this technology and trade in the opening of the historic relationship. Having acquired "the great countries of Oregon & California," Fillmore told the emporor, Americans with their new steamships can suddenly reach Japan "in less than twenty days. . . . Our object is friendly commercial intercourse, and nothing more. . . . Your empire has a great abundance of coal . . . which our Steamships, in going from California to China, must use." When Commodore Matthew C. Perry learned in 1852 that he was to head a mission to open Japan, he rushed up and down the Boston-Washington region to collect new American inventions and information from businesses so he could instruct the Japanese how to become industrialized. He later gave them their first telegraph as well as a miniature railroad that delighted Japanese officials who rode on it with gowns flying in the wind.[8]

Americans, however, also planned to "civilize" Japan. Until that happened, the Asians would resemble Native Americans who insisted on living outside the law. "You have to deal with barbarians as barbarians," a Whig senator from North Carolina declared, because Japan could not be expected to act like "the civilized portion of mankind." That view gained popularity after the Japanese acted rudely toward Perry during his first visit in 1853; but they then became cooperative a year later, when he returned with a much larger fleet. The U.S. secretary of the navy concluded that triumphs such as Perry's were "but an extension of popular virtue, republican simplicity and world-teaching example." A less enthusiastic senator from Florida, however, wondered whether Americans should only "take one continent at a time."[9]

The Japanese learned quickly. After intense internal debate, they followed the principle of jujitsu—that is, use the opponent's strength to control him. Soon after Perry departed, Japan set up an Institute for the Investigation of Barbarian Books so that it could learn how the West had become so strong technologically and militarily. On the other hand, Western philosophy and religion were clearly inferior and disruptive, so they were to be ignored.[10] By 1858, the Japanese willingly dealt with the American consul, Townsend Harris, more openly than they had with Perry. The 1858 treaty first opened five major ports to foreign trade and affirmed extraterritoriality rights. Diplomatic representatives were exchanged. In 1864, a small fleet of foreign warships, including a single U.S. vessel, shot their way back into Japan after foreigners were mistreated. But the Japanese adjusted rapidly. In 1868, the emperor returned to power. Under his rule the people resumed learning from foreigners while also playing them off against each other. The small, disciplined nation of islands learned the lessons so well that within a generation it challenged the West for supremacy on the Asian mainland.

Many Americans saw their successes in Japan as simply Manifest Destiny. A popular magazine caught the spirit and gave it proper historical perspective. "Twenty years ago the 'far west' was a fixed idea

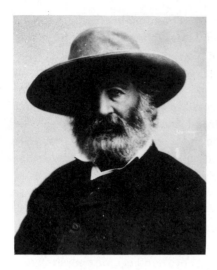

Walt Whitman (1819–1892) of New York is perhaps the greatest American poet and is certainly one of the nation's most original voices. He explored especially what he termed "the new empire" of the mid-nineteenth century that reached across the continent and toward Asia.

resting upon a fixed extent of territory," the journal wrote in 1852. But now "President Fillmore finds a 'far west' on the isles of the Japanese Empire and on the shores of China."[11] Poet Walt Whitman best expressed the belief that although U.S. territorial expansion had hit the wall of the Pacific Ocean, that was no reason to stop expanding. As Whitman said in his 1860 poem "The New Empire" (written to celebrate the first visit of Japanese diplomats to New York City), the Pacific could become a vast highway that opened to Americans an incredible future.

> I chant the world on my Western Sea; . . .
> I chant the new empire, grander than any before—as in a vision it comes to me;
> I chant America, the Mistress—I chant a greater supremacy;
> I chant, projected, a thousand blooming cities yet, in time, on those groups of sea-islands;
> I chant commerce opening, the sleep of ages having done its work— races, reborn, refresh'd. . . .[12]

SEWARD: PROPHET OF U.S.-RUSSIAN RELATIONS

No politician of the era better exemplified its spirit or more dominated its foreign policy than William Henry Seward of New York. "A slouching, slender figure; a head like a wise macaw, a beaked nose; shaggy eyebrows; unorderly hair and clothes; hoarse voice; offhand manner;

free talk, and perpetual cigar" was the firsthand description of Seward by Henry Adams.[13] Appearances could deceive. Despite the informality, Seward had one of the best-stocked minds of his time. His foreign policies, in the words of historian Ernest Paolino, "anticipated the direction of American foreign policy for the next generation and beyond."[14] Those policies arose from a deep, although not original, reading of history. As one of his biographers remarked, "He made the past his servant." When Seward first visited Washington in the 1840s, he was amazed at "how little study and how little learning men who have ambition on this great stage are content to arm themselves."[15]

A graduate of Union College in New York (at the age of nineteen in 1820), Seward was a lawyer and then the highly successful governor of New York before he entered the Senate as a Whig in 1849. He immediately opposed slave expansion. The New Yorker declared that "a higher law than the Constitution" should guide antislavery actions, a phrase that seemed to hint of revolution to many nonsoutherners as well as to slaveholders. By 1858, he warned of an "irrepressible conflict" that would continue until either slavery or freedom triumphed. These words did not come easily, for Seward, like his hero John Quincy Adams, believed in the nation's Manifest Destiny. But also like Adams, he opposed slave expansion so his own free-soil region could control the western lands—and Congress. Seward coveted Cuba, Central America, Mexico, and Canada. He even believed that, ultimately, so many Americans would live in the Southwest, the nation's capital should be moved from Washington to the Mississippi Valley—or perhaps even Mexico City. Realizing the political price of such expansion in the 1850s, however, he switched his expansionist enthusiasm to commerce and the Pacific trade.

Seward was the first U.S. official who developed a coherent Asian policy. It rested on a bedrock assumption: that the first step toward controlling Asia's markets required the spread of industry, railroads, and canals through the American heartland. "Open up a highway through your country, from New York to San Francisco," he proclaimed to the Senate in 1853. "Put your domain under cultivation and your ten thousand wheels of manufacture in motion. The nation that draws most materials and provisions from the earth, and fabricates the most, and sells the most of productions and fabrics to foreign nations, must be, and will be, the great power of the earth."[16] He was convinced that the Monroe Doctrine was already largely fulfilled. The United States was well on its way to dominating the Western Hemisphere. It was now "the Pacific Ocean . . . and the vast regions beyond" that were

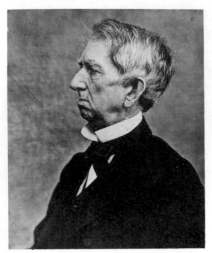

*William Seward (1801–1872) had been
a brilliant lawyer and governor of New
York before moving to the U.S. Senate
in 1849, where he became the leader of
the Whig and, later, Republican parties.
Lincoln defeated the outspoken antislave New Yorker for the White House,
but Seward left his mark as the prophet
(and later, between 1861 and 1869
when he served as secretary of state, as
the diplomat) for American expansionism into the Caribbean and, especially,
the vast Pacific Ocean regions.*

to "become the chief theatre of events in the world's great hereafter."[17]

An ambitious politician, a student of history, Seward was also a Whig
who urged the creation of a federal program of internal improvements
(such as national railroads) so that future Americans could use the
most efficient transportation. His radical antislave statements prevented him from capturing the Whig and then Republican party presidential nomination. But Abraham Lincoln appointed Seward to head
the Department of State in 1861, and in that post the New Yorker was
able to carry out some of his dreams. He worked out the tactics for
protecting both U.S. interests and freedom of action in Asia. The tactics included working for the territorial integrity of all Asian nations
(that is, not allowing Japanese or Europeans to colonize mainland
markets). He aimed at avoiding any political alliances but cooperated
with any nation that also wanted to maintain the open door.

Seward then drew a startling conclusion. The Americans' westward
push put them on a collision course with Russia. He hoped that the
meeting would be friendly. As secretary of state in 1861, he instructed
the new U.S. minister to St. Petersburg, Cassius Clay of Kentucky, that
"Russia, like the United States, is an improving and expanding empire.
Its track is eastward while that of the United States is westward." Seward
believed that "Russia and the United States may remain good friends
until, each having made a circuit of half the globe in opposite directions, they shall meet and greet each other in the region [Asia] where
civilization first began, and where, after so many ages, it has now become
lethargic and helpless."[18]

Such a breathtaking perspective was not new. Thirty years before, Alexis de Tocqueville, the acute French visitor, had prophesied that Americans and Russians, although "their starting point is different and their courses are not the same," seemed "marked out by the will of heaven to sway the destinies of half the globe."[19] In 1856, Commodore Perry, fresh from his triumph in Japan, warned that American and Russian expansion would continue until "the Saxon and the Cossack will meet once more" in Asia. "Will it be friendship? I fear not! I think I see in the distance the giants that are growing up for that fierce and final encounter: In the progress of events that battle must sooner or later inevitably be fought."[20] Seward was perhaps more optimistic than Perry. More important, the New Yorker could help control the growing relationship with Russia because of his power as secretary of state. Before Seward could realize his plans in Asia, however, he had to face a crisis at home that arose out of slavery and three centuries of imperial dreams.

CENTRAL AMERICA AND CUBA

An observer in the 1850s wondered why Americans fought each other so fiercely over such an issue as slavery in the desert regions of the southwest United States. It was a debate over "an imaginary Negro in an impossible place," this observer concluded. But he missed the context of the debate, for it occurred amid rampant expansionism. It seemed that it would be only a matter of time before regions north and south would fall to the irresistible magnet of U.S. Manifest Destiny.

In late 1853, the U.S. minister to Mexico, James Gadsden, following President Pierce's orders, approached Mexico to discuss the purchase of territory so that a U.S. railroad could have a clear southern route to the Pacific. The Mexican government, in need of money, agreed to sell a smaller area than Gadsden requested, some 45,000 square miles, in return for $15 million. The Gadsden Purchase ran into fierce antislave opposition in the Senate. The revised treaty then provided paying $10 million for 29,670 square miles, which included part of present-day Arizona and New Mexico. It marked the first time the Senate refused to accept land offered to it. Nevertheless, no one would have then guessed that the deal rounded out the boundaries of the continental United States. It marked the end of the conquest of an ocean-to-ocean empire.

At the time, however, it seemed one more step southward, with many more to follow. Just the first six months of 1854 exemplified how the aggressive Americans were on the move. During those months (the

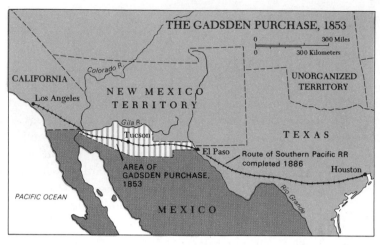

U.S. minister to Mexico, James Gadsden (a native of South Carolina) bought for $10 million what was finally an area of 29,670 square miles so that the southern states could have a transcontinental railway route. The Gadsden Purchase, accepted by the U.S. Senate despite violent northern opposition, rounded out the nation's continental boundaries in 1853–1854.

time when the bitter Kansas-Nebraska debates were shattering the Democratic party), Gadsden sent his treaty to the Senate; an American, William Walker, announced his plans to seize part of Mexico; the possibility of war with Spain over Cuba loomed; the Ostend Manifesto became public; the U.S. Navy shelled Nicaragua; and southerners launched new "filibustering" expeditions aimed at seizing Cuba and other Latin American territories for slavery.[21]

Americans seemed to be taking over Central America. Slaveholders hoped to acquire new territory and possibly even states. Merchants coveted control of the profitable, short isthmian passageways through Nicaragua and Panama that linked the two oceans. Even Republican free-soilers eyed Central America as the place in which free African Americans could be settled in a colonization scheme. Such resettlement would quiet the racial question at home—"Keep our Anglo-Saxon institutions as well as our Anglo-Saxon blood pure and uncontaminated," as a Republican declared—and would spread U.S. influence and values to Latin America.[22] The colonization plans finally collapsed because some Republicans did not want to lose cheap black labor. Moreover, the colonizers discovered that the cost and time needed to ship out all African Americans far exceeded the nation's available resources. In the 1850s, however, colonization remained a much-discussed solution to growing racial problems.

Nicaragua attracted special attention. The British had seized control of the eastern entry to a possible interocean canal route in the 1840s. One of the great U.S. adventurers, Cornelius Vanderbilt, appeared in 1848 to acquire from Nicaragua the right to monopolize transportation on the country's waters. U.S. power dramatically appeared in 1854. One of Vanderbilt's officials killed a Nicaraguan. Anti-American feelings ran high. The U.S. minister attempted to restore calm, only to have a bottle thrown at him. He asked Washington to teach the Nicaraguans a lesson. Commander George Nichols Hollins appeared at the Atlantic coast port of Greytown. Hollins demanded an apology and an indemnity from the Nicaraguans. The commander then loaded his ship's cannon and leveled the port's huts and buildings.

Hollins had scarcely sailed off before William Walker appeared. About five feet tall, very thin, a man consumed by the idealistic reform movements of the time (such as women's rights and the abolition of slavery), Walker had been a lawyer, then a journalist in New Orleans. By 1855, he had unsuccessfully tried to use a small private army to spread the blessings of democracy to parts of Mexico. Nicaraguan political factions asked him to help them fight their opponents. This "gray-eyed man of destiny," as he came to be known, assembled sixty men and, with Vanderbilt's help, conquered Nicaragua in 1855. The U.S. government moved to recognize Walker's regime officially. The self-styled disciple of democracy, however, made a fatal mistake. He allowed Nicaraguan land and mineral rights to be stolen by American business interests. Nicaraguans merely objected. Vanderbilt, whose interests were threatened, was not as passive. He set out to destroy Walker. The British gladly joined the crusade. In 1857, Walker fell. He could conquer Nicaragua but not Vanderbilt. The adventurer tried three more times to capture parts of Central America. In 1860, Honduran troops captured and shot him. The first U.S. clash with Nicaraguans had not been a happy occasion, as Nicaraguan school children forever after learned.

Cuba also became a target of U.S. expansionists. Southerners led the charge. "With Cuba and St. Domingo," the Charleston *Southern Standard* trumpeted, "we could control the productions of the tropics, and, with them, the commerce of the world, and with that, the power of the world."[23] A colorful and dangerous example of the South's determination was a secret society, the Knights of the Golden Circle, that pledged to extend slavery throughout the Gulf of Mexico. By 1860, the Knights claimed 65,000 members, three state governors, and several of President Buchanan's cabinet. But northerners also set their sights on the Caribbean. Some—particularly in New York City—especially desired Cuban trade. By 1855, U.S. commerce with the island had doubled in a decade until it was seven times greater than Great Britain's and even four times larger than Spain's—which owned Cuba. For their part, abolitionists wanted Cuba in order to open new markets for northern farmers and to end the slave trade in the region. The North's primary motive for coveting Cuba, however, was increased trade.

After the fiasco over the Ostend Manifesto in 1854, the issue died down, then revived with a rush in 1858. The Democratic party had suffered a severe blow. In 1857, the Supreme Court ruled in the *Dred Scott* decision that slavery could be taken into U.S. territories. (A territory was the stage just before a region reached statehood.) The Court added that the federal government had to protect the slaves, because they were property. Southern Democrats rejoiced. Northern Democrats, led by Stephen A. Douglas, opposed the Court's decision: they urged that the issue be settled in the territories through popular sovereignty. Southerners roundly condemned Douglas. Desperate Democratic leaders, led by inept, but expansion-minded President Buchanan, tried to use foreign policy to reunite the party. Polk's former secretary of the Treasury, Robert Walker, told the president: "Cuba! Cuba! (and Puerto Rico, if possible) should be the countersign of your administration, and it will close in a blaze of glory."[24]

Buchanan responded in 1858 by urging Congress to appropriate money to buy Cuba. Douglas and southerners came together to back the measure. But free-soilers blasted it. They were part of a rapidly growing Republican party that had come unexpectedly close to winning the presidency in 1856 and appeared to be in a position to take the House of Representatives in 1858. Seward, newly converted to the Republicans from the dying Whig party, helped lead the attack. In one of the more unique claims in American history, Seward announced that Cuba must some day become part of the United States because "every rock and every grain of sand in that island were drifted and washed out from American soil by the floods of the Mississippi, and the other estuaries of the Gulf of Mexico."[25] Some day—but not in 1858. The slave controversy, Seward believed, first had to be resolved. He received support from other Republicans, who argued that most Cubans were Roman Catholic and that the U.S. constitutional system could "only be maintained . . . on the principle of Protestant liberty."[26]

There was also the possible obstacle of the British fleet. London officials believed that Cuba would fall naturally into American laps, much
as John Quincy Adams had predicted thirty-five years earlier. But they
were determined not to allow the United States to conquer the island,
because it would allow southern slave expansionists to threaten British
holdings in the West Indies. In 1857, the British minister to Washington secretly suggested to London that Americans should have Cuba.
His superiors replied that he must have lost his senses. Giving Cuba to
the United States would resemble pleasing "an animal of Prey by giving him one of one's traveling companions. It would increase [the animal's] desire for similar food and spur him to obtain it."[27]

Out of the smoke and excitement of American expansionism in the
1850s, only the Gadsden Purchase actually emerged, although Cuba,
Central America, Canada, and Hawaii were heatedly discussed. In 1859,
the United States even made the McLane-Ocampo Treaty in which, in
return for a $4 million loan, the Mexicans would give their neighbor
extensive railroad routes and the right to intervene with force to provide police protection over all of Mexico. But the U.S. Senate rejected
the deal; and in other questions as well, the antiexpansionists carried
the day. These foreign-policy issues nevertheless shaped many of the
great debates and hopes of the decade as well as intensified southern
frustration and fears. Foreign-policy issues were a central cause of the
Civil War, for, while relatively few Americans urged total abolition of
slavery in all southern states, many determined never to allow slaveholders to establish their "peculiar institution" in the newly acquired
territories. Nor were the southerners to be allowed to conquer new
regions for their slave system. Foreign-policy issues had combined with
domestic controversy to form the combustible mixture that blew the
United States apart.

LINCOLN AND THE FOREIGN-POLICY
DREAMS OF 1860–1861

The Cuban issue resembled a monster in a science-fiction story that
repeatedly had knives driven through its heart but refused to die. Left
for dead by Seward and other Republicans in Congress during 1859,
the issue arose again a year later. This time Abraham Lincoln decided
to kill it once and for all. His decision helped drive the South out of
the Union.

Lincoln was a supreme politician who had carefully thought through the central problem of the relationship between foreign policy and slavery. Born in the slave state of Kentucky (and married into a slave-holding southern family), Lincoln moved to Indiana and then Illinois, where he ran successfully for office within seven months of his arrival. Only between 1849, when he returned to Illinois after serving a term in the U.S. House of Representatives, and 1854 did he not run for elected office. A lawyer for the new Illinois Central Railroad and a devout political follower of Henry Clay, Lincoln understood the industrializing corporate America that was transforming the nation's economy. As for slavery, he condemned all abolitionists "who would shiver into fragments the Union of these states" and "tear into tatters its now venerated Constitution." He also condemned, however, any measure that hinted of allowing slavery into the territories or newly acquired foreign areas. These lands were to be preserved for white men without slaves.

In 1858, Lincoln challenged Stephen A. Douglas in the Illinois Senate race. In their famous debates, Lincoln outlined his own views (expansion for none but free white men), then asked the "Little Giant" if he favored taking new territory regardless of how such a conquest might affect the slavery controversy. Douglas's amazing answer revealed his Young America expansionism:

> This is a young and growing nation. It swarms as often as a hive of bees, and . . . there must be hives in which they can gather and make their honey. . . . I tell you, increase, and multiply, and expand, is the law of this nation's existence. You cannot limit this great republic by mere boundary lines. . . . Any one of you gentlemen might as well say to a son twelve years old that he is big enough, and must not grow any larger, and in order to prevent his growth put a hoop around him to keep him to his present size. What would be the result? Either the hoop must burst . . . or the child must die. So it would be with this great nation.[28]

Lincoln barely lost the 1858 election. But by forcing Douglas to separate himself from many northern moderates and southern radicals, the loser became a national figure. In the 1860 Republican convention, he triumphed as a moderate over Seward. The 1860 election became a four-way race among Lincoln; Douglas, who gained the Democratic party nomination; John Bell of Tennessee, whose Constitutional Union party included remaining Whigs who hoped to find some compromise; and John Breckinridge of Kentucky, the nominee of the South's pro-slavery Democrats. Lincoln won a plurality of the popular vote and a majority of the electoral ballots to gain the presidency. The South prepared to secede. Congress met in short session during January–February 1861 to try to hold the Union together. John Crittenden of Kentucky fashioned a compromise that provided federal protection to slavery where it existed. Then, in the crucial clause, he proposed that "slavery or involuntary servitude" would be prohibited north of the old Missouri Compromise line of 36°30' but protected in all territory "now held, or *hereafter acquired*" (italics added).

Lincoln flatly rejected the Crittenden Compromise. "A year will not pass till we shall have to take Cuba as a condition upon which [the South] will stay in the Union," he warned friends. "There is in my judgment but one compromise which would really settle the slavery question, and that would be a prohibition against acquiring any more territory."[29] With those words, Lincoln not only separated himself from Douglas's belief that the American "bees" had to have new "hives" from which to swarm. He temporarily stopped four centuries of Amer-

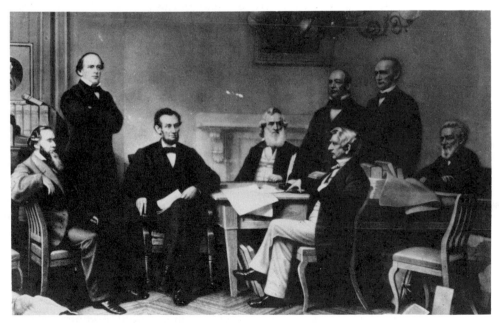

Abraham Lincoln (1809–1865) was considered a mere "prairie statesman" by leading Republicans. But he outmaneuvered them to win the presidency in 1860, then named some of them to his cabinet, where he could both watch and use them to restore the Union. Secretary of State Seward is seated in the right foreground. It took Seward awhile before he could accept his subordinate position.

ican territorial expansion. No American with his authority had ever taken such a position. Madison, Monroe, Polk, and Douglas, among many others, had argued that the preservation and prosperity of the American system depended on continued landed expansion. Lincoln took another tack. He believed that no expansion was preferable to expansion that enriched slavery and discriminated against freeholding whites.

The Crittenden Compromise never passed Congress. Lincoln took office in March 1861 as southern congressmen left Washington. The new cabinet debated the issue of trying to maintain the Union. The lead was taken by Secretary of State Seward, who had looked down on Lincoln as a "prairie statesman" and believed only he, Seward, could prevent a civil war. The New Yorker had urged compromise and moderation. He feared war. So did his supporters in the New York City mercantile community who acted as bankers and shippers for the great southern cotton crop. As early as January 1861, Seward thought he had hit upon a scheme to save the Union. As he privately told the British minister to Washington, he could unite America by declaring war against foreign powers who threatened to interfere with U.S. interests in the Caribbean. This scheme had one beneficial result. British officials decided to wait before trying to interfere in, or trying to gain benefits from, the growing sectional crisis.

But Lincoln continued to refuse to compromise on the territorial issue. The president then decided to force the question by overruling Seward and sending provisions to Fort Sumter, a Union-held island in Charleston Harbor. Lincoln's move would surely lead South Carolina to fire on the fort and start civil war. The desperate Seward then took a final gamble. On April 1, 1861, the secretary of state told Lincoln that Spain and France seemed to be threatening Santo Domingo and other areas in the Caribbean. Seward suggested that explanations be "demanded" from both European nations. If their answers were unsatisfactory, Lincoln should "convene Congress and declare war against them." Seward perhaps had in mind the conquest of Cuba. He then told the president that he (the secretary of state) should have all necessary power to conduct the diplomacy as well as the war that might result. Seward was convinced that the South would re-enter the Union to help fight such a conflict.[30]

Lincoln quietly buried the astonishing proposal. But Seward's idea was not new. He had been warning the British and others for months that a war for territorial expansion could resolve the domestic crisis. Americans, moreover, had gone to war in 1812 and 1846 to resolve internal as well as external problems. What was new in 1861 was Lincoln's determination not to use foreign policy as a salve for the temporary relief of the burning issue of slavery.

THE DIPLOMACY OF THE CIVIL WAR

As the North's blue- and the South's gray-uniformed armies prepared for battle in the spring of 1861, their leaders prepared to battle for European support. The Confederate nation's president, Jefferson Davis of Mississippi, had extensive political connections. He had been a U.S. Army officer, then married Zachary Taylor's daughter against Taylor's wishes. Davis also was experienced; during the 1850s he had led the South's fight in the Senate for landed expansion. A moderate among the secessionists, Davis had not at first sought the presidency. His wife recalled that when he received the telegram notifying him of the election, "he looked so grieved that I feared some evil had befallen our family."[31] Davis knew that the North's larger population and greater resources could grind down the South unless he obtained European aid. Russia and France, however, might neutralize each other's help. The tsar's government favored the North because Russia might need Union ports and support in case of possible war with Great Britain. Louis-Napoléon's France had nearly 700,000 textile workers dependent on southern cotton. Napoleon, moreover, had imperial dreams of his own for Latin America. He hoped to divide and contain North American expansion southward.

The key to Europe's response was, therefore, Great Britain. Economically, it was divided in its sentiments. The country's gigantic textile industry imported 80 percent of its cotton from the South. But the 1860 bumper crop had provided British mills with a two-and-a-half-year supply of the fiber. That breathing space allowed England to develop alternative supplies in India and Egypt. Moreover, a historic turn in Anglo-American trade had occurred in the mid-1840s. Lower British tariffs combined with spectacular new U.S. wheat crops (brought about in large part by such new technology as the McCormick reaper) to make England increasingly dependent on North American grain. King Corn began to checkmate King Cotton. Poor European grain harvests in 1860, 1861, and 1862 helped Lincoln by enriching U.S. farmers, who were becoming so efficient that they could feed both the giant Union armies and hungry Europeans. The British, in turn, found a vast market in the booming North for their manufactures. As Seward privately observed in early 1861, his section provided the "chief consumption of European productions," and more than a southern rebellion would be needed to "change these great features of American commerce."[32]

Aside from these economic magnets, powerful British liberals favored the North's battle to end slavery, especially after Lincoln's Emancipation Proclamation in September 1862. Because of their own self-interest, the British did not support the South. Divided economic and political opinion did not allow London officials to form a strong, united position. War with the Union could gravely endanger British shipping and, of course, Canada. Intervention might play into the hands of Louis-Napoléon, of whom the British were deeply suspicious as he constantly begged them to take the lead in helping the South. Moreover, with the humiliating northern military defeat at the first and second battles of Bull Run (near Manassas, Virginia) during 1861–1862, many Europeans believed a Union defeat was only a matter of time.[33]

Especially important in the British calculation was the issue of precedent. In April 1861, Davis, who had virtually no navy, commissioned privateers (privately owned ships that operated like pirates in preying on northern merchantmen). Lincoln retaliated with a blockade of the South. That act trapped Lincoln, for a blockade indicated an actual state of war. He had previously insisted that the South was not in a state of war with the North, but only in a state of rebellion. If a state of war was recognized, it could allow Europeans to deal with both sides equally. In May, London declared its neutrality, an act that also recognized the South's belligerent status. Seward and Lincoln, who had warned Europeans against such action, were angered. Seward severely warned France not to deal further with the South, or he would cut off all food exports that Frenchmen were "likely to need most and soonest." (While the crisis was building, however, Seward maintained close personal relations with the French minister to Washington by sending him fine cigars.)

The secretary of state also drafted a tough, even threatening, note (Dispatch Number 10) to the British. Lincoln calmed down Seward's rhetoric, and the new U.S. minister to Great Britain, Charles Francis Adams (John Quincy's son), watered down the wording before giving it to the British government. Adams's intelligence, calmness, and well-timed toughness made him one of the most successful diplomats in American history. A single major mistake in London could have changed the course of the Civil War.

Adams and Seward especially appealed to precedent and British self-interest. When the U.S. government intercepted neutral vessels en route to a neutral port and searched them for contraband, it committed an act that the British had repeatedly committed from 1793 through 1812. The British now did not strongly object as Lincoln repeated their earlier acts. In both the Revolutionary War and the War of 1812, the United States had depended on privateering, much to British displeasure. When Lincoln declared the South's privateering illegal, the British, who had considered it illegal years earlier, happily agreed. Finally, London honored Lincoln's loose blockade (the North did not have the ships needed to throw a tight blockade around the South's 3,500-mile-long coastline) because the British had used such a blockade in the past and would no doubt need to use it in the future.

After mid-1861, Seward settled down to conduct such successful diplomacy that historians have ranked him as the second greatest secretary of state in American history, just behind Seward's idol, John Quincy Adams. The New Yorker met and mastered four spectacular tests. The first occurred in November 1861, when hot-tempered Captain Charles Wilkes of the Union's navy learned that two Confederate diplomats, John Slidell and James Mason, had sailed for London on the British ship *Trent.* Wilkes stopped the ship, seized Slidell and Mason, then allowed the vessel to continue. The British protested and dispatched an ultimatum for the release of the two men. Seward knew that Wilkes had acted illegally. The Confederates had to be freed. But northern feelings ran high. Wilkes became a hero. Seward decided to release Slidell and Mason but, in a brilliant note to Great Britain, argued that Wilkes had been in the right. The secretary of state next neatly expressed gratefulness to the British for finally recognizing that their own acts of impressment before 1812 had been wrong. Seward thus averted war with Great Britain while stroking northern feelings. Journalist Richard Henry Dana wrote, "Seward is not only right, but sublime."[34]

A second crisis occurred in 1862, during the worst Union military setbacks. In March, the Confederate ironclad *Virginia* (formerly the *Merrimac*) fought a more powerful Union warship, the *Monitor,* to a standstill. The battle marked the first time that armored naval vessels had fired on one another. The stand-off demonstrated that the Confederate navy might not be as weak as many had assumed. On land, General Robert E. Lee's forces scored such impressive victories that Seward refused to discuss the Union's humiliations in his diplomatic correspondence.[35] Europeans, led by France, threatened to intervene and mediate a peace. Seward wrote the tsar, who was friendly to the

Union's cause, that Europe could "commit no graver error" than to become involved in the war.[36] A similar but toned-down version of this message also went to London.

Union general George McClellan, who had been overly cautious in fighting Lee, dramatically stopped the South's advance at Antietam, Maryland, in September. Lincoln meanwhile gained support in late 1862 by issuing the Emancipation Proclamation that freed all slaves in areas controlled by the Confederacy. Over the winter and early spring of 1863, a bolder general, Ulysses S. Grant, took great risks but succeeded in cutting off the Confederate force at Vicksburg, Mississippi. Grant's victory split the Confederacy and gave Lincoln control of the lower Mississippi. The triumph occurred, moreover, at the same time (July 1863) that northern troops won a bloody but decisive victory at Gettysburg, Pennsylvania. Concern over European intervention quickly declined in the North. Seward's diplomacy had gained time until the Union's greater resources could be mobilized to wear down Lee's brilliantly directed but undermanned forces. The Union's victories, especially at Antietam, Lincoln's well-timed Emancipation Proclamation, and Adams's shrewd use of these events were critical in forcing the British to pull back from any thought of helping the South.

Seward and Adams faced a third crisis in 1862–1863, when the Confederacy contracted with a British firm, the Laird Brothers, to build several ships. Before Adams could stop the construction, the *Alabama* and *Florida* slipped out of the shipbuilding yards and began attacking northern commerce. Insurance costs in the North rose as merchant shipping sank. A greater danger appeared when Laird began building armored rams that could break the North's blockade and attack northern coastal cities. Adams warned the British foreign secretary, Lord Russell, that if the Laird rams sailed, "it would be superfluous in me to point out to your Lordship that this is war." Aware that allowing the ships to leave was both bad policy and bad law, Russell had already stopped their launching. After the war, the British realized that outfitting these vessels set bad precedent; if the British themselves became involved in a war, their enemy could contract with U.S. shipbuilders to build such ships. To remove the precedent and improve tattered Anglo-American relations, the British paid the United States $15.5 million in 1872 to settle the *Alabama* claims.

A fourth crisis occurred in Mexico. In 1855, Santa Anna, who had tormented and teased both Texans and James K. Polk, finally lost power in Mexico City. He was replaced by Benito Juárez, whose ardent nationalism led him to suspend debts owed to Europeans. In 1861, a joint Spanish, British, and French force appeared to collect the debts, but the first two nations stopped cooperating when they learned that the French intended to control all of Mexico. In 1863, Napoleon III found another tool to achieve his plans for seizing Mexico, establishing a vast New World empire, and finally blocking the expansion of North American Protestants. The tool was an Austrian archduke, Maximilian, who, with his beautiful wife, Carlotta, was persuaded by Louis-Napoléon to lead a French force into Mexico. Seward strongly protested the Austrian's establishment of a monarchy during 1864, but he could do little else. With Lee's surrender at Appomattox Courthouse in Virginia on April 9, 1865, however, a huge, seasoned Union army was suddenly available to move south. General Philip Sheridan, who had trapped Lee at the final battle, led 50,000 soldiers to the Mexican border. Then, Seward again demanded that Maximilian leave Mexico. He carefully never mentioned the Monroe Doctrine, which Europeans refused to recognize, and instead rested his case on U.S. security interests—and, of course, on Sheridan's troops. But Seward only had to wait and watch as Juárez's guerrillas destroyed Maximilian's depleted army. Louis-Napoléon, concerned about the rise to power of Germany in the center of Europe, lost interest in Mexico and reneged on his earlier pledge not to desert the hapless archduke. In June 1867, a Mexican firing squad ended Maximilian's dreams. Carlotta spent most of the next sixty years insane and rambling around Europe in search of help to revive her empire.

Union armies, overwhelming northern resources, Lincoln's shrewdness and determination, Seward's diplomacy, and Adams's skill won the war. Ninety years after an independent United States had set out to settle a continental empire, the territory had been obtained, but at the cost of a civil conflict that took 600,000 lives. With the continent conquered and the issue of slavery decided, a new era opened. A different nation and a different foreign policy emerged. In historian Thomas Schoonover's words, "dollars not dominion" were to spread America's blessings.[37]

NOTES

1. Reginald Horsman, *Race and Manifest Destiny* (Cambridge, Mass., 1981), p. 228; David Potter, *The Impending Crisis, 1848–1861* (New York, 1976), pp. 181–182.

2. Eric Hobsbawm, "The Crisis of Capitalism in Historical Perspective," *Socialist Revolution* 6 (October–December 1976): 82–83. A superb analysis of this background is Kinley J. Brauer, "Diplomacy of American Expansionism," in *Economics and World Power . . .* , ed. William Becker and Samuel F. Wells, Jr. (New York, 1984), esp. pp. 56–58, 112–114.

3. Horsman, pp. 284–286.

4. Kenneth E. Shewmaker, "Daniel Webster and the Politics of Foreign Policy," *Journal of American History* 63 (September 1976): 314.

5. Donald S. Spencer, *Louis Kossuth and Young America* (Columbia, Mo., 1977), pp. 136–183.

6. David M. Pletcher, *The Diplomacy of Annexation: Texas, Oregon, and the Mexican War* (Columbia, Mo., 1973), p. 577.

7. Quoted in Akira Iriye, "America Faces a Revolutionary World," manuscript, in author's possession (1976), p. 2.

8. Eugene S. Ferguson, "The American-ness of American Technology," *Technology and Culture* 20 (January 1979): 18–19; Kenneth Shewmaker and Kenneth Stevens, eds., *The Papers of Daniel Webster. Diplomatic Papers, Volume 2, 1850–1852* (Hanover, N.H., 1987), pp. 255, 289.

9. William Neumann, "Religion, Morality, and Freedom: The Ideological Background of the Perry Expedition," *Pacific Historical Review* 23 (August 1954): 247–257.

10. John Paton Davies, "America and East Asia," *Foreign Affairs* 55 (January 1977): 368–394.

11. William Neumann, "Determinism, Destiny, and Myth in the American Image of China," in *Issues and Conflicts*, ed. George L. Anderson (Lawrence, Kan., 1959).

12. Walt Whitman, "A Broadway Pageant," in *Drum-Taps*, ed. F. DeWolfe Miller (Gainesville, Fla., 1959), pp. 62–64.

13. Henry Adams, *The Education of Henry Adams, an Autobiography* (Boston, 1918), p. 104.

14. Ernest N. Paolino, *The Foundations of the American Empire: William Henry Seward and U.S. Foreign Policy* (Ithaca, N.Y., 1973), p. 212.

15. Frederic Bancroft, *The Life of William H. Seward*, 2 vols. (New York, 1900), I, p. 153.

16. *Ibid.*, I, p. 469.

17. William H. Seward, *The Works of William H. Seward*, ed. George Baker, 5 vols. (Boston, 1853–1883), I, pp. 247–250.

18. *Ibid.*, V, p. 246.

19. Alexis de Tocqueville, *Democracy in America*, 2 vols. (New York, 1948), I, p. 434.

20. Hans Kohn, *American Nationalism, an Interpretive Essay* (New York, 1957), p. 175.

21. Potter, pp. 177–178.

22. Eric Foner, *Free Soil, Free Labor, Free Men* (New York, 1970), pp. 272–280.

23. Kohn, p. 117.

24. Bancroft, I, pp. 472–478.

25. Albert K. Weinberg, *Manifest Destiny* (Baltimore, 1940), p. 66.

26. Foner, p. 228.

27. Gavin B. Henderson, ed., "Southern Designs on Cuba, 1854–1857, and Some European Observations," *Journal of Southern History* 5 (August 1939): 385.

28. Harry Jaffa, *Crisis of the House Divided* (Seattle, 1973), p. 406.

29. David Potter, *Lincoln and His Party in the Secession Crisis* (New Haven, 1942), p. 223.

30. Bancroft, II, ch. 29. There are important comments and bibliography offered by Professors Kinley Brauer and Norman Ferris on Seward's proposal in *The Society for Historians of American Foreign Relations Newsletter* 13 (September 1982): 12–15.

31. Nathaniel W. Stephenson, "Jefferson Davis," in *Dictionary of American Biography*, ed. Allen Johnson and Dumas Malone, 21 vols. (New York, 1930–   ), V, p. 127.

32. Seward, V, pp. 210–211.

33. Brian Jenkins, *Britain and the War for the Union*, 2 vols. (Montreal, 1974–1980), II, pp. 61–105.

34. Foster Rhea Dulles, *Prelude to World Power: American Diplomatic History, 1860–1900* (New York, 1965), p. 11.

35. William H. Seward to Simon Cameron, 6 September 1862, Instructions, Russia, Record Group 59, National Archives, Washington, D.C.

36. Norman A. Graebner, "Northern Diplomacy and European Neutrality," in *Why the North Won the Civil War*, ed. David Donald (Baton Rouge, 1960), pp. 65–75.

37. T. D. Schoonover, *Dollars over Dominion* (Baton Rouge, 1978), p. 283.

FOR FURTHER READING

Consult the notes of this chapter and the General Bibliography at the end of this book; these materials are not repeated below. Above all, use the unparalleled *Guide to American Foreign Relations since 1700*, ed. Richard Dean Burns (1983), for pre-1981 materials. The following mostly deal with post-1981 publications. The best recent overview, with excellent bibliography is Bradford Perkins, *From Sea to Sea, 1776–1865*, in *The Cambridge History of U.S. Foreign Relations*, ed. Warren Cohen (1993).

K. Jack Bauer's *Zachary Taylor* (1985), sets the stage, especially with its examination of the 1850 debates that began under Taylor's presidency. Other major biographies are Larry Gara, *The Presidency of Franklin Pierce* (1991); and William C. Davis, *Jefferson Davis* (1991). The South's drive for expansion is interestingly and well told in Charles H. Brown, *Agents of Manifest Destiny* (1980), and Robert E. May, *John A. Quitman* (1985). The scene in the West and conflict with Native Americans can be explored in Robert M. Utley's *The Indian Frontier of the American West, 1846–1890* (1984), which also has a fine bibliography. James T. Wall, *Manifest Destiny Denied* (1982), is especially good on Nicaragua in the 1850s. Key is *The Papers of Daniel Webster: Diplomatic . . . 1850–1852*, ed. K. E. Shewmaker and K. R. Stevens (1987).

The entire era, and especially 1861–1868, is beautifully explored in James M. McPherson, *Ordeal by Fire: The Civil War and Reconstruction* (1982), with a superb bibliography. Herman Hattaway and Archer Jones, *How the North Won: A Military History of the Civil War* (1983), is detailed and focuses on Grant; Richard Current's *Speaking of Abraham Lincoln* (1983) is a series of important essays by a foremost Lincoln scholar; William Appleman Williams's *Empire as a Way of Life* (1980) is a stimulating analysis that is especially important for its original view of Lincoln. Also provocative and important are Norman Ferris, "William Seward and the Faith of a Nation," in *Tradi-*

tions and Values, ed. Norman Graebner (1985), and Gordon H. Warren, *Fountain of Discontent: The Trent Affair and the Freedom of the Seas* (1981). Warren F. Spencer has provided the definitive account on the title's subject and also much on the diplomacy in *The Confederate Navy in Europe* (1983), and interesting views by scholars in India are given in T. C. Bose's "The Diplomacy of the Civil War" and Dwijendra Tripathi's "Indian Cotton and Cotton Diplomacy," both in *American History by Indian Historians*, ed. Giri S. Dikshit, 2 vols. (1969), especially volume 2. On the Mexican crisis, the leading scholar is Thomas D. Schoonover, whose *Dollars over Dominion* (1978) should now be supplemented with his edition of *Mexican Lobby: Matías Romero in Washington, 1861–1867* (1986), a fascinating account of Washington politics during the Civil War as well as of U.S.-Mexican and U.S.-European relations. Another important foreign view is in Martin Crawford, *The Anglo-American Crisis of the Mid-Nineteenth Century: "The Times" of London and America, 1850–1862* (1987).

6

Laying the Foundations for "Superpowerdom" (1865–1896)

LEGACIES OF THE CIVIL WAR

Americans emerged from the dark shadows of the Civil War as a reluctantly united nation and, in the North, as a supremely confident people. Lincoln and Seward had exerted immense military power to force the South into unconditional surrender. At the same time, they had successfully managed the most delicate of foreign policies. These triumphs consolidated U.S. power and, in the words of historian David P. Crook, allowed the nation "to continue its headlong rush into superpowerdom."[1]

But something more than northern power triumphed. An incredible new industrial and communications complex also emerged from the conflict. This complex formed the launch pad for that "rush into superpowerdom" over the next thirty years. Many of the North's businesspeople had not wanted civil war, but once the South seceded, they moved quickly to pass probusiness legislation through Congress. They also took advantage of the nearly bottomless needs of the huge northern armies to make immense profits. When the North's humiliation at the first Battle of Bull Run in mid-1861 indicated that the war would be long, one northern financier confidently predicted a fortune for every person on Wall Street "who is not a natural idiot."[2] A young U.S. businessperson of 1860 lived in a nation that produced hardly any steel and little petroleum. Just forty years later, that person lived in the land that was the world's largest steel manufacturer and dominated the world's oil markets.

The Civil War provided the running start for such triumphs. Andrew Carnegie, the greatest iron and steel baron of the era, entered business during the war. Soon after oil pools were initially found in Pennsylvania during 1859, young John D. Rockefeller began combining his first five refineries during the Civil War. As early as 1865, oil ranked sixth on the list of U.S. exports. Rockefeller had begun the Standard Oil (later Exxon) global empire. The war spurred the same dramatic development in the businesses of carriages, sugar refining, and canning.

These businesses laid the foundations on which was built the world's economic superpower of the twentieth century. Such dominance resulted in part from considerable governmental aid. For example, Carnegie reaped huge profits partly because his steel business was protected against cheaper British steel by high tariff walls. From the 1840s until 1861, low tariffs had prevailed, but once the southerners left Washington, a series of tariff measures whipped through Congress. At first, the tariffs were to produce revenue to pay for the war effort, but by 1862, business lobbyists descended on the Capitol to bribe and cajole Congress into passing tariffs that protected their businesses from foreign competition. After the war, government expenses dropped, but the tariff walls remained high. By the 1890s, U.S. business had become so powerful that it could even vault over these walls to sell abroad and thus dominate world as well as American markets.

The manufacturers could move their goods on a rail system that had amounted to 31,000 miles in 1860, but 259,000 miles in 1900. Again, war and government action accelerated growth. In acts of 1862 and 1864, Congress gave railroad companies huge chunks of public land and easy credit to build transcontinental as well as shorter rail systems. By 1872, Washington had given private railroad builders 150 million acres, or an area equal to Maine, New Hampshire, Vermont, Massachusetts, Rhode Island, Connecticut, New York, and part of Pennsylvania combined. The Union Pacific Railroad doubled its original land grant by spending almost half a million dollars to bribe Congress. But few cared about the costs, either financial or moral. One industrialist pointed out the meaning of all this for U.S. foreign policy. Because of the vast rail system, he observed, "the drills and sheetings of Connecticut, Rhode Island, and Massachusetts and other manufacturers of the United States may be transported to China in thirty days; and the teas and rich silks of China, in exchange, come back to New Orleans, to Charleston, to Washington . . . to Boston in thirty days more."[3]

Despite the millions who served in the armies, labor remained cheap for the industrialists because of increased immigration. About 800,000 immigrants arrived between 1861 and 1865. Again, the government played a crucial role in helping private business. The 1864 contract labor law allowed business firms to send agents to Europe and Asia for laborers who were willing to sail to the New World. Seward had argued that Americans were happily following the example of other great empires: "The intermingling of races always was, and always will be, the chief element of civilization . . . [and] we emulate the sway of ancient Rome."[4] As secretary of state, Seward was able to encourage the entry of cheap Chinese labor to work on his favorite project, the transcontinental railroad. In 1868, he and Anson Burlingame (a former Massachusetts congressman and U.S. minister to China who now represented the Chinese government itself) wrote the so-called Burlingame Treaty that allowed the free immigration of each country's citizens.

With the cheap labor, great rail system, government grants, low taxes, and protected market, the number of industrial establishments rocketed upward some 80 percent during the 1860s until they hit 252,000. The number of industrial laborers soared 56 percent, to over 2 million. A new United States of factories and urban areas appeared. But despite the growing number of businesses, new concentrations of power also emerged. In key industries, giant corporations such as Standard Oil, Carnegie Steel, and Singer Sewing Machine began to swallow up small, individually owned businesses. The government gave corporations the right to raise large amounts of money through sale of stocks, but each investor had only limited liability if the business went sour. This almost magical power allowed a concentration of capital unimagined before the Civil War. As the *New York Commercial and Financial Chronicle* observed in 1866, "There is an increasing tendency in our capital to move in larger masses than formerly. Small business firms compete at more disadvantage with richer houses, and are gradually being absorbed into them."[5] These "larger masses" made the U.S. economy both highly efficient and a tough new competitor for the great banking and business combines of Europe. An industrializing America moved out to fight with the old giant empires in a prizefight ring that was global.

THE CONTEXT OF THE ERA: TRIUMPH AND TRAGEDY

The United States became a great world power between 1865 and 1900. It did so even as Americans endured severe economic depressions and

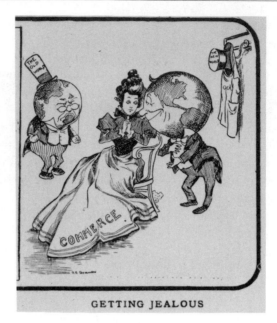

GETTING JEALOUS

In 1901, the Minneapolis Tribune *cartoonist caught the U.S. confidence that Americans were about to replace Europeans as the great world trading power. That confidence had begun to appear a generation earlier as the incredibly productive U.S. industrial and agricultural complexes came to dominate world markets—even in the middle of one of the worst economic depressions in history.*

widespread violence at home. Charles Dickens's opening for his novel, *A Tale of Two Cities,* perfectly applied to the United States of the post–Civil War era: "It was the best of times, it was the worst of times." It was the best of times because of the growing internal market (U.S. population more than doubled to 71 million between 1860 and 1900), the near-tripling of wheat production, the eightfold increase in coal production, the fivefold rise in steel and rail manufacturing, and the gushing of oil production by some twenty times to 55 million barrels in 1898. Total exports of all goods jumped from $281 million to $1.2 billion between 1865 and 1898, while imports rose from $239 million to $616 million. U.S. iron and steel products moved up the export list rapidly to threaten the traditional leaders—cotton and wheat.[6] Americans thus challenged Europeans for the world markets for highly profitable processed goods.

Beginning in 1874, moreover, U.S. exports regularly exceeded imports to produce a favorable balance of trade. With few exceptions (as during the economic panic of 1893–1894), the efficient Americans continued to sell more than they bought abroad—until 1971, when their comparative efficiency plummeted and they returned to their unfavorable merchandise trade balances of a century earlier. The profits gained from these post-1874 trade balances created even more efficient machines at home and fresh U.S. investments overseas.

But it was also the worst of times. In 1873, financial panic struck the country. Americans settled into a twenty-three-year-long depression that, with only a few brief upturns in the 1880s and early 1890s, became one of the most tragic in their history. Some twenty-three years of "boom" were nearly hidden in twenty-three years of "bust." For the depression was caused by the same production of U.S. factories and farms that raised the nation to the top of the slippery pole of international economic competition. Americans produced far more than they could consume. Prices consequently fell. But the increasingly mechanized industries continued to churn out more goods. Finally, laborers were put out of work in growing numbers. Strikes and riots gripped Chicago, Brooklyn, San Francisco, Cleveland, and other large cities. A perceptive British observer, Goldwin Smith, declared that "the youth of the American Republic is over; maturity, with its burdens, its difficulties, and its anxieties, has come."[7]

But even worse lay ahead. Nearly 24,000 labor strikes hit the United States between 1881 and 1900. One evolved into the Haymarket Riot of 1886, in which both strikers and police were killed in Chicago. Four supposed "anarchists" were hanged; another committed suicide. In 1894, President Grover Cleveland sent federal troops into Chicago to break up a railroad strike that had paralyzed much of the city. Not coincidentally, in 1886, the term *capitalism* had entered the American vocabulary as meaning "the concentration of wealth in the hands of the few; the power or influence of large or concentrated capital."[8]

The United States thus became a great world power as its system came under harsh attack at home. But the system was under attack because its productivity was so stunningly successful. Even with the doubling of U.S. population, certain businesses needed more and more overseas markets. The new iron and steel industry exported 15 percent of its goods by the turn of the century, sewing-machine makers 25 percent, oil refiners 57 percent of their illuminating oil. Farmers depended on volatile, unpredictable foreign markets to take as much as one-quarter of their wheat production. Between 70 and 80 percent of the cotton crop went abroad. As Russian and Argentine wheat fields enlarged in the late nineteenth century, and Egyptian and Indian cotton competed in world markets, Americans found out the hard way

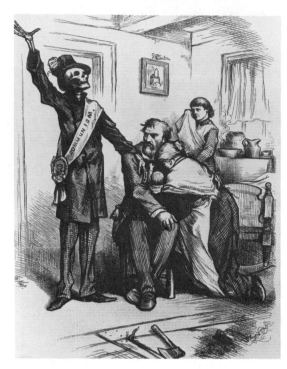

"Home, Sweet Home! There's no place like home!"
Destroyer of All: "Home ties are nothing. Family ties are nothing.
Everything that is—is nothing."

Thomas Nast did most of his drawings in the 1860s and 1870s, but he continues to rank as one of the greatest and most influential of political cartoonists. This powerful work of 1878 (just as Americans endured economic crises and a general labor strike) has two special characteristics: the depiction of a good American family trying to get along honestly, and the ghostly figure of "Communism" (with a "Free Love" button in his hat) cynically praising the home before he tries to destroy it. After the appearance of communism in the Paris Commune of 1871, most Americans hated the ideology and the social breakdown and violence associated with it. Anti-communism, as Nast shows, has deep roots in American society, especially during eras of great change.

how developments overseas directly affected their daily lives. Wheat prices received by U.S. farmers fell from $1.90 a bushel in 1860 to 57 cents in 1895. Cotton dropped below the 10-cents-a-pound break-even point to half that amount. Farmers went bankrupt, endured the agonies of moving west to find a new life, or moved their families into city tenements—all because they could not sell enough overseas.

These victims found little sympathy from their representatives in Washington. As the Civil War tariff and railway legislation vividly demonstrated, the political as well as economic system was coming under the control of the new corporate leaders. The officials who made foreign policy usually shared the views—and sometimes even the pocketbooks—of those who ruled the business community. Seward had observed that a political party was "in one sense a joint stock company in which those who contribute the most, direct the action and management of the concern." The politics were often not highly moral. But in terms of consolidating the power of the industrialists and others who shaped the new postwar United States, the politics were spectacularly effective. When Benjamin Harrison, a Republican, learned that he won the 1888 presidential election, he declared: "Providence has given us the victory." A Republican Pennsylvania political boss complained to a friend, "Think of the man. He ought to know that Providence hadn't a damn thing to do with it." Harrison "would never know how close a number of men were compelled to approach the gates of the penitentiary to make him President."[9]

The terrible shaking of the entire U.S. system between 1873 and 1897 even took some of the winners to the brink of a breakdown. John D. Rockefeller later recalled "how often I had not an unbroken night's sleep. . . . All the fortune I have made has not served to compensate for the anxiety of that period." Theodore Roosevelt, along with many others, turned for relief to "the strenuous life," as TR termed it in a famous speech of the 1890s. He urged Americans to "boldly face the life of strife" through "hard and dangerous endeavor. Oversentimentality, oversoftness . . . , and mushiness are the great danger of this age and this people," Roosevelt warned. "Unless we keep the barbarian virtues, gaining the civilized ones will be of little avail."[10] Americans took TR's advice and churned into furious activities during the 1880s and 1890s, especially in the new sports of baseball, football, and basketball. A rage for bicycle riding found men and women pedaling onto the roads. Indeed, a "new woman" appeared, one who rode bicycles, played tennis, and even attended golf clubs and racetracks. Bernarr Mac-Fadden's *The Power and Beauty of Superb Womanhood* (1901) displayed exercises so women could have the "muscular strength" to equal the hyperactive American male.[11] Thus, many Americans found outlets in feverish activities at home—and overseas.

Much of their energy focused on finding overseas markets for the U.S. glut of goods. Business needed an efficient global foreign policy to match industry's efficient global sales networks. A leading manufacturer was quoted in 1885 as saying that business most of all needed "an intelligent and spirited foreign policy" that would "see to it" that enough overseas markets were obtained, even if the use of military force was necessary.[12] Some Americans disagreed. Led by William Jennings Bryan in the 1890s, these dissenters argued that prices and employment could be improved by coining more silver (and not just gold) so that more money would be in circulation. But even these silverites accepted the common view that more foreign markets were required. They only shrewdly added that by using more silver, Americans would be able to capture those markets in areas where silver was widely used—as in China and Latin America. When the silverites and Bryan went crashing down to defeat in the 1896 presidential election, the all-purpose solution of more overseas markets continued to dominate American thought. Four years before, in 1892, U.S. foreign trade had already exceeded that of every country in the world except Great Britain. But it was not enough.

Some businesses found a new way to capture overseas markets. In the 1880s, it became possible for the first time to speak of U.S. multinational corporations. Such leading companies as Singer Sewing Machine, McCormick farm machinery, Standard Oil, and Kodak Camera directly invested overseas so they could more easily sell their products abroad. The 1890s economic depression spurred this movement. Sherwin-Williams Paint almost literally made good on its slogan "We Cover the Earth." By 1890, worried European officials warned of an "American invasion" into their economies. Articles appeared with the titles "The Americanization of the World" and "The American Invaders" to discuss the new multinationals. The largest firms did not require government help. But smaller companies did need support from the State Department. Consequently, a revitalized U.S. Consular Service and such business groups as the National Association of Manufacturers (formed during the depths of the 1894–1895 depression) appeared to work for the ambitious multinational corporations.[13]

The largest firms often handled their own foreign policy. By the 1890s, for example, John D. Rockefeller's Standard Oil controlled 70 percent of the world's oil markets. It quadrupled its sales abroad during the 1880s. William Herbert Libby, who directed Rockefeller's overseas invasion, bragged that petroleum had "forced its way into more nooks and corners of civilized and uncivilized countries than any other product in history emanating from a single source." But the Russian oil industry, with financial support from the great Rothschild banking house of France, rose to challenge Standard Oil. Rockefeller successfully fought back. A U.S. State Department consul in the Russian oil-producing area carefully kept Standard up-to-date on the competition's movements. Rockefeller opened new refineries in central Europe. And Standard set up a subsidiary that specifically targeted its efforts to undercut Russian moves in western Europe and the Far East. Long before other Americans fought a cold war with Russia, Standard Oil executives were engaged in their own bitter conflict.[14]

A CHRONOLOGY OF POSTWAR EXPANSION: THE ALASKA PURCHASE AND A BACKLASH

The U.S.-Russian confrontation, however, lay out of sight in a clouded future when Secretary of State Seward laid plans for an ambitious, post–Civil War foreign policy. Indeed, Russia, of all the major powers, seemed in 1865 to be the United States' best friend. Part of the tsar's fleet had made a dramatic, highly popular visit to the Union's ports during the Civil War—although Americans later learned (as Seward believed at the time) that the Russians actually cared less about the North's cause than finding refuge for their own ships in case of a war with the British. That war nearly occurred in the wake of a Polish uprising against Russia's rule in 1863. But Russian-American relations received a real boost in 1867, when the tsar decided to sell Alaska.

Alaska's fate had been decided by U.S. traders and merchants as early as the 1820s. By that date, the Russian Trading Company, charged with ruling and exploiting Alaska for the tsar, actually depended on U.S. sources—not Russian—for most of its necessities. By 1865–1866, the U.S. minister to St. Petersburg, Cassius Clay of Kentucky, pushed for Alaska as a route through which a U.S.-built telegraph line would link the two great countries. (The energetic fifty-six-year-old Clay worked for this project, that is, when he was not fighting off protective mothers of young girls he admired or when he was not challenging Russian nobles to duels with bowie knives.) The telegraph project was never completed, but Clay used information obtained from it to help persuade Russian officials to sell Alaska. Seward concluded the deal in Washington during March 1867. The United States agreed to buy the great expanse for $7.2 million.

But congressional opposition quickly arose. The price seemed extravagant for a frozen wasteland ("Walrussia" or "Seward's Ice Box," as Alaska became known). Seward and President Andrew Johnson, moreover, were hated by radical Republican leaders because the president wanted to bring the South back rapidly into the Union on easy terms. Seward finally triumphed for five major reasons. First, he and

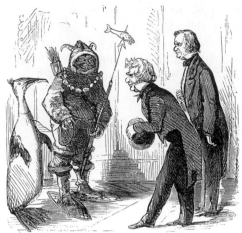

OUR NEW SENATORS.

Seward's purchase of Alaska from Russia turned out to be one of the all-time real-estate bargains, but he was ridiculed in 1867. Here a cartoonist has Seward telling the Alaskan representative to "bring . . . Mr. Seal along with you [to Washington]."

the Republican Senate leader, Charles Sumner from Massachusetts, emphasized the rich Alaskan mineral and animal resources awaiting exploitation by ambitious Americans. Second, they and others stressed that the purchase meant that the United States would partially block Great Britain's and Canada's access to the Pacific—would "cage the British Lion on the Pacific Coast," in one congressman's words—and perhaps make the annexation of Canada easier. Third, Alaska and the Aleutian Islands would serve, in the phrase of Republican House leader Nathaniel P. Banks of Massachusetts, as the "drawbridge between America and Asia." The rich China and Japan trade could be reached and protected more easily by the great circle route passing from San Francisco to Alaska to Asian markets. Fourth, Russia was a good friend. By working with her, Americans could remove a possible future source of conflict and cooperate with the friend against their common enemy— Great Britain. Finally, when the House of Representatives hesitated to appropriate the $7.2 million, the Russian minister in Washington apparently distributed about $73,000 as bribes to grease the passage. Seward, moreover, had already run up the Stars and Stripes over Sitka, Alaska—which allowed one congressman to proclaim: "Shall that flag which waves so proudly there now be taken down? Palsied be the hand that would dare remove it."[15]

Seward thus added 586,000 square miles, or an area nearly two and a half times the size of Texas, to the Union. The editor of *U.S. Railroad and Mining Register* crowed that the purchase ensured American greatness in the Pacific. But more, he added, both Americans and Russians "believe that in time not far remote Washington and St. Petersburg will be the political poles of the earth. . . . Never was international friendship deeper than between America and Russia."[16] Little could the ecstatic editor imagine what lay ahead for that "friendship."

Nor, in the flush of victory, could Seward and other expansionists imagine that Alaska was to be the last U.S. landed conquest for more than a generation. Seward had been able to annex the Midway Islands (about 1,200 miles west of Hawaii) in 1867 for possible use as a way station and cable point in the Asia trade. But he failed in efforts to obtain bases in Santo Domingo, Haiti, the Central American isthmus (for a future ocean-to-ocean canal), Hawaii, Greenland, and the Danish West Indies (Denmark's Virgin Islands) in the Caribbean. Congress was more interested in questions of the South and newly freed blacks than in distant territories. Such bases, moreover, could cost money, and the nation already was burdened with a huge Civil War debt. The House of Representatives actually passed a resolution in late 1867 opposing "any further purchases of territory" because of the country's "financial condition." Many also believed the nation already had enough land. As the *Chicago Tribune* phrased it, in the vast western regions "we have already more territory than we can people in fifty years."[17]

Americans, for the first time in their history, even lost interest in immediately annexing Canada. Radical Irish-Americans—Fenians— hoped to free Ireland from British rule by moving out of Buffalo, New York, to attack Canadian territory and thus stir up a U.S.-British war. Even Seward, who long lusted after Canada, disavowed the Fenians' bloody raids. After the 1867 North America Act, in which England granted autonomy to the new Dominion of Canada, some disgruntled western Canadians rebelled against the new regime and flirted with the idea of attaching their region to the United States. But Washington officials had lost their passion for such a romance. Their attention turned inward and then focused on the critical problem of finding overseas markets for their overproductive farmers and industrialists.

A CHRONOLOGY OF POSTWAR EXPANSION:
WINNING THE WEST

Americans obviously did not lose interest in foreign policy between the Civil War and the 1898 war. They only went about dealing with for-

eign policy differently. U.S. officials realized that they faced a new set
of problems. The most immediate problem was settling the vast western territories that had been conquered since 1803. Such settlement
was crucial for two reasons: to find new agricultural lands for the growing population and to develop the routes for the transcontinental railroads that would carry U.S. goods to Pacific ports, from which the goods
could find markets in Asia.

But settlement meant that tribes of Indians had to be moved or
destroyed. In this sense, the wars against the Native Americans between
1870 and 1890 marked the last step needed to unify and consolidate
the United States before Americans could go abroad to become the
superpower of the twentieth century. About 360,000 Indians lived west
of the Mississippi in 1850. They included the powerful Sioux, Chey-
ennes, and Comanches. White and black Americans numbered about
20 million. In 1860, 1.5 million whites lived in the West, but by 1890

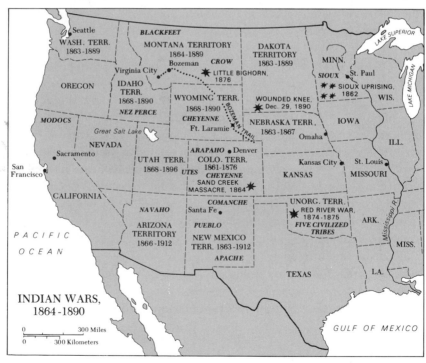

Between the Civil War and 1890, white Americans fought a seemingly contin-
ual war against the Indians to control land seized before 1848. Far from being
a quiet period in American settlement, it was one of the most active—especially
for the U.S. Army.

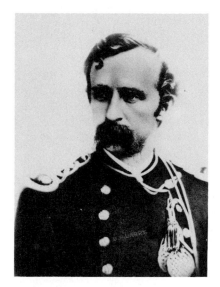

George Armstrong Custer (1839–1876) graduated at the bottom of his West Point class but fought bravely in the Civil War before leading two hundred of his troops into an Indian ambush in which he and his men were massacred. His name became synonymous with one of the few failures in nineteenth-century American expansion.

that number had multiplied six times. Native Americans had no idea that so many white people existed.

Many of the new settlers doubtless agreed with Theodore Roosevelt's view in his popular book, *The Winning of the West* (published in several volumes between 1889 and 1896), that "this great continent could not have been kept as nothing but a game preserve for squalid savages. . . . The man who puts the soil to use must of right dispossess the man who does not, or the world will come to a standstill."[18] In the early nineteenth century, Indians had been treated as "separate nations," but by 1871 Congress no longer viewed them as separate nations or made lasting treaties with them. Instead, U.S. officials simply passed laws to push Native Americans off desirable lands, created isolated reservations for the tribes, and—in the Supreme Court's words—saw the Indians not as "nations," but as "local dependent communities."

These views of Roosevelt and the government justified driving the Native Americans off their rich western lands. The victims not surprisingly struck back. Most notably they did so in 1876 at Little Bighorn in Montana, when 2,500 Sioux warriors, some with 16-shot repeating rifles, surrounded and slaughtered 260 men of George Custer's Seventh Cavalry. As later accounts described the horror, the cavalrymen were "bawling in terror, shooting themselves and each other." Then the "discovery of Custer's obliterated force: hills strewn with bloated pink, stripped, mutilated corpses and dead horses. Eyeballs and brains extracted and laid out on rocks, hearts impaled on poles."[19]

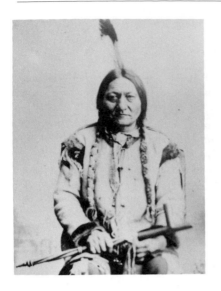

Sitting Bull (c. 1834–1890) was one of the great chiefs who resisted white American expansionism until he was captured after destroying Custer and his men at the Battle of Little Bighorn in 1876. He was made a part of a traveling Wild West show.

Between 1877 and 1890, however, such victims were usually red, not white. News of Custer's defeat reached the East as Americans celebrated the centennial of their independence. In the words of one popular magazine, they swore revenge by the time the next anniversary arrived in 1976, when nothing would remain of the "red man but a case of flint arrow-heads, stone hatchets, and moth-eaten trappings at the Smithsonian [a museum in Washington, D.C.]." Native Americans were systematically killed, starved by the extermination of the buffalo herds on which they depended for food and other needs, or pushed into desolate reservations. General Nelson A. Miles (who, in the 1898 war, headed the U.S. Army in its fight against Spain) tracked down Sitting Bull, who had destroyed Custer's forces, and the great Indian chief became an exhibit in the popular Buffalo Bill's Wild West Show. Sitting Bull later returned to his people, but a confrontation with white authorities developed, a gun discharged accidentally, and U.S. officials quickly killed the chief and seven Sioux, while the Indian's old circus horse mistook the gunfire for the Wild West Show and did tricks. The U.S. Army then surrounded another Sioux chief, Big Foot, and some 350 followers at Wounded Knee, South Dakota, reservation in 1890. Again, an accidental gunshot apparently set off full-scale firing. The U.S. troops lost 25 men (many of them victims of their own crossfire) but killed Big Foot and 150 others, including women and children.[20]

In historian Robert M. Utley's words, "The Indian frontier of the American West vanished in the smoke of Hotchkiss shells bursting over the valley of Wounded Knee Creek."[21] With the Native Americans crushed, whites settled more land in the thirty years after 1870 than they did in the previous three hundred years. Such settlement at once formed an immensely productive landed empire and a route from the East Coast to Asian markets. The U.S. Army meanwhile used the Indian wars as training for conflicts overseas. British observers thought the 25,000-man U.S. Army and its 2,000 officers one of the world's toughest fighting forces because of its battles with the Indians. Scholar Walter L. Williams has found that of the 30 U.S. generals who fought against Philippine rebels between 1898 and 1902, 26 (or 87 percent) had earned their spurs fighting Indians. Williams has also noted that the new legal terms devised after 1870 to control the Native Americans and take away many of their rights were simply transferred to Cuban, Philippine, and Puerto Rican affairs after 1898.[22] The post-1870 Indian wars were a key link between the whites' landed expansion to 1860 and their new overseas empire taken in 1898 and after.

A Chronology of Postwar Expansion: Africa and Latin America

U.S. overseas expansion had two main characteristics after 1870: it was almost entirely interested in markets (not in land), and it moved along not one but many routes to all corners of the earth. In Africa, for example, American interests had been almost nonexistent, except for the U.S.-sponsored colonization of free African Americans in Liberia that had occurred in the 1830s and 1840s. Even in Liberia, however, Washington officials refused to recognize the new nation, which declared its independence in 1847, until 1862. The slave controversy and antiblack feelings prevented recognition of the U.S.-created colony until that time. After 1862, relations remained slight.

In the 1870s, however, Commodore Robert Shufeldt led a pioneering voyage that gained new U.S. rights to coaling stations and trade in Africa and along the Persian Gulf. In 1884, private citizens who sought markets in Africa, and diplomat John Kasson, who well understood the need of fresh markets for U.S. goods, pushed Washington officials to send a delegation (led by Kasson) to participate in the Berlin Conference. This conference was called by the German government to resolve growing problems in the Congo. In that African region, the ambitions of the Belgian king, Leopold II, seemed on a collision course with other European colonial powers. The United States only wanted—and indeed obtained—a pledge by all the powers to an "open door" so that its goods could enter the Belgian Congo on fair terms. The U.S. delegation then helped Leopold block his European rivals, although the Belgian king was enforcing one of the most brutal colonial policies in all of Africa. Kasson's work at Berlin was strongly supported by the powerful Democratic senator from Alabama, John T. Morgan. Historian Joseph A. Fry, after studying Morgan's passionate expansionism, concludes that the Alabaman believed "the Congo's throngs of unclad natives seemed to offer an unlimited market" for the South's textile industry. Morgan also saw the region "as an ideal dumping ground for the South's surplus blacks."[23]

But not even Morgan's influence was enough. The new U.S. president, Grover Cleveland, took power in 1885 and disavowed Kasson's agreement because it could possibly become an entangling alliance. Five years later, U.S. opinion against Belgium was shaped by an extraordinary man. George Washington Williams had fought in the Civil War, had been a popular preacher, editor of a major black newspaper, the first African American ever elected to the Ohio legislature, and the first major black historian in the United States. After a trip to the Congo, his *Open Letter* of 1890 detailed twelve specific charges against Leopold's brutality, including enslaving "women and children" while neither educating nor economically developing the society. But even Williams could do little more than slow the growing belief of some Americans that a rich African market awaited them. By 1890, historian Milton Plesur relates, U.S. newspapers even predicted "that the whites would in time swallow up the African Negro in the same way the North American Indian had all but disappeared."[24]

The road to Latin American markets and bases seemed clearer and was certainly a more traditional path for U.S. expansion. In 1870, President Ulysses S. Grant tried to annex Santo Domingo partly at the request of several friends who had some highly corrupt business projects in that Caribbean country. Grant also wanted to ensure that no other power could control the country. He justified annexation in part by arguing that it would help quiet racial problems at home: Santo Domingo could support "the entire colored population of the United States, should it choose to emigrate." Americans' racism had usually restrained their expansionist impulses into the Caribbean, but the president now tried to turn racism into a reason for expansionism. He ran into a buzz saw of opposition. The powerful Sumner (who before the Civil War had been an Abolitionist on the slave issue), argued that as "an Anglo-Saxon Republic" the United States must not take in "colored communities" where the "black race was predominant." Secretary of State Hamilton Fish also opposed annexation in part for racial reasons. Maria Child, for forty years a vigorous opponent of U.S. expansionism (see p. 105), fought the president with quite different arguments. Child compared Grant's grab to a pre–Civil War "filibustering project." She feared that "this Republic will sink rapidly to degeneracy and ruin if we go on thus seizing the territory of our neighbors by fraud or force."[25] Grant finally gave up his plans, but he announced in 1870 that henceforth the Monroe Doctrine contained a new principle: "Hereafter no territory on this continent shall be regarded as subject to transfer to a European power." This "nontransfer" principle had appeared as early as 1811, when President James Madison applied it to Florida. But Grant's declaration first made the principle a formal part of the Monroe Doctrine.

Another, more promising chance to seize new territory occurred in Cuba. The Cubans had begun a revolution against decaying Spanish control in 1868. Some U.S. lives and property were lost in the fighting, but the major crisis arose in 1873, when Spain seized the *Virginius*, a ship under the U.S. flag that was carrying weapons to the rebels. The Spanish executed fifty-three crew members. Cries went up in the United States for revenge—that is, for taking Cuba. But Grant's cool-headed secretary of state, Hamilton Fish, knew that the ship had been breaking the law. Fish and other officials, moreover, wanted no part of the multiracial Cuban population. When one cabinet member raised the possibility of annexing Cuba, Fish squashed the idea by noting the terrible racial problems already existing in "South Carolina and Mississippi." Spain paid an $80,000 indemnity for the lives of the crew members. By 1878, it had been able to stop the revolution, but it had been a close call. Maria Child concluded, "I do believe if we could annex the whole world, we should [then] try to get a quarrel with Saturn, in order to snatch his ring from him."[26]

U.S. attention next turned to Central America. It focused on a new grave danger: in the late 1870s, the French began building an isthmian canal in Panama (a province of Colombia). The project directly threatened the 1850 Clayton-Bulwer agreement between the United States and Great Britain for joint construction of such a passageway. More pointedly, the French enterprise endangered the growing determination of Americans to build the canal by themselves. Seward had nearly obtained such a right from Colombia in 1869, only to have the Colombian legislature reject the treaty. When the French began their digging, the U.S. government warned sharply that it would never "consent to the surrender of this control [over an isthmian canal] to any Euro-

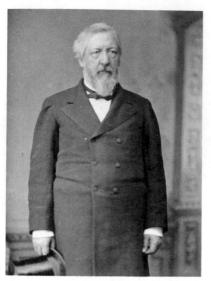

"The Plumed Knight from Maine" (nicely caught in this portrait), James G. Blaine (1830–1893) was secretary of state twice (1881 and 1889–1892), a defeated Republican presidential candidate (1884), and—of special importance—a skilled politician who understood the needs of the new American industrial complex and preached the need for U.S.–Latin American economic ties. Blaine foresaw U.S. relations with the Latin nations much as Seward foresaw U.S. relations with Asia in the twentieth century.

pean power or combination of powers." Secretary of State James G. Blaine entered office in 1881 and opened talks about building a canal in Nicaragua—as if the 1850 treaty did not exist. For most Americans the Clayton-Bulwer Treaty indeed did not exist. As one phrased it, Americans refused "to be bound hand and foot" by that "covenant of national disgrace." The French effort finally failed in the 1880s, a victim of enormous engineering problems as well as of the deadly mosquito-carried yellow fever. It was only a matter of time before Americans would try on their own. Indeed, during these year. U.S. military forces landed in Panama half a dozen times to restore order and protect American citizens threatened by armed uprisings against the Colombian government. The turn toward an ocean-to-ocean canal owned and operated by the United States occurred in the 1870s and 1880s, long before it was realized in Panama in 1903.[27]

Blaine personally exemplified the new U.S. approach to Latin America. A power in the Republican party (he was its presidential nominee in 1884), the "Plumed Knight from Maine" understood the needs of the fast-developing U.S. industrial system and the business leaders who built it—and who also contributed handsomely to his Republican party. As secretary of state, in 1881 he declared that his foreign policy must bring peace to, then increase U.S. trade in, Latin America. "To attain the second object the first must be accomplished," Blaine concluded. That conclusion meant more vigorous American intervention to ensure a secure marketplace. In 1890, again serving as secretary of state, Blaine spelled out his policy. His statement, which is a lesson in American history as well as diplomacy, serves as a summary of U.S. economic policy toward Latin America from 1865 until the late twentieth century:

> I wish to declare the opinion that the United States has reached a point where one of its highest duties is to enlarge the area of its foreign trade. Under the beneficent policy of [tariff] protection we have developed a volume of manufactures which, in many departments, overruns the demands of the home market. In the field of agriculture, with the immense propulsion given in it by agricultural implements, we can do far more than produce breadstuffs and provisions for our own people. . . . Our great demand is expansion. I mean expansion of trade with countries where we can find profitable exchanges. We are not seeking annexation of territory. At the same time I think we should be unwisely content if we did not seek to engage in what the younger Pitt so well termed annexation of trade.[28]

In 1889, the year before that speech, Blaine had called and then presided over the First International American Conference. He sought a customs union (a kind of vast, inter-American common market) and even a common currency to expedite U.S. exports southward. Blaine obtained neither objective, but the meeting did lead to the building of the Pan-American Highway system, linking the United States to nations in South America. The gathering also marked the beginning of the Pan-American movement that brought North and South Americans closer culturally and economically. Blaine's success helped lead, in 1890, to the first significant "reciprocity" tariff passed by the U.S. Congress. This legislation allowed certain Latin American products (especially coffee, hides, and sugar) to enter the United States freely as long as the nations that produced them allowed U.S. exports into their countries equally free from tariff restrictions. Under the 1890 reciprocity treaties, trade immediately boomed with Cuba and Brazil, among others.

Indeed, U.S. exports to Brazil rose $500,000 in three years, while imports from that country increased by an amazing $17 million. Then, in 1893, the friendly republican government in Brazil was threatened by an uprising led by promonarchical Brazilian naval units and encouraged by the British and other European powers. The U.S. administration of President Cleveland at first tried to remain neutral. But when U.S. exporters (including the Standard Oil Company) warned Cleveland that their trade could be endangered by a rebel victory, the president ordered naval units to protect U.S. shippers who wanted to unload goods in Brazilian ports. This order directly aided the government in the capital of Rio de Janeiro, because the government depended on revenue paid on the unloaded goods. Cleveland's action thus broke the back of the rebellion and protected the growing North American trade. When one rebel vessel challenged the U.S. warships escorting American merchantmen to the harbors, a U.S. warship fired a shell across the Brazilian vessel's bow and warned that any further challenge would result in the sinking of the rebel ship. The rebellion quickly ended. The grateful Brazilian government erected a statue to James Monroe, celebrated the Fourth of July, and even organized a serenade for the U.S. minister in Rio de Janeiro.[29]

Thus, the U.S. need to find more markets abroad had led to direct interference in internal Brazilian affairs. The story was less happy, but the conclusion much the same, when a rebellion threatened the pro-U.S. government in Chile during 1891. The U.S. minister, Patrick Egan, was a rambunctious Irishman who had the touch to be a successful politician in the United States but not a suave diplomat in Chile. His public support of the Chilean government led a mob to kill two U.S. sailors who were on shore leave in Valparaíso from the USS *Baltimore*. President Benjamin Harrison, a former Civil War hero, took a tougher line than even Egan and demanded an apology and indemnity. But Chile refused to pay for the mob's acts. As Harrison's anger grew, the two countries edged toward war. Some worried U.S. observers noted that Chile's navy was actually larger than the U.S. fleet, which had been allowed to rot after the Civil War. Blaine, in one of his last acts, and a new Chilean government then moved to cool the crisis. Chile finally paid an indemnity of $75,000 for the killing of the sailors.

The Chilean and Brazilian affairs displayed the new, active interventionism of the United States in Latin America. But nowhere did this vigorous policy appear more dramatically than in Venezuela during 1895–1896. For in that crisis, Washington officials challenged Great Britain, the world's leading power.

The showdown had begun long before, in the 1840s, when British policy makers claimed disputed territory lying between Venezuela and their colony of British Guiana. Little more happened, however, until the 1890s, when the British began to reassert their claim. Worried U.S. officials noted that the disputed land controlled the entry into the Orinoco, a vast waterway that could provide access to trade for a large section of South America. Rumors of rich mineral wealth in the region also appeared. President Cleveland especially focused on the British threat to the Monroe Doctrine. In 1895, he demanded that the London government of Lord Salisbury arbitrate the claim. Salisbury, one of Europe's great statesmen, was busy with Germany's threat to British interests in South Africa. He ignored Cleveland's message.

Infuriated, the president ordered his secretary of state, Richard Olney, to restate the U.S. position forcefully so that Salisbury would pay attention. Olney did so in a historic note of July 20, 1895. It claimed that the United States could enforce the Monroe Doctrine because the nation was now supreme in the Western Hemisphere. A surprised Salisbury became aware that his country and Cleveland's were rushing toward a conflict. He refused to recognize the legality of the Monroe Doctrine but did implicitly recognize Olney's spread-eagle claim that the "infinite resources [of the United States] combined with its isolated position render it master of the situation and practically invulnerable as against any or all other powers," as Olney had stated it in the note.[30] Salisbury agreed to arbitrate the dispute, and Venezuela indeed received the land controlling the Orinoco. The British prime minister finally bowed to U.S. demands because the gravest threat to his nation's interests came not in the New World, but from a rising Germany (especially the growing German fleet) and from explosive imperialistic rivalries with the French and Germans in Africa. Faced with those dangers, Salisbury shrewdly laid a foundation for Anglo-American friendship by agreeing to arbitrate the less important Venezuelan boundary.

For their part, Americans also replaced long-held British interests in Nicaragua during the 1890s. Indeed, throughout Central America—a region that London's power had shaped for half a century—U.S. companies and military power became overwhelming. By 1900, the United Fruit Company of Boston dominated Costa Rica's and Guatemala's economies. Soon, United Fruit's control of Central American affairs reached a point where the company was simply called "The Octopus." Sam "The Banana Man" Zamurray of New Orleans gained control of Honduras's economy after 1900, until that country became known as a banana republic. As early as the 1880s, a Guatemalan official recognized that the United States had become "the natural protector of the integrity of Central American territory."[31] But these moves into Central America only formed part of a larger expansionism that transformed the United States into the dominant power in the hemisphere between 1865 and 1896. Even Lord Salisbury had to admit the new extent of that power.

A CHRONOLOGY OF POSTWAR EXPANSION:
THE PACIFIC AND ASIA

When U.S. naval officers claimed the Midway Islands (so named because they were halfway between California and Japan) for the United States in 1867, they triggered a thirty-three-year surge of westward expansion over the Pacific Ocean. In 1867, Americans were trying to rebuild from the ruins of their civil war. By 1900, they had an army on the Asian mainland and had conquered a string of bases across the broad Pacific that linked that mainland to the United States.

The magnificent Hawaiian Islands were the first stop. As early as 1843, so many U.S. traders and missionaries worked there that wary British and French officials asked the United States to sign a treaty guaranteeing Hawaii's independence. The Americans not only refused, but a decade later tried to annex the islands—a move foiled by British opposition as well as by the growing division in Washington over the slavery and expansion issues. In 1867, Seward reopened the campaign to annex by shrewdly trying to seduce Hawaii into the U.S. orbit through a reciprocity treaty. Again, internal U.S. political fighting stopped Seward's move, but in 1875 Grant and Fish did negotiate such a trade treaty. The results were all that expansionists such as Seward and Grant could have desired. With the rich U.S. market at their disposal, Hawaiian planters, between 1876 and 1885, raised their sugar production from 26 million pounds to 171 million pounds. The planters utterly depended on the mainland as their exports to the United States quadrupled to $8.9 million in those ten years. By 1881, Blaine could call the islands "a part of the productive and commercial system of the American states."[32]

President Cleveland, mistakenly labeled by some historians as an antiexpansionist, worked hard to renew the reciprocity treaty in 1885. But domestic U.S. sugar interests hated Hawaiian competition and so opposed the agreement. The Hawaiians further sweetened the deal by giving the United States a lease on Pearl Harbor, an undeveloped but potentially spectacular naval base. Cleveland termed the islands "the stepping-stone to the growing trade of the Pacific." That phrase captured exactly how he and other officials saw Hawaii as a gateway to the great Asian commerce.[33] The Hawaiians, however, were soon shocked by the 1890 reciprocity treaties that allowed cheap Cuban sugar into U.S. markets. The islands' economy began sinking. By this time, the Americans who controlled the plantations also controlled the poli-

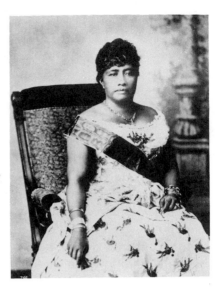

Queen Liliuokalani (1838–1917) was a determined and shrewd leader of her Hawaiian peoples. But in the early 1890s, she was unable to reverse the growing U.S. power on the islands, and in 1893 a coup, supported by the U.S. Navy, in effect ended her power despite President Cleveland's refusal to annex Hawaii at that point.

tics. They had demanded a constitution in 1887 that recognized their power. By the early 1890s, however, a strong-minded native monarch, Queen Liliuokalani, moved to neutralize the Americans' influence. Her attempt to reclaim power for the Hawaiians combined with the economic troubles to produce an American-led rebellion against her in January 1893. Washington's minister to Hawaii, John L. Stevens, actively helped by landing U.S. naval units to aid the rebels.

But now, Cleveland (just returned to the White House for a second term of 1893–1897) rejected the plea by the Americans in Hawaii for annexation. He knew the native Hawaiians had been coerced by U.S. force. Moreover, the president doubted that the U.S. Constitution could work when stretched across thousands of miles of water and imposed on such a non-Caucasian society. Cleveland also had enough problems at home. The 1893 stock-market collapse marked the lowest and most dangerous point in the twenty-five-year depression that had begun in 1873. But time was on the side of the pro-annexation group. Hawaii depended on U.S. markets. That dependence was tightened by an 1894 tariff bill restoring a favored place for the islands in the U.S. market. A new administration and new chance for a Pacific empire in 1898 finally allowed for the annexation of the islands. The annexation climaxed the expansionist drive that had begun more than half a century before.

The next stepping stone across the Pacific was Samoa. These beautiful islands, populated by Polynesians, had long served as an important stopping place for whaling vessels and traders (hence their early name, Navigators Islands). By the 1870s, their strategic location had attracted British and German attention. Into that rivalry stepped U.S. Naval Commander R. W. Meade. In 1871, Meade took the initiative to give Samoan chiefs American protection in return for their giving him a lease on the fine harbor of Pago Pago. The U.S. Senate did not accept that pact, but it ratified a similar treaty in 1878. Within a decade, the three Western powers were bitterly immersed in conflict over Samoa. By 1887, Cleveland's secretary of state, Thomas F. Bayard, asked for a conference before war possibly erupted. Bayard, a Delaware patrician with long political experience in an industrializing America, actually saw Samoa as an extension of the U.S. transcontinental railroad that carried U.S. goods to Asian markets. German Foreign Office officials angrily muttered that Bayard was extending the principles of "the Monroe Doctrine as though the Pacific Ocean were to be treated as an American lake."[34]

In 1887, Germany and Britain attempted to cut a deal over Samoa that threatened U.S. claims. Bayard refused to recognize the deal. At the same time, Germany began to bar U.S. meat imports (especially pork) on the grounds that they were tainted by a dangerous parasite. German-American relations, hardly in existence a generation before, suddenly became an intense rivalry over trade rights and access to the distant Pacific islands. The great German chancellor, Otto von Bismarck, had enough worries maintaining the new Germany that he had pieced together since 1860 through conquests and diplomacy. Wanting no war with Great Britain or the United States, in 1889 he called a conference in Berlin to discuss Samoa. Just before the meeting, a hurricane destroyed German and U.S. lives and vessels on the islands. Against this somber background, the Germans, British, and Americans agreed to divide the islands among themselves into a tripartite protectorate. They merely paid lip service to the Samoans' independence.

In 1899, the United States again found itself in a struggle with Germany and Great Britain over control of Samoan politics. British attention, however, was soon drawn off to that country's war in South Africa. London officials finally gave up all claims to Samoa. Germany and the United States then divided the islands between themselves, with the Americans retaining Pago Pago. The ending was peaceful, but, as historian Manfred Jonas observes, Germany, while giving in to U.S. claims, now viewed America as a rival. The Americans feared that German expansionism in Samoa might spread to the Caribbean. During this era, therefore, a "great transformation"[35] (as Jonas calls it) of the normally friendly U.S.-German relations began to strain the ties between Washington and Berlin. Within another generation, that strain would lead to war.

With the 1899 agreement on Samoa, the United States had added another key section in its bridge to Asia. The final destination was the Asian mainland itself, the quest of U.S. traders and missionaries for more than a century. Again, Seward had pointed the way. Since the 1840s, Americans had worked for an "open door" (that is, equality) for their trade in Asia. They did so, however, largely through "scavenger diplomacy"—coming behind the British Lion and taking from Asians whatever the Lion had left behind after its conquests. Seward dramatically changed that approach. In 1863 in Japan, and again in 1866 in Korea, the secretary of state worked alongside the British and French in their attempts to gain concessions. Thus, Seward added two new tactics to U.S. diplomacy in Asia: a willingness to use force, and a willingness to work with European powers to expand Western interests in Asia. These tactics shaped Washington's Asian diplomacy for the next eighty years.

Seward's policy, however, also created a problem—indeed, a contradiction—that bedeviled U.S. policy toward China over those next eighty years. For, in 1868, he signed with China's representative, Anson Burlingame, a treaty that allowed free immigration between the two nations. The agreement also pledged the United States not "to intervene in the domestic administration of China in regard to the construction of railroads, telegraphs, or other material internal improvements." Seward thus recognized China's control over its own internal development. But he refused to give up any claims on China's trade that might be made by the Western powers. While the United States thus recognized China's control of certain domestic affairs, it refused to recognize China as a fully sovereign country in control of its foreign commercial affairs. A month before he died in 1870, Burlingame wrote, "Let us try once, at least, to see what the Chinese will do if let alone by those who would Christianize them with gunpowder." Burlingame's hope was not to be realized. As his biographer, David L. Anderson, writes, Burlingame hoped to use the 1868 treaty to "replace coercion with cooperation" in U.S.-Chinese relations.[36] Instead, the United States merely mentioned Chinese sovereignty while working ever more closely with European powers to control Chinese affairs.

Seward especially got tough with Korea, the "Hermit Kingdom," over which China tried to claim control. Korea was strategically important, for it was at the gateway to the markets and raw materials of

Manchuria and northern China, as well as to eastern Russia itself. When the crew of the U.S. ship *General Sherman* mistakenly made its way into a Korean river, it was slaughtered by outraged Koreans. Seward quickly used his two new tactics. He prepared a U.S. naval attack, and asked the French to cooperate. But France, which had also lost citizens to Korean retaliation, refused to go along. In 1871, the Grant administration finally dispatched a fleet of five U.S. ships up the Han River. When Koreans fired on the ships, the Americans destroyed forts and killed more than two hundred people. Twelve Americans were killed, and the United States remained without any treaty with the tough Koreans. In 1876, Japan entered the scene by recognizing Korean independence from China. Korea now became a prize to be fought over by Japan and the Western powers.

The United States again took up the fight in 1882, when Commodore Robert Shufeldt forced Korea to sign a treaty opening itself to the Western world. An ardent expansionist, Shufeldt colorfully expressed his vision for American destiny in the Pacific:

> The Pacific is the ocean bride of America—China and Japan and Corea—with their innumerable islands, hanging like necklaces about them, are the bridesmaids, California is the nuptial couch, the bridal chamber, where all the wealth of the Orient will be brought to celebrate the wedding. Let us as Americans—let us determine while yet in our power, that no commercial rival or hostile flag can float with impunity over the long swell of the Pacific sea. . . . It is on this ocean that the East and the West have thus come together, reaching the point where search for Empire ceases and human power attains its climax.[37]

But the "bridesmaids"—Korea and China—were soon violated by Japan. The United States could do little about it. Americans certainly were concerned as Japanese power grew. Led by an extraordinary U.S. diplomat, Horace Allen, American interests in Korea temporarily increased. Allen, who nicely combined his Presbyterian missionary dedication with a robber-baron passion for making money, helped Americans develop Korean gold mines (perhaps the richest in Asia) and bribed authorities to obtain streetcar construction contracts.[38] But the U.S. attempt to split Korea from China backfired. Japan was the region's developing power, and it rightly saw Korea as vital to its own security.

As tension built between the rising Japanese and the declining Chinese empires, war finally erupted in 1894. Japan quickly forced China to quit Korea as well as give in to other demands. The Asian balance of power had shifted. Allen's and other U.S. enterprises were endangered by Japan. A prophetic U.S. senator, Anthony Higgins of Delaware, warned that when China "shall have arisen out of her defeat," she was likely to become the dominant military force of the globe. But most U.S. officials agreed with Secretary of State Walter Quintin Gresham in 1894: Japan was "the most civilized country" in Asia and, as such, could be trusted to respect the United States "as her best friend."[39] The friendship seemed to be reinforced strongly by trade. U.S. exports to China jumped from $3 million in 1890 to $7 million in 1896, but exports to Japan grew from $5 million to $8 million in those years. (The $22 million of imports from China in 1896 and $26 million of goods imported from Japan that year far outstripped U.S. exports to those two nations.)

THE 1865-TO-1896 ERA: A CONCLUSION

The race for the riches of Asia was accelerating. The race for dominance in Latin America, however, had ended. The United States had won that contest by 1896. This historic victory and the growth of American power in Asia signaled fundamental changes in U.S. diplomacy between 1865 and 1896, changes that shaped diplomacy throughout the twentieth century.

Most notably, the friends and enemies of 1865 exchanged places by the 1890s. During the century after 1776, the United States and England had fought two wars. Another conflict threatened during and after the Civil War, when the British built several ships, including the *Alabama*, for use by the Confederacy. After the war, infuriated Americans, led by Senator Charles Sumner, demanded that London pay millions for the damages that the ships had caused—or, as some Americans indicated, the annexation of Canada, which would be equally satisfactory as payment. As Anglo-American relations grew tense in the late 1860s, President Grant, who had come to despise the pompous Sumner, maneuvered the senator off the chairmanship of the powerful Foreign Relations Committee and made a deal with England. In the 1872 Washington Treaty, the British essentially apologized for releasing the *Alabama* and agreed to pay $15.5 million in the so-called *Alabama* claims. The United States, in turn, agreed to submit other disputes to arbitration. As a result of this agreement and long-held British claims against Americans, the United States finally paid England $7.4 million. Both U.S. and Canadian citizens gained free access to the St. Lawrence, St. John, and Yukon rivers, and also to Lake Michigan.[40]

In 1893, U.S. and British diplomats settled a long-festering dispute over the killing of female seals in the Bering Sea. The slaughter was destroying herds that provided rich, highly profitable furs. The United States, moreover, claimed control over the Bering Sea itself. Washington officials finally had to drop that claim, but in 1892–1893 Russians and Japanese, as well as Canadians, agreed with the American demand to protect the seals.

With these agreements of 1872 and 1892–1893, the air cleared between London and Washington. U.S.-British relations also were built on marriages of the children of American robber barons, who sought respectability, to those of British aristocrats, who sought dollars. But of special importance, in the Venezuelan crisis of 1895–1896, the British in fact recognized U.S. dominance in the Western Hemisphere, while in Asia the two English-speaking peoples shared a common commitment to the "open door" to China. Theodore Roosevelt caught this historic turn in 1898 when he wrote a friend: "I feel very strongly that the English-speaking peoples are now closer together than for a century and a quarter . . . ; for their interests are really fundamentally the same, and they are far more closely akin, not merely in blood, but in feeling and principle, than either is akin to any other people in the world."[41]

At the same time, however, relations with Russia, a long-time U.S. ally, turned worse. The tsars and the British monarchs were rivals, especially in the Near and Far East. As U.S.-British relations warmed, U.S.-Russian relations cooled. In Asia, the Russians, lagging far behind British and American industrial development, could not survive in an open-door type of economic competition. They favored outright colonization, which was precisely the policy the open-door approach opposed. Of special importance to many Americans, the tsar launched vicious attacks on Russian Jews in the 1880s. These pogroms, which had deep roots in the nation's history, occurred just as millions of European Jews migrated to seek opportunities in the United States. The attacks also appeared as many U.S. businessmen, including Jews, suffered discrimination when they tried to do business in Russia. U.S. opinion changed radically. "Russia's ambition is sleepless and insatiable," a Baltimore newspaper editor proclaimed in 1886. "It goes ahead step by step, through intrigue, through treachery, through diplomatic mendacity," and she cares not if "her people remain poor." The powerful Louisville newspaper publisher, Henry Watterson, put it simply: the

Russian had "proven his ability to fight like the European, and to deceive like the Asiatic."[42]

This historic switch in their international friendships was mirrored at home, when Americans realized in the 1890s that they had reached a turning point in their domestic life. The 1890 Census announced that the frontier line had finally disappeared. A young University of Wisconsin historian, Frederick Jackson Turner, explored the meaning of the Census finding. He did so in perhaps the most influential essay ever written on American history. In 1893, Turner argued that the U.S. economy and politics had been vigorous and successful because of the frontier. ("Economic power," Turner stated, in fact "secures political power.") The frontier had also produced "individualism" in the American character. Turner then had to conclude with a dramatic warning: "And now, four centuries from the discovery of America, at the end of a hundred years of life under the Constitution, the frontier has gone, and with its going has closed the first period of American history."[43]

To many Americans, the question now became: What can we find to replace the frontier so our economy, politics, and individualism can remain strong? That question took on a special urgency as strikes, riots, political radicalism, and bankruptcy struck the United States during the economic depression of the 1890s. Turner himself argued in 1896 that the frontier's disappearance created "demands for a vigorous foreign policy . . . and for the extension of American influence to outlying islands and adjoining countries."[44]

That conclusion had already been reached by Captain Alfred Thayer Mahan, who became perhaps the most influential military strategist in U.S. history. In 1886, Mahan was a bored, middle-aged naval officer. Then in a Lima, Peru, library he read that ancient Rome's control of the sea had secured its empire. Over the next quarter-century, in a series of widely read books and in lectures at the Naval War College in Newport, Rhode Island, Mahan built on that insight into Rome to construct a global foreign policy for the United States. He assumed that American surplus production required overseas markets. In order to obtain and protect those markets, the United States needed a great navy and fueling bases as rest stops for that navy. Beginning in 1886— and especially in 1890, when the first modern U.S. battleship was commissioned (and also the year when Mahan's first great book *The Influence of Sea Power upon History, 1660–1783,* appeared)—Americans built the Great White Fleet that fought the 1898 war and formed the basis of the twentieth-century U.S. Navy. Mahan pushed hard to annex an isthmian canal area, as well as bases in the Caribbean, Hawaii, and

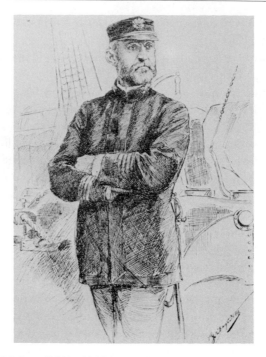

Alfred Thayer Mahan (1840–1914) was a friend of presidents and emperors because he knew how to use history to justify expansionism and the building of great navies. His seriousness, stiffness, discipline, and self-esteem are indicated in this portrait.

the distant Pacific to serve the fleet. He focused on the markets of Asia as the supreme prize.

To conquer that prize, he advised the United States to work with Great Britain and Japan (other seagoing powers who wanted the open door), and oppose Russia (a land-based power who opposed the open door). As a devout Christian, he believed that the seeking of this empire was "the calling of God." To do God's work, Mahan demanded a centralized government and powerful president. He blasted the democratic legacy of Thomas Jefferson, who "made a hideous mess in his own day, and yet has a progeny of backwoodsmen and planters who think what he taught a great success." Force was to be used freely, especially force in the form of large battleship fleets. The mere threat of such force, Mahan believed, prevented war. Anyway, he wrote, war had become merely "an occasional excess, from which recovery is easy."[45] Mahan enormously influenced U.S. officials, especially Presidents William McKinley and Theodore Roosevelt.

Other U.S. naval officers worked for a great navy because, in historian Peter Karsten's words, of "rank, discipline, and boredom."[46] Needing ships and action to gain personal promotion, they lobbied hard in Congress to build a new fleet with the most modern weapons. In 1883, the U.S. Navy was a pitiful collection of 90 woeful ships, 38 made of wood. Mahan and other officers, such as Mahan's mentor at the Naval War College, Stephen B. Luce, worked with Congress and such industrial giants as Bethlehem Steel and Andrew Carnegie to construct a great navy. It marked the success of the first military-industrial complex.[47] U.S. government dollars put laborers to work during the depression. Carnegie and other builders profited from highly subsidized government contracts.

The navy's officers obtained their fleet. And, in 1898, the United States moved to obtain what historian Frederick Drake calls "the empire of the seas."[48]

NOTES

1. David P. Crook, *Diplomacy during the American Civil War* (New York, 1975), p. 9.
2. Arthur C. Cole, *The Irrepressible Conflict, 1850–1865* (New York, 1934), p. 345.
3. Charles A. Beard and Mary Beard, *The Rise of American Civilization*, 2 vols. (New York, 1927), II, pp. 128–129.
4. William H. Seward, *The Works of William H. Seward*, ed. George Baker, 5 vols. (Boston, 1853–1883), III, pp. 498–499.
5. Thomas C. Cochran and William Miller, *The Age of Enterprise* (New York, 1942), p. 116.
6. David M. Pletcher, "Growth and Diplomatic Adjustment," in *Economics and World Power*, ed. William H. Becker and Samuel F. Wells (New York, 1984), pp. 120–124. For the agricultural side, the pioneering account is William Appleman Williams, *The Roots of the Modern American Empire* (New York, 1969).
7. Robert V. Bruce, *1877: Year of Violence* (Indianapolis, 1959), pp. 312–314.
8. Henry Nash Smith, *Mark Twain's Fable of Progress* (New Brunswick, N.J., 1964), pp. 8–9.
9. Cochran and Miller, p. 157.
10. David Healy, *U.S. Expansionism: The Imperialist Urge in the 1890s* (Madison, Wis., 1970), p. 115.
11. John Higham, "The Reorientation of American Culture in the 1890s," in *The Origins of Modern Consciousness*, ed. John Weiss (Detroit, 1965), pp. 26, 28.

12. Ralph Dewar Bald, Jr., "The Development of Expansionist Sentiment in the United States, 1885–1895, as Reflected in Periodical Literature" (Ph.D. diss., University of Pittsburgh, 1953), 266–267.

13. Mira Wilkins, *The Emergence of the Multinational Corporation* (Cambridge, Mass., 1970), pp. 68–69, 71.

14. Ralph W. Hidy and Muriel E. Hidy, *Pioneering in Big Business, 1882–1911: A History of Standard Oil* (New York, 1955), pp. 122–154.

15. Ronald Jensen tells the story well in *The Alaska Purchase and Russian-American Relations* (Seattle, 1975); see also Foster Rhea Dulles, *Prelude to World Power: American Diplomatic History, 1860–1900* (New York, 1965), pp. 53–56, and Fred H. Harrington, *Fighting Politician: Major General N. P. Banks* (Philadelphia, 1948), pp. 182–185.

16. *U.S. Railroad and Mining Register*, 6 April 1867, in "Alaska, 1867–1869" file, Papers of William H. Seward, University of Rochester, Rochester, New York.

17. Donald M. Dozer, "Anti-Expansionism during the Johnson Administration," *Pacific Historical Review* 12 (September 1943): 255–256; Charles S. Campbell, *The Transformation of American Foreign Relations, 1865–1900* (New York, 1976), p. 17. Seward and U.S. investors nevertheless moved significantly into Mexican affairs. Their important story is well told in Thomas Schoonover, *Dollars over Dominion* (Baton Rouge, 1978), pp. 252–254, 282–283 esp.

18. A superb analysis is Walter L. Williams, "U.S. Indian Policy and the Debate over Philippine Annexation," *Journal of American History* 66 (March 1980): 816; also Robert M. Utley, *The Indian Frontier of the American West, 1846–1890* (Albuquerque, 1984), p. 14.

19. Quoted in *Washington Post Book World*, 18 November 1984, p. 14; *Washington Post*, 29 December 1986, p. A3. A classic account is Stanley Vestal's *War-Path and Council Fire* (New York, 1948) on the Plains Indians.

20. Utley, pp. 186, 201, 251–257.

21. *Ibid.*, p. 261.

22. Williams, "U.S. Indian Policy," 828; Vestal, p. xi, quotes the British expert.

23. Joseph A. Fry, "John Tyler Morgan's Southern Expansionism," *Diplomatic History* 9 (Fall 1985): 329–346.

24. *The Gilded Age, a Reappraisal*, ed. H. Wayne Morgan (Syracuse, 1963), p. 167; Williams's story is beautifully told in John Hope Franklin, *George Washington Williams, a Biography* (Chicago, 1985), esp. pp. 202–203, 234–241.

25. Alexander DeConde, *Ethnicity, Race, and American Foreign Policy* (Boston, 1992), p. 46; Edward P. Crapol, "Lydia Maria Child: Abolitionist Critic of American Foreign Policy," in *Women and American Foreign Policy*, ed. E. Crapol (Westport, Conn., 1987), p. 13.

26. Richard H. Bradford's *The Virginius Affair* (Boulder, Col., 1980) is a fine account.

27. David Pletcher, *The Awkward Years* (Columbia, Mo., 1962), p. 105; Dulles, pp. 37–38; Campbell, pp. 15–18; Robert A. Friedlander, "A Reassessment of Roosevelt's Role in the Panamanian Revolution of 1903," *Western Political Quarterly* 14 (June 1961): 538–539.

28. James G. Blaine, *Political Discussions, Legislative, Diplomatic, and Popular, 1856–1886* (Norwich, Conn., 1887), p. 411; *New York Tribune*, 30 August 1890, p. 1.

29. The story is told and footnoted in Walter LaFeber, *The New Empire* (Ithaca, N.Y., 1963), pp. 210–218.

30. Richard Olney to Thomas F. Bayard, 20 July 1895, in *Foreign Relations of the United States, 1895*, 2 vols. (Washington, D.C., 1896), I, pp. 545–562; the classic account is Dexter Perkins's *The Monroe Doctrine, 1867–1907* (Baltimore, 1937), pp. 153–168.

31. Pletcher, *Awkward Years*, pp. 35–36.

32. *Foreign Relations of the United States, 1881* (Washington, D.C., 1882), pp. 635–639; Donald M. Dozer, "Opposition to Hawaiian Reciprocity, 1876–1888," *Pacific Historical Review* 14 (June 1945): 157–183.

33. *A Compilation of the Messages and Papers of the Presidents, 1789–1897*, ed. James D. Richardson, 10 vols. (Washington, D.C., 1900), VIII, pp. 500–501.

34. Quoted in LaFeber, p. 55.

35. Manfred Jonas, *The United States and Germany* (Ithaca, N.Y. 1984), pp. 48–49.

36. David L. Anderson, "Anson Burlingame: American Architect of the Cooperative Policy in China, 1861–1871," *Diplomatic History* 1 (Summer 1977): 239–256.

37. Quoted, with excellent analysis, in Frederick G. Drake, *The Empire of the Seas: A Biography of Rear-Admiral Robert N. Shufeldt* (Honolulu, 1984), p. 116.

38. The extraordinary story of Horace Allen is superbly told in Fred H. Harrington's *God, Mammon, and the Japanese* (Madison, Wis., 1944). Harrington published a reconsideration forty-two years later: "An American View of Korean-American Relations, 1882–1905," in *One Hundred Years of Korean-American Relations, 1882–1982*, ed. Yur-Bok Lee and Wayne Patterson (University, Ala., 1986).

39. Jeffrey M. Dowart, "The Pigtail War: The American Response to the Sino-Japanese War of 1894–1895" (Ph.D. diss., University of Massachusetts, 1971), 111–112.

40. Adrian Cook's *The Alabama Claims: American Politics and Anglo-American Relations, 1865–1872* (Ithaca, N.Y., 1975) tells this story well.

41. Theodore Roosevelt, *The Letters of Theodore Roosevelt*, ed. Elting E. Morison *et al.*, 8 vols. (Cambridge, Mass., 1951–1954), II, pp. 889–890.

42. Thomas A. Bailey, *America Faces Russia* (Ithaca, N.Y. 1950), pp. 147–148.

43. Frederick Jackson Turner, *The Frontier in American History* (New York, 1947), esp. pp. 32–37.

44. Frederick Jackson Turner, "The Problem of the West," *Atlantic Monthly* 78 (September 1896): 289–297.

45. Alfred Thayer Mahan, *Letters and Papers of A. T. Mahan*, ed. Robert Seager II and Doris D. Maguire, 3 vols. (Annapolis, 1975), II, pp. 506, 662; III, pp. 80, 484; William L. Livezey, *Mahan on Sea Power* (Norman, Okla., 1947), p. 263.

46. Two books by Peter Karsten are crucial here: *The Naval Aristocracy* (New York, 1972) and *Soldiers and Society* (Westport, Conn., 1978).

47. See especially B. F. Cooling, *Gray Steel and Blue Water Navy: The Formative Years of America's Military-Industrial Complex, 1881–1917* (Hamden, Conn., 1979).

48. Drake, p. xi.

For Further Reading

Begin with the well-organized pre-1981 references in *Guide to American Foreign Relations since 1700*, ed. Richard Dean Burns (1983); the notes of this chapter and the General Bibliography at the end of this book; the up-to-date bibliography in Robert L. Beisner, *From the Old Diplomacy to the New, 1865–1900* (1986); Walter LaFeber, *The American Search for Opportunity, 1865–1913*, in *The Cambridge History of U.S. Foreign Relations*, ed. Warren Cohen (1993); and the exhaustive list of works in Charles S. Campbell's *The Transformation of American Foreign Relations, 1865–1900* (1976). The Beisner and Campbell are also most helpful and provocative overviews, as is Richard Welch, Jr., *The Presidencies of Grover Cleveland* (1988).

For the context and perspectives on the "imperialist" debate, especially helpful are *Imperialism and After: Continuities and Discontinuities*, ed. Wolfgang J. Mommsen and Jurgen Osterhammel (1986); Tony Smith, *The Pattern of Imperialism: The U.S., Great Britain and the Late Industrializing World since 1815* (1982); Eric Hobsbawm, "The Crisis of Capitalism in Historical Perspective," *Socialist Revolution* 6 (October–December 1976): 77–96, especially on 1873–1896; William H. Becker, *The Dynamics of Business-Government Relations* (1982), for a more benign view of the relationship; Joseph A. Fry, *Henry S. Sanford: Diplomacy and Business in Nineteenth-Century America* (1982), for a fine case study; Tom E. Terrill's important analysis, *The Tariff, Politics and American Foreign Policy* (1973); and Edward Crapol's readable, significant study, *America for Americans* (1973), on Anglophobia.

Ideological and cultural influences are well analyzed in Michael H. Hunt, *Ideology and U.S. Foreign Policy* (1987), especially chapter III, tying internal and external racism together; Stuart Anderson, *Race and Rapprochement: Anglo-Saxonism and Anglo-American Relations, 1895–1904* (1981); Frank A. Cassell, "The Columbian Exposition of 1893 and U.S. Diplomacy in Latin America," *Mid-America* 67 (October 1985): 109–124; Robert W. Rydell, *All the World's a Fair: Visions of Empire at American International Expositions, 1876–1916* (1985), a fascinating account; and Donald C. Bellomy, "Social Darwinism Revisited," *Perspectives in American History* New Series, I (1984): 1–129, the best analysis. The frontier's impact is also noted in Brian W. Dippie, *The Vanishing American: White Attitudes and U.S. Indian Policy* (1982).

On specific geographical areas, the Latin American problems are explored in the Anderson and Cassell accounts noted above; Craig T. Dozier, *Nicaragua's Mosquito Shore* (1985); Joseph Smith, *Unequal Giants . . . 1889–1930* on U.S.-Brazil relations; Thomas Schoonover, "Imperialism in Middle America," a superb overview, in *Eagle against Empire*, ed. Rhodri Jeffreys-Jones (1983); Joyce S. Goldberg, *The Baltimore Affair: U.S. Relations with Chile, 1891–1892* (1986), now the standard account; and James F. Vivian, "U.S. Policy during the Brazilian Naval Revolt, 1893–1894: The Case for American Neutrality," *American Neptune* 41 (October 1981), a defense of U.S. policy. For Asia, see Phillip Darby, *Three Faces of Imperialism: British and American Approaches to Asia and Africa, 1870–1970* (1987), a fine comparative study; David L. Anderson, *Imperialism and Idealism: American Diplomats in China, 1861–1898* (1986); Yur-Bok Lee, *Diplomatic Relations between the United States and Korea, 1866–1887* (1970), which is the best on the subject, and also Lee's "Establishment of a Korean Legation in the United States, 1887–1890," *Illinois Papers in Asian Studies* 3 (1983). On Africa, begin with Darby's book noted above, and also Peter Duignan and L. H. Gann, *The United States and Africa: A History* (1984).

For individual administrations, Paul S. Holbo's *Tarnished Expansion: The Alaska Scandal, the Press, and Congress, 1867–1871* (1983) is most revealing; Clifford W. Haury, "Hamilton Fish and the Conservative Tradition," in *Studies in American Diplomacy*,

1865–1945, ed. Norman Graebner (1985), an interesting interpretation; Justus D. Doenecke, *The Presidencies of James A. Garfield and Chester A. Arthur* (1981), important on Latin America and Korea especially; Michael J. Devine, *John W. Foster: Politics and Diplomacy in the Imperial Era, 1873–1917* (1981), a good analysis of a key figure; and Charles W. Calhoun, *Gilded Age Cato: The Life of Walter Q. Gresham* (1988), the standard biography.

7

Turning Point: The McKinley Years (1896–1900)

THE SIGNIFICANCE OF THE LATE 1890s

As the twentieth century dawned, the United States stepped onto the world stage as a great power. Because of the triumphs scored between 1898 and 1900, it strode confidently now with Great Britain, France, Russia, Germany, and Japan—nations that possessed immense military strength and had used that strength for conquest. Never had a newly independent nation risen so far so fast as did the United States between 1776 and 1900.

Historians have argued not over whether the United States deserved great-power status by 1900 (all agree that it did), but whether Americans consciously intended to follow the expansionist policies after 1896 that projected them into such distant regions. Historian Ernest May believes that the United States had "greatness thrust upon it." But another scholar, Albert K. Weinberg, concludes that U.S. officials were no more passive at key moments than "is the energetic individual who decides upon, plans, and carries out the robbery of a bank."[1] The years 1896 to 1900 thus become critical for the student of U.S. foreign policy in the twentieth century. For if the nation entered the ranks of great world powers at this time, it is of central importance to know how it did so. By accident? Because of a few elite officials who pushed reluctant Americans overseas? Because of the U.S. system's domestic needs that forced that system to assume global responsibilities? The well-known saying "Just as the twig is bent, the tree's inclined" might have meaning for U.S. diplomatic history. The reasons why the United States moved outward so rapidly in the late 1890s help us understand why it grew from these roots (or twig) into a twentieth-century superpower.

McKINLEY AND McKINLEYISM

Americans living in the late 1890s understood that they were witnessing a historic turn. After the triumph over Spain in 1898 brought the United States new holdings in the Caribbean and the western Pacific, Assistant Secretary of State John Bassett Moore observed that the nation had moved "from a position of comparative freedom from entanglements into the position of what is commonly called a world power. . . . Where formerly we had only commercial interests, we now have territorial and political interests as well."[2]

Moore's boss, President William McKinley, presided over these changes. McKinley won the 1896 election over the highly popular Democrat, William Jennings Bryan. The affection Americans felt for McKinley ranked with the feelings they later had toward the popular Theodore Roosevelt, Franklin D. Roosevelt, and Dwight D. Eisenhower. A gentle, soft-spoken, highly courteous man, McKinley had long been known for the love and care he had lavished on his wife, an invalid who required much of his attention. Born in Niles, Ohio, in 1843, Major McKinley had been a Civil War hero, then parlayed his reputation and uncanny political instincts into a career in the House of Representatives between 1876 and 1890. By the end of his stay, no one on Capitol Hill better understood the new industrialized America. He dominated debates on the central issues of tariffs and taxes because he had mastered the facts and understood the powerful industrialists who made the country run. Moving on to the governorship of Ohio, he maintained order in an economically depressed state while nearby regions were wracked by riots. He was not reluctant to use state forces to control strikers, but he somehow did so while keeping the good will of the labor leaders. With the help of fellow Ohioan and millionaire steel industrialist Marcus Hanna, who ran a superbly organized campaign, McKinley moved to the White House. The new president named Ohio senator John Sherman as secretary of state and then rewarded Hanna by having him appointed to the empty Senate seat. The United States thus obtained a secretary of state who was aged, sometimes incapacitated, and too often senile; but in Hanna, McKinley enjoyed a

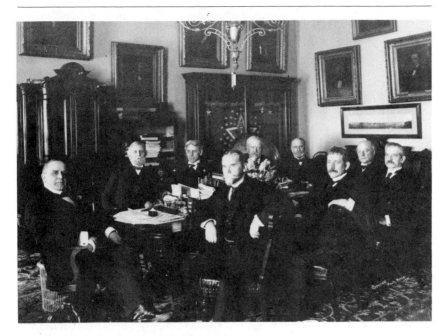

William McKinley (1843–1901) of Ohio was the last Civil War veteran to be president (enlisting at age seventeen, he had been a hero) but the first modern American chief executive. He also appointed a modern cabinet—that is, one made up of administrators who owed allegiance to the president. He is at far left. John Hay is at McKinley's right.

trusted power broker in the Senate who followed the president's every wish.

Anyway, McKinley intended to control foreign policy himself. An accomplished negotiator and an experienced politician whose antennae could instantly detect an opponent's weakness, the president knew how to conduct back-room talks and keep secrets. His State Department depended especially on Alvey A. Adee, a long-time professional who served in the department for fifty-five years until his death in 1924. Adee personally wrote or approved nearly every outgoing message. When he once bicycled past, a Washingtonian said, "There goes our State Department now." Though hard-of-hearing, Adee seemed to have learned everything that the president needed to know about international law and diplomatic history. The closed-mouth president, deaf Adee, and senile Sherman led to the complaint that "the President says nothing, the Assistant Secretary hears nothing, and the Secretary of State knows nothing."

Controlling foreign policy in the way that he did, McKinley became not only the first twentieth-century president, but the first modern chief executive. He developed new powers, especially in maneuvering and controlling Congress, while he kept the control of foreign policy in his own hands (and used the new devices of the telephone and typewriter while doing so). McKinley expanded the Constitution's commander-in-chief powers until, without congressional permission, he used it to dispatch U.S. troops to fight in China. His action set a precedent for the "imperial presidency" of the 1960s and 1970s.

McKinley and Hanna, moreover, cleverly used the backlash caused by the 1893–1897 economic crisis that had driven the Democrats from power in 1894 and 1896. The two men built a political coalition so powerful that only one Democratic presidential nominee would be elected between 1896 and 1932. The new politics had profound influence on presidential power. As a result of the 1890s political realignment, Republicans dominated the North and Democrats controlled the South. This division meant that contests between Republicans and Democrats declined in individual states, voters grew less interested, and many (especially black people in the South) were disfranchised.[3] The president thus broke free of the hard-fought party rivalry that had marked the 1876–1896 years. He enjoyed more freedom and a more dependable political base from which to conduct foreign policy. McKinley exploited these opportunities by becoming the first chief executive to appoint a staff member who dealt with newspaper reporters and prepared press handouts that publicized the administration's case. The Ohioan was even the first president whose inauguration was put on film.

The great Kansas journalist, William Allen White, observed that McKinley survived twenty years in the jungles of Ohio politics, "where survival values combined the virtues of the serpent, the shark, and the cooing dove." White believed that the president was too much "cooing dove," "too polite," for McKinley's "Prince Albert coat was never wrinkled, his white vest front never broken. . . . He weighed out his saccharine on apothecary scales, just enough and no more for the dose that cheers but does not inebriate." White further perfectly caught McKinley's genius for handling people, especially those in Congress. After rejecting one visitor's request for a favor, the president took the carnation he always wore in his coat and told the man to "give this to your wife with my compliments and best wishes." He did it so graciously that the visitor declared, "I would rather have this flower from you for my wife than the thing I came to get."[4]

At the same time, the president understood the brute truths of politics. Historian Henry Adams watched the president closely and described "what might be called McKinleyism; the system of combinations, consolidations . . . , realized at home, and realizable abroad."[5] Under McKinley, an industrialized America moved to Americanize new parts of the world.

Two Crises, One War

McKinley took the presidential oath in March 1897 as a revolution raged just ninety miles from U.S. shores. In 1894–1895, the U.S. tariff policy had kept out Cuban sugar from mainland markets. The island went into an economic tailspin. A revolution against Spanish colonialism had broken out between 1868 and 1878. It now re-emerged with greater force. By late 1895, the rebels claimed to have established a provisional government. Support for their cause swelled in the United States, but neither Cleveland nor McKinley would recognize the revolutionaries. To do so would have released the Spanish government from its responsibility for protecting $50 million of U.S. property in Cuba. Washington officials preferred to hold Spain fully responsible for protecting U.S. lives and property, while pushing the Madrid government to give Cuba enough autonomy so that the revolutionaries would stop fighting.

Spain, however, refused to move the island toward autonomy. Its once-great, four-hundred-year-old empire had rotted away until it amounted to little more than Cuba, Puerto Rico, a few scattered islands in the Pacific, and the Philippine Islands. No government in Madrid could surrender these last holdings and expect to remain in power. The Spanish instead took a tough approach. They dispatched 150,000 soldiers, who, under the command of General Valeriano Weyler (soon nicknamed "Butcher" Weyler by U.S. newspaper editors), tried to destroy rebel support by rounding up thousands of Cubans and placing them in barbed-wire concentration camps. The revolution nevertheless continued to spread. The insurgents burned U.S. property in the hope of forcing McKinley's intervention.

Nineteenth-century Americans had little respect for Spain. They had seized its North American empire piece by piece between 1800 and 1821. The Spanish, wrote one of the first American historians, the Reverend Jedidiah Morse, are "naturally weak and effeminate," and "dedicate the greatest part of their lives to loitering and inactive pleasures." "Their character," he sniffed, "is nothing more than a grave and specious insignificance."[6] In the 1890s, leading U.S. newspapers picked up Morse's views and demanded that the more civilized Americans help Cuba. The publishers were not unselfish. Technological breakthroughs in making paper and setting type had driven newspaper prices down to a penny or two a copy. These changes opened the possibility for mass distribution and the rich advertising fee that came with such a market. Two giants of the trade, William Randolph Hearst and Joseph Pulitzer, led the struggle to gain more newspaper readers. Each man sought subscribers through sensational front-page stories, and nothing was more sensational than events in Cuba—unless, of course, it was a U.S. war against Spain. Hearst especially promoted such a conflict. Congress picked up his beat and, in 1897, pressured McKinley to recognize the rebels.

The new president was moved by neither congressional demands nor the sensationalist "yellow journal" press. He feared that U.S. recognition would lead to war, a war whose costs could drag the United States back into the economic crises from which it was finally emerging in 1897. Businessmen and conservative politicians, both Republican and Democrat, warned that such a war could be paid for only by coining more silver. But more silver would cheapen the dollar and threaten U.S. credit overseas. McKinley, moreover, opposed war because it could lead to demands for annexing Cuba. Annexation would raise constitutional problems (for example, Can the Constitution safely stretch across water to take in new states without tearing apart?). Bringing Cuba into the Union would also incorporate a multiracial society at a

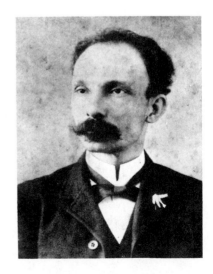

José Martí (1853–1895) was the father of the Cuban revolution that erupted in 1895, but he feared U.S. intervention as much as Spanish colonialism: "And once the United States is in Cuba," he asked, "who will drive it out?" A journalist in New York during the 1880s, he returned to Cuba in early 1895 to start the final phase of the uprising but was killed a month later by Spanish troops. Half a century later, he became a great hero of Fidel Castro.

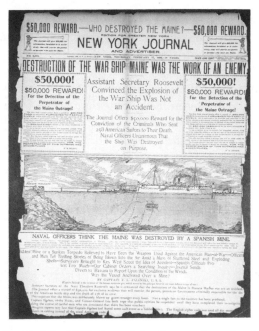

*"Yellow journalism" of the 1890s fanned the flames of war by giving Americans
immediate news of foreign-policy crises, especially if that news could be sensa-
tionalized to sell more newspapers.*

time when white Americans were already having problems dealing with
black Americans and millions of newly arrived immigrants. McKinley,
therefore, pressed Spain to grant enough reforms to undercut the revolutionaries. Madrid began to do so, even recalling "Butcher" Weyler
and offering the first steps toward autonomy. The president, however,
criticized the response as too little too late.

Spain had lost control. In late 1897, riots erupted in the Cuban capital of Havana. McKinley moved a warship, the *Maine*, into Havana
Harbor to protect U.S. citizens and property. In early February 1898,
a pro-war group in New York captured a letter in which the Spanish
minister to Washington, Dupuy de Lôme, called McKinley "weak and
a bidder for the admiration of the crowd." The minister also downplayed the importance of Spain's reforms. The little trust that Americans had in the Spanish evaporated. Six days later, on February 15, an
explosion shook the *Maine.* Settling into the muck of Havana Harbor,
the ship took more than 250 U.S. sailors to their deaths. In 1976, a
thorough investigation of the tragedy concluded that the vessel had
probably been destroyed by an internal explosion (perhaps in the engine

room) and not by some external device set by Spanish agents.[7] In 1898, however, Americans quickly concluded that a bomb had taken those lives, and the yellow journals and congressmen screamed for war. McKinley played for time by asking for an investigation. He feared, as he told a friend, that "the country was not ready for war." Military preparations had only begun. Economic dangers still loomed. He worried about the possible results of a victory: "Who knows where this war will lead us," he told a congressional leader. "It may be more than war with Spain."[8]

When making that remark, McKinley may have had in mind a second foreign-policy crisis that emerged in March 1898. It had begun with Japan's victory over China in 1894–1895 (see p. 182). In 1897, Germany blocked Japan from grabbing further territorial spoils. Using as an excuse the murder of two German missionaries, Berlin officials demanded as indemnity from China the port of Kiaochow (now Chiao Hsien). Located at an entrance to the rich Chinese province of Manchuria, Kiaochow controlled a trade route used by an increasing number of Americans. Other European powers and Japan then clamored for important parts of China's territory. The traditional U.S. open-door policy to all of China faced extinction. Great Britain, which shared much of Washington's concern about the open door, asked McKinley for help in stopping the other Europeans. The president sympathized with the British position, but he could not help. China was too far away, Cuba too close. McKinley had to deal with revolution before he could help protect the open door. Meanwhile, worried U.S. exporters and business newspapers began chanting a warning that, in the *Journal of Commerce*'s words, the Far East crisis threatened "the future of American trade."[9]

One possible escape from the dilemma had, however, already appeared. Rebels in the Philippines had begun war against Spanish rule. The islands could become a key military base from which to protect U.S. interests in Asia. McKinley, Captain Alfred Thayer Mahan, and Assistant Secretary of the Navy Theodore Roosevelt closely watched the Philippine struggle in early 1898. On February 25, when his superior was out of the office, Roosevelt sent a series of cables that ordered U.S. naval commanders to prepare their ships for fighting. The next day, the astonished secretary of the navy, John D. Long, rushed to the White House with the news that his assistant had single-handedly tried to push the country to the brink of war. McKinley ordered that all of Roosevelt's cables be recalled—except the order to Admiral George Dewey that his Pacific fleet prepare to attack the Philippines in case of war with Spain.[10] In actuality, Dewey had earlier received orders to attack the Philippines in case of war with Spain. The president, meanwhile, had been reinforcing Dewey's squadron. McKinley later soft-soaped critics of his Philippine policy by assuring them that he had involuntarily been pushed into conquering "those darn islands," which he could not even quickly locate on a map. His statement was good politics but bad history. The president knew very well before he went to war with Spain how much the Philippine base could mean to preserving the open door in China. The crisis caused by German and Japanese grabs of China's territory left him no alternative—unless he wanted to quit the century-long U.S. quest for Asian markets. And the president had no intention of doing that.

McKinley carefully prepared his policy to deal with the Cuban and Asian crises at once. After the *Maine*'s destruction, he moved rapidly to prepare the country for war. On March 9, he acquired $50 million from Congress to begin mobilization of the army and navy. On March 17, Republican senator Redfield Proctor of Vermont, one of McKinley's close friends, returned from a visit to Cuba and electrified Americans by announcing that he had changed his anti-war stand. A strong conservative, Proctor declared that his business contacts in Cuba had told him that Spain's reforms had failed. Property was being destroyed. Conservative Cubans wanted autonomy or U.S. annexation. Proctor's fears were underlined when State Department officials in Cuba warned McKinley that unless the fighting was stopped, "there might be a revolution within a revolution."[11] This meant that the rebellion threatened to take a sharp leftward turn that could threaten conservative property holders if the revolutionaries won. McKinley thus not only had to stop the fighting, but control the revolution itself.

On March 25, the president received a telegram from a close political adviser in New York City: "Big corporations here now believe we will have war. Believe all would welcome it as a relief to suspense."[12] This cable revealed that eastern business groups, long afraid of war, now felt that battle was preferable to the fears generated by Proctor's speech and the other events of February and March. New York business leaders had concluded that the United States could safely pay for a war without having to coin silver. Many midwestern and western business groups, as well as nationwide commercial journals who were frightened over the threat to the open door in Asia, had long supported war. The business community was uniting behind McKinley's military preparations.

Between March 20 and 28, the president sent a series of demands to

Spain. The Spanish would have to pay indemnity for the *Maine*, promise not to use the *reconcentrado* policy, declare a truce, and negotiate for Cuban independence through U.S. mediation, if necessary. In the end, Spain surrendered to all the demands except the last. No Madrid government could promise Cuban independence and remain in power. Spain stalled, no doubt hoping that once the rainy season began in Cuba during early summer, McKinley would ease the pressure until the weather cleared for fighting in the autumn. But the president decided to move quickly. On April 11, he sent his message to Congress. He asked for war on the grounds that the three-year struggle on the island threatened Cuban lives, U.S. property, and tranquillity in the United States itself.

The president did not want war. But he did want results that only war could bring: protecting property in Cuba, stopping the revolution before it turned sharply to the left, restoring confidence in the U.S. business community, insulating his Republican party from Democratic charges of cowardice in safeguarding U.S. interests, and giving himself a free hand to deal with the growing Asian crisis. For these reasons, McKinley took the country into war in April 1898.

"A SPLENDID LITTLE WAR . . ."

McKinley's war message triggered a bitter debate in Congress. Since 1895, many congressmen had supported the Cuban junto, which raised millions of dollars in the United States to support the rebels. A number of Americans invested heavily in Cuban bonds to purchase arms for the revolution. These pro-Cuban groups now insisted that McKinley recognize Cuban independence as part of the war declaration. The president instantly rejected the deal. Mistrusting the revolutionaries, he insisted on keeping his freedom of action in handling the island once the fighting ended. The Senate tried to impose the junto's policy on the president, but he blocked the measure in the House. Then, in a week of intense political infighting (during which the usually calm McKinley had to take sleeping potions so that he could rest), he forced the Senate to retreat. The president received exactly what he wanted: only a declaration of war. Theodore Roosevelt, angry because McKinley refused to rush into war, privately complained that the president had "no more backbone than a chocolate eclair" and added that the gentle Ohioan was a "white-livered cur." But as historian Paul Holbo notes, the central question by early April was not whether the country was going to war, "but who was to direct American policy."[13] The Senate fight demonstrated that the president could dominate Roosevelt, the Congress, and the powerful interests behind the Cuban junto.

Congress included in the war resolution the Teller Amendment. This provision declared that the United States was not entering the war to conquer territory. The Teller Amendment eased some consciences, but it actually aimed to protect American sugar producers from cheap Cuban sugar. (Senator Henry Teller, a Republican, came from the sugar-beet state of Colorado.) Historians later discovered, moreover, that Cuban leaders handed out $1 million in payment to lobbyists and perhaps to members of Congress who voted for the amendment. McKinley accepted the provision. He had no intention of annexing Cuba.[14] But he did want Hawaii—and quickly. The mid-Pacific islands could be vital bases for U.S. ships heading toward the Philippines. Wartime need, however, by no means explained why the United States annexed Hawaii in June 1898. The story begins earlier.

After 1893, when President Cleveland rejected requests from Americans in Hawaii for annexation, the United States paid little attention to the islands. That lack of interest dramatically disappeared in mid-1897, when McKinley received urgent messages that the Japanese were sending several warships to Hawaii. The Tokyo government was angry that its citizens who were attempting to enter the islands were being turned away. The reason for the rejection lay in numbers: in 1884, only 116 Japanese lived in Hawaii; but by 1897, their 25,000 people accounted for one-quarter of the entire population. The Japanese even outnumbered the Americans, Europeans, and native Hawaiians. If they obtained the vote, the power of the white planters who ruled the islands could be shattered. Hawaii could become a Japanese colony.

When Tokyo's two warships appeared in Hawaiian waters during early 1897, McKinley, who had long wanted to annex the islands, ordered U.S. vessels prepared for action. Captain Alfred Thayer Mahan privately warned Roosevelt in the Navy Department to be aware of "the very real present danger of war" with Japan.[15] To the delight of Roosevelt, Mahan, and other expansionists, the president sent a treaty for Hawaiian annexation to the Senate in June 1897. But he moved too quickly. The president could not line up the necessary 60 Senate votes for the two-thirds approval needed to ratify the pact. Americans wanted to think carefully before extending their Constitution that far into the Pacific. Domestic sugar producers especially assailed the pact; they feared Hawaiian sugar imports.

On May 2, 1898, a telegram reached Washington that Admiral George

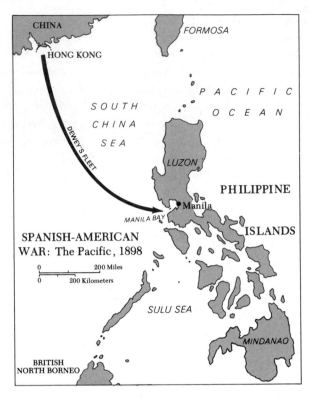

In the far west, the sailing of Dewey's fleet from Hong Kong to Manila made Americans a Pacific power. But U.S. interests had been growing in the region for a century.

Dewey's ships had destroyed the Spanish fleet in the Philippines. Two days later, McKinley again asked the Senate for Hawaiian annexation. He still did not have the needed 60 votes, so he resorted to the device of annexation through joint resolution of the House and Senate. (That same device had been used in 1846 to take Texas, see p. 108.) The majorities needed for passing the joint resolution were easily found in both houses. On August 12, 1898, Hawaii became a U.S. territory.

By then, the islands fit within a grander plan developing in McKinley's mind: "We need Hawaii just as much and a good deal more than we did California. It is manifest destiny," he had declared earlier in 1898.[16] The U.S. Minister to Siam, John A. Barrett, believed that "we need Hawaii to properly protect our cotton, flour, and richly laden ships which . . . will one day ply on the Pacific like the Spanish galleons of old," as they make themselves "masters of the Pacific seas." Mahan chimed in with his influential arguments about the need for mid-Pacific coaling stations on the route to Asia. The shortest route from California to China's markets was via the Alaskan coast. But, as historian Alan Henrikson has noted in a fascinating analysis, Mahan used Mercator, flat-world maps, not maps viewing the earth from the North and South Poles. Thus, the main U.S. Pacific base was developed at Pearl Harbor in Hawaii rather than on the more direct Alaskan–Aleutian Islands route.[17]

By early August, when Hawaii became a U.S. territory, Americans had already won the easiest conflict in their history. With the declaration of war in April, Dewey had set out from Hong Kong to engage the Spanish fleet in the Philippines. His small squadron appeared so weak that British officers at the Hong Kong Club observed sorrowfully: "A fine set of fellows, but unhappily we shall never see them again." When Dewey arrived at Manila Bay, however, he discovered seven armorless Spanish vessels. The Spanish commander was so certain of his fate that he simply moved his ships to the bay's shallowest waters so his men would not drown when their vessels were shot out from under them. Dewey then destroyed the Spanish flotilla, killing or wounding 400 men. No U.S. ship was badly hit, and only several Americans received scratches. After four hours of cannon fire, the United States had become a power in the western Pacific. "Our crews are all hoarse

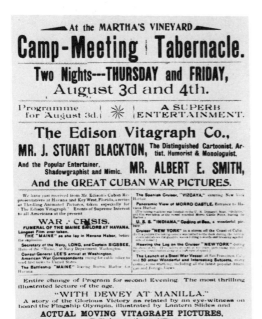

The 1898 meeting of empire, movies, and public education immediately after the "splendid little war" against Spain. Early, quite primitive motion pictures and slides brought home to Americans the thrill of the new overseas empire, as U.S. technology both won a war and then celebrated the winning.

from cheering," a U.S. official cabled Washington from Manila on May 4, "and while we suffer for cough drops and throat doctors we have no use for liniment or surgeons."

Washington officials also believed that Cuba would be captured by sea power. They, therefore, used much of the $50 million appropriated by Congress in March to prepare the navy, not the army, for action. As a result, the War Department bought few modern weapons or tropical clothing until after the fighting began. When McKinley ordered troops to prepare to invade Cuba and Puerto Rico, they had to wear heavy uniforms designed for northern climates. They ate provisions so badly prepared that one mainstay was accurately called "embalmed beef." Field weapons dated from the Civil War. As 180,000 volunteers trained to join the regular 30,000-man army, scandals rocked the War Department. Despite these disasters, in late May, General William R. Shafter began moving 16,000 troops from Tampa, Florida, to Cuba. His army traveled on 32 transports that could move no faster than 7 miles an hour. They sailed for 5½ days, much of it in well-lit vessels just off the Cuban coast, while the U.S. flagship crew enjoyed a band on deck that played ragtime.[18]

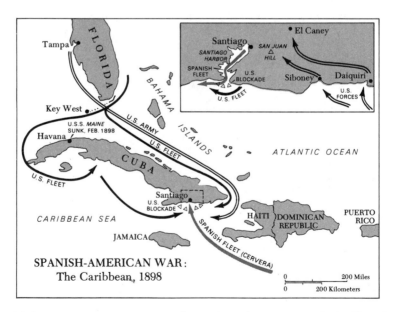

In the Caribbean, the war removed Spain from the region, made the United States the hemisphere's leading power, and opened an era of turbulent U.S.-Cuban relations.

The main U.S. fleet, including the three 10,000-ton battleships authorized in 1890, prepared to fight the Spanish fleet that was steaming across the Atlantic to Cuba. An important U.S. warship, the *Oregon*, arrived only after a highly publicized 68-day voyage from the Pacific around Cape Horn on the tip of South America to the Caribbean. It was a remarkable feat of seamanship that made Americans understand why they needed an isthmian canal cut through Central America. During the *Oregon*'s voyage, inhabitants of New York, Boston, and other coastal cities feared that their homes would be blasted by Spanish shells. They demanded protection, so McKinley sent a few broken-down Civil War coastal defense vessels, although he knew that the danger was nonexistent. The real question was whether the dilapidated Spanish squadron could even make it safely across the Atlantic. When it did, the U.S. fleet quickly cut off the four most respectable vessels in Santiago Harbor. As U.S. troops moved into Santiago by land, the Spanish ships tried to escape.[19] The twelve American vessels destroyed the entire fleet at the cost of one U.S. life. As Americans took target practice, one U.S. officer had to shout the famous order: "Don't cheer, men! Those poor devils are dying."

For nearly all Americans, the conflict gave war a good name. Fighting seemed easy and nearly cost-free. Journalist Richard Harding Davis concluded that "war as it is conducted at this end of the century is civilized."[20] No one benefited more from the conflict than Theodore Roosevelt. He left the Navy Department to organize friends (especially men he had met while living as a cowboy in South Dakota's Black Hills a decade earlier) into the "Rough Riders." Finally getting his long-sought chance to kill, TR determined to do it as a gentleman. For example, he ordered from Brooks Brothers clothiers an "ordinary Cavalry lieutenant Colonel's uniform in blue Cravenette" so that he would be properly outfitted. When he finally reached Cuba, he nearly destroyed his Rough Riders by leading them up the steep Kettle's Hill directly into hostile gunfire. Fortunately for TR, the Spanish weapons could not shoot accurately at slowly moving targets. Roosevelt emerged a national hero. He made certain his heroism was appreciated by publishing in 1899 *The Rough Riders*—a book that humorist Finley Peter Dunne ("Mr. Dooley," as he was known to newspaper readers) suggested could be entitled "Alone in Cubia."[21] But Richard Harding Davis's sarcasm at the time applied to the U.S. war effort as well as Roosevelt's: "God takes care of drunken men, sailors, and the United States."

TABLE 1

PRINCIPAL WARS IN WHICH THE UNITED STATES PARTICIPATED: U.S. MILITARY PERSONNEL SERVING AND CASUALTIES

War/conflict	Branch of service	Number serving	Casualties		
			Battle deaths	Other deaths	Wounds not mortal
Revolutionary War (1775–1783)	Total		4,435	—	6,188
	Army	—	4,044	—	6,004
	Navy	—	342	—	114
	Marines	—	49	—	70
War of 1812 (1812–1815)	Total	286,730	2,260	—	4,505
	Army	—	1,950	—	4,000
	Navy	—	265	—	439
	Marines	—	45	—	66
Mexican War (1846–1848)	Total	78,718	1,733	11,550	4,152
	Army	—	1,721	11,550	4,102
	Navy	—	1	—	3
	Marines	—	11	—	47
Civil War (Union forces only) (1861–1865)	Total	2,213,363	140,414	224,097	281,881
	Army	2,128,948	138,154	221,374	280,040
	Navy	—	2,112	2,411	1,710
	Marines	84,415	148	512	131
Spanish-American War (1898)	Total	306,760	385	2,061	1,662
	Army	280,564	369	2,061	1,594
	Navy	22,875	10	—	47
	Marines	3,321	6	—	21

Source: Department of Defense.

... FOR CONTROL OF CUBA AND PUERTO RICO

America's mood and future were better caught by the U.S. ambassador to France, Horace Porter. He wrote McKinley in November 1898 that European officials "express the opinion that we did in three months what the great powers of Europe had sought in vain to do for over a hundred years." These accomplishments included, Porter observed,

> having secured a chain of island posts in the Pacific, secured the Philippines, captured their trade, paved the way for a Pacific [telegraph] cable of our own, virtually taken possession of that ocean, and occupied a position at Manila ... only a couple of days in time from the Chinese coast with no fear of Chinese or Russian armies at our back yet near enough to protect our interest in the Orient.[22]

It all seemed miraculous. At the cost of 2,900 lives (with approximately 2,500 the victims of disease, not enemy gunfire) and only $250 million, the United States became a great world power. But if Americans were dreaming big dreams, McKinley refused to be carried away. He had only certain limited diplomatic objectives. In his first public statement on possible terms of peace, McKinley wrote in June 1898 that Cuba, Puerto Rico, and a Philippine naval base had to end up in U.S. hands. By late summer, he had actually rejected the opportunity to take control of Caroline Island and the Marianas, which Spain held in the Pacific.

In Cuba, the question became whether the island should be independent, annexed, or come under informal U.S. control. McKinley quickly ruled out immediate independence. His mistrust of the Cuban revolutionaries increased. Their ill-equipped, barefoot forces proved to be superb guerrilla fighters when working alongside U.S. troops but, in American eyes, became racial inferiors and thieves of U.S. food supplies when the fighting stopped. The U.S. forces "despise" the Cubans, one journalist reported. When General Shafter was asked about possible self-government, he retorted, "Why those people are no more fit for self-government than gun-powder is for hell."[23] McKinley also refused to annex the island. That solution could bring too many unpredictable mixed races into the Union. Moreover, annexation was not needed. Because Cuba was so close to U.S. shores, it, unlike the Philippines, could be controlled informally. The United States could use the island for its own purposes, but Cubans could have the headaches of day-to-day governing.

This imaginative policy was finally formulated by McKinley and his top military commander in Cuba, General Leonard Wood. The general convened a Cuban constitutional convention in late 1900 and instructed the delegates to establish their own internal laws. Washington required, however, that they include in their new constitution certain foreign-policy provisions: (1) the United States had the right to intervene as it wished to protect Cuba's independence; (2) the Cuban debt had to be limited so that European creditors could not use it as an excuse to use force to collect it—and perhaps take Cuban territory as compensation; (3) the United States demanded a ninety-nine year lease of the naval base at Guantánamo; and (4) an extensive sanitation program was to protect the Cuban people and make the island more attractive to U.S. investors. These provisions, drawn up by McKinley and his advisers, became known as the Platt Amendment after Republican Senator Orville Platt from Connecticut formally proposed them in Congress. Furiously attacking the proposals, the Cuban delegates refused to vote on them. Wood warned that he would keep them meeting until they did vote. He knew, moreover, that the Cubans needed immediate access to the American market for their sugar. Under intense U.S. pressure, the Cuban Constitutional Convention finally accepted the Platt Amendment in 1901 by a vote of 15 to 11. "There is, of course, little or no independence left Cuba under the Platt Amendment," Wood wrote Roosevelt.[24]

The McKinley and Roosevelt administrations then overcame tough opposition from high-tariff Republicans and sugar producers to negotiate and finally ratify a reciprocity treaty in 1903. The pact thoroughly integrated the U.S. and Cuban economies. Cuba's sugar and mineral wealth moved north, as American farm and industrial products flowed south. The U.S. sugar producers lost their fight when the giant American Sugar Refining trust, which wanted cheap sugar to refine for the home market, moved into Capitol Hill and bribed the necessary number of senators.[25] U.S.-Cuban trade skyrocketed from $27 million in 1897 to over $300 million in 1917.

The United States restored order to Cuba but assumed few responsibilities. "When people ask me what I mean by stable government, I tell them money at six percent," General Wood wrote to McKinley in 1900. That kind of "order," however, proved to be dangerous. As historian Lloyd Gardner notes, the Platt Amendment built into Cuba "a revolutionary impetus," because later critics of Cuban poverty could not effectively attack the island's own government, which had little control over the economy, but had to attack the United States.[26] As early as 1906, U.S. officials had to land troops to maintain order. The Platt Amendment continued to be the basis of U.S. policy in Cuba until 1934.

McKinley also took Puerto Rico away from Spain in 1898. The conquest was a surprise. Few Americans knew or cared about that island when war began. For that reason, however, McKinley's decision to annex it (as partial indemnity from Spain for U.S. war costs) raised little debate. The Puerto Ricans were not pleased. In a rare moment of Spanish colonial wisdom, Madrid officials had given Puerto Rico a large amount of autonomy, including its own elected legislature. McKinley destroyed that autonomy. General Nelson Miles, the U.S. military commander, conquered the country without opposition, then announced that the United States intended to give "the immunities and blessings of the liberal institutions of our government." But instead of granting such blessings, Congress passed the Foraker Act of 1900, which made Puerto Rico an "unincorporated territory" subject to the whim of Congress. For one of the few times since the 1787 Ordinance (see p. 33), the United States annexed a large territory with no intention of making the inhabitants U.S. citizens. Puerto Ricans had no guaranteed rights. As one of their newspapers complained in 1901, "We are and we are not a foreign country. We are and we are not citizens of the United States. . . . The Constitution . . . applies to us and does not apply to us."[27]

The U.S. Supreme Court proved the newspaper correct when it handed down a series of judgments between 1901 and 1904. In these historic decisions, known as the Insular Cases, the Court ruled that the Foraker Act was constitutional. The United States could annex an area, make it an "unincorporated" territory, and refuse to grant its people citizenship. Thus, the Constitution did not automatically "follow the flag," as many Americans had long believed. The territory's people were at Congress's mercy. The U.S. attorney general told the Court that the government had to have such power. In the future, he prophesied, a Puerto Rico–like situation might arise in Africa or even China, given the course of U.S. expansionism. The Constitution had to be interpreted to fit that expansionism. Later, the Insular Cases did provide a legal justification for the U.S. rule of Guam and other Pacific territories.[28]

Congress, meanwhile, passed tariff legislation that integrated Puerto Rico—and especially its increasing number of sugar plantations—into the U.S. economy. In 1850, the country's landholding had been fair

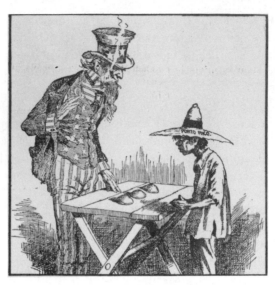

A cartoonist, who captioned this work "Find the Constitution," portrays in 1901 his belief that Americans were paying a high price to acquire overseas possessions. This is from the Philadelphia North American.

and equitable when compared with other countries in the Caribbean and Central America. By 1917, the best lands had fallen into the hands of a few wealthy owners who grew crops for export. In that year, the United States finally gave Puerto Ricans citizenship through the Jones Act. In 1947, the country won the right to elect its own governor. After that, Third World and Soviet-bloc countries in the United Nations regularly proposed resolutions condemning Washington's "colonial" policy. Puerto Ricans, meanwhile, divided among a small group demanding independence, a larger faction wanting U.S. statehood, and the largest number who preferred the tax and trade preferences obtained from the United States because of their commonwealth status. But Puerto Rico remained a poor country whose people increasingly sought work in the United States. Nearly a century after the 1898 conquest, Washington officials have not been able to devise a workable policy for development.[29]

. . . AND THE CONQUEST OF THE FILIPINOS

The best-known version of how McKinley decided to annex the Philippine Islands came from the president himself, when he talked with a group of Methodist church leaders in 1899:

I walked the floor of the White House night after night until midnight; and I am not ashamed to tell you, gentlemen, that I went down on my knees and prayed Almighty God for light and guidance more than one night. And one night it came to me in this way—. . . . (1) that we could not give [the Philippines] back to Spain—that would be cowardly and dishonorable; (2) that we could not turn them over to France or Germany— our commercial rivals in the Orient—that would be bad business and discreditable . . . ; . . . that there was nothing left to do but take them all, and educate the Filipinos, and uplift and civilize them, and by God's grace do the very best by them as our fellow-men for whom Christ also died. And then I went to bed, and went to sleep and slept soundly.[30]

It is a dramatic story, but few historians believe it. Recent scholarship reveals that the president's reasons were both more complex and fascinating. From the moment he had heard of Dewey's smashing victory in Manila Bay, the president wanted at least to annex that port for the use of U.S. commerce and warships. Indeed, he ordered troops to leave for the Philippines even before he received official word that Dewey won. It marked the first time a president had ever ordered U.S. soldiers outside the Western Hemisphere to fight. McKinley delayed deciding whether to annex all the Philippine islands, which stretched over 115,000 square miles. McKinley did not want the responsibility for governing them, especially since a strong Filipino revolutionary army, which had been effectively fighting Spain before 1898, intended to govern its own homeland. Nevertheless, as fighting continued in the summer of 1898, McKinley kept his options open: "While we are conducting war and until its conclusion we must keep all we get; when the war is over we must keep what we want."[31] On October 25, 1898, the president finally instructed the U.S. commissioners in Paris, who were negotiating peace terms, to demand all the islands. In return, the United States offered Spain $20 million.

McKinley made the decision for a number of reasons. He concluded that the Filipinos could not run their own country. Dewey had cabled him in mid-October that "the natives appear unable to govern." The problem was similar to the Cuban situation: the revolutionaries were divided among themselves, and one radical faction threatened property holdings. That difficulty led to a second reason for McKinley's decision: a civil war could allow those whom he termed "our commercial rivals in the Orient" (France, Germany, and Great Britain) to seize the islands. McKinley, moreover, had to make his decision just as the China cauldron began boiling again. Russia threatened to close Chinese ports, including Port Arthur, that were vital for U.S. commerce. Great

Britain considered quitting the open-door policy and joining the race for Chinese loot. To protect U.S. interests, the president needed a secure base. To use Manila for that purpose, however, required control of Luzon, Manila's home island. But to protect Luzon, McKinley learned, meant controlling the adjoining islands. As one U.S. army officer testified in mid-October, with "over 400 islands in the group . . . a cannon shot can be fired from one to another in many instances." Thus, the final and most important reason for McKinley's decision: to protect the naval base at Manila, he had to take all the islands.[32]

American public opinion had little to do with his decision. That opinion, as usual, was sharply divided. The *Presbyterian Banner* declared in August 1898 that the religious press, almost without exception, agreed on "the desirability of America's retaining the Philippines as a duty in the interest of human freedom and Christian progress." Three months later the same journal announced: "We have been morally compelled to become an Asiatic power. . . . America and Great Britain will see to it that China is not Russianized."[33] On the other side, many Americans, especially Democrats, feared extending the Constitution across the Pacific. Even McKinley's own cabinet was divided. His wartime secretary of state (and close friend from Ohio days), William R. Day, opposed annexation.

During a congressional campaign swing through the Midwest in October, the president decided he would test opinion on the annexation question. But he did so in an odd fashion. McKinley repeatedly brought crowds to their feet with rousing, patriotic speeches, such as one in Hastings, Iowa: "We want new markets, and as trade follows the flag, it looks very much as if we are going to have new markets." The president nevertheless seemed struck by how hard he had to work to arouse his audiences. As historian Ephraim Smith concludes, McKinley "seemed more concerned about the public's apprehension about accepting new responsibilities."[34]

Proof of that apprehension appeared on February 6, 1899, when the Senate accepted McKinley's peace treaty 57 to 27, a mere one vote more than the two-thirds needed to ratify. Until the final twenty-four hours, victory was in doubt. McKinley, aided by Republican Senate leaders, lobbied hard and distributed patronage plums with a free hand to obtain votes. Oddly, the president received unneeded last-minute help from his old Democratic opponent, William Jennings Bryan. The Democrat had fought annexation, then suddenly switched to urge Democratic senators to vote for the treaty. Bryan later argued that he wanted ratification so that the war would officially end, lives would be

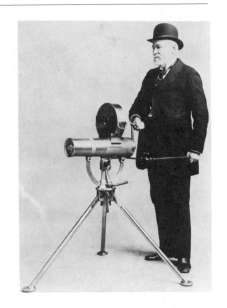

Richard Jordan Gatling stands by his Gatling Gun, the parent of the machine gun. Samuel Colt and others had developed a repeating rifle before the Civil War, but Gatling's 1862 patent led to the most famous rapid-fire weapon. Not used in the Civil War, the Gatling Gun was used to quell riots in New Orleans during 1868, to kill Indians during the 1870s–1880s campaigns, and, most famously, to help win the battle of Santiago, Cuba, against Spain in 1898, and to put down the Philippine revolt.

saved, and the Philippine mistake would then be corrected through diplomacy.[35] It was, however, one of Bryan's many unrealized dreams. Of even greater importance than Bryan's turn was the news that reached Washington on the evening before the vote: Filipino rebels had attacked U.S. soldiers. The revolt against American control had begun. McKinley immediately understood that he had won: a vote against his treaty could now be seen as a vote against supporting the U.S. soldiers embattled by the Filipinos.

The insurrection marked the first of many antirevolutionary wars fought by the United States in the twentieth century. The rebels were led by Emilio Aguinaldo (a moderate who had executed the more radical opponent within the revolutionary movement, Andres Bonifacio). They had originally welcomed the U.S. force that defeated Spain. Welcome turned to hostility when they learned that the Americans intended to remain. McKinley paid little attention to Aguinaldo until the rebel declared the creation of a Philippine republic in January 1899. The war that erupted the next month continued for three years. At first, U.S. officers believed that they could subdue the barefoot opponents with 20,000 or 30,000 men. Soon, the commanders asked McKinley for 40,000, then 60,000 regulars. In all, 120,000 U.S. troops finally fought in the Philippines. Nearly 4,200 were killed and 2,800 wounded. In turn, they killed outright 15,000 rebels, and estimates run as high as 200,000 Filipinos dying from gunfire, starvation, and the effects of

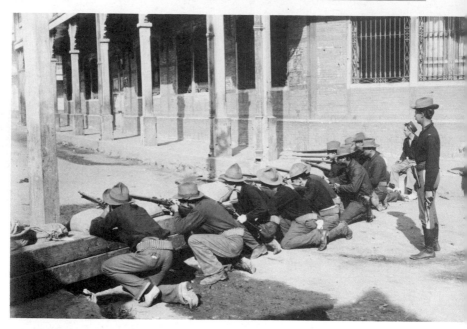

U.S. troops had to fight a vicious four-year war to defeat the Filipino resistance and consolidate the American hold over Manila's valuable port, where this picture of street fighting was taken.

concentration camps into which the United States crowded civilians so that they could not help Aguinaldo's troops.[36]

Viewing the Filipinos as they had viewed Native Americans, U.S. soldiers coined the term "gooks" to describe them. These racial views allowed the war to be fought even more savagely. As a young infantryman from New York reported home: "Last night one of our boys was found shot and his stomach cut open. Immediately orders were received . . . to burn the town and kill every native in sight. . . . About 1,000 men, women, and children were reported killed. . . . I am in my glory when I can sight my gun on some dark skin and pull the trigger."[37] When rebels massacred a squad of U.S. troops, an American commander ordered the killing of every male over the age of ten—an order, fortunately, that was quickly countermanded by his superiors.

The revolution was finally quelled after McKinley moved General Arthur MacArthur to top command in 1900. The new leader (father of General Douglas MacArthur, who governed the Philippines in the 1930s and was U.S. commander in the Pacific during World War II) took a different tack. He fought the war vigorously but also offered amnesty to rebels who surrendered. MacArthur worked closely with the islands' wealthy elite, who prospered by cooperating with the Americans. In 1901, U.S. troops captured Aguinaldo. The back of the revolt was broken, although fighting continued at reduced levels until 1913. After that, U.S.-trained and -directed Filipino forces fought a continual series of wars against rebels, wars that lasted from 1913 until at least the 1990s.[38] The Philippines have never remained pacified for very long. For his part, Aguinaldo finally had revenge by collaborating with Japanese forces, who drove the United States out of the Philippines in World War II.

Warriors such as Theodore Roosevelt argued that Americans had to remain in the Philippines to develop their own character and teach the natives self-government. Democratic senator Edward Carmack from Tennessee acidly observed that Roosevelt admitted that it had taken Anglo-Saxons one thousand years to learn self-government. Thus, "we are not to hold [the islands] permanently," Carmack quipped, "we want to experiment with them for only a thousand years or so." Famed sociologist William Graham Sumner was more pointed: "We talk of civilizing lower races, but we have never done it yet. We have exterminated them." Despite such criticisms, Carmack and Sumner could not slow McKinley's and Roosevelt's policies for taking the Philippines. After all, as Assistant Secretary of the Treasury (and banker) Frank Vanderlip observed, the Philippines were to be the U.S. Hong Kong so Americans could "trade with the millions of China and Korea, French Indo-China, the Malay Peninsula and the islands of Indonesia."[39]

McKinley's Triumphs in China

In 1899–1900, the president vividly demonstrated why the Philippines were vital for his foreign policy. At long last, he was free to fight the threat to the open door in China. The crisis had begun in 1897–1898 (see p. 200). By mid-1899, the Russians and Germans threatened to colonize and close off strategic areas of China. Meanwhile, the British, French, Japanese, and Americans scrambled to protect their trade and other interests. None of the powers was primarily concerned about the Chinese themselves. As Americans, for example, pressed for greater rights in China, they closed off Chinese rights of immigration obtained in the 1868 Burlingame Treaty.

By 1882, so many Chinese had found work in the United States that Americans were fearful. In that year, Congress passed the first anti-immigration measure in U.S. history when it stopped Chinese immigration for ten years. Anti-Chinese outbreaks nevertheless spread. In 1885, a mob killed twenty-eight Chinese in Wyoming. Observers feared even worse bloodshed would occur in California, where many Asian immigrants had settled. By the 1880s and 1890s, Americans were increasingly discriminating against immigrants just as the Americans themselves were moving out into other countries such as China and the Philippines. This historic turn was dramatized in 1886, when, in magnificent ceremonies, the United States dedicated the Statue of Liberty, placed in New York City Harbor as a gift from France. Not one speech in the ceremonies mentioned the lines Emma Lazarus had written for the statue: "Give me your tired, your poor, / Your huddled masses yearning to breathe free." Instead, the speakers stressed how Americans must go forth to spread liberty throughout other lands.[40]

In China, however, Americans seemed less interested in liberty for the Chinese than the liberty to sell goods for profit and save souls for Christianity. Economically, U.S. exports to China nearly quadrupled to $15 million between 1895 and 1900.[41] The Chinese took only 1 percent to 2 percent of total U.S. exports, but Americans focused on the potential (hundreds of millions of Chinese) and that market's rapid growth since 1895. Certain industries and sections in the United States depended utterly on the China market. No producers needed it more than those making textiles. That product ranked first among exports, with petroleum second, iron and steel products third. New England textile plants had overexpanded, then were badly stung by the 1873–1897 economic depression. Some moved to the South, but, as one spokesman warned, it was better to avoid "destructive competition" at home by developing markets abroad. "We want the open door," a Georgia senator exclaimed, "and a big one at that."[42] Historian Patrick Hearden concludes that by 1899, "the New South's rapidly growing China trade promised to keep the entire American cotton industry in a healthy condition."[43]

But no group surpassed the Christian missionaries' involvement in China. It was an era of extraordinary growth: between 1870 and 1900, Americans increased their Protestant overseas missions by 500 percent. In the single decade of the 1890s, U.S. missionaries in China doubled in number to over one thousand. This great movement arose in part out of the churches' determination to defy threats to their beliefs posed by new science and Darwinian challenges. The movement also sprang from colleges, where religious revivalism on such campuses as Oberlin, Cornell, and Yale produced the Student Volunteer Movement for Foreign Missions in 1887. By 1900, the Student Volunteers, who marched under the proud banner proclaiming "The Evangelization of the World in This Generation," had chapters in nearly every Protestant college. These groups reflected the profit seeking as well as soul seeking of the late nineteenth century. Some missionaries invested in foreign land and minerals; others preached morality and profit at once by asking that saved souls wear North Carolina textiles.[44] The missionaries patriotically represented their country as well as their religion. They also became more interested in mass conversion than in the slower saving of individual sinners from the fires of hell. Thus, they looked increasingly to the U.S. government for help and protection, especially as the other foreign powers crowded into Asia. This new approach was exemplified in 1896, when the U.S. government ordered a commission to travel to the Chinese government and insist on American rights. As Professor Thomas McCormick explains, "The commission consisted of the American Consul at Tientsin, a missionary, and a naval officer—the expansionist trinity."[45]

Women, especially a rising feminist movement, became an important source of missionary expansionism both at home and abroad. In 1880, about twenty women's foreign missionary societies existed. The number doubled by 1900. By 1915, 3 million women belonged to these forty societies. Some of the groups aimed to carry abroad the values of middle-class America. As one leader wrote, "The aim of this woman's work we conceive to be *in heathen lands*— . . . in bringing the women into His Kingdom, in the creation of Christian mothers." The "fathers and brothers" were to "strike vigorous blows at the brains of heathendom, to superintend large educational and evangelistic enterprises." But "to woman belongs the quiet, patient labour in the homes of the people." Women also understood, however, how they were to bring creature comforts and new values of an industrialized America to the "heathen." As one woman declared, foreign missionary work "should appeal to every broad-minded Christian woman who is interested in education, civics, sanitation, social settlements, hospitals, good literature, the emancipation of children, the right of women to health, home and protection; and the coming of the Kingdom of our Lord." As historian Patricia R. Hill observes, by this time, it seems, the Lord's kingdom tended to come at the end of the list.[46] American goods and social values went into China with the missionaries, both male and female.

The belief grew, as Secretary of State John Hay noted in 1900, that whoever understood China "has the key to world politics for the next five centuries."[47] No one tried harder to understand, or—after Seward—contributed more to U.S. policy in China than did Hay, the author of

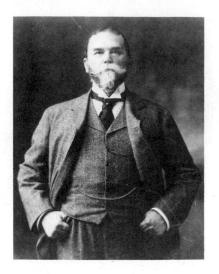

John Hay (1838–1905) was born in Indiana and had a distinguished career as secretary to Lincoln, an official in the Department of State, industrialist in Ohio, and U.S. ambassador to Great Britain before becoming a powerful secretary of state (1898–1905). A poet and novelist as well, Hay drafted the historic "open-door" notes of 1899–1900.

the 1899–1900 open-door notes. Nor did anyone better understand how U.S. business and politics related to policy in China. Born in Indiana in 1838, Hay went to Brown University, then used his midwestern political contacts to become Abraham Lincoln's secretary at the age of twenty-three. Hay grew to fear the mass, urbanized, industrialized society that developed after 1865. His fear multiplied when he entered the steel business in Cleveland and had to deal with the rising labor movement. He anonymously published a novel, *The Bread-Winners*, that remains one of the bitterest attacks ever made on the labor movement, especially the movement's foreign members. But he also worried that "the rich and intelligent" were so busy making money, they ignored the dangers: they "hate politics" and so "fatten themselves as sheep which could be mutton whenever the butcher was ready." Hay had no intention of becoming mutton. He supported McKinley in 1896, and the new president named him U.S. ambassador to Great Britain in 1897. Hay greatly admired England. He believed passionately that the British and Americans could save themselves and the best parts of their societies only by fighting Russia's, France's, and Germany's attempts "to divide and reduce China to a system of tributary provinces." McKinley knew Hay well and recalled him in 1898 to lead the fight for China as secretary of state.[48]

Hay's first initiative was an open-door note of 1899 that asked the other powers (especially Russia and Germany) to charge foreigners no more than their own citizens paid for shipping and railway privileges within so-called "spheres of interest" in China that each power claimed.

Hay's note also insisted that the general Chinese tariff apply to all the spheres of interest, and that China collect the duties itself. Chinese territorial integrity was to be reinforced. No other power rushed to agree with Hay's note, but none directly defied it either. Russia did not as yet believe that it had sufficient power to challenge the Americans, who were supported to some degree by Great Britain and Japan. Hay finally gained assent through an ingenious diplomatic tactic. He first gained agreement from the British and Japanese, who he knew were closest to his position, then obtained France's assent. Germany and Russia then had to agree or defy the other powers. The two nations did go along, but with considerable grumbling. With no U.S. military force in China and without making any political alliance with other powers, Hay had maneuvered them into declaring their agreement with U.S. open-door policy—a policy, as Hay neatly defined it, of "fair field and no favor" for anyone who wanted to compete in the China market. He and other knowledgeable Americans knew that with such ground rules, they could use their growing industrial power to undersell nearly any-

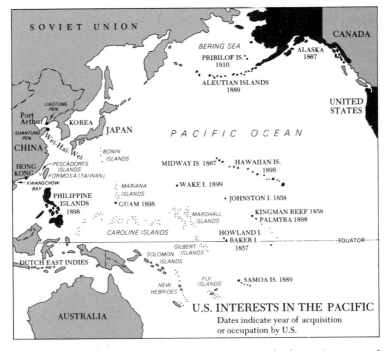

U.S. INTERESTS IN THE PACIFIC
Dates indicate year of acquisition or occupation by U.S.

By 1900, the new U.S. economic and military interests had stepping stones for crossing the Pacific to reach Asia. The dates indicate when the United States acquired its possessions.

one and capture much of China's market. That was, indeed, another sign of the high stakes for which McKinley and Hay played: they wanted to sell to all of China, not just a sliver or a sphere they might annex.

But the Chinese themselves refused to stand still while the powers exploited them. In early 1900, the empress dowager, head of the collapsing Manchu dynasty, encouraged a radical antiforeign and militaristic society known as the Boxers to attack foreigners and their property. By May, foreign compounds in Chinese cities were besieged. On May 29, U.S. minister Edwin Conger captured the terror when he cabled Washington from the capital of Beijing (Peking): "Boxers increasing. Nine Methodist converts brutally murdered at Pachow. The movement has developed into open rebellion. Chinese government is trying but apparently is unable to surpress it. Many soldiers disloyal."[49] The foreign powers, including the United States, sent in troops to protect their citizens. It became clear, however, that Russia, Germany, and even Japan were using the Boxers as an excuse to seal off parts of China into their own spheres of interest.

After McKinley ordered 5,000 U.S. troops to move from Manila into China, Hay used the force as a bargaining chip. He tried to pressure the other powers to agree to a policy of July 3, 1900, that became known as the second open-door notes. He asked all powers to declare directly that they promised to preserve "Chinese territorial and administrative integrity." This key point had only been implied in the 1899 notes. With the powers nervously eying each other as well as the Boxers, all of them fell into line behind Hay. McKinley and his secretary of state had pulled off a remarkable victory. By 1901, Russia seemed checked. The president had greatly increased his executive power by sending thousands of U.S. troops onto the mainland of China without bothering to consult Congress. And the foreign powers maintained the Manchu dynasty as the ruler of China, although that victory was short-lived. In 1911, internal conflict again erupted, and this time the dynasty disappeared amid the beginnings of the Chinese Revolution.

Hay understood both sides of U.S. policy in China: the American need for markets both commercial and religious, and the relatively little power the United States could exert in the region. In August 1900, a crisis flared when Russia again made threatening moves. This time, the British indicated that they might join the Russians. McKinley, in the middle of a tough re-election fight against Bryan, uncharacteristically panicked. He seriously considered carving off an area of China for the United States—that is, giving up the open-door policy and joining the other colonial powers. From a sickbed in New Hampshire, Hay

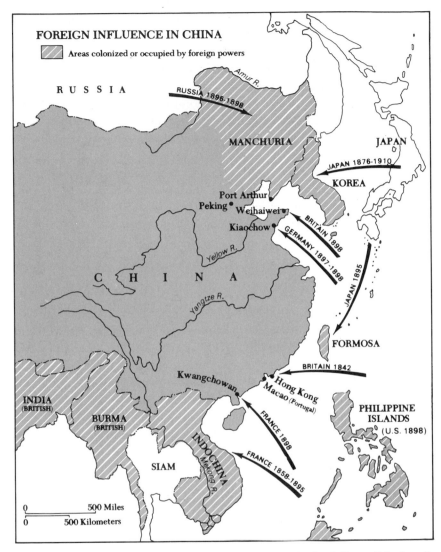

FOREIGN INFLUENCE IN CHINA

Areas colonized or occupied by foreign powers

RUSSIA

Amur R.

RUSSIA 1896-1898

MANCHURIA

JAPAN

JAPAN 1876-1910

KOREA

Port Arthur
Peking • Weihaiwei •
Kiaochow •

BRITAIN 1898

GERMANY 1897-1898

JAPAN 1895

Yellow R.

C H I N A

Yangtze R.

FORMOSA

BRITAIN 1842

Kwangchowan
• Hong Kong
Macao *(Portugal)*

PHILIPPINE
ISLANDS
(U.S. 1898)

INDIA
(BRITISH)

BURMA
(BRITISH)

FRANCE 1898

INDOCHINA

Mekong R.

FRANCE 1858-1895

SIAM

| 0 | 500 Miles |
| 0 | 500 Kilometers |

*China became an object of big-power competition and colonialism—"the bone"
amid the dogs, as a later U.S. official called China.*

convinced the president not to surrender the open-door approach. He
did so by giving McKinley a lesson in power politics:

> The inherent weakness of our position is this: we do not want to rob China
> ourselves, and our public opinion will not permit us to interfere, with an
> army, to prevent others from robbing her. Besides, we have no army. The

talk of the papers about "our preeminent moral position giving the authority to dictate to the world" is mere flap-doodle.[50]

Hay concluded that McKinley had no alternative but to remain in China and try to keep the powers *voluntarily* lined up behind the open-door policy. This could be accomplished not through U.S. military force, but only by playing power off against power, as Hay had done in 1899 and again in 1900. The secretary of state himself weakened only once. In late 1900, the U.S. War Department insisted that the navy needed a base in China. No doubt with some embarrassment, Hay asked the Chinese for a lease at Samsah Bay. Japan, which had plans of its own for China, quickly objected by throwing Hay's policy back at him: the U.S. request violated the open-door policy. The secretary of state dropped the request.

... AND A FINAL TRIUMPH AT HOME

By November 1900, the crisis in China had apparently passed—and none too soon. Throughout 1899–1900, Bryan and the Democrats had planned to club McKinley's re-election hopes with the issues of the bloody Philippine campaign and the volatile China crisis. Throughout the summer of 1900, both sides hotly debated foreign policy. The Democrats termed it "the paramount issue" in the election fight.

An "anti-imperialist" movement had grown rapidly after mid-1898 to oppose McKinley's policies. This movement was led by wealthy and upper-middle-class professionals (especially lawyers), mostly from the Northeast and Midwest. But it also included an increasing number of women. Historian Judith Papachristou estimates that in the five years after 1898 tens of thousands of women became foreign-policy activists: "Never before had American women involved themselves in foreign affairs in such a way and to such an extent." When the Anti-Imperialist League began to form at a meeting in Boston's Faneuil Hall during June 1898, more than half the audience was female. Women determined to have voting rights easily identified with Filipinos who were to be governed without their consent. Some anti-imperialists, both female and male, feared that extending the Constitution to the Philippines, Puerto Rico, and even Hawaii might change the basic provisions of the document and bring into the system certain races who were considered dangerous to traditional American values. Many anti-imperialists argued that these peoples were not ready for self-government; but if the United States tried to rule them, it would turn into an imperialist power and thus destroy its own democratic values. A South Carolina senator warned against "the incorporation of a mongrel and semibarbarous population into our body politic."[51]

That warning hit home in the North as well as the South. About 150 black people were lynched each year in the United States during the early 1890s. Race riots erupted in New York City in 1900, as well as earlier in southern states. It was not the time, Bryan and other anti-imperialists argued, to try to teach democracy to Filipinos with the tips of bayonets. Henry Blake Fuller caught the spirit with his anti-imperialist poetry of 1899. He dealt with the president of the United States as follows:

> G is for Guns
> That McKinley has sent,
> To teach Filipinos
> What Jesus Christ meant.

Fuller also provided a self-portrait of McKinley's vice-presidential running mate, Theodore Roosevelt, as anti-imperialists painted it:

> I'm a cut and thrusting bronco-busting
> Megaphone of Mars,
> And it's fire I breathe and I cut my teeth
> On nails and wrought-iron bars.[52]

Such extreme rhetoric could be discounted, but McKinley could not disregard Andrew Carnegie's large bankroll which financed many anti-imperialist activities.

The president directly challenged the anti-imperialists by naming Theodore Roosevelt to the Republican ticket. No one was more identified with, or more loudly defended, U.S. expansionism. Governor of New York in 1900, Roosevelt at first did not want to be only a vice-president. ("I would rather be professor of history in some college," he wrote a friend.) But he finally gave in, rightly noting that "it was believed that I would greatly strengthen the ticket in the West, where they regard me as a fellow barbarian and like me much."[53] While McKinley remained in Washington or in his hometown of Canton, Ohio, Roosevelt spun across the country, giving as many as ten speeches a day until he finally lost his voice on the eve of the election.

He blasted the anti-imperialist arguments. Because "the Philippines are now part of American territory," the only question was whether the Democrats planned "to surrender American territory." He attacked the anti-imperialists as antiexpansionist and thus, he charged, they had deserted the ideals of their own father—Thomas Jefferson—who had taken all of Louisiana. Dealing with the Indians, TR argued, established the needed precedents for dealing with the Filipinos, who were also "savages." If whites were "morally bound to abandon the Philippines, we were also morally bound to abandon Arizona to the Apaches." Bayonets were needed because "the barbarian will yield only to force." Other Republicans mocked Democrats who urged self-government in the Philippines or Hawaii by asking when the Democrats planned to extend the Declaration of Independence to southern black people. One observer commented on "Democrats howling about Republicans shooting negroes in the Philippines and the Republicans objecting to Democrats shooting negroes in the South. This may be good politics, but it is rough on the negroes."[54]

McKinley and Roosevelt decisively won the argument. By September, the president's policy in China and TR's attacks from the stump forced Bryan to reverse his campaign strategy. The Democratic nominee dropped foreign policy and began to emphasize Republican economic policy. His decision turned out to be politically fatal. The United States had emerged from its twenty-five-year depression to bask in prosperity in 1900. McKinley ran on the slogan "Let Well Enough Alone." He defeated Bryan more decisively in 1900 than he had four years before and even captured Bryan's home state of Nebraska. In the end, many anti-imperialists, including Andrew Carnegie, found that they could not tolerate Bryan's more radical economic program (especially after he dropped foreign-policy issues) and joined McKinley.

The president had led the United States into the small, select circle of great world powers. He did so not by following those powers and conquering large colonies. Between 1870 and 1900, Great Britain added 4.7 million square miles to its empire, France 3.5 million, and Germany 1.0 million. Americans, however, added only 125,000 square miles. They wanted not land, but more markets to free them of the horrors that had resulted from the post-1873 depression. Louisville newspaper publisher and Democratic party boss Henry Watterson explained what had occurred in 1898:

> From a nation of shopkeepers we became a nation of warriors. . . . We escape the menace and the peril of socialism and agrarianism, as England escaped them, by a policy of colonization and conquest. It is true that we

exchange domestic dangers for foreign dangers; but in every direction we multiply the opportunities of the people. We risk Caesarism certainly; but even Caesarism is preferable to anarchism.[55]

In September 1901, Watterson's "Caesar" traveled to Buffalo, New York, to explain to Americans the new world in which they lived. The president was greeted by a spectacular fireworks display that climaxed with the exclamation in the sky: "WELCOME MCKINLEY, CHIEF OF OUR NATION AND EMPIRE." As historian Edward Crapol summarizes, Americans were—finally—the equal of the British, and rapidly becoming more than equal.[56] The United States, McKinley told the Pan-American Exposition in Buffalo, now had "almost appalling" wealth. Consequently, "isolation is no longer possible or desirable." Americans had to frame new tariff and other policies to conquer world markets.

The next day, a deranged man shot and mortally wounded McKinley. That "wild man," as Marcus Hanna had called Theodore Roosevelt, suddenly became president of the United States. Once again, historian Robert Beisner notes, Americans were to test whether "a republic can prosper in a career of empire."[57] They would have to do so under the leadership of a person more flamboyant—and unpredictable—than McKinley.

NOTES

1. Ernest R. May, *Imperial Democracy* (New York, 1961), p. 270; Albert K. Weinberg, *Manifest Destiny* (Baltimore, 1940), p. 273.

2. Robert L. Beisner, *From the Old Diplomacy to the New, 1865–1900* (Arlington Heights, Ill., 1986), p. 89.

3. V. O. Key, "A Theory of Critical Elections," *Journal of Politics* 17 (February 1955): 12–15.

4. William Allen White, *The Autobiography of William Allen White* (New York, 1946), p. 292; Paul Boller, Jr., *Presidential Anecdotes* (New York, 1981), p. 189.

5. Henry Adams, *The Education of Henry Adams, an Autobiography* (Boston, 1918), p. 423. The best recent study of McKinley's extensive use of presidential powers is Lewis Gould, *The Presidency of William McKinley* (Lawrence, Kans., 1980).

6. Frances Fitzgerald, "Rewriting American History," *New Yorker*, 26 February 1979, p. 66. A Latin American view of the evolving U.S.-Cuban relationship is Manuel Moreno Fraginals, "Cuban-American Relations and the Sugar Trade," in *Diplo-*

matic Claims: Latin American Historians View the United States, ed. and trans. Warren Dean (Lanham, Md., 1985).

7. *Washington Post*, 21 July 1983, p. A23.
8. L. White Busbey, *Uncle Joe Cannon* (New York, 1927), p. 187.
9. *Journal of Commerce*, 14 March 1898, p. 1.
10. Theodore Roosevelt to George Dewey, 25 February 1898, Ciphers Sent, 1888–1898, Record Group 45, National Archives, Washington, D.C.; Charles S. Campbell, *The Transformation of American Foreign Relations, 1865–1900* (New York, 1976), pp. 279–280. Campbell's is the best-detailed analysis of the entire era and has a superb bibliography.
11. Fitzhugh Lee to William R. Day, 27 November 1897, Consular, Havana, and Hyatt to William R. Day, 23 March 1898, Consular, Santiago, Record Group 59, National Archives, Washington, D.C.
12. W. C. Reick to J. R. Young, 25 March 1898, Papers of William McKinley, Library of Congress, Washington, D.C.
13. Paul S. Holbo, "Presidential Leadership in Foreign Affairs: William McKinley and the Turpie-Foraker Amendment," *American Historical Review* 72 (July 1967): 1322–1334.
14. A superb analysis of the literature on McKinley and the war is Joseph Fry, "Essay Review: William McKinley and the Coming of the Spanish-American War," *Diplomatic History* 3 (Winter 1979): 77–97; John L. Offner, *An Unwanted War* (Chapel Hill, N.C., 1992), p. 189.
15. William Michael Morgan, "The Anti-Japanese Origins of the Hawaiian Annexation Treaty of 1897," *Diplomatic History* 6 (Winter 1982): 25–34.
16. *Washington Evening Star*, 11 January 1898, p. 1; 13 January 1898, p. 4; 19 January 1898, p. 14; also William Adam Russ, Jr., *The Hawaiian Republic, 1894–1898* (Selinsgrove, Pa., 1961), p. 240.
17. Alan K. Henrikson, "Maps, Globes, and 'The Cold War,' " *Special Libraries* 65 (October–November 1974): 445–454.
18. Frank Freidel, "Dissent in the Spanish-American War," in Samuel Eliot Morison *et al.*, *Dissent in Three American Wars* (Cambridge, Mass., 1970), pp. 74–75; the May 4 cable from Manila is in U.S. Senate Document no. 62, *A Treaty of Peace . . .* , 55th Cong., 3d sess. (Washington, D.C., 1899), p. 326.
19. Russell Weigley, *The American Way of War* (New York, 1973), pp. 183–184.
20. Frank Freidel, *The Splendid Little War* (Boston, 1958), p. 46.
21. Theodore Roosevelt, *The Letters of Theodore Roosevelt*, ed. Elting E. Morison *et al.*, 8 vols. (Cambridge, Mass., 1951–1954), II, p. 1099n.
22. Thomas J. McCormick, *The China Market* (Chicago, 1967), p. 224.
23. David F. Healy, *The United States in Cuba, 1898–1902* (Madison, 1963), pp. 34–36.
24. Leonard Wood to Theodore Roosevelt, 28 October 1901, Papers of Leonard Wood, Library of Congress, Washington, D.C.
25. Healy, pp. 204–205.
26. Lloyd Gardner, "From Containment to Liberation," in *From Colony to Empire*, ed. William Appleman Williams (New York, 1972), p. 220.
27. Richard M. Morse, "Embarrassing Colony," *New York Review of Books*, 6 December 1984, p. 17.
28. Louis Henkin, *Foreign Affairs and the Constitution* (Mineola, N.Y., 1972), pp. 268, 330.

29. The best analysis on post-1898 is now Raymond Carr, *Puerto Rico, a Colonial Experiment* (New York, 1984).

30. Lazar Ziff, *America in the 1890s* (New York, 1966), p. 221. The original account appeared after McKinley's death in the *Charleston Advocate* 68 (22 January 1903): 137–138; I am indebted to R. H. (Max) Miller for this citation.

31. H. Wayne Morgan, *America's Road to Empire: The War with Spain and Overseas Expansion* (New York, 1965), esp. chs. IV, V.

32. McCormick, pp. 168–187; Ephraim K. Smith, " 'A Question from Which We Could Not Escape': William McKinley and the Decision to Annex the Philippine Islands," *Diplomatic History* 9 (Fall 1985): 363–388; John Offner, "The U.S. and France: Ending the Spanish-American War," *Diplomatic History* 7 (Winter 1983): 1–22.

33. Julius W. Pratt, *Expansionists of 1898* (Baltimore, 1936), pp. 297–298.

34. Smith, 373.

35. William Jennings Bryan to Mrs. U. S. Wissler, 20 May 1900, Papers of William Jennings Bryan, Library of Congress, Washington, D.C. A fine discussion of this point and the context is given by Richard H. Miller in his edition of *American Imperialism in 1898* (New York, 1970), pp. 10–12.

36. Freidel, "Dissent in the Spanish-American War," p. 93.

37. A most compelling account, which includes this story, is David Haward Bain, *Sitting in Darkness: Americans in the Philippines* (Boston, 1984).

38. Russell Roth's *Muddy Glory: America's "Indian Wars" in the Philippines, 1899–1935* (West Hanover, Mass., 1981) is a good account of the post-1902 battles.

39. David Healy, *U.S. Expansionism: The Imperialist Urge in the 1890s* (Madison, 1970), pp. 237–238; Emily Rosenberg, *Spreading the American Dream* (New York, 1982), p. 43.

40. John Higham, *Strangers in the Land* (New Brunswick, N.J., 1955), pp. 14, 63.

41. U.S. Bureau of the Census, *Historical Statistics of the United States: Colonial Times to 1957* (Washington, D.C., 1960), p. 55.

42. Patrick J. Hearden, *Independence and Empire: The New South's Cotton Mill Campaign, 1865–1901* (DeKalb, Ill., 1982), pp. 127, 133.

43. *Ibid.*, p. 128.

44. Beisner, p. 83.

45. McCormick, p. 65.

46. Patricia R. Hill, *The World Their Household: The American Woman's Foreign Mission Movement and Cultural Transformation, 1870–1920* (Ann Arbor, 1985), pp. 3, 54, 112, 164; a fine case study is Joan Brumberg's *Mission for Life: The Story of the Family of Adoniram Judson . . .* (New York, 1980).

47. William Neumann, "Determinism, Destiny, and Myth in the American Image of China," in *Issues and Conflicts*, ed. George L. Anderson (Lawrence, 1959), p. 1.

48. This account is drawn from Walter LaFeber, "John Hay," in *Encyclopedia of American Biography*, ed. John A. Garraty and Jerome L. Sternstein (New York, 1974), pp. 502–503.

49. Edwin Conger to John Hay, 29 May 1900, Papers of William McKinley, Library of Congress, Washington, D.C.

50. John Hay to Alvey A. Adee, 14 September 1900, Papers of William McKinley.

51. Judith Papachristou, "American Women and Foreign Policy, 1898–1905: Exploring Gender in Diplomatic History," *Diplomatic History* 14 (Fall 1990), esp. pp. 493–500; *Congressional Record*, 55th Cong., 3d sess., 13 January 1899, p. 639.

52. Fred H. Harrington, "American Anti-Imperialism," *New England Quarterly* 10 (December 1937): 654–655.
53. Roosevelt, II, pp. 1244, 1291, 1358.
54. *Ibid.*, pp. 1404–1405; Walter L. Williams, "U.S. Indian Policy and the Debate over Philippine Annexation," *Journal of American History* 66 (March 1980): 819–826, 830–831; Martin Ridge, *Ignatius Donnelly* (Chicago, 1962), pp. 394–397.
55. Richard Hofstadter, *The Paranoid Style in American Politics and Other Essays* (New York, 1965), pp. 180–181.
56. Edward Crapol, "From Anglophobia to Fragile Rapprochement," unpublished paper in author's possession, p. 21.
57. Beisner, p. xviii.

FOR FURTHER READING

No text can hope to match the references for pre-1981 material in *Guide to American Foreign Relations since 1700*, ed. Richard Dean Burns (1983). Also consult this chapter's notes and the General Bibliography at the end of this volume. The bibliography that follows, as in all the bibliographies in this book, concentrates on post-1981 works.

Cultural influences are well explored in Stuart Anderson, *Race and Rapprochement: Anglo-Saxonism and Anglo-American Relations, 1895–1904* (1981), and Gary Marotta, "The Academic Mind and the Rise of U.S. Imperialism: Historians and Economists as Publicists for Ideas of Colonial Expansion," *American Journal of Economics and Sociology* 42 (April 1983). McKinley and the march toward war are nicely analyzed in John Offner, *An Unwanted War* (1992); Richard E. Welch, Jr., "William McKinley: Reluctant Warrior, Cautious Imperialist," in *Studies in American Diplomacy, 1865–1945*, ed. Norman Graebner (1985); Robert C. Hilderbrand, *Power and the People: Executive Management of Public Opinion in Foreign Affairs, 1897–1921* (1981), a pioneering account; Tennant McWilliams, *Hannis Taylor: The New Southerner as an American* (1978); David R. Contosta and Jessica R. Hawthorne, "Rise to World Power: Selected Letters of Whitelaw Reid, 1895–1912," in *Transactions of the American Philosophical Society* (1986), key on a major figure; Carl Parrini, "Charles A. Conant," in *Behind the Throne*, eds. T. McCormick and W. LaFeber (1993), essays in honor of Fred Harvey Harrington; and a superb study of Reid's influential newspaper in Richard Kluger, *The Paper: The Life and Death of the New York Herald Tribune* (1986). The best one-volume study of the war itself is David F. Trask, *The War with Spain in 1898* (1981).

Michael H. Hunt, "Resistance and Collaboration in the American Empire, 1898–1903: An Overview," *Pacific Historical Review* 48 (June 1979), provides interesting case studies of Cuba, China, and the Philippines; Hawaii is analyzed in Thomas J. Osborne, *Empire Can Wait: American Opposition to Hawaiian Annexation, 1893–1898* (1981), especially good on commercial interests; Cuba's revolt is seen as a prototype of later national wars for liberation in Louis A. Perez, Jr., *Cuba between Empires, 1878–1902* (1983); the Philippines are well explored in three key works: Stuart Creighton Miller, *"Benevolent Assimilation": The American Conquest of the Philippines, 1899–1903* (1983), which stresses racism; Kenton J. Clymer, *Protestant Missionaries in the Philippines, 1898–*

1916: An Inquiry into the American Colonial Mentality (1985); and *The Anti-Imperialist Reader: A Documentary History of Anti-Imperialism in the United States*, Vol. I: *From the Mexican War to the Election of 1900*, ed. Philip S. Foner and Richard C. Winchester (1984). For affairs in China, see James J. Lorence, "Organized Business and the Myth of the China Market: The American Asiatic Association, 1898–1937," in *Transactions of the American Philosophical Society* (1984); James Reed, *The Missionary Mind and American East Asia Policy* (1985); and the fascinating case study by Jane Hunter, *The Gospel of Gentility: American Women Missionaries in Turn-of-the-Century China* (1984).

New overviews include Jules R. Benjamin, *The United States and the Origins of the Cuban Revolution* (1990); Ivan Musicant, *The Banana Wars* (1990); Joseph A. Fry, *John Tyler Morgan and the Search for Southern Autonomy* (1992), a significant study of the South's expansionism; H. W. Brands, *Bound to Empire: The United States and the Philippines* (1992), a highly useful synthesis; Paul Gordon Lauren, *Power and Prejudice: The Politics and Diplomacy of Racial Discrimination* (1988); and Walter LaFeber, *The American Search for Opportunity, 1865–1913*, in *The Cambridge History of U.S. Foreign Relations*, ed. Warren Cohen (1993), which has additional bibliography.

8

The Search for Opportunity:
Rough Riders and Dollar Diplomats
(1901–1913)

THEODORE ROOSEVELT AND TWENTIETH-CENTURY U.S. FOREIGN POLICY

William McKinley was the first twentieth-century president, but no chief executive has better caught, exemplified, and gloried in the spirit of modern America than Theodore Roosevelt. As *Time* magazine wrote in 1979, "He was America." At the 1984 Republican convention in Dallas, a young follower of Ronald Reagan explained:

> People sometimes ask me who was the last great President. Some say Kennedy. I don't think so. . . . I say Teddy Roosevelt. He was a fighter, he was stubborn. He was almost a salesman for America. America was the greatest country in the world and he was willing to go to any lengths to prove it. And he had the qualities I was brought up on—that you do the best you can, whatever it is. . . . He *loved* life. And he loved America.[1]

No president has been more colorful. "Cowboy, crime-fighter, soldier, and explorer . . . ," David Healy writes, "he fulfilled as an adult the ambitions of every small boy."[2] Roosevelt, however, was also as complex as the nation he led. Raised in New York City by private tutors, a graduate of Harvard, having traveled abroad extensively, he came from America's aristocratic class. The author of a dozen books, an avid naturalist, a lover of art (if it was traditional), he better combined the scholar-in-politics than anyone since John Quincy Adams. But he had also been a cowboy in South Dakota's Black Hills in the 1880s (where he went to mourn after his first wife had died in childbirth), worked as a lowly ward politician amid the rank corruption of New York City, and became uncommonly popular with mass America.

An aristocrat, a scholar, and a politician, Roosevelt also loved killing. After an argument with a girl friend, the twenty-year-old vented his anger by shooting a neighbor's dog. When he killed his first buffalo in the West, Roosevelt danced wildly around the carcass while his Indian guide watched in amazement. As noted in earlier chapters, TR justified slaughtering Indians, if necessary; their life, he wrote, was only "a few degrees less meaningless, squalid, and ferocious than that of the wild beasts." But he had little more use for certain whites. In his history of New York City, he approved of the killing of thirty men who had joined antidraft riots during the Civil War. TR called the shooting an "admirable object-lesson to the remainder" of New Yorkers.[3]

Perhaps Roosevelt's inclination for war and killing was part of a common racism at the time that justified the removal of "inferior" peoples. Perhaps it arose from the belief that when a "civilized" people used force, it would be limited and improve human character: "No triumph of peace is quite so great as the supreme triumphs of war," TR believed. In this case, however, he meant war against less industrialized nations: "In the long run civilized man finds he can keep the peace only by subduing his barbarian neighbor." As for possible conflict between more "civilized" nations, however, "we have every reason . . . to believe that [wars] will grow rarer and rarer."[4] Perhaps TR's urge to subdue others simply came out of his legendary energy. France's distinguished ambassador to the United States, Jean Jules Jusserand, told Paris officials about hiking with the president through Washington's Rock Creek Park:

> At last we came to the bank of a stream, rather too wide and deep to be forded. . . . But judge of my horror when I saw the President unbutton his clothes and heard him say, "We had better strip, so as not to wet our things in the creek." Then I, too, for the honor of France removed my apparel, everything except my lavender kid gloves. . . . "With your permission, Mr. President, I will keep these on; otherwise it would be embarrassing if we should meet ladies."

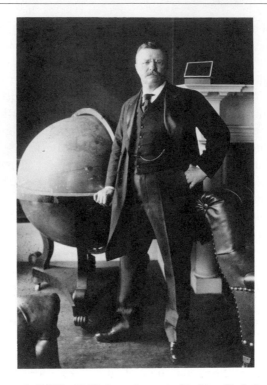

Theodore Roosevelt (1858–1919), born into an elite New York family (and also having experienced the life of a cowboy in the badlands of the Dakotas), became chief executive in 1901. He loved the presidency and the exercise of the new American power around the globe as much as most Americans loved him. Understanding that the U.S. mission often required the strenuous life of military force, Roosevelt declared that "I do not like to see young Christians with shoulders that slope like champagne bottles."

Other diplomats endured much the same experience in order to talk with the president of the United States. He once entertained a formal White House luncheon by using a judo hold to throw the Swiss Minister to the floor several times. An awed British official declared that Roosevelt was a combination of "St. Vitus and St. Paul . . . a great wonder of nature."[5]

Most of all, Roosevelt used force to bring about and maintain his central objective: order. Born in 1858, he grew to manhood amid the chaos of the Civil War and the post-1873 economic depression. He feared the danger posed by both the right ("the dull purblind folly of the very rich men," the "malefactors of great wealth"), and left-wing socialist and populist movements. He understood the need for reform;

but change had to evolve slowly, preferably under the guidance of a farseeing, honest broker with an aristocratic background. Roosevelt once said that he had become a modest reformer because "I intended to be one of the governing class." Only in that position could he preserve the best of American values by maintaining order and stability. A devotion to order especially explains TR's diplomacy. His policies abroad mirrored his politics at home. He opposed those whom he believed were reactionary (as tsarist Russia and, later, Kaiser Wilhelm's Germany), because by clinging to outdated beliefs they threatened to bring about catastrophic, radical change. But Roosevelt as strongly stood against those in Russia, China, and especially Latin America who worked for revolutionary change. TR, like the America of the Progressive Era that he led, sought a middle way.

He believed in the superiority of certain races, especially the Anglo-Saxon, because, in his view, they had organized, democratized, and especially industrialized and subdued "barbarians" more effectively than had other races. Roosevelt did not have great faith in Social Darwinism. (Social Darwinism enjoyed much popularity in his era and was used then and since to help explain why "lesser" peoples had to be controlled by the more "civilized." By applying Charles Darwin's studies on the evolution of lower animals to the evolution of human society, the Social Darwinians concluded that such "superior" races as the Anglo-Saxon resulted from unrestrained competition and individualism, and that the results were scientifically inevitable.) Roosevelt believed not in the Social Darwinians' inevitability, but in free will and an individual's (especially his own) ability to change society. He did not like rampant competition and individualism, for they too often had produced economic chaos, general disorder, and revolution.[6] He, instead, believed in regulating such competition so that disorder could be avoided. Roosevelt wanted order and peace, and for that he was prepared to go to war.

TR thus personally exemplified central themes of post-1890 U.S. foreign policy—a willingness to use force to obtain order, an emphasis on a special U.S. responsibility to guarantee stability in Latin America and Asia, and a belief that Anglo-Saxon values and successes gave Americans a right to conduct such foreign policy. He also hit upon a key theme of twentieth-century U.S. foreign policy when he declared in 1905: "The United States has not the slightest desire for territorial aggrandizement at the expense of any of its southern neighbors."[7] Americans wanted no more land.

After four hundred years, their quest for territorial expansion had ended in the twentieth century. Now they needed markets abroad. As Roosevelt's brilliant secretary of state, Elihu Root, announced in 1906, Americans had "for the first time accumulated a surplus of capital beyond the requirements of internal development."[8] Statistics bore out Root's announcement. Americans had invested overseas $0.7 billion in 1897, $2.5 billion in 1908, and, by 1914, $3.5 billion. Nearly half of those amounts went into Latin America, about 23 percent into Canada, 22 percent into Europe, and 5 percent to Asia (including the Philippines). William McKinley, almost until his dying breath, had preached the need for overseas markets to absorb products from American factories and farms. Roosevelt and Root agreed, but they now added the need for capital markets as well. They also believed that imaginative leadership could use this economic power to prevent disorder and revolution. American goods and capital could create happier, more stable societies in the Caribbean and Central America—even in distant Asia. Their successors, President William Howard Taft (1909–1913) and his secretary of state, Philander C. Knox, called this policy "dollar diplomacy."

THE AMERICAN SEARCH FOR OPPORTUNITY: A NEW PRESIDENCY FOR A NEW FOREIGN POLICY

Roosevelt bragged that he used the White House " as a bully pulpit." He led Americans and made them love it. But he also inherited a position whose powers had already multiplied during the post-1860 era. Roosevelt admired Lincoln's expansion of presidential powers during the Civil War. Even without a Civil War, however, TR believed that presidents had to follow what he termed the "stewardship" theory: "Occasionally great national crises arise which call for immediate and vigorous executive action." The president must then act "upon the theory that he is the steward of the people." It is "not only [his] right but his duty to do anything that the needs of the Nation demanded unless such action was forbidden by the Constitution or the laws."[9]

In 1890, the Supreme Court had almost accidentally moved to support this theory of large presidential powers. Deciding a case (In re Neagle) that actually had nothing to do with foreign policy, the Court declared that the president was not limited to carrying out congressional laws and treaties. His duty included enforcing "the rights, duties, and obligations growing out of the Constitution itself, our international relations, and all the protection implied by the nature of the govern-

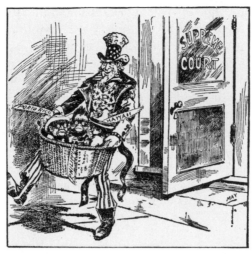

UNCLE SAM: "Now I can do what I please with 'em."

This cartoonist not only portrays the liberty that Uncle Sam took with the Constitution in order to control his new possessions, but catches as well some of the era's racism.

ment under the Constitution."[10] These were extraordinarily general, open-ended words, and they were obiter dicta—not binding or essential to the decision. But they were to be used later to justify the most vigorous presidential power, especially in "our international relations."

It was almost as if some members of the Supreme Court had looked into a crystal ball and had foreseen that a new foreign policy would soon require a new presidency. As late as 1897, some close observers wondered whether the Constitution could be adapted to a U.S. government that might soon have worldwide responsibilities. Captain Alfred Thayer Mahan warned that any projection of U.S. power overseas could smash up against constitutional restraints—"the lion in the path" of empire, as he vividly phrased it.[11] Apparently unfamiliar with the *Neagle* decision, Mahan believed that the ambitious president might simply have to ignore the Constitution in order to protect U.S. interests overseas. McKinley proved Mahan wrong. The president's handling of the 1898 war, the annexation of the Philippines, and the 1899–1900 China crises demonstrated the tremendous power a shrewd politician could exercise as chief executive of American foreign policy. The more Americans supported a vigorous foreign policy, the more they were going to get a vigorous presidency.

A young but already well-known political scientist best explained the effect of end-of-the-century foreign policy on presidential powers. The post-1898 "ownership of distant possessions and [the] many sharp struggles for foreign trade," Woodrow Wilson wrote in a widely used textbook, meant that "the President can never again be the mere domestic figure he has been throughout so much of our history." As the United States "has risen to first rank in power and resources," so the president "must stand always at the front of our affairs, and the office will be as big and as influential as the man who occupies it." Wilson prophesied:

> Men of ordinary physique and discretion cannot be Presidents and live, if the strain be not somehow relieved. We shall be obliged always to be picking our chief magistrates from among wise and prudent athletes—a small class.[12]

Roosevelt, the disciple of "the strenuous life," seemed perfect for the role. He believed that only the president could conduct foreign policy. Congress was too large and unwieldy. Public opinion, TR privately declared, was "the voice of the devil, or what is still worse, the voice of a fool." But he went to great lengths to ensure that public opinion was with him—or at least not against him. He, indeed, used the White House as a "bully pulpit," went on frequent speaking engagements, and carefully cultivated powerful journalists in Washington. When a New York State Supreme Court justice once tried to limit the president's power, TR dismissed him as an "amiable old fuzzy-wuzzy with sweetbread brains."[13]

More directly, Roosevelt used the president's power as commander in chief of the armed forces to dispatch U.S. troops as he saw fit in Latin America. Once when Congress refused to accept a treaty he had made, Roosevelt circumvented Congress with an "executive agreement." Such an agreement could be one of two types: authorized by congressional legislation, or—as became too common—made by a president on his own authority. A little-known device until the 1890s, presidents have used it since far more than treaties because an executive agreement is not submitted to Congress, as a treaty must be. It is an agreement between the president and another government. The real difference between the two is that treaties are binding on all parties as long as they are in force, but an executive agreement is technically binding only as long as the president who signed it is in power. That was good enough for Roosevelt. He judged (correctly) that future presidents would uphold his agreements—in part because they would want their successors to uphold their deals. Most notably, TR ignored Senate opposition by taking over the Caribbean country of Santo Domingo between 1905 and 1907. One angry congressman exclaimed that Roosevelt had "no more use for the Constitution than a tomcat has for a marriage license."[14]

But that was not entirely accurate. As a student of American history, Roosevelt had great respect for the Constitution. As a politician as well as student of his nation's history, however, he also had great respect for the need for American expansionism. And that turned out to be the problem. Americans, historian Robert Wiebe has argued, embarked on a "search for order" between 1865 and 1920. That well might have been so at home; given the long economic depression, general strikes, and social upheavals that struck the United States during those years, they understandably wanted peace and quiet. But it was not the case abroad. In their foreign policies, Americans valued a search for opportunity over the search for order. In Cuba, Hawaii, the Philippines, China, and Central America—and especially during the 1901–1913 years, in Cuba, Panama, the Dominican Republic, Nicaragua, China, and Mexico—Americans demanded opportunity for their trade, investment, and security needs. In every instance noted, the result in these countries was upheaval and, in several instances, revolution. But U.S. officials did not back off. They continued to demand economic and other rights, even if the demands climaxed in massive disorder. They valued those rights over the disorder the demands helped cause. At that point, Americans then demanded a new, more vigorous presidency to guarantee continued opportunities for their growing economic machine—and, if possible, to restore order in these foreign countries. The presidents, led by McKinley, Taft, and—most flamboyantly—Roosevelt, used military force to guarantee continued opportunity and, they hoped, order. Thus was born the twentieth-century "imperial presidency."[15]

In this new world for U.S. opportunity, Roosevelt was determined to use his considerable energy and powers to the limit. Thanks to Lincoln, the Supreme Court, McKinley, executive agreements, and the worldwide quest of Americans for opportunity, those limits stretched far. Roosevelt colorfully demonstrated Woodrow Wilson's insight: an aggressive foreign policy created a strong president. And vice versa.

East, North, and South to an Isthmian Canal

TR knew what he wanted to do with his new powers. He immediately moved to realize the American dream of a U.S.-controlled isthmian canal in Central America. First, however, he had to break the 1850 Clayton-Bulwer Treaty that made Great Britain a full partner in any canal project. Roosevelt and his first secretary of state (and close friend), John Hay, terminated that treaty. They did so while actually strengthening U.S.-British relations, despite events that tested the relationship. The tests occurred in South Africa, Alaska, and then Central America.

In South Africa, the British had become bogged down in a bloody struggle with the Boers between 1899 and 1902. The Boers (a Dutch word for "farmers") had settled at the southern tip of black Africa in 1652. The British seized the South African cape in 1795 and instantly clashed with the austere, Calvinist, isolated, and fiercely nationalistic Boers. In the 1830s, the Boers undertook the great trek north to escape British control. They created their own independent nation. Then, as diamonds and other mineral wealth were found in the 1870s, the Boers' region became a focal point for European colonial power rivalry, and the British moved in to reassert control. At that point, U.S. economic interests rapidly increased in the region. Between 1895 and the outbreak of the Boer War in 1899–1900, for example, U.S. exports to South Africa tripled to $20 million. Americans also believed that the British were more progressive and better able to "civilize" the black Africans, who represented the large majority of South Africans.

All-out war between the British and the Boers erupted in 1899. To everyone's astonishment, during "Black Week" of December, the Boer troops inflicted the worst military defeat on the powerful British forces in living memory. Most Americans, remembering 1776, sided with the Boers. But U.S. officials, while remaining officially neutral, strongly sided with the British. American bankers floated loans to pay one-fifth of England's war costs. Roosevelt and Hay were shaken by the British defeats. "It certainly does seem to me that England is on the downgrade," the president wrote privately. But he understood the need to champion Anglo-Saxon values. Roosevelt quietly supported the British and refused to send any aid to the Boers until London's armies turned the tide and won victory between 1900 and 1902. TR received few rewards for his help in South Africa. As historian Thomas Noer concludes, the United States supported Great Britain to ensure the entry of American goods through an open-door policy in South Africa, a policy that Roosevelt thought the British supported. But despite U.S. pressure and the growing interest of American blacks in South Africa after 1900, "this policy failed: British domination resulted in a decline of American economic influence and did little to improve the lot of the black African."[16]

British problems in Africa, however, did allow Roosevelt to score two victories closer to home. The first involved a disputed boundary between Alaska and Canada that became enflamed after gold was found in 1896. TR was furious at the Canadians for advancing what he considered to be an empty claim. "I'm going to be ugly," he warned his British friends. The president finally agreed to allow "six impartial jurists" to arbitrate the dispute. He showed his determination to have his way by dispatching troops to Alaska. Then he appointed three Americans who were neither "impartial" nor "jurists," but U.S. politicians who completely shared TR's views. The Canadian prime minister, Sir Wilfrid Laurier, rightly denounced the appointments as "an outrage." He named two Canadian members, and the British named their own lord chief justice—who promptly voted with the Americans and handed Roosevelt most of the land. The Canadians cried that they had been double-crossed. To the Americans and the British, however, maintaining their improving relationship was worth giving away what was a small, if valuable, slice of Canada. For not the first or last time, Canadian interests were sacrificed for the sake of U.S.-British friendship.[17]

The most significant victory over the British came after "Black Week" in South Africa. London officials reversed themselves and agreed to discuss doing away with the Clayton-Bulwer Treaty. The U.S. Senate, never reluctant to kick the British Lion as long as it was already badly wounded, pushed events along by introducing measures to build an American-owned canal regardless of the 1850 pact. In early 1900, Hay and the British ambassador to Washington signed the Hay-Pauncefote Treaty, which allowed the United States to build and own—but not fortify—an isthmian canal. The U.S. Senate indignantly rejected the treaty and told Hay to obtain the right to fortify as well. The secretary of state was furious with the Senate and especially with Democratic presidential nominee William Jennings Bryan, who led the opposition: "He struck at [the treaty] in mere ignorance and malice," Hay wrote a friend, "as an idiot might strike at a statue because he happened to have a hammer in his hand."[18] Hay nevertheless had no alternative, especially after the new president agreed with the Senate. A second Hay-Pauncefote Treaty was signed in November 1901. The United States gained the right to fortify the canal.

But where was the canal to be located? Official U.S. commissions between 1876 and 1901 recommended Nicaragua as the cheapest and most efficient route. Its rival, Panama (a province of Colombia), might have been cheaper, but the French company that owned rights to that route (Compagnie Universelle du Canal Interocéanique) demanded over

$100 million. By 1901–1902, however, as the second Hay-Pauncefote Treaty took effect, the company fell under the control of two shadowy, skilled lobbyists who changed the course of isthmian history. Philippe Bunau-Varilla was a Frenchman with extensive contacts in Panama and Washington. William Cromwell was senior partner in the influential New York law firm of Sullivan and Cromwell; he enjoyed access to powerful leaders in Washington politics and New York finance. The two men reduced their company's asking price to $40 million. Then, in June 1902, they pushed through Congress the Spooner Amendment, giving Roosevelt the right to pay $40 million to the company and purchase a six-mile zone in Panama from Colombia. The lobbying of the two men had received heaven-sent help when a Nicaraguan volcano suddenly erupted and endangered the proposed route. Bunau-Varilla quickly put a picture of the volcano (which the Nicaraguans had, unfortunately for themselves, printed on their postage stamps) on the desk of everyone in Congress.

The secretary of state negotiated the Hay-Herrán Treaty that gave Colombia $10 million plus $250,000 annually for the six-mile zone. The Colombian legislature, however, rejected the pact and demanded more money. In truth, the Colombians hoped to stall until 1904, when the French company's charter was to revert to Colombia. The Latin American country would then gain—and Bunau-Varilla and Cromwell lose—$40 million. Roosevelt blew up. All his considerable racism appeared. He refused to have those "banditti" in Latin America publicly humiliate and rob the United States. In truth, as Richard L. Lael observes in his important study of U.S.-Colombian relations, U.S. officials seemed ignorant of Colombia's deep problems as it emerged from a costly civil war, and "none of them seemed to realize, or seriously consider, the possibility that U.S. actions, as seen from Colombia, could legitimately be perceived as interventionist, dangerous, and imperialistic." Roosevelt instead spread the word that he would not be displeased if Panama revolted against Colombia. The Panamanians needed little encouragement. Since at least the 1880s, they had developed a strong nationalist movement that repeatedly tried to obtain independence. As Panama grew more restless, U.S. armed forces had become extraordinarily active. One estimate concludes that those forces had spent a total of about 200 days ashore in Panama in various forms of intervention during the second half of the nineteenth century. It was the longest U.S. occupation of any foreign area until 1898.[19]

Under Bunau-Varilla's guidance and with Washington's support, the Panamanians again revolted in November 1903. This time, the U.S.

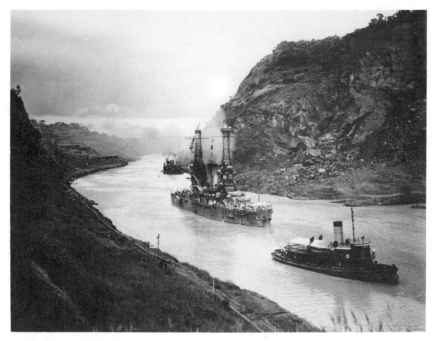

"Man's greatest liberty with nature," the cutting of the Panama Canal, was a crucial step in building twentieth-century U.S. military and economic power. In the photo, the battleship Ohio *sails through the passageway that opened in 1914.*

warships prevented Colombian troops from landing in Panama to quell the revolt. Roosevelt recognized the new nation two days after the rebellion started. He signed a treaty giving Panama $10 million plus $250,000 a year for rights to a ten-mile-wide strip that cut the country in half. The United States fully guaranteed Panama's independence. U.S.-Colombian relations did not return to normal until a treaty gave Colombia $25 million in 1921, two years after Roosevelt's death removed the loudest objection to making the pact.

Roosevelt and Hay found ingenious excuses for their actions in November 1903. They claimed that the 1846 treaty with Colombia gave the United States the right to maintain freedom of transit across the isthmus. The treaty did so, but certainly not against Colombia, which owned Panama and with whom the United States had made the 1846 pact. Nor did the treaty require Colombia to allow a canal to be built. Another rationale for the action was offered by TR's close friend, Oscar Straus, who claimed that the 1846 treaty was "a covenant running with the land"—regardless of whether Panamanians or Colombians owned

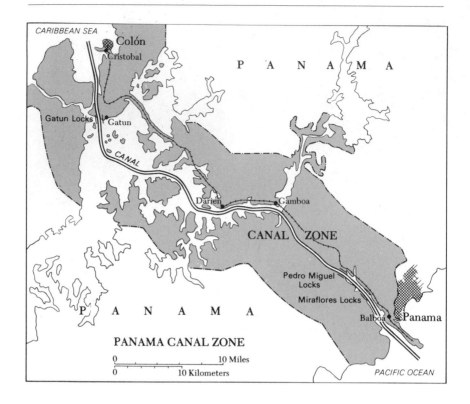

CARIBBEAN SEA

Colón
Cristobal

P A N A M A

Gatun Locks Gatun

CANAL

Darien Gamboa

CANAL ZONE

Pedro Miguel
Locks

Miraflores Locks

P A N A M A

Balboa Panama

PANAMA CANAL ZONE

0 ————————— 10 Miles
0 ————————— 10 Kilometers

PACIFIC OCEAN

the land. A State Department lawyer dismissed Straus's interpretation with the joke that it turned out to be a "covenant running (away!) with the land." The real reasons for Roosevelt's action were his determination to build a canal and the U.S. naval power that enforced his will. As for the Panamanians, they gained independence but lost part of their country. They soon claimed title over the ten-mile-wide strip, but the United States effectively closed it off and controlled the territory. John Hay justified U.S. rights with the phrase "titular sovereignty," a claim so vague that Washington officials could not define or defend it when Panamanians demanded the return of their land (and the canal) in the 1960s and 1970s.[20]

At a cabinet meeting, TR vigorously gave his reasons for taking the canal zone, then loudly challenged his advisers: "Have I defended myself?" Elihu Root answered, "You certainly have Mr. President. You have shown that you were accused of seduction and you have conclusively proved that you were guilty of rape." Roosevelt, of course, would never admit to having doubts about his act. He had overcome Colombia's opposition. He also overcame domestic opposition. But leading newspapers, led by the *New York Times* and the Hearst journals, claimed (in Hearst's words) that the "Panama foray is nefarious. Besides being a rough-riding assault upon another republic over the shattered wreckage of international law and diplomatic usage, it is a quite unexampled instance of foul play in American politics."[21]

Most Americans, however, overwhelmingly approved Roosevelt's actions. They cared about the canal, not about the means he used to acquire it. TR made "the dirt fly," as he put it, and in 1906 paid a personal visit to witness the construction. It marked the first time a president had ever left the United States while in office. Roosevelt saw miraculous engineering feats being performed as the waterway cut through Panama's mountains and lakes. The United States was completing the biggest construction job in history. He also watched medical history being made as American scientists discovered how to find and kill the mosquito that caused malaria and yellow fever, diseases that had destroyed the French effort in the 1880s. With the opening of the canal in 1914—"the greatest liberty Man has ever taken with Nature," in the words of British ambassador James Bryce—the distance between New York and San Francisco by boat shrank from 13,615 miles to 5,300 miles. U.S. merchants and warships now moved easily between the Atlantic and Pacific oceans. And Americans grew even more sensitive about disorder in the region surrounding their canal.

A Great Departure: The Roosevelt Corollary

Long before he obtained the canal area, TR understood the importance of the most hallowed of U.S. foreign policies, the Monroe Doctrine, and how it had to be enforced. "There is a homely adage that runs 'speak softly and carry a big stick; you will go far,' " he told the Minnesota State Fair audience in 1901. "If the American nation will speak softly and yet build and keep at a pitch of the highest training a thoroughly efficient navy, the Monroe Doctrine will go far."[22]

The danger to the doctrine no longer was British expansionism. London officials were preoccupied with Africa and Europe. The danger came from two other sources. The first, Germany, was not obvious and worried mainly U.S. military planners. Modern U.S. military planning began in 1900, when McKinley established the navy's General Board. (It was created largely so that war hero Admiral Dewey could occupy himself with war games instead of running against McKinley for the presidency.) In 1903, Secretary of War Elihu Root created the

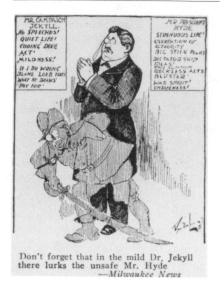

MR. CAMPAIGN JEKYLL. No SPEECHES! QUIET LIFE! COOING DOVE ACT! MILDNESS! If I DO WRONG BLAME LOEB THIS WHAT HE DRAWS PAY FOR!

MR. PRESIDENT HYDE. STRENUOUS LIFE! USURPATION OF AUTHORITY BIG STICK POLICY DICTATORSHIP? DEAS RECKLESS ACTS BLUSTER! WAR SPIRIT! UNSAFENESS!

Don't forget that in the mild Dr. Jekyll there lurks the unsafe Mr. Hyde
—*Milwaukee News*

This cartoon of 1904 from the Milwaukee News—*"Don't forget that in the mild Dr. Jekyll there lurks the unsafe Mr. Hyde"—is not only critical of Roosevelt the campaigner, but also indicates why cartoonists loved to draw the always active, colorful president.*

Army General Staff. That year, an interservice planning group, the Joint Army and Navy Board, was also set up. A global foreign policy needed sophisticated military planning. In the most sensitive region, the Caribbean, the planners grew to fear the growing navy and imperial ambitions of Kaiser Wilhelm's Germany. The kaiser was getting at cross-purposes in Europe, Africa, and Asia with England, TR's closest ally. Historians later discovered that in 1899, the kaiser actually ordered plans drawn up for possible war against the United States. A lack of ships forced him to stop the planning.[23]

The second danger to the Monroe Doctrine was well known, even blatant. Frequent revolutions in the smaller Caribbean–Central American nations were an open invitation for Germany and other powers to intervene to protect their citizens—and perhaps to stay indefinitely. Much as the United States feared Soviet involvement in Latin American revolutions after 1960, so Americans feared the European presence in the area long before the Russian Revolution of 1917. At first, in 1901–1902, Roosevelt thought that the Europeans were justified in intervening to protect their citizens and property and to collect just debts, as long as they did not remain. Then in 1902–1903, Germans, French, and British took TR at his word and used force to collect debts owed to them by Venezuela.[24]

An uproar ensued in the United States. It grew when the International Court of Justice at The Hague ruled that the Europeans acted within their rights. The U.S. State Department warned Roosevelt that the ruling put "a premium on violence" and undermined the Monroe Doctrine.[25] The Europeans had been careful not only to keep the president informed of their plans, but even to indicate their recognition of the Monroe Doctrine. Roosevelt nevertheless knew he was in a tight spot. He could not tolerate major European intervention in the region, but if he opposed it, the Europeans would demand that he make the Latin Americans behave properly. "These wretched republics cause me a great deal of trouble," he lamented.[26]

His moment of decision came in 1904. In Santo Domingo, whose harbors and customshouse Americans had been eying since at least 1870, U.S. business groups came into conflict with German and French interests. The U.S. minister to Santo Domingo, William F. Powell, used the threat of Germany to convince the U.S. government to intervene directly on behalf of American bankers and shipping companies. These foreign rivalries in turn triggered internal disorders. In late 1904, TR declared that he intended to stop the threat of possible revolution. He arranged the payment of debts to Europeans by seizing the customshouses. The president announced his policy to Congress in December 1904. Reviewing major themes of post-1865 as he gave a history lesson to Congress, TR stressed his belief in the obligations— and rights—of "civilized" nations as he outlined what became known as the Roosevelt Corollary to the Monroe Doctrine:

> It is not true that the United States feels any land hunger or entertains any projects as regards the other nations of the Western Hemisphere save such as are for their welfare. All that this country desires is to see the neighboring countries stable, orderly, and prosperous. . . . Chronic wrongdoing, or an impotence which results in a general loosening of the ties of civilized society, may in America, as elsewhere, ultimately require intervention by some civilized nation, and in the Western Hemisphere the adherence of the United States to the Monroe Doctrine may force the United States, however reluctantly, in flagrant cases of such wrongdoing or impotence, to the exercise of an international police power. . . . We would interfere with [Latin Americans] only in the last resort, and then only if it became evident that their inability or unwillingness to do justice at home and abroad had violated the rights of the United States or had invited foreign aggression to the detriment of the entire body of American nations.[27]

Roosevelt's action pleased U.S. businesses in the country as well as the president, Carlos Morales, whom they supported. But many Santo Domingans disliked the idea of the United States having a blank check to interfere in their affairs. Morales finally had to sign the treaty while

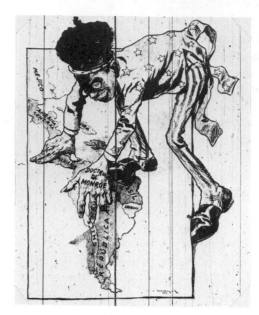

This Argentine cartoon, published in a Buenos Aires newspaper in early 1905, provides a growing Latin American view of U.S. foreign policy. An Uncle Sam figure, with the head of Theodore Roosevelt, reaches throughout the hemisphere with the heavy hand of the Monroe Doctrine. Santo Domingo is depicted as the small island below Cuba and between Uncle Sam's hands.

U.S. warships protected him from his own people. That, however, turned out to be the least of TR's problems, for next the treaty was rejected by the U.S. Senate: it refused to throw an American protectorate over the restless country. Roosevelt effectively thumbed his nose at the Senate by signing an executive agreement with Morales. U.S. government agents and bankers, led by J. P. Morgan and Kuhn, Loeb and Company, took over control of Santo Domingo. They paid off the debt owed the Europeans.

Roosevelt saw his action not as imperialism, but as work that a "policeman" must do to maintain order among less civilized people. As he privately wrote a friend in 1904:

> I want to do nothing but what a policeman has to do in Santo Domingo. As for annexing the island, I have about the same desire to annex it as a gorged boa constrictor might have to swallow a porcupine wrong-end-to. . . . I have asked some of our people to go there because, after having refused for three months to do anything, the attitude of the Santo Domingans has been one of half chaotic war towards us.[28]

The gorged-boa-constrictor analogy was appropriate, given that the United States was trying to digest Hawaii, the Philippines (which TR was beginning to see as "our Achilles heel" because it was so vulnerable to such powers as Japan), Puerto Rico, Cuba, and Panama. All had been brought within the American orbit within just six years.

But a gorged boa constrictor also wants peace and quiet. Roosevelt's corollary marked a historic break from Monroe's doctrine and anticipated U.S. policy toward Latin America for the rest of the twentieth century. It did so for five reasons. First, Monroe's message had supported Latin American revolutions, but TR's opposed them. Second, Monroe had urged nonintervention in those revolts by all outside parties, including the United States. Roosevelt, however, declared that he would directly intervene to maintain "civilized" order. Third, Monroe had seen U.S. economic power acting in a traditional marketplace— that is, buying and selling according to rules set by the home country. But Roosevelt used his economic power to control that marketplace and bring it under U.S., not home-country, control. (One senator who bitterly opposed TR's action sarcastically observed that the U.S. Navy rallying cry had been that of a commander in the War of 1812: "Don't give up the ship boys"; now, however, a U.S. naval officer could cry: "We have met the enemy and they are ours. Advance the bid on Dominican bonds.")[29] Fourth, because Monroe had argued for keeping out of internal Latin American affairs, he had no need for the use of military power. But Roosevelt's policy depended on force. Between 1898 and 1920, U.S. troops entered Latin American countries no fewer than twenty times. Those nations were seen less as neighbors in the hemisphere than problems to be managed militarily. Finally, because Monroe's policy had urged abstention, Congress had no role and the president did not have to be concerned about constitutional problems with the legislature. Roosevelt, however, followed a course that constitutionally required obtaining Congress's assent (to pursue such policies, for example, as making war on foreign nations or making treaties to operate their customshouses). But he simply ignored Congress when it opposed him. His actions drew power out of the legislative branch and pulled it into the executive.

The Roosevelt Corollary opened a new era in hemispheric relations. Latin Americans fully understood. They moved to curb TR's claims. In 1907, the so-called Drago Doctrine (named after Argentina's foreign minister Luis María Drago) became accepted international law. It declared that no nation could use force to collect debts. TR strongly opposed the Drago dictum and finally acquiesced only after it was radically weakened. In 1911, the United States even expanded its new version of the Monroe Doctrine. Republican senator Henry Cabot Lodge from Massachusetts, a close friend of Roosevelt's, learned that a Japanese company was angling to buy strategic Mexican territory. The Lodge Corollary, passed in a Senate resolution, declared U.S. opposition to the sale of any strategic area to a nonhemispheric company that might be an agent for a foreign government. The Japanese firm had earlier lost interest anyway, but the State Department used the resolution to discourage similar ventures after 1911. The Monroe Doctrine resembled U.S. industry and the president's powers: it grew larger all the time.

THE FATEFUL TRIANGLE: THE UNITED STATES, CHINA, AND JAPAN, 1900–1908

Roosevelt fervently believed that the American future rested on events in Asia—the new Far West—as well as on those in the Western Hemisphere. He had led the fight to take the Philippines and completely supported the open-door policy. His beliefs were bolstered by his close friend, Brooks Adams. Grandson of John Quincy Adams, Brooks was a brilliant eccentric who believed that he had discovered a historical "law" proving that the world's money center had moved ever westward over a thousand years. Following the sun, it had jumped from the Mediterranean to Paris and then to London. Now, he believed, it was poised once again to bestow greatness and wealth on a people. The only question was whether it would turn west to New York, or lurch east toward Germany and Russia. Brooks Adams saw the 1898–1900 triumphs "as the moment when we won the great prize. I do believe that we may dominate the world, as no nation has dominated it in recent time."[30]

But to reach, then remain at, the peak of world power, Americans had to conquer the world's greatest market and cheapest labor supply: China. And to do that, Adams told Roosevelt, the United States had to use its vast resources—but also strong government involvement—to build the cheapest, most efficient transportation system to carry its goods to Asia. "We must have a new deal . . . , we must suppress the states, and have a centralized administration, or we shall wobble over," Adams declared. Or, as he told TR, Americans "must command the terminus in Asia—if we fail in this we shall break down."[31] The president responded in July 1903 that he agreed: "We must do our best to prevent the shutting to us of Asian markets. In order to keep the roads to these terminals we must see that they are managed primarily in the interest of the country."[32] Out of such ideas emerged laws, pushed especially by Progressives such as TR, that created new central-government agencies to regulate the railroads and make the society more efficient.

In foreign policy, such ideas led Roosevelt, Hay, and Adams to try to guarantee an open door to the China market by supporting Japan (who seemed to agree with U.S. aims) and opposing Russia's attempts to colonize Manchuria and control Korea. Secretary of State Hay believed that if TR gave the Japanese "a wink," they would "fly at the throat of Russia in a moment." When some Americans feared such a "wink" might make Japan supreme in Asia and perhaps create disorder inside Russia, Hay dismissed the critics as members "of that highly respected family, the common or barnyard ass." Roosevelt warmly supported the historic 1902 alliance between Japan and Great Britain, which further isolated Russia in the Far East. And as the rivalry between Tokyo and St. Petersburg grew hot, TR sided with Japan.

In 1904, the Japanese launched a surprise attack that destroyed most of Russia's Pacific fleet. Americans supported Japan. Leading Jewish bankers who had vivid memories of Russia's recent anti-Semitic attacks provided war loans to Tokyo. The Japanese government worked through these bankers to float the first major foreign-government loan ever offered to American investors.[33] In the bright glow of Japan's early victories and TR's Latin American triumphs in 1903–1904, few doubted his policies. One who did, however, was Henry Adams. The brother of Brooks, a close friend of the president's, and perhaps the greatest of all American historians, Henry Adams eerily prophesied in 1904 that Americans—and the world—had stumbled down the wrong road:

> Everybody is interested, and excited, and all are anti-Russian, almost to a dangerous extent [he wrote privately]. I am the only—relative—Russian afloat, and only because I am half-crazy with the fear that Russia is sailing straight into another French revolution which may upset all Europe and us too. A serious disaster to Russia might smash the whole civilized world.[34]

In 1905, Henry Adams's prophesy began to come true. Revolution erupted in Russia. The tsar smashed it, but other European monarchs grew worried. They had asked Roosevelt to try to mediate a peace, and TR agreed, in part because he feared that Japan lacked the resources to fight a long war against Russia. He called the two sides to meet at

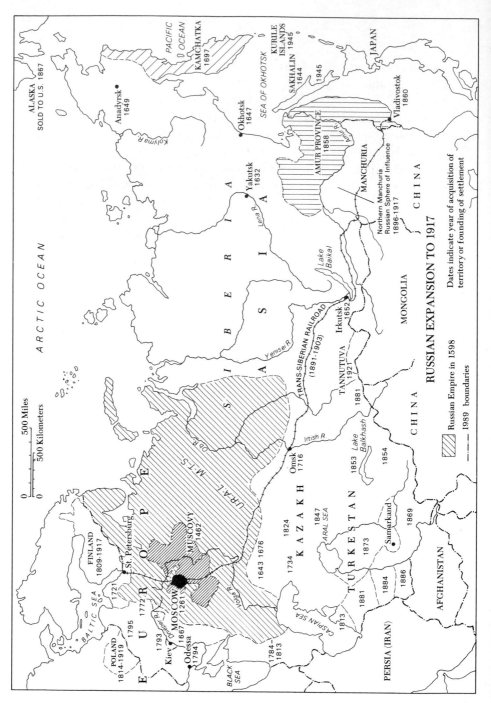

The American-Russian rivalry has deep roots. Early twentieth-century presidents mistrusted the Russians not only because of the tsars' autocratic system, but because of the history of Russian expansionism, shown on this map.

Portsmouth, New Hampshire, in late summer 1905. Although China's interests lay at the center of the talks, no Chinese were invited to participate. After the Japanese finally dropped their demand of a huge indemnity from the tsar, the two sides hammered out a peace treaty in September. Both nations agreed to respect China's territorial integrity (thus honoring the open door). But Japan emerged with controlling interest in Korea, key Chinese ports formerly belonging to Russia, the main railway in southern Manchuria, and the southern half of Sakhalin Island, formerly claimed by the tsar. The next month, Tokyo forced Korea to become a Japanese protectorate. Japan would remain in control until 1945. The Koreans appealed to TR for help, but he now refused to become involved.[35]

Instead, the president made a secret deal—the Taft-Katsura Agreement—in which Japan promised to keep hands off the Philippines, and TR recognized Tokyo's domination of Korea. He emerged from Portsmouth more anti-Russian than ever. "Bad as the Chinese are, no human being, black, yellow or white, could be as untruthful, as insincere, as arrogant—in short as untrustworthy in every way—as the Russians under their present system," he complained privately.[36]

But the Russo-Japanese War brought U.S. officials into a dangerous new world. The Chinese observed how an Asian people had humiliated a white race in conflict. Fresh antiforeign tendencies appeared when China stunned Roosevelt in 1905 by protesting U.S. immigration policy with a highly effective boycott of American goods.

A fascinating case study revealed some of the causes and results of the boycott. In the 1880s, James B. Duke learned about the invention of a machine that rolled cigarettes at high speeds. He decided—after glancing at an atlas's population chart—that only China had the population to buy so many cigarettes. By 1902, he was selling 1 billion cigarettes a year through his British-American Tobacco Company (BAT). He undercut both Chinese and Japanese competitors by using the newest technology and advanced sales techniques. When the boycott began in 1905, however, Chinese students and merchants alike targeted Duke's operation as a way of striking back at foreign control. The protestors turned BAT's advertising around by publishing posters showing a dog (which the Chinese considered a low form of life) smoking a BAT cigarette and saying, "Those who smoke American cigarettes are of my species." BAT, Standard Oil, and other U.S. firms urged TR to force the Chinese to end the boycott. But Roosevelt (who called people he deemed especially inefficient "Chinese") was bewildered by the boycott's efficiency. Finally, with its point made and pressure building, the

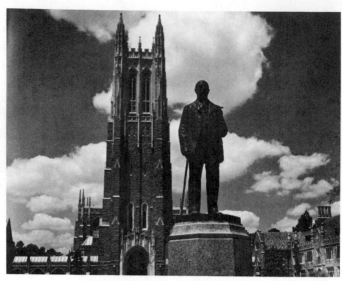

James Buchanan Duke (1856–1925) began working at the family's Durham, North Carolina, tobacco company in 1874. Some fifteen years later, the company controlled 50 percent of U.S. cigarette production, thanks to "Buck's" genius with machinery and marketing. He renamed it the American Tobacco Company, bought or drove off competitors, exploited the vast China market— until Chinese nationalism checked the company and the U.S. Supreme Court in 1911 dissolved Duke's monopoly. He gave generously to his hometown college, Trinity, which was renamed Duke University.

Chinese government ended the boycott. BAT quickly crushed its Chinese competitors who had appeared during the boycott, then set prices so high that by 1916 it enjoyed an 18 percent profit.[37] Three years later, in 1919, the Chinese Revolution began in earnest. The 1905 boycott, resembling the 1905 Russian revolt, had been a warning sign.

Roosevelt next had to confront a challenge from Tokyo. Japan closed off Korea to U.S. interests, then began moving into Manchuria itself. These direct threats to the open door were compounded by an uproar in the United States over Japanese immigration. In 1890, some 2,000 Japanese had lived in California. In 1900, the number reached 24,000 and the governor called the influx the "Japanese menace." The state prepared to pass an Asian exclusion bill, and in San Francisco, a city ordinance segregated Oriental children. Anti-Asian riots erupted. Fear of a U.S.-Japanese war spread. Tokyo officials were deeply angered at the discrimination, but Roosevelt could calm California only by stopping Japanese immigration. In a "gentlemen's agreement" of 1907, Japan said that it would no longer allow laborers to emigrate to the

United States provided that California stopped discriminating against Japanese.

A temporary calm set in, but TR knew that he was confronting an aggressive Japan. To show his resolve, he determined in 1907 to send the entire fleet of sixteen U.S. battleships around the world, with a special stop in Japan. Congressmen, anxious that the Japanese would sneakily attack the fleet as they had the Russian navy in 1904, threatened to withhold needed funds. Roosevelt responded that he had enough money to send the ships halfway around the world. If Congress wanted to bring them back, it could give him the funds. Congress surrendered. The fleet's visit to Japan was a huge popular success. Roosevelt, moreover, had dramatically shown the global reach of the new U.S. battle fleet.

But the trip's diplomatic effect was slight. Japan continued its pressure on Korea and Manchuria. In 1907–1908, a colorful twenty-seven-year-old U.S. consul in Manchuria, Willard Straight, set out to block Japan on his own. Raised on turn-of-century racism, Straight had turned against the Japanese after the Russo-Japanese War. "I now find myself hating the Japanese more than anything in the world," he wrote to a friend. Perhaps, he thought, it was due to the "strain of having to be polite and to seek favors from a yellow people." Straight worked with the great U.S. railroad builder, E. H. Harriman, to plan a railroad in Manchuria that would compete directly with the Japanese-held railway. The project was to be part of Harriman's round-the-world transportation scheme through which he hoped to obtain a stranglehold on global commerce. The Chinese naturally encouraged the Straight-Harriman scheme. China was following the traditional policy of playing off "barbarian against barbarian." But in 1905, the Japanese had secretly forced China to agree that no such competing rail line would be built in Manchuria. Straight, a close friend of Roosevelt's dashing daughter Alice, went to Washington to plead his case personally with the president.

Unfortunately for Straight (and the Chinese), the Japanese delegation arrived first and convinced Roosevelt (who actually needed little convincing) that it was no use challenging them. Instead of accepting the Straight-Harriman dream, TR agreed to a deal. In the Root-Takahira Agreement of 1908, he recognized Japan's pre-eminence in southern Manchuria. In return, Tokyo pledged to uphold the open door and independence of China, but carefully refused to agree to Chinese *territorial* integrity. (After all, southern Manchuria was supposedly a part of China.)[38]

In reality, Roosevelt had given up the open door in much of Manchuria. He had, however, avoided war with Japan and reached a shaky agreement with Asia's rising power. For a man who so loved war and killing, he had shown extraordinary sensitivity to the limits of U.S. power. This preacher of "the strenuous life" and the use of force against the "uncivilized" even won the Nobel Peace Prize for his efforts to end the Russo-Japanese War. In dealing with the Indians and Latin Americans, TR did use force to deal with weaker peoples. In Asia and Europe, however, he knew that the United States was outgunned. He, therefore, followed advice he had learned in the North Dakota frontier saloons: "Never draw unless you mean to shoot." Whether Roosevelt's successors in the White House could afford to follow this advice became a central question of twentieth-century American diplomacy.

Taft, Knox, and Dollar Diplomacy

TR's successor in the White House between 1909 and 1913, William Howard Taft, did not follow his example in Asia. The result was near-catastrophe for both Chinese and U.S. interests. Taft's failure was not due to lack of experience. He had been Roosevelt's secretary of war, headed the commission governing the Philippines, and traveled extensively in the Far East (including one venture during which he came to know Willard Straight). Nor was the failure due initially to Taft rebelling against Roosevelt. The Rough Rider hand-picked his successor, and one wit observed that TAFT stood for "Take-Advice-From-Theodore." But their relations cooled by 1911 as they clashed over a number of issues. TR even prepared to run against Taft for the presidency in 1912. Differences over foreign policy were major reasons for the cooling.

Part of Taft's failure was due to lack of energy. He weighed 300 to 320 pounds. And since his eating increased when his policies were in trouble, by 1911–1912 he was eating a great deal. He liked playing golf, sitting on the White House front porch and listening to the "music machine" (the new phonograph), and taking naps. Taft's real love was the law and the courts—their predictability, logic, and set of rules in which he had been trained. Foreign affairs (usually neither predictable nor logical) seemed messy. Five of his nine cabinet members were lawyers. Resembling the president, they thought cautiously, believed in following precedent, and admired tradition—even as the world rapidly changed around them. Taft was no moss-backed conservative. His

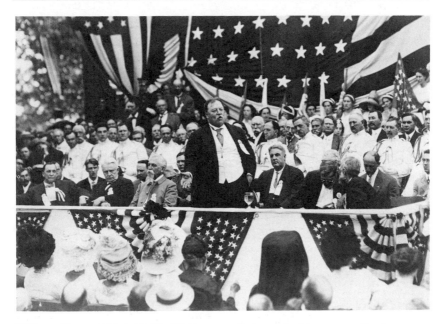

William Howard Taft (1857–1930) was a distinguished lawyer and jurist, a valued assistant and adviser to Theodore Roosevelt. But, contrary to the impression left by this photo, as president between 1909 and 1913 he was a weak politician and leader, although a famous advocate of building U.S. power in Asia and Latin America through what he termed "dollar diplomacy."

administration produced the amendment to the Constitution creating the income tax; created a Department of Labor; and successfully argued a series of antitrust cases against Standard Oil, U.S. Steel, and other giants that far surpassed TR's record as a "trust buster." Aware of the legal and economic complexities of American society, Taft had no similar understanding of foreign affairs. He only clung to certain principles: the open door in Asia, order in Latin America, and the belief that enough money (dollar diplomacy) could secure both.[39]

His secretary of state, Philander C. Knox, was a much thinner version of the president. A leading Pittsburgh corporation lawyer, Knox knew little about foreign policy. A British diplomat complained that Knox thought foreign relations resembled law practice: "To him a treaty is a contract, diplomacy is litigation, and the countries interested are parties to a suit." One advantage to this approach was Taft's and Knox's reorganization of the State Department so that it worked more like a corporation. They created a neat organization chart with specialists reporting upward to the secretary of state. The specialists were arranged

along separate geographical divisions (Straight became head of the Far
East Division for a short time) so that they could focus on the complexities of being a great world power. Neither Knox nor some of his
specialists, however, did enough homework. Many days, the secretary
worked at home until late morning, spent several hours at his office,
enjoyed a leisurely lunch, and then played golf much of the afternoon.
During one golf match, a partner suggested that Knox should travel to
China and see the growing crisis firsthand. "I'm just starting to learn
this game," he replied, "and I'm not going to let anything as unimportant as China interfere." Knox soon paid for such a schedule.

He and Taft believed more constructive foreign affairs could be
achieved by using the nation's rapidly growing capital resources and
downplaying Roosevelt's emphasis on military force. Branded at first
by critics as "dollar diplomacy," by 1912 the president himself took
credit for "substituting dollars for bullets. It . . . appeals alike to idealistic humanitarian sentiments, to the dictates of sound policy and strategy, and to legitimate commercial aims."[40] Dollar diplomacy, Taft
argued, could create orderly societies by helping develop the unindus-
trialized nations and, happily, make a nice profit for American investors.

DOLLAR DIPLOMACY IN ASIA

The Taft administration believed in the need to maintain the Asian
open door for U.S. goods and investment. U.S. officials understood
that because of this need, the Japanese and Russian domination of
Manchuria had to be checked. In 1907, the old enemies had made a
deal in which Russia and its Chinese Eastern Railroad effectively controlled northern Manchuria, and Japan and its South Manchurian
Railroad dominated southern Manchuria. Knox, however, refused to
surrender. The stakes were too high. He believed that whoever financed
the Chinese railway system would be the major voice in developing all
of the immense China market. Knox's most notable effort came in 1910.
He tried to break the Japanese-Russian hold on Manchuria by proposing a "neutralization" scheme. All the major foreign powers, he suggested, should pool their resources, buy the railroads, then operate them
in accordance with the open-door principle. The response was cold.
The British and French, who increasingly needed Russia's and Japan's
cooperation in protecting interests in Europe and southern Asia, pulled
away. The Russians and Japanese moved closer together to fend off

Knox. On July 4, 1910, the two nations signed a fresh treaty of friendship. Seven weeks later, Japan formally annexed Korea. As historian Michael Hunt notes, "By their own standards," the Taft-Knox policy "was bankrupt." Even the once-dominant U.S. cotton textiles were replaced in Manchuria by Japanese goods.[41]

U.S. dollar diplomacy came to the same sad end in China's heartland. In that region, British, French, and German capitalists planned to build the 563-mile-long Hukwang Railway between the capital of Beijing (Peking) and the great port of Canton. Knox demanded that U.S. bankers be included. J. P. Morgan, the Rockefeller-owned National City Bank, Kuhn, Loeb, E. H. Harriman, and other U.S. investors with previous involvement in China set up a group with State Department encouragement. The Chinese government, however, pulled back. It did not want the plan reopened and Americans—and then, no doubt, Japanese and Russians—brought in. Antiforeign riots again broke out. But the collapsing Chinese government could not hold off the United States. Much as China feared, Japan and Russia next forced their way into the deal. The Chinese government signed the contract, sold bonds it could never redeem, and soon disappeared in revolution.

His hopes to become an empire-builder in Asia destroyed, Willard Straight bitterly blamed the Chinese. The power of the Manchu dynasty is gone, he wrote a friend; "he [the Manchu emperor] didn't have his wings clipped," but instead the Chinese people "just naturally pulled out the feathers, and found that it was only a jack-daw with eagles' plumage after all. . . . Verily this is a nation of skunks." Straight, however, missed the main point. Foreign demands, including U.S. demands for increased economic opportunity, had fanned antiforeign feelings in China to a boiling point and had helped create the upheaval that drove the corrupt Manchu dynasty from power in 1912. Indeed, the Manchus, who had entered China from Manchuria in 1644, and in 1909 finally claimed full power, were themselves the targets of Chinese antiforeignism. The great China Revolution was underway. (The Taft demands for an open door for foreign opportunity cast long shadows. The new Nationalist government paid interest on the Hukwang Railway bonds until 1939. In 1983, nine Americans who still held the bonds won a $41.3 million claim in an Alabama court. The infuriated Communist government in Beijing (Peking) warned President Reagan that the claim, if pushed, could severely harm U.S.-Chinese relations. The legacy of the Hay-Taft policies in Asia lived on.)[42]

Roosevelt watched Taft's bumbling with growing alarm. He suggested that his successor make the best of a terrible situation by proposing that Japan develop Manchuria in return for California's right to exclude unwanted Japanese immigrants. When Taft showed no interest, TR warned that the president must not push too hard. The only way to maintain the open door in Manchuria, he wrote, was to fight Japan, and that would require a fleet as large as Great Britain's and an army as powerful as Germany's.[43] But Taft continued to believe that he had found a better way. During 1912, Knox tried to lead U.S. bankers into a six-nation consortium that was to provide a $300 million loan to the new Chinese republic. The bankers were not enthusiastic. Knox insisted. It was a last chance to prevent other powers, and perhaps Chinese nationalism itself, from closing the door. Taft's successor, Woodrow Wilson, pulled the Americans out of the consortium in 1913. It remained to be seen whether Wilson had a better plan for propping open the door.

DOLLAR DIPLOMACY IN LATIN AMERICA AND CANADA

Revolutions also threatened in Latin America. But here, as one U.S. Navy officer boasted, the Monroe Doctrine and American force held "this hemisphere in check against Cosmic Tendencies."[44] In 1906, Secretary of State Elihu Root declared that the United States had reached the point where it both needed Latin American markets and possessed the necessary "surplus of capital beyond the requirements of internal development" to develop in the hemisphere "the peaceful prosperity of a mighty commerce." South and North Americans, he argued, were made for each other. The South had the raw materials, the North the manufacturers. The South's people were "polite, refined, cultivated"; the "North American is strenuous, intense, utilitarian." Perhaps best of all, "Where we accumulate, they spend."[45] The United States thus had other reasons than the Panama Canal to insist on order in Latin America.

In 1906, for example, TR feared that the Cubans were acquiring "a revolutionary habit." He sent in U.S. troops to oversee elections that firmly established an orderly regime. In 1906–1907, Nicaraguan dictator José Santos Zelaya intensified a long-running feud with Guatemala by invading neighboring states. Partly because Zelaya introduced the machine gun to Central Americans, record numbers of people died each day of the war. Roosevelt and the Mexican dictator, Porfirio Díaz, twice intervened to stop the carnage and, on a U.S. warship, to arrange peace terms. In 1907, the United States also helped establish a historic

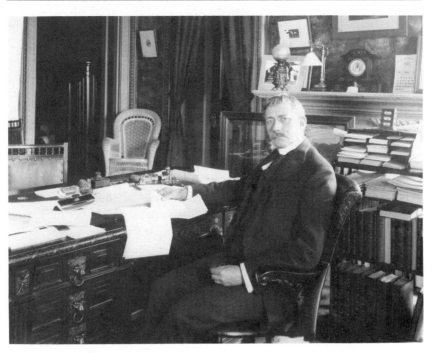

Elihu Root (1845–1937) of New York was probably the nation's top corporate lawyer during the era of the robber barons, secretary of war between 1899 and 1905 (when he made reforms that, in turn, made him "the father of the modern army"), and secretary of state (1905–1909). Root well understood, and described in his speeches, how the new U.S. economic power shaped the nation's overseas needs.

institution, the Central American Court. It was charged by the Central Americans to resolve outstanding regional problems peacefully. The court worked surprisingly well until 1914–1916, when Costa Rica won a decision against the United States. The Wilson administration disregarded the decision and effectively killed the court.[46]

In several Central American countries, U.S. investors themselves had for some years maintained order. Costa Rica was the most democratic nation in the region, in part because of its more equitable landholding. In 1872, a railroad builder from Brooklyn, New York, Minor Keith—described by one journalist as "an apple-headed little man with the eyes of a fanatic"—succeeded in building a major rail system in Costa Rica. He then developed banana plantations so that the trains would have cargo. Thus began the United Fruit Company of Boston, or "The Octopus," as Central Americans came to call it. By World War I, United Fruit controlled not only the banana market, but the rail systems, shipping, banking, and governments in Costa Rica and Honduras. The Roosevelt Corollary was not needed in those countries.[47]

Other countries were not as calm, however. Haiti was temporarily pacified in 1910 by an infusion of U.S. bank loans. In several Central American nations, TR's policies seemed to have had little good effect. Taft privately complained that he needed "to have the right to knock their heads together." Nicaragua's Zelaya was the worst offender. His persistent challenges to U.S. policies climaxed when rumors spread that he was going to give a non-American power the right to build an isthmian canal. In 1909, a revolutionary movement appeared on Nicaragua's east coast. It was helped along by U.S. diplomatic officials and U.S. Marines, who landed to protect the rebels. Zelaya caught two North Americans who were trying to blow up a boatload of his troops. Despite Knox's grave warning, the dictator executed both captives. Knox and U.S. naval commanders then pressured Zelaya to resign. Several changes of government later, U.S. bankers, with Knox's encouragement, were acquiring Nicaraguan banks and railroads in return for loans that kept the government afloat.

A new president, Adolfo Díaz (who had been a clerk in an American company in Nicaragua), finally offered to make his country a U.S. protectorate in return for more loans. Angry Nicaraguans revolted. Some 2,600 U.S. troops landed in 1912 to protect Díaz. The forces remained, reduced in number, until 1925, then had to return in 1926 for another seven-year stay.[48] Modern revolutionary Nicaragua began to arise out of Knox's dollar diplomacy.

The same approach led Taft into quite another kind of problem in U.S.-Canadian relations. Those ties had been quiet since the Alaskan boundary dispute of 1902–1903. The two countries enjoyed mostly prosperous years, and, consequently, the long-present interest on both sides of the boundary in possible annexation had declined. In 1909, Taft unintentionally stirred that interest again by proposing reciprocity treaties. Correctly analyzing the needs of an industrializing United States, he hoped through the reduced tariffs to lower costs of imported raw materials. Taft made the proposal only to have the powerful high-tariff wing of the Republican party rise in revolt. Roosevelt had refused to deal with the issue ("God Almighty could not pass a tariff and win the next election," he believed). But Taft waded in, compromised with the high-tariff interests in order to obtain a bill, and was promptly branded a traitor by low-tariff politicians.

The new tariff heavily discriminated against Canadian imports. Taft and Prime Minister Wilfrid Laurier quickly moved to avoid a trade war by signing a fresh U.S.-Canadian tariff agreement. From Washington's view, the deal could serve a stunning long-range goal: integrate Canada (and, through a similar treaty, Mexico) into a vast hemispheric industrial complex controlled by the United States. Between 1901 and 1908, U.S. investment in Canada had already increased four times to nearly $750 million, mostly in minerals, lumber, and other raw materials. Historian Robert Hannigan aptly calls the emerging U.S. policy "the new continentalism." It aimed, moreover, at changing Canadian-British trade to north-south trade. Careless U.S. politicians, however, began to spell out the probable result: the annexation of Canada. Infuriated and frightened Canadian Conservatives, fully supported by the British, killed the agreement. Dollar diplomacy failed in the north as well as the Far East, although President Ronald Reagan, seventy years later, would again push the idea of "the new continentalism" for many of the same reasons.[49]

The Irony of 1900–1913

After the easy triumphs of 1898–1901, U.S. officials encountered severe setbacks in Asia and the Western Hemisphere over the next dozen years. American power nevertheless continued to push outward, even in China and Canada. The United States also became involved in European affairs, an area it had largely bypassed since 1815.

These affairs centered on European attempts to colonize more of Africa. In two episodes, U.S. officials intervened to protect what they believed were threats to an open door in Africa. The first occurred in 1904–1906 in Morocco. In that country, where France claimed a sphere of influence, Germany challenged Paris officials by recognizing Moroccan independence. As war threatened, the European powers asked Roosevelt to repeat his success as mediator at Portsmouth. He hesitated, then agreed, rationalizing that an 1880 U.S.-Moroccan trade treaty gave the United States a strong economic interest in the country. Of at least equal importance, TR feared a possible European war. He convened the Algeciras Conference in 1906 at the Spanish port city. When the meeting protected French claims, Roosevelt, who strongly favored the growing British-French alliance, was secretly pleased.

Five years later, Taft won a more resounding victory for the open door in Liberia. That African country had been colonized, and was now controlled, by descendants of black slaves from the United States. After the Civil War, the U.S. government had shown no interest in the country. In dire financial straits, Liberia's land was being seized by surrounding colonies controlled by France and Great Britain. In 1910, Taft asked Congress to provide financial help and military protection. When the Senate rejected his plea, the president—following McKinley's and Roosevelt's examples—organized financial aid through private banks. The British and French were checked. The U.S.-supported black elite continued to rule. Historian Judson M. Lyon has placed the episode in perspective: Taft's proposals for Liberia were "almost identical" to those the president offered to Nicaragua and China. As a top State Department official believed, dollar diplomacy would bring order to these nations, while "extending the Open Door to as many regions of the world as possible."[50]

Taft's luck, such as it was, ran out in 1911, when he tried to negotiate arbitration treaties with France and Great Britain. The arbitration movement had gained popularity a decade earlier as it became apparent how brutal the next conflict among industrialized powers might be. The Hague Peace Conferences of 1899 and 1907 were one result. They produced the Permanent Court of Arbitration at The Hague as well as a set of rules for fighting wars, but little on how to avoid them.[51] Roosevelt supported the 1907 conference, although he had pointedly refused to submit the Alaskan boundary question to the court. In 1911, he became deeply angry when Taft made two bilateral arbitration pacts. TR was preparing to fight Taft for the 1912 presidential nomination, so his opposition was not dispassionate. Roosevelt's friends in the Senate carved up the treaties until Taft withdrew them. Nevertheless, between 1899 and 1911, the United States for the first time signed treaties with European and other nations that provided for peaceful resolution of disputes. Twenty-two pacts went into effect under Roosevelt, another twenty-one under Woodrow Wilson.

But the arbitration movement could not grow fast enough to stop World War I or even to prevent great powers such as the United States from using force to put down revolutions. In this sense, the American entry onto the world stage between 1898 and 1914 produced a most ironic result. For just as McKinley, Roosevelt, Taft, and, later, Wilson demanded order in Latin America, Africa, Asia, and even Europe, the world began to explode into revolution. Japan's victory over a white race in 1905 helped trigger anticolonial revolts in places as far apart as Vietnam, Persia, Turkey, and China. Russia experienced an ominous uprising in 1905. Mexico erupted in 1911–1913.

An understanding of twentieth-century U.S. foreign policy requires learning one central theme: just as Americans began to claim Great

Britain's title as the globe's greatest power and, at the same time, to demand an orderly world, the globe burst into revolution. The American claim was to be realized, but the demand was never met nor the revolutions ended.

Notes

1. V. S. Naipaul, "Among the Republicans," *New York Review of Books*, 25 October 1984, p. 17.
2. David Healy, *U.S. Expansionism: The Imperialist Urge in the 1890s* (Madison, Wis., 1970), p. 110.
3. The quotes and stories are found in Edmund Morris, *The Rise of Theodore Roosevelt* (New York, 1979), the best biography of TR's life until 1901, although weak on the historical context of 1895 to 1901; see especially pp. 98, 224, 463.
4. Healy, pp. 151–153.
5. Anne H. Oman, "Past and Present," *Washington Post Weekend*, 18 January 1985, p. 6; *Time*, March 3, 1958, p. 16; Nathan Miller, *Theodore Roosevelt, A Life* (New York, 1992) p. 387.
6. David Burton, *Theodore Roosevelt: Confident Imperialist* (Philadelphia, 1969), p. 137.
7. Albert K. Weinberg, *Manifest Destiny* (Baltimore, 1940), pp. 464–465.
8. Carl P. Parrini and Martin J. Sklar, "New Thinking about the Market, 1896–1904 . . . ," *Journal of Economic History* 48 (September 1983): 559–578, analyze, in a pioneering essay, the effects of surplus capital on U.S. foreign policy, especially in Asia from 1900 to 1904.
9. Arthur M. Schlesinger, Jr., *The Imperial Presidency* (Boston, 1973), p. 83.
10. Louis Henkin, *Foreign Affairs and the Constitution* (Mineola, N.Y., 1972), p. 309.
11. Alfred Thayer Mahan, *The Interest of America in Sea Power, Present and Future* (Boston, 1898), pp. 256–257, 268.
12. Woodrow Wilson, *Constitutional Government in the United States* (New York, 1908), pp. 78–80.
13. Lawrence Martin, *The Presidents and the Prime Ministers* (Toronto, 1982), p. 58.
14. Quoted in Morris, p. 3.
15. This argument is spelled out in Walter LaFeber, *The American Search for Opportunity, 1865–1913*, in *The Cambridge History of U.S. Foreign Relations*, ed. Warren Cohen (New York, 1993).
16. Howard K. Beale, *Theodore Roosevelt and the Rise of America to World Power* (New York, 1962), pp. 85–102, discusses the turn in TR's thinking toward England; see also Stuart Anderson, "Racial Anglo-Saxonism and the American Response to the Boer War," *Diplomatic History* 2 (Summer 1978): 219–236; Thomas J. Noer, *Briton, Boer and Yankee: The U.S. and South Africa, 1870–1914* (Kent, Ohio, 1978), pp. 5–20, 135, 186.
17. Martin, pp. 58–61.

18. John Hay to William McKinley, 23 September 1900, Papers of William McKinley, Library of Congress, Washington, D.C.

19. Richard L. Lael, *Arrogant Diplomacy: U.S. Policy Toward Colombia, 1903–1922* (Wilmington, Del., 1987), esp. p. xiv; Michael L. Conniff, *Panama and the United States* (Athens, Ga., 1992), pp. 33–34.

20. Dana G. Munro, *Intervention and Dollar Diplomacy in the Caribbean, 1900–1921* (Princeton, 1964), pp. 57–58; David S. Patterson, *Toward a Warless World: The Travail of the American Peace Movement, 1887–1914* (Bloomington, Ind., 1976), pp. 124–125.

21. Richard W. Leopold, *Elihu Root and the Conservative Tradition* (Boston, 1954), p. 178; *Public Opinion* 35 (19 November 1903): 645.

22. J. Bartlett, *Familiar Quotations* (Boston, 1981), p. 687.

23. Healy, pp. 112–113.

24. Dexter Perkins, *The Monroe Doctrine, 1867–1907* (Baltimore, 1937), p. 394.

25. *Ibid.*, pp. 419–421.

26. *Ibid.*, pp. 408–409.

27. The document is available in *The Record of American Diplomacy*, ed. Ruhl J. Bartlett, 4th ed. (New York, 1964), p. 539.

28. Theodore Roosevelt, *The Letters of Theodore Roosevelt*, ed. Elting E. Morison *et al.*, 8 vols. (Cambridge, Mass., 1951–1954), IV, p. 734.

29. Perkins, p. 440.

30. Daniel Aaron, *Men of Good Hope* (New York, 1961), p. 268.

31. Brooks Adams to Theodore Roosevelt, 17 July 1903, Papers of Theodore Roosevelt, Library of Congress, Washington, D.C.

32. Theodore Roosevelt to Brooks Adams, 18 July 1903, *ibid.*

33. This loan is analyzed in Grosvenor Jones, Chief, Investment and Financial Division, Bureau of Foreign and Domestic Commerce, to Herbert Hoover, 7 August 1926, Commerce, Off. Files, Box 130, Herbert Hoover Library, West Branch, Iowa.

34. Henry Adams to Elizabeth Cameron, 10 January 1904, in Henry Adams, *Letters of Henry Adams (1892–1918)*, ed. Worthington Chauncey Ford (Boston, 1938), pp. 419–420.

35. John Edward Wiltz, "Did the United States Betray Korea in 1905?" *Pacific Historical Review* 54 (August 1985): 243–270.

36. Paul A. Varg, *The Making of a Myth: The U.S. and China, 1897–1912* (East Lansing, 1968), pp. 83–88.

37. This fascinating story is told in Sherman Cochran, "Commercial Penetration and Economic Imperialism in China . . . ," in *America's China Trade in Historical Perspective: The Chinese and American Performance*, ed. John K. Fairbank and Ernest R. May (Cambridge, Mass., 1985), pp. 190–194, esp. for the boycott.

38. Michael H. Hunt, *The Making of a Special Relationship: The United States and China to 1914* (New York, 1983), pp. 204–208.

39. These paragraphs on Taft (and the ones on Knox that follow) are drawn from three good accounts: Walter Scholes and Marie Scholes, *The Foreign Policies of the Taft Administration* (Columbia, Mo., 1970), esp. pp. 1–31; Donald F. Anderson, *William Howard Taft: A Conservative's Conception of the Presidency* (Ithaca, N.Y., 1968); James Barber, *Presidential Character* (Englewood Cliffs, N.J., 1972), pp. 174–190, which has an interesting section on Taft.

40. Quoted in Lloyd Gardner *et al.*, *The Creation of the American Empire*, 2d ed. (Chicago, 1976), p. 280.

41. Michael H. Hunt, *Frontier Defense and the Open Door: Manchuria in Chinese-American Relations, 1895–1911* (New Haven, 1973), p. 228.

42. *Ibid.*, p. 241; Straight to Calhoun, 7 November, 1911, in Papers of Willard Straight, Cornell University, Ithaca, N.Y.; *New York Times*, 20 March 1983, p. E5.

43. Henry Pringle, *Theodore Roosevelt, a Biography* (New York, 1931), pp. 684–685.

44. Richard D. Challener, *Admirals, Generals, and American Foreign Policy* (Princeton, 1973), p. 20.

45. *Foreign Relations of the United States, 1906*, 2 pts. (Washington, D.C., 1909), pt. II, pp. 1457–1461.

46. The best account is Thomas L. Karnes, *The Failure of Union: Central America, 1824–1975* (Tempe, Ariz., 1976), pp. 200–202.

47. Thomas P. McCann, *An American Company*, ed. Henry Scammell (New York, 1976), pp. 15–30; William H. Durham, *Scarcity and Survival in Central America . . .* (Stanford, 1979), pp. 115–118; Mitchell Seligson, "Agrarian Policies in Dependent Societies: Costa Rica," *Journal of Interamerican Studies* 19 (May 1977): 218–224.

48. Walter LaFeber, *Inevitable Revolutions: The United States in Central America*, 2nd ed. (New York, 1993), pp. 47–51.

49. Robert Hannigan, "Reciprocity 1911: Continentalism and American Weltpolitik," *Diplomatic History* 4 (Winter 1980): 1–18.

50. Judson M. Lyon, "Informal Imperialism: The U.S. in Liberia, 1897–1912," *Diplomatic History* 5 (Summer 1981): 221–243.

51. The standard account remains Calvin D. Davis's prize-winning *The United States and the First Hague Peace Conference* (Ithaca, N.Y., 1962), esp. pp. 54–102, on the peace movement, and 207–212, on Roosevelt and the court.

For Further Reading

Pre-1981 references are most easily found in *Guide to American Foreign Relations since 1700*, ed. Richard Dean Burns (1983). Also see the notes to this chapter and the General Bibliography at the end of this book; those references are usually not repeated here.

Fresh overviews of Roosevelt and presidential power during these years can be found in Richard H. Collin, *Theodore Roosevelt, Culture, Diplomacy, and Expansion* (1985); John Milton Cooper, Jr., *The Warrior and the Priest: Woodrow Wilson and Theodore Roosevelt* (1983); Frederick W. Marks III, "Theodore Roosevelt and the Conservative Revival," in *Studies in American Diplomacy, 1865–1945*, ed. Norman A. Graebner (1985); Kathleen Dalton, "Theodore Roosevelt and the Idea of War," *Theodore Roosevelt Association Journal* 7 (Fall 1981), an interesting cultural perspective; Lawrence Margolis, *Executive Agreements and Presidential Power* (1985), a historical framework for TR's acts in 1904–1905; George Juergens, *News from the White House: The Presidential-Press Relationship in the Progressive Era* (1981).

Three recent economic-historical analyses are pathbreaking: Paul Wolman, *Most*

Favored Nation (Chapel Hill, N.C., 1992), on the tariff battles, 1897–1912; Emily S. Rosenberg, "Foundations of U.S. International Financial Power: Gold Standard Diplomacy, 1900–1905," *Business History Review* 59 (Summer 1985); and Vivian Vale, *The American Peril* (1984), on J. P. Morgan versus Great Britain. For Latin America, Lester Langley's *The Banana Wars* (1983, 1988) is a starting point for the Caribbean–Central American region; Louis A. Pérez, Jr.'s *Cuba under the Platt Amendment, 1902–1934* (1986) is now a standard account; Thomas Schoonover's "Imperialism in Middle America," in *Eagle against Empire*, ed. Rhodri Jeffreys-Jones (1983), places the U.S. drive for an isthmian canal amid the international scramble in a pioneering essay; J. Michael Hogan's *The Panama Canal in American Politics* (1986) is excellent on Roosevelt; Terence Graham's *The "Interests of Civilization": Reaction in the United States against the Seizure of the Panama Canal Zone, 1903–1904*, Lund Studies in International History (1983), well tells a story long needed to be told; Ivan Musicant's *The Banana Wars* (1990) provides an important overview; Leslie Manigat's "The Substitution of American for French Preponderance in Haiti, 1910–1911," in *Diplomatic Claims: Latin American Historians View the United States*, ed. and trans. Warren Dean (1985), is a critical view of a critical turn. On Canadian relations, R. A. Shields's "Imperial Policy and Canadian-American Commercial Relations, 1880–1911," *Bulletin of the Institute of Historical Research* 59 (May 1986), supplements the Hannigan essay listed in the notes.

Three good overviews of U.S.-Asian relations have been recently published: Michael H. Hunt's *The Making of a Special Relationship: The U.S. and China to 1914* (1983), especially important for its analysis of the Chinese side; James C. Thomson, Jr., Peter W. Stanley, and John Curtis Perry, *Sentimental Imperialists: The American Experience in East Asia* (1981), for its controversial view of U.S. motives; and Daniel M. Crane and Thomas A. Breslin, *An Ordinary Relationship: American Opposition to Republican Revolution in China* (1986), which puts the years 1911 to 1914 within a century of U.S. opposition to revolutions. The nonofficial dimension is studied in Key Ray Chong, *Americans and Chinese Reform and Revolution, 1898–1922: The Role of Private Citizens in Diplomacy* (1984), with emphasis on Sun Yat-sen's links to Americans. Raymond A. Esthus, *Double Eagle and the Rising Sun: The Russians and Japanese at Portsmouth in 1905* (1988), should become a standard account of the conference. A good overview of the entire era is Joseph A. Fry, "In Search of an Orderly World: U.S. Imperialism, 1898–1912," in *Modern American Diplomacy*, ed. John M. Carroll and George C. Herring (1986).

9

Wilsonians, Revolutions, and War (1913–1917)

THE WORLD OF WOODROW WILSON

It was Woodrow Wilson's fate to be the first U.S. president to face the full blast of twentieth-century revolutions. Wilson's responses made his policies the most influential in twentieth-century American foreign policy. "Wilsonian" became a term to describe later policies that emphasized internationalism and moralism and that were dedicated to extending democracy. Critics described them as unrealistic and especially unaware of power (by which the critics usually meant military power). Wilson's policies, however, now appear to be more complex and instructive than either his supporters or critics claimed. Many later presidents, including Lyndon Johnson, Richard Nixon, and Jimmy Carter, looked back to Wilson as the chief executive who had the largest vision of the nation's future and who had first confronted challenges that continued to plague them.

Born in Virginia in 1856, Wilson was the first native southerner to reach the White House since 1849. He had trained as a lawyer but failed miserably in his practice. The failure tended to make him mistrustful of lawyers and turned him toward an academic career. By 1912, Wilson had become a national figure. A respected political scientist and lecturer, he was president of Princeton and then the highly successful Progressive governor of New Jersey. His success came not only from his speaking ability, but also from a sharp, analytical mind that was as able to place problems in a historical context as any president's in the American experience.

A stern Calvinist, devout Presbyterian, Wilson believed he was guided by God's will. Wilson often appeared cold even to those whose support he needed. A leading Progressive journalist complained that the president's handshake was "like a ten-cent pickled mackerel in brown paper." The new chief executive even refused to attend his own inaugural dance. Privately, another Wilson sometimes appeared. This one loved vaudeville, baseball, told jokes in excellent dialect, wrote limericks, and loudly sang "Oh, You Beautiful Doll" when he courted his second wife in 1915; it now appears that he had an affair in Bermuda with a married woman during 1908. The tensions that resulted from such a background not only made him highly complex, but also caused him, starting in 1896 (when he was not yet forty), to suffer a series of small strokes. By 1916, he had to restrict his work time in the White House, and by 1919—during the critical days of the peace conference—he had to spend much time in bed recovering from flu and exhaustion.[1]

Wilson was not only a politician, but a scholar who developed policies out of an understanding of the nation's history. He knew that the large corporation was a staggering new fact of national life, but he nevertheless wanted to use government to reinforce traditional political and moral values. In his first inaugural address, Wilson repeatedly emphasized that "our duty is . . . to restore" and, again, "our work is a work of restoration." He demanded that the new corporate system be opened up so that "the little man on the make," as Wilson proudly called him, could have a chance along with the rulers of U.S. Steel. His view of history, especially his understanding that the nation's landed frontier had closed, nevertheless forced Wilson to conclude that "the days of glad expansion are gone, our life grows tense and difficult." The president had learned this directly from the great historian of the frontier, Frederick Jackson Turner. The two had met during the 1880s at Johns Hopkins University. Wilson believed that with the frontier "lost," a "new epoch will open for us."[2]

The implications for foreign policy seemed endless. U.S. producers, Wilson warned in 1912, "have expanded to such a point that they will burst their jackets if they cannot find a free outlet to the markets of the world."[3] A frontier of world markets had to be found to replace the lost landed frontier. The government, led by a strong president, must open and order those new frontiers. "The truth is that in the new order," Wilson announced, "government and business must be associated."[4]

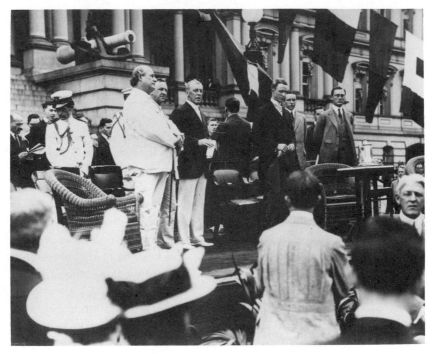

Woodrow Wilson's power as chief executive (1913–1921) arose in part from his oratorical ability. Here in white trousers, Wilson speaks in Washington during 1913 while at the far right his young assistant secretary of the navy, Franklin D. Roosevelt, and on the left his secretary of state, William Jennings Bryan, look on.

The young political scientist had been one of the first to understand the impact of the 1898 war on presidential power: "Foreign questions became leading questions again," and "in them the President was of necessity leader." Even before 1898, Wilson believed that at critical times, "the pleasure of the people" had to give way to presidential power: "He *exercises* the power, and *we obey*."[5]

He followed this principle in the White House. At times it worked. Between 1913 and 1916, he pushed through Congress a significant series of reform measures, including the 1913 Underwood Tariff that lowered rates significantly for the first time since 1894. At other times, however (as in the 1919 fight over the peace treaty), Americans refused to "obey" the president. As a student of British politics, he admired the parliamentary system in which the prime minister, as the leader of the majority party, almost automatically was assured victory. Wilson grew short-tempered with the more cumbersome American system. Until

1918, he nevertheless dealt effectively with Congress. One reason was his decision to appear before Congress (somewhat like the British prime minister) and deliver his annual and other special messages personally. Since the time of Jefferson, who knew he was not an orator, presidents had merely sent their messages to Capitol Hill via courier. Wilson changed all that, and as he was able to whip Congress into line, he sometimes paid little attention to public opinion. Public-opinion polls did not exist. He seemed to have read newspapers unsystematically. The man in charge of the White House mail room recalled that the president apparently cared little about incoming letters. During several diplomatic crises in 1914–1916 (such as the *Sussex* episode), Wilson almost totally isolated himself, then emerged to issue a policy—often personally pecked out on his own typewriting machine. Robert Lansing, his second secretary of state, noted that Wilson's "very nature resisted outbursts of popular passion. . . . He had the faculty of remaining impervious to such influences, which so often affect the minds of lesser men."[6]

His reading of history shaped foreign policy in yet another way. Wilson feared revolutionary change. He wanted order—or at least slow reform. The president believed that the American system had prospered because it avoided radical change. In 1889, he wrote that the year marked the centennial of both the U.S. Constitution and the French Revolution. "One hundred years ago," he concluded, "we gained, and Europe lost, self-command, self-possession." A people could not be "given" democracy, Wilson argued. It required "long discipline" and "a reverence for law."[7] Thus, for example, he doubted that Filipinos were fit for self-government. American ideas and goods, however, could prepare others for democracy—and could do so while making profits:

> Lift your eyes to the horizons of business [he told a U.S. business group visiting the White House] . . . let your thoughts and your imaginations run abroad throughout the whole world, and with the inspiration of the thought that you are Americans and are meant to carry liberty and justice and the principles of humanity wherever you go, go out and sell goods that will make the world more comfortable and more happy, and convert them to the principles of America.[8]

The landed frontier had closed, but, luckily, the world frontier now spread out before Americans. With some government help, ambitious, hard-working Americans ("the little man on the make") could find opportunities abroad. The president, in leading these efforts, wanted that world to be a safe and an orderly place in which Americans could compete equally—perhaps even a place in which all people, with enough time and help, would become much like Americans.

Wilson's views were reinforced by the few foreign-policy advisers he consulted. He first named William Jennings Bryan secretary of state not because Bryan knew much about foreign policy (he did not), but for his long service to the Democratic party. Bryan agreed with Wilson's emphasis on the need to help others with U.S. goods and values. Taft's dollar diplomacy, Bryan complained, tried to "till the field of foreign investment with a pen knife; President Wilson intends to cultivate it with a spade."[9] Bryan also shared many of Wilson's traditional values, although Bryan's came from a nineteenth-century rural America that seemed quaint to some. The secretary of state was "irresistably funny," young journalist Walter Lippmann wrote, "because he moves in a world that has ceased to exist."[10] But at a critical moment in 1915, Bryan resigned as a matter of principle because he believed that Wilson was no longer truly neutral in the European war. He was replaced by Robert Lansing, a New York lawyer who was well connected (his uncle had been a secretary of state in the 1890s; his nephew, John Foster Dulles, was to occupy the office during the 1950s). Lansing was pro-British and as worried as Wilson over revolutionary outbreaks.

The president's closest adviser never held a formal office. Colonel Edward M. House, born in Texas, educated in the Northeast, and reared in smoke-filled rooms of Democratic party bosses, befriended Wilson in 1911–1912 to ride his coattails into power. Independently wealthy, he traveled abroad to talk with the powerful. House was as stealthy and secretive as a cat. One official who thought he was a close friend only years later learned that House had tried to ruin him. The colonel "was an intimate," the official's son noted, "even when he was cutting a throat."[11] Wilson appreciated House's discretion as well as the colonel's large view of policy.

Much of that view appeared in a remarkable novel, *Philip Dru: Administrator*, which House published anonymously in 1912. Dru, as House portrayed him, was a West Point graduate who all Americans demanded had to assume near-dictatorial powers to save them from rich, short-sighted interests that were driving the people to revolution. By issuing brilliant decrees (note that Congress was not to be consulted), Dru saved the country and made it prosperous and happy again. He then turned to foreign policy. Here Dru and his creator began to converge. In both the novel and real life, House urged that a U.S.-British partnership had to be developed into which Germany would be

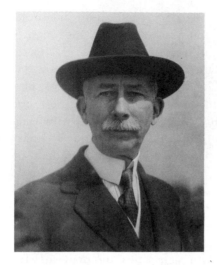

Politician, strategic thinker, and world-class flatterer, Edward M. House (1858–1938) came out of Texas politics and eastern drawing rooms to become Wilson's closest foreign-policy adviser, although he never held office. House's shrewdness and slyness come through in this portrait.

drawn. The three would then destroy the great threat to the West by driving "Russia back" (as the novel put it). Once Russia was properly contained, House believed that the three powers could then divide up, develop, and stabilize the rest of the world.[12] Such cooperation could halt the senseless fight over colonial areas as well as stop the growing militarization that threatened to bankrupt, if not destroy, Great Britain and Germany.

Wilson came to the White House with no direct experience in foreign policy. But with House close by and his own sense of history, the new president quickly developed strong, well-thought-out views to guide his decisions.

WILSON AND REVOLUTION: CHINA

In his first major diplomatic action, Wilson ditched Taft's dollar diplomacy in Asia. He pulled U.S. bankers out of the six-power consortium set up to stabilize China. Wilson withdrew not because he feared that the consortium would exploit the new Chinese republic that had arisen in 1911 from the ashes of the Manchu dynasty. Nor did he have any intention of deserting the open door. He fully understood that China was "the market to which diplomacy, if need be power, must make an open way," as he had written a decade earlier.[13]

Wilson rejected the consortium because he understood that the Russians and Japanese, who showed little regard for the open door, controlled the group. Moreover, while the United States was in the consortium, his hands would be tied. Wilson wanted to use growing U.S. economic power and go it alone in China. He also planned to bring in smaller U.S. bankers (those "little men on the make") and not depend on the few giants who had joined the original group. As historian Jerry Israel summarizes the president's policy, "Rather than a rejection of the open door goals, the American withdrawal . . . was an effort to speed up their attainment by the United States alone."[14]

The president was willing to pay a price. In a cabinet meeting, Wilson ordered that the U.S. Navy be on alert for a possible challenge from Japan, then reported one expert's advice that U.S. financial power by itself could build 10,000 miles of railroads in China. In May 1913, he recognized the new Chinese ruler, Yüan Shih-k'ai. Yüan had seized the revolution from its father, Sun Yat-sen, and then set about destroying its republicanism and making himself a monarch. Wilson never protested. He wanted only to work with any Chinese leader who promised stability and cooperation.

Fifteen months later, Wilson's dreams shattered as World War I erupted. Suddenly the British, French, Germans, and Russians—who Wilson assumed would check each other and the Japanese in China— were absorbed in Europe. Virtually alone, Japan swiftly moved to seize the exposed German colonies, including the key entry point at Shantung. Only the United States could possibly check Japanese power, but Wilson was preoccupied with European and Mexican affairs. U.S. bankers sent vast sums to both sides fighting in Europe and had none to spare for China. The president, moreover, deeply mourned when his first wife died in 1914, then quickly became involved in a passionate courtship with Edith Galt that led to marriage the next year. Willard Straight watched his hard work for the open door disappear in the wake of Japan's advance and privately cursed the president for making love, not war. Wilson seemed "somewhat similar to the white rabbit," Straight remarked to a friend, "with the sex instinct strongly developed but unwilling to protect its young."[15]

On January 18, 1915, Japan secretly pressed China to accept a document that became known as the Twenty-one Demands. Wilson found out about most of the demands, but because they largely involved areas in which Japan was already dominant, he did little. The Chinese, however, told Bryan that a final, secret set of the demands would give Japan influence in China's military and police as well as in the vital Yangtze River region of central China. When the Japanese ambassador blandly denied the accusation, Bryan believed him. But American missionaries

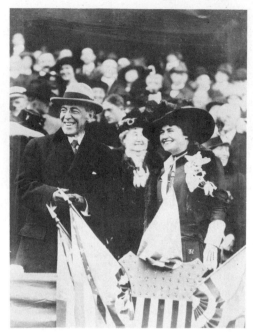

The president and his soon-to-be second wife, Mrs. Edith Galt, attend baseball's 1915 World Series. After Wilson's illness in 1919, she became a powerful figure who greatly influenced White House decision making.

in China and U.S. ambassador Paul Reinsch obtained evidence that Bryan had been lied to. In two tough notes in March and May 1915, Wilson told Japan to back down from the secret demands. Tokyo officials did so, but not because of U.S. pressure. Their own internal politics and British opposition forced them to retreat. Wilson had nevertheless repeated the historic U.S. commitment to Asia. As historian Noel Pugach observes, "In the historically important note of May 11, 1915, the United States declared to China and Japan that it would not recognize any agreement which impaired the right of the United States, the political or territorial integrity of China, or the Open Door." [16]

Wilson had hoped to enjoy both the open door and freedom of action in China. Now, with Japan on the loose, his policy was endangered. A century of U.S. policy in the region hung in the balance. Ambassador Reinsch urged the president to work with China against the Japanese. But Colonel House and Secretary of State Lansing (who replaced Bryan in June 1915) wanted Wilson to control Japan through cooperation— to work with, rather than fight, Tokyo. As the United States itself prepared to go to war in early 1917, Wilson believed that he had no choice.

The United States took two steps to cut a deal with Japan. First, in November 1917, the secretary of state negotiated the Lansing-Ishii Agreement. In it, the United States recognized that "territorial propinquity creates special relations between countries." This meant that the United States recognized Japanese dominance in such areas as southern Manchuria. But Japan, in turn, reaffirmed the open door. Lansing and Ambassador Kikujiro Ishii also agreed on a protocol that remained secret until 1938. It stipulated that neither side would use the war to gain privileges in China at the expense of other states. The protocol attempted to short-circuit anything more like the Twenty-one Demands.

Wilson's second step was to control Japan by repudiating his 1913 policy and, instead, creating a second consortium. The United States, Japan, Great Britain, and France would cooperate in investment projects in China. Japanese financiers could thus be more closely watched. Wilson was not coy about government-business relations. He promised "complete support" to U.S. bankers as he asked them to join the new group. That a revolutionary China might soon try to control its own affairs worried few officials in Washington.

WILSON AND REVOLUTIONS: MEXICO
(OR, PAINTING THE FENCE POST WHITE)

Until World War I demanded his attention, Wilson was immersed in the problems of revolutions in China, Mexico, and the Caribbean region. He understood that the upheavals arose out of such internal problems as poverty, oppression, and the failure of government to protect its citizens. He also realized that foreign intervention seldom cooled revolutionary fervor; the fervor only became more intense and antiforeign. But along with these views about internal causes, he concluded that revolutions could be caused by foreign corporate and banking interests that exploited smaller nations. By checking such interests and by cleansing a country's internal politics, revolution could be avoided. No better way existed to cleanse those politics and create a legitimate government, he reasoned, than democratic elections.

Determined to help other peoples become democratic and orderly, Wilson himself became the greatest military interventionist in U.S. history. By the time he left office in 1921, he had ordered troops into Russia and half a dozen Latin American upheavals. To preserve order in some countries, Wilson learned, required military intervention. He was not unwilling to use force. Journalist Walter Lippmann recalled

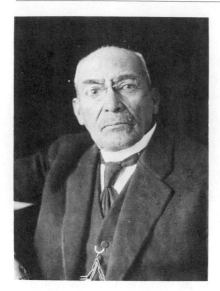

Victoriano Huerta took control of the Mexican Revolution in 1912–1913, only to run into Wilson's opposition. Their feud not only shaped U.S.-Mexican relations, but led to a historic change in U.S. recognition policy.

"one metaphor [Wilson] used to like to use a great deal illustrating his idea of how a progressive attitude was really conservative. He said 'If you want to preserve a fence post, you have to keep painting it white. You can't just paint it once and leave it forever. It will rot away.' "[17]

Some people, however, had concluded that their "fence posts" no longer served a useful purpose. They wanted the posts pulled up, not repainted. The Mexicans began reaching this conclusion in 1910–1911, when they rallied to Francisco Madero's attempt to overthrow the thirty-four-year-old dictatorship of Porfirio Díaz. Many U.S. interests were not pleased. Under Díaz's regime, U.S. investment in Mexico had sky-rocketed to nearly $2 billion, much of it in rich oil wells. Americans owned 43 percent of all the property values in Mexico—10 percent more than the Mexicans themselves owned.[18] Madero overthrew Díaz (who was rapidly becoming senile) but found that he had let loose forces he could not control. A number of armed groups tried to claim power. Unable to restore order, Madero was captured by a band led by Victoriano Huerta. The U.S. ambassador to Mexico, Henry Lane Wilson, was deeply involved in pushing Madero out of power, but he declared his surprise when Huerta's men killed Madero.

At this point, Woodrow Wilson entered the White House. Huerta not only had blood on his hands, but rumors circulated that he was supported by British oil interests that had long been in bitter competition with U.S. companies. London and other capitals soon recognized

Huerta's government. Wilson, however, refused. The president objected to Huerta's use of force to gain power. He feared that if the Mexican leader remained in power, other Latin American revolutionaries would follow his example. Wilson demanded that Mexico hold democratic elections. The president thus transformed U.S. recognition policy that went back to Jefferson's time. The United States had usually recognized any government that maintained internal order and agreed to meet foreign obligations (such as debts). Wilson added a third requirement: the new government had to come to power through a process acceptable to the United States. Most governments, of course, did not have America's democratic tradition. Indeed, he did recognize certain regimes (such as China's or Peru's) that made no pretense to being democracies. The belief grew that, in Mexico, the president used his demand for democratic elections only to get rid of the Huerta regime he so disliked.

The president began supporting Huerta's enemies, especially Venustiano Carranza, who led well-armed forces. Wilson sent a personal agent, John Lind, to tell Huerta that if he held an election in which he was not a candidate, a large loan might be available from U.S. oil, railway, and copper interests in Mexico.[19] Lind, a Minnesota politician who knew little about diplomacy, did not handle his mission well. Huerta turned down the attempt to bribe him and, with British support, conducted an election he handily won. (The election was so open, moreover, that even Lind reported he had cast a ballot.) Deeply angered, Wilson began to turn the screws on Huerta. He was determined, he said, that the Mexican government "be founded on a moral basis." Sir Edward Grey, the British secretary of state for foreign affairs, privately remarked that "it would require about 200,000 soldiers to put Mexico on a 'moral basis.' " Grey stepped back, however, after Wilson assured London that British interests in Mexico would be protected.[20]

Then, on October 27, 1913, Wilson warned, in a speech at Mobile, Alabama, that exploitative foreign "concessions" were no longer to be tolerated in Latin America. Claiming that his own nation's motives were pure ("the United States will never again seek one additional foot of territory by conquest"), the president said that Americans only wanted to be "friends" of other nations on terms "of equality and honor." He would oppose "foreign interests" that tried to "dominate" Latin America and so create "a condition . . . always dangerous and apt to become intolerable."[21] As the British and other foreign governments understood, the Mobile Address was Wilson's declaration that he now would try to throw out any foreign "concessions" that in his view created "intolerable" conditions. The British also began to realize that Huerta's days were numbered.

The president's opportunity arose suddenly in April 1914, when Huerta's agents arrested seven U.S. sailors who, while on shore leave, had wandered into a forbidden area. Huerta quickly apologized, but Wilson made a series of demands to satisfy American "honor." When Huerta rejected them, Wilson appeared before Congress to ask for the use of U.S. military force against Mexico. As Congress stalled and investigated the charges, the president learned that a German ship planned to unload arms for Huerta at Vera Cruz. Wilson ordered U.S. vessels to occupy the port. Firing broke out that killed 19 Americans and over 300 Mexicans. Latin American nations intervened to help restore peace and meet Wilson's real objective: Huerta's removal. In August 1914, Carranza assumed power. Wilson had apparently won—but only apparently. An ardent nationalist, Carranza refused to bargain with Wilson. The frustrated president now turned to aiding anti-Carranza forces, including Pancho Villa.

Carranza responded with one of the most momentous acts in the revolution. He announced plans for agrarian reform and, most notably, for Mexico's claim to all its subsoil mineral rights. In a stroke, the revolution had turned sharply to the left and threatened U.S. oil companies.[22] Wilson intensified his pressure on Carranza, but the Mexican leader succeeded in destroying most of Villa's forces. The president, involved in a continual series of crises arising out of the world war, most reluctantly recognized Carranza's government *de facto* in late 1915.

Villa responded by terrorizing Arizona and New Mexico in the hope that Wilson's military retaliation would undermine Carranza. When Villa murdered seventeen Americans in Columbus, New Mexico, and eighteen U.S. engineers in Mexico itself, Wilson demanded that Carranza allow U.S. troops to track down the killers. Carranza reluctantly agreed, but imposed limits on the movements of U.S. forces. In March 1916, 6,000 men under the command of Major-General John J. ("Black Jack") Pershing rode across the border. Pershing never captured Villa, but his forces did clash with Carranza's army when it tried to restrict Pershing's men. Forty Mexican and two U.S. troops died. Wilson was trapped. He knew the mission was failing. Carranza was firmly in power. But Wilson was determined to remove Carranza, and his determination was strongly reinforced by U.S. Roman Catholics, who feared the growing anticlericalism in the revolution. In early 1917, however, Wilson realized that he would have to enter the European struggle. He pulled out Pershing's forces and began coming to terms with Carranza.

The president had tried to stabilize and democratize the Mexican Revolution. Eighty percent of the people had never had a "look-in," he declared. "I am for that 80 percent!" He believed he knew what to do: "They say the Mexicans are not fitted for self-government," he had declared in early 1914, "and to this I reply that, when properly directed, there is no people not fitted for self-government." In "properly" directing the Mexican Revolution, however, Wilson twice invaded the country and killed Mexicans. Trying to repaint the old fence post proved expensive.

WILSON AND REVOLUTIONS: CENTRAL AMERICA AND THE CARIBBEAN

Upon entering office, Wilson declared that he wanted "orderly processes" in Latin America as well as stability in "the markets which we must supply."[23] But frequently, maintaining order meant maintaining the *status quo*. In much of Latin America, the *status quo* meant maintaining small elites who (as had Porfirio Díaz in Mexico) worked with foreign interests and exploited their own people. Only revolution or foreign intervention could overthrow such elites. "Democracy" often meant the continued power of those elites because they controlled elections. Wilson wanted elections, real change, order, and no foreign interventions—all at once. He never discovered how to pull off such a miracle. When he then chose order, Wilson and Bryan had to send troops into Haiti, Santo Domingo, and Cuba, as well as Mexico. Latin Americans began to call the U.S. Marines "State Department troops."

In 1913, the marines already were protecting the U.S.-created government in Nicaragua (see p. 262). President Adolfo Díaz's bankrupt regime needed money quickly. Bryan, who had made his political career by attacking bankers, had a novel idea. Why not, he asked Wilson, have the U.S. government lend the money to Nicaragua? The bankers and their exorbitant claims would be bypassed, banks and railways would remain in Central American hands, and it could "prevent revolutions, promote education, and advance stable and just government." Wilson rejected the plan. Substituting government funds for private bank loans would be too "novel and radical."[24] Bryan then resorted to the bankers, who already owned 51 percent of Nicaragua's national bank and railways. The bankers loaned Díaz another $1 million in return for the rest of the railways.

Díaz next asked that Nicaraguan (by which he meant his own) stability be guaranteed by extending the Platt Amendment's principles to the country. Bryan agreed to extend the protectorate, but the U.S. Senate rejected the plan. The secretary of state did sign the Bryan-Chamorro Treaty (finally approved in 1916) that gave Washington exclusive rights to build an isthmian canal through Nicaragua. In return, Díaz's regime received $3 million. The U.S. banks, U.S. government, and U.S. Marines controlled Nicaragua.

Wilson next ordered the marines to Haiti. That country, about the size of Maryland, had defeated the French colonials in 1804 to become the world's first black republic. Between 1843 and 1915, however, twenty-two dictators ruled Haiti in a highly corrupt version of a political revolving door. The last rulers in the line worked closely with German and French interests. Wilson disliked that connection. Moreover, the United States coveted the harbor of Môle St. Nicolas. When another revolt broke out in 1914, Bryan mentioned the Monroe Doctrine, told the Germans and French to stand aside, and asked Haiti for a treaty that handed over the country's vital interests to U.S. bankers. When the Haitians refused, Bryan landed marines, who carried $500,000 from the Haitian treasury back to New York City to protect, in the secretary of state's words, "American interests which were gravely menaced." With little financial support, the Haitian government began to collapse. Bryan demanded that elections be held. The Haitians refused. He then demanded that U.S. bankers be allowed to buy out the French interests and asked Wilson to have a U.S. warship available to obtain Haiti's attention.

The Haitians, meanwhile, were turning on President Vilbrun G. Sam, who thought he had assured himself a presidency for life by slaughtering over 160 of his imprisoned political opponents. A mob pulled Sam out of his hiding place in the French legation, hacked his body into pieces, placed parts on poles, then dragged the remaining trunk of the body through the dusty streets. Intent on teaching such mobs the meaning of democracy and order, Wilson dispatched the marines. A new government signed a treaty in August 1915 that granted the United States control over the country's foreign and financial affairs, and also the right to intervene whenever Washington officials thought it necessary. The marines remained for nineteen years.

The other part of Haiti's home island, Hispaniola, is occupied by the Dominican Republic. After 1904, when U.S. officials controlled its customshouses through the grace of the Roosevelt Corollary (see p. 247), the Dominican Republic remained stable until 1911. Renewed

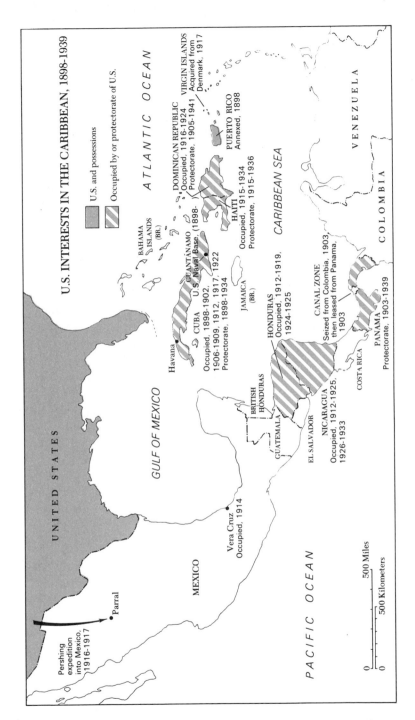

U.S. INTERESTS IN THE CARIBBEAN, 1898-1939

U.S. and possessions

Occupied by or protectorate of U.S.

ATLANTIC OCEAN

VIRGIN ISLANDS
Acquired from
Denmark, 1917

PUERTO RICO
Annexed, 1898

DOMINICAN REPUBLIC
Occupied, 1916-1924
Protectorate, 1905-1941

HAITI
Occupied, 1915-1934
Protectorate, 1915-1936

CARIBBEAN SEA

VENEZUELA

COLOMBIA

BAHAMA
ISLANDS
(BR.)

GUANTÁNAMO
U.S. Naval Base, (1898-

CUBA
Occupied, 1898-1902,
1906-1909, 1912, 1917, 1922
Protectorate, 1898-1934

JAMAICA
(BR.)

Havana

HONDURAS
Occupied, 1912-1919,
1924-1925

CANAL ZONE
Seized from Colombia, 1903,
then leased from Panama,
1903

PANAMA
Protectorate, 1903-1939

COSTA RICA

BRITISH
HONDURAS

GUATEMALA

EL SALVADOR

NICARAGUA
Occupied, 1912-1925,
1926-1933

UNITED STATES

GULF OF MEXICO

MEXICO

Vera Cruz
Occupied, 1914

Parral

Pershing
expedition
into Mexico,
1916-1917

PACIFIC OCEAN

500 Miles

500 Kilometers

The United States was active in the Caribbean throughout the post-1890s era, but, as the dates indicate, Wilson's administration was the most active.

disorder led Wilson in 1914 to demand the usual remedy: U.S.-sponsored elections. The government agreed to elections but not to the president's next demand—that U.S. bankers oversee the country's finances. In 1916, the government threatened to default on its debt. Eager to protect strategic routes in the Caribbean as well as to stop possible instability, Wilson landed the marines in May of that year. The U.S. military tried to rule the capital city of Santo Domingo, but guerrilla warfare tore the country apart between 1917 and 1922. U.S. investors took over large sugar and real-estate holdings. Racism fueled the anti-U.S. rebellion. (In a typical incident, a black shopkeeper brushed a U.S. soldier who screamed, "Look here, you damned Negro! Don't you know that no damned Negroes are supposed to let their bodies touch the body of any Marines?") By 1922, President Warren G. Harding's administration searched for an escape from the mess. The marines pulled out in 1925. A series of dictators again took over the country's affairs. As historian Kendrick Clements summarized, "Benevolent motives, backed by seemingly unlimited force, tempted the Americans to intervene where they were not wanted and where they did not understand the situation."[25] It would not be the last time in the twentieth century, unfortunately, that such a judgment could be made.

In June 1916, Wilson prepared a message to send to Congress. "It does not lie with the American people," he wrote, "to dictate to another people what their government shall be or what use shall be made of their resources." Secretary of State Lansing read the draft, then wrote in the margin: "Haiti, S. Domingo, Nicaragua, Panama." Wilson never sent the message. He did, however, keep U.S. troops in those places.[26]

THE UNITED STATES AND WORLD WAR I: LEGALITY VERSUS NEUTRALITY (1914–1916)

World War I began in August 1914. No one thought of it as a world war at first. The conflict seemed to resemble other crises that had arisen in the restless Balkans during 1908 and 1911–1913. These crises had been brought about by the slow collapse of the Austro-Hungarian and Ottoman empires. Circling the empires like vultures were two alliance systems—the Central Powers of Germany and Austria-Hungary itself, and the Entente (or Allied) powers of Great Britain, France, Russia, and, later, Italy. U.S. officials paid little attention to Balkan events. Nor, at first, did U.S. policy change in June 1914, when Archduke Francis Ferdinand of Austria was assassinated by a Serbian gunman.

When Austria tried to avenge itself against Serbia, however, Russia came to Serbia's side. Armies were mobilized, war declared, and bloodshed followed. Even then, many experts agreed with Captain Alfred Thayer Mahan's view that modern war was only an "occasional excess" from which recovery was easy. The huge arms build-up on both sides, these experts concluded, would deter either side from trying to push too hard.

By the autumn of 1914, it was clear that Mahan had been tragically wrong. As conflict expanded, all of Europe organized for war. Wilson issued a public statement urging Americans to be "neutral in fact as well as in name," "impartial in thought as well as in action." In reality, few could be neutral. Many recent Irish and German immigrants, for example, were anti-British. Many other Americans favored the Entente because of common language, the growth of economic ties, and the post-1895 warmth that cheered Anglo-American diplomats. That warmth rose considerably after British propagandists swamped the United States with stories of how the German "Huns" committed such atrocities as destroying the great library of Louvain when they invaded Belgium, killed in cold blood the famed British nurse Edith Cavell (who had, in truth, been acting as a spy), or, later, dispatched clumsy espionage agents to the United States itself.

Wilson's closest advisers quickly took sides. Colonel House had long hoped to work out U.S.-British-German cooperation. During the summer of 1914, House had been in Europe to sell these ideas to German and British leaders. As the war's shadows descended, the colonel feared that Wilson would have to choose between two evils: if the Central Powers won, German militarism would triumph; if the Allies won, then Russia could end up controlling central Europe. House chose to support the British and hoped that somehow the tsar could be held in check. Robert Lansing, then counselor in the Department of State, agreed. He was perhaps the most pro-British official in the administration's top echelons. Bryan took a more neutral position, although he was appalled by the German atrocities. Above all, the secretary of state did not want the United States to enter the war on either side.

It fell to Lansing to shape some of the first U.S. responses. When the war began, Wilson was recovering from the death of his first wife. The initial decisions, moreover, involved the U.S. response to the British naval blockade of German ports. As the administration's expert on international law, Lansing had some responsibility for drafting the proper response. By the end of 1914, he had strongly asserted U.S. neutral rights. But he had also gone far in recognizing the British right to stop

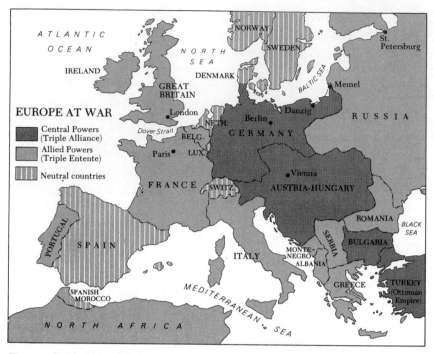

Europe divided bloodily between 1914 and 1918 as Americans (especially Wilson and House) had qualms about joining either the Central Powers or the Allies.

and search neutral (including U.S.) ships carrying munitions and other contraband (that is, weapons or other articles used to wage war) to the Central Powers. His position was good international law, but it also worked to Great Britain's advantage, especially when London officials began to expand the list of what they considered to be contraband.[27] The United States frequently protested British actions, but as Lansing later admitted, "I . . . prepared long and detailed replies" to complicate and prolong the controversies with London. Lansing hoped that as time passed, "the American people [would] perceive that German absolutism was a menace to their liberties."[28]

Lansing's tactics paid off. In February 1915, the Germans retaliated against the tightening British blockade with a submarine campaign aimed at Allied and neutral ships. The submarine (U-boat) was a shocking new weapon that brought sudden, unexpected death from the invisible depths of the Atlantic. There existed no body of international law to guide American responses to the U-boats. Wilson warned that he would hold Germany to "strict accountability" if U.S. ships were destroyed—although no one, including the president, knew exactly what this meant. The Germans took the position they had held for two years: they would call off their submarines if the British stopped trying to starve the Central Powers. Neither the British nor Wilson accepted that deal. Both believed that surface blockades were legal and traditional, but sudden submarine attacks illegal and uncivilized. In March 1915, the British passenger liner *Falaba* was sunk and one American life lost. In early May, the United States protested when one of its merchant ships was attacked and three lives lost.

Then, on May 7, a submarine sank the British liner *Lusitania*. Nearly 1,200 died, including 128 Americans. U.S. anti-German opinion grew white hot. Later investigation proved what the Germans claimed in 1915: the *Lusitania* was carrying a large cargo of munitions to Great Britain. Before it sailed, Germany had publicly warned that the ship was fair game. Wilson nevertheless prepared a note demanding that Germany pledge never again to attack a passenger liner. He insisted on the right of Americans to travel on any passenger ship they pleased. Bryan agreed on the need to protest but worried that the United States was moving slowly but surely into the Allied camp. He demanded that Wilson send an equally strong note to London protesting the British blockade. The president wavered and then, after discussing the problem with House (who was in London), refused Bryan's request. The secretary of state resigned.

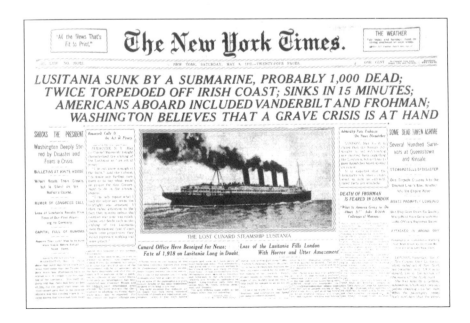

In his parting words, he not only questioned U.S. policy, but complained that Wilson had always allowed House to act as the real secretary of state. Louisville newspaper editor Henry Watterson expressed the popular reaction when he blasted Bryan's resignation: "Men have been shot and beheaded, even hanged, drawn, and quartered, for treason less heinous." Germany responded to Wilson's demand by apologizing for the *Lusitania* sinking and offering an indemnity. But the episode marked a turning point. Wilson had now decided to separate, openly and formally, British and German sea warfare. His demands of Germany were not to be related to his policies toward Great Britain's blockade. Bryan's resignation removed the most neutral member of the cabinet. Robert Lansing moved up to be secretary of state.[29]

In August 1915, a German submarine commander sank the British liner *Arabic* and killed two Americans. Berlin immediately disavowed the attack and apologized for the commander's action. Lansing warned that if Germany did not promise to stop attacking passenger liners (unless the passenger ships tried to escape or attack the subs), the United States "would certainly declare war." The kaiser's government finally made such a promise in the so-called *"Arabic* pledge." Merchant ships were not covered by the pledge; but in due time, Wilson would also have to close that loophole if he hoped to protect U.S. rights to travel and sell to both belligerents.

Wilson's decided tilt toward the Allies became especially notable when he had to decide whether U.S. bankers should be allowed to grant credits and loans to the belligerents. The stakes were high, for they involved nothing less than the health of the American economy. When the war began in mid-1914, the economy was entering a severe slump. The two key exports, wheat and cotton, depended on British and German markets. As the war demand shot upward, especially for these exports, the Allies and Central Powers discovered that they were quickly exhausting their cash reserves. They needed financial help, preferably loans from the Americans, who were—as Jefferson had put it a century before—"fattening upon the follies" of Europeans.

The administration at first decided against allowing loans. As Bryan declared, "Money is the worst of all contrabands because it commands everything else." But without money, the Europeans could not buy, and without their buying, the United States faced economic bad times. Wilson and Bryan decided to compromise. They quietly allowed bankers to offer credits (a transaction limited to a bank's own resources, in which the borrower usually uses the money only to buy specified goods).

They would not allow the bankers to float loans—that is, to offer securities on the public market to raise huge amounts of dollars to lend to the belligerents. The Americans who subscribed to the loans would then have to rely on British (or German) securities for repayment, a dependence that could make the lender exceptionally interested in having his or her borrower win the war.

By mid-1915, however, the bank credits proved inadequate to finance the multiplying trade in food and munitions. U.S exports by mid-1915 had more than doubled since mid-1914. The Allies and the Central Powers alike appealed for outright loans. After agonizing over the decision for a month, Wilson quietly reversed himself in September 1915 and allowed loans to be floated. (Bryan, it will be remembered, had resigned three months earlier.) The president changed his mind not only because he believed that both Germany and the Allies would have equal access to U.S. money markets, but above all because—as his secretary of the Treasury wrote—"our foreign commerce is just as essential to our prosperity as our domestic commerce."[30]

It turned out to be a pivotal decision. Bankers immediately floated the first Allied loan for $500 million. Although the amount was found only with difficulty, it opened the floodgates. The Allies, with their stronger links to U.S. banks, borrowed $2.5 billion over the next two years. (These loans were secured by British investments in American companies.) The Central Powers received less than one-tenth that amount. War-related U.S. exports doubled in the last half of 1915 to $2 billion (with most going to England and France), then doubled once more in 1916. Again, as Wilson's first major biographer observed, the president's decision to allow loans retreated from a position of " 'the true spirit of neutrality' to one based upon 'strict legality.' "[31] The decision also helped transform the United States from being one of the world's greatest debtors (it owed the world about $3.7 billion in 1914) to a creditor of $3.8 billion by the end of the war. This huge, quick movement of money between 1914 and 1918 helped turn the United States into the world's economic superpower of the twentieth century.

Wilson's dilemma was intense. He understood how U.S. submarine and financial policies were pushing him into the Allied camp. He certainly did not want a total German victory, but neither did he want an Allied triumph that destroyed the European balance of power and left Russia astride much of the continent. From the start of the conflict, he believed that he alone was in the best position to mediate a fair settlement and stop the bloodshed. Like a virtuoso, House played on Wilson's vision of himself as the great peacemaker. He convinced the president to allow him to act as Wilson's agent in Europe.

In early 1915, House sailed across the Atlantic to try to mediate an end to the war. He believed that a proper settlement would include German payment of reparations for invading Belgium and a general European disarmament. But it was too late. Too much blood had already been shed. The war aims on both sides had escalated. The Allies, moreover, had been negotiating secret treaties with Italy and Japan in which those powers promised to help the French and British in return for territory after the war. The stakes for victory were rising even as an entire generation of young Europeans was being slaughtered.

House, who seldom hid his pro-Allied biases, signed the so-called House-Grey Memorandum in February 1916 with British foreign secretary Sir Edward Grey. It attempted to seduce the Allies to a peace conference by promising that if they accepted, and if Germany refused to accept terms the Allies liked, the United States would then join the war with the Allies. When House reported his deal back to Washington, Wilson inserted the condition that Americans would "probably" join the war. Grey then rejected the proposal. He believed that it would be only a matter of time before Wilson would enter the war on London's side anyway.

The president was beginning to fear the same thing. In 1915, Wilson responded to this concern with his "preparedness campaign." Camps were set up to train American males for possible combat. Naval appropriation measures were readied. Wilson gave speeches warning his listeners that the nation had to be prepared to defend itself. Theodore Roosevelt, who had damned the president's every move because he would not take the nation into war against Germany, finally found a Wilsonian act he liked. TR justified preparedness on the grounds that it would firm the fiber of American men, especially the apparently more effete northeasterners, who responded to the call with unusual enthusiasm. Wilson, however, had other objectives. Although he wanted to counter Roosevelt's growing criticism, the president also wanted to show Germany that he meant business, as well as appease growing anti-German sentiment in the United States. Perhaps most important, he wanted to begin building military power so that he would have a strong base from which to mediate an end to the conflict. When he sat down at the peace conference, he hoped to have military leverage against both sides. In reality, as historian John W. Coogan concludes, Wilson, by late 1915, "had become a partner, and not always a silent partner, in the Allied economic campaign to strangle Germany."[32]

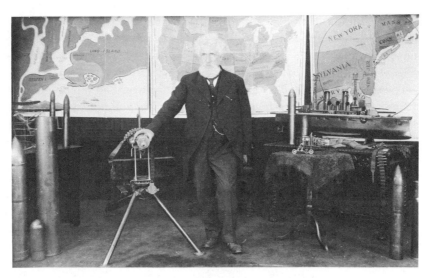

The Battle Cry of Peace, *one of the first movie spectaculars, was hugely popular in 1915–1916 and helped shape the debate over the preparedness campaign and U.S. neutrality. It was powerfully pro-war: foreign invaders (thinly disguised Germans) destroy New York City and Washington, kill the pacifists, and lead the women to commit suicide before they are ravaged. Theodore Roosevelt and Admiral George Dewey, among many others, strongly recommended the film. It was based on a book by Hudson Maxim, a munitions-maker and inventor of the Maxim Gun. As the picture shows, Maxim also starred in the film.*

THE DECISIONS FOR WAR (1916–1917)

On March 24, 1916, a German U-boat sank the French passenger liner *Sussex* and injured several Americans. Lansing and House urged that this violation of the *Arabic* pledge be met with a severing of diplomatic relations. Wilson refused. The president continued to believe that only as the great neutral could he end the war and establish a just peace. He did, however, take one more step toward Lansing's position by sending a note to Berlin demanding that the submarines not attack merchant ships (as well as passenger liners). If Berlin officials would not agree, Wilson threatened, the United States would sever relations. After intense internal debate, the Germans agreed, but they implied that Wilson must put equal pressure on the British blockade. Angry at the response, the president again separated the two issues. Berlin's *Sussex* pledge nevertheless gave the initiative—a diplomatic "blank check"—

to the Germans. If they decided that it was in their interest to launch an all-out submarine attack to win the war, Wilson would have little alternative but to join the conflict. He had lost even more of his freedom of action.

The president realized that his room for maneuver had rapidly shrunk. In the summer of 1916, he tried to balance his policies by vigorously protesting against Great Britain's interception of U.S. mail and its blatant discrimination against some 800 American companies that had dealt with the Central Powers. On the other hand, when both the House of Representatives and the Senate threatened to pass the McLemore Resolution, which prohibited Americans from traveling on belligerent ships, Wilson pulled out all stops to defeat the measure. The president refused to give in on the thorny neutral-rights issue. He insisted on the rights of U.S. citizens to move on the high seas as they wished. Because of Britain's control of those seas, however, his victory also required increased U.S.-Allied cooperation.

Wilson's hopes for creating a stable and open postwar world received their greatest jolt in May 1916, when the Allies met secretly in Paris to plan economic policies. They clearly foresaw that after the war, the United States would be the world's strongest and most competitive economic power. The British, French, Russians, and Italians, therefore, drafted a program to seal themselves off from the effects of that power. The Allies planned to use government subsidies, higher tariffs, and controlled markets to fight U.S. competition. Wilson and Lansing were stunned when they learned of the Paris economic conference. The president concluded that "our businessmen ought to organize their wits in such a way as to take possession of foreign markets." He told one business group that he very much favored the "righteous conquest of foreign markets."[33]

Clearly, however, White House pep rallies were not enough. The U.S. government would have to enter the contest by directly helping the business community to neutralize the weapons developed by the Paris conference. Wilson approached the problem from two directions. In the long run, he planned to insist on a peace that provided open marketplaces, competition, and the minimum of government involvement. In such an arena, he knew that U.S. business could more than hold its own. But this meant that it was all the more important that he attend the peace conference. More immediately, he sponsored legislation to allow U.S. business to gear up for the "righteous conquest." The Webb-Pomerene Act freed corporations from anti-trust laws, thus allowing them to combine legally to conquer foreign markets. The Edge

Act removed government restraints so that U.S. banks could rapidly set up overseas operations. Wilson thus refused to join the Allies in using government power to close off and protect markets. Instead, he aimed to release government controls so that U.S. businesses could more efficiently compete abroad. But he still needed to get to the peace conference to ensure that world markets remained open.[34]

By the autumn of 1916, the president had become so determined to beat down British maritime and economic power that he sponsored a huge appropriations bill to enlarge the navy. He aimed at nothing less than the world's greatest fleet within a decade. "Let us build a navy bigger than [Great Britain's] and do what we please," he told House in September.[35] At the same time, however, the United States continued to be drawn to the British side. The Allies were now spending $10 million a day in the United States for war goods. "There is a moral obligation laid up on us to keep out of this war if possible," Wilson believed. "By the same token there is a moral obligation laid up on us to keep free the courses of our commerce and our finance." The president was snared in an ugly trap.

When the Democrats nominated him for a second term in 1916, they coined the slogan "He Kept Us Out of War." Wilson knew, however, that the days of peace were probably numbered. In his acceptance speech, he grimly announced that Americans could not long remain neutral in a war-torn world. He began to discuss a postwar "universal association of nations" (an idea mentioned earlier by such Republicans as Roosevelt, Taft, and Lodge). Such an association could establish a just world and protect U.S. interests. After he defeated Republican nominee Charles Evans Hughes in the 1916 elections, Wilson made one more attempt to mediate an end to the war. Both the Allies and Central Powers finally rejected his offer. Each side had now enlarged its war aims—for territory, bases, indemnities—that only a total victory could provide. Wilson's hopes of acting as a neutral, honest broker had been dashed.

In January 1917, Germany decided to launch all-out submarine warfare. The debate had raged in Berlin since the *Sussex* crisis. Now the kaiser was convinced by his advisers that only a military victory could obtain his war aims of new territory, a neutral Belgium, naval bases in the Atlantic and Pacific, and perhaps even war indemnities from the Allies. The moment seemed right: war-torn Russia bloodily stumbled toward collapse, and German armies seemed on the point of victory on the eastern front. Now was the time to put full pressure on the West as well. The German naval command boasted that "England will lie on the ground in six months, before a single American has set foot on the continent." Civilian advisers were not so optimistic. Berlin military experts believed that, in any case, Americans could hardly do more to help the Allied side than they were already doing.[36]

Wilson realized that the United States was about to enter the war. But he remained torn between his belief that only as a neutral could he mediate a just peace and his fear that only if the United States became a belligerent could he be assured of a seat at the peace table. It was a terrible dilemma. On January 22, 1917, he appeared on Capitol Hill to announce U.S. postwar objectives. Wilson tried to cut through his growing dilemmas by pleading for "peace without victory"—that is, a peace in which neither side could dictate terms to the other. Equally important, he announced that the postwar settlement must protect U.S. interests. He directly attacked the old European balance of power that had failed to prevent the war and now, he feared, threatened to undermine the peace: "There must be not a balance of power, but a community of power; not organized rivalries, but an organized common peace."

Such a peace, he continued, had to include certain principles: (1) self-determination for all nations, large or small; (2) freedom of the seas—"the *sine qua non* of peace, equality and cooperation," as Wilson called it when he lashed out at both British and German maritime practices; (3) no more "entangling alliances" that created "competitions of power" instead of an open world. "These are American principles, American policies," the president declared. He thus announced that the United States was entering the blood-soaked conflict not out of the goodness of its heart, not out of mere idealism, but to protect its own self-interest. He drove this point home: "I am proposing as it were, that the nations should with one accord adopt the doctrine of President Monroe as the doctrine of the world: that no nation should seek to extend its polity over any other nation or people."[37]

The speech marked Wilson's last attempt as a neutral to define peace terms that he believed necessary for both U.S. interests and "every enlightened community." But the war-shocked Europeans could no longer afford to be so enlightened. One important British observer, Sir George Otto Trevelyan, privately dismissed the president's appeal: "The man is surely the quintessence of a prig." How dare he, Trevelyan argued, come in after three years of "this terrible effort" and ask both sides to put down their arms and meekly agree to American principles. French author Anatole France compared Wilson's "peace without victory" to "bread without yeast" or "a camel without humps" or "a town without brothel . . . in brief, an insipid thing" that would be "fetid, ignominious, obscene, fistulous, hemorrhoidal."[38] Germany responded by beginning total submarine warfare on February 1, 1917. All ships in war zones were now fair game. Two days later, Wilson broke diplomatic relations with Berlin.

But even as U.S. merchant ships were torpedoed in February and early March 1917, Wilson refused to walk his last mile to war. He knew that a strong anti-war group in Congress, led by powerful Progressives such as Republican senators Robert La Follette from Wisconsin and William Borah from Idaho, posed an obstacle. On the other hand, he did not want to appear to be giving in to his bitterest critics, Theodore Roosevelt and Henry Cabot Lodge, who had urged war since 1915. (Even after Wilson asked for war, TR dismissed the president's foreign policy as "nauseous hypocrisy.")

More important, Wilson worried that U.S. involvement in Europe would allow Japan to run wild in Asia. He told Lansing that " 'white civilization' and its domination in the world rested largely on our ability to keep this country intact."[39] The secretary of state, who wanted war, began to devise tactics to keep the Japanese in check so that Wilson could fight Europeans in better conscience (see p. 277). Above all, the president feared that becoming a belligerent would ruin his chance to broker a "peace without victory." On February 2, he told his cabinet that "probably greater justice would be done if the conflict ended in a draw." He feared that joining the Allies meant "the destruction of the German nation"[40] and the creation of a dangerous political vacuum in the middle of Europe.

By early March, however, Wilson knew he had no alternative. U.S. merchant ships were being sunk. On March 1, the news broke that British intelligence had intercepted the Zimmermann telegram. In the cable, dated January 16, the German foreign minister asked Mexico to ally with Berlin in return for getting back the Texas-to-California region after the United States was defeated. Wilson did not take the telegram too seriously (fortunately for him, neither did Mexico), but the British scored a major propaganda victory. Despite the telegram, however, the Senate killed Wilson's request of March 1 to arm U.S. merchant ships. He went ahead and armed them anyway on the basis of an almost forgotten eighteenth-century law.

On March 15, the Russian front nearly collapsed, and the tsar, Nicholas II, abdicated his throne. A more liberal provisional government took power. Americans were elated, not least because the new regime promised (foolishly, as it soon turned out) to continue to fight

Germany. The United States was the first government to recognize the new regime. Roosevelt, that caustic critic of things Russian, now told a New York audience that "Russia, the hereditary friend of this country," had chosen "enlightened freedom." Wilson even announced that Russia was "a fit partner" because it had been "always in fact democratic at heart." The liberal journal *New Republic*, long a critic of the autocratic tsar, went into rapture: "The war which started as a clash of empires in the Balkans will dissolve into democratic revolution the world over."[41] As historian Peter G. Filene writes, "Americans . . . imposed American terms" on Russia, which was, "in effect, to be a Slavic version of the United States."[42]

The dramatic turn in Russia did not convince Wilson to go to war on behalf of "democratic revolution." It did allow him, however, to argue that now all Allies were "fit" partners for Americans. On March 18, three U.S. ships were torpedoed and went to the bottom of the Atlantic. On March 20, Wilson met with his cabinet to make the decision for war. Public pressure had little to do with the decision. Most important, the president concluded that U.S. rights on the high seas had to be protected and that only by becoming a full belligerent could he attain his great objective: to be a full participant at the postwar peace conference. As he told the famed Progressive reformer Jane Addams (who opposed going to war), he had to fight or otherwise be content, when the peace conference gathered, merely to "shout" at the participants "through a crack in the door."[43]

On April 2, 1917, he asked Congress to declare war. Despite strong opposition from Borah and Republican congresswoman Jeanette Rankin of Montana, on April 6 the war resolution was approved by the Senate 82 to 6 and by the House 373 to 50. Most of the opposition came from the Midwest and the Rocky Mountain states, especially areas with heavy German immigrant populations. But Borah spoke for many when he declared: "I join no crusade; I seek or accept no alliances."

Wilson had learned that in such a conflict, the United States could no longer be both neutral and prosperous. Nor could it be neutral and hope to have a decisive voice in constructing the postwar peace. To practice peace, he had to wage war. Tragic choices had to be made. And they had to be made amid bloodshed and chaos that not even the wildest imagination had conceived in 1914. "We are living and shall live all our lives now in a revolutionary world," pro-Wilson journalist Walter Lippmann declared. In that world, Wilson led Americans onto the charred fields of Europe, where 50,000 would die so that the president could try to replace revolution with a democratic world based on

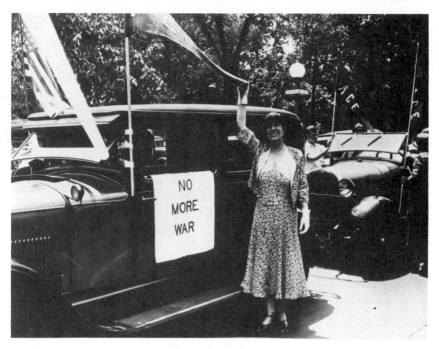

Jeanette Rankin (1880–1973) was a suffragist and then the first woman member of Congress in 1917. Raised on a Montana ranch, she voted against war in 1917, lost her election campaign because of her pacifism in 1918, then was re-elected in time to vote against war again in 1941—the only person who cast a vote against entering each world war.

American principles. It was a gamble for the highest stakes. The brilliant anti-war voice of Randolph Bourne cut to the core of Wilson's dilemma: "If the war is too strong for you to prevent, how is it going to be weak enough for you to control and mold to your liberal purposes?"[44]

NOTES

1. Edwin A. Weinstein, *Woodrow Wilson: A Medical and Psychological Biography* (Princeton, 1981); Paul F. Boller, Jr., *Presidential Anecdotes* (New York, 1981), p. 218.
2. David W. Noble, *The Progressive Mind, 1890–1917* (Chicago, 1970), p. 171.
3. William Diamond, *The Economic Thought of Woodrow Wilson* (Baltimore, 1943), pp. 132–133.

4. William Appleman Williams, *The Contours of American History* (Cleveland, 1961), p. 410.
5. Woodrow Wilson, *The Public Papers of Woodrow Wilson*, ed. Arthur S. Link *et al.* (Princeton, 1966–), VII, p. 352, italics in original; Woodrow Wilson, *Constitutional Government in the United States* (New York, 1908), pp. 58–59.
6. Robert Lansing, *War Memoirs of Robert Lansing, Secretary of State* (Indianapolis, 1935), p. 349.
7. Wilson, *Constitutional Government*, pp. 52–53; Lloyd Gardner, "The Cold War," manuscript, in the author's possession, has quote on 1889.
8. Diamond, pp. 136–139.
9. Lloyd Gardner, "A Progressive Foreign Policy, 1900–1921," in *From Colony to Empire*, ed. William Appleman Williams (New York, 1972), p. 225.
10. Paolo E. Coletta, *William Jennings Bryan* (Lincoln, Neb., 1964), p. 93.
11. Arthur Link, *Wilson*, 5 vols. (Princeton, 1947–), II, p. 95.
12. N. Gordon Levin, Jr., *Woodrow Wilson and World Politics* (New York, 1968), pp. 24–25, 37–38; [Colonel Edward M. House], *Philip Dru, Administrator: A Story of Tomorrow, 1920–1935* (New York, 1912), pp. 275–276.
13. Diamond, p. 133.
14. Jerry Israel, *Progressivism and the Open Door: America and China, 1905–1921* (Pittsburgh, 1971), p. 108.
15. Willard Straight to Henry P. Fletcher, 24 February 1916, Papers of Willard Straight, Cornell University Library, Ithaca, New York; excellent background for the U.S.-China relationship is in Daniel M. Crane and Thomas A. Breslin, *An Ordinary Relationship: American Opposition to Republican Revolution in China* (Miami, 1986), pp. 163–177.
16. James Reed, *The Missionary Mind and American East Asian Policy, 1911–1915* (Cambridge, Mass., 1983), is now a standard account; also, Link, III, pp. 269–270, 275–278, 280–285; Noel H. Pugach, *Paul S. Reinsch, Open Door Diplomat in Action* (Millwood, N.Y., 1979) p. 157.
17. Walter Lippmann Oral History, Columbia University Oral History Project, New York, p. 35.
18. Howard F. Cline, *The United States and Mexico*, 3d ed. (Cambridge, Mass., 1963), pp. 117–123, 130–134; Lloyd Gardner *et al.*, *The Creation of the American Empire*, 2d ed. (Chicago, 1976), p. 305.
19. Cline, pp. 144–146.
20. Peter Calvert, *The Mexican Revolution, 1910–1914* (Cambridge, Eng., 1968), p. 238.
21. *The Record of American Diplomacy*, ed. Ruhl J. Bartlett, 4th ed. (New York, 1964), pp. 540–541.
22. Lloyd C. Gardner, *Safe for Democracy* (New York, 1984), pp. 65–68. Mark T. Gilderhaus provides an important interpretation in "Wilson, Carranza, and the Monroe Doctrine: A Question in Regional Organization," *Diplomatic History* 7 (Spring 1983): 103–115.
23. Raymond Leslie Buell, "The United States and Central American Stability," *Foreign Policy Reports* 7 (8 July 1931): 177; Diamond, p. 151.
24. Wilson *Papers*, ed. Link *et al.*, XXVIII, p. 48; Diamond, p. 153.
25. Bruce J. Calder, *The Impact of Intervention: The Dominican Republic during the U.S. Occupation of 1916–1924* (Austin, Tex., 1984), is especially important on the anti-

U.S. guerrilla war; Kendrick Clements, *The Presidency of Woodrow Wilson* (Lawrence, Kans., 1992), p. 106.

26. Diamond, p. 154n.
27. Link, III, pp. 105–129.
28. Lansing, p. 112.
29. Two excellent analyses are Link, III, pp. 390–401, and Ernest R. May, *World War and American Isolation, 1914–1917* (Cambridge, Mass., 1959), chs. 6–7.
30. Diamond, p. 156; Link, III, pp. 62–64, 133–136, 606–625.
31. Ray Stannard Baker, *Woodrow Wilson: Life and Letters*, 8 vols. (Garden City, N.Y., 1935–1939), V, p. 187.
32. John W. Coogan, *The End of Neutrality: The U.S., Britain, and Maritime Rights, 1899–1915* (Ithaca, 1981), p. 193; John Garry Clifford, *The Citizen Soldiers* (Bloomington, Ind., 1972); Michael Pearlman, *To Make Democracy Safe for America* (Urbana, Ill., 1984). Clifford's and Pearlman's accounts are standard on prepardness.
33. Lloyd Gardner, "Commercial Preparedness, 1914–1921," manuscript (1966), in the author's possession.
34. Carl P. Parrini, *Heir to Empire: United States Economic Diplomacy, 1916–1923* (Pittsburgh, 1969), pp. 15–39.
35. Link, IV, p. 337.
36. May, ch. 18.
37. Link, V, pp. 265–274.
38. *Ibid.*, pp. 273–274.
39. Entry of 4 February 1917, in Diaries of Robert Lansing, Box #2 (Microfilm ed., reel #1).
40. Edward H. Buehrig, *Woodrow Wilson and the Balance of Power* (Bloomington, Ind., 1955), p. 144.
41. Christopher Lasch, *The New Radicalism in America, 1889–1963* (New York, 1965), pp. 198–199.
42. Peter G. Filene, *Americans and the Soviet Experiment, 1917–1933* (Cambridge, Mass., 1967), pp. 10, 12–14.
43. Link, V, ch. 9, has the full account. A fine brief discussion of the context is Lawrence E. Gelfand, "The Mystique of Wilsonian Statecraft," *Diplomatic History* 7 (Spring 1983): 87–101.
44. Ronald Steel, "Revolting Times," *Reviews in American History* 13 (December 1985): 588; David Green, *Shaping Political Consciousness* (Ithaca, N.Y., 1987), p. 83.

For Further Reading

Start with the well-indexed pre-1981 references in *Guide to American Foreign Relations since 1700*, ed. Richard Dean Burns (1983), and consult the notes to this chapter and the General Bibliography at the end of this book; these references are not usually repeated below. Good recent sources are David R. Woodward and Robert F. Maddox, *America and World War I: A Selected Annotated Bibliography of English-Language Sources* (1985), and Kendrick A. Clements, *Woodrow Wilson: World Statesman* (1987).

On Wilson, start with Kendrick Clements, *The Presidency of Woodrow Wilson* (1992); Akira Iriye, *The Globalizing of America, 1914–1945* in *The Cambridge History of U.S. Foreign Relations*, ed. Warren Cohen (1993). *Woodrow Wilson and a Revolutionary World, 1913–1921*, ed. Arthur S. Link (1982), has superb essays written by experts on the era, especially in regard to Mexico, Russia, Poland, and collective security. Link's magisterial *The Public Papers of Woodrow Wilson* (1966–   ) is nearly completed; while Link and Robert C. Hilderbrand have edited a special volume, *The Public Papers of Woodrow Wilson*, Vol. 50: *The Complete Press Conferences* (1985). Important documents, a fine introductory essay, and an excellent bibliographic essay are in *Wilson and Revolutions: 1913–1921*, ed. Lloyd C. Gardner (1982). Important interpretations are in Frederick S. Calhoun, *Power and Principle: Armed Intervention in Wilsonian Foreign Policy* (1986), a useful overview; Lloyd Ambrosius, "Woodrow Wilson and the Quest for Orderly Progress," in *Studies in American Diplomacy, 1865–1945*, ed. Norman A. Graebner (1985); Norman A. Graebner, *America as a World Power: A Realist Appraisal from Wilson to Reagan* (1984); Michael H. Hunt, *Ideology and U.S. Foreign Policy* (1987), for placing Wilson in the context of a U.S. ideology and an antirevolutionary framework; William H. Becker, *The Dynamics of Business-Government Relations: Industry and Exports* (1982), which de-emphasizes the role of government, as opposed to the thesis found in Burton I. Kaufman, *Efficiency and Expansion: Foreign Trade Organization in the Wilson Administration 1913–1921* (1974), a pathbreaking study. Wilson's particular genius is featured in Robert C. Hilderbrand, *Power and the People: Executive Management of Public Opinion in Foreign Affairs, 1897–1921* (1982). See Ernest C. Bolt, Jr., *Ballots before Bullets* (1977), on the war-referendum idea. Important studies of film include Michael T. Eisenberg, *War on Film* (1981); and Craig W. Campbell, *Reel America and World War I* (1985).

Specific studies on the entry into the war have recently included Melvin Small, "Woodrow Wilson and U.S. Intervention in World War I," in *Modern American Diplomacy*, ed. John M. Carroll and George C. Herring (1986); John W. Coogan, *The End of Neutrality: The U.S., Britain, and Maritime Rights, 1899–1915* (1981); Kendrick A. Clements, *William Jennings Bryan: Missionary Isolationist* (1982), using Bryan to point up larger themes in U.S. diplomacy; Paolo E. Coletta, "A Question of Alternatives: Wilson, Bryan, Lansing, and America's Intervention in World War I," *Nebraska History* 63 (Spring 1982), by Bryan's biographer; and Kathleen Burk, *Britain, America and the Sinews of War, 1914–1918* (1985), which uses J. P. Morgan as a focal point of the U.S.-British competition. The anti-war groups are superbly studied by Charles DeBenedetti, *The Peace Reform in American History* (1985), which sees World War I as a turning point; Sandi E. Cooper, *Patriotic Pacifism . . . 1815–1914* (1992); and *Peace Heroes in Twentieth-Century America*, ed. Charles DeBenedetti (1986), especially the chapters on Jane Addams and Eugene Debs.

In addition to the Calhoun book, noted above, the following are important for Wilson's interventionism in Latin America: Lester Langley, *The Banana Wars* (1983), with a helpful bibliography; Brenda Gayle Plummer, *Haiti and the United States: The Psychological Moment* (1992), now the standard overview; Lester Langley, *Mexico and the United States* (1991); Friedrich Katz, *The Secret War in Mexico: Europe, the U.S. and the Mexican Revolution* (1981), an exhaustive account; Berta Ulloa, "Tampico and Vera Cruz," in *Diplomatic Claims: Latin American Historians View the United States*, ed. and trans. Warren Dean (1985); Bruce J. Calder, *The Impact of Intervention: The Dominican Republic during the U.S. Occupation of 1916–1924* (1984); David Healy, "Admiral William B. Caperton," in *Behind the Throne*, eds. T. McCormick and W. LaFeber (1993), essays in honor of Fred Harvey Harrington; and, for a rather stunning contemporary view, Hiram Bingham, *The Monroe Doctrine, an Obsolete Shibboleth* (1913).

The relations with China are studied in Daniel M. Crane and Thomas A. Breslin, *An Ordinary Relationship: American Opposition to Republican Revolution in China* (1986); John Allphin Moore, Jr., "From Reaction to Multilateral Agreement: The Expansion of America's Open Door Policy in China, 1899–1922," *Prologue* 15 (Spring 1983); and most of the accounts listed in the second paragraph of this bibliography.

10

Victors without Peace
(1917–1920)

WILSON'S APPROACH TO WAR AND PEACE

President Wilson, as he informed Congress in his war message of April 2, 1917, intended to smash the "autocratic governments backed by organized force which is controlled wholly by their [the autocrats'] will, not by the will of the people." He emphasized, "We have no quarrel with the German people. We have no feeling towards them but one of sympathy and friendship."[1]

It seemed an odd way to go to war—that is, to express "friendship" for the people Americans were about to kill in large numbers. The words, nevertheless, fit Wilson's approach to the conflict. He believed that once the kaiser and other "autocrats" were destroyed, the "people" of Germany (and elsewhere) would create happier, democratic governments. Thus, he urged Americans to fight "to make the world safe for democracy." Once the "autocrats" disappeared, the mass of people would want to be democratic. Then, as he phrased it in his January 22, 1917, speech, the world could be rebuilt on "American principles."

There was idealism here, certainly, but also realism. Indeed, Wilson has become the most influential architect of twentieth-century U.S. foreign policy in part because he so eloquently clothed the bleak skeleton of U.S. self-interest in the attractive garb of idealism. Nothing, after all, could be more self-interested for Americans than to have the rest of the world act according to their principles. But the president also understood that Americans had little choice. They could no longer withdraw from world affairs. "Neutrality is no longer feasible or desirable" for the United States, he declared in his war message, "where the peace of the world is involved and the freedom of its peoples." The nation had learned this lesson the hard way between 1914 and 1917, when it mistakenly believed that it could have both neutrality and the freedom to sell anywhere it pleased. Wilson consequently hoped to make the competition play the game according to American rules. Making the "world safe for democracy" was the necessary first step.

The president, however, well understood the hurdles in his way. Most important, his closest allies disagreed with him. They wanted total victory, not "peace without victory," as he had asked. They made no distinction between the German people and their rulers. The French, who were losing one out of every two of their young men between the ages of fifteen and thirty to German machine guns, wanted vengeance. They saw little difference between the Germans who shot the weapons and the officials who gave the orders. Nor did the British intend to recognize "American principles" if one of them was freedom of the seas. London officials placed their trust in their great fleet, not in American principles. They and the French, moreover, depended on their far-flung colonial empires in Africa and Asia too much to agree to "democracy." The two European powers were not destroying an entire generation of their young men to give democracy to their imperial holdings in India or Indochina. Outspoken Americans such as Theodore Roosevelt and Henry Cabot Lodge wanted total Allied victory and total German defeat. Then, they argued, the victors could create a peace that suited them. They assumed that American and Allied war aims would be much the same. Wilson fought such views. He believed that such an approach could only produce more colonialism, more autocracy, and more wars.

The president, therefore, swept the United States into war not as an "Allied" power, but as an "Associated" power. He was doing what little he could to separate himself from the European conservatives who wanted total victory and a division of the spoils. When the president discovered that one U.S. government agency was trying to whip up war spirit by using slogans that included "Our Allies," Wilson sharply ordered the phrase changed to "our Associates . . . because we have no allies."[2]

Over There: The Western Front

The president's military policy fit this diplomatic approach. Wilson and his top military officials, led by General John J. ("Black Jack") Pershing, refused throughout 1917–1918 to allow the American Expeditionary Forces (AEF) in Europe to be integrated into Allied armies. Wilson insisted that they remain separate and under U.S. command. American armies were to be used for American, not necessarily British and French, war aims. One exception turned out to be the 200,000 African Americans who went to Europe. U.S. officers segregated and discriminated against them, to the displeasure of both the French and the black Americans. Finally, a large number of these troops were sent to fight with French forces, and they compiled a brilliant war record.

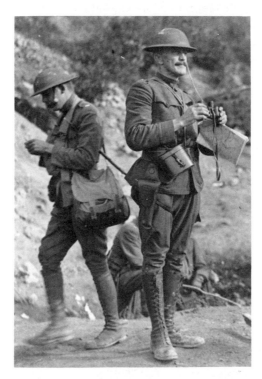

General John J. Pershing (1860–1948) led American troops in the bloody trench warfare of 1917–1918. A veteran of Indian wars and the war of 1898, and the leader of the U.S. military march into Mexico in 1916, Pershing quickly developed the American Expeditionary Force to fight on the western front. He became the nation's first general of the armies, a position that Wilson created to honor him.

Wilson insisted that U.S. forces fight on the single front of western Europe. The Allies also had to carry on campaigns in the east, where Russian troops fought with waning enthusiasm, and in Italy. Wilson cared little at first about these two fronts. In his view, they involved European imperial quarrels. He asked for a declaration of war against Austria-Hungary only in late 1917, after the Russian front had finally collapsed. Congress never did declare war against Bulgaria and Turkey, Germany's other two allies. Wilson wanted to focus on the kaiser's divisions, teach him not to sink U.S. ships, then create a democratic Germany.

The western European front, moreover, was closest to the United States and easiest for U.S. troops to reach. It was, however, a front on which British and French armies were approaching a critical point by early 1917. The carnage of trench warfare had long since become unfathomable. One young Frenchman had been unable to report for duty in August 1914 because of illness. By Christmas 1914, he was the only person still alive from his school class of twenty-seven boys. In early 1917, the British and French launched one more major offensive in the teeth of German machine guns and artillery to break through the kaiser's defenses before the Americans arrived. By late summer, the Allies had suffered 1 million casualties in this single offensive— which completely failed. Generals waited for fresh American troops to sacrifice on the battlefields. "We want men, men, men," French marshal Joseph Joffre proclaimed.

Wilson was able to place only half a million Americans under arms in 1917. U.S. officials aimed at a 2-million-man army but felt that they would need eighteen months to equip it. The Allies did not have that much time. Starvation was haunting France and Russia. Both eastern and western fronts were weakening. Under great pressure, a U.S. command under General Pershing was quickly set up in Europe during May 1917. By December, 200,000 Americans were in Europe but still in training. Nevertheless, they had to go into battle. The eastern front had collapsed, and, as the new Soviet government seized power, Russian armies evaporated. In the south, the Italians suffered a disastrous defeat at Kobarid (i.e., Caporetto), a village in Yugoslavia (later made famous by Ernest Hemingway in his novel, *A Farewell to Arms*), and were in headlong retreat toward Venice.

German commanders moved their troops from these collapsed fronts to France, where they launched a major assault on Allied positions in March 1918. By April, each side had suffered a quarter of a million casualties, but the kaiser's forces were just 40 miles from Paris. In

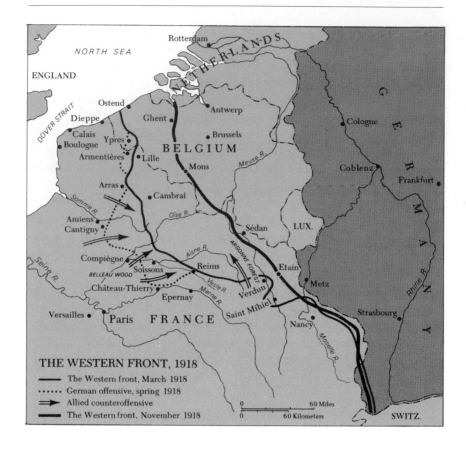

THE WESTERN FRONT, 1918

— The Western front, March 1918
····· German offensive, spring 1918
⇒ Allied counteroffensive
— The Western front, November 1918

May, the Americans entered combat in force. Their successful counterattacks were critical in turning back the Germans along the Marne River. Allied armies, moving along a broad front, were now spearheaded by a new weapon—the tank—which at last gave troops mobility and some protection. By September, 600,000 American troops launched a decisive campaign that broke through German lines. The U.S. and Allied armies continued to roll until the Germans asked for peace on November 11. The offensive was the largest military effort in U.S. history. Overall, during about a year of heavy fighting, 53,402 Americans had been killed, 204,000 wounded. Over 57,000 died from disease, especially from the 1918 influenza epidemic that ravaged Europe and the United States.[3]

U.S. naval policy also was fit into Wilson's broader diplomatic aims. The navy's mission was to carry troops to Europe and defeat German armies. To accomplish this mission, the command emphasized smaller, submarine-hunting ships that could efficiently work together in "convoys" (a new idea) that accompanied troopships through U-boat–infested waters. This policy flew in the face of traditional military beliefs, formulated by Mahan and other naval planners since the 1890s, that the navy should depend on huge battleships capable of winning major battles by destroying the opponent's surface fleet. The core problem in 1917 was not the German battleship fleet, but submarines. On the Atlantic, unlike in European trenches, Americans worked more closely with the British to establish the convoy system. The U.S. assembly lines, meanwhile, performed miracles. Philadelphia's Hog Island could produce a 7,500-ton ship every seventy-two hours, although, as historian Warren Kimball notes, "its most long-lasting significance may be the addition of a new word . . . —'hogie,' describing a sandwich popular among the Hog Island workers."[4]

Certainly, much of the prewar American planning turned out to be useless, given Wilson's diplomatic objectives. As late as 1915, U.S. war plans included invading Canada and protecting New York City from British naval attack. Americans had mostly prepared to fight defensively.[5] In 1917–1918, they instead had to ship huge armies across thousands of miles of dangerous water so that they could go on the offensive and make the world safe for democracy.

OVER THERE: IN SOVIET RUSSIA

When Wilson inserted that famous phrase "make the world safe for democracy" in his 1917 war message, Colonel House objected. He feared some people might take it literally: "It looked too much like inciting revolution."[6] Some Russians did, indeed, incite revolution, but it had little to do with Wilson's message. Instead, the immediate cause of the Russian government's collapse in early 1917 was the breakdown of its war effort and the collapse of its ruling elite. The country could no longer marshal the resources needed to fight a three-year all-out war. Tsar Nicholas II, a weak, besieged man, retreated into seclusion, where not even his military commanders could reach him. The Duma (Parliament) demanded that the tsar surrender his power so that a more popular and liberal government could wage the war. The tsar—or, more accurately, his strong-willed wife—refused. They were then swept from power by bread riots and an army mutiny. In July 1918, revolutionary forces executed them and their children.

The Duma established a provisional government that, by July 1917, was led by Aleksandr Kerensky, a moderate socialist. Wilson and Lansing liked Kerensky because he insisted on fighting Germany despite the continued disintegration of Russian armies. The whirl of revolutionary politics worried and confused U.S. officials. They received infrequent help from their ambassador to Russia, David R. Francis, an elderly Missouri politician who had no diplomatic experience but, according to rumor, considerable romantic experience with a beautiful woman who was a suspected German spy.

In mid-1917, Wilson decided to send a special mission to Russia. It was led by Elihu Root, Roosevelt's former secretary of state and a strong conservative who found little to like in the chaos and dirt of revolution. His major pleasure came from a case of Haig & Haig Scotch Whisky that he had had the foresight to take on the journey. When Kerensky pleaded for more money, Root responded tartly, "No fight, no loan." Kerensky's fighting days, however, were quickly winding down. After reading Root's report, Secretary of State Lansing feared the worst. Kerensky, Lansing believed, was caving in to "the radical element." The secretary wanted to help Russia, if possible, but concluded that it was heading straight into a "hideous state of disorder," comparable to the great French Revolution.[7]

Kerensky's regime was finally destroyed when one of his own generals tried to overthrow him. The Russian army had so decomposed, however, that its soldiers would not obey the general. At that point, on October 24 (according to the old Russian calendar, November 7 according to the new), the Bolsheviks, or radical socialists, seized power. They were led by V. I. Lenin. Months earlier, the Germans had allowed him to cross their lines when he was on a train traveling from Switzerland to Russia. German officials bet that if he gained power, Lenin would effectively take Russia out of the war. The Bolshevik leader and his military commander, Leon Trotsky, first consolidated their power by destroying the moderate socialists. Kerensky escaped, living much of the next half-century in Stanford, California.

The Bolsheviks destroyed landed estates and distributed the land to peasants, nationalized banks, placed factories under the workers' control, and, in an all-out attack on the church, confiscated its property. To Wilson's discomfort, Lenin published the Allies' secret treaties of 1915 that parceled out the conquests of war. Wilson had tried to ignore these agreements because they undercut his own plans for an open postwar world shaped by self-determination. The president grew even more alarmed as the Bolsheviks called for world revolution and mass opposition to fighting the war.

Wilson suddenly found himself trapped. The French and British conservatives, with their colonialism and secret treaties, were on one side. Now Lenin was on the other. The Russian leader, moreover, offered a radical program that directly challenged Wilson's liberal agenda and threatened to end the war effort, especially on the eastern front. The president's closest advisers were divided over how to escape the trap. Lansing believed that Lenin and Trotsky were "German agents" who had to be destroyed by force. Colonel House, however, wanted Wilson to try to keep the new Soviet regime in the war—and undercut Lenin's growing appeal to Europe's war-ravaged peoples—by declaring fresh, liberal war aims. Wilson had instantly despised and feared Lenin's radical government, but, as historian N. Gordon Levin notes, the president's inability to choose between Lansing's and House's advice soon "gave a somewhat erratic quality to Wilsonian efforts to contain Russian Bolshevik influence."[8]

The president confided to House that he really wanted to tell the Russians to "go to hell," but he initially accepted the colonel's advice to woo the Russians and the wobbling European liberals.[9] The result was the Fourteen Points speech to Congress on January 8, 1918. The president offered a more detailed vision of a Wilsonian postwar world. But it was specially shaped to answer Lenin's demands for revolution and an end to the war without territorial annexations on either side. The points included:

1. "Open covenants of peace, openly arrived at, after which there shall be no private international understandings of any kind." This directly struck at the Allies' secret treaties.
2. "Absolute freedom of navigation upon the seas . . . alike in peace and in war."
3. A worldwide open door: "The removal, so far as possible, of all economic barriers and the establishment of an equality of trade conditions among all the nations."
4. Reduction of armaments.
5. An "adjustment of all colonial claims," with the people in colonial areas having "equal weight" in deciding their fate with the colonial powers.
6. "The evacuation of all Russian territory and such a settlement of all questions affecting Russia as will secure the best and freest co-operation of the other nations of the world in obtaining for her an unhampered and unembarrassed opportunity for the independent determination of her own political development." Russia was to be welcomed "into the society of free nations under

institutions of her own choosing" and receive "assistance." "The treatment accorded Russia by her sister nations in the months to come will be the acid test of their good will." . . .

14. "A general association of nations must be formed under specific covenants for the purpose of affording mutual guarantees of political independence and territorial integrity to great and small states alike."

The president also demanded that Germany leave Belgian and French territory. He wanted territorial problems in Italy, the collapsing Austro-Hungarian Empire, the Turkish Empire, and "an independent Polish state" to be largely taken care of by the people in the regions—or, what he called in one case, "along clearly recognizable lines of nationality."[10] During the remainder of the war, he added thirteen more points to his plan, but the original fourteen proved to be the most important in the debate over peace terms that soon raged in Europe and the United States.

Lenin was not moved by Wilson's appeal. Looking first to his own and his country's survival, the Bolshevik was unswerving in his determination to make peace with Germany. On March 3, 1918, he signed the Treaty of Brest Litovsk, and did so despite German terms that in a moment destroyed centuries of Russian expansion. Poland, Finland, and the Baltic States were taken from the new government. Even the rich Russian breadbasket, the Ukraine, became independent. Russia had left the war—or, more accurately, had exchanged one conflict for another; for anti-Bolshevik forces, led by conservative White Russian armies, launched a civil war to overthrow Lenin's regime.

Wilson now faced another stark decision: whether to ignore the civil war or help the White armies. For the most part, the American public was savagely anti-Lenin and showed considerable confusion about Russian affairs by calling him and Trotsky "willing German tools." Russians, who had been "democratic at heart" a year before, now became mere "children" unfit for self-government. The *New York Times* reflected the frustration by predicting ninety-one times between 1917 and 1919 that the Bolsheviks must surely be ready to collapse.[11] Wilson shared the anger and frustration, but he knew that any direct attempt to overthrow Lenin would be difficult, if not impossible, especially since the Russian people would cluster around the Bolsheviks to fight foreign invaders. In April 1918, however, Japanese forces moved into Siberia. Tokyo officials claimed that they only wanted to ensure the operation of the Trans-Siberian Railroad and help anti-German forces in the region. The Japanese received support from the British and

French. The Europeans also pressured Wilson to intervene. The president turned down six such requests between January and May 1918.

The turn came in mid-1918. In May and June, 20,000 Czech soldiers, who had been fighting the Germans on the collapsed eastern front, began to move east to find transportation and fight elsewhere. When Soviet troops tried to disarm them, fighting broke out. The Czechs reached and occupied the Russian eastern port of Vladivostok, then asked the Allies for help. A State Department officer quickly saw the request as a " 'God-send.' " Lansing used it to convince the president to move into Russia. On July 6, Wilson surrendered. He agreed to send several thousand U.S. troops to Vladivostok to help the Czech soldiers and to guard Allied military stores. But Wilson also wanted it both ways: on the one hand, he announced that the forces must stay out of Russia's internal affairs and that he would have nothing to do with British or French intervention; on the other hand, the president planned to use the move as an excuse to send in a political mission that would test Lenin's "intentions."[12]

At almost the same time (July 1918), Wilson agreed to send several U.S. battalions to intervene in the northern Russian port of Murmansk. Working under British command and with British troops, this intervention was originally aimed at saving large amounts of Allied military supplies that had been landed to help the prerevolutionary Russian armies and to prevent a German takeover of the surrounding region. But the U.S. and British troops soon found themselves pressured by Soviet, not German, forces. All the while claiming that he did not want to interfere in Russia's internal affairs, Wilson intervened with U.S. troops not once, but twice—in eastern as well as in northern Russia.

In September 1918, three U.S. battalions arrived at Vladivostok. Wilson's motives were complex. He helped the Czechs, but he also moved the 10,000 U.S. soldiers into eastern Russia to watch Japanese ambitions in the region. By participating, the president believed that he could also moderate British and especially French plans to become more deeply involved in the Russian civil war. But he was clearly working with the anti-Bolshevik forces in that war himself. Wilson dispatched his army not only to help the Czechs, but to help determine internal Russian affairs—one major reason why U.S. troops remained in the country until 1920, long after Germany's surrender in November 1918. In 1918–1920, 222 Americans lost their lives in this intervention.

Wilson had ringed his intervention with many conditions so that he would not be seen as a political bedfellow of the British and French.

But at this point (January–July 1918), Wilsonian liberals and Leninist communists joined a battle that was to rage through most of the twentieth century. Lenin challenged the liberals' view of how the world worked and was to work. He argued that, contrary to Wilson's belief, socioeconomic classes could not coexist but were fated to fight to the death. To prove the evil intent of Wilson's "associates," Lenin published the secret treaties that made a mockery of self-determination. He asked for immediate self-determination, regardless of the effect on the war effort of the colonial empires. As historian Lloyd Gardner observes, Lenin had "absconded with the biggest piece of liberal theory: the principle of self-determination. Liberals were never able afterwards . . . to reclaim nationalism for their own. . . . Little wonder Wilson sweat blood over Russia."[13]

The president even began to lose young liberals in his own government. Russian experts in the State Department unsuccessfully opposed the growing antibolshevism in the administration.[14] They were led by William Christian Bullitt, a wealthy Main Line Philadelphian who was close to Colonel House. By September 1918, as the Allied intervention was clearly failing to weaken Lenin, Bullitt outlined the dilemma that would repeatedly face U.S. officials. The number of Allied troops, he argued, was not enough to overthrow the Bolsheviks, but enough to scare the Russians—perhaps, God forbid, even to drive them "into military alliance with Germany" against the Allies. What could be done? Perhaps, Bullitt wrote House, Japan should send in half a million men "to overthrow the Soviets," or, on the other hand, the United States could open relations with Lenin. The point was, he concluded, that affairs were so bad that "I do not know [what to do]. And you do not know. And the President does not know."[15]

But the president had let slip one conclusion after he heard that Lenin had made peace with Germany. The only way to deal with the kaiser, Wilson exclaimed, was "Force, Force to the utmost, Force without stint or limit, the righteous and Triumphant Force which shall make Right the law of the world, and cast every selfish dominion down in the dust."[16] It certainly was not "peace without victory." Trapped between the European conservatives who wanted to return to their 1913 world (without the German military) and the Russian Bolsheviks who rushed to create a classless world regardless of cost, Wilson tried to break free by using unilateral U.S. force, both in western Europe and in Russia. In Mexico's revolution five years earlier, Wilson had intervened twice with U.S. forces but had failed to put his own "good men" in office. Now it was to be seen whether he could succeed in another such venture—this time on a global scale, in a world torn between the "forces of order" and the "forces of movement," as Arno Mayer terms them.[17] Against his will and contrary to his intentions when he took Americans into war, Wilson had already been compelled to choose one of those sides as he traveled to the Paris peace conference of 1919.

PREPARING FOR PARIS

Despite his twists and turns forced by Lenin's challenge, Wilson knew what he wanted to accomplish at the peace conference. His general objective was to reconstruct the world along the lines of the Fourteen Points. He hoped to reach that new world through self-determination, free trade, and a league of nations that would be able to oversee and make necessary adjustments in the cumbersome mechanism of global power politics.

This neat package began to come undone as soon as the Germans approached Wilson in October 1918 and offered to surrender on the basis of the Fourteen Points. On close examination, many of the points were maddeningly general. Wilson had ordered a group of advisers, called The Inquiry, to elaborate his peace plan, but when it did produce specific proposals, the president often ignored them and went off on his own.[18] Colonel House, suddenly faced with the need to negotiate with Germany, desperately tracked down young Walter Lippmann in Paris and said: "You helped write these points. Now you must give me a precise definition of each one. I shall need it by tomorrow morning at ten o'clock."[19] Lippmann worked all night to produce a draft, but given the incredible complexity of the problems facing the victors, it was an ominous sign of how ill-prepared Wilson was to enter into tough, lengthy talks.

He had, moreover, already compromised two of the Fourteen Points. The British flatly refused to accept Point 2 on freedom of the seas. They would not endanger their fleet's ability to control their strategic water routes. Prime Minister David Lloyd George pointed out, moreover, that Wilson had fully cooperated with British maritime restrictions after the United States entered the war. The president backed down. On Point 6—the evacuation of Russia and the self-determination of its future—Wilson had failed his own "acid test" by intervening and maintaining U.S. forces in Russia.

The president hoped to overcome these problems through the force of his own personal popularity and eloquence, and also through the

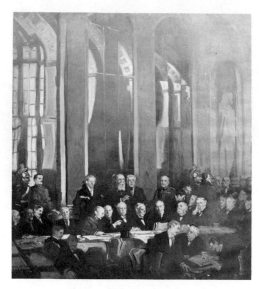

This painting by Johansen, Signing of the Treaty of Versailles, *not only pictures the Big Four in front, but catches the grandeur and historical significance of an occasion that would soon become the center of a heated debate in the United States.*

new, extraordinary power of the United States. Without doubt, Wilson did emerge from the war as the world's most popular and powerful individual. When he arrived in Europe in late 1918, millions of people greeted his triumphal tour by throwing flowers in his path. But his major opponents at Paris were to be not the German diplomats, but Lloyd George of Great Britain and the crusty, aged premier of France, Georges Clemenceau. Those two victors immediately realized that Wilson had made a near-fatal mistake in the 1918 U.S. congressional elections. He had asked Americans to give him a Democratic Congress to help him make the peace. Republicans struck back by crying that he impugned their patriotism and, after all they had done for the war effort, was accusing them of being un-American. The Republicans won the election and were able to put Wilson's archenemy, Henry Cabot Lodge, in control of the Senate Foreign Relations Committee that would have to accept or reject Wilson's work at Paris. The president then compounded his defeat by naming a peace commission, which he personally headed, that included not a single senator or Republican leader. In his defiance of Lodge, in his determination to dominate the commission, Wilson made a tactical blunder. If no Republican leader was to be involved as an architect, then the Republicans felt no responsibility for protecting the structure of the peace that Wilson brought back from Paris.

Meanwhile, Lloyd George's government won re-election by one of the largest margins in British history. In Paris, Clemenceau was given an overwhelming vote of confidence in the French Chamber of Deputies. Lloyd George suspected that Theodore Roosevelt better represented American, especially congressional, views, but the prime minister had to deal with Wilson. When the president threatened to appeal over Lloyd George's head to the British people on the freedom-of-the-seas issue, the prime minister called his bluff and dared him to try. Wilson dropped the challenge. Lloyd George called the president's threat an "unloaded blunderbuss" that intimidated neither him nor Clemenceau.[20]

The president also planned to use his country's new economic power as a weapon. During the war, he had held off pressing his postwar vision on the Allies because it would have led to disputes, perhaps even a crippling of the war effort. But Wilson did not mind. As he told Colonel House in mid-1917: "When the war is over, we can force [England and France] to our way of thinking, because by that time they will be financially in our hands."[21] And they were. By 1918, the Allies owed the United States over $3.5 billion. New York City was surpassing London as the world's financial center. But Wilson could never discover how magically to turn this power against the British and French (or the Bolsheviks).

The president did not help himself when, with the war's last shot, he pulled U.S. government representatives out of all the councils that had been established during the conflict to plan and finance the Allied war effort cooperatively. True to his pledge to build an open world, he refused to make any "special arrangements" to help Europeans rebuild their countries.[22] If they wanted help, they, like everyone else, had to go to New York private banks—not to Washington. Wilson was going to get the government out of the marketplace as rapidly as possible. That decision weakened his own economic leverage against Lloyd George and Clemenceau. Moreover, Wilson (and later presidents) learned that there were certain policies that just could not be purchased. Clemenceau's determination to ensure French security by crippling Germany had no price tag attached to it. Most nations do not place a purchase price on policies that they believe are required for their survival.

Such feelings were especially rampant in Europe after the horrors it had just experienced. Eight million soldiers and sailors had died. Over 1 million French soldiers had perished. Approximately 20 million civilians had died during the war and its immediate aftermath. More than 4,000 towns had been wiped off the map of France. Great Britain had suffered 900,000 troops killed and 2 million wounded. As Lloyd George put it, "Not a shack" had been destroyed in the United States. Americans, instead, had gotten much richer, even as the Europeans sacrificed millions of men and billions in treasure. "See that little stream?" novelist F. Scott Fitzgerald had a character say as he visited the site of the bloody Somme Valley battle. "We could walk to it in two minutes. It took the British a whole month to walk to it—a whole empire walked very slowly backward a few inches a day, leaving the dead behind like a million bloody rugs."[23]

Against that background of corpses and collapsing civilization, Clemenceau determined to protect French interests not with vague Wilsonian principles, but with boundary and economic agreements that protected France and crippled Germany. The Russian Revolution increased Clemenceau's concern. Not only did Lenin's victory threaten to radicalize much of Europe, but it destroyed France's valued prewar partner, tsarist Russia. Clemenceau had to find a new alliance arrangement. Wilson, meanwhile, sought agreement to his principles for an open, democratic world. While Clemenceau was driven by centuries of French history, Wilson believed, "If I didn't feel that I was the personal instrument of God I couldn't carry on."[24] After the peace conference, Lloyd George remarked, "I think I did as well as might be expected, seated as I was between Jesus Christ and Napoleon Bonaparte."[25] If it were true, moreover, that God helps those who help themselves, then even Wilson was in trouble. He failed to think through his own policies and suffered from severe, self-inflicted political wounds as he approached the conference table.

THE "BLACK CLOUD" OVER PARIS

Colonel House looked at war-devastated Europe, sized up the attractiveness of Lenin's message to millions of Europeans, then concluded, "We are sitting upon an open powder magazine and some day a spark may ignite it."[26] Sparks were everywhere. After the kaiser fled Germany in November 1918, the country came under a moderate Socialist government. In January 1919, Karl Liebknecht and Rosa Luxemburg tried to imitate Lenin's success. A Communist Germany was narrowly averted as right-wing troops smashed the attempted coup and killed Liebknecht and Luxemburg. Wilson had believed that Germany

TABLE 2

PRINCIPAL WARS IN WHICH THE UNITED STATES PARTICIPATED: U.S. MILITARY PERSONNEL SERVING AND CASUALTIES

War/conflict	Branch of service	Number serving	Casualties		
			Battle deaths	Other deaths	Wounds not mortal
World War I	Total	4,734,991	53,402	63,114	204,002
(6 Apr. 1917–11 Nov. 1918)	Army	4,057,101	50,510	55,868	193,663
	Navy	599,051	431	6,856	819
	Marines	78,839	2,461	390	9,520
World War II	Total	16,112,566	291,557	115,842	670,846
(7 Dec. 1941–31 Dec. 1946)	Army	11,260,000	234,874	83,400	565,861
	Navy	4,183,466	36,950	25,664	37,778
	Marines	669,100	19,733	4,778	67,207

Source: Department of Defense.

required major social change before it was ready for democracy, but communism was certainly not what he had in mind.

Radical Socialists did gain power in Hungary. In March 1919, moreover, Lenin established the Third International of the Socialist parties in an attempt to destroy the Second International, which moderate Socialists controlled. Western officials understood that the new organization was nothing less than Lenin's attempt to create a worldwide Communist party network under his control. In September, two Communist parties even appeared—with few members but much noise—in the United States.

The Big Three (i.e., Lloyd George, Clemenceau, and Wilson) had to work out a settlement amid spreading revolution. They also had to deal with the collapsing European empires in Asia, Africa, and the Middle East as nationalist leaders turned to Lenin as a model. While the victors met in Paris, Asians and Africans met in another part of the city to prepare their own demands. (One participant was young Ho Chi Minh, who between 1930 and 1969 led Vietnam against French, Japanese, and U.S. military forces to complete the task he had set upon in 1919.)

Ray Stannard Baker, Wilson's first major biographer and the president's friend, caught the picture. As the Big Three tried to reorder the world, there arose this "black cloud of the east, threatening to overwhelm and swallow up the world." Baker concluded that "Paris cannot be understood without Moscow." Lenin was never invited to the conference, but "the Bolsheviki and Bolshevism were powerful elements at every turn. Russia played a more vital part at Paris than [Germany]! For the Prussian idea had been utterly defeated, while the Russian idea was still rising in power."[27] As Lloyd George admitted, he found it nearly impossible to discuss Germany without mentioning Russia.

The French proposed to make the "black cloud" disappear through direct military action. Lloyd George objected. He had neither the finances nor the political support at home to embark on a crusade to overthrow Lenin. He confided, moreover, "I dread wild adventures in lands whose conditions are unknown, and," he added in a pointed reference to the last French army of Napoleon's that had marched on Moscow, "where nothing but catastrophe has awaited every Empire and every Army that has ever invaded them."[28] Wilson sided with Lloyd George on this point, but he refused to go along when the prime minister suggested recognizing Lenin's regime as a first step to dealing with it.

Wilson and Clemenceau only agreed to have their agents meet Lenin at the island of Prinkipo (now Büyükada), a site off the coast of Turkey, to discuss terms. The leaders in Paris chose the island so that Bolshevik diplomats could reach it without traveling through any European country in which they might spread their germs of revolution. Lenin agreed to talks and even offered to repay pre-1917 loans and give up territory if the Big Three would pledge not to interfere in Soviet affairs. He promised noninterference in other nations' domestic politics, but added that he could not control revolutionaries or propaganda in those countries. Clemenceau and Wilson disliked Lenin's response. Moreover, Russian exiles in Paris and agents of the White Russian Army lobbied hard to kill the Prinkipo talks. The meeting was never held.

Wilson, under great pressure from Colonel House and young liberals in the U.S. delegation, finally agreed to send William Bullitt to sound out Lenin in Moscow. Bullitt returned in April 1919 with terms that he believed held promise. Wilson, pleading that he was ill, refused to see him. The French ignored the young American. Bullitt and the other liberals began to move into opposition to the president. In reality, it was too late for Wilson to try to work out an agreement with Lenin. The president had chosen to try to contain Bolsheviks, not talk with them. He allowed his food administrator, Herbert Hoover, to help bring down the Hungarian Communist government by manipulating food supplies. When the Communists threatened Austria, Hoover again helped stop them by posting notices that such action would "jeopardize" Vienna's food supply.[29]

In 1920, Wilson announced that the United States would not officially recognize the Soviet government because the latter preached revolution and refused to honor international obligations. But Lenin refused to disappear. By late 1920, Trotsky's Red Army had smashed counterrevolutionary forces and had even driven into Poland before being pushed back. Lenin set up a deadly efficient secret police, the Cheka, to destroy internal opposition. Marxist-Leninist revolutionary ideology had been wedded to the power of the Russian state. The "black cloud of the east" was casting long shadows.

AT PARIS: THE PRICE OF THE COVENANT

Twenty-seven Allied and Associated nations began deliberations in Paris on January 12, 1919. The major decisions, however, were made by the most powerful: Wilson, Lloyd George, Clemenceau, and Italian Premier Orlando. This Big Four shrank to a Big Three after Orlando stalked out because of a dispute with Wilson over Italian claims.

The Big Four first tackled the question of the losers', especially Germany's, colonies. In the secret Treaty of London in 1915, the Allies had already divided many of these areas among themselves. Wilson, however, refused to agree. He urged that smaller nations be responsible for the former colonies under a League-of-Nations mandate. He ran into a stone wall of opposition from Japan (which wanted Germany's colonies in the Pacific north of the equator), Great Britain (which had its eyes on the Pacific colonies south of the equator as well as on oil-producing regions in the Middle East), and France. General Jan Christiaan Smuts of South Africa offered a compromise: the great powers would take over the colonies but under a League mandate. Wilson accepted this "mandate" principle.

Liberals quickly attacked him for allowing the victors to seize the spoils and even gain moral approval by doing it under the proposed League's banner. They also complained that Germany had nothing to say about these decisions, nor was it to be in any way compensated for these heavy losses. The policy certainly had nothing to do with self-determination. It seemed more like glorified imperialism. Even Smuts's South Africa emerged with control over the former German colony of South-West Africa. (Under the name of Namibia, the region would continue to be fought over more than half a century later.) Wilson wanted nothing for the United States, but the Allies insisted. He ended with a mandate over chaotic, starving Armenia and Constantinople in the disintegrated Ottoman Empire. Lansing estimated that it would take 50,000 U.S. troops to control this mandate. In 1920, the U.S. Senate disdainfully rejected the responsibility.

The president accepted the unfortunate mandate policy in part because he was intent on rushing on to discuss his League-of-Nations proposal. Lloyd George, Clemenceau, and most others disagreed. They urgently wanted to deal with Germany, which had been in limbo and had been threatened by a Communist takeover since the armistice two months earlier. Wilson persisted and won his point. Germany had to wait nearly four more months for a peace treaty that was written hurriedly and badly. The president, however, had convinced himself that the final treaty might, indeed, have problems, but that a properly created League of Nations could correct those problems over time.

Working largely on his own and with too little consultation with The Inquiry or other advisers, Wilson wrote out a covenant for the League in just ten days. He then left Paris on February 14, 1919, for a month of business in Washington. Wilson lobbied hard at home for his Covenant, including a lengthy, tough, give-and-take evening session with congressional leaders at the White House. He learned that the Monroe Doctrine had to be explicitly protected if the Senate were to accept the Covenant. Even then, a number of Republicans warned that they would accept the peace treaty, but not the Covenant. Wilson shot back that he intended to tie together the treaty and Covenant so tightly that the senators would have to accept both if they wanted either. On March 4, Senator Henry Cabot Lodge dropped his bombshell. He had circulated a Republican round robin, declaring the League, "as now proposed," unacceptable. Thirty-nine senators—well over the one-third needed to defeat Wilson's pact—signed Lodge's challenge.

With his hatred for Lodge refreshed, the president returned to Paris in March determined to undercut the round robin. He insisted that the Paris delegates specifically protect such U.S. interests as certain domestic issues (including immigration, tariff, and racial policies) and, above all, the Monroe Doctrine. They did so, but only after Wilson was reduced to making a series of trades that weakened both his moral authority and the principles in the Fourteen Points. He had already surrendered Point 2 (freedom of the seas) at British insistence. Perhaps, however, his most notable and costly decision was allowing Japan to remain in Shantung. Formerly under German authority, Shantung was part of China and included some 30 million Chinese. Japan was already bitter because Wilson and the European leaders had refused to agree to include a clause in the Covenant that would uphold racial equality. When Wilson also rejected their claim to Shantung, the Japanese threatened to leave both Paris and the proposed League. The president surrendered. He felt that it was more important to have Japan in the League than to uphold self-determination. It was a horrible dilemma, and his choice further alienated liberals (such as Bullitt) in the American delegation.

Wilson called Article 10 the "heart of the Covenant." It provided that each member pledge "to respect and preserve as against external aggression the territorial integrity and existing political independence of all Members of the League." This article, aiming at orderly change in the world community (and even then only when League members consented), became the center of Wilson's later struggle with the U.S. Senate. To enforce Article 10, the delegates accepted Article 16, which provided that if members were attacked, all other nations in the League would economically isolate the aggressor. The League could also recommend the use of military force.

AT PARIS: A "SANITARY CORDON"
INSTEAD OF A "SANITARY EUROPE"

The president obtained his Covenant, but the more important question was what kind of a world the new League would have to oversee. The answer to that depended on how the conference dealt with the traditional center of world power, Europe, and, specifically, how it treated Germany. Wilson and Clemenceau sharply differed. The "Tiger," as Clemenceau was appropriately known, wanted to dismember Germany so that its southwestern coal and iron regions would fall under French control. He also demanded that the Germans be held guilty for all the war's destruction and be made to pay reparations—hundreds of billions of dollars of reparations—for those damages. Such incredible payments would obviously cripple Germany's economy for decades. That was just fine with most French.

Wilson warned that Clemenceau's policy could only produce a sick, unbalanced Europe and more wars. The president had no hope of obtaining his healthy, open-trading world without a healthy and viable Europe at its center. Nor could Germany be dismembered without the principle of self-determination being made a total mockery. Above all, as he had earlier warned the British, "the spirit of the Bolsheviki is lurking everywhere." Germany was Lenin's prime target: "If we humiliate the German people and drive them too far, we shall destroy all form of government, and Bolshevism will take its place. We ought not to ground them to powder or there will be nothing to build up from."[30] The struggle with Clemenceau became so consuming that in early April, Wilson became seriously ill. Exhausted, he was confined to bed with a temperature of 103 degrees. The Tiger had little compassion. As the president stood his ground, Clemenceau bitterly accused him of being "pro-German." Wilson immediately ordered his ship, the *George Washington*, to prepare to sail back to the United States. He was ready to break up the conference. Cooler heads then prevailed, both men backed down, and deals were struck.

Clemenceau gave up his demand for French annexation of much of the German Rhineland and control of the remainder. In turn, Wilson and Lloyd George agreed that French armies could occupy the Rhineland for fifteen years. Most surprisingly, Wilson signed a security treaty with France that guaranteed its borders with Germany. Against the advice of many of his advisers, he thus signed the most entangling of alliances. But it was the price he willingly paid to keep western Ger-

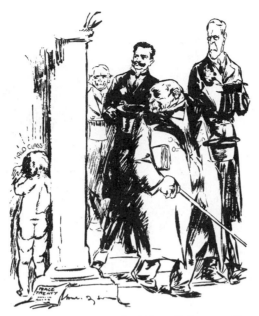

A cartoonist depicts a critical view of the "Tiger," Georges Clemenceau of France, who is saying that he thinks he hears a child crying. The "child" is the generation who would fight World War II. Wilson is at far right.

many in German hands. The defeated Central Powers were to be demilitarized and any necessary German military forces sharply limited. On the critical reparations issue, Germany was forced to sign a "war guilt" clause, but the total amount of payments was to be left to a reparations commission. Thus, Clemenceau won his principle, but Wilson believed the commission of experts would scale down the actual figure. The bill turned out to be $33 billion, far more than Germany was able to pay (especially after being effectively stripped of its colonies and parts of the Rhineland) but far less than Clemenceau had demanded.

With Germany's western boundaries settled, the Big Three turned to the highly sensitive question of its eastern regions—that is, the areas touching eastern and southern Europe where the distintegration of the Russian and Austro-Hungarian empires left only near-chaos. Wilson, of course, had a formula to propose. The boundaries of such new, independent nations as Poland and Czechoslovakia were to be settled by self-determination. But two problems plagued Wilson's approach. First, victors such as Japan and Italy cared more about acquiring nearby territory for their security and economic needs than about upholding vague principles. When Italy claimed a strip that was inhabited by

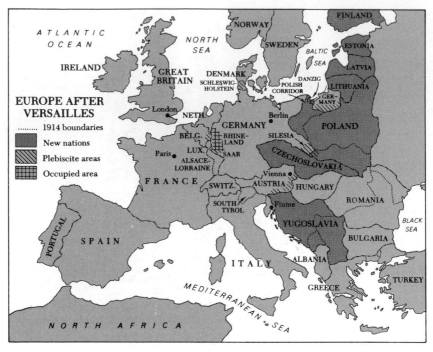

The victors at Versailles had pieced Europe back together after the devastation
of World War I but, in doing so, sacrificed the principle of self-determination in
order to create a Europe that they hoped could hold back bolshevism.

Yugoslavs (Croats), Wilson, operating on his belief that the masses were
more moral than their governments, went over Italian Premier Orlando's head and appealed directly to the Italian people. For Wilson, however, this Orlando had no dawn. The Italian leader angrily walked out
of Paris. The Italians not unnaturally chose their own government's
position over the American president's. Wilson backed off. Orlando
finally returned. After the peace conference concluded, the Italians and
Yugoslavs settled the dispute themselves.

Wilson's second problem was more general. If the principle of self-
determination was applied to eastern Europe, the nations might embrace
bolshevism. Hungary was already coming under the control of native
Communists. Wilson was forced again to choose between his principle
and European security. The result was a compromised eastern Europe.
Poland, for example, received special access to the Baltic Sea through
Danzig, which was made a free port although it was wholly German.
Only Lloyd George's and Wilson's determination prevented Clemenceau from giving Danzig to Poland directly. An area with several mil-

lion Germans also came under Czechoslovakia's control so that with this region—the Sudetenland—the Czech borders could be made more secure.

France brilliantly turned these arrangements to its advantage. It negotiated a series of pacts with the new nations in eastern and southern Europe to tie them into a security system dominated by Paris. But France's paper diplomacy—making treaties with Wilson to fix Germany's western boundary and with the smaller nations to contain Germany to the east—deceived. In reality, the Big Three placed the new, weaker states of Poland and Czechoslovakia between the two outcasts, Germany and Russia. The smaller states, thus, had to carry an enormous burden: containing both Russian and German ambitions as well as acting as a buffer to prevent bolshevism from moving westward to Germany. It, indeed, turned out to be a crushing burden. These states were too weak economically and politically to carry out such a policy.

Walter Lippmann, once an ardent Wilsonian but, by 1920, bitterly disillusioned by what he had witnessed in Paris, defined the problem when he returned to the United States: the Big Three had created a "sanitary cordon" to block Germany and Russia militarily, when they should have created a "sanitary Europe."[31]

IN WASHINGTON: THE DEFEAT OF THE COVENANT

Wilson came home determined to obtain Senate approval of his work at Paris. His determination seemed to rise as he was forced to compromise his original plans and as opposition gathered on Capitol Hill. Perhaps a majority of Americans wanted to join the League in 1919–1920. No one will ever know. It is certain, however, that two major groups of opponents awaited to attack Wilson's handiwork, and he played into their hands.

The first group of opponents earned the name "Irreconcilables." Numbering about twelve, they were led by old Progressive Republican senators such as William Borah of Idaho and Hiram Johnson of California. They opposed U.S. membership in any kind of organization resembling the League. This group especially feared being drawn in to defend the interests of such colonial powers as Great Britain and France. Instead, most Irreconcilables wanted to focus on problems at home and, when they did act abroad, to show sympathy for revolutions in Russia and China. They did not want to withdraw from the world, but, as Johnson declared, "I am opposed to American boys policing

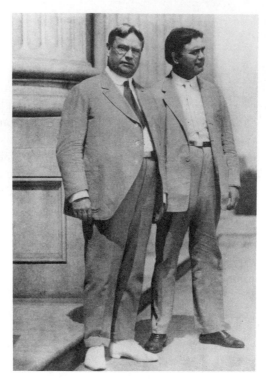

Hiram Johnson (on the left) was a powerful Progressive Republican senator from California. William Borah of Idaho led the opposition to war in 1917 and to the Versailles Treaty in 1919–1920. Borah, also a Progressive Republican, and Johnson led the Irreconcilables, who most bitterly fought Wilson's policies—including the president's refusal to recognize the Soviet Union.

Europe and quelling riots in every new nation's back yard."[32] Refusing to guarantee the badly drawn European borders, the Irreconcilables also condemned the Covenant, especially Article 10.

They were joined in that condemnation by a second group of opponents, the "reservationists," led by Senator Henry Cabot Lodge, the powerful Republican chairman of the Foreign Relations Committee. This group included such leading figures outside the Senate as Hughes, Taft, and Hoover. Lodge and Roosevelt had grown to hate Wilson personally; especially for what they believed to be the president's weak-kneed response to the Mexican Revolution and German submarine attacks. TR suddenly died in January 1919 at age sixty (he had never recovered from the death of his son, Quentin, on a European battlefield), and Lodge redoubled his opposition to Wilson's grand plan. But the senator also objected to the peace treaties on grounds of substance.

Along with the Irreconcilables and many liberals, the reservationists hated the deal on Shantung. When Lodge's committee considered the treaty, he pointedly substituted "China" in every spot in which Wilson had put "Japan" in dealing with the former German colonies in China. Wilson was furious. American missionaries and businessmen in China were delighted. The Lodge group also continued to believe that internal U.S. issues and especially the Monroe Doctrine were not adequately protected.

Above all, the reservationists feared Article 10. It locked the United States into having to act with the weakening European colonial powers. It also threatened Congress's power to declare war. When Wilson was asked directly whether the United States would have to act automatically if the League put Article 10 into effect, he tried to wiggle free: the commitment "constitutes a very grave and solemn moral obligation. But it is a moral, not a legal obligation, and leaves our Congress absolutely free. . . . It is binding in conscience only, not in law." His response was not good enough. Most of the Senate, as well as Wilson, took a "moral obligation" seriously. Under Article 10, the United States might—as Lansing had to admit before a congressional committee—support Japan's control of Shantung against valid Chinese claims, and Congress would have to go along with this "moral obligation." The famed economist, Thorstein Veblen, condemned the provision directly: it seemed "in effect to validate existing empires." Wilson vehemently denied that Article 10 opposed revolution, but he was never able to explain why. As historian William Widenor concludes, Article 10 was *"the* obstacle to ratification," because "the nature of the obligation assumed by Member States would determine what kind of organization the League would be."[33]

Neither the Irreconcilables nor the reservationists wanted to undertake that kind of obligation. But Lodge, who was certainly more sympathetic to British and French interests than was Borah, offered a compromise. He added fourteen points of his own to modify Wilson's Covenant. They aimed at removing any automatic U.S. commitment to the League's principles. Not surprisingly, the president refused such a compromise. He decided to go to the people. In September 1919, the president embarked on a cross-country speaking tour to whip up support for the League. Frustrated with the politics of Washington, he once again resorted to speechmaking so that his cause could transcend the grimy political arena. Working day and night, the sixty-three-year-old Wilson—already in questionable health from his angry encounters with Clemenceau—delivered thirty-six formal speeches in just twenty-three days. On September 26 at Pueblo, Colorado, he suffered a paralytic stroke. The broken president immediately returned to Washington. But assisted by his strong-willed wife, who rigidly controlled access to her husband, Wilson fought every attempt to compromise with Lodge. He received little help from House, with whom Wilson had broken after arguments in Paris. Lansing soon moved over to agree with many of Lodge's reservations. Disillusioned with Wilson (Lansing said that the president's mind was as clear as a pool ball), the secretary of state, in historian Dimitri Lazo's words, "encouraged" the Senate opposition with his "sarcastic commentary" about the treaty. In February 1920, Wilson fired him.[34] Such young liberals as Bullitt and Lippmann had already left the U.S. peace delegation and now actively opposed the president.

Historian Thomas Knock has noted that Wilson tried to put together a "progressive internationalist coalition"—a group of liberals who believed in self-determination, anti-imperialism, and even democratic socialism. But by November 1919, due in part to Wilson's own actions, hope for such crucial political support lay in ruins as the Senate prepared to vote on the Covenant.[35] The fear of bolshevism had spread to the United States, especially after a bomb exploded outside the home of Attorney General A. Mitchell Palmer in June 1919. Between November 1919 and January 1920, Palmer issued 3,000 arrest warrants and deported more than 500 aliens suspected of Bolshevist sympathies. The country was gripped by the "Red Scare." Wilson was not innocent of blame. During the war, his administration had helped inflame nationalist passions by passing an espionage act and a sedition act that allowed the government to arrest newspaper editors and others who were merely suspected of being critical of the war effort. Passions were out of hand. In Collinsville, Illinois, for example, a mob had decided that a town resident was a German spy and had then seized him, wrapped him in a U.S. flag, and murdered him. When Socialist party leader Eugene V. Debs condemned the war, he was jailed. Wilson kept him in prison until 1921, when President Warren G. Harding finally pardoned Debs. The administration's propaganda committee, directed by George Creel, played to fears of conspiracy and loudly protested Lenin's treachery in making peace with Germany. With few exceptions (historian Charles A. Beard of Columbia University was one), American intellectuals joined in the crusade.

Thus, the atmosphere was already poisoned when Wilson turned to Palmer in 1919 and ordered him not "to let this country see Red." In his 1919 tour, the president tried to gather support for his cause by

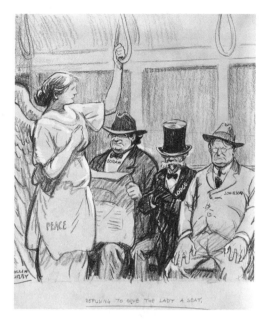

Captioned "Refusing to Give the Lady a Seat," this cartoon caricatures the three leading senators who opposed Wilson's handiwork at Paris and warns about the consequences of their opposition.

arguing that "there are apostles of Lenin in our own midst" and by warning about "the poison of disorder, the poison of revolt" that may actually have entered "into the veins of this free people." Wilson was trying to make the case that only his League could provide the antidote to this "poison." But, as historian Lloyd Gardner writes, Americans most feared that "the League would mean an increase in contacts with the poison-infected areas of the world." Or as Wilson himself cried, "This thing reaches the depths of tragedy."[36]

On November 19, in this supercharged environment, the Senate defeated the treaty containing Lodge's reservations 39 to 55. On Wilson's orders not to compromise, loyal Democrats joined the Irreconcilables to vote down the measure. Over the winter, however, public pressure built for reconsideration. Lodge's own opposition moderated. He was probably moving toward a deal with the Democrats when the Irreconcilables pulled him back, and Wilson once again refused to discuss such a deal. On March 19, 1920, the Senate again voted on the treaty that contained Lodge's reservations. This time a majority was in favor (49 to 35), but the number was short of the necessary two-thirds. Twelve Irreconcilables lined up with twenty-three diehard Wilsonian

Democrats to kill the measure, which again had a series of fifteen reservations attached. In 1921, the United States officially ended its role in the war by signing separate peace treaties with Germany and Austria.

Wilson actually hoped to recover from his paralysis and win an unprecedented third term in 1920 so that he could renew and win the fight for the League. Democratic party bosses never seriously considered his candidacy, throwing him a sop only by agreeing to make the campaign a "solemn referendum" on the Covenant. A U.S. presidential election is never a referendum on a single issue, however. Both the Republican ticket, led by Senator Warren G. Harding of Ohio, and the Democrats, headed by Ohio governor James Cox (with young New Yorker Franklin D. Roosevelt as the vice-presidential nominee), fudged the League issue until voters could not tell exactly where the candidates did stand.

Harding won an overwhelming victory by 7 million votes. The problem of restoring war-torn Europe and revolutionary Asia now fell to the Republicans. The League became a secondary issue, as well it might, for the central problem in 1919–1920 and after was not the Covenant, but the specific terms of boundaries, reparations, and mandates that the Paris peace conference produced. Historian Kendrick Clements believes that it is "perfect nonsense" to assume that U.S. membership in the League could have prevented the horrors of the 1930s.[37] Those catastrophes were rooted in the 1919 peace terms, not in the Covenant. Wilson bequeathed to Harding those treaties, a policy of containing (but not formally recognizing) the Soviet Union, and a world threatened with revolution. But the broken president was convinced that he only failed in part: "The world has been made safe for democracy. . . . But democracy has not yet made the world safe against irrational revolution."[38] It was up to Harding and, as it turned out, to all of his successors to deal with this more difficult problem of "revolution," both irrational and rational.

NOTES

1. *The Record of American Diplomacy*, ed. Ruhl J. Bartlett, 4th ed. (New York, 1964), pp. 456–457.
2. Dean Acheson, "The Eclipse of the State Department," *Foreign Affairs* 49 (July 1971): 598.

3. Allan R. Millett and Peter Maslowski, *For the Common Defense* (New York, 1984), pp. 344–346, 350–352, 356–358.
4. *Churchill and Roosevelt: The Complete Correspondence*, ed. Warren Kimball, 3 vols. (Princeton, 1984), I, p. 88. A useful short analysis on naval strategy is David F. Trask, "Woodrow Wilson and World War I," in *American Diplomacy in the Twentieth Century*, ed. Warren F. Kimball (St. Louis, 1980), pp. 7–10.
5. J. A. S. Grenville and George B. Young, *Politics, Strategy, and American Diplomacy, 1873–1917* (New Haven, 1966), pp. 330–336.
6. Christopher Lasch, *The New Radicalism in America, 1889–1963* (New York, 1965), pp. 200–201.
7. Robert Lansing, *War Memoirs of Robert Lansing, Secretary of State* (Indianapolis, 1935), pp. 337–338.
8. N. Gordon Levin, Jr., *Woodrow Wilson and World Politics* (New York, 1968), pp. 50–51; Lansing, pp. 343–345.
9. Edward M. Bennett, *Recognition of Russia: An American Foreign Policy Dilemma* (Waltham, Mass., 1970), p. 26.
10. *Record of American Diplomacy*, pp. 459–461.
11. Peter G. Filene, *Americans and the Soviet Experiment, 1917–1933* (Cambridge, Mass., 1967), pp. 24–25, 59.
12. Lloyd C. Gardner, *Safe for Democracy* (New York, 1984), pp. 186–191.
13. Lloyd C. Gardner, *A Covenant with Power: America and World Order from Wilson to Reagan* (New York, 1984), pp. 20–27. A noted account is George Kennan, *Russia and the West under Lenin and Stalin* (Boston, 1960), chs. 5–8.
14. Linda Killen, *The Russian Bureau: A Case Study in Wilsonian Diplomacy* (Lexington, Ky., 1983), chs. 3–4, especially tells an interesting story.
15. William C. Bullitt to Edward M. House, 20 September 1918, Papers of Colonel Edward M. House, Yale University, New Haven, Connecticut.
16. Arthur S. Link, *Woodrow Wilson: Revolution, War, and Peace* (New York, 1979), p. 85.
17. Arno Mayer's two seminal books on the subject are *Political Origins of the New Diplomacy, 1917–1918* (New Haven, 1959), and *Politics and Diplomacy of Peacemaking . . . 1918–1919* (New York, 1967).
18. The standard study is Lawrence E. Gelfand, *The Inquiry: American Preparations for Peace, 1917–1919* (New Haven, 1963).
19. Ronald Steel, *Walter Lippmann and the American Century* (New York, 1981), pp. 149–150.
20. David Lloyd George, *War Memoirs*, 6 vols. (London, 1933–1936), I, pp. 40–48.
21. William L. Langer, "Peace and the New World Order," in *Woodrow Wilson and the World of Today*, ed. Arthur P. Dudden (Philadelphia, 1957), p. 71.
22. Woodrow Wilson, *The Public Papers of Woodrow Wilson*, ed. Ray Stannard Baker and William E. Dodd, Jr., 6 vols. (New York, 1925–1927), V, p. 569; Michael J. Hogan, "The United States and the Problem of International Economic Control . . . 1918–1920," *Pacific Historical Review* 44 (February 1975): 93–94.
23. F. Scott Fitzgerald, *Tender Is the Night: A Romance* (New York, 1948), p. 117; and also Gordon A. Craig, "The Revolution in War and Diplomacy," in *World War I: A Turning Point in Modern History*, ed. Jack Roth (New York, 1967), p. 8, for the Fitzgerald reference. A fine, brief background on the war's costs is in Paul Dukes, *A History of Europe, 1648–1948* (London, 1985), pp. 362–364.

24. Felix Frankfurter, *Felix Frankfurter Reminisces* (New York, 1960), p. 161. A provocative analysis is Lloyd E. Ambrosius, "Woodrow Wilson's Health and the Treaty Fight," *International History Review* 9 (February 1987): 82.

25. Paul F. Boller, Jr., *Presidential Anecdotes* (New York, 1981), p. 220.

26. Geoffrey Barraclough, *Introduction to Contemporary History* (New York, 1964), pp. 213–214.

27. Ray Stannard Baker, *Woodrow Wilson and the World Settlement*, 3 vols. (Garden City, N.Y., 1922), I, p. 102; II, pp. 63–64.

28. Gardner, *Safe for Democracy*, p. 262.

29. Herbert C. Hoover, *The Ordeal of Woodrow Wilson* (New York, 1958), pp. 134–137, 140–141. The contradictions in Wilson's overall policy are superbly captured in Betty Miller Unterberger, "Woodrow Wilson and the Bolsheviks: The 'Acid Test' of Soviet-American Relations," *Diplomatic History* 11 (Spring 1987): esp. 87–90.

30. John L. Snell, "Document: Wilson on Germany and the Fourteen Points," *Journal of Modern History* 26 (December 1954): 366–368.

31. Walter Lippmann, "The Political Scene," in *New Republic*, "Supplement," 22 March 1919.

32. Filene, pp. 52–53.

33. Thomas J. Knock, *To End All Wars* (New York, 1992), p. 253; William C. Widenor, *Henry Cabot Lodge and the Search for an American Foreign Policy* (Berkeley, Calif., 1980), p. 338.

34. Dimitri D. Lazo, "A Question of Loyalty: Robert Lansing and the Treaty of Versailles," *Diplomatic History* 9 (Winter 1985): 52–53; also Henry W. Brands, Jr., "Unpremeditated Lansing: His Scraps," *Diplomatic History* 9 (Winter 1985): 25–33.

35. Knock, *To End All Wars*, esp. pp. 227–270.

36. Gardner, *Safe for Democracy*, pp. 258–260; Knock, *To End All Wars*, p. 245.

37. Clements is quoted in Luther Spoehr, "Films for Classroom Reviewed," *OAH Newsletter* 14 (May 1986): 17.

38. Ronald Steel, "Revolting Times," *Reviews in American History* 13 (December 1985): 591.

FOR FURTHER READING

The extensive list of pre-1981 publications can best be found in the well-annotated chapters 18 and 19 of *Guide to American Foreign Relations since 1700*, ed. Richard Dean Burns (1983). Those references and the sources in the notes to this chapter and the General Bibliography at the end of this book are not usually repeated below. Also important is David R. Woodward and Robert F. Maddox, *America and World War I: A Selected Annotated Bibliography of English-Language Sources* (1985); and Linda Kallen and Richard Lael, *Versailles and After: An Annotated Bibliography* (1983).

Useful overviews, with excellent bibliographical references, are Kendrick A. Clements, *The Presidency of Woodrow Wilson* (1992); Thomas J. Knock, *To End All Wars* (1992); and Lloyd E. Ambrosius, *Woodrow Wilson and the American Diplomatic Tradition* (1987). Important for the war at home are Charles DeBenedetti's several important books on the peace movement, especially *Peace Heroes in Twentieth-Century America* (1986), which he edited and which has good chapters on Debs and Addams; Nick Salvatore's prize-winning biography, *Eugene V. Debs* (1983); Stephen L. Vaughn, *Holding Fast the Inner Lines: Democracy, Nationalism and the Committee on Public Information* (1980). For the war abroad, Edward M. Coffman, *The War to End All Wars: The American Military Experience in World War I* (1987), is a standard by a distinguished military historian; Lester H. Brune, *The Origins of American National Security Policy: Sea Power, Air Power and Foreign Policy 1900–1941* (1981); and Gerald W. Patton, *The Black Officer in the American Military, 1915–1941* (1981), a helpful survey. Daniel Yergin's *The Prize* (1991) is a prize-winning account of the key role of oil.

Recent work on the peace settlement includes William C. Widenor, "The United States and the Versailles Peace Settlement," in *Modern American Diplomacy*, ed. John M. Carroll and George C. Herring (1986); Edwin A. Weinstein, *Woodrow Wilson: A Medical and Psychological Biography* (1981), a provocative analysis; the relevant chapters on post-1917 affairs in *Woodrow Wilson and a Revolutionary World, 1913–1921*, ed. Arthur S. Link (1982); and Arthur Link, *The Public Papers of Woodrow Wilson* (1966–   ), especially volume 55 on early 1919 (1987). The critical question of Germany is discussed in A. Lentin, *Lloyd George, Woodrow Wilson, and the Guilt of Germany* (1985), provocative; Klaus Schwabe, *Woodrow Wilson, Revolutionary Germany and Peacemaking, 1918–1919* (1985), provocative and exhaustive; Manfred Jonas, *The United States and Germany: A Diplomatic History* (1984), a good overview with useful bibliography. For French relations, see Henry Blumenthal, *Illusion and Reality in Franco-American Diplomacy, 1914–1945* (1986). Thomas N. Guinsburg, *The Pursuit of Isolationism in the U.S. Senate from Versailles to Pearl Harbor* (1982), is an important work on the fight in Washington. The intervention into Russia is reinterpreted by a leading scholar of that affair, Betty Miller Unterberger, "Woodrow Wilson and the Bolsheviks: The 'Acid Test' of Soviet-American Relations," *Diplomatic History* 11 (Spring 1987); and important new sources are Benjamin D. Rhodes, "A Prophet in the Russian Wilderness: The Mission of Consul Felix Cole at Archangel, 1917–1919," *Review of Politics* 46 (July 1984), and Rhodes's *The Anglo-American Winter War with Russia, 1918–1919* (1988).

More recent, important contributions include John Milton Cooper, Jr., and Charles E. Neu, eds., *The Wilson Era: Essays in Honor of Arthur S. Link* (1991), especially the Levering, Cooper, Neu, and Knock essays on 1917–1921; Betty M. Unterberger, *The United States, Revolutionary Russia and the Rise of Czechoslovakia* (1989); Christine A. White, *British and American Commercial Relations with Russia, 1918–1924* (1992); Sevan G. Terzian, "Henry Cabot Lodge and the Armenian Mandate Question, 1918–20," *Armenian Review* 44 (Autumn 1991), 23–37; and the important overview, Akira Iriye, *The Globalizing of America, 1914–1945*, in *The Cambridge History of U.S. Foreign Relations*, ed. Warren Cohen (1993).

11

The Rise and Fall of the American Structure for World Order (1920–1933)

Harding, Hughes, and Hoover

A bitter, disillusioned young Wilsonian, Walter Lippmann, wrote in November 1920 that the election of Warren Gamaliel Harding to the presidency was "the final twitch" of America's "war mind." Harding won not because many admired this mediocre Republican senator from Ohio, but because, in Lippmann's view, the people's "public spirit was exhausted" after the war effort. "The Democrats are inconceivably unpopular."[1] The new president's intellectual abilities were not high. Journalist H. L. Mencken wrote that Harding's use of language (which Mencken called "Gamalielese") was "so bad that a certain grandeur creeps into it." Alice Roosevelt Longworth, TR's tart-tongued daughter, recalled that "Harding was not a bad man. He was just a slob."[2]

But the president understood two facts that made U.S. foreign policies between 1920 and 1933 most instructive to later Americans. First, he knew that although the country wanted to return to "normalcy" (he meant to say "normality," but Gamalielese got in the way), the pre-1914 "old order" could never be rebuilt. Nor should it be rebuilt, Harding told Congress in 1922, because "out of the old order came the war itself." A new international system, built by American hands and money, and based on American principles, now had to be erected on the bloody ruins of the old European order. Second, Harding recognized his own weaknesses and looked for smart cabinet members to run the new foreign policy.

He found one such person in Charles Evans Hughes, who became secretary of state. A superb legal mind, a former governor of New York, and the 1916 Republican nominee for president, Hughes believed that Americans must seek "to establish a *Pax Americana* maintained not by arms but by mutual respect and good will and the tranquilizing processes of reason."[3] His views were shared, and with even greater passion, by the new secretary of commerce, Herbert Hoover, who became the personal symbol for the Republican policies of 1920 to 1933.

Raised in Iowa and orphaned before the age of ten, Hoover graduated in Stanford University's first class. The impoverished young geologist soon worked for mineowners in Australia, China, Latin America, and Russia. By 1919, the forty-five-year-old Hoover enjoyed a fabulous international reputation and a multimillion-dollar fortune. Hav-

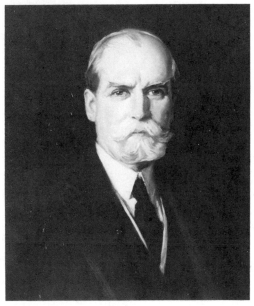

Charles Evans Hughes (1862–1948) was a professor of law who uncovered corrupt practices by "robber barons" in New York's utility and insurance industries, became the state's Republican governor, was defeated as the Republican nominee for the presidency in 1916, served as secretary of state (1921–1925), and then ruled as chief justice of the United States, where he opposed much of Franklin D. Roosevelt's New Deal legislation. This portrait, by H. C. Christy, captures the dignified but ruthless intelligence that put together the Washington conference treaties and the plan to rebuild Germany.

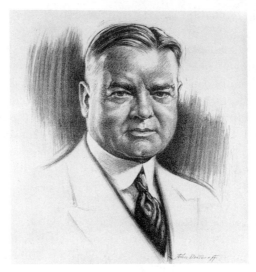

Herbert Hoover (1874–1964) was considered by many close observers as one of the ablest and most intelligent persons of his generation ("the damndest, smartest man I ever met," as one friend put it). Arising from poverty, he parlayed his engineering degree into a multimillion-dollar fortune, then became world-famous as a food administrator in World War I, secretary of commerce (1921–1929), president (1929–1933), and advocate of what he termed "American individualism." Known simply as "the Boss" to his close friends, Hoover's ideas shaped the 1920s—until he could not find the answers to deal with the economic depression and the 1931 Japanese invasion of Manchuria.

ing served brilliantly under Woodrow Wilson during the war and at the Versailles conference, Hoover broke with the president over Article 10 of the League of Nations charter. He insisted on complete U.S. freedom of action so that the nation could use its vast new power when and how it thought best. This did not mean following a policy of isolationism in world affairs. Instead, Hoover favored "independent internationalism," as historian Joan Hoff has called it[4]—that is, not retreating from the world (for that was impossible), but keeping American hands as free as possible to build a world order in which Americans could prosper.

Hoover believed that the ideas of "American individualism" had to govern world affairs as they had built the United States. In his view, state-controlled enterprise, whether it was of the conservatives in France or the radical Left in the Soviet Union, threatened the individual freedoms essential to happiness and peace. But to have "American individualism" in the new international arena, the United States had to realize that these freedoms were all intimately related: "I insisted that spiritual and intellectual freedom could not continue to exist without economic freedom," he wrote in his memoirs. "If one died all would die."[5]

Hoover finally accepted the cabinet post after Harding agreed that Hoover would be involved in key diplomatic decisions. The new secretary of commerce believed that individual freedom at home was closely linked with policy abroad: "I am thus making a plea for individualism in international economic life just as strongly as I would make a plea for individualism in the life of our own people," Hoover declared in 1921. But to assure such "individualism" abroad meant keeping the international arena open for individual enterprise. "Special privileges" (such as the European colonial empires in Asia and the Middle East) were not to be allowed. Hoover believed that, indeed, everything was at stake in foreign policy: "This system [of individualism] can not be preserved in domestic life if it must be abandoned in international life."[6] Most of all, he feared the effect of revolution, which, he noted, "is a tornado leaving in its path the destroyed homes of millions with their dead women and children." Historian Warren Cohen has noted the result: the old search for order at home, "so pronounced in the Progressive era, had become a search for world order."[7]

Rather than retreating from the world, Hoover and Hughes believed that they had to go out and restart the international economy so that freedom could be protected. It proved to be a heavier burden than they, or the American people, could carry. But Hoover was correct in his main point, for when the global system did collapse between 1929 and 1933 (as Hoover himself occupied the White House), individual freedom in the United States and elsewhere became gravely endangered.

New Rules for an Old Game:
The Washington Treaty System (1921–1922)

Hoover and Hughes knew that their first step had to be stopping the growing military competition. As the United States, Japan, and the western Europeans raced to build great navies, it seemed that the world was crazily returning to the competition that had helped trigger the world war. Moreover, military budgets sucked up money that would have been better used to develop world resources and build societies before some of them fell victim to radical revolution. Senators, led by Progressive Republican William Borah (Idaho), demanded meetings with Great Britain and Japan to discuss cutting military budgets. Hughes seized the initiative by inviting nine leading powers to Washington in late 1921 to discuss the arms race and such related problems as the smoking revolutionary cauldron of the Far East. He, pointedly, did not invite the Soviet Union or even extend it diplomatic recognition.

Hughes and his State Department advisers hoped to combine the disarmament problem with a more immediate danger that needed discussion: growing Japanese power in Asia. In historian Charles Neu's words, the 1919 peace conference had "left an ugly heritage in Japanese-American relations."[8] U.S. fears rose as Japan built the region's most powerful military machine. It did so, moreover, just as China, Russia, and smaller Asian countries spun into revolution. Popular books appeared in the United States with such subtitles as *The Rising Tide of Color* and *Must We Fight Japan?* Japan seemed to be the key diplomatic problem in Asia, and that problem worsened because Tokyo still enjoyed an alliance with Great Britain that had been made in 1902. If the United States and Japan did fight each other, Americans could find themselves fighting against the British fleet as well. Hughes demanded that the alliance be broken. When the British ambassador once made the mistake of referring to the 1902 treaty, he later remarked that he had "never heard anything like Mr. Hughes' excited tirade outside of a madhouse."[9]

Hughes not only intended to force naval disarmament and break up the Anglo-Japanese alliance, but he had a third objective, too: to make Japan dependent on the New York City money market. Especially after a severe postwar economic downturn hit them, the Japanese needed capital for both their military and their economic development of Manchuria and Korea. During May 1920, in a deal that perfectly demonstrated how the new U.S. economic power could work, New York banker Thomas Lamont agreed to open the city's vast resources to the Japanese. But, in return, they had to agree to honor open-door principles in China (except in southern Manchuria, which Japan had controlled since 1905). Thus, in return for New York dollars and rights in Manchuria, the Japanese promised to treat U.S. trade and investment fairly in most of China. As historian Carl Parrini observes, "Hughes had no intention of relying upon good faith alone." The secretary of state intended to use dollars to pressure Japan "to abide by the open door pledge."[10] He also intended to use the "Black Chambers," a secret U.S. code-breaking operation that allowed him to read the most sensitive instructions from Tokyo to the Japanese delegation in Washington. Hughes was ready for his master stroke.

He opened the Washington Conference with one of the most stun-

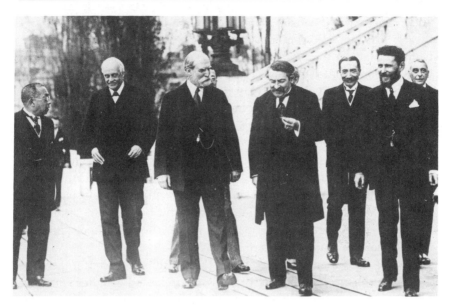

Secretary of State Charles Evans Hughes talked with French leader Aristide Briand at the historic Washington conference of 1921. Other foreign ministers included (from left), Prince Tekugawa of Japan, Arthur Balfour of Great Britain, and, at front right, H. E. Carlo Sanchez of Italy. The smiles no doubt belied the leaders' shock at Hughes's astonishing proposals at the conference.

ning speeches in diplomatic history. Hughes proposed to achieve real disarmament by offering to scrap thirty major U.S. ships, totaling 846,000 tons. He then turned to a shocked British delegation and told them that they should do away with 583,000 tons of their large warships. Hughes next instructed the surprised Japanese that they should destroy 450,000 tons of their capital ships. He asked for a final limit of 500,000 tons for the British and Americans, 300,000 for the Japanese, and 175,000 tons each for France and Italy. These limits were agreed to in the Five-Power Treaty.

Hughes set these numbers despite strong opposition from the U.S. War and Navy departments. The military warned that the figures gave Japan superiority in Asia. The secretary of state did not mind. Given Lamont's deal with Tokyo bankers, the Japanese had become a more trusted—and more controllable—ally in Asia.

To put a double lock on Japan, Hughes signed two other treaties at the Washington Conference. The Four-Power Treaty ended the Anglo-Japanese Alliance of 1902 and provided instead that in the event of an Asian crisis, the four powers (the United States, Japan, Great Britain, and France) would consult. They would not, in other words, necessarily act. The Nine-Power Treaty (signed by the four powers plus Italy, China, Belgium, the Netherlands, and Portugal) finally put the open-door principles into international law. The pact thus fulfilled a dream of U.S. officials since John Hay, if not John Quincy Adams. Japan signed the Nine-Power Treaty, however, only after adding a "security clause" that recognized Tokyo's influence in Manchuria. The Japanese, moreover, agreed with the crucial Five-Power agreement only after Great Britain pledged not to extend its fortifications at Hong Kong and the United States promised not to fortify bases in the Philippines, Guam, and Alaska any further. U.S. military officials again protested, and Hughes again turned them down. Any belief that Guam, for example, could become a key naval base was, he remarked, "nothing but a picture of the imagination."[11]

Despite the Japanese reservations, the Washington Conference was a success. Historian Thomas Buckley summarized Hughes's accomplishment: the United States "achieved a better position in relation to its competitors in the Pacific by a limitation of arms than it might have gained by arming; therein lay the wisdom of the American proposal."[12]

Many joined the U.S. military in criticizing the three Washington Conference treaties. Fearing a revived Germany, France angrily fought restrictions on its own naval power. China was bitter that the powers had given Japan control over much of Manchuria. Great Britain worried that with Tokyo's naval superiority in the region, the British fleet was no longer the determining military power along the Pacific rim. Even the Japanese military complained that they needed a 10:10:7 ratio (not 5:5:3) to protect their expanding empire. For the next decade they continually demanded more ships. But Harding, Hughes, and Hoover were delighted. The Americans considered China an inferior power that was cuddling too closely with the Soviet Union. As one U.S. delegate to the conference believed, China had not yet become "a full-fledged member of the family of nations." Besides, Americans had done their part by protecting China with the open-door principles. With Japan dependent on the U.S. money market and with the Nine-Power pledge in his pocket, Hughes believed that he had built the necessary base for a joint U.S.-Japanese effort to develop China and other profitable portions of Asia. Japan soon showed its good faith by agreeing to return the Shantung Peninsula to China and—finally—by pulling its last troops out of Siberia.

For its part, the United States did nothing at the conference that tied its hands or "endanger[ed] our freedom of action," as Harding privately observed.[13] Moreover, the building of smaller ships (submarines and destroyers) was not limited. Historian Akira Iriye correctly notes that the Washington treaties "did not mean that imperialism as such was gone,"[14] only that in China the century-long presence of Great Britain and Russia had been reduced while Japan and the United States had become the dominant powers. If only the Chinese would stand still and not get caught up in their own revolution. And if only the New York money market remained flush and open.

"CAPITAL . . . AND STATE CRAFT . . . GO HAND IN HAND": THE REPUBLICANS' SYSTEM

With the arms race under control, the Harding administration turned to rebuilding the war-devastated global system. U.S. officials had no doubt about their role. They would take the lead, and they knew just how they would rebuild: they would use their new economic wealth (not political or military power) to create a new, prosperous world that would be safe from the rivalries that had nearly destroyed everything in 1914. "Our international problems tend to become mainly economic problems," Hughes declared in 1922.[15] But the nation certainly had the resources to solve those problems. Americans had owed the world $3 billion when World War I started, but the world owed them more than $3 billion when the war ended. Gold and other international capital piled up in New York City. These riches meant, however, that somehow that money had to be recycled back to the poorer nations. Otherwise they could not buy U.S. goods.

This recycling, Washington officials agreed, had to be done by private bankers. The government should not become involved in the private marketplace. Too much government involvement led, as Hoover and other leaders constantly preached, to either socialism or fascism. But, these leaders quickly added, there did have to be close cooperation between bankers and government. Each needed the other: the bankers could carry out policies that benefited the entire country, while the government could quietly aid and protect the bankers overseas.

As Washington politicians and New York bankers worked together, critics cried that "Wall Street" was running the government. A top State Department official, Huntington Wilson, responded by explaining the new facts of international life. Critics have, "in the debauchery of their muck raking, been silly enough to insinuate that the Department of State was run by Wall Street," he observed. "Any student of modern diplomacy knows that in these days of competition, capital, trade, agriculture, labor and state craft all go hand in hand if a country is to profit."[16]

THE RULES FOR THE NEW REPUBLICAN SYSTEM

Hoover and Hughes set the ground rules for this cooperation. In 1921, they informed the bankers that money must not go to the Soviet Union or certain projects in China. These talks led to the greatest figure on Wall Street, J. P. Morgan, Jr., agreeing to keep Hughes "fully informed of any and all negotiations for loans to foreign governments."[17] Hoover tried to claim that this meant that the bankers would have to submit loan projects to him and Hughes for quiet, informal approval or disapproval. Thus, the money would go where the government wanted, but the government would not be directly responsible if anything went wrong with the loan.

The Hughes-Hoover policy on loans was perfectly in tune with the U.S. policy on war debts. Washington officials insisted that the war-scarred Europeans must repay the multibillion-dollar debt not only on grounds of principle ("They hired the money, didn't they?" President Calvin Coolidge growled), but because the debt was a weapon for U.S. officials. Hughes and Hoover could use the debt like a carrot and stick to force Europeans to behave. If the Europeans cooperated, the war debt might be discussed. But if, as they usually did, Europeans objected to U.S. policies, they could be threatened with quick collection of the debt.

Thus, Hoover and Hughes could use the debts and the loan-approval policy as sharp tools. When the British government tried to drive up the world price of rubber by controlling the British Empire's production, Hoover declared economic war. He was determined not to have the new, already rich American automobile industry held hostage by London. By using U.S. power over loans and war debts to threaten the British, and by encouraging such American producers as Firestone to enlarge their rubber plantations in Liberia and Southeast Asia, Hoover drove down the price from $1.21 a pound in March 1926 to 40 cents in just three months. He did much the same thing when Brazil tried to raise coffee prices and Germany attempted to corner the market on such vital raw materials as potash.[18] Hoover and Hughes were certainly not "isolationists." But, to use a later term, they delighted in playing "hard ball" diplomacy. They especially insisted that dollars not be spent on U.S. enemies (such as the Soviet Union) or on nonproductive enterprises (as war industry), but on friends and peaceful businesses—especially those who would buy American goods.

By the mid-1920s, however, the policy was no longer working. The bankers increasingly wanted to go their own way, even if it meant investing in the Soviet Union or in quick-profit schemes rather than in productive enterprises. For example, Hoover urged them to provide credit for U.S. exporters who were trying to conquer new foreign markets against stiff European and Japanese competition. The bankers, however, preferred to invest in more fly-by-night businesses abroad that promised a quick payoff. U.S. manufacturers, who needed credit, grew bitter. So did Hoover. But when he tried to tighten controls over the bankers, he ran into opposition from Secretary of the Treasury Andrew Mellon and President Calvin Coolidge (who entered the White House after Harding's sudden death in 1923). Mellon and Coolidge felt that government should not be so involved. The new president deeply disliked Hoover's activism. Whereas Harding had once called Hoover "the damndest smartest man I have ever met," Coolidge later groused that "that man [Hoover] has offered me unsolicited advice for six years, all of it bad."[19] While Hoover raced around Washington and seemed to be involved in everything, Coolidge liked to sleep eleven hours a day. (When writer Dorothy Parker was told in 1933 that Coolidge had died, she replied, "How can they tell?")

As these Washington officials fought each other, the bankers spun out of control—as did the economy. The history of the tariff during the 1920s became a classic example of how Americans tried to have everything and ended up with almost nothing. In 1922, the Fordney-McCumber Act raised tariff walls around American producers, who loudly demanded protection from cheap foreign goods. This act made little sense. Europeans could not repay their debts if they could not sell their goods in the rich U.S. market.[20] By 1928, the Hoover-Hughes policy of gently guiding the world into a happy, freer-market economy was in shambles. The two men had been unable to control Coolidge, Mellon, or the bankers.

Most Americans—as usual—paid no attention to these ominous storm clouds. People had never been wealthier or the nation more powerful. American holdings of the world's gold had doubled, and the United States was dominating the global economy. Europeans warned of the "Americanizing of the world" not only through the power of the almighty dollar, but through the new Hollywood motion pictures that spread U.S. culture across the world and whipped up a demand for the products shown in the films. A Belgian paper cried that Europe was threatened with more barbarism from the United States than from the Soviet Union. Famous British author George Bernard Shaw surveyed the source of this supposed barbarism and announced that "an asylum for the sane would be empty in America."[21]

But most Americans cared little about Shaw's comments. They instead tended to admire the new Italian leader, Benito Mussolini, whose loud approval of masculinity, athletics, efficiency, and activism seemed to be borrowed from American virtues. As historian David F. Schmitz notes, moreover, U.S. officials' desire for stability and a non-Bolshevist Europe led them to welcome Mussolini's seizure of power in 1922 and "to support Fascism in Italy" through the 1920s and 1930s "in direct contradiction with purported U.S. ideals."[22]

A CASE STUDY: EUROPE AND THE NEW RULES OF THE GAME

U.S. officials understood that European recovery was especially important. Secretary of State Hughes told the Brown University graduating class in 1921 that "the prosperity of the United States largely depends upon the economic settlements which may be made in Europe, and the key to the future is with those who make those settlements." Hughes knew that Americans held that key. Within Europe itself, Germany was the critical problem. Before 1914, it had been the dominant power on the Continent. As Hughes declared, "There can be no economic recuperation in Europe unless Germany recuperates."[23] Moreover, U.S. officials feared that if Germany were not well treated, it would turn to the Russian Bolsheviks for trade and sympathy.

The Germans, however, had been socked with a $33-billion bill for war reparations by the 1919 peace conference. The French were delighted. They believed that it would be generations before the debt-bound Germans could again threaten neighbors. But the reparations not merely weakened Germany, they almost suffocated it. In 1923, the country could no longer pay. The French struck back by sending troops into the strategic Ruhr Valley that they had long wanted. Germans responded by going on strike. European financial exchanges went haywire. Quietly, but decisively, Hughes moved.

The secretary of state put tremendous pressure on France by demanding payment of the debt that the French owed the United States. As the French franc sank in value, Paris officials had to come to New York and beg for $100 million in credit from J. P. Morgan & Company. With western Europe at his mercy, Hughes agreed to sponsor a meeting in 1924 to solve the crisis. The meeting was to be run, however, not by U.S. officials, but by private American bankers and businessmen. Thus, the government officials would not be directly responsible for the results, and—of special importance—Congress would not have to be consulted formally about the results of the meeting.

The major result was the Dawes Plan (named after Chicago banker and, later, vice-president of the United States, Charles G. Dawes, who pieced the deal together). Germany's reparations payments were sharply reduced to $250 million annually. They were to rise slowly over five years as the economy improved. To trigger that improvement, the Dawes Plan provided for an immediate $200-million loan to pump life into German production. U.S. private bankers were to provide half the amount, with the rest coming from foreign banks.

Suddenly, a snag appeared. J. P. Morgan, Jr., rightly feared that placing the Germans under new debt might make them angry about "the extent to which what was once a first-class power has been subjected to foreign control."[24] But after receiving more guarantees that secured the loan, Morgan went along. When Morgan floated the loan on the public U.S. market, it succeeded beyond anyone's wildest dreams. In a few days, over $1 billion was subscribed, or ten times the amount needed. Americans liked the idea of putting their dollars into German securities. By 1927–1928, money flooded into Germany faster than safe investments could be found for it. But the Dawes Plan had scored a stunning success. As one U.S. official in Europe reported home, "That America is the creditor nation and is trusted in all Europe even where she is despised . . . gives us a potential power to straighten out affairs over here."[25]

The Dawes Plan assumed that the $200 million would restart German industry so that the Germans could repay their debts. But it never worked out that way. Germany—and U.S. investors—became addicted to the loans. As historian Frank Costigliola explains, the Americans failed to see that their hope for a "limited, initial commitment" to ignite the German economy "would quickly and uncontrollably mushroom into a massive and ongoing obligation to keep the system working."[26] The Americans had to keep pouring new money in to support their old money. They had to run ever-faster to stay in the same place. Almost as bad, they entered into cutthroat competition with powerful British banks to see who could control German trade, Austrian and other European money markets, and, indeed, half the world's daily export trade, which London had financed and grown rich from before 1914.

As U.S. relations with Germany and France improved, U.S.-British ties became so bad that by 1927 a British diplomatic official privately warned that Americans had been treated "too much as blood relations, [and] not sufficiently as a foreign country."[27]

That very year, 1927, relations worsened when U.S., British, and Japanese officials met at Geneva, Switzerland, to try to limit the building of smaller warships (such as cruisers) that had not been dealt with at the Washington Conference. France and Italy refused to attend. The British and U.S. delegates so insulted each other that the *New York Times* reporter in Geneva was finally asked by his editor whether he was reporting from a disarmament conference or a battlefield. American arms manufacturers paid expensive lobbyists to ensure that the Geneva talks would fail.[28] But the problem went deeper than that. A declining Great Britain was desperately trying to protect its empire against upstart Americans whom it mistrusted and feared. Chancellor of the Exchequer Winston Churchill secretly told the British cabinet in 1927 that war with the United States was not "unthinkable."[29]

In one key region, however, Americans and British finally worked together. Before World War I, Great Britain dominated the Middle East's oil reserves. The riches had only been glimpsed (the incredible Saudi Arabian wells, for example, had not yet been discovered), but by 1921–1922, Western automobiles, industry, and battleships drank more and more barrels of petroleum. As a French leader put it, "Oil is as necessary as blood." U.S. oil companies appeared in the region of the former Ottoman Empire only after the war. Before that, they had produced their oil mostly in the Western Hemisphere. Now, led by John D. Rockefeller's Standard Oil, they fought for control of Middle East production as well.

The British and French at first tried to exclude U.S. companies. The Americans, joined by the State Department, loudly demanded an "open door" to the region's riches. After years of fighting and talking, five American companies (Gulf, Texaco, Mobil, Standard Oil of New York, all of which were led by Standard Oil of New Jersey) cut a deal with their competitors. They all sat down in 1928 and drew a red line around the area whose oil production they agreed to divide among themselves. This Red Line Agreement marked out the boundary for the world's greatest oil-producing regions, and it aimed to keep all other companies on the outside while "the open door," in historian Anthony Sampson's words, "proved to be a mysterious portal, with the habit of swinging shut again, just as the Americans had got inside." Or, as one of the 1928 participants declared, "Oilmen are like cats; you can never tell from the sound of them whether they are fighting or making love."[30] The Red Line Agreement proved so satisfying that the oilmen maintained this love affair until after World War II.

The Europeans tried to follow these economic settlements with political agreements. At Locarno, Switzerland, in 1925, Germany, France, and Belgium guaranteed each other's boundaries. Great Britain and Italy signed as guarantors. The "Spirit of Locarno" proved to be the peak of European diplomacy in the 1920s. The French, however, wanted more. Worried over possible German military revival, they asked the United States in early 1927 not for an alliance (which they knew Washington would refuse), but for a pact outlawing war between the two nations. It was a clever move. French premier Aristide Briand believed that such a pact would help France by preventing a repeat of 1914–1917, when Americans threatened to break with the French (and British) over neutral U.S. trading rights during wartime. American church groups quickly supported Briand's initiative. These groups had long unsuccessfully urged the Coolidge administration to join international organizations. (They had even held a "World Court Sunday.")

But Coolidge and his new secretary of state, Frank Kellogg, wanted nothing to do with Briand's idea. They feared that it would restrict American freedom of action and tie U.S. interests too closely to France. Kellogg instead made a counterproposal: a statement outlawing war that any nation could sign. Briand, bitterly disappointed, nevertheless could hardly object publicly to a statement opposing war, meaningless though it was. The Kellogg-Briand Pact of 1928, signed by most nations in the world, condemned war and pledged the signatories to settle disputes peacefully. (Within weeks, the U.S. Congress appropriated $250 million to build new warships.) The peace pact soon became known as a mere "international kiss." Dollars and the Washington treaty system of 1921–1922 remained the real weapons of U.S. foreign policy.

THE OUTCAST—SOVIET RUSSIA—
AND THE RULES OF THE GAME

The weapons seemed ever more effective, even in handling the great outcast, the Soviet Union. In 1920, the United States had refused to recognize the Soviets officially. During the next two years, however, U.S. officials were shocked into rethinking their position. Great Britain opened relations with Lenin's government in 1921. The next year, the two pariahs—Germany and the Soviet Union—stunned the world by signing a pact at Rapallo, Italy, that publicly recognized each other's interests. That pact also secretly cleared the way for the two nations to cooperate militarily.

Meanwhile, Lenin had announced his New Economic Policy (NEP) that invited capitalists to help develop Soviet resources. Western officials believed that he had seen the light and was turning the Soviet Union away from communism. Lenin was actually trying to develop the Communist economy as rapidly as possible, make westerners less interested in military interventions, and pit capitalist against capitalist for the profit of the Soviets. Secretary of Commerce Hoover declared the Soviet Union to be an "economic vacuum." U.S. business pushed forward to fill the vacuum with its goods. Relations further grew in 1921–1922, when Americans responded to a severe famine by setting up 18,000 feeding stations, sending $60 million in aid, and saving an estimated 11 million Soviet lives.

These openings, however, were not enough to warm Soviet-American political relations. The American Legion, the Roman Catholic church, and the American Federation of Labor (AFL) especially opposed any ties. AFL leader Samuel Gompers charged that even as the Bolsheviks were trying to undermine the U.S. government, short-sighted, greedy American bankers wanted to help Lenin for their own profit. Hoover and Hughes tried to ensure that the loans would not benefit the Soviet Union. But they fought a losing battle. Large corporations, led by General Electric, General Motors, and even Henry Ford's company, moved into the fertile Soviet market. W. Averell Harriman, the young, handsome heir to a huge railroad empire, opened extensive contacts and negotiated the rights to mineral resources estimated at $1 billion. The deal finally collapsed, but Harriman left the Soviet Union on friendly terms (and returned during World War II as the U.S. ambassador). In 1924, the Soviets set up Amtorg, a trading company located in New York City, to handle their business. By 1925, U.S.-Soviet trade reached $37 million but in the next five years jumped to $95 million, or twice the pre-1914 total of U.S.-Russian trade. Germany continued to be the Soviets' leading trading partner. The Americans, however, were closing ground—and doing so without the U.S. government even recognizing that the Soviet Union officially existed.[31]

Dollars seemed to be creating the new and better world everywhere. When the German economy slowed in 1928, U.S. officials again stepped in. During 1929, the Young Plan (named after Owen D. Young, head of General Electric, who negotiated the deal) further reduced German reparations. The $33 billion of 1921 shrank to $8 billion payable over fifty-eight years. Meanwhile, since 1925, U.S. banks had pumped nearly $1.25 billion of loans into Germany and had granted billions more in short-term credits. Americans directly invested $200 million into German plants.[32] Almost single-handedly, the United States had rebuilt Germany and much more of Europe besides.

"GOD, J. P. MORGAN AND THE REPUBLICAN PARTY" ARE NOT ENOUGH: THE COLLAPSE OF THE SYSTEM (1929)

By early 1929, newly elected President Herbert Hoover believed that continued prosperity was built into the nation's system. Even the usually critical journalist, Lincoln Steffens, agreed: "Big Business in America is producing what the Socialists held up as their goal: food, shelter, and clothing for all."[33] Naturally, Wall Street was optimistic. In 1927, a bull market made investors instant millionaires by shooting stock prices skyward. "There was a spirit of tremendous euphoria," one stockbroker recalled years later. "God, J. P. Morgan and the Republican party were going to keep everything going forever."[34] But the Great Bull Market was built on weakly supported loans as well as on a short-sighted and corrupt banking system.

In September 1929, investors found that they could not pay their loans and so began selling stocks. By October, the selling became a torrent. The money exchanges went crazy as prices dropped. Hoover, the bankers, and Harvard and Yale economists denounced the panic. They solemnly announced that the economy was sound. By the end of the year, however, stock prices had been chopped 50 percent. In March 1930, Hoover declared, "The crisis will be over in sixty days." John D. Rockefeller announced that such a bright future lay ahead that he and his sons were buying stocks. ("Sure," answered one observer, "who else [has] any money left?")[35] By the end of 1930, the economy slid downhill ever more rapidly. It had produced a gross national product (or the sum of all production and services in the economy) of $104 billion in 1929, but by 1933 it amounted to only $56 billion. In 1930 alone, 800 banks declared bankruptcy and ruined small savers who had trusted them. Unemployment was 3 percent, about 1.5 million people, in 1929, but 25 percent, or 12.6 million people, in 1933. And not only the average person suffered. A founder of General Motors, William C. Durant, lost his fortune and wound up operating a bowling alley in Flint, Michigan.

Few understood what was happening. Former President Coolidge exemplified the confusion: "The future may be better or worse," he actually told the nation. Coolidge added: "The final solution for unemployment is work."[36] But several problems became clear. First, the U.S. economy had tried to act as the foundation for the rebuilding of the world economy when, in reality, parts of that foundation were crumbling. The farm sector, for three hundred years the most important producer and buyer, was depressed throughout the 1920s. Textiles and mining were sick industries. Americans who made great profits in the decade did not use them to cure these trouble spots, but instead tried to make a quick killing in the stock market. Nor did the government help correct the foolishness. By the late 1920s, even the Hoover-Hughes attempt to police foreign loans had collapsed. Bankers went their merry way investing money wherever they saw a glimmer of profit. As Germany was flooded with too many dollars, the banks turned elsewhere and, if necessary, created markets: National City Bank of New York forced $90 million in loans on Peru in 1927–1928 by giving a $450,000 bribe to the son of Peru's president. In 1931, Peru defaulted on all the loans.

Even those kinds of opportunities began to dry up in 1928–1929, and so bankers put their funds in the stock market. Dollars had been the blood in the arteries of world commerce. As the dollars stopped flowing overseas by 1929, the economies of Canada, Japan, western Europe, and Latin America became severely ill. Nor could these countries easily buy Americans' cotton, wheat, and autos any longer. U.S. private lenders had supplied $355 million to foreigners in 1927 but only $191 million in 1933, and world trade dropped a full 40 percent in value. Congress responded by passing the Smoot-Hawley Tariff in 1931. It raised the average tariff on protected goods to 59 percent, the highest level in twentieth-century American history. Other nations had been repaying their debts to the United States or selling goods to Americans. Now the U.S. market was largely closed to the goods after the Smoot-Hawley Tariff passed. One expert reported that "in France our tariff was compared to a declaration of war, an economic blockade."[37]

By early 1931, President Hoover understood that he was in a world crisis and that it had to be handled in the global arena. He watched with horror as the Bank of England, the great financial backbone of the British Empire, lost $200 million in just two weeks. Great Britain finally went off the gold standard in September 1931. That standard had been pushed on London by the Americans in 1926 because they owned much of the world's gold and wanted to make the British dependent on it. Now Great Britain was freeing itself so that it could manipulate its own currency and declare economic war on the United States. Even worse threatened in Germany. Both the Communists and Adolf Hitler's National Socialists gained strength. The U.S. ambassador to Germany told Hoover that unless quick action were taken, revolution would overthrow Germany's democratic Weimar Republic.

Hoover responded with a proposal. In mid-1931, he declared that the United States would place a "moratorium" (temporary stop) on war debts owed to it by other nations such as France and Great Britain if, in turn, those nations quit taking war reparations out of Germany. Hoover hoped that this would give everyone time to come to their senses. But the French disagreed. They did not want Germany to escape the controls imposed by the reparations.

Other nations went off on their own. In 1932, the British met at Ottawa, Canada, with their Commonwealth members. They agreed to create an Imperial Preference System that gave each other's products preferred treatment (and pointedly discriminated against U.S. goods). Because many of the Commonwealth members, especially Canada and Australia, had been leading customers for Americans, U.S. officials were furious about the Ottawa deal. For the next fifteen years, these officials worked hard to destroy such economic blocs. Meanwhile, the Europeans met in 1932 to demand relief from paying their debts to New York. Nearly all had defaulted. The one that did not, Finland, forever held a special place in American hearts. In January 1933, Adolf Hitler came to power in Germany and repudiated the country's war debts and liberal trade policies. As historian Frederick C. Adams summarizes the situation at that point: "America found itself confronted by increased trade barriers and a united front of debtor nations."[38]

Hoover tried one other tactic to ease the crisis. As a Quaker and as an engineer who hated wasting resources on nonproductive goods, he had worked for disarmament. In Melvyn Leffler's words, "Hoover hoped that limiting armaments would reduce the burden of taxation and curtail the waste of human and capital resources without jeopardizing the nation's security."[39] In 1929, the president tried to lessen tension with the British by inviting Prime Minister Ramsay MacDonald to a fishing expedition (one of Hoover's greatest loves) at the president's hideaway in Virginia. The two leaders agreed to new ratios for warships and called for a major naval conference in 1930. The conference did agree on new figures and even gave Japan a higher ratio (10:10:7 instead of the old 10:10:6) on cruisers, but not on battleships. The economic crisis had now hit with full force. The Japanese demanded even more ships. The French and Italians also wanted more. These three nations prepared to quit the Five-Power Treaty of 1922.

The president had only one idea left. In 1932, he proposed a kind of diplomatic grand slam: a conference that would deal simultaneously with war debts, reparations, the economic crisis, and disarmament. He was correct in believing that these were linked. Nations were not willing to disarm until their economic security was assured. But their economies also needed relief from rising military budgets. The 1932 elections in the United States intervened, however, and Hoover went down to a humiliating defeat. The new president, Franklin D. Roosevelt, the former Democratic governor of New York, refused to tie his hands by accepting Hoover's proposal.

The disarmament issue soon became irrelevant. In 1933–1934, as Hitler consolidated his power, he tore off the restraints imposed in 1919–1920 on German rearmament. The Japanese had begun their march of armed conquest two years earlier.

COLLAPSE OF THE WASHINGTON TREATY STRUCTURE: ASIA AND WAR

War erupted when Japan invaded northern China in September 1931. U.S. officials were confused. They thought Japan had been brought under control by the Washington treaties and Tokyo's dependence on American dollars. By 1926, Japan had borrowed $200 million. Nearly 40 percent of its foreign loans rested in U.S. hands. It also bought more goods from Americans than from other people. In turn, Americans bought more than 40 percent of Japan's exports in the 1920s.[40]

Hoover was delighted with these figures. He was also happy, however, with the 1924 Immigration Law. The U.S. Congress decided to shut off the inflow of those it considered undesirable, both from eastern Europe and Asia, by sharply reducing immigration quotas. In part because of pressure from California, where anti-Japanese feeling was rampant, the law completely excluded Asians. Hoover privately agreed: "The biological fact makes mixture of bloods disadvantageous to Japan if it occurred there and to us if it occurs here." As he concluded, "We have set up a nation which must . . . be of a character that can evolve a consolidated race."[41] The humiliated Japanese bitterly protested. Dollars, however, helped in steadying relations—until 1929, when the dollars stopped. Japanese militants then used anti-U.S. feeling to gain support for their attacks on American interests.

Meanwhile, during the 1920s, the Republicans' dollar diplomacy also seemed to be working in China. Some $50 million of U.S.-Chinese trade in 1914 nearly quadrupled to $190 million by 1930. Those exchanges represented only 3 percent of total U.S. trade (and some $155 million of U.S. investment amounted to less than 5 percent of total U.S. foreign investment in 1930), but future profits seemed limitless. As a popular book title suggested, the Chinese had to be seen as *Four Hundred Million Customers.* Cigarette sales, for example, had grown from one each year per Chinese in 1900 to 19 per person in 1920. One of Hoover's top aides liked to observe: "Add one inch to the shirt tail of every Chinese and you will keep the cotton mills of the world busy for a year supplying the increased demand."[42]

Saving souls also seemed to be a growth industry. Some 1,000 Christian missionaries in 1900 had become nearly 3,000 by 1920. Since they had converted only 800,000 Chinese (out of a total population of 400 million), obviously much remained to be done. In 1926, Hoover's Commerce Department estimated that U.S. missionary and philanthropic groups had invested $69.3 million in China. It noted that the importance of the Rockefeller Foundation, which had given $34 million to establish a medical school in Beijing (Peking) and other funds for other Western-style colleges, "is not to be underestimated."[43]

The great question, however, was whether the Chinese wanted to be Westernized. On May 4, 1919, the flames of the revolution that had been lit eight years earlier suddenly blazed again when Beijing (Peking) students massively protested against the humiliations piled on China at the Paris peace conference. The May Fourth Movement was also fueled by foreign control of the nation's tariff collection and by British and Standard Oil monopoly of the kerosene trade used to light China's lamps. Sun Yat-sen, who had helped to overthrow the Manchu dynasty in 1911, again led the revolution. His Nationalist movement worked closely with the one nation willing to help revolutionaries—the Soviet Union. Indeed, the 1924 China-USSR agreement so stunned the Japanese that they quickly established relations with the Soviet Union in 1925. Now Americans were stunned. An Asiatic phalanx seemed to be rising. "That there is a menace to the entire West in such a combination seems self-evident," a U.S. diplomat warned.[44]

And as Chinese nationalism surged, Americans found it difficult to pose as protectors because the Chinese no longer wanted protection. Even worse threatened when the Chinese Communist party was officially founded in 1921. But Sun held real power, and by 1925 he had succeeded in achicving his two objectives: conquering various local "war lords" whose private armies controlled key regions, and destroying foreigners' special privileges. That year, Sun suddenly died. His power was seized by a young aide, Chiang Kai-shek, whose training by the Soviets and talent for intrigue were quickly mistrusted in Washington. After a series of military victories in 1926, however, Chiang was afraid that the Soviets and Communists were ready to eliminate him. In 1927, he beat them to the punch. He threw out the Soviet advisers and, with the help of gangster friends from the Chinese underworld, killed thousands of Communists and forced the rest into hiding.[45]

U.S. officials should have been pleased, but they were not. In 1925–1926, Chiang's success had intensified China's antiforeignism. That hatred of foreigners increased when British-led police and British and French troops killed sixty-five Chinese protesters. Foreigners, including missionaries, were sought out for revenge. By 1927, nearly 70 percent of the Protestant missionaries had left China. U.S. troops landed to help restore order in 1928 at Tianjin (Tientsin), 70 miles from the capital of Beijing (Peking). Soon, dance halls, bowling alleys, bars, gambling, and prostitutes (mostly Russian women in exile) were in evidence. A year later, the U.S. Marines were gone, but the memories—and unpaid bar bills signed by "Herbert Hoover" and "George Washington"—remained in Chinese minds.[46] Chiang's regime now demanded respect: "The time has come to speak to foreign imperialism in the language it understands," the Chinese foreign minister declared.[47] The foreign powers did restore tariff autonomy to China in 1928 but refused to give up other legal or military power they had exercised in a different China. Chiang and his Kuomintang (KMT) movement were feared as revolutionary and antiforeign.

This background must be understood if one hopes to grasp why the United States did nothing when Japan invaded Manchuria in 1931 and, in reality, tore up the Washington treaties before astonished American eyes. The invasion surprised Hoover and his secretary of state, Henry Stimson. Stimson was a wealthy New York lawyer who appreciated the Tokyo–New York dollar link. He (like his hero, Theodore Roosevelt) believed that Japan supported U.S. interests in Asia. As a conservative former governor general of the Philippines, Stimson viewed many Asians as inefficient and inferior, but he especially feared and disliked revolutionary Asians.

Stimson had agreed with Hoover's belief in September 1929 that "there is the most profound outlook for peace today that we have had

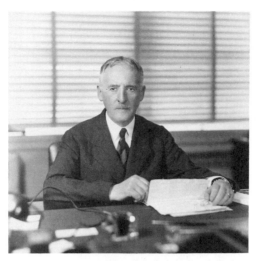

The life of Henry Stimson (1867–1950) in many ways was a history of American foreign policy between his service as secretary of war to President Taft (1911–1913) and to President Truman in 1945. In between, Stimson fought on the western front in World War I, acted as U.S. governor general of the Philippines in 1927–1929, became Hoover's secretary of state (1929–1933), then—after vigorously opposing German and Japanese expansion while growing wealthy from his law practice—received Franklin D. Roosevelt's appointment as secretary of war in 1940. As a godfather of the "American establishment," he strongly influenced many of the younger men who shaped U.S. economic and foreign policy after the 1930s. A Republican, Stimson exemplified the conservative, internationalist policies of U.S. diplomacy.

at any time in the last half century."[48] A month later the New York stock market collapsed. The Japanese, who had bet their economy and foreign policy on the dollar, now began to search for other alternatives. A liberal, pro-Western cabinet in Tokyo gave way to moderate groups and finally to a government in which militarists had a strong voice. The Chinese Revolution, moreover, directly threatened vast Japanese holdings in Manchuria and China proper. U.S. officials sympathized with Tokyo's predicament. They allowed Japan to increase its naval power at the 1930 naval conference. Hoover agreed with a journalist friend who wrote: "I think the Japs are our first line of defense in the Far East; and I am certainly glad they are well armed."[49]

On September 18, 1931, Japanese troops apparently set off an explosion on the South Manchurian Railroad that Japan had controlled since 1905. They then used the incident as an excuse to seize Manchuria once and for all. Hoover's mind was elsewhere. Americans were starving. Western Europe seemed on the edge of chaos. At first, Stimson

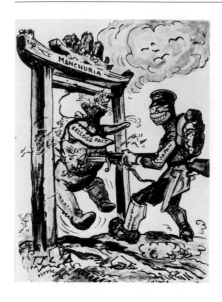

This cartoon by Cesare in Outlook *depicts how Japanese aggression in Manchuria in 1931–1932 destroyed the Kellogg Pact, ended a close U.S.-Japanese relationship, and violently shut a long chapter of the American open-door policy in Asia.*

thought the rail incident only a local crisis. Believing that because of his experience in running the Philippines he "knew something" about the "Oriental mind," the secretary of state decided not to pressure Japan and not to defend Chinese revolutionaries. As the U.S. ambassador to London told the Japanese, "The Chinese are altogether too cocky. What you people need to do is to give them a thoroughly good licking to teach them their place and then they will be willing to talk sense."[50] Japan agreed. By January 2, 1932, its army had seized key ports some 1,700 miles from where the war had started.

Stimson was now aware that he had misread the "Oriental mind" and desperately turned to a series of responses. He tried to wield the Kellogg-Briand Pact of 1928, but Japan paid no attention to its supposed moral force. Stimson hoped that the Japanese economy would crumble under war demands, but instead it improved. He hoped the League of Nations would stand up to Tokyo, but the League merely condemned the invasion. As for economic retaliation, Hoover bluntly refused. He feared that if the economic sanctions did not work, military involvement would have to follow, and he wanted none of that. Moreover, such sanctions would be the knockout blow to U.S.-Japan economic relations. "The result," in historian Gary Ostrower's words, "was confusion because Stimson wanted both to stop Japan militarily and expand relations with Japan economically."[51] (For its part, Japan quit the League in early 1933.)

On January 7, 1932, Stimson declared in the so-called "Hoover-

Stimson Doctrine" that the United States would not recognize Japan's control over Manchuria (or "Manchukuo," as Tokyo had renamed it). The Japanese militarists cared little. Eleven days later, their troops seized the great port city of Shanghai. On February 24, Stimson played his highest card. He sent an open letter to Senator Borah, who had strongly opposed Japan's actions. Stimson warned that unless Tokyo upheld the Nine-Power Treaty promise to observe the open door in China, Washington would not uphold the Five-Power Treaty limiting the building of warships. Thus, the United States threatened Japan with a war fleet in the Pacific—at least sometime in the future after the fleet was built. But this threat also had little effect. Stimson was now ready to get tougher with Japan. But Hoover flatly refused. Stimson fretted privately that the president was a good engineer who thought that foreign policy could be carefully calculated—"like building a bridge." Actually, the secretary of state told Hoover, "You . . . make your plans only for a certain distance," and the best rule is that "in case of doubt . . . march toward the guns."[52]

Hoover refused to march. He was afraid that a break with Japan could destroy all order in Asia. After all, he told his cabinet, Tokyo faced danger from "a Bolshevist Russia to the north and a possible Bolshevist China" on the flank. The president also told an aide that "just between ourselves, it would not be a bad thing if Mr. Jap should go into Manchuria, for with two thorns in his side—China and the Bolsheviks—he would have enough to keep him busy for awhile."[53] But the Soviets themselves were playing a two-faced game. They asked Japan for a friendship treaty, then secretly approached the United States to join them in "breaking [Japan] as between the two arms of a nut-cracker."[54] Hoover, however, could never diplomatically recognize a Soviet Union that, as Stimson complained, was always "violating the fundamental tenets of international intercourse."[55] The United States thus stood paralyzed amid the ruins of its economy and, therefore, the ruins of its entire postwar foreign policy.

GETTING "BLUE" OVER LATIN AMERICA

The 1922 treaty system implied that the military forces of certain powers would maintain order in their regions—for example, Japan in Asia and the United States in Latin America. The U.S. military was accompanied by bankers and traders seeking profit. They found it. Between 1924 and 1929, U.S. investments in Latin America more than doubled from \$1.5 billion to over \$3.5 billion, twice as much as Americans invested in any other geographical area. Much of the money was used to take over vital mineral resources such as Chile's copper and Venezuela's oil. Before 1914, most U.S. investors worked in the Central American–Caribbean region. But now they moved throughout the larger nations to the south. They were replacing the British, who had bankrolled South American development for a century. Washington officials believed that the dollars only produced happiness and order. "The number of rebellions per capita is highest in those republics where the per capita mileage of . . . highways is lowest," one wrote. "Romance may have been driven out by the cement mixer, but the mixer has paved the way for law and order."[56]

President Coolidge was not so sure. The more Americans invested, the more they seemed to be attacked by angry Latin Americans. Coolidge finally warned in 1925 that because "the person and property of a citizen are a part of the general domain of the nation, even when abroad," he had the right to send troops to protect that "domain."[57] Thus, U.S. Marines controlled Nicaragua, the Dominican Republic, Haiti, and Panama, and overshadowed many other nations. The easy excuse for sending in troops was the Monroe Doctrine. The founder of Christian Science, Mary Baker Eddy, spoke for millions of North Americans when she said in 1923, "I believe strictly in the Monroe Doctrine, in our Constitution, and in the laws of God."[58] Another motive was racism. U.S. officials running Haiti once had a Marine-trained band honor the Haitian president by playing "Bye, Bye Blackbird." Many of these officials were from the U.S. South and were sent to the Caribbean nations because they supposedly knew how best to handle black people.

By the late 1920s, Latin Americans were fighting such policies. They happily joined the League of Nations and were cool toward the idea of Pan-Americanism precisely because North Americans were not in the former and tried to dominate the latter. A leading Chilean newspaper warned in 1930 that the United States "Colossus" had "financial might" without "equal in history," and that its aim was "Americas for the Americans—of the North."[59] An earlier survey showed that of the twenty Latin American nations, all but six were controlled or heavily influenced by U.S. Marines, U.S. bankers, or both. In 1928, at the Havana Inter-American Conference, a resolution stated that "no state has a right to intervene in the internal affairs of another." When former Secretary of State Hughes tried to kill the resolution, he found only four

Latin American supporters—three of whose nations were run by U.S. military forces.

The State Department finally tried to deal with the growing condemnation in 1929–1930 by issuing a memorandum written by Undersecretary of State Reuben Clark. The Clark Memorandum declared that the Monroe Doctrine—or, more accurately, the Roosevelt Corollary to the doctrine (see p. 247)—should not be used to justify U.S. intervention. (Clark argued, however, that North Americans had other legal rights to protect themselves and their property abroad.) President Hoover scored a major success by announcing that he planned to withdraw the marines from the Caribbean and take a triumphant tour of South America.

But the turnaround came too late. Wall Street's collapse in 1929 meant in Latin America, as elsewhere, the collapse of what Hughes had called *Pax Americana.* Between 1929 and 1931, revolution struck seven hemispheric nations. By 1933, only Colombia, Uruguay, and Venezuela had escaped revolution. The United States, joined enthusiastically by the sitting governments, had refused in 1923 to recognize regimes that rose to power by force. In 1931, Stimson had to reverse that policy simply because the southern continent was in continual upheaval. The cement-mixer approach had not worked. "I am getting quite blue over the bad way in which all Latin America is showing up," Stimson wrote in his diary in 1932. They do not help themselves. "Yet if we try to take the lead for them . . . there is a cry against domination and imperialism."[60]

THOSE "BOLSHEVISTS" IN MEXICO AND NICARAGUA

Such a cry had been going up for years in two key nations, Mexico and Nicaragua. In Mexico, the long-festering dispute between U.S. officials and the revolutionary government finally stopped in 1923. An agreement was reached giving North Americans an indemnity for their lands seized by Mexico for redistribution to peasants. U.S. oil companies also received protection for their holdings. But these deals were never ratified by the U.S. Senate. In 1925, President Plutarco Calles bowed to rising protests in Mexico by trying again to tighten control over his country's rich oil reserves. Another crisis threatened U.S.-Mexican relations. This time, however, both sides quickly tried to find a compromise.

Coolidge and Secretary of State Kellogg hated what they saw as "Bolshevist" influences in the Mexican Revolution. They nevertheless listened to oil companies that wanted to make a deal. Coolidge consequently sent Dwight Morrow to negotiate a settlement in 1927. As a Wall Street lawyer, Morrow was acceptable to North Americans. As a smart, broad-minded negotiator who ordered a good-will visit to Mexico by his future son-in-law Charles Lindbergh (perhaps the world's most famous celebrity because he had been the first to fly across the Atlantic Ocean alone in 1927), Morrow became well liked in Mexico. The Calles government agreed to validate in perpetuity all titles to oil lands obtained before May 1917. The president's retreat soon paid off. When a revolt against Calles erupted in 1929, Hoover sent him arms and refused to deal with the rebels, who soon surrendered.

The Nicaraguan story did not have such a happy ending. U.S. troops had controlled the country since 1911–1912. In 1925, however, Coolidge concluded that order and the strength of pro-U.S. groups were sufficient to bring the boys back home. Within weeks, fighting again erupted. After a U.S. admiral tried to mediate aboard his warship, Adolfo Díaz emerged as a president acceptable to Coolidge. But again fighting broke out, with Mexico on the side of the anti-Díaz rebels. Crying that Russian bolshevism threatened Nicaragua, in 1926 Coolidge again landed the marines. Norman Davis, a leading Democrat and an experienced diplomat, blasted the decision: "By basing our policy with Latin America upon a fear of Bolshevism, we not only destroy our influence and prestige with Latin America, but we give great encouragement to the Bolshevists."[61] Coolidge nevertheless sent Henry Stimson in with the troops to work out an acceptable deal. Stimson talked both sides into laying down arms and cooperating with an election in 1928 held under U.S. supervision.

But one leader rejected Stimson's settlement. Augusto Sandino replied: "The sovereignty and liberty of a people are not to be discussed but rather defended with weapons in hand."[62] He organized a small guerrilla band to resist the marines. Sandino's well-to-do father, who gave his son a good education, had lost his political power when the marines appeared in 1911–1912. The son became further angered at the United States when he saw firsthand Woodrow Wilson's landing of U.S. troops in Mexico during 1914. By 1927, Sandino was less a revolutionary (he rejected the Marxism-Leninism of other Central American revolutionaries) than an anticolonialist. He simply wanted the United States out of his country.

His small army attacked U.S. troop camps. In 1927, the marine com-

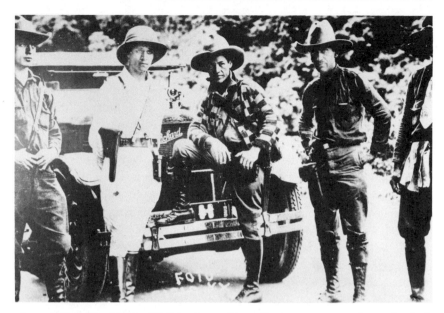

Augusto Sandino (1893–1934) is pictured here (in the center, wearing a checked shirt) with his aides in Nicaragua. Sandino led the resistance to the U.S. occupation of 1927–1933 and—as it turned out by the 1970s and 1980s—both opened a new chapter in U.S.–Central American relations and gave a bloody preview of the problems that Washington officials would have in dealing with Third World nationalist revolts.

mander responded to a Sandino attack on Ocotal by calling in five aircraft. In the first organized dive-bombing attack in the hemisphere's history, the planes bombed and machine-gunned the rebels with bloody results. Over one hundred Sandinistas were killed or wounded in minutes. But their leader survived. He found strong support in the mountains from peasants who had gained nothing from the long U.S. occupation. Sandino ruthlessly destroyed American property and often dealt with disloyal Nicaraguans by giving them a "gourd cut"—slicing off a part of the skull, exposing the victim's brain, and causing hours of convulsions and suffering before dying. "Liberty is not conquered with flowers," Sandino believed.[63]

By 1929, 5,500 marines were unable to capture the "bandits," as Stimson called the Sandinistas. But the troops were taking casualties and costing U.S. taxpayers millions of dollars. High-school debaters soon discussed the national debate topic of whether the marines should leave Nicaragua. Republican senator Burton K. Wheeler from Montana acidly declared that if the marines were really supposed to fight "bandits," they could best do it in Chicago. Another critic wrote that if the U.S. government actually thought it could impose democratic elections, it might try to begin in Philadelphia. A businessman warned that U.S. policy "has proved a calamity for the American coffee planters. . . . Today we are hated and despised" because the marines were sent "to hunt down and kill Nicaraguans in their own country."[64] Stimson was especially embarrassed to have to defend the marines in Nicaragua while he condemned the Japanese invasion of China.

He and Hoover decided to pull out the troops. But they left behind a U.S.-trained National Guard to maintain order. The guard's commander was Anastasio Somoza, a Philadelphia-educated Nicaraguan whose love of baseball and talent for cussing in English helped win Stimson's trust. As Sandino had promised, once the marines left in 1933, he laid down his arms. With a grant of amnesty, he began talks with the Nicaraguan government. After one session in February 1934, Somoza's henchmen seized Sandino and two of his closest aides, took them to a government airfield, and executed them. By 1936, Somoza had used the guard to claim dictatorial power. Elected civilians in Managua appealed to Washington for help. The State Department replied, apparently with a straight face, that it was contrary to U.S. policy to interfere in Nicaraguan affairs.[65]

But the story was not over. Sandino had presented a new challenge to the United States: a guerrilla leader who had strong mass support, an anticolonial ideology, and the military capacity to defy U.S. power. Some 136 marines lost their lives (including twelve who committed suicide in Nicaragua), but Sandino's success went far beyond battle casualties. He anticipated the problems that North Americans were to encounter later in China, Cuba, Vietnam, and, finally, Nicaragua itself after 1979, when the self-styled "Sandinista" revolutionaries would overthrow the Somoza dynasty and once again defy the United States.

Conclusion

North Americans did not retreat from the world in the 1920s. They, instead, tried nothing less than to restructure its affairs. The foundation of the new structure was the dollar, and atop it were piled the treaty systems of Washington, Locarno, Geneva, and Kellogg-Briand. The blueprint for the structure was based on the needs of Americans. They had become a great world power—indeed, the greatest economically. Hoover wanted them, however, to maintain their "American individualism" (to use the title of his widely read essay) as they circled a globe now shaped by new technology, industry, and national hatreds. World War I itself could never be repeated, the argument ran, because the world was going to be too integrated, too open, too Americanized for another such bloodletting. "We believed . . . that such a change [for peace] could now be predicated upon definite economic and evolutionary facts," Stimson wrote in 1933.[66]

By then, of course, the dollar had collapsed. The delicate treaty structure fell on top of it. In historian John M. Carroll's words, "The foundations of economic and political stability" laid during the 1920s were simply "swept away during the economic crisis of the 1930s."[67] Hitler, Japanese militarists, and the Somozas of the less-industrialized nations—not "American individualism"—threatened to restructure the world. Washington's response now came from the newly elected president, fifty-one-year-old Franklin D. Roosevelt, who searched through the wreckage of the 1920s for a new, workable blueprint. He never found it during peacetime.

NOTES

1. John Morton Blum, *Public Philosopher: Selected Letters of Walter Lippmann* (New York, 1985), pp. 136–137.
2. Paul F. Boller, Jr., *Presidential Anecdotes* (New York, 1981), pp. 229–230.
3. Charles Evans Hughes, *The Pathway of Peace* (New York, 1925), p. 159.
4. Joan Hoff Wilson, *Herbert Hoover: Forgotten Progressive* (Boston, 1975), pp. 168, 179.
5. Herbert C. Hoover, *Memoirs*, 3 vols. (New York, 1951–1952), II, p. 28.
6. David Green, *Shaping Political Consciousness: The Language of Politics in America from McKinley to Reagan* (Ithaca, N.Y., 1988), ch. 3.
7. Warren I. Cohen, *Empire without Tears: America's Foreign Relations, 1921–1933* (New York, 1987), p. 13; Herbert Hoover, *American Individualism* (Washington, D.C., 1922), p. 31.
8. Charles E. Neu, *The Troubled Encounter: The United States and Japan* (New York, 1975), pp. 100, 103.
9. Ira Klein, "Whitehall, Washington, and the Anglo-Japanese Alliance, 1919–1921," *Pacific Historical Review* 46, no. 2 (1968): 468–469; Lloyd C. Gardner, *Safe for Democracy* (New York, 1984), pp. 307–319, has a fine discussion.
10. Carl P. Parrini, *Heir to Empire: United States Economic Diplomacy, 1916–1923* (Pittsburgh, 1969), pp. 202–203.
11. The Washington treaties and Harding's rationale for them can be conveniently found in *The Record of American Diplomacy*, ed. Ruhl J. Bartlett, 4th ed. (New York, 1964),

pp. 486–497; the quote is from Lloyd Gardner, Walter LaFeber, and Thomas McCormick, *The Creation of the American Empire* (Chicago, 1973), p. 357.

12. Thomas Buckley, *The United States and the Washington Conference, 1921–1922* (Knoxville, Tenn., 1970), p. 187.

13. Andrew Sinclair, *The Available Man: The Life behind the Masks of Warren Gamaliel Harding* (New York, 1965), p. 244.

14. Akira Iriye, *After Imperialism: The Search for a New Order in the Far East* (New York, 1969), p. 20.

15. Charles Evans Hughes, "Some Aspects of the Work of the Department of State," *American Journal of International Law* 16 (May 1922): 358–359; a fine brief analysis is Justus D. Doenecke, "The Most-Favored-Nation Principle," in *Encyclopedia of American Foreign Policy*, ed. Alexander DeConde, 3 vols. (New York, 1978), II, p. 608.

16. Brenda Gayle Plummer, "Epilogue," in "Black and White in the Caribbean: Haitian-American Relations, 1902–1934" (Ph.D. diss., Cornell University, 1981).

17. Parrini, pp. 186–187.

18. Hoover, *Memoirs*, II, pp. 81–82.

19. Rexford G. Tugwell, *The Democratic Roosevelt* (Garden City, N.Y., 1957), p. 132.

20. Melvyn P. Leffler, *The Elusive Quest: America's Pursuit of European Stability and French Security, 1919–1933* (Chapel Hill, N.C., 1979), pp. 48, 170.

21. Ivy Lee, "The Black Legend: Europe Indicts America," *Atlantic Monthly* 143 (May 1929): 577–588.

22. David F. Schmitz, *The United States and Fascist Italy, 1922–1940* (Chapel Hill, N.C., 1988), pp. 1, 42; John P. Diggins, *Mussolini and Fascism: The View from America* (Princeton, 1972), tells this fascinating story.

23. Frederick C. Adams, *Economic Diplomacy: The Export-Import Bank and American Foreign Policy, 1934–1939* (Columbia, Mo., 1976), ch I, contains the quotes and a useful context.

24. Herbert Feis, *The Diplomacy of the Dollar, 1919–1923* (New York, 1950), pp. 40–42.

25. Leffler, p. 100.

26. Frank Costigliola, "The United States and the Reconstruction of Germany in the 1920s," *Business History Review* 50 (Winter 1976): 477–502, esp. 488.

27. D. Cameron Watt, *Succeeding John Bull: America in Britain's Place, 1900–1975* (Cambridge, 1984), p. 50.

28. *Ibid.*, p. 58–59.

29. *Ibid.*, p. 59. A similar U.S. view of Great Britain is nicely analyzed in Raymond G. O'Connor, *Perilous Equilibrium: The United States and the London Disarmament Conference of 1930* (Lawrence, Kans., 1962, 1969), pp. 13–14.

30. Anthony Sampson, *The Seven Sisters* (New York, 1975), pp. 58, 65; William Stivers, "A Note on the Red Line Agreement," *Diplomatic History* 7 (Winter 1983): 23, 30, 34.

31. William Appleman Williams, *American-Russian Relations, 1781–1947* (New York, 1952), pp. 193–201, 211–214; Joan Hoff Wilson, *American Business and Foreign Policy, 1920–1933* (Lexington, Ky., 1971), p. 105.

32. Manfred Jonas, *The United States and Germany, a Diplomatic History* (Ithaca, N.Y., 1984), pp. 182–183.

33. Arthur Schlesinger, Jr., *The Crisis of the Old Order, 1919–1933* (Boston, 1957), pp. 142–143.

34. *New York Times*, 23 September 1979, p. F8.

35. *Ibid.*

36. Boller, pp. 234–235.

37. Leffler, p. 198. The loan figures are in the U.S. Department of Commerce, *Historical Statistics of the United States, Colonial Times to 1957* (Washington, D.C., 1961), p. 564.

38. Adams, ch. II.

39. Leffler, p. 219.

40. Grosvenor Jones, Bureau of Foreign and Domestic Commerce, to Herbert Hoover, 7 August 1926, Commerce, Official Files, Box 130, Herbert Hoover Library, West Branch, Iowa; Iriye, p. 26.

41. "Draft" verbally stated to the president, 21 April 1924, Commerce, Official Files, Box 234, Hoover Library; Herbert Hoover to Mark L. Requa, 21 April 1924, Commerce, Official Files, Box 170, Hoover Library.

42. William L. Neumann, "Ambiguity and Ambivalence in Ideas of National Interest in Asia," in *Isolation and Security*, ed. Alexander DeConde (Durham, N.C., 1957), p. 136; William L. Neumann, "Determinism, Destiny, and Myth in the American Image of China," in *Issues and Conflicts: Studies in Twentieth Century American Diplomacy*, ed. George L. Anderson (Lawrence, Kans., 1959), pp. 11–12; C. F. Remer, *Foreign Investment in China* (New York, 1933), p. 274.

43. Grosvenor Jones, Bureau of Foreign and Domestic Commerce, to Herbert Hoover, 7 August 1926, Commerce, Official Files, Box 130, Hoover Library.

44. Pauline Tompkins, *American-Russian Relations in the Far East* (New York, 1949), p. 212.

45. John King Fairbank, *The Great Chinese Revolution: 1800–1985* (New York, 1986), pp. 182–183, 204–216.

46. *New York Times*, 12 July 1973, p. 14.

47. Foster Rhea Dulles, *China and America: The Story of Their Relations since 1784* (Princeton, 1946), pp. 166–167.

48. Robert H. Ferrell, *American Diplomacy in the Great Depression* (New Haven, 1957), p. 19.

49. O'Connor, p. 160n.

50. Ferrell, p. 146; Elting E. Morison, *Turmoil and Tradition: The Life and Times of Henry L. Stimson* (Boston, 1960), pp. 373–374.

51. Gary B. Ostrower, *Collective Insecurity: The U.S. and the League of Nations during the Early Thirties* (Lewisburg, Pa., 1979), p. 203; Armin Rappaport, *Henry L. Stimson and Japan, 1931–1933* (Chicago, 1963), pp. 148–149.

52. Morison, p. 313; Lloyd C. Gardner, *Economic Aspects of New Deal Diplomacy* (Madison, Wis., 1964), pp. 80, 111. There is also an important analysis in *The Diplomacy of Frustration: The Manchurian Crisis of 1931–1933 as Revealed in the Papers of Stanley K. Hornbeck*, ed. Justus D. Doenecke (Stanford, 1981), p. xii.

53. Richard N. Current, *Secretary Stimson: A Study in Statecraft* (New Brunswick, N.J., 1954), pp. 79, 87; Doenecke, ed., *The Diplomacy of Frustration*, p. 13.

54. Tompkins, ch. XII.

55. Morison, p. 312.

56. Julius Klein, *Frontiers of Trade* (New York, 1929), p. 39. Klein's view is well analyzed in Robert N. Seidel, *Progressive Pan Americanism*, Cornell University Latin American Studies Program Dissertation Series (Ithaca, N.Y., 1973), pp. 136–186.

57. Feis, p. 29.

58. Gaddis Smith, "The Legacy of the Monroe Doctrine," *New York Times Magazine*, 9 September 1984, p. 125.

59. Donald M. Dozer, *Are We Good Neighbors?: Three Decades of Inter-American Relations, 1930–1960* (Gainesville, Fla., 1959), pp. 4–7.

60. Gardner, *Economic Aspects of New Deal Diplomacy*, pp. 35–36.

61. Norman Davis to Claude A. Swanson, 14 January 1927, Box 53, Papers of Norman Davis, Library of Congress, Washington, D.C. Robert Freeman Smith found a poem written by Senator George Norris that satirized Coolidge's fear of Bolsheviks in the southern nations. (The form parodies a popular poem by James Whitcomb Riley.)

> "Once't there was a Bolshevik who wouldn't say his prayers, So Kellogg sent him off to bed, away upstairs; An' Kellogg heered him holler, and Coolidge heered him bawl, But when they turn't the kivers down he wasn't there at all. They seeked him down in Mexico, they cussed him in the press, They seeked him round the Capitol, an' evey'where I guess. But all they ever found of him was whiskers, hair and clout; An' the Bolsheviks 'ill get you ef you don't watch out."

(Robert Freeman Smith, "Republican Policy and the Pax Americana, 1921–1932," in *From Colony to Empire: Essays in the History of American Foreign Relations*, ed. William A. Williams [New York, 1972], pp. 256–257.)

62. Thomas W. Walker, *Nicaragua: The Land of Sandino* (Boulder, Col., 1981), p. 22.

63. Neill Macaulay, *The Sandino Affair* (Chicago, 1967), pp. 211–212.

64. Dozer, pp. 11–12.

65. Juan Sacasa, Emiliano Chamorro, Adolfo Díaz to Cordell Hull, 30 November 1936, in U.S. Department of State, *Foreign Relations of the United States, 1936*, 5 vols. (Washington, D.C., 1954), V, pp. 844–846.

66. Henry L. Stimson, "Bases of American Foreign Policy during the Past Four Years," *Foreign Affairs* 11 (April 1933): 383.

67. John M. Carroll, "Owen D. Young and German Reparations," in *U.S. Diplomats in Europe, 1919–1941*, ed. Kenneth Paul Jones (Santa Barbara, Calif., 1981), p. 60. The essays in this volume on the 1920s by Hogan, Jones, Costigliola, and Swerczek are also valuable.

FOR FURTHER READING

Check also the notes to this chapter and the General Bibliography at the end of this book; most of those references are not repeated here. But begin with *Guide to American Foreign Relations since 1700*, ed. Richard Dean Burns (1983), which is incomparable for helping those who wish to research specific topics. Because of Burns's work, the following references are almost entirely post-1981 publications.

The most helpful overviews on 1921–1933 are Warren I. Cohen, *Empire without Tears: America's Foreign Relations, 1921–1933* (1987), with lively writing and an excellent bibliography; Martin Sklar's pioneering, *The United States as a Developing Country* (1992);

Frank Costigliola, *Awkward Dominion: American Political, Economic, and Cultural Relations with Europe, 1919–1933* (1985), superb on Europe and especially cultural relations; Akíra Iriye, *The Globalizing of America, 1914–1945*, in *The Cambridge History of U.S. Foreign Relations*, ed. Warren Cohen (1993); John M. Carroll, "American Diplomacy in the 1920s," in *Modern American Diplomacy*, ed. John M. Carroll and George C. Herring (1986), a useful brief analysis; and two most important overviews by John Braeman: "Power and Diplomacy: The 1920s Reappraised," *Review of Politics* 44 (July 1982), and "The New Left and American Foreign Policy during the Age of Normalcy: A Re-examination," *Business History Review* 57 (Spring 1983). Cultural and economic expansion is nicely woven together in Emily S. Rosenberg's important *Spreading the American Dream* (1982), which covers 1890 to 1945 but is especially good on the "cooperative" state of the 1920s. On the peace movement, important accounts include Harold Josephson, "Outlawing War: Internationalism and the Pact of Paris," *Diplomatic History* 3 (1979), and George Peter Marabell, *Frederick Libby and the American Peace Movement* (1982).

Patrick Hearden, "Herbert C. Hoover and the Dream of Capitalism in One Country," in *Redefining the Past: Essays in Diplomatic History in Honor of William Appleman Williams*, ed. Lloyd C. Gardner (1986), is inclusive and gives additional sources; and the same can be said for Betty Glad, "Charles Evans Hughes, Rationalism and Foreign Affairs," in *Studies in American Diplomacy, 1865–1945*, ed. Norman Graebner (1985). An elite group whose origins tell much about 1920s policies is analyzed in Robert D. Schulzinger, *The Wise Men of Foreign Affairs: The History of the Council on Foreign Relations* (1984).

On Europe, the following are important (along with Costigliola, noted above): B.J.C. McKercher, *Anglo-American Relations in the 1920s* (1990); Michael Hogan, "Thomas W. Lamont and European Recovery," in *U.S. Diplomats in Europe, 1919–1941*, ed. Kenneth Paul Jones (1981), a book whose essays are most helpful for the entire interwar era; Peter H. Buckingham, *International Normalcy: The Open Door Peace with the Former Central Powers, 1921–1929* (1983); Henry Blumenthal, *Illusion and Reality in Franco-American Diplomacy, 1914–1945* (1986); Neal Pease, *Poland, the United States and the Stabilization of Europe, 1919–1933* (1986). Two crucial books on Middle East and oil policies are William Stivers, *Supremacy and Oil: Iraq, Turkey, and the Anglo-American World Order, 1918–1930* (1982), and Stephen J. Randall, *U.S. Foreign Oil Policy, 1919–1948* (1985), which stresses an "associational state" approach.

On the Far East, Roger Dingman, *Power in the Pacific: The Origins of Naval Arms Limitations, 1914–1922* (1976), is standard; Sandra C. Taylor, *Advocate of Understanding: Sidney Gulick and the Search for Peace with Japan* (1984), is important for far more than its excellent biography; Bernard D. Cole, *Gunboats and Marines: The U.S. Navy in China, 1925–1928* (1983), revealing for its analysis of divisions among U.S. officials; *The Diplomacy of Frustration: The Manchurian Crisis of 1931–1933 as Revealed in the Papers of Stanley K. Hornbeck*, ed. Justus D. Doenecke (1981), a pivotal source on a pivotal figure; William F. Wu, *The Yellow Peril: Chinese Americans in American Fiction, 1850–1940* (1982), interesting as cultural and diplomatic history.

On Latin America, see Robert Freeman Smith, "Thomas W. Lamont," in T. McCormick and W. LaFeber, eds., *Behind the Throne* (1993), essays in honor of Fred Harvey Harrington; Kenneth J. Grieb, *The Latin American Policy of Warren G. Harding* (1977), an important starting point; John H. Findling, *Close Neighbors, Distant Friends: United States–Central American Relations* (1987), very useful, inclusive, and with good sources for further research; Stephen G. Rabe, *The Road to OPEC: U.S. Relations with Venezuela, 1919–1976* (1982), superb on oil as well as Latin American policies; John A. Britton, *Carleton Beals: A Radical Journalist in Latin America* (1987), a much-needed biography of an outspoken critic; Kenneth A. Jennings, "Sandino against the Marines: The Development of Air Power for Conducting Counterinsurgency Operations in Central America," *Air University Review* 37 (July–August, 1986), a different perspective; and Michael Krenn's important *U.S. Policy Toward Economic Nationalism in Latin America, 1917–1929* (1990).

12

FDR and the Entry into World War II (1933–1941)

Franklin D. Roosevelt entered the White House in March 1933 as Americans reeled in shock from the economic crisis. The banking system lay in shambles, one of four workers had no job, formerly comfortable businessmen sold apples for 5 cents each on street corners, and dust storms choked those farmers not already driven off their land by bankruptcy. Hitler and Japanese expansionists began to shape world politics, while the League of Nations, mortally wounded by the U.S. and British refusal to support its call to action against Japan in 1932, stumbled slowly to its death.

No one could predict how Roosevelt might react to these crises. Born into a wealthy New York family, distantly related to Theodore Roosevelt, educated at an elite prep school and at Harvard (where his C average indicated that he spent most of his time editing the school newspaper), Roosevelt knew little about grass-roots America. But he moved successfully into New York state politics, then became assistant secretary of the navy under Woodrow Wilson. In 1920, the thirty-eight-year-old ran as vice-president on the Democratic party ticket that promised to support Wilson's League of Nations. The Democrats lost, but Roosevelt's future looked limitless—until he was struck down with polio in 1921. His legs were paralyzed for life, his political career apparently ruined. But, with the help of his wife Eleanor and close political friends, FDR fought back. He later said that global crises should be put in perspective: "If you had spent two years in bed trying to wiggle your big toe, after that anything else would seem easy."[1] In 1928, he won the governorship of New York and, four years later, defeated the hapless Herbert Hoover for the presidency. Roosevelt had gained the Democratic nomination, however, only after pleasing the party's isolationists by separating himself from the League and by delighting conservatives with his promises of a balanced budget.

FDR's consuming problem was how to lift the depression off American backs. His priority at first seemed clear: "I shall spare no effort to restore world trade by international economic readjustment," he declared in his inaugural address, "but the emergency at home cannot wait on that accomplishment." Foreign-policy aims were limited to a single paragraph of the speech. He only promised "the policy of the good neighbor—the neighbor who resolutely respects himself and, because he does so, respects the rights of others." During his first months in office, Roosevelt consequently searched for domestic solutions to the depression and downplayed foreign relations. Seeking relief at home, the president wanted no obligations overseas that might prevent him from doing whatever he thought necessary to ease the economic pressures in the United States.

A first target was the international gold standard. Often thought of as mysterious, magical, and impossible to understand (except by a chosen few in Washington or Wall Street), the gold standard actually worked quite simply. During the McKinley administration thirty-five years before, the United States had tied itself to the standard. Great Britain and other industrial powers also were linked to it. By doing so, these nations pledged to tie their national currencies (such as dollars or pounds) to their supply of gold. Because the gold supply was limited, the nations could not pay their debts merely by printing large amounts of money. The gold standard thus prevented inflation by preventing the printing of too much money. It also forced nations to curb their expenditures and balance their budgets. The gold standard supposedly kept expensive and dangerous military budgets from building up. Those nations that were creditors (and, thus, did not want to be repaid in cheaper, inflated dollars) and that had large supplies of gold were— not surprisingly—deeply in love with the gold standard.

Now it happened that the United States had become the world's great creditor in 1914–1917. In the 1920s it steadily added to an already large supply of gold. So Americans were especially charmed by the

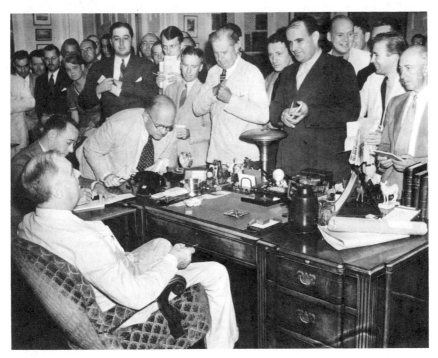

*In only the second photo he ever allowed taken of a White House press confer-
ence, FDR demonstrated how he informally and charmingly—but steadily and
successfully—handled reporters and got his message to the American people.
Here he tells the reporters, on August 25, 1939, that world war can still be
avoided.*

gold standard. By 1933, however, the standard was under attack. In
order to raise their prices (that is, print more money) and take control
of their economy away from the United States, the British, French, and
many others broke with gold. In mid-1933, FDR decided he could no
longer stick with it either. He wanted to be able to raise U.S. prices or
to go into debt—that is, have an unbalanced government budget—to
build large public projects such as dams and roads that would give
people work. His budget director, Lewis Douglas, and the young
undersecretary of the Treasury, Dean Acheson, resigned in protest.
Douglas even declared that breaking with the gold standard was "the
end of western civilization."[2] He feared that the United States had cut
itself off from the rest of civilization and that hordes of selfish Americans would descend on Washington to demand the printing of paper
money to pay for their own pet projects.

LONDON, FAILURE, AND HULL

The meaning of FDR's act for foreign policy was immediate. In 1932, Hoover had arranged a London Economic Conference to discuss cooperative efforts for increasing trade and reducing arms. As he left office, Hoover warned that only such international cooperation could maintain American individualism *and* world peace. For, he continued, if FDR tried instead to save the U.S. economy by increasing government's role in the society, the country would soon be on the road to socialism or fascism. The early New Deal confirmed some of Hoover's fears. Roosevelt did send a U.S. group to the London Economic Conference in the spring of 1933, but without instructions. When he learned that the conference wanted to tie the dollar and other currencies to a new international standard, FDR sent a telegram rejecting the deal. As the newspaper headlines proclaimed, he "torpedoed the conference." Roosevelt was determined to maintain control over the dollar—damn the foreign relations.

By late 1933, however, his domestic experiments had not worked. The depression continued to suffocate the economy. FDR knew that the nation stood at a historic turn. Something was fundamentally wrong with the system. In a 1932 campaign speech in San Francisco, he had used Frederick Jackson Turner's "frontier thesis" (see p. 185) to explain the crisis: "As long as we had free land . . . as long as our industrial plants were insufficient to supply our own needs, society chose to give the ambitious man free play and unlimited reward."[3] Now, the free land had mostly disappeared. The plants and farms produced great gluts of goods. His analysis implied that a radical solution was needed. But FDR was no radical. When his New Deal proposals failed to do the job quickly in 1933, he reversed himself and went back to the traditional American tactic of searching for markets abroad. "The plain truth is," wrote a journalist who knew him well, "that Roosevelt was perfectly ready to follow a political course that would have broken a snake's back."[4]

He already had a most traditional secretary of state in Cordell Hull. FDR had appointed him because Hull's long service in Congress helped ensure support from friends on Capitol Hill for whatever foreign policy the president wanted. But Hull was a tough sixty-two-year-old Tennessee mountaineer who uttered profanity with great skill gained from frequent use. He also knew his own mind, a mind shaped by his idol, Woodrow Wilson. Hull fervently believed that "unhampered trade

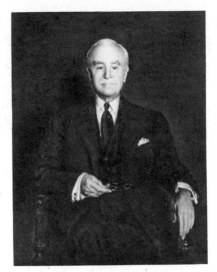

Cordell Hull of Tennessee (1871–1955) served as secretary of state longer than anyone else (1933–1944). President Roosevelt often ignored the former congressman's single-minded determination to create a freer-trade world that had no spheres of influence. But the stubborn, shrewd secretary of state nevertheless greatly shaped policy in the 1930s and the early cold war of the 1940s. He placed special emphasis on closer relations with Latin America.

dovetailed with peace; high tariffs, trade barriers, and unfair economic competition [dovetailed] with war." "A freer flow of goods," he emphasized, raised everyone's living standard, "thereby eliminating the economic dissatisfaction that breeds war." Widely read newspaper columnist Dorothy Thompson captured Hull: he was "a backwoods Tennessean, who looks very much like a gentle and long suffering saint. . . . Yet this quiet man is a person of considerable force; this restrained man is capable of complete and almost fanatical devotion to an idea [of the freest possible international trade] he believes in."[5]

Hull, therefore, thought FDR's attempt to make the country self-sufficient not only foolish, but dangerous. Self-contained economic blocs, Hull believed, meant international disagreement (as at the London conference) instead of cooperation, and such disagreement could lead to war. Hull served longer (1933–1944) than any other secretary of state in American history. He stuck so firmly to his Wilsonian course during those years that his policies are crucial if we are to understand the New Deal's foreign policy in the 1930s and the roots of the cold war in 1943–1945. FDR usually tried to avoid dealing with Hull and, instead, to keep foreign policy in his own hands. But after flitting around so that he could have "broken a snake's back," the president often ended by agreeing with Hull.

And so it was in 1934. FDR would not go back to the gold standard, but he had so cheapened the dollar (it was now at about half of its 1932 value) that the dollar was more competitive abroad. (In other words, foreigners could now buy many more dollars with their own currencies than they could have bought two years earlier and could use those dollars to buy more U.S. goods.) To push the glut of U.S. goods into foreign markets, Roosevelt and Hull devised two weapons that still remain in the U.S. economic arsenal: the Export-Import Bank (Ex-Im Bank) and the Reciprocal Trade Act (RTA).

The New Deal devised the first Ex-Im Bank to finance trade with Cuba and the Soviet Union. Before this time, private bankers had performed this job, but they had self-destructed between 1929 and 1933. Only the government had the resources to help U.S. merchants finance their overseas sales. But the bank's help was limited in 1934, when an angry Congress passed the Johnson Act forbidding private or public loans to the many governments that had defaulted on their debts to the United States. (The act passed despite strong European protests. As historian Benjamin Rhodes recounts, the British ambassador to Washington even recited the "forgive our debts" phrase from the Lord's Prayer to FDR's advisers, but to no avail.)[6] The bank, however, did obtain special permission to deal with the Soviet Union, and the Johnson Act did not affect foreign *individuals* who needed credit to buy U.S. goods.

In 1934, the Ex-Im Bank expanded so that it could help Americans trade with anyone. It especially scored successes in Latin America. Working through the bank, Roosevelt and Hull could control the flow of capital. If another nation needed dollars, it had to promise to buy U.S. goods and reduce its own barriers to North American investors and traders. Frederick Adams, the best historian of the bank, notes that such conditions increased trade, but "produced additional American interference in the internal affairs of neighboring states," and thus became a sophisticated version of the old "dollar diplomacy."[7]

The Reciprocal Trade Act of June 1934, one of Hull's pet projects, gave the president new powers to bargain for foreign markets. He could make a three-year treaty reducing the U.S. tariff by as much as 50 percent for another nation's goods, if that nation reciprocated by giving similar preferences to U.S. goods in its market. This approach became known as "unconditional-most-favored-nation," for Roosevelt could automatically extend tariff preferences unconditionally to all nations that cooperated. The act gave the chief executive vast new powers in foreign economic policy.

RTA was thus supposed to resemble a great wrecking ball knocking down tariff walls. When the president gave special breaks to one nation that had promised to reduce its tariff to Americans, those breaks automatically went to all other nations that also lowered their walls. The RTA also gave the president new powers to make the treaties without congressional assent. Those powers led one angry Republican senator to fume that RTA was "fascist" and "economic dictatorship come to America." But the Republicans had nothing better to offer.[8]

Again, RTA was especially effective in Latin America, where it helped integrate much of the Western Hemisphere's trade under Washington's control by exchanging the north's industrial goods for the south's minerals. In 1932, the United States accounted for one-third of Latin America's trade, but by 1938 it was involved in nearly half that trade. Globally, between 1934 and 1945, twenty-nine RTA treaties were made that reduced the U.S. tariff by nearly three-quarters. In the five years after the first act in 1934, U.S. exports rose more than $1.0 billion, and the nation's favorable trade balance (that is, more sales than purchases overseas) soared from $0.5 billion to nearly twice that amount.[9] A variation of RTA was passed in 1934 when, under the Tydings-McDuffie Act, Congress promised independence to the Philippines in ten years. (World War II delayed it until 1946.) American economic interests in the islands, especially the sugar growers, were protected by using reciprocity arrangements to tie the Philippine and U.S. markets closely together.

IMPROVING THE NEIGHBORHOOD

As the Ex-Im Bank and RTA illustrated, Roosevelt and Hull lavished special attention on Latin America. That region contained oil, sugar, coffee, and raw materials prized by North Americans, especially those who had $4 billion in investments in the region. Moreover, this "back yard" had been watched over since the 1823 Monroe Doctrine. When Roosevelt referred to the "good neighbor," he revived a phrase first applied by Henry Clay to Latin America in the 1820s, by the treaty of 1848 (even as that treaty seized one-third of Mexico from the Mexicans), and, more recently, by Hoover.

But FDR gave "neighbor" a special meaning by pulling the marines out of Haiti, ending the Platt Amendment that gave presidents the right to intervene in Cuba, opening new economic relations, and signing treaties with Panama in 1936 that finally recognized that nation's right to help operate and protect the great canal that cut the country in half. Not that everything went well. U.S. economic control in Haiti actually tightened to protect foreign investors and, in the later words of a top State Department official, "was an excessive drain on a country as poor as Haiti."[10] But Roosevelt shrewdly removed the U.S. political and military policies that had deeply angered Latin America since the 1890s. In the new atmosphere, he was able to increase U.S. economic influence. That influence accelerated after 1937, when Nazi Germany tried to infiltrate Latin America with trade deals and with such attractive services as those offered by its Lufthansa German Airlines. Washington responded by giving special help to Pan American Airlines and also by ordering the famous "G-men" of the Federal Bureau of Investigation (FBI) to expose Nazis and Communists alike in the region. A new State Department bureau appeared under the leadership of the young and ambitious Nelson Rockefeller (John D. Rockefeller's grandson) to expedite trade deals with Latin America. Rockefeller focused on the pivotal nation of Brazil, where he used the Ex-Im Bank to finance the vast $70-million Volta Redonda Steel plant project. He thus undercut growing German influence in Brazil.

The new economic ties were strengthened by historic political agreements. At the 1933 Pan-American Conference at Montevideo, Uruguay, Hull led the U.S. delegation that finally (if reluctantly) accepted the principle that no nation "has the right to intervene in the internal or external affairs of another." The U.S. Senate unanimously ratified the Montevideo pledge. In 1936 at Buenos Aires, Argentina, the inter-American conference tightened the pledge by declaring "inadmissible the intervention of any of [the Parties], directly or indirectly, and for whatever reason, in the internal or external affairs of any other of the Parties." The 1936 conference also provided for joint consultation in case of trouble.

When the American governments met next at Lima, Peru, in 1938, Hitler's shadow haunted the talks. The Lima Pact created machinery so that the region's foreign ministers could quickly consult in an emergency. After World War II began, the foreign ministers met with Hull in Panama during October 1939 and pledged to stand together to protect their neutral rights. A year later, they issued the Havana Declaration, announcing that they would defend any of the hemisphere's territories owned by non-Americans (for instance, Great Britain or France) so that other nations (such as Germany) could not seize them. In 1941, when the United States went to war, nearly all Latin Americans went with it (Argentina was the major exception). Hull later bragged with good reason that "the political line-up followed the economic line-up."[11]

Not all the good-neighbor policies turned out happily. Unappetizing dictators seized power in many Latin American nations and then held on to it with corruption and brutality. Anastasio Somoza of Nicaragua exemplified this type of leader, growing like a fungus on the debris of the depression. The Nicaraguan cracked down on the free press, broke up labor unions, and attacked the Roman Catholic church—that is, he tried to destroy anyone who threatened his personal power. But, in historian Lester Langley's words, at the same time he "kowtowed to the United States."[12] Somoza, who soon owned 15 percent of the country's land, declared that "Nicaragua is my farm." He nevertheless rode several blocks to work each day in a huge blue Cadillac protected by troops and aircraft. When Roosevelt welcomed the dictator on a state visit to Washington in 1939, a Mexico City newspaper charged that the good neighbor was becoming a "guarantee" for "the slavery of Latin American peoples."[13] But FDR, who with war on the horizon cared more about cooperation than guaranteeing democracy in Central America, privately dismissed such criticism with the alleged remark that Somoza "may be a son-of-a-bitch, but he's our son-of-a-bitch."

Other journals were friendlier. A Colombian newspaper wrote in 1938 that "from the 'Big Stick' to the 'Good Neighbor' was not only an evolution but a revolution." The "second Roosevelt," the editors thought, "has really been a good neighbor to Latin Americans."[14] One conclusion is certain: FDR and Hull changed the hemisphere's general mistrust of Washington in 1933 to general cooperation as they went to war in 1941. "That is a new approach I am talking about to these South American things," the president privately declared in 1940. "Give them a share. They think they are just as good as we are and many of them are."[15]

THE IMMEDIATE NEIGHBORHOOD: CUBA AND MEXICO

He followed this principle in dealing with pressing problems in Cuba and Mexico. Under U.S. control (although supposedly self-governing) since 1901, the Cubans were integrated into the North American economy by 1929. The small country was the fourth best U.S. customer, purchasing $200 million of goods and selling to the mainland all of its one-crop economy, sugar (owned mostly by North Americans). By 1933, however, Cuba's purchases had dropped 80 percent. Its sugar sales fell in half despite the price sliding to one-tenth of a cent per pound.[16]

By August 1933, internal discontent grew so rapidly that Hull sent his undersecretary of state, Sumner Welles (who had long been a close friend of FDR's), to help ease out the Cuban dictator Gerardo Machado. To Welles's dismay, however, Ramón Grau San Martín assumed power. Welles branded him "frankly communistic," and asked for U.S. military intervention. Hull rejected the request. He was supported strongly by Josephus Daniels, a North Carolina newspaperman under whom Roosevelt had served in the Navy Department and who now was the U.S. ambassador to Mexico. Daniels agreed with the secretary of state that "if we have to go in there again we will never be able to come out." Hull preferred to "walk from here to the South Pole than to have to intervene."[17]

U.S. diplomats began to pressure a young army sergeant, Fulgencio Batista, who with other officers had placed Grau San Martín in power. Welles held out the bait of economic aid to Batista, who soon placed Colonel Carlos Mendieta in power. A new commercial treaty and the Export-Import Bank helped shower economic benefits on the new regime. North Americans, meanwhile, increased their exports to Cuba by some 300 percent between 1934 and 1937. None of this exactly complied with the U.S. pledge at Montevideo in 1933 not to interfere in the affairs of other Latin American nations, but Roosevelt nicely deflected any criticism by abrogating the 1901 Platt Amendment that gave the United States the right to intervene in Cuba. He had just proven that the Platt Amendment was no longer necessary anyway: private political pressure and U.S. economic leverage seemed to be enough to make Cubans behave. Or so it appeared in 1934.

Mexican leaders, in Washington's view, had not behaved well since that nation's revolution began in 1911. A major problem was that the revolution had never been completed—that is, it never produced the equality, either political or economic, promised by its early champions. In 1934, a new president, Lázaro Cárdenas, pledged "Mexico for the Mexicans" and promptly strengthened labor unions so that they could strike against foreign corporations. In 1937, workers struck U.S. oil companies and demanded wage increases as high as 33 percent. The companies ignored court rulings upholding the unions. Cárdenas then retaliated by nationalizing the properties of the stunned foreign oil firms. He was also perhaps testing FDR to see whether the American president meant it when he accepted the nonintervention principle of the 1936 Buenos Aires meeting. Roosevelt apparently did, but Hull weakened.

Fearing that the seizure could trigger a chain reaction that would nationalize North American properties throughout the hemisphere, Hull sided with the oil companies, who demanded $262 million in compensation. Mexico insisted that $10 million was enough. Hull urged tough economic retaliation since "I have to deal with those Communists down there." But he was blocked by FDR, Ambassador Daniels, and Secretary of the Treasury Henry Morgenthau, who warned that if Cárdenas was driven to the wall, "we're just going to wake up and find that inside a year that Italy, Germany, and Japan have taken over Mexico."[18]

Morgenthau's fears were justified. When U.S. companies and banks tried to hurt Mexico, the Mexicans, in turn, boycotted U.S. goods and turned to Japan and Germany for products. Cárdenas leaked the news that Mexican oil might be sold to Hitler. After FDR tried several compromises that failed, in 1940 Sinclair Oil broke the solid front of U.S. companies and made a settlement. In November 1941, Washington and Mexico City finally agreed on $40 million in compensation for foreign-owned farmlands that had been seized and $29 million for the oil lands. Mexico's own national oil company, PEMEX, took over the fields. Nevertheless, U.S. influence steadily grew. Through a 1942 reciprocity treaty, Export-Import Bank activities, and U.S. purchases of silver (on which the value of the Mexican currency rested), Mexico's economy became quite dependent on North Americans. U.S. oil companies even continued to manage and market Mexican oil. Historian Clayton Koppes suggests that if the use of this economic power is seen together with U.S. support for client military figures in Nicaragua, the Dominican Republic, Cuba, and El Salvador (among other places), there appears "a combination of military, economic, and diplomatic levers" that demonstrated how "the Good Neighbor policy was United States hemispheric hegemony pursued by other means."[19]

GERMANS, JAPANESE, AND A ONE-ARMED NUTCRACKER

From his first moments in office, FDR was preoccupied with these German and Japanese threats. By May 1933, he personally warned Nazi officials about their violence against Jews. By 1934, German state control of trade clashed with Hull's reciprocal trade plans to open commercial channels. Hitler quit the League and all disarmament conferences while he built up an internal police (the future Gestapo) and a new army. The Americans watched with apprehension but did little. They believed that the British and French were responsible for maintaining peace in Europe. Growing U.S. public concern about European involvements (especially to help those cheaters who had refused

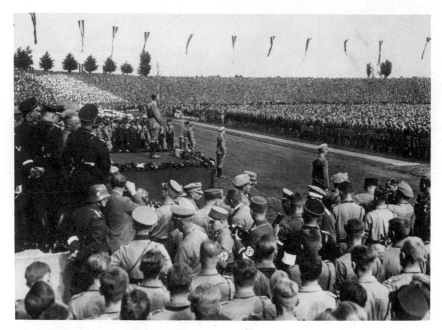

Adolf Hitler (1889–1945) mobilized Germany in the 1930s with a sweep and brutality that most Americans could not comprehend. Here he addresses thousands of Hitler youth at Nuremberg Stadium.

to pay their debts) also made FDR reluctant to become further involved.

Japan was a different story. Along with many other Americans, Roosevelt believed that the United States had rights in Asia that dated back a century. During his first year in office, FDR tried to cut off European loans to Japan. Then he obtained a $50 million credit from Congress so that besieged China could buy cotton, wheat, and airplane parts. He also spent $238 million as "public works" to begin building thirty-two warships, including two aircraft carriers. In April 1934, Japan struck back by issuing the so-called Amau statement: because Tokyo had the right to act alone to preserve Asian "peace and order," any outside interference, such as military aid to China, was unfriendly to Japan. Hull refused publicly to accept the Amau statement, but the United States did nothing else. Sino-Japanese battles quieted as Japan digested its conquests of the past three years.

One other bright signal flashed across the international skies in 1933–1934, but few could tell exactly what it meant. In November 1933, Roosevelt formally recognized the Soviet Union. He did so over vigorous objections from the American Legion, the American Federation of

Labor, the Daughters of the American Revolution, and—most significantly—his own State Department. In historian Thomas R. Maddux's words, the State Department was afraid that Moscow would "not live up to the standards of civilized society." Hull, of course, despised the state-run Soviet economy. He received ardent support from Robert Kelley, a long-time scholar of Russia who, as the ambitious son of a working-class Boston Irish family, had studied among the violently anti-Bolshevist Russian exiles living in Paris. By 1924, Kelley had convinced the State Department to train young experts so that they could deal with the Soviet danger. As head of the department's Eastern European Affairs desk, Kelley directed the education of the famous first class of experts, including George F. Kennan, Charles Bohlen, and others who were to shape post-1945 policy. "Without exception," historian Frederic L. Propas notes, these men "all emerged as hostile observers of the Soviet Union" in 1933.[20] Kelley warned his superiors that if recognized, the Soviets would never keep agreements, but instead foment revolution—as, he argued, they were then doing in Cuba.

FDR, however, apparently thought it strange that the United States did not recognize the existence of the world's largest nation. He received support from William C. Bullitt, still full of hatred for Wilson's supposed betrayal of Soviet-American relations at the Paris peace conference (see p. 319) and now an adviser to FDR. There were also strong economic reasons for recognition. Despite lack of diplomatic ties, U.S.-Soviet trade steadily rose in the 1920s but dropped sharply after 1931. A major reason was the Soviet five-year plans begun in 1928 by dictator Joseph Stalin to make the Soviet Union self-sufficient. But U.S. business noted that Germany, which did recognize the USSR and provided long-term credits, continued to profit from the trade. The Soviets, moreover, seemed to be enduring the depression better than the capitalists. The Soviets were paying a price, however. Stalin ordered the collectivization of agriculture. When peasants fought to hold their private plots, Stalin seized their grain, causing mass starvation. At least 10 million to 14 million Soviets died between 1929 and 1934. Roosevelt apparently knew little of the magnitude of these events. He might, however, have agreed with one U.S. economist who said that trade relations were needed because "the Russians are more dependable financially than Wall Street."[21]

Roosevelt also understood that a new U.S.-Soviet relationship could threaten to box in Japan—to put Tokyo between the arms of that "nutcracker" a Soviet official had asked for in 1931. Certainly, the Soviets responded quickly to FDR's opening because they hoped, above all, to

contain Japan.²² But the president, and especially the State Department, had no such commitment in mind. As FDR opened talks with
Soviet foreign minister Maxim Litvinov, the State Department set about
" 'reassuring' the Japanese," as one top official termed it.²³ Bullitt thus
went to Moscow as the first U.S. ambassador to the Soviet Union with
no aid for Stalin, but with great hopes. "A striking man: young, handsome, urbane, full of charm and enthusiasm, a product of Philadelphia
society and Yale . . . , and with a flamboyance of personality that is
right out of F. Scott Fitzgerald," George Kennan described his new
boss. Bullitt was "confident in himself, confident of the President's
support, confident that he will have no difficulty in cracking the nut of
Communist suspicion and hostility which awaits him in Moscow,"
Kennan continued.²⁴

But this nut was not cracked either. When Litvinov discovered that
the United States refused to help contain Japan, his own ruler, Stalin,
lost interest in Bullitt. Stalin instead tried to protect his flanks by working with France against Germany. The Soviets refused to pay the $150
million debt that they owed Washington. If they did pay, they would
have to pay vastly larger amounts owed to the British and French. Bullitt became angry. The anger turned to fury in 1935, when U.S. Communist party leaders appeared in Moscow at the Seventh Party Congress
to denounce the United States. Bullitt and Hull considered this a direct
violation of the Soviets' promise in 1933 not to spread anti-U.S. propaganda. Bullitt left the Soviet Union in 1936 and forever after worked
tirelessly against the Soviets.

"ISOLATIONISTS" VERSUS "INTERNATIONALISTS"

In 1935, Mussolini's Italy invaded Ethiopia in the hope of realizing
that dictator's crazy dream of resurrecting the Roman Empire of two
thousand years earlier. The League of Nations responded by asking
members to stop trading with Italy. The League, however, did not ask
the members to stop trading in the most important item, oil. And besides,
Great Britain, France, and the United States refused to get tough with
Mussolini. In 1936, Hitler tore up the Versailles peace treaty and the
Locarno agreement by seizing the Rhineland.

Americans were sharply divided over how they should deal with this
inflamed world. One group, the "isolationists," believed that the nation
should maintain complete freedom of action. In the words of historian
Wayne Cole, "Unilateralism and non-interventionism were central

themes in the thinking of most of them."[25] This group, however, did not want the United States to be entirely isolated. One of its leaders, Senator Borah, was willing to consider working with the Soviets in order to stop Japan. Indeed, many isolationists wanted to help China. They just opposed military involvements in Europe. They received support for their anti-European views in 1934–1935 when a congressional committee under Republican Senator Gerald P. Nye from North Dakota investigated the causes of American involvement in World War I. The Nye committee concluded that bankers and arms exporters (the "Merchants of Death") had, for their own profit, pushed the country into the conflict. In truth, the explanation for that involvement was much more complicated. (Nye himself, for example, thought that the entire American system, not just a few "Merchants of Death," was at fault.) But the public liked to label J. P. Morgan and the arms traders as the villains. Americans vowed never again to allow the profiteers to take them into world war. Pacifist groups also determined not to be misled again as they felt they had been by Wilsonian ideals ("make the world safe for democracy") in 1914–1917.[26]

"Internationalists," on the other hand, assumed that new technology (such as the airplane, now flying regularly across the Atlantic and Pacific) had drawn the world together and that U.S. prosperity depended on orderly world markets. Americans consequently bore responsibility for cooperating in the maintenance of a stable world that was in their own selfish interest. Historian Robert Divine notes that most internationalists were old-stock Protestants, felt close to Great Britain, and believed that America had replaced Britain as the world's great power. They cared about Europe while "they took Latin America for granted and neglected the Orient."[27] This group included executives of the great multinational, capital-intensive corporations—IBM, General Electric, Eastman Kodak, Standard Oil. They wanted an open world and low tariffs. Some firms, led by du Pont, Standard Oil, General Motors, and Union Carbide, even worked closely—sometimes secretly and illegally—with Nazi German firms until the late 1930s, or in some cases, even to 1941. At one point, Ford and General Motors subsidiaries actually produced half of Hitler's tanks in the 1930s.[28]

But the internationalists won few victories in the mid-1930s. U.S. officials, led by Hull, were frightened of the isolationists' strength in Congress. Roosevelt was also wary. In 1935, he had bowed to State Department and internationalist demands that the United States join the League's World Court. The president sent the appropriate agreement to the Senate for ratification. He quickly ran into a buzz saw of

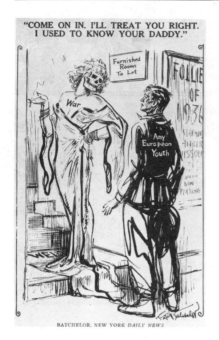

"COME ON IN. I'LL TREAT YOU RIGHT. I USED TO KNOW YOUR DADDY."

BATCHELOR, NEW YORK *DAILY NEWS*

As this 1936 cartoon indicates, Americans had vivid memories of 1914 through 1920 and were determined never again to follow in Europe's bloody footsteps. The cartoon shows an American view of Europe's morality, as well as its foreign policy, being corrupted once more.

opposition, led by publisher William Randolph Hearst and several Roosevelt-hating demagogues of the day: Father Charles E. Coughlin (the "radio priest") and Senator Huey ("the Kingfish") Long of Louisiana. Roosevelt refused to wage what he saw as a losing fight, and the agreement went down to a humiliating defeat.[29]

Worse lay ahead for FDR. The isolationists next whipped the 1935 Neutrality Act through Congress. According to the act, if the president declared that a war existed in the world, Americans could not ship arms or other weapons to any belligerent nation; U.S. ships could not deal in such arms traffic; and American travelers were warned that they sailed on belligerent ships at their own risk. The crises of 1914–1917 were not to be repeated. The 1936 Neutrality Act further restricted FDR's power. Professor Richard Harrison believes that "it was the most serious defeat Roosevelt ever suffered" in foreign policy.[30] The measure reaffirmed the earlier act and tightened it by prohibiting loans.

That act took effect as FDR prepared to run for his second term and as General Francisco Franco moved to overthrow the republic in Spain during 1936 to establish a fascistic regime. The United States government shed few tears for the Spanish people. Since 1931, Americans, especially such giant U.S. multinationals as International Telephone

& Telegraph, had fought the new Spanish republic's attempt to regulate them. Washington, therefore, believed (wrongly) that the republic was deeply infected by communism. In the best account of the relationship, historian Douglas Little concludes that because these economic and political conflicts had, "like a cancer, rotted Spanish relations" with the Americans and the British, Washington and London officials were willing to let the republic die "before the infection had a chance to spread."[31] FDR knew, moreover, that the republic's anticlericalism deeply angered the U.S. Roman Catholic hierarchy and the Vatican. Amid the election, he was content to follow British and French policies on Spain. These policies amounted to doing nothing to stop Franco. Three thousand Americans volunteered to fight for the republic (the Abraham Lincoln Battalion became the most famous American group), but they were not enough to stop the final fascist triumph in 1939. Meanwhile, Congress extended the 1936 Neutrality Act so the nation would not become involved in such civil wars as Spain's.

The 1937 Neutrality Act had a new wrinkle. Congress kept the main provisions of the earlier acts but, at the suggestion of financier Bernard Baruch, added a "cash and carry" clause. Belligerents could now purchase certain war materials from the United States if they paid for them promptly and carried them away in their own ships. As Robert Divine summarizes: cash and carry was "an ingenious method of preserving the profits of neutral trade while minimizing the risk of involvement in a major war."[32] It was, after all, tough for Americans to deny themselves overseas markets while they suffered from a crushing economic depression. Needs at home dictated policies abroad.

These needs worsened in 1937–1938, when Roosevelt reduced government spending to balance the budget and promptly threw the nation into the most severe economic tailspin in its history. Profits dropped 78 percent in nine months. With no new ideas, FDR tried to pump life into the system by sending Congress a $3 billion spending program in 1938. Part of the money was to build battleships. A leading New Dealer, Maury Maverick of Texas, explained that "the reason for all this battleship and war frenzy is coming out. . . . The Democratic administration is getting down to the condition that Mr. Hoover found himself. We have pulled all the rabbits out of the hat and there are no more rabbits."[33] In this gut-wrenching moment, FDR had to make three historic foreign-policy decisions during 1937–1938: how to deal with the Nazis' policy toward Jews, the Japanese invasion of China, and the Munich crisis.

AMERICANS AND THE HOLOCAUST

Hitler's hatred of Jews was well known in the United States by 1938. Vowing to "purify" Germany of its half a million Jews, he struck against them immediately after assuming power. By 1935, his Nuremberg Laws stripped them of citizenship. Teachers, doctors, and other professionals could not practice their craft, and half of all German Jews were unemployed. In early 1938, Hitler burned Munich's Great Synagogue, then sent 15,000 Jews to Buchenwald, the concentration camp whose name was soon to become synonymous with the most horrible crime that the Nazis committed.

Roosevelt responded by calling a conference of thirty-two nations in 1938 at Évian-les-Bains, France, to discuss which countries could accept Jews as émigrés. He believed that the United States could accept few: the depression and Americans' fear of allowing in more immigrants of any kind prohibited an open door, he concluded. None of the other larger, less-populated nations such as Brazil or Australia would accept many either. Only Holland, already densely populated, willingly took in large numbers. (Germany invaded Holland in 1940 and exterminated 75 percent of the Jews there.) Noting the world's reluctance to accept his "problem" and using as an excuse the assassination of a Nazi official in Paris by a Jew, in 1938 Hitler launched *Kristallnacht* (or "Crystal Night," so named for the shattered glass that littered the sidewalks after the destruction of Jewish businesses and homes). He sent 20,000 to 30,000 Jews to concentration camps. FDR expressed his shock, recalled the U.S. ambassador to Germany, and allowed 15,000 refugees on visitor permits to remain longer in the United States. But he would not do more—such as breaking trade relations with Hitler.[34]

The Nazis launched their "final solution" to the "problem" after they drove into the Soviet Union in 1941. Much of the Jewish population of eastern Europe (especially Poland) and the Soviet Union were packed into railroad freight cars and dumped at such camps as Buchenwald and Dachau to conclude, as Hitler called it, "the complete annihilation of the Jews." Certain names became engraved in memory as Russian Jews were slaughtered at Babi Yar in 1941 and during Purim in 1942 (small children were thrown into pits and Hitler's SS officers pitched candy to them as the victims were buried alive). The Germans tried to keep much of the brutality secret, but as early as autumn 1942, U.S. newspapers published reports of the horror. By late 1942, Rabbi Stephen S. Wise, chairman of the World Jewish Congress, declared that 2 million Jews had been slaughtered. The Roosevelt administration confirmed that figure. U.S. newspapers, however, placed the revelation on the inside pages. The *Atlanta Constitution* pushed it back to page 20, next to the want ads.[35] For the remainder of the war, the Allies did little, either to bomb the railways running to the concentration camps' gas ovens or to lower immigration bars so that Jews could find new homes.

There are many reasons why U.S. officials stood by as one of history's greatest atrocities unfolded. First, Americans simply desired no new immigrants of any type during economic bad times. Anti-Semitism reinforced that desire. Well-known German and Austrian Jews did enter the country (Albert Einstein, composer Kurt Weill, architect Walter Gropius, physicists Hans Bethe and Edward Teller among them). But an annual average of only 8,500 Jews were allowed into the country between 1933 and 1941. Between 1941 and 1945, the U.S. War Refugee Board rescued 200,000 Jews, but only 20,000 were allowed into the United States. Even then, the American record was better than the British or Soviet.

Second, the stories of the death camps seemed too terrible to be true. Americans remembered that World War I tales of torture had turned out to be propaganda. They swore that they would not be taken in a second time by "foreigners." When eyewitness stories reported millions being murdered in the death camps, one U.S. journalist responded, "We are from Missouri. We have to be shown."[36]

Third, top U.S. officials refused to deal with the issue. Some, such as the State Department's Breckinridge Long, who was responsible for handling immigration problems, were anti-Semitic and more concerned with diplomatic dealings with Hitler than dramatizing the plight of his victims. In 1933–1936, when Jewish and other groups demanded U.S. trade boycotts against Hitler, Hull refused to go against his belief that only good trade could lead to good political relations. During the war, officials refused to divert resources to liberate the death camps. Throughout the 1933–1944 period, U.S. and British officials especially feared that Germany would simply dump millions of Jews on them— or on Palestine—and they did not want to face such a dilemma. Top officials who were Jews, such as Secretary of the Treasury Henry Morgenthau and FDR's speechwriter, Samuel Rosenman, moved slowly, fearful of being branded "too Jewish." The *New York Times*, owned by a Jewish family, downplayed death-camp stories for the same reason. Nor did Congress want to help the refugees. When Democratic senator Robert Wagner of New York proposed bringing 20,000 more German

Jewish children into the United States, the Senate flatly refused to act on the Wagner bill.

Fourth, the Jewish community was itself divided. Zionists, dedicated to creating a Jewish state in Palestine, emphasized their cause rather than giving first priority to the rescue of east Europeans. Even leaders such as Rabbi Wise decided to move slowly rather than possibly further alienate the State Department, anti-Semitic Americans, and cautious Jews. Finally, as for Roosevelt himself, a distinguished historian concluded that FDR's "indifference to . . . the systematic annihilation of European Jewry emerges as the worst failure of his presidency."[37] By mid-1945, 6.5 million Jews had died in the Holocaust.

The Dilemma of "Quarantining" Japan (1937–1939)

Throughout the years 1933–1939, U.S. officials followed a century-old tradition by devoting more attention to Asia than to Europe. That attention riveted on the region in July 1937, when Japan reignited its war to conquer China. Tokyo was determined to create buffer states to protect its holdings in Manchukuo, to stop Chinese discrimination against Japanese goods, and—perhaps most importantly—to guarantee Japan's self-sufficiency by conquering mainland markets and raw materials. China, romanticized in the 1937 movie of Pearl Buck's best-selling novel, *The Good Earth*, had never been more popular among Americans. But U.S. officials, already dizzied by the recent economic downturn, were nearly paralyzed. As a top State Department figure had said in 1936, the United States had "no intention of using force for the preservation of the 'open door.' "[38] On the other hand, Japan's aggression and the closing off of Asian markets posed a deadly challenge to Hull's and FDR's hope for a more open world and set a dangerous precedent for other aggressors. But the Americans could not get tough: their military capabilities remained small, and Japan remained the third-best customer of U.S. goods.

FDR responded by refusing to issue the state-of-war declaration needed to trigger the application of the 1937 Neutrality Act. Applying the act would have favored Japan's stronger navy, which could "cash and carry" U.S. goods. The president next delivered a tough speech on October 5, 1937, in Chicago (virtually in the shadow of the Chicago Tribune Building, home of the nation's leading isolationist newspaper). He asked other nations to join in a "quarantine" to protect the world against the spreading "epidemic of world lawlessness."[39] A public uproar ensued, and, in a press conference, FDR—after being pressured by Hull, who feared isolationist feeling in Congress—blandly denied that the "quarantine speech" threatened anyone. Hull and FDR probably misread public opinion. Americans were more shocked and angry at Japan than ever before.[40]

Even the dying League of Nations aroused itself to seize upon FDR's speech and call a conference in Brussels, Belgium, to discuss how to stop Japan. After much anguish, the president sent a delegation to Brussels. The Japanese, not surprisingly, refused to attend a meeting called to condemn them. But the Soviets did appear and promptly asked the United States to cooperate against both Japan and Germany. The Americans coldly rejected the deal. Having refused the courtship of possible allies, the United States, in the words of historian Stephen Pelz, now faced a bitter choice: either to "run a hard-paced naval race with Japan" or "foresake its commitments in Asia."[41]

The corpse of the Brussels Conference was barely rigid before Japanese planes attacked a U.S. gunboat, the *Panay*, in China's Yangtze River on December 12, 1937. Two sailors died. Tokyo officials quickly condemned the attack as an error and apologized. But the next day Representative Louis Ludlow of Indiana seized the moment to push a constitutional amendment that would require a national referendum before the country could go to war. Fearing that the Ludlow Amendment could paralyze U.S. diplomacy, FDR pulled out all stops to defeat it.[42] Roosevelt then proposed a spending bill of $1.0 billion to increase the navy by 20 percent. He also prepared to fortify Guam and other Pacific bases. Undeterred, in November 1938, Japan proclaimed a Greater East Asia Co-Prosperity Sphere that was aimed against "bolshevism." More accurately, it announced Japanese determination to dominate Asia's resources. In April 1939, FDR sent fresh requests to Congress, including a $0.5 billion measure to create a 5,500-plane air force. The two close friends of the 1920s were now on a collision course.

Conjuring up the Ghost of Munich (1937–1939)

The United States was also on a collision course with another close friend of the 1920s. Germany seized Austria in March 1938. In September, Hitler demanded that Czechoslovakia surrender the German-populated Sudetenland that the Paris peace conference gave to the Czechs in 1919. U.S. newspapers condemned the dictator's act, but Washington officials were restrained. One key adviser, Adolf Berle, reminded FDR that many thought that the breakup of the Austro-Hungarian Empire in 1919 simply for the sake of self-determination had been a "mistake." William Bullitt added that French officials now called the Versailles Treaty of 1919 "one of the stupidest documents ever penned by the hand of man."[43]

U.S. policy was also shaped by growing mistrust of Great Britain, the nation that FDR and Hull believed should take the lead in European affairs. As Anglo-U.S. trade talks broke down in 1938, Hull considered telling the British "to go to hell," while London officials complained of the "bitterness and exasperation" of having to deal with the Americans.[44] Conservative prime minister Neville Chamberlain especially mistrusted what he believed to be Roosevelt's shallowness and bizarre economic and foreign policies. Chamberlain preferred striking a deal that would satisfy the Japanese and keep them away from the British imperial holdings of Hong Kong, Singapore, and India. Meanwhile, he planned to carry out a policy of appeasement—that is, allowing Hitler to rectify the 1919 treaty provisions—that would give the British military time to catch up with Germany's rising military power.

Roosevelt feared Chamberlain's policy in Asia. He believed that the weakened British hoped to push off on Americans the dirty job of containing Japan and—of special concern—protecting the British Empire. These mutual mistrusts and divergent interests explain why the two nations never cooperated to resist the Japanese between 1931 and 1941. In Europe, however, FDR supported Chamberlain's appeasement of Hitler. As the Czech crisis threw a dark shadow of war over Europe in September 1938, the president publicly asked Hitler for a peaceful settlement. Roosevelt especially hoped to use the Italian Fascist dictator, Benito Mussolini, as an honest broker to appease Hitler and prevent war. FDR privately told the British and French, who had guaranteed Czech borders, that he could not help them if conflict erupted.

Stalin, desperate to protect his dictatorship, signaled that if the French and British defended the Czechs, he would help them. Chamberlain and the French wanted no part of such a deal. The British prime minister feared communism, did not want Soviet armies marching through eastern Europe to reach the Czechs, and believed that the Soviet military was too weak to resist Hitler effectively. Instead, Chamberlain flew to Munich with French officials and surrendered the Sudetenland to Hitler—without Czechoslovakia's consent. Adolf Berle quietly breathed, "Thank God." FDR sent a two-word cable to Chamberlain: "Good man." But within days, Roosevelt realized the tragedy that had occurred. Hitler quickly launched "Crystal Night" against German Jews and then demanded the remainder of a now defenseless Czechoslovakia. Mussolini, whom FDR believed could be used to reason with Hitler, conquered Albania in March 1939. Increasing numbers of Americans condemned Chamberlain's appeasement policy. As columnist Dorothy Thompson acidly phrased it, he had somehow managed to go to Munich "on his knees at 200 miles an hour."[45]

But others believed that the Munich deal produced one good result. By giving Hitler what he wanted in the west, he could now turn and confront the Soviet Union, which seemed too weak to resist.[46] Stalin had ruthlessly carried out a bloody purge between 1934 and 1938 that not only killed millions of his real or imagined political opponents, but executed or imprisoned one-third of the Red Army officers and three of his top five marshals. Convinced that the British and French were trying to turn Hitler against him, Stalin secretly approached Berlin for a deal. He began by replacing his foreign minister, Maxim Litvinov, a Jew, with Vyacheslav Molotov, a gentile totally subservient to Stalin.

Western leaders ignored Stalin's signal. Chamberlain stuck to his appeasement policy. Roosevelt asked in April 1939 for a conference to deal with disarmament and equal access to world markets. Hitler's close adviser, Field Marshal Hermann Göring, told Mussolini that FDR's proposal must be evidence of "an incipient brain disease."[47] Hitler publicly humiliated the president by violently denouncing the idea. More pointedly, throughout the summer of 1939, the United States did not even bother to keep an ambassador in Moscow.

On August 23, 1939, Stalin and Hitler suddenly announced that they had signed a nonaggression pact. A stunned world at first refused to believe it. Fascists and Communists supposedly mixed no better than oil and water. But both men now needed time—Hitler to absorb western Poland and prepare an attack westward, Stalin to absorb eastern Poland and avoid a conflict with the superior Nazi armies. With the European harvest largely taken in, Hitler attacked Poland on September 1. The British and French, who had guaranteed Polish borders, had no choice but to declare war. Stalin followed through on his secret deal with Hitler by seizing eastern Poland and the three Baltic States of Latvia, Estonia, and Lithuania, which the Russian Empire had once ruled.

Forever after, "Munich" held powerful, but quite different meanings for Americans and Russians. To Americans, "Munich" meant the utter failure of appeasement, the uselessness of trying to stop aggressors with talk instead of force. To Russians, however, it meant—as Soviet leader Mikhail Gorbachev declared in 1985—"the ultimate political irresponsibility when the leading groupings of monopoly capital tried to manipulate the expansion of German fascism, directing it to the East." That policy, Gorbachev concluded, "brought a terrible tragedy to all the peoples of Europe."[48] The many-faced ghost of Munich would long haunt world affairs, but its first and worst shadow fell over the globe in September 1939.

AMERICA'S PHONY WAR OF 1939–1941

Hitler did not intend to repeat Germany's error of 1914–1917. Determined to keep the United States out of this war, he ordered his submarines not to attack passenger liners or U.S. ships. Roosevelt finally obtained repeal of the Neutrality Acts' arms embargo so that England and France could purchase weapons and ammunition from the United States.[49] Over the next two years, the president never resolved the key contradiction in his policy: the wish for no direct U.S. involvement in the war, but the belief that Germany and Japan had to be stopped before they stood astride Europe and Asia.

This contradiction sharpened in December 1939, when Stalin, determined to protect his northern cities, demanded a strategic buffer area from neighboring Finland. The Finns refused, and the Red Army invaded. FDR quickly condemned "this dreadful rape of Finland," but the Finns surprisingly battled the Soviets to a standstill in the Winter War of 1939–1940. Americans, led by Herbert Hoover, moved to help "brave little Finland," which had won their hearts by paying its debt to the United States after other debtors had stopped. But only about $10 million in aid went to the Finns. Roosevelt did place a "moral embargo" on airplanes, gasoline, and metals to the Soviet Union, but trade figures were telling: U.S. exports to the Soviet Union doubled to $29 million between November 1939 and January 1940. In March 1940, the Finns finally agreed to the border revision. The war ended, and Finland began moving closer to Hitler.

Meanwhile Germany absorbed Poland but did little else during the winter. The French, supposedly secure behind their heavily fortified Maginot line, and Chamberlain began to believe that it was all a "phony war." In April–May 1940, Hitler struck. His divisions knifed through Holland and Belgium to destroy the Maginot line from the rear. (The phrase "Maginot line mentality" afterward applied to a person or nation too rigid to respond to new challenges.) Chamberlain resigned in disgrace and was replaced by sixty-six-year-old Winston Churchill, who had long condemned appeasement. Hitler then tried to soften Great Britain with a blitz by his air force, which, during daylight and then nightly, bombed London and other major cities during the 1940–1941 winter. The Royal Air Force, however, made the Germans pay heavily for the raids. Unable to control the air, Hitler decided to delay a planned invasion of Great Britain.

Many Americans gave up on the British. "Saw Joe Kennedy [the U.S. ambassador to Great Britain and the father of John F. Kennedy]," Chamberlain told his diary in January 1940, "who says everyone in U.S.A. thinks we shall be beaten before the end of the month."[50] But other Americans vigorously disagreed. On May 15, 1940, journalist William Allen White helped found the Committee to Defend America by Aiding the Allies. The new group released studies showing the terrible impact on the U.S. economy of a Hitler victory, and it lobbied for a stronger defense and sending massive aid to the British. After Paris fell to the Nazis in June 1940, FDR, in a speech at the University of Virginia, pledged to help "opponents of force" with U.S. supplies. But he continued to downplay the idea that the United States might become militarily involved.[51] White's and FDR's actions helped produce one important result in mid-1940. Congress passed the first peacetime draft of young Americans in U.S. history and began the process that brought 15 million men and women into the armed services over the next five years.

As historians J. Garry Clifford and Samuel Spencer, Jr., show, the Selective Service Act climaxed a bitter three-month public debate that shattered much of the isolationists' strength.[52] The isolationists had come together in a group called "America First." Begun by Princeton students, supported by leading midwestern politicians, and bankrolled by executives of Quaker Oats, Montgomery Ward, Hormel meat packing, and Inland Steel, America First launched massive protest rallies. Lobbying efforts were led by Charles A. Lindbergh, the "Lone Eagle," who in 1927 first flew the Atlantic alone and became perhaps the nation's greatest hero. Lindbergh had personally analyzed Hitler's air force and, overrating its strength by a factor of ten, warned Americans not to get involved in Europe's quarrels. Great Britain's brave resistance and Lindbergh's remarks in 1941 that were widely viewed as anti-Semitic hurt the isolationists' cause. The isolationists were strongest in the farming areas of the Midwest and West, and also in Roman Catholic and Lutheran churches, where Irish-Americans, Italian-Americans, and German-Americans worshiped. But the farmers were also sensitive to chaos in international markets, and many Americans began to realize that two oceans might no longer protect them.[53]

These Americans were shocked by the new air power whose bombs lit the skies each night over Great Britain. The United States was no longer a fortress defended by ocean moats, but an island that could someday be attacked by planes flying over the arctic routes from northern Europe. When the globe was viewed from the poles, Americans were closer to Europe than to much of South America. New strategists, led by Sir Halford Mackinder and Nicholas Spykman, detailed the obvious military and political consequences of such a perspective.[54] By late 1940, growing U.S. fears were intensified by the media. Edward R. Murrow pioneered radio news when he broadcast the horrors and sounds directly into American homes from bombed London streets on the CBS network. Even children's programs joined in. On "Captain Midnight," a popular radio show, many segments were spent (between Ovaltine commercials) tracking and capturing the treacherous "Ivan Shark," who somehow seemed to be both Japanese and Communist.[55]

The isolationists were not able to kill a single major foreign-policy proposal of Roosevelt's in 1940–1941, although they did come close (for instance, on the Selective Service Act, which was renewed by a lone vote in 1941). Public-opinion polls showed that after the fall of France in June 1940, nearly 75 percent of Americans surveyed wanted to do more to help Great Britain. By early 1941, one poll revealed that two-thirds of those surveyed preferred to help the British than to stay out of the war. Roosevelt, who read highly detailed public-opinion analyses, knew of this growing internationalist sentiment, but he believed that Congress remained isolationist. When the British ambassador begged him to help in early 1940, FDR admitted that 40 percent of the people might support such help, but that he "could not get 25 percent of Congress."[56]

The president, moreover, had decided to break a tradition going back to George Washington and run for a hotly disputed third presidential term. He wanted as little public debate as possible over his foreign policy. Thus, when Churchill begged for some ships to protect the British Isles, FDR did not respond for six weeks. He finally (and ingeniously) worked out a deal that offered fifty aged U.S. destroyers to Great Britain in return for long-term leases to military bases located on British possessions between Newfoundland and Trinidad. Even then, Roosevelt made the deal only after he had received the pledge of his Republican opponent (Wendell Willkie of Indiana) not to make the swap a political issue. Roosevelt also moved only after his attorney general had made a questionable legal interpretation that justified the deal without forcing the president to ask Congress for permission. In September 1940, Japan moved to capture vital raw materials by entering the northern part of French Indochina. The Japanese, as historian Akira Iriye observes, assumed that U.S.-Japan relations would remain peaceful, and they had little "sense that the two nations were on a fatal march toward collision."[57] But FDR stunned Tokyo by cutting off iron and steel exports, a decision that was certain to drive the Japanese farther into Asia in quest of these resources. Nevertheless, in October 1940, FDR told a roaring Boston campaign audience, "I shall say it again and again: Your boys are not going to be sent into any foreign wars." Willkie was furious: "That hypocritical son of a bitch! This is going to beat me." Roosevelt overwhelmed Willkie 449 to 82 in the electoral college, 27 million to 22 million in the popular vote.[58] FDR now prepared to be bolder. "We must be," he told the nation in December 1940, "the great arsenal of democracy."

In September 1940, Germany, Italy, and Japan had signed the Tripartite Pact that formed the Axis bloc. Hitler clearly wanted to use Japan to keep the Americans busy in the Pacific. Churchill again begged from London's bombed rubble for massive U.S. aid. Vowing he wanted to "keep war away from our country and our people," Roosevelt proposed "lend-lease" to Congress: the United States would lend or lease goods to the British, who were then somehow to return the goods after the war. This, FDR declared, would avoid hard feelings about war debts by "leaving out the dollar mark." The plan resembled merely a "garden hose" lent to a neighbor whose house is on fire and to whom you say, "I don't want $15—I want my garden hose back after the fire is over." Or so the president argued. His supporters shrewdly had the plan proposed as House Resolution 1776, and Roosevelt lobbied hard for it. The $7 billion program survived violent attacks to pass by 100 votes in the House and by a 2-to-1 margin in the Senate on March 11, 1941. As the *New York Times* understood it, "the Battle of the Atlantic is on."[59] For FDR now had to ensure that the lend-lease goods survived the North Atlantic waters, where Hitler's U-boats were destroying 500,000 tons of British shipping each month.

THE REAL WAR (1941)

In taking this step, Roosevelt set precedents and created a long and bitter debate. The president believed, as he told advisers, that "public

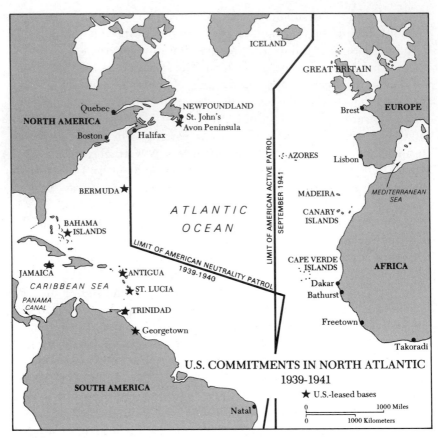

Between 1939 and 1941, FDR pushed U.S. naval power ever farther into the Atlantic to protect British ships and American exports from German submarine attacks.

opinion was not yet ready for the United States to convoy ships." He, therefore, decided to use his commander-in-chief powers, granted by the Constitution, to deploy U.S. warships without telling either Congress or the American people what he was doing.

As early as January 1941, U.S. and British military chiefs had secretly worked out joint plans to defeat the Axis. Canada, at war against Hitler, and the United States also set up a joint committee to coordinate war production. FDR, moreover, agreed to allow U.S. ships to patrol for German submarines 300 miles into the Atlantic. After subs sank nearly half of a twenty-two-ship British convoy during a single April night, Roosevelt instructed the U.S. fleet to patrol halfway across the Atlantic and report any subs to British ships (although he publicly said that the ships would report to Americans and warned journalists not to speculate about his policies). In April, he cast a U.S. protectorate over Greenland and the Azores. In July, he landed troops in Iceland to ensure the passage of Allied goods through these strategic areas. Secretary of War Henry Stimson asked FDR to tell Americans what he was doing, but the president refused. By November 1941, the United States had already spent billions in lend-lease goods for the British, Soviets, and Chinese, and had not even declared war yet. When isolationists questioned these actions, FDR secretly ordered the FBI to gather evidence that Lindbergh was a Nazi sympathizer (no such evidence was ever found), called Senator Nye a "boob," and complained that many critics were simply "wild Irish" who hated the British. Hull, meanwhile, became so saddened by the United States' inability to respond more fully that in cabinet meetings he kept muttering, "Everything [is] going hellward."[60]

But Hull's concern radically changed on June 22, 1941, when Germany invaded the Soviet Union in the largest land operation in history. Hitler and Stalin had squabbled over many issues, most notably who was to be dominant in the Balkans and the Black Sea region. Stalled in his plans to invade Great Britain, Hitler turned to the vast Eurasian landmass. Stalin, meanwhile, had gained maneuvering room on April 13, 1941, when he and the Japanese stunned the world—not the least Hitler—by signing a nonaggression pact. Both sides benefited. The Soviets no longer worried about their eastern border with Manchukuo, where shooting incidents between the Red Army and Japanese troops had occurred since 1934. Japan was free to strike south against British and U.S. holdings.

Stalin was, nevertheless, surprised by the Nazi invasion. "What have we done to deserve this?" Molotov innocently asked German officials. The dictator disappeared from sight for ten days and apparently almost suffered a nervous breakdown. Most Americans were equally puzzled. The State Department was unable to issue a statement for twenty-four hours, then published an announcement that blasted Soviet violations of human rights, but concluded that Washington supported any "forces opposing Hitlerism." Politicians were more direct. Senator Burton K. Wheeler declared, "Just let Joe Stalin and the other dictators fight it out." Democratic Senator Harry Truman from Missouri agreed: if Germany was winning, "we should help Russia and if Russia is winning we ought to help Germany . . . although I don't want to see Hitler victorious under any circumstances." The Soviets were equally suspicious of their new partners in the West. When a British official told a

Soviet leader how wonderful it was to be united in the common cause, the Soviet replied, "Perhaps."[61]

Hitler's divisions quickly advanced nearly to the gates of Moscow and Leningrad. U.S. Secretary of War Stimson and his military advisers concluded that the Soviets would last no longer than three months. But Churchill, who had long hated and fought bolshevism, now saw that the Red Army could prevent a Nazi invasion of Great Britain and demanded all-out support for the Soviet Union. FDR agreed. Overruling aides who thought that sending lend-lease supplies to the retreating Soviet troops was like pouring millions of dollars down a rat hole, the president demanded "a burr under the saddle" to "get things moving."[62] The first of some $12 billion in aid for the Soviet Union over the next four years left U.S. ports. The Red Army and its close ally, winter, finally stalled the Nazi armies in 1941–1942. The costs were enormous. Some 600,000 died in the Leningrad siege alone, many of starvation. Hitler had lost over 700,000 troops by late 1941, but he could not conquer Leningrad or Moscow.

FDR knew that a turning point had been reached. Rushing supplies to Churchill and Stalin could quickly lead to "shooting," he told the British ambassador in July 1941. The president was now "more hopeful" than he had been earlier.[63] In July, the Japanese turned south to seize the remainder of the French Empire in Indochina. Japanese politics, even the relatively moderate rule of Prince Fumimaro Konoye's faction, depended on foreign conquests rather than internal reforms. Roosevelt shocked Japan by freezing all Japanese assets in the United States (thus making it impossible, for example, for Japan to use its bank accounts in New York to buy U.S. goods) and persuaded Churchill to do the same in Great Britain. The president meant to place only a partial embargo on oil shipments to Japan. He did not want to push Konoye toward more conquest to obtain the vital resource. But a bureaucratic mix-up in Washington totally stopped oil shipments, and Roosevelt did not think that he could reverse the error without appearing to be retreating before Japanese aggression. Meanwhile, FDR accelerated military aid to Chinese forces fighting Japan.

Konoye, indeed, found his nation in a corner, stripped of oil and other goods that it depended on Americans to supply, and sucked into an endless war in China. In September, he proposed a summit meeting with FDR to discuss the crisis. The president was agreeable, but Hull insisted on prior Japanese concessions. Roosevelt finally declared that a summit could be held only if Japan agreed beforehand to pull back from China and Indochina, and pledge an open door in Asia. No Japanese government could accept such terms. The summit was never held.

SERGEANT YORK AND THE ANNOUNCEMENT OF THE AMERICAN CENTURY

By mid-summer 1941, leading Americans believed that the United States was actually in the war, although the country had not formally declared it. Hollywood seemed to be leading the way, despite bitter opposition from other media (especially some newspapers and radio commentators) to U.S. intervention in the conflict. The breakthrough for Hollywood was the midsummer 1941 film, *Sergeant York*, starring Gary Cooper. The story glorified the actual life of a former backwoods pacifist, Alvin York, who became a hero in World War I by single-handedly killing 20 German soldiers and capturing 132 others. As historians Clayton R. Koppes and Gregory D. Black observe, young male viewers "got the message that they, like York, should go off and fight for democracy. . . . *Sergeant York* capped an evolution in American motion pictures that took them from being fearful of political subjects to being aggressively interventionist."[64]

It was time to decide what Americans should fight for. This fascinating debate was led by Henry Luce, the powerful publisher of *Life*, *Time*, and *Fortune* magazines (which, not accidentally, had also widely publicized *Sergeant York*.) In a series of editorials published during the summer (and later collected in a small book, *The American Century*), Luce assumed that not only was the United States already involved in war, but that "only America can effectively state the aims of this war." Those aims had to include creating, under U.S. leadership, "a vital international economy" and "an international moral order." These were needed, Luce declared, because "Franklin Roosevelt failed to make American democracy work successfully on a narrow, materialistic, and nationalistic basis" between 1933 and 1939. Americans had to use their new power to create an international capitalist marketplace open to all, and which embodied the U.S. ideals of freedom, justice, and opportunity. Only then, Luce concluded, could American democracy itself survive. Thus, every American was called, he announced, "each in the widest horizon of his own vision, to create the first great American century."[65]

Luce spoke for a growing U.S. consensus, but a few strongly disagreed. Raymond Moley, a former FDR adviser but now angry with the

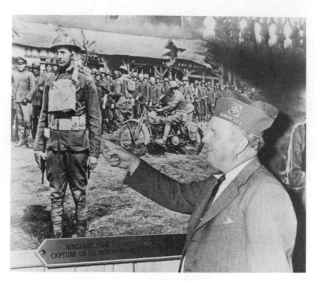

The real Sergeant Alvin York, one of World War I's heroes for single-handedly capturing 132 German soldiers, looks at the handsome Hollywood leading man, Gary Cooper, who played the lead in the 1941 film. Sergeant York *strayed rather far from the facts of York's Tennessee upbringing and battlefield exploits, but it was wildly popular, won Cooper an Academy Award for best actor, and played a part in the 1941 debates over U.S. neutrality policies.*

New Deal, warned that Americans had to resist this "temptation to drift into empire," because "an empire on which the sun would never set is one in which the rulers never sleep." Talk of "our century" was "childish" and could lead to "pure tragedy." One of Luce's own editors, John Chamberlain, questioned how Americans were sliding into war, then warned that "Luce's program requires a faith that can be sustained for short periods, when people are in the heroic mood." When those "short periods" end, Chamberlain believed, "Uncle Sam would . . . desert his trusting friends" abroad to take care of problems at home— and the American-century ideal could indeed become a tragedy.[66]

Roosevelt seemed to agree with Luce. On August 8, 1941, he secretly traveled to Newfoundland for his first meeting with Churchill. The president wanted nothing less than a joint declaration of war aims (although it was to be another four months before Americans formally declared war). After hard negotiating, FDR obtained a statement from the British that went far to meet the ideals of Hull, Luce, and himself. The Atlantic Charter told the world that the war was to be fought to protect self-government by all, freedom of the seas, a postwar "general security" system, freedom from fear and want, and a fair economic system that guaranteed equal access to world wealth to "all States, great or small, victor or vanquished." But Churchill bristled at the last point. He rightly understood that it was Roosevelt's and Hull's attempt to knock down the trade barriers around the British Empire, barriers that Churchill believed had to be reinforced against the U.S. powerhouse if a devastated Great Britain was to maintain its independence after the war. He insisted that a phrase be added: equal access would be guaranteed only "with due respect for . . . existing obligations." Thus, he tried to preserve Britain's colonial arrangements, such as the Imperial Preference System (see p. 351), already in place. FDR reluctantly agreed to this phrase.

Churchill, moreover, had his own ideas for the conference. He wanted the United States to enter the war immediately. Roosevelt was apparently amazingly candid, according to Churchill's account of the talks: "The President . . . said he would wage war, but not declare it" because of isolationist opposition in Congress, "and that he would become more and more provocative. If the Germans did not like it, they could attack American forces." FDR continued: "Everything was to be done to force an 'incident' that could lead to war."[67] None of these words of Roose-

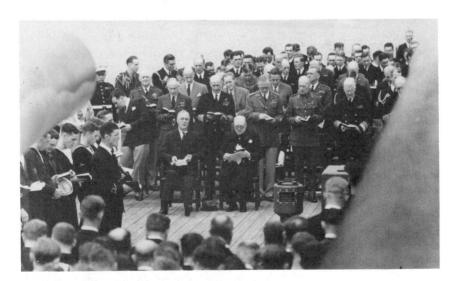

President Franklin D. Roosevelt and Prime Minister Winston Churchill (seated at the center left of the picture) met off Newfoundland in August 1941 to plan how to coordinate the fighting of World War II—although the United States was not yet formally in the war. In this photograph, the two leaders, their aides, and the crew of the British warship Prince of Wales *are singing a hymn at a church service.*

velt's were made public until more than thirty years later. Meanwhile, in August 1941, as historian Theodore Wilson notes, "the American people continued to hang in midair between the precipice of all-out aid to England and Russia and the rocks of war which lay below."[68]

But the rocks seemed to be getting rapidly closer. In early September, a U.S. destroyer, the *Greer*, tracked a German U-boat for three hours and signaled its location to British forces before the sub turned and attacked. The *Greer* escaped unharmed, but FDR used the incident to denounce Germany for an unprovoked attack. He never told Americans how the ship actually provoked the submarine. On September 11, 1941, he termed U-boats "the rattlesnakes of the Atlantic" and implied that, like such snakes, the subs were to be destroyed before they could attack. In October, three U.S. warships were torpedoed (one sank) while on convoy duty in the North Atlantic, and 172 men were lost. Roosevelt used the sinking to persuade Congress to repeal what remained of the Neutrality Acts' restraint upon his power to act as he saw fit.

PEARL HARBOR AND A "FEELING . . . OF RELIEF"

It seemed only a matter of time before war would erupt full-scale in the Atlantic. But when war came for Americans, it occurred 6,000 miles in another direction. Throughout October and November 1941, Hull negotiated with Japanese ambassador Kichisaburo Nomura to find a settlement for Asia. Actually, both sides were also preparing for war. After Prince Konoye rejected the U.S. conditions for a summit meeting, he lost power to an ardent militarist, General Hideki Tojo. Japan organized a secret attack to destroy U.S. bases in the Pacific. Talks in Washington did continue on three issues: Japan's possible repudiation of its Axis pact with Hitler; Japanese withdrawal from Indochina in return for American reopening of trade in oil and metals; and Hull's demand that Tokyo retreat from China and pledge the open door. Agreement was close on the first two issues. Japan, however, could not give up the fruits of its ten-year war in China. Thus, in historian Jonathan Utley's words, "Hull's insistence on total Japanese withdrawal from China would result in war."[69] By November 26, Tojo's government had given up on the talks and ordered the navy to launch the attack.

Hull and FDR knew about the Japanese decisions. U.S. intelligence had cracked the top-secret Purple Code in which the Japanese com-

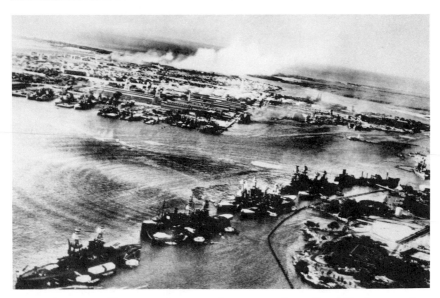

This is the view of Japanese airmen as they swooped over Pearl Harbor naval base on December 7, 1941, to destroy much of the U.S. Pacific Fleet. The ships appear to be lined up as if in a shooting gallery, but the important aircraft carriers had been sent to open sea days before and escaped the destruction.

municated their most sensitive messages. Hull, indeed, had used these so-called MAGIC intercepts to read the secret messages sent to Nomura before the ambassador even came in to negotiate. Roosevelt and Hull, however, did not know where Japan planned to attack. They assumed that the strike would occur in Southeast Asia and on the large U.S. base in the Philippines. The American military knew that it was not ready for an attack. As late as November 5, FDR's top military advisers begged him to fight only Hitler and not become involved in a two-front war—at least not until mid-1942, when U.S. defenses could be strengthened in the Pacific. But by late November, these military leaders knew that time had run out. On November 27, they told the U.S. commanders at Pearl Harbor naval base in Hawaii that Japan would probably attack in the next few days, but no one knew where.

Pearl Harbor seemed to be a logical target because much of the U.S. Pacific Fleet anchored there. In 1941, however, most Washington officials doubted that Japan had the power to strike the base. Incredibly, in early December they lost track of the Japanese fleet and knew only that it was somewhere in the west-central Pacific. U.S. aircraft carriers in Hawaii were ordered out to sea; but otherwise, Pearl Harbor, with five major battleships riding at anchor, was in a state of low alert on

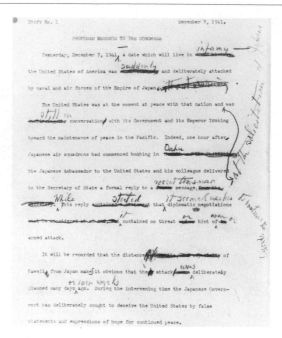

FDR's draft of his historic speech asking Congress to declare war against Japan. Note how most of his changes made the message simpler, more direct, and forceful.

the morning of December 7, 1941. About one and one-half hours before the Japanese planes struck, Washington officials intercepted coded messages from Tokyo that war was imminent. But even this vague signal was relayed to Pearl Harbor by slow commercial telegraph and arrived after much of the base, including three battleships, had been destroyed. A failure to collect sufficient intelligence left Pearl Harbor a sitting target. This failure was in large part due to top U.S. military officers who were jealous of other branches that grew with new technology (such as intelligence) and so had refused to give these branches funds to develop better intelligence collecting.[70]

Some of the U.S. military were humiliated, but top civilians reacted quite differently. "My first feeling," Secretary of War Stimson wrote in his diary on December 7, "was of relief that the indecision was over and that a crisis had come in a way which would unite all our people."[71] The next day, Roosevelt appeared before a joint session of Congress, declared December 7, 1941, "a date which will live in infamy," asked for a declaration of war against Japan, and swore to fight until total victory was won. The Senate approved the war resolution 89 to 0, the House 388 to 1. The lone dissenter was Jeanette Rankin of Montana, a pacifist and suffragist who, as a member of Congress, had also opposed war in 1917.

A great irony then became apparent. For nearly two years, FDR had prepared to fight Germany, but now he had to ask for war only against Japan. Roosevelt was not certain that a declaration of war against Germany was possible. On December 11, however, Hitler solved the dilemma by declaring war on the United States. He evidently did so because of his treaty ties to Japan; but more important were his beliefs that the Japanese had perhaps mortally wounded the Americans and that FDR's growing aid to the British and Soviets had to be stopped by force. Tokyo officials appreciated Hitler's support. They had few illusions and realized that they had no chance for victory if the war dragged on and the incredible U.S. industrial powerhouse had time to gear up to full blast.

THE LESSONS OF THE 1930s

The two major historical lessons of the era went far beyond the Pearl Harbor attack. The first was that, in the end, the United States admitted that its decades-long hope that Japan could be depended on to protect the open door in Asia had been a pipe dream. As diplomat John Paton Davies later wrote, in the U.S.-Japan-China triangle before 1941, "Japan was . . . the actor, China the acted upon. And the United States was the self-appointed referee who judged by subjective rules and called fouls without penalties, until just before the end of the contest. This provoked the actor into a suicidal attempt to kill the referee." The long, historical background that climaxed with this "suicidal attempt" has been well summarized by historian Michael Barnhart: "The Pacific War was, in essence, a conflict between two visions for East Asia. Each vision had a strong economic element. Japan's fundamental war aim was to establish the Greater East Asian Coprosperity Sphere as a self-sufficient and powerful unit with the Japanese Empire at its core. The United States," Barnhart notes, "sought, first, to thwart Japan's attempt and, second, to 'restore' the principles of . . . the Open Door." These two visions climaxed in the Pacific War.[72]

A second major lesson was that the Constitution's provisions that outlined how Americans were to go to war in an open, accountable process had broken down. Roosevelt secretly placed U.S. ships in areas where incidents could force Americans into war. He then misled the

American people about his actions. FDR also allowed the FBI to break the law by wire-tapping phones and opening mail of suspected Axis sympathizers; he also let the FBI spy on congressmen who merely criticized him. The president believed that Hitler posed a mortal threat to the United States. He also feared that openness would result in a violent isolationist backlash against his policies. Both those fears were valid, but the central question remains: whether those fears justified the damage to the constitutional restraints carefully placed by the Founders upon presidential power. Historian Robert Dallek notes how ironic it was that in his determination "to save democracy from Nazism, Roosevelt contributed to the rise of some undemocratic practices in the United States." Dallek adds, however, that the isolationists' failure to understand the Nazi menace might have pushed FDR into abuses of power that later presidents would repeat for less-exalted reasons. Amid the horrors of the Vietnam War a generation later, Democratic Senator J. William Fulbright of Arkansas made the link directly: "FDR's deviousness in a good cause made it much easier for [President Lyndon Johnson] to practice the same kind of deviousness in a bad cause."[73]

Americans felt the full impact of these two historical lessons much later. In 1941, Roosevelt had been purposely "vague" and had tried to "stifle national debate," as historian Richard Steele concludes. "The result was that when war did come, a great many Americans remained uncertain of the circumstances (beyond the Japanese attack on Pearl Harbor) that led them into global conflict."[74] They only knew that a history they did not understand must never be repeated—especially since before them, a glorious American century dawned over the limitless horrors of World War II. Or as Sidney Greenstreet explained to Humphrey Bogart in the classic film *Casablanca*, "Isolationism is no longer a practicable policy."

NOTES

1. Paul F. Boller, Jr., *Presidential Anecdotes* (New York, 1981), p. 266.
2. Frank Costigliola, *Awkward Dominion: American Political, Economic, and Cultural Relations with Europe, 1919–1933* (Ithaca, N.Y., 1985), ch. I; Arthur Schlesinger, Jr., *The Age of Roosevelt: The Coming of the New Deal* (Boston, 1959), pp. 199–201.
3. Lloyd C. Gardner, *Economic Aspects of New Deal Diplomacy* (Madison, Wis., 1964), p. 5, has the quote with a good analysis.

4. Joseph Alsop, *FDR, 1882–1945: A Centenary Remembrance* (New York, 1982), p. 112.
5. Cordell Hull, *The Memoirs of Cordell Hull*, 2 vols. (New York, 1948), I, pp. 81–82; "Pall-Mall Broadcast," 31 December, 1937, Papers of Cordell Hull, Library of Congress, Washington, D.C.
6. Benjamin D. Rhodes, "Sir Ronald Lindsay and the British View from Washington, 1930–1939," in *Essays in Twentieth Century American Diplomatic History Dedicated to Professor Daniel M. Smith*, ed. Clifford L. Egan and Alexander W. Knott (Washington, D.C., 1982), p. 72.
7. Frederick C. Adams, *Economic Diplomacy: The Export-Import Bank and American Foreign Policy, 1934–1939* (Columbia, Mo., 1976), pp. 224–225.
8. Schlesinger, pp. 253–255.
9. A useful discussion of the treaties' effect is in Dick Steward, *Trade and Hemisphere: The Good Neighbor Policy and Reciprocal Trade* (Columbia, Mo., 1975), pp. 208–220.
10. Laurence Duggan, *The Americas: The Search for Hemisphere Security* (New York, 1949), pp. 65–66.
11. Hull, I, p. 365. The 1930s agreements are excerpted in *The Record of American Diplomacy*, ed. Ruhl F. Bartlett, 4th ed. (New York, 1964), pp. 551–558.
12. Lester D. Langley, *The United States and the Caribbean, 1900–1970* (Athens, Ga., 1980), p. 203.
13. Donald M. Dozer, *Are We Good Neighbors?: Three Decades of Inter-American Relations, 1930–1960* (Gainesville, Fla., 1959), pp. 5–51.
14. *Ibid.*, pp. 35–37.
15. Gardner, p. 32.
16. *New York Times*, 19 November 1933, sec. 8, p. 3.
17. U.S. Department of State, *Foreign Relations of the United States, 1933*, 5 vols (Washington, D.C., 1952), V, pp. 389–414.
18. Gardner, p. 51.
19. Clayton R. Koppes, "The Good Neighbor Policy and the Nationalization of Mexican Oil: A Reinterpretation," *Journal of American History* 79 (June 1982): 80–81.
20. Thomas R. Maddux, *Years of Estrangement: American Relations with the Soviet Union, 1933–1941* (Tallahasee, 1980), p. 17; Frederic L. Propas, "Creating a Hard Line toward Russia: The Training of State Department Soviet Experts, 1927–1937," *Diplomatic History* 8 (Summer 1984): 222.
21. Richard W. Stevenson, *The Rise and Fall of Detente* (Urbana, Ill., 1985), p. 19.
22. "Summary of the Morning Newspapers, Tuesday, Nov. 7, 1933," Box 18, Papers of R. Walton Moore, Library of Congress, Washington, D.C. A good, brief analysis of the 1933 talks, especially in regard to USSR motives, is in U.S. Congress, House Committee on Foreign Affairs, *Soviet Diplomacy and Negotiating Behavior: Emerging New Context for U.S. Diplomacy*, House Document no. 96-239, 96th Cong., 1st sess. [prepared by Joseph G. Whelan], (Washington, D.C., 1979), pp. 65–83.
23. Stanley Hornbeck to Cordell Hull, 28 October 1933, and Stanley Hornbeck to William Phillips, 31 October 1933, which Phillips sent to Hull on 3 November, 711.61/333, RG 59, National Archives, Washington, D.C.
24. George Kennan, "Reflections: Flashbacks," *New Yorker*, 25 February 1985, p. 57.
25. Wayne S. Cole, "Senator Key Pittman and American Neutrality Policies, 1933–1940," *Mississippi Valley Historical Review* 46 (March 1960): 644n.; for background, see

Manfred Jonas, "Isolationism," in *Encyclopedia of American Foreign Policy*, ed. Alexander DeConde, 3 vols. (New York, 1978), II, p. 496.

26. Wayne S. Cole, *Senator Gerald P. Nye and American Foreign Relations* (Minneapolis, 1962), pp. 95–96. A new, most useful analysis of Nye's midwestern region is in Warren F. Kuehl, "Midwestern Newspapers and Isolationist Sentiment," *Diplomatic History* 3 (Summer 1979): 283–306. Kuehl believes that the region was more internationalist than most historians have believed.

27. Robert A. Divine, *Second Chance: The Triumph of Internationalism in America during World War II* (New York, 1967), pp. 21–23.

28. Manfred Jonas, *The United States and Germany, a Diplomatic History* (Ithaca, N.Y., 1984), p. 222. The thesis on labor-intensive versus capital-intensive firms that battled inside the New Deal is given in Thomas Ferguson, "From Normalcy to New Deal . . . ," *International Organization* 38 (Winter 1984): 41–94.

29. Gilbert N. Kahn, "Presidential Passivity on a Nonsalient Issue: President Franklin D. Roosevelt and the 1935 World Court Fight," *Diplomatic History* 4 (Spring 1980): 137–159.

30. Richard A. Harrison, "A Presidential Démarche: FDR's Personal Diplomacy and Great Britain, 1936–1937," *Diplomatic History* 5 (Summer 1981): 249.

31. Douglas Little, *Malevolent Neutrality: The United States, Great Britain and the Origins of the Spanish Civil War* (Ithaca, N.Y., 1985), p. 265.

32. Robert A. Divine, *The Illusion of Neutrality* (Chicago, 1962), pp. 165–166.

33. David Green, *The Shaping of Political Consciousness* (Ithaca, N.Y., 1988), ch. V.

34. Robert Dallek, *Franklin D. Roosevelt and American Foreign Policy, 1932–1945* (New York, 1979), pp. 166–168.

35. The background is well presented in Arnold Offner, *American Appeasement: U.S. Foreign Policy and Germany, 1933–1938* (Cambridge, Mass., 1969), esp. pp. 69–91, and Peggy Mann, "When the World Passed By on the Other Side," *Guardian*, 7 May 1978, pp. 17–18.

36. This example and others are given in a superb context in Deborah Lipstadt, *Beyond Belief: The American Press and the Coming of the Holocaust, 1933–1945* (New York, 1986).

37. David S. Wyman, *The Abandonment of the Jews* (New York, 1984), pp. x–xi, 80, 180–198, 311–340, 345–347; Gordon Craig, "Schreibt un Farschreibt!" *New York Review of Books*, 10 April 1986, pp. 7–11; Geoffrey S. Smith, "Isolationism, the Devil, and the Advent of the Second World War . . . ," *International History Review* 4 (February 1982): 87–88.

38. William L. Neumann, "Ambiguity and Ambivalence in Ideas of National Interest in Asia," in *Isolation and Security*, ed. Alexander DeConde (Durham, N.C., 1957), pp. 147–148.

39. The text is in *The Record of American Diplomacy*, pp. 577–580.

40. The pioneering study of this episode is Dorothy Borg, *The United States and the Far Eastern Crisis of 1933–1938* (Cambridge, Mass., 1964), and a good analysis of public opinion is also in Michael Leigh, *Mobilizing Consent, 1937–1947* (Westview, Conn., 1976), pp. 32–40.

41. Stephen E. Pelz, *Race to Pearl Harbor . . .* (Cambridge, Mass., 1974), p. 67; "4th Meeting, Brussels Conf.," Box 5, Meetings, November 1937, Papers of Norman Davis, Library of Congress, Washington, D.C.; Gardner, pp. 95–96.

42. A good brief context is given in Smith, 63–64. Especially good on the *Panay* is Irvine

H. Anderson, Jr., *The Standard-Vacuum Oil Company and U.S. East Asian Policy, 1933–1941* (Princeton, 1975), pp. 107–110.

43. Arnold A. Offner, "Appeasement Revisited: The United States, Great Britain, and Germany, 1933–1940," *Journal of American History* 64 (September 1977): 381–382.

44. D. Cameron Watt, *Succeeding John Bull: America in Britain's Place, 1900–1975* (Cambridge, 1984), p. 85.

45. Christopher D. Morley, *History of an Autumn* (Philadelphia, 1938), p. 7.

46. Offner, *American Appeasement*, pp. 215–216.

47. Jonas, *United States and Germany*, p. 234.

48. Excerpts of speech in *New York Times*, 9 May 1985, p. 10.

49. Robert A. Divine, *Roosevelt and World War II* (Baltimore, 1969), ch. II.

50. Ian Macleod, *Neville Chamberlain* (New York, 1962), p. 279.

51. Jonas, *United States and Germany*, pp. 245–246.

52. J. Garry Clifford and Samuel R. Spencer, Jr., *The First Peacetime Draft* (Lawrence, Kans., 1986).

53. Wayne S. Cole, *Roosevelt and the Isolationists, 1932–1945* (Lincoln, Neb., 1983), superbly presents the background (esp. p. 8).

54. Alan K. Henrikson has done crucial work on this subject, especially in "The Map as an 'Idea': The Role of Cartographic Imagery during the Second World War," *American Cartographer*, 2 April 1975, pp. 19–53.

55. Jim Harmon, *The Great Radio Heroes* (Garden City, N.Y., 1967), p. 232.

56. Philip Henry Kerr Lord Lothian to Foreign Office, 7 February 1940, FO 371 C5072 / 285 / 18, British Public Record Office, Kew, Eng. A good analysis of FDR's use of public opinion (and how it did not always restrain him) is in Hadley Cantril, *The Human Dimension: Experience in Policy Research* (New Brunswick, N.J., 1967), esp. pp. 35–42.

57. Akira Iriye, "The Role of the U.S. Embassy in Tokyo," in *Pearl Harbor as History*, ed. Dorothy Borg and Shumpei Okamoto (New York, 1973), p. 121.

58. A good context is in Dallek, pp. 247–251; Wayne Cole, "The Role of the U.S. Congress and Political Parties," in *Pearl Harbor as History*, ed. Borg and Okamoto, pp. 303–307; and the Willkie quote is cited by Robert A. Divine, *Foreign Policy and U.S. Presidential Elections, 1940–1948* (New York, 1974), pp. 82–83.

59. The quote and a most useful analysis is in Waldo Henrichs, "President Franklin D. Roosevelt's Intervention in the Battle of the Atlantic," *Diplomatic History* 10 (Fall 1986): esp. 313–314; Dallek, p. 255.

60. The Diary of Henry L. Stimson (microfilm), 27 May, 1941, Yale University; J. Garry Clifford and Robert Griffiths, "Senator John A. Danaher and the Battle against Intervention in World War II," *Connecticut History* no. 25 (January 1984): 55.

61. Laurence A. Steinhardt to Cordell Hull, 24 June 1941, U.S. Department of State, *Foreign Relations of the United States, 1941*, 7 vols. (Washington, D.C., 1958), I, pp. 174–175; Truman's quote is in *New York Times*, 24 June 1941, p. 7; the State Department and Wheeler statements are noted in Foster Rhea Dulles, *The Road to Tehran: The Story of Russia and America, 1781–1943* (Princeton, 1944), pp. 231–232.

62. "Memorandum for Wayne Coy" from FDR, 2 August 1941, President's Secretary File, Box 18, Russia, Papers of Franklin D. Roosevelt, Franklin D. Roosevelt Library, Hyde Park, New York.

63. Edward Viscount Halifax to Foreign Office, 7 July 1941, FO 954 / 29, British Public

Record Office; I am greatly indebted to Professor Warren Kimball of Rutgers—Newark for a copy of this document.

64. Clayton R. Koppes and Gregory D. Black, *Hollywood Goes to War* (New York, 1987), pp. 37–41.

65. Henry Luce, *The American Century* (New York, 1941), pp. 5–40.

66. *Ibid.*, p. 68; Moley is quoted in Frank Annunziata, "Raymond Moley and New Deal Liberalism," manuscript in possession of author, pp. 40–41.

67. British War Cabinet Minutes, 19 August 1941, CAB65 84 (41), British Public Record Office; I am indebted to Professor Warren Kimball and Professor Lloyd Gardner, Rutgers—New Brunswick, who discovered this document. A superb brief analysis can be found in *Churchill and Roosevelt: The Complete Correspondence*, ed. Warren Kimball, 3 vols. (Princeton, 1984), I, pp. 227–231.

68. Theodore A. Wilson, *The First Summit* (Boston, 1969), p. 267.

69. Jonathan G. Utley, *Going to War with Japan, 1937–1941* (Knoxville, Tenn., 1985), p. 162, with a good summary on pp. 178–181.

70. David Kahn, "U.S. Views of Germany and Japan in 1941," in *Knowing One's Enemies: Intelligence Assessment before the Two World Wars*, ed. Ernest R. May (Princeton, 1984), pp. 496–501.

71. Diary of Henry Stimson, 7 December 1941; *Churchill and Roosevelt*, I, p. 281.

72. John Paton Davies, "America and East Asia," *Foreign Affairs* 55 (January 1977): 381. A useful overview of recent scholarship on this topic by Japanese and Americans is Richard Leopold, "Historiographical Reflections," in *Pearl Harbor as History*, ed. Borg and Okamoto, pp. 1–24; Michael Barnhart, *Japan Prepares for Total War* (Ithaca, N.Y., 1988), p. 272. Barnhart's analysis is of great importance for both U.S. and Japanese policies.

73. Dallek, pp. 312–313; Clifford and Griffiths, 54. A great scholar of constitutional law wrote in late 1941: "Contrary to a common, but quite mistaken impression, no President has a mandate from the Constitution to conduct our foreign relations according to his own sweet will. If his power in that respect is indefinite, so is Congress' Legislative power, and if he holds the 'sword,' so does Congress hold the 'purse strings.' Simply from constitutional necessity, therefore, the actual conduct of American foreign relations is a joint affair." Edward S. Corwin, "Some Aspects of the Presidency," *Annals* 218 (November 1941): 122–131.

74. Richard W. Steele, "The Great Debate: Roosevelt, the Media, and the Coming of the War, 1940–1941," *Journal of American History* 71 (June 1984): 69.

FOR FURTHER READING

Begin with the notes to this chapter and the General Bibliography at the end of the book; these sources are usually not repeated here. For pre-1981 materials, there is nothing to match the usefulness of the *Guide to American Foreign Relations since 1700*, ed. Richard Dean Burns (1983), for either exhaustiveness or accessibility. Therefore, what follows deals mostly with post-1981 work.

Important overviews and further references can be found in Akira Iriye, *The Global-*

izing of America, 1914–1945, in *The Cambridge History of U.S. Foreign Relations*, ed. Warren Cohen (1993); Richard Dean Burns, "Cordell Hull and American Interwar Internationalism," in *Studies in American Diplomacy, 1865–1945*, ed. Norman Graebner (1985); Jane Karoline Vieth, "The Diplomacy of the Depression," in *Modern American Diplomacy*, ed. John M. Carroll and George C. Herring (1986); Kenneth S. Davis, *FDR* (1986), a biography on the 1933–1937 years; Thomas McCormick, "Adolf Berle," in *Behind the Throne*, eds. T. McCormick and W. LaFeber (1993), essays in honor of Fred Harvey Harrington; and David Green's pioneering *Shaping Political Consciousness: The Language of Politics in America from McKinley to Reagan* (1988), with an emphasis on the 1930s. The peace movement is well presented in Lawrence S. Wittner, *Rebels against War* (1984), with a new epilogue for a 1969 book. A new and crucial primary source is Larry I. Bland *et al.*, *The Papers of General George C. Marshall* (1981–   ), available to 6 December 1941.

The domestic debate is exhaustively presented in Wayne S. Cole, *Roosevelt and the Isolationists, 1932–1945* (1983), the summation of a life's work, with the use of important British and FBI records; Ellen Nore, *Charles A. Beard* (1983), on an outspoken critic and great historian; Justus D. Doenecke, "The Literature of Isolationism, 1972–1983: A Bibliographical Guide," *Journal of Libertarian Studies* 7 (1983), the crucial place to find more sources; Richard W. Steel, *Propaganda in an Open Society* (1985), key on FDR, 1933–1941. Leo V. Kanawada, Jr., *Franklin D. Roosevelt's Diplomacy and American Catholics, Italians, and Jews* (1982), on three key ethnic groups; and a sad story on a central figure is Betty Glad's *Key Pittman: The Tragedy of a Senate Insider* (1986).

On European policy, start with Melvin Small and Otto Feinstein, eds., *Appeasing Fascism* (1991); David F. Schmitz and Richard D. Challener, eds., *Appeasement in Europe* (1990); William R. Rock, *Chamberlain and Roosevelt* (1988), focuses on 1937 to 1940; C. A. MacDonald, *The United States, Britain and Appeasement, 1936–1939* (1981), is good on trade policies; Malcolm H. Murfett, *Fool-Proof Relations* (1984), is important for the British side in U.S.-U.K. naval cooperation, 1937–1940; David Reynolds, *The Creation of the Anglo-American Alliance, 1937–1941* (1982), is a standard in the field; *Essays in Twentieth Century American Diplomatic History Dedicated to Professor Daniel M. Smith*, ed. Clifford L. Egan and Alexander W. Knott (1976), has two useful essays: Brooks Van Everen's "Franklin D. Roosevelt and the Problem of Nazi Germany" and Benjamin D. Rhodes's "Sir Ronald Lindsay and the British View from Washington, 1930–1939." Patrick J. Hearden, *Roosevelt Confronts Hitler: America's Entry into World War II* (1987), is important for moving far beyond the FDR-Hitler confrontation; Theodore A. Wilson, *The First Summit* (1991), is a revised account of the Atlantic conference; Holger H. Herwig, "Miscalculated Risks: The German Declaration of War against the United States, 1917 and 1941," *Naval War College Review* 39 (1986), is suggestive; Jesse H. Stiller, *George S. Messersmith, Diplomat of Democracy* (1987), is a well-researched work on a central U.S. diplomat in Europe. In addition to David Wyman's standard works, Martin Gilbert, *Auschwitz and the Allies* (1981), analyzes the Allied inaction while the Holocaust developed.

For U.S.-Asian (especially Japanese) relations, the following are good in bringing together the best scholarship and suggesting further sources for research: *Diplomats in Crisis: U.S.-Chinese-Japanese Relations, 1919–1941*, ed. Richard Dean Burns and Edward M. Bennett (1975), with essays on Nomura, Hornbeck, and Grew, among others; Michael A. Barnhart, *Japan Prepares for Total War* (1988), noted above in the footnotes; Daniel Yergin's prize-winning account of the key role of oil in *The Prize* (1991); Jonathan C.

Utley, *Going to War with Japan, 1937–1941* (1985), good on Hull and the State Department; and two books widely discussed because of their divergent views of the Pearl Harbor attack: Gordon W. Prange's *Pearl Harbor: The Verdict of History* (1986), and Edwin T. Layton, *"And I Was There": Pearl Harbor and Midway—Breaking the Secrets* (1986). All of this is put into historical perspective with superb new research in the essays edited by Warren I. Cohen, *New Frontiers in American–East Asian Relations: Essays Presented to Dorothy Borg* (1983); and Akira Iriye and Warren Cohen, eds., *American, Chinese, and Japanese Perspectives on Wartime Asia, 1931–1949* (1990).

On U.S.-Soviet relations, a fine overview is Edward M. Bennett, *Franklin D. Roosevelt and the Search for Security* (1985), covering 1933 through 1939; *A Question of Trust— The Origins of U.S.-Soviet Diplomatic Relations: The Memoirs of Loy W. Henderson*, ed. George W. Baer (1986), by a hard-liner who was a key State Department official, covers the 1933 to 1938 years; James W. Crowl, *Angels in Stalin's Paradise* (1982), a critical study of two influential American reporters who covered the Soviet Union—Louis Fischer and Walter Duranty; Douglas Little, "Antibolshevism and American Foreign Policy, 1919–1939," *American Quarterly* 35 (1983), which ranges far beyond the U.S.-USSR relationship; and, for the war with Finland, Travis Beal Jacobs, *America and the Winter War, 1939–1940* (1981). A key book on a key subject is Louis A. Pérez, Jr., *Cuba under the Platt Amendment, 1902–1934* (1986); and a key dissenting view on U.S. policy is given in John A. Britton, *Carleton Beals: A Radical Journalist in Latin America* (1987).

13

World War II: The Rise and Fall of the Grand Alliance (1941–1945)

THE WASHINGTON CONFERENCE:
LAYING FOUNDATIONS IN THE GLOOM (1941–1942)

The most famous film of the early war years has become *Casablanca*, with Humphrey Bogart playing Rick Blaine, the American exile who owned a saloon in pro-Nazi French Morocco. The story takes place in 1941, just before the Pearl Harbor attack. U.S. audiences saw themselves when Rick is asked to help a leader of the anti-Nazi underground in Europe and snaps, "I stick my neck out for nobody."[1] It turns out, however, that, being a good American, the worldly Rick had already stuck his neck out: he had fought with the Ethiopians against the Italian invaders in 1935 and with the Spanish republic against Franco's fascists in 1936. And, in 1941, he finally agrees to save the life of the anti-Hitler underground agent. Americans, once aroused and fully committed, could not be distracted even by the beautiful Ingrid Bergman from risking their neck to defeat the Axis.

Casablanca's message reassured viewers, but in reality Americans seemed to have stuck out their neck too far by 1942–1943. They were trying to fight a worldwide, multifront war while suddenly having to deal with the most complex and far-reaching diplomatic decisions. No more had the Big Three (that is, the United States, Great Britain, and the Soviet Union) joined to fight the war, than they began to argue bitterly over the postwar peace. They did so, moreover, during days made so dark by German and Japanese victories that it was not clear in early 1942 which side would win the war.

In the Atlantic, U.S. ships became easy targets for Hitler's U-boats. With only 40 submarines available at one time, Germany sank an average of 100 Allied ships per month. U.S. and British crews destroyed 21 U-boats, which Hitler's plants replaced with 123 subs built in 1942. The subs' success threatened to starve an already war-shocked British people. It also made difficult any large U.S.-British operation to relieve the blood-soaked Russian front, where Nazi armies pressed their sieges of Leningrad and Moscow.

In the Pacific, Japanese forces struck with surprising ease and seized Hong Kong, Singapore, and Malaya from the British Empire. Americans were stunned at the humiliating defeat of Allied forces in Burma and the inability of Chiang Kai-shek (the leader of China) to protect either Burma or his own country from Japan. Preoccupied with destroying Mao's Communist forces in northern China, Chiang preferred to let the United States fight Japan. The U.S. commander attached to Chiang's headquarters, the tough, salty General Joseph W. ("Vinegar Joe") Stilwell, bluntly declared that in Burma "We got a hell of a beating . . . and it is humiliating as hell." When a reporter asked how it happened, Stilwell flashed, "We are allied to an ignorant, illiterate peasant son-of-a-bitch called Chiang Kai-shek."[2] Clearly, U.S. relations with its most important Asian ally, China, could be improved.

In the Pacific, the Japanese quickly took U.S. bases at Guam and Wake Island, then pressed the rich Dutch East Indies and Australia. In the Philippines, General Douglas MacArthur failed to protect his small air force, which Japanese bombers destroyed on the ground on December 8, 1941. Allowing his immense ego to overrule military judgment, MacArthur tried to fight the invaders with inadequate forces, who were largely wiped out. Some brave Filipino and U.S. troops held out on the natural fortress of Corregidor Island until May, when the Japanese took the survivors on a tortuous "death march" to prison camps. Meanwhile, MacArthur escaped to Australia, promising "I shall return." Roosevelt hoped that MacArthur could somehow do so with the inadequate army and navy that was at the general's command. The president, believing that Germany's power most threatened Allied survival, infuriated MacArthur by giving military priority to the European theater. U.S. bombers under the command of General James Doolittle did use aircraft carriers to bomb Tokyo in 1942. The surprise attack bolstered sagging U.S. morale but did little to damage Tokyo and even less to reverse the disastrous tide of the war in the Pacific. (Again, Hollywood improved on reality in three popular films—*Bombardier, Purple Heart,* and *Thirty Seconds over Tokyo*—which overlooked how three of Doolittle's pilots were executed as war criminals by Japan after they crash-landed in China.)[3]

Amid the gloom, Winston Churchill secretly traveled to Washington in December 1941 to discuss strategy with Roosevelt. As far as the public was concerned, the climax came on New Year's Day 1942, when the United States, Great Britain, the Soviet Union, and twenty-three other nations grandly announced a "Declaration of the United Nations" to fight to victory and make no separate peace with the Axis powers of Germany, Japan, and Italy. Secretly, however, the British and Americans argued long and passionately. Churchill, realizing that British power could not match America's, wanted separate military commands or at least key strategic decision makers located in London. FDR, advised by his army chief of staff, George C. Marshall, overruled Churchill.

Marshall was a different type of U.S. military leader. A graduate of Virginia Military Institute (not West Point), he had attended the new post–World War I Officers' Training Schools and represented the best of the crop: thoroughly professional, systematic, low-keyed, brilliant in developing and using younger staff (such as a Kansan, Dwight D. Eisenhower, who quickly became a Marshall protégé). He insisted on "unity of command." Thus, the top British and U.S. officers formed a Combined Chiefs of Staff located in Washington (not London) to handle the vast supplying of armies around the globe and to make broad strategic decisions. The Soviets were not included because Stalin did not want to become involved in the war against Japan. Marshall was less successful in stopping Churchill's drive for an invasion of North Africa. The prime minister eyed that region because British troops and imperial interests were already heavily involved. Marshall wanted to strike first at France. FDR sided with Churchill in 1942. He feared the Allies lacked the power to attack the Nazis on the European mainland.

But on a pivotal postwar question, Churchill had to give in. As historian Gabriel Kolko notes, U.S. officials assumed that "the key to the attainment of American postwar objectives for the world economy was Great Britain," because before 1939 the British and Americans together "accounted for about one-half of the total world trade."[4] Secretary of State Cordell Hull was at his Tennessee-mountaineer's toughest in trying to destroy the British Imperial Preference trading system (see p. 351) and do away with the hated closed "spheres of influence." Hull's weapon was the Lend-Lease Act's Article VII, which demanded that the British

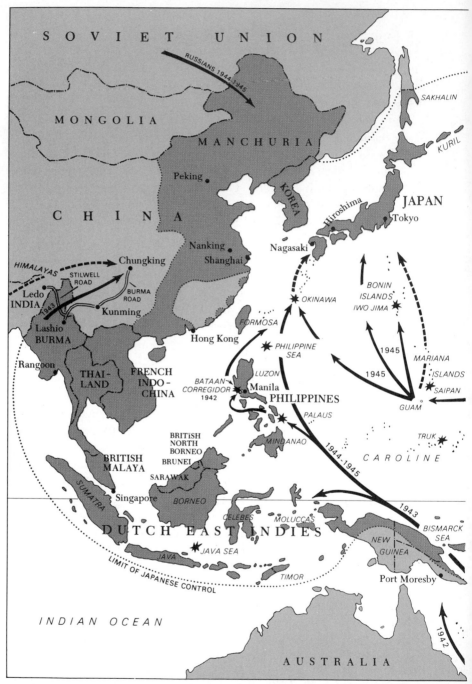

The United States recovered from the shock of Pearl Harbor to start an island-hopping campaign that was to climax with an invasion of Japan. Note how China is largely bypassed by U.S. war planners.

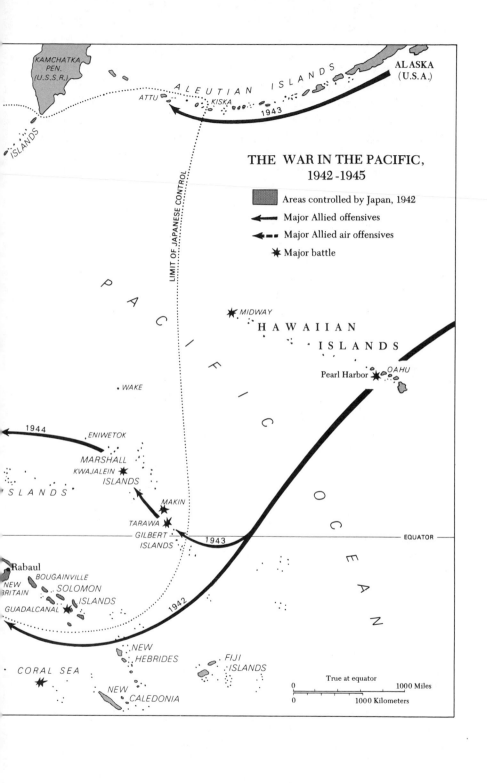

KAMCHATKA
PEN.
(U.S.S.R.)

A L E U T I A N   I S L A N D S

ALASKA
(U.S.A.)

ATTU   KISKA

1943

ISLANDS

THE WAR IN THE PACIFIC,
1942-1945

Areas controlled by Japan, 1942

Major Allied offensives

Major Allied air offensives

✳ Major battle

LIMIT OF JAPANESE CONTROL

P
A
C
I
F
I
C

O
C
E
A
N

✳ *MIDWAY*

H A W A I I A N

I S L A N D S

Pearl Harbor ✳ *OAHU*

• *WAKE*

1944

ENIWETOK

MARSHALL

KWAJALEIN ✳

ISLANDS

MAKIN

TARAWA ✳

GILBERT

ISLANDS

1943

EQUATOR

S L A N D S

Rabaul

BOUGAINVILLE

NEW
BRITAIN

SOLOMON

GUADALCANAL ✳

ISLANDS

1942

*NEW
HEBRIDES*

*FIJI
ISLANDS*

CORAL SEA

✳

*NEW
CALEDONIA*

True at equator

0   1000 Miles

0   1000 Kilometers

not create any more closed economic systems after the war. Fully real-izing that his nation would not be able to compete on equal economic terms with the United States, and fully understanding that FDR and Hull intended nothing less than to dismantle the British Empire, Churchill fought Article VII. In the end, however, he had to accept Hull's principle because British survival depended on U.S. help. The prime minister did try, however, to qualify his acceptance with reser-vations.

Churchill had more luck in handling Roosevelt's request that Great Britain give India immediate independence. The president was afraid that London's hold on the jewel of the empire would lead to revolution and instability throughout southern Asia. More immediately, he wanted Indians to fight Japan. The largest political group, Mohandas Gandhi's Congress party, refused to fight until Churchill guaranteed indepen-dence. Churchill bluntly rejected the demand, partly because he wanted to hold on to India, partly because he was afraid that independence would lead to civil war between the Hindu-dominated Congress party and the minority Moslem population that demanded its own nation. But FDR warned, in historian Kenton Clymer's words, that "if the West failed to support Indian nationalism, Japan would likely capture Asian nationalism generally and inspire a full-fledged anti-Western revolt."[5]

The president even sent special agents to push the British toward Indian independence. Churchill lashed back at one agent with "a string of cuss words . . . for two hours in the middle of the night," as a U.S. observer recorded. Proclaiming in November 1942 that "I have not become the King's First Minister to preside over the liquidation of the British Empire," Churchill threatened to resign. He finally was able to block independence until 1947.[6] But Hull could at least be pleased with London's acceptance of Article VII, for now, he believed, "the foundation was laid for all our . . . postwar planning in the economic" realm.[7]

AT WASHINGTON AND CASABLANCA: PREVIEWING THE COLD WAR (1942–1943)

Actually, only some of the "foundations" were laid. Hull himself pointed to the great obstacle to finishing the postwar structure when, shortly after Pearl Harbor, journalists asked him whether "Russia is to become our active ally, make peace with Germany and / or Japan, collapse, or what." Hull answered, " I wish I knew."[8] Certainly, he knew how Stalin had responded to the Atlantic Charter's call for self-determination and an open world marketplace. The dictator, even with his back to the wall before onrushing Nazi armies, had added a reservation that made his acceptance of the document meaningless.

Even worse occurred in late December, when British foreign minister Anthony Eden flew to Moscow. FDR and Hull were afraid that the British were trying to cut a secret deal with the Soviets. They warned Eden to make no postwar commitments. Stalin quickly asked Eden to guarantee the June 1941 boundaries—that is, to allow the Soviets to have the three Baltic States and a large slice of Poland. When Eden refused to agree, the dictator furiously declared that he thought the Atlantic Charter had been directed against Hitler, but it appeared now to be targeted against him. U.S.-British-Soviet relations were off to a bad start. They improved only slightly when Stalin's foreign minister, Vyacheslav Molotov, came to Washington to repeat Stalin's demands and ask, in addition, for an early invasion of western Europe so that pressure could be lifted from the Russian front. FDR and Hull held firm on postwar boundaries. Molotov finally dropped the territorial issue.

He apparently did so because the president did offer a second front "this year." Roosevelt further stroked Molotov by suggesting that after the war, "four policemen" (the Americans, British, Soviets, and Chinese) should walk the beat to keep order in their neighborhoods. This suggestion, however vague, was exactly what the Soviets wanted to hear because it could make them supreme in their neighborhoods of eastern Europe and northern Asia. When FDR asked whether the Soviets liked his idea, a delighted Soviet diplomat responded—apparently with a straight face—"anything for the common cause."[9] The president, however, soon had to break his promise for a second front because Churchill refused to agree and the West's military forces were too weak to mount a successful invasion. By mid-1942, the diplomatic outlook seemed nearly as bleak as the military situation.

Americans were so angry with Churchill's rejection of a second front in France that Marshall threatened to swing U.S. resources to the Pacific theater. In that region, on May 7, 1942, the Allies had stopped a possible Japanese invasion of Australia by destroying 100,000 tons of Tokyo's shipping at the Battle of the Coral Sea—the first naval battle waged largely by U.S. planes as well as ships. The U.S. Navy and Air Force, helped by brilliant intelligence work that intercepted messages and so could predict Japan's military plans, also won the Battle of the Midway Islands in June. Surprising victories stopped Japan's offensive and made possible U.S. landings on Guadalcanal (where seven Japanese troopships were sunk) and Tulagi. Costs were high. Ten thousand U.S. sailors died in the Solomon Islands actions alone. The Japanese lost 30,000 men. A counterattack put the last two U.S. aircraft carriers in the Pacific temporarily out of action, but the Japanese failed to stop the driving U.S. and Australian forces. MacArthur started an "island-hopping" campaign toward Tokyo.

Afraid that FDR might indeed divert resources to the Pacific, Churchill countered with a plan to send U.S. and British troops into action by invading North Africa.[10] Roosevelt finally agreed. Marshall and the U.S. military, however, bitterly protested. The general thought it a waste of resources. But later, he admitted that the military had "failed to see that the leader in a democracy has to keep the people entertained. That may sound like the wrong word, but it conveys the thought."[11] In other words, the president had to show Americans that U.S. soldiers were taking the offensive someplace in the European theater.

But FDR paid a high political price for invading North Africa. Vichy France controlled part of the region, while other points were held by Hitler's leading tank commander, Field Marshal Erwin Rommel, the famous "Desert Fox," who planned to conquer Egypt and the pivotal Suez Canal area. Roosevelt allowed the U.S. military commander, General Eisenhower, to try to save lives by making a secret deal with the Vichy French commander, Admiral Jean Darlan, so that the French would not resist the invaders. This attempt to work with fascist elements (FDR even called Darlan "my dear old friend") drew condemnation then and after the war. The British disliked Darlan for being pro-Nazi. Churchill, instead, wanted to deal with a tall, charismatic French general, Charles de Gaulle. A shrewd political operator who mystically believed that he personally embodied a thousand years of French history, de Gaulle had disavowed Vichy France and established Free French headquarters in London. Roosevelt, however, detested the vain, imperious de Gaulle, who correctly understood that FDR did not believe that the French people should play any major role (during or after the war), given their quick collapse in 1940 and their collaboration with Hitler. (Hull simply dismissed de Gaulle's Free French as "Polecats.")

The Americans again overruled Churchill and de Gaulle. FDR allowed Eisenhower to try to work with Darlan and invade North Africa in November 1942. Darlan then failed to keep up his part of the deal.

Eisenhower's forces met stiff resistance. French sailors blew up their ships rather than allow the Allies (or Germans) to take them. An assassin removed Darlan from the scene in December. The Americans' "Vichy gamble" became known as their "Vichy fumble." Hitler seized the rest of southern (Vichy) France. The only good news occurred in October 1942, when British and Australian forces stopped Rommel at the Battle of El-Alamein.

In January 1943, Roosevelt secretly traveled to Casablanca for summit talks with Churchill. The discussions focused on both military and diplomatic questions. Militarily, the Americans reluctantly agreed with the British that, contrary to their earlier assurances to Stalin, an invasion of France in 1943 would be too costly. They instead planned to invade Sicily and then Italy. On the diplomatic front, FDR again tried to destroy de Gaulle's Free French forces by combining them with the more pliable (and pro-U.S.) forces led by Henri Giraud. When de Gaulle refused to come when the President called, Roosevelt disgustedly wrote Hull: "We delivered our bridegroom, General Giraud, who was most cooperative on the impending marriage. . . . However . . . the temperamental lady DeGaulle . . . has got quite snooty . . . and is showing no intention of getting into bed with Giraud." When de Gaulle finally did appear, he was so mistrusted that Secret Service guards pointed tommyguns at him from hidden curtains when he talked with the president. Historian Frank Costigliola has noted how Americans since 1919 (most notably FDR in 1943–1945) characterized France "in terms that connoted a flighty, not-so-capable female: excessively emotional, hypersensitive, . . . licentious, too concerned with food, drink, fashion, sex, and love." Americans meanwhile saw themselves "in a 'masculine' mode—rational, calm, pragmatic, efficient, and wise." Such irrational biases poisoned U.S.-French relations even before their leaders sat down to talk.[12] De Gaulle emerged from the talks as powerful as ever.

FDR believed he accomplished much more at Casablanca on another diplomatic front. He dramatically announced in a press conference that this time the Allies would settle for nothing less than the "unconditional surrender" of Germany and Japan. Critics quickly cried that such a policy ruled out a negotiated peace and would drive the Axis to fight to the last soldier. But Roosevelt and Churchill were desperately trying to show Stalin that the absence of a second front did not mean that they were going to make a deal with Hitler. They were rightly concerned that the Soviet ruler himself might make another Moscow-Berlin arrangement at the West's expense. They pledged to fight to end the Nazi Empire, and they hoped Stalin would, too.

TEHRAN: THE MOMENTS OF TRUTH (1943)

Stalin's power rose significantly in 1943. During February, his troops began to cut off Hitler's Sixth Army that had already besieged Leningrad for sixteen months. The Soviets captured 300,000 Germans, including 25 generals. Stalin's armies, for the first time, also drove back the Germans without the aid of winter weather. At Kursk, in history's greatest tank battle, the Soviets triumphed during the summer despite Hitler's throwing into the fray 2,000 tanks and planes. Two-thirds of the territory lost to the Nazis soon fell back into the Soviets' hands. The Soviets had taken on 80 percent of the Nazi striking force, had stopped it, and were now turning it back—all without the help of the second front that FDR had promised. The Americans and British, meanwhile, put off their planned invasion of Sicily. "I think it is an awful thing," Churchill wrote FDR's closest adviser, Harry Hopkins, "that in April, May, and June, not a single American or British soldier will be killing a single German or Italian soldier while the Soviets are chasing 185 divisions around."[13] When the Allies finally invaded Sicily in July, their armies survived a German armored attack only through incredible bravery on the part of the U.S. Eighty-second Airborne Division. General George S. Patton's daring offensive finally broke the defenders' back. Eisenhower next led his forces into Italy. The Italians surrendered on September 8, 1943, but 11 German divisions quickly appeared and stopped Eisenhower's 14 divisions south of Rome.

Allied officials were deeply concerned. On August 22, 1943, an intelligence report for the U.S. Joint Chiefs declared that American "fundamental aims" in the war were "(1) to destroy the German domination of Europe, and (2) to prevent the domination of Europe in the future by any single power (such as the Soviet Union), or by any group of powers in which we do not have a strong influence. If we do not achieve *both* these aims," the report warned, "we may consider that we have lost the war." The authors of the report urged a massive landing of Allied troops in western Europe as soon as possible for diplomatic as well as military purposes. The next day, August 23, U.S. and British military chiefs approved a plan, code-named RANKIN, to inject troops into Germany immediately if it appeared that the Germans might collapse before the Soviet blows. As late as November, while traveling to Tehran to meet Stalin for the first time, Roosevelt discussed RANKIN and warned his advisers that there "would definitely be a race" for Berlin. As historian Mark Stoler concludes, U.S. officials had early "realized that the . . . 'second front' across the Channel could be used to aid the Soviets militarily and block their expansion at the same time."[14]

But such action would only solve half the problem. The other half was the organization of Europe *after* the Soviets were blocked and the war ended. Ivan Maisky, the Soviet ambassador to Great Britain, told Foreign Secretary Eden that "there were two possible ways" to handle Europe. Stalin, Churchill, and FDR "could agree each have a sphere of interest," or each could "admit the right of the other to an interest in all parts of Europe."[15] Maisky said he preferred the latter plan, but his boss, Stalin, no doubt wanted the former. On the American side, Secretary of State Hull preferred the second approach, while his boss, like Stalin, seemed to be moving toward the former with his "policemen" idea.

In truth, the president and Prime Minister Churchill had already made their choice. As their armies liberated part of Italy in early autumn 1943, Stalin demanded that he be involved in deciding occupation policy. FDR and Churchill refused. The British, who wanted to reinstall the Italian monarchy, did not want the Soviets stirring up Italy's large number of Communists. Churchill said it directly to Roosevelt: "We cannot be put in a position where our two armies are doing all the fighting but Russians have a veto and must be consulted."[16] The Soviets were effectively kept out of Italy.

Despite the obvious U.S.-British "sphere of influence," Hull—who opposed all spheres—refused to give up his dream. In October 1943, he flew across the Atlantic (for the first time and despite a lifelong problem with claustrophobia that made him terrified of airplanes). At the Moscow Conference, the secretary of state convinced the Soviets, British, and Chinese to agree to a "declaration" pledging them to join in a postwar international organization in which all would work cooperatively. An overjoyed Hull returned to tell Congress that the Four-Nation Declaration meant that "there would no longer be need for spheres of influence, for alliances, for balance of power," or for other bad things from "the unhappy past." Hull was as wrong, however, as he was happy. In Moscow, he had asked Stalin to agree to a plan in which the Allies would only act together in deciding how liberated areas were to be governed. This meant that Americans could have a veto power over Soviet actions in eastern Europe, and the Soviets could have similar power in Italy and western Europe. Doubtless vividly remembering how he had just been shut out of Italy, Stalin refused to agree. Hull accepted the rejection without protest. The other and larger half of the problem was now in full view: Stalin intended to control

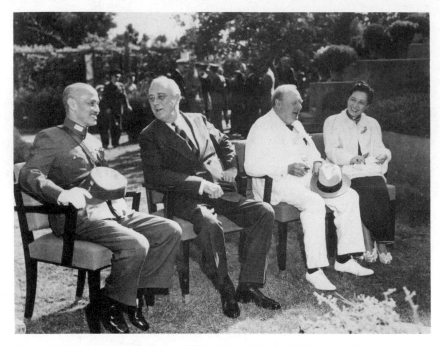

*Generalissimo Chiang Kai-shek, FDR, Churchill, and Madame Chiang at
Cairo in 1943. This meeting marked the high point of U.S.-Chinese relations,
which rolled downhill rapidly in 1944–1945. Given Churchill's mistrust of
Chiang, the prime minister is probably forcing himself to be sociable.*

eastern Europe as his own sphere of influence. FDR and Churchill had
actually set up such a sphere of their own already in Italy. But many
Americans, including Hull and key members of Congress, intended to
keep on pushing for an open, cooperative, democratic world without
spheres—at least in eastern Europe. They knew full well that the bricks
needed to build an open, liberal world order could not be made from
the straw of Communist regimes.

This was the dilemma that Roosevelt faced when he sailed to meet
Stalin and Churchill at Tehran in late 1943. (The president almost
missed the conference. En route, a destroyer in his convoy accidentally
released a torpedo that barely missed blowing up the president's ship.)
FDR first stopped at Cairo, Egypt, to meet Chiang Kai-shek and Churchill. Roosevelt was determined to treat the Chinese as one of the "four
policemen" despite Churchill's protests that the Chinese—especially
Chiang—were corrupt, weak, and attractive to Americans only because
they planned to replace the British as the dominant foreign power in
China after the war. All of those charges were true. But they only

strengthened Roosevelt's belief in his Far East policies. China had to be built up, he believed, so that it could be a worthy junior partner to the United States. To achieve this, the president pledged that he would supply 90 Chinese divisions so that they could launch a major offensive against Japan. Churchill growled that Chiang was no more than a "faggot-vote" that supported whatever Roosevelt wanted. Nevertheless, the president obtained a Cairo declaration that called for Japan's unconditional surrender and promised the return of strategic areas—most notably Formosa (or Taiwan)—from Japan to China. With good reason, Churchill feared that FDR's next step would be to encourage Chiang to push the British out of their imperial holdings at Hong Kong, Singapore, and even India after the war. U.S. military power in the Asian theater now surpassed Great Britain's. Roosevelt intended to use that power as well as America's great economic influence in China to create a postwar Asia that suited American, not British, interests.

Churchill and FDR then flew to Tehran to meet Stalin. For security reasons, Stalin insisted that the president stay in the Soviet Embassy. Roosevelt did so, but the rooms were no doubt bugged with listening devices. FDR had little to hide. He went out of his way to develop a warm relationship with the Soviet dictator and even teased Churchill in order to amuse Stalin. Quick agreement was reached on launching the second front in France during early 1944. The Big Three also concluded that they should dismember a defeated Germany. Roosevelt's one moment of indecision occurred when Stalin proposed that the postwar world be run by regional committees controlled by the "four policemen." The dictator was picking up Roosevelt's earlier idea, an idea that could give the Soviets domination in eastern Europe.

But Roosevelt now backed off. He faced the impossible job of squaring his "four policemen" approach with Hull's determination to have an open, international system. When Roosevelt could not reconcile the two U.S. policies, Stalin and Churchill agreed to put off discussion. The Soviet leader, however, noted Roosevelt's doubt that Congress would allow U.S. troops to be stationed in Europe after the war. The Tehran talks brought into the open the several key contradictions that haunted— even paralyzed—U.S. policy into the postwar years.

The most important decision at Tehran involved Poland. That unfortunate nation had spent most of the earlier three centuries suffering under Russian rule or, as between 1919 and 1939, clutching its independence while trying to fight off pressure from both Germans and Soviets. World War II nearly destroyed Poland. The United States lost 0.3 percent of its population (400,000 dead), the USSR 9 percent

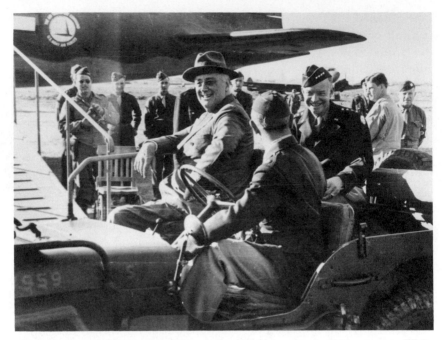

After the Tehran Conference of November 28–December 1, 1943, a jaunty FDR flew to Sicily to inform a smiling Dwight Eisenhower (who had commanded the Allied invasion of Sicily and Italy) that the general would lead the great invasion of France planned for mid-1944.

(15 million to 20 million), but Poland lost at least 14 percent of its population (5 million). Many of these were Jews who disappeared in the Holocaust.

After the Germans and Soviets invaded in 1939, two exile Polish governments formed. The London Poles represented the most pro-Western elements and were determined to regain their 1939 borders. The second group, the Lublin Poles, were pro-Communist, under Stalin's thumb, and, thus, willing to give the dictator those parts of eastern Poland he wanted. Stalin nevertheless kept his ties to the London group until April 1943. Then the Germans discovered in the Katyn Forest the bodies of 4,500 Polish military men who, Hitler claimed, had been massacred by the Soviets when the latter controlled the region in 1939–1940. Stalin naturally blamed the Germans for the slaughter. (But evidence, in 1943, and especially nearly a half-century later when Moscow finally released documents on the event, proved that Stalin had ordered the brutal executions.) When the London Poles demanded an investigation, Stalin seized the chance to break relations with them. Churchill asked the dictator to reconsider. Stalin refused, although he made a friendly gesture in mid-1943 by grandly disbanding the Comintern (the worldwide Soviet-run organization of Communist parties). He was attempting to assure westerners that he had no intention of subverting their governments. In reality, most Communist parties, including the American Communist party, continued to receive guidance from Moscow.

Churchill had little love for the London Poles, whom he found difficult, but he had a lifelong love for the British Empire. At Tehran, he was willing to make deals with Stalin. On the first night of the conference, Roosevelt went to bed after dinner, coffee, and cigars, but Churchill urged Stalin to stay up and discuss postwar affairs. The prime minister got straight to the point: using three matchsticks he showed how the Soviet Union could have part of eastern Poland and, in return, the Poles could move westward and take part of Germany. Stalin, to understate the case, was most pleased. When Roosevelt discovered what had occurred, he did not object. He only remarked that he could not then agree because of the possible political effect back home. Roosevelt was thinking of the large Polish–eastern European vote and his intention to run for a fourth term as president within eleven months.

Warren Kimball has assessed the Tehran talks by noting that they "avoided the hard questions" and performed "a kind of diplomatic papering over cracks in the wall." Nevertheless, they were "the most significant in the war" because the "postwar shape of Europe and East Asia was sketched out," a United Nations organization was agreed upon, and plans for the second front were finally launched.[17]

TO YALTA: BY WAY OF OMAHA BEACH (1944)

The course of the war would largely shape the final diplomatic settlement. Whoever killed the most Germans and Japanese and first reached the heart of Germany and Japan would hold high cards at the peace table. In early 1944, those high cards remained in the deck and were yet to be drawn. The Red Army drove west but encountered stiff resistance, including a fight to the death with Ukrainian nationalists who so hated both Nazi and Soviet leaders that they held out against the Soviets until 1947. In western Europe, massive Allied air raids tried to soften up Germany for the planned invasion. The Italian campaign

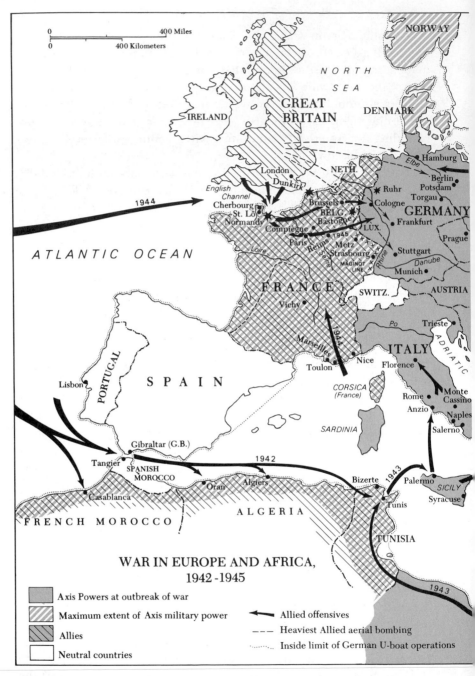

WAR IN EUROPE AND AFRICA, 1942-1945

▨ Axis Powers at outbreak of war	
▨ Maximum extent of Axis military power	◀━ Allied offensives
▨ Allies	‐ ‐ ‐ Heaviest Allied aerial bombing
☐ Neutral countries	⋯⋯ Inside limit of German U-boat operations

By late 1943, the German armies were in retreat from Soviet soil. In June 1944, the United States and British armies led the invasion that finally opened a second front on the shores of France. By early 1945, Hitler's Reich, which was to last a thousand years (so he claimed), was besieged from both east and west.

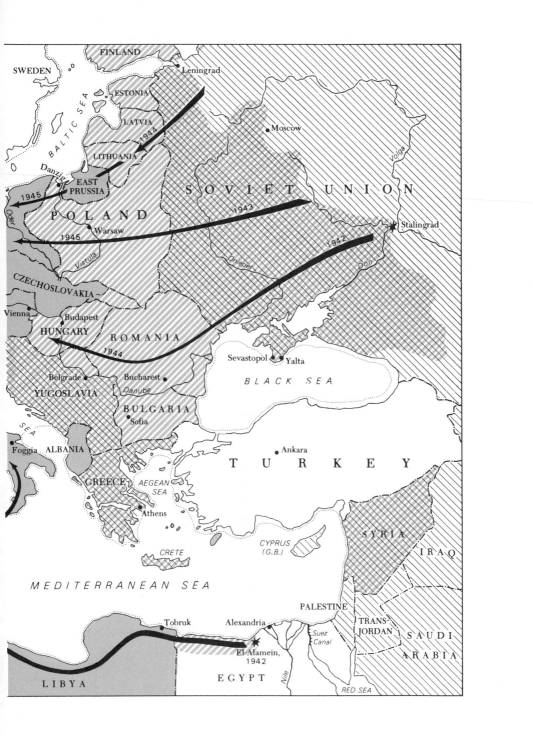

SWEDEN

FINLAND

Leningrad

BALTIC SEA

ESTONIA

LATVIA

Moscow

1944

LITHUANIA

Danzig

EAST
PRUSSIA

1945

Oder

POLAND

Warsaw

1945

Vistula

S O V I E T   U N I O N

1943

Volga

Stalingrad

1942

Don

Dnieper

CZECHOSLOVAKIA

Vienna

Budapest

HUNGARY

R O M A N I A

1944

Sevastopol

Yalta

B L A C K   S E A

Belgrade

Bucharest

Danube

YUGOSLAVIA

BULGARIA

Sofia

SEA

Foggia

ALBANIA

Ankara

T U R K E Y

GREECE

AEGEAN
SEA

Athens

CYPRUS
(G.B.)

S Y R I A

IRAQ

CRETE

M E D I T E R R A N E A N   S E A

PALESTINE

TRANS-
JORDAN

SAUDI
ARABIA

Tobruk

Alexandria

Suez
Canal

El-Alamein,
1942

Nile

LIBYA

E G Y P T

RED SEA

had bogged down, and the bomber pilots of the U.S. Air Force and the (British) Royal Air Force became heroes. Hollywood movies sang their praises. In *Desperate Journey* (1943), Ronald Reagan portrayed a captured U.S. flier who confused the Nazis by making up the names of airplane parts, such as "thermotrockles."[18] (Reagan, who spent the war in California portraying soldiers in films, later, as president of the United States, said that he had been "in uniform" between 1941 and 1945.) But Hollywood and the U.S. government told only part of the story. The U.S. Air Force lost over 40,000 crewmen and nearly 5,000 bombers in near-suicidal attacks against German industries. The Nazis lost only half as many airmen, yet their production continued to rise. Only by mid-1944, when new technology (such as radar-guided bombing) and long-range fighter planes were available, did the Allies gain full command of western Europe's skies.[19]

It occurred just in time. On June 6, 1944, 5,000 ships, 14,000 aircraft, and 100,000 troops launched the D-day invasion that centered on France's Normandy region. But the greatest amphibious invasion in history nearly failed. Dug-in German units, commanded by Field Marshal Rommel, inflicted 100,000 American casualties in the first month of fighting. The Allies were nearly driven back into the sea. Churchill's long-held fear that the English Channel would be "awash with corpses" came close to being realized. U.S. divisions, again with General Patton's Third Army tanks in the fore, worked with British troops to make a breakthrough. Paris was liberated on August 25, 1944. But then the Allies again bogged down as they overextended their supply lines and the Nazis fought ferociously. To add to the bad news, in mid-June 1944, Hitler's scientists began launching the V-1 and then the V-2 rockets on Great Britain. These pilotless missiles, which gave little warning before they exploded, struck fear into a British people already suffering from five years of war.

As he closely watched the invasion of Europe, Roosevelt also had to deal politically with the Allies. Free French leader Charles de Gaulle had destroyed all the rivals the president had sent to oppose him. Roosevelt wanted de Gaulle excluded from the invasion until Churchill noted that "it is very difficult to cut the French out of the invasion of France." The two leaders then instructed de Gaulle to broadcast their messages to the French people. The Frenchman refused to take orders. "He's a nut," FDR concluded. But de Gaulle got his way. He made the broadcast and told the French to follow his own orders. The tall general was beating Roosevelt in the high-stakes game of who was to control postwar France.[20]

To Yalta: By Way of Bretton Woods
and Quebec (1944)

Nor was the president able to control Churchill, despite the awesome economic and military power of the Americans. Between 1940 and 1944, U.S. industrial production shot up 90 percent, agricultural output 20 percent, and the total gross national production of all goods and services 60 percent. Most other economies, including the British, were devastated by war. U.S. leaders agreed with Will Clayton, former corporate executive and now State Department official, who warned in late 1943 that isolationism was dead. The nation's growing production and political interests demanded an open, orderly world, Clayton declared, or Americans would have to become an "armed camp, police the seven seas, tighten our belts, and live by ration books for the next century or so." Another of FDR's economic experts, Henry Grady, put the problem bluntly: "The capitalistic system is essentially an international system. If it cannot function internationally, it will break down completely."[21]

Roosevelt joined in by announcing that "Dr. New Deal" (which had emphasized domestic solutions) had been replaced by "Dr. Win-the-War." *Time* magazine, edited by Henry Luce, who had long argued that the New Deal failed to fix the U.S. economy, ran a sarcastic note in its "Milestones" section on January 3, 1944:

> Death Revealed. The New Deal, 10, after long illness; of malnutrition and desuetude. Child of the 1932 election campaign, the New Deal had four healthy years, began to suffer from spots before the eyes in 1937, and never recovered from the shock of war. Last week its father, Franklin Roosevelt, pronounced it dead.

As Clayton observed, U.S. officials now had to come up with an international plan to replace the New Deal, a plan that could keep the nation's economy pumping away so that the war-shocked world could be rebuilt and the U.S. system saved from a possibly fatal shock of another 1930s-like depression.

To solve these problems, U.S. leaders called a conference of the world's non-Axis nations at Bretton Woods, New Hampshire, in mid-1944. The meeting established two new organizations to ensure an open, capitalist postwar world. The first was the International Bank for

Reconstruction and Development (or the World Bank) that had a $7.6 billion treasury—nearly all from the United States—to help rebuild war-torn Europe and develop the newly emerging countries in Africa, Asia, and Latin America. By promoting growth and providing capital, the World Bank was to make less necessary state-controlled, perhaps socialistic, measures for development.

The second organization was the International Monetary Fund (IMF). Its $7.3 billion aimed to help nations suffering from high trade deficits. The IMF funds were to be used to stabilize those nations' currencies that were under pressure because of internal economic problems. The IMF hoped to prevent the highly destructive trade and currency wars of the 1930s (see p. 371). Moreover, Americans insisted at Betton Woods that the postwar economic system rest on gold and the U.S. dollar. Such insistence was not surprising. The United States controlled two-thirds of the world's gold. Washington officials dominated both the World Bank and IMF. They planned to use that power to create an open, international marketplace that did not need excessive state interference or high tariffs.[22]

Just as this economic structure was erected at Bretton Woods, the Allies also met at the Dumbarton Oaks estate in Washington, D.C., to build the political structure: the United Nations. The UN was to have a general assembly in which all the world's nations were represented. But the real power was to be in a twelve-member security council, with each of the five permanent members (the United States, the Soviet Union, Great Britain, France, and China) having a veto. The other seven seats on the council would rotate among all other members. Stalin agreed to join the UN but notably refused to join the World Bank and IMF.

Churchill and other British leaders had fought to redraw the U.S. plans at Bretton Woods. They knew that Roosevelt intended to use the new World Bank and IMF—as well as the all-powerful dollar—to force the British Empire to open up to American goods and investment. U.S. officials, however, simply steamrolled over London's objections. But an even worse clash occurred between Churchill and Roosevelt at a meeting in Quebec, Canada, in September 1944. The two bitterly argued over what to do with postwar Germany. At the Tehran Conference in late 1943, FDR had gone along with the idea of dividing Germany. At Quebec, however, Roosevelt was convinced by his secretary of the Treasury, Henry Morgenthau, not only to divide Germany, but rip all industry out of it (make it "pastoral") and heavily police it. The Morgenthau Plan aimed at creating an economic wasteland where the industrial hub of Europe once existed. Churchill hated the idea; he did not believe that the British economy could survive without a healthy Europe. He reluctantly went along after Morgenthau offered the British a $6.5 billion postwar credit. Roosevelt and Morgenthau were ready to pay a high price to make sure Germany would never rise again.

But back in Washington, Secretary of State Hull and Secretary of War Stimson were shocked. Hull later declared that nothing "angered me as much" as the Morgenthau Plan. Stimson and Hull told Roosevelt that an open, economically workable world could not exist without a healthy Europe. And a healthy Europe required a functioning Germany.[23] Roosevelt thought it over, then admitted that he had "pulled a boner" at Quebec. The president disavowed the Morgenthau Plan. Churchill wondered if the Americans knew what they were doing.

He had good reason to wonder—and fear. As historian Fraser Harbutt observes, after the Tehran Conference, FDR and his advisers "began to think of the Soviet Union" (not the weakening British Empire) "as their main postwar partner."[24] At Quebec, Roosevelt had so rudely brushed aside British concerns that Churchill finally blurted out, "Do you want me to beg, like Fala [FDR's dog]?" Moreover, how could Churchill (or Stalin) be certain that FDR could cooperate with them after the war even if the president wanted to do so? In 1943–1944, powerful figures in the United States, led by Senator Robert Taft, journalist Walter Lippmann, and historians Charles and Mary Beard, all issued warnings against the United States undertaking to police the world after the war. The Beards even went further. In books that sold millions of copies and reached 40 million Americans when Henry Luce published parts of them in his *Life* magazine, they argued that FDR had violated the Constitution in conducting foreign policy and that Congress had to regain its power.[25] In European eyes, such a change would make U.S. policy even more unpredictable. FDR won a fourth term as president in 1944 with a relatively unknown running mate, Senator Harry Truman of Missouri. But many wondered whether, with his sinking health, the president could live another term.

To Yalta, with a Detour at Moscow

Thus, Churchill had good reasons to worry about U.S. postwar policy. He determined to protect vital British interests in Greece by making a private deal with Stalin. As German troops were pushed out of that nation, civil war erupted between monarchical groups, whom Churchill supported, and Greek leftists. In May 1944, the British prime minister made an arrangement with Stalin: the British would control Greece, and the Soviets would control Romania. Hull quickly objected, pointing out that the deal created unacceptable "spheres of interest." The British were bitter. "As if there was ever such a sphere of influence agreement as the Monroe Doctrine!" complained one London official. Churchill privately groused that U.S. complaints about the evils of "power politics" were pure hypocrisy: "Is having a Navy twice as strong as any other power 'power politics'? . . . Is having all the gold in the world buried in a cavern 'power politics'? If not, what is 'power politics'?"[26] The prime minister cared little about labels but much about getting things worked out with Stalin.

His concern increased in August–September 1944, when the Red Army drove to the gates of Warsaw. The city's underground resistance rose up to destroy the Nazis and take the city before the Soviets entered. But the Red Army stopped, then sat outside the Polish capital for nearly two months as German troops turned and smashed the resistance. Stalin pleaded that his army was unable to advance because of supply and other military reasons, but he also damned the resistance as "a handful of power-seeking criminals" and refused to help U.S. and British attempts to drop supplies to the anti-Nazi forces. It seemed that Stalin would not tolerate any rival for power in Poland.

Churchill observed the Warsaw uprising's fate and the confusion in U.S. policy, then flew to Moscow in October 1944 to talk—as Stalin liked to call it—"practical arithmetic." FDR was told of the meeting and sent the U.S. ambassador, W. Averell Harriman, to the Soviet Union as an observer. But Churchill and Stalin also met privately without Harriman and worked out a trade: the Soviets would have 90 percent influence in Romania and 75 percent influence in Bulgaria and Hungary; in return, the British would have 90 percent influence in Greece; Yugoslavia was to be split 50–50. The prime minister added that all this must be explained diplomatically and that "the phrase 'dividing into spheres' [must not be used], because the Americans might be shocked." Churchill later wrote that Stalin never uttered "one word of reproach" when the British moved to smash the Greek leftists.[27]

The two men also agreed that Germany had to be dismembered and its heavy industry destroyed. Otherwise, Stalin noted, "every 25 or 30 years there would be a new world war which would exterminate the young generation. . . . [Thus,] the harshest measures would prove to be the most humane." The two leaders then quickly agreed on moving the Polish-Soviet and Polish-German boundaries westward, as the Tehran talks provided. Churchill pleaded with Stalin to bring the London Poles into agreement with the pro-Communist Lublin group. The Soviet dictator said that he would try. Both men agreed that the Polish leaders were difficult. Churchill: "Where there were two Poles there was one quarrel." Stalin: "Where there was one Pole he would begin to quarrel with himself through sheer boredom."[28]

Roosevelt raised no objection to the Polish arrangement, but he was not fully told by Churchill about the percentages deal. Earlier in the war, went one story, FDR was moving through the White House hallway when Churchill, who was on a brief visit, suddenly stepped, stark naked, out of a door. Roosevelt was visibly embarrassed, but Churchill quickly declared: "The Prime Minister of Great Britain has nothing to conceal from the President of the United States." This was not, however, quite true.

To Yalta: FDR's Rocky Road

Despite his smashing re-election victory over Governor Thomas E. Dewey of New York, October 1944 through February 1945 was FDR's

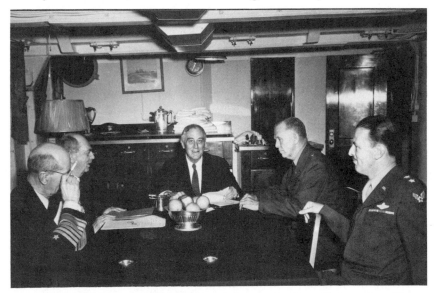

Franklin D. Roosevelt (1882–1945) loved ships and sailing. He vacationed by boating at Campobello Island on the U.S.-Canadian border, and he frequently sailed on the presidential yacht. Here he is aboard the USS Quincy, *off Malta, just before the February 1945 summit conference at Yalta. He is joined by his top military advisers (clockwise from lower left): Admiral Ernest J. King, Admiral William D. Leahy, General George C. Marshall, and General L. S. Kuter (representative for Air Force Chief of Staff General Henry "Hap" Arnold).*

winter of discontent. No doubt thinking of Churchill's and Stalin's plans, the president told a press conference in December that the Atlantic Charter's grand principles were "slipping away from us."[29]

Nor did the military campaigns in western Europe give him an advantage. Hitler suddenly counterattacked with 250,000 troops during mid-December. In the ensuing Battle of the Bulge, only courageous, last-ditch Allied resistance and a dry German supply line prevented a massive defeat. The Americans lost 100,000 men (the Germans 120,000) and were driven back from the German border. Meanwhile, a Soviet force of 7 million resumed its drive and in February, on the eve of the Yalta Conference, was only 50 miles from Berlin. At Churchill's prodding, bombing attacks were increased—partly to break German morale, partly to impress the Red Army with Western air power. The most infamous bomber attack occurred on February 13, 1945, when the magnificent—and militarily unimportant—city of Dresden was destroyed and 35,000 German lives lost. The next day, U.S. Mustang fighters machine-gunned refugees trying to flee the still-burning city. "There was a sea of fire covering in my estimation some 40 square miles," a British pilot recalled.[30] The systematic bombing of civilians, which had sickened and angered the West when it had occurred in China or Spain during 1937, now, just eight years later, had become an accepted act of war.

Allied forces in the Pacific also faced a difficult time. Proclaiming "I have returned," General MacArthur was recorded by movie cameras wading through knee-deep water as 200,000 U.S. troops invaded the Philippines in October 1944. But bad weather and suicidal Japanese resistance bogged down the invasion and finally forced MacArthur to fight a battle for the capital of Manila that cost 100,000 Filipino civilian lives in a single month. It was, historian Carol Morris Petillo writes, "one of the most destructive, albeit well-intentioned, armies of 'liberation' the world had ever seen."[31] The Japanese left little alternative. At Iwo Jima in February through March 1945, and at Okinawa during April through June, the struggle to control the small islands proved to be among the war's most costly. On Okinawa, the Americans lost 12,000 men in order to kill 80,000 Japanese entrenched in caves and bunkers. Such numbers doubtless haunted Roosevelt when he pressed Stalin to enter the war against Japan as quickly as possible. (See map, p. 416.)

The Allied position in China was also endangered. During mid-1944, the Japanese attacked General Stilwell's forces and threatened the entire south China theater, including bomber bases that FDR had hoped to use against Japan. The president begged Chiang Kai-shek to throw his

U.S.-supplied troops into the battle. Fearful of the Chinese Communists to the north, Chiang refused. A furious Stilwell marched into Chiang's office and, in the general's words, "hit the little bugger right in the solar plexus" with the demand that Chiang move immediately. The Chinese leader instead demanded Stilwell's recall. A discouraged Roosevelt ordered Stilwell home. The president realized that Chiang would neither protect U.S. interests in Asia nor responsibly help Americans dismantle the discredited European colonies in Asia.[32]

FDR most notably found himself in a fix over the French colonies in Indochina (especially Vietnam). He might consider the Free French leader, Charles de Gaulle, a "nut" and despise him for being so "snooty," but the arrogant French general had become FDR's best hope for maintaining order in both France and Vietnam against the Communist-led opposition. At stake, after all, were French cooperation in Europe and an overseas empire twenty-two times larger than France itself. Moreover, as Ambassador Harriman warned Roosevelt from Moscow, the Soviets were threatening to "become a world bully wherever their interests are involved. This policy will reach into China and the Pacific as well." By March 1945, FDR agreed to look the other way while de Gaulle moved to re-establish French colonial control over Indochina.[33]

But Roosevelt would not challenge Stalin directly. The president believed that he needed Soviet help against Japan and knew that he needed it to build a peaceful postwar world. Nor could the Red Army be overlooked. Of Germany's 13.6 million casualties in the war, the Russian front claimed 10 million, often in unimaginably brutal fighting. Henry Luce's *Life* magazine called Lenin "perhaps the greatest man of modern times" and the Soviets "one hell of a people" who, "to a remarkable degree . . . look like Americans, dress like Americans, and think like Americans." Such movies as *Mission to Moscow* and *North Star* led one critic to observe that "war has put Hollywood's traditional conception of the Muscovites through the wringer and they have come out shaved, washed, sober . . . Rotarians, brother Elks."[34] Roosevelt did hear, however, from some dissenters, including Secretary of the Navy James Forrestal, who complained to a friend in autumn 1944 that whenever an American tries to protect U.S. security, "he is apt to be called a god-damned fascist or imperialist." But

if Uncle Joe [Stalin] suggests he needs the Baltic Provinces, half of Poland, all of Bessarabia and access to the Mediterranean [through Turkey], all hands agree that he is a fine, frank, candid, and generally delightful fellow who is very easy to deal with because he is so explicit in what he wants.[35]

YALTA . . .

As Roosevelt sailed for the Soviet Black Sea resort city of Yalta and his final summit conference, he perhaps sympathized with Forrestal's frustration. But the president knew he could do little more. The reality was that Stalin and Churchill had already made their own deal to create spheres of influence in eastern Europe and the Mediterranean. FDR realized that he was not dealing with an irrational or a paranoid Soviet leader, but rather with Soviet leadership that, as Harriman explained, was totally preoccupied "with 'security' as Moscow sees it." Having been invaded at least four times since 1914 and having suffered the destruction of much of the western Soviet Union, he added, the Soviets wanted "puppet regimes in all contiguous countries" and a guaranteed "period of freedom from danger" to recover and industrialize.[36]

However, FDR also knew that Americans believed that they were fighting for self-determination and the Atlantic Charter principles. The State Department warned Roosevelt, moreover, that the Balkans and Poland had to have self-government, freedom for journalists, and "furtherance of legitimate economic rights, existing or potential." The Soviets would probably "exert predominant political influence" over eastern Europe, the State Department concluded, but the United States—for its own vital interests—had to have "trade . . . under the freest possible conditions." A conflict was brewing because "the United States is no longer so much a land of opportunity as a land looking for opportunity; and to an increasing extent Americans will seek it outside their own borders."[37]

How Roosevelt could ever maintain equal U.S. access to (for example) Romania while not undercutting Churchill's and Stalin's agreement of 90-percent Soviet control over that country, no one could say. Certainly, FDR's new secretary of state was of little help. Edward R. Stettinius had been a young corporation executive with slight experience in, and less talent for, international diplomacy. "A Secretary of State should be able to read and write and talk," a friend complained to Roosevelt. "He may not be able to do all of these, but Stettinius can't do any of them."[38] FDR, nevertheless, appointed him because Stettinius (unlike Hull) could be trusted to carry out orders without asking questions.

The Big Three efficiently settled certain problems at Yalta. With regard to the United Nations, Stalin dropped his demand for a veto over procedural questions in the Security Council and, in return, asked for two

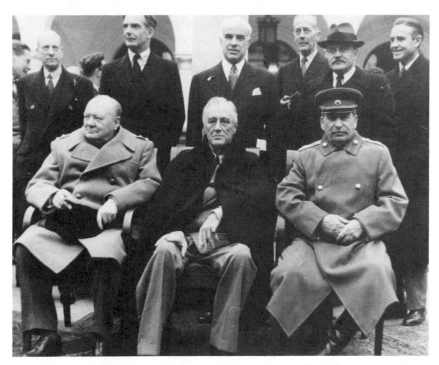

The conference at the Russian resort of Yalta, February 1945. Stalin is seated at the right, Roosevelt is in the center, and, on the left, with the ever-present cigar, is Churchill. Eden, Stettinius, and Molotov stand behind the chairs.

or three Soviet republics to have votes in the General Assembly, where all the world's nations were to be represented. FDR accepted this on the condition that, if he thought it necessary to get the UN Charter through the Senate, the same number of U.S. states could have similar voting rights. (Roosevelt never had to invoke this agreement.) Other questions, however, raised tempers and fears on both sides.

Most telling was the discussion about Poland. Stalin again asked that eastern Poland be "returned" to the Soviets. He had made the point clear in late 1944 by recognizing his Lublin Poles as the country's legitimate regime. FDR and Churchill had earlier granted Stalin's boundary demands, but now they asked that the boundary be modified and the new government be "more broadly based" by including Poles from London. They also asked for "free and unfettered elections as soon as possible." Churchill said that British "honor" was involved. FDR, for his part, did not refer to the State Department's argument for the need of an open eastern Europe. Instead, he insisted that the concessions were needed to please the 6 million to 7 million

Polish voters at home. Stalin blew up. Reminding them that the Soviet Union had been attacked through Poland, he declared that "it was a question both of honor and security." The dictator finally agreed to the loose phrases ("broadly based" governments and "free . . . elections"), but it was understood that Stalin interpreted such words differently than the two Western leaders.[39]

Stalin had once said that communism fit Germany like a saddle fit a cow. He now moved to dismember the cow. In discussing Germany, Churchill and FDR had (again) agreed to certain principles at Tehran fourteen months earlier. They had agreed, for example, on dismemberment. But two other questions about Germany caused problems. The three men had earlier given German land to Poland, but Churchill now questioned whether the Poles could handle such an area. The prime minister was probably beginning to see that such a transfer of land could anger many Germans and make Poland dependent upon the Soviets for protection against an angry Germany. (This boundary problem was only settled in 1970, when the West German government recognized the Polish borders that included a slice of pre-1939 Germany.) The second question involved Stalin's demands for $20 billion in reparations from Germany, with half going to the Soviets. Such reparations were to make Germans help pay for the 70,000 destroyed Soviet villages and the nearly 25 million homeless that the war produced. It would, of course, also make Germany weak for a long time. But the British opposed the $20 billion sum. Stalin again became angry. Roosevelt restored some calm by merely agreeing "in principle" to figures. Details were to be worked out later. Finally, to Stalin and FDR's disgust, Churchill succeeded in making France one of the occupying powers in Germany.

Stalin doubtless intended from now on to take whatever reparations he wanted from the German areas controlled by his Red Army. The only possible alternative might have been a $6 billion credit that his foreign minister, Molotov, asked from the United States in January 1945. The Soviets made other requests for varying amounts of money over the coming months, but nothing could ever be worked out. The Americans demanded in return, to use Ambassador Harriman's words, proper Soviet "behavior in international matters."[40] This meant that the Soviets were to allow an open eastern Europe and join the World Bank and International Monetary Fund. Stalin, however, was unwilling to sell out Soviet security, as he defined it, for any amount of money, no matter how large. FDR, for reasons best known to himself, never raised the issue of a loan to the Soviets at Yalta.

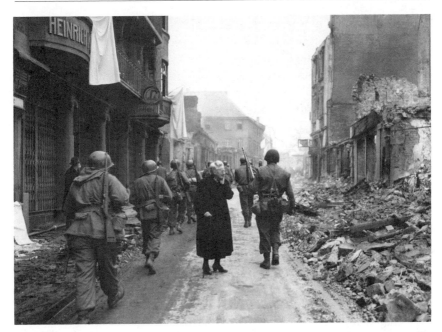

A German woman shows shock at the ruins of Bensheim as U.S. troops move by her. Taken in March 1945, the photo shows what had happened to Hitler's Reich just twelve years after he had assumed power. It also indicates the rebuilding job that faced the United States when it moved to restore West Germany's economy.

But Roosevelt did push a pet State Department project by asking that all agree on the Declaration of Liberated Europe. This declaration repeated the Atlantic Charter's principles; it also pledged the signers "to act in concert" in governing newly liberated countries. Taken literally, this could mean a U.S. veto over Soviet actions in, say, Poland. It was an attempt to take back much of what had been lost to the Soviets at Tehran, Moscow, and Yalta. But Molotov quickly insisted that a line be added stating that only *mutual consultations* were needed before an occupying power governed liberated countries. Thus watered down, the declaration lost its force, and the Soviets signed it.[41]

Finally, FDR (with little concern for Churchill's views) worked out a deal on the Far East. Stalin promised to fight Japan within three months after the German surrender. In return, Roosevelt agreed that the Soviets could (1) regain the Kuril Islands and the southern part of Sakhalin from Japan, (2) formally obtain a sphere of influence in Outer Mongolia, (3) work with China in running the valuable South Manchurian Railroad, and (4) have special rights in the Chinese ports of

Port Arthur and Dairen. By the early 1950s, Yalta had become a dirty word in American politics because many (especially Republicans) believed that FDR had sold out China at Yalta. But the reality was more complex and interesting. Roosevelt insisted on Stalin's making a formal deal with Chiang Kai-shek about the agreements reached at Yalta. The president thus maneuvered Stalin into working directly with Chiang instead of possibly recognizing the Chinese Communists. Moreover, the Soviet Union had long-standing claims to some of the concessions, such as the Kurils and Sakhalin, and would probably have the Red Army in position to seize rights in the other areas at the end of the war.

The American humorist Josh Billings (i.e., Henry Wheeler Shaw) once observed that "the glory is not whether you won or lost, but how you played a bad hand." Given the military problems in western Europe and Chiang's weakness in Asia—not to mention the earlier Stalin-Churchill percentage deal—FDR had won some glory. As historian Diane Clemens writes in her study of the conference, "The decisions at Yalta involved compromise by each nation, probably more by the Soviets than by the Western nations."[42] Roosevelt lost little at Yalta that had not already been agreed on earlier or had been taken by the Red Army. He worked to create ties between Stalin and Chiang. Roosevelt returned home knowing that the Atlantic Charter principles had been violated. But he believed that a basis had been laid for a victorious war effort and postwar cooperation by the Big Three. As journalist Walter Lippmann later observed, FDR never thought that he could simply "charm Stalin into agreeing with him. Roosevelt was a cynical man. . . . What he thought he could do was outwit Stalin, which is quite a different thing."[43]

. . . AND AFTER

Stalin clearly felt that the Yalta talks had confirmed the deal with Churchill at Moscow in 1944. The dictator set about reconstructing eastern Europe. Romania had been recognized by Churchill as part of the Soviet sphere. Stalin's agent told the Romanian king that a pro-Soviet government must assume power, then underlined the point by slamming the door so hard as he left the room that the plaster cracked. The State Department tried to help the king by insisting that Romanians should be governed by the Declaration of Liberated Europe. The Soviets replied that FDR and Churchill had done as they pleased in Italy, so now Stalin would do as he pleased in Romania.[44]

In Moscow, no agreement could be reached over how the Polish government was to be reorganized. The arguments grew bitter. "The map shows Mexico is nearer to America while Poland is nearer to us," Soviet Foreign Minister Molotov lectured the Americans, "and what happens in Poland is more important to Russia than to you."[45]

Danger also flared in Switzerland. U.S. secret agents led by Allen Dulles opened surrender talks with Nazi generals. Stalin learned about the meetings and strongly complained to FDR and Churchill. He implied that Dulles was attempting to arrange a secret Munich-type surrender so that Nazi armies would be free to turn against the Soviet Union. FDR had to send several messages to reassure the dictator. Meanwhile, Red Army troops drove on Berlin. General Eisenhower's Western forces were pushing toward the capital as well, but he ordered them to swing south. It was one of the most controversial decisions in the war. Eisenhower justified allowing the Soviets to take Berlin because, first, the Big Three had already agreed to put Berlin in the Soviet occupation zone and, second, he feared that fighting the 200 miles to the capital would kill far too many of his troops to capture a city that he would have to leave anyway.

Churchill, dismayed by Stalin's actions and facing a difficult election campaign at home, began prodding FDR to get tough with the Soviets. The prime minister was trying to eat his cake and have it, too—that is, maintain his Moscow deal of 1944 that gave him a free hand in Greece, while pushing Roosevelt to demand that Stalin allow Romania and Poland to be more open. FDR responded slowly—in part because he was ill at his vacation retreat in Warm Springs, Georgia, and in part because he apparently doubted that Stalin was breaking the rubber-band-like Yalta agreements. The president, moreover, wanted the reluctant Soviets to attend a conference in San Francisco to establish the new United Nations. He had to move carefully. On April 6, he told Churchill that no one must think that "we are afraid. Our armies will in a very few days be in a position that will permit us to be 'tougher.' "[46] Exactly what these words meant will never be known. Six days later the president died from a massive stroke.

HARRY TRUMAN AT POTSDAM

The new president, Harry Truman, had been a senator from Missouri and a compromise nominee for the vice-presidency at the 1944 Democratic party convention. He knew little about foreign policy, and FDR

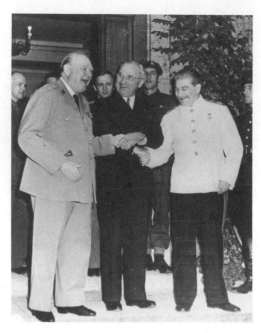

*Churchill, Truman, and Stalin during one of the few light moments at the con-
ference at Potsdam (just outside Berlin, Germany), July 17–August 2, 1945.
Churchill was soon voted out of office. U.S. and Soviet leaders would not hold
hands again for ten years.*

did absolutely nothing to educate him. The British ambassador to
Washington called the new president "an honest and diligent medio-
crity" and noted the "Missouri County court-house calibre" of his personal friends.[47] Truman, however, did not listen to those Missourians,
but to Ambassador Harriman and such poker-playing friends as Secretary of the Navy Forrestal, who believed that the time had arrived for
a showdown with Stalin.

A cabinet meeting on April 23 was crucial. Truman listened to sev-
enty-eight-year-old Secretary of War Henry Stimson, who warned that
the Soviets had rights in Poland and were needed to defeat Japan.
General George Marshall supported Stimson. But the president then
followed Harriman's and Forrestal's tough advice. Clearly, the inexperienced leader did not want to be thought of as insecure. Moreover,
Truman knew little as yet about the 1943–1945 deals that had been
reached on eastern Europe. He summoned Foreign Minister Molotov
to the White House and "in words of one syllable," as Truman later

reported, told the Russian that unless Stalin began behaving better, Americans would turn anti-Soviet. Molotov supposedly protested that he had never been talked to like that in his life. Truman shot back that if Molotov carried out his agreements, he would not be talked to like that. The president later bragged to a friend that he had given Molotov "the straight one-two to the jaw." But the insecure Truman then asked his friend, "Did I do right?"[48]

Perhaps Truman had doubts because Stalin had refused to budge. The dictator responded with a "one-two" of his own. He reminded Truman that "Poland has the same meaning for the security of the Soviet Union as . . . Belgium and Greece [has]" for British security. Privately, the dictator prophesied that the Germans would be "on their feet" in fifteen years, "and then we'll have another go at it." Next time, he would not be caught unprepared: "Everyone imposes his own system as far as his army can reach. It cannot be otherwise."[49]

Truman backed off to reassess the situation. Germany surrendered on May 7, 1945. Hitler and his mistress, Eva Braun, committed suicide several days earlier as Soviet troops swept over Berlin. But Truman still needed Stalin's help against Japan. The president agreed to meet in a summit conference at Potsdam (Germany) in July 1945. Churchill looked forward to the talks, only to have Clement Attlee's Labour party stun the British leader in a national election. Attlee replaced Churchill as prime minister midway through the Potsdam Conference.

In preparing for the conference, Truman did not give up hope of blocking the Soviets in eastern Europe. Indeed, he believed it to be essential. As he told advisers, all of Europe must be united because the eastern sections grew cattle and wheat while the west's "big industries" produced iron and steel. Each had to have the other for an orderly, prosperous Europe. Truman believed as well that Germany had to be unified and Poland at least open to U.S. "trade, investments and access to sources of information," as the State Department put it.[50]

The Big Three talks at Potsdam revolved around the endless problem of Germany. Truman and the State Department now concluded that the dismemberment plan accepted at Tehran and Yalta was wrong. Germans would never accept it, except through force, and Germany could, thus, "keep the world in lasting perturbation."[51] Moreover, a prosperous, orderly Europe required a prosperous, orderly Germany at its center, much as an apple could not be good if its core were rotten. Truman now even flatly opposed giving German territory as compensation to Poland. Stalin bitterly complained, but his policy actually put Truman in a corner. The president could either have a united Germany under the control of occupying powers or a divided Germany with Soviet influence limited to just one zone. Because the first alternative threatened to spread Stalin's power throughout much of central Europe, Truman finally chose the second alternative. He signaled this choice by changing the U.S. position on reparations. The president backed away from the $20 billion figure that had been discussed at Yalta. He instead insisted on a percentage arrangement that mentioned no specific figures. In reality, Truman's new policy prevented the Soviets from taking reparations out of the U.S., British, and French occupation zones. After all, a percentage of nothing was nothing. Potsdam, in truth (but not through mutual agreement), settled three key German problems: dismemberment went forward; reparations from the western zones to the Soviet Union were soon stopped; and, over Truman's and Attlee's objections, Stalin insisted that the new Poland have German territory.

A DIFFERENT WORLD:
THE ATOMIC BOMB AND JAPAN'S SURRENDER

On July 18 at Potsdam, Truman casually told Stalin that a new weapon had been exploded at a test site in New Mexico two days before. The program that climaxed with the explosion of an atomic bomb had begun in 1939, when two scientists, Albert Einstein and Leo Szilard—both refugees in America from Hitler's genocidal campaign against Jews— told Roosevelt that it was "conceivable" that a "new type" of an "extremely powerful" bomb could be released from the atom of uranium ore.[52] By the time of the Pearl Harbor incident, Americans worked with British and Canadian scientists to develop the weapon. In early 1942, FDR tried to cut the other two nations from the project. Churchill fought back and regained British access to the work, but the British rightly suspected the Americans of wanting to keep the secret to themselves. "The salad is heaped in a bowl permanently smeared with the garlic of suspicion," one London official observed in early 1945.[53] Roosevelt never seriously considered bringing Stalin into the project. As historian Barton Bernstein concludes, FDR followed "the strategy of excluding the Soviets from knowledge of the bomb and of reserving the options of using it in the future as a bargaining lever, threat, military counterweight, or even a weapon against the Soviets."[54]

Truman continued this policy. His secret "Interim Committee" of scientists and government officials, chaired by Secretary of War Stimson, discussed how to use the new bomb to make "Russia more manageable in Europe." Throughout the Manhattan Project at Los Alamos, New Mexico, where the bomb was made, top officials assumed that the bomb had to be built (especially because they knew that Hitler's scientists were working on one, too). They also assumed that it was being built at a cost of $2 billion to be used. Truman wondered aloud to Stimson how the weapon might help settle the Polish, Romanian, Yugoslav, and Manchurian problems on his terms. There is evidence that the president scheduled the Potsdam Conference on dates he believed the bomb was to be tested so that he would be able to use it as a diplomatic lever against Stalin. When the president learned at Potsdam that the weapon indeed worked, he "was tremendously pepped up," Stimson recorded. Churchill noted that Truman was "a changed man" as he suddenly got tougher with Stalin.

The president had set his sights high. He had earlier declared that he might not get "100 percent" of what he wanted from Stalin, but he would get "85 percent." He could never figure out, however, how to use the new bomb to obtain even that figure. This first attempt at "atomic diplomacy"—that is, waving the bomb without making overt threats and hoping that the Soviets would give in—never worked. Even when Truman mentioned the new bomb to Stalin at Potsdam, the Soviet dictator was, to the president's surprise, unmoved. And with good reason. Documents found in Moscow after the Soviet Union's collapse in 1991 revealed that Stalin's spies had penetrated the Manhattan Project, which was developing the U.S. bomb, and had been feeding information back to the Kremlin since late 1941. One analysis even suggests that "Stalin could well have been better informed about the making of the U.S. atom bomb than Truman himself." In any case, the dictator only reacted by secretly instructing Soviet scientists to speed up their own work.[55]

The director of the scientists at Los Alamos, J. Robert Oppenheimer, watched the giant mushroomlike cloud rise over the New Mexico desert and remembered a Hindu text: "Now I am become death, destroyer of worlds." Another scientist declared, "I am sure at the end of the world—in the last millisecond of the earth's existence—the last man will see what we saw."[56] Several scientists pushed U.S. officials to warn Japan with a demonstration of the weapon on a deserted Pacific island, not on a Japanese city. The suggestion was rejected—the weapon might not work properly, U.S. officials feared, and only two bombs were available to help end the war.

Truman later declared that he dropped the bombs on Japan to avoid "a half million" Americans dying in an invasion of the home islands. Others used the figure of 1 million possible casualties. In reality, at the time, Truman had reports that the U.S. losses would probably be 40,000 to 50,000.[57] U.S. planes using incendiary bombs were already burning entire cities. On March 9–10, a single such attack on Tokyo "scorched and boiled and baked to death" 84,000 people, as a U.S. Air Force officer described the results.[58] Japanese officials approached the Allies for surrender terms that would preserve the religious figure of the emperor. Truman rejected this offer because he wanted unconditional surrender. Stalin rejected it because he wanted to declare war and to claim Japanese territory.

Few had moral qualms about dropping atomic bombs on Japan's cities. World opinion had been horrified by Fascist and Japanese bombing of civilians in 1937–1938 but, by 1945, accepted the slaughter of 80,000 or more civilians on a single night without a murmur. The Japanese especially seemed fair game. As Truman liked to note, their attack on Pearl Harbor earned them any penalty that Americans could inflict. In a key work on the racial hatred between Americans and Japanese, historian John Dower quotes a 1946 remark of an American who believed his country hated Japan with "emotions forgotten since our most savage Indian wars." One of FDR's advisers publicly declared in April 1945 that he favored "the extermination of the Japanese in toto." Journalists who worked in both war theaters noted how Germans were hated but treated like human beings, while Japanese were treated as if they were jungle beasts. Popular motion pictures of the war defined Japanese as "monkey people," "ringtails," and "rats" usually prefixed by "yellow." Hollywood films sometimes (as in Alfred Hitchcock's classic *Lifeboat* of 1944) noted differences between bad Nazis and good Germans, but movies almost never showed a good Japanese. Such racial hatred and fears had allowed Roosevelt to incarcerate nearly 112,000 Japanese-Americans in concentration camps in early 1942. (They remained there even though their sons in a Japanese-American unit fighting in Italy were among the bravest and most honored of U.S. military forces.) Meanwhile, Tokyo officials stressed their nation's divine origin and racial purity while belittling other less-civilized Asians and, especially, the multiracial, "liberal," "barbarian," and "soft" Americans.[59]

In addition to U.S. moral views about using the atomic bomb, Truman felt that, because of the weapon, he did not need (or want) the Soviets to invade Manchuria and Japan. Or, as Stimson put it, "I hope to hell [Stalin] doesn't come in."[60] A U.S. B-29 bomber, the *Enola*

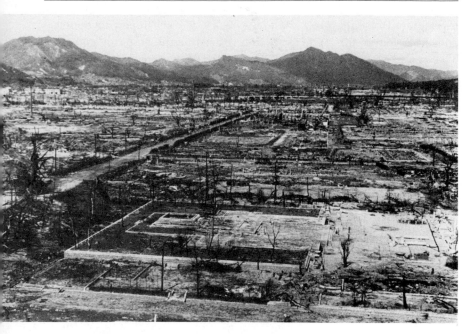

The beginning of a new era in human history and the end of World War II: Hiroshima at Ground Zero in August 1945 after the United States dropped the first atomic bomb.

Gay, dropped the world's first atomic bomb on Hiroshima at 8:15 A.M. on a hot, humid August 6, 1945. Within a second, a 650-foot fireball seared everything in its path; every brick building within a mile disappeared; every wooden structure within 1.2 miles blew apart; and, within thirty minutes, a firestorm was triggered whirled by a 40-mile-an-hour wind and accompanied by black, radioactive rain. By 4:00 P.M., 80,000 had died; 120,000 more suffered from burns and other effects of radiation. A physician recalled that patients "had no faces! Their eyes, noses, and mouths had been burned away, and it looked like their ears had melted off. It was hard to tell front from back."[61]

On August 8, almost three months to the day after Germany's surrender, Stalin declared war on Japan. On August 9, the United States dropped the second atomic bomb; this fell on Nagasaki. Another 65,000 Japanese immediately died. Truman now wanted Japan to surrender quickly, especially before Soviet troops approached the Japanese home islands. But for the next four days the president's advisers argued heatedly over whether to allow even a greatly limited Japanese emperor to remain in power. Stimson wanted to compromise and end the conflict immediately. Secretary of State Byrnes, however, hoped to appease American hatred for Japan by further restricting the emperor's powers. The result was a vague U.S. response to Tokyo's peace feelers that made some Japanese militarists decide to fight to the end. Between August 10 and 14, wave after wave of U.S. planes destroyed Japan's cities and killed thousands of civilians. A third atomic bomb was to be readied by August 19, but Truman never had to make the decision to use it. On August 14–15, the emperor, fearing that his nation would be "annihilated," overruled the militarists and accepted a U.S. position that implied the continuation of his imperial institution, but in greatly reduced form. Truman now approved the condition. If he had so accepted the emperor's continued role earlier, much death and destruction might have been avoided. Historian Martin Sherwin concludes that "*neither* bomb may have been necessary; and certainly . . . the second one was not."[62]

CONCLUSION

On September 2, 1945, General MacArthur sailed into Tokyo Bay on the USS *Missouri*. He watched as Japanese officials signed the papers of surrender. World War II was over. Another war, however, had already begun in a world remade by fourteen years of global destruction and two atomic bombs.

This different world demanded new thoughts. One view was formulated by David Lilienthal, a close adviser of Truman: "The fences are gone. And it was we, the civilized, who have pushed standardless conduct to its ultimate." A quite different view was much later expressed by Phyllis Schlafly, a leader of conservative Republicans: "The atomic bomb is a marvelous gift that was given to our country by a wise God."[63] In the new war and the different world, Americans would have to choose between foreign policies those two statements suggested.

It was already clear, however, that the gigantic U.S. power, even the atomic bomb, could not resolve the problems and contradictions that had developed in foreign policy. On the one hand, FDR and Truman had hoped to construct an open, liberal world along the lines of the Atlantic Charter principles. On the other hand, they had to recognize Stalin's determination to control eastern and perhaps central Europe, especially because the Red Army had the power to support such determination. Because both superpowers hoped to be dominant over a united (but weak) Germany, neither power could take the chance that the other might actually end up controlling this hub of Europe. As historian Frank Ninkovich phrases it, "The immense force of the global superpower confrontation had, like the collision of two geological plates, created a new mountain barrier whose most formidable massif was a divided Germany."[64] Nor could the Americans reconcile their commitment to self-government with their standing by as the British and French moved back into their Asian and African colonies. Truman faced a dangerous, incredibly complex world, even while he believed that he held the power in his hands to obtain at least "85 percent" of what he and most Americans wanted.

Notes

1. Bernard F. Dick, *The Star-Spangled Screen* (Lexington, Ky., 1985), pp. 21–22, 167–171.
2. E. J. Kahn, Jr., "Profile," *New Yorker*, 8 April 1972, p. 64; Allan R. Millett and Peter Maslowski, *For the Common Defense: A Military History of the United States of America* (New York, 1984), pp. 401, 415.
3. Important on the MacArthur-Philippine connection is Carol Morris Petillo, *Douglas MacArthur, the Philippine Years* (Bloomington, Ind., 1981), esp. pp. 201–205; also see Dick, p. 132.
4. Gabriel Kolko, *The Politics of War: The World and U.S. Foreign Policy, 1943–1945* (New York, 1968), p. 280.
5. Kenton J. Clymer, "The U.S. and the Decolonisation of Empire in Asia," in *American Studies in Malaysia*, ed. K. S. Nathan (Kuala Lumpur, Malaysia, 1986), p. 14.
6. *Churchill and Roosevelt: The Complete Correspondence*, ed. Warren Kimball, 3 vols. (Princeton, 1984), I, pp. 446–447, quotes the American observer (Harry Hopkins); D. Cameron Watt, *Succeeding John Bull: America in Britain's Place, 1900–1975* (Cambridge, 1984), p. 234.
7. Cordell Hull, *The Memoirs of Cordell Hull*, 2 vols. (New York, 1948), II, p. 1153.
8. "Private Memorandum" of conversation with Cordell Hull, 11 December 1941, Black Book #I, Papers of Arthur Krock, Princeton University.
9. Robert A. Divine, *Roosevelt and World War II* (Baltimore, 1969), pp. 59–61.
10. Joseph L. Strange, "The British Rejection of Operation Sledgehammer: An Alternative Motive," *Military Affairs* 46 (February 1982): 6–14.
11. Eric Larrabee, *Commander in Chief: Franklin Delano Roosevelt, His Lieutenants, and Their War* (New York, 1987), p. 9.
12. Frank Costigliola, "The Image of France in the United States," unpublished manuscript in author's possession, pp. 1–6.
13. *Churchill and Roosevelt*, II, p. 148.
14. "Joint Chiefs of Staff Memorandum for Information No. 121," 22 August 1943, in *Records of the Joint Chiefs of Staff*, Soviet Union, Pt. I, 1942–1945, p. 11. I am indebted

to Richard Mandel for a copy of this memorandum; Mark A. Stoler, "The 'Second Front' and American Fear of Soviet Expansion, 1941–1943," *Military Affairs* 39 (October 1975): 136–140.

15. Vojtech Mastny, *Russia's Road to the Cold War* (New York, 1979), pp. 107–108.

16. *Churchill and Roosevelt*, II, pp. 487–488; Kolko, pp. 37–39.

17. *Churchill and Roosevelt*, II, p. 612.

18. Dick, p. 201.

19. Millett and Maslowski, pp. 438–440.

20. This section draws from Frank Costigliola's important and highly readable analysis, *France and the United States* (New York, 1992), Ch. I; and from Walter LaFeber, "Roosevelt, Churchill, and Indochina, 1942–1945," *American Historical Review* 80 (December 1975): 1277–1295.

21. Lloyd C. Gardner, *Economic Aspects of New Deal Diplomacy* (Madison, Wis., 1964), p. 308, has the Clayton quote; also note p. 344.

22. A good, succinct overview is in David Baldwin, "The International Bank in Political Perspective," *World Politics* 18 (October 1965): 68–81.

23. Hull, II, pp. 1614–1615.

24. Fraser Harbutt, "Churchill, Hopkins, and the 'Other' Americans . . . ," *International History Review* 8 (May 1986): 261.

25. "Beard's Republic," *Life*, 20 March 1944, p. 36.

26. Christopher Thorne, *Allies of a Kind: The U.S., Britain and the War against Japan, 1941–1945* (New York, 1978), p. 515; Daniel Yergin, *Shattered Peace: The Origins of the Cold War and the National Security State* (Boston, 1977), p. 64.

27. Winston S. Churchill, *The Second World War*, 6 vols. (Boston, 1948–1953), VI, p. 293; "Record of Meeting at the Kremlin," 9 October 1944, PREM 3 / 4347, British Public Record Office, Kew, Eng. I am indebted to Professor Warren Kimball for a copy of this document.

28. "Record of Meeting at the Kremlin," 9 October 1944, PREM 3 / 4347, British Public Record Office; the context is well analyzed in Warren F. Kimball, "Naked Reverse Right . . . ," *Diplomatic History* 9 (Winter 1985): 1–7.

29. *Washington Post*, 23 December 1944, p. 17.

30. A good analysis of how the military background shaped the Yalta discussions is in Diane Shaver Clemens, *Yalta* (New York, 1970), pp. 82–95; for a retrospective on the Dresden bombing, see the *New York Times*, 30 January 1985, p. 2.

31. Petillo, pp. 221–228, esp. quote on p. 224.

32. Larabee, pp. 509–578; see also Jonathan Spence, who puts Stilwell's experience in the context of three hundred years of China's experience in *To Change China* (New York, 1980), pp. 263–264.

33. U.S. Department of Defense, "U.S. Policy, 1940–1950: Summary," in *United States–Vietnam Relations, 1945–1967*, 12 vols. (Washington, D.C., 1971), I, pp. IA1–A4. These are the original "Pentagon Papers." W. Averell Harriman to Harry Hopkins, 10 September 1944, Harriman File, Box 96, Papers of Harry Hopkins, Franklin D. Roosevelt Library, Hyde Park, New York.

34. Clayton R. Koppes and Gregory D. Black, "What to Show the World: The Office of War Information and Hollywood, 1942–1945," *Journal of American History* 64 (June 1977): 98–99; *Churchill and Roosevelt*, I, p. 421.

35. Gaddis Smith, *American Diplomacy during the Second World War, 1941–1945* (New York, 1965), p. 128.

36. U.S. Department of State, *Foreign Relations of the United States: The Conference at Malta and Yalta, 1945* (Washington, D.C., 1955), pp. 450–451.

37. *Ibid.*, pp. 234–235, 237.

38. Martin Weil, *A Pretty Good Club: The Founding Fathers of the U.S. Foreign Service* (New York, 1978), p. 183.

39. U.S. Department of State, *Malta and Yalta*, pp. 668–669, 677–678, 898; Smith, pp. 138–139, 148–149.

40. Herbert Feis, *Churchill, Roosevelt, Stalin: The War They Waged and the Peace They Sought* (Princeton, 1957), pp. 645–646. A good summary of the discussion over Germany is in Clemens, pp. 275–282.

41. U.S. Department of State, *Malta and Yalta*, pp. 977–978.

42. Clemens, p. 290.

43. Oral History of Walter Lippmann, Columbia University, p. 217.

44. "Daily Staff Summary," 19 March 1945, Lot File, RG 59, National Archives, Washington, D.C.; Mastny, pp. 250–258.

45. "Daily Staff Summary," 6 April 1945, Lot File, RG 59, National Archives.

46. A good analysis is Kimball, "Naked Reverse Right," 14–24; the documents and editorial comment are in Kimball, *Churchill and Roosevelt*, III, p. 617; and *Roosevelt and Churchill*, ed. Francis L. Loewenheim, Harold D. Langley, and Manfred Jonas (New York, 1975), pp. 704–709.

47. Watt, p. 105.

48. Martin Sherwin, *A World Destroyed* (New York, 1975), p. 172; Harry S. Truman, *Memoirs*, 2 vols. (Garden City, N.Y., 1955–1956), I, p. 80; Henry L. Stimson and McGeorge Bundy, *On Active Service in Peace and War* (New York, 1949), p. 609.

49. Milovan Djilas, *Conversations with Stalin* (New York, 1962), p. 114.

50. U.S. Department of State, *Foreign Relations of the United States: The Conference of Berlin (The Potsdam Conference), 1945*, 2 vols. (Washington, D.C., 1960), I, p. 715. For Truman's view of how Europe had to be united, there is an important analysis in Lloyd C. Gardner, *Architects of Illusion: Men and Ideas in American Foreign Policy, 1941–1949* (Chicago, 1970), pp. 78–81.

51. U.S. Department of State, *The Conference of Berlin*, I, pp. 456–461.

52. The standard account is Sherwin, esp. pp. 14–21.

53. Watt, p. 97.

54. Barton J. Bernstein, "Roosevelt, Truman, and the Atomic Bomb: A Reinterpretation," *Political Science Quarterly* 90 (Spring 1975): 31.

55. Sherwin, pp. 220–228; *Washington Post*, October 4, 1992, p. A1.

56. George Kistiakowsky, quoted in the *New York Times*, 12 December 1983, p. E18.

57. Barton J. Bernstein, "A Postwar Myth: 500,000 U.S. Lives Saved," *Bulletin of Atomic Scientists* 42 (June/July 1986): 38–40.

58. John Dower, *War without Mercy* (New York, 1986), pp. 40–41.

59. *Ibid.*, pp. 33, 54–55, 240–259; Clayton R. Koppes and Gregory D. Black, *Hollywood Goes to War* (New York, 1987), pp. 277–315. Dick, p. 230; Geoffrey S. Smith, "Doing Justice: Relocation and Equity in Public Policy," *Public Historian* 6 (Summer 1984): 83–97, a good brief analysis of the Japanese-American experience.

60. Bernstein, "Roosevelt, Truman, and the Atomic Bomb," 44n.

61. Robert Karl Manoff, "American Victims of Hiroshima," *New York Times Magazine*, 2 December 1984, p. 118.

62. Sherwin, p. 237; a most important analysis is Barton J. Bernstein, "The Perils and

Politics of Surrender: Ending the War with Japan and Avoiding the Third Atomic Bomb," *Pacific Historical Review* 46 (February 1977), pp. 1–27.

63. Paul Boyer, "The Fences Are Gone," *Reviews in American History* 10 (September 1982): 453; *The Progressive, No Comment* (Madison, Wis., 1983), p. 35.

64. Frank A. Ninkovich, *Germany and the United States* (Boston, 1988), p. 73.

FOR FURTHER READING

References for specific topics can also be found in this chapter's notes and in the General Bibliography at the end of this book; these references usually are not repeated below. The following focuses on post-1981 works because the pre-1981 accounts are presented in full, with helpful comments, in the *Guide to American Foreign Relations since 1700*, ed. Richard Dean Burns (1983).

For the overall war effort, Robert Leckie, *The Wars of America*, rev. and updated ed. (1981), is readable and useful; Eric Larrabee, *Commander in Chief: Franklin Delano Roosevelt, His Lieutenants, and Their War* (1987), is exhaustive and beautifully researched; *America Unbound*, ed. Warren F. Kimball (1992); and Warren F. Kimball, *The Juggler* (1991), on FDR's wartime planning, provide details and new perspectives on the war's diplomacy; Michael S. Sherry, *The Rise of American Air Power* (1987), is important because it ranges far beyond the strategic-bombing campaign itself into the American psyche. The domestic side of foreign policy is delineated in H. Schuyler Foster, *Activism Replaces Isolationism: U.S. Public Attitudes, 1940–1975* (1983), by a former State Department official who supervised the public-opinion polling; Susan M. Hartmann, *The Home Front and Beyond: American Women in the 1940s* (1982); Deborah Gesensway and Mindy Roseman, *Beyond Words: Images from America's Concentration Camps* (1987), a powerfully presented account; John J. Bukowczyk, *And My Children Did Not Know Me: A History of the Polish-Americans* (1987); Clayton R. Koppes and Gregory D. Black, *Hollywood Goes to War* (1987), is superb on the war's movies.

For new approaches to U.S.-Asian relations (in addition to John Dower's prize-winning *War without Mercy*, cited in the notes), important accounts include Arne Westad, *Cold War and Revolution: Soviet-American Rivalry and the Origins of the Chinese Civil War, 1944–1946* (1993), with superb use of Chinese sources; Akira Iriye, *Power and Culture: The Japanese-American War, 1941–1945* (1981); John J. Sbrega, *Anglo-American Relations and Colonialism in East Asia, 1941–1945* (1983); Dennis Merrill, *Bread and the Ballot: The U.S. and India's Economic Development, 1947–1963* (1990), a major account; Kenneth Chern, *Dilemma in China, 1945* (1980), good on the U.S. debate; Gary R. Hess, *The United States Emergence as a Southeast Asian Power, 1940–1950* (1986), a fine overview; *Child of Conflict: The Korean-American Relationship, 1943–1953*, ed. Bruce Cumings (1983), a collection of superb essays; Marc S. Gallichio, *The Cold War Begins in Asia* (1988).

Scholars of U.S.-European relations have recently produced valuable work, especially on U.S.-British ties and how those ties related to the outbreak of the cold war. Warren Kimball's three volumes of Churchill-Roosevelt correspondence, cited in the notes, are the place to begin, and his work can be well supplemented with Randall B. Woods, *A*

Changing of the Guard ... 1941–1946 (1991); Terry H. Anderson, *The United States, Great Britain and the Cold War, 1944–1947* (1981), which sees FDR as being highly aggressive at the end of his life; Robert M. Hathaway, *Ambiguous Partnership: Britain and America, 1944–1947* (1981), which argues that there never was a real partnership; Alan P. Dobson, *U.S. Wartime Aid to Britain, 1940–1946* (1986), highly detailed on the nature of the aid; Henry B. Ryan, *The Vision of Anglo-America* (1987), which explores 1943 through 1946 to outline the ideal as well as the real world of each nation; and, of special importance, Lawrence Wittner's analysis of how Americans finally joined the British in a crucial region, *American Intervention in Greece, 1943–1949* (1982). For France, Raoul Aglion, an associate of de Gaulle's, provides one view in *Roosevelt and de Gaulle: A Personal Memoir of Allies in Conflict* (1988); and a good overview is Henry Blumenthal, *Illusion and Reality in Franco-American Diplomacy, 1914–1945* (1986). U.S.-Italian relations are well analyzed in James Edward Miller, *The United States and Italy, 1940–1950* (1986). In addition to David Wyman's standard work on the Holocaust (see Chapter 12, above), important for the wartime years is Leonard Dinnerstein, *America and the Survivors of the Holocaust* (1982).

Other works that focus on East-West (i.e., Soviet-U.S.) relations and the wartime origins of the cold war include Edward M. Bennett, *Franklin D. Roosevelt and the Search for Victory: American-Soviet Relations, 1939–1945* (1990); Robert L. Messer, "World War II and the Coming of the Cold War," in *Modern American Diplomacy,* ed. John M. Carroll and George C. Herring (1986), a most useful overview; Robert A. Pollard, *Economic Security and the Origins of the Cold War* (1986), a detailed account; Michael T. Ruddy, *The Cautious Diplomat: Charles E. Bohlen and the Soviet Union* (1986), readable and important on a key State Department expert; *Witnesses to the Origins of the Cold War,* ed. Thomas T. Hammond (1987), interviews with U.S. diplomats who were in eastern Europe; Hugh DeSantis, *The Diplomacy of Silence* (1980), on Foreign Service officers involved with Soviet policy between 1933 and 1947; Keith Sainsbury, *The Turning Point* (1985), now a standard study on the 1943 summit conference, with superb use of British sources; Paul D. Mayle, *Eureka Summit* (1987), which, like Sainsbury, uses British materials well and sees the Tehran Conference as the war's diplomatic turning point; Russell D. Buhite, *Decision at Yalta* (1986), a critical view of FDR's diplomacy; P. G. H. Holdich, "A Policy of Percentages?: British Policy and the Balkans after the Moscow Conference of October 1944," *International History Review* 9 (Feb., 1987), on the pivotal 1944 Churchill-Stalin deal. For the Soviet side, William Taubman, *Stalin's American Policy* (1982), is a useful introduction; Joseph G. Whelen, *Soviet Diplomacy and Negotiating Behavior* (1982), is a mind-boggling, detailed, and irreplaceable analysis; *History of Soviet Foreign Policy, 1917–1945,* ed. B. Ponomaryov, A. Gromyko, and V. Khvostov (1974), remains perhaps the best Soviet view; while *The Impact of World War II on the Soviet Union,* ed. Susan J. Linz (1985), provides an important context.

Five superb books have recently been published on U.S.–Middle East relations and oil policies: Irvine Anderson, *ARAMCO, the U.S., and Saudi Arabia* (1981), which covers the 1933-to-1950 origins of the relationship; David S. Painter, *Oil and the American Century: The Political Economy of U.S. Foreign Oil Policy, 1941–1954* (1986), now a standard overall study; Aaron David Miller, *Search for Security* (1980), a pioneering analysis on U.S.-Saudi relations between 1939 and 1949; and Michael Stoff, *Oil, War, and American Security* (1980), especially important on the attempt to bring the U.S. government into the oil marketplace; and Daniel Yengin, *The Prize* (1991).

On Latin America, the place to begin is David Green's *Containment of Latin America*

(1971); and a new, useful work is Leslie B. Rout, Jr. and John F. Bratzel, *The Shadow War* (1986), which analyzes how five hundred German spies in Latin America brought unilateral U.S. responses, especially through the FBI. A fine overview is Randall Bennett Woods, *The Roosevelt Foreign Policy Establishment and the Good Neighbor* (1979), on the United States and Argentina.

Some of the effects of technology on diplomacy are examined in Alexander S. Cochran, Jr., " 'Magic,' 'Ultra,' and the Second World War," *Military Affairs* 46 (April 1982), a good overview of publications on intelligence operations; the ultimate technology is examined in a blockbuster of a book, Richard Rhodes, *The Making of the Atomic Bomb* (1987); and see John S. Gilkeson, Jr., *Gathering Rare Ores: The Diplomacy of Uranium Acquisition, 1943–1954* (1987).

Robert C. Hilderbrand, *Dumbarton Oaks* (1990), is now the standard volume on the origins of the United Nations.

14

The Cold War, or the Renewal of U.S.-Russian Rivalry (1945–1949)

TRUMAN AND A NEW WORLD

For President Harry Truman, events in 1945–1946 resembled a spaceship that rocketed him from a known world to a quite different universe. The end of the war in August 1945 brought wild celebration throughout the Allied camp. To most observers, the Big Three relationship of the United States, Great Britain, and the Soviet Union seemed so solid that many agreed with Eric Johnston, president of the U.S. Chamber of Commerce, who prophesied: "Russia will be, if not our biggest, at least our most eager consumer."[1] Truman privately (and colorfully) doubted it: "Our agreements with the Soviet Union have been a one-way street," the president complained, and the Soviets "could go to hell."[2] But the Soviets only remained in central and eastern Europe. They refused to cooperate economically, as Johnston and Truman had once hoped. In 1945, one set of U.S. policies, devised during the war by Franklin D. Roosevelt and Cordell Hull to create an open, cooperative, unified world, rapidly dissolved in the acidic aftermath of the Yalta and Potsdam disagreements.[3] No new policies were yet available.

At home, Truman had to spend much of 1945–1946 replacing FDR's advisers with officials whom he knew and trusted. Meanwhile, the nation's incredibly productive factories and farms, turning out an unbelievable 50 percent of the world's goods and services, required new markets. With their huge wartime savings, Americans also demanded new and more goods. The question became whether Truman, as head of the most powerful nation in recorded history, could navigate the spaceship so that everyone could reach the new postwar world safely.

THE VICTOR IN A HOSTILE WORLD: EUROPE

No one doubted the amazing extent of U.S. power. Americans dominated world trade, alone held the secret of the atomic bomb, and controlled the oceans with their fleets, while much of the rest of the world, including the Soviet Union, shoveled away the rubble that had once been towns and cities. The war, however, also destroyed a large portion of Germany and Japan, which for decades had been the industrial and military hubs around which their regions of the world revolved. Those two nations, moreover, had been the walls to stop any expansion of Soviet influence.

Another problem also arose from the destruction. Western Europe and Great Britain, as well as eastern Europe, turned sharply left in an effort to find the resources needed for massive rebuilding. Communists flourished, but so did Socialists. Thus, in mid-1945, the British Labour party replaced Churchill's Conservatives, who were in power. Some European right-wing leaders had collaborated with the Nazis and were totally discredited. The most important partners of the United States, in other words, were moving left and away from capitalist models just as Americans wanted more open markets and less government involvement.[4]

Great Britain dramatized the problem. For centuries it had been dependent on imports (even of meat and butter) but now found overseas markets as well as British factories devastated by war. U.S. leaders had long realized that they were going to replace the British as the great world power. But there was a price to be paid. As one Washington official observed in 1944, in every alliance one partner wears boots and spurs while the other wears a saddle. "We are obviously wearing the boots," he noted; but "if we want to stay in this fortunate position, we have to find some way to feed the horse."[5] The way was temporarily found in late 1945, when the United States forgave much of London's lend-lease debt. Then Washington gave Britain a $3.75 billion credit with low interest, but in return cold-bloodedly required the British to spend the money in the United States and open the British Empire to American competition.[6]

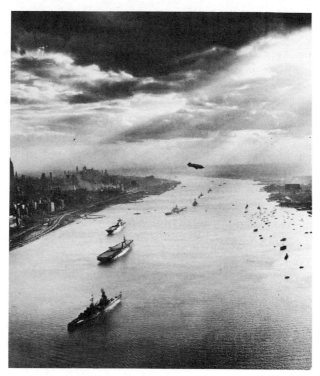

Awesome U.S. power at the end of World War II. On Navy Day, October 27, 1945, millions of New Yorkers joined the president to hail the return of the fleet. The climax of the celebration was a review of a seven-mile line of men o'war anchored in the Hudson River as 1,200 navy planes roared overhead.

The next question was whether the other member of the Big Three would play by such rules, voluntarily or otherwise. Observers could point out that Stalin's European empire did not equal in size the empire of Tsar Alexander I at the end of the Napoleonic Wars in 1815. The United States, moreover, enjoyed overwhelming naval and air superiority. With its gigantic fleet of 70,000 vessels (equal to the rest of the world's navies combined) and 100,000 planes, and its monopoly on the atomic bomb, Americans felt justified in demanding that their soldiers be returned home. Truman, however, had dropped his only two available atomic bombs on Japan in 1945; and, in Europe, Stalin—although he quickly discharged 9 million Russians so that they could help rebuild the economy—poised 30 divisions against 10 U.S., British, and French divisions in central Europe. If the United States launched an atomic attack, Stalin was apparently prepared to overrun and hold hostage much of Europe.[7]

Truman simply could not figure out how to transform his atomic monopoly and economic superiority into a foreign policy that could push Stalin back and reunite Europe. His secretary of war, Henry Stimson, who was about to retire after nearly forty years of public service, had once thought that the A-bomb could be used to break down "Russia's secret police state." By September 1945, however, Stimson had second thoughts. He believed that the bomb could not be used as "a direct lever to produce the change" and urged Truman to negotiate the best settlement possible with Stalin. If we, instead, only wear "this weapon rather ostentatiously on our hip," Stimson warned, "suspicions" and "distrust" would mount. But the president was not willing to settle for Stimson's approach.[8]

As for U.S. economic power, the Soviets refused to cooperate with the U.S.-controlled international economic institutions constructed at Bretton Woods (see p. 431). "At first sight," a top Soviet official remarked, the U.S. plans at Bretton Woods "looked like a tasty mushroom, but on examination they turned out to be a poisonous toadstool."[9] Americans might think the "open door" and "equal opportunity" for their dollars and trade the best principles for an international system, Soviet foreign minister Molotov declared in 1946. But, he continued, the United States was so strong that if these principles prevailed, American dollars would take over most European businesses. The radio in these countries would then broadcast not native languages, but "one American gramophone record after another." "Was this what we fought for when we battled the fascist invaders?" Molotov asked.[10]

U.S. officials thus failed when they tried to use dollar loans as a lever to push back Soviet influence in Poland—or even in Czechoslovakia, where an independent government held on despite increasing Soviet pressure. Truman also failed when he demanded new elections in Romania and Bulgaria. Stalin, however, moved cautiously in eastern Europe through much of 1945–1946. He allowed pro-Western factions to share power in parts of the region. The dictator wanted to do nothing that would force Truman to take retaliatory measures. But by late 1946, Soviet stubbornness drove even the British Labour party's foreign minister, Ernest Bevin, over the brink during one conference. A smart, tough, husky former dock worker, Bevin, tired of hearing Molotov defend Soviet policies and attack British proposals, rose to his feet, clenched his fists, and lurched toward the Soviet foreign minister, shouting, "I've had enough of this, I'ave," before security guards moved in.[11]

Although frustrated in eastern Europe, Truman enjoyed tremen-

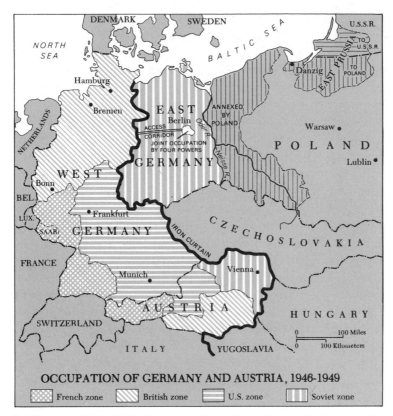

Divided Europe, 1946–1949. Note the vulnerable positions of Berlin and Czech-oslovakia.

dous power in western Europe. He could treat the U.S. occupation zone in Germany as he pleased. By early 1946, the few German reparations that had gone to the Soviets were stopped. JCS 1067 (Joint Chiefs of Staff Directive 1067) of April 1945 had instructed the U.S. military governor, General Lucius Clay, to limit Germany's industry severely as well as to destroy all hints of Nazism. By mid-1945, however, U.S. officials concluded that the plan must have been made "by economic idiots." Clay ditched JCS 1067 and allowed industry to rebuild so that American taxpayers would not have to feed and clothe Germans. He also urged that the four occupation zones merge into a single unit. Neither the French, who turned livid whenever German recovery was mentioned, nor the Soviets agreed with Clay, but the general's plans moved ahead anyway.

Secretary of State James Byrnes, in a speech given in Stuttgart, Germany, in September 1946, emphatically stated U.S. determination to retain control over at least western Germany's affairs. Byrnes had grown frustrated after endless wrangling with Molotov ("Old Iron Pants"), especially when the Soviets played to German opinion by urging that a unified Germany be created. Molotov wanted Soviet access to the industrially rich western regions of such a united Germany. Byrnes's speech undercut Molotov by declaring that the German-Polish boundary remained an open question (a remark that surprised and pleased the Germans, who hated giving their land to Poland). The secretary of state then announced that Germany could only be unified through democratic elections and a "national council" (in which the three Western powers could outvote the Soviets 3 to 1). Byrnes emphasized U.S. intentions to stay in central Europe. Not surprisingly, Stalin turned aside Byrnes's proposals. Germany remained divided as Americans and Soviets remained in Germany.[12]

Meanwhile, Soviet and U.S. agents were secretly wooing German scientists to the Soviet Union or America to work on supersensitive missile and bomb projects. Truman gave the order that no active supporters of "Nazism or militarism" be employed on these projects. But under Project Paperclip, about 765 German scientists entered the United States between 1945 and 1955. Some of them were later charged with having experimented on humans during the war and for using slave labor in Nazi Germany.[13] At this point, however, the growing cold war led Soviets and Americans to hire, not imprison, former Nazis.

THE VICTOR IN A HOSTILE WORLD: ASIA

Truman had better luck rebuilding Japan. He simply froze out all other powers (especially the British and Soviets) and installed General Douglas MacArthur to run the country as U.S. interests dictated. MacArthur immediately established his authority. With Japanese cities still burning, he landed, unarmed, at Yokohama airport (the bravest of "all the amazing feats in the war," Churchill declared) and drove into the city. Some 30,000 Japanese troops with fixed bayonets lined his route, but they had their backs to him—the same position they assumed when their emperor passed. MacArthur imprisoned or hanged military war criminals, planted democratic political processes in a new constitution, placed severe limits on industrial recovery of the old (and huge) corporate combines called *zaibatsu*, and started a successful land-reform program.

China did not present as happy a picture. Chiang Kai-shek's Kuomintang (KMT or Nationalist) party was engaged in a battle to the death with Mao Zedong's (Mao Tse-tung's) Communists. U.S. officials had sided with Chiang. But such experienced Foreign Service Officers (FSOs) as John Stuart Service, John Carter Vincent, and John Paton Davies (the "three Johns," as their critics soon called them) pushed hard to work with Mao for two reasons: their belief that he might win the long civil war, and their fervent hope that U.S. aid and friendship could separate Mao from any close ties with the Soviet Union, which they hated and feared. While on the so-called "Dixie Mission" of 1944, some of the FSOs had come to know the Communists well. They watched Mao's troops consolidate their power with the peasants in the north and enjoyed playing softball with the Communists.

The advice of the FSOs was countered, however, by General Patrick J. Hurley, FDR's personal representative to Chiang. Hurley knew little about China (when he landed in China, the native Oklahoman greeted his startled hosts with a Cherokee war cry) and cared little about learning. One expert sent to brief Hurley on China instead had to listen to a 45-minute monologue not "connected by any readily discernible pattern of thought," as the expert recalled.[14] But Hurley knew what he wanted: to eject British interests from China, to keep the Soviets out, and to ensure that Chiang triumphed over Mao. Roosevelt backed Hurley, and the president even rejected feelers from Mao for a top-level Chinese Communist visit to Washington.

By November 1945, however, Chiang's power was being threatened by Mao's successes. Meanwhile, the Soviets were moving into Manchuria to disarm Japanese troops and to seize industrial plants for use in the Soviet Union. Truman made a series of decisions. First, he ordered some of the 1 million Japanese troops in Manchuria and northern China to remain until they could be replaced by Chiang's or U.S. forces. Next, he sent his own troops into the region. By late 1946, 110,000 U.S. soldiers tried to police parts of northern China. Finally, he overruled Hurley and decided to send a mission to work out a deal between Chiang and Mao. Hurley dramatically resigned on November 27, 1945. He blamed the FSOs for siding with the Communists. The FSOs, however, had a more realistic policy than Hurley believed.

Truman sent his own hero, General George Marshall, to work out a military truce and political settlement. The president backed Marshall with the 110,000 U.S. troops and a pledge of $800 million in aid to buy Chiang's cooperation. Truman clearly assumed that Chiang, not Mao, was to be the undisputed leader of China. The Marshall mission quickly gained the trust of both sides and worked out a military truce and a political settlement that recognized the Communists' grass-roots strength. A plan to integrate the KMT and Communist armies reflected Chiang's 3-to-1 superiority in manpower. Nevertheless, the armies continued to fight over Manchurian positions. After one struggle around Changchun in February 1946, Chiang declared that the Communists had broken the truce. He launched a full-scale military campaign. Marshall warned Chiang not to do so. Despite the KMT's overwhelming superiority in men and firepower, Marshall knew that Chiang's forces were overextended and badly led.

By mid-1947, Mao's armies were cutting off and chopping up chunks of the KMT's best forces. Chiang assumed that he could ignore Marshall's advice, as he had Stilwell's in 1944, because the United States had no choice but to support him. Chiang's confidence increased when Henry Luce's powerful *Life* magazine began attacking Marshall's policies. But Chiang had made a fatal error. Marshall could only stand by and watch while both the KMT forces and the Chinese economy dissolved. Under the KMT's corrupt leadership, inflation skyrocketed until prices in mid-1948 were 3 million times those of late 1945. In January 1947, Truman and Marshall decided to terminate the general's mission. They blamed both sides for the failure but singled out Chiang for not cooperating and for using bad military judgment.[15]

Under pressure from pro-Chiang supporters in the U.S. Congress, Marshall (now secretary of state) sent General Albert C. Wedemeyer to investigate the situation in mid-1947. Wedemeyer's report recommended massive U.S. economic aid and as many as 10,000 American advisers to work with KMT troops. Knowing firsthand that such help would not be enough, Marshall rejected Wedemeyer's report. But he also unfortunately kept it secret and so gave new ammunition to those who later claimed that he and Truman had "lost" China (as if it were theirs to lose) and then tried to hide their sin. By this time, moreover, the Soviets had withdrawn from Manchuria and posed no direct threat to China. In all, as historian Steven Levine concludes, Marshall "had no intention of pulling [Chiang's] chestnuts from the fire."[16]

Truman came under harsh attack for retreating from China. General MacArthur had long argued that Asia had to be seen as the new American West, an extension of the four-hundred-year-old frontier: "Europe is a dying system," he had declared in 1944. "The lands touching the Pacific with their billions of inhabitants will determine the course of history in the next ten thousand years." In 1948, MacArthur announced that "to our western horizon we must look for . . .

yet untapped opportunities for trade and commerce."[17] The general spoke for many who wanted to carry on the long U.S. tradition embodied in John Hay's open-door notes and Henry Luce's "American Century" vision.

DEAN ACHESON'S AMERICAN CENTURY

But that tradition carried little weight with the most influential diplomat of the Truman presidential years and, in Secretary of State Henry Kissinger's words of 1976, "the greatest Secretary of State of the 20th-century."[18] Dean Acheson rightly entitled his memoir of 1941 through 1953 *Present at the Creation.* His outlook and policies, as much as any others, shaped U.S. diplomacy during these critical cold-war years.

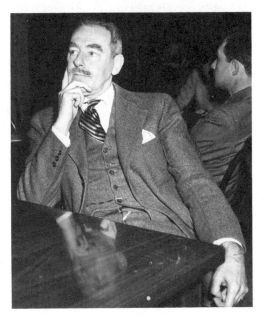

Dean Acheson (1893–1971) was, as this photograph suggests, an elegant and thoughtful man who was perhaps the most important secretary of state in the twentieth century. He was a leader in creating the Bretton Woods institutions, the Truman Doctrine, the Marshall Plan, NATO, NSC-68, the hydrogen-bomb project, and pivotal policies toward Vietnam and the People's Republic of China. By the end of his term as secretary of state (1949–1953), he was highly unpopular—in part because of his personal elegance, which, in the eyes of some congressmen, made him more British than American, and in part because he was viewed as not sufficiently tough on communism, especially in Asia.

He was born in 1893. His Canadian mother's family derived its wealth from banking and whiskey interests; his father was an Episcopal rector. Acheson's perception of what was "decent and civilized" came from "an image of upper middle class life in England, Canada, and the eastern United States in the late Victorian era—and he measured other men and nations by that perception," in the words of biographer Gaddis Smith.[19] That perception was reinforced by education at exclusive private schools, Yale, and Harvard Law School. He closely studied British history and admired London's use of its financial and military power to create the long post-1815 era of peace. As assistant secretary of state specializing in Anglo-American economic relations between 1941 and 1945, Acheson saw firsthand how the British were going bankrupt. He assumed that the United States would take top place in the world.[20] He also assumed, as he rose to undersecretary of state (1945–1947), that the alliance with the Soviet Union could continue into peacetime, but only if the Soviets accepted the guidelines he had helped write at the Bretton Woods Conference of 1944. Acheson's attitude toward the Soviets grew very tough in 1946 as the two nations clashed over German, Japanese, Iranian, Turkish, and atomic-energy questions.

But throughout all these years he held tightly to beliefs that guided his foreign policy. Seeing himself as a realist, he thought that "there are moral problems and real problems." Foreign policy's real problems, Acheson once observed, were not "a lot of abstract notions," but involved "what you do—these business transactions, credit through central banks, food things . . .—all this makes foreign policy." He wrote that "industrial productivity" formed the most important source of national power.[21] He constantly warned in 1944–1945 that Americans either had to find open markets and liberal international trade or they would find themselves again facing the economic horrors of the 1930s. Since the Soviets refused to open their empire or join the Bretton Woods system, Acheson turned to a reliance on military power. He concluded that Stalin could only be dealt with from "positions of strength," to use one of Acheson's more famous phrases. His understanding of history shaped his view of the present. Among other lessons that history taught, Acheson concluded, was that American survival could not be entrusted to merely the rule of law. "Law," he once declared, "simply does not deal with such questions of ultimate power." Or again: "The survival of states is not a matter of law," but of power.[22]

As Acheson tried to teach Americans the importance of economics and power, he also told them where they could find protection. Certainly, they should not look to the United Nations, which was a mere

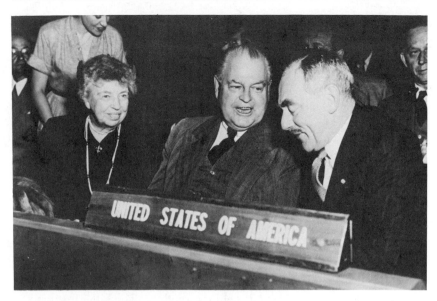

Eleanor Roosevelt (1884–1962) became a powerful voice for international coop-
eration, human rights, and critics who believed that the Truman-Acheson poli-
cies toward the Soviet bloc were too dependent on military confrontation. In the
late 1940s and early 1950s, she was an influential member of the U.S. delega-
tion to the United Nations—an organization she devoutly believed in, as did
Warren Austin (center), the first U.S. ambassador to the United Nations, but for
which Secretary of State Dean Acheson (seated at right) sometimes had an ill-
concealed contempt.

"forum." Speeches in the UN counted for little: "In the Arab proverb,
the ass that went to Mecca remained an ass, and a policy has little
added to it by its place of utterance." Nor did he have much hope for
the U.S. Congress. A senator, Acheson complained, too easily gets
excited, and his mind does not work "in a normal way. . . . He is a
violent partisan" and ignorantly "goes in swinging." Acheson lamented
that Congress listened to a usually uninformed public opinion. Americans had become "a somewhat hypochrondiac type" and "ascertain
our state of health by this mass temperature taking of public opinion
polls," he complained in 1946.[23] For its part, Congress mistrusted the
brilliant Acheson. One senator had to admit that Acheson was "the
kind of lawyer I'd like if I were guilty as hell." But another senator
complained that Acheson talked to him arrogantly, "as if a bit of fish
had got stuck in his mustache." Yet another referred to the elegantly
dressed official as "that goddam floorwalker."[24] Even friends admitted
that he handled Congress and the press badly because "he sometimes

talks over their heads. . . . He knows so much more than they do that it embarrasses them and they don't like it."

As undersecretary of state (1945–1947) and then secretary of state (1949–1953), Acheson enjoyed Truman's total support. They were an odd couple, this down-home president from a Missouri political machine and the highly polished member of elite eastern schools and law firms. But they admired and worked closely with each other. Acheson could lose patience on those rare occasions when the president failed to take his advice. ("Truman is like a boy you tell not to stick peanuts up his nose," Acheson complained to a friend, and "the minute you turn around, there he is sticking peanuts up his nose.")[25] But Acheson knew that his own power totally rested on his "constituency of one"—the president. He respected Truman's political talents, his hard work, his decisiveness, and especially his willingness to take Acheson's advice. In return, the State Department official was completely loyal as well as ruthless in carrying out Truman's policies. When once asked the trait a secretary of state most needed, Acheson replied, "The killer instinct."[26]

THE AWFUL YEAR OF 1946: EUROPE AND THE MIDDLE EAST

Acheson's changed attitude toward the Soviets in 1946 reflected the more general change of U.S. foreign policy. He focused on events in the European region because he and most U.S. officials believed that the American future depended not on vague Asian frontiers—conjured up by General MacArthur's word magic—but on Europe. For in that region, Americans had historically looked first for their trade, culture, and—as two world wars in twenty-four years bloodily demonstrated— most vital security interests. Moreover, not only were the Red Army's divisions concentrated in eastern Europe, but large Communist parties in war-devastated France and Italy were poised to seize power. Byrnes and Molotov fought bitterly at foreign ministers' meetings until they finally agreed on peace treaties for Finland and Italy that Americans liked, and for Romania, Hungary, and Bulgaria that the Soviets could accept.

Europe was the site of continual diplomatic talks in 1946, but the Mediterranean–Middle East region threatened to become an actual U.S.-Soviet battleground. Iran posed the first danger. That country was occupied by the British, Soviets, and Americans during the war to ensure a route for lend-lease goods to the Soviets. After 1941, the three powers scrambled for postwar rail and, especially, oil concessions until a truce was declared in 1944. The Tehran Conference Declaration of 1943 agreed that the three powers would withdraw within six months after the war's end. The Americans pulled out in January 1946 and the British on March 2. But Red Army troops remained. Moscow demanded oil rights as well as a pro-Communist regime in the Azerbaijan Republic that bordered the Soviet Union. Stalin perhaps again thought that he was only collecting earlier tsarist claims. A 1907 treaty had recognized dominant Soviet interests in northern Iran, and this recognition had been confirmed by post-1917 pacts.

The British, however, had long fought to block any Soviet penetration into the Middle East. Truman picked up that British commitment. As reports reached Byrnes of Soviet tanks moving toward the Iranian border in early March 1946, he sent warnings to Moscow. The secretary of state then went to the United Nations and, in the new organization's first major crisis, focused world attention on the Soviet move. It was not a good start for the UN. Most importantly, a shrewd Iranian government delegation met with Stalin to work out a deal: the Communist Tudeh party would have certain rights in Azerbaijan, and the Soviets could have oil concessions—subject, however, to the withdrawal of the Red Army from Iran and to the approval of the Iranian legislature. Stalin withdrew his troops; the Iranians then seized and executed a number of Tudeh party leaders; the legislature refused to ratify the agreement—and Iran, under a new, young shah, seemed firmly in the Western camp.[27]

In Iran, as well as most other places, FDR's "four policemen" were now down to one. The U.S. policeman next moved his beat into the highly sensitive and strategic Straits, which linked the Mediterranean Sea to the Black Sea and to the Soviet Union itself. The Montreux Convention of 1936 had given Turkey control of The Straits. But for centuries the Russians had sought access through the Black Sea to the warm-water Mediterranean. At Tehran in 1943 and again at Moscow in 1944, Churchill promised Stalin such access. A month after the Yalta Conference in 1945, Stalin tried to cash Churchill's blank check by denouncing Turkey (which had worked with Hitler) and demanding some control over The Straits. But when Stalin next presented the blank check at the Potsdam Conference in July 1945, he discovered that the new cashier, Harry Truman, had other plans. The president cleverly asked that all "inland waterways" bounded by more than two states be placed under international control. With this simple move, Truman blocked Soviet control of The Straits and threatened to open much of eastern Europe by putting the Danube under multinational (instead of Red Army) control, but neatly protected Turkey's domination of The Straits, the U.S. hold on the Panama Canal, and the British authority over the Suez Canal because only a single country bordered those waterways.

Protesting that the new cashier was changing the rules in the middle of the deal, Stalin tried other tactics. In early 1946, he made demands directly on Turkey. Truman thought of sending an aircraft carrier to the region, but tension eased. Then on August 7, 1946, Stalin demanded from the Turks joint control of The Straits. Acheson warned Truman that the Soviets aimed to dominate Turkey; then Greece, the Middle East's oil, and "India and China" could fall next. Only "force of arms" could stop Stalin. Truman agreed with this early version of the so-called "domino theory." The president replied, "We might as well find out whether the Russians [are] bent on world conquest now as in five or ten years."[28] With tough U.S. backing, Turkey turned down Stalin's demand. A month later, the U.S. Navy announced that its newly dispatched fleet, led by the giant aircraft carrier *Franklin D. Roosevelt,* was to remain permanently in the eastern Mediterranean.[29]

THE AWFUL YEAR OF 1946:
ATOMIC ENERGY AND HENRY WALLACE

The American people knew of these crises but realized neither the extent nor danger for the Big Three relationship. In 1946, Truman did not use the crises to damn the Soviets publicly. Nor did he try to mobilize the American people to fight a cold war. He instead tried to come to terms with major changes in his own foreign and domestic affairs.

In foreign policy, Stalin challenged the fundamentals of U.S. plans in a speech of February 9, 1946. The dictator announced that the Soviet Union planned to turn inward and rebuild itself with more five-year plans that demanded sacrifice from his people. Stalin thus rejected once and for all any possibility of entering the Bretton Woods economic arrangements. Apparently for that reason, U.S. Supreme Court Justice William O. Douglas called Stalin's speech "the Declaration of World War III."[30] A month later, former Prime Minister Winston Churchill declared at Westminster College in Fulton, Missouri, that "an iron curtain has descended" to cut off the world from the "police governments" in eastern Europe. With Truman looking on, Churchill thanked God for entrusting the atomic bomb to the Anglo-Saxon people and demanded an alliance of the English-speaking nations for the coming "trial of strength." Truman had no intention of weakening his nation's policies by tying them to Britain's rapidly declining power. But the president agreed with Churchill's view of the Soviet threat. In Moscow, Stalin angrily responded that Churchill was with the "war-mongers" who followed the "racial theory" that only those speaking English could "decide the destinies of the entire world."[31]

Against this grim backdrop, Truman had to deal with a U.S.-Soviet agreement of December 1945 to discuss possible international control of atomic energy. The deal had been made by Secretary of State Byrnes with Stalin. Truman knew little of Byrnes's bargaining in Moscow until the secretary of state returned. The president then blew up. He ordered Byrnes to meet him on the presidential yacht in Chesapeake Bay even "if he [had] to swim," as one aide phrased the order, and then gave Byrnes "the trimming of his life." Within eleven months, Byrnes was replaced by Marshall. But Truman still had to deal with the atomic-energy agreement negotiated by Byrnes.

He appointed a committee headed by Dean Acheson and David Lilienthal (the respected administrator of the Tennessee Valley Authority) to draft a policy. The Acheson-Lilienthal Plan provided for an international body to control the raw materials and the production facilities used for atomic energy. It assumed that the United States was far ahead in the field and could build bombs quickly, so the authors worried little about what might occur if the Soviet Union violated the agreement and began to build its own atomic weapons.

Truman then asked Bernard Baruch to present the plan at the United Nations. That was a mistake. A seventy-six-year-old multimillionaire, Baruch's fame rested not only on real administrative talents, but also on hired public-relations agents and his large contributions to as many as sixty members of Congress. He knew nothing about atomic-energy policy. Nevertheless, Baruch changed the Acheson-Lilienthal Plan by inserting a voting procedure that would give the United States control over every step—even the establishment of atomic power for peaceful purposes *within* the Soviet Union. Not surprisingly, when he presented this "Baruch Plan" in June 1946 at a dramatic UN session, the Soviets soon rejected it. Suddenly aware that a historic chance to control atomic power had been ruined, leading U.S. journalists blasted Baruch for "inflexible diplomacy." Truman, now besieged by crises abroad and at home, admitted privately that appointing Baruch was "the worst blunder I ever made. . . . But we can't fire him now, not with all the other trouble." Before the end of 1946, however, Baruch had resigned. Con-

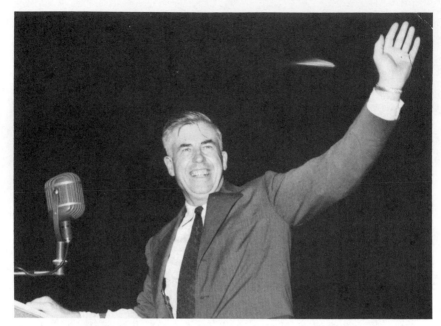

Henry Wallace (1888–1965) had been FDR's popular secretary of agriculture (1933–1940), then vice-president (1941–1945), and secretary of commerce (1945–1946) until President Truman fired him in mid-1946 after Wallace criticized the growing U.S. and British confrontation with the Soviets. Running as a Progressive against Truman in 1948, Wallace was not only defeated badly, but his loss helped discredit left-liberal analyses of the growing cold war and led to the American consensus on how to fight that war. A native of Iowa, Wallace retired after 1948 to become a gentleman farmer.

gress passed the Atomic Energy Act, which essentially outlawed any exchange of atomic-energy information. The world remained embarked on an uncontrolled atomic-arms race.[32]

One U.S. official publicly objected. Henry A. Wallace had been FDR's vice-president from 1941 to 1945 (until he was replaced, at Roosevelt's request, by Truman) and was widely admired as an ardent New Dealer. As secretary of commerce, Wallace gave a speech at New York's Madison Square Garden in September, 1946, in which he condemned the arms race and blamed U.S. as well as Soviet policy. Wallace urged a return to economic cooperation between the two powers. He hoped that Stalin would open eastern Europe to U.S. trade and investment. Byrnes and Republican Senator Arthur Vandenberg from Michigan, who were at the time suffering through negotiations with the Soviets in Europe, immediately demanded that Truman fire Wallace. The president was trapped. He badly needed Wallace's wide political support. But amid the uproar, he also privately blasted his secretary of commerce as one of "the Reds, phonies, and the 'parlor pinks' [who] . . . are becoming a national danger."[33] He removed Wallace, who now prepared to challenge Truman for the presidency in 1948.

Truman endured a bad year in 1946. In addition to problems with Byrnes and Wallace at home, even leading scientists came out against the president's policies. In late 1945, they began publishing the *Bulletin of Atomic Scientists* each month "to preserve our civilization," as one scholar said, "by scaring men into rationality."[34] But for Truman, the worst blow came in November 1946, when congressional elections gave Republicans a majority of 6 members in the Senate and a stunning 127 in the House. The president's public-approval rating that had stood at 87 percent in mid-1945 now sank like a stone to a historic low of 32 percent.

Then, in early 1947, Truman and Acheson used foreign policy to pull off a political miracle. They were so successful, moreover, that other presidents have tried to repeat the original miracle ever since.

CREATING THE POSTWAR WORLD:
KENNAN AND THE LONG TELEGRAM

The miracle actually began in February 1946, when the longest telegram in State Department history began to clatter over the department's Telex machines. It was sent from Moscow by forty-two-year-old George Frost Kennan, the chargé d'affaires in the U.S. Embassy. The cable was the result of an urgent State Department request for an explanation of Stalin's "election speech."

Kennan had long waited for the opportunity to educate U.S. officials. A native of Milwaukee and educated at Princeton, the quiet, bookish Kennan joined the Foreign Service in the 1920s. Fluent in Russian and German, and an authority on classic nineteenth-century Russian literature as well as twentieth-century politics, he trained as a member of the initial group of U.S. experts on the Soviet Union in the American listening post of Riga, Latvia. In 1933, he helped William Bullitt open the first U.S. Embassy in the Soviet Union. For much of the next twelve years, Kennan lived in the Soviet Union and eastern Europe. He loved the Russian people and many of their pre-1917 traditions. But Kennan strongly disliked the Bolshevist Revolution. As he witnessed Stalin's bloody purges of the 1930s, the ever-growing police state, and the ris-

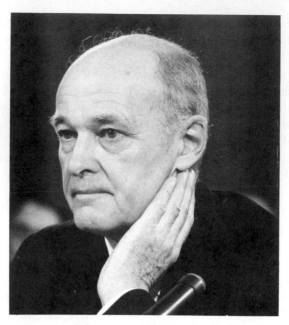

*George Frost Kennan (1904–   ) became the nation's best-known expert on
Soviet affairs and was the famous "X" who wrote the containment policy in
1946–1947. A reserved, conservative graduate of Princeton, Kennan loved traditional, nineteenth-century Russian literature and society but feared Stalinist
Russia. Highly mistrustful of public opinion, he wanted diplomacy controlled by
professional diplomats (like himself)—until after 1949, when U.S. diplomacy
became, in his view, overmilitarized. He then left the State Department to
become a prize-winning historian who appealed to public opinion to support
détente with the Soviets and a mutual withdrawal of the two superpowers from
central Europe.*

ing disputes with the United States, he became a bitter critic of Soviet
policies. By 1945, the young Foreign Service officer believed that Roosevelt's hopes of cooperation with Stalin were hopelessly naïve. Kennan, however, did not want to go to the other extreme and declare war
on the Soviets to free eastern Europe. Believing that the Soviets were
unable to conquer—and, at present, uninterested in conquering—what
Kennan considered to be the great power bases in the world (western
Europe, Japan, and the United States), he urged U.S. officials to remain
cool and prepare for a long political struggle.

He detailed his argument about "containing" the Soviets in the long,
secret telegram of February 22, 1946. In July 1947, he published a
public version, "The Sources of Soviet Conduct," under the name of
"X"—a disguise that fooled no one.[35] Why was Stalin so uncoopera-

tive? Because, Kennan answered, the dictator needed to portray the West as evil in order to justify his own control over the Russian people. Kennan said nothing about the U.S. and Allied military invasions of Russia in 1918–1920 nor about Washington's refusal to deal diplomatically with the Soviets until 1933. He instead stressed that because of the Soviet leadership's internal needs, the Soviet Union viewed the West as an enemy and would exert constant pressure to reduce Western power. He believed, however, that the Communists, unlike Hitler, were in no hurry and had no timetable. The Soviets would have to "be contained by the adroit and vigilant application of counterforce at a series of constantly shifting geographical and political points." If Americans could be patient and work to ensure the long-run prosperity and stability of their own system, then Marxism would be disproved and "containment" end in a great climax: "either the break-up or the gradual mellowing of Soviet power." (A self-described "conservative," Kennan doubted whether Americans could create and stay with such a long-term policy. But he kept these doubts mostly to himself in the 1940s.)

The Long Telegram of 1946 and the "X" article a year later caused a sensation. Kennan was recalled from Moscow and became a powerful voice in Washington. "Containment" became the magic term of U.S. foreign policy. Then and later, Kennan puzzled over why he and his ideas suddenly became so famous. Other State Department officials were also analyzing Soviet actions and coming up with explanations different from Kennan's. One policy paper, for example, claimed that because U.S. power was so much greater than the Soviet power, Truman could safely try to work out a long-term settlement with Stalin—including the possible sharing of atomic secrets.[36] But such views were discarded. Kennan's analysis was accepted for a number of reasons.

First, Kennan's timing was perfect. Stalin had just stunned Washington with his "election speech" and his policies in Iran, Turkey, and Germany. Kennan immediately provided a detailed explanation for the dictator's actions. Second, Kennan's explanation was attractive because it entirely blamed the Soviet Union for the growing cold war. The alternative views suggested that the United States had also made some errors, but Washington officials did not want to hear about what they had been doing wrong since 1917. Third, "X's" suggestion that the Soviet Union be contained, and no longer negotiated or compromised with, perfectly fit Truman's and Acheson's view of Soviet issues. Of course, diplomatic talks did not end between the two superpowers in

1946–1947. But at that point, U.S. officials depended more on economic and military power than on diplomacy to deal with the Soviets, and Kennan's containment theory justified the use of such power.

That turn was nicely marked in September 1946, when Truman's special counsel in the White House, Clark M. Clifford, wrote a long policy paper for the president. Using the Long Telegram as his starting point and after talking with top officials throughout the government, Clifford concluded that the Soviets believed that a war with the capitalists was going to occur. "The language of military power is the only language" Moscow understands, he told Truman. "The main deterrent to Soviet attack on the United States, or to attack on areas of the world which are vital to our security," will not be negotiations, but "the military power of this country."[37] Truman, tired of dealing with Stalin abroad and Henry Wallace at home, was ready to act on the Kennan-Clifford advice.

CREATING THE POSTWAR WORLD:
THE TRUMAN DOCTRINE

His chance came on a wintery morning in late February 1947, when a British official drove to the new State Department building in the Foggy Bottom section of Washington. The official told Acheson that Great Britain had to pull out of Greece and Turkey. The bankrupt British admitted that they could no longer aid the conservative Greek government that had been fighting left-wing forces since 1944–1945. Nor could the British any longer help Turkey's military forces, which had come under Soviet pressure.

Acheson knew about the Greek problem. Since the Nazis had withdrawn from Greece in 1944, the British had tried to restore a monarchy. But leftist forces, headed by Communists, had fought back and had gained much support—in part because they had led the courageous underground resistance against the Nazis. By early 1947, the United States had contributed $200 million and many advisers to help the British. The leftists, however, gained strength with the help of a Communist neighbor, Marshal Tito (Josip Broz), the leader of Yugoslavia. In return, Tito hoped to include parts of Greece in a Balkan federation under his rule. Stalin had been very cool to Tito's plans. The Soviet dictator disliked Tito's personal imperialistic ambitions. Stalin wanted to run the Communist camp himself. Moreover, he had promised Churchill in 1944 to stay out of Greek affairs and had kept the promise, as even Churchill admitted.

Stalin's hands-off policy made things difficult for Truman and Acheson. They could not publicly accuse the dictator of interference in Greece because it was not true. But if they warned of Tito's interference, few Americans would care. They also faced a second problem. To prop up the Greek and Turkish governments could cost hundreds of millions of dollars. The new Republican Congress, however, intended to cut taxes for the folks back home, not increase taxes to spend dollars in countries most Americans cared little about. Congress was especially suspicious about spending large amounts for the apparent rescue of the British Empire. Americans had mistrusted that empire since 1776. And, finally, Truman had become unpopular throughout the country.

Acheson solved all these problems in a few minutes in late February. He and Truman had concluded that the British retreat opened a historic opportunity to launch an offensive against the Soviet Union. They could have solved the problem, after all, by sending Greece leftover military equipment from U.S. stockpiles from World War II. Or they could have turned the Greek problem over to the United Nations. Instead, they decided to go for broke. Acheson explained why to suspicious congressional leaders that late February afternoon. The crisis, he argued, had little to do with the British Empire but everything to do with whether Americans would contain communism. If the United States backed away, he warned, then, "like apples in a barrel infected by one rotten one, the corruption of Greece would infect Iran and all to the east." The "infection" could communize Africa, then Europe, until the United States virtually stood alone. "The Soviet Union was playing one of the greatest gambles in history at minimal cost," Acheson told his listeners. "We and we alone" could "break up the play." A stunned silence followed until the Republican foreign-policy leader, Senator Vandenberg, told Truman that if the president said that to Congress, "he would be supported."[38]

Another version had Vandenberg telling Truman that he should "scare hell out of the American people." Acheson tried to do that when writing Truman's speech that the president gave before Congress on March 12, 1947. In a brilliant move, the speech simply divided the world between "free peoples" and governments that relied upon "terror and oppression . . . the suppression of personal freedoms." Which side, Truman asked Congress in so many words, are you on? No third choice was given. Nor did the speech note that the Greek regime and the Turkish government were known for corruption and brutal oppression.

"No government is perfect," Truman admitted. He, nevertheless, demanded that Americans now choose between two "ways of life."

The president never mentioned the Soviet Union by name in the speech. Instead, he asked Congress to oppose a certain ideology wherever it appeared in the world. The commitment could be open-ended, and that deeply worried some officials. Secretary of State George Marshall and his closest adviser on Soviet affairs, Charles Bohlen, objected to Acheson's draft of the speech because it contained "a little too much flamboyant anti-communism." Even Kennan disliked such sweeping language. He especially opposed sending military aid to Turkey, which bordered the Soviet Union. Stalin might react to that aid as Truman would if Soviet military supplies suddenly appeared in Mexico. But most importantly, Kennan attacked Acheson's key assumption: the "rotten apple" theory (a version of the later "domino" theory). Kennan believed that Communist "infection" could not spread through the Middle East, for example, where devout Moslems hated the Soviets and godless communism. Nor was communism attractive enough or the Red Army strong enough to infect regions beyond.

Truman and Acheson overruled these objections. They wanted a broad call to action, not a precise analysis of the world situation. The Republicans, one delighted Democrat declared, were now to be "smoked out," for they would either have to quit posing as anti-Communists or else hand Truman the money he requested. Within weeks, the president received the $400 million he had asked for, $250 million for Greece and $150 million for Turkey. U.S. aid poured into Greece, as did 350 U.S. advisers. But the well-led leftists actually increased their strength. By late 1947, the crisis had grown until Washington officials debated whether to send in several divisions of U.S. troops. That decision could have involved the Americans in a morass resembling their later involvement in Vietnam. But that ultimate decision never had to be made. In June 1948, Tito and Stalin publicly and violently split apart. Tito fought off Soviet attempts to overthrow him, but the Yugoslav had no time to continue helping the Greek Left. By 1950, the civil war was over. In historian Lawrence Wittner's words, however, U.S. policies had helped fasten "right-wing governments and policies" on Greece.[39]

Americans also long felt the aftereffects of Truman's speech. The president's success made him increasingly popular and put him on the road to his surprising re-election in 1948. In late March 1947, he ordered a federal loyalty program—the first such program in U.S. peacetime history—to uncover possible Communists in government. The attorney general, moreover, for the first time published lists of suspected subversive organizations. Truman's order increased his power by pushing Congress to follow his lead in fighting communism. A "Red Scare" developed, a scare that Truman soon lost control of to less responsible politicians.

And there were other aftereffects. Americans, who before the speech were concerned about economic problems at home, now became excited about foreign-policy issues.[40] They were more willing to support strong anti-Communist action by the president. U.S. military and economic influence in Greece, Turkey, and the rich oil-producing areas of the Middle East also grew by leaps and bounds. The idea developed, moreover, that if Americans could win such a victory in Greece, they could win anywhere—say, in Vietnam or Korea, two areas where U.S. officials became more active in late 1947. From Truman to Ronald Reagan, presidents repeatedly revived the Truman Doctrine's specific words to justify their policies in such places as Lebanon, Southeast Asia, and Central America. As Senator J. William Fulbright wrote in the 1970s, "More by far than any other factor the anti-communism of the Truman Doctrine has been the guiding spirit of American foreign policy since World War II."[41]

CREATING THE POSTWAR WORLD: THE MARSHALL PLAN

The most spectacular spinoff of the early 1947 crisis was the Marshall Plan, a \$13 billion program that rebuilt war-devastated western Europe between 1948 and 1952. In doing so, it helped integrate that key region into a U.S.-controlled alliance against the Soviets. The roots of the Marshall Plan went back to World War II. In 1944–1945, leading U.S. business groups warned that if Americans hoped to avoid a terrible postwar depression, they had to double their merchandise exports to the then-unbelievable figure of \$10 billion. To do that, however, Europeans—virtually bankrupted by war—would have to receive loans from the United States so that they could buy American exports. In 1946, a young State Department official, Paul Nitze, estimated that the Europeans quickly needed as much as \$8 billion. The most dangerous problem, as Nitze (a former Wall Street investment broker) and business leaders saw it, was not the threat of Soviet invasion, but a European economic collapse that could turn the pivotal region toward socialism, paralyze the U.S. economy, and threaten the entire capitalist system.[42]

The State Department began developing a rescue plan at the same time (February–March 1947) that it formulated the Truman Doctrine.

Indeed, just six days before he announced his doctrine, Truman gave a speech at Baylor University that outlined the economic crisis. Not only their trade, but their very freedom was at stake, Truman told his listeners. "For, throughout history, freedom of worship and freedom of speech have been most frequently enjoyed in those societies that have . . . a considerable measure of freedom of individual enterprise." All those freedoms were, indeed, "indivisible." Nations had to cooperate to keep trade open—and not allow trade to be controlled by government interference (as in Socialist or Communist states) or tariff wars: "We must not go through the [nineteen] thirties again."[43]

The State Department's Policy Planning Staff, directed by Kennan, drew up a plan that was publicly revealed by Secretary of State George Marshall at Harvard University on June 5, 1947. Marshall warned that American prosperity depended on European recovery. That recovery, in turn, depended on a long-term program whose "initiative, I think, must come from Europe" itself. He pointedly did not exclude Soviet participation.[44] Privately, Kennan had urged Marshall to "play it straight" with the Soviet Union and exclude no one—that is, no one who would participate on certain U.S. conditions. Western Europeans and a large Soviet delegation traveled to Paris in mid-1947 to discuss the plan. Within days, however, the Soviets angrily left. Stalin had refused to agree to two particular U.S. conditions: a pooling of resources (that might, for example, use Soviet resources to help rebuild parts of western and central Europe) and open accounting so that Americans could see where their money was being spent.

Seventeen western European nations did agree to the conditions and estimated that they needed $27 billion. Truman and the U.S. Congress reduced that to $17 billion, and the final amount spent was nearly $13 billion—enough, as Marshall Plan administrator Paul Hoffman said, to "get Europe on her feet and off our backs."[45] The $13 billion was a huge amount. If Americans had wanted to repeat the plan in the late 1980s, the equivalent, relative to their gross national product, would have cost them $180 billion.

The largest amounts went to Great Britain, France, and Germany. In other words, most dollars went not to the nation with the largest Communist party (Italy), but to the key industrial nations whose recovery could lift living standards throughout the region. The effect on Communist parties was nevertheless quickly felt. The French, understanding U.S. feelings and needing dollars, kicked the Communist members out of the ruling ministry. Another result also soon appeared: the Soviets feared the sudden U.S. involvement in European recovery,

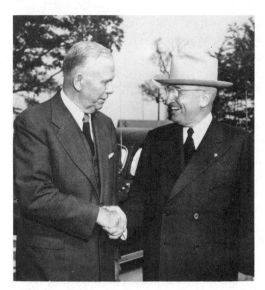

President Harry Truman (1884–1972), at right, believed General George Marshall (1880–1959) to be second only to George Washington as the greatest American. As Truman's secretary of state (1947–1949), Marshall (at left) helped fashion the Marshall Plan for rebuilding western Europe and, as secretary of defense (1950–1951), directed the U.S. effort in the Korean War. He won the Nobel Peace Prize in 1953 for the Marshall Plan. But Marshall's many accomplishments did not mean that Truman took the general's advice on such issues as the Truman Doctrine's wording or the recognition of Israel.

especially the rebuilding of a powerful West Germany. In the 1990s, a U.S. scholar, Scott D. Parrish, examined the newly opened Soviet archives to discover how Stalin and his advisers saw the Marshall Plan. Parrish concluded: "Conceived by American policymakers primarily as a defensive measure to stave off economic collapse in Western Europe," the Marshall Plan "proved indistinguishable to the Soviet leadership from an offensive attempt to subvert the security interests of the Soviet Union. The upshot was the Cold War."[46] Stalin ordered a retreat behind the iron curtain and, through Soviet-controlled trade pacts, set up a Molotov Plan to try to tie together the Communist bloc. Red Army troops cracked down on anti-Communists in Hungary. A massive ideological campaign led by Andrei Zhdanov forced a brutal conformity on eastern Europe. When Poland and Czechoslovakia hinted that they were interested in joining the Marshall Plan, Stalin ordered their leaders to forget it. In March 1948, a Red Army–supported coup overthrew what remained of Czech democracy and independence. The coup stunned the West. Truman immediately seized the opportunity to appear before Congress on March 17, 1948, and demand the passage of money bills required for the Marshall Plan. An anxious Congress soon granted his wish.

The Marshall Plan was nevertheless perhaps the greatest postwar success of U.S. diplomacy. Through it, as historian Michael J. Hogan writes, "American leaders sought to recast Europe in the image of American neocapitalism"—that is, a capitalism that combined freer trade (rather than government controls) and open-market forces. But it also demanded close cooperation between labor, owners, and government. Hogan calls this approach "corporatism." As he concludes, the Marshall Plan created "an integrated European market—one that could absorb German power, boost productivity, raise living standards, lower prices, and thus set the stage for security and recovery on the Continent."[47]

In 1947–1948, U.S. officials quickly moved to ensure that trade would remain as open and free as possible. They worked with twenty-two other nations to create the General Agreement on Tariffs and Trade (GATT). The twenty-three creators promised to abide by the most-favored-nation trade principle. That principle forced any lower tariff or trade favor given by one nation to another to be given automatically to all the other nations in GATT. The principle thus acted like a sledge hammer to knock down tariff walls and government restraints on trade. Within fifteen years, sixty-three nations controlling 80 percent of world trade belonged to GATT.[48] Using the Marshall Plan and GATT as tools, U.S. officials created a new, vast marketplace.

Truman had not been able to rip through Stalin's iron curtain and turn the entire globe into an open, capitalist trading system. But the president certainly was doing well on his side of the curtain. The Marshall Plan proved so successful that long afterward, experts preached the need for "another Marshall Plan" to solve problems in the Middle East or Vietnam or Central America. Marshall's approach, however, could only work in western Europe. Only there did a skilled labor force, a great potential industrial economy, and largely stable political societies exist. But there was a price to be paid even for this success, for the Marshall and Molotov plans sealed the division of Europe. The "two worlds" that James Monroe and other Americans had discussed during the previous 180 years now starkly appeared. Those worlds, however, were not Monroe's New and Old, but Truman's "free" and "totalitarian." Republican Senate leader Robert Taft of Ohio noted the result in 1947: "We apparently confront the Moscow challenge on every front and on every issue. It is a total 'war of nerves' at least."[49]

CREATING THE POSTWAR WORLD: LIPPMANN'S LAMENTS,
TRUMAN'S TRIUMPHS

As cold-war tensions rose, so, too, did Truman's popularity and power. In 1947, he proposed, and Congress passed, a national-security act that greatly enlarged and centralized presidential power. The former War Department and Navy Department were combined into a powerful Defense Department. The first secretary of defense was James Forrestal, a hard-line anti-Soviet official who championed Kennan and Kennan's containment theory.

The 1947 act also created the Central Intelligence Agency (the CIA) to coordinate the government's intelligence operations and give the president quick, clear information. In 1948, after the fall of Czechoslovakia to communism, Truman gave the CIA authority to conduct covert political operations—or what State Department official Dean Rusk later called the "back alley war" against communism. The secret order authorizing covert "sabotage" and "subversion" also allowed for lying, if necessary. Operations were to be "so planned and executed that . . . if uncovered the U.S. Government [can] plausibly disclaim any responsibility for them." In 1948, the CIA ran its first secret operation by intervening with money and men in Italy's elections to ensure a Christian Democratic victory over a Communist challenge. The CIA's involvement was soon discovered and condemned, especially by Italians. The irony was that the Communists would doubtless have lost even if the CIA had not intervened.[50]

The 1947 act also established the National Security Council (NSC) in the White House. Its director was to coordinate foreign-policy information and decisions for the president. At first, the NSC was a paper-shuffling agency. By the 1960s, it had become a separate and, in some ways, more powerful State Department that developed and carried out policy secretly and at the president's pleasure.

Truman was scoring victories but also coming under heavy political fire. Republican senator Robert Taft and New Deal liberal Henry Wallace became well-known critics. Taft objected that "if we assume a special position in Greece and Turkey, we can hardly . . . object to the Russians continuing their domination" in eastern Europe.[51] But the most interesting attack came from Walter Lippmann, once Woodrow Wilson's young adviser and now a conservative and the most respected of American journalists.

In a series of newspaper columns, later published in book form as

The Cold War, Lippmann tore apart Kennan's containment theory and the Truman Doctrine. Any attempt to contain communism worldwide, Lippmann warned, would wreck the Constitution by necessarily creating an all-powerful president as commander in chief. It would also hurt the U.S. market economy by regimenting it to fight the Soviets. Containment, moreover, threatened whatever good the United Nations might do, for the world organization would either have to be "cast aside like the League of Nations" or "transformed into an anti-Soviet coalition. In either event the U.N. will have been destroyed." Most importantly, he feared that Kennan's theory would militarize U.S. foreign policy instead of seeking peaceful settlements. Indeed, it would militarily link Americans to their "puppets" and "clients" on Soviet borders, whom U.S. officials would neither understand nor control. Lippmann, on the other hand, strongly approved of the Marshall Plan.[52] It aimed at economic cooperation with America's natural and traditional allies in Europe. And it did so (unlike "X's" plan) with a limited, well-planned approach.

Lippmann's attack on containment was prophetic. But within a year, his hope that the Marshall Plan could mean a revived Europe was nearly destroyed. For reviving western Europe required reviving Germany—or at least West Germany, which had been the economic generator of the region. And reviving West Germany revived the Soviet fear that a third war with a new German state could lie ahead. Truman refused to change course. Given his view of U.S. economic and security needs, he had no choice. The western zones of Germany occupied by U.S., British, and French troops were in sad shape. Their economy, indeed, rested on Lucky Strikes; the popular cigarettes were used in trade because dollars were not available and the German currency was worthless. One journalist asked sarcastically if Truman intended to revive the country by lending 50-million cartons of Lucky Strikes.[53] In June 1948, the United States suddenly introduced a new and stronger German currency that was clearly designed to undergird a unified, perhaps independent West German state.

On June 24, the Soviets cut rail and other surface traffic that linked western Germany to the western-controlled zones of Berlin, the old capital city now located deep within Communist-dominated eastern Germany. "How long do you plan to keep it up?" a top U.S. official asked a Soviet general. "Until you drop your plans for a West German Government," the Soviet replied. In March, the U.S. military governor, General Lucius Clay, had sent a secret cable that rocked Washington by warning that war "may come with dramatic suddenness."

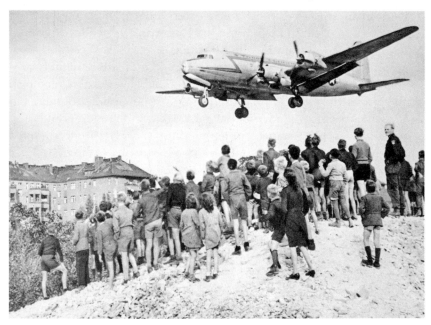

The massive airlift of supplies into crowded and besieged West Berlin in 1948–1949 was a political risk and logistical challenge that Truman and the air-force fliers braved and won. In more than 200,000 flights the pilots landed 1.5 million tons of supplies.

Clay had sent the telegram, it turned out, not because he was afraid of a Soviet attack, but merely because he had hoped to help his superiors scare Congress into appropriating more money for the military—especially for the aircraft industry, which, led by Lockheed, was pushing hard for military contracts. Secretary of Defense Forrestal, who was attracted to the idea of conspiracies like metal filings were attracted to a magnet, and who believed that the U.S. government moved only when pushed by a crisis, seized the opportunity. He helped turn Clay's telegram into a sudden war scare. Within two months Forrestal's budget for spending on military airplanes shot up 57 percent, and the Pentagon budget rose 30 percent. "No President before or since—not even Ronald Reagan at his most influential [in the 1980s]," writes historian Frank Kofsky, "has ever come close to expanding military expenditures so dramatically."[54]

The fake crisis in March quickly passed after the Pentagon budget ballooned, but the June crisis in Germany turned out to be real. If the United States retreated from Berlin, Secretary of State Marshall told Truman, it meant the "failure of the rest of our European policy."[55]

The president declared that he was determined to remain in Berlin, but he would not do so by fighting the Red Army. Instead, he ordered an airlift to fly over that army and feed the 2.2 million West Berliners. Truman, however, did dispatch sixty B-29 planes, which could carry atomic bombs, to British bases as a signal to Stalin. (Probably unknown to the Soviet dictator, Truman had only five operational bombs and never sent any of them to Great Britain.) Against tremendous odds and despite crashes and horrible winter conditions, Western pilots landed almost minute by minute in the tiny West Berlin airfield to deliver 1.6 million tons of food and fuel over the next 320 days. In May 1949, Stalin lifted the blockade.

Presidential counsel Clark Clifford had earlier told Truman that there was "considerable political advantage" in fighting the Kremlin. "In times of crisis," Clifford noted, "the American citizen tends to back up his President."[56] Sure enough, the public's approval of Truman's foreign policy rose amid the Berlin crisis and as the 1948 presidential election approached. Truman made certain that he kept the support of one key Democratic party group—the American Jewish community— by recognizing the new state of Israel on May 14, 1948, just fifteen minutes after the state declared itself to be in existence. The recognition was astonishing because Arab nations, which were good friends of the United States and whose oil was important to the West's ability to conduct the cold war, violently opposed Israel's existence. Within hours after the new state appeared, Arab armies launched a full-scale offensive to end the state's life. (The Israelis stopped the offensive during bloody fighting over the next six months until a UN-sponsored truce was called.)

Truman's recognition of Israel was even more remarkable because he ignored bitter opposition from Secretary of State Marshall (whom the president revered) and Defense Secretary Forrestal. These officials were afraid that recognition could turn the Arab oil producers against the United States. They also believed that close Soviet-Israeli ties might turn the new nation into a pro-Communist outpost in the Middle East. Marshall, instead, favored a UN-supervised trusteeship over Palestine that would have Jews and Arabs within one country, not a partitioned region with an independent Israel. State Department officials even warned Truman that Soviet Jewish agents were being infiltrated into Israel.

The president, however, listened to Clark Clifford and others who urged recognition of a separate Jewish state. Truman had long respected pro-Israeli Jews in the United States. In addition to his hope of offsetting Soviet influence, the president doubted whether Arabs and Jews could live under a trusteeship. Warren Austin, the U.S. ambassador to the UN, innocently pleaded for Jews and Arabs to act as brothers and settle their differences "in a true Christian spirit." But only worse warfare flared. Jewish voters, moreover, were crucial in New York, Ohio, Illinois, and California, and Truman certainly understood the politics. "In all of my political experience," he told a friend in 1948, "I don't ever recall the Arab vote swinging a close election."[57] The president ended up with the best of both worlds, for while he recognized Israel, the State Department and U.S. oil companies redoubled efforts to cement their ties with Arab oil producers.

As the 1948 presidential campaign accelerated, the Republican candidate, Governor Thomas E. Dewey of New York, was heavily favored over Truman—so heavily, indeed, that Dewey decided to wage only a light campaign that said little about foreign policy. Dewey believed that by avoiding a partisan position, he would be able to develop a bipartisan foreign policy with Democrats after he replaced Truman in the White House, a replacement that seemed as certain in 1948 as the New York Yankees winning the pennant.

But Truman put on a dazzling political display. He accelerated containment policies in both Europe and Asia, while telling voters that he was the one who could assure peace but that his opponent, Dewey, was a Neanderthal "isolationist" of the 1930s who could not be trusted to fight communism. As for his opponent on the Left, Henry Wallace of the new Progressive party, Truman compared him to traitors who have sold out their country. As historian Robert Divine notes, Truman used his control over foreign policy to stand firm in the Berlin crisis and make "shrewd use of the peace issue," while exploiting his recognition of Israel. The president won the most stunning political upset in twentieth-century American politics by carrying twenty-eight of the forty-eight states. He destroyed the Progressives (who won not a single electoral vote) by linking Wallace with Stalin and Molotov.[58] And Cleveland upset New York to win baseball's American League pennant.

CREATING THE POSTWAR WORLD: ALLIANCES WITH LATIN AMERICA

Truman rounded out his containment policy with two military alliances. The first, involving Latin America, did not mark a historic break in U.S. foreign policy. The second, involving western Europe, did.

U.S.-Latin American relations were never closer than during World War II, nor were they ever more one-sided. Washington gave the southern nations $450 million in lend-lease aid, but 80 percent went to Brazil—long the closest U.S. partner in the region. For their part, Latin Americans sent 50 percent of their exports to North America to help the war effort. But they received low, controlled prices for those exports. Moreover, the income turned out to be worth less after the war as inflation drove up the prices of the U.S. goods that the Latin Americans wanted to buy. Sending their goods to Europe and Asia during and after the war, North Americans simply ignored Latin America. As early as 1942, Chile's president warned that by exporting valuable copper and iron to U.S. factories but getting nothing in return, Chile was "like the 'work horse' who carries an abundance of fresh hay but is not allowed to eat it." After the conflict, Bolivia's foreign minister was asked what North American businessmen had left behind from the war effort. He replied, "empty tin cans, . . . broken-down Frigidaires, rural air strips from which their airplanes took off with their household goods, their office employees, and their blondes. In the tin and wolfram mines, cavities in the ground and cavities among the democratic workers who left their lungs behind in the tunnels in order to save democracy."[59]

One nation rebelled. Argentina, long suspicious of both U.S. and Brazilian policies, remained neutral in the war until 1944. In early 1945, Washington's pressure finally forced the Argentines to break with Germany (otherwise they would be kept out of the UN). But the nation's leader, Colonel Juan Perón, continued to defy the United States. Perón and his charismatic wife, Evita, were very popular, especially with the labor unions. The State Department believed that the Peróns were fascists. In 1946, the U.S. ambassador to Buenos Aires, Spruille Braden, made the mistake of openly opposing Perón's candidacy in the presidential elections. Perón told Argentines that they had to choose between "the pig Braden or the patriot Perón" and won a landslide victory that humiliated the State Department. But that setback was an exception. With no other real political or economic alternative in the growing cold war, most Latin Americans marched to Washington's orders. Those orders were nicely exemplified during the UN conference of 1945, when a U.S. senator grew angry after several Latin American nations defied Washington's wishes. "Your God-damned peanut nations aren't voting right," the senator told a State Department official. "Go line them up."[60] They lined up.

By using such pressure, the United States controlled a sphere of influence in Latin America as surely as the Soviets controlled their sphere in eastern and central Europe, but by quite different means. Henry Stimson worried in 1945 about U.S. officials who were "anxious to hang on to exaggerated views of the Monroe Doctrine and at the same time butt into every question that comes up in Central Europe." But not even Stimson was willing to give up either U.S. rights under the Monroe Doctrine or the U.S. belief that it had the right to intervene in central Europe.[61]

To consolidate U.S. power in the hemisphere (and to show that they were paying some attention to the region), U.S. officials, led by Secretary of State Marshall, traveled to Brazil in 1947 and signed the Rio military pact. This alliance continued the process begun in the 1930s to make the enforcement of the Monroe Doctrine a more collective, multilateral effort instead of a U.S. solo. The signatories agreed that "an armed attack by any state against an American state shall be considered an attack against all the American states." Each state would "assist in meeting the attack" whenever two-thirds of the nations voted to do so, although no one had to respond militarily unless it wished. The pact also tightened relations between U.S. and Latin American military forces. In historian David Green's words, it helped establish "Latin American dependence upon the United States" by creating "a militarily closed hemisphere under United States domination."[62]

The Rio Treaty did not satisfy Latin Americans. They wanted a new economic deal with the United States so that they could enjoy better access to U.S. markets. Washington officials flatly refused. They argued that their resources must go to Europe and that if the Marshall Plan worked, the Latin Americans would benefit by having new European markets. As the U.S. ambassador to Brazil declared, Europe suffered from "a case of smallpox," while Latin America only had "a common cold." A compromise was finally reached. At a meeting of American states at Bogotá, Colombia, in the spring of 1948, Secretary of State Marshall offered $500 million of Export-Import Bank help. It was far less than the southern nations wanted. But the parties also signed the historic charter of the Organization of American States (OAS) that created a new institution to handle hemispheric relations. Most important was the charter's Article 15, which the Latin Americans inserted over U.S. objections: "No State or group of States has the right to intervene, directly or indirectly, for any reason whatever, in the internal or external affairs of any other State." As the OAS charter was signed, massive rioting—caused in part by food shortages and aimed at the United States—erupted in Bogotá. Public buildings were destroyed, over a thousand people were killed, and the U.S. delegates were at times unable

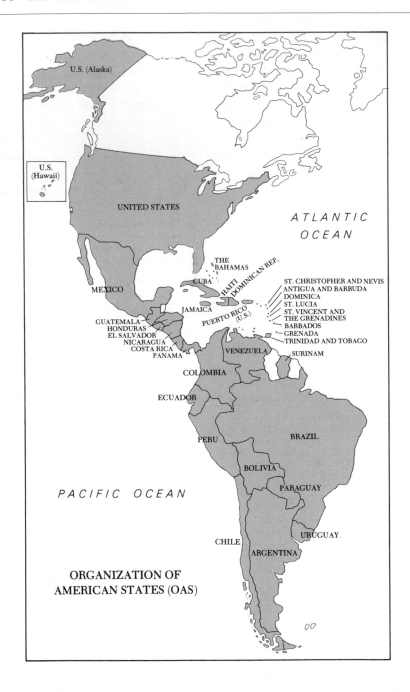

U.S. (Alaska)

U.S.
(Hawaii)

UNITED STATES

ATLANTIC
OCEAN

THE
BAHAMAS

CUBA

HAITI

DOMINICAN REP.

MEXICO

JAMAICA

PUERTO RICO
(U.S.)

ST. CHRISTOPHER AND NEVIS
ANTIGUA AND BARBUDA
DOMINICA
ST. LUCIA
ST. VINCENT AND
THE GRENADINES
BARBADOS
GRENADA
TRINIDAD AND TOBAGO

GUATEMALA
HONDURAS
EL SALVADOR
NICARAGUA
COSTA RICA
PANAMA

VENEZUELA

SURINAM

COLOMBIA

ECUADOR

PERU

BRAZIL

BOLIVIA

PARAGUAY

PACIFIC OCEAN

URUGUAY

CHILE

ARGENTINA

ORGANIZATION OF
AMERICAN STATES (OAS)

to leave their embassy.[63] Unfortunately, the riots, not Article 15, better previewed the next forty years of U.S.–Latin American relations.

CREATING THE POSTWAR WORLD: NATO

As historian Roger Trask notes, the Rio Treaty and the OAS were models "for a host of later Cold War collective defense treaties and regional organizations. They were among the earliest examples of [Truman's] implementation of the containment policy."[64] None of the treaties turned out to be more important than the one that created the North Atlantic Treaty Organization (NATO) of 1949. It was the first U.S. military alliance with Europe in 171 years.

But the 1949 pact differed from that first one made with France in 1778. Earlier, the United States was a very junior partner at the mercy of a great world power. In 1949, the United States was the greatest of all world powers. It could now dominate an alliance by using its partners to carry out U.S. foreign-policy aims. By 1948–1949, these aims in Europe were to contain the Soviet Union and to restore West German independence and economic power. The two objectives were closely related (a restored West Germany could best help contain the Soviet Union), but other western Europeans greatly feared German recovery. They not only agreed with Moscow that Germany should remain divided ("I love Germany so," a Frenchman wrote sarcastically. "Every day I thank God that there are two of them").[65] They also feared that U.S. policy was creating a powerful, armed West Germany.

Europeans moved to protect themselves. In March 1947, France and Great Britain signed the Treaty of Dunkirk to provide for their mutual defense. A year later, after the Communist takeover of Czechoslovakia and U.S. moves to build up West Germany, five European nations— Great Britain, France, the Netherlands, Belgium, and Luxembourg— signed the Brussels Pact to extend their mutual defense. U.S. officials now actively encouraged such cooperation. They saw it as the military side of the Marshall Plan. They also knew that it provided the reassurance needed as Germany recovered. In 1948, the Senate passed Senator Vandenberg's resolution that the United States become involved on the Continent, but within the broad framework of the UN Charter so that there would be no direct defiance of the world organization.

In April 1949, the NATO Treaty was signed by twelve nations—the United States, Canada, Great Britain, France, Italy, Denmark, Portugal, Norway, Iceland, Belgium, the Netherlands, and Luxembourg.

Truman's new secretary of state, Dean Acheson, signed for the United States. It was appropriate, for the pact created tight North Atlantic ties and a new military "position of strength," both of which Acheson believed to be fundamental. The partners pledged close political and economic collaboration, and "to develop their individual and collective capacity to resist armed attack." Most importantly, they agreed in Article 5 "that an armed attack against one or more of them . . . shall be considered an attack against them all." Each party would then "individually and in concert with the other Parties [take] such action as it deems necessary, including the use of armed force." The United States thus pledged to become involved in future European wars. In ratifying the treaty by an 82-to-13 vote in July, however, Vandenberg and the Senate carefully protected their own freedom of action—and tried to restrict the president's—by declaring that the constitutional "relationship" between the two branches of government remained the same. That is, Congress assumed it would continue to have the power to declare war.[66]

NATO nicely served the interests of all its members. It "kept the Russians out, the Americans in, and the Germans down," as one analysis phrases it. The French had finally succeeded in bringing Americans onto the Continent to help guarantee European security. But the United States gained the most. North Americans received valuable military bases in Europe. U.S. officials suddenly had a key role in deciding such internal European questions as "the length of military service required of each nation's troops" and even "recommendations of how much of a nation's gross national product should be dedicated to the alliance," in historian Lawrence Kaplan's words. U.S. military personnel flooded into Europe. In Norway, the sixty North Americans working with NATO were more numerous than the entire Norwegian Foreign Office.[67]

WINNING THE COLD WAR

By mid-1949, Truman and Acheson basked in the successes of their foreign policy as well as the warmth of a Washington summer. After a treacherous, unsure start in 1945–1946, Truman's doctrine, Marshall's plan, Kennan's containment theory, and Acheson's rotten-apple argument set U.S. policy on a straight course. U.S. officials did not think small. In historian Melvyn Leffler's words, they aimed for nothing less than "a strategic sphere of influence within the Western Hem-

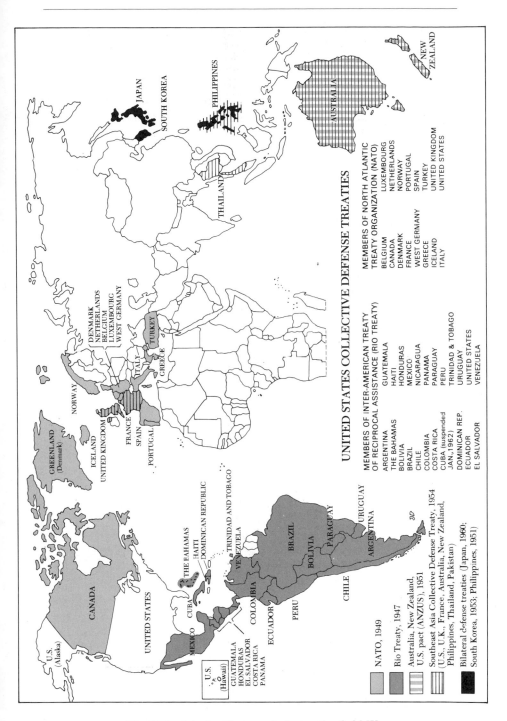

The U.S. global military web during the Cold War.

isphere, domination of the Atlantic and Pacific oceans, an extensive system of outlying bases to . . . project American power . . . , access to the resources and markets of most of Eurasia, denial of those resources to a prospective enemy, and the maintenance of nuclear superiority."[68] And they had hit all these targets by 1948. Truman's 1948 election triumph seemed both a sweet approval of past policies and a guarantee of future success.

The two cornerstones of postwar U.S. policy—a recovered West Germany and a resurrected Japan—seemed firmly in place even though both had been mortal and hated enemies of North Americans just several years earlier. Shortly after NATO came into being, the independent Federal Republic of Germany appeared. Some were afraid that Acheson's next step would be to flesh out NATO's small ground forces with West German troops. He strongly denied any such intention. Anyway, as Charles Bohlen privately told Acheson, the Soviets had already been "forced . . . from the offensive in Germany to an almost terrified defense of their control in the Eastern zone."[69]

Asia also seemed to be brightening. China might be falling to communism, but Truman could do nothing about that. In any event, the Communists would probably require decades to consolidate their power. Japan, not China, had long been the hub of Asia, and Japan was firmly in U.S. hands. That nation was again industrializing (although much too slowly), moving toward political independence, cracking down on Communist labor unions, and allowing the rebuilding of the giant Japanese corporations that could make the nation self-sufficient and a worthy friend of Washington's.

All seemed well in that summer of 1949. Truman was emerging as the winner in the cold war. Then, suddenly, in September, North Americans found themselves in new and possibly greater danger than ever before. Communists had completed their conquest of China in weeks, not decades. Much worse, the Soviets exploded their own atomic bomb. A new era had begun.

NOTES

1. Walter Z. Laqueur, "Brezhnev," *New York Times Magazine*, 17 June 1973, p. 52.
2. Diane Shaver Clemens, *Yalta* (New York, 1970), pp. 269–270.
3. Melvyn P. Leffler, "Adherence to Agreements: Yalta and the Experiences of the

Early Cold War," *International Security* 11 (Summer 1986): 88–123, a most important recent work on the disagreements, lays heavy responsibility on the United States.

4. David Reynolds, "The Origins of the Cold War: The European Dimension, 1944–1951," *Historical Journal* 28, no. 2 (1985): 500.

5. Robert M. Hathaway, *Ambiguous Partnership: Britain and America, 1944–1947* (New York, 1981), pp. 316–317.

6. Lloyd C. Gardner, *Architects of Illusion: Men and Ideas in American Foreign Policy, 1941–1949* (Chicago, 1970), ch. 5.

7. Thomas Wolfe, *Soviet Power and Europe, 1945–1970* (Baltimore, 1970), p. 33.

8. Henry L. Stimson and McGeorge Bundy, *On Active Service in Peace and War* (New York, 1949), pp. 638–650.

9. Frank Roberts to C. F. A. Warner, 19 September 1946, FO 371 N12380 / 97 / 38, Public Record Office, Kew, England.

10. V. M. Molotov, *Problems of Foreign Policy: Speeches and Statements, April 1945–November 1948* (Moscow, 1949), pp. 210–216.

11. Charles E. Bohlen, *Witness to History, 1929–1969* (New York, 1973), p. 255.

12. John Gimbel, *The American Occupation of Germany: Politics and the Military, 1945–1949* (Stanford, 1968), pp. 15–16; also see Gardner, pp. 250–256, for a good, brief discussion.

13. *Boston Globe*, 2 March 1985, p. 4; Clarence G. Lasby, *Project Paperclip: German Scientists and the Cold War* (New York, 1971), is a standard account; a new interpretation is John Gimbel, "U.S. Policy and German Scientists: The Early Cold War," *Political Science Quarterly* 101, no. 3 (1986): 433–451.

14. E. J. Kahn, Jr., "Profile," *New Yorker*, 8 April 1972, p. 61; for superb brief analyses of the FSO-Hurley fight, see Gary May, *China Scapegoat: The Diplomatic Ordeal of John Carter Vincent* (Washington, D.C., 1979), pp. 109–155; Akira Iriye, *The Cold War in Asia* (Englewood Cliffs, N.J., 1974), esp. pp. 82–83.

15. Harry S. Truman, *Memoirs*, 2 vols. (Garden City, N.Y., 1955–1956), II, pp. 90–92; the most recent authoritative account is Forrest Pogue, *George C. Marshall: Statesman, 1945–1959* (New York, 1987), pp. 54–143.

16. Steven I. Levine, "A New Look at American Mediation in the Chinese Civil War: The Marshall Mission and Manchuria," *Diplomatic History* 3 (Fall 1979): 374.

17. Tang Tsou, *America's Failure in China, 1941–1950*, 2 vols. (Chicago, 1963), II, p. 469.

18. *New York Times*, 27 October 1976, p. 44.

19. Gaddis Smith, *Dean Acheson*, vol. XVI of *The American Secretaries of State and Their Diplomacy*, ed. Samuel Flagg Bemis and Robert H. Ferrell (New York, 1972), p. 3.

20. This is discussed in David S. McClellan, *Dean Acheson: The State Department Years* (New York, 1976), pp. 30–31.

21. Dean Acheson, *Power and Diplomacy* (Cambridge, Mass., 1958), p. 29; Oral History Interview of Dean G. Acheson, 18 February 1955, Harry S. Truman Post-Presidential Papers, Truman Library, Independence, Mo.; Thomas L. Hughes, "Foreign Policy: Men or Measures?" *Atlantic* 234 (October 1974): 53.

22. Richard J. Barnet, *Roots of War* (New York, 1972), p. 121.

23. *The Pattern of Responsibility*, ed. McGeorge Bundy (Boston, 1952), p. 17; Princeton Seminar transcripts, 22–23 July 1953, Papers of Dean G. Acheson, Truman Library.

24. *Harper's Magazine* 211 (November 1955): 20; Gregg Herken, *The Winning Weapon: The Atomic Bomb in the Cold War, 1945–1950* (New York, 1980), p. 356.

25. Martin Weil, *A Pretty Good Club: The Founding Fathers of the U.S. Foreign Service* (New York, 1978), p. 258.

26. Roger Hilsman, *The Politics of Policymaking in Defense and Foreign Affairs* (New York, 1971), p. 168.

27. An original, comprehensive analysis is Mark H. Lytle, *The Origins of the Iranian-American Alliance, 1941–1953* (New York, 1987), esp. pp. xiii–xix, 156–170. Also, a key essay is Richard Pfau, "Containment in Iran, 1946: The Shift to an Active Policy," *Diplomatic History* 1 (Fall 1977): 359–372.

28. Thomas G. Paterson, *Soviet-American Confrontation: Postwar Reconstruction and the Origins of the Cold War* (Baltimore, 1973), pp. 192–193; James Forrestal, *The Forrestal Diaries,* ed. Walter Millis (New York, 1951), p. 192.

29. Dean Acheson, *Present at the Creation: My Years in the State Department* (New York, 1969, 1987), pp. 195–196.

30. Arnold A. Rogow, *James Forrestal* (New York, 1963), p. 204n.

31. William H. McNeill, *America, Britain and Russia: Their Cooperation and Conflict, 1941–1946* (New York, 1953), p. 658; Walter Bedell Smith, *My Three Years in Moscow* (Philadelphia, 1950), pp. 52–53.

32. Important analyses are Jordan A. Schwarz, *The Speculator: Bernard M. Baruch in Washington, 1917–1965* (Chapel Hill, N.C., 1981), pp. 495–505; Herken, pp. 160–190; and also David Lilienthal to Bernard Baruch, 14 April 1948, David F. Lilienthal File, Atomic Energy, Papers of Bernard Baruch, Princeton University, Princeton, N.J.

33. Allen L. Yarnell, *Democrats and Progressives: The 1948 Presidential Election as a Test of Postwar Liberalism* (Berkeley, 1974), p. 17; Henry A. Wallace, *The Price of Vision: The Diary of Henry A. Wallace, 1942–1946* ed. John M. Blum (Boston, 1973), pp. 589–601; Forrestal, pp. 206–209.

34. Urs Schwarz, *American Strategy: A New Perspective* (Garden City, N.Y., 1966), pp. 68–69; the standard account is Alice Kimball Smith, *A Peril and a Hope: The Scientists' Movement in America, 1945–47* (Chicago, 1965).

35. "X," "The Sources of Soviet Conduct," *Foreign Affairs* 25 (July 1947): 566–582; "Long Telegram" excerpts are in George Kennan, *Memoirs, 1925–1950* (Boston, 1967), pp. 547–559.

36. "The Bohlen-Robinson Report," *Diplomatic History* 1 (Fall 1977): esp. 397; a good analysis is in Robert L. Messer, "Paths Not Taken: The U.S. Department of State and Alternatives to Containment, 1945–1949," *Diplomatic History* 1 (Fall 1977): 297–319.

37. The Clifford Report can be found in Arthur Krock, *Memoirs* (New York, 1968), pp. 419–482.

38. Acheson, *Present at the Creation,* pp. 218–219.

39. Lawrence Wittner, *American Intervention in Greece, 1943–1949* (New York, 1982), p. 312. The Truman speech is in *The Record of American Diplomacy,* ed. Ruhl J. Bartlett, 4th ed. (New York, 1964), pp. 723–727; it is also given, with a commentary, in Walter LaFeber, "The Truman Doctrine," in *The Course of U.S. History,* ed. David Nasaw (Homewood, Ill., 1986), from which much of this section is drawn.

40. *Public Opinion Quarterly* 11 (Winter 1947–1948): 658.

41. J. William Fulbright, *The Crippled Giant* (New York, 1972), pp. 6–24.

42. U.S. Congress, House, 80th Cong., 1st and 2d sess., *United States Foreign Policy for a Post-War Recovery Program,* 2 vols. (Washington, D.C., 1948), I, pp. 68–81; Rich-

ard Freeland, *The Truman Doctrine and the Origins of McCarthyism* (New York, 1972), esp. chs. I and II, is a pioneering account; David W. Eakins, "Business Planners and America's Postwar Expansion," in *Corporations and the Cold War*, ed. David Horowitz (New York, 1969), pp. 143–168.

43. U.S. Government, *Public Papers of the Presidents of the United States: Harry S. Truman, 1947* (Washington, D.C., 1963), pp. 167–172.

44. The speech and an important contemporary analysis are in Joseph M. Jones, *The Fifteen Weeks* (New York, 1955), esp. appendix; also Pogue, pp. 197–217, 525–528.

45. Reynolds, 512.

46. *Los Angeles Times*, January 25, 1993, p. A4; I am indebted to Milton Leitenberg for this reference.

47. Michael J. Hogan, "American Marshall Planners and the Search for a European Neocapitalism," *American Historical Review* 90 (February 1985): 44–72, esp. 45.

48. Justus D. Doenecke, "The Most-Favored-Nation Principle," in *Encyclopedia of American Foreign Policy*, ed. Alexander DeConde, 3 vols. (New York, 1978), II, p. 608.

49. Arthur Vandenberg, *The Private Papers of Senator Vandenberg*, ed. Arthur H. Vandenberg, Jr. (Boston, 1952), p. 374.

50. Gregory F. Treverton, "Covert Action and Open Society," *Foreign Affairs* 65 (Summer 1987): 996–997, has the quote; Rusk's quote is in Lyman B. Kirkpatrick, Jr., "Intelligence and Counterintelligence," in *Encyclopedia of American Foreign Policy*, ed. Alexander DeConde, 3 vols. (New York, 1978), II, pp. 422–423. The standard account on CIA intervention in the Italian election is now James Edward Miller, *The United States and Italy, 1940–1950* (Chapel Hill, N.C., 1986), esp. pp. 248–252; an important detailed analysis is Eric Edelman, "Incremental Involvement: Italy and U.S. Foreign Policy, 1943–1948" (Ph.D. diss., Yale, 1981).

51. Lawrence S. Kaplan, *The United States and NATO: The Formative Years* (Lexington, Ky., 1984), p. 35.

52. Walter Lippmann, *The Cold War* (New York, 1947), esp., pp. 15–29, 52–59; a classic biography is Ronald Steel, *Walter Lippmann and the American Century* (New York, 1980), esp. ch. XXXIV–XXXV.

53. Richard J. Barnet, *The Alliance: America-Europe-Japan, Makers of the Postwar World* (New York, 1983), p. 40.

54. Frank Kofsky, *Harry Truman and the War Scare of 1948* (New York, 1993), ch. I; Forrestal, pp. 387, 395; Barnet, p. 46; Michael Howard, "Governor-General of Germany," *Times Literary Supplement*, 29 August 1975, pp. 969–970.

55. Forrestal, pp. 454–455, 459.

56. Yarnell, p. 37.

57. Francis O. Wilcox, *Congress, the Executive and Foreign Policy* (New York, 1971), p. 138; the Austin quote is in George T. Mazuzan, *Warren R. Austin at the U.N, 1946–1953* (Kent, Ohio, 1977), p. 99; for Marshall's opposition, see Pogue, pp. 337–375.

58. The best analysis of the foreign-policy issues is Robert A. Divine, *Foreign Policy and U.S. Presidential Elections, 1940–1948* (New York, 1974), pp. 167–276, esp. pp. 173, 262; also Yarnell, pp. 77–78.

59. Donald M. Dozer, *Are We Good Neighbors?: Three Decades of Inter-American Relations, 1930–1960* (Gainesville, Fla., 1959), ch. IV, pp. 200–201; an important analysis of the economic dimension by a top official is Laurence Duggan, *The Americas* (New York, 1949), esp. pp. 123–126.

60. Dozer, p. 200.

61. "A sphere of influence is an area into which is projected power and influence of a country primarily for political, military-strategic, or economic purposes, but sometimes cultural purposes may be added. States within the area are usually nominally independent, but the degree of influence may be so great as to leave little independence; or it may be so indirect and restrained as to permit considerable independence." John P. Vloyantes, *Spheres of Influence* (Tucson, Ariz., 1970), p. 2; Paul Keal, *Unspoken Rules and Superpower Dominance* (New York, 1983), p. 15.

62. David Green, *The Containment of Latin America* (Chicago, 1971), p. 260; the treaty's context and terms are outlined in Graham H. Stuart and James L. Tigner, *Latin America and the United States*, 6th ed. (Englewood Cliffs, N.J., 1975), esp. pp. 70, 80–85, 138.

63. Pogue, pp. 386–393.

64. Roger R. Trask, "The Impact of the Cold War on United States–Latin American Relations, 1945–1949," *Diplomatic History* 1 (Summer 1977): 284.

65. Barnet, p. 248.

66. The treaty and the Senate's declaration are in *The Record of American Diplomacy* pp. 733–736; especially important is Kaplan, chs. I and VI.

67. Lawrence S. Kaplan, "The Treaties of Paris and Washington, 1778 and 1949," in *Diplomacy and Revolution*, ed. Ronald Hoffman and Peter J. Albert (Charlottesville, Va., 1981), p. 182; the analysis quoted is by Allan R. Millett and Peter Maslowski, *For the Common Defense: A Military History of the United States of America* (New York, 1984), p. 483.

68. Melvyn P. Leffler, "The American Conception of National Security and the Beginnings of the Cold War, 1945–48," *American Historical Review* 89 (April 1984): 379, a most important essay.

69. Charles E. Bohlen to Dean G. Acheson, 9 June 1949, Bohlen Records, Box 1, Lot File, RG 59, U.S. Archives, Washington, D.C.

FOR FURTHER READING

References to specific topics can be found in the notes to this chapter and in the General Bibliography at the end of this book; most of these references are not repeated below. Three other bibliographies are important. Most detailed is the *Guide to American Foreign Relations since 1700*, ed. Richard Dean Burns (1983). J. L. Black, *Origins, Evolution, and Nature of the Cold War: An Annotated Bibliography* (1985), is exhaustive. Justus D. Doenecke, *Anti-Intervention: A Bibliographical Introduction to Isolationism and Pacifism from World War I to the Early Cold War* (1987), is indispensable, especially for references to dissenters of cold-war policy such as Senator Robert Taft.

Two new overviews are of significance, for their bibliographies as well as interpretations: Melvyn P. Leffler, *A Preponderance of Power* (1992), now the standard account for 1945–1952; and Warren Cohen, *America in the Age of Soviet Power, 1945–1991*, in *The Cambridge History of American Foreign Relations*, ed. Warren Cohen (1993). Especially helpful is Edward Crapol, "Some Reflections on the Historiography of the Cold War," *The History Teacher* 29 (1986–1987). Important biographies that cover these years include

Townsend Hoopes and Douglas Brinkley, *Driven Patriot: The Life and Times of James Forrestal* (1992); Kai Bird, *The Chairman: John J. McCloy* (1992); Thomas Alan Schwartz, *America's Germany* (1991), a fine examination of U.S. policy through an analysis of McCloy; Jean Edward Smith, *Lucius D. Clay* (1990), key on Germany but also on Clay's criticism of Kennan; H. W. Brands, *Inside the Cold War: Loy Henderson. . . .* (1991), an interesting perspective; Deborah Welch Larson, *Origins of Containment: A Psychological Explanation* (1985), for its biographical examinations; *Without Precedent: The Life and Career of Eleanor Roosevelt*, ed. Joan Hoff-Wilson and Marjorie Lightman (1984); Ronald Pruessen's standard biography, *John Foster Dulles* (1982), taking Dulles to 1952; Mark G. Toulouse, *The Transformation of John Foster Dulles* (1985), especially for the religious influences, 1947–1952; the key biographical studies of Kennan, Acheson, Lovett, McCloy, and others in Walter Isaacson and Evan Thomas, *The Wise Men: Six Friends and the World They Made* (1986); and David McCullough's popular *Truman* (1992).

On the outbreak of the cold war, key studies include U.S. Institute of Peace, *Origins of the Cold War: The Novikov, Kennan, and Roberts "Long Telegrams" of 1946* (1991), which contains important documents; James L. Gormley's succinct *The Collapse of the Grand Alliance, 1945–1948* (1987); Robert L. Messer, *The End of an Alliance* (1982), pivotal on the Truman-Byrnes relationship, as is Patricia Dawson Ward's important *The Threat of Peace* (1979); John Lewis Gaddis, *Strategies of Containment* (1982), with a suggestive overview; U.S. Department of State, *The State Department Policy Planning Staff Papers, 1947–1949*, with valuable introductions by Anna Kasten Nelson, 3 vols. (1983); Steven L. Rearden, *History of the Office of the Secretary of Defense*, Vol. I: *The Formative Years, 1947–1950* (1984), beautifully researched; Robert Conquest, *Stalin* (1991), the most recent one-volume biography; Michael M. Boll, *Cold War in the Balkans* (1984), important for its case study of Bulgaria; Robert A. Gason, "American Foreign Policy and the Limits of Power: Eastern Europe, 1946–1950," *Journal of Contemporary History* 21 (July 1986), a good overview; Edward J. Sheehy, *The U.S. Navy, the Mediterranean and the Cold War, 1945–1947* (1992), on the naval build-up; Scott L. Bills, *Empire and Cold War: The Roots of U.S.–Third World Antagonism, 1945–1947* (1990), on the Eurocentric U.S. view toward the third world between 1945 and 1947; and Chester J. Pach, Jr., *Arming the Free World* (1991), crucial for origins of military aid program, 1945–1950. The U.S. side of the nuclear-arms race is covered in Gregg Herken, *The Winning Weapon: The Atomic Bomb in the Cold War, 1945–1950* (1980), while the Soviet build-up is best traced by David Holloway's 2nd edition of *The Soviet Union and the Arms Race* (1984). Excellent biographies of Kennan provide important insights into the cold war's origins: Anders Stephanson, *Kennan and the Art of Foreign Policy* (1989); Walter L. Hixon, *George Kennan: Cold War Iconoclast* (1989); David Mayers, *George Kennan and the Dilemmas of U.S. Foreign Policy* (1989); Barton Gellmann, *Contending with Kennan* (1984); and Wilson D. Miscamble, *George F. Kennan and the Making of American Foreign Policy, 1947–1950* (1992).

On domestic issues, no one has better analyzed the impact of public opinion during these years than Thomas G. Paterson, "Presidential Foreign Policy, Public Opinion, and Congress: The Truman Years," *Diplomatic History* 3 (Winter 1979); Michael J. Heale's *American Anti-Communism* (1990) is a 140-year overview; Stephen J. Whitfield's *The Culture of the Cold War* (1990) is especially good on the late 1940s; Fred Inglis, *The Cruel Peace: Everyday Life and the Cold War* (1992); Thomas Hill Schaub, *American Fiction in the Cold War* (1991), especially on "liberal narratives" of the 1940s–1950s; Frank Ninkovich, *The Diplomacy of Ideas: U.S. Foreign Policy and Cultural Relations,*

1938–1950 (1981); and *For Better or Worse: The American Influence in the World*, ed. Allen F. Davis (1981). The last two references analyze how Americans exported their beliefs.

For U.S.-European relations, Frank Costigliola, *France and the United States: The Cold Alliance since World War II* (1992), is important and a delight to read, as is Frank Ninkovich, *Germany and the United States* (1988); *Power in Europe: Great Britain, France, Italy and Germany in a Postwar World, 1945–1950*, ed. Josef Becker and Franz Knipping (1986), is seminal for its European viewpoint and sources; *The Special Relationship: Anglo-American Relations since 1945*, ed. William Roger Louis and Hedley Bull (1986), is a distinguished overview; John W. Young, *Britain, France, and the Unity of Europe, 1945–1951* (1984), is a pivotal study on the subject; C. J. Bartlett, *The Special Relationship* (1992), is a political analysis of post-1945 Anglo-American relations; Richard A. Best, Jr., *"Co-operation with Like-minded Peoples": British Influences on American Security Policy, 1945–1949* (1986); Terry H. Anderson, *The United States, Great Britain and the Cold War, 1944–1947* (1981), stresses continuity from Roosevelt to Truman.

Many of the above citations are important for the Truman Doctrine and the Mediterranean. Lawrence S. Wittner, *American Intervention in Greece, 1943–1949* (1982), is indispensable and superb on these subjects. Other important studies include Howard Jones, *A New Kind of War: America's Global Strategy and the Truman Doctrine in Greece* (1989), placing Greece in U.S. global strategy; Theodore A. Couloumbis, *The United States, Greece and Turkey* (1983), good for the entire postwar era; and G. M. Alexander, *The Prelude to the Truman Doctrine: British Policy in Greece, 1944–1947* (1984), which gives the British side well.

On the Marshall Plan, reconstruction, Germany, and NATO, the starting place is Michael Hogan's *The Marshall Plan: America, Britain, and the Reconstruction of Western Europe, 1947–1952* (1987); other important works include Alan S. Milward, *The Reconstruction of Western Europe, 1945–1951* (1984); Sallie Pisani, *The CIA and the Marshall Plan* (1992); Carolyn Eisenberg, "U.S. Policy in Post-War Germany: The Conservative Restoration," *Science and Society* 46 (Spring 1982), a most important overview; John H. Backer, *Winds of History: The German Years of Lucius DuBignon Clay* (1984), to be used with the superb Smith and Schwartz biographies noted above; Daniel F. Harrington, "The Berlin Blockade Revisited," *International History Review* 6 (February 1984), a useful analysis and bibliography; Lawrence Kaplan, *The United States and NATO* (1984), by the leading U.S. scholar on the alliance; Jeffrey Diefendorft, *et al.*, eds., *American Policy and the Reconstruction of West Germany, 1945–1955* (1993). Along with the Edelman and Miller studies listed in the notes, a good volume on U.S.-Italian economic relations is John Lamberton Harper, *Reconstruction of Italy, 1945–1948* (1986). Extremely important is material on Truman and the CIA covered in Rhodri Jeffreys-Jones and Andrew Lownie, eds., *North American Spies* (1991).

On Asia, begin with the important essays in *Uncertain Years: Chinese-American Relations, 1947–1950*, ed. Dorothy Borg and Waldo Heinrichs (1980); Gordon H. Chang, *Friends and Enemies* (1990), on post-1948 U.S.-Chinese relations; Russell D. Buhite, *Soviet-American Relations in Asia, 1945–1954* (1981), one of the few attempts to set this in the larger context. American occupation policy in Japan is well traced in Michael Schaller, *The American Occupation of Japan* (1985); Kyoko Inoue, *MacArthur's Japanese Constitution* (1991), is a fascinating study of the language; Richard B. Finn, *Winners in Peace* (1992), is on MacArthur and Yoshida as key players; Toshio Nishi, *Unconditional Democracy: Education and Politics in Occupied Japan, 1945–1952* (1982), is a critical

Japanese view. A series of well-written and well-researched books give excellent over-views: Michael Schaller's *MacArthur* (1989); Howard Schonberger, *Aftermath of War* (1989), which is on Japan; Patricia Neils, *China Images in the Life and Times of Henry Luce* (1990); Marc S. Gallicchio's important *The Cold War Begins in Asia* (1988), espe-cially on Vincent and the China Hands; Paul G. Lauren, ed., *The China Hands' Legacy* (1987); June M. Grasso, *Harry Truman's Two-China Policy, 1948–1950* (1987), to be used with Nancy Bernkopf Tucker's definitive *Patterns in the Dust* (1983); and Gary May, *China Scapegoat* (1982), another good analysis of Vincent. A superb study is Den-nis Merrill, *Bread and the Ballot* (1990), on U.S.-Indian relations after 1947.

Hemispheric, Middle East, and African relations are discussed in the following works. A key Canadian official's view is John W. Holmes, *The Shaping of Peace* (1982), on Canada and the world, 1943–1957, especially Canada's relations with the United States; Thomas M. Leonard, *The United States and Central America, 1944–1949* (1984); Joseph Tulchin's important *Argentina and the United States* (1990), especially for the Perón showdown; and Lester Langley, *The United States and Mexico* (1991). A pathbreaking account is Thomas Borstelmann, *Apartheid's Reluctant Uncle* (1993), on U.S.–South African relations, 1945–1952, while the context is well presented in Thomas J. Noer, *Cold War and Black Liberation: The United States and White Rule in Africa, 1948–1968* (1985). For the Middle East, David S. Painter, *Oil and the American Century: The Political Economy of U.S. Foreign Oil Policy, 1941–1954* (1986), is good on the 1941–1954 years; Steven L. Spiegel, *The Other Arab-Israeli Conflict: America's Middle East Policy from Truman to Reagan* (1985), is important on domestic politics; Cheryl Rubenberg, *Israel and the American National Interest* (1986), is a critical analysis; Michael J. Cohen, *Truman and Israel* (1990), is very good, especially on the defeat of the Arabists in the State Depart-ment; and David Schoenbaum's *The United States and the State of Israel* (1993), is an important overview.

15

The Big Turn: The Era of the Korean War (1949–1952)

TWO SHOCKS AND A NEW WORLD

In early summer 1949, Americans could believe that victory in the cold war was within their grasp. They like their wars, hot or cold, the same way they like their baseball: easily understood, brief, and with a definite score at the end so that it is clear who won. By the end of 1949, however, two events—the conquest of China by Communist forces and the explosion of the first Soviet atomic bomb—so shocked Americans that they were still dealing with the results decades later.

Truman and Acheson had long known that China was lost. "We picked a bad horse," the president wrote privately in 1949. Chiang Kai-shek's (Jiang Jieshi's) Nationalist (Kuomintang or KMT) government "was one of the most corrupt and inefficient that ever made an attempt to govern a country."[1] Acheson and the president tried to prove that point by publishing a State Department white paper with vast numbers of diplomatic documents from 1844 to 1949. The white paper argued that the KMT was rotten and—more importantly—that nothing more the United States might have done could have saved Chiang. Republicans attacked Acheson for letting Chiang be driven back to the island of Taiwan by Mao Zedong's (Mao Tse-tung's) Communist armies. No serious critic, however, ever urged the only policy that might have saved the KMT: dispatching a mammoth U.S. force to China.

Giving up on Chiang as he fled to Taiwan did not mean embracing

Mao. The Soviets had played no important role in the Communist victory, but in June 1949 Mao declared that the Chinese would now "lean" toward the Soviets. At the same moment, U.S. and Chinese Communist diplomats cautiously sounded each other out about possible contacts. State Department officials encouraged further exchanges, but Truman killed the idea. The president apparently was furious with Mao's public statements, mistrusted the Communists, and feared political uproar in Washington from the Republicans. Nevertheless, as historian Nancy Bernkopf Tucker persuasively argues, Truman and Acheson carefully kept open the possibility of recognizing Mao's new government.[2] U.S. trade with the Chinese even continued well into 1950. But closer relations would require time and the capture of Taiwan by the Communists so that Chiang's embarrassing presence would finally disappear. U.S. officials believed that Communist conquest of Taiwan would occur within a year.

The possibility thus existed in 1949–1950 for the United States and the new China to recognize each other diplomatically. If it had occurred, some of the most humiliating and bloody pages in U.S. (and Chinese) history could have been prevented. But neither side moved. Mao bitterly mistrusted the country that had backed Chiang. Top Communist officials told historian Warren Cohen many years later that the last real chance of working out a deal with the Americans had occurred in 1945. When, however, both President Roosevelt and President Truman decided to stick with Chiang, the chance for friendship disappeared. By 1949, in Cohen's words, Mao was not interested in "reaching out to the United States."[3] The Chinese leader had to consolidate his control over the nation's vast expanse. He also had to get along with his giant next-door neighbor, the Soviet Union.

In Washington, Truman's anticommunism and mistrust of Mao were reinforced by those in Congress who demanded support for Chiang. One hope for friendly relations disappeared in November 1948, when the Chinese arrested and put on public trial the U.S. consul, Angus Ward, for alleged espionage activities. In January 1950, despite Acheson's direct warning, the Communists seized U.S. diplomatic buildings in the capital of Beijing (Peking). And in February 1950 came the great blow: Mao traveled to Moscow and signed an alliance with Stalin. The treaty emerged only after weeks of bitter talks (especially over Stalin's demands for territory that the Chinese considered theirs). But the West was stunned as these two powerful land masses were locked together by a joining of Communist hands.

Not even that historic event, however, proved to be as shocking as

Truman's announcement, in September 1949, that the Soviets had exploded an atomic weapon. U.S. airplanes had picked up radioactive evidence of the explosion in August. U.S. officials spent days planning how to break the news to the country. After all, many experts had predicted that Soviet scientists were not good enough to come up with such a bomb for years. Only a few U.S. scientists, led by Hans Bethe and Frederick Seitz, warned that such a secret could not be kept hidden and that Stalin could have a bomb by 1950. The Soviets were well on their way to building their own bomb, but Soviet scientists admitted in 1993 that U.S. secrets given them by a British spy, Klaus Fuchs (see below, p. 509), helped them develop a bomb two years earlier than they expected.[4] Truman broke the news in a quiet, understated announcement. But the real meanings could not be quieted: Americans and their allies were now as open to mass destruction as the Soviets had been. It "changed everything," Acheson later observed. And Truman "realized it ten seconds after it had happened, and within a month he had put the machinery of government into operation to work things out."[5]

NSC-68: WHY AND HOW THE U.S. WILL FIGHT THE COLD WAR

The U.S. response was NSC-68 (National Security Council paper 68). "This is the fundamental paper that still governs" American policy, Acheson said in 1955, and it continued to provide the United States with a plan for fighting the cold war for years to come. Many of its ideas became firmly fixed in the American mind and U.S. policy, even though it was classified top secret until 1975.

The paper was written as a result of Acheson's painful realization, in late 1949, that the cold war had entered a new stage. Fresh tactics had to be found to fight the Soviets. And fresh ideas had to be found as well to mobilize Americans so that they would wage—and pay for—that fight. Since 1947, Truman had enjoyed good relations (so-called "bipartisanship") with Congress in foreign policy. "Politics," the happy phrase went, "stopped at the water's edge." But Truman's smashing victory in 1948, Republican mistrust and dislike of Acheson, and the loss of China had made bipartisanship a dirty word to many Republicans. Acheson even had problems within his own inner circle. George Kennan wrote an anguished private letter asking that the secretary of state not allow the nation to respond to the Soviet explosion with a massive arms race, one that might include the building of a new,

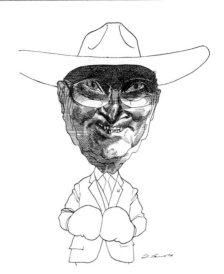

Artist David Levine catches the jaunty, combative Harry Truman, complete with sharp teeth and boxing gloves. This is the Truman who was ready to tell the Russians "to go to hell" in 1945, who became the "Give-'em-Hell Harry" in the 1948 presidential campaign, and who surprised the world with his aggressive reaction in Korea throughout 1950.

incredibly destructive "super" hydrogen bomb. Kennan, the director of the State Department's Policy Planning Staff, asked instead for a full review of U.S. policy to search for other alternatives. For some time, Acheson had been worried that Kennan was losing his appetite for standing up to the Soviets. Kennan seemed to prefer negotiations, patient talks, and turning away from an arms race. Acheson preferred "positions of strength." Kennan resigned. Acheson named Paul Nitze, a veteran hard-liner, to replace Kennan and supervise the writing of NSC-68. There was to be a fundamental review of U.S. policy, but its conclusions would be quite different from those reached by Kennan.

The final draft, which Truman initialed in April 1950, began with a series of assumptions. If you accepted these assumptions, you had little choice but to accept the policy recommendations that followed. First, NSC-68 assumed that with the destruction of German and Japanese power, and the decline of Great Britain and France, world power was being contested for only by the United States and the Soviet Union. Second, the Soviets' top priority was establishing "absolute power" over their homeland and eastern Europe, but they were being driven by communism, "a new fanatic faith" that "seeks to impose its absolute authority over the rest of the world." Third, "conflict" between the two superpowers was thus "endemic." With growing numbers of "terrifying weapons of mass destruction, every individual faces the ever-present possibility of annihilation." Fourth, the "inescapably militant" dictatorship could nevertheless be checked. Because the Soviets depended on military power to carry out their "fundamental design" in the world, they could be stopped, in turn, by U.S. military power. Finally, if this military pressure worked, there was hope, because the Kremlin's weakest link was its "relations with the Soviet people." The mass of those people supported the Kremlin leaders only out of fear. Once the United States showed that it could contain and drive back Communist power, it would also "foster the seeds of destruction within the Soviet system." NSC-68 thus aimed not just at containing the Soviet system, but destroying it.

The paper then discussed tactics. It briefly considered several options (a U.S. retreat to the Western Hemisphere or, at the other extreme, the quick launching of war on the Soviet Union) and rejected them in favor of a rapid, massive military build-up. Most importantly, Americans had to create a large and expensive conventional force of troops and weapons so that they could stop a Soviet invasion in a limited war instead of having to fight a nuclear war of "annihiliation." As part of this effort, vast alliance systems were to be established. Moreover, not only were more "atomic weapons . . . necessary," but a new "thermonuclear" bomb of much greater explosive power had to be built—especially to "bring increased pressure on the U.S.S.R." Such a plan required huge sums of money, but Acheson and Nitze believed that Americans could increase their military spending by four times (from $13 billion to about $50 billion). Massive spending, unheard of in peacetime, could actually help the U.S. economy, they argued, because that economy was slowing and might face a depression unless it was spurred on by much larger military budgets. As historian Melvyn Leffler concludes, "What was new about NSC-68 was that Nitze simply called for more, more, and more money . . . to achieve the goals already set out. He envisioned higher taxes, and he thought that domestic social and welfare programs might have to be curtailed."[6]

Until this vast rearming occurred, no diplomatic talks with Stalin could be useful. He only understood power. However, if the Soviets were so militant that the United States had to conduct a long build-up before negotiating, there might not be any talks for years or decades. There was also the danger that such a build-up to fight a militarized cold war could undermine the U.S. constitutional system. Conservative journalist Walter Lippmann had made such an argument two years earlier (see p. 484). But that danger did not bother Nitze and Acheson. To the contrary, NSC-68 declared that anything goes: "The integrity of our system will not be jeopardized by any measures, covert or overt, violent or nonviolent, which serve the purposes of frustrating the Kremlin design." That optimism was to be severely tested.

In secret discussions, some U.S. officials strongly attacked these policies. Secretary of Defense Louis Johnson, for example, questioned whether the nation could (or should) spend such money to fight a global conflict. Thus, it was Acheson's State Department, not the military, that led the drive in 1949–1950 to militarize U.S. foreign policy. Even within the State Department, however, George Kennan and Charles Bohlen attacked NSC-68. These two top experts on the Soviets not only felt that Stalin had little intention of conquering the world, but had no capability of doing so. Stalin had far too many problems at home and in eastern Europe. Kennan especially feared that the militarization of U.S. foreign policy would destroy possible diplomatic solutions and, instead, lock the world into a horror-filled, decades-long cold war. Acheson overruled these and other objections. He obtained Truman's assent to the document in April 1950, but Truman wanted to know the exact cost of NSC-68 before he gave final approval.

THE DECISION TO BUILD THE "SUPER": ATOMIC POLICY (1945–1952)

In January 1950, however, Truman had already accepted one key conclusion of the paper. A thermonuclear, or hydrogen, bomb had to be built. He made the decision after long, intense wrangling among his advisers, but he believed that he had no other option. Because the Soviets might build one, the United States had to build one first.

Since 1945, moreover, U.S. military plans had assumed that such weapons would be used to resist any Soviet aggression. Of course, some embarrassing problems appeared in these early years. Secret U.S. war plans of 1946–1947 assumed that in a war, the United States would win by destroying seventeen key Soviet cities with atomic bombs. The problem was that the U.S. Air Force had no more than a dozen bombs. Moreover, these were disassembled weapons that were stored in New Mexico and that required nearly forty men over two weeks to put together. As late as mid-1947, Truman and his closest advisers did not know officially how many such weapons they had.[7]

These weird policies began to change with the Berlin crisis of 1948. Truman then had to think seriously about responding with atomic bombs. Tests earlier that year, moreover, had produced a technological breakthrough that allowed cheaper construction of more—and more efficient—bombs. The president also locked himself into dependence on the weapons when he insisted that the military budget be tightly controlled. Running for election in 1948, he wanted to give voters a balanced budget. But the decision forced him to move away from more expensive conventional forces and rely on the bomb. Late in 1948, the administration finally prepared a top-secret paper on the use of such weapons. In the event of war, the paper concluded, the bombs must be ready for quick deployment, and only the president should decide when and where to use them. Congress and the American people might consider this "annihilation without representation," but no alternative existed. In 1949 Truman told his advisers, "Since we can't obtain international control we must be strongest in atomic weapons."[8]

He thus ordered more atomic bombs to be built. Experts, however, concluded that in the foreseeable future the president would never have enough to bomb the Soviets into submission. At this point, scientists, led by Edward Teller, tried to convince Truman that an even more destructive weapon could be built. The atomic bomb worked on the principle of fission, in which a nuclear explosion is created by splitting atoms. The new bomb was to work on the principle of fusion, in which a fission explosion served only as the trigger to force light atoms to fuse together to form heavier atoms and thus set off a thermonuclear blast, which resembles the process that creates heat from the sun. Energy in atomic bombs was measured in kilotons, or a force equal to thousands of tons of TNT. But the energy in the superbomb was to be measured in megatons, or millions of tons of TNT.

Teller quickly met strong opposition from scientists led by J. Robert Oppenheimer, who had directed the U.S. effort to build the atomic bomb in 1942–1945. The opponents did not believe such a superbomb could be built. Even if it could be constructed, they argued, it would lead to an endless arms race. Scientific advice was so united in opposing the "super" that, as scientist Hans Bethe recalls, "we were really shocked when President Truman decided in favor of a crash program."[9] Teller's determination, Truman's growing dependence on such weapons, and the arguments appearing in the NSC-68 drafts shaped the president's January 1950 decision. The opponents next begged Truman in 1952 not to test the new weapon. They argued that since testing was necessary to produce a usable bomb, if neither the Americans nor the Soviets tested, an all-out arms race could be stopped. Nevertheless, the United States tested the "super" in 1952. The Soviets set theirs off a year later. And within twenty-five years, at least five more countries had tested such a weapon.

McCarthy, Acheson, and the Call to Action

As NSC-68 and the hydrogen bomb were being born, Acheson decided to deliver a series of speeches in early 1950 to warn Americans of the new dangers—indeed, to scare them into supporting new, more active policies. Too long, he noted later in the 1950s, U.S. officials were merely "trying to guess where each play [of the Soviets] would come through the line." But "no team can win a pennant this way. No team can win a pennant unless the hometown rooters give it every possible financial and moral support."[10]

But Acheson suddenly discovered "the hometown rooters" giving cheers he disliked. In January 1950, headlines announced that Alger Hiss had been convicted of perjury. Hiss was a symbol of the "Eastern Establishment"—an elegant, Ivy League–educated State Department official who had been with Roosevelt at Yalta in 1945. Journalist Whittaker Chambers claimed that in the 1930s Hiss had been a fellow Communist party member who passed secret government documents to him. Hiss denied it, but a young California Republican congressman, Richard Nixon, pursued him until documents hidden in a hollowed-out pumpkin on Chambers's farm convinced a jury that Hiss had lied when he denied that he had been a Communist. Nixon, overnight a national hero, declared that a "conspiracy" existed to keep Americans from "knowing the facts."[11] He hinted that communism had scored recent successes because of traitors within the U.S. government. Acheson, who barely knew Hiss, nevertheless loyally declared out of friendship for Hiss's family that "I do not intend to turn my back on Alger Hiss" and was promptly damned by congressional and newspaper critics. That same month (January 1950), a spy ring was discovered. It included Klaus Fuchs, a British scientist who had helped develop the atomic bomb and who had passed secrets to Soviet agents. (Fuchs was arrested in England, sentenced to a fourteen-year prison term, and died in East Germany in 1988.)

That same month, a virtually unknown Republican senator from Wisconsin, Joseph McCarthy, searched anxiously for an issue to win re-election in 1952. After discarding several possibilities, he seized on the issue in the headlines. At Wheeling, West Virginia, McCarthy charged that 205 Communists had infested the State Department. He had no evidence and, when pushed for proof, quickly changed the numbers to 81, 57, and, finally, "a lot." A Senate investigation con-

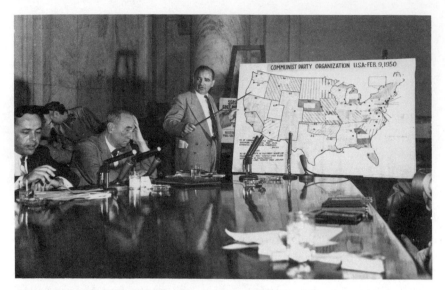

*Joseph McCarthy (1908–1957), the junior senator from Wisconsin (1946–1957),
gave his name to an era ("McCarthyism") by conducting a search for Communists within the U.S. government that uncovered no security risks, but nearly
destroyed the spirit of the Foreign Service, especially among experts on Asia.
The senator succeeded in driving out the critics of U.S.–Far Eastern policies—
including those officials who wanted to work more closely with Communist
China in order to split it from the Soviets. As this photo shows, McCarthy often
used charts and documents to bolster his arguments. But on close examination,
the visual aids usually proved far less than he claimed.*

cluded that McCarthy's accusations were empty, but a phenomenon
had been launched. "McCarthyism" became a name for the 1950–
1955 era. The term meant a ruthless search for Communists, a search
usually conducted without evidence but publicly and in a manner that
destroyed the reputations of its targets. Those targets ranged from government officials to college teachers to Hollywood actors and script
writers. Highly partisan (he dubbed the Democrats the "Commicrat
Party"), McCarthy actually had little interest in policy, only in headlines. As journalist Richard Rovere observes, "He was an essentially
destructive force, a revolutionist without any revolutionary vision." In
waging his fight, McCarthy used what Rovere calls the "multiple lie"—
that is, lies of so many parts and made so rapidly that no one could
keep track of the charges.[12]

The time was perfect for McCarthy's tactics in early 1950. Even
Acheson was traveling around the country to warn the populace about
communism. After the secretary of state spoke at a U.S. governors'

conference, one listener reported that Acheson "scared the hell out of us" as he discussed the international scene. McCarthy, however, saw Communists within the government, while Acheson feared them outside the country. Even then, however, Acheson tried to educate Americans about both the reality of the danger and the limits of U.S. power. In a soon-to-be-famous speech at the National Press Club in January 1950, the secretary of state stressed two points. First, he declared that the United States intended to defend Japan. The U.S. "defensive perimeter runs along the Aleutians to Japan," he said, and then "to the Philippine Islands." Beyond that "perimeter" (for example, in Korea), Americans could make no guarantees, although they would work "under the Charter of the United Nations" to help resist any other "armed attack." Second, Acheson urged that faith be placed in Asian nationalism, not communism. He believed that nationalism would someday turn China against the Soviet Union. He noted the historic territorial disputes between those two giants, then stated: "We must not deflect from the Russians to ourselves the righteous anger, and the wrath, and the hatred of the Chinese people which must develop."[13] On the other hand, Acheson had no intention of recognizing Mao's regime in the near future.

To Acheson's mind, the central problem was Soviet power. He made many speeches during the spring of 1950, he told a friend, to convince Americans that they were involved in "a cold war" that "is in fact a real war and that the Soviet Union has one purpose and that is world domination."[14] Public-opinion polls showed that Americans were responding slightly, but neither they nor their president were ready to spend additional billions of dollars as the secret NSC-68 paper demanded. The spy trials and economic problems at home reduced Truman's personal popularity dramatically. Affairs looked bleak to Acheson by June 24, 1950.

KOREA: THE UNEXPECTED WAR

That all changed during the next forty-eight hours. Late on June 24, Acheson received the message that North Korean troops had moved in force across the thirty-eighth parallel that separated Communist North Korea and U.S.-supported South Korea. By late June 25, Truman had committed the United States to stopping the invasion. A three-year war began, a war that took 33,000 American lives, twice that number of South Korean lives, and between 1 million and 2 million North Korean and Chinese lives. The bloodshed opened a new page in the cold war. "I think we can sum it up this way," Acheson observed in 1953, "that Korea moved a great many things from the realm of theory and brought them right into . . . the realm of urgency." The war "confirmed in our minds the correctness of the analysis of NSC 68." In addition, the war meant that "the USSR was willing to use forces in battle to achieve objectives."[15] Suddenly, a worldwide military confrontation with the Soviet Union loomed.

U.S. officials were stunned that the showdown seemed to start in Korea, of all places. In 1905, the rising Japanese Empire had seized that country because, as the saying went, Korea formed "a dagger pointed at the heart of Japan." At the Tehran Conference of 1943, the Big Three promised to create a united and free Korea after the war. In truth, however, U.S. Army officers (including a future secretary of state, Dean Rusk), concluded in 1944–1945 that to avoid conflict between U.S. and Soviet armies of occupation, the thirty-eighth parallel should serve as a temporary dividing line. During the next five years that line became the permanent boundary between the two Koreas.

From the moment of Japan's surrender in 1945, both Koreas were seething, anxious problems for U.S. officials. Left-wing groups, intent on creating a mass-based, independent government, started uprisings against the U.S. occupation in late 1945. Right-wing groups armed in opposition, usually with the help of American authorities. A virtual civil war raged, a war so intense that by 1950 it had claimed about 100,000 lives. But amid the fighting, two governments emerged. In the north, the Soviets helped establish Kim Il Sung's Communist regime and, in 1948, began to withdraw their troops. In the south, the United States demanded reunification through nationwide elections supervised by the United Nations. Kim and the Soviets would have none of that, so elections in the south during 1948 produced a right-wing regime led by Syngman Rhee. Since 1919, Rhee had been a leader in the Korean independence movement. By 1948, however, U.S. officials had grown to mistrust his corruption and dependence on Washington's support. The Americans, however, could find no better alternative.[16]

They could, nevertheless, reduce their relations with Rhee. Truman's military advisers told him in 1948–1949 that Korea "is of little strategic value to the United States and that commitment to United States use of military force in Korea would be ill-advised."[17] As Soviet and U.S. troops left in 1949, even General MacArthur believed that the defense of South Korea was beyond U.S. capability. Secretary of State Acheson repeated that belief in his Press Club speech of January

1950 but did so (as noted above) with careful reservations. The Soviets continued to train and supply North Korea's army. The United States did the same for Rhee's troops, but at a much slower pace.

Kim Il Sung, watching his own military build-up while Rhee suffered ever-larger political problems in the south, concluded that the moment was ripe for a strike. The North Korean Communist believed his armies could move so rapidly that U.S. forces could not arrive in time to save Rhee. Kim traveled to Moscow twice and finally persuaded Stalin to approve the attack. Documents released in Moscow more than forty years later, however, showed that Stalin was most reluctant to go along with Kim. The Korean War, contrary to Truman's and Acheson's (and most Americans') belief, was not triggered by a militarily aggressive Stalin who commanded a monolithic Communist Empire. Instead, the Communist bloc was already fragmented, and Stalin had begun to worry deeply about the challenge that Mao's China posed to Soviet interests. The Soviet dictator feared that if he did not go along with Kim's ambitious plans, the North Korean would turn to Mao for help, and the Soviets would lose the little leverage they had on the Koreans. Stalin also feared, with good reason, that Truman was pulling Japan into a U.S. military alliance that could threaten the eastern Soviet Union. A Communist Korea could help neutralize that threat. Stalin therefore went along with Kim, but with no enthusiasm—and carefully protected himself by telling Kim the Koreans were on their own. If they ran into trouble, Stalin was not going to bail them out.[18]

Truman was tending to family business in Missouri when the invasion began. On his plane ride back to Washington, the president determined to reverse years of U.S. policy in Korea. He would stand and fight. Acheson and most (but not all) of his top aides agreed for several reasons. First, as Truman declared publicly, the invasion "makes it plain beyond all doubt that communism has passed beyond the use of subversion to conquer independent nations and will now use armed invasion and war." Force had to be met with force. Second, not just Korea, but U.S. interests everywhere seemed to be at stake. For if Stalin and Kim won in Korea, Truman believed, the Soviets would next hit more pivotal U.S. interests, especially those in Japan and western Europe. The president reached these conclusions largely through his use (once again) of history. He and his top advisers believed that Soviet policy resembled Japan's attempt to take China piece by piece in the 1930s or Hitler's similar attempt to conquer Europe. If Stalin was "appeased," as Japan had been in 1931 and Hitler had been in 1936–1938, world peace would be threatened.[19]

Truman realized that the inexperienced 95,000-man South Korean force alone could not drive back the 135,000-man North Korean army. The president also felt that the entire world's security was at risk. He asked the United Nations to support his policies. On June 25, the Security Council passed a U.S. resolution condemning the invasion and calling for a cease-fire and the withdrawal of North Korea's armies to the thirty-eighth parallel. The resolution passed only because the Soviets had earlier walked out of the Security Council to protest the exclusion of Communist China from the UN. The speed of Truman's response had taken Stalin by surprise. Forty-eight hours later, the South Koreans were in headlong retreat while suffering 50 percent casualties in the early fighting. On June 27, the Security Council passed a new U.S.-written resolution that asked members to help South Korea "repel the armed attack and to restore international peace and security in the area."[20]

Truman had already ordered U.S. naval and air power into action. The president also appointed MacArthur to be the U.S. commander of the operations. The general then took control of the entire UN effort, although he always received his orders from Washington, not the United Nations. Nevertheless, the North Koreans rolled on. Truman finally ordered U.S. combat troops into action on June 30. They and the South Koreans, supported by unchallenged U.S. air and naval units, held on grimly to a small area (the Pusan Perimeter) and then, in July and August, actually began to move to the offensive. Meanwhile, Stalin, surprised by Truman's sharp response, showed how little stomach he had for the war by ordering Soviet ships, bound for North Korea with supplies, to turn around and come back home before they might encounter U.S. ships.

THE BIG TURN OF 1949–1950: PRESIDENTIAL POWER AND THE UN

The events of 1949–1950 that included the Korean invasion transformed U.S. foreign policy. Presidential power, the United Nations, West Germany, Japan, even Vietnam—all were profoundly affected.

Truman vastly increased presidential power by sending U.S. troops to fight in Korea without following the Constitution's requirement that Congress declare war. Following Acheson's advice, the president justified his action by referring to his commander-in-chief powers (that is, his constitutional authority as the commander of U.S. military forces).

He also used the United Nations resolutions as justification for sending U.S. troops. Other presidents had used their commander-in-chief authority to deploy forces without consulting Congress, but none had involved Americans in such a long-term, costly war simply on the basis of this authority.

Truman and Acheson decided not to ask Congress to declare war because, they feared, such a declaration could easily lead to an all-out effort resembling World War II. They, instead, hoped to keep the conflict limited and short. The president accepted a reporter's suggestion that it was only a "police action," not a war. Truman also said that U.S. force merely had to defeat "a bandit raid." His confidence grew in early July 1950, when the Soviets defined the struggle as a civil war between the two Koreas. The great powers, Moscow urged, should stay out of it. Clearly, Stalin had no intention of becoming directly involved. But that raised a greater danger in Truman's mind: Korea was perhaps a trap to draw in U.S. forces while the Soviets struck in the most vital areas of Europe or the Middle East. "We are fighting the second team," Acheson warned, "whereas the real enemy is the Soviet Union."[21] Thus, he and the president wanted no congressional declaration of war on North Korea because the real war might soon erupt elsewhere. In that case, Truman told a reporter privately, the United States would abandon Korea because he wanted any showdown to come in western Europe, "where we can use the bomb."[22]

Meanwhile, Congress, at Truman's request, created ever-larger power for the president's use. During the summer of 1950, U.S. ground forces rose from 630,000 to 1 million. A volunteer army disappeared, and a military draft began to call up eighteen-year-olds. Congress did all this with remarkably little complaint. Only the Republican Senate leader, Robert Taft of Ohio, repeatedly declared that if Truman got away with sending troops to Korea without Congress's approval, the president "could send troops to Tibet . . . or to Indo-China or anywhere else in the world, without the slightest voice of Congress in the matter."[23] Until the war began to go bad in late 1950, however, most of Congress did not want to challenge the president's powers.

Taft also blasted Truman's use of the UN resolutions as a justification for sending Americans to faraway Korea. But the president and Acheson moved to increase the UN's authority. They knew that when the next crisis arose, the Soviets would probably be back in the Security Council to veto any attempt to stop a Communist invasion. The United States, therefore, proposed that if, in the future, the Security Council could not act, the General Assembly (where no veto power existed)

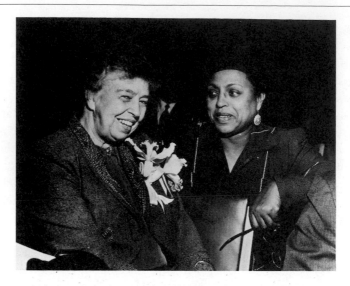

As the U.S. delegate to the United Nations General Assembly, Eleanor Roosevelt was world famous for her support of human rights and especially the rights of minorities everywhere in the world. Between 1950 and 1952, an alternate U.S. delegate was Judge Edith S. Sampson (1901–1979), shown at right with Mrs. Roosevelt. Judge Sampson was the first African-American woman elected to the Illinois court system. In the late 1940s and 1950s, as the cold war intensified, she was president of the "World Town Hall Seminar," which educated Americans about foreign-policy issues. She also traveled around the world (often at her own expense) to tell other peoples about the situation of African Americans and to answer the anti-American propaganda of Moscow radio.

could pass resolutions asking UN members to take collective action, including the use of force. This "Uniting for Peace" resolution passed in October 1950. It changed the UN. In the future, the organization could be mobilized by the United States regardless of the Soviet veto— if, that is, U.S. officials controlled a majority of the vote. They did enjoy such support in 1950. But what might occur if that majority turned neutral or even favored the Soviet case, the Americans apparently did not worry enough about in 1950.[24]

The world organization continued to be popular among Americans despite the Soviet veto. Much of this popularity was due to the work of Eleanor Roosevelt. During the 1930s and World War II, she had emerged first as a strong voice for the New Deal at home and then for cooperation abroad. After her husband's death in April 1945, Truman appointed Mrs. Roosevelt to the U.S. delegation to the United Nations. Her lectures, newspaper columns, and especially her work in drafting the UN's Declaration of Human Rights made Mrs. Roosevelt a major foreign-policy figure. She condemned the Truman Doctrine and other U.S. military acts that she believed undercut the UN's mission.[25] Rather than arguing with her (a dangerous venture for any Democratic politician), Truman used her popularity and the UN authority—but selectively, and when it was in his interest to do so.

THE BIG TURN OF 1949–1950: REMARRYING CHIANG ON TAIWAN

Truman built on decades of precedent when he multiplied his presidential powers. When making another crucial decision in June 1950, however, he broke sharply with the past. The decision involved Formosa (or Taiwan, as the Chinese preferred to call it), the large island off the China coast that Japan had controlled between 1905 and 1945. When the Korean War erupted, it was a last refuge for Chiang Kai-shek's failed forces. Some congressmen demanded that Truman protect Chiang. But the president was sick of the KMT leader; he agreed with Republican senator Arthur Vandenberg from Michigan, who said in August 1949 that sending aid to Chiang was "like sticking your finger in the lake and looking for the hole."[26] A group of U.S. military officers, led by MacArthur, also hoped to save the Nationalists. But when a senator asked in closed-door hearings whether Acheson thought it "inevitable" that the Communists would seize Taiwan, the secretary of state replied, "My own judgment is that it is."[27]

On January 5, 1950, Truman told a press conference that the United States did not want "Formosa or . . . any other Chinese territory," nor did he have any plans "at this time" to set up military bases on Taiwan. U.S. military and economic aid would not be sent to Chiang. The Korean War completely changed U.S. policy. On June 27, Truman announced that the United States opposed any Communist attempt to occupy Taiwan. He ordered the U.S. Seventh Fleet to seal off Formosa from Mao's troops. The new turn was forced by the Pentagon, which argued that the region around Taiwan formed a vital strategic area for the protection of U.S. forces in Korea. Acheson agreed for different reasons: he believed that communism must not be rewarded with new conquests, feared that if he opposed the decision he would be outgunned by the military, and understood that congressional "China-Firsters" were ready to attack him. By the end of 1950, U.S. military missions worked with Chiang's troops, and economic aid reopened.[28]

American allies, led by Great Britain, harshly criticized the new U.S.

commitment. They believed Chiang to be a lost cause and recalled the 1943 Cairo Declaration, signed by President Roosevelt, that recognized Taiwan as part of China. Acheson responded that Roosevelt never meant *this* China.

THE BIG TURN OF 1949–1950: JAPAN

With China's conquest by communism, the recently defeated Japanese became the key to U.S. policy in Asia. Acheson termed Japan "the workshop of Asia." By 1949–1950, U.S. policy makers saw it as the "stabilizer" of Asia. Historian Michael Schaller notes that Japan was to be the centerpiece of a "Great Crescent" of vital U.S. interests that stretched from the Alaskan boundary far along the vast Pacific rim to southern Asia.[29]

To make Japan the centerpiece of their policies, however, U.S. officials had to solve several problems. The first was a severe dollar shortage that threatened to paralyze the Japanese economy. The Korean War temporarily solved the problem by pouring billions of dollars into Japan, which served as the main base for UN forces. The nation's economy took off. Few booms in history match the Japanese economic expansion of 1950–1951.

Another problem was how to give Japan its independence but keep U.S. military bases on both the home islands and Okinawa, the strategic Japanese-populated island in the western Pacific. In early 1950, Acheson asked John Foster Dulles to find a solution to this dilemma. A leading Republican, Dulles helped restore some of the bipartisan spirit in Washington. An experienced diplomat and a famed international lawyer, Dulles had the necessary background. In early 1951, he solved the problem by convincing the government of Shigeru Yoshida—a shrewd and daring prime minister who was the key founding father of postwar Japan—to make a deal. The Japanese could have full independence if, in return, they agreed to create a small "self-defense" army and sign a ten-year treaty (that could be renewed) guaranteeing U.S. bases in Japan and Okinawa. Dulles pulled off the deal, moreover, while excluding the Soviets from any involvement.

Finally, when Yoshida indicated that he was thinking of opening trade relations with Japan's old economic partner, China, Dulles quickly stopped it. Any arrangement between Japan and the Communists could upset U.S. plans and anger Congress. In the so-called Yoshida Letter, the Japanese government indicated that it would work with Chiang and not with Mao. Yoshida signed the letter despite his belief that geography and economic need would soon force Japan and China to work together. As historian Howard Schonberger concludes, the deal brought Japan into "the American-sponsored economic and political blockade" of China but frustrated and angered the Japanese.[30]

In completing the peace treaty, Dulles encountered strong opposition from Australia and New Zealand, who, with fresh memories of Japanese invaders half a dozen years before, feared a revived Japan. The United States responded by creating the ANZUS (Australia, New Zealand, and the United States) Treaty in 1951. It provided for collective security in the region. The pact clearly signaled that Americans had replaced the British as the protector of Australia and New Zealand, both of whom were members of the British Commonwealth.

In all, Dulles and Acheson pulled off a most successful work of diplomacy. Ronald Pruessen, as Dulles's major biographer, writes that the Japanese peace treaty "is justifiably seen as a major landmark in the diplomatic history of the post–World War II era" and that Dulles was a "supervisor" of the pact's construction.[31] One more foundation stone was now required to complete the structure in the Pacific. It turned out to be one of the costliest pieces of work in U.S. history.

THE BIG TURN OF 1949–1950:
INDOCHINA AND SOUTHEAST ASIA

Long before the Korean War, U.S. officials concluded that if Japan were to recover, it needed Southeast Asia's markets and raw materials (including rich stores of tin, oil, natural rubber, and rice). Between 1931 and 1945, the Japanese had, indeed, tried to conquer that region. Now, as Dulles and others in Washington believed, if Southeast Asia were not open to their enterprise, the Japanese would turn to Communist China or would have to dump their goods on the U.S. market. But (as usual) there were problems. Much of Southeast Asia was underdeveloped and needed economic aid. In his so-called Point Four proposal of 1949, Truman suggested a "bold new program" to make U.S. science and technology available for such "underdeveloped areas" as Southeast Asia. However, Congress's reluctance to spend money, coupled with the Korean War's expenses, stunted Point Four's good idea from the start.

Most importantly, the region was in political turmoil. European colonial powers had controlled much of the area since the nineteenth century. Japan's occupation profoundly shook the colonial hold and encouraged nationalisms to emerge. In such nations as Malaya, Indochina, and Indonesia, that nationalism was often headed by leftists whom Americans feared. In Indonesia (Southeast Asia's largest country)—or the Dutch East Indies, as it had long been known—nationalists moved to overthrow the shell of Dutch colonialism. The United States mostly stood aside until 1947–1949, when it became clear that the Dutch could not maintain control and—of special importance—that further warfare could alienate the rising nationalists from the West's interests in the cold war. The United States then got tough. In historian Robert McMahon's words, Washington's pressure, "more than any other factor . . . compelled the Dutch to make key concessions."[32] The new sovereign nation of Indonesia appeared in 1949.

The story was less happy in Indochina. France's colonial hold on Vietnam, Laos, and Cambodia slipped under military blows struck by nationalists led by Ho Chi Minh. Because of those setbacks and U.S. pressure, the French promised autonomy to that country in early 1949, but the promise was empty because foreign policy and defense were to remain under France's control. Ho fought on. Paris officials then brought in an Indochinese, Bao Dai, to put a native face on the French-controlled government. But Bao Dai, who notably liked to spend his time on the French Riviera, could not compete with Ho's popularity and growing power.

The United States generally backed France despite at least eight requests from Ho to Washington for support of Vietnam's independence. None of these requests was answered. U.S. intelligence reported in late 1948 that Ho was not anti-American and that little evidence existed that he was under Moscow's control. That view changed, however, as China became Communist and Acheson became secretary of state. Ho must be an "outright Commie," Acheson cabled U.S. diplomats in Indochina in May 1949. The "question whether Ho [is] as much nationalist as Commie is irrelevant. All Stalinists in colonial areas are nationalists."[33] Acheson, moreover, needed France's help for his plans to build NATO and a revived West Germany. To obtain that help, the secretary of state actively supported the French war against Ho. U.S. involvement deepened in late 1949, when Acheson concluded that the victorious Chinese Communists might turn south in search of new lands to conquer.[34]

Japan's need for Southeast Asia sealed the U.S. commitment to France.[35] On March 10, 1950 (more than three months before the Korean War began), Truman sent the first major U.S. military aid to Indochina. Acheson knew that a chance was being taken, but he believed it necessary. The Korean outbreak led Truman to send much more help to the French. Ho was, after all, "a Moscow-trained Communist," and he already controlled in various degrees "more than two-thirds" of Vietnam. "Unavoidably, the United States is, together with France, committed in Indochina."[36] Or so the top U.S. policymakers believed.

Acheson saw no other way out. The situation was bad, but the stakes were great. As a joint State Department–Defense Department mission reported to him in December 1950: "America without Asia will have been reduced to the Western Hemisphere and a precarious foothold on the western fringe of the Eurasian continent. Success will vindicate [and] give added meaning to America and the American way of life."[37]

THE BIG TURN OF 1949–1950: REARMING WEST GERMANY

But Acheson also determined to hold and expand that "precarious foothold" on the "western fringe" of Eurasia. The new NATO military alliance was of little help. In early 1950, its badly equipped 12 divisions faced 27 ready Soviet divisions. Even before the Korean conflict, Acheson hinted to the new West German government that West Germany might have to rearm because only its people could provide the troops NATO needed. But Acheson could do little more. Although the Pentagon wanted West Germany to rearm, Acheson's State Department was badly split. Some officials feared the French, not to mention the Soviet, reaction if West Germans again held arms.

War in Korea forced a decision. If Communists used force in Asia, Acheson reasoned, they might well use it in central Europe. Moreover, the western Europeans were frightened of a possible Soviet move and they had to be reassured. Most importantly, however, the time was ripe to flesh out NATO. At a meeting with the French and British foreign ministers at the Waldorf-Astoria Hotel in New York City during September 1950, Acheson suddenly proposed West German rearmament. He urged that it be controlled, however, by placing the Germans within an integrated European army. No separate national German force would be created.

The stunned French foreign minister, Robert Schuman, had a habit of talking slowly (so slowly, one observer noted, that his voice sounded like a motor running out of gas). But on this occasion, Schuman rapidly made it clear that France wanted to kill the U.S. plan. Acheson, in turn, made it equally clear that West Germany would be rearmed. If the French did not wish to help set the controls on Germany, the Americans would go ahead on their own. In October 1950, the cornered French proposed the Pleven Plan: all forces, including West German, were to be integrated into the smallest possible unit of a European army, and the force was to be almost entirely controlled by Europeans (not by Americans, whom Paris officials suspected were dangerously pro-German). Thus, the argument took shape. It was to last four more years, but the West Germans were finally rearmed.[38]

Meanwhile, Truman acted alone to beef up NATO. In late 1950, he announced "substantial increases" in U.S. troop strength in Europe. Republicans, led by Senator Taft, exploded. They argued that the war was in Asia, not Europe, and that Truman was using Korea as an excuse to lock the United States into a declining Europe. They also condemned him for abusing his commander-in-chief powers again and ignoring Congress's wishes. A compromise was soon worked out: only four U.S. divisions were to be sent; Truman named General Dwight D. Eisenhower, hero of both Republicans and Democrats, to be NATO's supreme commander; and the president indicated that he would not again send troops without consulting Congress. He also agreed with Congress's and the Pentagon's wish that Greece and Turkey be brought into NATO, and that closer ties be established with Spain. Truman did not like the last part. He despised Spain's dictator, General Francisco Franco, who had cooperated with Hitler during the war. But containing the Soviets did demand a price, so as Truman swallowed hard, U.S.-Spanish relations grew warmer.

As for West Germany, its aged chancellor, Konrad Adenauer, especially profited from the U.S. proposals. Adenauer cleverly denied wanting his nation armed so soon after World War II. In truth, he was like a boy wanting to be coaxed to eat ice cream. As the top U.S. official in West Germany, John McCloy, pushed Adenauer to accept rearmament. Adenauer, in turn, demanded more independence, a navy, a German general staff, and equal rights in any European force. In one agreement alone, McCloy made 122 concessions to obtain the German leader's cooperation. The joke soon circulated that "Adenauer is the real McCloy."[39] In Paris, however, no Frenchman joked about the sharp turn taken by the United States toward Germany.

THE BIG TURN OF 1949–1950:
ROLLBACK AND THE START OF A TWENTY-YEAR
U.S.-CHINA CONFLICT

The new U.S. policies climaxed in late summer 1950, when Truman decided to cross the thirty-eighth parallel (which had separated North and South Korea since 1945), liberate North Korea, and drive to the very borders of China. The American policy of containment was to be replaced by a new idea of rollback. The Communists were to be removed, not merely contained, and Truman intended to roll them back to the borders of the two Communist giants themselves, the Soviet Union and China.

It was a historic gamble, but the odds seemed to favor the president. By mid-July 1950, General MacArthur's UN forces had stopped the North Korean invasion. Washington officials divided over the next step. Dean Rusk, assistant secretary of state for the Far East, and John Foster Dulles wanted to go on and take North Korea. They were joined by military officials from the Pentagon. Paul Nitze and George Kennan warned, however, that crossing the thirty-eighth parallel could anger European allies (who wanted no further Asian involvement) and cause the Chinese or Soviets to react. Truman and Acheson decided to go ahead with the new strategy as long as MacArthur did not meet heavy resistance, especially from Chinese troops.[40]

The president decided that he need not fear a Soviet response. Stalin had carefully distanced himself from the conflict. Nor did the president fear a massive Chinese move into Korea. Mao's troops, after all, had just emerged from a long, bitter civil war, and they had no air force to protect them against U.S. bombing. But Truman did fear attacks from Republicans and other critics at home. Senator Joseph McCarthy was again riding high by late summer. In July, Julius Rosenberg was arrested for passing atomic secrets to the Soviets. (He and his wife, Ethel, were later executed amid bitter dispute over their guilt.) Panic was setting in. When five people wrote "PEACE" on a wall in Brooklyn, a judge sent them to jail because he suspected that they were Communists.[41] By autumn, polls showed that nearly two-thirds of Americans wanted to drive the Communists out of all of Korea. On September 11, 1950, Truman approved instructions giving MacArthur permission to cross the thirty-eighth parallel.

Any doubts about the crossing disappeared four days later when

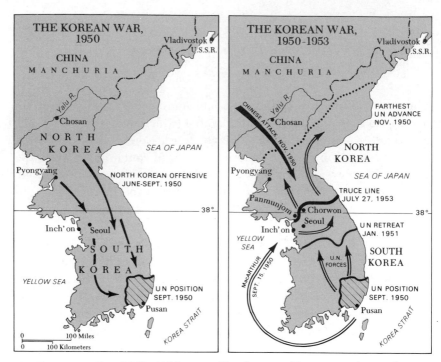

The Korean conflict (1950–1953) was a bloody yo-yo-like war, as the northern Communists nearly expelled the U.S.–South Korean forces and, in November, the UN forces nearly conquered all of North Korea only to have the Chinese human-wave attacks nearly seize all of Korea in early 1951. A two-year stalemate then ensued largely along the original dividing line between North and South Korea—the thirty-eighth parallel.

MacArthur surprised the North Korean force with a brilliant landing at Inch'on. He had cut them off, although main Communist forces slipped through and lived to fight again. The general triumphed despite warnings from Washington that the Inch'on operation was too dangerous and should not be attempted. His top field commander later wrote that MacArthur's reputation became so glorious after Inch'on that if, in another invasion, he had "suggested that one battalion walk on water to reach the port, there might have been someone ready to give it a try."[42] On October 7, the UN passed a U.S.-written resolution permitting MacArthur's army to push into North Korea. Such allies as the British, French, and Canadians had strong reservations, but Acheson overrode them and the allies reluctantly went along.

By mid-October, the UN force rapidly drove toward the Chinese-Korean border. To double-check the risks, Truman flew 6,000 miles to confer with MacArthur on Wake Island. The general assured the president that "we are no longer fearful of [Chinese] intervention." If Mao's troops did enter Korea, U.S. air power ensured that "there would be the greatest slaughter."[43] Throughout August to early October, Chinese officials warned UN forces against marching to the Yalu River that formed the China-Korea border. Truman and Acheson discounted the warnings. As the U.S. First Cavalry Division drove across North Korea, however, the first Chinese troops appeared on October 16. After a ten-day pause in which Mao was probably checking the U.S. reaction, MacArthur's attack continued. On October 26, the Chinese began to move in force. MacArthur marched on and, in defiance of Truman's orders, allowed U.S. and other non-Korean troops to approach China's borders. On November 24, the general announced an "end-the-war offensive." The boys, he declared, were to be home by Christmas.

The Chinese, however, had decided they would pay any price to prevent a permanent U.S. force on their northeast border of Manchuria. Fragmentary documents released by the Chinese in the early 1990s revealed that on October 13, 1950, Mao wrote Prime Minister Zhou Enlai (Chou En-lai): "If we do not send troops, allowing the enemy to press to the Yalu border and the arrogance of reactionaries [that is, Mao's political enemies] at home and abroad to grow, this will be disadvantageous to all sides. Above all it will be most disadvantageous to Manchuria; all of the South Manchurian electricity will be threatened." Mao concluded "we must enter the war" even if Truman ordered the bombing of Chinese cities. Otherwise, as the Chinese leader wrote on October 2, "Korean revolutionary power will suffer a fundamental defeat and the Americans will run more rampant. . . ." Mao's most frightening moment occurred, not because of Truman, however, but because of his supposed friend, Stalin. With a Chinese offensive scheduled for October 15, Stalin, at the last minute, refused to supply the air cover and supplies Mao believed he needed. The Soviets wanted no part of a confrontation with the United States. Perhaps Stalin also figured that if Mao's forces were crushed by MacArthur's, the main challenge to his own control of international communism would also be crushed. Mao quickly reassessed the situation and decided that the offensive nevertheless had to be ordered. It began on October 19, 1950, as 260,000 Chinese troops began to move into Korea.[44]

On November 26, hundreds of thousands of Chinese troops stormed UN positions in waves. Some 20,000 U.S. and South Korean soldiers were trapped at the Chosin Reservoir by 120,000 Chinese as a deadly winter began. The First Marine Division fought its way out over 78 miles of narrow road that was made a living hell by deep ravines, 2,500-foot cliffs, and 30-degrees-below-zero blizzards. A medic tending wounded soldiers dipped his fingers in blood to keep them warm. One company went into battle with 225 men, came out with 7, and lost 4 commanding officers in an hour.[45]

The marines finally got out, bringing their wounded with them, but with heavy losses. Throughout North Korea, Chinese "volunteers" (Mao's government carefully tried to maintain the fiction that its own troops were not directly involved) cut MacArthur's overextended supply lines and smashed UN forces. When the general demanded an air attack on China's home bases and the bridges across the Yalu, Truman allowed only the southern half of the bridges to be bombed. Nothing in China proper was to be attacked. The president feared that such strikes could bring the Sino-Soviet alliance into play and create all-out war between the two superpowers. Moreover, so much air power would be needed to bomb China effectively that U.S. forces in Europe would be denuded and leave that most vital of all regions open to Soviet attack.

The last days of 1950 were among the worst in American history. UN casualties in just two days rose to over 11,000. In a November 30 press conference, Truman mentioned that the use of the atomic bomb in Korea had always been under consideration. A stunned world response led the White House to downplay the remark. Behind the scenes, however, officials were, indeed, seriously debating whether to give China a warning to withdraw or else face the "prompt use of the atomic bomb."[46]

The British prime minister, Clement Attlee, quickly flew to Washington to stop any policy that was to end in an atomic fireball. Attlee was reassured about that possibility, but he failed to persuade Truman and Acheson that a political compromise had to be reached with China. Acheson strongly argued that Chinese military aggression must not be rewarded with political concessions (for example, China's entry into the United Nations). U.S. credibility in Europe, Acheson added, would be badly damaged if U.S. credibility in Korea were not defended. His comments meant that there would be more war. Attlee's remarks meant that the closest U.S. allies doubted the wisdom of Truman's policies. By late December, Chinese and North Korean troops drove back across the thirty-eighth parallel. UN forces finally stabilized the battlefront with a successful spring offensive in 1951, but costly fighting continued for another two years. And for the next twenty years, the United States and China were to be bitter enemies. A century of the open-door policy had somehow climaxed in a generation of hatred.

McCarthy and MacArthur

The Korean War gave new life to McCarthyism. Republicans won major congressional victories in the 1950 elections, and observers noted that key politicians who had opposed McCarthy went down to defeat. Of special interest was Helen Gahagan Douglas's loss to Richard Nixon in a no-holds-barred Senate contest in California. McCarthy's crusade soon spread to other causes. Book burners, for example, tried to ban the story of Robin Hood (which, after all, preached the Communist doctrine of taking from the rich and giving to the poor). Racists seized on McCarthyism to argue, in the words of one Washington state legislator, that "if someone insists there is discrimination against Negroes in this country . . . there is every reason to believe that person is a communist." In lighter moments, when college men began to leap into

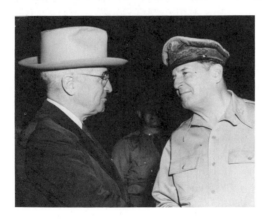

President Truman and General MacArthur had little liking for each other (contrary to this picture). But Truman flew thousands of miles to meet with the general at Wake Island in October 1950, only to receive bad information and worse advice from MacArthur about possible Chinese intervention. As Truman privately described the meeting: "We arrived at dawn. Gen. MacArthur was at the airport with his shirt unbuttoned, wearing a greasy ham and eggs cap that evidently had been in use for twenty years. . . . The General assured the President that the victory was won in Korea . . . , and that the Chinese Communists would not attack." (Longhand Notes, 1950, PSF: Long Hand Notes, 1945–1952, Box 333, Harry S. Truman Papers, Harry S. Truman Library, Independence, Missouri.)

women's dormitory rooms to conduct panty raids, one observer declared that this was the only outlet for student energy because McCarthyism had imposed "a vast silence" on students and had made serious work impossible.[47] As McCarthy continued to flay Acheson for "losing" China, Truman defended his secretary of state by responding, "If communism were to prevail," Acheson "would be one of the first, if not the first, to be shot by the enemies of liberty and Christianity."[48] It was not one of the more profound debates in American history.

In this context of McCarthyism and war with China, the president raised a political fire storm by firing General MacArthur. Since mid-1950, the general had publicly disagreed with Truman's policies of fighting a limited war, not bombing China itself, and not allowing Chiang Kai-shek's Nationalist exiles on Taiwan to become involved in the fighting. MacArthur's miscalculations about a possible Chinese invasion shook the president's confidence in his commander.

In March 1951, Truman took steps to open truce talks with North Korea, but MacArthur undercut the president by declaring that North Korean and Chinese armies should surrender before they collapsed. Truman was furious but did little. During early April, Republican leader Joseph W. Martin, congressman from Massachusetts, released a letter from MacArthur. It declared that "we must win. There is no substitute for victory." Truman now had enough. He carefully consulted with his top military officers (the Joint Chiefs), who agreed that MacArthur should be recalled. They concluded he had undercut his civilian commander in chief and, of special importance, was losing the confidence of his own troops in Korea. As MacArthur's replacement, Truman named General Matthew Ridgway, a hero of World War II, the top field commander in Korea, a soldier who was totally loyal to his civilian superiors. As Truman nicely explained privately, "I was sorry to have to reach a parting of the way with the big man in Asia but he asked for it and I had to give it to him."[49]

The American people also "gave it to him" on his return—huge ticker-tape parades, rallies, pro-MacArthur hysteria in cities from San Francisco to Boston. But as is often the case when Americans respond wildly to a supposed hero, they cooled off after listening closely to what he said. In the public "MacArthur hearings" of spring 1951, Americans could listen to a congressional investigation of the war. The general eloquently described the terrible bloodshed that, in his view, demanded total victory. But tough questioning revealed that such a victory was impossible without all-out war with China. Moreover, he wanted power placed in military hands and taken from civilians. MacArthur dis-

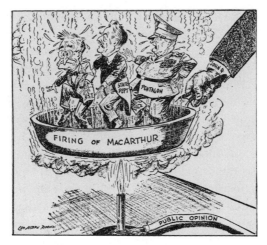

A cartoonist critical of Truman's decision to fire MacArthur in April 1951 warns that public opinion will make the president suffer for his act. Note the duck-tailed figure resembling Acheson.

missed any possibility of Soviet intervention despite the Sino-Soviet alliance. He had not been in the United States for more than thirteen years, and his answers indicated that he was out of touch with American feelings.

In rebuttal, Acheson and top U.S. military officials blistered MacArthur's position by emphasizing that a costly all-out war with China had to be avoided. Such a conflict would lose the support of the European allies. The chairman of the Joint Chiefs, General Omar Bradley, condemned MacArthur's desire for total war in Asia as "the wrong war, at the wrong place, at the wrong time, and with the wrong enemy."[50]

On April 19, 1951, in an eloquent speech before a hushed joint session of Congress, MacArthur presented his case for winning. He then recalled an old West Point song that said, "Old soldiers never die, they just fade away." Much to Truman's relief—and MacArthur's surprise—the general did exactly that.

CONCLUSION: THE BIG TURN OF 1949–1951

The twenty months between the announcement of the Soviet A-bomb explosion in September 1949 and the fading away of MacArthur in June 1951 marked a major turn in American diplomatic history. NSC-68 provided the guidelines for the next generation of U.S. policy. The document urged a quadrupling of defense expenditures. When Truman achieved that goal with a $50 billion figure in 1952, the modern defense budget was born. The nation made its first significant military commitments to both Vietnam and Taiwan. West Germany was put on the road to rearmament. Japan became independent and agreed to allow long-term U.S. military bases on its territory. Power in the United Nations began moving from the Security Council (where the Soviets could use their veto) to the General Assembly. Presidential power soared as Truman, without obtaining a congressional declaration of war, took Americans into a long war on the Asian mainland. Civilian control of the military was reaffirmed in the MacArthur-recall episode.

But Truman and Acheson also suffered telling setbacks. Americans were to pay dearly for extending containment to Vietnam and Taiwan. In the nearer term, Truman's exercise of presidential powers and his dismissal of MacArthur triggered a political reaction that made it impossible for him to seek re-election in 1952. The war, moreover, had unleashed McCarthyism. Hollywood films recorded the turn. The pro-Soviet *Song of Russia* of World War II was replaced by *The Red Menace* (1949) and *I Was a Communist for the FBI* (1951), in which Communists usually appeared slovenly, overly fat, or effeminate—but always dangerous.[51] On the Senate floor, McCarthy unleashed vicious attacks on Acheson and Marshall. In one speech, the senator made up the story of a wounded Korean veteran, "Bob Smith, from Middleburg, Pa.," who had been trapped at the Chosin Reservoir:

> His hands and his feet are still in the hills on this side of the Yalu—a tribute to the traitorous Red Communist clique in our State Department, who have been in power ever since before the days of Yalta. I suggest that when the day comes that Bob Smith can walk, when he gets his artificial limbs, he first walk over to the State Department. . . . He should say to Acheson: "You and your lace handkerchief crowd have never had to fight in the cold, so you cannot know its bitterness. . . ." He should say to him, "Dean, thousands of American boys have faced those twin killers [of bullets and freezing] because you and your crimson crowd betrayed us."[52]

Such attacks soon drove some of the most experienced and knowledgeable officers out of the Foreign Service. Former Secretary of State James Byrnes tried to defend one victim by saying that since the officer "was reared in the state of Georgia, he could not be expected to have any Communist tendencies."[53] But that defense did not work either.

McCarthyism, the Truman-Acheson-MacArthur errors in trying to take North Korea, the Chinese invasion—all combined into a highly perilous venture. "The Korean war," historian William Stueck writes, "stands as the most dangerous armed conflict" in the entire post-1945 era. Several times between November 1950 and early 1953, Stueck notes, U.S. officials discussed expanding the war beyond Korea, "which would have made a direct confrontation with the Soviet Union difficult to avoid."[54] In 1952, Republican presidential nominee Dwight D. Eisenhower swept into the White House with the assurance that he would stop the war but protect U.S. interests. The Republican platform promised to "end neglect of the Far East which Stalin has long identified as the road to victory over the West." That proved to be a big job, even after Stalin suddenly disappeared from the scene.

NOTES

1. Margaret Truman, *Harry S. Truman* (New York, 1973), pp. 449–450.
2. Nancy Bernkopf Tucker, *Patterns in the Dust: Chinese-American Relations and the Recognition Controversy, 1949–1950* (New York, 1983).
3. Warren Cohen, "Conversations with Chinese Friends," *Diplomatic History* 11 (Summer 1987): 283–289. Parts of this argument are outlined in Cohen's widely used text, *America's Response to China*, 2d ed. (New York, 1980), pp. 200–207.
4. Jeremy Bernstein, *Hans Bethe, Prophet of Energy* (New York, 1980), p. 88; *New York Times*, 14 January 1993, p. A12.
5. Oral History interview of Dean Acheson, 16 February 1955, Harry S. Truman Post-Presidential Papers, Harry S. Truman Library, Independence, Mo.
6. NSC-68 can best be found in a well-edited version, and with the important supporting documents, in U.S. Department of State, *Foreign Relations of the United States, 1950*, 8 vols. (Washington, D.C., 1977), I, pp. 234–292; Melvyn Leffler, *A Preponderance of Power* (Stanford, 1992), p. 356.
7. David A. Rosenberg, "American Atomic Strategy and the Hydrogen Bomb Decision," *Journal of American History* 66 (June 1979): 62–67; David Alan Rosenberg, "The Origins of Overkill: Nuclear Weapons and American Strategy, 1945–1960," *International Security* 7 (Spring 1983): 11–15.
8. Rosenberg, "The Origins of Overkill," 21–22.
9. Bernstein, p. 94.
10. Princeton Seminar, 10–11 October 1953, Papers of Dean Acheson, Harry S. Truman Library.
11. Stephen E. Ambrose, *Nixon: The Education of a Politician, 1913–1962* (New York, 1987), pp. 205–206.

12. Richard N. Rovere, *Senator Joe McCarthy* (New York, 1959), pp. 8, 110.
13. Gaddis Smith, *Dean Acheson, The American Secretaries of State and Their Diplomacy*, Vol. XVI, ed. Samuel Flagg Bemis and Robert Ferrell (New York, 1972), p. 135, analyzes the speech.
14. U.S. Department of State, I, pp. 206–209.
15. Princeton Seminar, Acheson Papers.
16. This story is well told in Bruce Cumings's pioneering *The Origins of the Korean War* (Princeton, 1981), esp. chs. IV–VI and X–XII, on the 1945–1947 years, and *Child of Conflict: The Korean-American Relationship 1943–1953*, ed. Bruce Cumings (Seattle, 1983), in which Cumings, Stephen Pelz, John Merrill, and James I. Matray contribute key essays on pre-June 1950 events.
17. Richard E. Neustadt and Ernest R. May, *Thinking in Time: The Uses of History for Decision-Makers* (New York, 1986), pp. 34–35.
18. Nikita Khrushchev, *Khrushchev Remembers*, ed. and trans. Strobe Talbott (Boston, 1970), pp. 367–373; the newly released documents are discussed in *Los Angeles Times*, 25 January 1993, p. A4. I am indebted to Milton Leitenberg for this reference.
19. Glenn D. Paige, *The Korean Decision, June 24–30, 1950* (New York, 1968), pp. 132–133, 174–177; Smith, pp. 185–186.
20. The important UN and U.S. documents of late June 1950 can be found in *The Record of American Diplomacy*, ed. Ruhl J. Bartlett, 4th ed. (New York, 1964), esp. pp. 768–769.
21. Steven L. Rearden, *The Evolution of American Strategic Doctrine: Paul H. Nitze and the Soviet Challenge* (Boulder, Col., 1984), p. 30; Neustadt and May, p. 43.
22. Arthur Krock, *Memoirs* (New York, 1968), p. 260.
23. Robert A. Taft, *A Foreign Policy for Americans* (New York, 1957), pp. 21–36.
24. A good recent account of the resolution is in Ronald W. Pruessen, *John Foster Dulles: The Road to Power* (New York, 1982), pp. 426–431.
25. Blanche Wiesen Cook, "Eleanor Roosevelt and Human Rights," in *Women and American Foreign Policy*, ed. Edward M. Crapol (New York, 1987), esp. pp. 107–117.
26. Arthur Vandenberg, *The Private Papers of Senator Vandenberg*, ed. Arthur H. Vandenberg, Jr. (Boston, 1952), p. 536.
27. U.S. Congress, Senate, Foreign Relations Committee, 81st Cong., 1st and 2d sess., 1949–1951, *Reviews of the World Situation: 1949–1950*, Historical Series (Washington, D.C., 1974), p. 184.
28. A useful analysis, placed within the context of the Korean War, is William W. Stueck, Jr., *The Road to Confrontation: American Policy toward China and Korea, 1947–1950* (Chapel Hill, N.C., 1981), esp. pp. 137–143, 196–198.
29. Michael Schaller, *The American Occupation of Japan: The Origins of the Cold War in Asia* (New York, 1985), pp. viii–ix, 298; Richard J. Barnet, *The Alliance: America-Europe-Japan, Makers of the Postwar World* (New York, 1983), p. 94.
30. Howard Schonberger, "Peacemaking in Asia . . . ," *Diplomatic History* 10 (Winter 1986): 73; a distinguished Japanese view is in Chihiro Hosoya, "Japan's Response to U.S. Policy on the Japanese Peace Treaty . . . ," *Hitotsubashi Journal of Law and Politics* 10 (December 1981): 15–27.
31. Pruessen, pp. 459, 494–495.
32. Robert J. McMahon, "Anglo-American Diplomacy and the Reoccupation of the Netherlands East Indies," *Diplomatic History* 10 (Winter 1978): 23; and McMahon's

fine analysis, *Colonialism and Cold War: The United States and the Struggle for Indonesian Independence, 1945–49* (Ithaca, N.Y., 1981), esp. pp. 315–316; and also an early classic account, George McTurnan Kahin, *Nationalism and Revloution in Indonesia* (Ithaca, N.Y., 1952).

33. This document can be conveniently found in *Vietnam: A History in Documents*, ed. Gareth Porter (New York, 1979, 1981), pp. 79–80.

34. Thomas McCormick, "Crisis, Commitment, and Counterrevolution, 1945–1952," in *America in Vietnam: A Documentary History*, ed. William A. Williams *et al.* (New York, 1985), pp. 97–99.

35. *Ibid.*, esp. pp. 82–87, 104–111, for the key documents on the Japan–Southeast Asia connection, with commentary and editorial notes.

36. *Vietnam: A History in Documents*, p. 86.

37. U.S. Department of State, VI, pp. 164–173; quoted and analyzed in Lloyd Gardner, *Approaching Vietnam: From World War II through Dienbienphu* (New York, 1988), ch. III.

38. Barnet, pp. 123–137.

39. *Ibid.*, pp. 57–58.

40. Dean Acheson, *Present at the Creation: My Years in the State Department* (New York, 1969), pp. 452–455.

41. David M. Oshinsky, *A Conspiracy So Immense: The World of Joe McCarthy* (New York, 1983), pp. 172–173.

42. Matthew B. Ridgway, *The Korean War* (Garden City, N.Y., 1967), p. 42.

43. Omar Nelson Bradley, *Substance of Statements Made at Wake Island Conference on October 15, 1950* (Washington, D.C., 1951), esp. p. 5.

44. Allen S. Whiting, *China Crosses the Yalu* (New York, 1960), pp. 155–159; the Chinese documents and an analysis are in *The Korea Herald*, 27 February 1992, pp. 1, 5. I am indebted to Milton Leitenberg for this reference. Also of major importance is Jian, Chen, "The Sino-Soviet Alliance and China's Entry Into the Korean War," a paper published by the Woodrow Wilson Center's Cold War International History Project (Washington, D.C., 1992).

45. Michael Kernan, "The Chosin Survivors," *Washington Post*, 1 December 1984, p. D1.

46. Rosemary Foot, *The Wrong War: American Policy and the Dimensions of the Korean Conflict, 1950–1953* (Ithaca, N.Y., 1985), pp. 114–118.

47. Rovere, p. 9; Nora Sayre, *Running Time: Films of the Cold War* (New York, 1982), p. 11.

48. Press release, statement by the president, 19 December 1950.

49. Harry Truman to Dwight Eisenhower, 12 April 1951, 1916–1952 Files, Box 108, Papers of Dwight D. Eisenhower, Dwight Eisenhower Library, Abilene, Kans.

50. U.S. Congress, Senate, Committee on Foreign Relations and Committee on Armed Services, *Hearings: Military Situation in the Far East* (Washington, D.C., 1951), pp. 32, 45, 66–68, 86–87 (esp. for MacArthur's views), and 924–926 (for Acheson's reply); Allan R. Millett and Peter Maslowski, *For the Common Defense: A Military History of the United States of America* (New York, 1984), pp. 489–490.

51. Sayre, p. 80.

52. *Congressional Record* (Senate), 82d Cong., 1st sess., 24 May 1951, 97, pt. 4, p. 5779.

53. Gary May, *China Scapegoat: The Diplomatic Ordeal of John Carter Vincent* (Washington, D.C., 1979), p. 207.

54. William Stueck, "The Korean War as International History," *Diplomatic History* 10 (Fall 1986): 291; the same point is made in Coit D. Blacker, *Reluctant Warriors: The U.S., the Soviet Union, and Arms Control* (New York, 1987), pp. 71–72; and for comments on U.S. plans to use the A-bomb in Korea, see Bruce Cumings to the editor, *New York Times*, 21 June 1984, p. A22.

FOR FURTHER READING

For further reading on specific topics, consult this chapter's notes and the General Bibliography at the end of the book; these references are usually not repeated below. Most important, begin with the well-annotated entries in *Guide to American Foreign Relations since 1700*, ed. Richard Dean Burns (1983), which is exhaustive on the pre-1981 publications. See also references in chapter 14. The following are largely post-1981 accounts.

Good overviews can be found in Melvyn P. Leffler's magisterial *A Preponderance of Power* (1992); and Warren Cohen, *America in the Age of Soviet Power, 1945–1991*, in *Cambridge History of American Foreign Relations*, ed. Warren Cohen (1993); Robert J. Donovan, *Tumultuous Years: The Presidency of Harry S. Truman, 1949–1953* (1982); the early chapters in Lawrence Freedman, *The Evolution of Nuclear Strategy* (1983); Joseph M. Siracusa, *Rearming the Cold War: Paul H. Nitze, the H-Bomb and the Origins of a Soviet First Strike* (1983); and one of the most important primary sources, U.S. Congress, Senate, Foreign Relations Committee, 81st Cong., 1st and 2d sess, *Reviews of the World Situation: 1949–1950*, Historical Series (1974), in which Acheson and others become frank behind closed doors. Excellent on the subject is Ernest R. May, ed., *American Cold War Strategy: Interpreting NSC-68* (1993), as is David McCullough, *Truman* (1992).

On Asia, especially China, a useful overview is Carol Morris Petillo, "The Cold War in Asia," in *Modern American Diplomacy*, ed. John M. Carroll and George C. Herring (1986); Nancy Bernkopf Tucker, *Patterns in the Dust* (1983), is standard on U.S.-China relations, 1949–1950; June M. Grasso, *Harry Truman's Two-China Policy, 1948–1950* (1987), is key on the Truman-Taiwan relationship and based on new documents; Leonard A. Kusnitz, *Public Opinion and Foreign Policy: America's China Policy, 1949–1979* (1984), has extensive data. Joseph Camilleri, *Chinese Foreign Policy: The Maoist Era and Its Aftermath* (1980), is most important on the Chinese policies; and William A. Walker, *Opium and Foreign Policy* (1991), is a fascinating, pioneering study. The effect on the U.S. Foreign Service and foreign policy is analyzed in *The "China Hands" Legacy: Ethics and Diplomacy*, ed. Paul Gordon Lauren (1987), especially essays by May, Iriye, Hsu, Davies, Wylie; a fine case study of a central figure is Gary May, *China Scapegoat: The Diplomatic Ordeal of John Carter Vincent* (1979).

Thomas C. Reeves, *The Life and Times of Joe McCarthy* (1982), is a good narrative. *Beyond the Hiss Case: The FBI, Congress, and the Cold War*, ed. Athan G. Theoharis (1982), is crucial for understanding both the time and U.S. government policies, as is Ronald Radosh and Joyce Milton's widely noted *The Rosenberg File* (1983).

Recent research has focused on initial U.S. commitments to Vietnam to give important insights into U.S. policy more generally in Asia (especially Japan) and, indeed, worldwide. Seminal are William S. Borden, *The Pacific Alliance: U.S. Foreign Economic Policy and Japanese Trade Recovery, 1947–1955* (1984); Andrew J. Rotter, *The Path to Vietnam: Origins of the American Commitment to Southeast Asia* (1987); Gary R. Hess, *The U.S. Emergence as a Southeast Asian Power, 1940–1950* (1986); and, for an exhaustive bibliography, *The Wars in Vietnam, Cambodia and Laos, 1945–1982*, ed. Richard Dean Burns and Milton Leitenberg (1984), with excellent cross references. One result is traced through from the Japanese perspective in Michael M. Yoshitsu, *Japan and the San Francisco Peace Settlement* (1982).

For Korea, the background is well provided in Yur-Bok Lee and Wayne Patterson, *One Hundred Years of Korean-American Relations, 1882–1982* (1986), and three indispensable books from Bruce Cumings: *Child of Conflict: The Korean-American Relationship, 1943–1953* (1983), which he edited and wrote with leading scholars, and *The Origins of the Korean War*, whose first volume on 1945–1947 appeared in 1981, and whose second volume, *The Roaring of the Cataract* (1990), is a classic study of the 1947–1952 events. Excellent on the war's diplomacy is Rosemary Foot, *The Wrong War* (1985), critical of U.S. policy. Important and useful overviews, with good bibliographical references, include Barton J. Bernstein, "New Light on the Korean War," *International History Review* 3 (April 1981); Robert Jervis, "The Impact of the Korean War upon the Cold War," *Journal of Conflict Resolution* 24 (December 1980); and Arthur A. Stein, *The Nation at War* (1980), especially useful for its suggestive approach to how the war affected U.S. society. The war's battles and attendant politics are well examined in Callum A. MacDonald, *Korea: The War before Vietnam* (1987), which ranks with the Cumings and Foot volumes as one of special importance; Bevin Alexander, *Korea: The First War We Lost* (1987), by a combat historian in the war; and Roy E. Appleman, *East of Chosin* (1987), a distinguished military history of the darkest days for U.S. forces. The role of India and Indian scholars' views on the war, U.S.-Chinese relations, and U.S.-Indian relations are central to understanding the diplomacy of the conflict and can be found in *American History by Indian Historians*, ed. Norman H. Dawes (1964); but also consult Dennis Merrill's important *Bread and the Ballot* (1990), on U.S.-Indian economic relations.

16

The Era of Eisenhower: The Good Old Days (1953–1960)

When Dwight D. Eisenhower entered the White House in January 1953, he was better prepared to handle foreign policy than any other twentieth-century president. Texas-born son of pacifist parents, "Ike" had graduated from West Point. He then lived in Asia, Latin America, Europe, and Africa as well as in Washington during the early 1930s, where, as a lobbyist for the U.S. Army, he came to know Congress well. During World War II, he commanded the greatest amphibious invasion force in history and became a world hero by liberating much of western and central Europe from Nazism. Meanwhile, he displayed rare political talent by dealing successfully with Roosevelt, Stalin, Churchill, and de Gaulle. After the war, Eisenhower served as U.S. Army Chief of Staff, president of Columbia University, and then supreme commander of Allied forces in NATO.

He was more than certain of his own abilities, but in public he called himself just "a farm boy from Kansas," where he had grown up.[1] That approach, together with his famous grin and soldierly bearing, made him the trusted father figure of the 1950s. As television ownership expanded from 9 percent of U.S. homes in 1950 to 87 percent in 1960, Eisenhower knew how to exploit the new technology. A father figure could be politically popular when the most-watched television program, "I Love Lucy," showed the laughs and happiness enjoyed by a supposedly typical American family. Ike's low-keyed manner, his apparent preference for the golf course over the White House, led observers to consider him a "national sedative." After the frenzy of 1947–1952, however, Americans were ready for a sedative.[2]

Harry Truman, who had grown to dislike Eisenhower, growled that "The general doesn't know any more about politics than a pig knows about Sunday." But Ike's vice-president, Richard Nixon, saw a different Eisenhower—a "complex," even "devious man" who approached problems from many "lines of reasoning" and preferred to be "indirect" rather than obvious and direct.[3] Nixon knew firsthand. He was never completely trusted by Eisenhower, nor did he ever fully know where he stood with the president. Nixon also learned that Ike's grin hid a boiling temper that had moved entire armies. "My God," an aide remarked after watching one explosion, "how could you compute the amount of adrenalin expended in those thirty seconds? I don't know why long since he hasn't had a killer of a heart attack."[4] Eisenhower did suffer a severe heart attack in 1955. But despite this, Americans so trusted him that they re-elected him by a landslide in 1956 in his second race against the eloquent Democratic party nominee, Adlai Stevenson of Illinois.

Eisenhower remained popular in part because foreign-policy setbacks were usually blamed on his sour, militantly anti-Communist secretary of state, John Foster Dulles. Ike's sparkle radiated next to "Dull, Duller, Dulles." One British observer reflected widespread opinion when he concluded that Dulles was not "a likeable or well-balanced personality."[5] But as Dulles himself said, his foreign policy did not aim at "winning a popularity contest. . . . I prefer being respected to being liked."[6] He was most respected by the only one who really counted: Eisenhower. The president knew that this son of a Presbyterian minister in Watertown, New York, had been closely involved with U.S. diplomacy since the first decade of the century. "Foster has been studying to be Secretary of State since he was five years old," Ike commented.[7] The president trusted Dulles to be his agent abroad. The secretary of state spent so much time going to and from airports that critics exclaimed, "Don't do something, Foster, just stand there!" But Eisenhower always controlled the policy. For his part, Dulles recalled how his uncle, Secretary of State Robert Lansing, had been fired for crossing Woodrow Wilson, and so was careful never to repeat such a mistake with Eisenhower. When both were in Washington, they often got together privately for a late-afternoon drink at the White House to exchange views.

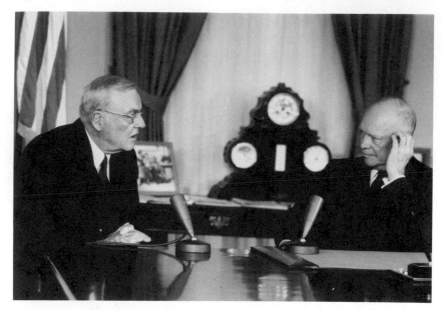

President Dwight D. Eisenhower (1890–1969), at right, and Secretary of State John Foster Dulles (1888–1959) formed the most experienced foreign-policy team in recent U.S. history. They presided over American power as it reached its peak and, by 1958–1960, was beginning a relative decline.

Besides Eisenhower's trust, Dulles enjoyed the confidence of both liberals and conservatives within the Republican party. Eisenhower thus used Dulles as lobbyist in Congress as well as a political lightning rod to deflect criticism from the presidency. Dulles worked hard shaping opinion. Privately, he could explain his policies by giving hard-headed geopolitical reasons. But publicly, he used the moral and religious reasons that he believed Americans preferred to hear, even though he was often laughed at by observers at home and overseas for mouthing platitudes. Dulles was the first secretary of state to allow reporters to quote him directly and, later, to allow television to cover his press conferences.

Eisenhower and Dulles dominated Congress, although they had to overcome two early problems to do so. The first problem was Senator Joseph McCarthy's shrill anticommunism. In one of the worst moments of his life, Eisenhower had refused to criticize McCarthy in the 1952 campaign, even though the senator had grossly defamed General George Marshall, the man who had championed Eisenhower's military career. In 1953–1954, the president kept his distance from McCarthy. And in mid-1954, the senator went too far by accusing Ike of being soft on communism and then by trying to conduct a witch hunt within the U.S. Army. In late 1954, with the elections safely past, the Senate finally found the political courage to censure McCarthy's conduct. His political power faded.

Eisenhower's second problem with Congress was the Bricker Amendment. This proposed addition to the Constitution, pushed by conservative Republican Senator John Bricker of Ohio, aimed at limiting the president's power to make executive agreements with foreign countries. More generally, its supporters wanted to ensure that no international agreements (such as those passed in the United Nations to improve the rights of women or blacks) could become law in the United States without congressional approval. Bricker mirrored the long Republican frustration with Roosevelt's deals at Yalta and Tehran. Eisenhower, who was not about to surrender any of his power, began to wonder if Bricker's supporters "had lost all their brains." Ike won a key Senate test by only one vote in 1954. But, by the end of the year, his hard lobbying in Congress made the amendment a dead issue.[8]

After that, Eisenhower controlled Congress. He held regular afternoon meetings with Democratic leaders, usually over a much-appreciated bourbon and branch water, and courted Republican leaders— even those, such as Senator William Knowland of California, for whom he had little respect. (In Knowland's case, Ike noted in his diary, there seemed to be no final answer to the question: "How stupid can you get?")[9] Eisenhower's popularity was such that polls revealed a majority of liberals thought him a liberal, and a majority of conservatives believed that he agreed with them. Thus, he and Dulles ably fashioned a bipartisan foreign policy. But, as is usually the case in American politics, bipartisan policy actually meant ever-greater presidential power.[10]

Eisenhower, nevertheless, had to work within some limits. McCarthy was dying (he passed away in 1957), but McCarthyism remained alive. Dulles tried to please fervent anti-Communists by allowing one of them, Scott McLeod, to oversee State Department personnel. As a result, hundreds left the Foreign Service, and morale and standards sank. (A bitter Dean Acheson said privately that "Dulles's people seem to me like [Russian] Cossacks quartered in a grand city hall, burning the paneling to cook with.") Asian policy especially suffered. The Committee of One Million, which appeared in the early 1950s, was a well-financed pressure group formed to help Chiang Kai-shek's (Jiang Jieshi's) exiles on Taiwan and to ensure that the United States never deal with the Chinese Communists. This "China lobby" included Republican conservatives such as Knowland as well as Democratic lib-

erals such as Senator Hubert Humphrey of Minnesota. Thus, the president had to deal with China policy gingerly.[11]

The atmosphere of the 1950s was captured in *Invasion of the Body
Snatchers*, a popular movie of the decade that tells of normal Americans being taken over by alien forces that duplicate the bodies but kill
the emotions of their victims, thus creating a society of docile, seemingly content humanoid beings. Subtly capitalizing on Americans' fears
of communism, the film drew huge audiences. A more important movie
of the 1950s, however, was *High Noon*. In it, a brave frontier marshal
(Gary Cooper) decides, despite great personal fear, to stand up to a
band of ugly, vicious villains, although the cowardly townspeople and
even his new wife (Grace Kelly) urge him to run away. The film was
written by Carl Foreman, who himself became a victim of Hollywood
McCarthyism.[12] Given the climate of the 1950s, however, whether Gary
Cooper's brave lawman represented Dwight Eisenhower or Senator
McCarthy depended on the politics of the viewer. But few doubted that
a lot of ugly villains threatened American happiness, and their numbers seemed to increase dangerously as the decade wore on.

EISENHOWER AND DULLES ABROAD:
CAPITALISM AND NUCLEAR WARS

The new president followed two principles in shaping his foreign policy. First, communism must not be allowed to expand. Second, capitalism must not go bankrupt in trying to contain communism.

Nothing, not even communism, seemed to obsess Eisenhower as much
as his fear that capitalists would ruin their system by spending too much
on defense. A sometime reader of Marx and Lenin, the president warned
that those Communists might be correct: capitalists were too "selfish,"
too willing to spend and profit now at the cost of "long-term" interest
and thus "in the long run would destroy any free economic system."[13]
Military spending that leads to inflation and waste should not be thrown
into budgets but into civilian goods. "Unless we can put things in the
hands of people who are starving to death we can never lick Communism," he told his cabinet. Worse, a militarized U.S. economy "would
either drive us to war—or into some form of dictatorial government"
and perhaps even force "us to *initiate* war at the most propitious
moment."[14] After beating back demands from Congress and private
corporations for more military spending, Ike privately exclaimed, "God

help the nation when it has a President who doesn't know as much about the military as I do."[15]

Eisenhower, therefore, searched for a cheap way to contain communism. He found it in the nation's huge nuclear superiority over the Soviets. He and his top advisers worked out the policy during mid-1953 in Operation Solarium, named for the White House sun room where the secret discussions were held. The group considered three ways to deal with the Soviet Union: continued containment largely through conventional means; telling the Soviets that nuclear weapons would be used if the Soviet Union tried to take more territory; and, finally, using all-out economic and propaganda campaigns to roll back communism. Eisenhower decided on a combination of the first two: containment and reliance on nuclear weapons, instead of fighting expensive and unpopular conventional wars (as Truman did in Korea).[16] He and Dulles also planned to build new alliance systems so that every non-Communist part of the world would be a responsibility of the United States and its allies. But above all, nuclear weapons gained new importance. As historian David A. Rosenberg concludes: "Where Harry Truman viewed the atomic bomb as an instrument of terror and a weapon of last resort, Dwight Eisenhower viewed it as an integral part of American defense, and, in effect, a weapon of first resort."[17]

This policy became known as "massive retaliation." Dulles defined it as the "free world's" ability to "retaliate, instantly, by means and at places of our own choosing." Trying to match Communists "man for man, gun for gun," he warned, meant "bankruptcy."[18] Instead, Americans should get "more bang for the buck," as the 1950s phrase went, not more expensive conventional weapons. Eisenhower, thus, had it both ways. To reduce expenditures in 1954, he cut Truman's military budget of $50 billion to $34 billion largely by reducing the number of men in the army. But to contain communism, he increased the number of nuclear warheads from 1,000 in 1953 to 18,000 by early 1961. Although U.S. superiority was already overwhelming, one additional nuclear weapon soon rolled off the American production line each day. Eisenhower also exploited new technology. In 1955, the huge B-52 bomber appeared. The eight-engine giant was the first true jet bomber designed to carry nuclear weapons (although it later became famous for destroying hundreds of square miles of Vietnam in mere minutes with conventional bombs). The two-stage ballistic missile, Polaris, capable of being fired from a submerged submarine, provided a capability in 1960 to launch a nuclear attack from deep within the oceans.

Nuclear testing by both superpowers produced an ever-larger weapon

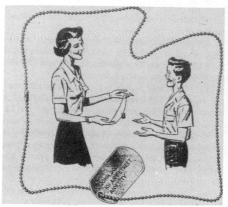
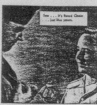
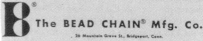

The cold war comes home. Schools prepared for possible nuclear war in the early 1950s by having students wear "dog-tags" so they could be identified after the attack.

(equal to 400 Hiroshima-type bombs). It also produced deadly radio-active fallout. As early as 1953, milk in Albany, New York, was found to contain sixteen times the normal amount of this radiation. U.S. officials lied or hid information about the effects of testing. The world shuddered in 1954, when it learned that twenty-three members of a Japanese fishing boat, the *Lucky Dragon*, innocently sailed into a U.S. nuclear testing area in the Pacific and within days became deathly ill from radiation poisoning. Testing, nevertheless, continued on both sides. American education leaders prepared school students for possible nuclear war. Youngsters in New York City, San Francisco, and elsewhere wore identification necklaces so they could be better identified in case of attack. Schools were redesigned, and windows eliminated, to protect students against radiation and fallout from nuclear war. There was no panic; instead "the threat of atomic war was domesticated," in the words of historian JoAnne Brown, and Americans were to accept the possibility of all-out nuclear conflict as part of their daily lives. By 1958, larger bombs produced so much radiation that it could more gravely threaten Americans in a future war than could enemy weapons—or so reported a U.S. Navy commander. Overruling strong objections from the Pentagon and such scientists as Edward Teller, Eisenhower, on his own, stopped testing in October 1958. Khrushchev halted Soviet testing the next month.[19]

By 1955, the president realized that growing crises in Vietnam and the Middle East might remain limited and not escalate into a direct confrontation with the Soviets. Experts, including Henry Kissinger of Harvard University, warned that the United States would face many such crises in the Third World and had to learn to fight effective "limited wars," short of an all-out nuclear exchange with the Soviet Union. But Eisenhower was determined not to become trapped in another Korea-type war that, in historian Barton Bernstein's phrase, could "drain America's resources . . . split the NATO alliance, and impair [Eisenhower's] popularity at home."[20] In 1955, the president said it directly: nuclear bombs were to be considered conventional weapons and "used just exactly as you would use a bullet or anything else."[21]

He even claimed to have secretly followed that policy in Korea. During the 1952 campaign, Eisenhower blasted the Democrats for mishandling the war. He scored a triumph by announcing that if elected, "I shall go to Korea" (although he never said what he would do after he arrived). Eisenhower did travel to Korea and decided to get tough with China. In February 1953, he announced the so-called "unleashing" of Chiang Kai-shek, who could now threaten to attack the mainland. But the crisis peaked in early summer 1953, when Eisenhower found the peace talks tied up. South Korean president Syngman Rhee refused to surrender his dream of ruling all Korea. He tried to kill the talks by freeing thousands of Chinese prisoners whom China's government wanted returned home. The Communists broke off the talks and began a military offensive. The president and Dulles hinted, through Indian officials close to the Chinese, that unless the Communists signed a truce, the United States would "not be limited" in its use of weapons. Public-opinion polls showed that a majority of Americans wanted atomic shells used. The effect of the warning is unknown. The Chinese later denied they were frightened by it. Strong evidence exists that they and the Soviets had actually decided to end the war immediately after Stalin's death three months earlier. But U.S. officials believed that the threat broke the logjam. In any case, in mid-summer both sides signed a truce, and the war finally stopped.[22]

That was not the last time Eisenhower considered "massive retaliation." In 1955, he and his advisers agreed that if China invaded Indochina, they would ask Congress for a declaration of war and then use "new weapons" on China itself. In 1958, when the Chinese shelled the small offshore islands held by Chiang Kai-shek, Eisenhower moved "tactical" nuclear weapons into place. During the Berlin crisis of 1958–1960, U.S. fighter-bombers went on regular airborne alert. Some planes carried weapons 1,000 times more powerful than the 1945 bombs. The U.S. Navy flew bombers loaded with nuclear weapons off China's coast—partly to see how Chinese radar reacted.[23]

Supporters claimed that the threat of "massive retaliation"—or, as Dulles called it, "going to the brink of war"—made the Soviets and Chinese behave. But it did not achieve Dulles's goal of "liberating" the Soviet bloc. During the 1952 campaign, he and Eisenhower had urged such "liberation," although Eisenhower emphasized that it must be done "only by peaceful means."[24] Their chance arose in spring 1953. Stalin had suddenly died in March. Frustrated East Berlin workers seized the opportunity to strike and even riot against the Communist regime. Red flags were ripped down as the protests threatened to spread. U.S.-government-sponsored radio programs egged the workers on. But when Soviet tanks suddenly appeared to smash the riots and execute the leaders, the United States did nothing except issue protests.

British Prime Minister Winston Churchill dramatically proposed that the Big Four leaders (the United States, USSR, Great Britain, and France) meet at a summit conference to discuss—and perhaps even settle—the most dangerous problems. The new Soviet leaders were clearly trying to find more effective policies (for example, they called for a Korean peace), and Churchill thought the time ripe to work with them. Eisenhower flatly refused to meet with the Soviets unless the new leaders agreed beforehand to surrender key Soviet positions on German, eastern European, atomic-energy, and Asian issues. That demand, of course, effectively killed Churchill's plan. After all, Ike told the prime minister, "Russia was . . . a woman of the streets and whether her dress was new, or just the old one patched, there was the same whore underneath."[25]

EISENHOWER AND DULLES ABROAD: REVOLUTIONS AND THE CIA

"Massive retaliation" might control the whore, but Eisenhower and Dulles knew that her supposed children—the growing number of revolutionaries in the newly emerging nations—required other kinds of action. Eisenhower understood that using nuclear weapons to defeat these rebels was as wildly out of proportion as burning down buildings to control ants. He, therefore, devised a second policy to deal with communism: covert operations handled by the Central Intelligence Agency. The policy's attractions were many: cheapness, secrecy, speed, and no need to deal with Congress. Eisenhower alone supervised the CIA's activities, working closely with its director, Allen Dulles, the secretary of state's brother. Both the president and the director had extensive experience running such covert operations during World War II. Within eighteen months after entering the White House, Eisenhower and Dulles used the CIA to destroy supposed revolutionaries in two nations.

The first was Iran. In 1951, Mohammad Mosaddeq had risen to power in that country. Described by Dean Acheson as a "pixie" with a bald, "billiard-ball head," Mosaddeq was a shrewd politician and fervent nationalist. He challenged the monopoly over his country's oil long held by the British-controlled Anglo-Iranian Oil Company. The company had exploited Iran for decades, allowing the country to have about 20 percent of the profits from its own oil. That cozy deal, however, had been jarred in 1950, when the U.S. oil company, Aramco, gave Saudi Arabia 50 percent of the profits from Saudi oil. Mosaddeq demanded the same. The British refused. In 1952, as the Iranians moved toward seizing the British company's resources, the Truman administration tried to mediate. Acheson sympathized with Mosaddeq.[26] But U.S. policy changed sharply when Dulles replaced Acheson.

The new administration feared Mosaddeq's nationalism and agreed with British warnings that he was becoming dangerously dependent on Iran's Communist party, the Tudeh. With Washington's approval, the large international oil companies cooperated to prevent Iranian oil from reaching world markets. Mosaddeq found that he could produce oil but not sell it. In early summer 1953, he asked Eisenhower for economic help. The president responded that he would be happy to provide aid after Mosaddeq reached agreement on the oil dispute. With his power slipping, Mosaddeq called a public referendum to approve his policies, then fixed the results to gain more than 95 percent of the vote, a figure Eisenhower associated with Communist elections. Having tried and failed to remove Mosaddeq, the young Mohammad Reza Shah Pahlavi, who had replaced his father as ruler of Iran, left the country suddenly for a "rest cure." As pro-Mosaddeq mobs took to the streets, Eisenhower and the British decided to move.

CIA agents found supporters in the capital of Tehran, especially in the military, then bought off other Iranians and arranged massive street demonstrations that threw the city into chaos. Mosaddeq was arrested, and the shah returned to claim his throne. (He offered a toast to the top CIA agent: "I owe my throne to God, my people, my army, and to you.") As frosting on an already rich cake, the major U.S. oil companies forced the British company to cut them in on the production of Iran's oil. Allen Dulles declared that Iran had been saved from a "Communist-dominated regime." But historian Mark Lytle offers a more accurate judgment. Knowing "almost nothing about Iran," U.S. officials overthrew a nationalist and "revered" figure, Mosaddeq. Afterward, the shah "would always seem beholden to the United States," and so both he and Americans would become targets of nationalists and Moslem fundamentalists in Iran. It was, Lytle concludes, "interventionism of the worst kind."[27]

In the poorer Central American nation of Guatemala, the CIA again overthrew a nationalist regime in the name of anti-communism. Until 1944, the ruling Guatemalan elite made up 2 percent of the population but held more than 60 percent of the land. The poorest 50 percent of the people held only 3 percent of the land but depended on the land for their food. Half the population were Indians who earned less than $100 annually and suffered brutal discrimination. In 1944, a student–middle-class revolt overthrew a corrupt, stagnant dictatorship and installed a reform-minded government. Jacobo Arbenz Guzmán came to power in 1951 after perhaps the fairest election in the country's history. He and his wife, the beautiful and wealthy Mariá Vilanova, who was determined to aid the nation's poor, especially set out to help the landless and the Indians. Among other measures, Arbenz planned to give them land by seizing 234,000 acres from the United Fruit Company (UFCO), the Boston-based "Octopus" that controlled much of the region's fruit production, transportation, and even governments. He singled out UFCO simply because it owned 42 percent of the country's arable land but was using less than 10 percent of it. Arbenz offered to pay for the land, but UFCO demanded much more.

The Dulles brothers, whose old law firm had close ties with UFCO, were afraid that the seizure of U.S. property would be copied by other governments in Latin America. But most of all, they and Eisenhower concluded that Arbenz's action indicated that Guatamala was turning Red. The country's Communist party did grow in popularity, especially in the poor rural areas and among union workers. Only four Communists, however, sat in the fifty-six-member Congress. Arbenz and his top advisers, moreover, were not Communist, nor, certainly, were the most powerful national institutions—the Roman Catholic church and the army.

Dulles, nevertheless, flew to an inter-American conference in Caracas, Venezuela, in March 1954 and demanded the condemnation of "international Communism." He obtained the resolution. But when, in May, he asked for help from the Organization of American States in taking action, the Latin Americans refused—especially after Dulles admitted that it was "impossible to produce evidence clearly tying the Guatemala Government to Moscow."[28] Deciding to go it alone, Eisenhower ordered the CIA to train Guatemalan exiles to overthrow Arbenz. The frightened Guatemalan government accepted a shipload of arms from the Soviet bloc.

That was enough for Eisenhower. In June, the CIA-led exiles moved from bases in Honduras and Nicaragua to eliminate Arbenz. The exile army nearly failed, but at the decisive moment Eisenhower ordered American-flown planes to drop small sticks of dynamite on the capital, Guatemala City. Arbenz's army then deserted him, and that desertion was the turning point. (Learning directly from this experience, Fidel Castro in Cuba during the 1960s and the Sandinista revolutionaries in Nicaragua during the 1980s made the army and their revolutionary government a single unit so that they would not be victimized as Arbenz had been.)

As Arbenz fled, the exile leader, General Carlos Castillo Armas, became president and put hundreds of Arbenz's followers in front of firing squads until the reform movement was destroyed. In 1957, one of his own palace guard murdered Castillo Armas. He was the first in a long line of military dictators who brutalized and exploited Guatemala during the next three decades. Nevertheless, in 1954, John Foster Dulles concluded that the country had been saved from "Communist imperialism" and that Castillo Armas's victory added "a new and glorious chapter to the already great tradition of the American States." He never mentioned the CIA's role. Others disagreed. Historian Richard Immerman concludes that Arbenz's attempt to end "social and economic injustice" was stopped by CIA action that "made moderation impossible" in Guatemala.[29] Philip C. Roettinger, a U.S. Marine colonel who helped overthrow Arbenz, wrote in 1986 that it turned out to be "a terrible mistake. . . . Our 'success' led to 31 years of repressive military rule and the deaths of more than 100,000 Guatemalans."[30]

Eisenhower, nevertheless, had used the CIA to install new governments in Iran and Guatemala. The agency did not stop there, however. Although its 1947 charter forbade it from engaging in "security functions" within the United States itself, from the 1950s onward the CIA opened letters that Americans mailed overseas (some 13,000 such letters a year by 1959) and wire-tapped journalists and other private citizens.[31] Meanwhile, Eisenhower's popularity jumped. As a leading journalist wrote in 1954, "That man has an absolutely unique ability to convince people that he has no talent for duplicity."[32]

"YOU BOYS MUST BE CRAZY":
EISENHOWER AND INDOCHINA (1953–1954)

U.S. officials had little time to celebrate the overthrow of Arbenz because, at the same moment, they were confronting a major crisis in Southeast Asia. During that crisis, they learned that in some cases neither "massive retaliation" nor the CIA could achieve U.S. policy objectives. It was the first in a long line of lessons that Vietnam taught those Americans who cared to learn.

The reasons that had moved U.S. officials to become involved in Vietnam during 1949–1950 (see p. 519) only became more powerful after 1952. Chinese communism had to be contained. With the British fighting revolutionaries in Malaya and the Philippine government facing a rebellion, U.S. leaders believed that Ho Chi Minh's Communists in Vietnam had to be defeated or no place in the region would be safe. With massive U.S. help, the Filipinos did contain their revolutionaries. The British, on their own, began winning in Malaya, thus convincing U.S. officials that Ho could also be beaten. Southeast Asia, moreover, had both the strategic materials (such as oil and tin) and locations (for air and naval bases) that the West required for its cold-war build-up. The area seemed especially important because, in American eyes, its markets and raw materials were necessary for Japan's stability. If Southeast Asia became Communist, a top-secret National Security Council paper concluded, it could mean "Japan's eventual accommodation to Communism." Eisenhower later finished that thought: "Should Japan go communist (in fact or in sympathy) the U.S. would be out of the Pacific, and it [i.e., the Pacific] would become a communist lake."[33]

The president tied all this together in a famous press conference that took place on April 7, 1954, when he speculated about the results if Indochina turned Communist:

> First of all, you have the specific value of a locality in its production of materials that the world needs. Then you have the possibility that many human beings pass under a dictatorship that is inimical to the free world. Finally, you have broader considerations that might follow what you would call the "falling domino" principle.

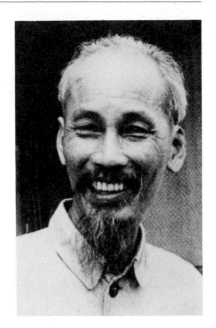

Ho Chi Minh (1890–1969), the father of the Vietnamese revolt against France (1946–1954), led the fight against U.S. intervention until his death. His career as a revolutionary reached back to 1919–1920, when he met with other Third World leaders in Paris while Woodrow Wilson vainly tried to create a world that was "safe for democracy."

> You have a row of dominoes set up, you knock over the first one, and what will happen to the last one is a certainty that it will go over very quickly. . . .
>
> It takes away, in its economic aspects, that region that Japan must have as a trading area or Japan, in turn, will have only one place to go—that is, toward the Communist areas in order to live.
>
> So the possible consequences of the loss are just incalculable to the free world.[34]

In addition, the French had to be helped in Asia or they would be even weaker and less cooperative partners in western Europe. The United States poured over $4 billion into the French attempt to defeat Ho between 1950 and 1954. The money did little good. Neither French arms nor French-controlled Vietnamese governments could stop the revolution. During early 1954, France's commander decided to fight a climactic battle at Dien Bien Phu, near the northern Vietnamese border. It was one of the great errors of twentieth-century military history. The French garrison occupied the bottom of a valley while Ho's Vietminh armies bombarded the garrison by moving artillery to the heights—a feat the French did not think the shabby-looking Communist army could pull off.

Eisenhower privately called the French "a hopeless, helpless mass of protoplasm." Dulles, nevertheless, warned publicly in late March

1954 that Vietnam had to be saved even if it "might involve serious risks." He and Eisenhower secretly spelled out those risks in early April, when the president asked congressional leaders for authority to use, if necessary, U.S. forces to save the French position. Led by Democratic Senator Lyndon Johnson from Texas, the congressmen refused to go along unless the British also joined. They warned that there must be "no more Koreas with the United States furnishing 90 percent of the manpower."[35] Prime Minister Churchill, who considered the French effort a lost cause, flatly rejected any plan for intervention.

Eisenhower knew that Vietnam was pivotal, but he refused to go in alone. "Unilateral action . . . would destroy us," he later observed privately. "If we intervened alone in this case we would be expected to intervene alone in other parts of the world."[36] Both Dulles and U.S. military officials then put forward the idea of saving the French by using small nuclear weapons. "You boys must be crazy," Eisenhower replied. "We can't use those awful things against Asians for the second time in ten years. My God."[37] His army chief of staff, Matthew Ridgway, had helped convince Eisenhower that even nuclear weapons would not work without sending in a U.S. ground force afterward. And that was something neither Eisenhower nor Ridgway would seriously think of doing.

On May 7, 1954, Dien Bien Phu fell. Against Dulles's wishes, the French traveled to Geneva, Switzerland, where an international conference met to settle the war. China's sharp, urbane foreign minister, Zhou Enlai (Chou En-lai), attended. Against his will, Dulles also went, although he made it clear that he would meet with Zhou (Chou) only if their "cars collide." The Geneva Conference finally produced two agreements. The first, signed by the French and Ho's Vietminh, provided for a cease-fire, the temporary division of Vietnam along the seventeenth parallel, and regrouping French forces south of the line while the Vietminh moved north. This agreement emphasized that the seventeenth parallel was not to be seen as "constituting a political or territorial boundary." The second agreement, or Final Declaration, provided that neither north nor south would join a military alliance or allow foreign bases. General elections were to be held in 1956. Neighboring Laos and Cambodia were to be neutral. Unwilling to deal away half of Vietnam to communism and have his picture taken as he did it, Dulles refused to have the United States sign the Geneva Accords. He did issue a separate statement that agreed with the general principles and promised not to "disturb them" by the "threat or the use of force."[38]

PICKING UP THE PIECES IN ASIA (1954–1961)

But Eisenhower and Dulles then devised a dual policy to contain China and Ho Chi Minh. First, they used economic and political pressure to push out the French and bring in Ngo Dinh Diem to lead the South Vietnamese. Diem had never worked for the French, but he had collaborated with the Japanese occupation and, since 1950, had lived in Europe and the United States rather than fight in the nationalists' struggle. His Roman Catholic beliefs set him apart from the Buddhists, who made up more than 90 percent of Vietnam's population. Those beliefs, nevertheless, made him popular with many Americans. To oversee Diem, Dulles installed two U.S. advisers: General J. Lawton Collins and Colonel Edward Lansdale. Within a year Collins felt that Diem had neither the public support nor the talent to pull South Vietnam together. But Lansdale, who had played a major role in containing the Philippine revolutionaries, believed that he and Diem could repeat that triumph and make South Vietnam a nation. Eisenhower finally went along with Lansdale. From the start of Diem's rule, the United States set out to protect him by ignoring key agreements made at Geneva. The seventeenth parallel was not to be temporary (as the Geneva Accords provided), but was to become a permanent boundary between North and South Vietnam. Dulles and Diem, moreover, had no intention of holding the promised elections in 1956 because they feared Ho would win.[39] Thus, the United States not only became committed to South Vietnam, but—as the phrase soon went—to "sink or swim with Ngo Dinh Diem."

The second Eisenhower-Dulles response was to create the Southeast Asia Treaty Organization (SEATO) in September 1954. Its odd assortment of members included the United States, France, Great Britain, New Zealand, and Australia. The only Asian countries that joined were the Philippines, Thailand, and Pakistan (which hoped to use SEATO against its bitter enemy, India). Each nation agreed that in case of an armed attack against a Southeast Asian state or territory, it would respond "in accordance with its constitutional processes." Dulles clearly told the U.S. Senate: "We do not intend to dedicate any major elements of the United States Military Establishment to form an army of defense in this area."[40] In reality, the other members contributed little to SEATO either, and the organization became militarily irrelevant, although for the next dozen years U.S. officials used this supposed *col-*

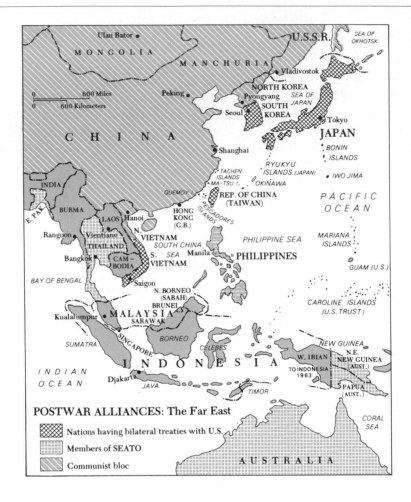

POSTWAR ALLIANCES: The Far East

Nations having bilateral treaties with U.S.

Members of SEATO

Communist bloc

lective security pact to justify the *unilateral* American commitment to Vietnam.

Between 1954 and 1961, Eisenhower, indeed, committed the United States to Vietnam. U.S. Army advisers taught Vietnamese soldiers how to fight a conventional war (as in Korea), not counterrevolutionary tactics. Diem proved to be a weak ruler. He was afraid to carry out needed reforms because he would lose support of rich and powerful Vietnamese. By 1961, he was among the top five recipients of U.S. foreign aid in the world, but his economy was failing. The year before, his army had proved to be inept when fighting resumed with Ho's Vietnamese Communists or Vietminh. In 1957, the first American, Captain Harry Cramer, had died in the war. But as a U.S. expert in Vietnam wrote in 1961, "American aid has built a castle on sand." George Herring, author of the standard one-volume history on U.S. involvement in Vietnam, concludes that only by leaving office in 1961 did Eisenhower avoid suffering "the ultimate failure of his policies in Vietnam."[41]

Between 1954 and 1958, however, Eisenhower and Dulles felt that they had taught the Communists, especially the Chinese, a lesson. The Americans could point not only to holding firm in Vietnam, but also to successes in the so-called offshore-islands crises. Those islands (especially Quemoy and Matsu) were tiny spots just off China's coast but claimed by Chiang Kai-shek. In August 1954, the Communists called for liberation of the islands and began shelling them. Dulles and Chiang then signed a mutual defense alliance, but it said nothing about defending the offshore islands.

In early 1955, Eisenhower asked Congress for broad authority to use U.S. forces in the area at his discretion. In an amazing display of trust, within five days both houses of Congress overwhelmingly gave Eisenhower such power. In that short time, Congress surrendered to the president its constitutional power to decide when and for which reasons war might be declared. The resolution set a historic precedent for later grants of power by Congress to the president that Congress regretted. But the shelling of the islands quieted. In 1958, the Chinese Communists again threatened Quemoy and Matsu. This time, Eisenhower moved nuclear weapons into place in case Mao's armies tried to move toward the offshore islands and Taiwan. Fortunately, the crisis again passed.

The consequences of the offshore-islands crises were many. Congress helped build the "imperial presidency" (as it was soon known). Eisenhower further militarily allied the United States with Chiang. The president again threatened to use nuclear weapons against Asians. U.S. officials concluded that the Chinese Communists would stop their expansionism only when confronted with massive force. Finally, perhaps the crises helped widen the split developing between the Chinese and Soviets. Mao became angry when Moscow showed no interest in going to war with Americans over something as small as the offshore islands. Dulles indeed now concluded that by being tough, he could show Mao how undependable the Soviets were and thus split the two Communist powers. Historian David Mayers concludes that the U.S. military pressure seemed "to have contributed," as Eisenhower and Dulles hoped, "to the weakening" of the Sino-Soviet partnership until it finally fell apart between 1957 and 1961. But history played an interesting joke, for the split did not occur as U.S. officials had predicted. They thought Mao might be a new Tito (see p. 478) and move closer to the United States. Instead, U.S.-China relations worsened while, incredibly, U.S.-Soviet relations warmed. Observers began to suggest, only half-humorously, that a Soviet leader might be the new Tito.[42]

THE "AGONIZING REAPPRAISAL": EISENHOWER, DULLES, AND EUROPE

Those Soviet leaders were smashing into a number of problems. Stalin's death in early 1953 left them with a leadership crisis and a set of foreign policies that had grown stagnant by the early 1950s. Nikita Khrushchev gained power by 1955 and drew up fresh policies. A British official wondered, "How can this fat, vulgar man with his pig eyes and ceaseless flow of talk, really be the head" of the Soviet Empire?[43] But Khrushchev, born in a lowly miner's family, had shown ruthlessness in purging anti-Stalinists in the Ukraine during the 1930s and in trying (unsuccessfully) to improve Soviet agriculture later. As he clawed his way to the top, moreover, he shrewdly understood that Stalin's brutal policies had alienated the growing number of newly emerging peoples and had even helped the United States arm a frightened western Europe. By 1954–1955, Khrushchev was flying around the globe, trying to woo India, Burma, and other neutral countries.

As for Europe, the Soviets began to wonder whether a relaxation of tension would reassure the westerners and perhaps loosen up the NATO alliance. At one point (on April Fool's Day 1955), the Soviets even offered to join NATO to show their good will. The new approach seemed to work. In August 1954, France finally and flatly rejected the U.S. plan to rearm West Germany. Warning that the security of the Western world was at stake, Dulles announced that the United States would have to undertake an "agonizing reappraisal" of its foreign commitments if France did not change its mind. Translated, Dulles's phrase meant either that the United States would go home and leave Europe to Soviet mercies or—much more likely—go ahead and arm the Germans without French participation. A solution to the crisis finally occurred to British foreign minister Anthony Eden during his Sunday morning bath. West Germany was to be rearmed, but increased controls would be imposed, including the prohibition of German-produced nuclear weapons. To reassure the French further, Eden reversed historic British policy and pledged to station four divisions of British troops on the mainland of Europe to help protect France against aggression. In December 1954, the French accepted the deal. But Dulles

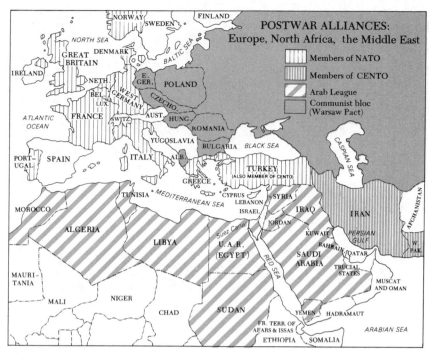

By 1955, with the rearmament of West Germany by NATO and the Soviet creation of the Warsaw Pact alliance, Europe seemed divided into two camps. But that division became confused in 1956 with the Suez Canal affair and the anti-Soviet uprisings in Hungary and Poland.

and Eisenhower had also compromised. They had hoped that their plans for a new European Defense Community (EDC) would further integrate the Europeans militarily, while allowing a cutback of U.S. military spending in NATO. Eden's plan, however, killed the EDC while attaching the new German military to NATO. As historian Brian R. Duchin observes, Eisenhower's decision to accept Eden's plan "placed security above fiscal economy."[44]

Khrushchev made the best of it. He certainly did not like West German rearmament, but he loved a divided Germany. Thus, he established diplomatic relations with the West Germans in 1955. At the same time, he built up the Communist East German Army. Most importantly, in May 1955, he broke a ten-year logjam by agreeing to pull Soviet troops out of Austria and to allow that nation to regain independence. He demanded in return that Austria remain neutral. After signing the treaty, Molotov and Dulles—Old Ironpants and Old Sourpuss—even appeared on a balcony to wave handkerchiefs in cel-

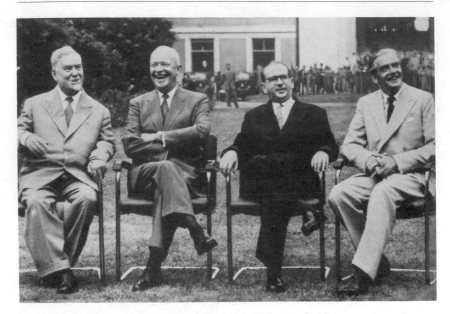

*Given the intensity of the cold war and their failure to hold a summit confer-
ence for ten years, the mood seemed jovial when the Big Four (Bulganin of the
USSR, Eisenhower of the United States, Faure of France, and Eden of Great
Britain) convened at Geneva in the summer of 1955. Although the photo typifies
the famous "spirit of Geneva," there were no significant diplomatic results to be
celebrated.*

ebration. That breakthrough led, in turn, to a four-power summit
meeting at Geneva in mid-1955, the first summit since the Potsdam
Conference of a decade before. The meeting produced nothing of
importance except good will. But given the events of the previous ten
years, the world gratefully accepted even that result.[45]

A TURN: SUEZ AND HUNGARY, 1956

In the following year, world affairs nearly fell apart, then regrouped,
and marched off in dramatically different directions. Crises in eastern
Europe and the Middle East, at first disconnected, suddenly came
together in November and opened a new chapter in the cold war's
history.

In early 1956, Khrushchev continued to try to reform and make more
efficient the Soviet system. He shocked the Twentieth Communist Party
Congress in Moscow by condemning Stalin's brutalities against party

members and the Communist system. (He carefully did not criticize Stalin's crimes against the Soviet people because Khrushchev himself had been involved in some of those.) The new leader then reversed Stalinist policy and urged "peaceful coexistence between states with differing political and social systems." The effect of his words was electric. The CIA director, Allen Dulles, suggested that perhaps Khrushchev was merely drunk when he made the speech. But peoples in the Soviet bloc quickly tried to pull down leaders associated with Stalin and demanded more open and democratic societies. Protesters in Poland attacked Communist party headquarters. In Hungary, street protests turned anti-Soviet. Khrushchev now appeared unsure and confused in responding to these challenges.[46]

Meanwhile, another crisis brewed in the Middle East. Egyptian army officers had begun pushing the British out of the Suez Canal area in 1954. The following year, the Egyptians turned to the Soviet bloc for a supply of arms. Eisenhower and Dulles did not approve, but they understood. Throughout 1955, Egyptian and Israeli forces had been involved in sharp border skirmishes. Moreover, Dulles had long condemned British colonialism for alienating such people as the Egyptians and driving them toward the Soviets. He decided to pull the Egyptians back by helping finance the building of the Aswan Dam on the Nile. The dream of their new leader, General Gamal Abdel Nasser, the dam was to help tame the river and create rich lands for cotton, among other crops.

But within six months, Dulles changed his mind. He had hoped that in return for the money, Nasser would move toward peace with Israel and end the dangerous fighting between Egyptian and Israeli armies. Nasser refused. To do so could be his ruin both within Egypt and throughout an Arab world that refused to recognize the existence of the Jewish state. Moreover, Congress cooled as it saw that Egyptian cotton would compete with the U.S. crop and that Nasser was becoming friendly with China.[47] In a rather crude move, Dulles announced that the United States would not fund the dam just when Nasser's foreign minister was flying to Washington to sign the contract. Furious, Nasser seized and nationalized the Suez Canal to obtain his own funds and to defy the West.

The Egyptian leader now controlled the waterway through which the West's oil supply flowed. British prime minister Anthony Eden and the French secretly decided to use force to regain the canal. Paris officials especially hoped that destroying Nasser would stop the aid going to Algerian revolutionaries who were killing many French soldiers and

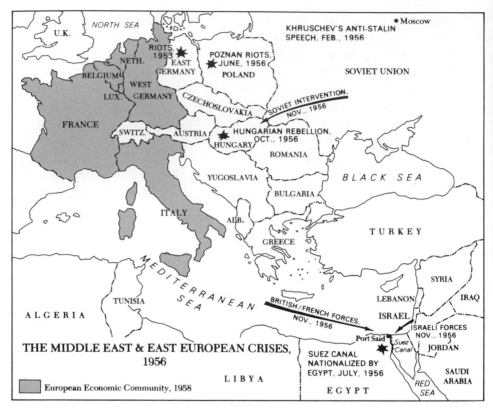

THE MIDDLE EAST & EAST EUROPEAN CRISES, 1956

European Economic Community, 1958

The international arena changed dramatically in 1956, and the cold war entered a new phase—in the Middle East and in eastern Europe, but also within the Western alliance itself.

destroying what remained of the French Empire. For their own reasons, Israelis agreed to cooperate with Paris and London. Although kept in the dark by the British, Dulles and Eisenhower knew from intelligence reports that something was afoot. Warning Eden to be restrained, the two Americans worked to find a compromise between the British and the Egyptians.

But it was too late. On October 29, 1956, Israel, according to plan, attacked Egypt and drove toward the Suez. Then, however, the plan collapsed. Eden and the French delayed sending in their forces. When they did so, their armies moved slowly. Eisenhower's famous temper exploded: "It's the damnedest business I ever saw supposedly intelligent governments getting themselves into." He was afraid that the Soviets would use the crisis to provide massive help to Nasser. U.S. officials angrily told the British "to comply with the goddamn cease-fire [resolution passed by the U.N.] or go ahead with the goddamn invasion. . . . What we can't stand is [the] goddamn hesitation waltz while Hungary is burning!"[48]

For as the Middle East became engulfed in war, Khrushchev had seized the chance to smash protests in Poland and Hungary with Soviet tanks. Proccupied with Suez (and the final hours of his own re-election campaign), Eisenhower did not know how to respond. He rejected sending U.S. troops or supplies because Hungary was "as inaccessible to us as Tibet." He rejected a suggestion of using atomic weapons because "to annihilate Hungary . . . is in no way to help her."[49] His only answer was to focus on the Middle East and end the war before Khrushchev moved in to help Nasser. In one phone conversation, the furious president reduced the British prime minister to tears. U.S. officials threatened to cut off oil to Great Britain and ruin the British currency unless the war stopped. By November 5, Khrushchev was proclaiming that he would use Soviet missiles for "country busting" in western Europe, unless the British and French left Egypt. Eisenhower warned him to back off and by mid-November restored some order to the Suez area as the British-French-Israeli forces retreated.

But the world would not be the same afterward. By defying Great Britain and France, Nasser helped trigger immense pride and ambitions in the newly emerging nations. By turning the screws on the Brit-

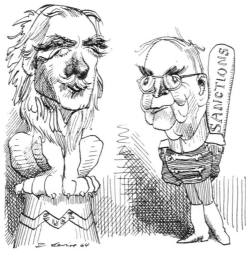

David Levine's cartoon nicely captures how, by the Suez crisis of November 1956, U.S. Secretary of State Dulles was taming and caging the once-feared British lion (here with Prime Minister Anthony Eden's face).

ish and French after they had deceived him, Eisenhower—with Eden's
blundering help—badly split the Western alliance. Not just the United
States suffered, however. By having to impose order and restore hard-
line Communist leaders in Poland and Hungary through sheer force,
Khrushchev had to admit just how fragmented and anti-Russian the
Soviet bloc had become. Since 1945, the globe had been described as
"two camps." But with the 1956 crises, the two camps splintered into
many camps. Eisenhower faced a different world as he began his second term.

EUROPE IS EUROPEANIZED AS THE U.S. ECONOMY IS LESS U.S. (1957–1960)

The Suez disaster was followed in October 1957 by the Soviet launching of Sputnik I, the first small, human-made satellite placed in orbit
around the earth. The Soviet triumph convinced most Americans that
Soviet science was equal to, if not ahead of, U.S. science. It also made
them believe that, indeed, Khrushchev could now "direct rockets to
any part of the globe," as the Soviets bragged. In 1957, Eisenhower
suffered a small stroke. His speech never fully recovered. The next
year, charges of corruption riddled the White House staff. In 1959,
John Foster Dulles died after a two-and-a-half-year fight with cancer.
Against this background, the president had to deal with an angry Europe
and a revolutionary, newly emerging bloc of nations—and do so, moreover, with a sliding U.S. economy.

Great Britain and France had been humiliated by the Suez fiasco.
The episode marked the true end of the British Empire and destroyed
French chances to put down the Algerian rebellion. France's failures
finally led to the demand that the tall, arrogant figure of General Charles
de Gaulle be returned to power in 1958. De Gaulle began to pull France
out of Algeria. Then he moved to restore French authority and independence. De Gaulle told Eisenhower that the French and British should
be involved in U.S. decisions about the Western alliance, especially
those involving nuclear weapons. Eisenhower ignored the request. The
United States was not going to give up its freedom of action, especially
to down-on-their-luck colonial nations. De Gaulle responded by accelerating development of a French nuclear bomb. The British did the
same with their own bomb. As a London official told an American,
"Since the events of last year [in Suez] we cannot be entirely confident
of America."[50]

The Europeans also moved on the economic front. In 1950, the French had proposed a European Coal and Steel Community to tie together the basic French and German industries. The French hoped, thereby, to control German recovery and to gain access to rich West German raw materials. In 1957, the French and West Germans took the next step: they formed the Common Market (the European Economic Community or EEC) in a historic agreement with four other states—Italy, Belgium, the Netherlands, and Luxembourg. The EEC aimed at eliminating tariffs between members and making the region a United States of Europe for traders and investors. Members did, however, erect a tariff against outsiders—for example, against the British, who refused to join, and the Americans.

In 1957–1958, U.S. investors began flooding the promising, rich EEC with dollars. The Americans had grown wealthy from their post-1945 trade and had money to invest abroad. U.S. corporations, moreover, flocked to Europe to get inside the new tariff wall and sell to the vast EEC market. American private investment overseas shot up from $11.8 billion in 1950 to nearly $30 billion by 1959. Historically, this investment had gone into Canada and Latin America. (U.S. business owned three-fourths of the oil and gas as well as half of the manufacturing plant of the Canadians.) But after 1957, the investment tripled in western Europe to $6 billion within three years. The United States was taking over large parts of Europe's economy in an "American invasion."

Just as suddenly, the Americans—by far the richest people in history—discovered that they were beginning to run out of money. They were not only sending billions abroad for investment, but billions overseas to contain communism. Until 1957, these vast expenses had been paid for by a large trade surplus. (Americans each year were selling about $7 billion more abroad than they bought.) After 1957, this surplus slid to under $4 billion and, for a moment in 1959, actually moved into the red as Americans bought more abroad than they sold. The moment passed, but it returned in 1971 to stay. Thus, the late 1950s marked a historic turning point in U.S. economic and diplomatic history. For the first time since the 1870s, Americans found that they could not compete as they wanted in world markets. They were suddenly spending more overseas than they earned. U.S. officials could cover this deficit in only two ways: by printing more dollars or by shipping out gold bars from their reserves. By 1960, the U.S. gold supply, which led the world in 1945 with a total of nearly $25 billion, sank to $19 billion and, by 1968, to $10 billion. Not enough gold remained to

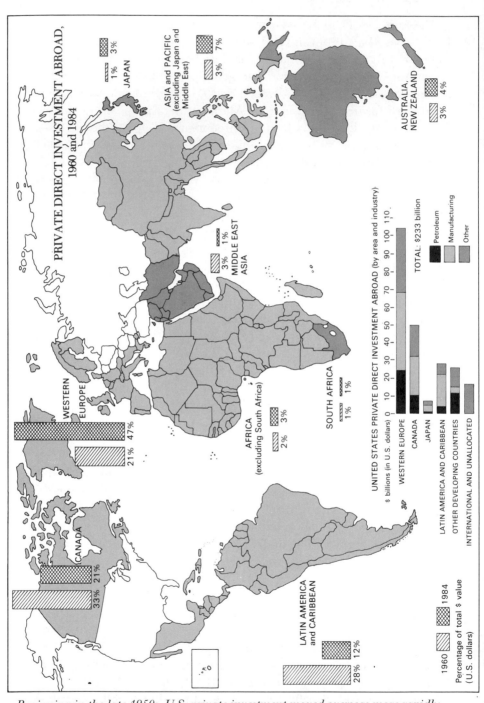

PRIVATE DIRECT INVESTMENT ABROAD, 1960 and 1984

JAPAN
1% 3%

ASIA and PACIFIC (excluding Japan and Middle East)
3% 7%

AUSTRALIA, NEW ZEALAND
3% 4%

MIDDLE EAST ASIA
3% 1%

WESTERN EUROPE
21% 47%

CANADA
33% 21%

AFRICA (excluding South Africa)
2% 3%

SOUTH AFRICA
1% 1%

LATIN AMERICA and CARIBBEAN
28% 12%

1960

1984

Percentage of total $ value (U.S. dollars)

UNITED STATES PRIVATE DIRECT INVESTMENT ABROAD (by area and industry)
$ billions (in U.S. dollars)   0 10 20 30 40 50 60 70 80 90 100 110

TOTAL: $233 billion

Petroleum
Manufacturing
Other

WESTERN EUROPE
CANADA
JAPAN
LATIN AMERICA AND CARIBBEAN
OTHER DEVELOPING COUNTRIES
INTERNATIONAL AND UNALLOCATED

Beginning in the late 1950s, U.S. private investment moved overseas more rapidly, especially into western Europe, where observers warned of an "American invasion." By the mid-1980s, however, Americans owed other nations more than foreign nations owed Americans.

support the dollar bills Americans used every day, let alone support the dollars moving overseas.

For most Americans, however, the dollar's dilemma was not the bad news. They were being flooded with cheaper and better goods from West Germany (such as Volkswagens) and Japan. The United States economy slowed and stumbled into a recession in 1958–1959. In retrospect, it is clear that these years marked part of another historic turn— the turn in the United States from an industrial (iron, steel, autos) to a service (insurance, investment, communications) economy. It was going to be a tough adjustment for many Americans. And it could not have come at a worse time. For they faced a slumping economy at home just when they were confronting challenges from Japan and western Europe, and major threats from the Soviet Union and revolutions in the newly emerging world.[51]

EISENHOWER, HIS DOCTRINE, AND CRISIS (1957–1960)

Between 1945 and 1960, approximately 40 nations with 800-million people revolted against their colonial masters. This political earthquake shook the United Nations. Its original 51 members exploded to 100 and then to 114 by 1965. The United States could no longer assume support from a majority in the UN. A growing gap appeared between the prosperous United States and the poor, newly emerging world, where only one out of seven persons earned more than $450 per year (in India the average worker got 15 cents a day), where drinkable water and medical care were rare, and where money needed for trade and development disappeared into Japanese and Western pockets because of unfavorable trade balances.

Eisenhower and Dulles emphasized that communism could not be stopped unless the West outraced the Communists economically. But the Soviets were "increasing their own productivity at the rate of about 6 percent per annum, which is about twice our rate," the secretary of state complained. In newly emerging areas such as India, Southeast Asia, and Latin America, "there is little, if any, increase. That is one reason why Communism has such great appeal" and "slogans of 'liberty, freedom' " do not. The U.S. ambassador to the United Nations, Henry Cabot Lodge, bluntly told Eisenhower's cabinet in 1959 that Americans should quit pushing "the specific word 'Capitalism' which is beyond rehabilitation in the minds of the non-white world." Lodge then asked the big question: "The U.S. can win wars but the question is can we win revolutions."[52]

Dulles hoped to solve that problem—at least in part—by bringing the new nations into a U.S. alliance system. When a top State Department official asked him if "we are opposed to any neutrals," Dulles answered, "Yes." After all, he went on, the Soviets believe that "a neutral is one who does not participate in [U.S.] collective security arrangements." Dulles wanted to try to lock the newly independent peoples into SEATO, OAS, and various Middle East arrangements (such as the Baghdad Pact). But he knew that this was not enough. Eisenhower finally enlarged the Export-Import Bank funding, agreed to easier World Bank loans to the new nations, and even set up new regional development banks (for Latin America and the Middle East) to provide economic carrots.

The president also used a stick (often held by the CIA). In Africa, Ghana's independence from the British Empire in 1957 helped trigger the appearance of a dozen new African nations over the next four years. Many had not been prepared for self-rule by their colonial governors. The Belgian Congo had long been notorious for exploiting its black subjects (see p. 172), and when it became independent in 1960, Eisenhower instantly viewed its leader, Patrice Lumumba, as a possible Communist. Lumumba was an ardent nationalist, not a Communist, but CIA agents saw little difference and prepared plans to eliminate the Congolese leader. In Indonesia, the Eisenhower team also sent in the CIA when Dulles thought that President Achmed Sukarno was turning leftward. A long-time hero and leader of Indonesia, Sukarno was also a nationalist, colorful and effective, who used Communists for his own purposes. But Allen Dulles, director of the CIA, tried to overthrow him with $10 million of support for anti-Sukarno rebels. It was a plan patterned after the 1954 CIA coup in Guatemala. Eisenhower publicly claimed that the U.S. policy was only "careful neutrality," but Sukarno's forces shot down a CIA plane, damned the U.S. involvement, and then destroyed the rebellion. Relations between the United States and Southeast Asia's largest nation sank to a new low in 1959–1960.

Eisenhower's policies worked better in the Middle East, but only in the short run. The Suez disaster set off major political changes in the region, including the rise of General Nasser to hero's status among many Arabs. He worked with Syria and Jordan to spread his pan-Arab policies, which, Secretary of State Dulles feared, had strong Soviet support. Dulles privately condemned Nasser as "an expansionist dic-

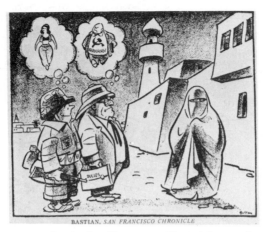

BASTIAN, *SAN FRANCISCO CHRONICLE*

Bastian, the cartoonist for the San Francisco Chronicle, *catches the complexities of Middle Eastern politics of July 1958, when Dulles and Eisenhower landed U.S. troops on Lebanon's beautiful beaches in an effort to contain what they feared was Arab radicalism that had appeared in Egypt and Iraq.*

tator somewhat of the Hitler type" who "will get help from the Soviet Union."[53] Eisenhower asked Congress to give him authority to use force, whenever he thought it necessary, to prevent "international communism" from conquering the Middle East. Some Democratic senators protested giving such a blank check to the president, but Eisenhower, as usual, won. Congress passed the so-called Eisenhower Doctrine of 1957, which allowed him to use armed forces to help any nation resist "armed attack from any country controlled by international communism." Congress, again giving the president an enormous amount of power, never tried to define what it meant by "international communism."

The doctrine had little effect on Nasser's popularity. Jordan finally broke with Nasser (and received massive military help from the United States as a reward). But Egypt and Syria formed the United Arab Republic in early 1958. On July 13, 1958, the weak Iraqi kingdom fell to nationalist army officers who admired Nasser. Eisenhower was afraid that Lebanon would be next. That nation's Maronite Christian officials were under fire from the much larger Moslem majority. On July 14, with little hesitation or preparation, Eisenhower ordered 5,000 U.S. troops to land on Lebanon's beautiful beaches and maintain order. The president never invoked the Eisenhower Doctrine. Everyone understood that nationalism, not communism, was on the march. But the president was afraid that the dominoes were falling in a strategic area where the last to fall could land on U.S. companies that controlled the world's largest oil reserves. It was too late, however, to restore the Iraqi kingdom or the U.S.-created treaty system (the Baghdad Pact) in which Iraq was the key link. U.S. troops finally left Lebanon in October. They also left a Middle East that was greatly changed since the Suez crisis, one much less friendly to the United States.[54]

Castro and the Threat to the Monroe Doctrine (1957–1960)

Latin America was also building up to an explosion by the late 1950s. Dulles had trouble blaming this crisis on communism. The Soviets had little interest or contact in the region. Local Communist parties sometimes had large memberships, but they were politically irrelevant, ignored by Moscow, and closely watched by powerful Latin American army officers.

The central problem was economic. With the end of the Korean War, demand and prices slumped for Latin American raw materials. The region's imports rose much more rapidly than exports. Money grew ever scarcer. Economic hard times struck as the U.S. economy slowed; the proven rule was that when the North American economy sneezed, Latin Americans got pneumonia. The slowdown hit as the area's population growth rate was 2.5 percent annually, one of the world's highest. The number of Latin Americans would double to 360 million in just thirty years. U.S. businesses moved into the region but invested mostly in Venezuelan oil. These North American companies, nevertheless, accounted for 10 percent of Latin America's gross national product and a full 30 percent of its exports, figures that set the Southern Hemisphere apart from Africa or even Southeast Asia. In those parts of the world, problems could be blamed on European colonialism. But in Latin America, where few colonial enclaves existed, the economic problems were often pinned on U.S. control of the export economies.

U.S. officials usually tried to keep the lid on these boiling problems by working with Latin American military officers. Eisenhower even awarded medals to two of the area's worst dictators: Manuel A. Odría of Peru and Marcos Pérez Jiménez of Venezuela. Pérez Jiménez was overthrown in January 1958. Four months later, Vice-President Nixon visited Caracas, Venezuela. Earlier in his trip through the region, he had encountered hostile crowds, but in Caracas mobs spit on Nixon and his wife, Pat, then stopped and tried to overturn his limousine.

One Secret Service man sitting next to Nixon pulled his revolver and said, "Lets get some of these sons-of-bitches." Nixon ordered him to "put that away," at least until the mob tried to enter the car itself. The driver finally managed to get the car to safety. Meanwhile, Eisenhower mobilized U.S. military units for a possible parachute drop to rescue the vice-president. Nixon returned to Washington shaken but unscathed.[55] He urged that new policies be pushed, but no one could think of fresh approaches that would be both non-revolutionary and cheap.

As the debate wandered on, U.S. power was suddenly challenged in the most surprising place in Latin America: Cuba, which Washington had controlled since the war of 1898. By the late 1950s, North Americans owned nearly all of its mines and cattle ranches and half of its sugar—the three products on which the nation's economy rested. After 1934, U.S. officials had stood aside as General Fulgencio Batista took control of the island. He reigned over a highly corrupt society marked by Mafia rule, rampant unemployment, and widespread prostitution. On July 26, 1953, a twenty-six-year-old lawyer-politician, well educated in Roman Catholic schools and embittered by the U.S.-Batista alliance, tried to overthrow the government.

Fidel Castro was captured, jailed (where he organized prisoners and read Shakespeare, Kant, Lenin, Einstein, novels, and books on Franklin D. Roosevelt), released in 1955, and then went to Mexico where he gathered support for another try. He and eighty other revolutionaries landed in Cuba in 1956 but were nearly wiped out by Batista's forces. The rebels were down to sixteen soldiers when their fortunes turned around. Long-suffering peasants joined them. Batista's troops could not exterminate Castro's followers. When the dictator claimed he had done so, newspapers (especially the *New York Times*) published interviews with Castro that made him an international hero. By late 1958, U.S. officials finally took Castro's threat seriously as he scored military victories. They tried to stop his Twenty-sixth of July Movement by bringing to power someone who thought like, but was more popular than, Batista. It was too late.[56] On New Year's Day, 1959, the raggedy rebel soldiers marched victoriously into Havana.

The triumphant Castro was determined to change Cuban society. That meant breaking ties with the United States so that he could control his nation's resources. He understood the special need for a massive land-reform program (0.5 percent of the population owned one-third of the land, much of which lay unused). Castro later claimed that he had been a Marxist-Leninist since he had read their works

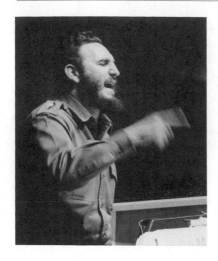

Fidel Castro (1926–   ) led the Cuban revolution that deposed a pro-U.S. government in 1959. An effective guerrilla leader, Castro also proved adept at mobilizing the Cuban people with his speeches, some of which continued for hours.

years before, but the evidence is more complex. He had received little help from the inept Cuban Communist party and later used the party only to carry out his own program. When Castro visited the United States in April 1959, Eisenhower refused to meet him, but Vice-President Nixon held a long talk with Castro and came away believing that the Cuban was not a Communist.[57] Nevertheless, relations rapidly fell apart. U.S. economic help slowed. In early 1960, Castro agreed to sell sugar to the Soviets in return for oil and industrial goods. He then demanded that the U.S. oil firms in Cuba refine the oil. The companies were bitter but agreed to do so until the State Department told them to refuse. Castro seized the oil companies. Eisenhower shut off the U.S. market on which Cuban sugar had depended since the 1890s. Khrushchev moved in to buy more sugar. In March 1960, Eisenhower secretly ordered the CIA to prepare plans for overthrowing Castro. The Cuban leader rapidly moved to confiscate privately owned firms, both foreign and domestic. Eisenhower responded by cutting off all U.S. trade to Cuba except medicine and some food staples. By the time the president left office in January 1961, U.S.-Cuban relations had broken.

Historian Richard Welch believes that "Castro only became a Marxist sometime between fall 1960 and fall 1961." Welch also concludes that U.S. policy did not fully determine the course of Castro's policies, but U.S. responses gave the Cuban revolutionaries excuses for centralizing their power and accelerated "the formation of the Cuban-Russian alliance." To use Lodge's phrase, the United States had not been able to "win revolutions" even 90 miles off its own coast. In mid-1960, Khrushchev publicly boasted that the Monroe Doctrine was dead. Privately he predicted that "Castro will have to gravitate to us like an iron filing to a magnet."[58]

Sputnik versus U-2: The U.S.-Soviet Rivalry (1957–1960)

The Soviet leader had also caused Eisenhower other bad nights. In October 1957, Soviet missiles had sent Sputnik into space. A month later they sent up another satellite, this time with a dog on board. Eisenhower's public-opinion rating sank an astonishing 22 percent. The Soviets actually seemed to be beating the land of Henry Ford at the American game of technology and invention. For the first time since World War II, the United States mobilized schools and factories to fight a war, this time in technology and science instead of on battlefields. "It was Us versus Them," a journalist recalled of the post-Sputnik days. "It was the American way of life, not to mention tailfins, Wrigley's Spearmint gum, Wednesday night bowling and attending the church of your choice, going against the godless horde."[59]

Even before Sputnik mania set in, Eisenhower secretly appointed a special committee, headed by H. Rowan Gaither, Jr., of the Ford Foundation, to study U.S. security needs. In a report written largely by Gaither and Paul Nitze, the Gaither committee warned the president that the United States would lose the cold war in the near future unless he pumped up defense spending by $11 billion to some $48 billion. Using phrases that indicated that the nation's survival was at stake, Gaither's group also argued that spending such money would boost employment and help avoid economic recession. When the committee's conclusions leaked to newspapers, they worsened the panic already caused by Sputnik.[60]

But Eisenhower refused to panic. He flatly rejected most of Gaither's recommendations. When the committee urged the creation of fallout shelters to protect Americans against atomic radiation (at the cost of $100 per American, or $30 billion over five years), the president said that no defense existed against such a war. He was afraid that another $10 billion for defense would fuel inflation and undermine the economy. The retired general called military hardware this "negative stuff." Nor did he change his mind when leading Democrats, smelling the 1960 presidential race just ahead, blasted Eisenhower for letting the nation's guard down. Senators Stuart Symington of Missouri, John F. Kennedy of Massachussetts, and Lyndon Johnson of Texas led the attack. Aiming at the 1960 Democratic nomination as well as at Eisenhower, they warned of a large "missile gap" in Khrushchev's favor unless the president spent more money. Eisenhower privately called them "sanctimonious hypocritical bastards."[61]

The president felt strongly about the accusations because he knew no missile gap existed—or, more accurately, that one existed and that it overwhelmingly favored the United States. He knew this because since June 1956 he had secretly approved flights of a new plane, the U-2, piloted by CIA agents at 70,000 feet to take pictures of Soviet military installations. The plane supposedly flew too high to be shot down by Soviet missiles, although from the start Khrushchev apparently knew that the U-2s were flying over his territory. Using cameras that, from a distance of 11 miles, could photograph the license-plate numbers on a Soviet official's car, Eisenhower learned that Khrushchev had decided not to rush ahead and build missiles. The Soviet leader apparently was waiting for new missiles to be developed, meanwhile using Sputnik as a way to bluff Americans into thinking that the USSR had a massive strategic force. Knowing that it was a bluff, Eisenhower refused to listen to demands for much larger military budgets. He did, however, go along with a $2.5 billion rise, especially for the air force. Instead, Congress gave him $8 billion more in 1958. Eisenhower, meanwhile, could not make public the information gleaned by the secret U-2 flights or by the first spy satellites circulating in outer space that he authorized in 1960. Once again, politics could not keep pace with technology.[62]

Khrushchev tried to use his bluff to win a great prize: Berlin. Fearful that West Germany would obtain nuclear weapons, he floated the Rapacki Plan (named after the Polish foreign minister) to create a nuclear-free zone in central Europe. In the United States, George Kennan supported such a disengagement, only to be bitterly attacked by Dean Acheson (Kennan's boss in the State Department during 1949–1950), who wanted no part of negotiations with Moscow: "Mr. Kennan has never . . . grasped the realities of power relationships, but takes a rather mystical attitude toward them." (Columnist James Reston observed: "Next to the Lincoln Memorial in moonlight the sight of Mr. Dean G. Acheson blowing his top is without doubt the most impressive view in the capital.") Dulles privately thanked Acheson for blasting Kennan. The Rapacki Plan consequently had a short life, so in late 1958 Khrushchev issued an ultimatum. Calling West Berlin a "malignant tumor" inside the Communist bloc, he demanded the Western powers evacuate the city within six months. Believing that abandoning 2 million Germans in West Berlin would ruin the entire U.S. position in Europe, the president said the United States would not leave. He then underlined his point by warning that he had no intention of fighting a ground war against the massive Soviet army in central Europe. The war would be nuclear. He would, however, be happy to talk with Khrushchev about it, if Moscow removed its six-month ultimatum.[63]

Khrushchev, who lusted after an invitation to visit the United States for the first time, quickly accepted. His trip to the president's retreat at Camp David, Maryland, and to a midwestern farm went well. (A visit to Hollywood to see the filming of *Can-Can* went less well; Khrushchev was shocked by the brief costumes and sexy dancing.) A "spirit of Camp David" emerged. The Soviets announced a cut in their army by 1 million men, and a thaw began to melt the cold war. A summit conference was scheduled in Paris for May 1960, after which Eisenhower planned to make a triumphal tour of the Soviet Union.

On the eve of the summit, the Soviets finally shot down a U-2 plane. Eisenhower, believing the pilot had died, lied, saying that it was only a weather plane that had gone off-course. With great glee Khrushchev then produced the live pilot, Francis Gary Powers, who had already confessed to the spy mission. Humiliated, Eisenhower told his secretary that he was "very depressed" and "would like to resign." Khrushchev went to Paris, attacked Eisenhower, and short-circuited the summit. The Soviets again upped the pressure on West Berlin. The cold war returned in force. But the question remains: Why, in the midst of the most promising era of U.S.-Soviet relations since 1945, did someone in the CIA or the White House allow the U-2 to make this final, fateful mission? That question has never been answered.[64]

THE EISENHOWER ERA AS FANTASY AND FACT

In looking back, the 1950s seem one of the happiest, most stable, and most secure eras in American history. At the time, however, the United States was a troubled nation, made nearly paranoid by McCarthyism, revolutions in the newly emerging world, and imagined "missile gaps," as well as by the shadow of economic recession. Hope seemed to lie in the military, CIA, and FBI. Hollywood's science-fiction films (which were new in postwar movie making) mirrored the great fear of technology, communism, and the unknown. In *The Thing*, for example, scientists were ignorant or evil (if not pro-Soviet), while the military personnel knew that the only way to deal with the creature from outerspace was to kill it. The memorable last line of the film could be understood as a political warning: "Tell the world—Watch the skies, everywhere—Watch the skies!"[65]

Eisenhower, however, seemed a center of calm and reason. His popularity, journalist James Reston wrote in 1955, had become "a national phenomenon, like baseball." The president tried to use his great appeal to control defense spending and, above all, to protect the U.S. economy. In truth, by early 1961 the U.S. nuclear stockpile had tripled in just two years to 18,000 weapons. The Pentagon's plans were now aimed at striking not the twenty to thirty Soviet targets picked out in 1948, but more than 2,500 such targets in 1960. U.S. nuclear weapons were stationed in at least four overseas countries. As for the economy, in 1960, the head of the Federal Reserve Board warned that gold and dollars were so rapidly exiting the country that "this is the first time in my lifetime that the credit of the United States has been questioned." Eisenhower meanwhile set important precedents by using the CIA to try to overthrow nationalist, popular governments in Iran, Guatemala, and Indonesia. Dulles fashioned a far-flung network of alliances that, in Eisenhower's words, committed Americans "to support the defense of almost every free area . . . facing the Sino-Soviet complex."[66]

With these foreign policies, Eisenhower helped transform the Republican party from one led by conservative senator Robert Taft—who feared overextended commitments, mistrusted presidential power, and especially disliked NATO—to one led by Richard Nixon and Ronald Reagan, who believed that such global commitments and increased presidential power were both necessary and natural. Eisenhower's popularity and prestige helped make possible Nixon's and Reagan's expansive policies.

But Eisenhower is especially remembered for his farewell speech of January 1961. About to turn the White House over to John F. Kennedy, the old soldier, on national television, warned his audience that there would be "a recurring temptation" to solve crises through "some spectacular and costly action" that promised to be "the miraculous solution to all current difficulties." Such a miracle cure, Eisenhower declared, did not exist, nor could "a huge increase" in defense spending find it. He was worried that the nation would, nevertheless, bow to the pressures of vast powers "new in American experience": the "immense military establishment and a large arms industry." Americans "must guard against the acquisition of unwarranted influence, whether sought or unsought, by the military-industrial complex. The potential for the disastrous rise of misplaced power exists and will persist."[67]

Eisenhower, thus, left some interesting advice to his young successor. But he also left a powerful CIA, nuclear superiority based on a huge stockpile of weapons of mass destruction, and global commitments that depended on that "military-industrial complex." In the words of historian H. W. Brands, Jr., by emphasizing anticommunism and increased collective security, Eisenhower left "a debt of commitments that would outstrip American capabilities"; and by waging the cold war "by covert and admittedly repugnant means," and by failing to take "serious steps toward disarmament," Eisenhower left behind a record that could "eventually damage America's interests."[68] It was now up to Kennedy to choose.

Notes

1. Stephen E. Ambrose, *Eisenhower*, Vol. II: *The President* (New York, 1984), pp. 18–19.
2. Robert Wright, "Eisenhower's Fifties," *Antioch Review* 38 (Summer 1980): 277–290.
3. Douglas Brinkley, *Dean Acheson: The Cold War Years, 1953–71* (New Haven, Conn., 1992), pp. 8–9; Fred I. Greenstein, *The Hidden-Hand Presidency: Eisenhower as a Leader* (New York, 1982), pp. 9, 69.
4. Paul Boller, Jr., *Presidential Anecdotes* (New York, 1981), p. 292.
5. Sir Maurice Peterson to N. M. Butler, 10 April 1947, FO 371 AN 1480/28/45, British Public Record Office, Kew, Eng.; Ambrose, p. 21.
6. *U.S. News & World Report*, 24 January 1958, p. 104.
7. Robert J. Donovan, *Eisenhower: The Inside Story* (New York, 1956), p. 162.
8. A good and slightly different view is Duane A. Tananbaum, "The Bricker Amendment Controversy: Its Origins and Eisenhower's Role," *Diplomatic History* 9 (Winter, 1985): 73–93; "Legislative Leadership Meeting, Jan. 11, 1954, Supplementary Notes," Legislative Meetings, January–February 1954 File, Box 1, Ann Whitman File, Papers of Dwight D. Eisenhower, Dwight Eisenhower Library, Abilene, Kans.
9. Michael R. Beschloss, *Mayday: Eisenhower, Khrushchev, and the U-2 Affair* (New York, 1986), p. 83.
10. Anna K. Nelson, "John Foster Dulles and the Bipartisan Congress," *Political Science Quarterly* 101 (Spring 1987): pp. 43–44, 64.
11. Brinkley, p. 17; Stanley D. Bachrack, *The Committee of One Million: "China Lobby" Politics, 1953–1971* (New York, 1976).
12. Nora Sayre, *Running Time: Films of the Cold War* (New York, 1982), pp. 176, 201.
13. Diary entry of 2 July 1953, from the personal diaries of Dwight D. Eisenhower, made available by Francis L. Loewenheim, professor of history, Rice University, who found it at the Eisenhower Library.
14. Lloyd C. Gardner, *A Covenant with Power: America and World Order from Wilson to Reagan* (New York, 1984), p. 51; Donovan, pp. 3, 9.
15. Beschloss, p. 153.

16. William B. Pickett, "The Eisenhower Solarium Notes," *Society for Historians of American Foreign Relations Newsletter* 16 (June 1985): 1–8; Robert A. Divine, *Eisenhower and the Cold War* (New York, 1981), pp. 33–39.

17. David Alan Rosenberg, "The Origins of Overkill: Nuclear Weapons and American Strategy, 1945–1960," *International Security* 7 (Spring 1983): 27.

18. Samuel F. Wells, Jr., "The Origins of Massive Retaliation," *Political Science Quarterly* 96 (Spring 1981): 31–52; John Foster Dulles, "A Policy of Boldness," *Life*, 19 May 1952, p. 151.

19. JoAnne Brown, "A is for Atom, B is for Bomb: Civil Defense in American Public Education, 1948–1963," *Journal of American History* 75 (June 1988), pp. 80–88; Robert A. Divine, *Blowing on the Wind: the Nuclear Test Ban Debate, 1954–1960* (New York, 1978), esp. pp. 4–11, 100–101, 182–193, 281–295; *Washington Post*, 27 December 1983, p. A9; Robert Divine, "Early Record on Test Moratoriums," *Bulletin of Atomic Scientists* 42 (May 1986): 24–26.

20. Barton J. Bernstein, "Foreign Policy in the Eisenhower Administration," *Foreign Service Journal* 50 (May 1973): 30.

21. Lawrence Freedman, *The Evolution of Nuclear Strategy* (New York, 1983), pp. 77–78.

22. The standard account of the war is now Burton I. Kaufman, *The Korean War* (New York, 1986), esp. pp. 251–342, on ending the conflict; also see Ambrose, pp. 51–52; and especially Michael Carver, "Across the Dividing Line," *Times Literary Supplement*, 11–17 December 1987, p. 1368.

23. Walter Pincus, "Early Postwar Era . . . ,"*Washington Post*, 22 January 1985, p. A8; Wells, 37.

24. Divine, *Eisenhower and the Cold War*, ch. I, details the debate over "liberation."

25. John Colville, *Winston Churchill and His Inner Circle* (New York, 1981), p. 139; the best account of the debate in the summer of 1953 is M. Steven Fish, "After Stalin's Death: The Anglo-American Debate over a New Cold War," *Diplomatic History* 10 (Fall 1986): esp. 343,353.

26. Dean Acheson, *Present at the Creation: My Years in the State Department* (New York, 1969), pp. 652–659.

27. Mark Hamilton Lytle, *The Origins of the Iranian-American Alliance, 1941–1953* (New York, 1987), pp. 192–203, 205–218; Barry Rubin, *Paved with Good Intentions: The American Experience and Iran* (New York, 1980), pp. 45–90. A remarkable firsthand account by the key CIA agent is Kermit Roosevelt, *Countercoup* (New York, 1979).

28. Blanche Wiesen Cook, *The Declassified Eisenhower* (New York, 1981), pp. 269–270, 276.

29. Richard H. Immerman, *The CIA in Guatemala: The Foreign Policy of Intervention* (Austin, Tex., 1982), pp. 190–201; Robert J. McMahon, "Eisenhower and Third World Nationalism: A Critique of the Revisionists," *Political Science Quarterly* 101, no. 3 (1986): 467. The Dulles quote is in Peter Lyon, *Eisenhower, Portrait of the Hero* (Boston, 1974), p. 627.

30. Philip C. Roettinger, "For a CIA Man, It's 1954 Again," *Los Angeles Times*, 16 March 1986, pt. V, p. 5; an important recent account, put in the 1944–1985 context, is Robert Trudeau and Lars Schoultz, "Guatemala," in *Confronting Revolution*, ed. Morris J. Blachman (New York, 1986), esp. pp. 25–28.

31. Jonathan Schell, *The Time of Illusion* (New York, 1976), p. 59.

32. Beschloss, p. 104.

33. "Legislative Leadership Meeting, June 21, 1954, Supplementary Notes," Legislative Meetings Series, Box 4, Eisenhower Library; *The Pentagon Papers*, Senator Gravel ed., 4 vols. (Boston, 1971), I, pp. 83–84.

34. U.S. Government, *Public Papers of the Presidents of the United States: Dwight D. Eisenhower, 1954* (Washington, D.C., 1958), pp. 382–383.

35. George C. Herring and Richard H. Immerman, "Eisenhower, Dulles, and Dienbienphu," *Journal of American History* 71 (September 1984): 356–357; Colville, p. 140.

36. Divine, *Eisenhower and the Cold War*, pp. 45–51.

37. Ambrose, p. 184. The most thorough and useful analysis of the 1953–1954 U.S. decisions is now Lloyd Gardner, *Approaching Vietnam: From World War II through Dienbienphu* (New York, 1988), esp. chs. IV–VIII

38. The Geneva agreements and the U.S. statement are in Department of State, *American Foreign Policy, 1950–1955: Basic Documents* (Washington, D.C., 1957), pp. 750–788; a good brief discussion is in George Herring, *America's Longest War: The United States and Vietnam, 1950–1975*, 2d ed. (New York, 1986), pp. 37–42.

39. George McT. Kahin, *Intervention: How America Became Involved in Vietnam* (New York, 1986), pp. 70–81.

40. The U.S. creation of SEATO as a means for containing communism is a central theme in Gardner, *Approaching Vietnam;* U.S. Congress, Senate, Committee on Foreign Relations, 83d Cong., 2d sess., 1954, *Hearings . . . on the Southeast Asia Collective Defense Treaty* (Washington, D.C., 1954), pt. I, pp. 16–17; important documents and commentary are in Lloyd Gardner, "Dominoes, Diem, and Death, 1952–1963," in *America in Vietnam*, ed. William Appleman Williams *et al.* (New York, 1985), esp. pp. 172–179.

41. Herring, pp. 71–72; Kahin, p. 88, has the 1961 quote by the U.S. expert.

42. David Mayers, "Eisenhower's Containment Policy and the Major Communist Powers, 1953–1956," *International History Review* 5 (February 1983): 83; and Mayers's detailed analysis in his *Cracking the Monolith* (Baton Rouge, La., 1986), esp. pp. 135–150; Gordon H. Chang, *Friends and Enemies* (Stanford, 1990), p. 144.

43. Beschloss, pp. 103–104.

44. Anthony Eden, *The Memoirs of Anthony Eden: Full Circle* (Boston, 1960), pp. 60–71, 167–194; Brian R. Duchin, "The 'Agonizing Reappraisal,' " *Diplomatic History* 16 (Spring 1992), p. 220.

45. Richard J. Barnet, *The Alliance: America-Europe-Japan, Makers of the Postwar World* (New York, 1983), pp. 574–596; an authoritative French view is Pierre Mélandri, *Les États-Unis face à l'unification de l' Europe: 1945–1954* (Paris, 1980).

46. Adam B. Ulam, *Expansion and Coexistence: The History of Soviet Foreign Policy, 1917–1967* (New York, 1968), pp. 574–596.

47. Nelson, 58; Chester L. Cooper, *The Lion's Last Roar: Suez, 1956* (New York, 1978), p. 94.

48. Cooper, pp. 181–182; Beschloss, p. 137.

49. Ambrose, p. 367. The best detailed analysis of the Suez (and eastern bloc) crisis is Donald Neff, *Warriors at Suez* (New York, 1981), esp. pp. 342–414, on how events in the two regions collided.

50. Cooper, pp. 259–260.

51. A superb analysis of the change in the late 1950s is Burton Kaufman, *Trade and Aid* (Baltimore, 1982), esp. pp. 152–182; Harold Vatter, *The American Economy in the 1950s: An Economic History* (New York, 1963), pp. 259–264.

52. "Minutes of Cabinet Meeting, November 6, 1959," p. 2, Cabinet Meetings of President Eisenhower (microfilm), Eisenhower Library; H. W. Brands, Jr., "Blueprint for Quagmires, or Keeping the SOBs on Our Side," *Society for Historians of American Foreign Relations Newsletter* 17 (March 1986): 5.

53. "Remarks of the Secretary," Opening Session, Western European Chiefs of Mission Meeting, Paris, 9 May 1958, Conference Dossiers, Papers of John Foster Dulles, Princeton; off-the-record remarks to U.S. ambassadors to Europe, Paris, 9 May 1958, NATO Ministers' Meeting, Conference Dossiers, *ibid.*

54. Steven L. Spiegel, *The Other Arab-Israeli Conflict: Making America's Middle East Policy, from Truman to Reagan* (Chicago, 1985), pp. 82–93; documents on the doctrine and the invasion are in *The Record of American Diplomacy*, ed. Ruhl J. Bartlett 4th ed. (New York, 1964), pp. 842–848.

55. Stephen E. Ambrose, *Nixon: The Education of a Politician, 1913–1962* (New York, 1987), pp. 476–477.

56. Tad Szulc, *Fidel: A Critical Portrait* (New York, 1986), pp. 284, 314–315, 381; Wayne S. Smith, *The Closest of Enemies: A Personal and Diplomatic Account of U.S.-Cuban Relations since 1957* (New York, 1987), esp. ch. I.

57. Jeffrey J. Safford, "The Nixon-Castro Meeting of 19 April 1959," *Diplomatic History* 4 (Fall 1980): 425–431; Saul Landau, "Asking the Right Questions about Cuba" (1987), manuscript in author's possession.

58. Richard E. Welch, Jr., *Response to Revolution: The United States and the Cuban Revolution, 1959–1961* (Chapel Hill, N.C., 1985), pp. 10, 26; Arkadi Shevchenko, *Breaking with Moscow* (New York, 1985), p. 105.

59. Unnamed *Washington Post* columnist quoted in the *Nation*, 21 December 1985, p. 687.

60. Ambrose, *Eisenhower: The President*, p. 434; the text is available in U.S. Congress, Joint Committee on Defense Production, 94th Cong., 2d sess., 1976, *Deterrence and Survival in the Nuclear Age* [the Gaither Report of 1957] (Washington, D.C., 1976), esp. pp. 12–23.

61. Beschloss, p. 154; a sample of Johnson's criticism is in *U.S. News & World Report*, 17 January 1958, pp. 100–102.

62. Beschloss, pp. 5, 392; Douglas Kinnard, *The Secretary of Defense* (Lexington, Ky., 1980), pp. 60–61.

63. Brinkley, p. 82; Barry M. Blechman and Stephen S. Kaplan, *Force without War: U.S. Armed Forces as a Political Instrument* (Washington, D.C., 1978), pp. 374–377; Beschloss, pp. 162, 378.

64. Beschloss, pp. 254, 317.

65. Sayre, pp. 191–198.

66. Dwight D. Eisenhower, *The White House Years*, 2 vols. (Garden City, N.Y., 1963–1964), II, pp. 364–365; Rosenberg, p. 66; Godfrey Hodgson, *America in Our Time* (New York, 1976), p. 7, a useful and readable survey of the post-1945 years.

67. The text is in *Eisenhower as President*, ed. Dean Albertson (New York, 1963), pp. 162–163.

68. H. W. Brands, Jr., *Cold Warriors: Eisenhower's Generation and American Foreign Policy* (New York, 1988), p. 211, also 195, 199–200.

For Further Reading

Materials for further reading on specific topics may be found in the notes of the relevant sections of this chapter and also in the General Bibliography at the end of this book. The best place to look next is *Guide to American Foreign Relations since 1700*, ed. Richard Dean Burns (1983), more helpful on pre-1981 works than any textbook could be. References that follow are consequently mostly post-1981 publications. References in the notes and General Bibliography are generally not repeated below.

A useful bibliographical source is R. D. Bohanan, *Dwight Eisenhower: A Selected Bibliography of Periodical and Dissertation Literature* (1981). For overviews of the 1950s and more references (other than the Ambrose and Divine volumes listed in the notes), helpful are Jeff Broadwater, *Eisenhower and the Anti-Communist Crusade* (1992), an important analysis that stresses Ike's anti-communism even after McCarthy was discredited; Gary W. Reichard, *Politics as Usual: The Age of Truman and Eisenhower* (1987), especially good for interpretations; *Reevaluating Eisenhower: American Foreign Policy in the Fifties*, ed. Richard A. Melanson and David Mayers (1987), with interpretive essays; John Lewis Gaddis, *Strategies of Containment* (1982), critical and places the 1950s in a larger containment context; Frederick C. Mosher, David W. Clinton, and Daniel G. Lang, *Presidential Transitions and Foreign Affairs* (1987), good case studies on 1952 and 1960; Burton I. Kaufman's important and pioneering *Trade and Aid: Eisenhower's Foreign Economic Policy, 1953–1961* (1982); Walt W. Rostow, *Eisenhower, Kennedy and Foreign Aid* (1985), an insider's account.

The Eisenhower Presidential Library at Abilene, Kansas, has been an exemplary leader in declassifying and making available its rich resources. University Publications of America has microfilmed many of these resources. Subjects include the Dulles-Eisenhower telephone conversations, NSC meetings, cabinet meetings, and, of particular interest, twenty-eight reels (with printed guide) of *The Diaries of Dwight D. Eisenhower, 1953–1961.* Two sets of important letters are available in published form in *Ike's Letters to a Friend, 1941–1958*, ed. Robert W. Griffith (1984); and Peter G. Boyle, *The Churchill-Eisenhower Correspondence, 1953–1955* (1990).

Good work has appeared on specific subjects and geographical regions. On Korea, Edward C. Keefer, "President Dwight D. Eisenhower and the End of the Korean War," *Diplomatic History* 10 (Summer 1986), provides both synthesis and interpretation; on Vietnam (in addition to the key volumes by Gardner and Herring cited in the notes), the dean of U.S.–Southeast Asia scholars, George McT. Kahin, has published *Intervention: How America Became Involved in Vietnam* (1986); Louis A. Peake's *The United States in the Vietnam War, 1954–1975: An Annotated Bibliography* (1984), has 1,200-plus well-organized entries, along with a chronology; and David L. Anderson's *Trapped by Success* (1991) is good on Vietnam policy, 1953–1961. On the Offshore Islands crises, Thomas E. Stolper, *China, Taiwan, and the Offshore Islands* (1985), is especially important for the Chinese side.

For U.S.–Western European relations, see especially Frank Costigliola, *France and the United States* (1992); Frank Ninkovich, *Germany and the United States* (1988); *The*

Special Relationship: Anglo-American Relations since 1945, ed. William Roger Louis and Hedley Bull (1986), is crucial on the English-speaking partners; Alfred Grosser, *The Western Alliance: European-American Relations since 1945* (1980), gives a distinguished western European viewpoint; a French view is in Bernard Lewidge, *De Gaulle et les Americains* (1984); Robert Rhodes, *Anthony Eden: A Biography* (1987), exploits Eden's private papers and, along with David Carlton's biography of Eden, can be used to gain insight into the decline of British power from 1935 to 1956; Diane B. Kunz's important *Economic Diplomacy of the Suez Crisis* (1991); Evelyn Shuckburgh, *Descent to Suez: Foreign Office Diaries, 1951–1956*, ed. John Charmley (1986), gives a British insider's view of the sad story; and Peter L. Hahn, *The U.S., Great Britain and Egypt, 1945–1956* (1991), is the standard account. The historic agreement on Austria is well analyzed in Audrey Kurth Cronin, *Great Power Politics and the Struggle over Austria, 1945–1955* (1986). A too-often-overlooked analysis is Bennet Kovrig's important and provocative *The Myth of Liberation: East-Central Europe in United States Diplomacy and Politics since 1941* (1973). On the Middle East, other than the volumes dealing with Suez noted above, William J. Burns, *Economic Aid and American Policy toward Egypt, 1955–1981* (1985), is especially good on U.S. domestic politics, as is Steven L. Spiegel, *The Other Arab-Israeli Conflict: Making America's Middle East Policy, from Truman to Reagan* (1985); and Cheryl Rubenberg, *Israel and the American National Interest* (1986), which is more critical of those domestic politics. Two key accounts are David W. Lesch, *Syria and the United States* (1992), and Douglas Little, "Cold War and Covert Action, The U.S. and Syria, 1945–1958," *Middle East Journal* 44 (Winter 1990). On Africa, Martin Meredith, *The First Dance of Freedom: Black Africa in the Postwar Era* (1985), is a starting point, as is Peter Duignan and L. H. Gann, *The United States and Africa: A History* (1984), important for its sweeping historical framework; Madeline Kalb, *The Congo Cables: The Cold War in Africa from Eisenhower to Kennedy* (1982); and for a revealing case study, see Harold G. Marcus, *Ethiopia, Great Britain, and the United States, 1941–1974: The Politics of Empire* (1983), rich in its use of British materials and questioning of Western policies. On the Cuban Revolution and on U.S. policy in Latin America more generally, Morris Morley's *Imperial State and Revolution: The United States and Cuba, 1952–1985* (1987) is important, as is Louis A. Perez, Jr., *Cuba and the United States* (1990). W. LaFeber, "Thomas C. Mann," in *Behind the Throne*, eds. T. McCormick and W. LaFeber (1993)—essays in honor of Fred Harvey Harrington—gives an overview on Latin American policy. A standard account is now Piero Gleijeses, *Shattered Hope* (1991), which is on U.S.-Guatemalan relations.

Nuclear strategy in the 1950s has received much attention. In addition to the Divine volumes listed in the notes, and Divine's *Eisenhower and Sputnik* (1993), a good overview is provided in George T. Mazuzan, "American Nuclear Policy," in *Modern American Diplomacy*, ed. John M. Carroll and George C. Herring (1986); Walter A. McDougall's magisterial and prize-winning *The Heavens and the Earth: A Political History of the Space Age* (1985); Samuel F. Wells, Jr., "The Origins of Massive Retaliation," *Political Science Quarterly* 96 (Spring 1981), which traces the roots back to Truman; *The Structure of the Defence Industry: An International Survey*, ed. Nicole Ball and Milton Leitenberg (1983), especially Judith Reppy and David Holloway on the United States and the USSR since 1945; Howard Ball, *Justice Downwind: America's Atomic Testing Program in the 1950s* (1986); Milton S. Katz, *Ban the Bomb: A History of SANE, the Committee for a Sane Nuclear Policy, 1957–1985* (1986), provides important social as well as political history; Richard Pfau, *No Sacrifice Too Great: The Life of Lewis L. Strauss* (1984), a fine biography that focuses on the *Oppenheimer* case; and Barton J. Bernstein's view of the same subject in "Sacrifices and Decisions: Lewis L. Strauss," *Public Historian* 8 (Spring 1986). In addition to the work of David Holloway and Adam Ulam, George W. Breslauer, *Khrushchev and Brezhnev as Leaders* (1982), is important for a glimpse inside the Kremlin; and T. Michael Ruddy, *The Cautious Diplomat: Charles E. Bohlen and the Soviet Union, 1929–1969* (1986) examines a key figure, if sometimes a distant one. An important interpretive overview is Lloyd C. Gardner, "The Atomic Temptation," in *Redefining the Past: Essays in Honor of William Appleman Williams,* ed. Lloyd C. Gardner (1986). A key perspective is Stuart W. Leslie, *The Cold War and American Science: The Military-Industrial-Academic Complex at MIT and Stanford* (1992).

17

JFK and LBJ: From the New Frontier through the Great Society to Vietnam (1961–1969)

KENNEDY

The 1960s were characterized by violence, domestic rioting, near-nuclear war, assassinations, and economic failure. The decade also was a time of unmatched progress in civil rights; in peaceful relations between Soviets and Americans; in long-needed programs to help schools, the sick, and the elderly; and in music (the Beatles) and technology (the first person, Neil Armstrong, walked on the moon in 1969). One view of the 1960s was recalled a quarter of a century later by a distinguished American historian: "Unparalleled power, unprecedented wealth, unbridled self-righteousness—it all struck me as an ominous combination full of potential dangers to the republic."[1]

Another view emerged from a 1979 public-opinion poll revealing that 33 percent of Americans wished that John F. Kennedy, of all U.S. presidents, "were President today." JFK received more than twice the support given the second choice (Franklin D. Roosevelt).[2] Remembered as "decisive," no doubt he was also recalled as a handsome man with a beautiful wife and family who perfectly used the relatively new medium of television. He represented in his own career the American-dream marriage between the glamor of Hollywood (where his father invested in movies and JFK dated actresses) and the power of Washington.

Born in 1917, raised in both Boston's Irish-Catholic neighborhoods and high society's vacation spots in Florida and Cape Cod, Kennedy first gained attention in 1940, when he published his Harvard senior thesis, *Why England Slept.* He argued that deep forces in democracy and capitalism had paralyzed the West in the 1930s. Democratic leaders, in his view, had disastrously failed to meet Hitler's challenge. During World War II, he became a hero when Japanese ships destroyed his torpedo boat and he rescued other sailors before the survivors were found by U.S. vessels. Elected to the House of Representatives in 1946 and the Senate in 1952, Kennedy was not a Democratic party power. His votes on economic issues earned him his reputation as a liberal, but he was more conservative on civil liberties (his public attitude toward Senator Joseph McCarthy was not critical) and on many foreign-policy issues. He condemned a "sick" Roosevelt for giving away too much at the 1945 Yalta Conference, blasted Truman for supposedly losing China to the Communists, and urged always higher defense spending.[3] Between 1956 and 1960, he used his family's great wealth to help set up an organization outside the Democratic party's machine, whose senior members considered his youth and his Roman Catholicism to be handicaps in a presidential race.

A City on the Hill on the New Frontier

Kennedy, nevertheless, won the nomination and faced Vice-President Richard Nixon in the 1960 campaign. Each man took a hard line on foreign policy. Kennedy was tougher on Castro than was Nixon, and the vice-president was more adamant about defending the Chinese offshore islands than was Kennedy. Neither impressed Harry Truman or Dean Acheson, who considered Nixon too sleazy and Kennedy too young and more concerned with image than substance. "The best campaign cheer," Acheson wrote friends, is that "anyway, they can't elect both of them."[4] But Nixon's poor appearance in the first televised debate between two presidential candidates, an economic downturn, and southern votes gathered by JFK's vice-presidential nominee, Lyndon B. Johnson of Texas, had more to do with Kennedy's paper-thin margin of victory than did foreign-policy issues.

The new president saw himself as a man of action. His movie hero was John Wayne, his favorite reading included Ian Fleming's novels about superagent James Bond. His campaign theme was "the New Frontier" on which he believed Americans must embark. In his inaugural address, the key line was "And so, my fellow Americans: ask not what your country can do for you—ask what you can do for your country." He believed that Americans would "bear any burden" to win "the freedom of man."[5] Scholars had recently predicted that the technological society would put an end to ideological debates (such as communism versus capitalism), and Kennedy believed that the nation was moving beyond them as well to form a new consensus on national— and especially foreign—policies.

He had good reasons for reaching such a conclusion. In 1961, a commission funded by the Rockefellers (led by Nelson Rockefeller, the Republican governor of New York) published *Prospects for America*,[6] which called for a rapid military build-up to close the supposed missile "gap" that favored the Soviets, more money and men needed to fight expensive conventional (not just nuclear) wars, and more resources poured into newly emerging nations before the Soviets could obtain footholds. Republicans shaped the Rockefeller report (the staff director was a young Harvard professor, Henry Kissinger). But Democrats, including Dean Rusk, also signed it. From now on, the cold war was to be waged against communism abroad, not argued about at home.

Or so many on the New Frontier believed. Leaving Boston in 1961 to move into the White House, Kennedy quoted the famous words of John Winthrop to the Massachussetts Bay settlers in 1630: "We must always consider that we shall be as a city upon a hill—the eyes of all people are upon us." Such overblown rhetoric was too much for one Republican. Kennedy is making a "frightful call to arms," while building a huge government "that is Big Brother to us all." "Under the tousled boyish hair cut it is still old Karl Marx." Thus wrote Hollywood actor Ronald Reagan to Richard Nixon.[7]

THE CONSENSUS PRESIDENCY

The new administration believed that a strong, popular, glamorous presidency supported by key Republicans would allow Kennedy to ignore such critics as Reagan and dismiss—or control—public opinion. As the president's top aide, Theodore Sorensen, phrased it, public opinion "is frequently hampered by myths and misinformation." It is "promiscuous and perfidious in its affection, and always difficult to distinguish. For it rarely speaks in one . . . united voice."[8] Voices that did emerge in 1961 strongly supported their own version of anti-communism. For example, the Committee to Warn of the Arrival of Communist Merchandise on the Local Business Scene was formed that year in Miami and quickly spread to forty-six states. It attacked merchants who sold communist-made products (such as hams from Poland) by posting signs saying, "Always buy your Communist products at _____."[9]

Kennedy moved to cement the anti-Communist consensus by reappointing the ultraconservative J. Edgar Hoover as director of the Federal Bureau of Investigation (FBI) and Allen Dulles as director of the Central Intelligence Agency (CIA). After consulting extensively with Republicans, he appointed Dean Rusk as secretary of state. Rusk was not a Republican, but a quiet Democrat who had been president of the Rockefeller Foundation. Between 1949 and 1953, he had served as Dean Acheson's top assistant for Far Eastern affairs and was known as violently anti-Chinese—or, as he put in in a 1951 speech, he believed that the Maoist "regime may be a colonial Russian government. . . . It is not the government of China."[10] Rusk was a secretive, capable bureaucrat who was rightly proud of his rise to power from a childhood spent in the poor Georgia back country.

Rusk's State Department had quadrupled from 6,200 persons in 1941 to over 24,000 in the 1960s. It had to act on some 1,300 incoming telegrams every day and send out over 1,000.[11] The cautious Rusk and his careful professionals moved too slowly for the on-the-move Kennedy crowd that relaxed by playing bruising games of touch football. The president appointed McGeorge Bundy to head the National Security Council (NSC). A Harvard professor and member of a well-connected New England family, Bundy had long been close to Republicans. With Kennedy's approval, he changed the NSC until it became a small, fast-acting State-Department-in-the-White-House that could immediately respond to the president's desires. And, unlike Rusk, Bundy could not be called before Congress to testify. The NSC could act more secretly as well as more rapidly.

To head the Defense Department, Kennedy named Robert McNamara. A Republican and the young president of the Ford Motor Company, McNamara had a mind like a computer and the firm belief that if you could find the right numbers, you could find the right foreign policy. To make the Pentagon more efficient, McNamara brought in "whiz kids" from leading universities. These experts from "think tanks" of M.I.T., Columbia, Princeton, California, and Harvard had worked closely with the military to develop a more efficient generation

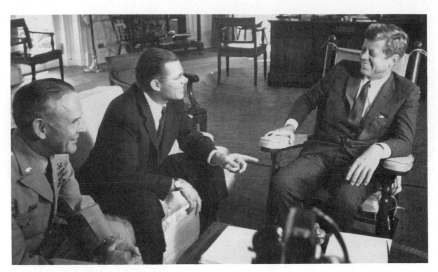

*President John F. Kennedy (1917–1963) confers with Secretary of Defense
Robert S. McNamara (center) and General Maxwell Taylor (left) as the two
advisers brief the president on the war in Vietnam. The resulting instability in
the nations involved forced American diplomacy to focus increasingly on the so-
called Third World.*

of technology for U.S. forces as well as computerized accounting methods so that the Pentagon could deliver more bang for the buck. Foreign
policy was to be removed as far as possible from politics and made
more scientific.[12]

THE CONSENSUS ECONOMY

The president gave the key Treasury position to C. Douglas Dillon,
another Republican and head of one of the world's most powerful
investment banking houses. Kennedy worried that unless the economy
was pumped up, his foreign policy would collapse. "If we cannot keep
up our export surplus," he warned, dollars would not be available "to
meet our overseas military commitments." And if Americans had to
"pull back," they might repeat the tragic story of the ancient Romans,
whose success "depended on their will and ability to fight successfully
at the edges of their empire." Kennedy was not certain that "we were
yet in a position" to fight on those edges of the American Empire.[13]
He ordered Dillon to strengthen the economy.

But the new Treasury secretary hoped to do it without radical measures. Neither of the two great drains on the economy—military spending and private overseas investment—was to be cut. Indeed, Kennedy asked that both be jumped to ever-higher levels. The new costs were to be paid by cutting and reforming the tax structure so that the economy would speed up and produce more government revenue. The export of gold to pay for U.S. trade deficits was to be stopped by a variety of economic tinkering. And, above all, world markets were to be opened to U.S. goods. In 1962, Congress passed the most far-reaching trade bill since the 1930s. It gave the president the power to cut U.S. tariffs 50 percent for nations that would welcome more American goods. It also established under the president a special trade representative who was to open more international markets for U.S. producers. This measure led to a "Kennedy round" of trade talks in which other nations did, indeed, agree to open global trade, although the prosperous European Economic Community, under French president Charles de Gaulle's prodding, never opened itself to American goods as Washington officials had hoped.

The Kennedy team also tried to find dollars by setting up an office in the Defense Department to sell weapons abroad for profit. *Forbes* business magazine noted that, in the 1930s, such salesmen of weapons were called "merchants of death," but "times have changed." The government itself now helped sell arms to assist "non-communist countries . . . and also to close the dollar gap." Unfortunately, as *Forbes* admitted, arms sometimes also went to non-Communists who hated each other—such as India and Pakistan, who used the weapons to fight against one another. Nevertheless, such giant firms as General Dynamics and Lockheed sold about $1 billion worth of arms abroad each year.[14]

The Kennedy policies helped create a U.S. economic boom between 1961 and 1967. But it was not enough. American overseas commitments and costs rose faster than even the booming economy could pay for. By mid-1963, despite growing political troubles worldwide, Kennedy told a French visitor that he was most worried about the dollar's weakness.[15] The greenback was less and less able to pay for defending the free world. The president's attempt to create a political consensus also stumbled. He had brought experts to power, and "they may be every bit as intelligent as you say," the salty, powerful Speaker of the House, Sam Rayburn, told Vice-President Johnson, "but I wish just one of them had run for sheriff once."[16]

THE CHALLENGE: LATIN AMERICA AND THE ALLIANCE FOR PROGRESS

A series of crises quickly challenged Kennedy's ability to fight the cold war. The first arose in the less-industrialized world. The president was especially sensitive to these nations because, in January 1961, Nikita Khrushchev delivered a ringing declaration that revolutions in such countries were the wave of the future; the Soviet system—not the American—was best able, he proclaimed, to ride that wave.

The new nations in Asia, Africa, and Latin America helplessly watched the prices of their raw materials sink 22 percent between 1950 and 1964 as compared to the prices of manufactured goods they bought from Europeans, Japanese, and Americans.[17] The rich were getting richer, the poor poorer—and more numerous. The world population of 2.8 billion in 1960 was projected to reach 7.0 billion by the year 2000. John Spanier estimated that India's population increase each year equaled a city the size of New York, and the Asians were doubling their birth rate over that of Europeans, while Latin Americans were roughly doing the same over that of North Americans.[18]

In his January speech, Khrushchev pointed to Castro's victory in Cuba as a sign that the "onslaught of the imperialists" was being destroyed with a triumphant "war of national liberation."[19] Kennedy was not pleased. During the presidential campaign, he had blasted Eisenhower for losing Cuba and urged military intervention by U.S.-supported Cuban exiles to remove Castro. But the president realized, too, that parts of Latin America were, indeed, ripe for Castroism. Poverty multiplied, and U.S. aid was insignificant. Between 1946 and 1960, the United States gave about $60 billion in foreign aid, but less than 7 percent of it went to Latin America, and most of that directly benefited U.S. corporations operating in the region.[20] On March 13, 1961, Kennedy proposed to Latin American ambassadors the Alliance for Progress. Over the next ten years, $100 billion ($20 billion from North Americans and $80 billion from Latin Americans) had to be made available for development. U.S. aid would thus multiply many times. But, in return, Kennedy asked for land and tax reforms so that the money would benefit the poor and middle classes. In 1962, he warned of the consequences if the alliance failed: "Those who make peaceful revolution impossible will make violent revolution inevitable."[21]

The alliance was organized at Punta del Este, Uruguay, in August

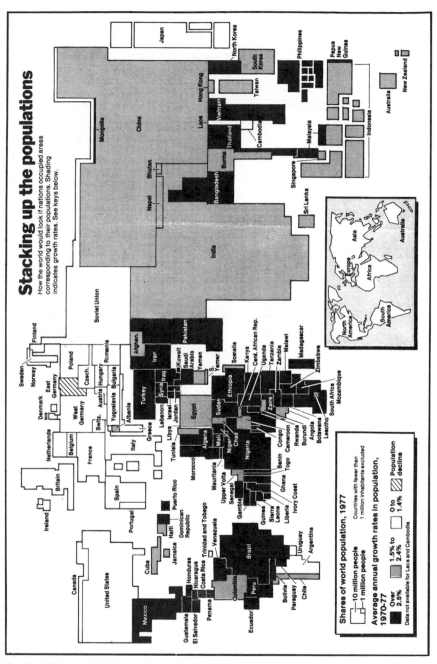

Stacking up the populations

How the world would look if nations occupied areas corresponding to their populations. Shading indicates growth rates. See keys below.

Shares of world population, 1977

- 10 million people
- 1 million people

Countries with fewer than 1 million inhabitants excluded

Average annual growth rates in population, 1970-77

- Over 2.5%
- 1.5% to 2.4%
- 0 to 1.4%
- Population decline

Data not available for Laos and Cambodia

In the 1960s and 1970s, awareness grew about the impact of the increasing population on dwindling resources. The U.S.'s Alliance for Progress was a key program created to handle the problem. (Source: *Michael Kidron and Ronald Segal*, The State of the World Atlas. *Used by permission, Simon & Schuster.)*

1961, when the hemisphere's nations—except for Cuba, which abstained—pledged to make the reforms in return for the billions. But the plan soon broke down, and by 1970 Latin America was worse off than in 1961. The reasons for the failure were many. First, most southern nations were ruled by small, rich elites, or oligarchs, who controlled the best lands. They had little intention of giving up their land to the landless or heavily taxing themselves. The oligarchs, thus, took the dollars but also kept their wealth. To make the alliance work first required political change to remove these elites. But U.S. officials wanted nothing to do with throwing out or weakening these stable, pro-Washington oligarchs.

Second, Congress directly ordered no U.S. funds to be used to carry out the heart of the program—that is, land redistribution to the poor. Taking from the rich and giving to the poor may have sounded good to Robin Hood, but it sounded too much like socialism to Congress.

Third, most Roman Catholic Latin Americans rejected birth-control methods needed to curb the population increase. They were supported by Latin American politicians, who warned that birth control was a Yankee plot to keep southern nations weak. And with high infant mortality as well as the need for many cheap hands in the villages, southern Americans believed they needed large families to survive.[22]

Fourth, the Latin elites put alliance funds not into staple foods (such as beans) to feed the poor, but into export crops (such as cotton and coffee). Thus, the elites profited from their export trade, while the poor starved.

Fifth, U.S. officials were never able to create a plan or an organization to resolve these problems. The officials wanted slow reform and believed that measures proven effective under the Marshall Plan (1948–1952) in western Europe (see p. 479) could work in Latin America. But Latin American economies were radically different from democratic European societies that only needed capital to rebuild war-devastated industries. In Latin America, fundamental change, not just money, was needed.

By the mid-1960s the alliance did reach its target of an annual 5.5 percent growth rate in the region. But of every $100 of new income produced, only $2 went to the poorest 20 percent of the people. Anger and frustration grew until terrorism and revolution burst out in Venezuela, Colombia, Bolivia, and Guatemala. Latin American military forces often responded brutally. By 1970, military rule had replaced thirteen constitutional governments since 1960, usually by forceful overthrow. Kennedy was rarely downbeat, but just before his death in November

1963 he admitted he was "depressed" by the alliance's sad turn of affairs.[23]

The Challenge: The Bay of Pigs

One month after announcing the Alliance for Progress, Kennedy launched an invasion of Cuba at the Bay of Pigs to overthrow Castro. In 1960, Eisenhower had ordered the CIA to train several hundred Cuban exiles for a military offensive. The agency believed that a small invasion would trigger an uprising against Castro, just as the invasion of Guatemala in 1954 caused the overthrow of that government (see p. 546). By April 1961, the invasion force had grown to 1,500, but Kennedy had decided not to provide U.S. air cover. He feared that if the United States became directly involved, Khrushchev would perhaps retaliate by invading West Berlin.[24]

Nevertheless, the president pressed ahead, despite warnings from his military advisers, because the CIA believed that there would be an anti-Castro uprising. Moreover, Kennedy did not want to kill Eisenhower's plan, especially after he had condemned Eisenhower for being too soft on Castro. In early April, White House aide Arthur Schlesinger, Jr., wrote a public white paper to justify an invasion on the ground that Castro had betrayed the Cuban Revolution. The white paper was mostly propaganda, especially since Castro himself had largely defined that revolution. Meanwhile, a CIA agent refused to tell the anti-Castro underground inside Cuba when the invasion would begin, thus revealing another weakness in the plan. "I don't trust any goddamn Cuban," the agent declared. The leader of the CIA operation, Richard Bissell, knew little about Cuba and its people, and, as it turned out, even less about the Bay of Pigs (where the CIA thought that photos of sharp coral reefs that wrecked landing craft revealed only seaweed). When Kennedy told Dean Acheson of the plan, even this crusty old Cold Warrior was astounded: you didn't need to consult such accountants as "Price Waterhouse to discover that 1,500 [invading] Cubans weren't as good as 250,000 [Castroite] Cubans," Acheson told the president.[25]

Without air cover, without a historical justification, without trust, and without intelligence, the invasion began on April 17. Within hours, it was wiped out by Castro's forces. No uprising occurred. Castro had learned the real lesson of the 1954 Guatemala operation—he made the government and the army one and the same. Thus, his army, unlike

Guatemala's, never deserted his government. In all, the Bay of Pigs invasion was the perfect failure. Kennedy was humiliated. But the consensus held. Public-opinion polls gave him the highest ratings of support during his entire presidency immediately after this disaster. "It's just like Eisenhower," Kennedy joked. "The worse I do the more popular I get."[26] But he knew that one more such failure and his presidency could be finished.

He and his brother, Attorney General Robert Kennedy, secretly set up a $100 million plan—code-named Operation Mongoose—employing several thousand people to wage a covert war against Castro. The president ordered the CIA to sabotage the Cuban economy. The agency also planned to kill Castro, plans apparently worked out in cooperation with U.S. mob figures. One plan was to give Castro exploding cigars. Another plan was to spread the word in Cuba that the Lord's Second Coming was about to occur, but that the Lord hated Castro. On the day of the Lord's supposed appearance, a U.S. submarine would surface along the coast, set off fireworks, and so frighten the Cubans that they would then overthrow Castro. One CIA agent labeled this bizarre plan "Elimination by Illumination."[27]

To paraphrase Shakespeare, however, the problem was not in the stars but in Kennedy's foreign policy. He and the CIA actually made Castro more popular and powerful than ever. In a televised speech of April 20, 1961, the president took full responsibility for the invasion fiasco and called on Americans to rally around him to fight a new kind of cold war in, among other places, Vietnam.[28]

THE CHALLENGE: VIETNAM (1961–1963)

In 1961, Southeast Asia seemed to be swinging like a huge pendulum, slowly but surely toward neutralism, perhaps communism. The British had largely destroyed a Communist rebellion in their former colony of Malaya, but newly independent (and renamed) Malaysia remained weak and vulnerable. India and Indonesia also seemed open to Communist-bloc pressure. The three former French colonies of Indochina— Vietnam, Laos, and Cambodia—appeared to be falling slowly to Communist rebels despite nearly $1 billion in U.S. aid that poured into the area between 1955 and 1961, and despite 658 U.S. advisers in Vietnam and 300 more in Laos.

Even before the Bay of Pigs embarrassment, Kennedy had determined to stand firm in Southeast Asia. Vividly recalling the vicious attacks (including his own) against Truman for "losing" China, Kennedy did not plan to become a similar political victim in the 1960s. Moreover, the need of Japan (by far the most important U.S. ally in Asia) for Southeast Asian markets and raw materials rose along with the skyrocketing Japanese economy. But the picture in Vietnam itself was grim. As elderly General Douglas MacArthur told the young president in late 1961, "The chickens are coming home to roost, and you live in the chicken house."[29]

Kennedy's most pressing problem was in Laos, the narrow, strategically located nation that the 1954 Geneva Conference had supposedly neutralized. But Laos became a vital highway (the Ho Chi Minh Trail) along which Ho's North Vietnamese Communist forces moved covertly into South Vietnam. Moreover, by 1961, the United States had ignored the Geneva agreement and established a friendly regime of General Phoumi Nosavan. Laos's Communists, the Pathet Lao, and neutralist forces countered by seizing key areas. As he left the White House, Eisenhower emotionally warned Kennedy that Laos was the gateway to all of Southeast Asia, and if it fell, the new president could forget about saving the rest of the region.[30] (See map, p. 552.)

In April 1961 (amid the Bay of Pigs failure), Kennedy sent the U.S. Seventh Fleet and a helicopter force to the area. He obtained a cease-fire between Phoumi and the Communists, but far-right forces—supported by the CIA—kept on fighting. The Communists retaliated and seemed on the brink of a major victory. Kennedy sent air power and U.S. Marines into areas bordering Laos. Both sides then agreed to talk and, in July 1962, made a pact that again neutralized Laos. All foreign troops were to leave. But the Pathet Lao continued to seize territory, and the North Vietnamese continued to protect the Ho Chi Minh Trail. Americans both armed the neutralist right-wing government and bombed Communist forces. In 1964, a right-wing faction seized control of the government. The CIA returned to Laos in force.[31]

Throughout his ordeal, Kennedy's allies refused to give much help. They believed that the West's power in Laos was small, almost nonexistent. One day on a yacht cruising down the Potomac, the president tried to convince the elegant, cool British prime minister, Harold Macmillan, to send help. Macmillan refused to waste scarce British resources in Laos. Amid the argument, they saw a local college team rowing a small racing scull down the river. "What have we here?" asked Macmillan. "The Laotian Navy?"[32]

By the end of Kennedy's presidency, Vietnam had become more important than Laos. When he entered the White House, the president found Vietnam still governed by the authoritarian, inefficient regime of Ngo Dinh Diem. Reforms, especially crucial land reform, had stopped. Between 1958 and 1960, Ho Chi Minh's northern Communists had begun organizing revolts against Diem and had discovered that many of the South's peasants were willing to join. With Ho's help, the National Liberation Front (NLF or Vietminh) became the rebels' political arm in 1960. It included non-Communist as well as Communist leaders. China helped by accelerating economic aid to Ho.

In April 1961, a special U.S. military mission told Kennedy that Diem only controlled 40 percent of South Vietnam. Shortly after this report (and the Bay of Pigs invasion), the president sent 500 more U.S. advisers to help Diem. The president especially took a strong personal interest in the new Special Forces, or Green Berets, that he had helped develop (he even paid special attention to such details as the design of their uniform) to fight revolutionaries in such places as Vietnam. Kennedy broke the 1954 Geneva agreement, which provided that no more than 685 military advisers were to be in South Vietnam. As historian Stephen Pelz concludes, "Between January and May [1961] Kennedy had committed the United States to save South Vietnam."[33]

At this point, the president dispatched Vice-President Johnson to examine the growing crisis. Johnson publicly called Diem the "Churchill of today," but Diem rejected the U.S. request that American troops be sent in to help fight the war. Determined to keep control of his own army, Diem only wanted U.S. advisers to train his soldiers. But, as Kennedy's top military adviser, General Maxwell Taylor, recalls, "We eventually broke down [Diem's] resistance."[34] In October 1961, a mission led by Taylor and Walt Rostow of the State Department reported back to the president that only a major increase in the U.S. effort could save Diem. Kennedy took their report seriously. Taylor had belonged to a group known as the Never Again Club—top military officers experienced in the Korean War who swore that U.S. troops should never again be sent to fight in Asia without, if necessary, nuclear weapons. But Kennedy also knew that sending more troops could be dangerous. "The troops will march in," he said privately, "the bands will play; the crowds will cheer; and in four days everyone will have forgotten. Then we will be told we have to send in more troops. It's like taking a drink. The effect wears off and you have to take another." Historian Lloyd Gardner comments: "Prompted by the advisers he had appointed . . . , Kennedy took the first drink. How could he do otherwise?"[35]

Rejecting one U.S. military request that 40,000 men be sent, he nevertheless ordered in 10,000 troops during 1962–1963. By 1963,

Kennedy had placed more than 16,000 U.S. soldiers in South Vietnam and had tripled military aid to the area to $185 million. But it was not nearly enough. Diem's regime continued to flounder, especially when powerful Buddhist leaders protested the war as well as Diem's governmental policies. As more U.S. soldiers died, the American media began to pay attention. Kennedy and the military tried to restrict media coverage and to remove critical journalists, but with little success.[36]

Even his acclaimed win in the Cuban missile crisis of October 1962 (see p. 597) did not help Kennedy. He, indeed, concluded that while that victory taught the Soviets a lesson, the Chinese—now bitter enemies of the Soviets—would want to humiliate both superpowers by gaining control of Southeast Asia. "The Chinese are perfectly prepared, because of their lower value of human life," he privately told a French official in 1963, "to lose hundreds of million [of people] if necessary . . . to carry out their militant and aggressive policies." It is now clear that Kennedy became so obsessed with his fear that China was developing a nuclear weapon that, after the Cuban missile crisis, he approached Khrushchev with the suggestion that military strikes might be used to destroy the Chinese nuclear facilities. As he phrased it in instructions to the U.S. diplomat (W. Averell Harriman) who was to discuss this with the Soviet leader: "You should try to elicit Khrushchev's view of means of limiting or preventing Chinese nuclear development and his willingness either to take Soviet action or to accept U.S. action aimed in this direction." As the historian of this remarkable episode, Gordon Chang, concludes, "The Kennedy administration came dangerously close to answering in the affirmative the question . . . : 'Should we bomb Red China's bomb?' " Only Khrushchev's cold response to Kennedy's approach perhaps prevented a U.S. attack on China.[37]

But as the president became more fixated on the Chinese threat to Asia, he seemed to become more confused, at least publicly, about how to deal with his collapsing policy in Southeast Asia. In a television interview of September 1963, Kennedy declared, "In the final analysis it is their [the Vietnamese'] war." A week later, however, the president told another television audience that "I believe" in the domino theory. China (which "looms so high") could seize the region, so "I think we should stay" in Vietnam. "We should not withdraw."[38]

Washington officials saw Diem as the problem. After eight years of U.S. training, his much larger army was humiliated by a mere battalion of Vietminh at a key battle in the village of Ap Bac during 1963. Three Americans died in the fight. Diem's army then fired into a crowd

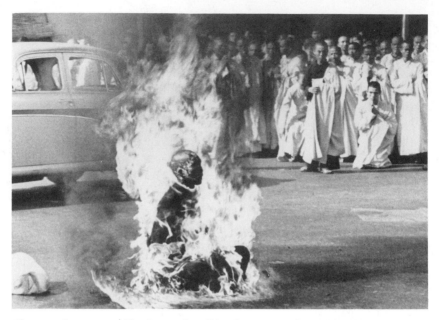

Dismissed as a mere "barbecue show" by the sister-in-law of South Vietnam's leader, Ngo Dinh Diem, the self-immolation by Buddhist monks who protested Diem's rule created a major crisis for Kennedy's policy in Vietnam in mid-1963.

of Buddhists who were defying a government ban on parading religious banners. Riots erupted in mid-1963. In protest, Buddhist monks burned themselves to death while U.S. television cameras rolled. Americans were doubly shocked when Diem's sister-in-law, Madam Nhu, described the scene as a "barbecue show." The U.S. policy of "Sink or Swim with Ngo Dinh Diem and Let's Have No Poo about Madam Nhu" now began to change. Kennedy demanded that Diem hurry reforms and listen to U.S. advice. Frustrated South Vietnamese generals saw their chance and prepared to overthrow Diem. U.S. officials did nothing to stop the coup and, indeed, gave signals that the generals interpreted as a green light. On November 1, 1963, Diem and his brother Ngo Dinh Nhu were captured and killed by the generals. (Madame Nhu was out of the country.) Three weeks later, President Kennedy was assassinated in Dallas, Texas.

Historians have since argued whether, as some of his aides have claimed, Kennedy intended to pull U.S. troops out of Vietnam once he was safely re-elected in 1964. Filmmakers have also entered this argument, led by Oliver Stone, whose highly popular movie, *JFK*, starred Kevin Costner. Stone's Kennedy intended to leave Vietnam, and, as a result, was assassinated by right-wing conspirators who intended to put Lyndon Johnson in the White House so the United States would remain in Southeast Asia. The evidence for Stone's argument is, to say the least, weak. If Kennedy had any thoughts about getting out, he had to drop them after Diem's murder because, after that, the military situation in Vietnam fell apart, U.S.–South Vietnamese forces were faced with defeat, and the United States now had heavy responsibility for the new South Vietnamese regime it had helped put in power. The number of U.S. advisers continued to grow on the battlefields, and in Washington Kennedy placed great faith in the very advisers who later pushed Johnson to increase the American commitment. Kennedy's closest aide, Theodore Sorensen, later said that the president viewed the war as "this nation's severest test of endurance and patience," and that "He was simply going to weather it out, a nasty, untidy mess to which there was no other acceptable solution." But it was now Lyndon Johnson's war. The warning given by U.S. Department of State official Chester Bowles to Kennedy in 1961 seemed prophetic: "We are headed full blast up a dead end street."[39]

THE SUPERPOWERS: FROM VIENNA AND TANKS IN JULY

Vietnam was not the only "chicken" that came "home to roost" in Kennedy's White House during 1961. Khrushchev renewed his 1958 demands that the Allies turn West Berlin over to the Communist East German regime. Kennedy was determined not to give way on the German question. He agreed with a top adviser that without West Germany, "Western Europe is an eggshell."[40]

The two leaders met in Vienna during June 1961. It was a frosty affair. (When a frustrated JFK asked the Soviet leader whether the latter ever admitted to having made a mistake, Khrushchev only replied, "Certainly"—in 1956 "I admitted all of Stalin's mistakes.")[41] Kennedy warned that neither side should try to upset the balance of power, especially in the newly emerging world. Khrushchev retorted that the Soviets would continue to support "wars of national liberation." The two men engaged in a heated ideological debate. Kennedy returned home worrying that it was "going to be a long winter."

But the president also knew by mid-1961 that the so-called missile gap did, indeed, exist—overwhelmingly in his favor. The U.S. Samos II spy satellites revealed that instead of the 400 intercontinental ballistic missiles (ICBMs) that Kennedy feared the Soviets possessed, a mere

4 existed. The president dug in his heels when Khrushchev threatened in July to move on Berlin. On national television Kennedy warned that the United States would tolerate no changes. To make his point, he ordered 150,000 reservists to active duty, tripled the number of draft calls for young men, and asked for an immediate $3.2 billion to spend on defense. (Eisenhower's arms budget of nearly $46 billion in 1960 was on its way to becoming $54 billion by the end of 1963.) Most ominously, the president demanded $207 million for more civil defense in anticipation of possible nuclear war. "In the coming months," Kennedy told Americans, "I hope to let every citizen know what steps he can take without delay to protect his family in the case of attack." As historian Douglas Brinkley comments, "JFK had made the Berlin crisis a test of both his and America's courage and determination."[42] And the president had overwhelming superiority in nuclear weaponry to back him up in the test.

As tension thickened in early August 1961, East Germans (especially the better educated) left their Communist home in ever-greater numbers. On August 13, Khrushchev suddenly solved the problem by building a cement-block wall, topped with barbed wire and sentry houses, to seal off East Berlin (and, later, most of East Germany) from the West. No longer could skilled East Germans leave for work in western Europe. The wall was built on Soviet-controlled territory. Kennedy could only have destroyed it by invading East Germany. He instead sent Vice-President Johnson to buck up West German morale. West German officials angrily demanded more and better U.S. protection. Talks between Kennedy and aged Chancellor Konrad Adenauer were so bitter that they agreed to burn the record of their meeting. In June 1963, the president nevertheless made a triumphant visit to West Berlin. Before the wall he told a huge crowd, "All free men, wherever they may live, are citizens of Berlin, and, therefore, as a free man I take pride in the words, *'Ich bin ein Berliner'* [I am a Berliner]."

Despite American rhetoric, the wall stood and the military build-up accelerated on both sides. Kennedy's NSC adviser, McGeorge Bundy, told him during the 1961 crisis that if force had to be used, "the current plan calls for shooting off everything we have in one shot."[43] To gain flexibility, the president ditched Eisenhower's plan to depend on nuclear weapons. Instead he listened to Paul Nitze, whose NSC-68 in 1950 (see p. 504) had urged a conventional force build-up. Kennedy, thus, could make a "flexible response." But he and McNamara also continued developing their nuclear stockpile of ICBMs. The United

States was running the arms race against itself, for Khrushchev had decided to await new technology.

By 1962, Kennedy and top Pentagon officials realized the extent of their force superiority. They began to discuss openly the possibilities of a U.S. first strike (to which the Soviets could not respond) or making nuclear war more attractive by using their new, more accurate weapons to hit only military targets (a "counterforce" strategy) instead of civilian targets. Furious Soviet officials denied that such targets could be so neatly separated. Khrushchev halted his three-year nuclear test ban in September 1961 by exploding huge (if primitive) weapons. Kennedy also resumed testing, despite the U.S. lead and pleas from the British that he not do so. Meanwhile Khrushchev angrily asked his advisers, "Why [do] Americans have so many bases around the Soviet Union and we have no bases near the United States?"[44]

... To the Cuban Missile Crisis (1962)

Resembling the U.S.-USSR nuclear relationship, U.S.-Cuban relations had also worsened since the Bay of Pigs. In early 1962, Kennedy was able to have Cuba expelled from the Organization of American States (OAS) and an economic embargo imposed on the island. Castro moved closer to Khrushchev. By mid-1962, estimates placed more than 20,000 Soviet advisers inside Cuba. Reports circulated that Soviet missiles and IL-28 jet bombers were in place. Sensing a political victory in the 1962 congressional elections, Republicans cried that Kennedy stood by while missiles were being placed in Cuba to level "the American heartland." The president responded that defensive missiles (that is, ground to air) were acceptable, but ground-to-ground weapons were not. He believed that the Cubans had the former but not the latter missiles. In truth, Kennedy was finding himself cornered. His CIA Director, John McCone, had warned the president in August 1962 that Khrushchev might move missiles and bombers into Cuba. McCone was the only Kennedy adviser who gave the warning, but the president became so worried about the political implications that he ordered McCone to change the wording of his report. McCone believed that Kennedy feared if information of the arrival of Soviet bombers in Cuba "got into the press, a new and more violent Cuban issue would be injected into the [1962 political] campaign and this would seriously affect his independence to act." When in September, the CIA warned

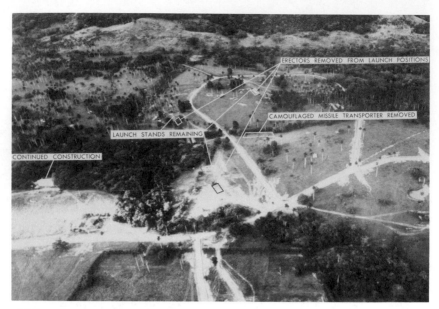

A U.S. reconnaissance spy-plane photo of Soviet missile sites in Cuba during the tensest moments of the October 1962 crisis.

Kennedy that a surface-to-surface missile system might be moving into Cuba, the White House ordered the information kept completely away from the American public.[45]

On October 14, 1962, however, a U-2 plane filmed medium-range (1,000 mile) missiles on Cuban launching pads. Intermediate (2,000 mile) missiles also appeared to be under construction. Documents released nearly thirty years later in Moscow revealed why Khrushchev took the gamble of his life. To his closest advisers, he gave two reasons: first, the Americans intended to invade Cuba with their own forces ("we had good information on this account"); and second, "since the Americans have already surrounded the Soviet Union with a ring of their military bases and various types of missile launchers, we must pay them back in their own coin . . . so they will know what it feels like to live in the sights of nuclear weapons." There was also a third reason: Castro so strongly wanted nuclear protection against the United States that, ultimately, he was willing to incinerate his island if only Khrushchev would strike the United States first. In June, Fidel's brother, Raul, had flown to Moscow to work out the plan. By October 14, missiles and warheads were in Cuba when the U-2 spotted the sites.[46]

Two days later, Kennedy convened a special group of top officials, soon known as the ExComm (Executive Committee), to discuss policy in strict secrecy. One member (Sorensen) doubted that the missiles "significantly alter[ed] the balance of power." McNamara agreed with Sorensen, but the top military officials (the Joint Chiefs of Staff) argued that the power balance was substantially changed. The usually cautious Rusk decided at one point that instead of going "down with a whimper," it might be "better to go down with a bang." ExComm finally sorted out four possible options: handle the issue diplomatically and make no military response; trade off U.S. missiles in Turkey for the removal of Soviet missiles in Cuba; attack the missile sites by air and, if necessary, follow up with a U.S. invasion; or set up a blockade (or "quarantine") that would cut off Cuba and squeeze Khrushchev and Castro into removing the missiles. President Kennedy finally chose the last option, in part because if it did not work he could then escalate to a military option. Dean Acheson (brought in as a special adviser), was so bitterly disappointed that Cuba and the Soviet bases were not going to be bombed immediately that he resigned from ExComm.[47]

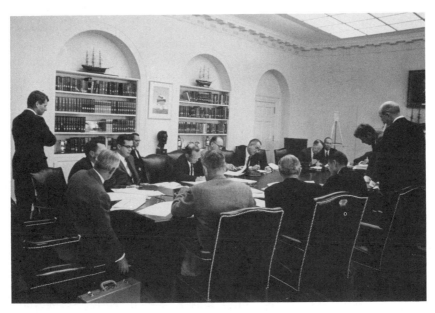

The ExComm (Executive Committee) group that advised President Kennedy during the missile crisis of 1962. Secretary of State Rusk stands at the right, the president bends down in front of Rusk, Vice-President Johnson is across the table from the president, Attorney General Robert Kennedy paces at left. The president's top aide, Theodore Sorensen (seated third from the left), later wrote: "I saw first-hand how brutally physical and mental fatigue can numb the good sense as well as the senses of normally articulate men."

In a dramatic television speech of October 22, the president announced the naval "quarantine," demanded the removal of the missiles, and warned that if any of the weapons were launched against the United States, he would fully respond—against the Soviet Union itself. Within forty-eight hours, the western European allies endorsed his policy. The OAS unanimously supported the blockade. The U.S. Strategic Air Command (SAC) went on its biggest airborne alert, with part of the B-52 bomber force, loaded with nuclear bombs, in the air at all times. Five army divisions prepared to invade Cuba. Unknown to McNamara, the SAC commander raised his forces to the next-to-highest level of alert in a clear, uncoded order so the Soviets could read it (which they did). The commander, as a later observer phrased it, rubbed "the Soviets' noses in their nuclear inferiority." Khrushchev never ordered his forces to go on alert. "We had a gun at his head and he didn't move a muscle," a U.S. Air Force general recalled.[48] On October 24, twelve of the twenty-five Soviet ships headed for Cuba changed course to return home. The remaining vessels carried no missiles.

But the most dangerous moments of the crisis lay ahead. In a rambling letter of October 26, Khrushchev indicated that he would dismantle the missiles in return for Kennedy's pledge never to invade Cuba. When told of the message, Acheson declared that the Soviet leader was "either tight or scared" and urged that the president get even tougher with Khrushchev. On the twenty-seventh, a quite different note arrived from Moscow: a demand that fifteen U.S. Jupiter missiles be removed from Turkey in return for dismantling the Cuban weapons. Kennedy had, months before, moved to take out the old, unneeded Jupiters; but any removal now could appear to give Khrushchev a major public victory. And just as Khrushchev's tougher note arrived, Kennedy learned that one of his U-2 planes had been shot down over Cuba and its pilot killed. McNamara believed that new orders had been given to Soviet and Cuban soldiers on the island, perhaps in preparation for war. At that moment, Kennedy received yet another piece of bad news: the Soviet technicians had moved the warheads closer to the missiles, possibly in preparation for a strike. That Saturday, the twenty-seventh, ExComm held a bitter meeting. Its members were exhausted as they approached a decision about attacking Cuba, a strike that would obviously kill many Soviets and perhaps provoke a response. McNamara realized, as he later said, that one missile "directed at Miami or New York or even Washington might have killed a million or 2 million people."[49]

Kennedy finally accepted a suggestion from his brother, the attorney general, to ignore the last note from Moscow and accept Khrushchev's suggestion of October 26. A virtual ultimatum cabled to Moscow demanded that the Soviets immediately stop work on the missiles. But Kennedy also gave vague assurances that there would be no invasion of Cuba. Moreover, he sent Robert Kennedy to inform a Soviet diplomat privately that the president had ordered the removal of the Jupiter missiles at NATO bases in Turkey and Italy. The attorney general further told the diplomat that if the Cuban missiles were not dismantled in forty-eight hours, the United States would take military action. Then, as Rusk revealed a quarter-century later, the president apparently moved to make certain there would be no war. He gave UN Secretary General U Thant a statement that the Jupiters would be removed if the Cuban weapons were dismantled. The statement was to be made public if Khrushchev rejected the ultimatum. "I am not," Kennedy said privately, "going to go to war over worthless missiles in Turkey." U Thant never had to use the statement. Khrushchev was ready to deal. On the twenty-sixth, the Soviet leader received a secret letter from Castro begging Khrushchev to launch a nuclear strike on the United States if Kennedy tried to invade Cuba. Castro seemed prepared to go down in flames. Khrushchev further learned of incidents that were erupting between Soviet and Cuban military. He considered the shooting down of the U-2 dangerously irresponsible. It was time to end the crisis. On October 28, he accepted Kennedy's public offer of taking out the missiles in return for a no-invasion pledge. The world stepped back from nuclear annihilation. Castro angrily castigated Khrushchev, refused to receive the Soviet ambassador to Cuba, and did his best to prevent a UN team from verifying that the missiles had indeed been taken down.[50]

How close the two superpowers came to the ultimate war became clear only a quarter-century later when American and Soviet documents began to be declassified. It was then revealed that Khrushchev had also placed in Cuba Luna missiles with nuclear warheads that had a range of twenty-five miles. If U.S. forces invaded, and communications with Moscow were cut, the Soviet commander in Cuba had the authority, on his own, to use these nuclear weapons against the invaders. When McNamara heard this in 1992 he was deeply shaken: "No one should believe that U.S. troops could have been attacked by tactical nuclear warheads without the U.S. responding with nuclear warheads. And where would it have ended? In utter disaster." Instead of utter disaster, Kennedy escaped with a spectacular victory. It later became apparent that he had even left a loophole in his no-invasion pledge: he promised no invasion if the missiles were removed and if "Cuba itself commits no aggressive acts against any of the nations of the Western Hemisphere." That loophole could have allowed his successors in the White House to invade Cuba in the 1960s, 1970s, and 1980s, given the belief of many Americans that Castro was indeed stirring up revolution in the hemisphere. In Moscow, Khrushchev's power never recovered. In early 1963, he dolefully complained in a secret, rambling, thirty-page letter to Castro that the Chinese were attacking him for not treating the United States like "a paper tiger, dung." As the Sino-Soviet split widened and Soviet-Cuban relations worsened, Khrushchev's Politburo finally removed him from power in October 1964 for public failures both abroad and at home (especially in collective agriculture). Meanwhile, Kennedy drew the most important lesson from the missile crisis: "Domestic issues can only lose elections, but foreign policy issues can kill us all."[51]

THE FALLOUT FROM THE MISSILE CRISIS

The effects of the crisis were felt far into the future. First, the Soviets made up their minds that "you Americans will never be able to do this to us again," as a top Soviet diplomat declared in late 1962.[52] The Moscow government launched a massive military build-up that within a decade pulled it close to U.S. nuclear strength. Khrushchev was replaced by a new group led by Leonid Brezhnev and Aleksei Kosygin—conservative, unimaginative, but usually predictable bureaucrats who jacked up military budgets.

Second, at home, the Democrats won the 1962 elections, but the missile crisis contributed little to the win. Kennedy came under strong attack from such Republicans as Arizona Senator Barry Goldwater and columnist William F. Buckley, Jr., for supposedly selling out the Monroe Doctrine with a no-invasion pledge that allowed Soviet influence to remain in the Western Hemisphere. The issue continued to boil. Twenty years later, conservatives urged the repudiation of the supposed 1962 pledge because the Communists brought in new jets and used Cuba as a base for supporting revolution in the region.[53]

Third, during the weeks after the missile crisis, the Western alliance, oddly, nearly shattered. European leaders had publicly supported Kennedy in the dark days of October, but, in President Charles de Gaulle's words, they were "informed" rather than "consulted" about U.S. policy. Europeans feared that they had gotten uncomfortably close to annihilation without representation. The snub was compounded when

Kennedy pushed a "grand design," one that would integrate U.S.-European economic and political policies so that the partners could pay more of the U.S. defense costs. When the Europeans saw that he had no intention of allowing them to help shape U.S. nuclear decisions, they blotted out the "grand design." But even worse occurred in late 1962, when Kennedy told London officials that they would not receive the U.S.-built Skybolt missile for use in British jet bombers. Eisenhower had promised them the Skybolt, and Great Britain had planned its air force around it. Now it was suddenly gone because the Americans thought the weapon not cost-efficient. The British then accepted other arms that made them even more dependent on the Americans.

De Gaulle had seen enough. He had long agreed with a British official who spit out, "The United States didn't want a partner. They wanted a satellite." He built up his own nuclear arsenal so that France would be independent of U.S. plans. De Gaulle never believed that in a future crisis the United States would risk nuclear war merely for French interests. He also announced that France would formally leave NATO by 1966. Then came his final blow: in early 1963, the stumbling British economy tried to find help by joining the European Common Market, but de Gaulle killed London's application. The British, he declared, were a "Trojan horse" for Washington, which, he feared, would use the horse to take over the entire Common Market. De Gaulle, one frustrated U.S. official complained, "is the most goddamn undealable-with human being that's ever existed."[54] Kennedy left the Western alliance much weaker than he had found it.

A fourth result of the missile crisis was the growing American fear that others would copy de Gaulle. The crisis revealed that at the moment of truth, neither superpower consulted its allies nor wanted to go to war. Thus, the stand-off allowed the allies—especially the newly emerging nations—to have more freedom from the superpowers. Washington officials privately warned that U.S. policy had to stop this fragmentation, this splintering of Western cooperation, by stepping up American commitments.[55] This reasoning led to greater involvement in Vietnam during 1963, and also to Kennedy's determination to contain China's influence in the newly emerging nations.

Fifth, one part (perhaps the most important) of U.S. foreign policy markedly improved. Both Americans and Soviets had learned the horror of teetering on the brink of nuclear war. In a June 1963 speech at American University in Washington, D.C., Kennedy asked that the cold-war rhetoric and policies be changed so such crises could be avoided. Khrushchev responded cooperatively. In August 1963, the two nations signed their first arms-control pact, an agreement in which the above-ground testing that was causing lethal radiation in milk and other foods was prohibited. The two powers also wanted a deal that would discourage nuclear testing by new competitors (such as the French and Chinese). Besides, weapons for Kennedy's new "flexible response" military plans could be tested below-ground. Indeed, below-ground testing went on at an ever-faster rate. But at least a first step had been taken in arms control. Kennedy took that step, however, only after fighting and compromising with those Pentagon, CIA, and Senate opponents who feared any arms deal at all with Communists. When the president next made a major wheat sale to the Soviets, Richard Nixon (now practicing law while raising himself from the political dead) warned that "the [Soviet] bear is always most dangerous when he stands with his arms open in friendship."[56]

Finally, after the crisis, Kennedy secretly entered into indirect talks with Fidel Castro, even as the CIA's Operation Mongoose tried to destroy Castro's regime and as the president showed warm support for the anti-Castro Cuban exiles in Miami. Castro opened the exchange, Kennedy responded, and both sides wrote out an agenda for the talks just before Kennedy was shot in Dallas on November 22, 1963.[57]

Henry Kissinger suggested a dozen years later that "the Kennedy period will be seen as the last flowering of the previous era rather than as the beginning of a new era."[58] Between 1961 and 1963, confidence in U.S. power and in a glamorous, active presidency had never been higher. That confidence resembled a star that beamed brightest just as it began to burn out.

LBJ: AT HOME AND THE GULF OF TONKIN

Many believed the new chief executive, Lyndon Baines Johnson of the Texas hill country, would never burn out. He seldom saw movies because he "didn't like to be alone in dark places," an aide said. "Talking on the telephone was the way he unwound." On the phone or in person, LBJ was usually giving someone "the treatment." As described by one Texas politician, "Lyndon got me by the lapels and put his face on top of mine and he talked and talked and talked. I figured it was either getting drowned or joining." His vice-president, Minnesota Democrat Hubert Humphrey, was often poked in the chest and once pulled his trouser leg up to show cuts where Johnson had kicked him while yell-

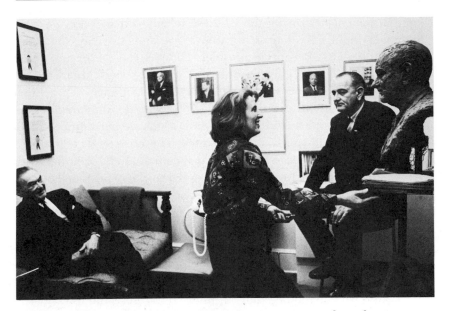

Walter Lippmann (1889–1974), at left in the picture, was perhaps the most influential American journalist in the twentieth century. As a young man he was a leading theorist of Progressivism; later he became a theorist of American conservatism. Refusing to serve in government after his disillusionment with Woodrow Wilson (see p. 325), he nevertheless was an intimate of many presidents, including Lyndon Johnson, sitting here for a bust of himself in April 1965. But as Lippmann became a key conservative critic of the Truman Doctrine in 1947 (see p. 483), so he became an early and leading critic of Johnson's policies in Vietnam, until the two men became bitter enemies in 1966–1967.

ing, "Get going now!" Despite, or because of, "the treatment," and because of a rare political intuition, Johnson had become perhaps the most powerful majority leader in the U.S. Senate's history before Kennedy asked him to run as vice-president. With his aggressiveness came immense pride and possessiveness in his state's, his nation's, and his own power. When he invited dignitaries to his Texas ranch, they were met by a fleet of large cars and helicopters, including, one foreign leader recalled, one "helicopter for the liquor—the United States is a great power." "You will never work for or with a more complicated mind than Lyndon Johnson so long as you live," Robert McNamara told a White House aide.[59] One way or another, the new president believed he could control any person, any situation.

He grew up politically in the 1930s, when Munich was a bad name (see p. 386). World War II seemed to be proof that Americans could, when they put their minds to it, run world affairs. He attacked Harry

Truman for not destroying the Chinese in the Korean War and condemned Dwight Eisenhower for allowing a supposed "missile gap." Within hours after becoming president, he pledged, "I am not going to be the President who saw Southeast Asia go the way China went."[60] Sometimes, however, he scored with remarkable patience. When Fidel Castro shut off the water supply to the U.S. base in Guantánamo Bay, many screamed for retaliation. Johnson only dispatched equipment so that the base could purify its own water. The crisis ended; the base remained. In Panama, the Panamanians' demand to fly their flag with the American banner in the canal zone led to riots and bloodshed in early 1964. In December 1964, LBJ agreed to negotiate a historic pact to replace the 1903 treaty that divided Panama in half. The new pact needed fourteen more years of talk, but Johnson had taken the crucial first step.

During the 1964 presidential campaign, however, Johnson was less patient. This was partly due to conservative Republican nominee Barry Goldwater, who demanded tough military responses. And it was partly due to the weakness of the post-Diem governments in South Vietnam. Regime replaced regime as if they were in a revolving door. The war could not be waged effectively because of this weakness. Nor—of special importance—could Johnson think of negotiating a settlement with Ho Chi Minh's Communist regime in North Vietnam while holding such a weak hand. Amid this frustration, North Vietnamese torpedo boats attacked a U.S. warship on August 2 in the Gulf of Tonkin. Two days later, another attack supposedly occurred.

Johnson's response proved historic. He ordered U.S. planes to bomb the north's ships and bases. Then LBJ asked Congress to pass a Gulf of Tonkin resolution giving him the right "to take all necessary measures to repel any armed attack against the forces of the United States and to prevent further aggression." The resolution sailed through the House by a vote of 416 to 0 but encountered trouble in the Senate from Oregon Democrat Wayne Morse and Alaskan Democrat Ernest Gruening, who warned that the measure gave the president a blank check to use force as he wished in Southeast Asia. This charge was denied by Arkansas Democrat J. William Fulbright, chairman of the Senate Foreign Relations Committee, who urged that the president be trusted. The Senate then passed the resolution 88 to 2 on August 7, 1964. Over the next four years, evidence appeared that the Gulf of Tonkin attack was not unprovoked. The U.S. ships were accompanying sabotage operations against North Vietnam. Moreover, the second attack had probably never occurred.[61]

Johnson, nevertheless, had it both ways in 1964. He lambasted Goldwater as a dangerous fanatic and pledged that "we are not about to send American boys 9 or 10,000 miles away from home to do what Asian boys ought to be doing for themselves."[62] Meanwhile, he ordered air attacks on North Vietnam. As usual, foreign policy mattered little in most voters' minds. (One survey showed 25 percent of Americans did not know that China was a Communist country or that U.S. soldiers were fighting in Vietnam.)[63] Johnson, emphasizing the need for a "Great Society" at home made up of government programs for helping the young, old, poor, and minorities, buried Goldwater in a political landslide.

LBJ AND LATIN AMERICA: THE JOHNSON DOCTRINE IN ACTION

Johnson knew that he was dealing with a boiling furnace in trying to handle the newly emerging world. But he could figure out neither how to escape to a safe distance nor how to turn the fire down. The president noted in 1966 that eight years before, thirty-four important conflicts had erupted in the world, but in 1965 some fifty-eight had occurred—more than half in nations whose people earned less than $100 annually. In Latin America, the Alliance for Progress was creating an immense foreign debt, military rulers, and revolutions, not progress. LBJ continued to support publicly the alliance and change, but his speechwriter thought that LBJ's words seemed like "a lot of crap to me."[64] Johnson feared revolution and had grown to mistrust the alliance. He wanted stability and order. U.S. training for Latin American police and military was increased.

"I know my Latinos," said Thomas Mann, LBJ's top adviser on Latin America. "They understand only two things—a buck in the pocket and a kick in the ass."[65] Johnson used the bucks in Brazil and the kicks in Peru and the Dominican Republic. Throughout the twentieth century, huge, rich, strategically located Brazil had been Washington's closest Latin American partner. By 1964, however, the government of João Goulart, like its neighbors, was in deep economic trouble. When Goulart could not carry through internal belt-tightening, Johnson cut off U.S. aid. Inflation went out of control. Goulart then moved to seize U.S. properties. Encouraged by officials from the U.S. Embassy, the Brazilian military overthrew Goulart, while Washington ordered its fleet to stand off the coast in case it were needed. But the Brazilian military required no help and established a brutal twenty-year dictatorship.

Ironically, once in power, the generals often defied the United States by dealing with revolutionary African regimes and refusing to promise Washington that they would not build nuclear weapons.[66]

But Johnson continued to send aid to the generals while cutting off money to Peru's civilian government. The Peruvians were trying to gain control of their country's major oil company, a firm owned by Standard Oil of New Jersey. Robert Kennedy, now a senator from New York, observed: "What the Alliance for Progress has come down to then is that you can close down newspapers, abolish congress, jail religious opposition [such as in Brazil] . . . and you'll get lots of help, but if you fool around with a U.S. oil company, we'll cut you off without a penny." A State Department official agreed, "That's about the size of it."[67]

LBJ also delivered a kick to the Dominican Republic. Since the 1930s a U.S. Marine-trained dictator, Rafael Trujillo, had ruled the country and supported Washington's policies. In 1956–1958, however, his brutal police agents carried out kidnappings and murders of Trujillo's opponents in the United States. His methods at home seemed to be creating conditions for another Castro to come to power. President Eisenhower sent weapons to the Dominican military who opposed Trujillo. In May 1961, they gunned down the elderly dictator as he drove to visit his twenty-year-old mistress. Juan Bosch, a moderate, won election to the presidency. By 1963–1964, the military had deposed Bosch and regained power.

The Dominican military, however, divided into factions. Bosch's group also maneuvered to regain power. In April 1965, one military group tried to overthrow the government. Civil war erupted. Bosch's supporters gained strength, a turn that frightened U.S. officials, who wrongly believed that Bosch was a mere front for communism. On April 28, 1965, a panicked U.S. Embassy told Johnson that "Castro-type elements" might win. If that occurred, a top aide told LBJ, "it will be the worst domestic political disaster any administration could suffer." The president sent 22,000 U.S. and OAS troops to the Dominican Republic to stop the fighting and install a conservative regime. He claimed on television on May 2, 1965, that a "communist dictatorship" threatened—a threat "the American nations cannot, must not, and will not permit."[68]

This Johnson Doctrine (the president could use military force whenever he thought communism threatened the hemisphere) caused an angry uproar in both Latin America and the United States. The doctrine directly contradicted the nonintervention clause in the OAS char-

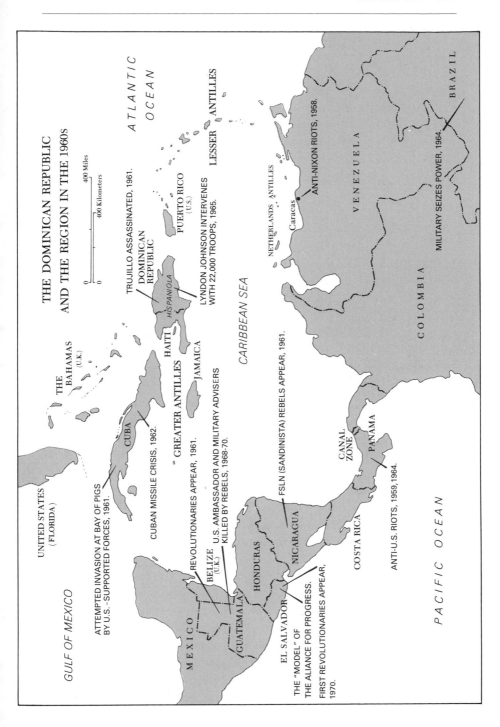

THE DOMINICAN REPUBLIC
AND THE REGION IN THE 1960s

400 Miles

400 Kilometers

ATLANTIC
OCEAN

UNITED STATES
(FLORIDA)

GULF OF MEXICO

THE
BAHAMAS
(U.K.)

CUBA

ATTEMPTED INVASION AT BAY OF PIGS
BY U.S.-SUPPORTED FORCES, 1961.

CUBAN MISSILE CRISIS, 1962.

GREATER ANTILLES

REVOLUTIONARIES APPEAR, 1961.

HAITI

HISPANIOLA

DOMINICAN
REPUBLIC

TRUJILLO ASSASSINATED, 1961.

PUERTO RICO
(U.S.)

LYNDON JOHNSON INTERVENES
WITH 22,000 TROOPS, 1965.

LESSER   ANTILLES

JAMAICA

CARIBBEAN SEA

NETHERLANDS ANTILLES

Caracas

ANTI-NIXON RIOTS, 1958.

VENEZUELA

BRAZIL

MILITARY SEIZES POWER, 1964.

COLOMBIA

U.S. AMBASSADOR AND MILITARY ADVISERS
KILLED BY REBELS, 1968-70.

BELIZE
(U.K.)

MEXICO

GUATEMALA

HONDURAS

FSLN (SANDINISTA) REBELS APPEAR, 1961.

NICARAGUA

EL SALVADOR

THE "MODEL" OF
THE ALIANCE FOR PROGRESS.
FIRST REVOLUTIONARIES APPEAR,
1970.

COSTA RICA

CANAL
ZONE

PANAMA

ANTI-U.S. RIOTS, 1959, 1964.

PACIFIC OCEAN

ter signed in 1948 by the United States. The roar grew louder in Washington when reporters discovered that the dozen or so inept, isolated Communists in the Dominican Republic posed no danger. If they were Marxists, they seemed closer to Groucho than Karl. Congress (now including the powerful Senator Fulbright) and other Americans concluded that LBJ had deceived them. Their anger increased between 1965 and 1972, when the new government in the small nation could neither stop hundreds of political killings each year nor curb rampant corruption. But for Johnson, much worse lay ahead.

LBJ AND VIETNAM: THAT "BITCH OF A WAR"

In December 1963, Defense Secretary McNamara declared, "We have every reason to believe that [U.S. military] plans will be successful in 1964." By late 1964, however, the South Vietnamese government and army were falling apart, while Americans were killed by terrorists in the South Vietnamese capital of Saigon. Johnson had not yet decided how to respond. He passionately wanted his Great Society at home more than a war 10,000 miles away. But he wondered whether Americans would support him in Washington if he appeared weak in Vietnam. His closest advisers, led by McNamara and NSC director McGeorge Bundy, believed that an escalated response by the world's greatest power would compel Ho Chi Minh's Communist forces to retreat. They also argued that LBJ had to move rapidly or the chaotic Saigon government would collapse.

These arguments moved Johnson to action in February 1965, when communist guerrillas killed 7 Americans and wounded 109 at the U.S. base at Pleiku. He first ordered air strikes against North Vietnam. Then he announced in April a $1 billion aid program and, in May, dispatched two U.S. Marine combat divisions. Only American soldiers, he believed, could now pump life into South Vietnam. In July, U.S. troop numbers jumped from 75,000 to 125,000. By late 1965, Americans had found two military leaders who promised to provide the needed political stability: Premier Nguyen Cao Ky and President Nguyen Van Thieu. Neither had the nationalist, anti-French background of Ho Chi Minh, but they were the most acceptable leaders whom U.S. officials could find. By the end of 1965, 160,000 U.S. troops were in Vietnam.

Johnson made this Far Eastern commitment for many reasons, reasons that tell us much about the entire course of post-1945 U.S. foreign policy. First, he believed that every president since Roosevelt had made

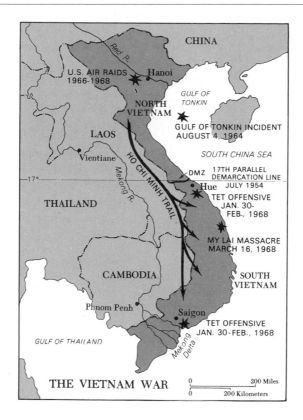

THE VIETNAM WAR

a commitment to protect Vietnam. American "credibility" was, therefore, at stake worldwide. If Communists won in Asia, he said in 1966, they can "succeed anywhere in the world."[69]

Second, he believed that China posed the great threat. Quoting Theodore Roosevelt, that Americans now lived in the "Pacific era," Johnson declared that "over this war—and all Asia" lay "the deepening shadow of Communist China," which "is helping the forces of violence in almost every continent." China was to be contained by Americans fighting in Vietnam. U.S. fear grew as Chinese scientists exploded a first, small atomic bomb in 1964 and, within three years, set off a hydrogen bomb one hundred times larger than the first bomb.

Third, his view of history appeared when Johnson raised the ghost of the 1930s: "We learned from Hitler at Munich that success only feeds the appetite of aggression."

Fourth, Johnson increasingly saw links between winning "the only woman I really loved" (the Great Society programs at home) and the "bitch of a war" in Asia. Losing could be costly. Truman's problems at home with the McCarthyites and witch hunts after the fall of China in 1949, LBJ believed, "were chickenshit compared with what might happen if we lost Vietnam."

Fifth, Johnson assumed that the incredible U.S. power could do the job—and do it alone, if necessary. Merely by picking up the phone, he could send hundreds of thousands of soldiers across the ocean. They would be accompanied by the genius of American technology. Helicopters, experimented with in France as early as 1914, had only run medical missions in the Korean War, but they now gave U.S. soldiers battlefield mobility and protection never before known. The air force and scientists united to defoliate huge jungle areas, where guerrillas liked to hide. ("Only we can prevent forests," ran one air unit's motto.) When critics noted how the French had failed to win in Indochina, a Pentagon official shot back, "The French also tried to build the Panama Canal."

Finally, Johnson believed that if he escalated slowly and did not demand too much of Americans and their economy, they would support his policy. The president, therefore, refused to ask for a congressional declaration of war that could justify a full-scale effort. With good reason, he believed that Americans would support a strong president who fought communism. "We did not put on big bond drives or [have] movie actors going around the country whopping up war-fever," Rusk later said, "because there's too much power in the world to let the American people become too mad." The plan, Rusk declared, "was not to let the situation go down the chute—the chute into a larger war."[70] Johnson, thus, tried to find a middle way that gained Americans' support but avoided war with China and the Soviets.

LBJ AND VIETNAM: THE MISCALCULATIONS

By 1966–1967, each of these reasons had crumbled. First, allies, indeed, began to doubt U.S. "credibility." But they did so because LBJ insisted on pouring resources into a bottomless war that these partners did not believe could be won. Moreover, many observers doubted that any links existed between Communist advances in Asia and those in, say, Latin America. Each region had its own peculiar conditions.

Second, experts on Asia noted that for a thousand years Vietnamese nationalists such as Ho had fought (not embraced) China. In 1946, Ho had even preferred to work with France: "It is better to smell the French dung for awhile than eat China's all our lives." Mao's government, moreover, had sunk into bitter infighting followed by a "cultural revolution" in 1966–1967 in which young Chinese tried to restore revolutionary fervor in the nation. Instead, they nearly drowned China in chaos. At the same time, nationalists in a number of newly emerging nations (even Castro's Cuba) killed or drove out pro-Chinese Communist factions. On the other hand, China did move 50,000 men into North Vietnam, partly to operate base complexes but mostly to warn Johnson that an invasion of the North could (as in Korea) lead to a larger war. Johnson and McNamara admitted that if U.S. power was not limited, it could "trigger Chinese intervention on the ground."[71] Having gone to war to contain China, Johnson now found that Chinese threats were being limited around the world—except in a pocket of North Vietnam, where the Chinese effectively contained U.S. power.

Third, Ho's (or Mao's) nationalism was not the same as Hitler's worldwide ambitions. The rugged peasants in the Communist army hardly compared with Hitler's armored divisions, and the 1930s bore little resemblance to the nuclear world of the 1960s.

Fourth, the Great Society sank as war expenses rose. Johnson and Vice-President Humphrey repeatedly said that the U.S. economy could produce "both guns and butter." But by 1967, it could not turn out as many guns and as much butter as the Johnson policies demanded without imposing new taxes (which the president feared for political reasons) or creating severe weaknesses in the economy. War costs shot upward from $8 billion in 1966 to $21 billion in 1967. Dollars flew out of the United States to pay for both the war and growing American private investments abroad (which rose from $49 billion in 1960 to $101 billion in 1968). The nation's export trade could not pull those dollars back. Instead, U.S. producers were finding that they could no longer compete with Japanese and German products. Americans were spending so much money abroad that the dollar, the backbone of the world's financial system, began to weaken. Confidence in that backbone started to disappear. The long U.S. economic slide had begun, and it had been heavily greased by the Vietnam War's costs.[72]

Fifth, the power of American technology proved to be less potent than the willingness of the North Vietnamese to die for their cause. As Johnson sent in more troops, Ho moved about 1,000 of his soldiers into the south each month in 1964, but 4,500 per month in 1965, and 5,000 each month in 1966. Secretary of State Rusk noted in 1971 that the Communists suffered the loss of over 700,000 (the equivalent, given the size of the two populations, of killing 10 million Americans), but "they continue to come." Johnson and the U.S. military could come up with no better policy. Journalist Walter Lippmann condemned LBJ for "conducting the war like a gambler who, when he loses one round, doubles his bet in the hope of recovering what he has lost." McNamara's faith in statistics was undercut by figures that were misleading or cooked up to please Washington officials. U.S. troops in Vietnam called such statistics MEGs—Mostly Exaggerated Guesses. American ignorance of Vietnamese history and customs seemed so limitless that it could never be made up by U.S. technology. For example, when the Communists destroyed much of the South's rice harvest, the United States rushed in California and Louisiana rice, only to find that the Vietnamese hated American rice so much that they used it instead of dirt to fill their sandbags.[73]

LBJ AND VIETNAM: AT HOME

Johnson certainly had problems but they did not include his power as president. In 1966, columnist James Reston marveled at LBJ's incredible authority: not even the leader of the Soviet Union enjoyed "such freedom of action in foreign affairs." Power over Vietnam policy was centralized in a Tuesday luncheon group that included the president, Rusk, McNamara, and NSC director Walt Rostow and that, one macabre joke went, began with prayer and ended with selecting bombing targets. When Congress complained that the Constitution gave it, not the president, the authority to declare war, Assistant Attorney General Nicholas Katzenbach told Congress flatly that the constitutional clause was "an outmoded phraseology." That remark, Minnesota Democratic Senator Eugene McCarthy declared, was "the wildest testimony I have ever heard. There is no limit to what he says the President could do." As a result of this exchange, McCarthy decided to challenge Johnson for the 1968 presidential election.[74]

An anti-war movement in colleges was soon marked by "teach-ins" conducted by faculty and outside lecturers. A "new Left" bloomed, differing from the "old Left" of the 1930s by being less ideological, less interested in economics, and more devoted to community and social changes as well as to opposing the war. A counterculture appeared that cared more about music and political activism than about shaving and being well dressed. These groups thought critically about subjects long uncriticized by most of American society. A landmark was Stanley Kubrick's film, *Dr. Strangelove,* in which the U.S. presidency, nuclear war, and the American military (in the figure of "General Jack D. Rip-

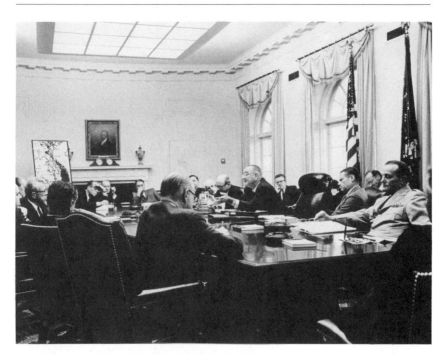

President Johnson discusses his policy on Vietnam with his top advisers. Johnson sits at center right. Secretary of Defense McNamara is to his left and Secretary of State Rusk to his right.

per") were made to appear as foolish as the Soviet characters. All authority seemed open to question.[75]

Johnson had once courted college students, but by 1967–1968 their protests made it impossible for him to visit campuses and some cities safely. "To him," one aide said, these students "appeared to be extra-terrestrial invaders—not only non-American but nonearthly."[76] Some 250 students from twenty-five medical schools signed a pledge that they would not serve in Vietnam. The protests gained a new dimension when students joined forces with civil-rights demonstrators to obtain full rights for blacks and other minorities. Johnson had worked hard for civil rights, but it was too late. Urban riots began in mid-1964. In 1965, the Los Angeles black ghetto of Watts erupted in violence, and thirty-four persons were killed. By 1968, Tampa, Newark, Cincinnati, Atlanta, and Detroit (where forty-three died) had burned, and finally the nation's capital itself exploded in flames during April 1968, after civil-rights and anti-war leader Martin Luther King, Jr., was assassinated.

The war had come home. U.S. military vehicles moved onto Capitol

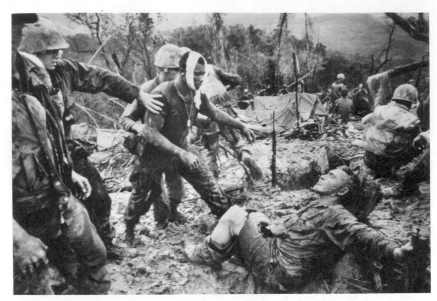

A marine, despite his wounds, reaches out for another marine during a lull in the bloody battle of October 1966 over Hill 484 in South Vietnam. This stunning photo was taken after U.S. soldiers had barely driven back North Vietnamese troops.

Hill and the grounds of the White House to protect the government's leaders from the violence. Violence seemed to breed more violence. From July 1965 to December 1967, U.S. planes dropped more bomb tonnage on Vietnam than the Allies dropped on Europe during all of World War II. More than 344,000 of Ho's forces were killed in these months, but their strength actually rose from 187,000 to 261,000. The war's frustrations, especially the inability to tell a Vietnamese peasant from a deadly enemy, led to wholesale destruction. After the village of Ben Tre was burned, a U.S. officer declared, "It became necessary to destroy the town in order to save it." The war abroad and at home also linked up when the veterans began to return. As one medical aide put it, "It's not at all like a John Wayne movie. The most distressing, the most grotesque are those with an arm or a leg blown off," and "you realize what despair, what deformity, what suffering they're going to have."[77]

Leaders such as George Kennan and Senator Fulbright (chairman of the Senate Foreign Relations Committee) also opposed the war. So did retired military leaders such as Generals Matthew Ridgway (hero of the Korean War) and David Shoup (former Marine Corps commandant). Johnson grew furious at allied leaders who took advantage of visits to the United States to condemn the conflict. When Canadian prime minister Lester Pearson did so in 1965, LBJ got Pearson alone, grabbed him by the shirt collar, and yelled, "You pissed on my rug!"[78] But the attacks continued, especially after the 1967 national election in South Vietnam, which was obviously rigged. Political opponents were imprisoned so that Thieu and Ky could retain their hold on the government.

But Johnson continued to hope. He could be encouraged because, until early 1968, U.S. television largely reported the war uncritically and gave weight to the administration's views.[79] In January 1968, both LBJ and his top commander in Vietnam, General William Westmoreland, said with good evidence on their side that the war was being won. Then, in late January 1968, it all changed. Taking advantage of a holiday lull during the lunar New Year (Tet), the Communists launched

---

I went to Vietnam to heal
and came home silently wounded.
I went to Vietnam to heal
and still awaken from nightmares
about those we couldn't save.
I went to Vietnam to heal
and came home to grieve for those
we sent home blind, paralyzed,
limbless, mindless.
I went to Vietnam to heal
and discovered I am not God.

To you whose names are on this wall
I am sorry I couldn't be God.
If I were God, if there were a God,
there would be no need for such a wall.

But I am not God, and so I go on
seeing the wounded when I hear a
chopper, washing your blood from my hands,
hearing your screams in my sleep, scrubbing
the smell of your burned bodies from my clothes,
feeling your pain, which never eases,
fighting a war that never ends.

—Dusty [a former nurse in
Vietnam 1966–1968]

A poem written by a survivor of Vietnam in memory of eight U.S. nurses who did not survive. The poem captures the feelings of many veterans who returned from the war but could never leave it behind.

a massive offensive in which hand-to-hand combat actually occurred in the U.S. Embassy compound in Saigon. Ho's troops took tremendous losses (probably 30,000 dead), and after being repulsed they were again devastated when they tried a second offensive. But U.S.–South Vietnamese losses were also high.

Americans were stunned that the Communists could launch such a massive campaign after Johnson and Westmoreland claimed that the war was being won. The U.S. positions in the cities and villages had clearly been weakened. American television, led by the country's most respected newsman, Walter Cronkite of CBS News, now publicly questioned whether the conflict could ever be won. Critics zeroed in on ineffective South Vietnamese troops, who, a U.S. military adviser declared, "are leaderless and gutless."[80]

General Westmoreland publicly claimed a great victory, but news then leaked that he had asked the president for 206,000 more U.S. troops. Badly shaken, Johnson called in a group of "Wise Men," senior retired officials led by Dean Acheson and McGeorge Bundy. At first strong supporters of the war, by March 1968 they believed that the cost had soared too high. They received strong support from Clark Clifford, the new secretary of defense. Clifford and the Wise Men especially feared the effect of a prolonged war on a stumbling U.S. economy. When a top U.S. general argued that the Americans must never retreat, but admited that a "classic military victory" was impossible, Acheson roared, "Then what in the name of God are five hundred thousand men doing out there? Chasing girls?" Acheson reviewed the evidence and told Johnson that he (the president) had been badly misled by his military advisers. Some officials opposed sending more troops overseas because of the fear that the troops would be needed to put down uprisings within the United States itself.[81]

On March 31, 1968, LBJ declared on national television that he was limiting the bombing of North Vietnam as part of an appeal for peace talks with Ho Chi Minh. The president then stunned the country by announcing that in order to concentrate on ending the war, he would not be a candidate for re-election. The war claimed the Johnson administration as its ultimate victim.

OTHER COSTS OF VIETNAM: U.S. RELATIONS WITH AFRICA, THE MIDDLE EAST, AND THE SOVIET UNION

Johnson had become obsessed with the war. Unable to sleep, he visited the White House War Room in the middle of the night to learn whether

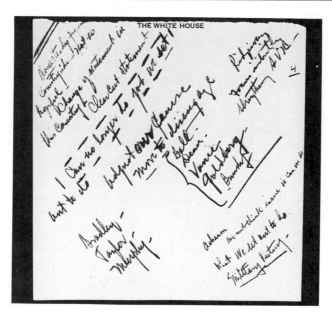

President Johnson's doodling during the crucial March 25, 1968, meeting with his "wise men" on Vietnam. Note Johnson's highlighting of Acheson's comment to the group that the United States "can no longer do job we set out to do."

the bombers he had ordered out had returned safely. Such obsession prevented the administration from dealing more effectively with other troubles—and opportunities—in the world.

Along with Southeast Asia and Latin America, Africa was transformed between 1958 and 1968. Dominated by European colonial powers in the mid-1950s, within a decade it was a huge continent of independent nations (see map, p. 664). As usual, the United States publicly supported this anticolonial movement. President Kennedy spent much time greeting heads of the new states and obtaining aid for them.

There was, however, a glaring, embarrassing contradiction at the center of U.S. policy in Africa. It was South Africa, where a white minority of 4 million oppressed some 20 million blacks through a system of apartheid (rigid, legal, police-enforced racial separation.) Apartheid had begun in 1948 when the white Nationalist Party responded to the worldwide explosions of anticolonialism and demands for racial equality, which appeared during and after World War II, by turning inward and brutally putting down any talk of racial moderation in South Africa. Under Harry Truman and Dwight Eisenhower, U.S. policy accepted apartheid because officials cared much more about South Africa's strategic location and, above all, its rich uranium mines so necessary to the making of nuclear weapons. Moreover, the segregation of the races was accepted by Americans in the late 1940s and early 1950s. As historian Tim Borstelmann explains the growing U.S.–South African partnership in trade and military planning, "A country in which white people held the preponderance of power and people of color were widely disenfranchised, impoverished, and physically intimidated could not have seemed strange to representatives of the United States" at that time. U.S. racism and anticommunism meshed together perfectly in the relationship with South Africa. That tie did not begin to loosen until nearly a decade after the 1954 U.S. Supreme Court decision, *Brown* v. *Board of Education*, that finally outlawed racial segregation in the United States. President Kennedy, understanding the contradiction in professing democracy and supporting South African apartheid, finally cut off arms sales and government loans to the white government. It would, however, be another quarter-century before Washington's policies finally helped pull down apartheid.[82]

But Kennedy and Johnson also used the CIA and other weapons to fight black nationalists whom they believed to be pro-Communist. The Congo became the example. In June 1960, this West African nation (later renamed Zaire), finally broke free of an especially incompetent, ruthless, and exploitative Belgian colonialism. Strategically located, the Congo was rich in tin, copper, gold, cobalt, and diamonds. Its Katanga Province (later Shaba Province) produced the tantalum the United States needed to build aircraft. Prime Minister Patrice Lumumba was a charismatic socialist who kicked out remaining Belgian troops and frightened the 100,000 remaining Europeans. With Belgian support, however, Moise Tshombe declared Katanga and its riches an independent province. Although Eisenhower sympathized with the Belgians, he supported the United Nations team that tried to work out peace terms. The UN group was led by Ralph Bunche, a black American who had won the Nobel Peace Prize for his extraordinary diplomacy in the Middle East. The Soviets then tried to enter the scene by accusing Bunche of being a mere frontman for U.S. interests. Soviet military advisers appeared to help Lumumba as the Congo fragmented.

With CIA help, Colonel Joseph Mobuto's soldiers captured and killed Lumumba in January 1961, just as Kennedy moved into the White House. The new president sympathized with African nationalism but was in no mood to watch the Soviets make any gains in Africa. Through CIA and U.S. military aid, he helped Mobutu gain power. When rebels seized some 3,000 foreigners as hostages in late 1964, U.S. and Belgian troops rescued them and helped crush the rebellion. By 1965, the United States had replaced Belgium as the dominant foreign power.[83]

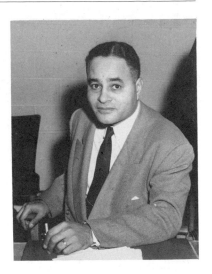

Ralph Bunche (1904–1971), the grandson of a slave, was born in Detroit, was educated at UCLA and Harvard, became a teacher at Howard University, joined the State Department, then gained fame as the United Nations official who successfully mediated the 1949 Arab-Israeli War, a success that brought him the Nobel Peace Prize. He led the UN effort to find peace in the Congo in the early 1960s. This photo was taken during his service with the United Nations.

Mobutu took his place as a virtual (if elected) dictator whose regime became increasingly corrupt but more pro-Western. Johnson wanted to augment U.S. aid to Mobutu and other new African leaders, but Vietnam's costs prevented it.

Kennedy and Johnson could do even less to help preserve peace in the Middle East. JFK hoped to follow an "even-handed" approach in dealing with the bitter dispute between Egypt and Israel. He did not want to give up the advantage of Israel's military power or the support of Jewish voters at home, but he did want to work with Egypt's General Gamal Abdel Nasser so that the general would not look to the Soviets for help. Kennedy's plan, however, fell apart in 1962–1963. When the small Middle East kingdom of Yemen became embroiled in revolution, Nasser sent 75,000 troops to help the revolt. Saudi Arabia (the region's greatest oil producer and Washington's closest Arab friend) quickly intervened in Yemen to stop Nasser. The United States first pressured Nasser to step back but then decided not to oppose his policy. The Saudis quickly squeezed U.S. oil firms. Israel and Great Britain protested Kennedy's tilt toward Egypt. The president reversed course, declared Nasser untrustworthy, and sent air power to defend the Saudis. By the time of his death, JFK had fully moved U.S. policy to a pro-Israel, pro-Saudi, anti-Egypt position.[84] Kennedy pledged to use the U.S. Sixth Fleet to protect Israel, if necessary, and for the first time sold a large amount of arms (antiaircraft missiles) to the Israelis.

Johnson, long a close friend of American Jewish groups, moved even closer to Israel. The first U.S. shipments of tanks and Skyhawk bombers went to the Israelis in 1965–1966. But intensifying problems in Vietnam and at home forced LBJ to stand on the sidelines in 1967, when Nasser moved to cut off a vital ocean route to Israel. Egypt ordered a UN peacekeeping team out of the Sinai Peninsula, then moved 100,000 troops close to Israel's borders. The most Johnson could do—and did do—was to tell the Israelis that if they struck Egypt, he would not restrain them as Eisenhower had done at Suez in 1956. The Israeli troops suddenly attacked on June 5, 1967. In the spectacular Six-Day War, they destroyed much of Nasser's army and air force. They also crippled Egypt's allies, Jordan and Syria. Israel then seized the West Bank of the Jordan River (claimed by Jordan), the Sinai, and the Gaza strip, as well as all of the great city of Jersualem. Israel had won near-total victory, but the question of whether more than half a million Palestinian Arabs on the West Bank would have to remain in Israel now haunted Middle Eastern diplomacy. For the next six years, the United States could do little to help solve that explosive issue.

Nor could Johnson do as much as he had hoped to improve U.S.-USSR relations. After the Cuban missile crisis, the United States continued its nuclear build-up, while the Soviets built up even faster to catch up with the Americans. By 1967, the president, and especially Defense Secretary McNamara, feared that the race was getting out of hand. The United States had 1,054 ICBMs, and the Soviets approached 900 in their arsenal. Also ominous was a Soviet antiballistic missile (ABM) system that could possibly make Communist cities less vulnerable to U.S. missiles. Johnson accelerated U.S. development of an ABM, and the Americans also stepped up work on Multiple Independent Reentry Vehicles (MIRVs)—nuclear warheads that were launched on a single missile and, in flight, separated to fly off in as many as ten different directions to hit targets. Thus, two new arms races threatened.

In a speech at Montreal in 1967, McNamara warned that "bridges" had to be built to Moscow, even to Beijing (Peking), to stop the arms build-up. He was worried that the growing number of conflicts in the newly emerging world could dangerously escalate and begged that money for arms be spent instead on erasing the poverty that produced these conflicts. He, Johnson, and Soviet president Aleksei Kosygin met for a hastily planned summit conference at Glassboro, New Jersey, in 1967. McNamara again passionately argued for controls on arms and especially on ABM development (which, he feared, could lead to the building of more offensive weapons that would simply overwhelm any ABM system).

Kosygin refused to agree with McNamara, but the two sides signed a historic treaty to halt the proliferation of their nuclear weapons (to third powers such as China or the two Germanies, for example). In 1968, fifty-seven other nations also signed the nonproliferation pact. Direct air service opened between New York and Moscow. Johnson planned to visit Moscow in 1968 to help continue thawing the cold war. Before he could do so, however, in August 1968 the Soviets invaded Czechoslovakia.

The Czechs had begun economic and political reforms that frightened the conservative, military-based Communist governments of eastern Europe. If they were not stopped, the reforms could sweep through the bloc like a warm, unwelcome breeze. Soviet leader Leonid Brezhnev justified using force to stop the "Prague spring" (as it became known in the West) with a "Brezhnev Doctrine": Communist governments were justified in using force to preserve communism where it was already established. Johnson canceled his trip. Cold-war temperatures dropped dangerously. The arms races sped on.

JFK, LBJ, *Bonnie and Clyde*

John Kennedy did not leave behind a bitterly divided society. "Our country is not divided today, not split into warring groups—thank goodness," President Johnson said in June 1964.[85] The tall, dynamic Texan tried to ensure national unity (and compassion) with his Great Society programs.

Despite his successes, however, by 1969 the nation was ripped apart by anti-war and pro-civil-rights riots. In April 1968, Martin Luther King was murdered in Memphis, Tennessee, and cities exploded. Smoke from blocks of burning buildings curled above the Capitol. King had become the victim of the violence he had spent his life exposing—both in the United States and more recently Vietnam. For by 1966–1967, he believed that "racism and militarism" were interrelated problems in America that could not be solved while "the heart of the administration is in that war in Vietnam."[86] Senator Robert Kennedy had reached the same conclusion, but in June 1968 he was also assassinated in Los Angeles just after winning the California Democratic primary election. Street protests at the Democratic convention in Chicago and brutal retaliation by the city's police prevented Johnson from attending his party's nomination of Vice-President Hubert Humphrey for the top job.

Artists reflected the effects of these divisions on American society.

Writer Susan Sontag called the white race the cancer of history. In 1967, Hollywood produced a highly popular film, *Bonnie and Clyde*, the story of two uneducated bankrobbers whom the film portrayed as more innocent than the unjust, violence-ridden society that drove them to crime.[87] Violence seemed the only effective response to a violent society that devastated square miles of Southeast Asia and square blocks of American cities.

Kennedy, however, had left behind much of the foreign policy that led to this devastation. The "most important decision" Kennedy made, Secretary of State Rusk recalled, was breaking the troop limits set by the 1954 Geneva Accords and committing "about seventeen- or eighteen-thousand [U.S. troops] before his death."[88] Kennedy's decision in 1961–1962 to build on the tremendous U.S. nuclear superiority, rather than negotiating arms agreements, led to an accelerated arms race in which the Soviets would catch up to America within a decade. JFK's glamor, the "Camelot" of the Kennedy White House, enlarged and added purple hues to an already "imperial presidency" in foreign policy. Johnson carried on these Kennedy legacies until the Tet offensive in Vietnam and the rioting at home forced a reassessment. Then, as historian Larry Berman puts it, the war had become "at once, a human and a national tragedy in the United States."[89] Johnson finally

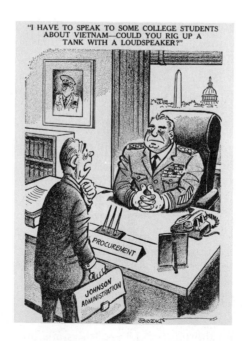

"I HAVE TO SPEAK TO SOME COLLEGE STUDENTS ABOUT VIETNAM—COULD YOU RIG UP A TANK WITH A LOUDSPEAKER?"

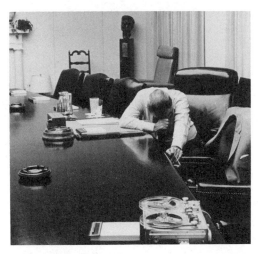

President Lyndon Johnson buries his head in his arm at the cabinet table as he sits alone listening to his son-in-law's taped descriptions of the death and destruction witnessed during his tour of duty in Vietnam. Taken by Jack Knight-linger on July 31, 1968, the photo caught not only the feelings of the president, but those of many Americans after nearly four years of intensified war.

decided to restrict the bombing, but he never wavered in his determination to keep South Vietnam non-Communist.

LBJ's decision to open peace talks came too late to save Hubert Humphrey. In a tight race, Republican Richard Nixon defeated the vice-president by 0.7 percent of the popular vote. Vietnam played a major, but not decisive, part in Humphrey's defeat. More important, polls revealed, was the desire of the average American ("the housewife in Dayton, Ohio," as one pollster said) to be able to walk down a street without crime and violence—and to live again in a country of law and order, not Bonnies and Clydes.[90] Nixon had solemnly promised to end the war in both Vietnam and on American streets.

NOTES

1. C. Vann Woodward, *Thinking Back: The Perils of Writing History* (Baton Rouge, La., 1986), p. 103.

2. Thomas E. Cronin, "Looking for Leadership, 1980," *Public Opinion* 3 (February–March, 1980): 18.

3. James MacGregor Burns, *John Kennedy: A Political Profile* (New York, 1960), pp.

40–42, 79–84, 88–95; John F. Kennedy, *Why England Slept* (New York, 1940), esp. pp. 215–216, 224–231.

4. Douglas Brinkley, *Dean Acheson: The Cold War Years, 1953–71* (New Haven, 1992), p. 112.

5. Henry Fairlie, *The Kennedy Promise: The Politics of Expectation* (Garden City, N.Y., 1973), p. 116; *Washington Post*, 29 August, 1976, p. E3. The New Frontier and related concepts and phrases are placed in context in Arthur Schlesinger, Jr., *A Thousand Days* (Boston, 1965), pp. 4–5, a detailed, highly favorable biography of Kennedy.

6. Rockefeller Brothers Fund, *Prospects for America* (Garden City, N.Y., 1961).

7. Stephen E. Ambrose, *Nixon: The Education of a Politician, 1913–1962* (New York, 1987), p. 546.

8. Theodore Sorensen, *Decision-Making in the White House* (New York, 1963), pp. 45–48.

9. Bruce W. Jentleson, "From Consensus to Conflict: The Domestic Political Economy of East-West Energy Trade Policy," *International Organization* 38 (Autumn 1984): 640.

10. Dean Rusk, "Chinese-American Friendship," *Department of State Bulletin*, 21 May 1951, pp. 846–847.

11. Barry Rubin, *Secrets of State* (New York, 1985), p. 95.

12. David Halberstam, "The Programming of Robert McNamara," *Harper's* 242 (February 1971): 44; *National Observer*, 6 December 1965, p. 1.

13. Frank Costigliola, "The Failed Design: Kennedy, de Gaulle, and the Struggle for Europe," *Diplomatic History* 8 (Summer 1984): 229.

14. *Forbes*, 1 February 1966, pp. 15–16.

15. Oral History interview of Couve de Murville, 20 May 1964, John F. Kennedy Presidential Library, Boston, Mass.

16. *Newsweek*, 19 November 1973, p. 90.

17. *New York Times*, 22 November 1965, p. 43.

18. John Spanier, *American Foreign Policy since World War II* (New York, 1965), pp. 176–177.

19. W. W. Rostow, *The Diffusion of Power* (New York, 1972), p. 52.

20. *New York Times*, 12 July 1960, p. 7.

21. U.S. Government, *Public Papers of the Presidents of the United States: John F. Kennedy, 1962* (Washington, D.C., 1963), p. 223. Documents on the Alliance for Progress and its implementation are in *The Record of American Diplomacy*, ed. Ruhl J. Bartlett, 4th ed. (New York, 1964), pp. 868–874.

22. Pat M. Holt, "The Political Aspects," in U.S. Congress, Senate, Committee on Foreign Relations, 91st Cong., 1st sess., 1969, *Survey of the Alliance for Progress* (Washington, D.C., 1969), pp. 14–16.

23. Theodore C. Sorensen, *Kennedy* (New York, 1965), pp. 535–536.

24. Barton J. Bernstein, "Kennedy and the Bay of Pigs Revisited Twenty-four Years Later," *Foreign Service Journal* 62 (March 1985): pp. 535–536.

25. Review of Peter Wyden's *Buy of Pigs* (New York, 1979), in *Business Week*, 23 July 1979, p. 17; Brinkley, p. 127.

26. Michael R. Beschloss, *Mayday: Eisenhower, Khrushchev, and the U-2 Affair* (New York, 1986), p. 303; Schlesinger, p. 292.

27. *Washington Post*, 12 September 1976, p. L5.

28. Speech excerpts and analysis can be found in Lloyd Gardner, "Dominoes, Diem, and Death, 1952–1963," in *America in Vietnam*, ed. William Appleman Williams *et al.* (New York, 1985), pp. 189–191.

29. Paul Boller, Jr., *Presidential Anecdotes* (New York, 1981), p. 301; *New York Times*, 14 February 1965, p. E9.

30. Stephen E. Pelz, " 'When Do I Have Time to Think?': John F. Kennedy, Roger Hilsman, and the Laotian Crisis of 1962," *Diplomatic History* 3 (Spring 1979): 223, quoting Clark M. Clifford, "A Viet Nam Reappraisal: The Personal History of One Man's View and How It Evolved," *Foreign Affairs* 47 (July 1969): 604.

31. Gareth Porter, "After Geneva: Subverting Laotian Neutrality," in *Laos: War and Revolution*, ed. Nina S. Adams and Alfred W. McCoy (New York, 1970), pp. 179–212.

32. *Washington Post*, 28 November 1980, p. C4.

33. Stephen E. Pelz, "John F. Kennedy's 1961 Vietnam War Decisions," *Journal of Strategic Studies* 4 (December 1981): 370–371.

34. Maxwell D. Taylor, *Responsibility and Response* (New York, 1967), p. 57.

35. Gardner, p. 143.

36. James Aronson, *The Press and the Cold War* (New York, 1970), pp. 182–183.

37. Oral History interview of William Tyler, 7 March 1964, John F. Kennedy Presidential Library; Chester L. Cooper, *The Lost Crusade: America in Vietnam* (New York, 1970), p. 171; Gordon H. Chang, *Friends and Enemies* (Stanford, 1990), pp. 240–252.

38. Gardner, pp. 198–201, has the interviews; Leslie H. Gelb, "Kennedy and Vietnam," *New York Times*, 6 January 1992, p. A31.

39. Pelz, "Kennedy's Vietnam Decisions," p. 378.

40. W. Averell Harriman quoted in Frank Costigliola, "The New Atlantic Community" (1987), manuscript in the author's possession, p. 13.

41. Boller, p. 303.

42. Brinkley, p. 147; Kennedy's speech in Berlin is in U.S. Government, *Public Papers of the Presidents of the United States: John F. Kennedy, 1963* (Washington, D.C., 1964), pp. 524–525; Costigliola, "The Failed Design," pp. 240–241.

43. Scott D. Sagan, "SIOP-62: The Nuclear War Plan Briefing to President Kennedy," *International Security* 12 (Summer 1987): 23n.

44. *New York Times*, 14 October 1987, p. A10.

45. Walter Pincus, "CIA Records Offer Behind-the-Scenes Look at Cuban Missile Crisis," *Washington Post*, 19 October, 1992, pp. A10–A11.

46. Foreign Broadcast Information Service, *Daily Report Annex: Soviet Union*, 17 January 1989, pp. 6–11.

47. Marc Trachtenberg, "The Influence of Nuclear Weapons in the Cuban Missile Crisis," *International Security* 10 (Summer 1985): 148–149; Elie Abel, *The Missile Crisis* (Philadelphia, 1968), pp. 70, 81, 118–119.

48. J. Anthony Lukas, "Class Reunion: Kennedy's Men Relive the Cuban Missile Crisis," *New York Times Magazine*, 30 August 1987, p. 51; Trachtenberg, p. 161; Laurence Chang and Peter Kornbluh, eds., *The Cuban Missile Crisis, 1962: A National Security Archive Documents Reader* (New York, 1992), pp. 150–154.

49. Chang and Kornbluh, eds., *The Cuban Missile Crisis*, pp. 197–199; Lukas, p. 58; Walter Pincus, "Standing at the Brink of Nuclear War," *Washington Post*, 25 July 1985, pp. A1, A10.

50. The recorded discussion of the 27 October meeting is in McGeorge Bundy, transcr., and James G. Blight, ed., "October 27, 1962: Transcripts of the Meetings of the ExComm," *International Security* 12 (Winter 1987–1988): esp. 48, 58, 87–88; Chang and Kornbluh, eds., *The Cuban Missile Crisis*, pp. 226–229, 230–232; the Castro letter was originally printed in *Le Monde*, and then reprinted in the Louisville *Courier-Journal*, 2 December 1990, pp. D1, D4.

51. Letter to the editor from Bruce J. Allyn and James G. Blight, *New York Times*, 2 November 1992, p. A18; *Washington Post*, 7 January 1992, p. A12; *New York Times*, 22 January 1992, p. A30. *New York Times*, 14 October 1987, p. A10; Rubin, p. 98.

52. Charles E. Bohlen, *Witness to History, 1929–1969* (New York, 1973), p. 495.

53. Gaddis Smith, "The Legacy of the Monroe Doctrine," *New York Times Magazine*, 9 September 1984, p. 128; Thomas G. Paterson and William J. Brophy, "October Missiles and November Elections . . . ," *Journal of American History* 73 (June 1986): 87–93, 112–119; Stephen S. Rosenfeld, "That Cuban Missile Understanding," *Washington Post*, 2 April 1982, p. A17.

54. Costigliola, "The Failed Design," 234–235, 237; Stewart Alsop, "The Collapse of Kennedy's Grand Design," *Saturday Evening Post*, 6 April 1963, pp. 78–81; Alexander Werth, *De Gaulle, a Political Biography* (New York, 1966), pp. 331–333.

55. Walt W. Rostow, "Domestic Determinants of U.S. Foreign Policy: The Tocqueville Oscillation," *Armed Forces Journal* 27 June 1970, p. 16D.

56. Theodore Draper, *Present History* (New York, 1983), pp. 197–198; U.S. Congress, Senate, Committee on Foreign Relations, 88th Cong., 1st sess., 1963, *Nuclear Test Ban Treaty* (Washington, D.C., 1963), pp. 422–427.

57. Oral History statement by William Attwood, 8 November 1965, John F. Kennedy Presidential Library; Terence Ripmaster, "The Kennedy Assassination in U.S. History Books," *The Third Decade: A Journal of Research on the John F. Kennedy Assassination* 3 (May 1987): 4–6.

58. *Department of State Bulletin*, 12 May 1975, p. 606.

59. Robert Divine, "The Johnson Literature," in *Exploring the Johnson Years*, ed. Robert Divine (Austin, Tex., 1981), pp. 3–4, 13; *Washington Post*, 29 August 1976, p. E3; Boller, p. 310; Lawrence Martin, *The Presidents and the Prime Ministers* (Toronto, 1982), p. 220.

60. *Who We Are: An Atlantic Chronicle of the United States and Vietnam*, ed. Robert Manning and Michael Janeway (Boston, 1969), pp. 16, 216.

61. The documents may be found in *America in Vietnam*, pp. 234–239; U.S. Congress, Senate, Committee on Foreign Relations, 90th Cong., 2d sess., 1968, *The Gulf of Tonkin: The 1964 Incidents* (Washington, D.C., 1968).

62. U.S. Government, *Public Papers of the Presidents of the United States: Lyndon B. Johnson, 1964* (Washington, D.C., 1965), pp. 1390–1391, 1441.

63. Barry Hughes, *Domestic Context of American Foreign Policy* (San Francisco, 1978), p. 57.

64. Oral History interview of Harry McPherson, tape #4, p. 13, Lyndon B. Johnson Presidential Library, Austin, Tex.; U.S. Government, *Public Papers of the Presidents of the United States: Lyndon B. Johnson, 1966* (Washington, D.C., 1968), p. 936.

65. Samuel Baily, *The United States and the Development of South America, 1945–1975* (New York, 1976), pp. 58, 118–119, 215–216.

66. Phyllis Parker, *Brazil and the Quiet Intervention, 1964* (Austin, Tex., 1979), pp. xi, 58, 63, 68–70, 81, 92–99, 102–103; Thomas E. Skidmore, "U.S. Policy toward Bra-

zil: Assumptions and Options," in *Latin America: The Search for a New International Role*, ed. Ronald G. Hellman and H. John Rosenbaum (New York, 1975), pp. 198–200.

67. Arthur Schlesinger, Jr., "The Alliance for Progress: A Retrospective," in *Latin America*, p. 80.

68. *New York Times*, 3 May 1965, p. 10; "Report for the President" from Jack Valenti, 30 April 1965, CO 1-8, White House Central Files, Lyndon B. Johnson Library.

69. Sources of the quotations in this and the next four paragraphs can be found in (in order): U.S. Government, *Public Papers of the Presidents, 1966*, p. 762; *New York Times*, 13 July 1966, p. 2; U.S. Government, *Public Papers of the Presidents of the United States: Lyndon B. Johnson, 1965* (Washington, D.C., 1966), pp. 395, 794; George C. Herring, "The War in Vietnam," in *Exploring the Johnson Years*, p. 27; Richard E. Neustadt and Ernest R. May, *Thinking in Time: The Uses of History for Decision-Makers* (New York, 1986), p. 86; Michael Herr, *Dispatches* (New York, 1977), p. 154; Neustadt and May, p. 86.

70. Oral History interview of Dean Rusk, recorded in 1969, released in 1987, Lyndon B. Johnson Library; a splendid detailed analysis of the crucial 1965 decision can be found in Larry Berman, *Planning a Tragedy* (New York, 1982), esp. pp. 31–129, and also in George McT. Kahin, *Intervention: How America Became Involved in Vietnam* (New York, 1986), pp. 286–401.

71. Oral History interview of Rusk; Allen S. Whiting, *The Chinese Calculus of Deterrence: India and Indochina* (Ann Arbor, Mich., 1975), pp. 182–189.

72. William S. Borden, *The Pacific Alliance: U.S. Foreign Economic Policy and Japanese Trade Recovery, 1947–1955* (Madison, Wis., 1984), pp. ix, 3–17, 37–41, 218–222; "Economic Report of the President," *Department of State Bulletin*, 26 February 1968, p. 280.

73. Murray Fromson, "The American Military in Vietnam: 1950s," in *Vietnam Reconsidered: Lessons from a War* ed. Harrison E. Salisbury (New York, 1984), p. 39; John E. Mueller, "The Search for the 'Breaking Point' in Vietnam," *International Studies Quarterly* 24 (December 1980): 497, has the Rusk quote; *New York Times*, 23 April 1965, p. 42, on the "MEGs"; *New York Herald Tribune*, 28 December 1965, p. 18, has the Lippmann quote.

74. *New York Times*, 18 August 1967, p. 14; *ibid.*, 2 February 1966, pp. 7–8; David C. Humphrey, "Tuesday Lunch at the Johnson White House," *Diplomatic History* 8 (Winter 1984): 81–101, a helpful overview.

75. Nora Sayre, *Running Time: Films of the Cold War* (New York, 1982), pp. 218–219.

76. George Reedy, *The Twilight of the Presidency* (New York, 1970), pp. 96–97.

77. *New York Times*, 3 March 1968, p. 6.

78. Martin, p. 2.

79. Daniel C. Hallin's *The "Uncensored War": The Media and Vietnam* (New York, 1986) is a full, critical account.

80. *New York Times*, 28 February 1968, p. 27.

81. *Vietnam: A History in Documents*, ed. Gareth Porter (New York, 1979, 1981), pp. 354–357; for U.S. business opposition by 1967, there is a good account in Bruce M. Russett and Elizabeth C. Hanson, *Interest and Ideology: The Foreign Policy Beliefs of American Businessmen* (San Francisco, 1975), pp. 59–96; Brinkley, p. 261.

82. Thomas Borstelmann, *Apartheid's Reluctant Uncle* (New York, 1993), esp. pp. 195–202.

83. *New York Times*, 5 July 1966, p. 15; Henry Jackson, *From The Congo to Soweto* (New York, 1982), pp. 25–45.

84. Douglas Little, "From 'Even-Handed' to 'Empty-Handed': JFK, Nasser, and U.S. Policy in the Middle East, 1961–1963" (1985), manuscript in the author's possession; *Egypt, a Country Study*, ed. Richard Nyrop (Washington, D.C., 1982).

85. U.S. Government, *Public Papers of the Presidents . . . 1964*, p. 777.

86. David J. Garrow, *Bearing the Cross* (New York, 1986), pp. 551–573.

87. Richard Dorfman, "Conspiracy City," *Journal of Popular Film and Television* 7, no. 4 (1980): 435–436.

88. Oral History interview of Rusk.

89. Berman, p. xiii.

90. *Washington Post*, 1 October 1969, p. A23; Richard M. Scammon and Ben J. Wattenberg, *The Real Majority* (New York, 1970), pp. 38–49; William L. Lunch and Peter W. Sperlich, "American Public Opinion and the War in Vietnam," *Western Political Quarterly* 32 (March 1979): 21–44.

FOR FURTHER READING

Begin with *Guide to American Foreign Relations since 1700*, ed. Richard Dean Burns (1983), which no text can match for pre-1981 references. (Consequently the listing below notes post-1981 references almost entirely.) Also consult the chapter's notes and the General Bibliography at the end of this book for specific topics; those references are usually not repeated below.

An important overview and bibliography are in Warren Cohen, *America in the Age of Soviet Power, 1945–1991*, in *The Cambridge History of American Foreign Relations* series, which Cohen edited (1993). Good surveys on Kennedy include James N. Giglio, *The Presidency of John F. Kennedy* (1991), with a useful bibliography; Herbert S. Parmet's *JFK: The Presidency of John F. Kennedy* (1983), and Warren Cohen's *Dean Rusk* (1980), a searching biography of an enigmatic man; the enigmatic man's own remembrances, Dean Rusk as told to Richard Rusk, *As I Saw It* (1990); Lloyd Gardner's essay on McGeorge Bundy in *Behind the Throne*, eds. T. McCormick and W. LaFeber (1993), essays in honor of Fred Harvey Harrington; Montague Kern, Patricia Levering, and Ralph B. Levering's *The Kennedy Crisis: The Press, the Presidency, and Foreign Policy* (1983), an excellent analysis; David P. Calleo's *The Imperious Economy* (1982), perhaps the best available examination of international economic policy from 1960 to 1980; Charles Lipson's *Standing Guard: Protecting Foreign Capital in the Nineteenth and Twentieth Centuries* (1985), especially provocative on the 1960s; Michael R. Beschloss, *The Crisis Years: Kennedy and Khrushchev, 1960–1963* (1991), the major account of the Soviet-American rivalry during those years; Desmond Ball's *Politics and Force Levels* (1981), a powerful argument that Kennedy unnecessarily escalated the arms race; Bernard J. Firestone's *The Quest for Nuclear Stability: John F. Kennedy and the Soviet Union* (1982), which focuses on the nuclear test ban.

On specific topics and regions, C. J. Bartlett's useful survey, *The Special Relationship* (1992) explores how U.S.-British relations deteriorated in the 1960s; Frank Costigliola's

The Cold Alliance (1992) is the standard, and highly readable, account of post-1945 U.S.-French relations. On Asia (besides the separate Vietnam accounts noted below), Timothy P. Maga's *John F. Kennedy and the New Pacific Community, 1961–1963* (1990) is a succinct account that deemphasizes Vietnam in the regional context; Harold A. Gould and Sumit Ganguily, eds., *The Hope and the Reality: U.S.-Indian Relations from Roosevelt to Reagan* (1992), is important on Kennedy. On Cuba and Latin America, Graham H. Stuart and James L. Tigner's *Latin America and the United States,* 6th ed. (1975), is an encyclopedic account that is a superb starting place; W. Michael Weiss, *Cold Warriors and Coups D'état* (1992), is important for the U.S.-Brazil relationship to 1964; Bruce Palmer, *Intervention in the Caribbean: The Dominican Crisis of 1965* (1989), is a standard account; Trumbull Higgins's *The Perfect Failure* (1987) is fine on the Bay of Pigs; Morris Morley's *Imperial State and Revolution: The United States and Cuba, 1952–1985* (1987) provides a highly critical context for the missile crisis and after. On the missile crisis itself, Robert A. Divine, ed., *The Cuban Missile Crisis,* 2nd ed. (1988), is a good place to start for further references and interpretations; Raymond L. Garthoff, *Reflections on the Cuban Missile Crisis,* rev. ed. (1989), is by a former U.S. official and an expert on Soviet affairs; James G. Blight, *On the Brink* (1990), superbly brings together the then-latest U.S. and Soviet recollections; Dino A. Brugioni, *Eyeball to Eyeball* (1992), is by a technician who interpreted the U-2 pictures; James A. Nathan, ed., *The Cuban Missile Crisis Revisited* (1992), is a set of especially important essays (notably Barton Bernstein's and Philip Brenner's); and Chang and Kornbluh, eds., *The Cuban Missile Crisis, 1962* (1992), cited in the footnotes, is the authoritative set of correspondence and documents published by the National Security Archive. On Africa, Zaki Laidi, *The Superpowers and Africa: The Constraints of a Rivalry, 1960–1990* (1990), is a useful interpretive overview; while Peter Duignan and Lewis H. Gann's *The United States and Africa: A History* (1984) provides a historical context; and Richard D. Mahoney's *JFK: Ordeal in Africa* (1983) is important for the early 1960s; Thomas J. Noer's *Cold War and Black Liberation: The U.S. and White Rule in Africa, 1948–1968* (1985) is now the standard on the entire era; William Attwood's *The Twilight Struggle: Tales of the Cold War* (1987) is important for both its African and Cuban sections. On the Middle East, Seth P. Tillman's *The United States and the Middle East* (1982) is a thoughtful and important analysis; James W. Harper's "The Middle East, Oil, and the Third World," in *Modern American Diplomacy,* ed. John M. Carroll and George C. Herring (1986), is both a good overview that sees a decline in the U.S. ideological drive and useful for its bibliography; Steven L. Spiegel's *The Other Arab-Israel Conflict* (1985) critically looks at domestic policy making.

For the Johnson presidency, in addition to materials given in the notes and in the paragraph above on specific geographical areas, a most useful place to begin for further reading is Staff of the Lyndon Baines Johnson Library, *Lyndon B. Johnson: A Bibliography* (1984); Clark Clifford's *Counsel to the President* (1991); Vaughn D. Bornet's *The Presidency of Lyndon B. Johnson* (1983) is an overview with a chapter on Vietnam; Göran Rystad's *Prisoners of the Past?: The Munich Syndrome and Makers of American Foreign Policy in the Cold War Era* (1982) is good on both JFK and LBJ, but especially the latter; Glenn T. Seaborg, with Benjamin S. Loeb, *Stemming the Tide: Arms Control in the Johnson Years* (1987), provides most useful information from an insider; Michael McGwire's *Military Objectives in Soviet Foreign Policy* (1987) is important for its emphasis on the 1966–1967 Soviet changes; Karen Dawisha's *The Kremlin and the Prague Spring* (1984) is now the standard account of the Soviet intervention in 1968. A fascinating interpretation of the 1965 Dominican Republic intervention is put in a larger and provocative context in Frank Brodhead and Edward S. Herman's *Demonstration Elections* (1984), which compares that intervention with Vietnam.

Vietnam materials are overwhelming in number and variety of topics. Useful places to begin (other than entries cited in the notes of this chapter and in the General Bibliography) include George C. Herring, "The Vietnam War," in *Modern American Diplomacy*, ed. John M. Carroll and George C. Herring (1986); Herring's abridged edition of *The Pentagon Papers* (1993); *The Wars in Vietnam, Cambodia and Laos, 1945–1982*, ed. Richard Dean Burns and Milton Leitenberg (1984), with over 6,200 entries for further reading; Benjamin R. Beede, *Intervention and Counterinsurgency: An Annotated Bibliography of the Small Wars of the United States, 1898–1984* (1985); *Vietnam As History*, ed. Peter Braestrup (1984), papers and discussions by fifty experts; Loren Baritz's *Backfire: A History of How American Culture Led Us into Vietnam and Made Us Fight the Way We Did* (1985), the best social history of the conflict; Larry Berman's fine *Lyndon Johnson's War* (1991); Gabriel Kolko's *Anatomy of a War* (1985), especially important for its analysis of U.S. economic policies; Ellen J. Hammer's *A Death in November: America in Vietnam, 1963* (1987), a definitive account of Ngo Dinh Diem's overthrow; Andrew F. Krepinevich, Jr.'s *The Army and Vietnam* (1986), which contradicts Harry Summers, Jr.'s *On Strategy: A Critical Analysis of the Vietnam War* (1981), a much discussed critique of U.S. military (and political) strategy; William Rust, *Kennedy in Vietnam* (1985); David DiLeo's excellent *George Ball, Vietnam. . . .* (1991); Ronald Spector, *After Tet* (1992); and David W. Levy, *The Debate over Vietnam* (1991).

Dissenters are discussed and exemplified in Kenneth Heineman, *Campus Wars: The Peace Movement at American State Universities in the Vietnam Era* (1993); Todd Gitlin's *The Sixties* (1987); James Miller's *Democracy Is in the Streets* (1987); George Ball's *The Past Has Another Pattern* (1982); William C. Berman's *William Fulbright and the Vietnam War* (1988), which uses Fulbright papers; Eugene Brown's *William Fulbright: Advice and Dissent* (1984), another good biography; Melvin Small's *Johnson, Nixon, and the Doves* (1988); Lawrence S. Wittner's *Rebels against War: The American Peace Movement, 1933–1983* (1984), an updated edition of a fine work; *Peace Heroes in Twentieth-Century America*, ed. Charles DeBenedetti (1986), especially on Martin Luther King and the Berrigans; David J. Garrow's *Bearing the Cross: Martin Luther King and the Southern Christian Leadership Conference* (1986); Steven M. Gillon's *Politics and Vision: The ADA and American Liberalism, 1947–1985* (1987), on the dilemma of the Democrats' liberal wing; and Douglas Pike's *Vietnam and the Soviet Union* (1987), which surveys the entire relationship. In a category by itself as an account of the war is Neil Sheehan, *A Bright Shining Lie: John Paul Vann and America in Vietnam* (1988).

18

Coming to Terms with History:
The Nixon-Kissinger Years
(1969–1976)

OF OUTHOUSES AND COWBOYS

Richard Nixon, most so-called experts concluded in the early 1960s, was politically dead. After losing the races for the presidency in 1960 and the California governorship in 1962, he angrily told reporters that they would not "have Nixon to kick around anymore." But private law practice did not calm this most restless and fascinating of post-1945 politicians. By 1968, he was back at the top of the political heap. His determination was never in doubt. While attending Whittier College, he decided to win a contest to find the largest outdoor wooden toilet to throw into the flames of the annual bonfire rally. The all-time champion had been a three-holer, but Nixon had somehow located a four-holer and hauled it to the rally. "Picture the systematic intensity that went into this achievement," biographer Garry Wills suggests.[1]

The young Nixon also played a fair, if risky, game of poker. In the navy during World War II, he won thousands of dollars, which helped him launch his political career as a California congressman. In 1950, he won election to the Senate. After serving as Dwight Eisenhower's vice-president (1953–1961) and spending the 1960s on the "rubber chicken circuit," speaking at endless Republican dinners for local candidates, Nixon was the best known and most owed of the party's candidates. With his wide experience and contacts, he should have been superbly equipped to rebuild the national consensus destroyed by the Vietnam War and to govern the country effectively.

But throughout, as Henry Kissinger later observed, there was the problem of how this true loner, who had few close friends, could "become a politican. He really dislikes people."[2] Nixon admired films made by Clint Eastwood and John Wayne about strong, lonely, one-of-a-kind men. His all-time film favorite was *Patton*, in which (according to him) a brash but brave and brilliant U.S. general accomplished what better-liked military officers could not. (Some critics felt that the film only showed how war allowed a mentally unbalanced person to gain life-and-death power over others.)[3] Nixon's instincts for politics, resembling George Patton's for battles, were well developed, if flawed. By the late 1960s, he understood that the Vietnam War signaled the breakdown of U.S. postwar domination. Other powers—the Soviet Union, China, Japan, even newly emerging states—were creating a new world arena in which Americans faced tough competition. Nixon especially believed that, during the 1960s, Americans "saw a break-down in frankly what I could call the leadership class of this country."[4] He concluded that history had taken a sharp turn and that he was now the most capable person to steer the U.S. system around that turn.

The vehicle for making the turn had to be foreign policy. Domestic affairs were petty and boring—simply "building outhouses in Peoria," as Nixon once phrased it.[5] Foreign relations, unlike internal affairs, also allowed the president much freedom of action. He ensured his control over diplomacy by placing an equally secretive Harvard professor, Henry Kissinger, at the head of his National Security Council (NSC). Kissinger later liked to picture himself as a "lone cowboy" who bravely rode into town to battle evil international forces. In reality, he had risen to power by working closely with Harvard's international-affairs groups, New York's prestigious Council on Foreign Relations, and the rich, ambitious governor of New York, Nelson Rockefeller, who had challenged Nixon for the Republican nomination. Kissinger exemplified the "eastern establishment" that had long controlled U.S. foreign policy. Resembling many others in that "establishment," he had disliked and mistrusted Nixon. When Rockefeller lost the nomination, however, Kissinger moved easily into the victor's camp. "Nixon had a consuming need for flattery and Kissinger a consuming need to provide it," one journalist recalled.[6]

But Nixon also picked Kissinger for other, more important reasons. Both agreed that they alone should control foreign policy. In their view, neither the State Department nor Congress had the imagination or will to take the daring new initiatives needed. Nixon appointed an old friend (and distinguished lawyer), William Rogers, as secretary of state, precisely because Rogers knew little about diplomacy. He could be counted on to be loyal and keep the State Department preoccupied with minor matters while Nixon and Kissinger conducted policy. Both men also feared the right wing of American politics more than the left wing. Nixon had been identified with that right wing in the 1950s, but to protect himself from it further, he named the former governor of Maryland, Spiro Agnew, as his vice-presidential running mate. In the 1968 campaign, Agnew blasted Democratic candidate Hubert Humphrey as having been "soft on Communism and soft on law and order over the years." Between 1969 and 1973 (when he had to resign his office due to charges of corruption and fraud), the vice-president delighted in attacking the supposed "liberal" media.

For his part, Kissinger quickly cut everyone but the president out of policy making. He loved to conduct supersecret, so-called "back channel" diplomacy with leaders of the other major powers, especially the Soviets. In a secret report of June 12, 1969 (only released in Russia in 1993), Soviet Ambassador to the United States Anatoly F. Dobrynin described Kissinger to Kremlin officials:

> Kissinger himself, an intelligent and erudite man, is at the same time vain and prone in conversations with me . . . , especially when we have dinner alone, to brag of his influence. At our last conversation, for example, he declared without excess modesty that in all Washington only two people can answer precisely at any given moment about the U.S. position on this or that issue: President Nixon and he, Kissinger.

Determined to monopolize policy making, and with "absolutely paranoid suspicions" about the bureaucracy, as one aide described it, the NSC director even wire-tapped the telephones of his own staff. While Agnew and Nixon wanted to treat reporters "with considerably more contempt" (in the president's words), Kissinger cultivated and shaped stories written by leading journalists. His abilities, as well as an intellectual background that too often awed his listeners, enabled him to sell the administration's policies through the media from the top down—even as Agnew regularly condemned the media. It all was brilliantly orchestrated.[7]

If, then, as Kissinger wrote, "the acid test of a policy . . . is its ability to obtain domestic support,"[8] he and Nixon seemed to control the levers necessary to obtain that support—at least during their first term in power.

. . . AND WOODROW WILSON AND ELEPHANTS

Nixon had another reason for naming Kissinger to head the NSC. Both men thought in broad, conceptual terms. Both believed the United States had reached a historic turn. Both agreed on the outlines of a new, workable foreign policy. In mid-1970, Kissinger placed the American crisis in perspective. During a private discussion with reporters, he declared that after Vietnam, no president would again repeat John F. Kennedy's inaugural address that had asked Americans to "fight any foe, support any friend." Instead, Kissinger continued, "a new phase" of policy had to begin, one which assumed that Americans would no longer rush out to stop "aggression wherever it occurred."[9] At the same time, however, U.S. interests would somehow have to be protected. It was a terrible tightrope to walk.

One answer was simply to reduce U.S. overseas interests and commitments. By 1969, Americans had 302 major and 2,000 secondary military bases abroad. Perhaps those incredible numbers could be cut. Nixon and Kissinger, however, did not want to reduce those commitments drastically. They believed that to retreat would, among other things, fly in the face of four hundred years of American history. As a German-Jewish émigré in the 1930s, and as a scholar of European history, Kissinger knew that "in Europe the frontier repelled; in America it beckoned." Citing "the great historian [Frederick Jackson] Turner," Kissinger declared that Americans' experience with their frontier gave them a sense of triumph over nature that held meaning for "all mankind. America was not itself unless it had a meaning beyond itself. This is why Americans have always seen their role in the world as the outward manifestation of an inward state of grace."[10] In other words, Americans now had the world as their frontier (much as they once had the Ohio River or Rocky Mountains as their frontier), and to retreat from it meant that they would be the first Americans to fail, the first to deny the greatness of their own past. Obviously, a great deal was suddenly at stake.

Nixon believed that Woodrow Wilson ("our greatest President of this century") provided "the greatest vision of America's world role." Wilson "wasn't practical enough" in conducting diplomacy, Nixon added, but clearly understood how the United States had to lead a

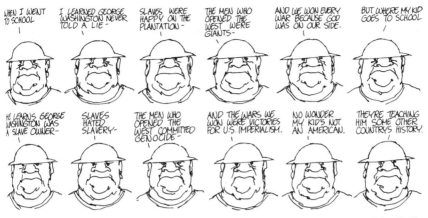

WHEN I WENT TO SCHOOL

I LEARNED GEORGE WASHINGTON NEVER TOLD A LIE—

SLAVES WERE HAPPY ON THE PLANTATION—

THE MEN WHO OPENED THE WEST WERE GIANTS—

AND WE WON EVERY WAR BECAUSE GOD WAS ON OUR SIDE.

BUT WHERE MY KID GOES TO SCHOOL

HE LEARNS GEORGE WASHINGTON WAS A SLAVE OWNER—

SLAVES HATED SLAVERY—

THE MEN WHO OPENED THE WEST COMMITTED GENOCIDE—

AND THE WARS WE WON WERE VICTORIES FOR U.S. IMPERIALISM.

NO WONDER MY KID'S NOT AN AMERICAN.

THEY'RE TEACHING HIM SOME OTHER COUNTRY'S HISTORY.

Jules Fieffer

collective effort (in Wilson's famous phrase) to make the world safe for democracy. In a 1967 essay, Nixon had sketched out his plans to lead such an effort. First, Asians were to help themselves more and rely on the United States less. But Americans had to play a great role by reaching "westward to the East" and by working with Japan to build "a Pacific community." Second, after more changes occurred inside China, it, too, could help build this community. That was a stunning proposal from the man who, since 1949, had damned "Red" China (and those U.S. officials who had "lost" China).[11]

Kissinger and Nixon began to see that (in the professor's words) "the greatest need of the contemporary international system is an agreed concept of order," and that China—after a decade of turmoil and major economic and diplomatic failures—might be ready to support such order. The two Americans most feared not communism, but disorder—especially revolutionaries who wanted to destroy order. Kissinger even thought order more important than justice. After all, he argued, order could lead to justice, but justice did not necessarily lead to order. He and Nixon believed that the Soviets and Chinese were both interested in peace and order as well as better relations with the United States (especially to obtain U.S. technology and wheat). The real enemies to world peace were North Vietnam, Cuba, and revolutionaries in Africa and other newly emerging areas that wanted to destroy the order that the United States had created and had benefited from since 1945.[12]

Nixon and Kissinger concluded that U.S. interests could be protected (and with less expense to financially squeezed Americans) by having Japan, China, and even the Soviet Union work with the United States—especially against revolutionaries. The country had gone through a kind of hell in the 1960s, but it had hung on to remain the world's greatest power, although that power was slipping. "Living next to you is in some ways like sleeping with an elephant," Canada's prime minister Pierre Trudeau told Americans in 1969. "One is affected by every twitch and grunt."[13] If Nixon succeeded, the elephant would sleep more soundly but roam more widely when awake, especially in a world viewed as a frontier for American opportunity. But first the Vietnam War had to be resolved.

VIETNAM AND THE NIXON DOCTRINE (1969–1972)

As early as 1966, Kissinger publicly admitted that the Vietnam conflict could not be won militarily. In his first day in office in 1969, top-secret studies informed Nixon that the United States could not win the war. The Pentagon believed that, under the best of conditions, it would take eight to thirteen years just to control all of South Vietnam. Those "best of conditions" had never been found in the region. U.S. troop strength stood at 543,000. The war's cost to Americans had leaped to $30 billion annually.[14] Some 14,600 U.S. troops had died in 1968 alone. Nixon decided to withdraw—but slowly and on his terms. By the time he finished in 1973, another 26,000 Americans and at least 1 million more Southeast Asians had perished in the conflict.

Nixon's plan rested on Vietnamization and the Nixon Doctrine. Through Vietnamization, the president planned to withdraw his forces slowly, replacing them with well-supplied Vietnamese. The idea had first appeared in the 1950s, when U.S. officials wanted "good Asians" to fight "bad Asians." It had not worked, but Nixon now determined to support Vietnamization with other strategies. He wanted to sit down with the Communists and negotiate a cease-fire and mutual U.S.–North Vietnamese withdrawal from South Vietnam, Cambodia, and Laos. Then he planned to launch massive bombing raids on the North until the Communists agreed to withdraw. It seemed to be an offer they could not refuse.

The president placed this approach into a much broader policy. The Nixon Doctrine, presented at Guam in mid-1969, indicated that the United States would help "the defense and development of allies and friends" but "cannot—and will not—conceive all the plans, design all the programs, execute all the decisions and undertake all the defense of the free nations of the world." Others would have to grab the oars

TABLE 3

PRINCIPAL WARS IN WHICH THE UNITED STATES PARTICIPATED: U.S. MILITARY PERSONNEL SERVING AND CASUALTIES

War/Conflict	Branch of service	Number serving	Battle deaths	Casualties Other deaths	Wounds not mortal
Korean Conflict (25 Jun. 1950–27 Jul. 1953)	*Total*	5,720,000	33,643	20,617	103,284
	Army	2,834,000	27,709	9,429	77,596
	Navy	1,177,000	466	4,043	1,576
	Marines	424,000	4,268	1,261	25,744
	Air Force	1,285,000	1,200	5,884	368
Vietnam Conflict (4 Aug. 1964–27 Jan. 1973)	*Total*	8,744,000	47,312	10,705	153,303
	Army	4,368,000	30,899	7,269	96,802
	Navy	1,842,000	1,605	919	4,178
	Marines	794,000	13,070	1,749	51,392
	Air Force	1,740,000	1,738	766	931

Source: Department of Defense.

and help row. By announcing that he would begin to pull U.S. troops out of Vietnam, Nixon showed that he meant business with his doctrine. He also planned to cut back the inflated military budget by ordering American forces to have only the capability to fight 1.5 wars (for example, a major conflict in Europe and a lesser one in a newly emerging area) instead of the present capability to wage 2.5 wars. By late 1972, he had pulled out all but 3,000 U.S. troops from Vietnam as well as one-third of the 60,000 American soldiers in South Korea, 12,000 from Japan, and 16,000 from Thailand.

But, in Kissinger's words, "we could not simply walk away from an enterprise involving two administrations, five allied countries, and thirty-one thousand dead as if we were switching a television channel." Nor, as the president vowed privately, would he bow to New York's Wall Street and legal communities who advised "scuttling Vietnam at any price." Nixon combined the troop withdrawal with an incredible bombing campaign that, on average, dropped a ton of bombs each minute on Vietnam between 1969 and early 1973. Democratic Senator J. William Fulbright from Arkansas agreed with the *Washington Post* that Nixon had become "the greatest bomber of all time."[15] Meanwhile, the CIA's Phoenix program weakened the Communists by killing at least 21,000 supposed enemy civilians who worked in the villages of South Vietnam. The North's government, however, continued to refuse to accept a divided Vietnam.

Kissinger flew secretly to Paris to talk with the North's negotiator, Le Duc Tho—"gray-haired, dignified," as the American described him, with perfect manners and "large luminous eyes [that] only rarely revealed the fanaticism" that had led him at the age of sixteen to fight the French. Nixon decided that the North's representative was stalling in the talks until the Communists could rebuild their forces. The president discussed the bombing of harbors and even considered using nuclear weapons. He pulled back at the last minute from expanding the bombing in October 1969, when a massive anti-war rally marched on Washington. Nixon announced that he had ignored the marchers and had coolly watched a televised Ohio State football game. In truth, the frightened president had ordered 300 troops armed with light machine guns to protect him in the White House.[16]

CAMBODIA, LAOS, AND KENT STATE

Vietnamization was not working. Nixon was furious that the Communists used trails through Cambodia and Laos to supply their troops in the south. The 6.5 million people of Cambodia, a beautiful country the size of Oklahoma, had been spared most of the war's horrors. Although its leader, Prince Sihanouk, had broken relations with the United States in 1965, he said nothing when Nixon bombed the Communist bases in Cambodia. Nixon did so secretly—a secret kept, that is, from Congress and the American people but not from Southeast Asians who were the targets. The air strikes forced the Communists farther inside Cambodia, and the nation became more unstable. In March 1970, Sihanouk was overthrown by his prime minister, General Lon Nol, who was more willing to work with the Americans.

The new regime was corrupt and incompetent, but Nixon seized the chance and launched an invasion of eastern Cambodia on April 30, 1970, to destroy the camps of some 40,000 Communists. It was a sudden, highly risky expansion of the war. Even the old cold warrior, Dean Acheson, had his doubts. Nixon, Acheson told a friend, was the only horse he knew who would run back into a burning barn.[17] On national television, the president warned that when "the chips are down," the United States must not act "like a pitiful helpless giant." But the invasion failed. U.S. and South Vietnamese troops could not find and destroy the Communist forces. By late 1970, those forces had grown until they spread over at least one-third of Cambodia. By early 1974, they controlled the entire country—or what remained of a starving population that soon became virtually enslaved by the brutal, Communist Khmer Rouge.[18]

Nixon failed at home as well. The Cambodian campaign, known as a "sideshow" to the main event in Vietnam, triggered a massive protest when American students in nearly 450 colleges went on strike. Many students marched on Washington to lobby both the administration (some of Nixon's advisers, but not Kissinger, sympathized with the protesters) and Congress. The president called the students "bums" who are "blowing up the campuses." Then, in early May, the Ohio National Guard fired on anti-war protesters at Kent State. Four students died. Ten days later, two black students were shot to death by Mississippi state police during protests at Jackson State College. The nation went into shock. On the night of the Kent State shootings, Nixon could not sleep, made fifty-one phone calls, and led Kissinger to conclude that the president was "on the edge of a nervous breakdown."[19] Amid the chaos, several thousand hard-hat construction workers paraded in New York City to support the president and beat up members of anti-war groups. But other New Yorkers, including Wall Street banking leaders, flew to Washington to warn Nixon that the threat of a wider war was threatening a stock-market collapse and a possible financial panic.[20]

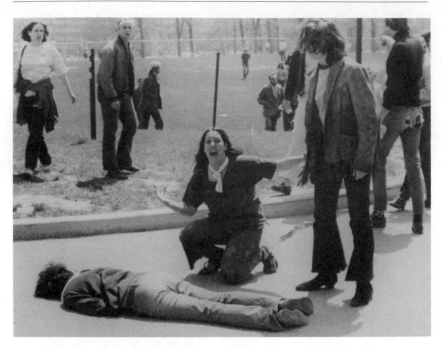

This photograph captures the horror of the shootings at Kent State University on May 4, 1970, when the campus erupted in protest against President Nixon's invasion of Cambodia. A young woman screams over the body of Jeffrey Glenn Miller.

The president announced that the U.S. soldiers in Cambodia would be out by June 30, 1970. Congress voted to prohibit U.S. combat troops or advisers from re-entering Cambodia. Sixteen years after the United States had become enmeshed in Southeast Asia, Congress, for the first time, had been able to find the votes to limit the president's power to make war in the region.

That ability, nevertheless, remained awesome. Nixon grew frustrated as he continued to withdraw U.S. troops from Vietnam, but the Vietnamese soldiers could not fill the gap left by the Americans. He decided to try to buck up his collapsing Vietnamization policy by attacking neighboring Laos, along whose supposedly neutral territory the Communists marched their troops into South Vietnam. The size of Oregon and with only 3 million people, Laos had been promised neutrality by both sides since 1954; both sides had repeatedly broken the promise. Since 1964, and especially 1968, giant U.S. B-52 bombers secretly bombed the Ho Chi Minh Trail in massive attacks. The CIA covertly armed 15,000 Meo tribesmen to fight 30,000 Laotian Communist troops. The Communists, nevertheless, continued to gain ground. Laos became a case study of how bombing did not have the desired effect on peasant revolutionary forces. The attacks only produced thousands of dead Laotians and hundreds of thousands of desperate refugees. In February 1971, Nixon tried to drive back the Communists with an invasion of Laos. This time only South Vietnamese troops, not Americans, went in. Vietnamization, however, failed miserably. The South Vietnamese broke and retreated before Communist attacks. By late 1971, the pro-Communist groups held more of Laos than before.

THE GREAT TURNAROUND: THE DRAFT PROVIDES POLITICAL ROOM

By February 1971, when Laos was invaded, Nixon faced failure on nearly every side. In addition to problems with Vietnamization, he endured riots at home, Democratic victories in the 1970 elections, defeats in attempts to obtain conservative Supreme Court appointments, and rapid decline in public support. In mid-1971, the *New York Times* obtained 7,000 pages of secret documents, the so-called Pentagon Papers, that revealed the innermost decisions that had led to deepening U.S. involvement in Vietnam between the 1940s and 1968. Ordered in 1967 by Secretary of Defense Robert McNamara, who was determined to learn from this tragic past, the Pentagon Papers did not include documents from the Nixon years. But the record revealed enough embarrassing errors in policy and blatant attempts to lie to the American people that the anti-war movement received additional fuel.

Nixon and Kissinger, moreover, were terrified that new leaks would reveal their own secrets, especially the bombing of Cambodia and Laos. The Pentagon had even falsified computer records to ensure that Americans would remain ignorant of the bombing. When the *New York Times* published a story about the bombing in May 1969, Kissinger quickly placed secret wiretaps on his own assistants to uncover the leak. He never did discover who was leaking the information to the media, but by 1971 the president had set up a White House "plumbers" unit that used former and present CIA agents to discover and stop leaks. In 1972, one plumbers group was arrested when it broke into the Watergate Hotel office complex in Washington to tap Democratic party telephones. The discovery led to the downfall of Richard Nixon in 1974, after he tried to cover up the crime. It all seemed to prove correct a

Chinese official's remark to Kissinger: "One should not lose the whole world just to gain South Vietnam."[21]

Between 1971 and 1974, however, the president opened a startlingly new chapter in U.S. foreign policy, a chapter that historian Lloyd Gardner has entitled "The Great Nixon Turnaround."[22] The president began by correctly estimating that he could stop much of the anti-war protesting. As one of his aides phrased it, "If there is one thing the Americans are more sick of today than fighting in the jungles abroad, it is fighting in the streets and campuses at home."[23] Many polls showed that Americans did not want to lose Vietnam, but neither did they want to send thousands of their sons and daughters to die for such a country. The U.S. military agreed. Its morale and fighting ability were being destroyed by the war. One general later recalled walking through a train station "when a well-dressed, middle-aged woman came up, called me names I couldn't repeat and spit on me."[24] Nixon went far in stopping such protests by announcing that the draft was to end in 1973. A much reduced military would find its soldiers through a lottery system and volunteers. College campuses began to quiet down. The president had created some political breathing space. To help Vietnamization, he increased the bombings. Americans now said little.

THE GREAT TURNAROUND: THE ECONOMY

They were complaining loudly, however, about the rising rates of inflation and unemployment in 1971. The U.S. economy seemed about to collapse. True, its annual gross national product (GNP) had passed the $1 trillion mark in 1970 for the first time. True, U.S. exports incredibly quintupled between the 1950s and 1970s to $107 billion, excluding services, and now accounted for the sale of nearly 20 percent of U.S. factory and farm production. But not even those staggering figures were enough to pay for global U.S. defense commitments and overseas investment. Americans were spending more than they could produce and sell.

Since the Bretton Woods agreements of 1944 (see p. 431), the world's economy had largely rested on the dollar because Americans could back up the dollar with their dynamic economy and $15 billion to $24 billion in gold. By 1970–1971, however, they had spent too many dollars. Some $40 billion was held overseas, but only $10 billion in gold remained in the United States to support it. Foreigners began to doubt that the dollars they held were truly "as good as gold." That doubt

U.S. MERCHANDISE TRADE BALANCE, 1967–1984

Source: U.S. Department of State, *Atlas of U.S. Foreign Relations* (December 1985).

turned to near panic in 1971, when figures revealed that, for the first time since 1893–1894, the United States had imported more goods (such as oil and automobiles) than it had been able to sell abroad. It marked a moment of historic importance. Foreigners and Americans alike started to cash in their dollars for gold and other securities. Nixon recalled that, in 1958, the United States had "all the chips" in the "great poker game" of international economics, and that no one else could play unless the Americans passed out some of their chips. By the early 1970s, he sorrowfully noted, "the world [was] a lot different."[25] Others were now building up their pile of chips as the American pile disappeared.

The president had several choices. First, he could save dollars by reducing U.S. defense commitments even below the level promised by the Nixon Doctrine. He and Kissinger, however, were determined to expand, not reduce, the nation's influence. Second, he could limit U.S. investment abroad. Between 1958 and 1968, American manufacturers had moved into the new European Common Market, or had sought cheap labor in Asia, by increasing their overseas capacity by an amazing 471 percent, compared with a 72 percent expansion at home. (Ford, for example, made 40 percent of its cars abroad.) American multinational corporations were reshaping the world but bringing too few dollars back to the United States. Nixon, however, refused to interfere in this marketplace. He knew that if he tried, the corporations could ignore him and continue to operate out of overseas offices, where they would be out of his reach.

He decided upon a third choice: he would force allies to help the U.S. economy. At Kansas City in mid-1971, Nixon declared that the world now contained "five great economic superpowers"—the United States, Japan, USSR, China, and the European Common Market. (As historian Alan Henrikson notes, "This was an admission [by Nixon] of the descent of the United States from superiority to parity, from being *the* center to being *a* center.")[26] Because "economic power will be the key to other kinds of power" in the late twentieth century, Nixon warned, Americans had to get their economic act together or they would go the way of ancient Rome. In August 1971, he tried to stop the erosion of U.S. power by placing ninety-day controls on wages, prices, and rents. But that was only a Band-Aid. As the election approached, he could not safely demand more from Americans. Indeed, he even slashed income taxes. So he demanded more from allies who depended on U.S. goods and military protection. He turned the job over to a tough Texan, Secretary of the Treasury John Connally. "My basic approach," Connally declared, "is that the foreigners are out to screw us. Our job is to screw them first."[27]

Nixon's and Connally's "new economic policy" imposed a 10 percent surcharge on U.S. imports. Japan and Canada quickly felt the shock. So did western Europeans and newly emerging nations. Nixon did not care. He privately condemned the Japanese because, he believed, they had cheated on a deal that he had made with them: they were to get back the Pacific island of Okinawa (which U.S. bombers had used as a major base since 1945) and, in turn, were to reduce the flood of their textile exports to the United States. But the Japanese government did not deliver on its end of the deal. By early 1971, a secret U.S. analysis reflected Nixon's fury by concluding that Japan had to be considered a potential enemy. As for the western Europeans, they were making political and economic deals with the Soviets but not lowering their tariffs on U.S. goods. Nixon determined to keep their feet to the fire until they promised to help support the dollar.

In an agreement made at Washington's Smithsonian Institution in late 1971, the allies finally agreed to accept a cheaper dollar (a dollar that also cheapened U.S. goods and so made them more competitive) and more expensive Japanese and European currencies. Nixon typically called it the "greatest monetary agreement in the history of the world." But the following year, the dollar again sank. A second deal was needed to prop it back up. The U.S. economy had contracted a fundamental sickness. The Smithsonian agreement, however, did help improve conditions enough to aid Nixon's re-election victory in 1972. It also enabled him to deal from greater economic strength as he made historic journeys to China and the Soviet Union.

THE GREAT TURNAROUND: CHINA

In July 1971, Nixon told an astonished world that he planned to travel to China. According to opinion polls, 56 percent of Americans continued to see China as the world's most dangerous nation.[28] Moreover, some 50,000 U.S. lives had been lost in Vietnam supposedly to contain Chinese Communist power. Few Americans, however, could challenge Nixon from the right. Since 1949, he had led the attacks on Democrats for "losing China." He could travel to Beijing (Peking) without political fears. As for Vietnam, the rationale for the U.S. commitment had gone through a strange, little-noted change. By 1971, the Soviets were becoming the great ally of the Communist Vietnamese (who historically feared the Chinese anyway). The greatest hatred in the region was not between Communists and U.S.-supported "dominoes," but between the Communists themselves as the Chinese tried to block growing Soviet influence on their southern borders. Instead of using Vietnam to contain China, Nixon concluded that he had better use China to contain Vietnam.

The Chinese had been through a kind of hell and were ready to change policies. In 1966, Mao had ordered a "cultural revolution" to shake up the society. Wild teen-aged Red Guards killed suspected conservatives and sent intellectuals and government officials to work in the fields with fertilizers (urine and feces). By 1969, when Mao finally put a brake on the Red Guard, the society and his foreign policy were in chaos. Moreover, a massive million-man build-up by the Soviet and Chinese armies along their common border of some 5,000 miles erupted in shooting and the death of both Chinese and Soviet troops in 1969. Hatred between the two Communist powers became red-hot. ("Who do they think they are!" exclaimed Soviet Ambassador to the United Nations Yakov Malik. "We'll kill those yellow sons of bitches!") If John F. Kennedy had contemplated attacking Chinese nuclear facilities in 1963 only to have the Soviets refuse to cooperate, now the Soviets seemed

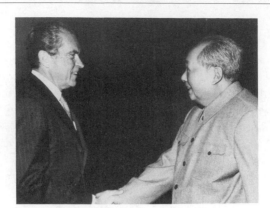

Richard Nixon (1913–　) surprised the world and began to reorient U.S. foreign policy toward China when, in 1972, he flew to Beijing (Peking) and shook hands with a man he had long attacked—Mao Zedong (Tse-tung) (1893–1976), the leader of the Chinese Revolution.

ready to attack while the United States pulled back. Assessing the crisis, Mao and his brilliant prime minister, Zhou Enlai (Chou En-lai), decided to reverse their policies toward the United States. They sent friendly signals to Nixon. The president responded during the border fighting by publicly signaling to the Soviets to back off. He even privately considered the use of nuclear weapons in case the Soviets tried to invade China. Premier Zhou (Chou) invited a U.S. table-tennis team to play Chinese teams. Nixon then relaxed the trade embargo and stopped military flights over China. In another border war of 1971, the United States publicly "tilted" toward Pakistan, which was pro-Chinese, and against Pakistan's enemy, India, which had moved closer to the Soviets. Nixon even stood with Pakistan when its army overthrew an elected government and unleashed a brutal attack against East Pakistan (which, with India's help, became the independent nation of Bangladesh). In return for U.S. support, the Pakistanis helped Kissinger travel secretly to Beijing (Peking) to plan the president's visit.

In February 1972, Nixon became the first U.S. president to step on Chinese soil. He seemed awestruck by what he was doing (when visiting the Great Wall of China he could only say, "This is a great wall"). At a state banquet, he told Zhou (Chou) in a public toast that "our two peoples tonight hold the future of the world in our hands"—which, no doubt, was news to the Soviets. But the final Shanghai communiqué, issued by Nixon and Zhou (Chou) on February 27, was indeed a turning point. In a thinly veiled reference to Soviet power, they declared that they would oppose anyone trying "to establish hegemony" in "the

Asia-Pacific region." They also agreed to broaden their relations through scientific, cultural, and economic exchanges as well as some political ties. (Full diplomatic recognition did not occur until 1979). On the most divisive point of Taiwan, the Chinese continued to claim the island, and the United States carefully announced it would "reduce its forces and military installations on Taiwan as the tension in the area diminishes."[29] In the meantime, U.S. ties with the island remained.

Between 1971 and late 1973, U.S.-China trade made a great leap forward from $5 million to $900 million annually. Excluding special grain deals, it even surpassed U.S.-Soviet trade. Thus, Nixon had also successfully moved to block Japan's attempts to monopolize China's foreign concessions. But most of all, as a watchful French official said, the president "wanted to show the Russians. This was the biggest purpose of the trip [to China], and it was very successful."[30]

THE GREAT TURNAROUND: THE SOVIETS AND VIETNAM

The president thus approached his second historic meeting in 1972 from a good position. As Soviet leader Leonid Brezhnev openly admitted the year before, the Soviets' badly run economy had slowed to a crawl. It needed a jump-start from foreigners, especially from U.S. technology and American-built ("turnkey") truck and car factories. For its part, the United States could use the Soviet Union's rich mineral resources. (Americans, Nixon's secretary of commerce complained, used up their own resources "like a drunken sailor" who now begins to feel "the hole in the bottom of his pocket.") Brezhnev also needed some arms controls so that more money could go into the basic economy. By 1972, the United States and the USSR had enough nuclear weapons to explode 15 tons of radioactive TNT on every man, woman, and child on earth. World military expenses ran $200 billion annually, a figure greater than the combined gross national product of Africa and southern Asia. Governments spent two-and-one-half times the amount on arms that they spent on health.[31]

Nixon had his own reasons for meeting Brezhnev. Besides wanting to ease the growing American economic strain by making trade and arms deals, he hoped for a television spectacular on the eve of the 1972 presidential campaign. He also hoped to regain the diplomatic initiative and put Vietnam behind him. In 1969–1972, for example, he had lost that initiative in central Europe when West Germany's popular chancellor, Willy Brandt, ended a quarter-century-long argument by recognizing the existence of the East German Communist government. Brandt also signed pacts that finally accepted eastern European boundaries drawn by the Red Army in 1945. The chancellor believed that Communist rule could better be penetrated—and all Germany reunited—by a policy of détente, or a lessening of tension, than by aggressive anticommunism. Nixon and Kissinger did not like Brandt's play to the Soviet Union (for one thing, the Americans had little control over it), but they did not try to stop him. Nixon just decided to make his own deals with Brezhnev. In the president's view, the West Germans and others (including Middle Eastern and Asian governments) too easily played off Americans against Soviets.

Unlike Eisenhower and Kennedy, Nixon and Kissinger held power when the United States could no longer build up to such military superiority that it could simply face down the Soviets. The Soviet nuclear force approached parity with the American, and Brezhnev used this new power to extend his influence into such areas as Egypt and Vietnam. The two Americans believed that a new means for controlling the Communists had to be found. In their hands, détente was to be the containment of Soviet power by different—and cheaper—means.

Nixon also hoped that Brezhnev would help him escape from Vietnam with some honor. It was a badly misplaced hope. Although the Soviets heavily supplied Vietnam, they had little control over the Hanoi government. Documents discovered in Moscow in the early 1990s indeed showed that the Vietnamese ruthlessly used the Soviets—not least when Vietnam's gunboats positioned themselves next to Soviet vessels as the gunboats blasted away at U.S. planes. The Vietnamese dared the Americans to bomb them when the bombs could well hit Soviet ships instead. Brezhnev (like Stalin and Khrushchev before him) simply could not fully control smaller members of their supposed "fraternal socialist camp." Indeed, on March 30, 1972, as Nixon prepared for his Moscow trip, North Vietnam launched a massive attack against South Vietnamese and what remained of U.S. troops. The president viewed the attack, led by Soviet-built tanks, as a direct challenge to his entire policy and, more personally, as an attempt to embarrass him before the world. He responded with a renewed bombing campaign (code-named Operation Linebacker, reflecting Nixon's love for football) that devastated targets never before hit. Using laser-guided bombs of 500 to 3,000 pounds, the planes destroyed bridges, railroads, and other military and civilian targets with great precision. On May 8, U.S. planes dropped mines in Haiphong harbor, where Soviet ships were anchored. The Soviets made no response. At home, telegrams poured into the White House supporting Nixon's action. (Later, however, his aides admitted they had used about $8,400 from CREEP—the Committee to Re-elect the President—to send the telegrams to themselves and to place a phony advertisement in the *New York Times* congratulating the president.)[32] Abroad, Brezhnev never let out a peep of protest. Soviet interests overrode North Vietnamese lives.

Brezhnev did show his displeasure by giving Nixon a cool reception when the president arrived in the Soviet Union on May 22, 1972. And, of course, the Soviets bugged the U.S. delegation's hotel with listening devices. When Nixon casually mentioned to a secretary he'd like an apple, in ten minutes a hotel maid appeared with the fruit. But the two leaders got along well personally. Brezhnev, like nearly all Soviets, was terrified of a potentially powerful China on his border. He tried later to convince Nixon that "we the whites" and "we Europeans" should control the Chinese before they became "a superpower."[33] Nixon rejected that approach but used the USSR's fear of China as a high card in his negotiations.

The discussions produced four historic agreements at the summit. The first was SALT I (Strategic Arms Limitations Talks), which limited the number of offensive intercontinental ballistic missiles to 1,410 land-based missiles and 950 submarine-launched missiles on the Soviet side, and, for the United States, 1,000 land-based missiles and 710 submarine-launched weapons. The Americans more than made up the gap with their allies' nuclear deterrents in western Europe, the greatly superior fleet of U.S. bombers (450 to 150 USSR planes), and especially with the astonishing MIRVs (Multiple Independent Re-entry Vehicles). Hoping to take advantage of U.S. technology, Nixon refused to accept any limits on these "space buses," as Pentagon officials called them. His refusal proved to be a crucial mistake. The Soviets not only soon produced MIRVs of their own, but had larger missiles (such as their huge SS-18) on which they could place as many as ten warheads.

A second agreement (actually a part of SALT I) involved defensive antiballistic missile systems (ABMs). Since the late 1960s, U.S. officials had warned the Soviets not to continue to deploy such systems because it would force the United States to build more and larger nuclear weapons to overcome these defenses. Thus, ABMs would speed up—not slow—the arms race. Brezhnev finally accepted the reasoning. In the ABM treaty, both sides agreed to limit themselves to one defensive system for their capitals and a second to defend an area containing ICBM launchers. Both powers abided by the deal (indeed, the United States never even bothered to build a system to protect Washington) until the 1980s. Then President Ronald Reagan tried to destroy the ABM pact so that he could test his Strategic Defense Initiative (SDI or Star Wars) that he hoped would form a defensive shield.

The third agreement was the "Basic Principles of U.S.-Soviet Relations." Not a treaty, it attempted to set up ground rules to make superpower competition less dangerous. Both sides pledged to avoid confrontation and to coexist peacefully. They also promised to renounce claims to privileges in other regions (which U.S. officials—but certainly not Brezhnev—interpreted to mean the end of the Brezhnev Doctrine [see p. 623]).

Nixon and Kissinger not only hoped to tie the Soviets closer to U.S. interests, but to pressure Brezhnev to observe the other agreements. Thus, they presented him with a fourth deal: new U.S.-Soviet economic exchanges. As Kissinger later noted, U.S. trade and technology "would be a carrot for restrained [Soviet] political behavior."[34] This "carrot" became known as "linkage"—that is, telling the Soviets that progress in one area of diplomacy was linked to their behavior in another area. U.S.-Soviet trade did triple between 1971 and 1973 to about $650 million (with American exports accounting for a rich $546 million of the total). But in 1972–1973, half the trade occurred when the Soviets cleverly and secretly entered the American grain market to buy up at low prices wheat and corn that U.S. taxpayers had paid farmers high subsidies to produce. As U.S. grain dealers made a fortune and Brezhnev obtained shiploads of cheap farm products, Nixon did nothing. American bread prices increased. U.S. politicians grew furious at the way Americans had been taken by Communist buyers. When the president agreed to give the Soviets favored-trade treatment in a new reciprocity deal, the U.S. Senate rebelled.

The Senate, despite reservations by anti-Soviet "hawks," had accepted both SALT I and the ABM accord by an 88-to-2 vote. But in 1974, led by "superhawk" Washington Democrat Henry Jackson, the Senate tied the Jackson-Vanik Amendment to the reciprocity treaty. The amendment stated that most-favored-nation status would be extended to the Kremlin only when it allowed more Jews to leave the Soviet Union. Working quietly, Nixon and Brezhnev had increased the number of Jewish emigrants (usually to Israel or the United States) from 400 annually in 1968 to 35,000 in 1973. Human-rights advocates worldwide, including such prominent Soviet citizens as Nobel Prize–winning physicist Andrei Sakharov, demanded that the remaining thousands of Jews who wanted to leave should now have their wish granted. Suddenly, in 1973, Brezhnev imposed a tax, making emigra-

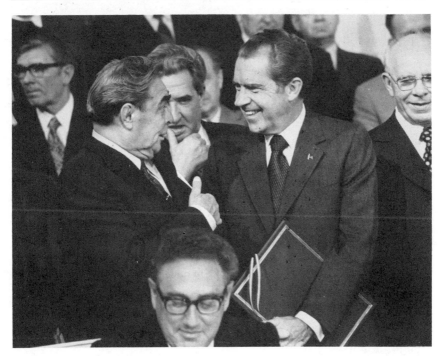

Soviet leader Leonid Brezhnev met with President Nixon in 1972, 1973, and 1974 (when this photo was taken, with Secretary of State Kissinger in the foreground). The meetings opened the first important era of U.S.-USSR détente but did not save Nixon's presidency. Kissinger recalled Brezhnev as "quintessentially Russian" in that he combined "crudeness and warmth," and was both "brutal and engaging. . . . Having grown up in a backward society nearly overrun by Nazi invasion, he . . . seemed to feel in his bones the vulnerability of his system." (Henry Kissinger, White House Years [Boston, 1979], p. 1141.)

tion from the Soviet Union more difficult. The Jackson-Vanik Amendment followed. Democratic senator Adlai Stevenson, Jr., from Illinois attached another amendment to the treaty sharply limiting the credit that U.S. agencies (such as the Export-Import Bank) could provide to increase U.S.-Soviet trade. The Soviets angrily denounced the entire treaty. The number of Jewish émigrés dropped 40 percent in 1975.

The results of the first major effort at détente were mixed. Of the 105 treaties that the United States and Soviet Union made between 1933 and 1980, 41 were drawn up between May 1972 and May 1974. Several were historic in slowing the arms race. But in the United States, the Pentagon demanded more money to build more efficient and destructive Trident submarines, new bombers, and better missiles. In the Soviet Union, Brezhnev also modernized his forces and cracked down on dissent until one lonely critic cried that "we [in the Soviet Union] are living on a moonscape. There is no one left. We are all alone on the moon."[35] Americans grew embittered, and Kissinger saw one reason for it: "It is an uncomfortable experience for Americans to deal with a country of roughly the same strength. We have never had to do this in our history."[36] In the short run, however, Nixon profited. As he rolled over Democrat George McGovern in the 1972 presidential election, eight of ten Republicans believed that Nixon's greatest achievements in office were his foreign policies. "You would argue that [the president] is not a moral leader," Kissinger told novelist Norman Mailer, a loud Nixon critic, ". . . but perhaps you go along with me that he has political genius." Mailer replied, "Absolutely."[37]

DÉTENTE'S TURNAROUND: CHILE

In 1973–1974, Nixon's political skills were put to the ultimate test and failed. The U.S. Congress held hearings on the Watergate break-in. At the same time, a series of foreign-policy events began to undermine the president's authority.

The key events occurred not in U.S.-Soviet relations, but in relations with the newly emerging nations, those outer edges of U.S. power where that power was most easily eaten away. Kissinger was ultrasensitive to the danger. "The peace of the world will be threatened, when it is threatened," he observed, "not primarily by strategic forces [of the superpowers] but by geopolitical changes, and to resist those geopolitical changes we must be able to resist regionally."[38] This fear had led to the "Basic Principles" agreement at the summit in which the United States tried to obtain Brezhnev's pledge to accept the *status quo* in the world. For their part, the newly emerging nations, eager to develop and gain control over their own destinies, were determined to change the *status quo* as fast as possible.

The first post-summit challenge occurred in Chile. In 1970, Salvador Allende Gossens, a middle-aged, experienced politician, used his Popular Unity party (a coalition of his own Socialist party and other Marxist groups) to run for the presidency. Determined not to have a second Cuba and intent on showing Brezhnev that the United States could control its own hemisphere, Kissinger saw Allende as "a challenge to our national interest."[39] Just before the election, Nixon ordered the CIA to prevent the Socialist's victory, even if it cost $10 million.[40] A two-track policy was launched. Track 1 cut off outside aid to Chile, with the aim of squeezing the nation's economy until it "screamed," to use Nixon's word. Track 2 secretly put the CIA into contact with extreme right-wing army officers who would use force to prevent an Allende victory.[41] But it was too late. Allende, with 36 percent of the vote, won by a paper-thin margin. The U.S. ambassador cabled home: "Chile voted calmly to have a Marxist-Leninist state, the first nation in the world to make this choice freely and knowingly." U.S. officials then turned to overthrowing the newly elected president. They systematically cut off international as well as American aid. By September 1973, the CIA had reported spending $8 million in anti-Allende activities, much of this money used in cooperation with the Chilean military. Allende did not help himself. Mismanagement worsened an already declining economy. He was unable to counter either his opponents' or the CIA's success with both the army and the middle class (especially housewives), who took to the streets to protest shortages. In September 1973, the army attacked the president's offices. Allende, the U.S. ambassador to Chile claimed, apparently committed suicide during the struggle.[42] But the circumstances of his death remain murky. Many, including his closest family members, believe he was murdered.

The United States had again helped overthrow an elected government. Nixon did so for many reasons. Several of his closest supporters, including Donald Kendall of Pepsi-Cola and Harold Geneen of International Telephone & Telegraph, urged the president to get rid of Allende before their extensive Chilean holdings were nationalized. U.S. intelligence and military agencies also feared the loss of their stations in Chile. But, above all, Nixon and Kissinger saw Allende as a threat to their order in the hemisphere. "I don't see why we have to let a country go Marxist just because its people are irresponsible," Kissinger was quoted as exclaiming.[43]

But the price turned out to be high. Word spread of the deep CIA involvement, a congressional investigation was held, and the result was a scathing indictment of the Nixon-Kissinger policies. In Chile itself, the brutal dictatorship of General Augusto Pinochet Ugarte locked into power. Pinochet's brutality even bloodied the streets of Washington, D.C., in 1976, when his agents killed Orlando Letelier, Allende's foreign minister and an outspoken critic of the new dictatorship. An American woman was also killed in the bomb attack.

Pinochet's legacy for North Americans was explored in the popular film, *Missing*, of 1982. The leading character, a U.S. citizen played by actor Jack Lemmon, discovers that his son has been one of some 10,000 victims of Pinochet's police. The son apparently knew too much about plans drawn up by the Chilean military and U.S. advisers to topple Allende. Until that point, Lemmon's character uncritically accepted the American way of life: "I can no longer abide the young people of our country who live off their parents and the fat of the land and then they find nothing better to do than whine and complain." But when he concludes that U.S. officials have tried to cover up the killing of his son, he confronts the U.S. ambassador. The official, however, tells Lemmon: "We're here to protect American interests. Over 3,000 U.S. firms do business here and that is your, our interest. . . . I'm concerned with the preservation of a way of life. . . . You can't have it both ways."[44]

Elsewhere in the hemisphere, Nixon did (and apparently cared) little. With his attention fixed on the Soviet Union and China, the aid he sent Latin America was mostly supplies to the armies that maintained order by force. Many South American nations, led by Argentina and Brazil, turned against these policies and increased trade with Europe and Japan. Soviet trade, especially in the Argentine wheat market, leaped forward. Despite (or because of) Allende's overthrow, Nixon and Kissinger faced losing control of a most important region.

DÉTENTE'S TURNAROUND: THE MIDDLE EAST

Both the Soviets and Americans nearly lost control of their allies in the Middle East during 1973. The result was a military alert that brought the world closer to nuclear war than at any time since 1962.

The crisis began on October 6, 1973, when Egyptian and Syrian forces launched a devastating surprise attack against Israel in an attempt to regain the land lost to Israeli armies in the 1967 war (see p. 622). Both attacking forces received massive supplies and military intelligence from the Soviet Union, although Brezhnev carefully kept the Soviet military out of any direct involvement. He did not have to urge on Anwar el-Sadat, who became Egypt's leader after Nasser suffered a fatal heart attack in 1970. Sadat was determined to avenge Egypt's 1967 humiliation. But he had also grown fearful of Soviet involvement in his country and had expelled 10,000 Soviet advisers in 1972. He clearly wanted to move closer to the United States. Nixon and Kissinger ignored the signals until Sadat took matters into his own hands by invading Israel on Yom Kippur, the most solemn Jewish holy day.

After suffering severe losses, the Israeli army counterattacked and, by October 20, was driving toward Egypt. Kissinger and the Soviets arranged a cease-fire. But Israel surrounded and began to starve out

Sadat's best troops. Brezhnev, mistakenly believing that Kissinger had tricked him with the cease-fire policy, supported Sadat's plea for joint U.S.-USSR intervention to stop the fighting. Nixon coldly turned down the offer. He was not about to allow the Soviet Union to become a power broker in the Middle East. Brezhnev then threatened to move unilaterally to save Sadat's troops. On the night of October 24, Kissinger and other senior officials responded by telling the Soviets to stay out of the region. They made the point clear by ordering U.S. forces worldwide to move to a stage 3 alert—halfway up the ladder to launching a nuclear attack. With the Watergate scandal engulfing him, a nearly broken-down Nixon isolated himself in another part of the White House but was apparently kept informed. After some anxious hours had elapsed, it became clear that Soviet forces were not going to go on alert or try to move into the Middle East.[45]

Kissinger, however, did not desire a total Israeli victory. By manipulating U.S. supplies, he pressured Israel into breaking its encirclement of the Egyptian army. Kissinger, whom Nixon had made secretary of state in September 1973, now had what he wanted: a Middle East in which neither side—Israel or the Arab nations—had won total victory but in which both depended on him to mediate a peace. His peace efforts received help at the United Nations, where Israelis, Arabs, and other members agreed on UN resolutions 242 (passed in 1967) and 338 (passed in 1973), which called for direct talks, Israeli withdrawal, and recognition of "the territorial integrity of every state in the area." In return for withdrawing, Israel was to be recognized by the Arabs. But withdraw from where? That was the question that Kissinger had to answer while assuring Israeli officials that their nation's security would not be endangered by withdrawal.

In several rounds of exhausting "shuttle diplomacy," Kissinger flew between the Egyptian and Israeli capitals until his plane was known as the "Yo-Yo Express" because it was up and down so often. By the end of 1975, he had persuaded the Israelis to give up strategic passes and oil fields in the Sinai desert (located between Israel and Egypt). In return, Sadat promised to deal with Israel peacefully. It marked a historic breakthrough: the Israelis retreated from land gained by military conquest for the first time, and Egypt recognized Israel's right to exist. Kissinger also negotiated the Israelis' withdrawal from Syrian territory, although they remained in the strategic Golan Heights. The Syrians, with extensive Soviet aid, became the leading anti-Israeli power in the Middle East. Tensions soon rose as Kissinger failed to move Israel from its occupation of the West Bank of the Jordan River, where 1 million

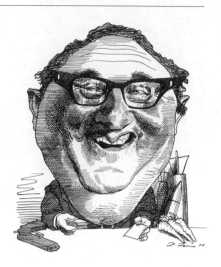

*David Levine caricatures the Henry
Kissinger of 1974 as a card dealer who
keeps both a gun and carrots in reserve.
At the time, the secretary of state was
trying to settle critical problems in the
Middle East, Africa, Southeast Asia,
and the North Atlantic alliance, even as
the Nixon administration collapsed.*

Palestinian Arabs lived. The Israelis had seized the land from Jordan
in their 1967 triumph. In 1968, the Palestine Liberation Organization
(PLO) was formed under the leadership of Yasir Arafat. The PLO was
dedicated to an Arab state in Palestine, which the Israelis interpreted
as meaning the destruction of their own homeland. In 1974, Arab states
recognized the PLO as the sole representative of the Palestinians. The
West Bank problem became a festering boil that soon infected internal
Israeli, as well as broader Middle Eastern, politics.

The Israelis had, nevertheless, gained much, including the U.S. pledge
to send billions of dollars each year in military aid and to protect their
security. But relations also warmed between Washington and Cairo,
where Sadat began receiving U.S. aid. Relations between Washington
and Moscow, however, grew worse by the day.

DÉTENTE'S TURNAROUND: THE ARAB OIL EMBARGO

For Americans, the most dramatic result of the Yom Kippur War of
1973 was a quick doubling, and then a near-doubling again, of the
price that they paid for gasoline and oil. Costs shot up, and inflation
soared as Arab oil producers cut back production in an effort to pressure Israel to meet their demands for a return to the pre-1967 boundaries. Because Washington was Israel's strongest supporter, the Arabs
tried to cut off oil completely to the United States.

In perspective, the oil embargo marked an important turn in U.S.
economic and diplomatic history. Resembling other such turns, it had

deep roots. Just twenty years before, in the early 1950s, Americans had produced at home all the oil they needed. By 1960, however, their booming factories and wasteful automobiles made them dependent on foreign sources for one of every six barrels of oil they used. By 1973, one of every three barrels they consumed came from abroad. Few worried. Supply seemed assured, and Arab or Venezuelan oil was cheaper then the U.S. product. But signs had appeared. In 1959–1960, the U.S.-dominated petroleum companies (the so-called "Seven Sisters") were awash in oil and tried to cut back prices paid to producers. Led by Venezuela, Iran, and Saudi Arabia, the producers formed OPEC (Organization of Petroleum Exporting Countries) in 1960 to restore higher prices. They failed to obtain more money. But one of OPEC's members, Libya, scored a breakthrough in 1970.

The year before, a group of young army officers, led by Mu'ammar al-Qadhafi, had overthrown the disorganized pro-U.S. Libyan monarchy. Qadhafi and his followers disliked U.S. military bases (although many of the men had been trained in the United States) and especially Western influences. (As Moslems, they condemned drinking, smoking, gambling, and prostitutes—all of which were known to appear around U.S. bases.) A major oil producer, Libya also had large cash reserves. Qadhafi knew that U.S. consumers, U.S. companies, and U.S. allies needed his petroleum. He succeeded in squeezing a higher price from the American companies pumping Libyan oil.[46] Thus, an OPEC member had forced the once all-powerful companies to pay producers higher prices.

When OPEC successfully enforced the embargo of 1973–1974, the

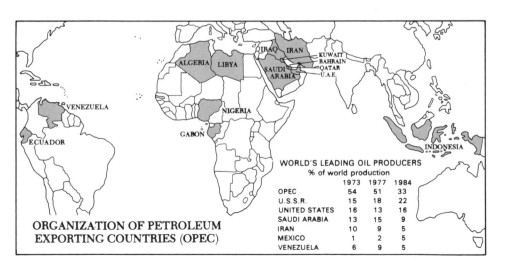

ORGANIZATION OF PETROLEUM EXPORTING COUNTRIES (OPEC)

WORLD'S LEADING OIL PRODUCERS
% of world production

	1973	1977	1984
OPEC	54	51	33
U.S.S.R.	15	18	22
UNITED STATES	16	13	16
SAUDI ARABIA	13	15	9
IRAN	10	9	5
MEXICO	1	2	5
VENEZUELA	6	9	5

West and Japan were, nevertheless, surprised and badly shaken. As a result, first, the United States appeared highly vulnerable—not to the pressures of the other superpower, but to the oil-producing machines of small Middle Eastern countries. Second, Nixon and Kissinger found some relief from the shah of Iran, who quietly shipped large amounts of oil to Americans. Since 1972, Nixon had depended on the shah to be the guardian of U.S. interests in the Persian Gulf region. Until the late 1960s, that guardian had been the British, but they had to pull back. Nixon then went to the shah in 1972 and simply pleaded, "Protect me."[47] The astonished shah was delighted to do so. He came through handsomely in the 1973 crisis but demanded several pounds of flesh in return, including much higher prices for his petroleum and massive U.S. arms shipments. Those shipments amounted to over $9 billion between 1973 and 1977. The Americans and the shah had become intimate allies.

Third, as enormous amounts of money moved to the Middle East producers, the West's bankers gladly moved in to help the producers invest these billions. Huge amounts were lent to oil consumers (Argentina, the Philippines, Peru, South Korea), to countries intent on rapid industrialization (Poland, Brazil), and even back to the oil producers themselves (Mexico, Venezuela). When the world economy slowed between 1975 and 1982, many of these nations were buried under an unpayable debt that threatened the world's financial system.

Finally, the oil crisis helped sink détente. The Soviets actually exported ten times more oil to the United States in 1973 than they had in 1972 (and, of course, charged top price). But they had also worked closely with the Egyptians, whose attack on Israel triggered the crisis. U.S. officials angrily believed that in the spirit of détente Brezhnev should at least have warned Washington about the attack. Nor did the U.S. move to a stage 3 nuclear alert improve relations. Détente could not prevent either superpower from acting in its own interest in the newly emerging world, whether the opportunity lay in Egypt or Chile.

DÉTENTE'S TURNAROUND: THE ALLIES AND A BAD "YEAR OF EUROPE"

Kissinger believed that during the 1973 crisis, the closest U.S. allies had acted like traitors. He deeply feared the western Europeans' warmer relations with the Soviets. The once-formidable NATO alliance, he later wrote, was so bogged down in disputes that it was merely "an acciden-

tal array of forces in search of a mission."[48] U.S. and European producers, especially farmers, tore into each other for alleged trade
discriminations. Kissinger knew that he and Nixon had ignored Europe
to follow their own agendas in Vietnam, Moscow, and Beijing (Peking).
So in mid-1973, he announced that it was to be "the year of Europe."
The historic relationship was to be restored. The western Europeans,
however, believed that little substance lay below his rhetoric. Since
1963–1965 (if not since the Suez fiasco of 1956), U.S. attention had
been diverted from the Atlantic and Japan, and toward the newly
emerging nations and the superpowers' concerns. As the president of
France sarcastically informed Nixon, "For Europeans every year is the
year of Europe."[49]

Then, during the 1973 Mideast crisis, Nixon asked the NATO allies
to make their military bases available to U.S. planes flying supplies to
Israel. All except Portugal refused. Even West Germany turned Nixon
down. The Europeans, who received 80 percent of their oil from the
Arab producers, and the Japanese, who received over 95 percent, openly
defied the president. In the most serious break in the post-1949 alliance system, these allies made their own deals to obtain Middle East
oil. "I don't care what happens to NATO," Kissinger reportedly blurted
out, "I'm so disgusted."[50] Anti-Tokyo feelings also rose as the ever-
efficient Japanese increased their exports to ever-eager U.S. buyers until
the trade balance in Japan's favor more than quadrupled between 1973
and 1977 to $8.1 billion.

The alliance's slide continued in 1974–1975, when the long-lived
dictatorships of Franco in Spain and Salazar in Portugal ended in death.
Strong Socialist and Communist factions appeared in both nations.
Kissinger, assuming the worst, concluded that without secret CIA help,
the two nations would swing toward Moscow. Western European moderates, led by Christian Socialists and Social Democrats, disagreed.
Believing the Spanish and Portuguese peoples capable of finding their
own way to democracy, the European leaders checked Kissinger's moves.
The Europeans were proven correct as moderates came into power in
both Spain and Portugal, although not without overcoming threats from
both the military right wing and the Communist factions. Kissinger
refused to raise his estimate of the allies: "All of Europe will be Marxist within a decade," he reportedly declared in 1976.[51]

Canada, neighbor and leading trading partner of the United States,
also turned bitter. In 1968, Pierre Trudeau became prime minister. A
playboy bachelor, Harvard-educated, wealthy, and athletic, he would
have been a perfect match for John Kennedy but was an ill-fit for Rich-

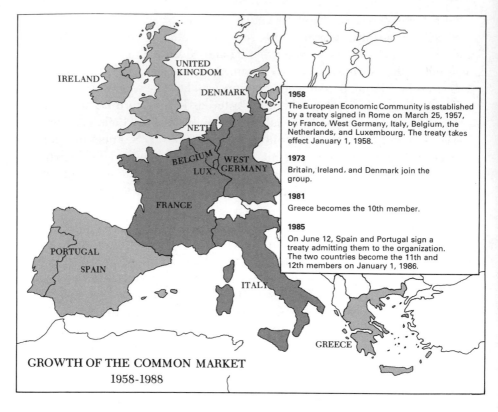

1958

The European Economic Community is established by a treaty signed in Rome on March 25, 1957, by France, West Germany, Italy, Belgium, the Netherlands, and Luxembourg. The treaty takes effect January 1, 1958.

1973

Britain, Ireland, and Denmark join the group.

1981

Greece becomes the 10th member.

1985

On June 12, Spain and Portugal sign a treaty admitting them to the organization. The two countries become the 11th and 12th members on January 1, 1986.

GROWTH OF THE COMMON MARKET
1958-1988

ard Nixon. Relations soured when Washington, without consulting Ottawa, set off a nuclear device in the Aleutian Islands that threatened to spread (but did not) a radioactive cloud over much of Canada. When the unattached Trudeau met Nixon, the president publicly greeted "the Prime Minister and his lovely wife." But nothing shook the relationship like Nixon's 1971 import tax. With 70 percent of their exports going to Americans, Canadians were hurt more severely than any other people by Nixon's actions. For its part, Canada had taken in thousands of American men who moved north to resist the military draft. Trudeau, faced with a difficult economy and a declining NATO, next cut back his nation's commitment to the military alliance.[52] By 1976, U.S.-Canadian relations approached a twentieth-century low.

DÉTENTE'S TURNAROUND: AFRICA

The Nixon-Kissinger view held that Africa, like the allies, had to play second fiddle to the more important U.S. relations with China and the

Soviet Union. Black Africa was so unimportant (and racism so strong in the Nixon White House) that at one point the president told Kissinger, "Henry, let's leave the niggers to Bill [Secretary of State William Rogers] and we'll take care of the rest of the world."[53] In 1970, this attitude was made policy in the National Security Council's secret paper, National Security Study Memorandum 39 (or NSSM 39). It declared that the United States should help the many new black African nations but place primary emphasis on relations with the white government of South Africa and the white colonial government of Portugal. This approach was labeled the "Tar-Baby option" by a State Department dissenter who believed (correctly) that it would stick Americans to a lost Portuguese cause.

South Africa's attractions were its highly effective military force, its rich holdings of minerals, its strong economy (where the rate of return on U.S. investment was above 17 percent annually), and its strategic location at the tip of Africa. These lures overcame U.S. qualms about South Africa's brutal apartheid policy under which 22-million blacks and 5 million other nonwhites were now forcefully segregated and discriminated against by 5 million ruling whites. Portugal's value was its bases in the eastern Atlantic, for which Washington paid nearly $500 million each year. The Portuguese spent the money trying to stop anticolonial wars in Angola, Mozambique (where a Marxist government soon came to power), and Guinea.[54]

Nixon and Kissinger had again bet on the wrong horse. By 1974, the Portuguese had lost the fight in the key nation, Angola. Some 170,000 whites could no longer rule 4.6 million blacks. The African nation became a case study of how local problems in emerging countries were turned into a global confrontation between the Americans and the Soviets. Three factions, all black, fought to rule the newly independent Angola. Agostinho Neto's MPLA had long received Soviet and Cuban aid. That aid, however, was reduced after 1972, and Neto vowed to protect the U.S.-owned Gulf Oil Company, which produced the revenues on which the economy rested. Opposed to Neto were the FNLA (supported by the United States and China) and Jonas Savimbi's UNITA (backed by South Africa). In early 1975, the three factions agreed to settle differences through an election. But since at least mid-1974, the CIA had bankrolled the FNLA; and now the FNLA, with secret U.S. support, destroyed the agreement by attacking the stronger MPLA. Kissinger later said that he had intended to show China how to be tough with Soviet-backed groups. But the Soviets and Cubans responded with 230 military advisers to help Neto, who seized power. The fighting

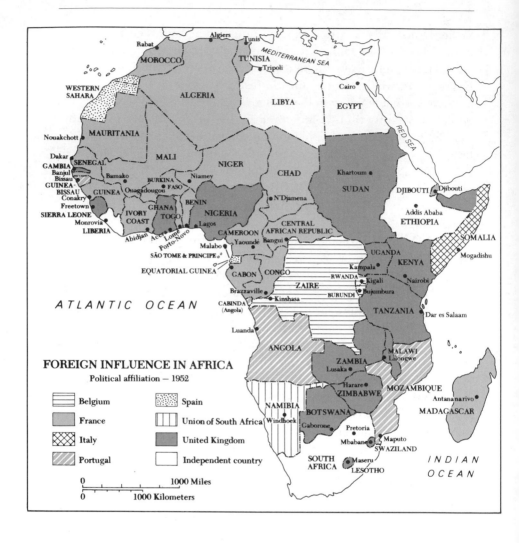

FOREIGN INFLUENCE IN AFRICA
Political affiliation — 1952

Belgium

France

Italy

Portugal

Spain

Union of South Africa

United Kingdom

Independent country

0   1000 Miles

0   1000 Kilometers

escalated until South African troops, CIA agents, and over 20,000 Cubans were involved. Some of the Cuban troops protected Gulf Oil property. The Chinese decided to make a quick escape from the entire mess.

Kissinger insisted that the United States had to respond to the Communists' escalation. Massive arms shipments flowed from both superpowers—Soviet aid to Angola, Uganda, and Somalia; American aid to Kenya, Zaire, and Ethiopia. Africa became a bloody arena for superpower confrontation and brutal wars. But there seemed to be little understanding of, or concern about, the local causes of the wars. In Ethiopia, for example, a radical regime came to power and, for its own domestic reasons, switched to the Soviet side in 1976 even though the United States had just delivered $100 million worth of advanced jet fighters. As in a game of musical chairs, Kissinger then clutched Ethiopia's enemy, Somalia, as a U.S. ally, although Somalia had just been supported by Moscow.[55]

The U.S. Congress was shocked. Vietnam had made it leery of Third-World wars. And, in 1974, it passed a law (the Hughes-Ryan Amendment) that tried to curb CIA activities. The agency obviously had paid little attention to the law during the Angolan affair. So Congress next passed the Clark Amendment, which prohibited U.S. military assistance to either side in Angola. Kissinger railed against the law, but Congress held fast. Since 1970, Kissinger and Nixon had chosen whites over blacks, a military policy over a negotiated settlement, and a focus on superpower rivalry over a focus on local conditions. Kissinger could no longer convince Congress that U.S. policy made sense. Unlike the Tar Baby of Uncle Remus's famous story, Congress seemed to be freeing itself from the Angolan (if not South African) Tar Baby. But because of African affairs, the superpowers had become more tightly locked into a new cold war.

Détente's Turnaround: The Last Days of the Vietnam War and Nixon's Imperial Presidency

"America's longest war," as historian George Herring calls the conflict in Vietnam, meanwhile ended with a series of bangs. The first and biggest bang went off in late 1972. After nearly three years of talks, Kissinger believed that he had an agreement with North Vietnam to end the conflict. "Peace is at hand," he announced in late October 1972. But the South Vietnamese government refused to accept the deal because it was afraid that the Communists would obtain even more power in the South. Nixon, in the last days of his re-election fight, deserted Kissinger's agreement so that it would not appear that he (Nixon) was deserting South Vietnam. When Kissinger returned to the talks after the election and demanded nearly seventy changes, the North Vietnamese refused.[56]

The president then decided to show his willingness to use force. He unleashed the heaviest bombing raids of the war. Nixon declared that he "did not care if the whole world thought he was crazy" dropping so many bombs, because "the Russians and the Chinese might think they were dealing with a madman and so [they] had better force North Viet-

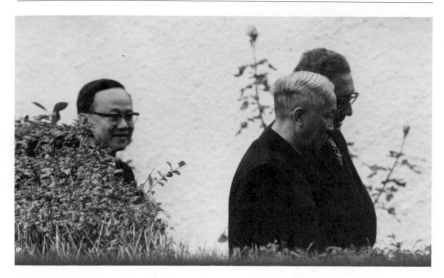

Henry Kissinger and North Vietnam's envoy, Le Duc Tho, walk together in Paris in February 1972 during their protracted talks to end the war. The two men shared the Nobel Peace Prize in 1973 for their efforts. But because the war continued, Le Duc Tho refused to accept his share of the prize.

nam into a settlement before the world was consumed in a larger war." Only 24 percent of Americans polled opposed this "madness." Congress did nothing to stop Nixon.[57]

In January 1973, Kissinger and the North Vietnamese finally reached an agreement. In the view of some experts, the settlement could have been obtained months—perhaps even years—earlier.[58] First, a cease-fire went into effect, and Nixon agreed to pull out all U.S. combat forces in sixty days. Meanwhile, the Communists were to withdraw from Laos and Cambodia. Second, all U.S. prisoners were to be released. Third—and of special importance—the United States recognized the "unity and territorial integrity of Vietnam," but South Vietnam's "right to self-determination" was also recognized by both sides. Finally, the pro-U.S. Thieu government was to remain in power pending an election in which Communists could participate. To obtain Thieu's acceptance this time, Nixon secretly told him that if the Communists violated the pact, "You can count on us" to protect the South.[59]

Congress was not told of Nixon's secret assurance, but that legislative body had long since quit trusting the president. In 1971, it had finally repealed the 1964 Gulf of Tonkin Resolution (see p. 606). In early 1973, the House and Senate forbade Nixon to bomb Indochina after July 1 of that year. In the War Powers Resolution of late 1973,

Congress passed a law that (1) asked the president to consult with Congress before committing troops to combat areas, and (2) required that if he did send troops, he must withdraw them within ninety days unless Congress expressly approved the commitment. Nixon angrily vetoed the act, but Congress passed it over his veto.

Congress had finally begun curbing the powers of King Richard. With the 1972 Watergate break-in and his attempt to cover up that criminal act, Nixon was personally guilty for the loss of his power. But the changing nature of the presidency went much deeper. Cold-war issues were developing less in the military arena (where the president as commander in chief can take the lead) and more in the economic arena (where the Constitution gives Congress greater control). The changing nature of the cold war produced a changing relationship between a once-all-powerful president in foreign policy and a now more active Congress. House and Senate attempts at limiting the CIA and military ventures in Africa also signaled this change.

Despite Nixon's pledge to Thieu, South Vietnam fell on April 30, 1975, twenty-one bloody years after Eisenhower had tied the United States to the anti-Communist regime. In March 1974, the last U.S. combat troops had left. In August 1974, Nixon, facing impeachment,

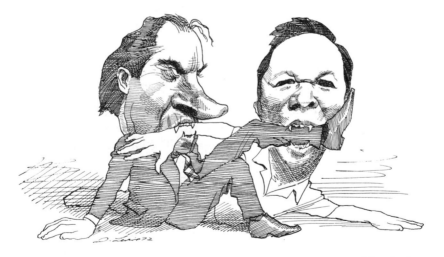

As David Levine illustrates in this cartoon, Nixon's most serious problem by late 1972 was no longer with the North Vietnamese (who had largely agreed to peace terms), but with his ally, Nguyen Van Thieu, leader of South Vietnam, who disliked the terms and forced Nixon to re-enter negotiations. The president finally stopped the biting and clawing by secretly guaranteeing Thieu in 1973 that the United States would use force, if necessary, to protect Thieu's regime under the peace agreement.

became the first U.S. president to resign his office. In October, North Vietnam's leaders concluded that even if the Americans re-entered the war, Thieu's government could not be saved. The Communists launched a major offensive in March 1975. They believed that a two-year war would follow. Instead, the South Vietnamese army, now left on its own, melted away. Kissinger and the new president, Gerald Ford, pleaded that Congress had a "moral obligation" to send $300 million more in military aid. Congress refused. It was afraid that the money would only be wasted or end up in Communist hands. Moreover, Congress knew that, according to CIA estimates, the Thieu regime had already received $3.3 billion in 1973–1974—as opposed to the North's $730 million from its Communist partners—but was no longer able to use aid effectively.[60] The Communists ended the war with the capture of Saigon, the South's capital (now renamed Ho Chi Minh City).

Kissinger blamed the Watergate scandal, congressional opposition, and the Communist breaking of the 1973 agreements as the reasons for the final collapse. "If we didn't have this damn domestic situation," he complained in 1973, "a week of bombing would put this Agreement in force."[61] But in quieter moments, Kissinger admitted that there was another reason for the North's triumph: "Because there were always more Vietnamese prepared to die for their country than foreigners, their nationalism became the scourge of invaders and neighbours alike."[62]

By the end, the costs of the civil war had become enormous. About 58,015 Americans died (more than half after 1968), and 150,303 more were wounded. Some groups suffered more than others. Hispanics, who made up 7 percent of the U.S. population, suffered 20 percent of the battle deaths. African Americans, with 11 percent of the population, also suffered 20 percent of the deaths. The largest number of U.S. deserters were minorities and blue-collar whites who knew little about Vietnam until they arrived there. The middle class, especially whites, used lawyers and college deferments to escape the war. On the other side, 2 million Vietnamese died. Twice that number were wounded. The U.S. government, moreover, had broken numerous laws during the conflict. Although the CIA charter forbids it from conducting covert activities within the United States, the agency (acting on presidential orders) infiltrated college student groups and other organizations suspected of not being sufficiently patriotic. By 1971, the CIA was opening nearly 8,000 private letters. In Operation Chaos, the agency kept secret computer files on 7,500 Americans (and indexes on 300,000 more),

---

Dear 'Smitty,

Perhaps, now I can bury you; at least in my soul. Perhaps, now, I won't again see you night after night when the war re-appears and we are once more amidst the myriad hells that Vietnam engulfed us in.

We crept 'point' together and we pulled 'drag' together. We lay crouched in cold mud and were drenched by monsoons. We sweated buckets and endured the heat of dry season. We burnt at least a thousand leeches off one another and went through a gallon of insect repellent a day that the bugs were irresistibly attracted to.

When you were hit, I was your medic all the way, and when I was blown 50 feet by the mortar, you were there first. When I was shaking with malaria, you wiped my brow.

We got tough, 'Smitty. We became hired guns, lean and mean and calloused. And after every ambush, every firefight, every "hot" chopper insertion you'd shake and get sick.

You got a bronze star, a silver star, survived 18 months of one demon hell after another, only to walk into a booby trapped bunker and all of a sudden you had no face or chest.

I never cried. My chest becomes unbearably painful and my throat tightens so I can't even croak, but I haven't cried. I wanted to, just couldn't.

I think I can, today. Damn, I'm crying now.

> 'Bye Smitty,
> Get some rest

A letter left by a Vietnam veteran at the Vietnam Veterans Memorial in Washington, D.C.

---

despite the CIA director's knowledge that it was illegal. These operations marked "a step toward the dangers of a domestic secret police," in the words of a Senate report.[63]

The war did produce a victor other than North Vietnam: the Soviet Union. Fearful of its ancient enemy China, North Vietnam turned increasingly to Moscow for help. By the late 1970s, the Soviet navy had taken over the strategic Vietnamese bases built in the 1960s by the United States. Moscow's power leapfrogged over much of Asia to become a presence in Southeast Asia, as well as to surround further with Red Army might the nervous Chinese. To obtain all this, the Soviets lost few lives and little money. "Somewhere in the world," a U.S. official groused in 1974, "there must be a school where foreign governments learn to con Americans."[64] The problem, however, lay much closer to home, where Americans were ignorant of their own and others' histories, and, consequently, ignorant of the limits of their own power.

DÉTENTE'S TURNAROUND:
THE FORD PRESIDENCY (1974–1977)

Gerald Ford had to pick up the tattered remnants of a failed foreign policy. A graduate of the University of Michigan, where he had been a star football player, Ford was a likable, unpretentious, ardent Republican who, without displaying excess talent, rose to the leadership of the House of Representatives. In mid-1973, Nixon tapped him to replace the disgraced Agnew as vice-president. One observer wrote that "few men are better qualified than Ford for a job that demands practically nothing of the man who holds it."[65] In August 1974, he suddenly became president. If the departing Nixon liked the movie *Patton*, Ford's favorite was the cotton-candy *That's Entertainment, Part 2*. When pressed to explain the declining U.S. economy, the new president declared, "Things are more like they are now than they've ever been."[66]

But the new chief executive also showed an openness, an ability to identify with the person on the street, that sharply separated him from Nixon. Americans had finally grown suspicious of power, even their own. That suspicion was made evident in the popularity of such movies between 1969 and 1976 as *Z*, *All the President's Men*, and *Three Days of the Condor*, which showed society's most powerful figures engaged in secret conspiracies (such as the Watergate scandal) to overturn democratic systems.[67] Ford's apparent innocence and directness restored some confidence in White House authority. His attempt to use that authority in foreign policy, however, produced few successes.

First, he and Kissinger made a last-ditch attempt to save South Vietnam in April 1975. When that try failed, Ford traveled to Hawaii and announced a Pacific Doctrine. Despite the tragedies in Vietnam, he declared, the United States remained a Pacific power. In a new variation of Frederick Jackson Turner's frontier thesis (see p. 185), the president declared, "The center of political power in the United States has shifted westward. Our Pacific interests and concerns have increased." He demanded an "equilibrium" of power to protect U.S. interests in the region. Ford focused on the growing American "commercial involvement" in Asia, thus acknowledging the rising commitment to Pacific rim markets. For the first time in four hundred years, U.S. economic interests in Asia were becoming larger than those in Europe. Yet Ford's doctrine also acknowledged that U.S. power was much less than it had been a generation earlier. Americans needed help from partners in Indonesia, Japan, and the Philippines.[68] That need had

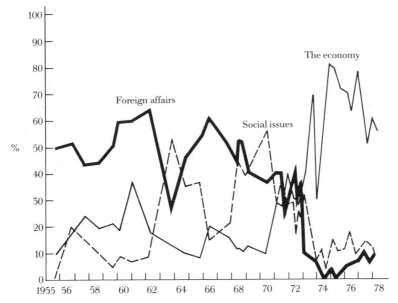

This graph from Public Opinion *(May / June 1978) illustrates what Americans considered to be their "most important problem facing the country today" (between 1955 and 1978). Note the sharp changes in 1964–1968, when the Vietnam War reached its peak, and then the increasing concern over the economy with the Arab oil embargo of 1974.*

been one reason why Nixon and Ford said nothing after Philippine ruler Ferdinand Marcos imposed a corrupt martial-law regime on his people in 1972. Of special importance, the economic relationship along the Pacific rim was being defined by Japanese efficiency, not by Americans.

Second, Ford and Secretary of State Kissinger made a major effort at reviving détente. They met with Brezhnev in the Soviets' Pacific coast city of Vladivostok during November 1974. Building on the last two Nixon-Brezhnev summits of 1973–1974, the Americans and Soviets agreed to place a ceiling on the number of strategic nuclear missiles and big bombers. A later meeting was to turn this general agreement into a treaty with specific numbers. In 1975, U.S. and Soviet astronauts worked together for the first time in a dramatic Apollo-Soyuz space flight. Later that year, thirty-five nations (led by the United States and the USSR) met at Helsinki, Finland, to make historic agreements in four areas (called "baskets"). One basket provided that force would not be used to change frontier boundaries, an agreement the Soviets had wanted to make with the United States since the Red Army redrew

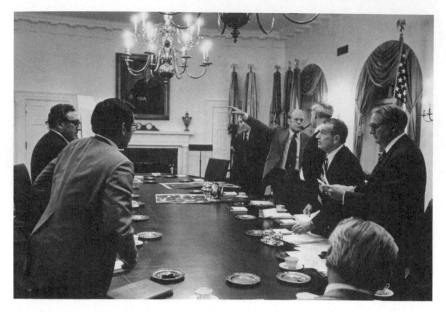

President Gerald Ford (1913–   ) points during a meeting held to discuss the Mayaguez *crisis in 1975. The president talks with Secretary of Defense James Schlesinger. Secretary of State Kissinger is at left.*

European boundaries between 1944 and 1948. In return, the Soviets had to agree to a basket that recognized the right of peoples to enjoy human freedoms, including the freedom to move across national borders. When, however, "Helsinki Watch" groups appeared in the Soviet Union to ensure that these rights would be respected, they were brutally beaten and imprisoned. The Helsinki baskets, which seemed to offer hope for détente, turned into another reason to believe that détente was dying, if not dead. As he ran for election in 1976, Ford outlawed the use of the word *détente* by his staff. Kissinger lamented that it "is a word I would like to forget."[69]

Third, Ford effectively revived the president's commander-in-chief power during a crisis in 1975. On May 12, Communist Cambodian vessels captured a U.S. freighter, the *Mayaguez*, and imprisoned its thirty-nine-member crew. Determined to show their muscle, Ford and Kissinger ordered the bombing of a Cambodian port, then dispatched troops to rescue the crew. Unknown to them, the Cambodians were already releasing the prisoners. An accidental explosion killed forty-one of the U.S. troops. Ford had, indeed, made his point: the Vietnam failure did not lessen U.S. willingness to use force. He did so, moreover, while refusing to recognize formally that Congress's 1973 War

Powers Act in any way limited his power to dispatch troops without consulting Congress. But Americans had paid a high and unnecessary price for the Ford-Kissinger adventure.

ADJUSTING TO A NEW WORLD

After an era of unequaled U.S. dominance in world affairs between 1945 and the 1960s, Americans began to discover the limits of their power. The unfavorable international trade balances of the late 1950s and early 1960s flashed a first sign. The Vietnam tragedy became the clearest indication that the tide had turned. Nixon and Kissinger faced the task of gently convincing Americans that the 1945-to-1960s years were unnatural. No people have ever taken readily to the idea that they had to give up power. Many Americans, whose ignorance of history especially left them unprepared to face such a challenge, not surprisingly refused to accept the realities of the new world.

Nixon failed in part because of the corruption, indeed crime, that undermined his presidency. Tapes on which he recorded White House conversations revealed a man who had no hobbies and no real friends except Miami businessman Bebe Rebozo, who would spend hours drinking with Nixon while feeding his ego and paranoia ("You're doing a great job," or "Your enemies are out to get you.") Two drinks could spin the president off into a slurred, sometimes reckless speech; once he simply fell asleep while in the middle of a phone conversation with a close aide. He covered insecurity with racism; in private conversation (but recorded on tape), Jews were "kikes" and blacks were "niggers," while the detested journalists were "press pricks." Believing himself surrounded by enemies, by 1973–1974 the president seemed to feel closer to the enemies in Moscow than the enemies in Washington. As for Kissinger, he had publicly warned that, in a democracy, obtaining public support was a statesman's "acid test." Historian Robert Beisner concludes that "Kissinger failed the 'acid test' . . . because he stepped outside the constraints imposed by the American political tradition without reshaping that tradition itself."[70] The same conclusion applies to Nixon.

These personal and political failures became especially disastrous for Nixon and Kissinger because through détente, they had planned to contain Soviet power, but at lower cost than in the past.[71] Détente, however, required that Americans no longer view the Soviets simply as evil aggressors, but as friendly enough to be negotiated with—but dangerous enough to be guarded against. After thirty years of a fierce cold war, this subtle policy turned out to be too much to ask from a society whose historic dealings with Indians, Mexicans, Spaniards, Chinese, and Russians had hardly been subtle. Nor was U.S. tolerance helped by Brezhnev's policies, which stressed détente with the United States, military support for "wars of liberation," and, at home, the exiling of dissenters to Siberian prisons.

Many Americans, disappointed with Nixon and détente, and tired of helping such ungrateful people as the western Europeans and Vietnamese, began to retreat to a position that critics termed "neo-isolationism." The respected conservative journalist Walter Lippmann gave his view of the problem: "Well, neo-isolationism is the direct product of foolish globalism. If you think you can run the world and then you find out you can't, you withdraw to what you can run." In 1975, the governor of Louisiana heard Kissinger describe how Americans were going to help developing countries around the world and retorted: "I hope we can do it for them a helluva lot better than we have been able to do it for ourselves, because we haven't done it in this country yet. And I think Americans and the world ought to come to grips with that reality."[72]

It was not unlike the late 1920s, when a postwar world structure, carefully constructed under U.S. guidance, rested on American economic power. When that power buckled, the structure began to collapse. Nixon and Kissinger had worked to prop up the structure, but the foundations—the U.S. economy and their domestic support—crumbled under their touch. It was now left for Jimmy Carter and Ronald Reagan to design fresh policies for this different world or to try to go *Back to the Future* (as a popular film of the 1980s was entitled) in an attempt to retrieve the lost American power of the 1950s.

NOTES

1. Garry Wills, *Nixon Agonistes* (Boston, 1970), p. 160.
2. Lawrence Martin, *The Presidents and the Prime Ministers* (Toronto, 1982), p. 259.
3. Ralph H. Wolfe quoting Ted Sennett in "Review Essay," *Journal of Popular Film and Television* 12 (Summer 1984): 89.
4. Interview of Richard Nixon, *Washington Star*, 10 November 1972, p. 1.
5. Garry Wills, *Reagan's America* (New York, 1987), p. 344.
6. Seymour Hersh, *The Price of Power* (New York, 1983), p. 40.

7. Dobrynin's 1969 report is in *New York Times*, 8 February 1993, p. A8. *New York Times*, 31 May 1987, p. 24; *ibid.*, 26 January 1974, p. 19; Theodore Draper, "Kissinger's Apologia," *Dissent* 27 (Spring 1980): 253.

8. Henry A. Kissinger, *A World Restored: Castlereagh, Metternich, and the Problems of Peace, 1812–1822* (London and New York, 1957, 1964), pp. 326–330.

9. *New York Times*, 6 July 1970, p. 2.

10. Henry A. Kissinger, *American Foreign Policy*, exp. ed. (New York, 1974), pp. 182–183.

11. Richard M. Nixon, "Asia after Vietnam," *Foreign Affairs* 46 (October 1967): 111–125; Wills, *Nixon Agonistes*, pp. 20–21.

12. Kissinger, *American Foreign Policy*, p. 57; J. L. S. Girling, " 'Kissingerism': The Enduring Problems," *International Affairs* 51 (July 1975): 325n; the justice-versus-disorder reference is in John G. Stoessinger, *Henry Kissinger: The Anguish of Power* (New York, 1976), pp. 12–14.

13. Martin, p. 241.

14. Henry Kissinger, *White House Years* (Boston, 1979), p. 235; Hersh, pp. 50–51; Theodore Draper, *Present History* (New York, 1983), p. 153.

15. The Kissinger quote is in Kissinger, *White House Years*, pp. 227–228; Douglas Brinkley, *Dean Acheson: The Cold War Years, 1953–1971* (New Haven, 1992), p. 269; J. William Fulbright, *The Crippled Giant* (New York, 1972), p. 74.

16. Hersh, p. 130; Kissinger, *White House Years*, p. 441.

17. Garry Clifford, "Present before and after the Creation," *SHAFR Newsletter* 16 (March 1985): 2–3.

18. The best account is William Shawcross, *Sideshow: Kissinger, Nixon, and the Destruction of Cambodia* (New York, 1979), esp. pp. 128–160.

19. Jonathan Schell, *The Time of Illusion* (New York, 1976), pp. 100–101.

20. Leonard Silk, *Nixonomics* (New York, 1972), p. 144.

21. Draper, "Kissinger's Apologia," 248.

22. Lloyd C. Gardner, *The Great Nixon Turnaround: America's New Foreign Policy in the Post-Liberal Era (How a Cold Warrior Climbed Clean Out of His Skin)* (New York, 1973).

23. *Washington Post*, 28 February 1971, p. B3.

24. *Wall Street Journal*, 17 November 1986, p. 17.

25. *Department of State Bulletin*, 5 November 1973, p. 555.

26. Alan K. Henrikson, "America's Changing Place in the World: From 'Periphery' to 'Centre,' " in *Centre and Periphery: Spatial Variation in Politics*, ed. Jean Gottmann (Beverly Hills, Calif., 1980), p. 92. Nixon's five-bloc speech is in U.S. Government, *Public Papers of the Presidents of the United States: Richard Nixon, 1971* (Washington, D.C., 1972), pp. 805–813.

27. Quoted by Frederick Adams in "Why Certain Ideas Count," *Reviews in American History* 11 (September 1983): 440.

28. Leonard A. Kusnitz, *Public Opinion and Foreign Policy: America's China Policy, 1949–1979* (Westport, Conn., 1984), p. 138.

29. A good succinct background, including the Malik quote, is in Gordon H. Chang, *Friends and Enemies* (Stanford, 1990), esp. p. 285. The text of the communiqué and Kissinger's press conference are in *New York Times*, 28 February 1972, p. 16.

30. André Malraux, quoted in C. L. Sulzberger, *The World and Richard Nixon* (New York, 1987), p. 7.

31. *Washington Post*, 1 June 1972, p. F2.
32. *Los Angeles Times*, 25 January 1993, p. A4; Carl Bernstein and Bob Woodward, *All the President's Men* (New York, 1974), pp. 265–266.
33. Sulzberger, pp. 199–200. A superb overview of these agreements and the talks leading to them is U.S. Congress, Senate Committee on Foreign Affairs, 96th Cong., 1st sess., 1979, *Special Studies Series on Foreign Affairs Issues*, Vol. I: *Soviet Diplomacy and Negotiating Behavior: Emerging New Context for U.S. Diplomacy* (Washington, 1979), pp. 444–491. This study was prepared by Dr. Joseph G. Whelan of the Congressional Research Service.
34. Kissinger, *White House Years*, p. 1250.
35. *New York Times*, 23 December 1974, p. 16.
36. *Department of State Bulletin*, 1 March 1976, p. 269.
37. Norman Mailer, *St. George and the Godfather* (New York, 1972), p. 119. The term "détente" comes from the Latin *tendere*, meaning "to stretch," by way of the Old French *destente*, which was a device that held and then released the tensed string of cross-bows. When bows gave way to guns, *détente* became the modern French word for "trigger." In both French and English, it came to signify a relaxation of tension. (*New York Times*, 28 June 1974, p. 2.)
38. Interview of Henry Kissinger in *U.S. News & World Report*, 15 March 1976, p. 28.
39. Kissinger, *White House Years*, pp. 653–654.
40. *Ibid.*, p. 673.
41. Hersh, pp. 275–276.
42. Nathaniel Davis, *The Last Two Years of Salvador Allende* (Ithaca, N.Y., 1985), pp. 278–306.
43. Kissinger, *White House Years*, p. 673; Hersh, pp. 260, 267–269 (on Kendall and Geneen); Roger Morris, *Uncertain Greatness* (New York, 1977), pp. 240–241.
44. Stephen Prince, *Visions of Empire* (New York, 1992), pp. 90–93.
45. Scott D. Sagan, "Lessons of the Yom Kippur Alert," *Foreign Policy* no. 36 (Fall 1979): 160–174.
46. Carl Solberg, *Oil Power* (New York, 1976), pp. 203–204; James E. Akins, "The Oil Crisis: This Time the Wolf Is Here," *Foreign Affairs*, 51 (April 1973): 462–465, 470–472.
47. Gary Sick, *All Fall Down: America's Tragic Encounter with Iran* (New York, 1985), pp. 16–17.
48. Draper, *Present History*, p. 81.
49. Richard J. Barnet, *The Alliance: America-Europe-Japan, Makers of the Postwar World* (New York, 1983), p. 320.
50. *Ibid.*, pp. 324, 328; *Washington Post*, 27 October 1973, p. A7.
51. Quoted by Flora Lewis in the *New York Times*, 16 February 1976, p. 1.
52. Martin, pp. 236–237, 242–243.
53. Hersh, p. 111.
54. *The Kissinger Study of Southern Africa/NSSM 39/(SECRET)*, ed. Mohamed A. El-Khawas and Barry Cohen (Westport, Conn., 1976), esp. pp. 19–54, 86–100.
55. The superb analysis is John A. Marcum's *The Angolan Revolution*, Vol. II: *Exile Politics and Guerrilla Warfare (1962–1976)* (Cambridge, Mass., 1978); and for a fine, succinct analysis by a leading expert on the region, see Gerald J. Bender, "Angola, a Story of Stupidity," *New York Review of Books*, 21 December 1978, pp. 26–36.
56. *Vietnam: A History in Documents*, ed. Gareth Porter (New York, 1979, 1981), pp.

419–420; George Herring, *America's Longest War: The United States and Vietnam, 1950–1975*, 2d. ed. (New York, 1986), esp. pp. 250–256.

57. Barry B. Hughes, *The Domestic Context of American Foreign Policy* (San Francisco, 1978), p. 39; the Nixon quote is in Thomas L. Hughes, "Foreign Policy: Men or Measures?" *Atlantic Monthly* 234 (October 1974): 56.

58. Leslie Gelb, "The Kissinger Legacy," *New York Times Magazine*, 31 October 1976, pp. 82–83; the terms are outlined in the *New York Times*, 28 January 1973, p. E1.

59. *Washington Post*, 7 January 1979, p. A25.

60. *Vietnam: A History in Documents*, p. 445.

61. Henry Kissinger, *Years of Upheaval* (Boston, 1982), pp. 302, 318–319, 326, 338.

62. *Ibid.*, p. 12.

63. *New York Times*, 19 May 1976, p. 14; Lyman B. Kirkpatrick, Jr., "Intelligence and Counterintelligence," in *Encyclopedia of American Foreign Policy*, ed. Alexander DeConde, 3 vols. (New York, 1978), I, pp. 426–427; casualties suffered by minority groups are analyzed in comments by Frank Walker and Ruben Treviso in *Vietnam Reconsidered: Lessons from a War*, ed. Harrison E. Salisbury (New York, 1984), esp. pp. 184, 206.

64. *Washington Post*, 28 July 1974, p. A7.

65. Richard Rovere in the *New Yorker*, 3 December 1973, p. 173.

66. Mark Green, "Presidential Truth and Consequence," *Nation*, 29 October 1983, p. 385; on the film preferences, see the *Washington Post*, 29 August 1976, p. E3.

67. Richard Dorfman, "Conspiracy City," *Journal of Popular Film and Television* 7, no. 4 (1980): 436–437.

68. *Department of State Bulletin*, 29 December 1975, p. 914.

69. *Ibid.*, 1 December 1975, p. 767; Richard W. Stevenson, *Rise and Fall of Détente* (Urbana, Ill., 1985), p. 172.

70. Robert Beisner, "History and Henry Kissinger," *Diplomatic History* 14 (Fall 1990), p. 526; Seymour Hersh, "Nixon's Last Coverup: The Tapes He Wants the Archives to Suppress," *The New Yorker*, 14 December 1992, pp. 93–94.

71. *Department of State Bulletin*, 12 May 1975, p. 609.

72. *Washington Post*, 10 October 1971, p. C5; *Department of State Bulletin*, 6 October 1975, p. 522; two useful French views on the U.S. problems are Michel Tatu, *Eux et nous: Les relations est-ouest entre deux détentes* (Paris, 1985), by a distinguished journalist, and Denise Artaud, *La Fin de l'inocence: Les États-Unis de Wilson à Reagan* (Paris, 1985), which provides the larger framework.

For Further Reading

For specific topics, also consult the notes of this chapter and the General Bibliography at the end of the book. For sources published before 1981, use *Guide to American Foreign Relations since 1700*, ed. Richard Dean Burns (1983), whose exhaustive annotated lists of reading cannot be matched by any text and makes possible noting mostly post-1981 publications below. References listed in the notes usually are not repeated here.

For general analyses of the Nixon years, Kissinger's two volumes of memoirs and

Seymour Hersh's detailed critique of Kissinger's policies (all listed in the notes) can be supplemented with Richard Nixon, *RN: The Memoirs of Richard Nixon* (1978); Stephen E. Ambrose, *Nixon*, 3 vols. (1987–1992); Walter Isaacson, *Kissinger* (1992), which is the most detailed biography; Franz Schurmann, *The Foreign Politics of Richard Nixon: The Grand Design* (1987), focusing on Nixon himself and critical of his Third-World policies; Harvey Starr, *Henry Kissinger: Perceptions of International Politics* (1984); Robert D. Schulzinger, *Henry Kissinger* (1989), a fine study; David P. Calleo, *The Imperious Economy* (1982), which remains the best critical overview of the post-1960 economic policies; John S. Odell, *U.S. International Monetary Policy: Markets, Power, and Ideas as Sources of Change* (1982), stressing post-1965 years; and Terry L. Deibel, *Presidents, Public Opinion and Power: The Nixon, Carter, and Reagan Years* (1987), a helpful brief account.

On Soviet relations, the place to begin is Raymond L. Garthoff's detailed *Détente and Confrontation* (1985); Alexander L. George et al., *Managing U.S.-Soviet Rivalry: Problems of Crisis Prevention* (1982), with excellent essays (especially George Breslauer's on détente); Richard Pipes, *U.S.-Soviet Relations in the Era of Détente* (1981), a conservative, critical argument; Robert S. Litwak, *Détente and the Nixon Doctrine* (1984), a more balanced analysis; Robert C. Gray and Stanley J. Michalak, Jr., *American Foreign Policy since Détente* (1984), a series of essays, especially useful on the world economic context; Philip J. Fungiello, *American-Soviet Trade in the Cold War* (1988); Gerard Smith, *Doubletalk: The Story of SALT I* (1985), by the U.S. negotiator of SALT I, who is highly critical of Kissinger; Paul B. Stares, *The Militarization of Space: U.S. Policy, 1945–1984* (1985), by far the best on the subject; Philip Hanson, *Trade and Technology in Soviet-Western Relations* (1981), which can be used with *The Politics of East-West Trade*, ed. Gordon B. Smith (1984), good on technology and agriculture. For Soviet policy and motivations, along with Garthoff, noted above, start with Jonathan Steele, *Soviet Power: The Kremlin's Foreign Policy—Brezhnev to Andropov* (1983), a superb survey; Harry Gelman, *The Brezhnev Politburo and the Decline of Détente* (1984); Adam Ulam, *Dangerous Relations: The Soviet Union in World Politics, 1970–1982* (1983), readable and critical; *Soviet Decisionmaking for National Security*, ed. Jiri Valenta and William C. Potter (1984), especially Garthoff's essay on SALT and Golan's on the 1973 war; and Galia Golan, *Soviet Policies in the Middle East* (1990).

For Asian affairs, a brief, suggestive essay by a professional diplomat is Leslie H. Brown, *American Security Policy in Asia*, Adelphi Papers No. 132 (1977), focusing on the Nixon Doctrine; Robert G. Sutter, *The China Quandary: Domestic Determinants of U.S. China Policy, 1972–1982* (1983), based on over one hundred interviews of officials; David Shambaugh *Beautiful Imperialist: China Perceives America, 1972–1990* (1991); *Soviet Policy in East Asia*, ed. Donald S. Zagoria (1984); Thomas R. H. Havens, *Fire across the Sea: The Vietnam War and Japan, 1965–1975* (1987), a first-rate study on Japan's turn, and also its anti-war movement; I. M. Destler, Haruhiro Fukui, Hideo Sato, *The Textile Wrangle: Conflict in Japanese-American Relations, 1969–1971* (1979), excellent on perhaps the pivotal event; Kunio Muraoka, *Japanese Security and the United States*, Adelphi Papers No. 195 (1973), a Japanese diplomat's view of the Nixon 1971 shocks.

On Vietnam, Gabriel Kolko's *Anatomy of a War* (1985) is a richly researched book on the entire post-1945 era; Harry G. Summers, Jr., *On Strategy: The Vietnam War in Context* (1981), one of the more widely discussed critiques of U.S. military policy; Timothy J. Lomperis, *The War Everyone Lost—and Won* (1984), viewing the war as both revolution and conventional war; Ole Holsti and James R. Roseneau, *American Leadership in World Affairs: Vietnam and the Breakdown of Consensus* (1984), much quantitative evidence to provide the context; John Hellmann, *American Myth and the Legacy of Vietnam* (1986), on U.S. self-image in novels, films, and memoirs; Nguyen Tien Hung and Jerrold Schecter, *The Palace File* (1986), important for the Nixon-Thieu correspondence; Truong Nhu Tang with David Chanoff and Doan Van Toai, *A Vietcong Memoir* (1985), by a North Vietnam insider; Melvin Small, *Johnson, Nixon, and the Doves* (1988), quantitative evidence on the anti-war movement's influence; and Anthony Campagna, *The Economic Consequences of the Vietnam War* (1991).

Other specific topics and areas are analyzed in the following accounts. On Latin America, Stephen G. Rabe, *The Road to OPEC: U.S. Relations with Venezuela, 1919–1976* (1982), is standard on U.S.-Venezuela, most helpful on OPEC's rise; James E. Petras and Morris Morley's *The United States and Chile* (1975) remains a most powerful critical account; Seymour Hersh's *The Price of Power,* listed in the notes, which is detailed in condemning the Kissinger approach to Chile; William F. Sater, *Chile and the United States* (1990), for an overview; and John Dinges and Saul Landau, *Assassination on Embassy Row* (1980), the best account of the Letelier assassination and the Chilean government's (and some Americans') complicity in the event. On Canada, Charles F. Doran, *Forgotten Partnership: U.S.-Canada Relations Today* (1984), key on the oil-gas question; William Diebold, "Canada and the United States: Twenty-five Years of Economic Relations," *International Journal* 39 (Spring 1984). On the Middle East, see William R. Polk, *The Arab World,* 2nd ed. (1991), an overview with a useful bibliography; Seth P. Tillman, *The United States in the Middle East* (1982), an authoritative, critical analysis, especially good on Arab relations; Daniel Yergin, *The Prize* (1991), on the U.S., oil, and the Middle East; Steven L. Spiegel, *The Other Arab-Israeli Conflict* (1985), emphasizing U.S. domestic ideas and background; James W. Harper, "The Middle East, Oil, and the Third World," in *Modern American Diplomacy,* ed. John M. Carroll and George C. Herring (1986); Noam Chomsky, *The Fateful Triangle: The U.S., Israel, and the Palestinians* (1984), a provocative critique of U.S. policy toward the Palestinians. The *Mayagüez* crisis is analyzed in Richard G. Head, Frisco W. Short, and Robert G. McFarlane, *Crisis Resolution* (1978). On Africa, two good (and critical) overviews are Henry Jackson's *From the Congo to Soweto: U.S. Foreign Policy toward Africa since 1960* (1982) and Ali A. Mazrui's *Africa's International Relations* (1977).

The best overall view of the Ford presidency can be found in the Schulzinger, Korb, and Finger essays in *Gerald R. Ford and the Politics of Post-Watergate America,* 2 vols, ed. Bernard J. Firestone and Alexej Ugrinsky (1993).

19

Back to the Future:
The Carter-Reagan Years (1977–1988)

JIMMY CARTER: THE SEARCH FOR A FOREIGN-POLICY
CONSENSUS

By 1976, Americans had learned firsthand every day how their power
had relatively declined since the 1950s. They could do little about having to pay Arab sheiks and other foreign producers four times more for
gasoline. U.S. prices doubled between 1968 and 1978, not only driving
up the cost of their groceries, but making their goods less competitive
in the tough global marketplaces. Thousands of American workers faced
unemployment in such old "rust belt" industries as steel and autos.
Their nuclear forces continued to be superior to the Soviets, but Brezhnev was closing the gap, and, in any case, gaps meant little when a
nuclear exchange could trigger nearly 50,000 warheads. Traditional
cold-war alliances with western Europe and Japan were tattered. Many
African and Latin American countries moved toward revolution. The
strong and respected (if not always liked) presidency of Truman and
Eisenhower collapsed into Nixon's forced resignation and Ford's confusion.

To reverse such a flow of history was like trying to change the flow
of a great river. Jimmy Carter, who had been educated at the U.S.
Naval Academy as an engineer, believed he could do it. After all, few
had thought this little-known former governor of Georgia could win

the White House. When he had told his mother that he was going to run for president, even she asked, "President of what?"[1] With brilliant organization, dogged work, and the message that he, as a Washington outsider, could best clean up the mess in the Capital, the Georgian had won it all. Carter was helped by Republican nominee Ford's major errors (in one televised debate, Ford even made the astounding remark that "no Soviet domination" of Poland existed), but the Georgian also made his share of mistakes. Perhaps the best known occurred when this born-again Baptist tried to win *Playboy* readers by telling the magazine that "I've committed adultery in my heart many times."[2] After losing a lead of thirty points in early public-opinion polls, Carter won by attacking Republican economic policy and by riding on the coattails of Democratic candidates running for the House and Senate.

Thus, from the start, the new president found himself in a weak position. Members of Congress owed him little. He had, moreover, run against the Washington power blocs. Now he found that he had to work with those blocs. He also discovered that the Democratic party was of little help. No "party loyalty or discipline" existed, Carter later wrote. "It was every member for himself, and the devil take the hindmost."[3] It was partly his own fault. His campaign had been too "Jimmyist" and not enough "Democratic," as one observer noted. But the president's dilemma also came from a long decline in political-party institutions—and their replacement by special-interest-group politics—that posed special dangers. In 1977, some political scientists grew so concerned that they held a rally at Washington's Jefferson Memorial and warned: "Our political party system, first inspired by Thomas Jefferson, is in serious danger of destruction. Without parties, there can be no organized and coherent politics. When politics lacks coherence, there can be no accountable democracy."[4]

Carter had won the election but now found that he had trouble governing effectively. The new president tried to help solve this dilemma by appointing as his top foreign-policy advisers two respected members of the New York–Washington "establishment." Cyrus Vance became secretary of state. A New York City lawyer, Vance had served with distinction at sub-cabinet positions in earlier Democratic administrations. A low-keyed, colorless, intelligent, and experienced diplomat, he concluded that the Nixon-Kissinger détente policy had collapsed because, by focusing so much on the Soviet Union and China, that policy had failed to understand, in Vance's words, "the explosive forces of change in the developing world." Problems in that world, he stressed, had to be dealt with "on their own terms and not through the prism of East-

West competition."[5] Vance had learned this the hard way: he had been involved in making Vietnam policy during the 1960s, when U.S. officials thought that they were dealing with Chinese or Soviet expansionism but were really facing Vietnamese nationalism. As far as the Kremlin was concerned, Vance emphasized arms control. Although human rights and economic relations were important, reducing nuclear arsenals was "a life or death" issue, in his words. It had to be handled by itself, not "linked," as many Americans wanted, to Soviet good behavior on human-rights questions or Third-World issues.

Carter named another New Yorker, Zbigniew Brzezinski of Columbia University, as the National Security Council director. The two had known each other since 1973, when Brzezinski and New York banker David Rockefeller set up the Trilateral Commission, a private group of American, western European, and Japanese businesspeople, officials, and academicians who, Rockefeller hoped, could coordinate the capitalist world's policies in the face of the newly emerging nations' challenges. Carter was brought into the commission as a representative southerner and soon considered Brzezinski "my teacher" in foreign policy.

Brzezinski differed with Vance over two key points. First, unlike the reserved secretary of state, the NSC director was brash, colorful, and happy to talk with reporters—much to the displeasure of Vance, who believed that he (Vance) should be the president's sole foreign-policy voice. Second, Brzezinski's gut response to foreign-policy difficulties often was to blame the Soviets. The son of a prewar Polish diplomat, his family had little love for Russians. He believed that the Soviet system was doomed to stagnation and was afraid that Kremlin leaders would try to save themselves through adventurism and expansion abroad. When problems erupted in Africa or Asia, therefore, he (unlike Vance) saw Moscow's hand at work and often urged direct military responses. Brzezinski became highly infatuated with China and the possibility of using the "China card" against the Soviets.[6] Vance thought this a bad bet. He already had suffered through one disaster in the 1960s, when Americans tried to pit Asians against Soviets.

JIMMY CARTER: THE SEARCH FOR A FOREIGN POLICY

As the final decision maker, Carter had placed himself between two men with quite different foreign-policy views. The president had little experience in overseas questions. He tried to decide policy through incredibly hard work (Brzezinski noted with amazement how Carter would turn a short briefing into an intense seven-hour session) and by mastering every detail. One experienced Washington observer believed that "Carter's an engineering officer" and, thus, has "to know how every single engine or pump works. . . . He looks upon government as machinery to be improved, to be lubricated."[7] This implied that Carter had no larger framework, no set of fundamental beliefs (such as Nixon's détente or Acheson's "positions-of-strength") that he could use to make decisions. He lacked "a historical memory," one official noted, that was needed to judge. Carter realized this weakness. In 1979, he told a reporter that he had read more history since becoming president than in all his earlier life.[8] But by then, it was too late.

As a result, he seemed to go in many directions at once. In the 1976 campaign, he condemned Kissinger as a "Lone Ranger" who acted without regard for Congress or allies. But Carter also consulted with few in Washington and handled western European and Japanese problems so inconsistently that the alliances were gravely weakened. He pledged to reduce expensive U.S. commitments to such peripheral (and increasingly wealthy) areas as South Korea; but after pulling out 6,000 troops, he reversed course and reaffirmed the commitment to South Korea. He promised to cut defense spending by $5 billion to $7 billion; but after six months in office, he moved to increase it. In a remarkable speech at the University of Notre Dame in 1977, Carter memorably said: "Being confident of our own future, we are now free of that inordinate fear of Communism which once led us to embrace any dictator who joined us in that fear." He asked instead that U.S. policies stress human-rights, environmental, and development issues, not simple anticommunism. Within twenty-four months, his own policy increasingly revolved around anticommunism. A veteran journalist wrote as early as February 1977 that Carter acted less like the captain of a ship of state than like a "frantic . . . white-water canoeist."[9]

The president tried to make his policies more coherent in two ways. First, he toyed with the Trilateral Commission approach. Besides Brzezinski and Vance, the president employed twenty other members (or nearly one-third of the entire U.S. membership on the commission) in his administration. After the trauma of Vietnam, Carter hoped that trilateralism would restore the confidence of American leaders and renew cooperation within the Western-Japanese capitalist community. But trilateralism proved an empty dream. As U.S. officials condemned Japan's huge $12 billion trade surplus with the United States, the Japanese belittled the Americans' refusal to save and make their economy

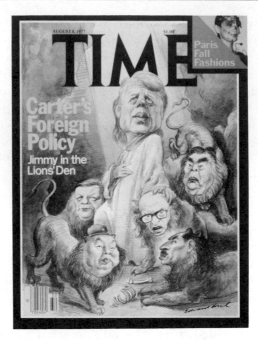

Time *magazine's cover of August 8, 1977, catches Jimmy Carter's early—and many—foreign-policy dilemmas. Clockwise from the lower left, the "lions" surrounding the pious Carter are Mao Zedong of China, Helmut Schmidt of West Germany, Leonid Brezhnev of the Soviet Union, Menachem Begin of Israel, and Anwar el-Sadat of Egypt. Note that some of the "lions" are eying each other (not Carter) for attack.*

more competitive. Some Americans responded by slitting tires on Japanese-made automobiles or by reverting to World War II racism in calling them "those little Yellow people," to use the words of one Michigan congressman. When the Japanese and West Germans most reluctantly agreed to try to help the sliding U.S. economy in 1977, the operation was termed Coordinated Reflation Action Program (or, appropriately, CRAP) and utterly failed. Each nation's domestic pressure groups prevented such international teamwork. West German chancellor Helmut Schmidt bluntly declared that the Americans had given up their economic leadership in the early 1970s, and he saw no one in New York or Washington "training for the job." Carter recorded privately that in a "bitter" discussion of economic issues, Schmidt "got personally abusive toward me."[10]

Trilateralism also came apart in the Middle East, where the United States tried to take a tough line against Arab oil producers and anti-Israeli forces. The Europeans and Japanese—who had great need for oil but had no Jewish political pressure groups at home—refused to follow Washington's line. Trilateralism collapsed as well in the handling of East-West issues. Carter dealt with Brezhnev bilaterally, using increasingly tough economic sanctions against the Soviets. The western Europeans, however, grew deathly afraid whenever Russians and Americans began talking alone behind closed doors. But both Europeans and Japanese continued their profitable trade with Moscow and refused to cut off the new financial arrangements (especially those for developing oil and gas fields) that they made with the Soviet bloc.

Most significantly, Americans and Europeans wrangled over nuclear defense. Since the 1950s, the Soviets, who could not hit the United States with precision, had aimed nuclear missiles at Europe to hold it hostage against a possible U.S. attack on the Soviet Union. Americans promised to defend Europe with U.S.-based missiles and, after 1962, with small "tactical" nuclear weapons in Europe itself. As Brezhnev's military closed the nuclear gap, however, western Europeans grew uneasy—especially West Germany, which was banned from having its own nuclear weapons. They were no longer certain that a U.S. president would defend Hamburg if it meant the obliteration of Chicago. Their unease grew in the mid-1970s, when Moscow began deploying 180 mobile, more precise SS-20 missiles, each with three independently targeted warheads aimed at Europe. Pressured at home and personally disdainful of Carter ("who knows everything and understands nothing"), Chancellor Schmidt warned that European security was being undermined.

Carter responded in part by announcing that he would develop a neutron bomb. It could counter a Soviet conventional attack by killing people with radiation but not destroying property. A top German official called the bomb a "symbol of mental perversion," but Schmidt reluctantly promised to support Carter. The president then changed his mind and ditched the neutron bomb, apparently for moral reasons. Schmidt was furious. So were Washington hawks such as the Committee on the Present Danger, led by Paul Nitze, who warned that Carter's indecisiveness was giving the Soviets a nuclear advantage. The president then promised to install 572 Pershing II and ground-based cruise missiles in Europe to counter the SS-20s. These missiles had little effect on the military balance. The United States already had 7,000 tactical nuclear weapons in Europe; Carter made the commitment for political reasons—and especially to appease Schmidt. Massive antinuclear protests erupted in Europe in 1980–1981. To blunt the protests, Carter and other Western leaders announced that they would install the Pershing IIs but also open talks with the Soviets in the hope that the intermediate weapons on both sides would be mutually withdrawn. The withdrawal would not occur for a decade.

Long before, in early 1978, one U.S. official announced the obvious: "The trilateral idea is dead."[11] At its postwar low in 1973–1974, the Western alliance had sunk even lower by 1981.

Carter also attempted to give coherence to his foreign policies by declaring in his inaugural address that he had an "absolute" commitment to human rights. The president condemned the U.S. policy that supported "right-wing monarchs and military dictators" as long as they were anticommunist. (He doubtless had in mind Kissinger's backing of Chile's military rule and Africa's conservative white-minority governments.) By stressing "moral principles," he believed that repressive governments could be reformed before left-wing revolutionaries replaced them.[12] Carter concluded, moreover, that this emphasis could help restore Americans' confidence in their own idealism, which had been lost in the muck of Watergate and Vietnam. Congress approved. It had, indeed, begun demanding improved human rights in the Communist bloc and Third-World nations as early as 1973–1974. Brzezinski agreed because he saw that preaching human rights could put the Soviets on the defensive.

Carter appointed a talented, feisty human-rights activist, Pat Derian, as assistant secretary of state for human rights and humanitarian affairs. She worked near-miracles in pushing repressive military regimes in Argentina and Brazil toward democracy, but elsewhere her efforts often hit stone walls. Some of the walls were built by Carter himself. Demands that the South Korean dictatorship allow more human rights were largely silenced when the president realized that the demands might destabilize or alienate such a strategically located country. China's government regularly imprisoned dissidents. But instead of effectively protesting, Carter (at Brzezinski's urging) sent new technology to the Chinese. When El Salvador's military butchered opponents, Carter cut off military aid. The Salvadorans ignored him. When their regime was threatened by revolutionaries in 1980–1981, he turned aid back on despite evidence that four U.S. churchwomen had been raped and killed by Salvadoran military in 1980.

Carter's commitment to human rights was, therefore, not "absolute." "The real problem," a U.S. diplomat noted, "was that the human rights policy was not a policy but an attitude."[13] When the "attitude" threatened to undercut governments important to U.S. strategic or economic interests, it was dropped. Brzezinski, however, used the policy more consistently against the Soviets. When they jailed leading dissidents, the White House temporarily stopped the sale of computers to Moscow. The Soviets, who naïvely believed that Carter was using human rights only as a "bargaining chip" to obtain other concessions from them, became angry and condemned the policy as mere "propaganda." Such allies as West Germany and France also disapproved. They saw no profit intervening in Soviet internal affairs and disrupting their growing trade with the Soviet market.[14]

Carter never solved these contradictions in his trilateral and human-rights approaches. He did score two diplomatic triumphs, however, through hard work and by following Vance's advice to deal with the newly emerging world on its own terms.

A Victory: The Panama Canal Treaties

Almost from the moment in 1903 that the United States claimed complete control over the Canal Zone that cut their country in half, Panamanians had tried to share, if not remove, that control. Their efforts intensified as U.S. officials established camps for training Latin American police and military, and built large air-force bases. Bloody anti-U.S. riots led Lyndon Johnson to take the first step toward sharing power in 1964–1967. Despite loud complaints (one conservative senator objected to having "a country with one-third the population of Chicago kick us around"), Henry Kissinger, in 1974, agreed in principle to transfer ultimate control of the canal to Panama. He realized that the great waterway, beautifully engineered and still durable, was also highly vulnerable to sabotage and other kinds of stoppages. It was also being bypassed by huge oil tankers and container ships that could not pass through the Canal locks and often did not need to use it anyway given alternative ship-train routes.

Carter had the political courage to complete the treaties in September 1977 and then push them through the Senate in the spring of 1978. He spent much of his small political capital in the effort—so much, some observers believed, that his influence over Congress, which was never great, became almost invisible. He won the fight despite bitter opposition of conservatives led by former California governor Ronald Reagan, who claimed that the treaty was "appeasement" and proved that the United States was collapsing like a corrupted ancient Roman Empire. Carter received strong support from other conservatives, including columnist William Buckley, Jr., and film star John Wayne, who regularly sailed his yacht in Panamanian waters. In addition, State Department officials spanned across the country on over 1,500 occasions to sell the treaties in an intense, nationwide debate.

The first treaty, which outlined U.S. rights after the year 2000, when Panama will assume control of the canal, passed with one vote to spare, 68 to 32, in early 1978. The second pact, stipulating how Panama was gradually to obtain authority over the waterway during the next twenty-two years, passed by the same vote. But the Senate accepted the agreements only after inserting a "reservation" proposed by Arizona Democrat Dennis DeConcini. It stated that if the canal were to close after 2000 for any reason, the United States had the right to intervene to open it. Panamanians rioted, and their government declared that it would never grant such a right. The Senate then rewrote the DeConcini reservation: the United States could intervene to keep the canal open, but Americans did not have the right of intervention.[15] With that wondrous word magic, both sides accepted the treaties. It had been the second-longest treaty debate in the Senate's history. But Carter and the Senate leadership had avoided more bloodshed and the possible closing of the canal. He scored the most significant victory in U.S.– Latin American relations since Franklin D. Roosevelt's good-neighbor policies four decades earlier.

A VICTORY: THE CAMP DAVID ACCORDS

The president pulled off an even more remarkable diplomatic feat in the Middle East. Kissinger's diplomacy had produced a delicate truce in 1975. That same year, however, Lebanon began to be torn apart by the terrorist acts of the Palestine Liberation Organization (PLO), which claimed to represent millions of homeless Palestinians. As the country fell apart, Syria (which received large amounts of Soviet supplies), Egypt, and Israel jockeyed dangerously for control of Lebanon. Meanwhile, PLO-Egyptian-Syrian fury grew as Israel's hard-line government of Menachem Begin consolidated its power over the Jordan River's West Bank, where the Palestinians hoped either to have their own homeland or settlements linked to Jordan. (See map, p. 727.)

Carter angered Begin by calling for a Palestinian homeland. Israel saw such a homeland on the West Bank as a grave threat to its existence, especially if that homeland came under PLO control. Carter then frightened Egypt's leader, Anwar el-Sadat, by agreeing with the Soviets to sponsor a Mideast peace initiative. Sadat was afraid that

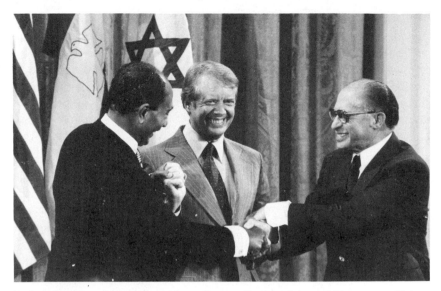

Before the flags of the three nations, Jimmy Carter celebrated his greatest diplo-matic triumph as president: Prime Minister Anwar el-Sadat of Egypt (at left) and Prime Minister Menachem Begin of Israel clasp hands after signing the Camp David Accords in September 1978.

Egypt would be isolated as the Soviets supported Syria and other Arab states while the United States backed Israel. In a dramatic and historic decision, Sadat personally flew to Israel and talked with Begin, whose nation Egypt had never fully recognized. Sadat's and Begin's refusal to deal with the Soviets undercut Carter's peace plan. The region then threatened to go up in flames when Begin sent troops into Lebanon to secure Israel's borders and destroy the PLO. Washington pres-sured the Israelis to retreat, but everyone feared another, greater explosion.

The President boldly—and desperately—invited Sadat and Begin to discuss a settlement at his Camp David retreat in Maryland. Both Israel and Egypt depended on U.S. aid, but Sadat also faced threats of retal-iation by other Arab states if he gave away too much to the Israelis. Begin was restrained by his view of his nation's security needs, includ-ing the West Bank and Gaza. At different times, Carter prevented both men from walking out of the talks with threats of cutting aid or prom-ises of more concessions (and sometimes even by holding long, quiet discussions about the Bible with Begin). In March 1979, Israel and Egypt signed their first peace agreement in history. Sadat agreed to recognize Israel's government; Begin pledged to turn the Sinai desert region over to Egypt. Carter and Sadat believed that they also had an Israeli pledge to freeze Jewish settlements on the West Bank and negotiate a deal on this explosive area. But Begin later denied that those vaguely worded provisions promised any such thing. He refused to retreat from the West Bank, and the issue continued to fester. The three men had, nevertheless, achieved a great deal, if perhaps not enough.

DEFEAT: CARTER, AFRICA, AND ANDREW YOUNG

Carter enjoyed a high point of his presidency in early 1979 with the Camp David Accords. His last two years in office were pockmarked by a series of devastating setbacks. He had not discovered how to stop the leakage of U.S. power or, especially, how to bring order to disorderly—even revolutionary—areas. Nor had he discovered how to reconcile Vance's and Brzezinski's differing policies.

African problems centered on two areas: the Horn (or the central eastern coast) and southern Africa. The Horn is a key strategic region controlling the Indian Ocean–Suez Canal route sailed by giant oil tankers. It encompasses five countries containing 70 million of the world's poorest people. Between 1974 and 1977, a Marxist regime had risen to power in Ethiopia. Neighboring Somalia saw the chance to seize disputed territory in the Ogaden desert region long held by Ethiopia. The Ethiopians turned to the Soviets, who airlifted in supplies and 13,000 Cuban troops. Somalia, holding the most valuable strategic location, asked for U.S. aid. Carter demanded that it first retreat from the Ogaden, which Somalia did. But guerrilla warfare and the Cubans remained. Brzezinski urged Carter to send a U.S. fleet to the area to tell the Soviets to pull out the Cubans or else U.S.-USSR arms talks would stop. Vance hotly disagreed. He wanted no such "linkage," and he was supported by the U.S. ambassador to the United Nations, Andrew Young, the highest-ranking black man in the administration and a close friend of the president. Carter dispatched NSC officer David Aaron to Ethiopia to stop a possible Ethiopian counterattack. (Aaron recalled that the Ethiopian leader, Mengistu Haile Mariam "kept lions, live lions, right under his office. Each time my voice rose to make a point, it was drowned by the roar of beasts beneath my feet. With my eyes glued to the floor, searching for a trap door, I almost missed his offhand assurance that Somalia would not be invaded.")[16] But nothing else worked out: the war continued; the Soviet-Cuban presence was

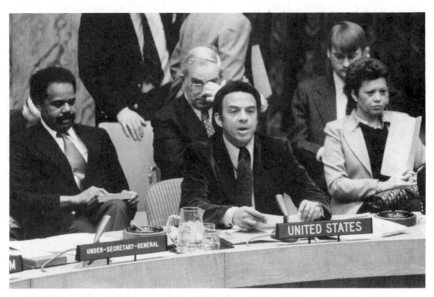

Andrew Young (1932–   ) served as Carter's ambassador to the United Nations until he was dismissed for talking with PLO representatives. A native of New Orleans, educated at Howard University, Young worked closely in the 1960s with Martin Luther King, Jr., and was notably successful in quietly negotiating agreements with the white power structure in cities that Dr. King pushed to desegregate. Eloquent, skilled in negotiations, Young brought strong black support to Carter's presidency and greatly improved U.S. relations with black African nations.

firmed up by a twenty-year USSR-Ethiopian alliance; and the episode further poisoned the superpower relationship.

Young did score some victories. Nigeria, an African power and the second largest exporter of oil to America, had refused to deal with Kissinger because of his Angolan policies (see p. 663). But the Nigerians cooperated with Young. The UN ambassador, however, could not persuade Carter to recognize the Angolan government, especially after Cuban troop strength rose to 20,000 to help the Angolans put down a rebellion. Nor could he toughen U.S. policy toward South Africa's white apartheid government. Carter's tongue-lashing of South Africa's human-rights abuses against the majority black population did not help the blacks, but did make the white South Africans determined not to help the president in handling other regional questions. Historian Thomas J. Noer has concluded that Carter's record "in southern Africa was one of naiveté and failure." By late 1979, Young was gone. He broke a U.S. policy of not dealing with the PLO in any manner when he met secretly with PLO observers at the UN. Protests, led by pro-Israeli voices, erupted. The protests sharpened because Young and TransAfrica (a leading black political action group in Washington) had pointedly condemned growing Israeli–South African relations. With Young forced out, Vance lost one of his most important allies in the battle against Brzezinski.[17]

DEFEAT: SOMOZA FALLS, SANDINISTAS RISE, SALVADORANS KILL

Proud of his Spanish-language ability and some trips south of the border, Carter hoped to pull U.S.–Latin American relations out of the quicksand of the previous decade. The 1977 treaties with Panama were a major step forward. Also in 1977, he and Fidel Castro agreed to thaw U.S.-Cuban ties by lifting some travel and economic restrictions. Diplomatic "Interests Sections" opened in Havana and Washington, although no formal diplomatic recognition occurred. By 1979, however, the relationship had again cooled, and Carter's policies turned sharply toward a renewed cold-war stance (as they had in Africa).

Most notably, the United States and Nicaragua were becoming deadly enemies. This seemed odd. Since the 1930s, the Somoza dynasty had made Nicaragua a warm friend of Washington's. But the Somozas also milked their country until they controlled its most profitable industries as well as 5 million acres of fine land (an area roughly equal to El Salvador). As the peasants and middle class lost out, revolutionaries taking their name from the martyred Augusto Sandino (see p. 360) began organizing with Castro's support in 1961. Originally consisting of only three men, the Sandinistas made little headway until Kennedy's Alliance for Progress sharpened class divisions, the government's response to a terrible 1972 earthquake revealed Anastasio ("Tacho") Somoza's incompetence and corruption, and several daring raids into the capital city of Managua demonstrated the power and rising popularity of several hundred Sandinistas. In early 1978, Tacho's troops foolishly gunned down Pedro Joaquín Chamorro, a respected newspaper publisher and Somoza critic. Working from a strong rural base, the Sandinistas expanded their authority. They were joined by moderate middle-class leaders who were sick of Somoza's greed, use of torture on political prisoners, and air bombing of barrios (slum areas) to root out Sandinista sympathizers. (See map, p. 722.)

Carter could not decide what to do. His top State Department experts urged the removal of Somoza. They wanted to install moderate leaders

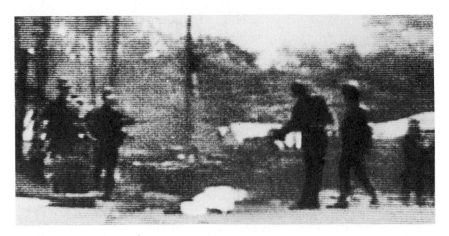

In mid-June 1979, Bill Stewart, an ABC-TV reporter, was covering the Sandinista revolt in Nicaragua when troops of dictator Anastasio Somoza stopped him. Kneeling, he held his hands out to show he was unarmed, but the soldiers shot him in cold blood. They did not know that Stewart's colleagues were filming the atrocity. The pictures finally led many Americans to understand the nature of the Somoza regime and why the Sandinistas had waged a nearly twenty-year revolution that finally triumphed the following month. (Courtesy ABC News NYT Pictures)

before the revolutionaries seized power. That advice, however, was countered by Tacho's powerful friends in the U.S. Congress and Carter's hope that somehow elections could bring in a new, friendly regime. How legitimate elections could be held amid a revolution and after the Somozas had corrupted every balloting for thirty years was difficult to figure out. As usual, most people in the United States paid little attention and took Central America for granted. This began to change on June 20, 1979, when Somoza's troops seized an ABC-TV reporter, Bill Stewart, made him kneel in the street, then shot him in the head. The cold-blooded murder was captured on film by other reporters, and the scenes horrified U.S. viewers. (In the popular, important film, *Under Fire* [1983], actor Gene Hackman plays a reporter whose murder resembles Stewart's. In the film, Hackman's one-time lover, Joanna Cassidy, breaks down and cries. A Nicaraguan nurse reminds Cassidy that thousands of Nicaraguans had been murdered by the Somozas, then adds bitterly, "Maybe we should have killed an American journalist fifty years ago.") Carter nevertheless continued to equivocate, and as he did so, the Sandinistas launched their "final" offensive in May 1979. In June, Carter asked the Organization of American States to intervene and establish a moderate government. Not one Latin

American nation supported the U.S. plan. On July 19, the Sandinistas completed their "triumph" by marching into Managua. Tacho and his mistress escaped to Miami, then to Paraguay, where he was obliterated in a car bombing.[18]

About 50,000 Nicaraguans had died (equivalent to 4.5 million U.S. citizens), and Somoza had stolen nearly all of the national treasury. Carter moved to reconcile the Sandinistas by asking Congress to send $75 million in economic aid. Congress, however, refused to act on the request until spring 1980. The Sandinistas, meanwhile, looked for help (in health and educational as well as military aid) to Castro, who had long backed them. The new leaders also declared their independence in the cold war by refusing to vote for U.S. resolutions at the UN. They opened relations with western Europe, Canada, and the Soviet bloc. The Sandinistas held tightly to power. Promised elections were pushed back to 1984. Moderate leaders quit the government. Nicaragua was not a Communist nation; 60 percent of the economy remained in private hands, and the Roman Catholic church remained strong and loudly critical of the Sandinistas. But neither was the nation any longer an unquestioning friend of Washington's.

Next door, El Salvador threatened to follow in Nicaragua's revolutionary footsteps. Since the 1930s, the Salvadoran oligarchs (or "the fourteen families") had formed an alliance with the military to preserve their monopoly of Salvadoran wealth. In one of the region's richest and most efficient nations, 10 percent of the 4.6-million Salvadorans had to migrate to other countries to find land and food for survival. Eighty percent of children under five years of age suffered from serious malnutrition. A revolutionary movement took root in the 1960s, but the military had kept it in check with "death squads" that killed suspected critics. When Carter condemned the brutalities and cut off military aid, the Salvadorans went elsewhere for equipment. By 1979, however, five revolutionary groups expanded their control and formed the Farabundo Martí National Liberation Front (FMLN). More moderate military officers tried to institute reforms after seizing power in 1979, but the oligarchs and conservative military reasserted themselves. In 1980, José Napoleón Duarte, educated at the University of Notre Dame in Indiana, returned from exile to head the government. A moderate who had been tortured by the military in 1972, the popular Duarte now tried to stop both the FMLN on the Left and the death squads on the Right.

But he found himself depending on the military for his own survival. Death squads had murdered the archbishop of San Salvador while he was saying mass in March 1980 and, in December, raped and murdered four U.S. churchwomen. Carter cut off aid to Duarte. The rebels announced their own "final" offensive. Duarte appealed for help, and Carter now responded. The Salvadoran military stopped the FMLN drive. The war became a low-intensity struggle marked by incredible brutality. It wrecked the Salvadoran economy in a Central America that had suddenly become an arena for a new cold war.

Defeat: Carter, the Shah, and the Ayatollah

By 1980, U.S. control of Central American affairs was at its lowest point in a century. U.S.-Iranian relations had also reached their nadir. Since the end of World War II, and especially since 1973, the ruling shah had been the central U.S. military and economic partner in the region. But he also alienated his own people by westernizing and overmilitarizing Iranian society. Powerful fundamentalist Shiite Moslems, led by their religious leaders, the ayatollahs, bitterly objected. The shah used force to keep the fundamentalists in line. After they tried to seize power in 1963, he exiled their leader, Ruhollah Khomeini, to Iraq and then Paris, where the shah hoped Khomeini would be forgotten. It was the shah, however, who had forgotten the wonders of telephones and audio cassettes, which Ayatollah Khomeini used to mobilize his millions of supporters. The shah had also forgotten an old saying: "Stepping on an ayatollah is like stepping on a Persian rug: it only increases in value."

The Iranian ruler was sitting on a powder keg. Two-thirds of the population was under age thirty; the urban settlements had quadrupled to 20 million after 1955; 15 percent of the nation tried to live around the capital of Tehran, where slums lacked proper sewage or water facilities; vast oil wealth was not trickling down, especially not to a restless student generation; and the government bureaucracy was bloated and corrupt. Even the military was losing status, despite the shah's squandering of $18 billion on arms purchases (mostly from the United States) between 1974 and 1978. As the Shiite leaders gained support, the shah's secret police, Savak, imprisoned 50,000 people.[19] Iranians flocked to the security and absolute beliefs of the ayatollahs for refuge.

Most U.S. officials knew or cared little about these changes. Accepting Brzezinski's awkward description of Iran as a "regional influential," the president said nothing about Savak's brutality and reaffirmed

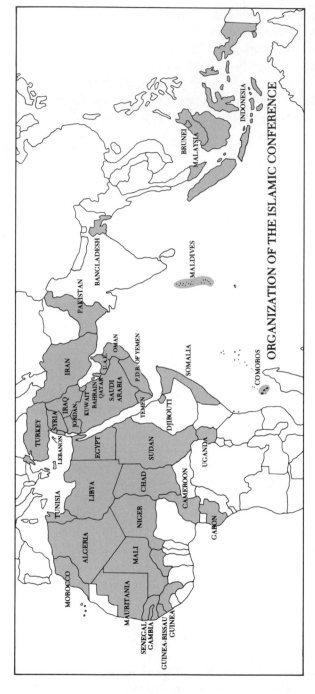

ORGANIZATION OF THE ISLAMIC CONFERENCE

Islam, the religious faith of Moslems, dominates much of Africa and the Middle East, and was electrified by the triumph of Islamic fundamentalists in the Iranian revolution of 1979. Moderate Moslems, as well as much of the rest of the world, worried that the fundamentalism might spread into neighboring states.

Richard Nixon's dedication to the shah. In a New Year's Eve toast in 1977, Carter praised the shah for making Iran "an island of stability" and also for "the admiration and love which your people give you."[20] U.S. intelligence agents had obeyed the shah's wishes that they maintain little contact with his opposition; so as strikes and street protests grew to fever pitch in 1978, neither the shah nor U.S. officials understood what was happening.

As his reign wobbled, the shah hesitated, in part because of growing ill-health from a cancer that had struck him in 1974. He especially feared ordering the Shiite-infiltrated military to fire on other Shiites. Carter also hesitated as his advisers were bitterly divided on the issue. Vance and the U.S. ambassador to Iran, William Sullivan, opposed any use of force. They wanted to work with the opposition to effect a transitional government. Brzezinski, however, opposed any deals with revolutionary religious fanatics. He urged working with the military to keep the shah in power. During the last days of the shah's rule, Carter told Sullivan to follow Brzezinski's plan. The ambassador wired back that the president of the United States must be "insane." The revolution had moved far past the point where Americans could set its course. In February 1979, the military made its deal with the ayatollahs, the shah fled, and the nearly eighty-year-old Khomeini took power.[21]

In mid-1979, the shah asked to enter the United States for treatment of his cancer. His close friends, Henry Kissinger and David Rockefeller, as well as Brzezinski, pressured Carter to approve the request. Carter prophetically observed that he "did not wish the Shah to be here playing tennis while Americans in Tehran were being kidnapped or even killed." But the president took pity and allowed the shah in.[22] Within a month, Khomeini's followers seized the U.S. Embassy in Tehran and held fifty-three Americans hostage. As the Iranians paraded and mocked the hostages before worldwide television, U.S. officials were helpless. American anger riveted on Khomeini, even to the point of creating ABC-TV's popular late-night program, "Nightline," originally aired to keep daily watch on the crisis. Allies condemned the seizure but refused to use force to free the Americans. Vance assured them that only negotiations, not force, would be employed. In April 1980, however, the cornered, frustrated Carter—in the middle of a bitter re-election campaign and urged on by Brzezinski—ordered a daring helicopter rescue of the hostages. Vance resigned. He was the first secretary of state to resign on a matter of principle in sixty-five years. On their way into Tehran, two helicopters had mechanical problems. Another hit a U.S. C-130 plane and crashed in the Iranian desert. Eight Americans perished. The Iranians displayed the burned corpses for television. Khomeini finally released the hostages on January 20, 1981, and timed the release so it occurred several minutes after Carter left office. After thirty-five years, U.S. influence over a pivotal Middle East nation had ended.

Iran's turmoil drove up the price of oil 60 percent in 1979. U.S. infla-.tion, running at a dangerous 7 percent annual rate since 1975, nearly doubled to 13 percent. The world economy threatened to spin out of control as oil-poor nations went ever-deeper in debt. Amid this chaos, Carter found himself at flashpoint with the Soviets.

Defeat: Carter, SALT II, and Afghanistan

That crisis did not come out of the blue. Both Brezhnev's aged regime and the Soviet economy were slowing down like an unwound clock. Soviet economic growth had sunk toward an actual 0 percent in 1979–1980. Brezhnev suffered foreign-policy reverses in relations with southern Asia and especially China and the Middle East. The appearance of the violently anti-Communist Khomeini on their boundary must have given top Moscow officials very long nights, especially as religious fundamentalism threatened to infect the large Moslem population inside the Soviet Union. Communism produced no new ideas to deal with these problems. One Soviet scholar believed, "You can read any book [on ideology] in 20 minutes" because it merely repeated all other books on the subject. The Soviets, however, did excel at building military equipment and space programs. "This place is like a banana republic," a U.S. journalist declared privately in Moscow, "but this one can incinerate us."[23]

Carter and Brezhnev had hoped to expand détente. But the president's human-rights policy defending Soviet dissidents and Moscow's involvement in Angola and Ethiopia had stalled the relationship. In 1977, moreover, Carter, pushed by Brzezinski and other "hawks," tried to go beyond the SALT II agreement made by Brezhnev and Gerald Ford in 1975. Carter's proposal to reduce nuclear weapons was mostly aimed at reducing the heaviest missiles (on which Soviet forces relied), and Brezhnev bitterly rejected the deal. As tempers cooled, Brzezinski again seized the initiative and persuaded Carter to establish formal diplomatic relations with China, now the Soviet Union's archenemy. Over Vance's objections about the timing, Carter did so on New Year's Day, 1979. A new trade agreement gave China economic privileges not granted the Soviets, and Sino-American trade boomed to $4 billion in 1980 (with three-fourths being profitable U.S. exports).

Both leaders, however, needed a new SALT deal—Brezhnev for economic reasons, Carter for a badly needed political push toward the 1980 elections. At the Vienna summit in June 1979, they struck a SALT agreement. It capped strategic nuclear launchers at 2,400 (with a future reduction to 2,250), and no more than 1,320 were to be MIRVed. To help obtain the U.S. Senate's consent, Brezhnev allowed 50,000 Jews—the highest number ever—to leave the Soviet Union in 1979. But the United States did not respond cooperatively. U.S. officials refused to give Moscow the same trade privileges that they had just given Beijing (Peking). More important, SALT II came under scathing attack. Led by the Committee on the Present Danger and its best-known spokesman, Paul Nitze, the opponents warned that the treaty allowed the Soviets to keep 300 missiles and warheads that were much larger than the Americans' weapons. Defenders of the deal, led by Carter's arms negotiator, Paul Warnke, responded that only the treaty's limits on numbers of actual warheads could prevent the Soviets from using their big missiles as Nitze feared. Such arguments as Nitze's convinced the Senate to move slowly in debating SALT II.[24]

The formal debate, indeed, never occurred. On December 25–27, 1979, 80,000 Soviet troops invaded neighboring Afghanistan. Soviet influence had long been dominant there, but the fiercely independent 14 million Moslems who lived in the mountainous country the size of Texas had no intention of becoming another Bulgaria. A coup in 1973 and another in 1978 threw into turmoil the pro-Communist faction that ruled the country. Soviet involvement rapidly grew. When U.S. ambassador Adolph Dubs was kidnapped by rebels in 1978, Afghan forces, advised by Soviet officers, killed Dubs in an attack on the kidnappers. Washington strongly protested to Moscow. But neither the Afghan regime nor Brezhnev's officials could restore order. In the later view of both Vance and Brzezinski, the Soviets had probably concluded by this time that they had more to gain in Afghanistan than in the rapidly souring U.S.-USSR relationship.[25] When Red Army troops finally invaded Afghanistan, Brezhnev claimed that the Afghan leader, Hafizullah Amin, had invited them in. But they quickly killed Amin and tried to overrun the country. The Russians ran straight into a fanatical Islamic resistance of the mujahedeen, Afghan peasant fighters who were as brutal as they were effective. Soon, 115,000 Soviet troops found themselves enmeshed in a costly war that could not be won.

U.S. IMPORT DEPENDENCE AND IMPORT SOURCES IN THE 1970s
(1977 estimates except where noted)

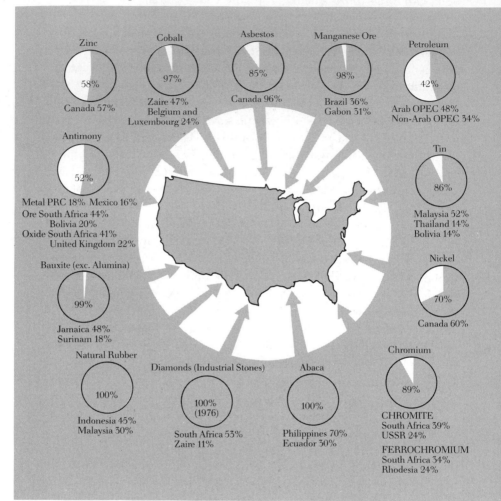

Source: U.S. State Department, *The Trade Debate* (May 1978).

THE CARTER RESPONSE AND DEFEAT (1980)

The president declared that the invasion was "the gravest threat to peace" since 1945. It was estimated that the Soviets had used military force as an instrument of foreign policy at least 190 times since 1945. (The same estimate concluded that the United States had done so on over 200 occasions.)[26] But now Soviet forces had actually moved beyond the boundaries established between 1944 and 1948. Carter struck back by shutting off grain and high-tech exports that had been flooding into the Soviet Union. He ordered young men to register for a military draft and requested that U.S. athletes not participate in the 1980 Summer Olympic Games in Moscow.

Most dramatically, in his January 1980 State of the Union Address, he announced a Carter Doctrine: "An attempt by any outside force to gain control of the Persian Gulf region" would "be repelled by any means necessary, including military force." Brzezinski helped convince Carter to follow this policy by emphasizing that it would be modeled on the historic 1947 Truman Doctrine—a doctrine that had long enjoyed almost automatic support from Americans (see p. 476). Critics such as Richard Betts warned that the similarity was slight and, above all, that Carter, unlike Truman, might have to reach "for the nuclear crutch" even as Nitze and others warned of a growing U.S. inferiority.[27] U.S. military and medical aid, nevertheless, began flowing directly to the Afghan rebels.[28]

Carter now seemed to abandon any idea of military parity with the Soviets. He wanted to obtain superiority: "The United States will remain the strongest of all nations." Even earlier, he had made a pivotal decision to produce and deploy the MX, a new and supposedly more accurate intercontinental missile with ten warheads, and to protect the new weapons by placing them on two hundred huge "race tracks" around which they would continually move so that the Soviets could not have a fixed-site target. And even while he was asking the Senate to accept SALT II, he was also asking approval for the largest new U.S. weapons program in nearly thirty years. In 1980, he signed Presidential Directive 59, drawn up mainly by Brzezinski and Defense Secretary Harold Brown. PD-59 planned to give U.S. officials the massive arms needed to fight a controlled, prolonged nuclear war and to win the exchange on every level of escalation that would probably occur over a period of months, not days or hours. After cutting $36 billion in domestic spending, Carter added $47 billion in new weapons systems. The Pentagon budget jumped from $170 billion in 1976 to $197 billion in 1981 (in 1986 dollars). To buck up both the allies and the stumbling U.S. economy, Carter also nearly doubled arms sales between 1977 and 1980 to $15.3 billion. Historian Gaddis Smith calls Carter's policies of 1979–1980 the "return to militarism."[29]

Carter's defense budgets formed the roots of Ronald Reagan's policies in the 1980s. But that did not save Carter from scathing attack. Allies in western Europe and Japan continued their rich trade with the

Soviets and ignored Carter's pleas for economic sanctions. Argentine and Canadian wheat farmers sold to the Soviet Union the wheat it needed. As U.S. farmers and companies lost direct access to USSR markets, George Shultz (once Nixon's Treasury secretary and soon to be Reagan's secretary of state), damned Carter for "light switch" diplomacy that made international trade so unpredictable. By mid-1980, in a public-opinion poll, 75 percent of Americans gave Carter an over-all negative rating, and 82 percent disliked his foreign-policy record. Much of this anger came from his handling of Iran, but it also arose from his decision to allow into the country 100,000 Cuban refugees— a decision that especially infuriated American blacks, Hispanics, and southerners, who were having economic troubles of their own. The president, one politician declared, "couldn't get the Pledge of Allegiance through Congress."[30]

Historian Burton Kaufman summarized Carter's position in 1980: "His domestic and foreign policies were largely in ruin; the economy seemed incurable; the hostage crisis was dragging on with no end in sight; major differences had surfaced between the United States and its allies over Iran and Afghanistan; a Congress controlled by his own party had rebuked him; . . . and he had the lowest approval rating of any president ever." *Business Week* drew a conclusion: The "Pax Americana that shaped modern history since World War II is fast disintegrating. . . . Even America's closest allies in Europe and Asia are now its fiercest competitors."[31]

REAGAN

The Republican presidential nominee in 1980, Ronald Reagan—former movie actor and California governor—rode Carter's troubles and the nation's pessimism to victory. Americans must ask themselves, Reagan declared, "Is the United States stronger and more respected than it was 3½ years ago? Is the world today a safer place in which to live?"[32] He not only captured the White House, but, for the first time in twenty-eight years, Republicans gained control of the Senate (although not the House).

Reagan's triumph had many sources. The politics of key Western nations (especially Great Britain and West Germany) responded to the shocks of the 1970s by polarizing between Right and Left, and then giving majorities to the Right. Many in the United States especially were alienated by the results of the counterculture and Great Society programs of the 1960s. Such experiences had caused "a social-political hangover," one prominent left-wing critic argued in 1980.[33] To regain their confidence that the nation had a unique role to play in world affairs (the need for "a new Wilsonianism," as one Reaganite referred to the revival of Woodrow Wilson's old dreams), Americans supported much larger military budgets and more CIA operations.[34]

Many observers considered Reagan dangerous. He knew little about foreign policy and seemed lazy and easily confused. He introduced Liberia's head of state, Samuel Doe, as "Chairman Moe." He had little curiosity or apparently little interest in mastering details. The respected journalist, Lou Cannon, who had followed Reagan since the 1960s, wrote that no one could recall when the president had last read a book. He cited Reagan's own joke: "It's true hard work never killed anybody, but I figure, why take the chance?" No one, however, denied the president's talent in keeping his several central beliefs before Americans, and his political brilliance and determination in making them accept his ideas. With "strength, patriotism, and charm," Cannon noted in 1987, Reagan "remains . . . secure in his convictions as well as his ignorance."[35]

Some of these convictions produced serious problems. As a television pitchman for General Electric in the 1950s, Reagan had a standard speech that warned of "encroaching government control." His hero became Calvin Coolidge, who cut income taxes in the 1920s. But Reagan also intended to increase military spending sharply and to impose a conservative social agenda. One result was that the government's debt rose by more than $1 trillion between 1981 and 1987 (or more debt in 6 years than the U.S. government had accumulated during the previous 190 years). Another result, in the *Washington Post*'s words, was a "steady infiltration of the Defense Department into U.S. factories and laboratories." Research programs in many industries and universities increasingly depended on the national government to give thumbs up to their requests.[36] The government's share of the gross national product rose, not fell.

Nevertheless, Reagan's popularity remained high. He knew he was going to succeed, he told a reporter in 1980, "for one simple reason. . . . The American people want somebody in command." Moreover, he believed he knew one way to command. Once, he recalled, he believed because he was "only an actor" he could not be a politician. Now he wondered "how you could be President and not be an actor." Since the time of John F. Kennedy, Hollywood's illusions and Washington's politics had seemed to be converging. In Reagan's presidency, they met. They would never again be easily separated.[37]

THE REAGAN FOREIGN-POLICY STRUCTURE: FOUR CORNERSTONES

The first cornerstone of Reagan's overseas policies rested on his insight that Americans wanted someone who appeared to be in command. Extending presidential powers to the fullest, he swamped the imperial Congress of 1973 to 1980 with a revived imperial presidency. As an accomplished actor, he did this by using his considerable talents on television and radio. But he also gained power by defining U.S. policies in military terms (in which case he could use his constitutional commander-in-chief authority) rather than in economic terms. As the military budget soared, economic foreign aid dropped. Congress seldom fought back successfully, even though public opinion on such issues as arms talks and Central American policy often supported congressional positions. Congress was too fragmented, its members too frightened of being fingered by Reagan as the villains if their alternative policies did not work out. When a presidential spokeswoman claimed that "there are some in Congress who would actually welcome a Marxist victory in El Salvador," she was revealing not the truth, but a well-tested tactic that pushed frightened fence-sitters in Congress over to the president's side. Like his predecessors, Reagan refused to recognize the restraints placed on him by the 1973 War Powers Act (see p. 666). In 1983, the Supreme Court helped him by issuing a decision that declared unconstitutional one of those congressional restraints.[38]

A second cornerstone of his foreign policies was an ardent, outspoken anticommunism that focused on Soviet power. Since at least 1917—and especially since the Truman Doctrine of 1947—anticommunism had been a most potent political medicine when presidents spooned it out in large doses. If that medicine had lost some of its punch during Nixon's détente years, it had regained its strength in 1978–1981. Reagan went further than any recent president in administering it. In a 1980 interview, he declared that "the Soviet Union underlies all the unrest that is going on. If they weren't engaged in this game of dominoes, there wouldn't be any hot spots in the world." In his first presidential press conference, he said that Moscow rulers reserved "the right to commit any crime, to lie, to cheat." He later told a West Point audi-

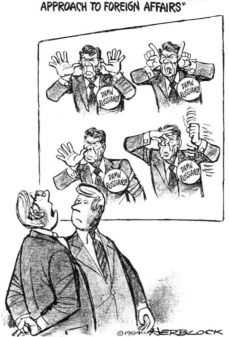

During the President's first term in office, Washington Post *cartoonist "Herblock" (Herbert Block) caught President Ronald Reagan's single-minded focus on fighting and destroying the "evil empire," as Reagan called the Soviet Union. The second term was to be quite different.*

ence that the Soviet Union was "an evil force" and repeated to a Christian fundamentalist gathering that the Soviets were "the focus of evil in the modern world . . . an evil empire."[39]

Until 1982, Reagan also defined China as an enemy of the United States. He opposed talks with Beijing (Peking) and condemned Nixon and Carter for moving closer to China or for implying that the Chinese should have something to say about Taiwan's fate. Reagan had to retreat from this position by 1983, however. U.S.-Soviet relations were so bad, and the American need for Chinese cooperation and markets so great, that he swallowed his earlier words and traveled to the People's Republic in 1984 to strengthen U.S.-Chinese ties. His anticommunism thus focused on the Soviets. The highly popular *Rambo* movies captured the moment as the make-believe hero single-handedly, and with the use of awesome fire power, destroys Communists (especially in Vietnam) who are backed by the Soviets. The Soviets responded with their own Rambo, a Soviet commando leader in the highly popular film, *Solo Voyage*, who stops a group of supersecret and slightly crazy U.S. agents from starting a nuclear war between the two superpowers. Neither side lacked imagination in defining the other side as evil or in making money from such work.

A third cornerstone was a distinction between "authoritarian" governments (which Reagan supported in South Africa, the Philippines, and Argentina) and "totalitarian" regimes (which he opposed in the Soviet Union and China). The distinction had been drawn for him by Jeane J. Kirkpatrick in a 1979 essay, and it led to her appointment as the U.S. ambassador to the UN in 1981. Kirkpatrick argued that although "authoritarians" suppressed freedoms in the political area, they were stable, had demonstrated the possibility of evolving into more democratic regimes, kept their economy open to foreign investors, and usually supported the United States. "Totalitarians," however, were Communists (or Fascists), demonstrated little likelihood of becoming more democratic, hated American-style capitalism, and opposed U.S. interests. If Jimmy Carter had acted on these insights, Ambassador Kirkpatrick believed, he would have kept the shah of Iran and the Somoza dictatorship in Nicaragua in power. Her neat formula allowed Reagan to support right-wing systems and oppose those on the Left. It also allowed him to reverse Carter's human-rights policies. Carter had stressed the sanctity of human life and freedom from starvation and torture. Reagan said that he also supported human rights, but he meant such political freedoms as the right to vote in elections. Authoritarian regimes were often glad to allow meaningless votes, but they had not wanted to listen to Carter's protests about the mistreatment of their people.

Kirkpatrick's distinction, however, soon appeared to have fatal problems. In 1982, "authoritarian" Argentina (whose military leaders she strongly supported) attacked the nearby Falkland Islands (or Malvinas), which Great Britain had colonized in 1830. To her dismay, Reagan decided to work with the closer and more democratic British ally, which did succeed in holding on to the islands. Contrary to her formula, moreover, U.S. officials discovered that it was necessary to work more closely with totalitarian China. And when authoritarian regimes in the Philippines and Haiti began to topple, Reagan at first tried to shore them up and then—despite Kirkpatrick's warnings—followed the advice of Secretary of State George Shultz and helped both countries remove the authoritarian rulers in an effort to create more represen-

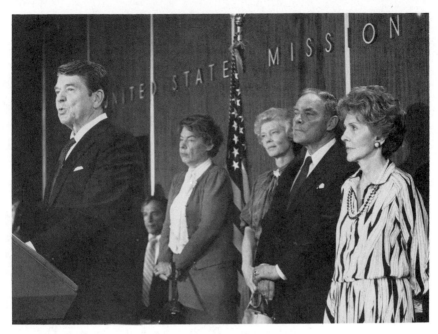

President Ronald Reagan (1911–) was educated at Eureka College in Illinois, broadcast Chicago Cubs baseball games, became a notable Hollywood actor, served as governor of California, and then won the presidency in 1980. In this photo, the new president visits the United Nations to introduce his closest foreign-policy advisers who are standing behind him: (from left) Jeane Kirkpatrick (1926–), U.S. ambassador to the UN; Mrs. and Secretary of State Alexander Haig (1924–); Nancy Reagan (1923–).

tative and stable regimes. By 1985, Kirkpatrick's ideology had proven to be both unworkable and unpopular, especially because it placed U.S. support behind some of the world's most oppressive rulers in South Africa, the Philippines, and Latin America.[40]

The final cornerstone of the Reagan foreign policies was the most obvious and, in dollar terms, most costly. He pledged to "rearm" the United States by jacking up military spending over five years from Carter's projection of $1.1 trillion to $1.5 trillion. The plans included a massive nuclear build-up that threatened to destroy the limits set in 1979 by Carter's and Brezhnev's SALT II agreement. The administration also planned to create a 600-ship navy that revolved around 13 to 15 aircraft-carrier battle groups. The navy, which would be of little use in all-out war with the Soviets, was clearly being planned for actions in the newly emerging nations. The fleet, along with expensive Rapid Deployment Forces, was particularly aimed at winning low-intensity conflicts (or LICs) in such Third-World regions as Central America and the Middle East. In the words of one leading study by Michael T. Klare and Peter Kornbluh, the new forces and the LIC plans represented "a strategic reorientation of the U.S. military establishment, and a renewed commitment to employ force" against "Third World revolutionary movements and governments."[41]

Reagan increased military spending 40 percent between 1980 and 1984, while cutting taxes. He had also promised to balance the budget, a claim that his 1980 Republican rival and later vice-president, George Bush, had called "voodoo economics." But Bush was proved correct as the administration's spending fastened the trillion dollars of debt on the country. That spending, moreover, came under sharp questioning by 1984–1985, as the Central Intelligence Agency admitted that it had far overestimated Soviet defense expenditures after 1976. It also became clear that even when Carter had left office in 1981, the United States was the equal of—and usually superior to—the Soviets in nearly every important defense category.[42]

By 1985, defense spending finally slowed, but resources were also being shifted to high-cost research for the president's Strategic Defense Initiative (SDI or Star Wars, as some critics derided it). Announced in a surprise presidential speech of March 1983, Reagan hoped that SDI would be a space-based defense system forming a high-tech defensive shield over Americans and their allies against incoming missiles. Defense Secretary Caspar Weinberger revealed a major objective of SDI (and, indeed, a major reason for the entire defense build-up): a hope that Americans could return to the more secure days of the 1940s, when they had absolute nuclear superiority. "If we can get a system which is effective and which we know can render their weapons impotent," he told Congress, "we would be back in the situation we were in, for example, when we were the only nation with the nuclear weapon and we did not threaten others with it."[43]

Critics of SDI argued that such absolute security could never be scientifically achieved. Nor did they believe that Americans wanted their existence turned over to hair-trigger, novel computers that would have to operate Star Wars just seconds after a supposed Soviet attack. Many feared that if one side mounted a defensive shield, the other side would plan simply to overwhelm it with vast numbers of missiles—a planned response that could set off a limitless arms race. Others drew back when they concluded that the massive military spending distorted the economy and made U.S. goods less competitive in the world marketplace. Many Americans were especially dismayed that Reaganites seemed to treat even nuclear war lightly. T. K. Jones, a Defense Department official, declared that if such a war broke out, Americans only had to "dig a hole, cover it with a couple of doors, and then throw three feet of dirt on top. . . . If there are enough shovels to go around," he believed, "everybody's going to make it." But even the president sometimes seemed confused about the protection that SDI would provide for its $1-trillion cost: "My concept of the strategic defense system has been one that, if and when we finally achieve what our goal is, and that is a weapon that is effective against incoming missiles, not a weapon system that is effective against incoming weapons, missiles."[44] Or so the president said in 1985.

THE GREAT DEBATE OVER THE USE OF FORCE

Perhaps, then, it was not surprising that the military build-up produced bitter debates inside as well as outside the administration. The most important erupted between Weinberger and Shultz. The secretary of defense spoke for the U.S. military that certainly wanted more modern weapons. But the military also wanted no more involvements such as Vietnam, which had nearly destroyed the morale of, and public trust in, the military. In a November 1984 speech, Weinberger consequently asked that U.S. forces not be sent into conflict unless six criteria were met: (1) the war was vital for U.S. or alliance interests; (2) it was to be fought "wholeheartedly, and with the clear intention of winning"; (3) objectives were to be clearly defined; (4) reassessments of the commitment were constantly to be made; (5) popular and congressional support of the commitment were reasonably certain; and (6) use of arms was the last resort to protect U.S. interests.

Secretary of State Shultz attacked such thinking. Believing that "diplomacy not backed by military strength is ineffectual," he warned that at critical moments, foreign policy might require quick military action without the six assurances. Indeed, such moments had already arisen in 1982 when Shultz persuaded Reagan to back U.S. policy with force in the Middle East, and in 1983 when the administration overthrew the government on the Caribbean island of Grenada. In both instances, the Pentagon was reluctant to commit forces, much to Shultz's frustration. On the other hand, the two secretaries also clashed over arms talks with the Soviets. Weinberger feared such talks. He preferred trying to outspend and outarm the Soviets. Shultz, however, pushed hard after 1983 for a deal to reduce nuclear arms. He believed

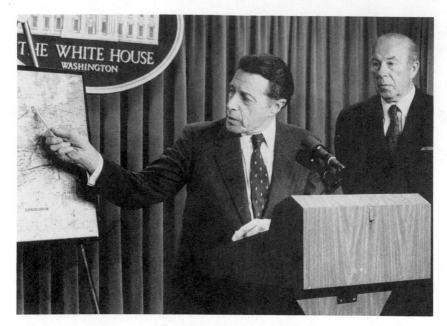

Secretary of Defense Caspar Weinberger (1917–   ) and Secretary of State George Shultz (1920–   ) are shown here briefing the press in 1986 after the U.S. raid in Libya. The two men were not always this close. Indeed, after Shultz replaced Haig as secretary of state in mid-1982, he and Weinberger often strongly disagreed over foreign policy. When Weinberger resigned in 1987, Shultz had become the most powerful foreign-policy official in the Reagan administration.

that such an agreement would reassure allies who feared the nuclear build-up and would also cut some defense spending. The two men never resolved their differences. Weinberger resigned in 1987 before he had to support a treaty, negotiated by Shultz, that eliminated the U.S. and Soviet intermediate-range missiles stationed in Europe. The president joked that "sometimes in our administration, the right hand doesn't know what the far-right hand is doing."[45]

The debate over whether and how the United States should use military force naturally used the Vietnam War as a reference point. Reagan and others who wanted to use force condemned the preoccupation with the Vietnam defeat. This fundamental, historic debate was, as usual, reflected in films. In 1968, *The Green Berets,* starring John Wayne, had shown a Vietnam conflict that more resembled the so-called "good war" of 1941–1945 than the actual savage, complex struggle then occurring in Southeast Asia. By the mid-1980s, however, a series of films, led by *Apocalypse Now, The Deer Hunter, Coming Home, Platoon,* and *Full Metal Jacket,* among others, showed the horror, brutalities, and personal consequences of the U.S. involvement in Vietnam. Unfortunately, these films were notably weak in picturing Vietnam and Vietnamese. They viewed the war narrowly as about people and values in the United States, while usually ignoring the millions of people in Vietnam who had perished in the thirty-year conflict. But within their narrower focus, many popular films for the first time began to raise questions about the use of U.S. power abroad—and the price that might have to be paid at home.[46]

SHIFTING SANDS: THE ECONOMY

Historian Paul Kennedy noted an especially disturbing result of the arms build-up when he traced the rise and inevitable decline of empires over the past five hundred years: "Great Powers in relative decline instinctively respond by spending more on security, thereby diverting potential resources from investment and compounding their long-term dilemma."[47] That insight applied to the relative decline of both U.S. and Soviet economic power in the 1970s and 1980s. But it seemed especially ominous for the future of the U.S. system and the international capitalist order to which it had given birth after 1945.

Even as the stock market soared between 1982 and 1987, Americans found their economy shifting beneath them in dangerous, even historic, ways. For fifteen of the sixteen years between 1970 and 1986, they suffered trade deficits (that is, they bought more goods from abroad than they sold abroad). This development was historic because between 1894 and 1971 they had always sold more than they bought from other nations. (See the graph on p. 645.) Nevertheless, until 1981, this dangerous trend was disguised because U.S. investments overseas (in foreign businesses, stocks, and branches of U.S. corporations) had produced so much income that it helped wipe out the merchandise trade problem.

But in 1981, that changed. As the Reagan budget deficits climbed to an unheard-of $200 billion each year, Americans had to borrow from foreigners to pay for the deficit. By 1985, their borrowing, especially from the Japanese and western Europeans, became so heavy that, for the first time since 1914, Americans actually owed more money overseas than they were owed from abroad. After seventy-one years, they had become a debtor nation—like Mexico, Brazil, and many Third-

World countries. Indeed, by 1988, they had borrowed until they owed more than $400 billion to foreign lenders and were the world's most indebted people. "It will be recorded of us in the 1980s," New York Democratic Senator Daniel Patrick Moynihan wrote, that "America borrowed a trillion dollars from the Japanese and gave a party." The nation's top banker, Paul Volcker, chairman of the Federal Reserve Board, warned that "we are obviously in danger of losing control over our own economic destiny." As the U.S. domestic debt soared toward another trillion dollars in the 1990s, young Americans faced a lifetime of paying Japanese and other non-U.S. creditors, while cutting back not only on their own spending, but on spending for their national defense.[48]

This washing away of the economy had many causes. Americans spent far more than Japanese and western Europeans on military power (in part, to defend the Japanese and western Europeans), and so had less to spend on improving their civilian productivity. Americans only saved about one-third as much as did Japanese, so Japan had more money for new investment (and for investment in land, factories, and apartment houses in the United States). Reagan slashed taxes in 1981, supposedly so Americans could save more, but they instead spent more on themselves while their savings rate dipped 25 percent. For 350 years, farm exports had been the backbone of U.S. trade. But those exports sank from $43.7 billion in 1981 to $26.3 billion in 1986. Foreign buyers were too deeply in debt themselves or working hard to become self-sufficient in food to buy American goods. The United States could no longer compete in key sectors of the world economy.

Reagan tried to stimulate the economy in part by reducing trade barriers between the United States and Canada, who were already the world's largest trading partners. He envisioned a massive free-trade community of Canada, the United States, and Mexico. He finally signed a preliminary agreement with Canada in 1987, and in 1989 a giant free-trade area of the United States and Canada began to take shape. Nevertheless, bitter debate erupted on both sides of the border over the question of whether all North America and Mexico would become a giant common market.[49]

The Reagan military plans became a prime target for those who hoped to discipline spending. The Pentagon budget was reduced in real dollars during the later 1980s. In the words of Alexander Haig, who in 1981–June 1982 had been Reagan's first secretary of state, "This administration threatens in eight years to be the largest defense spender and the largest defense cutter simultaneously, and that's the worst kind

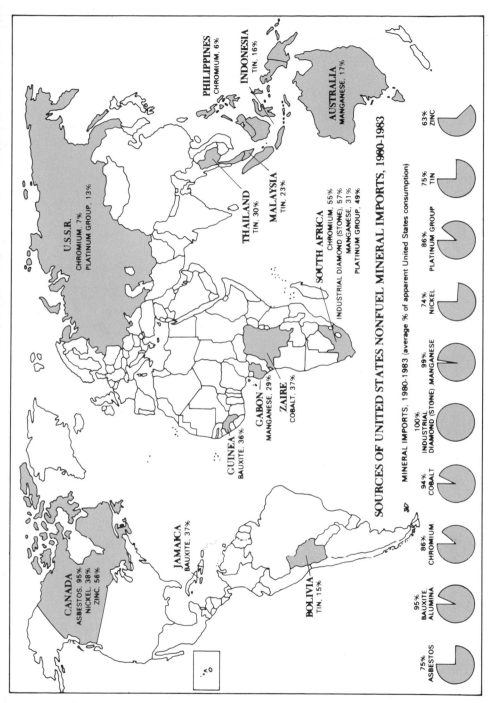

By the 1980s, Americans were heavily dependent on other nations for the essential minerals that made the U.S. economy go. Note especially the American dependence on minerals from South Africa and the Soviet Union.

of defense policy there is." Nevertheless, military spending remained near $300 billion. The Defense Department was the nation's largest purchaser of goods and services. It employed one-quarter of American scientists and engineers. An "iron triangle" of the Pentagon, defense industries, and members of Congress whose constituents depended on military spending kept arms budgets at near-record levels despite the cuts and the effects on the economy.[50]

THE SUPERSTRUCTURE: THE REAGAN DOCTRINE (OR WILSONIANISM UPDATED)

The administration, indeed, required new, expensive military power to reach a prized foreign-policy goal: the so-called Reagan Doctrine. The president best defined it in his 1985 State of the Union message:

> Freedom is not the sole prerogative of a chosen few; it is the universal right of all God's children. . . . [Peace and prosperity flourish] where people live by laws that ensure free press, free speech, and freedom to worship, vote, and create wealth. Our mission is to nourish and defend freedom and democracy, and to communicate these ideals everywhere we can. . . . We must stand by all our democratic allies. And we must not break faith with those who are risking their lives—on every continent, from Afghanistan to Nicaragua—to defy Soviet-supported aggression and secure rights which have been ours from birth. . . . Support for freedom fighters is self-defense.[51]

The doctrine's roots went back at least to Woodrow Wilson's faith that the world could "be made safe for democracy" by direct United States involvement. Now, U.S. officials told the Soviets that the 1968 Brezhnev Doctrine (which stated that Soviet socialist regimes must be considered permanent and guaranteed by force, if necessary) was dead and that "it's a new ball game." The Soviets concluded that traditional U.S. containment policy was out and that a rollback policy was in.[52]

It sounded attractive. Americans were to go on the offensive in the newly emerging nations by supporting indigenous anti-Communist groups. Thus, there would not be a costly Vietnam but, instead, cheap supplying of the "freedom fighters," probably with covert CIA aid. Large U.S forces would supposedly not be needed. With this approach, U.S. political debate could also be quieted. Out of sight meant out of mind, Reaganites hoped. The new CIA director, William Casey, took on the

During the 1980s, a vigorous debate erupted over whether the Soviet Union and the United States had entered an era of inevitable "decline." Some argued that on the basis of their severe economic problems and their overspending on military budgets, the two great powers, and especially the Soviets, were following the examples of the Dutch, Spanish, French, and British who had created great empires and then had become overextended until they finally lost their empires and global power. Washington Post cartoonist "Herblock" (Herbert Block) raises the question of whether U.S. political leadership had declined in the 200 years after the decisive 1781 victory of the American revolutionaries at Yorktown, Virginia.

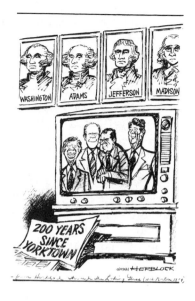

job with gusto. A Republican party power and self-made millionaire, Casey had probably been happiest during World War II, when he was operating spy missions inside Nazi Europe.[53] Casey believed that Congress did not need to know about some of his operations (despite laws requiring such disclosures), and he apparently did not even at times inform the president. Critics pointed out other problems with the Reagan Doctrine as well. Both George Kennan and Robert W. Tucker (who had advised Reagan in 1980), warned that it was too open-ended and ideologically explosive. It could deeply involve Americans in a country where they had few interests.[54]

The Reaganites disagreed. They were willing to engage in an ideological—even a covert military—war for the sake of democratic "universalism and moralism," as one phrased it. The president and Secretary of State Shultz, moreover, were furious and frustrated because of terrorist attacks on U.S. citizens, including the killing of an American and a Turkish citizen in a West Berlin nightclub bombing. When Reagan claimed to have evidence linking the bombing to Libya's leader, Mu'ammar al-Qadhafi, the president ordered fifty-five U.S. planes to bomb Libyan shore facilities and Qadhafi's living quarters in April 1986. Qadhafi escaped, but the casualties were not light. Two American flyers and at least thirty-seven Libyans lost their lives. (Later evidence indi-

cated that Syria, not Libya, had instigated the nightclub explosion.)
But the Reagan Doctrine's key targets became Afghanistan, Angola,
Kampuchea (Cambodia), and Nicaragua.

The greatest success appeared in Afghanistan. Some 115,000 Soviets troops could not control the country after their 1979 invasion. The
Soviets suffered at least 40,000 casualties in fighting against the mujahedeen by 1987. Many survivors returned home as drug addicts and
alcoholics. U.S. support of the rebels leaped upward (nearly doubling
to at least $400 million in 1984–1985 alone) and included Stinger missiles with which the mujahedeen rebels shot down Soviet helicopters.
After three aged Soviet leaders died in power between 1982 and 1985,
Mikhail Gorbachev assumed the top job in Moscow. Gorbachev had
supported the invasion, but he saw that the conflict was draining
resources required for his top priority: revitalizing the slowing, inefficient Soviet economy. The war threatened to have no end. In early
1988, he declared that Soviet troops planned to leave Afghanistan,
although a pro-Moscow regime and Red Army advisers were to remain.

Reagan's policy in Afghanistan enjoyed strong congressional support, but such a consensus did not exist on Angola. Having tried to
overthrow the Marxist Angolan government since 1975 (see p. 663),
U.S. officials found themselves supporting Jonas Savimbi's guerrilla
forces. In 1985, the president had successfully pushed Congress to repeal
the Clark Amendment, which had prohibited U.S. involvements in the
quarrel. But then the Reagan Doctrine ran into problems. For one, the
Angolan government continued to work closely with U.S. oil companies (especially Chevron and Texaco), welcomed Western investment,
and modified its socialist controls. For another, Savimbi made little
headway on his own, but he was embarrassingly successful in blowing
up U.S.-owned oil facilities in 1986, just one month after he had received
American military aid. Perhaps most important, Savimbi's main support came from the white South African government. It repeatedly used
the continent's most powerful military to attack neighboring black states
that supported the blacks inside South Africa who fought to end the
apartheid system.

The white South Africans were hated throughout the region. U.S.
interests were not helped by being allied with them and Savimbi.
Nevertheless, the Reaganites asked Congress for funds to help Savimbi
and also to follow a policy of "constructive engagement" toward the
South African regime. Reagan's policy condemned apartheid, but it
also condemned Jimmy Carter's attempts to use political and economic pressures to change the apartheid system. Reagan hoped instead

---

SULLIVAN PRINCIPLES

In 1977, Reverend Leon Sullivan—a Baptist minister in Philadelphia and General Motors Corp. director—formulated a set of principles for fair employment practices in South Africa. He encouraged U.S. companies with investments in South Africa to implement these principles in their South African facilities and thus break down the apartheid regulations.

- Nonsegregation of the races in all eating, comfort, and work facilities;
- Equal and fair employment practices for all employees;
- Equal pay for all employees doing equal or comparable work for the same period of time;
- Initiation and development of training programs that will prepare blacks, coloreds, and Asians in substantial numbers for supervisory, administrative, clerical, and technical jobs;
- Increasing the number of blacks, coloreds, and Asians in management and supervisory positions;
- Improving the quality of employees' lives outside the work environment in such areas as housing, transportation, schooling, recreation, and health facilities.

In 1987–1988, after more than 150 U.S. corporations in South Africa adopted the Sullivan Principles, Reverend Sullivan concluded that South African society had not sufficiently changed and urged the corporations to withdraw from South Africa.

---

to work quietly with South Africa to provide it with economic and political security so that the whites would be willing to give the blacks (who formed 72 percent of the population) more freedom to move, live, and work as they pleased. By 1984, however, the whites proposed a new constitution that gave no significant new rights to blacks. When protests erupted, the government imposed martial law, killed more than a thousand blacks over a period of fifteen months, and threw out foreign television crews when they tried to report the events.

A storm of protest erupted in American corporate stockholders' meetings and on college campuses, where pressure built to force large U.S. firms working in South Africa to "divest" and quit cooperating with the white government. A number of firms (including Ford and IBM) did pull out, but their plants kept running, often under South African white management. Of the 350 American companies operating in South Africa in 1980, nearly 200 remained by 1988. In 1986, an angry U.S. Congress began replacing Reagan's policy with tough economic sanctions against the South African government.[55] Within four years these sanctions seemed to have an effect. The white government began to ease apartheid and even to release the leading black leader, Nelson Mandela, from a long jail term.

In other trouble spots, the Reagan Doctrine proved irrelevant. In 1986, after fourteen years of dictatorship, Ferdinand Marcos lost his grip on the Philippines. He could not stop a growing pro-Communist insurgency on the nation's outlying islands—at least not without further oppressing a people from whom he had already stolen over $1 billion. U.S. officials had said little. They believed that they needed the huge American bases at Subic Bay and Clark Field. Marcos happily leased the bases for an annual rent of $500 million. In 1981, Vice-President George Bush toasted Marcos: "We love your adherence to democratic principle and to the democratic processes." Many Filipinos disagreed, especially after Marcos's military gunned down leading political opponents. By February 1986, Marcos could no longer deal with either the rebels or rising demands for a fair election. Running against Corazon Aquino (the wife of one of his murdered opponents), Marcos won, but the vote was so corrupt that street demonstrations and—at the last minute—White House pressure forced him to leave the country. Reagan had supported the dictator nearly to the end. Aquino won power, but she proved ineffective in blunting the growing rebel movement that by 1987 operated in sixty-three of the nation's seventy-three provinces. U.S. financial problems prevented Reagan from giving her the aid she needed to breathe life into the devastated Philippine economy.[56] The Reagan Doctrine's determination to roll back Communist gains oddly seemed to be failing in a nation that had been closely allied with the United States since 1898.

THE REAGAN DOCTRINE, LATIN AMERICA, AND THE TICKING TIME BOMB

The doctrine's most hotly debated action occurred in Central America. The president tried to keep leftist guerrillas from seizing power in El Salvador, while he attempted to prevent the Sandinista government from remaining in power in Nicaragua. But these crises were only two of many dangerous developments that threatened U.S.–Latin American relations.

Tiny El Salvador presented Reagan with his first test case. The revolutionary FMLN offensive had miserably failed in early 1981 (see p. 695), and the rebels wanted to discuss a settlement. The president rejected any such deal. As his new NSC adviser, Richard Allen, put it, U.S. military force in the hemisphere "has always been the basis for the development of a just and humane foreign policy, and it's some-

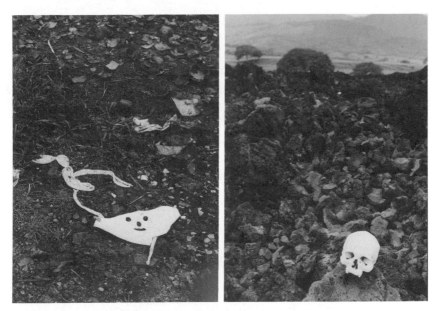

El Playón, a lava bed outside of El Salvador's capital, San Salvador, has been used for years as the dumping grounds for those seized, tortured, and killed by Salvadoran police, security squads, and right-wing vigilantes. Between 40,000 and 50,000 Salvadorans (equivalent to nearly 3 million U.S. citizens) have been murdered in this manner. They have been critics, or merely suspected critics, of the military-dominated Salvadoran government and have especially been targeted by large landowners who are determined to hold on to their wealth. The Reagan administration strongly supported the Salvadoran government while trying—unsuccessfully—to stop the torture and killing. The picture on the left shows masks at El Playón once worn by death-squad members. The picture on the right shows the remains of one of the nearly 50,000 victims.

thing we can be proud of." Reagan's first secretary of state, Alexander Haig, assured him, "Mr. President, this is one you can win."[57] With enough military help, the 17,000-man Salvadoran army could not only destroy the 4,000 guerrillas, but show the Soviets that the Reagan administration did not intend to be the "wimp" that Reagan had accused Carter of being. U.S. advisers and the CIA moved into El Salvador in large numbers, while thousands of Salvadoran soldiers were brought to the United States for training.

But the president's policy floundered. Guerrillas more than doubled in number, controlled large sections of the country, carried out attacks within the capital of San Salvador, and wrecked key sectors of the economy. Reagan's approach stressed the need for democratic elections in a nation that had never known democracy. When elections were held in 1982, right-wing military factions, closely associated with the secret "death squads" that had slaughtered tens of thousands of Salvadorans, nearly seized the presidency. They were stopped only when U.S. officials intervened to nullify the election results and install a more moderate politician as president. In 1984, new elections, more closely supervised by the United States and financed by as much as $1.5 million in CIA funds, brought the U.S.-educated José Napoleón Duarte back to power. Duarte was the one figure both Salvadorans and North Americans could rally around, and the U.S. Congress was willing to trust him with funds. By 1988, Washington pumped $1.5 million per day into El Salvador to keep Duarte and the decimated Salvadoran economy afloat.

The effort resembled rolling a huge boulder uphill. The money built little, especially as the richest Salvadorans sent their money to safe overseas banks. Duarte's key reform—land redistribution to the peasant masses, who depended on but had no land—stopped as the right-wing death squads killed officials and peasants who tried to carry out the reform. In 1985–1986, the FMLN lost ground to the U.S.-supplied military, but they then carried out daring raids, including the murder of four U.S. soldiers in San Salvador. Duarte, whom the constitution prevented from running again in 1989, lost much of his control. In late 1986, hundreds of university students burned the U.S. flag and threw rocks at Duarte in one of the largest anti–United States protests in years. On the other side, the death squads stepped up their work. Frightened Salvadoran courts released military figures implicated in the murder of North Americans and Salvadorans. In 1988, right-wing groups linked with the death squads won nationwide legislative elections as Duarte's party went down to a crushing defeat. The war intensified, the people suffered, the dying continued.[58]

Reagan focused his Central American effort on Nicaragua, where the revolutionary Sandinistas had seized power in 1979 from the U.S.-supported Somoza dictatorship. The Sandinistas kept nearly 60 percent of the economy in private hands, but they were determined to carry out fundamental reform and break the long North American grip on their country's affairs. They nationalized banks and some land (mostly Somoza's old holdings), as well as foreign trade. They also set up neighborhood committees to carry out the revolution and, according to critics, to intimidate those who questioned the revolution. The Sandinistas rapidly improved both literacy and health conditions, but they also lost support of more moderate (especially business) groups that had backed the revolution. The new government turned to Cuba, then the Soviet bloc, for military supplies, advisers, and health and education aid—although western Europe, other Latin Americans, Japan, and Canada also sent much economic help.

From the start, Reagan's policy seemed to aim at either overthrowing the Sandinistas (make them cry "uncle," as the president said at one news conference) or forcing them to share power with U.S.-financed "Contras," who had begun fighting the government in 1981. Key Contra military leaders had belonged to Somoza's regime, but the United States—contrary to its own laws—allowed them to train in Florida to prepare to overthrow a government that Washington itself recognized. In November 1981, the president signed a secret order permitting the CIA to spend at least $19 million to train and lead the Contras. The United States also built large bases in Honduras from which the Contras could launch attacks and where up to 30,000 U.S. soldiers and sailors carried out maneuvers after 1983 to frighten the Sandinistas. The president called the Contras "freedom fighters" and compared them to the "founding fathers" of 1776. The *Boston Globe*, noting the many reports of how Contras destroyed health facilities and killed women and children in their attacks, called them "an unlikely collection of cattle rustlers, terrorists, members of a discredited dictatorship, profiteers [whose leaders lived comfortably in Miami] and mercenaries." The CIA privately called them its "unilaterally controlled Latin assets."[59]

But the CIA and the Contras could not deliver a victory. Bitter disputes erupted within the Reagan administration between State Department area experts, who believed that Sandinista power could be better (and certainly more cheaply) contained through diplomatic negotiations, and other civilians—especially in the Pentagon and the White House—who favored escalating the fighting. The U.S. military, fearing another Vietnam and considering Nicaragua a small sideshow, mostly agreed with the State Department. In 1983, Reagan tried to quiet this fight in Washington by appointing a special commission, headed by Henry Kissinger, to investigate the problem. The commission recommended increased aid to the Contras, continued support of the Salvadoran government (but tied to demands that the Salvadorans quit killing political opponents), and a massive aid program to rebuild the war-devastated Central American nations. Reagan followed the first recommendation, tied aid to human rights only after Congress forced him to do so, and failed to work out any effective economic-aid program. The CIA finally took matters into its own hands in late 1983 by mining Nicaraguan harbors and attacking oil and airport facilities. An angry Congress responded by cutting off military aid to the Contras in

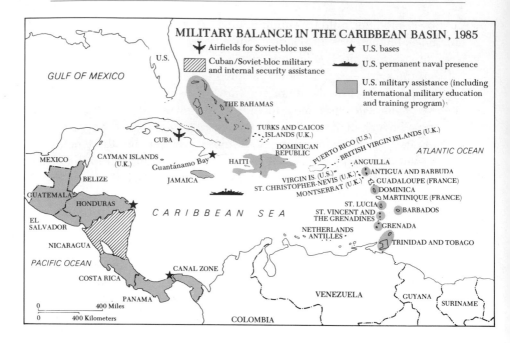

MILITARY BALANCE IN THE CARIBBEAN BASIN, 1985

✈ Airfields for Soviet-bloc use   ★ U.S. bases

▨ Cuban/Soviet-bloc military and internal security assistance   ⬛ U.S. permanent naval presence

⬛ U.S. military assistance (including international military education and training program)·

1984. Reagan officials retaliated by publicly encouraging private Americans to send money for the overthrow of the Nicaraguan government and by diverting CIA and other funds to the same effort.

Nevertheless, the Sandinistas stopped the Contras in the field and held an election in 1984 that many observers (but not U.S. officials) considered open and fair. Sandinista leader Daniel Ortega Saavedra was elected president. In 1985, Ortega imposed martial law on the land, held as many as 4,000 political prisoners (critics claimed that there were 12,000 such prisoners), and closed opposition media. Washington's policy seemed to be at a dead end. "None of our options hold much promise," a U.S. official gloomily concluded in 1985.[60] But Reagan doggedly continued to pressure Congress for Contra military aid, and in 1986 he won. As the Nicaraguan economy suffered from Sandinista mismanagement and U.S. strangulation (Reagan succeeded in cutting off nearly all international lending to Managua, except for Soviet-bloc aid), the Contras' numbers grew. They, nevertheless, had little chance of defeating the well-trained, experienced Sandinista army, and suffered 400 dead and wounded each month by 1987.

One hope for peace suddenly appeared in mid-1987, when President Oscar Arias Sanchez of Costa Rica convinced the other four Central American presidents (including Ortega) to sign a peace plan. It included (1) a cease-fire throughout the region; (2) negotiations between governments and rebels, especially in El Salvador and Nicaragua; (3) a cutoff of aid from outside sources to rebel forces (that is, a cutoff of U.S. aid to the Contras and Soviet-bloc aid to the FMLN in El Salvador); and (4) the promise that all nations would move toward elections and "political pluralism." Arias won the 1987 Nobel Prize for Peace, but Reagan was much less impressed. He objected that the plan allowed the Soviets to continue helping the Sandinista government. (It also allowed him to continue helping the Salvadoran government.) He believed that the Sandinistas would never accept real political pluralism. When Reagan consequently insisted on more military aid for the 10,000 to 12,000 Contras, Arias warned that such aid could destroy all hopes for peace because the Sandinistas would never allow more freedom within if they were so threatened from without. Arias announced that "the contras . . . are the problem, and not the solution."[61]

The peace process edged along, but Reagan and other Contra supporters determined to keep the rebels alive and fighting—by private gifts, if necessary. Meanwhile, the war that had already taken 40,000 Nicaraguan lives between 1981 and 1987 stopped in early 1988 as the Contras and Sandinistas began peace talks. North Americans now faced the question of whether they would continue to try to impose their policies on their "backyard" as they had throughout the twentieth century, or whether—since those policies had not prevented the worst death and destruction in 350 years of the region's history—they would allow, for the first time in the twentieth century, Central Americans such as Arias and Ortega to determine Central American affairs.

U.S. officials' fixation on Nicaragua gave them little time to deal with other dangers in the region. Reagan's policy turned Honduras into a huge staging base for U.S.-Contra operations. The second poorest nation in the hemisphere, this one-time "banana republic" lived less by bananas than by U.S. aid (which soared from $3 million annually to over $100 million in seven years) and by catering to the American military's need for places of relaxation and prostitution. Terrorism and anti-U.S. protests broke out for the first time in the 1980s, but the Honduran army maintained order. Elsewhere, the Reaganites bragged that ten Latin American military rulers gave way to democratic governments during the 1980s. Such rushes of democracy were not new: they had appeared in the late 1950s, only to revert to military control within a decade. Credit was, nevertheless, due in the 1980s to Carter's human-rights policies, Reagan's preaching about the need for democracy, and the Latin American military's realization that it could no longer govern the economically sick system in such pivotal nations as Brazil and Argentina.

But this apparent turn toward democracy hid the time bomb that was ticking throughout the region. Latin American nations (led by the giants Brazil, Argentina, and Mexico) owed hundreds of billions of dollars for debts that had piled up during the 1960s and 1970s. To pay the debts meant taking resources out of their own populations and perhaps causing revolts. Not paying the debts threatened the U.S. banks and international lenders that made the loans. Per-capita Latin American income sank 10 percent between 1980 and 1988. Inflation raged at over 150 percent annually in Mexico, Brazil, and Argentina. Growth rates plummeted as population (especially of those under age sixteen) rose. The Reagan administration at first trusted the marketplace to find solutions. When that failed, it could come up with nothing else to turn off the ticking bomb. One of Brazil's solutions was to become a leading arms dealer, making fat profits by selling weapons to nations (such as Libya) that Reagan strongly disliked.[62]

In one tiny Caribbean island, however, Reagan had his way. Grenada had become independent of Great Britain in 1974, then was ruled by a highly corrupt anti-Communist regime until 1979, when Maurice Bishop forcefully replaced it with a leftist government that soon cooperated with Fidel Castro. Between 1981 and 1983, Bishop opened secret talks with the United States. He offered to call elections and discuss Washington's concerns, but Reagan finally refused to talk with Bishop in mid-1983. When a more radical Bernard Coard overthrew and killed Bishop, then fired into pro-Bishop protesters, U.S. officials determined to invade. The official reason for the October 25, 1983, invasion was to protect 595 U.S. medical students supposedly endangered by Coard's forces. The more important reason was the opportunity to use U.S. fire power quickly and successfully on behalf of the Reagan Doctrine—especially after 241 U.S. troops had been killed by terrorists two days before in Lebanon. The invasion, however, suffered embarrassing problems of logistics and a failure of the Eighty-second Airborne Division (supposedly the crack U.S. fighting force) to overcome 700 Cuban engineers who fought back. American troops even discovered that they had to use 1977 tourist maps that had such points of interest as nutmeg factories on it instead of the grid coordinates needed in battle. After the invasion force was increased from 1,900 to 6,000, had lost 19 dead (116 wounded), and had killed 24 Cubans and 45 Grenadan soldiers, it finally conquered the island.[63]

By the late 1980s, the good-neighbor policy was only a historical memory. As historian Mark T. Gilderhus observes, "Unlike Carter administration officials who understood the [Latin American] problem as a North-South issue pitting the less-developed against the developed world, the Reagan administration presented the turmoil as an East-West issue. Indeed, [to Reagan] it appeared as a classic Cold War confrontation conducted by surrogates in which the Communists sought strategic advantage by destabilizing countries on the southern flank of the United States. . . ." Twenty-five years after the Alliance for Progress had begun in 1961, the head of the Organization of American States declared, "On the whole, the region is worse off than it was 25 years ago."[64]

THE REAGAN DOCTRINE, THE MIDDLE EAST, AND THE IRAN-CONTRA AFFAIR

U.S. policy struggled in Latin America. But "in the history of the American Republic it is unlikely that any issue of foreign relations has confounded and frustrated the nation's policy makers more completely, repeatedly, and over a longer period of time than the problems of the Middle East in the years since World War II," as historian Seth Tillman observes.[65] Washington officials had never been able to figure out how to achieve all—or even any—of their objectives: Israel's security; Egypt's stability and acceptance as a leader by other Arab nations; self-determination and a territorial settlement accepted by millions of displaced Palestinians; placating the strong anti-Israeli feelings in oil-rich Arab kingdoms, especially Saudi Arabia; and containment of Soviet influence, particularly as it worked through Syria, which disliked Egypt and hated Israel. It was a minefield of religious, racial, and national rivalries that could explode instantly.

One explosion had occurred in 1982. The Palestine Liberation Organization (PLO) had finally settled in Lebanon. The PLO was involved in skirmishes along the border with Israel, then shot the Israeli ambassador to Great Britain. In June 1982, Israel invaded Lebanon, drove out the PLO, and tried to establish a friendly Maronite Christian regime. But Lebanese politics collapsed, and brutalities escalated. Secretary of State Shultz and President Reagan sent in U.S. troops to work with western Europeans in enforcing a cease-fire. The Israelis found themselves entrapped. They were attacked by Shiite Moslems and then shocked by bloody Christian massacres of Palestin-

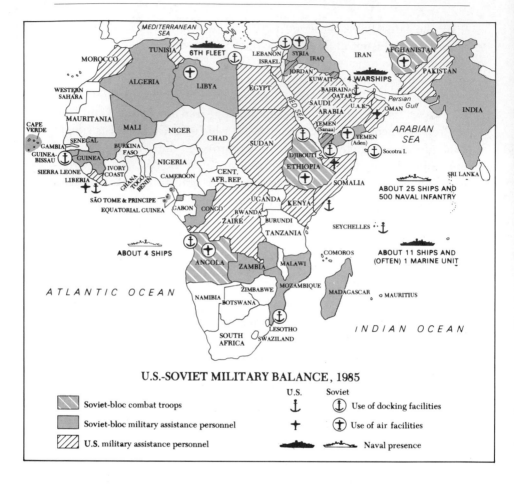

U.S.-SOVIET MILITARY BALANCE, 1985

	U.S.	Soviet	
▨ Soviet-bloc combat troops	⚓	⊕	Use of docking facilities
▦ Soviet-bloc military assistance personnel	✚	✚⊕	Use of air facilities
▨ U.S. military assistance personnel	▬	▬	Naval presence

Map labels include: MEDITERRANEAN SEA, TUNISIA, 6TH FLEET, LEBANON, SYRIA, IRAQ, IRAN, AFGHANISTAN, MOROCCO, ISRAEL, JORDAN, KUWAIT, PAKISTAN, ALGERIA, LIBYA, EGYPT, BAHRAIN, QATAR, 4 WARSHIPS, WESTERN SAHARA, SAUDI ARABIA, U.A.E., OMAN, Persian Gulf, INDIA, MAURITANIA, MALI, NIGER, CHAD, YEMEN (Sanaa), YEMEN (Aden), ARABIAN SEA, CAPE VERDE, GAMBIA, SENEGAL, BURKINA FASO, SUDAN, DJIBOUTI, Socotra I., GUINEA-BISSAU, GUINEA, NIGERIA, ETHIOPIA, SRI LANKA, IVORY COAST, SIERRA LEONE, LIBERIA, GHANA, TOGO, BENIN, CAMEROON, CENT. AFR. REP., SOMALIA, ABOUT 25 SHIPS AND 500 NAVAL INFANTRY, SÃO TOMÉ & PRINCIPE, EQUATORIAL GUINEA, GABON, CONGO, UGANDA, KENYA, RWANDA, BURUNDI, SEYCHELLES, ZAIRE, TANZANIA, ABOUT 11 SHIPS AND (OFTEN) 1 MARINE UNIT, ABOUT 4 SHIPS, ANGOLA, ZAMBIA, MALAWI, COMOROS, ATLANTIC OCEAN, ZIMBABWE, MOZAMBIQUE, MADAGASCAR, MAURITIUS, NAMIBIA, BOTSWANA, INDIAN OCEAN, SOUTH AFRICA, LESOTHO, SWAZILAND

ians in Israeli-controlled camps. A shaken Menachem Begin resigned as Israel's prime minister.

Afraid that the chaos and Israeli withdrawal would permit Syria to move into Lebanon, Reagan—who had said in early 1983 that he wanted to "expedite" the departure of the U.S. forces in the region—implied that the troops would remain as long as necessary to restore order. In April 1983, despite (or because of) their presence, a powerful bomb wrecked the U.S. Embassy in Beirut, killing 46 people, including 16 Americans. Reagan had condemned earlier presidents for sending U.S. troops into Vietnam "with one hand tied behind them." But he now placed the Marines in a virtually indefensible position on the outskirts of Beirut. On October 23, 1983, Moslem terrorists drove a vehicle packed with explosives into the marines' barracks and killed 241 men. Reagan declared that "the United States will not be intimidated by terrorists" and later announced that Americans would never "cut and run."[66] But the marine position could not be defended, U.S. policy was bankrupt, and the president faced a re-election campaign. In early 1984, he pulled out the troops. Lebanon became a chaotic battlefield.

Another explosion in the region had occurred in 1980, when Iraq's Sunni Moslem government attacked Khomeini's Shiite Moslems in neighboring Iran. The United States sympathized with Iraq, but neither side could defeat the other despite exceptionally brutal and bloody fighting. By 1985, however, Iranian-backed terrorists had seized a number of U.S. hostages in the Middle East, including State Department and CIA personnel. In 1979–1981, Carter had negotiated with the Iranians to gain the release of U.S. hostages. But Reagan swore loudly and often (especially when running against Carter in 1980 and Carter's former vice-president, Walter Mondale, in the 1984 election) that he would never "be intimidated by terrorists" or negotiate with them. His passion rose higher as Americans died in terrorist attacks on airplanes, airports, and even cruise ships.

In August–September 1985, however, the president worked through Israel to send TOW antitank missiles and other military equipment to

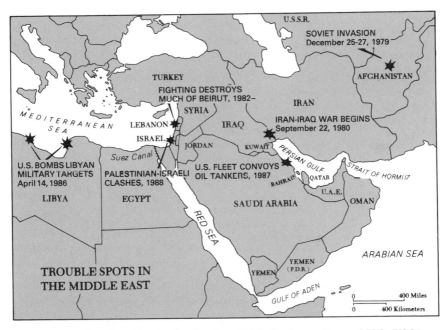

The Middle East became the focal point of U.S. foreign policy and U.S.-USSR competition in the 1980s, much as central Europe and then Asia had been such focal points in the 1940s, 1950s, and 1960s.

Khomeini's regime in a highly secret operation. Clearly, the shipments were sent to gain the release of hostages. As the weapons continued to flow to Iran in several shipments over the next fourteen months, some hostages were released. But new ones were then seized. Under Reagan's orders, his NSC adviser, Robert McFarlane, secretly went to Tehran (carrying, for some reason, gifts of a chocolate cake and a Bible) to negotiate with the Iranians. Nothing resulted. When the weapons shipments and mission were revealed in November 1986 by a Lebanese journal, Reagan told stunned Americans that the policy was aimed at opening contact with Iranian "moderates," although who the moderates might be in Khomeini's fundamentalist regime was never made clear. It turned out, moreover, that the president had followed the arms-for-hostages policy despite strong protests from Secretary of State Shultz and Secretary of Defense Weinberger.

Three weeks after this revelation, Attorney General Edwin Meese announced that money obtained from the arms sales to Iran had been secretly sent to the Contras for use in Nicaragua. This diversion of funds had occurred in 1985–1986 despite Congress's ban on the sending of lethal aid to the Contras. The scheme was apparently the brainchild of William Casey, head of the CIA, whose budget was rising even faster than the Defense Department's budget. The CIA was literally out of both the president's and Congress's control. Casey worked through Lieutenant Colonel Oliver North, an aide in the White House NSC who had fought in Vietnam and was haunted by the U.S. failure.[67] North determined that such a failure would never occur in Central America. Working with Casey as well as with General Manuel Antonio Noriega, head of the Panamanian government (and later indicted as a leading international drug trafficker), North directed secret supply missions to the Contras. Some equipment was paid for by Iranian arms sales, others by North's effective multimillion-dollar fund-raising among conservative Americans.

During the summer of 1987, joint Senate and House special committees conducted nationally televised hearings on the schemes. As they organized, a special commission headed by former Texas Republican Senator John Tower, which Reagan had asked to investigate the role of the White House in the Iran-Contra affair, made its report. The Tower commission concluded that the NSC staff was responsible for the chaotic policy and that the president was out of touch with the foreign policies of his own White House. The House-Senate investigation confirmed much of the Tower commission's report. North testified that he had largely worked under Casey's direction, but he had also kept the new NSC director, Admiral John Poindexter, informed of the plan. Poindexter testified that he never told the president about the diversion plan. Casey never testified at all. He had died of a brain tumor months earlier and took to the grave whatever he had told his close friend Ronald Reagan about the plan.

North became a hero to much of the television audience for his defense of the Reagan Doctrine, even if the defense meant breaking the law. His attractiveness wore off, however, as second thoughts appeared. North, after all, admitted that he had illegally destroyed government documents that might have contained damning evidence. He also admitted that he had made statements to Congress that were "false," "evasive and wrong." The *Army Times* condemned North for having "paraded a travesty of military values before a credulous national television audience." Retired Colonel Harry Summers damned North and the others for selling weapons to Iran that might well be used against U.S. soldiers, and for starting down the "slippery slope" by placing their wishes above those of Congress or the president—"for at the bottom of that slope is military dictatorship" in the United States.[68]

The State Department's point man on Central America, Assistant Secretary of State Elliott Abrams, had also lied to Congress when he told it, in November 1986, that no third-party funds were going to the Contras, even though he personally had begged for some of those funds from the sultan of Brunei. Abrams became an outcast on Capitol Hill (Minnesota Republican Senator David Durenberger said that he would trust Abrams no further "than I can throw Oliver North"), but Reagan and Shultz kept him in the State Department. Democratic congressman Lee Hamilton from Indiana, chairman of the House investigation committee, summarized the affair by declaring that the "policy was driven by a series of lies— . . . lies to our friends and allies, lies to the Congress, and lies to the American people." Hamilton concluded that "the policy achieved none of the goals it sought. The Ayatollah got his arms, more Americans are held hostage today [and] subversion of U.S. interests throughout the region by Iran continues."[69] Reagan's confusion throughout the three-year affair was exemplified when reporters asked him if the late William Casey had engaged in secret CIA activities without the president's knowledge. Reagan replied, "Not that I know of." In the end, 11 members of the Reagan administration were convicted or pleaded guilty. Two of these convictions (including North's) were overturned on technical grounds. Several others were saved from trial by presidential pardons issued by George Bush.[70]

But he was not finished with the Middle East. In early 1987, his administration concluded that Iran threatened the oil exports of Kuwait (which was pro-Iraq in the Iran-Iraq war). The Kuwaiti exporters depended on free movement of their tankers through the Persian Gulf. The president put Kuwaiti tankers under the American flag and used a U.S. fleet to protect them against attacks by Iranian gunboats. Behind that decision lay Reagan's and Shultz's determination to reassert their power in the region as well as to try to intimidate Khomeini. Reagan had been told that the nine U.S. warships in the area were sufficient for the job. Within two months, however, he had to send forty-one combat vessels to the region and spend $10 million to $20 million each day on the operation. Even then, the Iranians disabled a number of U.S. and non-U.S. flagships. Americans and Iranians were virtually at war with each other. In 1987, a missile from Iraq—which Reagan was supporting in its war with Iran—killed 37 sailors on a U.S. ship. In mid-1988, a U.S. naval commander mistook an Iranian airliner for an attack jet and shot it down, killing 290 innocent civilians. The passageway was kept open, and the U.S. Navy, with the help of a few allies, continued to carry off a difficult and dangerous task. Critics believed that, given Iranian policy and naval strength, the passage would have remained open without such a U.S. commitment.[71]

REAGAN, THE SOULLESS EMPIRE, AND THE INF TREATY

The president viewed all foreign policy through the telescope of the U.S.-Soviet conflict. Like nearly all Americans, he despised and belittled the Soviet system. "Sometimes I think Adam and Eve must have been Russian," he repeatedly told audiences. "They didn't have a roof over their heads, nothing to wear, only one apple between them, and they called it paradise." In more serious moments in the 1960s he said he would refuse even to negotiate with them because "how do you compromise with men who say we have no soul, there is no hereafter, there is no God?" Critics replied that talks were necessary simply because although each side had the nuclear weapons to incinerate the other, neither had the power or resources to impose its will on the other.

Reagan received little contrary advice from his closest advisers. William Clark served as NSC adviser during much of the president's first term, and while he was a close personal friend, Clark knew little about foreign policy and had even less experience in it. His one conviction was that the Soviet Union was "a bizarre and evil episode of history whose last pages are even now being written."[72] Another powerful official, Assistant Secretary of Defense Richard Perle, had more sophisticated views, but they ended up at the same place: the Soviets could be handled through a major arms build-up; no serious talks should be held on arms control and little talk held on anything else except human rights inside the Soviet Union. Not one top Reagan official between 1981 and 1984 had significant experience dealing with the Soviet Union.

By 1983, Reagan's policies were beset by at least two contradictions. If, as he planned, he did exert immediate short-term pressure against Moscow, he had to do it through economic sanctions. Military build-ups took time, and no responsible official considered threatening Brezhnev with nuclear war. To exert economic pressure effectively, however, required extensive government controls in the marketplace— exactly the kind of controls that Reagan had promised to avoid. Condemning Carter's grain embargo and turnoff of some high-technology items in 1980, Reagan promised American voters that he would impose no such restraints. After hesitating, he did lift the grain embargo. When, however, the Communist government in Poland imposed martial law in late 1981 to control economic crisis and loud political dissent from the Solidarity labor movement, Reagan stopped food shipments to the Poles. He found himself fattening the Soviets and starving the Poles. When he did allow goods to go into Poland again, the president's right-wing supporters damned him for trading with the Communists. Reagan discovered that he could not fight communism without compromising his free-enterprise principles.

But a second contradiction also existed. When he tried to pressure the Soviets by stopping the sale of U.S. high-tech and oil-gas drilling equipment to them, his closest allies in western Europe and Japan continued to send these items to the Soviets. These allies considered the Soviets' gas and oil supplies to be more dependable than the Middle East's. Furious, Reagan tried to stop the trade by intervening in the internal affairs of the allies and met angry reaction. After he replaced Haig in mid-1982, Secretary of State Shultz finally began to change Reagan's and Clark's policies by lifting many of the trade restraints and no longer bothering the allies about the issue. The alliance not only strengthened, but, in 1987, U.S. business was selling new items such as personal computers to Moscow, and, in turn, the Soviets signed a long-term agreement to buy American grain.

As he began running for re-election in 1984, Reagan had not scored one important diplomatic success. During the previous year, his announced intention of building SDI (Star Wars) and, in September 1983, the Soviet shooting-down of South Korean Airliner 007, which

Major reasons for détente. The dot in the center square represents all of the fire power used in World War II, including the atomic bombs dropped on Hiroshima and Nagasaki. The 6,000 dots in the rest of the squares represent the comparative destructive power of the nuclear weapons that existed in the 1980s. Just two squares on the chart represent enough fire power to destroy all of the large- and medium-sized cities of the world.

killed 269 including a U.S. congressman, poisoned superpower relations. The Soviets claimed that the airliner, which was 350 miles off course, had intentionally strayed over some of their most sensitive military installations for the purposes of U.S. intelligence. The president countered that it was not an intelligence mission, and even if it had strayed off course, the Soviets should never have fired on a civilian airliner. U.S.-USSR relations reached their lowest point since the worst days of the cold war in the early 1950s.

Then, as both sides began to worry about rushing down a dead-end road that ended in a superpower confrontation, they searched for side exits. Reagan began softening his rhetoric. "The fact that neither of us likes the other system is no reason to refuse to talk," he noted in early 1984, which he then defined as "a year of opportunities for peace."[73] Not wanting to frighten Americans during an election year, the president also declared that his military build-up had reached the point where negotiations could now be profitably held. (He, doubtless, also realized that major budget problems prevented any such future arms build-up.) Shultz's State Department fought endless battles to check Perle and others in the Pentagon and White House who wanted to ignore the informal SALT II arms limits (signed in 1979) and to force the allies to get tough with Moscow. On at least two occasions, Shultz kept Reagan on the path to negotiations by threatening to resign if the president ditched efforts to cap the arms race.

By 1985, the Soviets were also ready to talk. During the three years after Brezhnev's death in 1982, they had endured two more elderly, ill leaders. After they died, fifty-four-year-old Mikhail Gorbachev came to power in early 1985. Trained as a lawyer and an agricultural expert, he had no personal ties to the Stalinist years (as had his three predecessors) and slowly but surely brought to power others of his age and outlook. Gorbachev's policy was driven by several insights. He realized that the Soviet economy could not continue business as usual. It had fallen behind Japan as well as the United States and was slipping so badly that it had begun to resemble a poor African economy—"an Upper Volta with missiles," as even Gorbachev allegedly remarked. Few worked hard or imaginatively, drunkenness abounded, productivity dived. Industry had been denuded of investment capital to pay for the military build-up during the 1960s and 1970s. Gorbachev determined not to tinker, but to begin fundamental restructuring (or *perestroika*). He planned to do it by lessening tensions, curbing military deployments, and opening the society to outside competitiveness (or *glasnost*). These decisions led to Gorbachev's second insight: the United States had also declined in economic power and no longer served (as it had during the Nixon years, for example) as the single source of high technology and expertise needed by the Soviets. He could find better and more dependable sources of such technology in Japan and West Germany. But even a declining America could offer something no one else could match: a break in the arms race and overall improvement in super-power relations so that Gorbachev could concentrate on the top priority of reviving the Soviet economy and society.[74]

In 1983, the Soviets had walked out of arms talks in Geneva because Reagan had insisted on continuing to deploy intermediate Pershing IIs and cruise missiles in western Europe (see p. 685). By early 1985, however, the Kremlin returned to the talks. In April, Gorbachev made the first of several proposals to cap, then cut back, the intermediate missile forces on both sides in Europe. At Geneva during November 1985, in the first summit meeting in six years, the two men agreed in principle on an intermediate-force (INF) deal, renewed cultural and academic exchanges, created a Risk Reduction Center to analyze how to avoid risks of a nuclear war, and decided to cooperate to prevent the spread of nuclear forces. The summit marked a giant step forward for both sides. At a hastily convened second summit in Reykjavík, Iceland, in October 1986, an INF deal was nearly struck until Gorbachev wanted it linked to some limits on the SDI program. Reagan refused; the talks collapsed. Gorbachev was bitter, especially as relations threatened to refreeze. The Soviet leader believed he had been misled by the Americans. In a Politburo meeting (whose minutes were only declassified in 1993), Gorbachev declared, "Yes, Reagan appears a liar." But he nonetheless urged his Soviet colleagues not to "stop before [taking] the most decisive measures."[75] Gorbachev, however, needed immediate relief for an economy staggering under Communist inefficiency, and that meant, in turn, imposing some kind of controls on military spending.

In early 1987, he dropped the linkage between limiting INF and his demand for limits on Reagan's beloved SDI program. The two superpowers agreed to a heretofore unimaginable deal: a "double-zero option"—that is, the elimination of both intermediate missiles (600 to 3,400 miles) and short-range missiles (300 to 600 miles). Perle and other hard-liners had actually suggested the "double-zero option" during 1981–1982 negotiations in the firm belief that the Soviets would never accept it. Gorbachev not only accepted it, but agreed to historic verification measures in which, for the first time, officials and scientists on each side were to inspect the other side's highly sensitive military and scientific installations.[76]

At a third summit, in Washington during December 1987, Gorbachev and Reagan signed the historic agreement. It marked the first time that the actual number of nuclear weapons had been reduced (about 4 percent of all such missiles) and that an entire class of arms had been dismantled. The Soviets took out about 1,500 of their warheads from Europe; the United States, less than half that number. The two leaders made much of the completed INF treaty at their summit meeting in Moscow in May 1988. The summit produced no other major result, although it was the leaders' fourth such meeting in just three years.

Hope also rose that superpower clashes in the newly emerging nations would now cool. As a top State Department official noted, Gorbachev had told the Twenty-seventh Party Congress earlier in 1987 that Soviet friends in the Third World must build socialism "mainly by their own efforts." Gorbachev made no specific offers of military and economic help to those nations.[77] The Soviet leader clearly wanted to get out of Afghanistan (while protecting USSR security interests). At the Washington summit, he even told Reagan that he was willing to discuss a

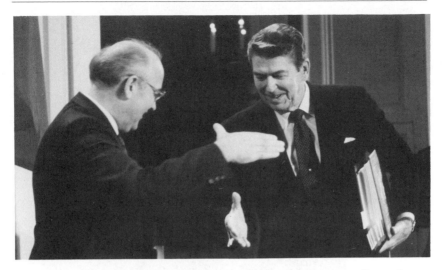

Soviet leader Mikhail Gorbachev (1931–) flew to Washington in December 1987, worked the press and U.S.-citizens-in-the-street like a talented American politician, then shook hands with President Reagan after the two men signed the INF (Intermediate Nuclear Force) treaty that removed both nations' intermediate nuclear weapons from central Europe.

cutoff of Soviet aid to the Sandinistas in Nicaragua. Reagan made no response to the offer.

LEGACIES OF THE 1980s

The post-1985 events were the most hopeful in years. If the ardent anti-Communist wing in American politics (represented by Reagan) and a younger Soviet leadership realizing the necessity of reconciling foreign hopes to domestic needs (as represented by Gorbachev) could strike such deals, the future could be more promising and exciting for young Americans and Soviets than ever before in the history of U.S.-Soviet competition. But the obstacles seemed huge. For more than a century, Americans had not gotten along with Russians, whether those Russians were under Communist or tsarist rule. Moreover, the earth was a revolving powder keg. Its inhabitants spent $930 billion—or $1.8 million per minute—on military goods in 1987. Americans accounted for $293 billion of this amount, the USSR $260 billion. A single U.S. Trident submarine, armed with twenty-four missiles, alone carried the destructive force of eight World War II conflicts.[78] In other parts of the

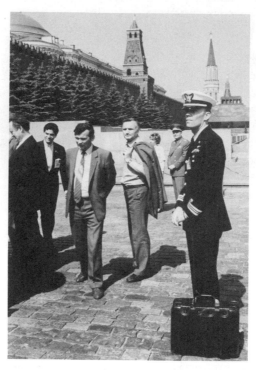

*This photo, taken while President Reagan met with Gorbachev in Moscow dur-
ing the May–June 1988 summit, nicely captures both the progress of U.S.-Soviet
relations in the mid-1980s and the irony of the nuclear competition between the
superpowers. Lieutenant Commander Woody Lee is manacled by a leather
strap to the briefcase (known as "the football") that contains the codes to be
used by President Reagan if he decides to launch nuclear weapons. Lee, whose
job it is to be close to the president at all times and to protect "the football" with
his life, is standing in Moscow's Red Square—on which, presumably, many of
the U.S. nuclear missiles are targeted.*

world, and even in the United States, the gap widened between rich
and poor.

As the world's leading power, Americans had their own problems in
dealing with this complex, explosive planet. When Americans celebrated the bicentennial of their Constitution (the world's oldest such
written charter), they suffered the embarrassment of watching an inept
imperial executive out of control in the Iran-Contra scandal and a
Congress unable to supervise foreign policy because of the splintering
of the entire political-party system. And although Americans depended
increasingly on foreign nations for goods and even economic survival,
polls showed them to be abysmally ignorant of national and interna-

tional affairs. In 1925, Walter Lippmann had predicted that Americans would fail in this task: "The public will arrive in the middle of the third act and will leave before the last curtain, having stayed just long enough perhaps to decide who is the hero and the villain of the piece."[79]

But Americans faced another problem as well. After enjoying the luxury of applying their unchallenged economic resources to dealing with both their internal and external problems throughout the twentieth century, they suddenly found this power wasting away in the 1970s and 1980s. The world's great moneybags between 1914 and 1970, the United States, after 1971, lost much of its ability to compete in the world marketplace and then, between 1981 and 1987, shockingly turned into the world's greatest debtor.[80] The legacies of the Reagan years were both hopeful and ominous.

Notes

1. Paul Boller, Jr., *Presidential Anecdotes* (New York, 1981), p. 340.
2. The quote and a good analysis of the effect is in Gerald Pomper *et al.*, *The Election of 1976* (New York, 1977), p. 68.
3. Jimmy Carter, *Keeping Faith* (New York, 1982), p. 80.
4. *New York Times*, 14 November 1978, p. 14; the best analysis of interest-group politics is Theodore Lowi's *End of Liberalism* (New York, 1979); William Lee Miller, *Yankee from Georgia: The Emergence of Jimmy Carter* (New York, 1978), pp. 82–83 for the "Jimmyist" reference.
5. Cyrus Vance, *Hard Choices* (New York, 1983), esp. pp. 23–24.
6. Zbigniew Brzezinski, *Power and Principle* (New York, 1982), pp. 8, 42–44; Richard Burt, "Zbig Makes It Big," *New York Times Magazine*, 30 July 1978, p. 20; Stanley Hoffmann, "In Search of a Foreign Policy," *New York Review of Books*, 29 September 1983, p. 51.
7. Quoted in Hedrick Smith, "Problems of a Problem Solver," *New York Times Magazine*, 8 January 1978, pp. 30 ff.
8. Interview of Don Oberdorfer, *Washington Post*, 18 February 1979, p. C4.
9. Richard E. Neustadt and Ernest R. May, *Thinking in Time: The Uses of History for Decision-Makers* (New York, 1986), p. 68; the Notre Dame speech is in U.S. Government, *Public Papers of the Presidents of the United States: Jimmy Carter, 1977*, Book 2 (Washington, D.C., 1978), pp. 954–962.
10. Carter, p. 112; *Washington Post*, 16 March 1979, p. 1; Richard J. Barnet, *The Alliance: America-Europe-Japan, Makers of the Postwar World* (New York, 1983), pp. 385–386, 388–390.
11. *New Yorker*, 1 May 1978, p. 109; Barnet, pp. 372–377; for a good overview of early trilateralism, see the *Washington Post*, 16 January 1977, p. A1; a useful background

on the Pershing II decision is Fred Kaplan's "How Politics Led to the Euromissiles," *Boston Globe*, 8 March 1987, p. 1.

12. Carter, pp. 142–143.

13. *New York Times*, 13 February 1981, p. A8.

.14. Tom J. Farer, "Reagan's Latin America," *New York Review of Books*, 19 March 1981, p. 15; Banning Garrett and Mark Paul, "Trading on Human Rights," *Inquiry*, 18 September 1978, pp. 1–15.

15. J. Michael Hogan, *The Panama Canal in American Politics* (Carbondale, Ill., 1986), pp. 6–7, 194–195; Carter, pp. 161–162.

16. David Aaron, "Playing with Apocalypse," *New York Times Magazine*, 29 December 1985, p. 26.

17. Thomas J. Noer, *Cold War* and *Black Liberation* (Columbia, Mo., 1985), p. 249; *New York Times*, 14 June 1978, p. A3; Henry Jackson, *From the Congo to Soweto* (New York, 1982), pp. 152–162.

18. Stephen Prince, *Visions of Empire* (New York, 1992), p. 104; the contradictions and hesitations of the Carter policies are revealed by an insider in Robert Pastor's *Condemned to Repetition* (Princeton, 1987), esp. pp. 13–14, 50–66, 74–79, 153–176.

19. Useful overviews are in Gary Sick's *All Fall Down: America's Tragic Encounter with Iran* (New York, 1985), pp. vii–49; Abul Kasim Mansur, "The Crisis in Iran," *Armed Forces Journal International* 116 (January 1979): 27–33.

20. U.S. Government, p. 2221; Vance, p. 323.

21. Brzezinski's view can be found in *Power and Principle*, esp. pp. 355, 388–393; Vance's in *Hard Choices*, esp. pp. 340–341; an insider's expert view is given in Sick, pp. 99–101, 138–140, 160–161.

22. Brzezinski, pp. 474–475; Carter, pp. 452–453.

23. Author's conversation in Moscow, 12 November 1980; *New York Times*, 29 June 1979, p. A6; *New York Times*, 6 November 1977, p. E5; William Pfaff, "Reflections," *New Yorker*, 16 August 1976, p. 58.

24. Both sides are argued succinctly in *Newsweek*, 21 May 1979, p. 43; Fred Kaplan, *The Wizards of Armageddon* (New York, 1983), pp. 377–384; Adam Ulam, *Dangerous Relations: The Soviet Union in World Politics, 1970–1982* (New York, 1983), pp. 236–241.

25. Vance, pp. 388–389; Brzezinski, p. 353; especially important is Melvyn P. Leffler, "From the Truman Doctrine to the Carter Doctrine," *Diplomatic History* 7 (Fall 1983): 245–266; *New York Times*, 22 February 1979, p. A7.

26. *Washington Post*, 2 March 1981, p. A5.

27. Richard K. Betts, *Nuclear Blackmail and Nuclear Balance* (Washington, D.C., 1987), p. 11; Brzezinski, pp. 443–446.

28. Tad Szulc, "Putting Back the Bite in the CIA," *New York Times Magazine*, 6 April 1980, p. 28; Milton Leitenberg, "United States Foreign Policy and the Soviet Invasion of Afghanistan," *Arms Control* 7 (December 1986): 271–290.

29. Gaddis Smith, *Morality, Reason and Power: American Diplomacy in the Carter Years* (New York, 1986), pp. 9, 81–84; *Washington Post*, 27 February 1986, p. A11; *ibid.*, 29 March 1981, p. 82; Jeffrey Richelson, "PD-59, NSDD-1 and the Reagan Strategic Modernization Program," *Journal of Strategic Studies* 6 (June 1983): 125–146. I am especially indebted to Max Miller and Milton Leitenberg for analyses of PD-59 and its links to the Reagan policies.

30. *Washington Post*, 30 July 1980, p. A12, has the polls; Business Week Team, *The*

Decline of U.S. Power (Boston, 1980), p. 15; Boller, p. 344; *Economist*, 14 June 1980, p. 73.

31. Burton I. Kaufman, *The Presidency of James Earl Carter, Jr.* (Laurence, Kan., 1993), p. 179; Business Week Team, pp. 1–2.

32. Text of Reagan's 1980 acceptance speech, *New York Times*, 18 July 1980, p. A8.

33. Irving Howe, quoted in the *New York Times*, 28 December 1980, p. E5.

34. *New York Times*, 14 December 1980, p. E5; Charles Krauthammer columns, *New Republic*, 4 March 1985, p. 25, and 8 September 1986, pp. 17–24.

35. *Boston Globe*, 24 August 1987, p. 15.

36. *Washington Post*, 1 March 1985, p. A7.

37. Terry Deibel, *Presidents, Public Opinion and Power: The Nixon, Carter and Reagan Years* (New York, 1987), p. 48; George F. Custen, *Bio-Pics* (New Brunswick, N.J., 1992), p. 205.

38. I. M. Destler, "Dateline Washington: Life after the Veto," *Foreign Policy* no. 52 (Fall 1983): 181–186; I. M. Destler and Eric Alterman, "Congress and Reagan's Foreign Policy," *Washington Quarterly* 7 (Winter 1984): 91–101; Theodore Lowi, *The Personal President* (Ithaca, N.Y., 1985), pp. 15–20.

39. Strobe Talbott, *The Russians and Reagan* (New York, 1982), pp. 32–33; *Wall Street Journal*, 3 June 1980, p. 1.

40. Jeane J. Kirkpatrick, *Dictatorship and Double Standards* (New York, 1982), esp. pp. 2–52 for the essay; Judith Elwell, "Barely in the Inner Circle: Jeane Kirkpatrick," in *Women in American Foreign Policy*, ed. Edward P. Crapol (New York, 1987), pp. 153–171; John Pearson, "Flawed Rationale," *Business Week*, 6 September 1982, p. 10; an Argentine view is in J. R.-Lallemant, *Malvinas, Norteamèrica en guerra contra Argentina* (Buenos Aires, 1983).

41. *Low Intensity Warfare*, ed. Michael T. Klare and Peter Kornbluh (New York, 1988), p. 3.

42. *New York Times*, 10 January 1984, p. A23. An early, thorough critique of Reagan's defense expenditures is in the various papers in Ronald V. Dellums with R. H. Miller and H. Lee Halterman, *Defense Sense* (Cambridge, Mass., 1983).

43. Union of Concerned Scientists, *The Fallacy of Star Wars* (New York, 1984), p. 28.

44. Jeremy Bernstein, letter, *New York Times Book Review*, 1 December 1985, p. 44; Kaplan, *Wizards of Armageddon*, p. 88; Robert Dallek, *Ronald Reagan: The Politics of Symbolism* (Cambridge, Mass., 1984), pp. 146–147.

45. *Washington Post*, 29 September 1986, p. A2; *New York Times*, 30 November 1984, p. 86; News Release, Office of Assistant Secretary of Defense (Public Affairs), "The Uses of Military Power," 28 November 1984, no. 609–84.

46. Prince, *Visions of Empire*, pp. 117–151.

47. Paul Kennedy, "The (Relative) Decline of America," *Atlantic* 254 (August 1987): esp. 34.

48. *New York Times*, 21 December 1986, p. E11; *New York Times*, 20 May 1987, p. D2; *Washington Post*, 18 June 1985, p. E1.

49. *Washington Post*, 21 May 1987, p. F4; *Economist*, 25 October 1986, p. 13; *New York Times*, 2 February 1986, p. E4.

50. *Washington Post*, 20 October 1987, p. A4; *Washington Post*, 17 January 1986, p. 50.

51. U.S. Government, *Weekly Compilation of Presidential Documents*, XXI, 11 February 1985, pp. 145–146.

52. Talbott, pp. 72–73.

53. Bob Woodward, *Veil: The Secret Wars of the CIA, 1981–1987* (New York, 1987), pp. 50–53.
54. Stephen S. Rosenfeld, "The Guns of July," *Foreign Affairs* 64 (Spring 1986): 701–705; *New York Times*, 21 February 1986, p. A14.
55. Thomas J. Downey, "Reagan's Real Aims in South Africa," *Nation*, 8 February 1986, pp. 138–140; *Washington Post*, 31 July 1986, p. A2.
56. *New York Times*, 26 February 1986, p. A16; a good account of post-1972 U.S. involvement is Raymond Bonner's *Waltzing with a Dictator* (New York, 1987).
57. Garry Wills, *Reagan's America* (New York, 1987), p. 47; Penny Lernoux, "El Salvador's Christian Democrat Junta," *Nation*, 1 December 1980, p. 63; *Washington Post*, 14 October 1981, p. A14.
58. *Washington Post*, 4 January 1988, p. A21, on the return of the death squads; *ibid.*, 12 November 1986, p. A21, on the protests; *ibid.*, 25 January 1982, p. A1; *New York Times*, 5 March 1983, p. 4.
59. *Boston Globe*, 15 May 1987, p. 14; *New York Times*, 28 December 1981, p. A16.
60. The quote is in the *Boston Globe*, 25 January 1985, p. 19; also James Chace, "The End of the Affair," *New York Review of Books*, 8 October 1987, p. 28.
61. *Washington Post*, 10 December 1987, p. A48.
62. Abraham F. Lowenthal, *Partners in Conflict: The U.S. and Latin America* (Baltimore, 1987), pp. 103–130; *New York Times*, 4 January 1988, p. 17; *Washington Post*, 16 June 1985, pp. C1, C4.
63. *New York Times*, 28 October 1983, p. A9, contains the text of Reagan's speech on the invasion; Max Holland's "The Origins of the Problem," *New York Times*, 30 November 1986, p. E15, has important background.
64. *Washington Post*, 19 March 1986, p. A30; Mark T. Gilderhus, "An Emerging Synthesis?" *Diplomatic History* 16 (Summer 1992), 149–150.
65. Seth P. Tillman, *The United States in the Middle East* (Bloomington, Ind., 1982), pp. 275–276.
66. *New York Times*, 9 February 1984, p. A12, has a useful record of Reagan's quotes, 1982 to 1984.
67. Sidney Blumenthal, "Dateline Washington: The Conservative Crackup," *Foreign Policy* 69 (Winter 1987–1988): 183–184.
68. The *Army Times* is quoted in the *Washington Post*, 6 August 1987, p. A20; Summers's views are inserted by Congressman Ronald Dellums in the *Congressional Record*, 100th Cong., 1st sess., 14 July 1987, 133, p. E2885.
69. U.S. Congress, House and Senate Select Committees, 100th Cong., 1st sess., 1987, *Report of the Congressional Committees Investigating the Iran-Contra Affair with Supplemental, Minority, and Additional Views* (Washington, D.C., 1987), esp. pp. 11–22, 195–209, 352–353, 375–384. I am deeply indebted to Max Miller for the copy of this complete report.
70. *Washington Post*, 5 October 1987, p. A2; Scott Spencer, "Laurence Walsh's Last Battle," *New York Times Magazine*, July 4, 1993, pp. 28–33.
71. Michael H. Armacost, "U.S. Policy in the Persian Gulf and Kuwaiti Reflagging," U.S. Department of State, *Current Policy*, no. 978, 16 June 1987; *New York Times*, 2 August 1987, p. 1.
72. The Reagan quotes are in George W. Ball's "White House Roulette," *New York Review of Books*, 8 November 1984, p. 5. The Clark quote is in Steven R. Weisman,

"The Influence of William Clark," *New York Times Magazine*, 14 August 1983, pp. 17–20.

73. *New York Times*, 17 January 1984, p. A9.

74. This section has been especially informed by Paul Marantz's "Gorbachev's Road to Reykjavík and Beyond," ms. in the author's possession (1987), esp. 6–8; and the analysis in the U.S.Congress, Joint Economic Committee, 100th Cong., 1st sess., 1987, *Gorbachev's Economic Plans*, 2 vols. (Washington, D.C., 1987), esp. chs. I, II, IV, VII, and X. I am, again, indebted to Max Miller for making these volumes available.

75. *New York Times*, 8 February 1993, p. A8.

76. *Treaty between the United States of America and the Union of Soviet Socialist Republics on the Elimination of Their Intermediate-Range and Shorter-Range Missiles* (Washington, D.C., 1987), pp. 4–6, 12–18.

77. Michael Armacost, "U.S.-Soviet Relations: Coping with Conflicts in the Third World," U.S. Department of State, *Current Policy*, no. 879, 26 September 1986, p. 3.

78. Ruth Leger Sivard, *World Military Expenditure, 1987–1988*, 12th ed. (Washington, D.C., 1987), pp. 5–9; Coit D. Blacker, *Reluctant Warriors: The United States, the Soviet Union and Arms Control* (New York, 1987), p. 1.

79. Quoted in Steven R. Weisman, "Can the Magic Prevail?" *New York Times*, 29 April 1984, p. 54.

80. Stanley Hoffmann, "The New Orthodoxy," *New York Review of Books*, 16 April 1981, p. 26.

FOR FURTHER READING

See also the notes to this chapter and the General Bibliography at the end of the book; references in those sections are usually not repeated here. *Guide to American Foreign Relations since 1700*, ed. Richard Dean Burns (1983), has some useful sources for the late 1970s. Recent overviews include Warren Cohen, *America in the Age of Soviet Power*, in *The Cambridge History of American Foreign Relations* ed. Warren Cohen (1993); Saul Landau, *The Dangerous Doctrine* (1988); *Estrangement: America and the World*, ed. Sanford J. Ungar, (1986), especially the David Watt essay; Fred Halliday, *The Making of the Second Cold War*, 2d ed. (1986), a critical view; Robert O. Keohane, *Neorealism and Its Critics* (1986), a stimulating framework; two books on the economic dilemmas: Alan Wolfe, *America's Impasse* (1981), and Bernard D. Nossiter, *The Global Struggle for More* (1987); David Green's imaginative *Shaping Political Consciousness: The Language of Politics in America from McKinley to Reagan* (1988); Edmund Muskie *et al.*, *The President, the Congress, and Foreign Policy* (1986).

On the Carter administration, a starting place for a fine overview (and excellent bibliography), is Burton I. Kaufman, *The Presidency of James Earl Carter, Jr.* (1993). Other than the Carter, Brzezinski, and Vance memoirs listed in the notes, David S. McLellan's *Cyrus Vance* (1985) should be read along with Gaddis Smith's work that is noted. *Tri-*

lateralism ed. Holly Sklar (1985), is an important, critical set of essays; Strobe Talbott's *Endgame* (1979) is crucial for the politics of SALT II.

On the Reagan years, Lou Cannon's *President Reagan: The Role of a Lifetime* (1991) is standard; Robert Dallek's *Ronald Reagan* (1984) gives an interpretive overview, as does Michael Schaller's *Reckoning with Reagan* (1992); Michael P. Rogin's *Ronald Reagan: The Movie* (1987) analyzes provocatively the relationship between films and politics; Thomas Ferguson and Joel Rogers's *The Hidden Election . . . 1980* (1981) is special, most notably for Bruce Cumings's essay; Alexander M. Haig, Jr.'s *Caveat* (1984) is a bitter memoir by Reagan's first secretary of state. David K. Kyrig, ed., *Reagan and the World* (1990), has good essays on geographical areas.

On U.S.-Soviet competition and the arms race, Raymond L. Garthoff's *Détente and Confrontation* (1985) is a standard, encyclopedic reference; a respected journalist's view is in Michel Tatu, *Eux et nous: Les relations est-ouest entre deux détentes* (1985); Alexander L. George *et al.*, *U.S.-Soviet Security Cooperation* (1988), provide twenty-one case studies on maintaining balance of power; *The Making of America's Soviet Policy*, ed. Joseph S. Nye (1984), goes far beyond bureaucratic politics; Stephen A. Garrett's *From Potsdam to Poland* (1986) is important, especially in noting the influence of ethnic groups on U.S. policy; Don Oberdorfer, *The Turn* (1991) is by a correspondent with access to top officials; *U.S.-Soviet Relations: The Next Phase*, ed. Arnold L. Horelick (1986), provides analyses by leading experts on key areas of contention. Anthony Arnold's *Afghanistan* (1981) places the invasion in post-1919 perspective; Bruce Jentleson's *Pipeline Politics* (1986) is a pivotal study on the declining U.S. ability to use economic sanctions. Ronald E. Powaski's *March to Armageddon* (1987) surveys the arms race since the outbreak of World War II; Strobe Talbott's *Deadly Gambits* (1984) is a fascinating analysis of nuclear-arms politics inside the early Reagan administration; Stephen J. Cimbala's *The Reagan Defense Program* (1986) has useful statistics and analyses; Ronald V. Dellums, R. H. Miller, and H. Lee Halterman's *Defense Sense* (1983) provides essays with an alternative policy to Reagan's; Robert Scheer's *With Enough Shovels* (1982) contains eye-popping interviews with Reagan and his civil-defense officials; Paul Stares's *Space and National Security* (1987) is standard for SDI and its background; Sidney Drell *et al.*, *The Reagan Strategic Defense Initiative* (1985), gives a useful, critical overview; and Dan Caldwell, *The Dynamics of Domestic Politics and Arms Control* (1991), is on the SALT II debate.

On other specific regions, *Perspectives on a U.S.-Canadian Free Trade Agreement*, ed. Robert M. Stern (1987), is important for an often-overlooked part of U.S. foreign policy. U.S.-European relations are studied in *The Atlantic Alliance and Its Critics*, ed. Robert W. Tucker and Linda Wrigley (1983); Diana Johnstone, *The Politics of Euromissiles* (1985); Antony J. Blinken's *Ally versus Ally* (1987), studies in depth the 1982 gas-pipeline dispute. On the Middle East, William B. Quandt's *Camp David* (1986) and Shibley Telhami, *Power and Leadership . . . : The Path to the Camp David Accords* (1990), are excellent accounts; *The Middle East since Camp David*, ed. Robert D. Freedman (1984), is a valuable overview on all the players; Itamar Rabinovich's *The War for Lebanon* (1984, 1986), is a most useful and important account that stresses the historical context; Cheryl A. Rubenberg's *Israel and the American National Interest* (1986), takes a critical look; Edward Tivnan's *The Lobby: Jewish Political Power and American Foreign Policy* (1987), is on a most effective foreign-policy pressure group; Seymour M. Hersh, *The Samson Option* (1991), is on U.S. policy and Israel's nuclear bomb; R. K. Ramazani's *The U.S. and Iran* (1982), is short but superb, especially on the shah's manipulation of Americans; *The Iranian Revolution and the Islamic Republic*, ed. Nikki R. Keddie and

Eric Hooglund (1986), has important essays on U.S. policies; Robert Huyser's *Mission to Tehran* (1987), is by Carter's last emissary; but start with Michael A. Palmer's overview, *Guardians of the Gulf* (1992), which is on U.S. policy in the Persian Gulf from 1833–1991. On China, Robert G. Sutter's *The China Quandary* (1983) studies 1972 to 1982 with the help of many interviews; Leonard A. Kusnitz's *Public Opinion and Foreign Policy* (1984) ends with 1979 and sees public opinion as crucial in shaping key approaches to China. Robert Shaplen's *The Unfinished Revolution* (1987) should be used with Raymond Bonner's *Waltzing with a Dictator* (1987) to understand U.S.-Philippine relations since the 1960s. There are some excellent studies on U.S.-African relations: Sanford J. Ungar's *Africa* (1985), is a superb overview; Gerald J. Bender *et al.*, *African Crisis Areas and U.S. Foreign Policy* (1985); *Politics and Government in African States*, ed. Peter Duignan and Robert H. Jackson (1987), are on key African nations; Christopher Coker's *The United States and South Africa, 1968–1985* (1986), is a succinct, helpful interpretive survey; Anthony Sampson's *Black and Gold* (1987), is a readable analysis focusing on U.S. corporations in South Africa; David A. Korn's *Ethiopia, the United States, and the Soviet Union* (1986), is on a key problem area, as is Jeffrey A. Lefebvre, *Arms for the Horn: U.S. Security Policy in Ethiopia and Somolia, 1953–1991* (1991).

The material on Latin American relations is rich. Three special studies have informed this chapter: Abraham F. Lowenthal's *Partners in Conflict* (1987) and two books by Lars Schoultz—*Human Rights and U.S. Policy towards Latin America* (1981) and *National Security and U.S. Policy toward Latin America* (1987). *The United States and Latin America in the 1980s*, ed. Kevin J. Middlebrook and Carlos Rico (1986), has Latin American as well as North American views presented; Henry Kissinger's *The Report of the President's National Bipartisan Commission on Central America* (1984) is the administration's view, for the most part; *Central America: Anatomy of Conflict*, ed. Robert S. Leiken (1984), is a detailed criticism of the Kissinger commission's assumptions; PACCA, *Changing Course* (1984), criticizes the Kissinger commission and offers a "blueprint" for an alternative policy; Walter LaFeber's *Inevitable Revolutions: The United States in Central America* (1984, 1993) tries to put Central American policies in the context of two hundred years of U.S. relations with the region; Karl Bermann's *Under the Big Stick* (1985) is a superb volume on the United States and Nicaragua since 1848, as is John Booth's *The End and the Beginning* (1982, 1985); Mary B. Vanderlaan's *Revolution and Foreign Policy in Nicaragua* (1986) beautifully relates internal Nicaraguan change in the 1980s to U.S. policies; *Reagan versus the Sandinistas*, ed. Thomas W. Walker (1987), has excellent essays and is only the latest from Walker, who has also published other important studies in the 1980s on the Sandinistas; E. Bradford Burns's *At War in Nicaragua* (1987) is a readable overview by a dean of U.S. scholars of Latin America; *Trouble in Our Backyard*, ed. Martin Siskin, (1984), has important critical essays, especially those by Womack and Montgomery; *El Salvador: Central America in the New Cold War*, ed. Marvin Gittleman *et al.* (1982), is a valuable collection of documents and essays on the entire region; Tommie Sue Montgomery's *Revolution in El Salvador* (1982) has the best account; David N. Farnsworth and James W. McKenney's *U.S.-Panama Relations, 1903–1978* (1983) is especially strong on Panamanian politics; William J. Jorden's *Panama Odyssey* (1984) is a detailed account by the U.S. ambassador in the 1970s; Michael L. Conniff's *Panama and the United States* (1992) gives a fine overview; Tom Barry *et al.*'s *The Other Side of Paradise: Foreign Control in the Caribbean* (1984) provides an excellent critical perspective; Morris Morley's *Imperial State and Revolution* (1987) is the standard (and provocative) study of the United States and Cuba since the early 1950s; Louis A. Perez, Jr.'s

Cuba and the United States gives the best one-volume overview (1990); Carla Anne Robbins's *The Cuban Threat* (1983) is by a journalist who knows Cuba well; *American Intervention in Grenada*, ed. Peter M. Dunn and Bruce W. Watson (1985), has excellent overview essays, especially by George Quester; Hugh O'Shaughnessy's *Grenada* (1985) is a most valuable critique by a British journalist who was there; Reynold A. Burrowes's *Revolution and Rescue in Grenada* (1988) provides a good account and is kinder to U.S. policy than most; Peter H. Schuck and Rogers M. Smith's *Citizenship without Consent* (1985) has an important legal and historical analysis on illegal aliens. Latin American views are in *Estados Unidos: Una visión latinoamericana*, ed. Luis Maira (1984); *La Política de Reagan y la crisis en Centroamérica*, ed. Luis Maira (1982), a good collection of papers; SELA (Sistema Económico Latinoamericano), *América Latina/Estados Unidos* (1983, 1986), a series on economic relations during the debt crisis; Francisco López Segrera, *El Conflicto Cuba–Estados Unidos y la crisis Centroamericana* (1985), for a larger context. A good account is George D. Moffett III's *The Limits of Victory* (1985), which is on the Panama treaties.

On the Iran-Contra debacle, Theodore Draper's *A Very Thin Line* (1991) is a superb starting place; Malcolm Byrne and Peter Kornbluh, eds., *The Iran-Contra Affair* (1993), has key documents; Joseph E. Persico's *Casey* (1990) is the biography of the CIA director; Caspar Weinberger's autobiography, *Fighting for Peace* (1990), is bland, but George Shultz's autobiography, *Turmoil and Triumph* (1993), is detailed and highly important on the range of 1980s foreign policies as well as on Iran-Contra, which Shultz opposed.

On the growing debate over immigration, starting points include Bill Ong Hing's *Making and Remaking Asian America Through Immigration Policy, 1850–1990* (1992); Barbara M. Yarnold's *Refugees Without Refuge* (1990), which is on U.S. asylum policy; Roger Daniels's *Asian America: Chinese and Japanese in the United States Since 1850* (1988).

20

New World Order to World Disorder: Bush and Clinton (1989–1993)

FROM DOROTHY TO LULA

"We meant to change a nation, and instead we changed a world," Ronald Reagan declared in his televised "farewell address" on January 11, 1989. "Countries across the globe are turning to free markets and free speech." The outgoing president placed this remark into historical context: "I've thought a bit of the shining 'city on a hill.' The phrase comes from John Winthrop, who wrote it [in 1630] to describe the America he imagined. . . . And how stands the city on this winter night? More prosperous, more secure and happy than it was eight years ago."[1]

Some observers were not as certain. *Commonweal*, a Roman Catholic journal, noted that in the president's "farewell" there were "No warnings here . . . . Nothing about racism. Nothing about the global environment. Nothing about national addictiveness, nuclear mismanagement, homelessness, the financial IOU's we are leaving to our children. And certainly nothing about corruption in government or the growing gap between rich and poor." The respected "TRB" column in the sometimes liberal *New Republic* agreed: the last years of Reagan's rule were marked by "an ongoing struggle among advisers for the soul of a man who was virtually brain dead. The fact that things worked out no worse than they did is either a tribute to the institutional sturdiness of the presidency or proof of the existence of God."[2]

These bitter assessments of the most popular president of the previous quarter-century symbolized the mixed legacy of his policies. The oldest person ever to serve as chief executive, Reagan belonged to a cold-war era that began to end after Mikhail Gorbachev gained power in the Soviet Union in 1985–1986. The world suddenly became more complex, unpredictable, even strange—as when Americans and their vigorously anti-Communist president began cooperating with the Soviets on issues that had once bitterly divided them. Popular films again captured some of the transition in American history from an earlier era when, even on the verge of world war, Americans seemed to be more optimistic and certain than they were in the late 1980s. In *The Wizard of Oz*, released in 1939, Dorothy, the Scarecrow, the Tin Man, and the Cowardly Lion journeyed through danger down "the yellow brick road" to find their search fulfilled, their hopes realized. The story was as old and as upbeat as the white settlers' quest for land and political sufficiency in the West during the several previous centuries. Sam Shepard (one of the country's most popular playwrights and actors) and David Lynch (director of the widely watched television show "Twin Peaks" and of several well-known films, especially *Wild at Heart*) showed a much different American character between 1988 and the early 1990s. *Wild at Heart* revealed the former western frontier region now full of characters such as Sailor and Lula, who lacked aim or values and moved through a society that was breaking down. Sailor laments that it is too bad a person "can't just visit that old Wizard of Oz and get some advice." Lula later observes, "Seems we sort of broke down on the yellow brick road."[3] The popularity of Lynch and Shepard seemed difficult to reconcile with President Reagan's confidence that it "is morning in America."

Reagan's successor in the White House, George Bush, did come to symbolize some of the confusion and, finally, the lost hope that Lynch's characters portrayed. George Herbert Walker Bush grew up in a prominent Connecticut family (his father was a wealthy banker and U.S. Senator) during the late 1930s and early 1940s when *The Wizard of Oz* and the political commitments of *Casablanca* were popular. Just turned eighteen when he entered Naval Flight School in 1942, he survived a plane crash in 1944 and continued to fight the Japanese. His historical hero was that most all-American of presidents, Theodore Roosevelt. Bush said he admired TR because Roosevelt had left (as did Bush) a comfortable life in the East to live, and make much of his political fortune, on the frontier, and because he (like Bush), loved "the strenuous life" of outdoor activity and athletics. One of the new president's first acts in 1989 was to hang Roosevelt's portrait in the Cabinet Room of the White House.[4]

Also resembling TR, Bush paid special attention to foreign policy. Few came to the job with a better diplomatic background. After successfully building a fortune in Texas oil, and helping create a Republican party in hostile Texas politics, Bush served in Congress, directed the U.S. Liaison Office in China, was head of the Central Intelligence Agency, and then became Reagan's vice-president—a position from which he helped shape U.S. policy, especially in Latin America and Asia.

One of the few people who could approach the broad political experience Bush brought to the presidency was his new secretary of state, James Baker. A wealthy lawyer from an old Texas family, Baker had helped Bush build the Texas Republican party. He managed Reagan's spectacular 1980 electoral victory, then served as a highly skillful White House chief of staff, secretary of the Treasury, and the brains behind Bush's come-from-behind victory in 1988 over Democratic nominee Michael Dukakis. In the State Department he surrounded himself with a small, young, fiercely loyal staff, only a few of whom had any diplomatic experience. The question became whether, for all their great political abilities, Baker and his young staff had the necessary sense of history and broad vision to deal with the new, incredibly complex, post–cold-war world that suddenly began to take shape.

Despite his experience, Bush proved to be of little help to Baker in working out what the new president called "the vision thing." His first, much-awaited foreign-policy statement in the spring of 1989 only asked for more of the same U.S. policies. A product of the cold-war era, he would be the last president who had served in World War II; he seemed almost reluctant to see the post-1941 era end. Such reluctance was part of a natural caution that restrained Bush from making commitments to fresh policy departures. Part of that reluctance was probably rooted in 1975–1976, the years of Gerald Ford's presidency, when Bush was director of the CIA. His national-security adviser, General Brent Scowcroft, was Ford's NSC adviser, and his secretary of defense, Richard Cheney, served as Ford's White House chief of staff. Bush, Scowcroft, and Cheney never forgot how Ford was associated with the Nixon-Kissinger détente policy toward the Soviets, then lost the 1976 election as détente became a dirty word in American politics (see p. 672). Bush never wanted to repeat that political disaster. A tough, cold-war-like approach seemed safest. "I will never apologize for the United States of America, ever. I don't care what the facts are," he declared in 1988.[5]

"THE END OF THE MIDDLE AGES" IN CENTRAL AMERICA?

In one bloody area, however, Bush did break free of, while learning from, cold-war history. He and Baker realized that Reagan's tough military policies had not resolved the long, terrible wars in Nicaragua, El Salvador, and Guatemala. Those conflicts indeed threatened to infect the other two Central American nations of Costa Rica (the most democratic and literate society in Latin America), and Honduras. Moreover, Americans polled in the 1980s consistently opposed Reagan's use of force. Even Congress had grown tired of this failed approach by the mid-1980s. When Reagan officials tried secretly to avoid Congress's restraints on them, the result—the Iran-Contra debacle (see p. 725)— set off a U.S. political, constitutional, and diplomatic crisis.

Bush and Baker wanted to resolve these Central American problems so they could move on to more profitable and popular diplomatic ventures. They suddenly were doubly blessed in 1989. The peace plan of Costa Rican President Oscar Arias picked up speed. The Nicaraguan Sandinista government accepted the peace plan's key provisions: a military cease-fire, a de-escalation of military-force numbers, and the holding of open elections. The Sandinistas fully expected to win such elections over their Contra foes and more moderate opponents led by popular newspaper publisher Violeta Chamorro. Then Mikhail Gorbachev tired of throwing scarce Soviet resources into bottomless Central American wars. He also reduced his help to Fidel Castro's Cuba, which had long supported the region's revolutionaries. Bush and Baker proposed a deal: They agreed to accept the results of the Nicaraguan election in early 1990 if Gorbachev would cut aid to the Sandinistas and warn them that they too had to accept the results. It seemed to be a highly risky deal for Bush.[6]

But he won. The Sandinistas lost the 1990 elections—the victims of their inability to create a growing economy amid civil war, and also of Gorbachev's deal with the Americans. It became clear later, moreover, that the United States had not only spent $9 million openly during the election, but the CIA had spent millions more covertly to ensure Mrs. Chamorro's victory.[7] The Sandinistas surrendered power to Chamorro's National Opposition Union (UNO). The Contras, with U.S. aid, dismantled their bases. After nearly a decade of war, peace broke out. The people, however, found little comfort. When Chamorro tried to create a consensus by allowing the Sandinistas to continue to control the army and police, she was harshly attacked by her own supporters and the United States. Bush and the Congress cut back on economic aid. Political murders began again. Some six hundred Contras returned to northern jungle areas to prepare for a new civil war. As Chamorro's hold weakened and the economy slid, the Sandinistas' well-organized party hoped to regain power in the 1996 elections.[8]

Bush also profited when Arias, and then the United Nations, brokered a truce in El Salvador's decade-long bloodbath. The war had stalemated as the revolutionary FMLN obtained less support from the disintegrating Soviet bloc, and the United States finally pressured its Salvadoran military allies to make peace in January 1992. The army was reduced, and the FMLN slowly laid down its arms. Most dramatically, a commission studying the brutalities of the war forced the removal of thirty-four army officers, including the minister of defense. A UN Truth Commission verified that while both the FMLN and the military had committed horrible crimes, the U.S.-supported and trained military was especially guilty of uncivilized acts, including the murder of an archbishop while he said mass in 1980, the rape-murders of 4 U.S. churchwomen in 1980, the massacre of 200 civilians in 1981, and the killing of 6 Jesuit priests in 1989. U.S. officials had lied throughout the 1980s to cover up these crimes so Congress would continue to send nearly $5 billion of aid to the Salvadoran military. Reporters who had written accurately about the crimes, and were then attacked as liars by the Reagan administration, were now vindicated by the UN Commission.[9]

Guatemala, after thirty years of war in which the United States had fully supported the military government, had suffered 150,000 dead, another 50,000 "disappeared" (that is, unaccounted for), and one million displaced (many of whom had gone to the United States). In 1990, this war also wound down, although fighting between the revolutionaries and the army continued. Bush cut off $3.2 million in U.S. aid after an American was killed in 1990, probably by government forces. World attention focused on Guatemala when Rigoberta Menchú won the Nobel Peace Prize in 1992. Born to a peasant Indian family, she saw two of her brothers die of malnutrition, a not-uncommon occurrence in Guatemala. Her father had been burned to death by the army when he peacefully protested the military's repression. Her mother was tortured, raped, and killed; her body, the daughter recalled, was found "tied to a tree and partially devoured by animals." Menchú refused to become directly involved on either side in the war, but instead she eloquently condemned the atrocities while living in exile. The Guatemalan military and U.S. officials denounced her actions as supporting

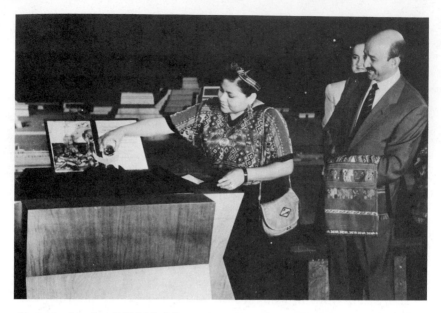

*After winning the 1992 Nobel Peace Prize for her opposition to the militaristic
Guatemalan regime, Rigoberta Menchú placed her Nobel medallion in a
Mexico City museum where it would remain, she announced, until her native
Guatemala became peaceful. President Carlos Salinas de Gortari and Cecilia
Ocelli de Gortari watched Menchú, who had been forced by the Guatemalans
to seek refuge in Mexico City.*

the revolutionaries. The Nobel citation declared she was "a vivid symbol of peace and reconciliation."[10]

A Salvadoran leader hoped that "it is the end of the Middle Ages in
El Salvador." Nearly all Central Americans prayed they could say the
same for their own nations. A historical verdict for U.S. foreign policy
was given by Honduran President Rafael Callejas: "Most of the U.S.
money came to sustain the wrong policies. We lost a decade."[11]

THE INVASION OF PANAMA

In another part of the region during late 1989, Bush sent not U.S.
money, but 24,000 troops to overthrow the Panamanian dictatorship
of General Manuel Antonio Noriega. On the surface, such massive use
of force was puzzling. Since 1903, the United States had dominated
Panama. Since the mid-1970s, Bush, first as director of the CIA and
then as vice-president, had personally worked closely with Noriega.

The Panamanian had cooperated with Bush in providing intelligence and by fighting against Central American revolutionaries. Not that Noriega was a nice man. A sadist who tortured and assassinated political opponents, he also cooperated with major drug traffickers (who profited enormously from U.S. buyers), and openly corrupted elections to maintain his power. The Reagan administration was nevertheless willing to overlook Noriega's crimes—until 1986–1987, when he quit cooperating so fully with U.S. military policies in Central America. By 1989, Bush and Noriega taunted each other publicly. Often derided as a "wimp" for his indecision, Bush seemed to live up to the term in the autumn of 1989, when he moved too slowly to help Panamanian military officers who were trying to overthrow Noriega. Noriega smashed the revolt.

Tension thickened between Noriega's forces and the 13,000 U.S. troops stationed in Panama, supposedly to protect the canal. In mid-December, Panamanian forces killed an American soldier who, they claimed, tried to run a roadblock in front of Panama's military headquarters. Then a U.S. naval officer and his wife were attacked and abused. Bush decided to show that he was not a wimp. On December 19–20, 11,000 more U.S. troops flew in and overthrew, then finally captured, Noriega. At least 300 Panamanian civilians died in the bombardment, 3,000 were wounded; 23 U.S. servicemen were killed, 324 more wounded; 18,000 Panamanians lost their homes.[12]

Bush gave four major reasons for the invasion: first, the threat to U.S. personnel in Panama; second, the danger Noriega posed to the Panama Canal's security; third, the general's deep involvement in drug traffic headed for North American streets; and fourth, the need to create democracy in Panama. As a former naval officer, Bush seemed to feel especially strong about the first point.

Critics quickly raised questions about these reasons. As to the first, special investigating committees of the New York City Bar Association concluded that Bush could have removed the threat to U.S. personnel by moving or isolating them (as often was done in other countries when Americans were threatened), instead of ordering an invasion that caused many civilian casualties. As to the second, the Bar Association and other investigators discovered no threat posed by Noriega to the canal. He had carefully avoided threatening it. As to the third point, Noriega's involvement with the drug trade was real, but less so than Bush alleged. Moreover, despite the capture of Noriega, by 1991–1992 more cocaine than ever was moving through Panama's so-called "trampoline" route that acted as a springboard for flying drugs into the United

States. Packets of cocaine washed up on Panamanian beaches. Those who lived along the ocean in Panama City itself observed "Little boats . . . with the stuff and then fine cars, sometimes Mercedes-Benzes, come to take it away." If the Bush administration cared about this traffic in 1989, it seemed to care much less in 1991. Finally, instead of a functioning democracy, Panamanian politics seemed headed toward chaos and corruption by 1992. The civilian government installed by Bush was threatened with destruction by its own military and was finally saved again by U.S. troops. Noriega meanwhile was taken to Florida. After a lengthy and highly criticized trial, he was sentenced to long terms in a U.S. jail for his drug trafficking.[13]

A central reason for Bush's strong action seemed to be his determination to escape both Noriega's taunting and the wimp label. The president also demonstrated to other possible opponents that he was not reluctant to use massive military power. The effect of the invasion on Panama is less clear. As New Year's Day of the year 2000 approaches (that is, the moment when, according to the 1977–1978 treaties, the United States will turn over the great canal to Panamanian control), the passageway's importance declines. Larger warships cannot use it, and alternative carriers (such as oil pipelines and giant railway container cars) have become more popular. But the canal's strategic and economic usefulness remains significant, even as its future remains endangered.

THE HISTORIC TURN OF THE LATE TWENTIETH CENTURY: BUSH AND GORBACHEV

The president was finally decisive, awesomely so, in destroying Noriega. He was less decisive in dealing with his greatest foreign-policy problem—indeed, the most historic event in the last half of the twentieth century: the collapse of the Soviet Union and, consequently, the end of the cold war.

As Bush entered the White House, Soviet leader Mikhail Gorbachev knew he was burdened by an increasingly weak economy and, indeed, a disintegrating society. Generations of Communist rigidity and corruption had taken a heavy toll, but Gorbachev and his foreign minister, Eduard Shevardnadze, were the first Soviet leaders to act on those facts. After signing historic agreements with Reagan (see p. 734), in late 1988 Gorbachev announced major cuts in the Soviet military, began pulling troops out of the eastern European Communist bloc, and moved to end the disastrous ten-year intervention in Afghanistan. For these acts, he won the Nobel Peace Prize in 1990.

The scene was set for a dramatic response by Bush. But the new president spent the first half of 1989 making an extensive, and finally bland, policy analysis of U.S.-Soviet relations. Having known only the cold war in their lives, the president and his top advisers (NSC adviser Brent Scowcroft and Secretary of State James Baker) feared chaos and dangerous unpredictability if the cold war suddenly ended. They also feared what Scowcroft called "the clever bear syndrome," that is, that Gorbachev was lulling the West to sleep while secretly preparing to launch a new, more devastating cold war. Bush and Baker even privately condemned Reagan for having made too many deals with Gorbachev. In other words, they believed Ronald Reagan had been too soft on communism. Having little knowledge of, or apparent interest in, the broad historical background, Bush, Scowcroft, and Baker became limited by the only history they knew—that of the cold war. Vice-President Dan Quayle ridiculed Gorbachev as just a Stalinist "in Gucci shoes." Bush's press secretary called the Soviet leader, "a drugstore cowboy." (That remark led a knowledgeable State Department official to comment, "Some cowboy. Some drugstore!")[14]

Gorbachev, however, believed he had no alternative but to continue putting an end to the cold war. In mid-1989, the Soviets agreed to U.S. positions on key arms disputes. Gorbachev also suddenly and dramatically refused to send Soviet troops into Poland, Hungary, or Czechoslovakia to prop up falling Communist regimes. He told the Polish Communists in the summer of 1989 that they had to make their own deals with their political opposition. Soon, to the West's surprise, Poland's anti-Communist Solidarity party won open elections and began claiming power. Gorbachev, it is clear, was also surprised. He remained a devout Communist. But he believed that good Communists in the USSR and its East European satellites saw the light as he did—that is, they would scale down the cold war, reform their inefficient economies, revitalize their societies, and continue to hold power. Poland's experience, however, proved that Gorbachev was a dreamer.

His, and Bush's, greatest shock lay just ahead. By October 1989, Hungary and Czechoslovakia had followed Poland in overthrowing Communist rulers. Romania's dictatorship fell, as well, in late 1989. East Germany's hard-line Communists, however, tried to crack down on internal dissenters, only to find that East Germans were escaping in large numbers to West Germany through the Hungarian and Czech gaps in the iron curtain. At 11:17 P.M., on November 9, 1989, a new

East German government decided, with Gorbachev's support, to recognize new realities by opening the Berlin Wall. Within seventy-two
hours this blood-stained, twenty-eight-year-old symbol of the cold war
was being battered down by giant jackhammers, and also by small
hammers wielded by aspiring capitalists who sold small pieces of the
wall to eager U.S. and European buyers.

The changes in Poland forced the president to believe that "There's
big stuff, heavy stuff going on here." As he watched the Berlin Wall
come down, he finally concluded that the Soviets have "got to be really
serious—more serious than I realized." Bush now fully embraced Gorbachev and, in skillful diplomatic strokes, helped the Soviets prepare
for the unthinkable: the reunification of the powerful 62 million West
Germans with the 16 million East Germans. Gorbachev fought against
German reunification, for, among other things, it would be the ultimate humiliation for the Soviets who had sacrificed so greatly (including 20 million lives) to win World War II. Since the late 1940s, Western
leaders had said they supported a united Germany, but now that it
suddenly became a real possibility, they had second thoughts. West
German Chancellor Helmut Kohl was nevertheless determined to make
his place in history, despite estimates that it would cost his people a
half-trillion dollars over ten years to raise the East German living standards. Realizing the inevitable, Bush helped bring Gorbachev around
to accepting unification, and even the inclusion of the new Germany
in NATO, by assuring him that U.S. troops would remain in Europe to
help keep Germany under control, if such restraint were needed. He
also pieced together a $24 billion aid package for Gorbachev, although
the Soviets received only a small fraction of it. It was Kohl, however,
who controlled the unification process in early 1990. While Bush (like
most Americans and western Europeans who had vivid memories of
World War II) had qualms about a new, united, powerful Germany,
and while the British and French governments actually pleaded with
Gorbachev not to allow unification, the German Chancellor flew to
Gorbachev's summer home and negotiated the pivotal deals. Kohl
accepted a long-term U.S. military presence in Europe, gave Gorbachev $15 billion, and—most important—guaranteed the new Ger-
many's acceptance of the boundaries imposed by the triumphant Allies
in 1945. The Chancellor, that is, gave up all claims to parts of Poland
that had once belonged to Germany.[15]

As these agreements took effect in mid-1990, Bush finally admitted
that the cold war had ended. Gorbachev agreed: "We are no longer
adversaries." The events were mind-boggling. For decades, the Soviets
had tried to push the United States out of Europe. But Gorbachev,

faced with a rising Germany and a declining Soviet military power, now told the president, "It's important for the future of Europe that you are in Europe, so we don't want to see you out of there." Bush agreed; he knew that NATO was one of the few remaining points through which the United States could influence European affairs. Nevertheless, the 300,000 U.S. troops in Europe declined to 180,000 by 1993 and seemed to be headed toward 100,000. The Soviet retreat from eastern Europe was even more rapid. In early 1991 Gorbachev issued the stunning announcement that the Warsaw Pact—the Moscow-directed military alliance through which the Red Army had policed eastern Europe since 1955—would be dissolved in April 1991. The Communist bloc's economic alliance, Comecon, also disappeared.[16]

For obvious reasons, Bush now saw Gorbachev as "really the best hope" for U.S. policies. The president had become convinced that without Gorbachev, the Soviet Union, with its 30,000 nuclear weapons, would fragment and finally split apart. He seemed as terrified of this possibility as were Soviet leaders. At a press conference, Bush declared that the "enemy" was not Germany (or the Soviet Union, or Japan, as many Americans believed). "No, the enemy is unpredictability. The enemy is instability." This view took Bush to dangerous ground. The three Baltic states (Latvia, Lithuania, and Estonia) had been conquered by Stalin in 1939–1940, although the United States had never formally recognized Soviet control. In 1990–1991, the Baltic peoples moved toward independence. Gorbachev resisted. In early 1991, fifteen Lithuanian protesters were killed by Red Army units. Bush refused to condemn the Soviet action or undercut Gorbachev. At the same time, several other of the fifteen republics making up the Soviet Union also demanded their independence. They were led by Ukraine and Georgia. In August 1991, Bush flew to Ukraine's capital, Kiev, to lecture the parliament that it should remain under Gorbachev's guidance. Critics, who wanted to seize this golden opportunity to dismantle the Soviet empire, condemned what they labeled Bush's "Chicken Kiev" speech.[17]

Three weeks later, Gorbachev was nearly destroyed by a right-wing coup. He was saved, temporarily, by his political enemy, Boris Yeltsin.

The Historic Turn in the Late Twentieth-Century: Bush and Yeltsin

Yeltsin was the tall, white-haired, rough-edged Russian who was strongly reform-minded—in part because he came from a poor peasant family

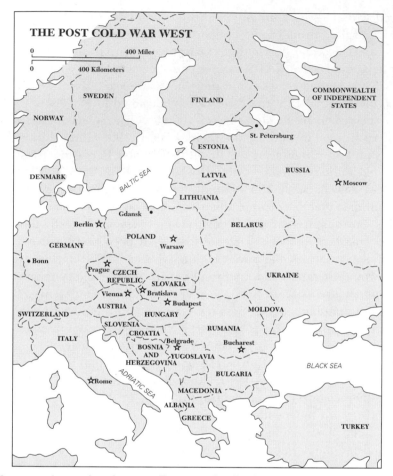

THE POST COLD WAR WEST

The map of central and eastern Europe radically changed three times during the twentieth century: 1919, 1945, and 1990–1991. This map shows the vital region in 1993. Note the newly united Germany. Estonia, Latvia, Lithuania (the three Baltic States), Belarus, Ukraine, and Moldova had—along with the giant republic of Russia—been part of the Soviet Union before 1989 but now moved toward independence. Note also Croatia and Bosnia and Herzegovina, once part of Yugoslavia but now areas for brutal wars in 1992–1993 among Croatian Christians, Muslims (especially in Bosnia), and Serbian Eastern Orthodox Christians. Prague (Czech Republic) and Budapest (Hungary) were becoming cultural and business centers of eastern Europe.

(which for warmth had slept on their hut's floor with the farm animals). His father was arrested during Stalin's bloody purges in the 1930s.[18] In 1987, Gorbachev threw Yeltsin out of the Soviet government for being too reform-minded. The two men became bitter oppo-

nents. Yeltsin clawed his way back. In early 1990 he won election to
the new Russian Parliament. In June 1991, he won 57 percent of the
vote to become the Russian Republic's first elected president in its history. He enjoyed much stronger democratic credentials than did Gorbachev, whose election to the Soviet presidency had been by votes of
the old Communist party hacks who were now trying to stop his programs of change.

Yeltsin was becoming a hero in Russia, but not in Washington. In
1989, Scowcroft reluctantly agreed to talk with Yeltsin, brought him
quietly into the White House through a side door so few would notice,
then fell asleep while Yeltsin talked at length. Rumors spread that the
Russian was publicly drunk. Bush agreed with Scowcroft that Yeltsin
was a "boor" and that Gorbachev seemed so much more civilized. Bush,
however, relied too much on his taste for personality. Several overriding events proved to be more important. Yeltsin had a strong democratic base, and Gorbachev did not. Yeltsin, moreover, realized that
the Soviet Union was coming apart and was willing to make deals with
the emerging republics. Gorbachev meanwhile worked to keep the old
Soviet Empire together. When the Red Army killed the fifteen Lithu-
anians in 1991, Yeltsin flew to the scene to sympathize with the victims. "That son of a bitch," Gorbachev cried—and Yeltsin had to return
secretly to Moscow after fears spread that his plane was to be sabo-
taged. Finally, Yeltsin wanted to dismantle the Soviet military more
rapidly than did his rival. As Yeltsin built his democratic base, Gorbachev tried to save his power by appointing old Communists and militarists. These were the people who then tried to overthrow him in
August 1991.[19]

Bush nevertheless stuck doggedly with Gorbachev, even as the Soviet
leader's popularity sank with the economy. Without an economic plan,
and unable to deal with a mushrooming "Moscow Mafia" (one Russian likened the situation to that in Chicago during gangster Al Capone's
days in the 1920s), Gorbachev floundered as inflation soared and the
people lost the security they at least had received from the old, stagnant, Communist regime. A Soviet economist found "it strange to hear
Americans talk about the 'possibility' of an economic crash. The crash
has already happened when, as now, there are deep shortages of 95
percent of all goods." Experts on Soviet affairs in both the Pentagon
and the CIA warned Bush and Scowcroft that they were on the wrong
side of a historic turn. These experts urged that the United States and
its allies at least push Gorbachev and Yeltsin to work together so the
strongest possible political team could ease the USSR's political and

economic tensions. Bush and Scowcroft refused. They compared Gorbachev to Lincoln in 1861 heroically trying to keep the Union together. Not so, the Pentagon and CIA responded; he resembled those in 1776 who fought vainly against revolutionary change and the overriding need for a new constitution in the United States.[20]

In April 1991, the CIA warned that an anti-Gorbachev coup by right-wing hard-liners could occur. Scowcroft dismissed the warning as "simplistic" and believed the agency was a hotbed of Yeltsinistas. On August 19–20, the hard-liners struck. They put Gorbachev under house arrest, although he refused to sign a letter of resignation as they demanded. Key elements of the army, however, refused to follow the coup-plotters' orders. Yeltsin and his followers held out in the "white house" a short distance from the Kremlin. New technology helped undermine the plotters: CNN televised the events, and Yeltsin's determined opposition, throughout the world. American culture also played a small part; McDonald's, with its largest outlet in the world in Moscow, trucked hamburgers and coffee to the "white house." Disorganized, often quite drunk, unsupported by enough of the military, the plotters finally quit. One committed suicide. Gorbachev returned to Moscow, but as Bush said privately, "I'm afraid he may have had it." Yeltsin was the hero. The reformer took power, stripped Gorbachev of his office, launched an economic reform program and—in a historic moment on December 25, 1991— decreed that the Soviet Union ceased to exist. Yeltsin nevertheless controlled an impressive nation: Russia, whose vastness stretched across ten time zones and some of the world's richest mineral resources. He hoped to work out new relationships, moreover, with the eleven other increasingly independent republics.[21]

The Soviet Union was dead at age seventy-four. Gorbachev and Bush had been unable to control its final illness. Bush quickly moved to work with Yeltsin. The two men signed the Start II treaty that cut their nuclear weapons by two-thirds so that each held 3,500 warheads and bombs. The United States continued to work on the $24 billion aid package. It was, however, again too late. Three years had been lost. As Yeltsin tried to push Russia's huge bureaucracy-burdened economy into a free-market system, prices skyrocketed 350 percent in weeks. Inflation began to soar toward a 2,000 percent annual level (Americans worry when their inflation rate goes above 4 percent). Food and other necessities grew scarce. Even with the $24 billion and another $12 billion that the new, French-created European Bank for Reconstruction could invest, the West on its own could not significantly help turn around the Russian economy.[22]

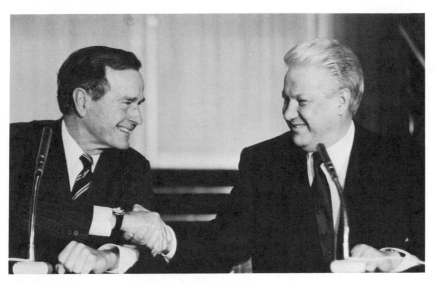

The smiles of President George Bush and President Boris Yeltsin were appropriate. The U.S. and Russian leaders had just signed in Moscow a historic START-II treaty that for the first time sharply reduced the strategic nuclear weapons on both sides. The smiles, however, also hid a personal relationship between the two men that had in 1989–1991 been tense and even bitter as Bush had strongly supported Yeltsin's rival in Moscow, Mikhail Gorbachev. The picture was snapped on January 3, 1993—less than three weeks before Bush was due to leave office.

One Western banker complained that trying to start a business in Moscow was "like trying to irrigate a desert with a garden hose." Throughout the cold war, the CIA and military intelligence, for their own budgetary purposes, had consistently overestimated Soviet economic capacity—which, it turned out, on a per capita basis was more equal to Mexico's than to the economies of the United States or western Europe. Although many Western businesses (such as McDonald's, Pizza Hut, Pepsi-Cola, and several oil companies), found profits, others, in the words of a U.S. newspaper, "go away complaining about unappetizing meals that cost $75 and shabby $200-a-night rooms in [Moscow] hotels where 25-watt bulbs and prostitutes are part of the decor." The number of homeless and beggers increased dramatically.[23] Some of the more ambitious Russians seized the opportunity to find (or steal) Western goods and become rich by charging exorbitant prices. Russians, whose history was filled with such (indeed, worse) crises, nevertheless still found humor in their situation: a Moscow mother asks what her small child hopes to be after growing up. The child replies, "A foreigner."

THE POST–COLD-WAR DISORDER: WAR WITH IRAQ

With the Soviet Union (or much of it) now calling itself the Commonwealth of Independent States, the State Department's Soviet Desk retitled itself EUR/ISCA—that is, "Europe—Office of Independent States and Commonwealth Affairs." Some critics believed a better title for Bush's Soviet advisers was EUR/OBE, or "Europe—Overtaken By Events."[24] During the 1990–1991 conflict with Iraq, however, the president's cultivation of Gorbachev paid off.

Since the 1970s, Soviet military advisers had trained and helped supply Iraqi dictator Saddam Hussein's military. In 1980–1981, when Iraq began one of the bloodiest, most brutal, and longest twentieth-century wars by attacking Iran, the United States and some of its allies (notably West Germany and France) also began sending aid to the Iraqi dictator. Informed estimates of this aid between 1983 and 1988 run as high as $34 billion, with half coming from the Soviets. The Reagan administration also gave Saddam Hussein valuable intelligence information. By 1988, with the Iranians and Iraqis exhausted, the war halted. Nearly bankrupted by the conflict, Saddam Hussein pushed his fellow Arab oil producers to cut production and thus increase both oil prices and his income. Led by Saudi Arabia and Kuwait, they refused. The dictator did not take opposition kindly. He had slaughtered his political opponents in cold blood, sometimes with his own hand, as he moved toward power after 1968. Now he demanded that Kuwait give him strategic islands and oil fields that had been in dispute since British colonial officials (who then controlled the region) had drawn arbitrary boundaries between Kuwait and Iraq in 1922. Kuwait also refused these demands.[25]

Saddam Hussein prepared again for war. He apparently believed, with good reason, that the Soviets would continue to support him. He thought the Americans were paralyzed by memories of Vietnam. In any case, as he prepared to launch the attack on August 2, 1990, the U.S. ambassador to Iraq, April Glaspie, assured him the United States "had no opinion" on these boundary struggles. She said this on direct instructions to her from the Bush-Baker State Department. (Later, she unfairly became the scapegoat for this disastrous policy and suffered severely professionally and personally.) The Iraqi dictator was already on record as declaring he hoped to see all Israel in flames. He also had used poison gas in trying to destroy the Kurds, a minority people concentrated in northern Iraq. Bush, however, was so determined to have normal relations with Saddam Hussein that when the U.S. Congress moved to impose economic sanctions on Iraq in response to the dictator's brutalities on his own people, Bush blocked the attempt. If Bush had not blocked the sanctions, U.S. farmers, as well as arms merchants, would have been upset. American rice growers, for example, sold one-fifth of their exports to Iraq as part of an overall $1 billion in U.S. agricultural shipments to that country.[26]

On August 2, 1990, Iraq seized Kuwait in a lightning military operation. Saddam Hussein now controlled about 20 percent of the world's known oil reserves. U.S. officials feared he was poised to conquer Saudi Arabia; he then would have 40 percent of the reserves, as well as control of a close U.S. military ally. A surprised Bush hesitated, then (pushed especially by Britain's tough Prime Minister, Margaret Thatcher, whose nation depended heavily on Kuwaiti money), the president vowed to defend Saudi Arabia and liberate Kuwait. Over the next six months, Bush gave various reasons for this commitment: the naked Iraqi seizure of territory (he compared Saddam Hussein to Hitler); the threat posed to world oil prices; the opportunity to destroy Iraq's growing capacity to produce nuclear and chemical weapons; the need to uphold the UN's pledge to resist aggression; and the bitter personal betrayal he felt after trying to work with the Iraqi leader. Bush notably argued that with the end of the cold war "a new world order" was emerging, but that it could be stillborn, with a more dangerous world appearing unless aggressors such as Saddam Hussein learned their lessons now.[27] (In reality, neither Bush nor any of his advisers was ever clear about what this "new world order" meant. The term had been mentioned in an informal discussion by NSC Adviser Scowcroft shortly after the Iraqi invasion. When Pam Olson, of CNN television, asked a Bush adviser what was going on, he responded that "the new world order" was at stake. She used the term on television and it promptly became identified with Bush's policy and worldview—although neither then nor later did he ever bother to define it. It became one of those terms that many people used, but none knew exactly what it meant.)

The most spectacular successes of Bush's presidency followed. He pieced together an effective alliance of nations, including some (such as Israel on the one hand, and Saudi Arabia and Syria on the other) that were violent political enemies. He gained full support from the United Nations which, for the first time in its history, acted as its founders of 1944–1945 had planned. It could resist Iraqi aggression because for the first time the Soviets, under Gorbachev, cooperated with rather than blocked UN action. Bush's personal diplomacy paid dividends, for Gorbachev rejected advice from his pro-Iraqi military (which predicted a great victory for Saddam Hussein over the U.S. forces). Gorbachev tried to work out a peace plan and delay the start of the U.S. offensive, but he never directly opposed Bush's actions. The president was also shrewd, if rather devious, at home. He shipped 250,000 men and women to Saudi Arabia and other bases immediately after the Iraqi invasion, but then waited until after the November congressional elections before he doubled those forces. The doubling of the troops signaled an early military confrontation. Having avoided a divisive political debate in the election campaign, he went to Congress in January 1991 and demanded that it pass a resolution supporting his use of force. Bush was the first president since Franklin D. Roosevelt in 1941 to honor, however loosely, the Constitution's requirement that Congress must declare war. Intense debate followed. Opponents argued that by sending in a half-million troops, Bush had put them in an impossible position to debate a war resolution; clearly, war was inevitable anyway. They also argued that economic pressures would force Saddam Hussein to give in without the need to go to war. The resolution authorizing the president to use force narrowly passed the Senate (52–47) and more easily passed the House (250–183).[28]

The great question became whether U.S. and allied forces could destroy Iraq's battle-hardened troops without suffering heavy casualties. Such casualties could lead, as they had in the Vietnam conflict, to Americans demanding an immediate peace. Secretary of Defense Richard Cheney told a Middle East official, "The military is finished in this society, if we screw this up."[29] U.S. military officers, however, had closely studied and learned from the Vietnam debacle. By using overwhelming force at the start, and by aiming at definite objectives, they believed U.S. forces could achieve quick victory and avoid a political backlash.

This strategy was best argued by General Colin Powell, chairman of the Joint Chiefs of Staff. The first African American to hold this highest of military positions (and the first as well to hold the job of NSC adviser—from 1987–1989), Powell had been educated at City College of New York and George Washington University. He served two tours in Vietnam. When not rapidly moving up the military ladder (or pursuing his hobby of restoring Volvos), Powell studied Vietnam's lessons.[30] He steadily opposed committing U.S. forces unless (as in Panama,

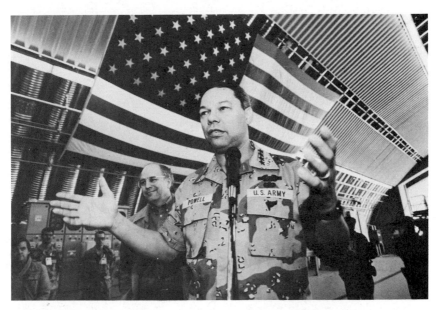

General Colin Powell and Secretary of Defense Richard Cheney (behind Powell's arm) visited a U.S. base in Saudi Arabia during February 1991—just before the all-out ground assault against Iraqi forces. Powell, the first African American to serve as the President's National Security Adviser and then as Chairman of the Joint Chiefs (1989–1993), proved to be a brilliant strategist in fighting the war, but in other instances also acted as a restraint on both Presidents Bush and Clinton when they considered the use of U.S. forces in later crises.

and now in Iraq), he believed a quick, relatively cost-free victory that achieved specific targets (such as the liberation of Kuwait), could be won. Bush agreed both to commit overwhelming power and not to second-guess Powell once fighting began.

On January 16, 1991, U.S. planes and missiles, many launched from ships in the Persian Gulf, massively attacked Iraq. The Iraqis responded with Soviet-built Scud missiles that caused fatalities in Israel and Saudi Arabia. U.S.-built Patriot missiles destroyed some of the Scuds (often captured in spectacular television pictures instantly shown in the United States via satellites), although apparently not more than twenty-four of the eighty-six Scuds that Iraq launched were actually hit. Overall, the U.S. air and missile attacks were less effective than the Bush administration claimed during the conflict.[31] Saddam Hussein's installations for developing nuclear and chemical weapons, for example, were not destroyed. Nevertheless, the Iraqi military suffered severe damage. A

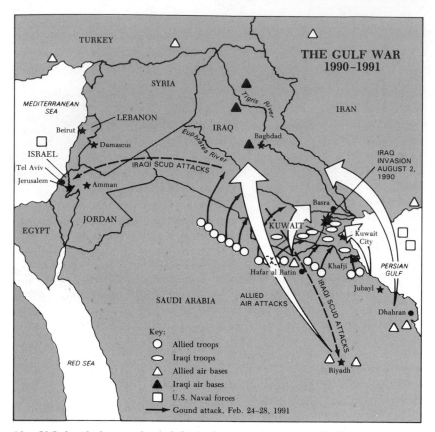

After U.S. battleships and amphibious forces in the Persian Gulf made a feint at landing at Kuwait City, the half-million troops in the coalition forces moved along the ground out of Saudi Arabia to cut off Iraqi forces in Kuwait and southern Iraq. The war lasted less than 100 hours in February 1991, although U.S. airpower failed to destroy one of its key targets: chemical and nuclear plants in central and northern Iraq.

month later, the allied ground forces attacked Kuwait and southern Iraq. Saddam Hussein had promised to wage "the mother of all battles," but in only a hundred hours his troops were either destroyed or retreating to the capital of Baghdad.

Kuwait was freed, but it turned out that many of the dictator's best troops survived. In one of several miscalculations at the end of the fighting, U.S. officers allowed Iraqi helicopter forces to escape. These forces were later used again to attack the Kurdish people in northern Iraq.[32] Bush and Powell had no intention of widening the war's objectives by driving to Baghdad and destroyng Saddam Hussein's regime, nor would any of their Arab allies have approved such a drive. Many of the Arab people on the streets of such nations as Jordan, Egypt, and even Saudi Arabia sympathized with Saddam Hussein's struggle against the Western forces. A direct attempt to overthrow him could lead to severe political disturbances within those and other Middle East nations. The Iraqi dictator therefore was able to intensify efforts to build nuclear weapons, hold off UN teams that tried to inspect his nuclear plants, and launch new attacks on the Kurds and other internal enemies until U.S. and UN forces finally had to try to protect these victims. Meanwhile, the United States moved to implement the "new world order" in the Middle East by building the region's greatest military presence. That power rested on new base agreements with Kuwait and other Arab countries to support the long-term stationing of 24,000 U.S. troops,

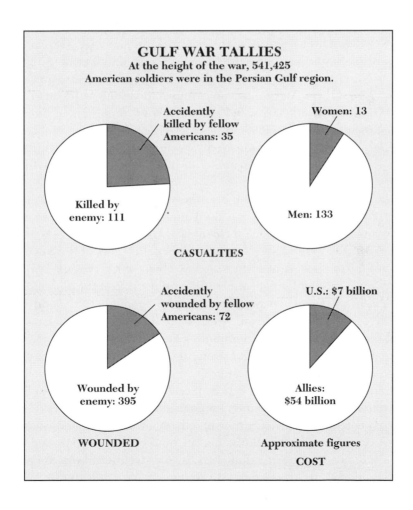

GULF WAR TALLIES
At the height of the war, 541,425
American soldiers were in the Persian Gulf region.

Accidently
killed by fellow
Americans: 35

Killed by
enemy: 111

Women: 13

Men: 133

CASUALTIES

Accidently
wounded by fellow
Americans: 72

Wounded by
enemy: 395

WOUNDED

U.S.: $7 billion

Allies:
$54 billion

Approximate figures
COST

26 warships, and more than 150 planes.[33] These agreements marked a long step since 1946, when U.S. officials had debated whether to put even one U.S. warship in the eastern Mediterranean.

THE NEW DISORDER: BUSH TO CLINTON

George Bush thought of himself as the foreign-policy president, much as Richard Nixon had thought of himself twenty years earlier. And like Nixon, Bush was removed from office before he wanted to leave, albeit in a more regular process of election. Bush was justly proud of many foreign-policy accomplishments: triumphing over Iraq; initiating the first comprehensive peace process to end the nearly half-century war between Israel and its neighbors; pushing negotiations that established the world's richest free-trade area comprising Canada, Mexico, and the United States; handling the Soviet collapse and German unification; signing the most radical nuclear-arms reduction agreements in history; improving, in a controversial move, relations with China even after Communist officials killed pro-democracy protesters in Beijing's Tiananmen Square in 1989; and helping bring an end to several bloody Central American revolutions. In a speech at Texas A & M University in late 1992, he boasted that many of "these once seemed a dream. Today they are concrete realities."[34]

Critics, as usual, nevertheless found weaknesses. When Bush and other Republicans claimed that the United States (or, more precisely, the Republican party) "won" the cold war, George Kennan—the father in 1947 of the tough U.S. "containment" policy toward the Soviets—called the claims "intrinsically silly." To believe Americans had such power over another "great country on another side of the globe is simply childish," Kennan wrote. In truth, he concluded, "Nobody—no country, no party, no person, 'won' the cold war. It was a long and costly political rivalry, fueled on both sides by unreal and exaggerated estimates of the intentions and strength of the other party." It resulted in the weakening, if not near-bankruptcy, of both sides.[35] Others believed that the true victors were not U.S. foreign policies, but U.S. political institutions, which absorbed technological changes and overcame the lies and corruption of McCarthyism, Nixon's Watergate, and Reagan's Iran-Contra scandal. The Soviet Union, on the other hand, rotted from the inside out. Some critics attacked Bush as well for having no policy for handling Americans' greatest economic competitor, the Japanese;

for being too kind to the Chinese totalitarians; and for largely ignoring world environmental problems.[36]

Bush's challenger in the 1992 presidential campaign, Democratic governor Bill Clinton of Arkansas, attacked the president on all these issues. He emphasized, however, the weak U.S. economy that, Clinton claimed, Bush had mishandled and ignored. A talented politician, Clinton was single-minded, even cynical, in his pursuit of power. Among his "laws of politics," he said, were "There's no such thing as enough money," and "When someone tells you it's nothing personal, it means they're fixing to screw you." He promised "to focus like a laser beam" on the economy. This approach shaped his foreign-policy plans, Clinton declared, because now that "the Cold War is won," "we have entered a global economy." After defeating Bush and third-party candidate Ross Perot of Texas, Clinton observed in his January 1993 Inaugural Address: "There is no longer division between what is foreign and what is domestic—the world economy, the world environment, the world AIDS crisis, the world arms race—they affect us all."[37]

Clinton also echoed Woodrow Wilson: Americans must "organize and lead a long-term Western strategy" to advance "democracy," especially in the former Soviet Union. He, like Wilson, also stressed the need to use military power, if necessary, to advance this cause. He attacked Bush for being too reluctant to commit U.S. forces to stop the brutalities and starvation of the Muslim population in a disintegrating Yugoslavia controlled by Christian Serbs. He also stressed that stronger governmental action was needed to help Americans prepare themselves for intense competition in the new global marketplace. In 1972, the young Bill Clinton, fresh from a Rhodes Scholarship at Oxford, England, had worked for George McGovern's presidential campaign. In 1992, however, Clinton's aides made clear that he had then worked only for the end of the U.S. involvement in Vietnam, not for broader "isolationist" foreign policies that McGovern had been accused of supporting.[38]

CLINTON'S WORLD: THE PROBLEM OF ASIA

The world, of course, had changed considerably since Woodrow Wilson preached the need for Americans to support international democracy. Just how complicated the globe had become was shown when the new president and his top advisers—Secretary of State Warren Christopher and National Security Adviser Anthony Lake—turned toward

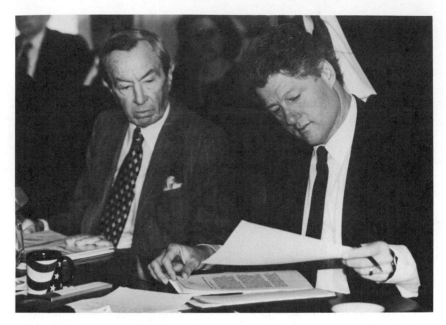

Bill Clinton, at right, had won the presidency in 1992 by promising to focus on domestic issues. But once he entered office in January 1993, he found that he had to work closely with his secretary of state, Warren Christopher (at left) to deal with crises in Russia, Yugoslavia, U.S.-Japan relations, the planned U.S.-Canada-Mexico common market, Somalia, Haiti, and Angola—among others. The American economy was now so tightly integrated within the world economy that Clinton could not improve conditions at home (for example, find more jobs for U.S. workers) without dealing with foreign policy.

Asia. In that region Japan's economic powerhouse had tormented key U.S. producers for more than twenty years. China was emerging as an economic and major military force, complete with nuclear weapons; an unpredictable Communist North Korea hurriedly built its own nuclear weapons. And the world's largest democracy, India, erupted again in a murderous struggle between the majority Hindus and the minority Muslims. Christopher had been a successful Los Angeles lawyer, an able deputy secretary of state in the Carter administration, and a masterful negotiator who gained the release of the U.S. hostages in Iran during 1980–1981 (see p. 698). But he had little experience in Asian affairs.

Lake, once a professional Foreign Service officer, had served courageously in Vietnam and had resigned when Nixon expanded the war in 1970–1971. After working in the Carter State Department, he spent the 1980s teaching at Mount Holyoke College and raising beef cattle.

Lake was the idea man, the conceptualizer, among Clinton's closest advisers. The NSC director believed the foreign-policy debate in the 1990s was between those (such as George Bush) who saw the world in traditional balance-of-power terms, and those (such as Clinton and himself) who had a "neo-Wilsonian view" that led to using U.S. power to promote democracy around the world. Indeed, in President Carter's State Department, Lake had worked successfully to use economic pressure against white-ruled Rhodesia until that African nation was finally governed by the black population that had a huge majority. But Lake was also greatly affected by the misuse of power in Vietnam, and—like General Powell and other military leaders—swore never to make that kind of mistake again. Lake wrote that the Vietnam Veterans Memorial in Washington, with its list of 58,000 dead, "perfectly represents America's collective memory of its longest war." This memory of Vietnam shaped the Clinton administration's response to crises in Yugoslavia, Africa, and elsewhere.[39]

Asia was explosive largely because, as historian Bruce Cumings noted, while Europe had entered the post–cold war era, "East Asia remains decidedly" in the cold-war era.[40] China and North Korea remained Communist controlled. China, however, was more dangerously complicated. Its Communist leaders had built the nation's economy in the 1980s by encouraging free-market enterprise. The nation's annual economic growth rate soared toward 12 percent. Even Japan's rate had slowed to about half of China's. U.S.-Chinese trade boomed, although China enjoyed a large favorable balance. This growing gap led U.S. critics to demand that China open itself to more American goods, and that its Communist leaders allow more democracy and personal expression. Beijing officials, however, wanted no part of political democracy. It threatened their own power and also threatened to fragment their vast country. Clinton and his advisers had to decide whether to push for more democracy and possibly lose valuable trade just as the long-mythical "China market" seemed to materialize, or push for more trade and give up Clinton's emphasis on democracy.

The new president also faced another dangerous choice because China was rapidly building its military forces to the level, one expert declared, of a "regional superpower." It was developing a modern navy while buying advanced fighter planes and missiles from Russia. Neighbors, such as Taiwan, South Korea, and Indonesia, grew nervous. Even as the Taiwanese, once a part of China (which the Chinese still claimed as part of their empire), invested heavily on the Communist mainland, they also rushed the building of their own military. Japan, long reluctant to overcome its "nuclear allergy" and again become a military power, boosted its spending until it possessed the region's best navy and air force—although both were to be used only for the close defense of the home islands. Uneasiness grew in the region as the United States, faced with tighter defense budgets and Philippine nationalism, abandoned its advanced naval and air bases in the Philippines. Americans had maintained them since 1898. U.S. forces now moved back to Guam. Clinton thus faced the problem of protecting U.S. interests in an explosive, dynamic Asia with fewer American resources.[41]

Asia also exemplified another danger for Clinton. A growing consensus of scientists concluded that the world's delicate environmental balance was gravely threatened by a rapidly rising population, increased carbon emissions that caused global warming (and thus melted icecaps that could raise the oceans to dangerous levels), depletion of the ozone layer (and a consequent rise of skin cancers), the mass destruction of valuable forests, and the erosion of topsoil until farming in such areas as Haiti, parts of Africa, and Central American regions was impossible. These dangers haunted the entire globe, even the relatively prosperous United States. But as the huge populations of China (1.5 billion), India (1 billion), and Indonesia (150 million) grew and developed economically, Asian environmental problems increasingly became a worldwide threat. Merely putting modern refrigerators in each Chinese home, for example, could drive up the release of ozone-destroying chlorofluorocarbons to extremely dangerous levels.[42] How Clinton and other world leaders could meet demands for rapid economic development from Asia, Africa, and Latin America, yet protect human life (and the crops and animals needed to help sustain that life), stood at the center of post–cold war problems.

Finally, since 1947 the Washington-Tokyo relationship had been the most important in U.S.-Asian policy. The rapid economic and military changes of the 1980s, especially the rise of China and the declining importance of American military power, placed a heavy strain on that relationship, as did the intense, often bitter economic competition between Americans and Japanese. The new U.S. leaders had to figure out how to strengthen this relationship—or create a fundamentally different policy toward Asia.

CLINTON'S WORLD: THE PROBLEM OF THE BLOCS

Since 1945, the world had been neither peaceful nor unchanging. It nevertheless retained a kind of order and predictability because two superpowers dominated its military and economic life. Each super-power had learned to fear and, to some extent, understand the other. After 1990, that order was gone. Nationalist, ethnic, and religious con-flict, once held in check by the superpowers, now erupted. Such con-flict even broke out with a dangerous intensity inside the former Soviet Union itself.

The new order seemed not to be orderly at all. Instead, it seemed to be going off in two quite different, perilous directions. One direction was growing regional economic blocs. That is, as the military and eco-nomic blocs of the two superpowers disappeared, they were being replaced by three major economic blocs: the twelve-nation European Community (EC), the U.S.-Canada-Mexico free-trade area being negotiated to create a huge American common market, and the less-formal-but-nevertheless-potent Asian development area powered by Japanese capital. These units were soon called the Deutsche-mark bloc (because of Germany's enormous economic power in the EC), the dol-lar bloc, and the yen bloc.

By the time Bill and Hillary Rodham Clinton entered the White House in 1993, however, they found each of the blocs in trouble. In Europe, the new, united Germans threatened to grow so powerful and indepen-dent that first Denmark, then Great Britian, pulled away. A top British official charged that the EC was merely "a German racket designed to take over the whole of Europe," with the French acting as Germany's "poodles." The EC was supposed to be largely unified by 1993, but instead it was bogged down amid nationalist disputes. In the Americas, Canadians believed they were being exploited by their 1989 free-trade treaty with the United States. They even forced out of power the prime minister who had negotiated the treaty. U.S. citizens, especially in organized labor, meanwhile condemned the proposed U.S.-Mexican agreement because it allowed too many industries to move to Mexican regions where wages were low (Mexican laborers received in a day the wages U.S. laborers received in an hour) and environmental standards were below those in the United States. Pro-treaty forces estimated that by opening Mexico to U.S. goods, a net of 175,000 jobs would be cre-ated in the United States.[45] But Clinton insisted that he would accept the U.S.-Mexico treaty only after safeguards were added to help Amer-ican labor and protect the environment. Japan's bloc meanwhile was hurt by a Japanese economic downturn and rising power centers in Taiwan and China.

Hopes that the new economic world would be more orderly seemed to be disappearing as the blocs ran into trouble. Of equal importance, the long-running talks (begun in Uruguay in 1986), among more than a hundred nations for the purpose of opening world markets to greater international trade also seemed to have hit a dead end. Just as Americans depended increasingly on the global marketplace for their jobs, that marketplace was threatened with the specter of trade wars that reminded some observers of the terrible 1930s.

CLINTON'S WORLD: THE NEW WORLD DISORDER

Hence the post-1990 world headed off in another, more dramatic direction: toward fragmentation, intense nationalism, and deeply scarred and bloody ethnic and religious wars. Freed of Stalinist restraints, not only did the fifteen former Soviet republics move toward independence, but such major republics as Armenia, Georgia, and Russia began to split apart themselves. Where one nuclear power once stood, now four (Russia, Belarus, Ukraine, Kazakhstan) housed these weapons, although the Russian military supposedly continued to control all the triggers. The former Soviet military disintegrated until its ability to restart a long cold war disappeared. Some 60 to 70 percent of young men ordered to report for service simply refused to show up. But danger remained amidst the disorder: the Russian military "can do nothing much in Moscow," one expert believed, "but they can wipe out New York."[44]

In Yugoslavia, Africa, and parts of the former Soviet Union, the spreading conflicts posed a critical foreign-policy problem for Clinton: Should he intervene in these struggles if they threatened to spin out of control? And if so, how capable would U.S. military power be in solving such crises? After all, the military, led by General Powell and his Vietnam-trained generation, willingly fought only wars that promised quick victories. As many foreign armies had discovered over the centuries, quick victories were not to be found in Russia or Yugoslavia. As for Africa, the United States paid little attention to the great continent after the white South African government finally, after forty years, began to end apartheid and treat the black majority better, although by no means equally. Analyst Marguerite Michaels noted that the end of the cold war "set America free to pursue its own interests in Africa—and found that it did not have any." U.S. investments between 1985 and 1993 tripled in Latin America, quintupled in East Asia, but actually declined in Africa.[45]

So why, on December 4, 1992, did President Bush, with President-elect Clinton's strong support, suddenly send 21,000 U.S. troops into

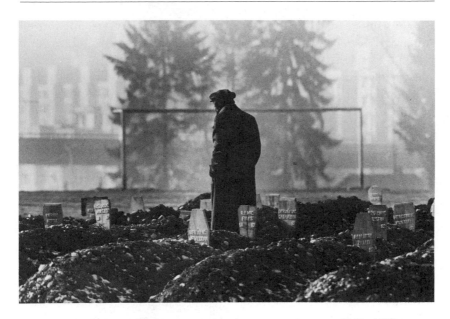

A New World Order? After the collapse of the Soviet empire in 1989–1991, many hoped for "a new world order," as President Bush phrased it in 1991. Instead, nationalist, ethnic, and religious wars erupted in parts of the globe. The worst occurred in Yugoslavia during 1992, when the country splintered and religious groups (especially Eastern Orthodox Christians and Muslims) fought each other. As the casualties mounted into the tens of thousands in the Bosnian capital of Sarajevo, this soccer field had to be turned into a cemetary—and a place where an elderly man mourned the death of his wife of some fifty years. She had been killed by the random shelling and sniper fire. Neither the United States nor the Europeans could figure out how to end the horror without sacrificing their own soldiers. U.S. Secretary of State Warren Christopher called Yugoslavia a "problem from hell."

the East African nation of Somalia? This episode exemplified the kinds of questions that promised to plague (and tax) Americans in the new era of disorder.

In the 1980s, first Moscow, then Washington poured weapons into this poor, but strategically located, nation of 5 million souls in order to keep Somalia's dictator, Mohamed Siad Barre, friendly. In 1991, the cold-war aid dried up and Siad Barre fled. He left behind enough U.S. and Soviet arms "to fuel hostilities for 100 years" in Somalia, one Pentagon official noted. In early 1991, two factions used these weapons to kill each other as each tried to seize power. The country spiraled downward into banditry, wholesale looting, mass destruction, and finally spreading starvation. United Nations personnel who tried to feed the people were repeatedly attacked. U.S. television crews soon showed American viewers fly-covered, starving children with rail-thin legs and bloated stomachs. Some 300,000 people died, with 2 million more starving. Demands rose that Bush and other world leaders act. The United Nations seized the moment and, for the first time in its history, became directly involved militarily in a nation's internal affairs without that nation's consent. It was a historic turn. Bush thus dispatched the U.S. troops (joined by 2,000 French soldiers and military units from a dozen other nations.)[46]

Bush aimed to end the starvation by protecting food supplies from the many armed bandits. (One puzzled U.S. soldier was told how to tell friends from enemies: the "good guys" were very thin and the "bad guys" were fat.) It was a mission of mercy, the arrival of "the cavalry" as in movie westerns, declared General Powell. Questions, however, plagued Bush and Clinton. First, should U.S. forces be used for such missions when no direct American strategic or political interest was involved? That question became more pressing as U.S. soldiers were killed and a planned two-month mission stretched far longer. Second, how could Americans and other UN members decide when intervention was necessary? Starvation was not limited to Somalia. It was perhaps worse in parts of the Sudan, Liberia, and Yugoslavia. Some critics believed Somalia was singled out because it was defenseless and easy for U.S. forces to reach. Critics also believed Somalia gained attention simply because television highlighted the starvation there. U.S. policy and lives, in other words, were becoming dependent on decisions made in the offices of CNN, ABC, NBC, and CBS. When the troops waded ashore, they fought their way, not through Somali resistance, but through hundreds of reporters, cameras, and giant strobe lights that turned the night into day.[47]

Another question involved the United Nations. Freed of Soviet-bloc opposition, the UN took on some fourteen peacekeeping operations (including Somalia), with its blue-helmeted forces that represented many nations. These operations had even received the Nobel Peace Prize in 1988, especially for efforts in the Middle East and Africa. The question became whether Americans, who historically have greatly mistrusted an international organization unless they controlled it, would accept such peacekeeping responsibilities if future UN policies ran against U.S. interests. China, after all, held a veto in the UN, as did the Russians. Secretary of State Christopher, moreover, believed that Germany and Japan would become the sixth and seventh permanent members of the Security Council, and thus also would hold veto power.

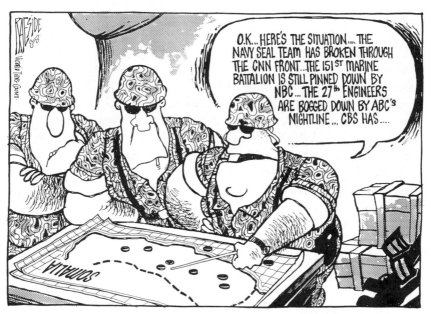

Raeside's cartoon caught the influence that the media exerted on U.S. policy toward Somalia and, in particular, on the military landings—landings that occurred in December 1992 amid ranges of television cameras and lights controlled by scores of reporters who occupied the landing sites ahead of the troops.

United Nations power could fragment, much as power was already fragmenting in the world the UN represented. Indeed, by mid-1993, UN efforts in Somalia were threatened by disputes among the U.S., French, Pakistani, and Italian forces that made up the UN peacekeepers. When Somali strongmen, angry at the UN presence, killed thirty-five peacekeepers, U.S. gunships strafed and bombed the strongmen's bunkers—only to have the Italians condemn Clinton's use of force as resembling "Rambo's" and demanding that diplomacy replace force.[48]

Clinton's World: The American Age

Answering these questions assumed that Americans can respond meaningfully and rationally to the problems of the growing disorder in the world. Americans are, after all, the only remaining superpower. Only they can militarily intervene nearly anywhere on the globe. They enjoy an economy that is twice the size of its nearest competitor. Their culture of films, fast food, jeans, sports, music, and language permeates other important countries, even those, such as Japan and France, that are intensely protective of their own national cultures. It would seem, therefore, that Americans should indeed be worldly wise, careful, and rational.

Shrewd observers, however, have expressed doubts about this assumption. Perhaps the shrewdest, the French visitor Alexis de Tocqueville, wrote in the 1830s that the American democratic system was splendid for developing a continent, but he did not believe the individualistic, open, rapidly changing society could conduct an effective foreign policy.[49] In the 1920s, Walter Lippmann, agreed (see p. 737).

Between 1947 and 1990 Tocqueville's and Lippmann's fears were removed by the Truman Doctrine. This 1947 doctrine created such a strong anti-Communist consensus that U.S. officials could simply assume public support when they confronted the Soviet bloc. In 1990–1991, however, the consensus disappeared along with the Soviet bloc. George Bush could not build a new consensus. The Republican party, which had brilliantly used anticommunism to paper over its internal disputes on such domestic issues as abortion, began to divide. Clinton played on those divisions by stressing domestic issues in his campaign.

The question nevertheless remained whether the new president could build a consensus for his foreign policies. He made two early attempts. First, he urged Americans to rally behind the advancement of democracy and self-determination. When Secretary of State Robert Lansing had heard Woodrow Wilson's cry for self-determination in 1918, he worried that "the phrase is simply loaded with dynamite. It will raise hopes that can never be realized. It will, I fear, cost thousands of lives. What a calamity that the phrase was ever uttered!" Lansing's fears were borne out in eastern Europe after 1990. Even Secretary of State Christopher warned in 1993 that unless something was done, "We'll have 50,000 countries rather than the hundred plus we now have."[50]

Clinton's second attempt to build a consensus arose from his economic policies. He declared that, contrary to Reagan's and Bush's beliefs, government had to play a strong role in supporting U.S. economic interests. The new president found, however, that many such interests existed, and some bitterly clashed with others. For example, industrialists and investors, as noted above, supported the free-trade treaty that allowed them to build plants in Mexico, but U.S. laborers fought the treaty.

President Clinton's hope that Americans would support active economic policies overseas also hit other obstacles. There was, for instance, a question of how far Americans could even shape such policies. The world economy was increasingly dominated by giant multinational

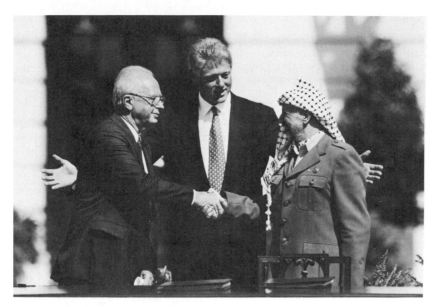

*A handshake marked a high point of early post–cold war history and symbol-
ized the hope to end generations of war in the Middle East. In September 1993
Prime Minister Yitzhak Rabin of Israel (on left) and Yasir Arafat, chairman of
the Palestinian Liberation Organization (PLO) gingerly shook hands on the
sun-drenched White House lawn after their foreign ministers signed a historic
peace treaty. President Bill Clinton helped pull the once-mortal enemies
together for the handshake. The treaty provided that Israel withdraw its troops
from Gaza and the West Bank city of Jericho, then later from other populated
West Bank areas. Palestinians in these areas would move toward more self-government. Israel would retain military supremacy in surrounding territory. The
PLO's one-time pledge to destroy Israel would be replaced by joint PLO-Israeli
groups to work out common problems. Clinton promised to tackle the pivotal
problem of raising some $4 billion (mostly from allies) to ease the West Bank–
Gaza economic crises. Rabin's eloquence captured the moment: "We who have
seen our relatives and friends killed before our eyes; we who have attended their
funerals and cannot look into the eyes of their parents . . . we say to you [Pales-
tinians] today, in a loud and clear voice: enough of blood and tears. Enough."*

corporations (Honda, General Motors, Nike, Sony, Ford, IBM) that
easily moved across national boundaries. Many a multinational produced more goods than did dozens of nations. Over a trillion dollars a
day moved through world financial markets. A nation, even the United
States, would try to control that tide of money only at its own financial
peril.

Such private economic power could help develop countries, but it could also help push them into disorder. Most notably, as the cold war's vast military needs ended, producers and merchants of military arms sold their weapons in regions where the new wars erupted. In 1987, the United States sold $6.5 billion in arms abroad. By 1992, the figure nearly quadrupled to $24 billion. Taiwan, Kuwait, Saudi Arabia, and South Korea were among the heavy buyers. China and Russia also sold massive amounts of arms, especially to such anti-U.S. countries as Iran. As one U.S. banker put it, "We're unlikely to sacrifice economic interests to take the moral high ground in curbing arms sales."[51]

Americans liked stability. But they also liked modern capitalism, and they wanted other peoples to emulate their economic system. They had problems, however, in seeking both stability and capitalism. Modern, multinational capitalism could be quite disorderly. As the conservative journal, the *Economist* of London, phrased it, in 1993 Russia again "is convulsed by a revolutionary idea imported from the West. The idea this time is not Marxism but the market. Yet the upheaval could end once more in disaster."[52] A disaster had already occurred in China. Dynamic fresh ideas, especially private enterprise, clashed with the government's Communist ideology. One result was the government's killing of protesters in Tiananmen Square in 1989. As noted earlier in this book, Americans had actually experienced similar disasters themselves. Between the 1840s and 1900 a new U.S. industrial and financial capitalism had produced strikes that were put down with armed force, massive social dislocation, violent protests in major cities, and, some would argue, the Civil War. In the 1990s, President Clinton dealt with an even more dynamic and independent capitalism that breached national boundaries—just as ethnic and religious hatreds exploded within those boundaries.

Clinton represented a new generation, the Vietnam generation, that now took the reins of government. But key problems seemed to resemble less the 1960s than the 1920s, or the late nineteenth-century-to-1914 era. After forty years of cold war, history seemed to be beginning again. Americans had to come to terms with that history. What we are and what we would like to be, the conservative British philosopher Michael Oakeshott warned, is a creature of what we have been.[53] Understanding and building on that past is necessary, or else a famous American conservative, Henry Adams, might have the last word:

> Modern politics is, at bottom, a struggle not of men but of forces. The men become every year more and more creatures of force, massed about central power-houses. The conflict is no longer between the men, but between

the motors that drive men, and the men tend to succumb to their own motive forces.[54]

James Madison and other founders raised grave doubts about Adams's pessimistic view that individuals could not control the "motors" of their own society. Out of a fragmented country, Madison and his colleagues created a more coherent and prosperous nation. In 1829, Madison wrote that he did not expect the system he helped create to last forever. But to note the way he and others went about their work in 1787, especially how they studied and learned from history, is an appropriate way to end as well as begin the story of the American age.

NOTES

1. Paul Boyer, ed., *Reagan as President* (Chicago, 1990), pp. 264–267.
2. *Ibid.*, pp. 270–281.
3. This is drawn especially from Caryn James, "Today's Yellow Brick Road Leads Straight to Hell," *New York Times*, 19 August 1990, p. H1.
4. *New York Times*, 22 March 1989, p. A25.
5. George Bush, *Bushisms*, compiled by the editors of *The New Republic* (New York, 1992), p. 60.
6. Michael R. Beschloss and Strobe Talbott, *At the Highest Levels* (Boston, 1993), p. 193; Walter LaFeber, *Inevitable Revolutions*, 2nd ed. (New York, 1993), pp. 339–353.
7. William I. Robinson, *A Faustian Bargain: U.S. Intervention in the Nicaraguan Elections and American Foreign Policy in the Post-Cold War Era* (Boulder, Colo., 1992), pp. 111–119.
8. *Washington Post*, 15 November 1992, p. A31; *New York Times*, 16 February 1993, p. A1.
9. *New York Times*, 16 March 1993, p. A20; *Washington Post*, 16 December 1992, p. A1; *Washington Post*, 13 March 1993, p. A1; *Washington Post*, 14 March 1993, p. C1.
10. *New York Times*, 17 October 1992, p. 5; *Washington Post*, 17 October 1992, p. A18; Rigoberta Menchú, *I, Rigoberta Menchú . . .* (London, 1984).
11. *Washington Post*, 16 December 1992, p. A24.
12. *Ibid.*, 22 November 1992, in *Central America NewsPak*, 16–29 November 1992, p. 2.
13. The background is in Michael L. Conniff, *Panama and the United States* (Athens, Ga., 1992), esp. pp. 149–168; and Andrew Zimbalist and John Weeks, *Panama at the Crossroads* (Berkeley, Calif., 1991), pp. 142–156. The most thorough investigation is the New York Bar Association Committees' report in *The Record of the Association of the Bar of the City of New York* 47 (October 1992), esp. pp. 607–609, 634–

651, 674–678, 692–693; also *New York Times*, 13 August 1991, p. A1, on later drug traffic; *Washington Post*, 10 April 1992, p. A35, for a summary of the Noriega trial.

14. Beschloss and Talbott, *At the Highest Levels*, pp. 9–13, 27–28, 34, 43–45; Don Oberdorfer, *The Turn* (New York, 1991), pp. 333–334; David Remnick, "Dumb Luck; Bush's Cold War," *The New Yorker*, 25 January 1993, p. 106.

15. Frank Costigliola, "German Reunification, NATO, and the Problem of U.S. Leadership, 1989–1990," forthcoming, in *Contemporary European History*, 1994; Beschloss and Talbott, *At the Highest Levels*, pp. 169–170, 184–187; Stephen F. Szabo, *The Diplomacy of German Unification* (New York, 1992), pp. 41–51, 62–65, 95–112; *Newsweek*, 25 December 1989, p. 33; *Washington Post*, 14 September 1990, p. A18; *New York Times*, 1 July 1990, p. 6.

16. Oberdorfer, *The Turn*, p. 381; *New York Times*, 7 July 1990, p. A1.

17. Beschloss and Talbott, *At the Highest Levels*, pp. 176–177, 192.

18. John Morrison, *Boris Yeltsin* (New York, 1991), pp. 33–35.

19. Beschloss and Talbott, *At the Highest Levels*, pp. 296–309; also Morrison, *Yeltsin*, pp. 56–73, for background.

20. Beschloss and Talbott, *At the Highest Levels*, p. 349; author's interviews in Moscow, June 1989, March 1991; *Washington Post*, 30 May, 1990, p. A8.

21. *Washington Post*, 22 March 1993, p. A12; *Washington Post*, 17 February 1993, p. A42; Beschloss and Talbott, *At the Highest Levels*, pp. 421–441; Remnick, "Dumb Luck," pp. 106–108.

22. *Washington Post*, 22 March 1993, p. A12.

23. *Ibid.*, 6 June 1990, p. A17; *New York Times*, 4 February 1991, p. D6.

24. Christopher Madison, "Catch-up Diplomacy," *National Journal*, 22 February 1992, p. 448.

25. Judith Miller and Laurie Mylroie, *Saddam Hussein, The Crisis in the Gulf* (New York, 1990), esp. chaps. 1–4; Daniel Yergin, *The Prize* (New York, 1991), pp. 770–775; Theodore Draper, "The Gulf War Reconsidered," *New York Review of Books*, 16 January 1992, pp. 46–51; *Washington Post*, 7 August 1990, p. A14.

26. Micah L. Sifry and Christopher Cerf, eds., *The Gulf War Reader* (New York, 1991), pp. 119–133 for the Glaspie-Saddam Hussein exchange; Draper, "Gulf War Reconsidered," pp. 51–53; *New York Times*, 9 August 1990, p. D19.

27. Yergin, *The Prize*, pp. 775–779.

28. A good contemporary analysis is Elizabeth Drew, "Letter from Washington," *The New Yorker*, 4 February 1991, pp. 86–88; representative views can be found in Sifry and Cerf, *The Gulf War Reader*, pp. 234–264, 269–289, which also gives the joint resolution's text of January 12, 1991.

29. Michael A. Palmer, *Guardians of the Gulf: A History of America's Expanding Role in the Persian Gulf, 1833–1991* (New York, 1992), p. 196.

30. *New York Times*, 17 August 1990, p. A1; the best analysis of Powell, and his reluctance to use force in Iraq, is Bob Woodward, *The Commanders* (New York, 1992).

31. *Economist*, 2 May 1992, pp. 53–54.

32. Laurie Mylroie, "Iraq's Real Coup," *Washington Post*, 28 June 1992, p. C1.

33. *Washington Post*, 20 January 1993, p. A4; *Washington Post*, 5 September 1992, p. A15.

34. The text is in *New York Times*, 16 December 1992, p. A25.

35. *New York Times*, 28 October 1992, p. A21.

36. Wade Huntley, "Point of View," *Chronicle of Higher Education*, 31 March 1993, p. A40; *New York Times*, op-ed by James Webb, "What Foreign Policy?," 1 December 1991; *New York Times*, 14 June 1992, p. 10.

37. *Washington Post*, 19 September 1992, p. A10; *Washington Post*, 6 November 1992, p. A11; *Washington Post*, 21 January 1993, p. A26, for the inaugural address.

38. "Remarks Prepared for Delivery. Governor Bill Clinton. Foreign Policy Association. New York—April 1, 1992," unpublished; *New York Times*, 4 October 1992, p. 28.

39. *New York Times*, 3 January 1993, p. 16; Lake, "Vietnam War," in Joel Krieger, et al., eds., *The Oxford Companion to the Politics of the World* (New York, 1993) p. 958.

40. Bruce Cumings, "Trilateralism and the New World Order," *World Policy Journal* 8 (Spring 1992), p. 210.

41. *Washington Post*, 1 December 1992, p. A30; *Economist*, 20 February 1993, pp. 19–22; *New York Times*, 18 March 1993, p. A23; *New York Times*, 11 January 1993, p. A1.

42. *Washington Post*, 3 May 1992, p. A1; *Washington Post*, 15 May 1990, p. A4.

43. Gregory F. Treverton, *America, Germany, and the Future of Europe* (Princeton, 1992), pp. 180–181; *Washington Post*, 11 October 1992, p. C7.

44. *Washington Post*, 24 March 1993, p. A24.

45. *New York Times*, 7 March 1993, p. E4.

46. *Washington Post*, 4 December 1992, p. A20; *Washington Post*, 1 December 1992, p. A1; Richard J. Barnet, "Still Putting Arms First," *Harper's Magazine* (February 1993), pp. 59–65.

47. Stephen John Stedman, "The New Interventionists," *Foreign Affairs* 72 (No. 1, 1992–1993), esp. pp. 2–4; *New York Times*, 13 December 1992, p. E3; *New York Times*, 8 December 1992, p. C20; *Washington Post*, 4 December 1992, p. A24.

48. Samuel W. Lewis, "Point of View: The Decade of the 1990s," *United States Institute of Peace Journal* III (March 1990), p. 2; *New York Times*, 9 December 1992, p. A17; *New York Times*, 22 July 1993, p. A23.

49. Alexis de Tocqueville, *Democracy in America*, 2 vols. (New York, 1948), I, pp. 234–236.

50. *New York Times*, 7 February 1993, p. 1; *New York Times*, 22 September 1993, p. A13.

51. *Ibid.*, 4 October 1992, p. F5.

52. *Economist*, 13 March 1993, p. 17.

53. Quoted in Henry Jackson, *From the Congo to Soweto* (New York, 1982), p. 39.

54. Henry Adams, *The Education of Henry Adams* (Boston, 1918), p. 421.

FOR FURTHER READING

Begin by consulting the footnotes for this chapter and the General Bibliography at the end of the book. References given in those two places are usually not repeated here. A number of useful overviews have been published on the end of the cold war and possible consequences: Michael J. Hogan, ed., *The End of the Cold War* (1992); Nicholas X. Rizopoulos, ed., *Sea-Changes* (1990), especially the McNeill, Strange, Hoffmann essays for background; James Chace, *The Consequences of the Peace* (1992), good notably on economic consequences; William G. Hyland, *The Cold War Is Over* (1991), by an experienced expert on Russia; Robert Jervis and Seweryn Bailer, eds, *Soviet-American Relations after the Cold War* (1991), especially the Dallek essay on U.S. responses; John Lewis Gaddis, *The United States and the End of the Cold War* (New York, 1992), which gives more credit to Reagan than do many observers.

For Russian-American relations, a key source is U.S. Congress, House Committee on Foreign Affairs, *Special Studies Series on Foreign Affairs Issues*. Volume III: *Soviet Diplomacy and Negotiating Behavior—1988–1990: Gorbachev-Reagan-Bush Meetings at the Summit* (1991). Also very helpful are Fred Halliday, *From Kabul to Managua* (1989), on the background; Lubomyr Hajda and Mark Beissinger, eds., *The Nationalities Factor in Soviet Politics and Society* (1990); Timothy Garton Ash, *The Magic Lantern* (1990), wonderful on the opening of eastern Europe; Charles Gati, *The Bloc That Failed* (1990), by a respected scholar on eastern Europe; Michael A. Freney and Rebecca S. Hartley, *United Germany and the United States* (1991), with helpful documents as well as commentary; John R. Lampe, *et al.*, *Yugoslav-American Relations Since World War II* (1991), for background to the tragedy; Francis Fukuyama, *The End of History and the Last Man* (1992), the widely read argument on what it all means.

On specific regions, the following are helpful as starting points: Jan S. Adams, *A Foreign Policy in Transition: Moscow's Retreat from Central America and the Caribbean, 1985–1992* (1992); John Booth and Thomas Walker, *Understanding Central America* (1993); Brenda Gayle Plummer, *Haiti and the United States* (1992), a superb, concise background for understanding the immigrant question and Haiti's upheaval in 1990–1993; Kevin Buckley, *Panama: The Whole Story* (1991), to be used with Conniff, noted in the footnotes; Michael Clough, *Free at Last? U.S. Policy Toward Africa and the End of the Cold War* (1992); Zaki Laidi, *The Superpowers and Africa, 1960–1990* (1990). For the trade relationships, as well as the political relationships, Frank Costigliola, *The Cold Alliance* (1992), is an excellent analysis of U.S.-western European economic developments since 1945, and the best account of U.S.-France relations during the cold war and after; René Schwok, *U.S.-EC Relations in the Post–Cold War Era* (1991), has good background; Sidney Weintraub, *A Marriage of Convenience* (1990), is excellent on U.S.-Mexico relations; Sidney Weintraub, *et al.*, *U.S.-Mexican Industrial Integration* (1991), is an excellent overview; Robert Bothwell, *Canada and the United States* (1992), examines the political effects of economic ties; Kenneth B. Pyle, *The Japanese Question* (1992), is an excellent and concise discussion of the historical background; Paul Krugman, ed., *Trade with Japan* (1992), is a thorough analysis; Akio Morita and Shinturo Ishihara, *The Japan That Can Say "NO"* (1990), is a widely noted, controversial Japanese view; William Dietrich, *In the Shadow of the Rising Sun* (1991), well analyzes why the United States faces such tough Japanese competition.

On the Persian Gulf War, the best overviews are Stephen R. Graubard, *Mr. Bush's War* (1992), and Jean Edward Smith, *George Bush's War* (1992), which is also quite critical; Michael A. Palmer, *Guardians of the Gulf* (1992), is an excellent history of 1833–1991; Kenneth R. Timmerman, *The Death Lobby* (1991), brilliantly reveals how Saddam Hussein was armed by the West; Abdul-Reda Assiri, *Kuwait's Foreign Policy* (1990), is a Kuwaiti view of a nation that was not especially friendly to the United States until August 1990; General Norman Schwarzkopf, with Peter Petrie, *It Doesn't Take a Hero* (1992), is the U.S. general's best-selling account; Alexander George, *Forceful Persuasion* (1992), beautifully explores nonmilitary alternatives in the Iraqi and other crises.

Warren Cohen, *America in the Age of Soviet Power*, in *The Cambridge History of American Foreign Relations*, ed. Warren Cohen (1993) is superb on the pre-1992 background and has an excellent bibliography.

For the Clinton administration. Charles F. Allen, *The Comeback Kid* (1992), is an initial start on a biography of Clinton.

U.S. Presidents and Secretaries of State

Presidents	Secretaries of State
George Washington of Virginia (1789–1797)	Robert R. Livingston of New York (1781–1783 under Continental Congress)
	John Jay of New York (1784–1789 under Continental Congress)
	Thomas Jefferson of Virginia (1789–1793)
	Edmund Randolph of Virginia (1794–1795)
John Adams of Massachusetts (1797–1801)	Timothy Pickering of Pennsylvania (1795–1800)
	John Marshall of Virginia (1800–1801)
Thomas Jefferson of Virginia (1801–1809)	James Madison of Virginia (1801–1809)
James Madison of Virginia (1809–1817)	Robert Smith of Maryland (1809–1811)
	James Monroe of Virginia (1811–1817)
James Monroe of Virginia (1817–1825)	John Quincy Adams of Massachusetts (1817–1825)
John Quincy Adams of Massachusetts (1825–1829)	Henry Clay of Kentucky (1825–1829)
Andrew Jackson of Tennessee (1829–1837)	Martin Van Buren of New York (1829–1831)
	Edward Livingston of Louisiana (1831–1833)
	Louis McLane of Delaware (1833–1834)
Martin Van Buren of New York (1837–1841)	John Forsyth of Georgia (1834–1841)

William Henry Harrison of Ohio (1841)

Daniel Webster of Massachusetts (1841–1843)

John Tyler of Virginia (1841–1845)

Abel P. Upshur of Virginia (1843–1844)

John C. Calhoun of South Carolina (1844–1845)

James K. Polk of Tennessee (1845–1849)

James Buchanan of Pennsylvania (1845–1849)

Zachary Taylor of Louisiana (1849–1850)

John M. Clayton of Delaware (1849–1850)

Millard Fillmore of New York (1850–1853)

Daniel Webster of Massachusetts (1850–1852)

Edward Everett of Massachusetts (1852–1853)

Franklin Pierce of New Hampshire (1853–1857)

William L. Marcy of New York (1853–1857)

James Buchanan of Pennsylvania (1857–1861)

Lewis Cass of Michigan (1857–1860)

Jeremiah S. Black of Pennsylvania (1860–1861)

Abraham Lincoln of Illinois (1861–1865)

William H. Seward of New York (1861–1869)

Andrew Johnson of Tennessee (1865–1869)

Ulysses S. Grant of Illinois (1869–1877)

Hamilton Fish of New York (1869–1877)

Rutherford B. Hayes of Ohio (1877–1881)

William M. Evarts of New York (1877–1881)

James A. Garfield of Ohio (1881)

James G. Blaine of Maine (1881)

Chester A. Arthur of New York (1881–1885)

Frederick T. Frelinghuysen of New Jersey (1881–1885)

Grover Cleveland of New York (1885–1889)

Thomas F. Bayard of Delaware (1885–1889)

Benjamin Harrison of Indiana (1889–1893)

James G. Blaine of Maine (1889–1892)

John W. Foster of Indiana (1892–1893)

Grover Cleveland of New York (1893–1897)

Walter Q. Gresham of Indiana (1893–1895)

Richard Olney of Massachusetts (1895–1897)

William McKinley of Ohio (1897–1901)

John Sherman of Ohio (1897–1898)

William R. Day of Ohio (1898)

John Hay of the District of Columbia (1898–1905)

Theodore Roosevelt of New York (1901–1909)

William Howard Taft of Ohio (1909–1913)

Woodrow Wilson of New Jersey (1913–1921)

Elihu Root of New York (1905–1909)
Robert Bacon of New York (1909)
Philander C. Knox of Pennsylvania (1909–1913)
William Jennings Bryan of Nebraska (1913–1915)
Robert Lansing of New York (1915–1920)
Bainbridge Colby of New York (1920–1921)

Warren G. Harding of Ohio (1921–1923)

Calvin Coolidge of Massachusetts (1923–1929)

Herbert C. Hoover of California (1929–1933)

Franklin D. Roosevelt of New York (1933–1945)

Charles Evans Hughes of New York (1921–1925)
Frank B. Kellogg of Minnesota (1925–1929)
Henry L. Stimson of New York (1929–1933)
Cordell Hull of Tennessee (1933–1944)
Edward R. Stettinius of Virginia (1944–1945)

Harry S. Truman of Missouri (1945–1953)

James F. Byrnes of South Carolina (1945–1947)
George C. Marshall of Pennsylvania (1947–1949)
Dean G. Acheson of Maryland (1949–1953)

Dwight D. Eisenhower of New York (1953–1961)

John Foster Dulles of New York (1953–1959)
Christian A. Herter of Massachusetts (1959–1961)

John F. Kennedy of Massachusetts (1961–1963)

Lyndon B. Johnson of Texas (1963–1969)

Richard M. Nixon of California (1969–1974)

Gerald R. Ford of Michigan (1974–1977)

Jimmy Carter of Georgia (1977–1981)

Dean Rusk of New York (1961–1969)

William P. Rogers of Maryland (1969–1973)
Henry A. Kissinger of the District of Columbia (1973–1977)
Cyrus R. Vance of New York (1977–1980)
Edmund Muskie of Maine (1980–1981)

Ronald Reagan of California (1981–1989)

Alexander Haig of Maryland (1981–1982)

George Shultz of California (1982–1989)

George Bush of Texas (1989–1993)

James A. Baker of Texas (1989–1993)

William Clinton of Arkansas (1993–   )

Warren Christopher of California (1993–   )

General Bibliography

AFGHANISTAN: Anthony Arnold, *Afghanistan* (1981); Stanley Wolpert, *Roots of Confrontation in South Asia* (1982).

AFRICA: *Africa Contemporary Record: Annual Survey and Documents* (1968–   ); Peter Duignan and Lewis H. Gann, *The United States and Africa* (1984); Henry F. Jackson, *From Congo to Soweto* (1982). (See also individual countries.)

ANGOLA: John A. Marcum, *The Angolan Revolution*, 2 vols. (1969, 1978). (See also AFRICA.)

ARGENTINA: Joseph Tulchin, *Argentina and the United States* (1990); Arthur P. Whitaker, *The U.S. and the Southern Cone* (1976). (See also LATIN AMERICA.)

ATLASES: Gerard Chaliand and Jean-Pierre Rageau, *Strategic Atlas* (1985); Michael Kidron and Dan Smith, *The State of the World Atlas* (1981); Harry F. Young, *Atlas of U.S. Foreign Relations* (1983).

AUSTRALIA: Glen St. John Barclay, *Friends in High Places: The Australian-American Security Relationship since 1945* (1985).

BIBLIOGRAPHY: *Guide to American Foreign Relations since 1700*, ed. Richard Dean Burns (1983); Linda Killen and Richard L. Lael, *Versailles and After: An Annotated Bibliography of American Foreign Relations, 1919–1933* (1982). (See also individual topics.)

BRAZIL: Frank D. McCann, *The Brazilian-American Alliance, 1937–1945* (1972); Robert Wesson, *The U.S. and Brazil* (1981). (See also LATIN AMERICA.)

CAMBODIA: William Shawcross, *The Quality of Mercy* (1984); William Shawcross, *Sideshow* (1979). (See also VIETNAM.)

CANADA: Charles Doran, *Forgotten Partnership* (1985); *Canada and the United States*, ed. Charles F. Doran and John H. Sigler (1985); Seymour Martin Lipset, *Continental Divide* (1990); Lawrence Martin, *Presidents and the Prime Ministers . . . 1867–1982* (1982).

CENTRAL AMERICA: John Booth and Thomas Walker, *Understanding Central America* (1993); *The Central American Crisis*, ed. Kenneth M. Coleman and George C. Herring (1991); Walter LaFeber, *Inevitable Revolutions* (1993); Thomas M. Leonard, *Central America and U.S. Policies, 1820s–1980s* (1985). Ralph L. Woodward, *Central America* (1986). (See also individual countries.)

CENTRAL INTELLIGENCE AGENCY: John Ranelagh, *The Agency* (1987); Bradley F. Smith, *The Shadow Warriors* (1983); Gregory F. Treverton, *Covert Action* (1987).

CHILE: James Petras and Morris Morley, *The U.S. and Chile* (1975); William F. Sater, *Chile and the United States* (1990).

CHINA: Warren Cohen, *America's Response to China* (1990); John K. Fairbank, *The U.S. and China* (1983); Michael H. Hunt, *The Making of a Special Relationship: The U.S. and China to 1914* (1983); Arnold Xiangze Jiang, *The U.S. and China* (1988); Michael Schaller, *The U.S. and China in the Twentieth Century* (1990).

COLOMBIA: Richard Lael, *Arrogant Diplomacy . . . 1903–1922* (1987).

COMMUNISM: Hoover Institution, *Yearbook on International Communist Affairs* (1966–   ). (See also individual countries.)

CONGRESS: John Rourke, *Congress and the Presidency in U.S. Foreign Policymaking* (1983); *Congress and American Foreign Policy*, ed. Göran Rystad (1982); *To Advise and Consent*, 2 vols., ed. Joel Silbey (1990).

CONSTITUTION: Louis Fisher, *Constitutional Conflicts between Congress and the President* (1985); Louis Henkin, *Foreign Affairs and the Constitution* (1975); Charles A. Lofgren, *Government from Reflection and Choice* (1986); John H. Sullivan, *The War Powers Resolution* (1982).

CONTAINMENT: *Containment*, 2 vols., ed. Terry L. Deibel and J. L. Gaddis (1986); J. L. Gaddis, *Strategies of Containment* (1982).

CUBA: Philip S. Foner, *A History of Cuba in Its Relations with the U.S.* (1962–   ); Morris H. Morley, *Imperial State and Revolution* (1987); Louis A. Perez, Jr., *Cuba: An Annotated Bibliography* (1988); Louis A. Perez, Jr., *Cuba and the United States* (1990); Robert F. Smith, *The U.S. and Cuba* (1969).

CULTURE AND PHILANTHROPHY: Edward H. Berman, *The Influence of the Carnegie, Ford, and Rockefeller Foundations on American Foreign Policy* (1983); Morrell Heald and Lawrence S. Kaplan, *Culture and Diplomacy* (1977); Frank A. Ninkovich, *The Diplomacy of Ideas . . . 1938–1950* (1981); Ron Robin, *Enclaves of America; The Rhetoric of American Political Architecture Abroad, 1900–1965* (1992).

DEPARTMENT OF STATE: Robert U. Goehlert and Elizabeth Hoffmeister, *The Department of State and American Diplomacy* (1986) [bibliography]; Barry Rubin, *Secrets of State* (1985); Richard H. Werking, *The Master Architects: Building the U.S. Foreign Service, 1890–1913* (1977).

DICTIONARIES: John E. Findling, *Dictionary of American Diplomatic History* (1980).

DOCUMENTS: Ruhl Bartlett, *The Record of American Diplomacy* (1964); U.S. Department of State, *Foreign Relations of the United States* (1861–   ); U.S. Superintendent of Documents, *Monthly Catalog of U.S. Government Publications* (1895–   ).

DOMINICAN REPUBLIC: Rayford W. Logan, *Haiti and the Dominican Republic* (1968).

ECONOMICS: *Economics and World Power*, ed. William H. Becker and Samuel F. Wells, Jr. (1984); Joan Edelman Spero, *The Politics of International Economic Relations*, (1981); *Economic Coercion and U.S. Foreign Policy*, ed. Sidney Weintraub (1982); Mira Wilkins, *The Emergence of the Multinational Enterprise* (1970); Mira Wilkins, *The Maturing of the Multinational Enterprise* (1974); William A. Williams, *The Tragedy of American Diplomacy* (1988).

EGYPT: William J. Burns, *Economic Aid and American Policy toward Egypt, 1955–1981* (1985). (See also MIDDLE EAST.)

EL SALVADOR: Cynthia Arnson, *El Salvador* (1982); Raymond Bonner, *Weakness and Deceit* (1984); *El Salvador*, ed. Marvin E. Gettleman *et al.*, (1981); Tommie Sue Montgomery, *Revolution in El Salvador* (1982). (See also CENTRAL AMERICA.)

ENCYCLOPEDIAS: *Political Handbook of the World*, ed. Arthur S. Bank (1975–   ); *Ency-*

clopedia of American Foreign Policy, 3 vols., ed. Alexander DeConde (1978).

ETHIOPIA: David A. Korn, *Ethiopia, the U.S., and the Soviet Union* (1986). Jeffrey S. Lefebvre, *Arms for the Horn . . . 1953–1991* (1991). (See also AFRICA.)

ETHNIC GROUPS: *Ethnic Groups and U.S. Foreign Policy*, ed. Mohammed E. Ahrari (1987); Paul Findley, *They Dare to Speak Out* (1985); Edward Tivnan, *The Lobby* (1987); Stephen A. Garrett, *From Potsdam to Poland* (1986) [on Polish ethnic groups]. (See also RACE AND ETHNICITY.)

EUROPE: Richard Barnet, *The Alliance* (1984); *American Historians and the Atlantic Alliance*, ed. Lawrence Kaplan (1991); Pierre Mélandri, *Les États-Unis face à l'unification de l'Europe: 1945–1954* (1980); *The Dissolving Alliance*, ed. Richard L. Rubenstein (1987). (See also individual countries.)

EXECUTIVE AGREEMENTS: Diane Shaver Clemens, "Executive Agreements," in *Encyclopedia of American Foreign Policy*, ed. Alexander DeConde (1978); Lawrence Margolis, *Executive Agreements and Presidential Power in Foreign Policy* (1986). (See also CONSTITUTION.)

FRANCE: Frank Costigliola, *The Cold Alliance* (1992); Julian G. Hurstfield, *America and the French Nation* (1986).

GERMANY: Manfred Jonas, *U.S. and Germany* (1984); Frank Ninkovich, *Germany and the United States* (1988); *Germany and America*, ed. Hans L. Trefousse (1981).

GREAT BRITAIN: *The Special Relationship . . . since 1945*, ed. William R. Louis and Hedley Bull (1986).

GREECE: *Greek-American Relations*, ed. Theodore A. Couloumbis and John O. Iatrides (1980); Lawrence S. Wittner, *American Intervention in Greece, 1943–1949* (1982).

GRENADA: *American Intervention in Grenada*, ed. Peter M. Dunn and Bruce W. Watson (1985); Gordon K. Lewis, *Grenada* (1987).

GUATEMALA: Jim Handy, *Gift of the Devil* (1985); Richard Immerman, *The CIA in Guatemala* (1982). (See also CENTRAL AMERICA; LATIN AMERICA.)

HAITI: Tom Barry *et al.*, *The Other Side of Paradise* (1984); Brenda Gayle Plummer, *Haiti and the United States* (1992). (See also LATIN AMERICA.)

HUMAN RIGHTS: Natalie Kaufman, *Human Rights Treaties and the Senate* (1990); A. Glenn Mower, *The U.S., UN, and Human Rights* (1979); Lars Schoultz, *Human Rights and U.S. Policy toward Latin America* (1981).

IMPERIALISM: Philip Darby, *Three Faces of Imperialism . . . 1870–1970* (1987); Michael W. Doyle, *Empires* (1986); *Imperialism and After*, ed. Wolfgang J. Mommsen and Jurgen Osterhammel (1986); Vivian Triás, *Historia del imperialismo norteamericano*, 3 vols. (1975–1977).

INDIA: H. W. Brands, *India and the United States* (1990); Gary R. Hess, "Global Expansion and Regional Balances . . . ," *Pacific Historical Review* 56 (May 1975): 159–195 [a valuable bibliographical essay]; Dennis Merrill, *The United States and India . . . 1947–1962* (1990); Kilaru Ram Chandra Rao, *India, U.S. and Pakistan* (1985).

INDIANS (NATIVE AMERICANS): Brian W. Dippie, *The Vanishing American* (1982); Francis Paul Prucha, *The Indians in American Society* (1985).

INDONESIA: Michael Leifer, *Indonesia's Foreign Policy* (1983).

INTELLIGENCE: *Knowing One's Enemies*, ed. Ernest R. May (1985). (See also CENTRAL INTELLIGENCE AGENCY.)

INTERNATIONAL LAW: Calvin D. Davis, *The U.S. and the First Hague Peace Conference* (1962); Calvin D. Davis, *The U.S. and the Second Hague Peace Conference* (1976); *International Law: A Contemporary Perspective*, ed. Richard Falk *et al.* (1985); Daniel

Patrick Moynihan, *The Law of Nations* (1990); D. P. O'Connell, *The International Law of the Sea* (1982).

Iran: James A. Bill, *The Eagle and the Lion* (1988); Mark H. Lytle, *The Origins of the Iranian-American Alliance, 1941–1953* (1987); R. K. Ramazani, *The United States and Iran* (1982).

Iraq: See Middle East; Oil; Persian Gulf.

Ireland: Donald H. Akenson, *The U.S. and Ireland* (1973).

Isolationism: Wayne S. Cole, *Roosevelt and the Isolationists* (1983); Justus D. Doenecke, *Anti-Intervention: A Bibliographical Introduction to Isolationism and Pacifism from World War I to the Early Cold War* (1987); Manfred Jonas, *Isolationism in America* (1966).

Israel: Cheryl Rubenberg, *Israel and the American National Interest* (1986); David Schoenbaum, *The U.S. and Israel* (1993); (See also Middle East.)

Italy: Alexander DeConde, *Half-Bitter, Half-Sweet* (1971); H. Stuart Hughes, *The U.S. and Italy* (1979).

Japan: *The U.S. and Japan in the Postwar World*, ed. Akira Iriye and Warren Cohen (1989); Charles E. Neu, *The Troubled Encounter* (1975); William L. Neumann, *America Encounters Japan* (1963).

Korea: *One Hundred Years of Korean-American Relations*, ed. Yur-Bok Lee and W. Patterson (1986); Chae-Jin Lee and Hideo Sato, *U.S. Policy toward Japan and Korea* (1982).

Labor: Philip S. Foner, *U.S. Labor . . . and Latin America (1846–1919)* (1988); Ronald Radosh, *American Labor and U.S. Foreign Policy* (1969).

Latin America: Cole Blasier, *The Hovering Giant* (1975); Lester Langley, *America and the Americas* (1990); Lester Langley, *Americans and the Caribbean in the Twentieth Century* (1980); John T. Reid, *Spanish-American Images of the U.S., 1790–1960* (1977); Harold Molineau, *U.S. Policy toward Latin America* (1986); (See also Central America; individual countries.)

Law: See International Law.

Lebanon: Itamar Rabinovich, *The War for Lebanon* (1986). (See also Middle East.)

Liberia: Katherine Harris, *The U.S. and Liberia* (1985); Hassan B. Sisay, *Big Powers and Small Nations* (1985).

Libya: P. E. Haley, *Qaddafi and the U.S. since 1969* (1984).

Malaysia: *The United States and Malaysia*, ed. Pamela Sodhy (1988).

Manifest Destiny: Albert K. Weinberg, *Manifest Destiny* (1935).

Mexico: George W. Grayson, *The U.S. and Mexico* (1984); Lester Langley, *Mexico and the United States* (1991); W. Dirk Raat, *Mexico and the United States* (1992); Alan Riding, *Distant Neighbors* (1984); Josefine Zoraida Vazquez and Lorenzo Meyer, *The U.S. and Mexico* (1985). (See also Latin America.)

Middle East: L. Carl Brown, *International Politics and the Middle East* (1984); Thomas Bryson, *U.S.–Middle East Diplomatic Relations, 1784–1978* (1979) [an annotated bibliography]; William R. Polk, *The Arab World Today* (1991); Steven L. Spiegel, *The Other Arab-Israel Conflict* (1985); William Stivers, *America's Confrontation with Revolutionary Change in the Middle East, 1948–1983* (1986); Seth Tillman, *The U.S. in the Middle East* (1982). (See also individual countries.)

Military: Benjamin R. Beede, *Intervention and Counterinsurgency . . . 1898–1984* (1985) [annotated bibliography]; *The Wars in Vietnam, Cambodia, and Laos, 1945–1982*, ed. Richard D. Burns and Milton Leitenberg (1984) [annotated bibliography]; John Whiteclay Chambers, *To Raise an Army: The Draft Comes to America* (1987); *A Bibli-*

ography of American Naval History, ed. Paolo E. Coletta (1981); Kenneth J. Hagan and William R. Roberts, *Against All Enemies* (1986); *American Historians and the Atlantic Alliance*, ed. Lawrence Kaplan (1991); Ariel E. Levite, Bruce W. Jentleson, Larry Berman, *Foreign Military Intervention* (1992); Peter Maslowski and Richard Millett, *The Common Defense* (1984); Paul B. Stares, *The Militarization of Space* (1985).

MISSIONS: William R. Hutchison, *Errand to the World* (1987); James Reed, *The Missionary Mind and American East Asia Policy, 1911–1915* (1986).

MONROE DOCTRINE: Dexter Perkins, *A History of the Monroe Doctrine* (1963).

NETHERLANDS, THE: *A Bilateral Bicentennial: A History of Dutch-American Relations, 1782–1982*, ed. J. W. Nordholt *et al.* (1982).

NICARAGUA: Karl Bermann, *Under the Big Stick* (1986); Peter Kornbluh, *Nicaragua, the Price of Intervention* (1987); Thomas W. Walker, *Nicaragua* (1991). (See also CENTRAL AMERICA; LATIN AMERICA.)

NORWAY: Sigmund Skard, *The U.S. in Norwegian History* (1976).

NUCLEAR ARMS: Coit D. Blacker, *Reluctant Warriors* (1987); Lawrence Freedman, *The Evolution of Nuclear Strategy* (1983); Institute for Strategic Studies (London), *The Military Balance* (1959–   ); Ronald Powaski, *March to Armageddon* (1987); Gordon C. Schloming, *American Foreign Policy and the Nuclear Dilemma* (1987). (See also MILITARY.)

OIL: David S. Painter, *Oil and the American Century* (1986); Stephen J. Randall, *U.S. Foreign Oil Policy, 1919–1984* (1985); Michael B. Stoff, *Oil, War, and American Security* (1980); Daniel Yergin, *The Prize* (1991).

PAKISTAN: *U.S.-Pakistan Relations*, ed. Leo E. Rose and Noor A. Husain (1985); M. S. Venkataramani, *The American Role in Pakistan, 1947–1958* (1982). (See also INDIA.)

PANAMA: Michael L. Conniff, *Panama and the United States* (1992); David N. Farnsworth and James W. McKenney, *U.S.-Panama Relations, 1902–1978* (1983); George D. Moffett III, *Limits of Victory* (1985); Walter LaFeber, *The Panama Canal* (1990). (See also LATIN AMERICA.)

PEACE MOVEMENTS: *Peace Heroes in Twentieth-Century America*, ed. Charles DeBenedetti (1986); Charles DeBenedetti, *The Peace Reform in American History* (1980); Justus D. Doenecke, *Anti-Intervention* (1987) [annotated bibliography]; Lawrence S. Wittner, *Rebels Against War . . . 1933–1983* (1984).

PERSIAN GULF: *The Persian Gulf States*, ed. Alvin J. Cottrell (1980); Charles A. Kupchan, *The Persian Gulf and the West* (1987); Michael A. Palmer, *Guardians of the Gulf: A History of America's Expanding Role in the Persian Gulf, 1833–1992* (1992); *The Gulf War Reader*, ed. M. L. Sifry and C. Serf (1991). (See also MIDDLE EAST; OIL.)

PERU: Frederick B. Pike, *The U.S. and the Andean Republics* (1977). (See also LATIN AMERICA.)

PHILIPPINES: Raymond Bonner, *Waltzing with a Dictator* (1987); H. W. Brands, *Bound to Empire* (1992); *Reappraising an Empire*, ed. Peter W. Stanley (1983).

POLAND: Stephen A. Garrett, *From Potsdam to Poland* (1986); Piotr Wandycz, *The U.S. and Poland* (1980).

PRESIDENT: E. S. Corwin, *The President* (1957); Theodore Lowi, *The Personal President* (1985); Edmund Muskie *et al.*, *The President, the Congress and Foreign Policy* (1986). (See also CONGRESS; CONSTITUTION.)

PUBLIC OPINION AND THE PRESS: Bernard C. Cohen, *The Public's Impact on Foreign Policy* (1973); W. A. Dorman and Mansour Farhang, *The U.S. Press and Iran* (1987); Ralph B. Levering, *The Public and American Foreign Policy, 1918–1978* (1978).

PUERTO RICO: Raymond Carr, *Puerto Rico* (1984); *Time for Decision*, ed. George Heine (1983).

RACE AND ETHNICITY: Alexander DeConde, *Ethnicity, Race, and American Foreign Policy* (1992); Paul Gordon Lauren, *Power and Prejudice (1988).*

RUSSIA AND THE SOVIET UNION: Michael Beschloss and Strobe Talbott, *At the Highest Levels* (1993) [covers 1988–1992]; John L. Gaddis, *Russia, the Soviet Union and the United States* (1990); Raymond L. Garthoff, *Détente and Confrontation* (1985) [covers 1969–1984]; Colin White, *Russia and America* (1988).

SAUDI ARABIA: Irvine H. Anderson, *Aramco, the U.S. and Saudi Arabia* (1981); Benson Lee Grayson, *Saudi-American Relations* (1982); David E. Long, *The U.S. and Saudi Arabia* (1985). (See also MIDDLE EAST; OIL.)

SOMOLIA: Jeffrey A. Lefebvre, *Arms for the Horn . . . 1953–1991* (1991).

SOUTH AFRICA: Thomas Borstelmann, *Apartheid's Reluctant Uncle* (1993); Christopher Coker, *The U.S. and South Africa, 1868–1985* (1986); *The Anti-Apartheid Reader*, ed. David Mermelstein (1987); Thomas J. Noer, *Cold War and Black Liberation . . . 1949–1968* (1985); Anthony Sampson, *Black and Gold* (1987). (See also AFRICA.)

TERRORISM: Augustus Norton and Martin Greensburg, *International Terrorism* (1980) [annotated bibliography].

THAILAND: Robert J. Muscat, *Thailand and the United States* (1990).

TURKEY: Theodore A. Couloumbis, *The U.S., Greece and Turkey* (1983). (See also MIDDLE EAST.)

UNITED NATIONS: Seymour M. Finger, *American Ambassadors at the UN* (1987); Thomas M. Franck, *Nation against Nation* (1985); Evan Luard, *A History of the UN* (1982); Edmund Jan Osmanczyk, *The Encyclopedia of the UN and International Agreements* (1985); Giuseppe Schiavone, *International Organizations: A Dictionary and Directory* (1983).

URUGUAY: Arthur P. Whitaker, *The U.S. and the Southern Cone* (1976). (See also LATIN AMERICA.)

VENEZUELA: Sheldon B. Liss, *Diplomacy and Independence* (1978); Stephen G. Rabe, *The Road to OPEC: U.S. Relations with Venezuela, 1919–1976* (1982). (See also LATIN AMERICA; OIL.)

VIETNAM: Loren Baritz, *Backfire* (1985); *The Wars in Vietnam, Cambodia, and Laos, 1945–1982*, ed. Richard Dean Burns and Milton Leitenberg (1984) [an annotated bibliography of 6,200 entries]; Lloyd Gardner, *Approaching Vietnam* (1988); George Herring, *The Longest War* (1986); George Kahin, *Intervention* (1986); Paul M. Kattenburg, *The Vietnam Trauma in American Foreign Policy, 1945–1975* (1980); Gabriel Kolko, *Anatomy of a War* (1985); Gareth Porter, *Vietnam* (1980) [extensive documents]; Neil Sheehan, *A Bright Shining Lie: John Paul Vann and America in Vietnam* (1988); William A. Williams *et al.*, *America in Vietnam* (1985) [documents and introductions].

Acknowledgments for the
First Edition

Along with the usual but ever more sincere thanks to Sandra, Scott, and Suzanne LaFeber for making the past years and the writing of this book worthwhile, I am deeply indebted to Ed Barber of W. W. Norton & Company and Gerry McCauley for the encouragement that made the book possible. The growing length of the manuscript was unforeseen, but not Ed Barber's patience, sound advice, and humor, and they made the enterprise bearable. I am also indebted to Linda Puckette and Carol Flechner of Norton for special help in preparing the manuscript for publication, and to indexer Anne Eberle.

Lloyd Gardner of Rutgers University critiqued the entire manuscript and continues to set the example as both a committed scholar and friend. Robert Divine of the University of Texas also read all the pages, as he has of much else I have drafted, and his friendship has been especially important during the past several years. The historical profession lost what it cannot afford to lose when R. H. Miller left it to join Congressman Ron Dellums's staff. Max Miller not only read all of this book, but conducted a private four-year seminar by providing detailed comments and volumes of research materials. I am much indebted to Diane Clemens of the University of California and William Widenor of the University of Illnois, both of whom gave large sections of the manuscript close and most helpful readings. Milton Leitenberg, whether in Sweden or Washington, provided important studies of his own and others on East-West relations. Despite the Carter-Reagan attempts to close off documents from scholars, there remain some to whom we owe a huge debt for their professionalism and practicing belief that a democracy can survive only when the government's actions can be examined. These persons include David Langbart of the National

Archives, David Humphrey of the Lyndon Johnson Presidential Library, and Dennis Bilger of the Harry S. Truman Presidential Library.

Eric Edelman and Dan Fried of the Department of State, and John Greer, now a lawyer, are scholars, valued friends and detached critics. The best ideas in this book are probably largely stolen from those named above or from Fred Harvey Harrington and Tom McCormick, both of the University of Wisconsin, and William Appleman Williams of Oregon State; those three are very special as scholars and friends.

Persons associated with Cornell University have, as always, been irreplaceable. Marie Underhill Noll's encouragement is even more valued now because she is also a neighbor. David Maisel, Arthur Kaminsky, Peter Schuck, Jeff Bialos, David Wechsler, Laurie Keenan, Stephen Arbogast, Dan Weil, Mark Lytle, Eric Alterman, Douglas Little, Frank Costigliola, Fred Adams, Frederick Drake, Bob Seidel, David Green, Gayle Plummer, Rich Johnston, and Kathy Harris are former students who now enjoy much success in their various professions but are never too busy to provide valuable advice and reading materials. Rick Mandel, David Jackson, Colleen Curtin, Agnes Sagan, and Jessica Wang have been imaginative research assistants. Cathy Hendley typed the final draft carefully and against deadlines. Jackie Hubble kindly helped with the typing when the deadlines were pressing. The Cornell University Libraries continue to be unsurpassed in resources and accessibility; I owe Alain Seznec, David Corson, Caroline Spicer, Janie Harris, and Martha Hsu particular thanks.

Five friends in the History Department read much of this book in various forms and provided important materials which often resulted from their own scholarship. This book is dedicated to them. They first came to Cornell to help teach the introductory American history course, and they have remained to become distinguished scholars, noted teachers, superb colleagues, and—of special importance—close friends. They and other friends who are Americanists—Margaret Washington, Stuart Blumin, Paul Gates, Fred Somkin, Dan Usner, Glenn Altschuler, Nick Salvatore, Bob Harris, and, in a special category, Ted Lowi—have made Ithaca a stimulating place in which to study American history.

Walter LaFeber
March 1988

Photo Credits

P. 13: National Portrait Gallery, Smithsonian Institution; p. 20: Bibliothèque Nationale, Paris; p. 22: New-York Historical Society, New York; p. 31: Department of State; p. 44: American Philosophical Society; p. 49: Warder Collection; p. 53: Historical Pictures Service; p. 59: Metropolitan Museum of Art; p. 60: Courtesy Department of Library Services, American Museum of Natural History; p. 64: Library of Congress; p. 72: Metropolitan Museum of Art, Gift of I.N. Phelps Stokes, Edward S. Hawes, Alice Mary Hawes, Marion Augusta Hawes, 1937 (37.14.34); p. 77: National Archives; p. 83: Pennsylvania Academy of Fine Arts; p. 102: National Portrait Gallery, Smithsonian Institution; p. 103: Library of Congress; p. 115: National Archives; p. 128: Metropolitan Museum of Art, Gift of I.N. Phelps Stokes, Edward S. Hawes, Alice Mary Hawes, Marion Augusta Hawes, 1937 (37.14.2); p. 128: Metropolitan Museum of Art; p. 130: National Archives; p. 131: National Archives; p. 139: UPI-Bettmann; p. 151: *Public Opinion*, January 17, 1901; p. 156: Granger Collection; p. 160: State Historical Society of North Dakota; p. 161: State Historical Society of North Dakota; p. 164: Library of Congress; p. 169: Public Archives of Hawaii; p. 176: Warder Collection; p. 183: National Portrait Gallery, Smithsonian Institution; p. 186: Brown Brothers; p. 187: New-York Historical Society, New York; p. 193: Charles Musser, *The Emergence of Cinema: The American Screen to 1907* (New York: Scribner's, 1990); p. 199: *Literary Digest*, January 26, 1901; p. 201: Smithsonian Institution; p. 203: Library of Congress; p. 207: Library of Congress; p. 220: Library of Congress; p. 228: Library of Congress; p. 231: *Public Opinion*, September 1, 1904; p. 241: Library of Congress; p. 245: Library of Congress; p. 255: Franklin D. Roosevelt Library; p. 258: National Portrait Gallery, Smithsonian Institution; p. 260: Library of Congress; p. 263: Library of Congress; p. 271: *The New York Times*; p. 280: UPI-Bettmann; p. 288: National Archives; p. 297: National Portrait Gallery, Smithsonian Institution; p. 305: *Daily Herald;* p. 308: Warder Collection; p. 311: Library of Congress; p. 317: Department of State; p. 318: National Portrait Gallery, Smithsonian Institution; p. 321: Wide World Photos; p. 337: Historical Pictures Service; p. 338: Cesare, *Outlook;* p. 343: National Archives; p. 352: Franklin D. Roosevelt Library; p. 354: National Portrait Gallery, Smithsonian Institution; p. 361: UPI-Bettmann; p. 365: C. D. Batchelor, © 1936 New York News Inc., reprinted with permission; p. 381: Franklin D. Roosevelt Library; p. 383: National Archives; p. 384: Franklin D. Roosevelt Library; p. 394: Franklin D. Roosevelt Library; p. 404: Franklin D. Roosevelt Library; p. 407: Franklin D. Roosevelt Library; p. 417: Franklin D. Roo-

Index

Italicized page numbers refer to drawings and photographs.